DIAGNOSTIC PATHOLOGY

Neuropathology

SECOND EDITION

BURGER | SCHEITHAUER
KLEINSCHMIDT-DEMASTERS | RODRÍGUEZ | TIHAN
ERSEN • RUSHING

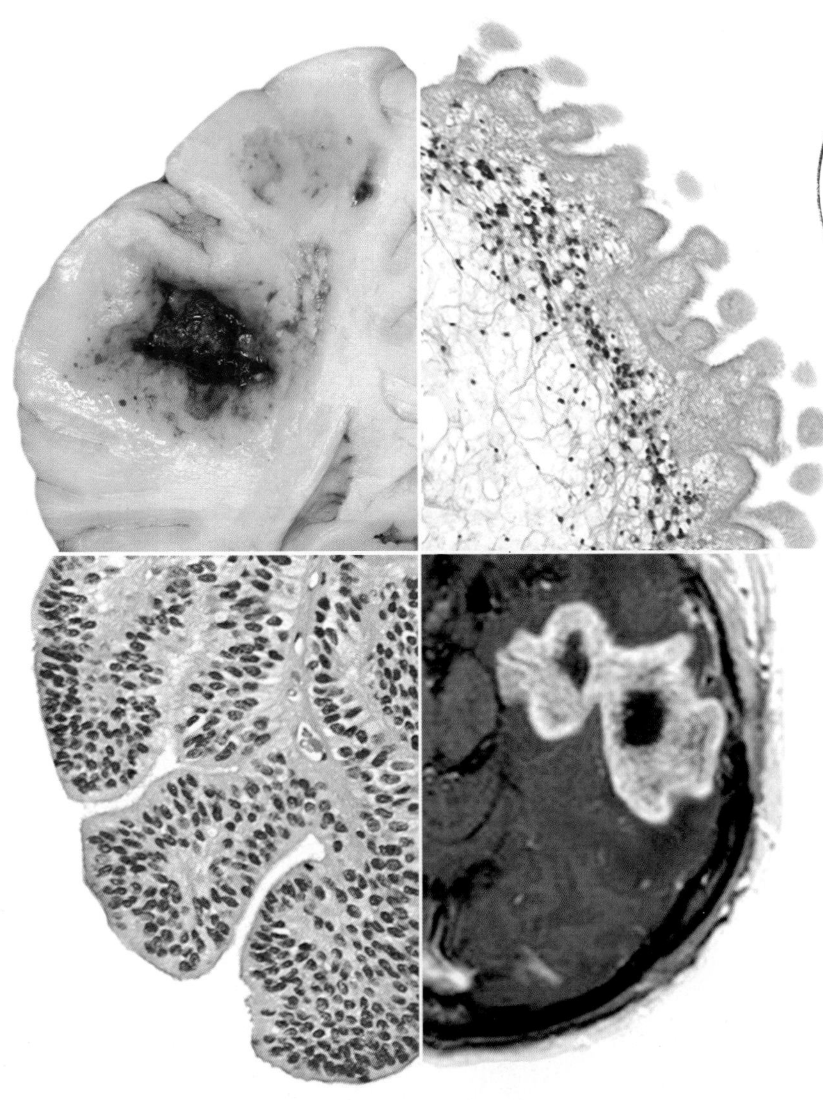

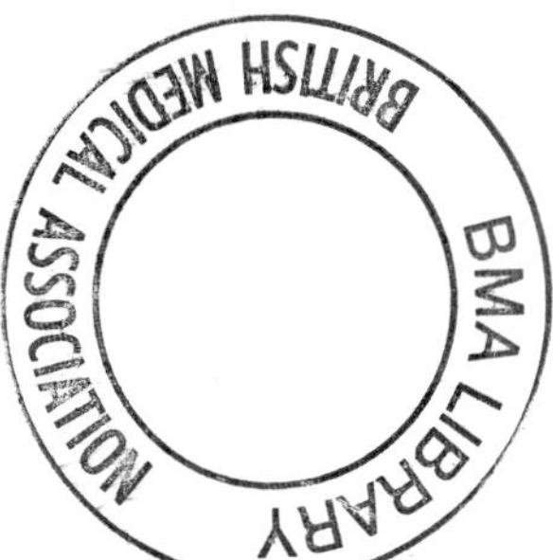

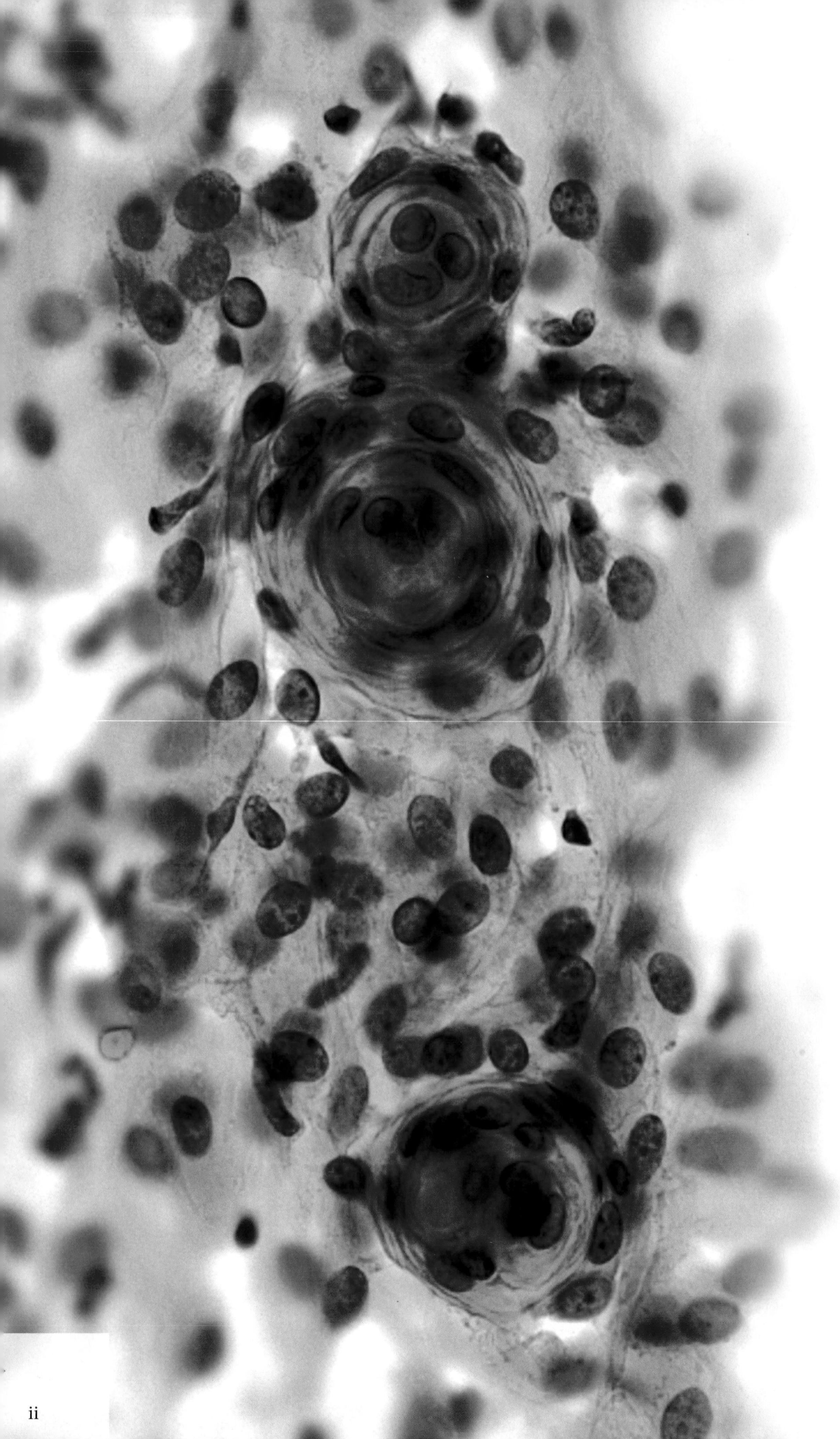

WITHDRAWN FROM
LIBRARY
BMA

BRITISH MEDICAL ASSOCIATION
1000451

DIAGNOSTIC PATHOLOGY

Neuropathology

SECOND EDITION

B. K. Kleinschmidt-DeMasters, MD
Professor of Pathology, Neurology, and Neurosurgery
Director of Neuropathology
University of Colorado School of Medicine
Aurora, Colorado

Fausto J. Rodríguez, MD
Associate Professor of Pathology and Oncology
The Johns Hopkins University School of Medicine
Baltimore, Maryland

Tarik Tihan, MD, PhD
Professor of Pathology
UCSF Department of Pathology, Neuropathology Division
San Francisco, California
Visiting Professor, Koc University School of Medicine
Istanbul, Turkey

ELSEVIER

1600 John F. Kennedy Blvd.
Ste 1800
Philadelphia, PA 19103-2899

DIAGNOSTIC PATHOLOGY: NEUROPATHOLOGY, SECOND EDITION ISBN: 978-0-323-44592-4

Notices

Knowledge and best practice in this field are constantly changing. As new research and experience broaden our understanding, changes in research methods, professional practices, or medical treatment may become necessary.

Practitioners and researchers must always rely on their own experience and knowledge in evaluating and using any information, methods, compounds, or experiments described herein. In using such information or methods they should be mindful of their own safety and the safety of others, including parties for whom they have a professional responsibility.

With respect to any drug or pharmaceutical products identified, readers are advised to check the most current information provided (i) on procedures featured or (ii) by the manufacturer of each product to be administered, to verify the recommended dose or formula, the method and duration of administration, and contraindications. It is the responsibility of practitioners, relying on their own experience and knowledge of their patients, to make diagnoses, to determine dosages and the best treatment for each individual patient, and to take all appropriate safety precautions.

To the fullest extent of the law, neither the Publisher nor the authors, contributors, or editors, assume any liability for any injury and/or damage to persons or property as a matter of products liability, negligence or otherwise, or from any use or operation of any methods, products, instructions, or ideas contained in the material herein.

Publisher Cataloging-in-Publication Data

Names: Kleinschmidt-DeMasters, Bette. | Rodríguez, Fausto J. | Tihan, Tarik.
Title: Diagnostic Pathology : Neuropathology / [edited by] B.K. Kleinschmidt-DeMasters, Fausto J. Rodríguez, and Tarik Tihan.
Other titles: Neuropathology.
Description: Second edition. | Salt Lake City, UT : Elsevier, Inc., [2016] | Includes bibliographical references and index.
Identifiers: ISBN 978-0-323-44592-4
Subjects: LCSH: Nervous system--Diseases--Diagnosis--Handbooks, manuals, etc. | Pathology, Surgical--Handbooks, manuals, etc. | MESH: Nervous System Diseases--pathology--Atlases. | Brain Neoplasms--pathology--Atlases. | Cerebrovascular Disorders--pathology--Atlases.
Classification: LCC RC347.B86 2016 | NLM WL 17 | DDC 616.8′047--dc23

International Standard Book Number: 978-0-323-44592-4

Cover Designer: Tom M. Olson, BA

Printed in Canada by Friesens, Altona, Manitoba, Canada

Last digit is the print number: 9 8 7 6 5 4 3 2 1

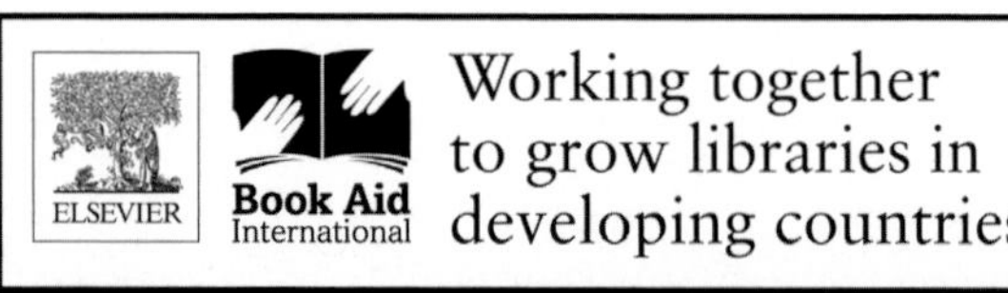

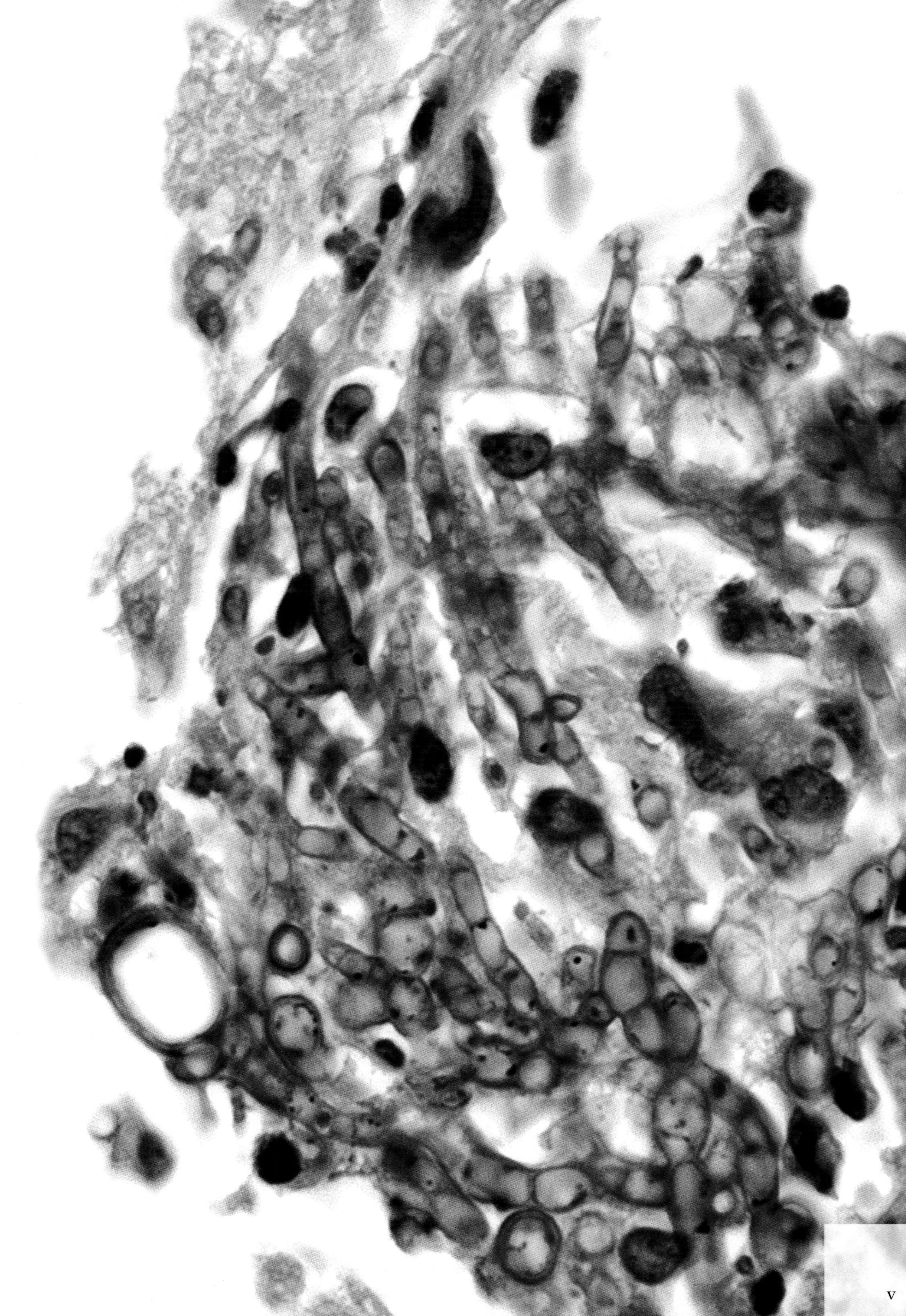

Dedications

The bell rings, and it is teaching time!! The little porcelain bell chimes with a soft melodious tone, and everyone around the six-headed microscope is aware of the impending words of wisdom that hardly come out of the master's lips at other times. The ensuing statement, whether advice or an observation, better be recorded in your mind's hard drive since it will be of use many times as you face the same challenges in your own ventures. This little bell has accompanied all the sign-out sessions of Dr. Peter C. Burger at Johns Hopkins Hospital since the time I began working with him as an assistant professor in 1997. Many years later, the bell still chimes and brings awe and smiles to all those around that microscope. It has been a unique privilege to have worked with Peter C. Burger, undoubtedly one of the giants and keen observers of surgical neuropathology. Hundreds of publications, numerous books, lectures, and other scholarly works can only underscore a part of an academician's life that has inspired, motivated, provoked, and enticed numerous pathologists and other scientists.

There is little need to reiterate the timeline and accomplishments of Dr. Burger here but much necessity to pay tribute to my quiet mentor, who does not like to be in the limelight nor cares to talk about himself or his accomplishments. An occasional jape about his prowess on correct diagnosis or uncanny observational skills is all you can hear from him about decades of hard work. This whimsical statement often compels you to remember the crucial issues in a particular case and recall how he reached the diagnosis that may have eluded many skilled diagnosticians.

My entire career in neuropathology is a dedication to my Captain, as he has forced us to be far better than we can be. I have to tell him that none of the cups of coffee along with the good wisdom we have shared have been forgotten. This book is still the product of Peter C. Burger and Bernd W. Scheithauer to the very last sentence. Their vision, teachings, and passion for diagnostic neuropathology drives all of us to be worthy of the high standards they have established. Despite all the gloom and doom in this world, the efforts my two mentors have put into this book represent our faith in the good of humanity and our desire to see our patients cured of their ailments.

TT

It has been an enormous pleasure to participate in this project started by two extraordinary men, who had an enormous influence in shaping how I practice medicine today. Bernd had a consistent presence during my formative years in pathology and neuropathology, an energetic motivator with his boundless enthusiasm for diagnostic neuropathology. Peter is a wonderful colleague and mentor and a continuous source of wisdom and advice in my professional and nonprofessional life. We are proud to preserve their voice and teachings as we carry this evolving project into the future and incorporate the recent exciting developments that are transforming our daily practice.

FJR

The original "footprints" of Peter Burger and Bernd Scheithauer, the initial senior authors of this text, remain throughout this second edition of their book. While I have never had the privilege of working directly with either Peter or Bernd, their "walk" has been directly extended by two of their most talented "academic descendants" (a.k.a. trainees), Tarik and Fausto. Together, the three of us have attempted to leave what was perfect in the first edition but update what was necessary in the current edition. We did this work as a direct tribute to both Peter and Bernd; we hope the reader will be pleased with the result and find the information useful in their practice.

BKKD

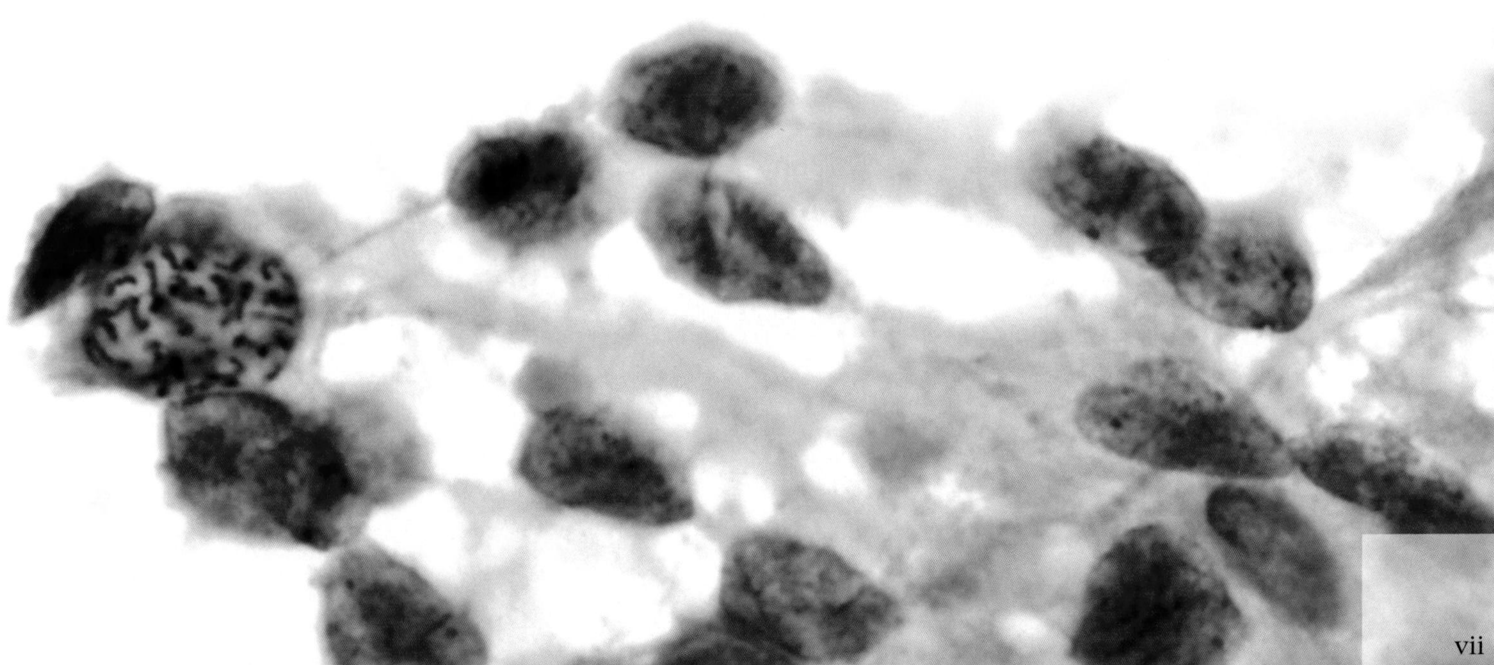

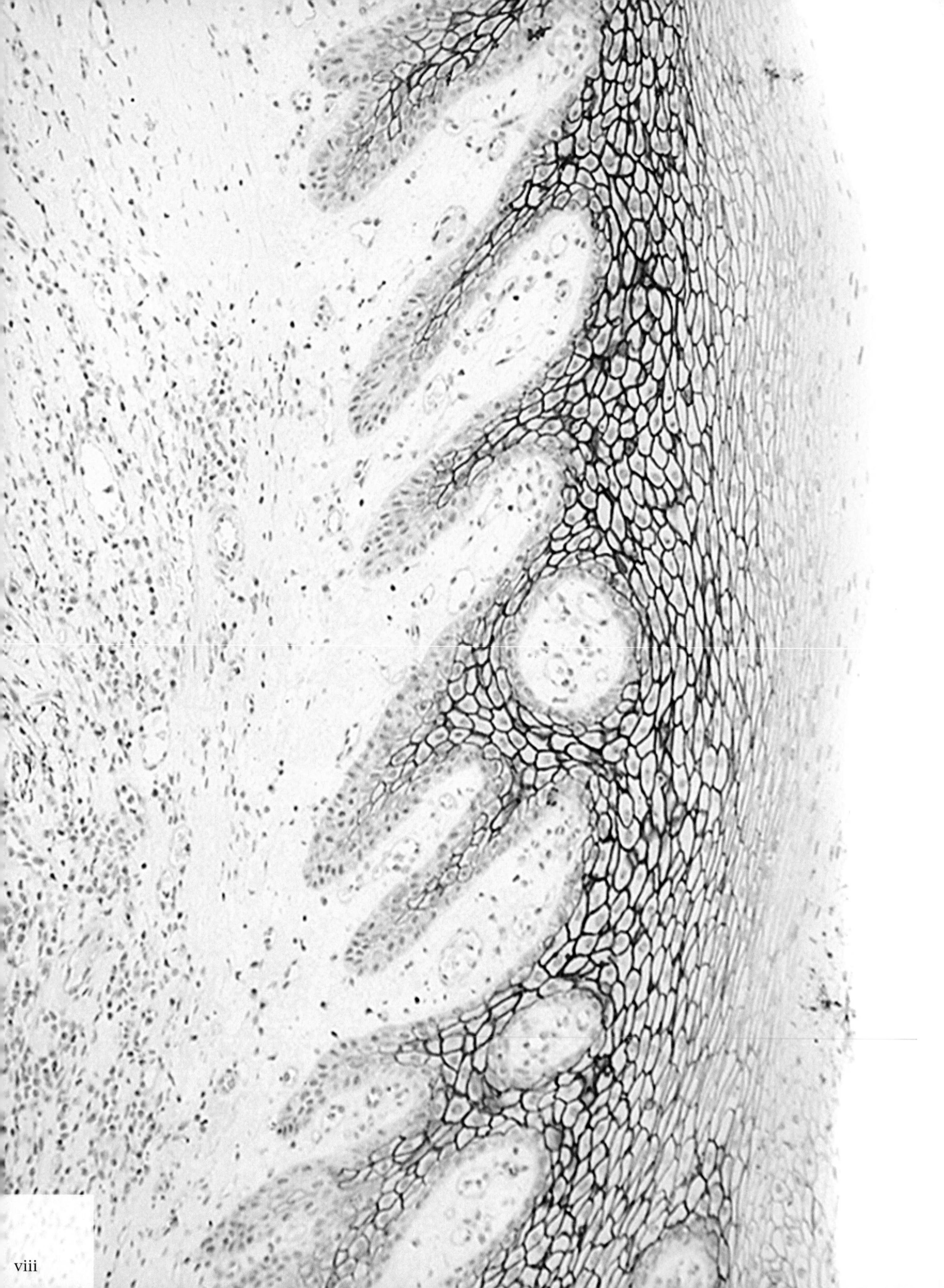

Contributing Authors

Peter C. Burger, MD
Professor of Pathology
Department of Pathology
The Johns Hopkins University School of Medicine
Baltimore, Maryland

Bernd W. Scheithauer, MD
Professor Emeritus of Pathology
Consultant Emeritus in Pathology and Laboratory Medicine
Mayo College of Medicine
Rochester, Minnesota

Ayca Ersen, MD
Assistant Professor of Pathology
Department of Pathology
Dokuz Eylul University
Izmir, Turkey

Elisabeth J. Rushing, MD
Professor of Neuropathology
Institute for Neuropathology
University of Zurich
Zurich, Switzerland

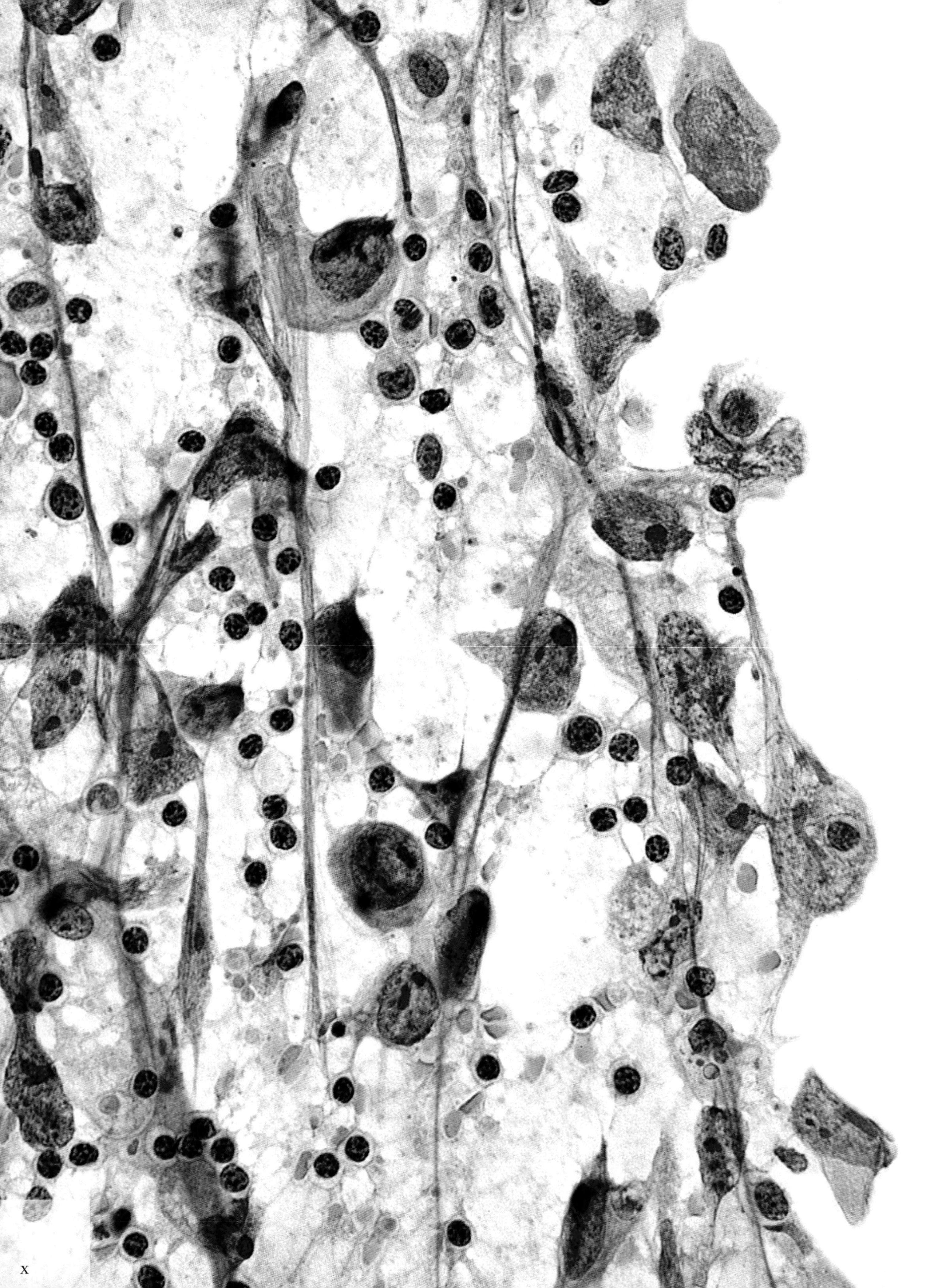

Preface

Until only two decades ago, it was quite sufficient to diagnose surgical neuropathology material based on routine hematoxylin and eosin (H&E)-stained sections, and the information gleaned from these sections was often sufficient to characterize tumors and categorize nonneoplastic processes. This practice has been sufficient for the clinicians in a majority of the diseases. The routine H&E stain still constitutes the critical starting point for surgical neuropathology today.

Yet, the explosion of new methods and models, advances in radiological, clinical, morphological, and molecular aspects of diseases, as well as the increasing options for different treatment modalities require frequent updating of "classical" textbooks and revision of diagnostic algorithms. The revision of this book was prompted by this necessity and the desire to continue the remarkable works of two giants in diagnostic neuropathology. Like the original work, the collaborative effort of the authors provides a pragmatic, visually satisfactory, and user-friendly reference for the everyday surgical pathologist.

Much is changing in the world of CNS neoplasia, and the modifications in this book reflect the changing times and the adoption of the "integrated diagnosis" that merges the old with the new methodology to provide a better guide for our colleagues.

Many chapters have been substantially updated, and all have been revised with new images and additional information. There is a new contributor to many chapters, and the readers will notice a change in the listing of authors for chapters with extensive revisions. This book remains the product of collaborative work, hours of deliberation, and careful consideration of the practical facts and key issues that will immediately attract the reader's attention. Our goal was to provide a reference that can be used in daily signout sessions and for teaching activities of our colleagues. We hope that the practicing pathologists at all levels—residents, fellows, academicians, and private practitioners—will find this work equally fun and useful and easy to navigate.

We are, as we always will be, grateful to our mentors, whom we owe the ability to carry on their journey with the hopes that our students will see even wider horizons. We are also grateful to all those countless workers in our divisions and in Elsevier, who tirelessly tried to make this book come alive. The search for better understanding and cures continues.

B. K. Kleinschmidt-DeMasters, MD
Professor of Pathology, Neurology, and Neurosurgery
Director of Neuropathology
University of Colorado School of Medicine
Aurora, Colorado

Fausto J. Rodríguez, MD
Associate Professor of Pathology and Oncology
The Johns Hopkins University School of Medicine
Baltimore, Maryland

Tarik Tihan, MD, PhD
Professor of Pathology
UCSF Department of Pathology, Neuropathology Division
San Francisco, California
Visiting Professor, Koc University School of Medicine
Istanbul, Turkey

What Is New and WHO Is Changing

There have been a number of discoveries since 2007 that are likely to be added in the next revision of the WHO classification of CNS tumors, and some are highlighted below. Some changes are significant, while others are minor but helpful developments. Furthermore, the use of "integrated diagnosis" that incorporates molecular pathological findings is being proposed as the standard reporting format.

Diffuse Astrocytomas

There seems to be a distinct difference between the molecular characteristic of adult and pediatric (age < 15) diffuse astrocytomas, and they will need to be considered in separate categories.

A. Adult Diffuse Astrocytomas; grouped into two distinct categories based on the presence of *IDH1/2* mutation

- **a.** ***IDH1/2* mutant diffuse astrocytomas**
  - **i.** Often coexist with ATRX mutation or loss of protein expression (on immunohistochemistry) and *TP53* mutation
  - **ii.** IDH mutant grade IV glioblastomas were shown to have better prognosis than IDH wild-type anaplastic (grade III) astrocytomas
  - **iii.** No significant prognostic difference was found between *IDH1/2* mutant WHO grade II and grade III diffuse astrocytomas
  - **iv.** *IDH1/2* mutant glioblastomas correspond to secondary glioblastoma
- **b.** ***IDH1/2* wild-type diffuse astrocytomas**
  - **i.** Uniformly have worse prognosis compared to all other diffuse gliomas
  - **ii.** Harbor genetic alterations more typical of glioblastomas (e.g., *EGFR* amplification &/or *PTEN* deletion)
  - **iii.** Often have intact ATRX expression and wild-type *TP53* gene
  - **iv.** *IDH1/2* wild-type glioblastomas correspond to primary glioblastoma
  - **v.** Frequently have *TERT* promoter mutations
- **c.** **Granular cell diffuse astrocytomas behave as glioblastoma, regardless of histological grade**

B. Pediatric Diffuse Astrocytomas and Glioblastomas

- **a.** **Pediatric high-grade astrocytomas (anaplastic astrocytomas, glioblastomas) lack *IDH1/2* mutation and mostly lack EGFR and PTEN alterations**
  - **i.** Most diffuse intrinsic pontine gliomas behave adversely, regardless of histological grade; many have mutations in genes encoding histone proteins (*H3F3A*, *HIST1H3B*, others)
  - **ii.** *H3K27M* increasingly identified in midline gliomas, especially thalamic and brainstem, as well as some spinal cord, in both children and adults; can be tested by IHC

Oligodendrogliomas

Oligodendroglial tumors are defined by presence of both co-deletion of chromosomes 1p and 19q and *IDH1/2* mutations.

- It has been suggested that tumors formerly classified as glioblastoma with oligodendroglioma component by the WHO that also harbor 1p/19q co-deletions be considered anaplastic oligodendroglioma, WHO grade III
- Diagnosis of mixed oligoastrocytoma is discouraged (based on data showing almost all are either genetically oligodendroglioma (i.e., *IDH1/2* mutant, co-deletion of 1p, 19q, no ATRX mutation [i.e., no loss of nuclear ATRX by IHC] OR *IDH1/2* mutant, no co-deletion, ATRX +/- *TP53* mutations, not both and not an admixture of cells with both)
- Frequent *TERT* promoter mutations
- There are rare tumors in the pediatric population histologically similar to adult oligodendrogliomas without the above molecular changes; their nature is yet to be understood
- A distinct group of tumors currently termed "diffuse leptomeningeal oligodendroglial-like neoplasms" or DOLN harbor *KIAA-BRAF* duplications and 1p deletion, and may be considered a new entity

Other Pertinent Developments

- Pilomyxoid astrocytoma still remains a variant of pilocytic astrocytoma, but grading has been questioned, and a suggestion to omit WHO grading has been proposed
- Primitive neuroectodermal tumor no longer recognized terminology: Tumors formerly designated supratentorial or CNS PNET are now designated Embryonal Tumor, NOS
- Peripheral neuroectodermal tumor no longer recognized terminology: Tumors formerly designated pPNET are now simply Ewing sarcoma
- Chordoid glioma now recognized to express nuclear TTF-1, similar to other infundibular region lineage tumors (pituicytoma, spindle cell oncocytoma, granular cell tumor of neurohypophysis)
- Some supratentorial ependymomas are characterized by C11orf95-RELA fusion (testing may be performed by PCR or FISH for break-apart probes) and aggressive behavior; these tumors also show strong L1CAM positivity on immunohistochemistry
- TTF1 nuclear positivity is shared by pituicytoma, spindle cell oncocytoma, granular cell tumor of neurohypophysis, which suggests a common origin
- SOX10 positivity is seen in melanocytic and peripheral nerve sheath tumors and is useful in distinguishing them from other mesenchymal neoplasms
- STAT6 nuclear IHC expression (parallels STAT6:NAB2 fusion) in solitary fibrous tumor/hemangiopericytoma family of neoplasms distinguishes them from other spindle cell tumors, such as meningiomas or schwannoma
- SSTR2A strong diffuse positivity is somewhat better than EMA positivity in the diagnosis of meningiomas
- SF-1 (steroidogenic factor 1) now defines gonadotroph adenoma, distinguishes it from hormone negative SF-1 negative null cell adenoma
- Pit-1 expression in pituitary adenomas links all types of GH, PRL, TSH, and admixed hormonal combinations

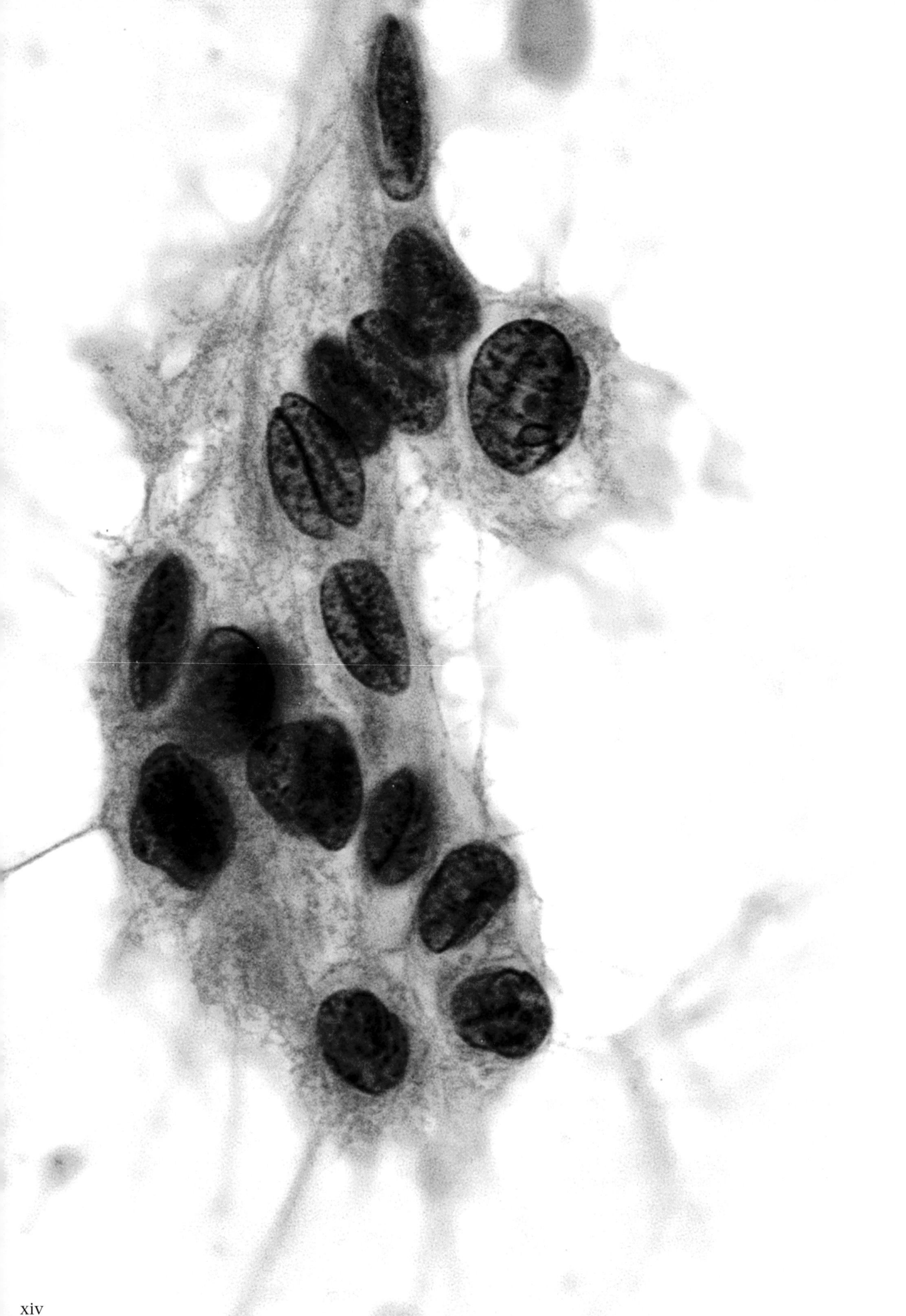

Acknowledgments

Text Editors

Arthur G. Gelsinger, MA
Nina I. Bennett, BA
Tricia L. Cannon, BA
Terry W. Ferrell, MS
Lisa A. Gervais, BS
Karen E. Concannon, MA, PhD
Emily C. Fassett, BA

Image Editors

Jeffrey J. Marmorstone, BS
Lisa A. M. Steadman, BS

Illustrations

Laura C. Sesto, MA
Lane R. Bennion, MS
Richard Coombs, MS

Art Direction and Design

Tom M. Olson, BA
Laura C. Sesto, MA

Lead Editor

Sarah J. Connor, BA

Production Coordinators

Angela M. G. Terry, BA
Rebecca L. Hutchinson, BA

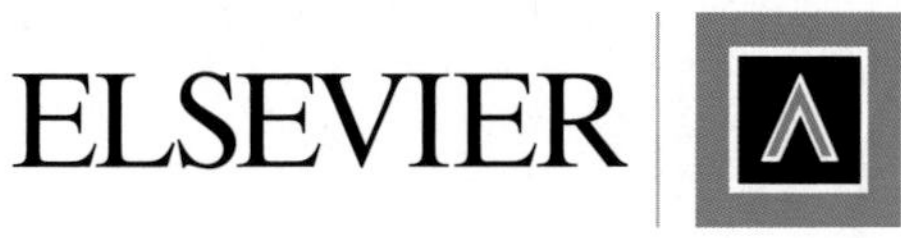

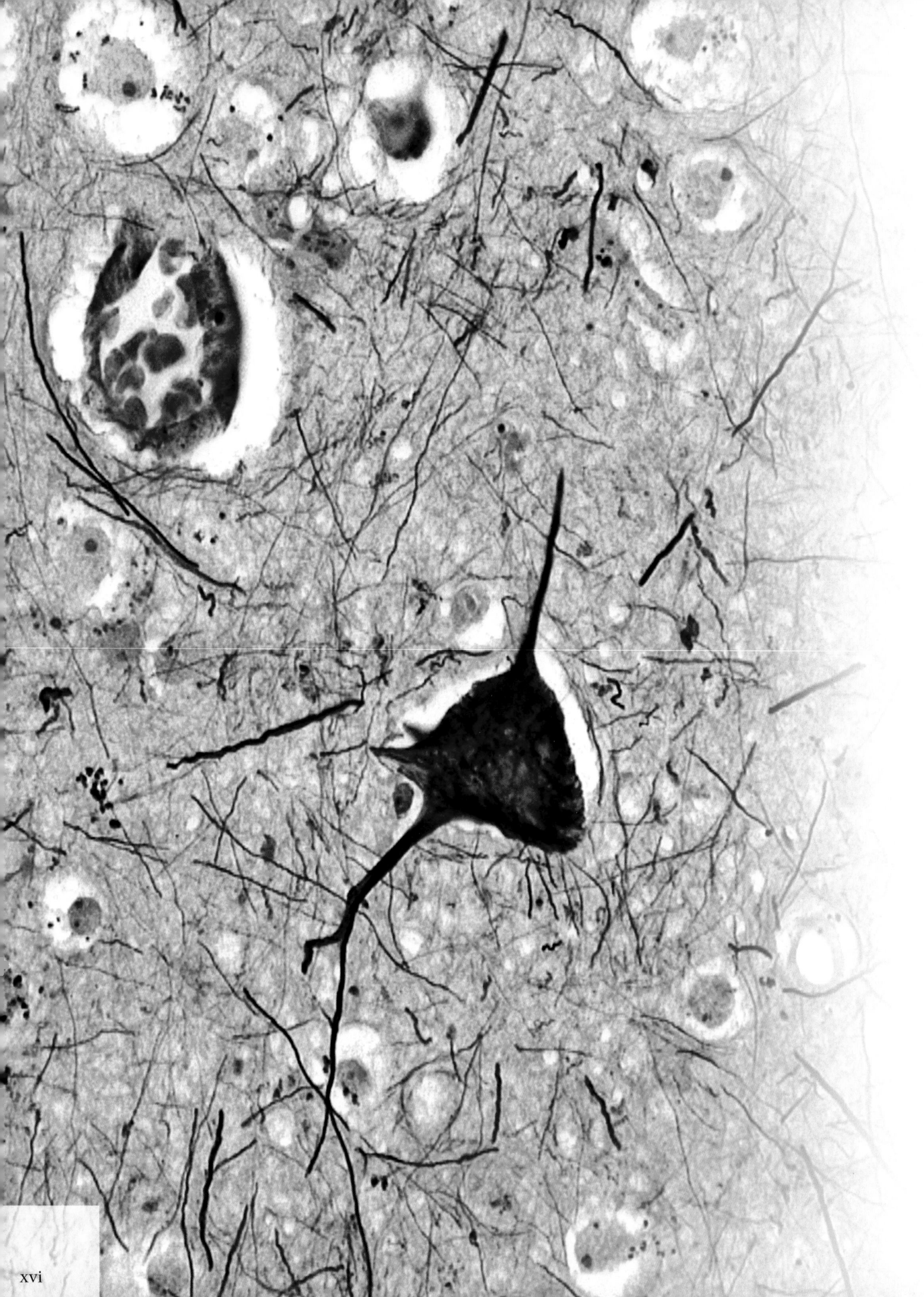

Sections

TABLE OF CONTENTS

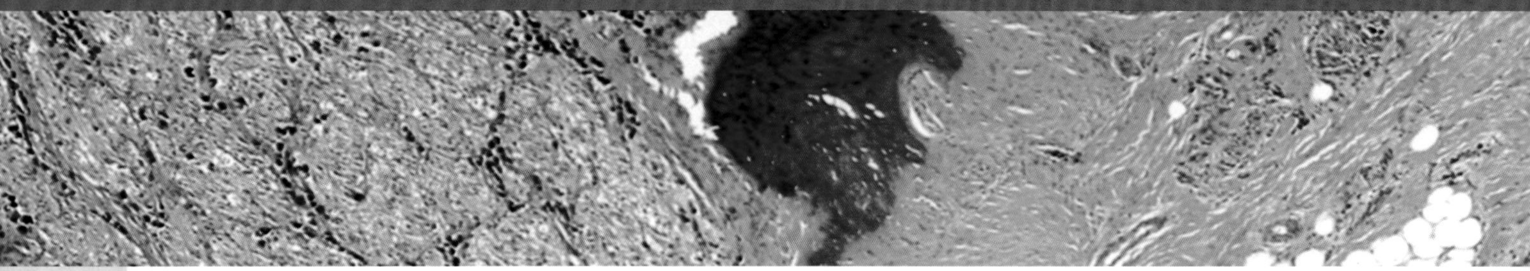

Part I: Neoplastic

SECTION 1: BRAIN AND SPINAL CORD

INFILTRATIVE ASTROCYTIC NEOPLASMS

OLIGODENDROGLIAL NEOPLASMS

LOCALIZED ASTROCYTIC NEOPLASMS

TUMORS OF EPENDYMA AND RELATED CELLS

CHOROID PLEXUS NEOPLASMS

NEURONAL AND GLIONEURONAL NEOPLASMS

PINEAL PARENCHYMAL NEOPLASMS

TABLE OF CONTENTS

TABLE OF CONTENTS

TABLE OF CONTENTS

DIAGNOSTIC PATHOLOGY

Neuropathology

SECOND EDITION

BURGER | SCHEITHAUER
KLEINSCHMIDT-DEMASTERS | RODRÍGUEZ | TIHAN
ERSEN • RUSHING

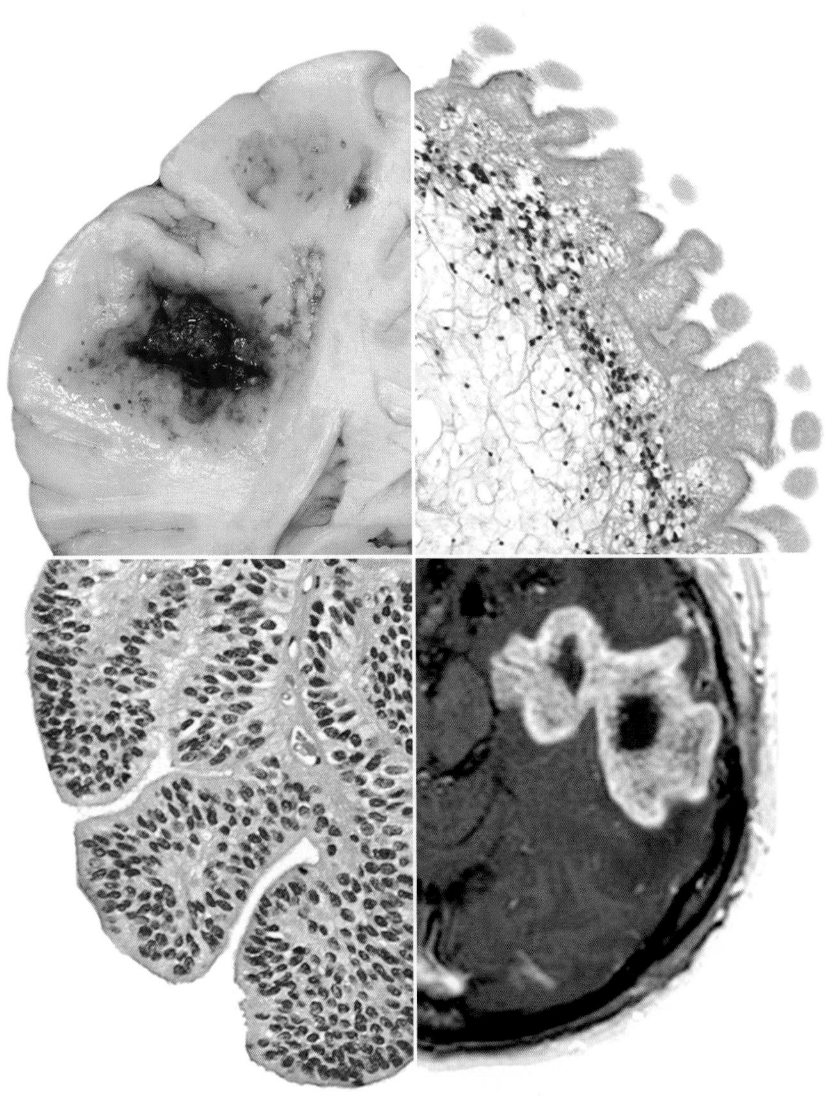

PART I
SECTION 1

Brain and Spinal Cord

Infiltrative Astrocytic Neoplasms

Oligodendroglial Neoplasms

Localized Astrocytic Neoplasms

Tumors of Ependyma and Related Cells

Choroid Plexus Neoplasms

Neuronal and Glioneuronal Neoplasms

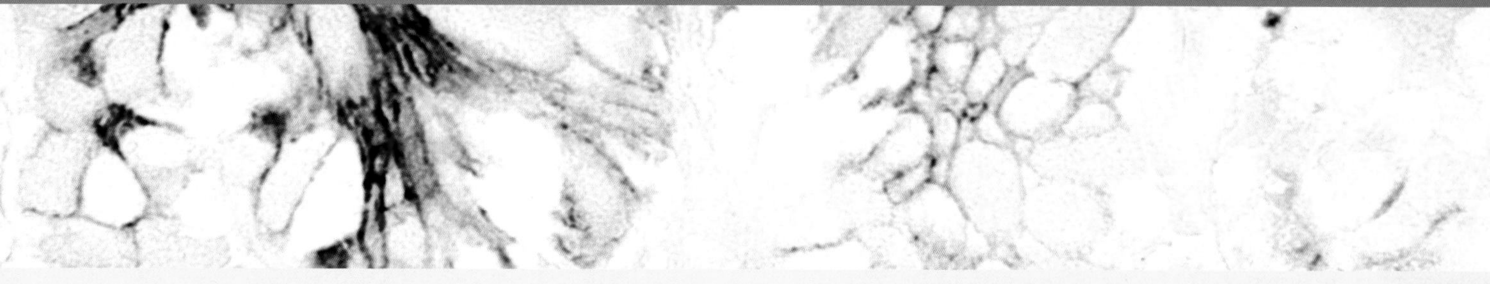

Pineal Parenchymal Neoplasms

Embryonal Neoplasms

Germ Cell Neoplasms

Hemangioblastoma

Lymphomas and Hematopoietic Neoplasms

Metastatic Neoplasms

Diffuse Astrocytoma

KEY FACTS

TERMINOLOGY

- Infiltrating glioma with astrocytic differentiation
- Mutations in *IDH1/2, ATRX, TERT,* and *TP53* and co-deletion of 1p/19q correlate better with tumor biological and clinical behavior than do stratifications based only on histological features

IMAGING

- Ill-defined or relatively discrete area of T1 hypointensity and T2/FLAIR hyperintensity

MICROSCOPIC

- Cell distribution more irregular than in oligodendroglioma
- Hypercellularity, but may be very slight
  - Particularly in cases with prominent intratumoral edema
- Nuclear atypia
- Cytoplasm inconspicuous (naked nuclei) in comparison to fibrillar or gemistocytic
- No mitoses, particularly in small specimens
- One may suffice for grade III in very small specimen

ANCILLARY TESTS

- IDH-1 usually (+) in adolescents and adults (85%)
- IDH-1 immunohistochemistry identifies only mutant protein resulting from most common mutation
  - R132H: Arginine to histidine at position 132
- Olig2(+) (almost all)
- Ki-67: Low labeling index
- No codeletion of chromosomes 1p and 19q
- Many with *IDH1/2* mutation have strong nuclear p53(+) &/or loss of nuclear ATRX
- Diffuse astrocytomas by definition, devoid of 1p/19q codeletion
- Pediatric gliomas have differing genetic features than adult gliomas

Axial MR: Mesial Temporal Tumor

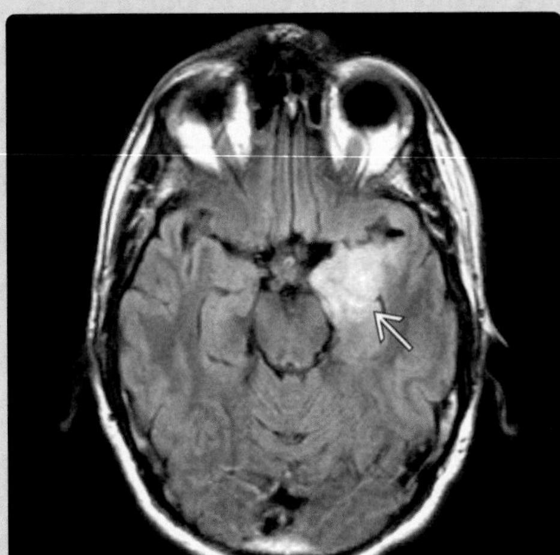

Microcysts

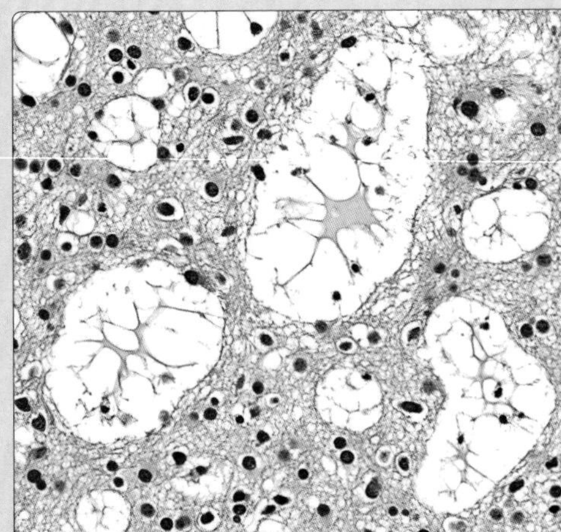

(Left) *FLAIR brightness in diffuse astrocytomas ➡ is due to intratumoral edema &/or myxoid matrix.* **(Right)** *Hypercellularity, a modest degree of nuclear pleomorphism, and occasional microcysts are common features of grade II diffuse astrocytomas.*

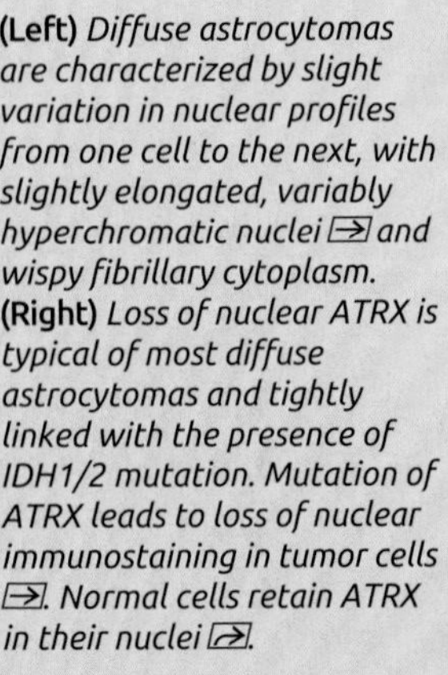

(Left) *Diffuse astrocytomas are characterized by slight variation in nuclear profiles from one cell to the next, with slightly elongated, variably hyperchromatic nuclei ➡ and wispy fibrillary cytoplasm.* **(Right)** *Loss of nuclear ATRX is typical of most diffuse astrocytomas and tightly linked with the presence of IDH1/2 mutation. Mutation of ATRX leads to loss of nuclear immunostaining in tumor cells ➡. Normal cells retain ATRX in their nuclei ↪.*

Slight Variation in Nuclear Profiles

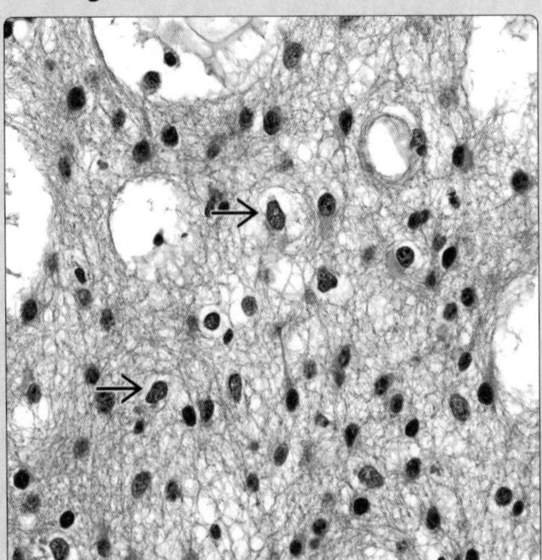

Loss of Nuclear ATRX

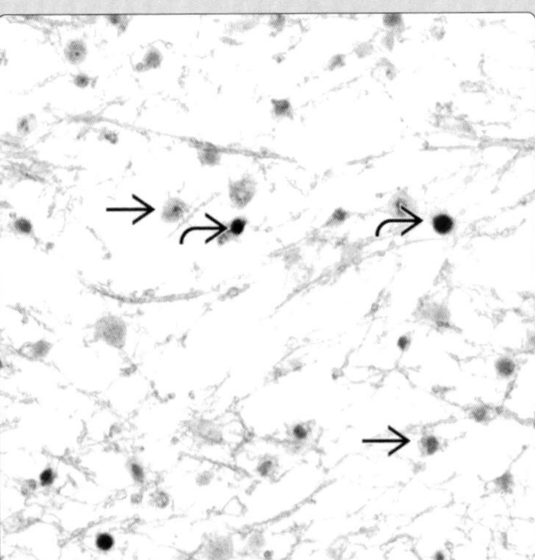

TERMINOLOGY

Definitions

- Infiltrating glioma with astrocytic differentiation
- Defined as nonoligodendroglial infiltrating glioma
- Includes
  - *IDH1/2*-mutated diffuse adult gliomas without 1p/19q codeletion and usually with *p53* &/or *ATRX* mutations
  - Uncommon adult *IDH1/2* wild-type tumors behave as glioblastoma
  - Pediatric diffuse pontine gliomas have differing genetics, especially *H3F3A K27* mutations
  - Pediatric patients < 14 years with diffuse gliomas in other sites do not have *IDH1/2* mutations
- WHO grade II

CLINICAL ISSUES

Epidemiology

- Age
  - Adults (usually < 50 years) and children
- Sex
  - Slight male predominance

Site

- Cerebral hemispheres (children and adults)
- Thalamus (children and adults)
- Brain stem
  - Typically children
  - Usually pons
- Cerebellum (usually adults, uncommon)
- Spinal cord (children and adults, uncommon)

Presentation

- Seizures with cerebral hemispheric lesions
- Neurological deficits uncommon, location dependent
- Signs and symptoms of increased intracranial pressure, usually only with ventricular obstruction

Treatment

- Surgical approaches
  - Stereotactic biopsy
  - Resection
    - Partial is rule
    - Complete with margins, unlikely
  - Often none for pontine astrocytomas
    - Usually diagnosed from clinical and radiological features
    - Pretreatment biopsy in some centers
- Adjuvant therapy
  - Some cases, not standard
- Radiation
  - Variable depending on site, size, symptomatology, and patient age
- Observation, in many cases

Prognosis

- Recurrence and frequent progress to higher grade astrocytoma within 10 years; incidence unclear
- Better in children
- Incidence of anaplastic transformation unclear, but higher than for oligodendroglioma grade II
- Unclear benefit of total excision with negative margins over conventional gross total resection
- Those adult gliomas with *IDH1/2* mutations have significantly better prognosis than those without
  - *IDH1/2* wild-type adult diffuse gliomas resolve into other entities
  - Many *IDH1/2* wild-type adult diffuse gliomas behave adversely, akin to glioblastoma
    - 78% diagnosed as molecular equivalent of conventional glioblastoma (GBM) using methylation arrays, copy number
    - 9% showed genetic features akin to pediatric diffuse pontine gliomas with *H3F3A* mutation
    - 8% showed methylation profile similar to those with *H3F3A* mutation (but without the mutation)
    - *H3F3A*-mutated group in adults tumors of infratentorial and midline localization
- Diffuse intrinsic pontine gliomas often have poor prognosis despite apparent low-grade histological features
  - Prognosis relates more to mutational status than mitotic rate, presence or absence of microvascular proliferation &/or necrosis
  - Patients with tumors harboring K27M mutation in H3.3 (*H3F3A*) may not respond clinically to radiotherapy as well, relapse significantly earlier, and exhibit more metastatic recurrences than those in H3.1 (*HIST1H3B/C*) mutation

IMAGING

MR Findings

- Ill-defined or relatively discrete area of T1 hypointensity and T2/FLAIR hyperintensity
- Usually expansion of affected areas
- No enhancement
- Large cyst (some, e.g., gemistocytic types)
- Engulfment of basilar artery in pontine lesions

MACROSCOPIC

General Features

- Ill defined; blurring of gray-white junction
- Variable mass effect
- Large cyst (some, e.g., gemistocytic types)
  - Exception to rule that macrocystic CNS tumors are well circumscribed
- Enlarged pons; often partially surrounds basilar artery

Texture

- Variable
  - Soft, gelatinous
  - Firm

MICROSCOPIC

Histologic Features

- Infiltrative, diffuse
  - Trapped axons in white matter best seen on immunostain for neurofilament protein
  - Gray matter/secondary structures: Perineuronal satellitosis, subpial infiltration, and perivascular aggregation
    - All less common than in oligodendroglioma

- Fibrillary astrocytoma
  - Irregular cell distribution compared to oligodendroglioma
  - Hypercellularity: Slight to moderate in cases with tumoral edema
  - Microcysts: None to prominent
  - Cytoplasm
    - Scant (naked nuclei) in hypocellular tumors
    - Moderate with processes of fibrillary astrocytes
    - Prominent but not gemistocytic
    - Fine fibrillary background (some cases)
  - Nuclei
    - Atypia in all cases; degree can overlap with that of anaplastic astrocytoma
  - Nuclear enlargement, irregularity, hyperchromasia
  - Pleomorphic giant cells (uncommon)
  - Mitoses
    - Absent or rare in sizable specimens
    - Threshold for grade III (anaplastic astrocytoma) not sharply defined
    - New data suggest using old 2007 WHO grading criteria, no significant difference in patient age or prognosis for *IDH1/2*-mutated tumors formerly considered WHO grade II or WHO grade III
    - *IDH1/2* wild-type adult gliomas using old 2007 WHO grading criteria (i.e., > 1 mitotic figure identified = WHO grade III) also correlate poorly with prognosis
      - *IDH1/2* wild-type adult gliomas behave like glioblastoma
  - Calcifications (occasional)
    - Rarely dense cortical, gyriform pattern of oligodendroglioma
- Gemistocytic astrocytoma: Variable but prominent gemistocytes
  - Uncommon in pure form
  - Usually 20% or more of tumor cells; occasionally 50% or more
  - Regional variation in number of gemistocytes
  - Angular, polygonal cells
    - Glassy pink cytoplasm
    - Stout processes form coarse fibrillar background
  - Generally uniform, peripheral nuclei
  - Scattered large, round, dark nuclei with little cytoplasm (small cells)
    - Proliferating component
    - Small cell subpopulation with higher Ki-67 index compared to low index in gemistocytic element
  - Frequent perivascular lymphocytic infiltrates
  - Generally rare or no mitoses; low Ki-67 labeling index despite lesion propensity for anaplastic transformation
    - If *IDH1/2* mutated, however, grading by number of mitotic figures is not as important, ie., using old WHO 2007 grading criteria, no substantial differences between WHO grades II and III *IDH1/2* mutated gliomas in terms of demographics or prognosis

ANCILLARY TESTS

Cytology

- Tissue fragments in smear preparations
- Mild to moderate nuclear pleomorphism and hyperchromasia
- Naked nuclei in hypocellular lesions
- Prominent cytoplasm in gemistocytic lesions
- Cytoplasmic processes/fibrillar background

Immunohistochemistry

- IDH-1 (mutant IDH-1 protein, R132H)
  - Adolescents and adults (+) in almost all cases (85%)
  - Children < 14 years old usually (-)
  - Antibody only covers the common mutation; tumors with other *IDH1* mutations at same site but with different amino acid substitutions (or with *IDH2* mutations) still have favorable prognosis but must be identified by mutational analysis
- Olig2(+) (almost all)
- GFAP
  - Variable reactivity depending in part on amount of cytoplasm
  - Cells with naked nuclei negative
  - Gemistocytes
    - Peripheral cytoplasm or all of cytoplasm (+)
- p53
  - Diffuse strong nuclear positivity (about 1/4)
  - Higher in gemistocytic types
- Ki-67 variable (usually < 4%)
- Many adult diffuse gliomas with *IDH1/2* mutation also have loss of nuclear ATRX
  - Nuclear ATRX is either completely lost in all tumor nuclei or retained, not different in different subsets of cells from same tumor
  - Use neuronal or endothelial cell nuclei as internal control for area of slide being interpreted
  - Do not attempt to interpret area(s) of slide without positive internal control(s)
- Pediatric gliomas have differing genetic features than adult gliomas
  - Some pediatric gliomas may also show loss of nuclear ATRX but do not have *IDH1/2* mutation or *IDH1* R132H IHC(+)
  - More pediatric gliomas with *H3F3A* mutation and H3F3a K27M IHC(+) even if histologically low grade
- Increasing number of midline young adult gliomas of brainstem, thalamus, spinal cord also show H3F3A K27M IHC(+) &/or loss of nuclear ATRX
  - Mutations in *IDH1/2* and histones mutually exclusive

Genetic Testing

- Mutations in *IDH1*, 85% in adolescents and adults
  - Early event
  - R132H (arginine to histidine, position 132)
  - Other amino acid substitutions occurring at same site uncommon (~ 1/10 to 1/6 of overall *IDH1* mutations)
- Gain of chromosome 7
- No codeletion of chromosomes 1p and 19q

Genetic Testing

- Gain of chromosome 7 in most cases

DIFFERENTIAL DIAGNOSIS

Normal Brain

- Low cellularity and even cell distribution
- No microcysts
- No atypia
- Very low to zero Ki-67 index
- IDH-1(-), p53(-)

Nonspecific Gliosis

- Evenly spaced hypertrophic fibrillary or gemistocytic astrocytes
- Hemosiderin, in some cases, rare in untreated astrocytoma
- Low Ki-67 index
- IDH-1(-)
- Negative to weak p53
- Intact chromosome 7

Demyelinating Disease

- Sharp border, usually
- Numerous macrophages
- Perivascular lymphocytes
- Multinucleated reactive astrocytes (Creutzfeldt cells)
- Loss of myelin (H&E/LFB stain), spared axons
- IDH-1(-)
- Weak to moderate p53 (scattered cells)
- Intact chromosome 7

Anaplastic Astrocytoma (Grade III)

- Higher cellularity but not always
- Greater cytological atypia usually
- Mitoses: Rare to numerous
- Higher Ki-67 rate, usually ≥ 5%, but overlap at lower end of range

Oligodendroglioma

- More uniform cell distribution
- Cytological monomorphism
    - Round nuclei with open chromatin and distinct nucleoli
- Generally more prominent perineuronal satellitosis and subpial concentration
- Perinuclear halo ("fried egg" cells)
    - Back-to-back arrays
- Little fibrillar background
- Prominent perineuronal satellitosis
- Intracortical (gyriform) calcification
- 1p/19q codeletion (ie., have LOH 1p, 19q)
- No *p53* mutation but p53 immunostaining may be seen
- No gain of chromosome 7

Pilocytic Astrocytoma

- Circumscribed and contrast enhancing, usually
- Compact architecture but infiltrative periphery, especially in cerebellum and optic nerves
- Biphasic pattern
    - Spongy microcystic tissue with eosinophilic granular bodies
    - Compact piloid tissue with Rosenthal fibers
- Glomeruloid vasculature, in some cases
- Activation of MAPK pathway, incidence site dependent
- IDH-1(-)

DIAGNOSTIC CHECKLIST

Clinically Relevant Pathologic Features

- Infiltrative nature usually precludes complete resection

Pathologic Interpretation Pearls

- Always consider alternative possibility of reactive lesion, e.g., gliosis or demyelinating disease
- IDH-1: Immunohistochemical marker of infiltrating gliomas, both astrocytic or oligodendroglial
- IDH-1 immunostaining directed only against mutant protein resulting from most common mutation; other *IDH1/2* mutations must be diagnosed by mutational testing
- Loss of nuclear ATRX typical of diffuse astrocytomas, not oligodendrogliomas or reactive gliosis

SELECTED REFERENCES

1. Cancer Genome Atlas Research Network et al: Comprehensive, integrative genomic analysis of diffuse lower-grade gliomas. N Engl J Med. 372(26):2481-98, 2015
2. Castel D et al: Histone H3F3A and HIST1H3B K27M mutations define two subgroups of diffuse intrinsic pontine gliomas with different prognosis and phenotypes. Acta Neuropathol. ePub, 2015
3. Feng J et al: The H3.3 K27M mutation results in a poorer prognosis in brainstem gliomas than thalamic gliomas in adults. Hum Pathol. ePub, 2015
4. Foote MB et al: Genetic classification of gliomas: refining histopathology. Cancer Cell. 28(1):9-11, 2015
5. Liu Q et al: Genetic, epigenetic, and molecular landscapes of multifocal and multicentric glioblastoma. Acta Neuropathol. 130(4):587-97, 2015
6. Reuss DE et al: Adult IDH wild type astrocytomas biologically and clinically resolve into other tumor entities. Acta Neuropathol. 130(3):407-17, 2015
7. Reuss DE et al: IDH mutant diffuse and anaplastic astrocytomas have similar age at presentation and little difference in survival: a grading problem for WHO. Acta Neuropathol. 129(6):867-73, 2015
8. Reuss DE et al: ATRX and IDH1-R132H immunohistochemistry with subsequent copy number analysis and IDH sequencing as a basis for an "integrated" diagnostic approach for adult astrocytoma, oligodendroglioma and glioblastoma. Acta Neuropathol. 129(1):133-46, 2015
9. Aihara K et al: H3F3A K27M mutations in thalamic gliomas from young adult patients. Neuro Oncol. 16(1):140-6, 2014
10. Sahm F et al: Farewell to oligoastrocytoma: in situ molecular genetics favor classification as either oligodendroglioma or astrocytoma. Acta Neuropathol. 128(4):551-9, 2014
11. Venneti S et al: A sensitive and specific histopathologic prognostic marker for H3F3A K27M mutant pediatric glioblastomas. Acta Neuropathol. 128(5):743-53, 2014
12. Bjerke L et al: Histone H3.3. mutations drive pediatric glioblastoma through upregulation of MYCN. Cancer Discov. 3(5):512-9, 2013
13. Gerges N et al: Pediatric high-grade astrocytomas: a distinct neuro-oncological paradigm. Genome Med. 5(7):66, 2013
14. Gielen GH et al: H3F3A K27M mutation in pediatric CNS tumors: a marker for diffuse high-grade astrocytomas. Am J Clin Pathol. 139(3):345-9, 2013
15. Kannan K et al: Whole-exome sequencing identifies ATRX mutation as a key molecular determinant in lower-grade glioma. Oncotarget. 3(10):1194-203, 2012
16. Khuong-Quang DA et al: K27M mutation in histone H3.3 defines clinically and biologically distinct subgroups of pediatric diffuse intrinsic pontine gliomas. Acta Neuropathol. 124(3):439-47, 2012
17. Wu G et al: Somatic histone H3 alterations in pediatric diffuse intrinsic pontine gliomas and non-brainstem glioblastomas. Nat Genet. 44(3):251-3, 2012
18. Pollack IF et al: IDH1 mutations are common in malignant gliomas arising in adolescents: a report from the Children's Oncology Group. Childs Nerv Syst. 27(1):87-94, 2011
19. Capper D et al: Application of mutant IDH1 antibody to differentiate diffuse glioma from nonneoplastic central nervous system lesions and therapy-induced changes. Am J Surg Pathol. 34(8):1199-204, 2010
20. Capper D et al: Characterization of R132H mutation-specific IDH1 antibody binding in brain tumors. Brain Pathol. 20(1):245-54, 2010

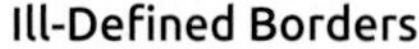

Ill-Defined Borders

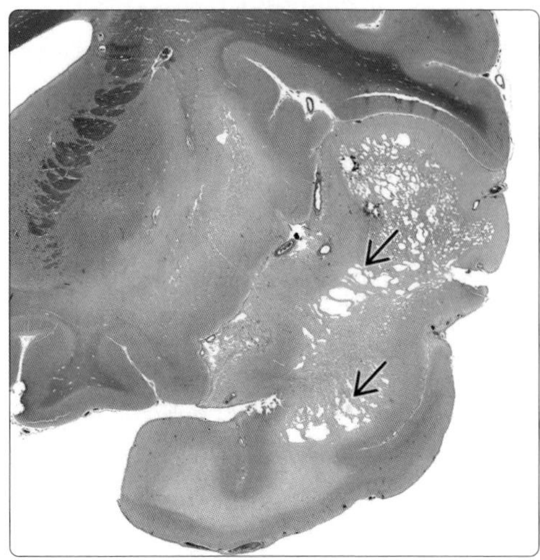

Pontine Glioma

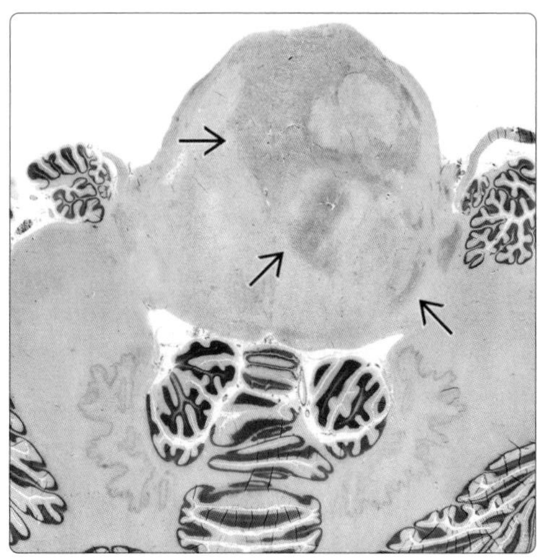

(Left) *A whole-mount section stained with H&E/Luxol fast blue illustrates a temporal lobe tumor's ill-defined borders and extensive microcystic change* →. **(Right)** *A whole-mount section of pons and cerebellum, stained with cresyl violet, illustrates diffuseness and varying degrees of cellularity in grade II astrocytomas* →. *In children, such lesions are usually treated on the basis of clinical and radiological findings alone. Most of these diffuse intrinsic pontine gliomas have a poor prognosis, whatever the grade.*

Spinal Cord Astrocytoma

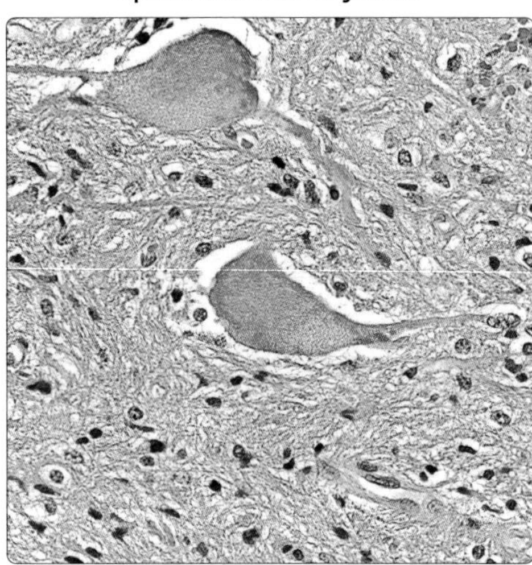

Infiltrative, With Preserved Axons

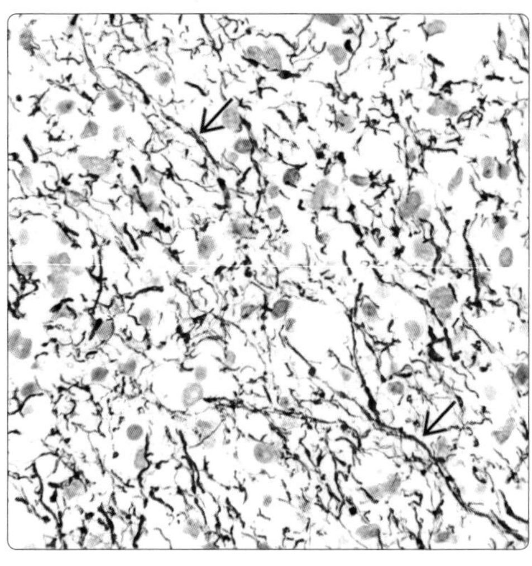

(Left) *Diffuse astrocytomas infiltrate tissues and surround neurons, as in this spinal cord example. The difficulty in distinguishing such cases from gliosis is obvious.* **(Right)** *Tumor cells enmeshed among axons stained for neurofilament protein* → *illustrate the infiltrative nature of diffuse astrocytomas. Intratumoral axons are also seen variably in such macroscopically discrete lesions as pilocytic astrocytoma.*

Mimicking Ganglioglioma

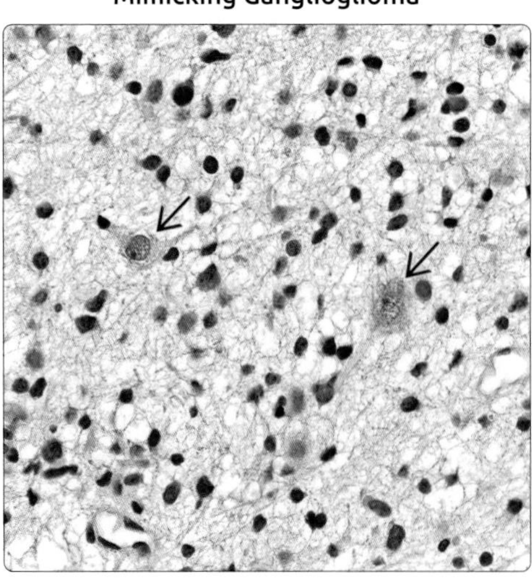

Perineuronal Satellitosis, Minimal

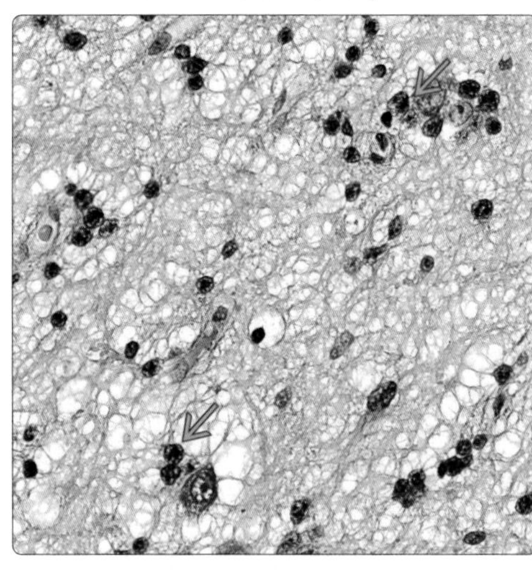

(Left) *The combination of diffuse astrocytoma and normal ganglion cells* → *should not be mistaken for ganglioglioma.* **(Right)** *Perineuronal satellitosis* → *is usually restrained in diffuse astrocytomas. This and other forms of secondary structure are more prominent in oligodendrogliomas. Tumor cells are larger and cytologically more atypical than normal satellite oligodendroglia.*

Gliomatosis Cerebri

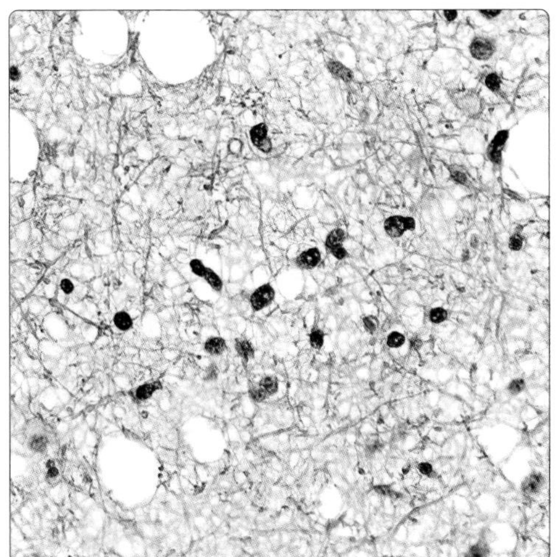

Paucicellular

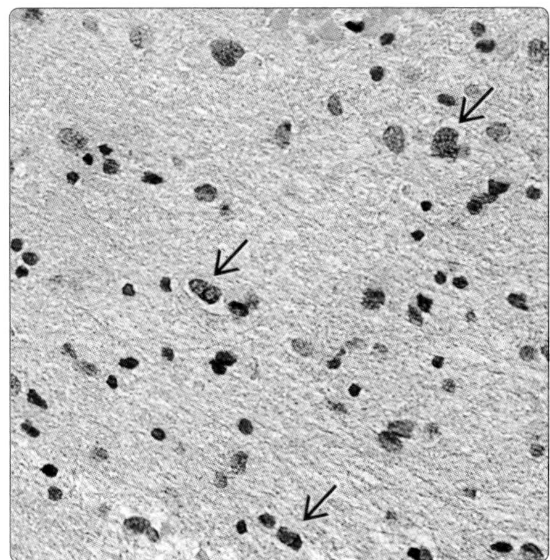

(Left) *In spite of impressive tumor size shown by neuroimaging, gliomatosis cerebri may have few tumor cells.* **(Right)** *Paucicellular lesions such as this are at the threshold of what can be diagnosed astrocytoma on histology alone. Positive immunostaining for IDH-1 would substantiate the diagnosis, but a negative reaction would not exclude a tumor. The degree of nuclear pleomorphism and hyperchromatism ➔ is typical of diffuse astrocytomas.*

Elongated Nuclei

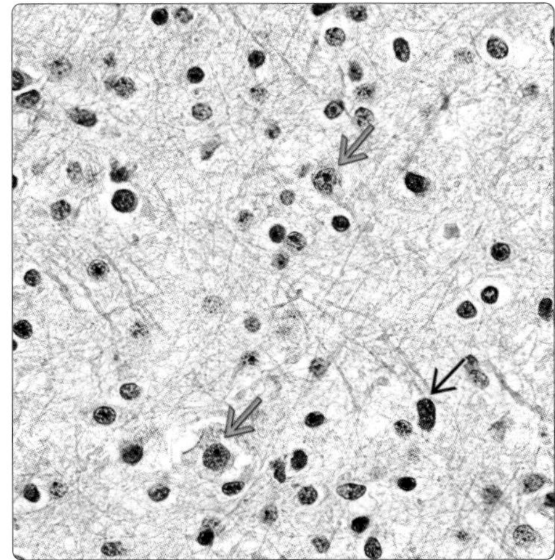

Subtle Nuclear Elongation

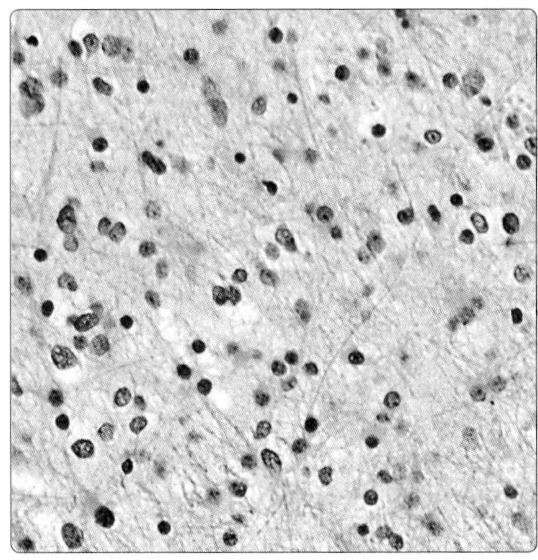

(Left) *While overall somewhat round, scattered elongated cells ➔ suggest that the tumor is astrocytic, not oligodendroglial. Trapped neurons are present ➔.* **(Right)** *This degree of cellularity clearly exceeds that of reactive gliosis. Unlike in subacute gliosis, little cytoplasm is seen. Most nuclei show subtle elongation, but the possibility of oligodendroglioma would certainly arise.*

Dark Angular Nuclei

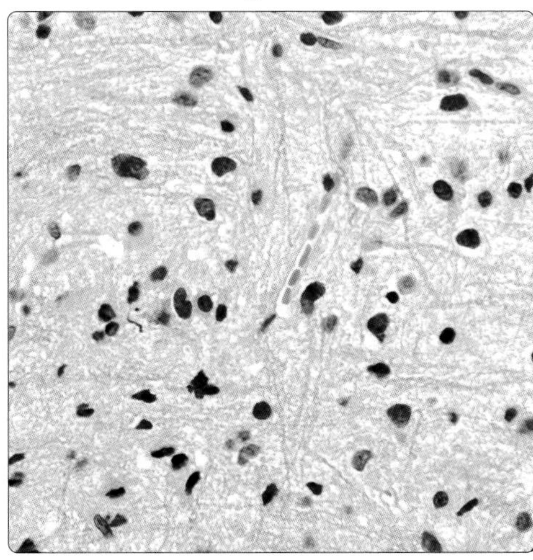

Prominent Cytoplasm

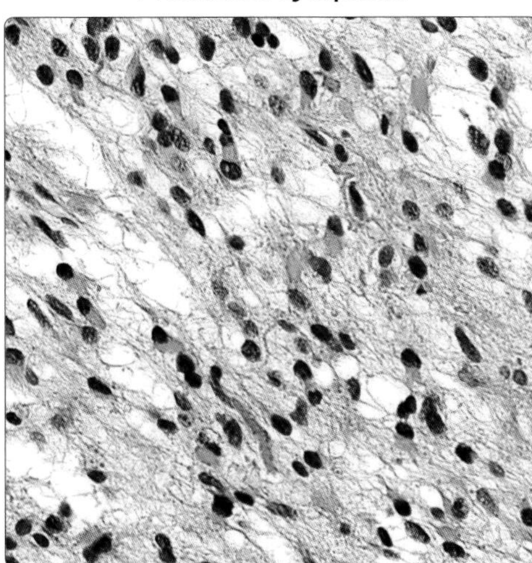

(Left) *Dark, elongated, and sometimes angular nuclei without apparent nucleoli are typical of infiltrating astrocytomas of any grade. As here, cytoplasm is often inconspicuous, if discernible at all (naked nuclei).* **(Right)** *Paranuclear pink cytoplasm and processes create a fibrillar background and help identify this tumor as astrocytic.*

(Left) *The combination of gemistocytes and vacuolated tumor cells somewhat resembles the reactive astrocyte-macrophage mixture of demyelinating disease, but the sheer number of gemistocytes is greater than in reactive gliosis. Some of these gemistocytes also resemble "mini" gemistocytes present in some oligodendrogliomas.* **(Right)** *A loose cobweb of processes is present in some astrocytomas. Dark angulated nuclei ⇨ are typical of diffuse astrocytoma.*

Gemistocytes

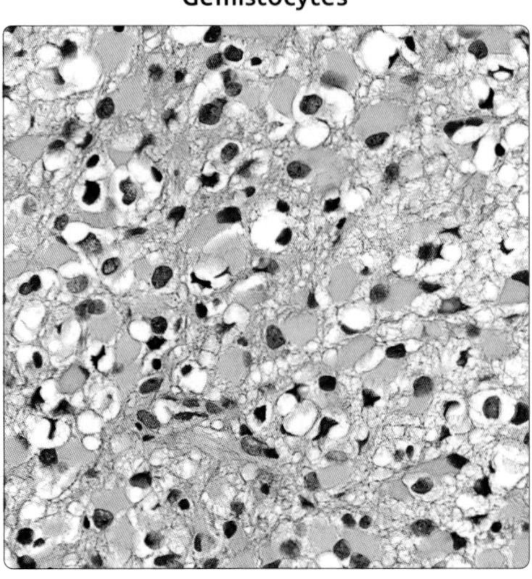

Dark Angulated Nuclei

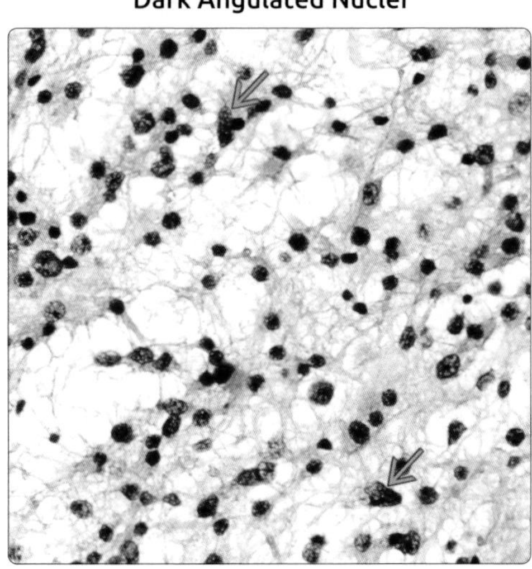

(Left) *Focal round nuclei with clear halos add an oligodendroglioma quality to many astrocytomas. The degree of hyperchromasia and shape of the nuclei are helpful features. Immunohistochemistry for ATRX and p53 as well as studies for 1p/19q deletion would be appropriate.* **(Right)** *Nuclei of fibrillary astrocytomas are darker, more angulated, and more irregularly distributed than those of oligodendroglioma.*

Mimicking Oligodendroglioma

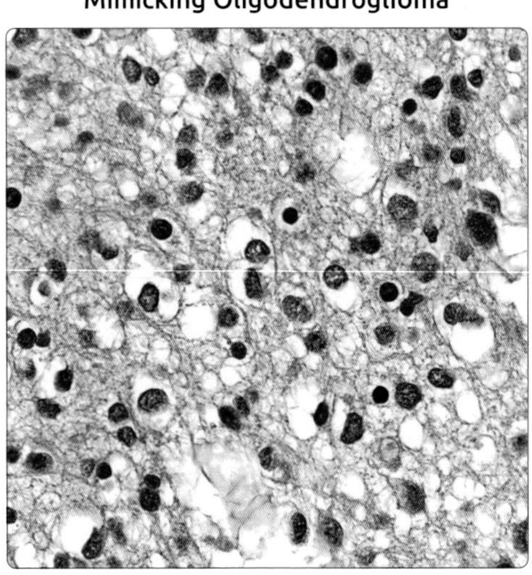

Fibrillary Astrocytoma

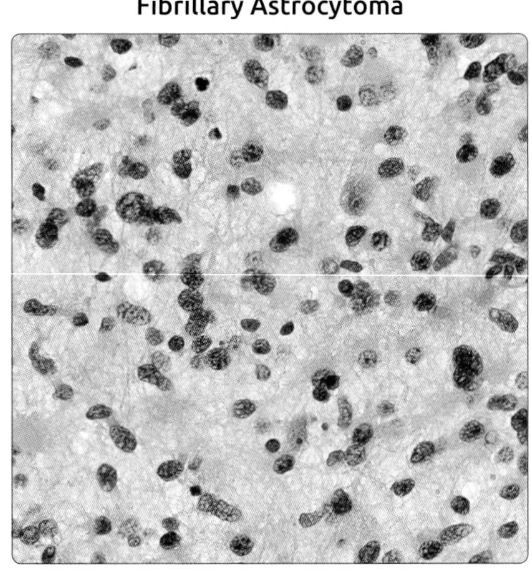

(Left) *Somewhat hyperchromatic nuclei without nucleoli and uneven cell distribution are typical of infiltrating astrocytomas. These tumor cells do not have enough cytoplasm to be gemistocytes.* **(Right)** *This degree of cellularity and atypia raises suspicions of grade III astrocytoma, but mitoses were very rare in a generous specimen. Dark, angulated nuclei ⇨ help distinguish this neoplasm from oligodendroglioma. Apoptosis ⇨ is not a grading parameter.*

Prominent Fibrillary Cytoplasm

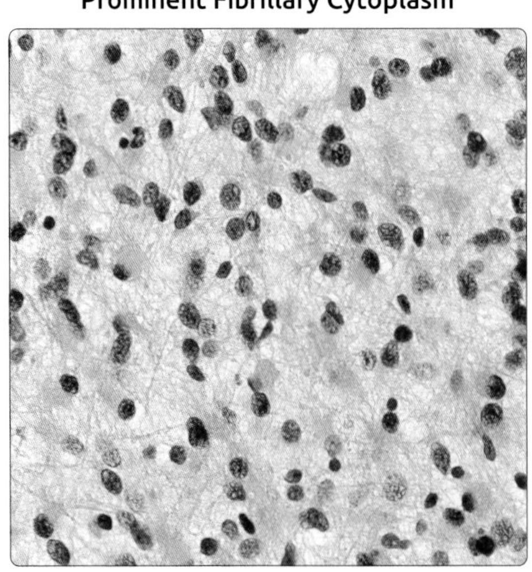

Apoptosis

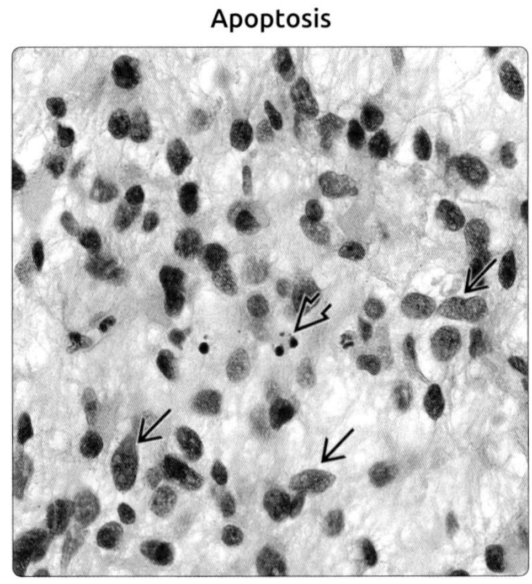

Perivascular Lymphocytes

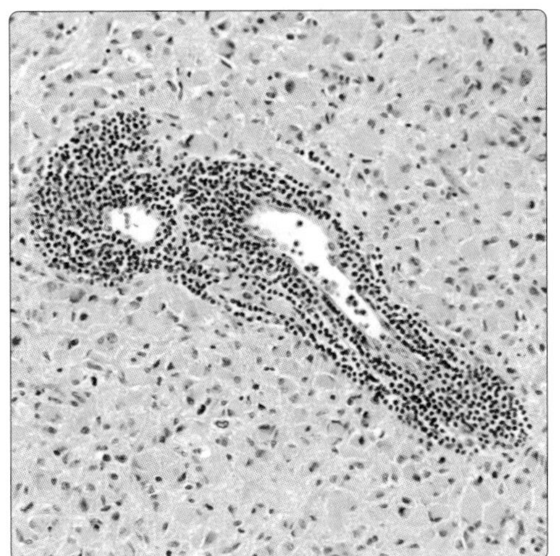

Gemistocytic Astrocytoma

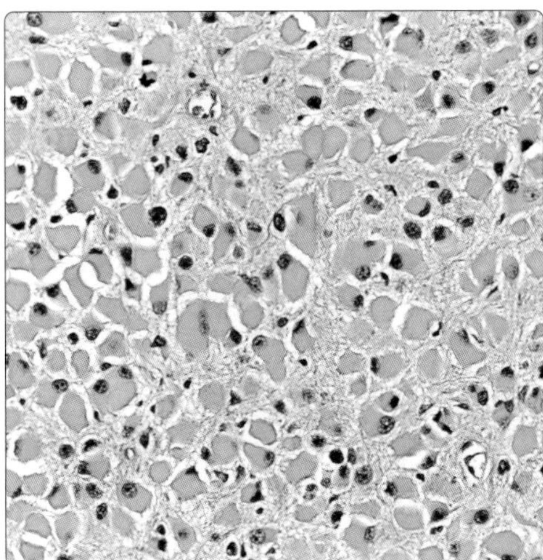

(Left) *Gemistocytes and perivascular lymphocytes are topographically linked. While this lesion is too cellular and cytologically atypical to be reactive gliosis, the possibility of demyelinating disease still needs to be considered.* **(Right)** *Gemistocytes are polygonal cells with peripherally displaced nuclei and glassy cytoplasm, as well as coarse processes. Despite the tumor's aggressive behavior, mitoses are usually hard to find.*

Admixed Nongemistocytic Tumor Cells

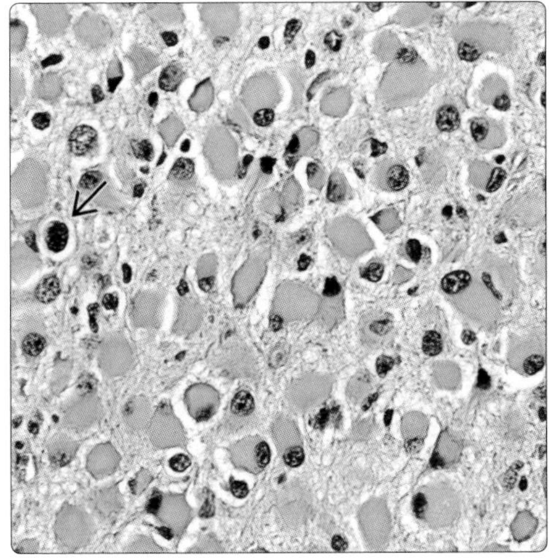

Heterogeneous Features

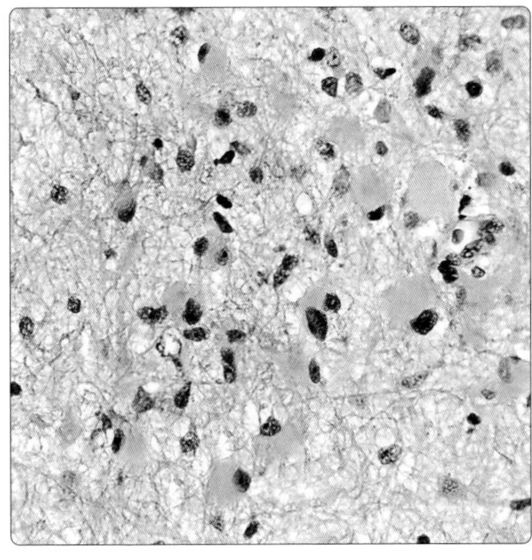

(Left) *Scattered cells with round, especially hyperchromatic nuclei* ➔ *are the principal proliferating element in gemistocytic astrocytoma.* **(Right)** *Some tumors have fibrillary astrocytes, gemistocytic astrocytes, and transitional forms. While there is no fixed percentage of gemistocytes required for the designation gemistocytic, a threshold of 20% is often used.*

Microcysts With Faint Mucoid Contents

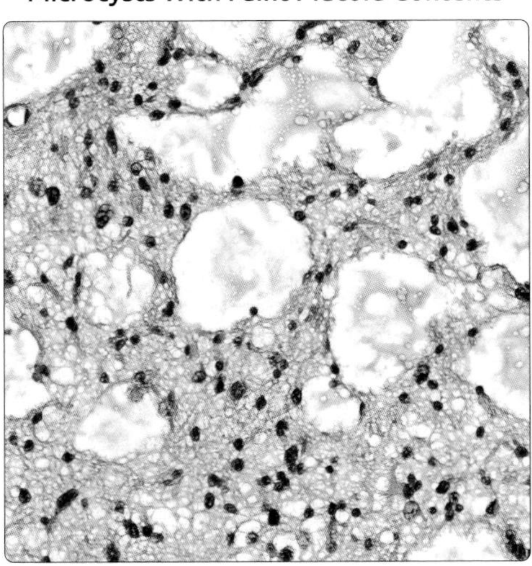

Rounder Nuclei

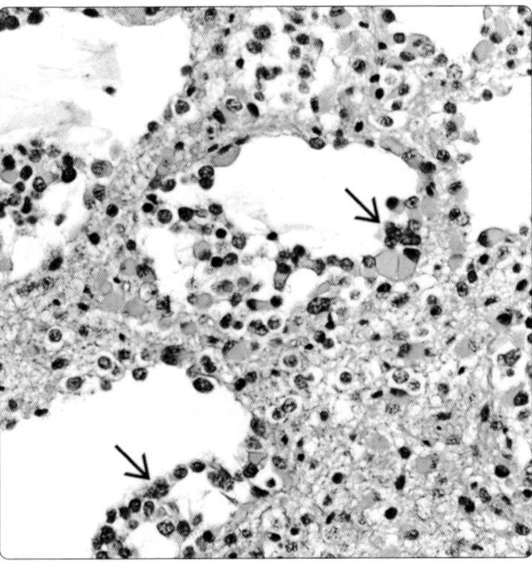

(Left) *Microcysts, often filled with a faintly basophilic mucoid substance, are not uncommon in astrocytomas or oligodendrogliomas. The dark, angulated nuclei in this case are typical of infiltrating astrocytomas.* **(Right)** *Round cells cling to the wall of microcysts* ➔ *in occasional astrocytomas of either grade II or III, having an oligodendroglioma quality. Significant immunoreactivity for nuclear p53 &/or loss of nuclear ATRX is common in these tumors, which are not codeleted for chromosomes 1p and 19q.*

(Left) *Irregular, dark nuclei with inconspicuous nucleoli sit in a fibrillar background. Nuclei of oligodendroglioma would be rounder and less dense. The process-rich background would also be absent.* **(Right)** *Gemistocytes vary in their immunoreactivity for GFAP but are often centrally negative, having only rim-like positivity. Others are entirely negative.*

Smear, Astrocytoma

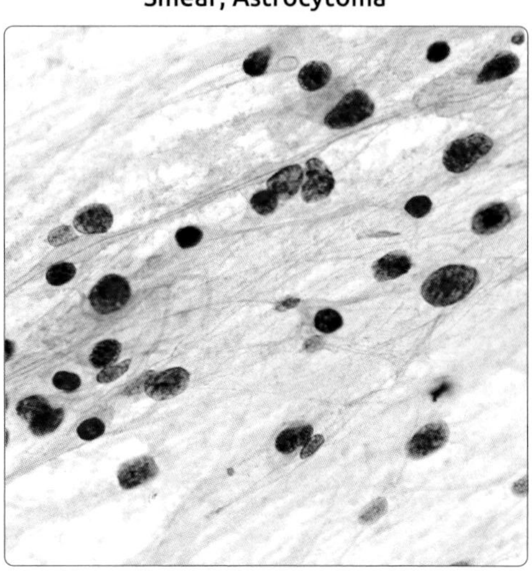

Rim-Like GFAP

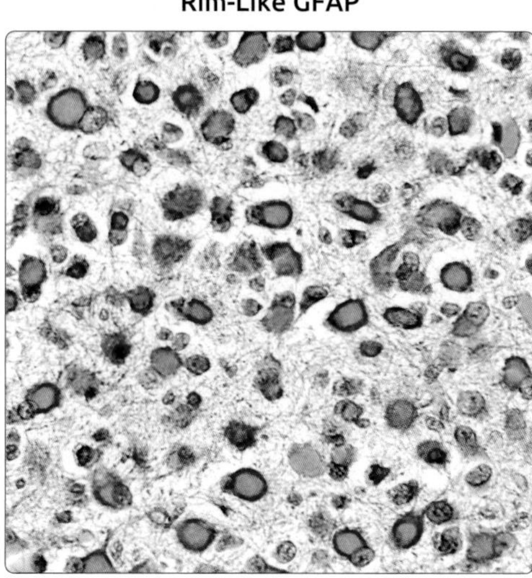

(Left) *Strong diffuse nuclear immunostaining for p53 is present in ~ 25% of diffuse astrocytomas. Although not a molecular test per se, such staining is highly unlikely in a 1p/19q codeleted oligodendroglioma. Also unlikely in an oligodendroglioma is loss of nuclear ATRX.* **(Right)** *Nuclear immunostaining for Olig2 helps identify tumor cells as being of astrocytic or oligodendroglial lineages. Unfortunately, despite the name, this immunostain is not specific for tumors of oligodendroglial lineage.*

Nuclear p53

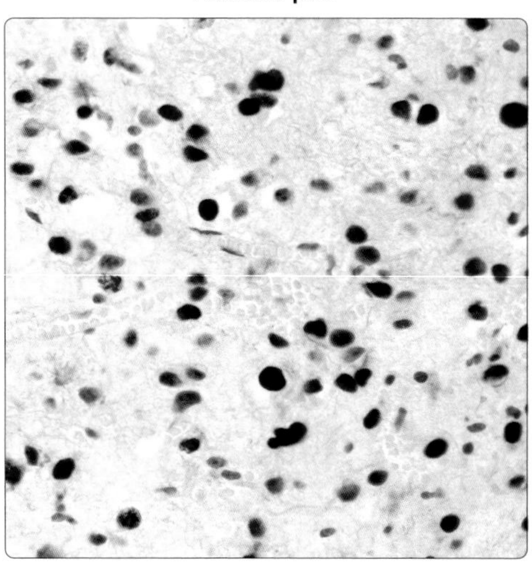

Olig2 in Astrocytoma

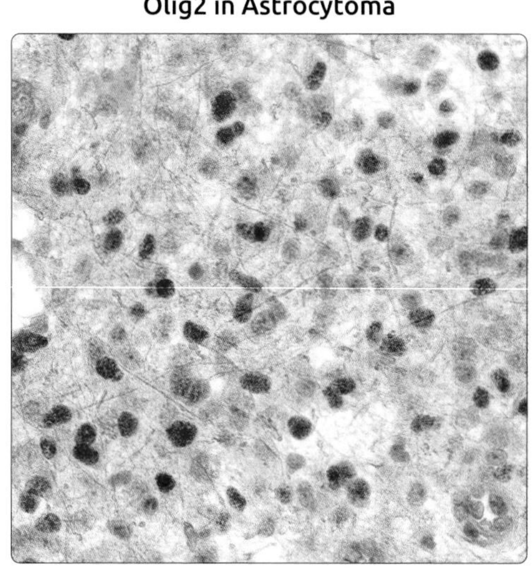

(Left) *Cytoplasmic and, to a lesser extent, nuclear staining for mutant IDH-1 is present in almost all adult grade II diffuse astrocytomas. However, this antibody will only pick up 85% of astrocytomas with IDH1/2 mutation.* **(Right)** *Loss of nuclear ATRX is often seen in IDH1-mutated diffuse astrocytomas. Indeed, if loss of nuclear ATRX is detected but IDH-1 immunohistochemistry is also negative, mutational analysis for IDH2 or noncanonical (i.e., non-R132H) IDH1 mutations should be performed.*

IDH-1

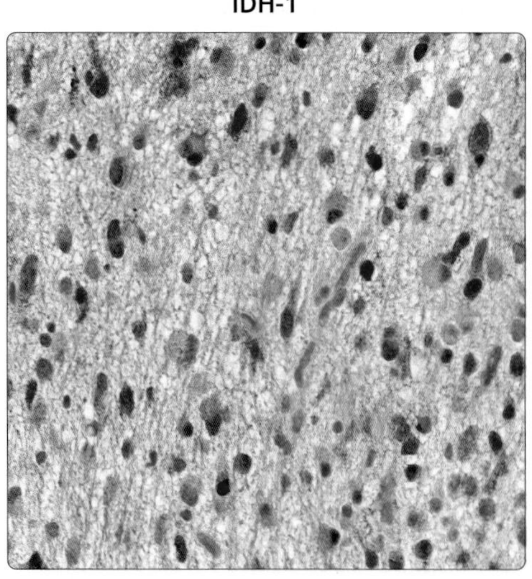

Loss of Nuclear ATRX

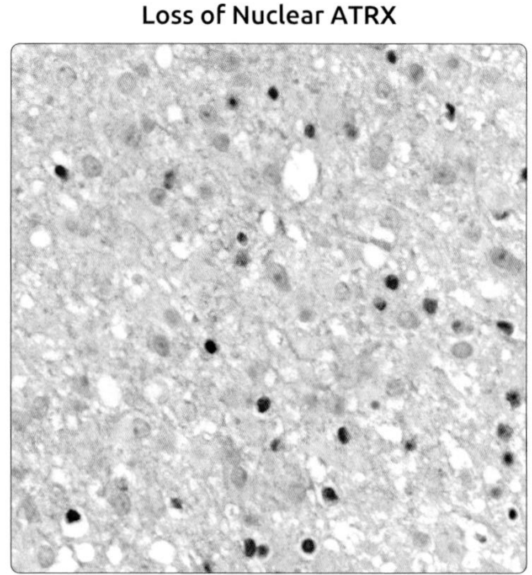

ATRX Retained in Normal Cortex, Endothelial Cells

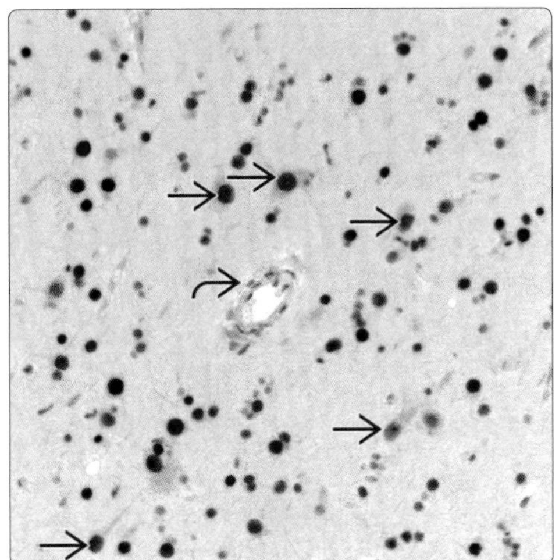

ATRX in Nonneoplastic Neuronal Nuclei

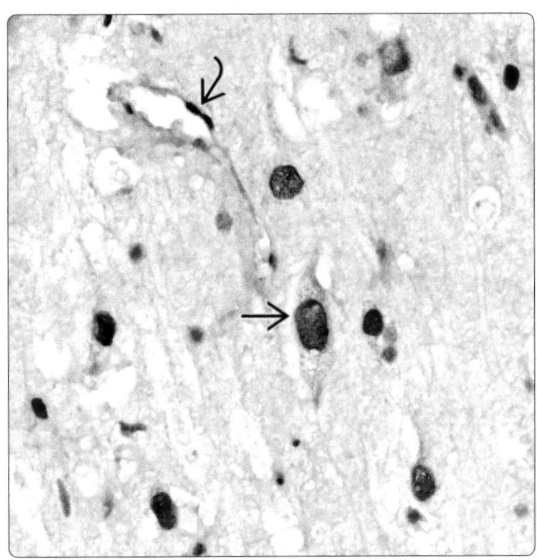

(Left) *If diffuse astrocytomas have mutated ATRX, immunostaining is lost in tumor nuclei. In contrast, normal nontumor cells such as cortical neurons ➡ and endothelial cell nuclei ➦ retain nuclear IHC. This serves as an internal control for immunostain fidelity.* **(Right)** *ATRX IHC should always be interpreted in the area(s) of the slide where a positive internal control exists, such as nonneoplastic neurons ➡ or endothelial cell nuclei ➦. Tumor cells are usually either completely ATRX negative or positive.*

Gain of Chromosome 7

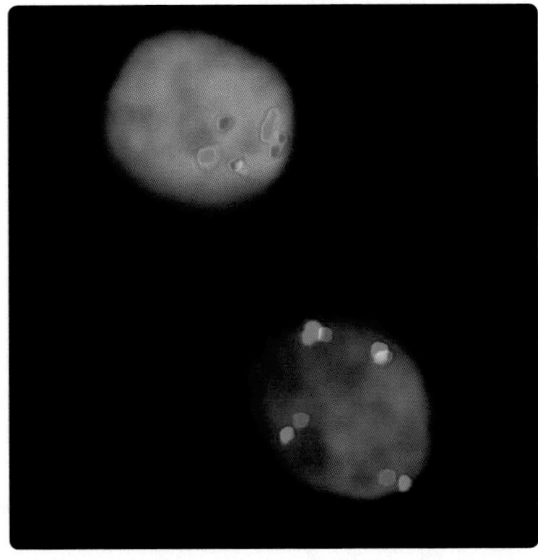

Diffuse Astrocytoma With Nuclear ATRX Loss but No *IDH1/2* Mutation

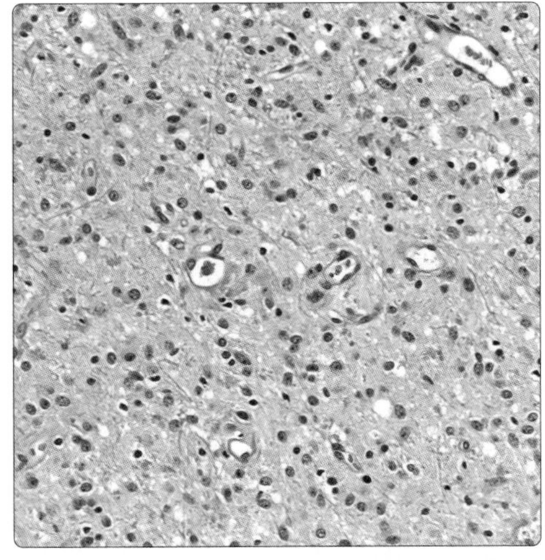

(Left) *Gain of chromosome 7 is common in diffuse astrocytomas and rare in oligodendrogliomas. It is apparent here on FISH analysis as multiple signals for chromosome 7. Such gain is to be distinguished from amplification, which is seen in glioblastoma. (Courtesy M. Rosenblum, MD.)* **(Right)** *Young adult gliomas, particularly those in midline sites, may have loss of nuclear ATRX but no IDH1/2 mutation. Some of these additionally have histone H3.F3A K27M mutation.*

Reactive Gliosis, Encephalitis

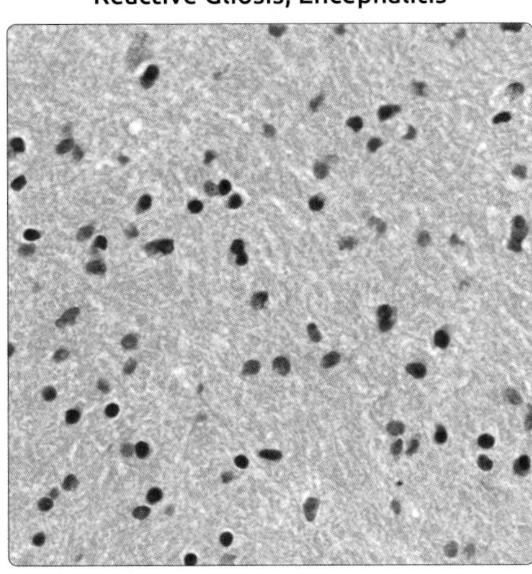

GFAP, Reactive Astrocytosis

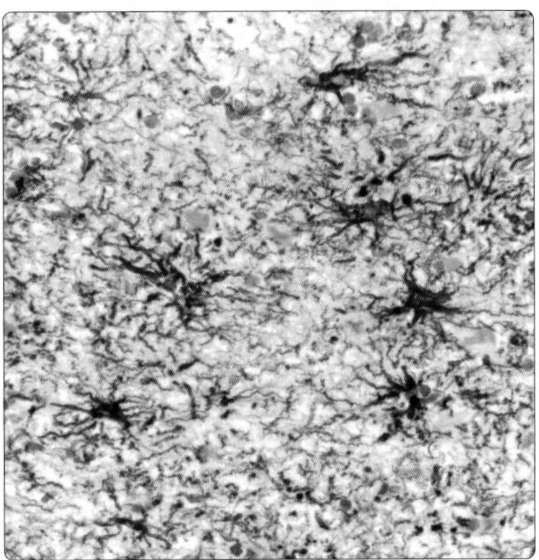

(Left) *This minimally hypercellular biopsy shows little or no cytological nuclear atypia but was submitted as a low-grade glioma for consultation. All immunohistochemical markers that might suggest glioma (IDH-1, absence of diffuse nuclear p53, retention of nuclear ATRX) were negative. Patient proved to have reactive gliosis & encephalitis.* **(Right)** *Reactive stellate GFAP(+) astrocytes in a case of encephalitis are identifiable by their long stellate, tapering processes and near-equidistant placement.*

Anaplastic Astrocytoma

KEY FACTS

TERMINOLOGY

- Mitotically active infiltrating astrocytoma

CLINICAL ISSUES

- Poor prognosis; most patients succumb within 5 years

IMAGING

- Enhancement
  - Minority of cases patchy
  - Rim or ring pattern, indicates incompletely sampled glioblastoma (GBM)

MICROSCOPIC

- Broad category, overlaps at extremes with grade II astrocytoma and GBM
- Mitoses
  - No defined number per 10 HPF
  - WHO: Grade III
  - 1 usually considered sufficient in small stereotactic biopsy
  - WHO: 1 insufficient in large specimen

ANCILLARY TESTS

- IDH1 R132H (+), most cases
  - Cases with *IDH1/2* mutation often have strong nuclear p53 &/or loss of nuclear ATRX
  - Immunohistochemistry for mutant IDH1 protein does not recognize all *IDH1* mutations or any (rare) *IDH2* mutations
- IDH-1(-)
  - Associated with poor prognosis, similar to GBM
  - Undersampled primary glioblastoma, in some cases

DIAGNOSTIC CHECKLIST

- Exclude mimics, e.g., reactive gliosis, pilocytic astrocytoma, and pleomorphic xanthoastrocytoma
- Be careful in diagnosis; grade III astrocytomas treated with radiation and chemotherapy

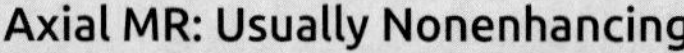
Axial MR: Usually Nonenhancing

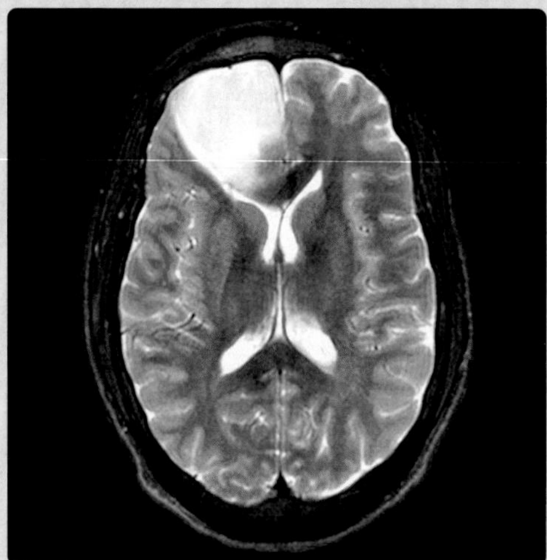

Multiple Mitoses

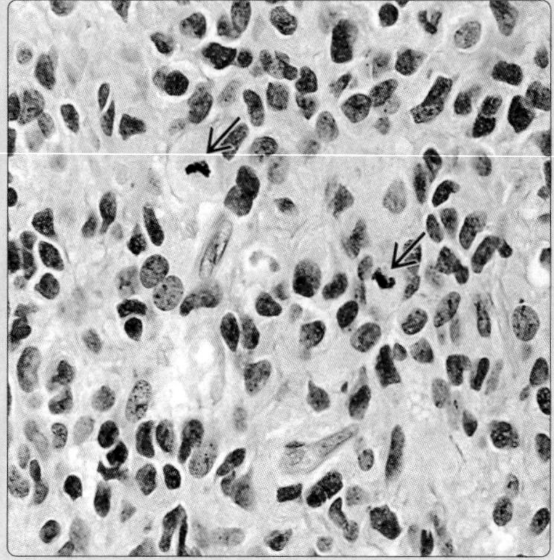

(Left) *T2WI MR shows anaplastic astrocytomas as white, edematous areas with variable mass effect. Despite their reputation to the contrary, most do not enhance.* **(Right)** *Nuclear pleomorphism confirms the tumor's astrocytic nature, and mitoses ⇒ indicate grade III.*

Small Cell Astrocytoma

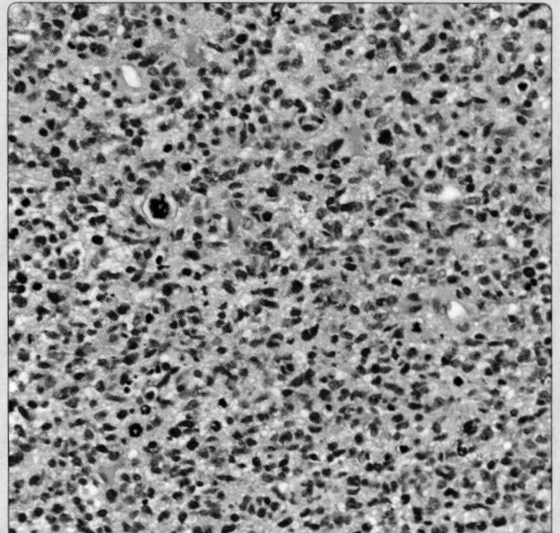

Ki-67 Elevated

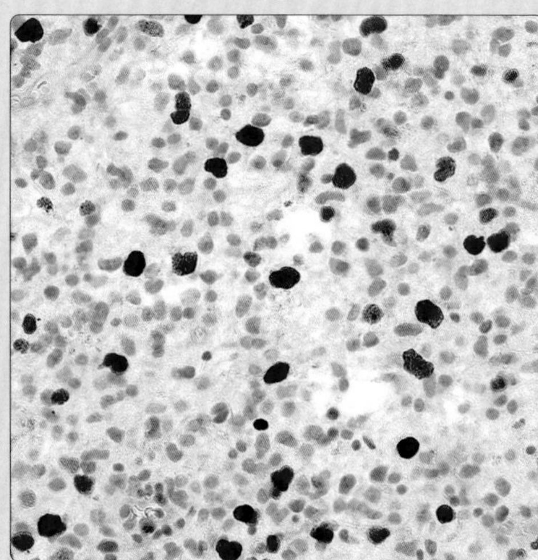

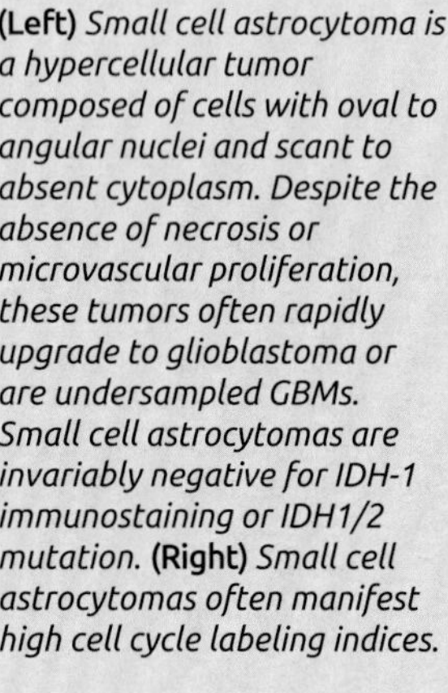
(Left) *Small cell astrocytoma is a hypercellular tumor composed of cells with oval to angular nuclei and scant to absent cytoplasm. Despite the absence of necrosis or microvascular proliferation, these tumors often rapidly upgrade to glioblastoma or are undersampled GBMs. Small cell astrocytomas are invariably negative for IDH-1 immunostaining or IDH1/2 mutation.* **(Right)** *Small cell astrocytomas often manifest high cell cycle labeling indices.*

TERMINOLOGY

Abbreviations

- Anaplastic astrocytoma (AA)

Definitions

- Mitotically active infiltrating astrocytoma
- Can appear de novo or arise from grade II astrocytoma
- Common form of gliomatosis cerebri
- Incidence relative to astrocytoma grade II dependent on number of mitoses required
- WHO grade III

CLINICAL ISSUES

Site

- Cerebral hemispheres (children and adults)
- Thalamus (children and adults)
- Brain stem
  - Usually pons
  - Typically children
- Cerebellum (usually adults) rare
- Spinal cord (usually children and adults) uncommon

Presentation

- Seizures with superficial cerebral lesions
- Neurological deficits vary with location
- Signs and symptoms of increased intracranial pressure

Treatment

- Drugs
  - Temozolomide, in most cases

Prognosis

- Poor; most patients succumb within 5 years
- Often progress to glioblastoma (GBM)
- Especially poor, equivalent to that of GBM, when negative for *IDH1/2* mutation

IMAGING

MR Findings

- FLAIR/T2 bright
- Generally ill defined
- Variable mass effect
- Enhancement
  - None, most cases; patchy, minority
  - Rim pattern, indicates incompletely sampled GBM

MACROSCOPIC

General Features

- Tissue expansion (in most cases)
  - Ill defined, lower range of grade
  - Fleshy, highly cellular at upper range of grade
  - Hypertrophy of pons with partial engulfment of basilar artery

MICROSCOPIC

Histologic Features

- Broad category, overlaps at extremes with grade II astrocytoma and GBM
- Infiltrative
  - Many intratumoral axons
  - Overrun neurons, subpial accumulation, but usually not as prominent as in oligodendroglioma
- Cellularity, variable
  - Generally moderate to high
  - Can overlap with GBM or astrocytoma grade II
- Cell types
  - Fibrillary, naked nuclei to moderate cytoplasm with fine processes
  - Gemistocytic: Abundant cytoplasm
  - Small cell
    - Monomorphous, cytologically bland cells
    - Scant cytoplasm and processes
- Nuclei
  - Highly variable degree of atypia
    - Bland, overlapping with grade II astrocytoma, or
    - Markedly atypical overlapping with GBM
- Mitoses (rare to abundant)
  - 1 usually considered sufficient in small specimen, such as needle biopsies
  - WHO: 1 insufficient in large specimen, but no codified number
- Calcifications (uncommon)
- Perivascular lymphocytes, usually with gemistocytes
- Neuronal differentiation uncommon
  - Rosetted synaptophysin (+) islands of neuropil, surrounded sometimes by Neu(+) neurocytes (rare)
  - PNET-like tissue (rare, more often in glioblastoma)

ANCILLARY TESTS

Cytology

- Tissue fragments ± fibrillar processes
- Prominent cytoplasm in gemistocytic lesions
- Moderate nuclear hyperchromasia and pleomorphism
- Mitoses, but may be difficult to find

Immunohistochemistry

- p53 diffusely (+) in minority of cases
- Olig2(+)
- IDH1 R132 H(+) in most cases
  - Immunohistochemistry for mutant IDH1 protein does not recognize all *IDH1* mutations or *IDH2* mutations
- IDH-1(-)
  - Associated with poor prognosis, similar to GBM
  - Undersampled primary glioblastoma, in some cases
- Ki-67: Usually in 5-15% range
- Loss of nuclear ATRX often seen in tumors with *IDH1/2* mutation
- Retention of nuclear ATRX in adult tumors without *IDH1/2* mutation

DIFFERENTIAL DIAGNOSIS

Reactive Gliosis

- Low to medium cellularity
- Generally uniform cells with no or minor cytological atypia (chronic)
  - Radial processes
  - Cytoplasm moderate (subacute) to minor (chronic)

- Low Ki-67 rate

Demyelinating Disease

- Usually sharp border
- Macrophages, many, and perivascular lymphocytes
- Few, if any, mitoses
- Astrocytes with micronuclei (Creutzfeldt cells)

Progressive Multifocal Leukoencephalopathy

- Associated with immunosuppression
- Macrophage background
- Viral cytopathic effect, bizarre astrocytes
- Immunostaining or in situ hybridization (+) for SV40, JC virus
- Few, if any, mitoses

Astrocytoma Grade II

- Mitotically less active
- ↓ cytological atypia and ↓ Ki-67 rate, but overlap

Glioblastoma

- Enhancement with central necrosis
- Microvascular proliferation &/or necrosis

Anaplastic Oligodendroglioma

- Uniformly distributed round, uniform cells
- Often areas of classic oligodendroglioma grade II
- 1p/19q codeletion, in most cases

SELECTED REFERENCES

1. Appin CL et al: Molecular pathways in gliomagenesis and their relevance to neuropathologic diagnosis. Adv Anat Pathol. 22(1):50-8, 2015
2. Reuss DE et al: ATRX and IDH1-R132H immunohistochemistry with subsequent copy number analysis and IDH sequencing as a basis for an "integrated" diagnostic approach for adult astrocytoma, oligodendroglioma and glioblastoma. Acta Neuropathol. 129(1):133-46, 2015
3. Cryan JB et al: Clinical multiplexed exome sequencing distinguishes adult oligodendroglial neoplasms from astrocytic and mixed lineage gliomas. Oncotarget. 5(18):8083-92, 2014
4. Haberler C et al: Clinical Neuropathology practice news 2-2014: ATRX, a new candidate biomarker in gliomas. Clin Neuropathol. 33(2):108-11, 2014
5. Sahm F et al: Farewell to oligoastrocytoma: in situ molecular genetics favor classification as either oligodendroglioma or astrocytoma. Acta Neuropathol. 128(4):551-9, 2014
6. Kannan K et al: Whole-exome sequencing identifies ATRX mutation as a key molecular determinant in lower-grade glioma. Oncotarget. 3(10):1194-203, 2012
7. Perry A et al: Small cell astrocytoma: an aggressive variant that is clinicopathologically and genetically distinct from anaplastic oligodendroglioma. Cancer. 101(10):2318-26, 2004
8. Teo JG et al: A distinctive glioneuronal tumor of the adult cerebrum with neuropil-like (including "rosetted") islands: report of 4 cases. Am J Surg Pathol. 23(5):502-10, 1999
9. Daumas-Duport C et al: Grading of astrocytomas. A simple and reproducible method. Cancer. 62(10):2152-65, 1988
10. Burger PC et al: Glioblastoma multiforme and anaplastic astrocytoma. Pathologic criteria and prognostic implications. Cancer. 56(5):1106-11, 1985

Significant Nuclear Atypia

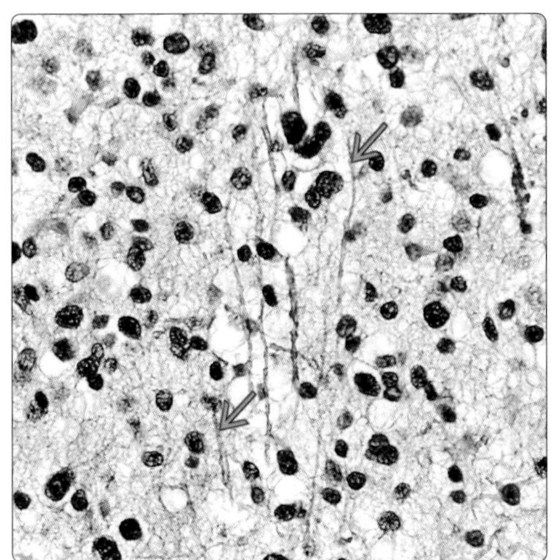

Infiltrating Tumor Cells Amongst Axons

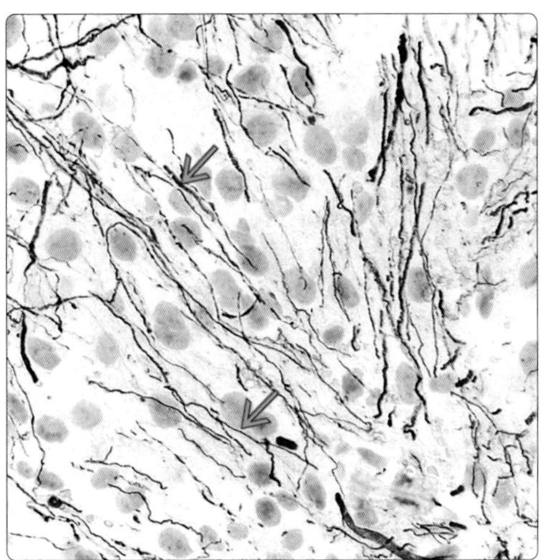

(Left) *The irregular, dark (almost black) nuclei intercalated among axons ➡ are common in infiltrating astrocytomas, either grade II or III. The degree of atypia in this case is common in grade III astrocytomas, but it may be present in some that are grade II as well. Atypia is not a grading parameter. Mitoses elsewhere in the tumor established grade III.* **(Right)** *Tumor cells infiltrate between axons stained for neurofilament protein ➡.*

Angular Hyperchromatic Nuclei

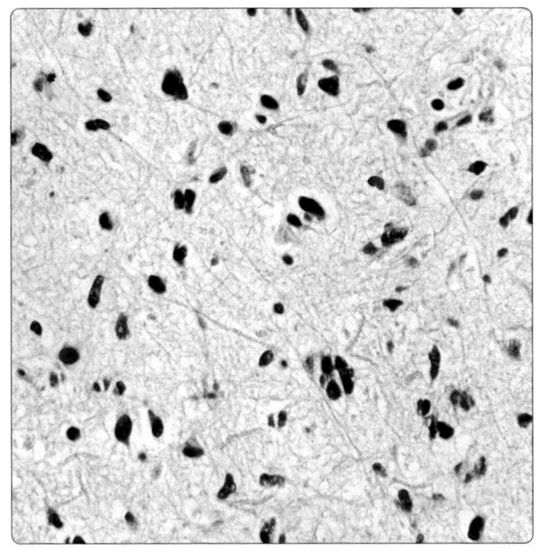

Multiple Mitoses

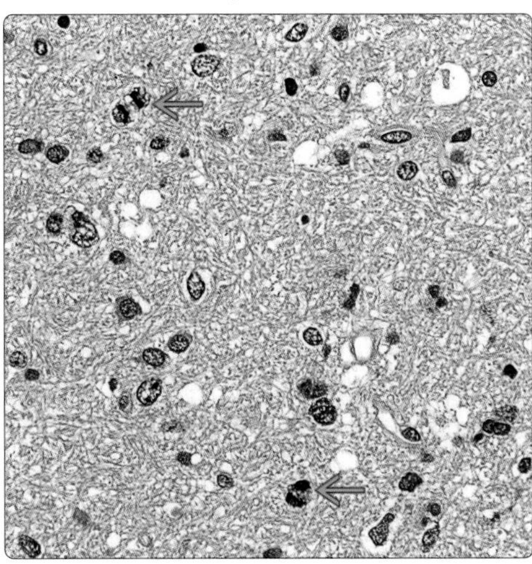

(Left) *Given the nuclear hyperchromatism and angulation, this infiltrating glioma is clearly not oligodendroglioma. The diagnosis of grade III astrocytoma depends on mitotic activity, which was present elsewhere in the specimen.* **(Right)** *Cellularity may be low in grade III gliomatosis cerebri, but multiple mitoses ➡ may be present. Such cases usually have few Ki-67 positive cells per unit area but a significant index when the latter is computed per tumor cell.*

Perinuclear Halos Simulating Oligodendroglioma

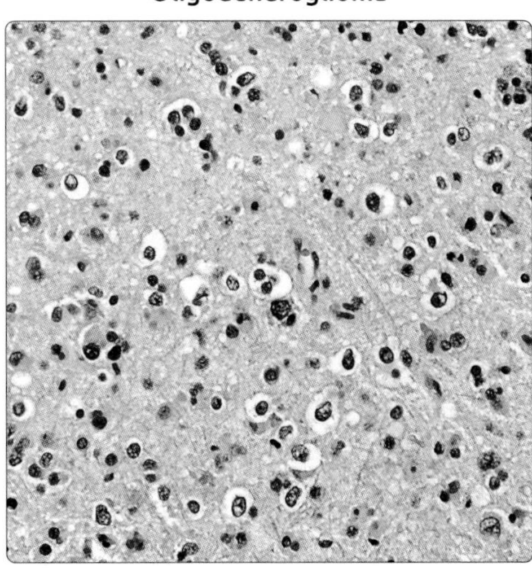

Atypia Not Grading Criterion

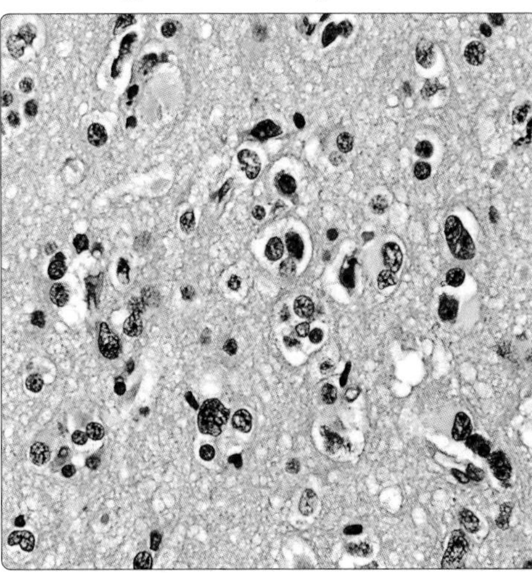

(Left) *Perinuclear halos and some round nuclei lend an oligodendroglioma quality, but the pleomorphism, hyperchromatism, and uneven cell distribution are not typical features of oligodendroglioma.* **(Right)** *The degree of atypia here, while common in anaplastic astrocytomas, is not in itself a criterion for grade III.*

(Left) *While more characteristic of oligodendrogliomas, perineuronal satellitosis ➡ may occur in infiltrating astrocytomas of any grade (grade III in this case).* **(Right)** *The irregular nuclei of these infiltrating cells help identify the lesion as astrocytoma. The mitosis ➡, if accompanied by others in a large specimen, establishes grade III.*

Perinuclear Satellitosis

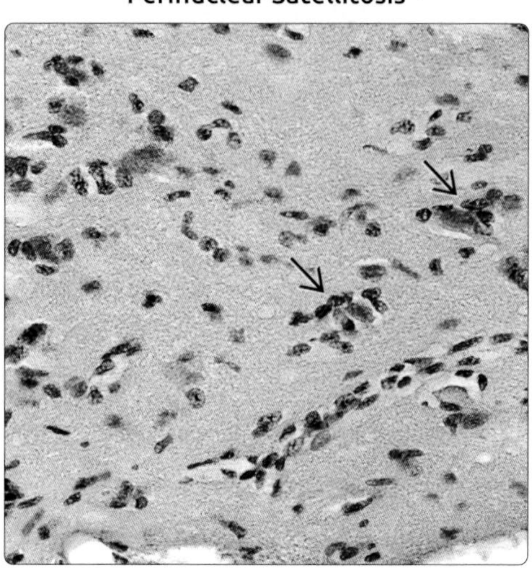

Irregular Tumor Nuclei

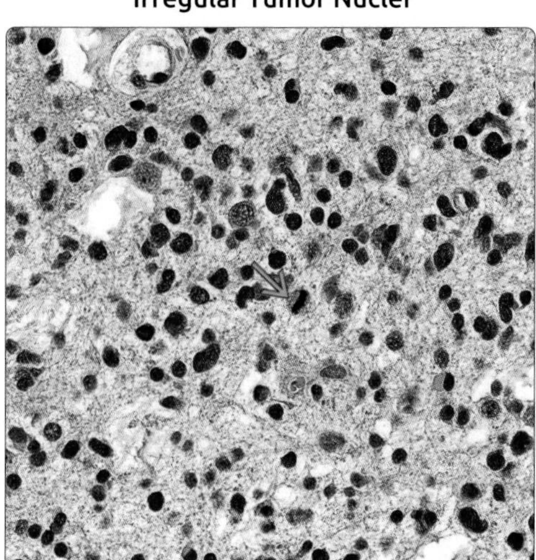

(Left) *Cytological atypia may not be extreme in grade III astrocytomas. As a diagnostic criterion, the presence of mitoses ➡ ruled in this case. Without them, this would have been fibrillary astrocytoma grade II.* **(Right)** *This degree of atypia could be present in either astrocytoma grade II or III. Without mitotic activity ➡, the lesion would be grade II.*

Relatively Mild Cytological Atypia

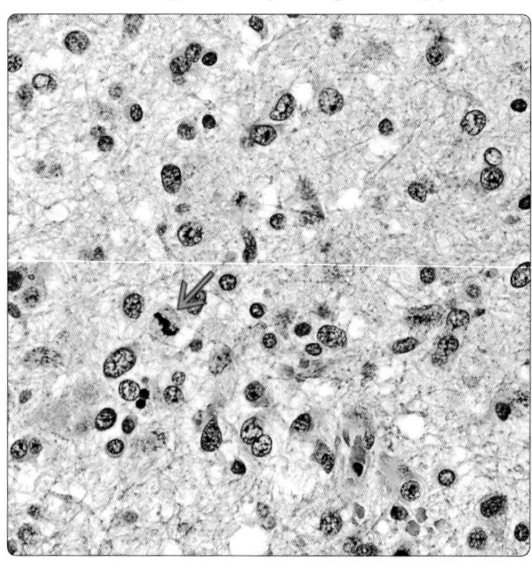

Hyperchromatic Nuclei

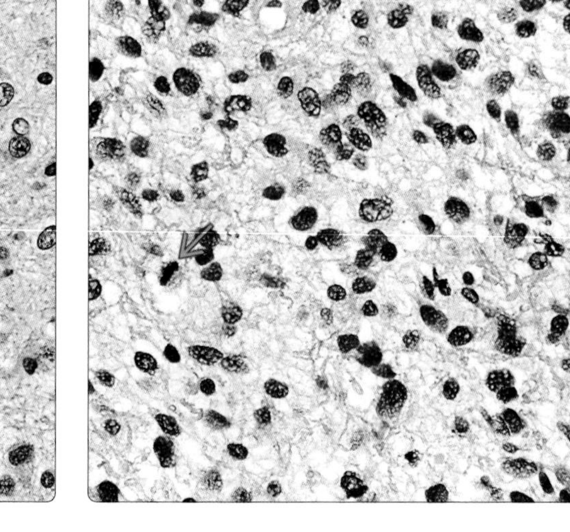

(Left) *High cellularity, uneven cell distribution, and nuclear hyperchromatism comprise a neoplasm that lacks only mitoses to be anaplastic astrocytoma. Mitotic figures were present elsewhere (not shown). The glassy cytoplasm with short stubby processes is typical of many astrocytomas.* **(Right)** *Nuclei with this degree of elongation and hyperchromatism ➡ can only be those of an astrocytoma, grade III in this case due to mitotic activity elsewhere.*

Uneven Cell Distribution

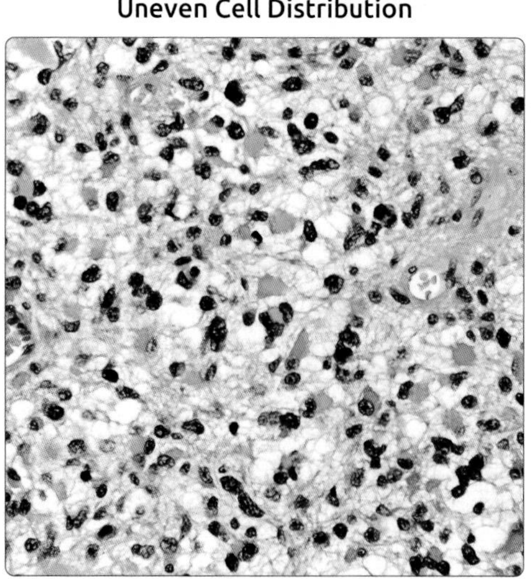

Nuclei Too Elongated for Oligodendroglioma

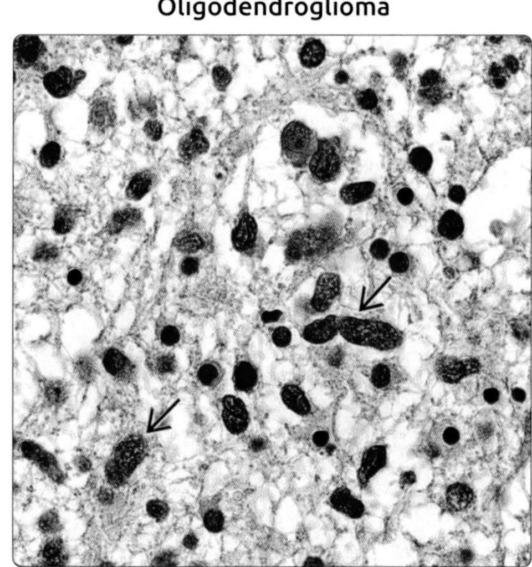

Gemistocytic Astrocytoma

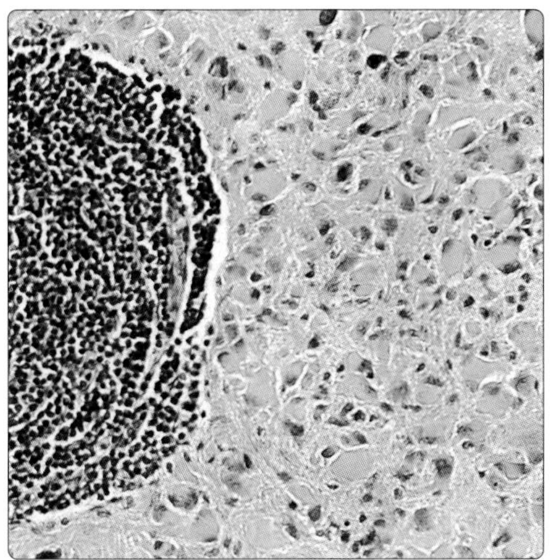

Interspersed Less-Differentiated Cells

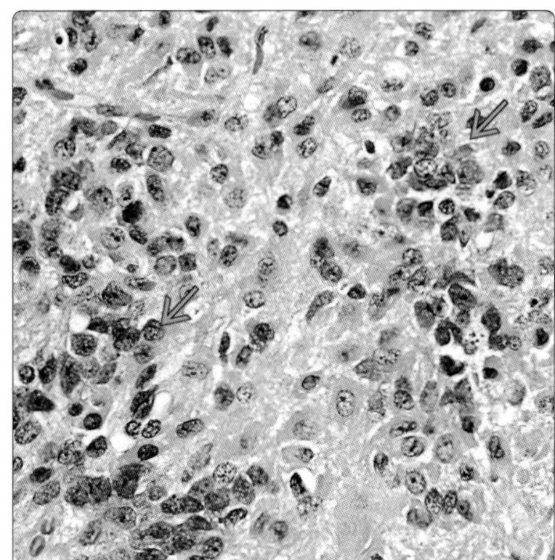

(Left) *Gemistocytic astrocytomas can be either grade II or grade III. The degree of pleomorphism in this case almost ensures that the requisite number of mitoses for a classification of grade III is present. Perivascular lymphocytes are almost always associated topographically with gemistocytes.* **(Right)** *Nests of smaller, less differentiated cells* ➙ *corroborate the supposition that this gemistocytic astrocytoma is grade III.*

Extreme Cytological Atypia

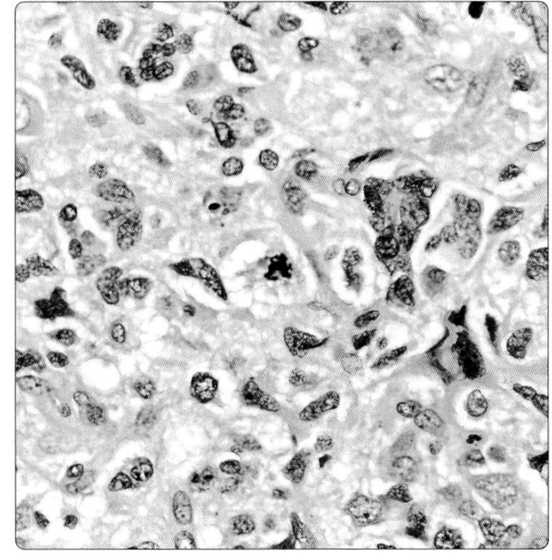

Small Cell Astrocytoma

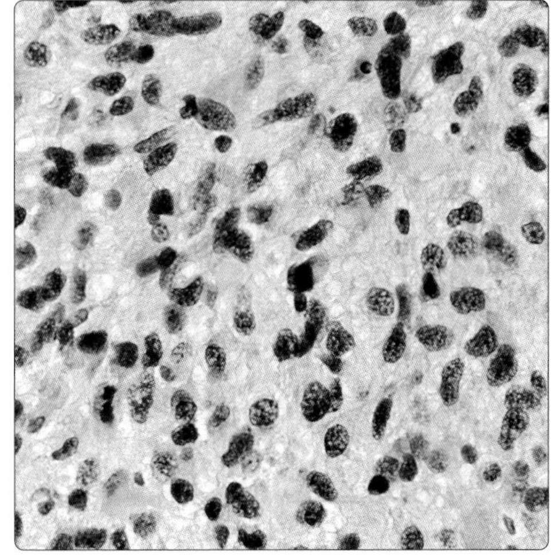

(Left) *The presence of a contrast enhancement in a rim pattern would be radiological evidence that this high-grade lesion is a glioblastoma. Note the extreme cytological atypia in this case.* **(Right)** *Small, elongate tumor cells of some highly cellular anaplastic small cell astrocytomas are cytologically identical to those of the small cell glioblastoma. These highly cellular grade III lesions usually acquire the rim pattern of enhancement typical of glioblastoma within weeks (i.e., transform to WHO grade IV rapidly).*

Primitive Neuroectodermal Component

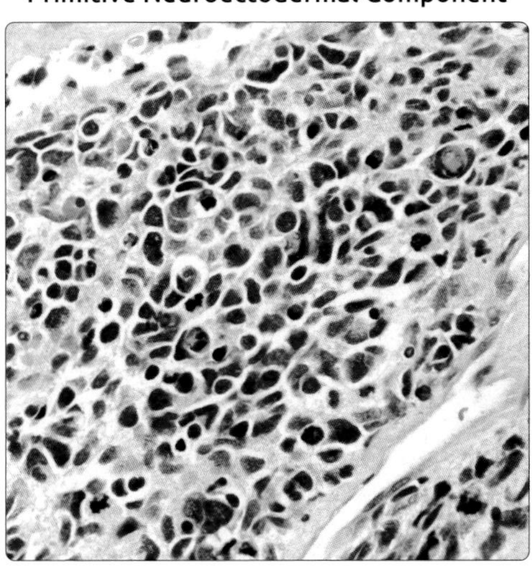

Synaptophysin, PNET Component

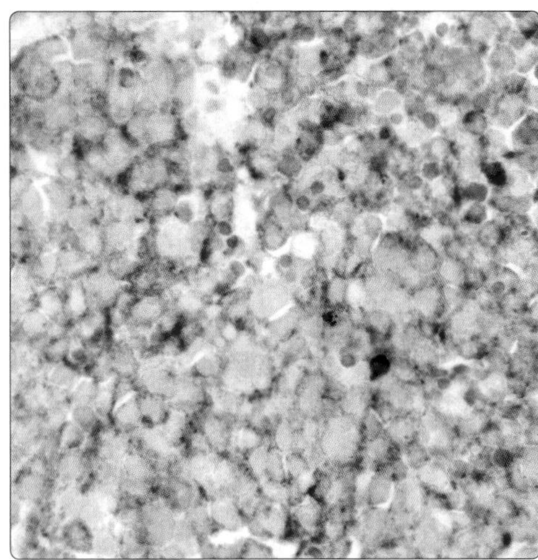

(Left) *As with glioblastomas, anaplastic astrocytomas and even rare grade II astrocytomas sometimes contain colonies of primitive neuroectodermal tumor-like tissue. Marked hyperchromatism, cell-cell wrapping, and nuclear molding are defining features.* **(Right)** *Primitive neuroectodermal-like tissue in infiltrating gliomas is synaptophysin immunoreactive. Such tissue is usually intensely and diffusely p53 positive as well.*

(Left) *In anaplastic astrocytomas with neuropil-like rosettes, circular finely fibrillar areas are demarcated by tumor cells ⇨ that will stain for neuronal markers. The rosettes' fibrillar cores will be synaptophysin immunoreactive.* **(Right)** *Rosetted areas of neuropil are synaptophysin immunoreactive. While there are exceptions, such islands usually occur in high-grade gliomas, typically astrocytic.*

Neuropil-Like Rosettes

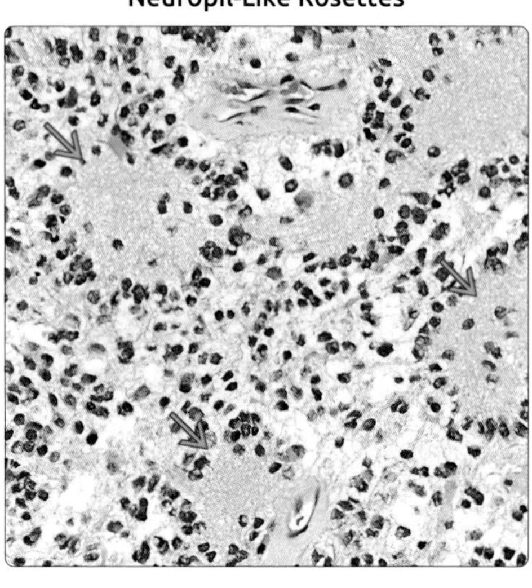

Synaptophysin, Neuropil-Like Rosettes

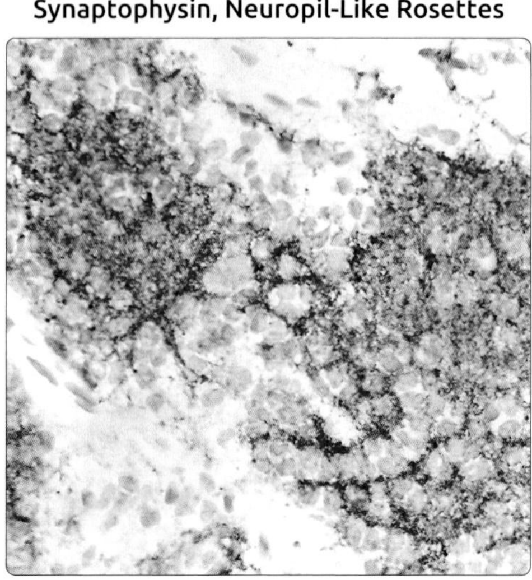

(Left) *Cytoplasm and, to a lesser extent, nuclei, are immunoreactive for IDH-1 in most anaplastic astrocytomas. These tumors are not biologically or prognostically similar to glioblastoma and have a more favorable prognosis than IDH-1(-) WHO grade III anaplastic astrocytomas.* **(Right)** *When anaplastic astrocytomas are negative for IDH-1, there is a more unfavorable prognosis; however, one caveat is that the IDH-1 R132H antibody does not recognize all IDH1 mutations or any IDH2 mutations.*

IDH-1(+)

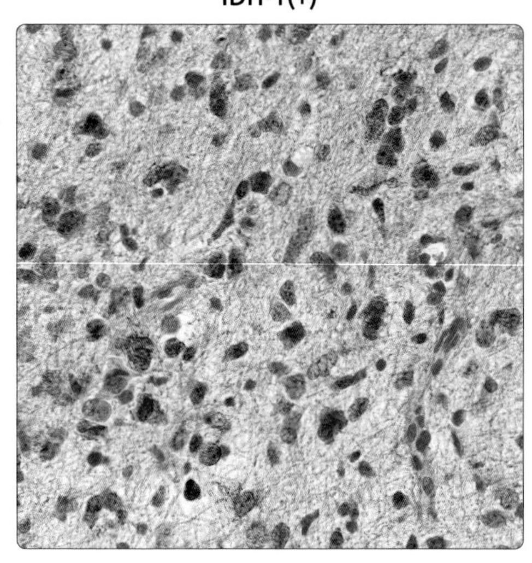

IDH-1(-)

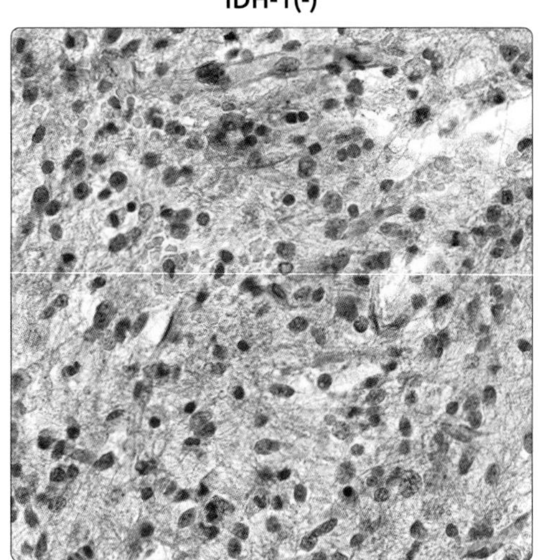

(Left) *Diffuse, strong nuclear immunoreactivity for p53 helps distinguish anaplastic astrocytoma from its oligodendroglial counterpart. A negative result has little diagnostic significance, however, since positivity is present in only a minority of astrocytomas, grade II or III. Nuclear ATRX can also be utilized; it is often lost in grades II and III astrocytic, but not oligodendroglial tumors.* **(Right)** *While there is no defined cutoff, Ki-67 indices are generally above 5%. It is approximately 12% here.*

p53

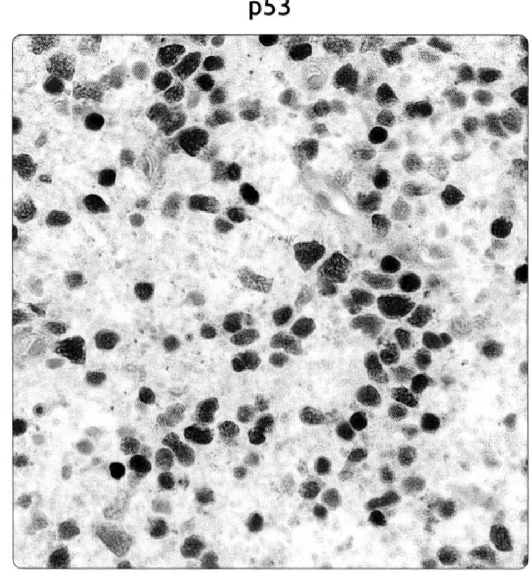

Ki-67

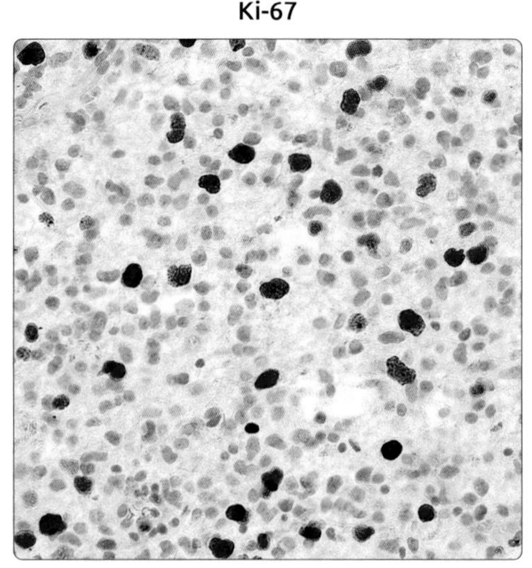

Interspersed Reactive Astrocytes

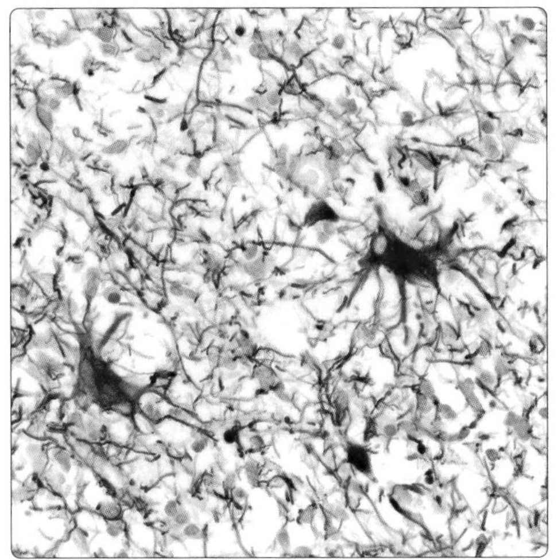

Strong GFAP

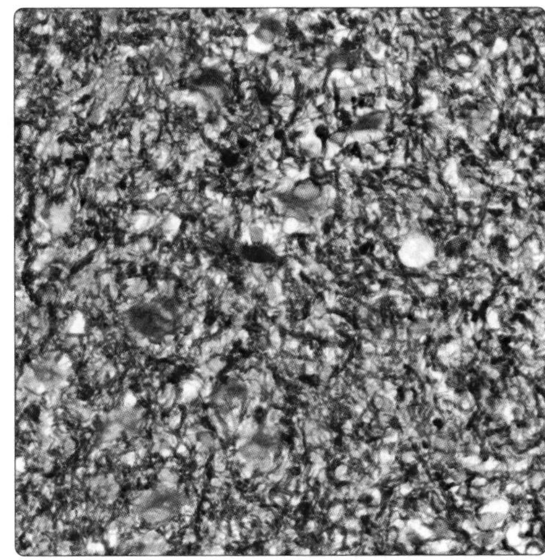

(Left) *Small cell astrocytoma often shows very little GFAP immunoreactivity within the tumor cells, but interspersed stellate reactive astrocytes with long tapering processes may be strongly highlighted by this immunostain.* **(Right)** *Some anaplastic astrocytomas may manifest abundant amounts of eosinophilic cytoplasm, which translates into strong diffuse immunoreactivity for GFAP in multiple tumor cells.*

Nuclear ATRX Lost

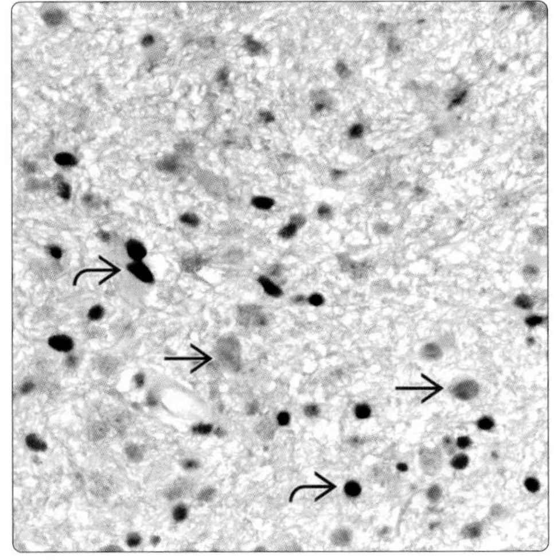

Bizarre Mitoses

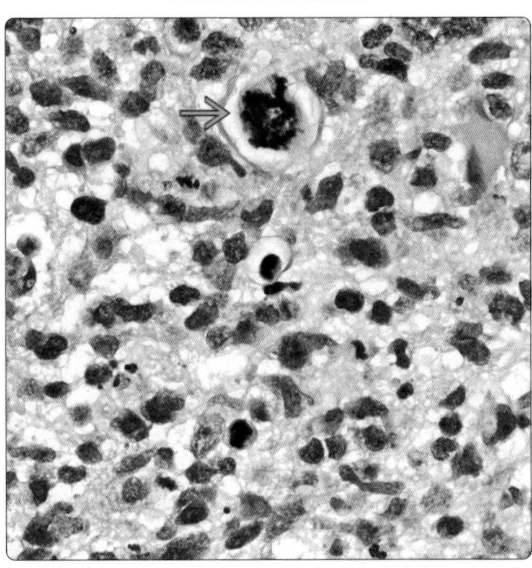

(Left) *Anaplastic astrocytomas with IDH1 mutation will often also show mutation of ATRX, which will result in loss of nuclear ATRX immunostaining in the tumor cells →. In contrast, entrapped normal cells retain nuclear immunoreactivity ↪. Anaplastic oligodendrogliomas retain nuclear ATRX.* **(Right)** *Despite the importance of > 1 mitosis in cementing the diagnosis of anaplastic astrocytoma, bizarre mitoses ⇒ do not receive extra weight in grading criteria.*

Smear, Anaplastic Astrocytoma

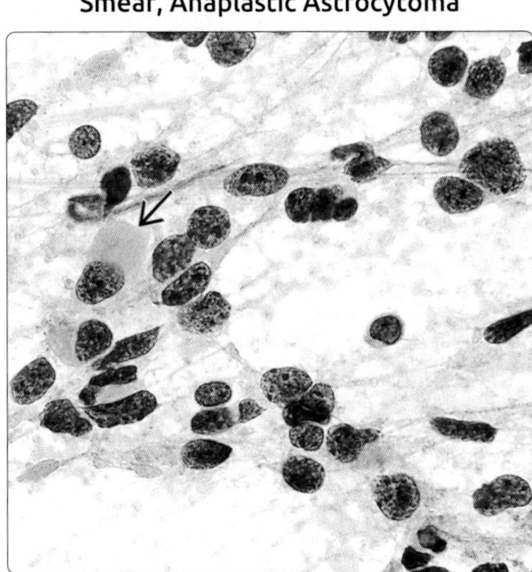

Smear, Prominent Eosinophilic Cytoplasm

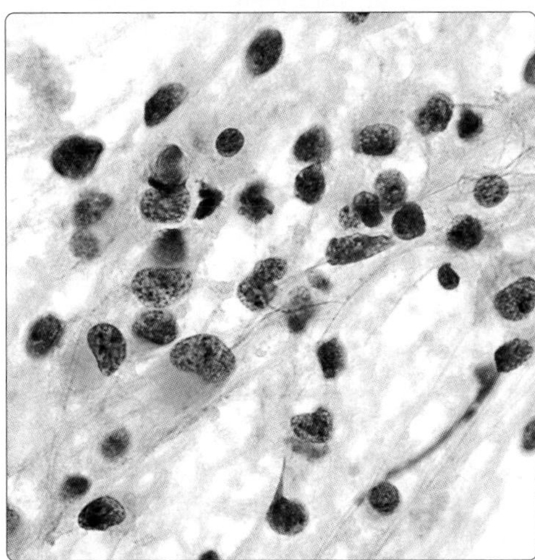

(Left) *While there is a cell resembling a gliofibrillary oligodendrocyte →, the irregular, dark nuclei without discernible nucleoli are typical of astrocytic, not oligodendroglial tumors. The coarse chromatin is also very astrocytic.* **(Right)** *Prominent pink cytoplasm, fibrillar background, and the character of the nuclei help establish this as an infiltrating form of astrocytoma.*

Glioblastoma

KEY FACTS

CLINICAL ISSUES

- Most common primary brain tumor
- Any age, but usually > 40 years
- Primary and secondary types
- Pseudoprogression, apparent posttreatment recurrence due to radiation/chemotherapy effects can be difficult to distinguish clinically and radiologically from active tumor recurrence
- Prognosis poor, most patients succumb ≤ 3 years

IMAGING

- Almost always enhancing in ring or rim pattern

MICROSCOPIC

- Anaplastic astrocytic neoplasm with necrosis &/or microvascular proliferation
- Multiple tissue patterns
  - Typical: Mixture of small- and medium-sized cells, fibrillary and gemistocytic astrocytes
  - Small cell
  - Giant cell
  - With oligodendroglioma component
  - With neuronal component
  - With PNET-like tissue
  - Treatment effects (pseudoprogression)
  - Myxoid
  - With mesenchymal metaplasia (gliosarcoma)
  - Acute necrosis with neutrophilic inflammation

ANCILLARY TESTS

- Methylation of *MGMT* inactivates this enzyme (~ 30%)
  - Favorable prognostic and predictive factor
  - Can change to (+) or (-) after treatment
- Presence of mutant IDH1(+) (or *IDH1/2* mutation) strongly predictive of more favorable prognosis than IDH1(-)

(Left) *Glioblastoma multiformes (GBMs) typically have an irregular, contrast-enhancing rim around a dark necrotic center.* **(Right)** *GBMS, recurrent in this case, are mass-producing with the potential to force the medial temporal lobe over the edge of the tentorium ➔ and compress the brain stem. The cause of death in other cases is less clear, and not always due to local effects of the neoplasm. Note the variegated appearance of an admixed necrotic and viable tumor.*

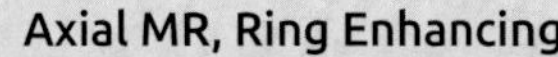

Axial MR, Ring Enhancing

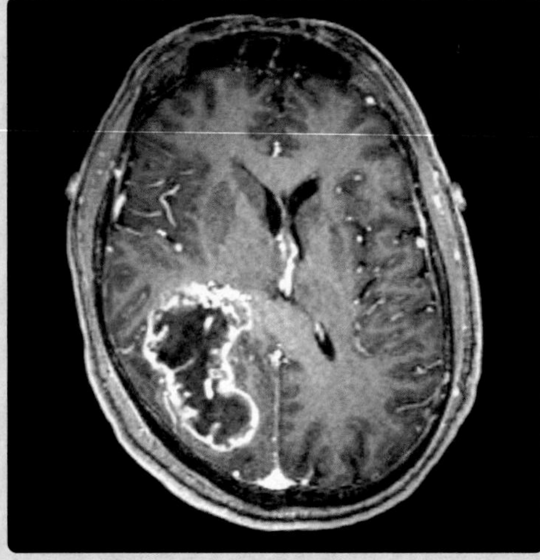

Multiforme Appearance

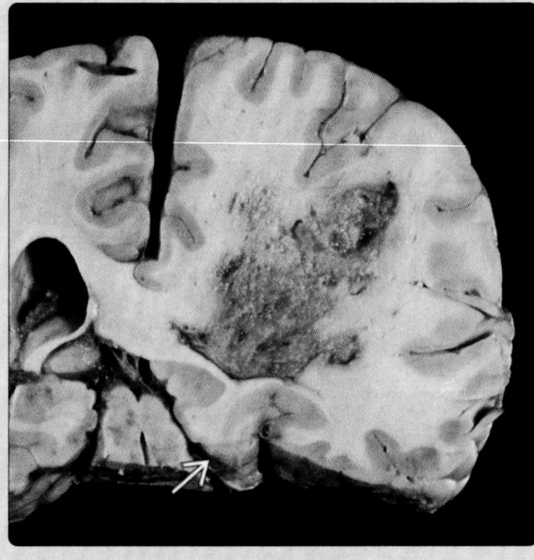

(Left) *H&E/myelin-stained section emphasizes the GBM's classic rim of viable neoplasm ➔ around a necrotic center.* **(Right)** *Vascular thromboses ➔ are often identified in GBMs, although their presence per se are not part of the grading criteria.*

Necrotic Center

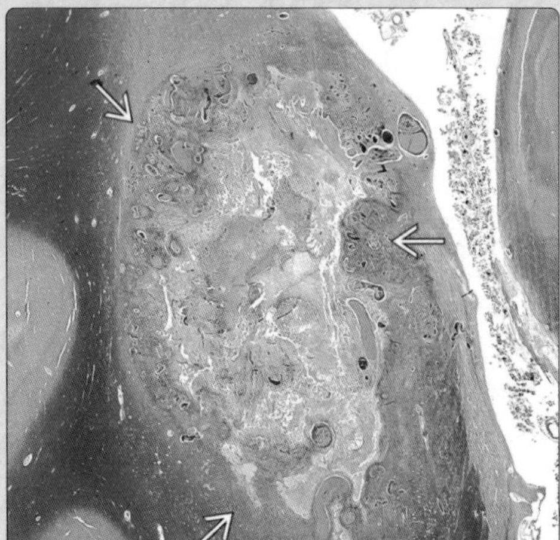

Vascular Thromboses

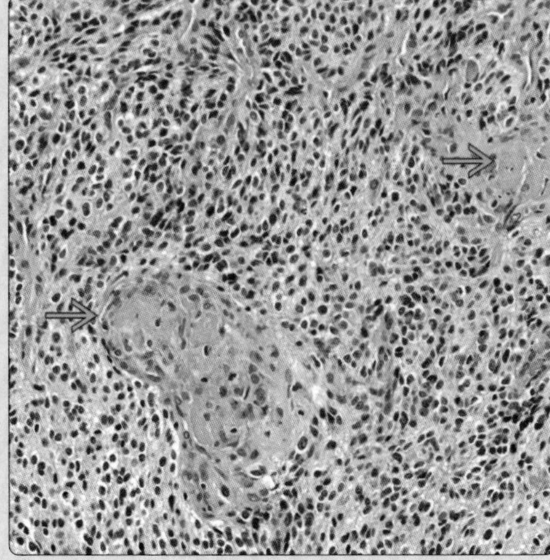

TERMINOLOGY

Synonyms

- Glioblastoma multiforme (GBM)

Definitions

- High-grade glioma with predominant astrocytic differentiation
- WHO grade IV
- Primary glioblastoma
  - Lower grade, arises abruptly without precursor lesion, symptom duration < than 3 months
    - ~ 95% of all GBMs
- Secondary glioblastoma
  - Tumor arising from previously lower grade astrocytoma
    - ~ 5% of GBMs

ETIOLOGY/PATHOGENESIS

Unknown

- Almost always unknown

Prior Radiochemotherapy

- Unrelated tumors
  - Pituitary adenoma
  - medulloblastoma
  - acute lymphoblastic leukemia (in children)

Inherited Cancer Syndrome

- Neurofibromatosis 1 (uncommon)
- Turcot syndrome with defects in DNA mismatch repair genes (rare)

CLINICAL ISSUES

Epidemiology

- Incidence
  - Glioma (most common)
- Age
  - Any, but usually > 40 years
  - Exception is pediatric GBMs, including diffuse intrinsic pontine glioma of infants and children
- Sex
  - Primary glioblastoma
    - Slightly more common in men
  - Secondary glioblastoma
    - Slightly more common in women

Site

- Cerebral hemispheres
  - Including thalamus and basal ganglia (usually adults, but sometimes children)
- Corpus callosum (either primarily or by extension)
- Visual pathways (optic chiasm); adults, rare
- Brain stem (especially pons); usually children
- Cerebellum (children and adults, rare)
- Spinal cord (children and adults, uncommon)

Presentation

- Generally acute; < 3 months in primary type
- Longer duration with secondary type
- Specific clinical expressions
  - Seizures; mass effects such as headache and herniation; site-dependent focal neurological deficits
- Pseudoprogression
  - Apparent posttreatment recurrence due to radiation/chemotherapy effects
    - Difficult to clinically and radiologically distinguish from active tumor recurrence

Treatment

- At presentation
  - Radiation and chemotherapy (temozolomide)
- At suspected recurrence
  - Chemotherapy with active recurrent tumor
    - Bevacizumab [vascular endothelial growth factor (VEGF) blocker] (some cases)
  - No additional treatment with pseudoprogression
- Pediatric pontine examples usually treated on basis of clinical and radiological features (without biopsy)

Prognosis

- Poor
  - Most patients succumb ≤ 3 years
- Ameliorating factors
  - Young age: < 45 years old and better preoperative performance score
  - *MGMT* methylation status
  - Proneural gene expression profile
- Relationship of primitive neuroectodermal tumor (PNET)-like tissue to outcome unclear, but prone to CSF dissemination

IMAGING

MR Findings

- Almost always enhancing in ring or rim pattern
- Solitary (typical)
- Multicentric (uncommon)
  - Unilateral, often histologically contiguous
  - Bilateral (uncommon)
- Prominent T2/FLAIR hyperintensity (white) signal around enhancing area
- Mass effect
- Pontine types often partly surround basilar artery

MACROSCOPIC

General Features

- Most GBMs widely infiltrate brain but show limited tendency for CSF metastases, at least in life
- Diffuse instrinsic pontine gliomas show leptomeningeal spread in 1/3 at autopsy; subventricular spread, diffuse parenchymal infiltration to distant areas of brain (i.e., frontal lobe)

Cerebral Hemispheres

- Generally subcortical
- Symmetric with corpus callosum involvement (butterfly glioma)
- Sometimes circumscribed; superficial dura attached and firm, similar to meningoma or metastasis
  - Especially giant cell, epithelioid, and rhabdoid types
- Variegated, with gray cellular areas

- Central necrosis
- Thrombosed vessels ("black veins")

Brainstem (Usually Pons)

- Enlarged ("hypertrophy"); sometimes symmetric
- Central necrosis

Spinal Cord

- Irregular enlargement
- Involvement of pial surface (most cases)

MICROSCOPIC

Histologic Features

- Borders/growth pattern
  - Generally ill-defined, infiltrative with secondary structures: Perineuronal satellitosis, perivascular concentration, subpial concentration
  - Occasionally well circumscribed (at least partly), especially in giant cell variant, epithelioid, rhabdoid, and any type involving meninges
- Patterns of spread
  - Direct, local; often along white matter pathways, especially corpus callosum, but also anterior commissure, middle cerebellar peduncle
  - Subependymal
  - Intraspinal leptomeninges (drop metastasis)
  - Systemic
    - Bone marrow, liver, lymph node (rare)
- Necrosis
  - Includes tumor cells and vessels
  - Coagulative, few macrophages
  - ± pseudopalisading
- Vascular proliferation
  - Glomeruloid, mass of multiple small vessels
  - Endothelial proliferation (multilayered, intraluminal)
- Thrombosis of small vessels
- Mitoses
  - Variable
    - Many in small cell variant
    - Few in "quiescent," posttreatment tumors
- Apoptosis, especially in areas of pseudopalisading
- Component cell types
  - Fibrillary astrocytes
  - Gemistocytes
  - Polymorphic, medium-sized astrocytes
  - Small cells (in most glioblastomas, but exclusive or largely so in small cell variant)
    - Highly infiltrative
    - Bipolar
    - Cytologically bland
    - Mitotically active
  - Epithelioid (uncommon)
    - Sharp cell borders
    - Glassy cytoplasm
    - Round, open nuclei with nucleoli
  - Rhabdoid (rare)
    - Discrete cell borders
    - Eccentric oval nuclei with prominent nucleoli
    - Prominent paranuclear filament whorl
  - Granular
    - Coarse, intracytoplasmic lysosomes
    - Bland nuclei
    - Resemble macrophages
  - Lipidized; closely simulates adipose tissue (rare)
- Perivascular lymphocytes (especially in gemistocytic tumors)
- Microglia, CD68(+), may be numerous
- Pattern variation
  - Often mixture of fibrillary and gemistocytic astrocytes
  - Small cell
    - Homogeneous sheets of small cells mimicking oligodendrocytes at low magnification
    - Microcalcifications (occasional)
    - Vague perivascular pseudorosettes (occasional)
    - Preceded in some cases by small cell astrocytoma without necrosis or vascular proliferation
  - Giant cell
    - Compact; often little evidence of infiltration
    - Large, bizarre multinucleate cells
    - Fibrous stroma
    - Perivascular lymphocytes in some cases
    - Little, if any, microvascular proliferation or pseudopalisading necrosis
  - GBM with oligodendroglioma component
    - Foci of classic oligodendroglioma (often minor)
    - Necrosis
    - As yet not fully characterized
    - Viewed by some as better considered grade IV mixed glioma (oligoastrocytoma)
  - GBM with neuronal immunophenotype
    - Immunohistochemical discovery (especially in giant cell types)
    - No known prognostic significance
    - Not in itself basis for diagnosis of glioneuronal tumor
  - GBM with primitive neuroectodermal component
    - Highly cellular, often circumscribed PNET foci
    - Small cells in some; large cells in others
    - Anaplastic PNET in some cases with large cells, abundant apoptosis, cell-cell wrapping
    - Homer Wright (neuroblastic) rosettes in some cases
  - Myxoid
  - GBM with mesenchymal differentiation (gliosarcoma)
  - GBM with epithelial differentiation (most often in gliosarcoma); squamous, &/or glandular
  - Acute necrosis with PMNs
    - Acute neutrophilic inflammation (little viable tumor)
    - Can raise consideration of bacterial brain abscess (especially on frozen sections, small samples)
  - Infarctive
    - Extensive macrophage-rich necrosis
- Primary vs. secondary types
  - Clinical diagnosis depending on length of symptoms, < 3 months, and lack of history of lower grade astrocytoma
  - Usually separate areas of lower and precursor higher grade astrocytoma, but not defining feature
  - Pediatric GBMs nearly always are primary; only rarely arise from lower grade glioma
- Treatment effects (pseudoprogression)
  - Paucicellularity

- Fibrinoid necrosis of vessels, tumoral, and parenchymal necrosis without peripheral palisading
- Little, if any, vascular proliferation
- Nuclear pleomorphism
- Hyalinized vessels
- Calcification
- Few mitoses
- May be difficult to assign common intermediate cases into pseudoprogression or true tumor progression category

ANCILLARY TESTS

Cytology

- Tissue fragments with fine fibrillar background, individual and clustered cells
- Mixture of cell types in accordance with histological subtypes and tissue patterns
- Cellular/nuclear pleomorphism common in irradiated tumors
- Mitoses (but may be few)
- Vascular proliferation
- Necrosis

Immunohistochemistry

- GFAP(+)
  - Most cases, generally in proportion to abundance of cytoplasm
  - Adipocyte-like cells (+) in lipidized variant
- Cytokeratins
  - AE1/AE3(+) (many cases)
  - CAM5.2(-)
- Olig2(+)
- Mutant IDH1
  - Secondary glioblastomas (+)
  - Primary glioblastomas (-)
- EMA(+), cytokeratins (+) in rare tumors with epithelial metaplasia
- INI1 (loss of nuclear staining) (rhabdoid type); conventional glioblastoma in same tumor with retained staining
- p53
  - More often in secondary and giant cell types
  - Uncommon in primary type
- Ki-67
  - Variable in classic lesion
  - Very high in PNET-like components
- Macrophage markers (CD68, CD163, HAM56)
  - Many (+) cells (some cases)

Genetic Testing

- EGFR/RAS/NF1/PTEN/P13K pathway: 60% of primary and 33% of secondary GBM
  - *EGFR* amplification in ~ 40% of all GBMs (usually primary, rarely secondary)
    - *EGFR* deletion mutant *vIII* (~ 50% of amplified cases)
- TP53/MDM2/MDM4/p14ARF pathway: 50% of primary and 70% of secondary GBM
- P16INK4a/CDK4/RB1 pathway: 50% of primary and 50% of secondary GBM
- *IDH1* mutation (secondary GBM)
- Methylation of *MGMT* (~ 30%)
  - Favorable prognostic and predictive factor
  - Can change to (+) or (-) after treatment
- Amplifications
  - *EGFR*
    - ~ 80% of small cell type
    - Rare *EGFR* in giant cell type
  - *MYC* amplification in PNET elements (some cases)
- Microsatellite instability (higher incidence in pediatric GBM)
- Loss of chromosome 10, especially 10q
- Gain of chromosome 7
- Pediatric GBMs have different genetics than adult GBMs
  - Diffuse intrinsic pontine gliomas (DIPGs)
    - *H3.3* mutations at K27 position occur at median age of 11 years, in midline locations (pons/thalamus)
      - DIPGs mutated for *K27M-H3.3* have adverse behavior even if low grade by histological criteria (i.e., behavior of WHO grades II and III tumors = WHO grade IV)
      - DIPGs wild type for *K27M-H3.3* survive slightly longer
  - Mutations *ATRX, DAXX, TP53, H3.3*
    - *H3.3* mutations at G34 position occur in teenagers, in cerebral hemispheres
  - Pediatric GBMs rarely have *IDH1/2* mutations and are absent in patients < 14 years

DIFFERENTIAL DIAGNOSIS

Anaplastic Oligodendroglioma

- Cytologically monomorphous
- Round nuclei
- Mini gemistocytes and gliofibrillary oligodendrocytes
- Often associated areas of grade II oligodendroglioma
- 1p/19q codeletion

Anaplastic Ependymoma

- Discrete, but focally infiltrative in some cases
- Monomorphous
- Perivascular pseudorosettes
- True rosettes (uncommon)
- EMA(+)
  - Dot-like and microlumina (most cases)
  - Surface staining of rosettes and canals

Metastatic Neoplasm

- Sharp border
- Epithelial or melanocytic features
- Necrosis sparing vessels; collars of viable tumor
- Little vascular proliferation, except in renal cell
- Epithelial or melanocytic markers (+)
- Perivascular lymphocytic infiltrates in adjacent brain

Primary CNS Lymphoma

- Homogeneous contrast enhancement (no dark necrotic center) in immunocompetent patients with lymphoma
- Angiocentricity, resulting in patchy lymphoma cell distribution
- Typical cytological features (e.g., round or notched nuclei, prominent nucleoli, scant cytoplasm)
- Abundant apoptosis
- Ring enhancement in immunodeficient patients with lymphoma

- Necrosis in AIDS-associated examples
- No vascular proliferation
- B-cell > T-cell type

Medulloblastoma (Cerebellum)

- Nodules/reticulin in nodular-desmoplastic type
- Minimal or no glial differentiation
- Synaptophysin (+)
- Necrosis less common, usually no pseudopalisading
- Microvascular proliferation rare

Primitive Neuroectodermal Tumor (Supratentorial)

- No origin in malignant glioma
- Synaptophysin (+)
- Nodular architecture (some cases)

Acute/Subacute Infarct

- Ischemic, red neurons
- Hypertrophic, but usually minimally hyperplastic, vascular cells
- Macrophages in subacute and chronic phases

Abscess

- No cytologically malignant cells
- Acute inflammation
- Prominent lymphoplasmacytic infiltrate
- Fibroblastic proliferation/capsule in organizing lesion

SELECTED REFERENCES

1. Appin CL et al: Molecular pathways in gliomagenesis and their relevance to neuropathologic diagnosis. Adv Anat Pathol. 22(1):50-8, 2015
2. Kleinschmidt-DeMasters BK et al: BRAF VE1 immunoreactivity patterns in epithelioid glioblastomas positive for BRAF V600E mutation. Am J Surg Pathol. ePub, 2015
3. Wu G et al: The genomic landscape of diffuse intrinsic pontine glioma and pediatric non-brainstem high-grade glioma. Nat Genet. 46(5):444-50, 2014
4. Brennan CW et al: The somatic genomic landscape of glioblastoma. Cell. 155(2):462-77, 2013
5. Kleinschmidt-DeMasters BK et al: Epithelioid GBMs show a high percentage of BRAF V600E mutation. Am J Surg Pathol. 37(5):685-98, 2013
6. Capper D et al: Characterization of R132H mutation-specific IDH1 antibody binding in brain tumors. Brain Pathol. 20(1):245-54, 2010
7. Colman H et al: A multigene predictor of outcome in glioblastoma. Neuro Oncol. 12(1):49-57, 2010
8. Donev K et al: Expression of diagnostic neuronal markers and outcome in glioblastoma. Neuropathol Appl Neurobiol. 36(5):411-21, 2010
9. Kleinschmidt-DeMasters BK et al: Epithelioid versus rhabdoid glioblastomas are distinguished by monosomy 22 and immunohistochemical expression of INI-1 but not claudin 6. Am J Surg Pathol. 34(3):341-54, 2010
10. Ohgaki H et al: Genetic alterations and signaling pathways in the evolution of gliomas. Cancer Sci. 100(12):2235-41, 2009
11. Perry A et al: Malignant gliomas with primitive neuroectodermal tumor-like components: a clinicopathologic and genetic study of 53 cases. Brain Pathol. 19(1):81-90, 2009
12. Watanabe T et al: IDH1 mutations are early events in the development of astrocytomas and oligodendrogliomas. Am J Pathol. 174(4):1149-53, 2009
13. Rodriguez FJ et al: Epithelial and pseudoepithelial differentiation in glioblastoma and gliosarcoma: a comparative morphologic and molecular genetic study. Cancer. 113(10):2779-89, 2008
14. Ohgaki H et al: Genetic pathways to primary and secondary glioblastoma. Am J Pathol. 170(5):1445-53, 2007
15. Hegi ME et al: MGMT gene silencing and benefit from temozolomide in glioblastoma. N Engl J Med. 352(10):997-1003, 2005
16. Ohgaki H et al: Genetic pathways to glioblastoma: a population-based study. Cancer Res. 64(19):6892-9, 2004
17. Perry A et al: Small cell astrocytoma: an aggressive variant that is clinicopathologically and genetically distinct from anaplastic oligodendroglioma. Cancer. 101(10):2318-26, 2004
18. Burger PC et al: Cytologic composition of the untreated glioblastoma with implications for evaluation of needle biopsies. Cancer. 63(10):2014-23, 1989

Butterfly Glioma

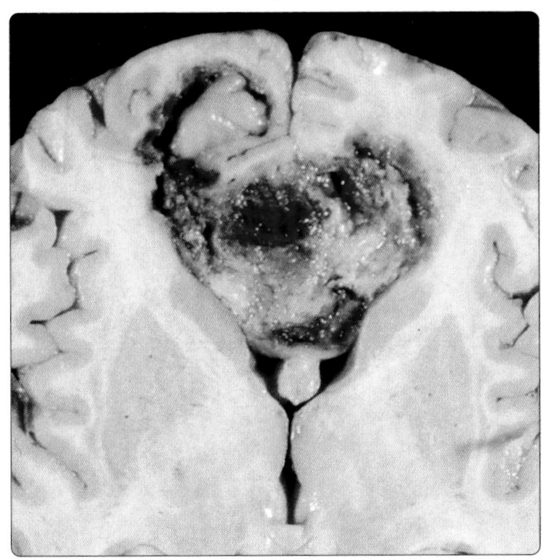

Mimicking Metastasis

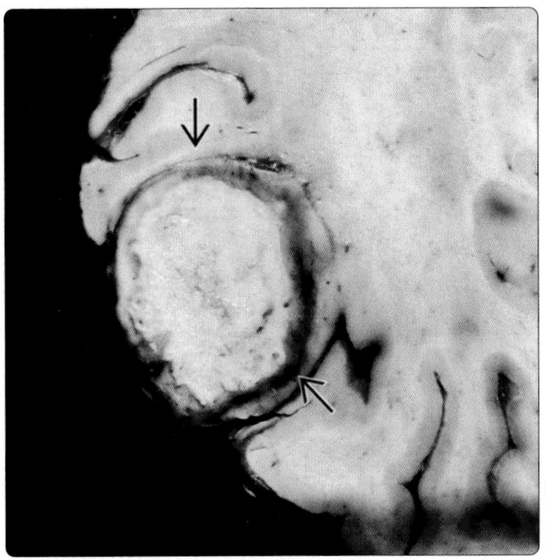

(Left) *Symmetric, variegated glioblastomas in the corpus callosum create the classic butterfly appearance. Central necrosis is typical of GBMs at any site. (Courtesy R. McComb, MD.)* **(Right)** *Well-circumscribed, giant cell GBM ➙ may grossly mimic meningioma or metastasis, especially when the glioma occurs superficially, as in this case. Gliosarcomas, which are often well circumscribed, may also simulate metastasis and meningioma.*

Pseudopalisading Necrosis

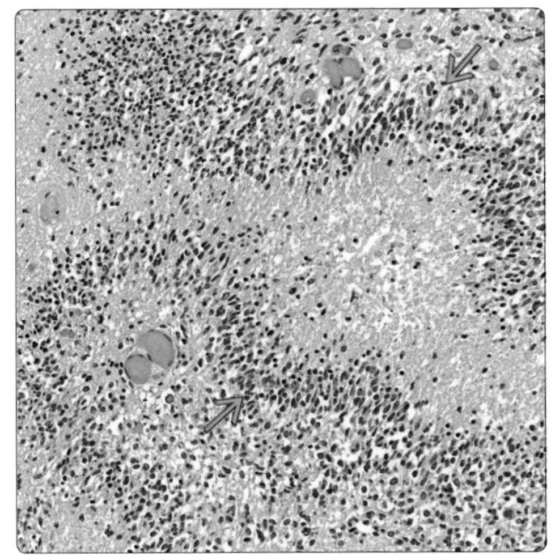

Apoptosis in Pseudopalisading

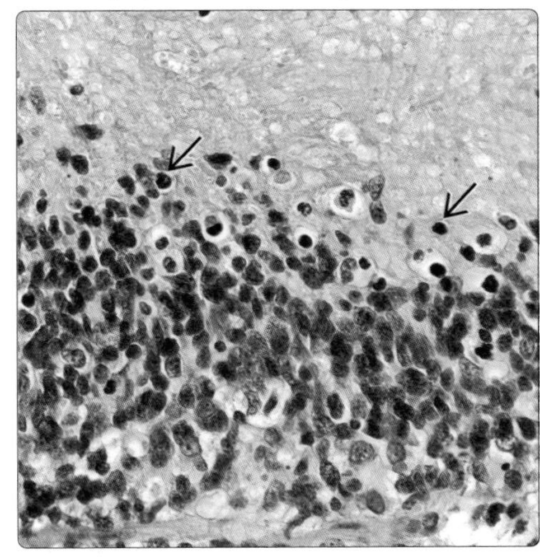

(Left) *A sinuous, hypercellular band of cells ➙ traces the border of necrotic zones in what is known as pseudopalisading.* **(Right)** *Apoptosis ➙ is common in areas of pseudopalisading, especially the zone immediately bordering the lesion's necrotic core. Pseudopalisading is not present around necrotic areas in all glioblastomas. The presence of zonal necrosis or pseudopalisading necrosis have equal weight in grading criteria.*

Zonal Necrosis

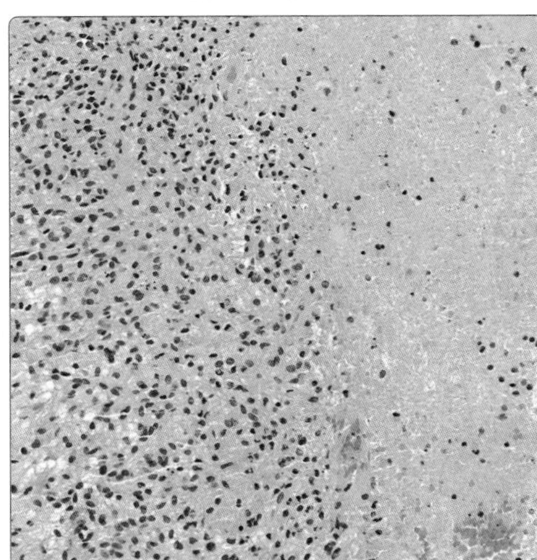

Acute Necrosis, Neutrophils

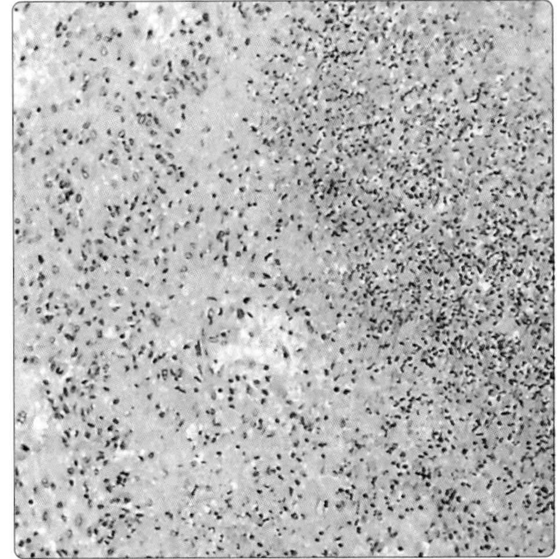

(Left) *Necrosis in GBM involves both tumor cells and blood vessels. Coagulative zonal necrosis, shown here, is absent in sporadic CNS lymphomas, wherein cell death largely involves apoptosis. As seen in this case, necrosis in GBMs does not necessarily have pseudopalisading. Either type of necrosis serves equally as grading criterion.* **(Right)** *There is enough acute inflammation and necrosis in some glioblastomas to suggest an inflammatory/infectious process rather than a neoplasm. Finding unequivocal tumor cells may be difficult.*

(Left) *Glomeruloid vascular proliferation ⇒ is a classic histological feature in GBM, but also occurs in other primary CNS neoplasms (particularly low-grade lesions such as pilocytic astrocytoma).* **(Right)** *Multilayered intravascular endothelial cells ⇒ represent a more prognostically important form of vascular proliferation than the more common glomeruloid type.*

Microvascular Proliferation

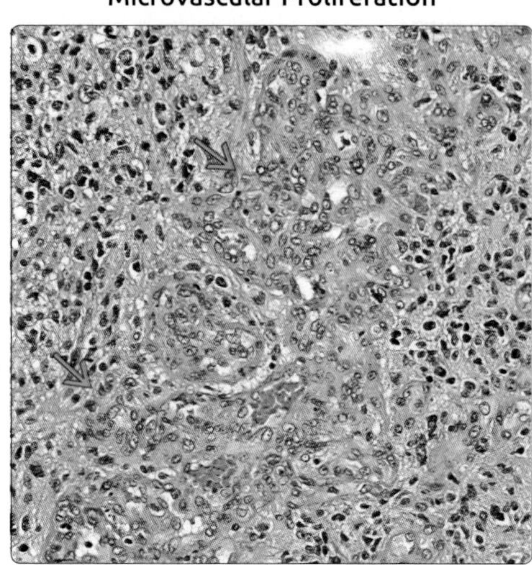

Multilayered Endothelial Cells

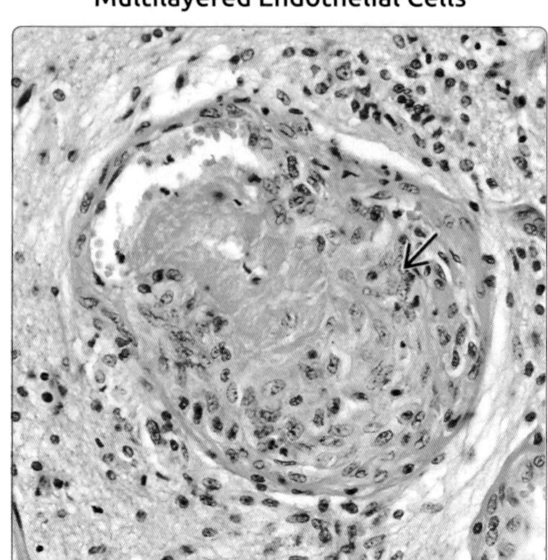

(Left) *Thin-walled, telangiectatic vessels are nonspecific findings not to be equated with microvascular proliferation. They do not contribute to grading criteria.* **(Right)** *Known by the surgeon as black veins, thrombosed vessels are common in glioblastoma.*

Telangiectatic Vessels

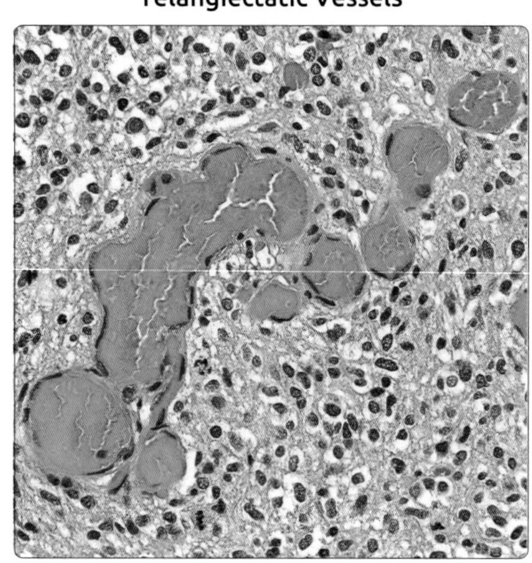

Thrombosed Veins

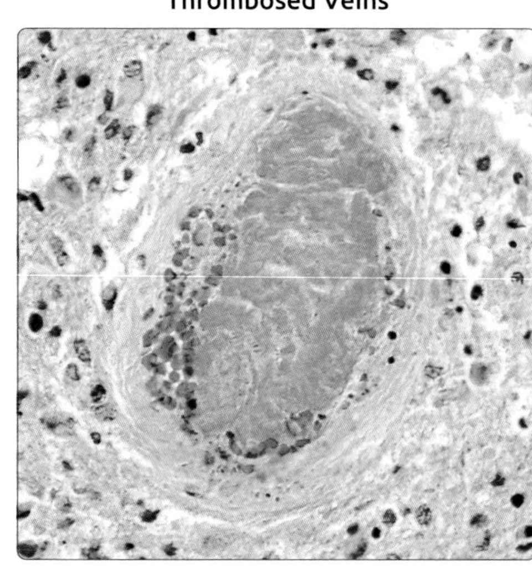

(Left) *Paucicellular infiltrating areas in some GBMs may suggest an inflammatory infiltrate with activated microglia. In a lesion without a cellular, centrally necrotic epicenter, the tissue pattern is consistent with gliomatosis cerebri.* **(Right)** *While not generally as prominent as in oligodendrogliomas, perineuronal satellitosis ⇒ is not uncommon in GBM.*

Mimicking Microglia

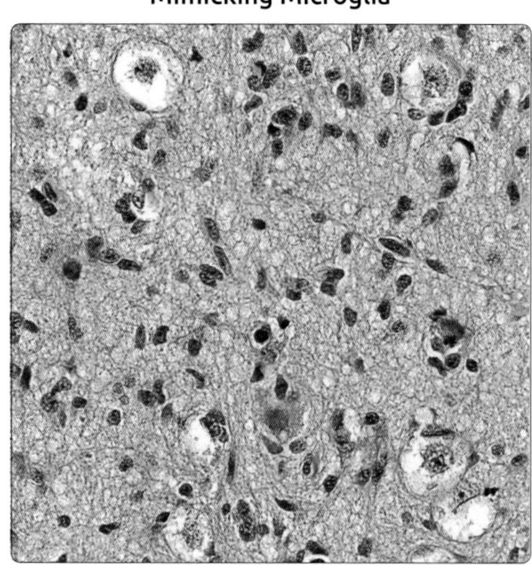

Modest Perineuronal Satellitosis

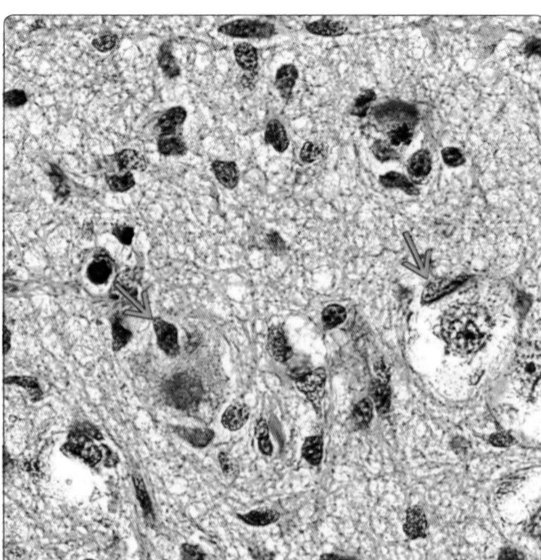

Heterogeneous Population

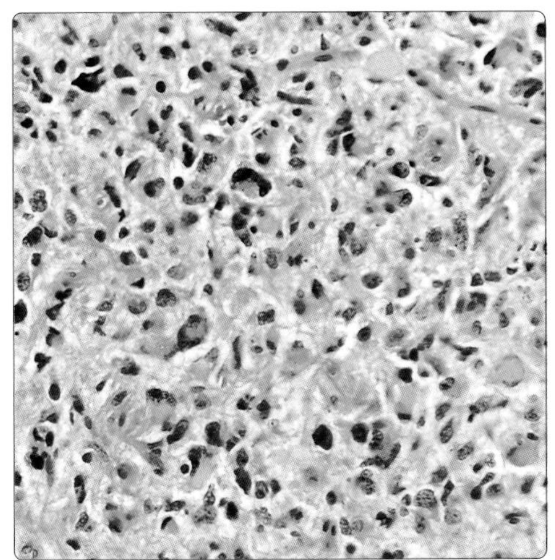

Tumor Cell Heterogeneity

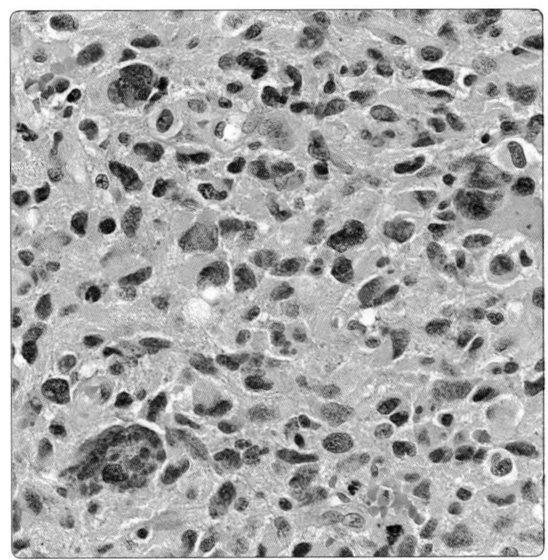

(Left) *A polymorphous population of astrocytes is common in GBM. With mitoses, but without microvascular proliferation &/or necrosis (of either zonal or pseudopalisading type), the lesion would be an anaplastic astrocytoma grade III.* **(Right)** *Polymorphous large and small cells intermingle in a common tissue pattern of GBM. In the presence of either necrosis or microvascular proliferation, the diagnosis would be glioblastoma. GBMs can be multiforme in both their gross and microscopic appearance.*

Pleomorphic Cells

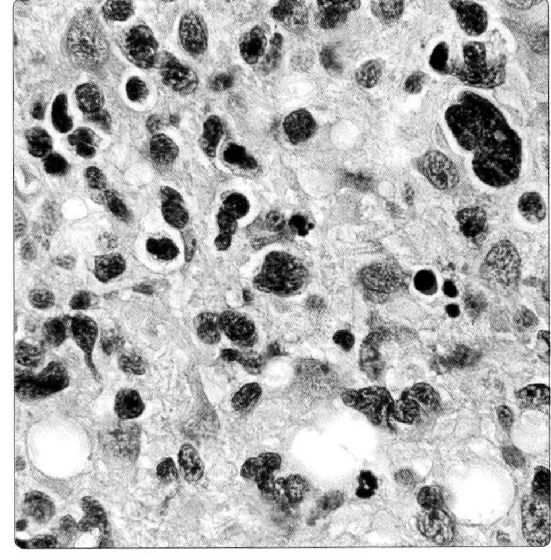

Round Nuclei

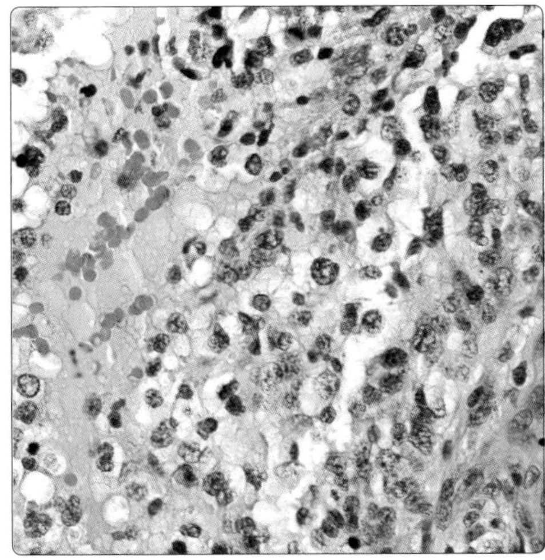

(Left) *While sizable, cells such as these are not as large &/or bizarre as those of giant cell glioblastoma, nor are they the dominant cell type as in giant cell GBM.* **(Right)** *A few round cells with perinuclear halos in a GBM are insufficient for the diagnosis of glioblastoma with an oligodendroglial component. The latter entity requires at least some area with a more classic oligodendrocytic appearance.*

Elongated Nuclei

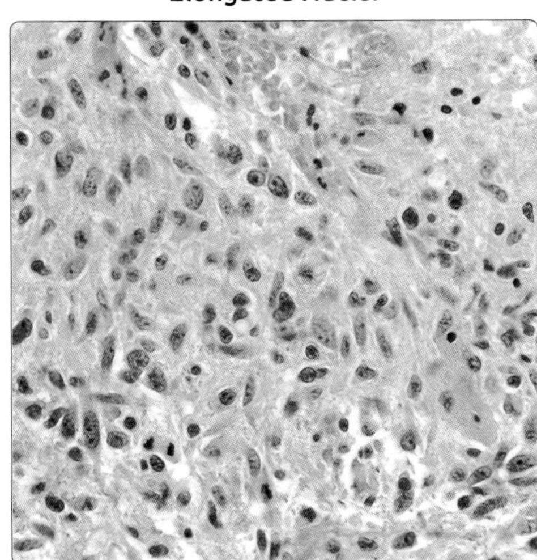

Gemistocytic Features

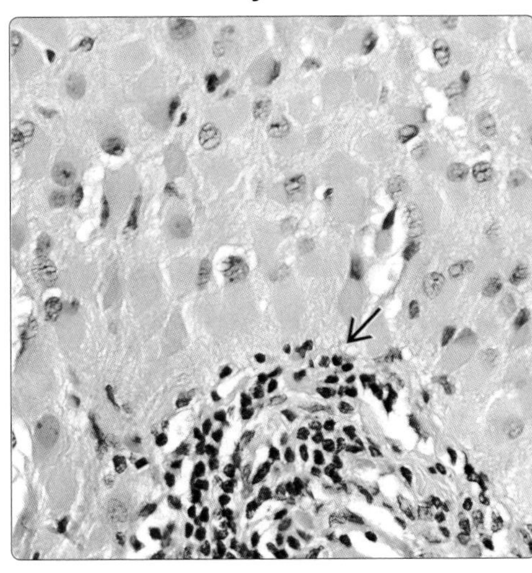

(Left) *Small tumor cells with this degree of elongation are astrocytic, not oligodendroglial.* **(Right)** *A gemistocytic astrocytoma precursor is present in some glioblastomas. Such tumors support a clinical impression of secondary glioblastoma. Perivascular lymphocytes* ⇒ *are present in most gemistocytic astrocytomas.*

(Left) *Small cell glioblastomas are remarkably uniform in both cell size and distribution. Although the cells are often a bit elongate rather than round, anaplastic oligodendroglioma enters into the differential diagnosis. Molecular studies for 1p and 19q would be prudent.* **(Right)** *While more common in oligodendrogliomas, calcifications ⇒ are also present in some glioblastomas, especially the small cell type.*

Small Cell GBM

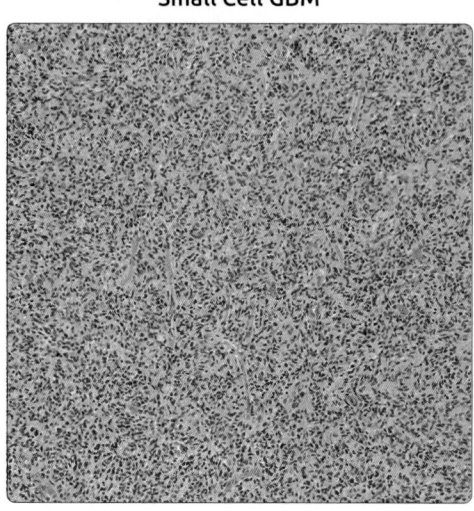

Calcification in Small Cell GBM

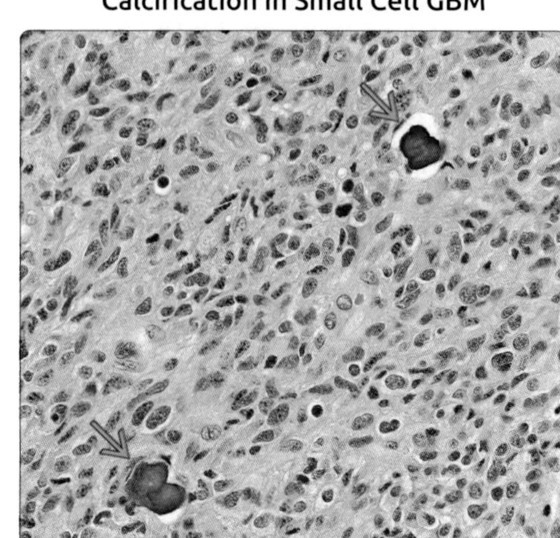

(Left) *Perivascular formations ⇒ superficially resembling ependymal pseudorosettes are not uncommon in small cell glioblastomas.* **(Right)** *Individual small tumor ⇒ cells at the infiltrating margin of a glioblastoma can be difficult to identify as neoplastic on the basis of cytologic features alone. A high Ki-67 labeling index would be supportive, but not definitive, evidence of neoplasia.*

Perivascular Structuring

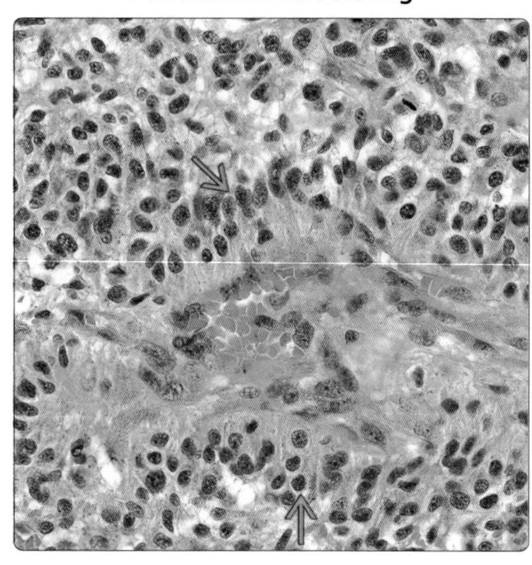

Rare Infiltrating Cells

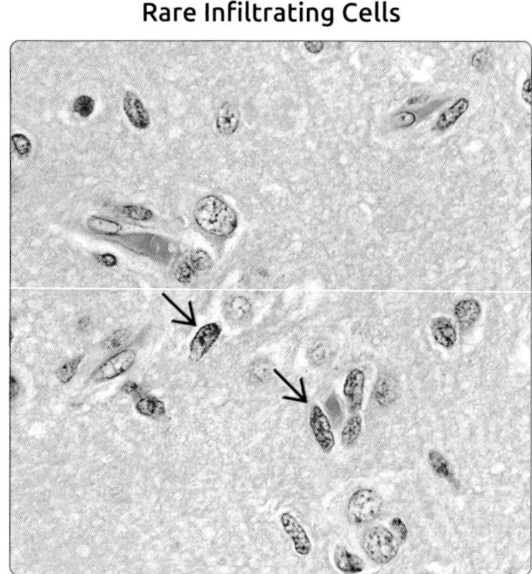

(Left) *Gross extremes of size, pleomorphism, and multinucleation mark the giant cell glioblastoma. This uncommon tumor is to be distinguished from conventional GBM with focal, large, even giant cells, which are more infiltrative and consist predominantly of smaller cells.* **(Right)** *Mitoses may be numerous in giant cell glioblastomas ⇒, but are difficult to find in others. Microvascular proliferation is often absent.*

Giant Cell GBM

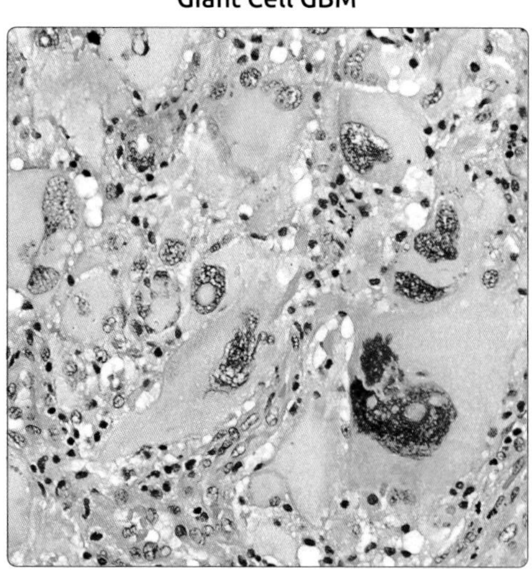

Giant Cell GBM

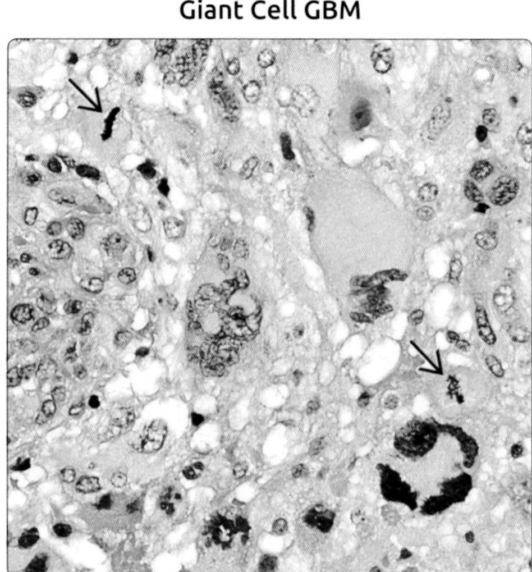

Giant Cell GBM

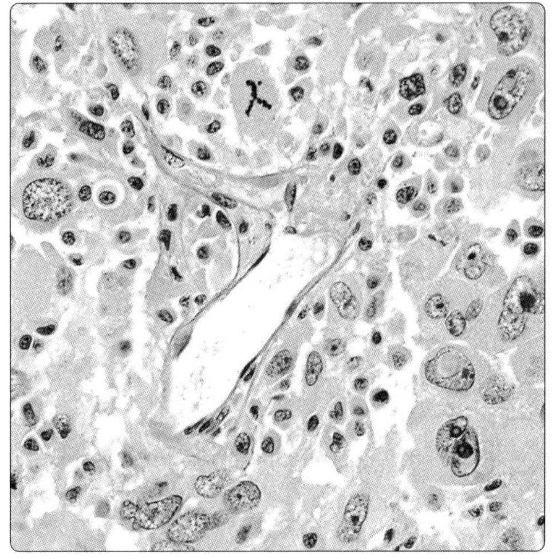

Giant Cell GBM, Necrosis Without Pseudopalisading

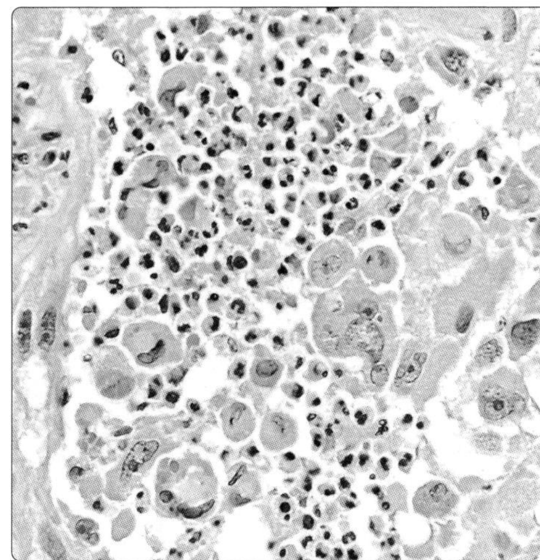

(Left) *Some cells in giant cell GBM may be large, but not giant. The compact giant cell variant often shows little tissue infiltration.* **(Right)** *Necrosis in giant cell glioblastoma is usually associated with little, if any, pseudopalisading. Vascular proliferation is also typically absent.*

Mimicking Metastasis

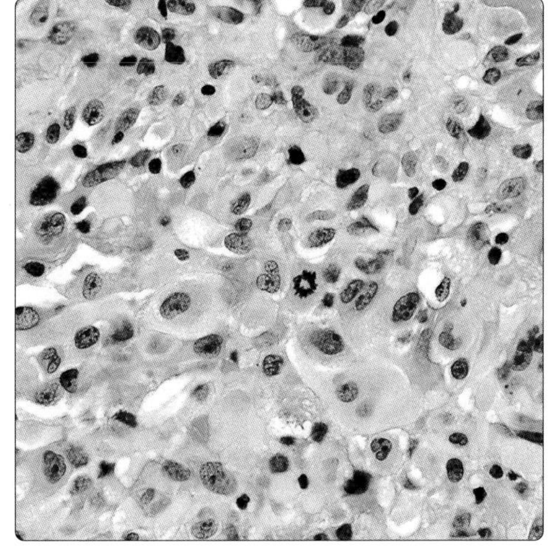

Epithelioid GBM

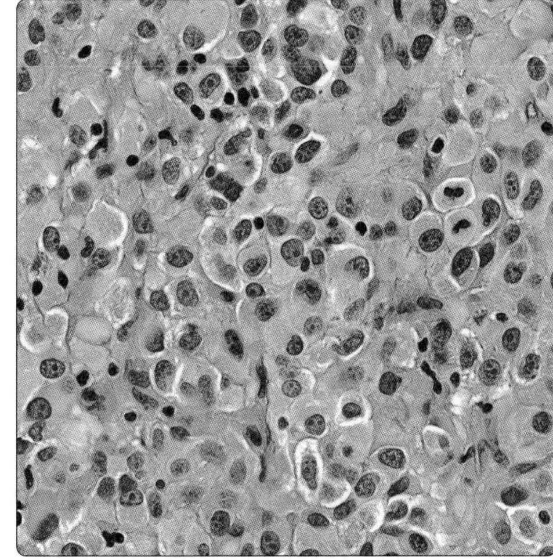

(Left) *Immunostaining for GFAP, as well as for epithelial and melanocytic markers, may be required in GBMs (such as this case) that are cytologically intermediate between carcinoma and glioma.* **(Right)** *Epithelioid tumor cells with plump cytoplasm and sharp cell borders simulate metastatic carcinoma or melanoma. Immunohistochemistry &/or identification of classic GBM elsewhere in the tumor usually resolves the issue. The distinction is difficult to achieve in some cases, however.*

Simulating Melanoma

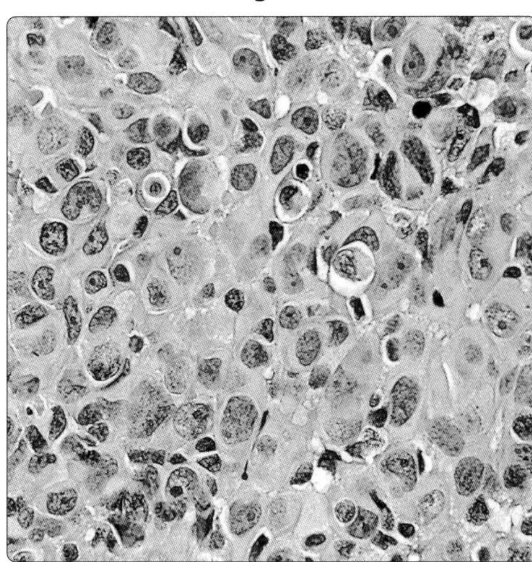

Simulating Carcinoma

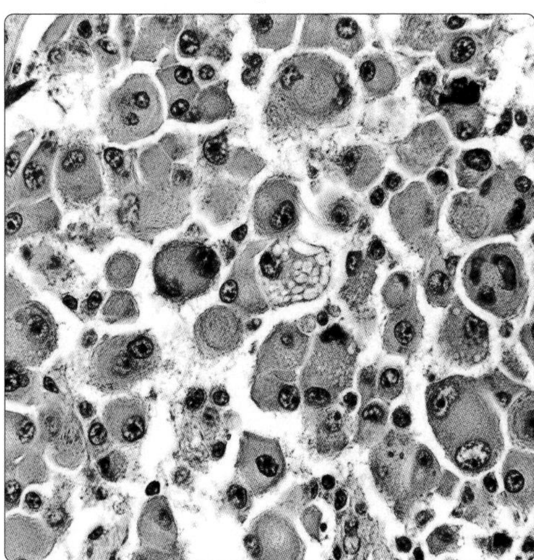

(Left) *GBMs with well-circumscribed cells may simulate a metastatic carcinoma or melanoma. An anaplastic PNET-like tissue component would also come to mind. These nuclei are too pleomorphic to be those of lymphoma (other than the rare anaplastic variant).* **(Right)** *Dyscohesive cells with prominent, well-circumscribed cytoplasm can closely resemble those of metastatic carcinoma and melanoma.*

(Left) *Up to 50% of epithelioid GBMs harbor BRAF V600E mutations, while this is very uncommon in other GBM types. The mutant BRAF protein can be detected by immunohistochemistry.* **(Right)** *Rare glioblastomas consist, in part, of focal areas with rhabdoid cells* ⇨ *similar to those of atypical teratoid/rhabdoid tumors.*

BRAF(+) Epithelioid GBM

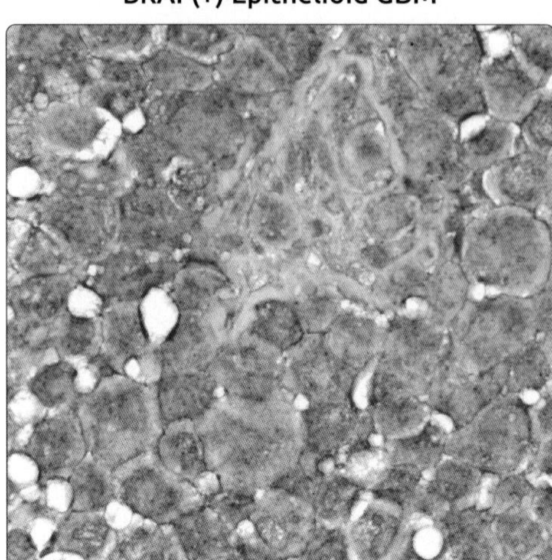

Rare Rhabdoid Component

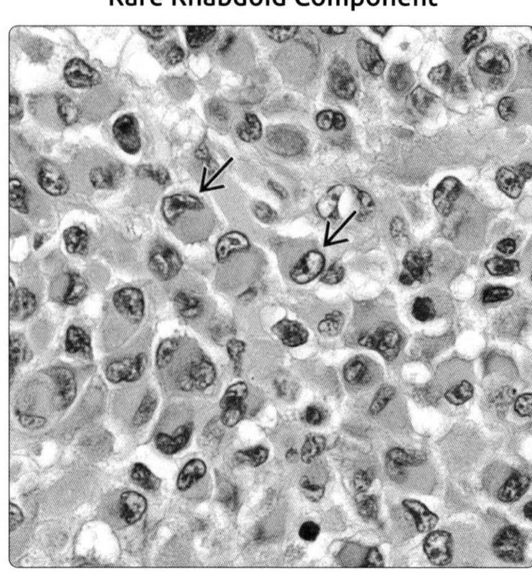

(Left) *Rhabdoid cells in some GBMs show "loss of retention" of immunostaining* ⇨ *for INI1 (i.e., no staining of nuclei). Surrounding more conventional glioblastoma cells have the nuclear staining* ⇨ *expected of nonrhabdoid tumors.* **(Right)** *A minority of GBMs feature a compact, mesenchyme-like, but glial, spindle cell component. Unlike mesenchymal metaplasia in GBM (gliosarcoma), this tissue is reticulin-poor.*

Rare Rhabdoid GBM

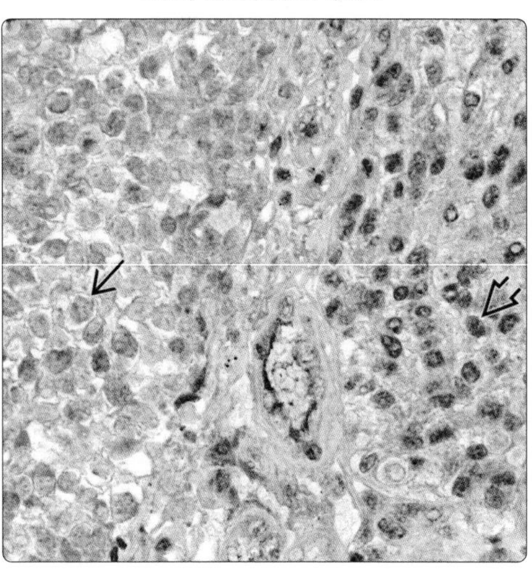

Spindle Cell Features

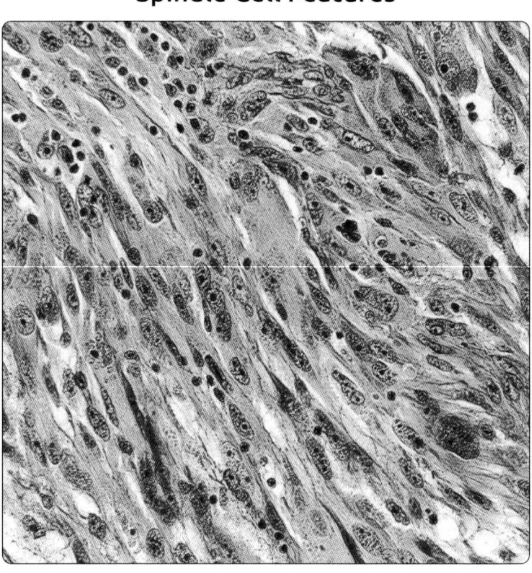

(Left) *Spindle cells in a background of a basophilic, mucinous matrix lend a mesenchymal quality to some GBMs.* **(Right)** *Metaplasia to true epithelial tissue is present in a very small percentage of GBM. Both glandular* ⇨ *and squamous differentiation* ⇨ *are present in this case. Epithelial metaplasia is more common in gliosarcomas than in conventional GBM.*

Increased Mucinous Matrix

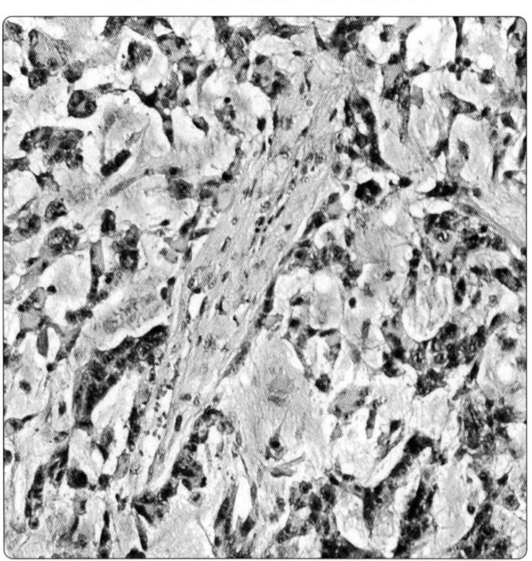

Epithelial Metaplasia

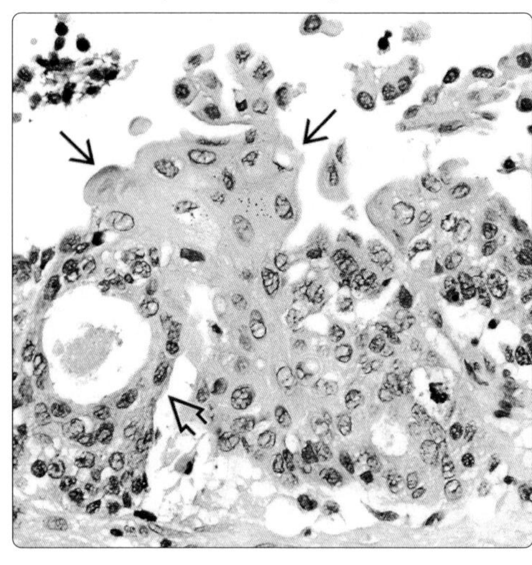

Squamous Metaplasia

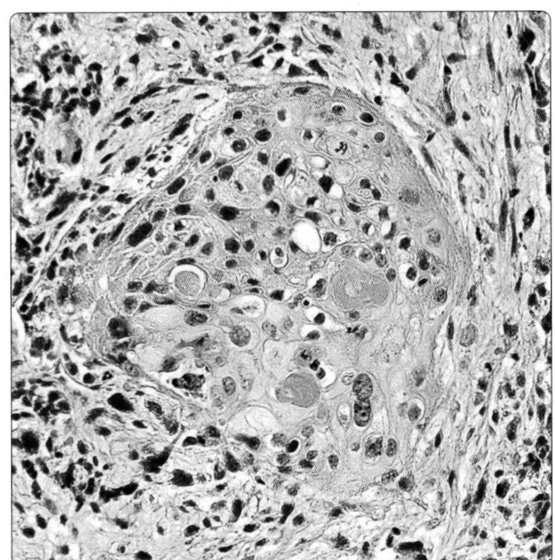

Glandular Metaplasia

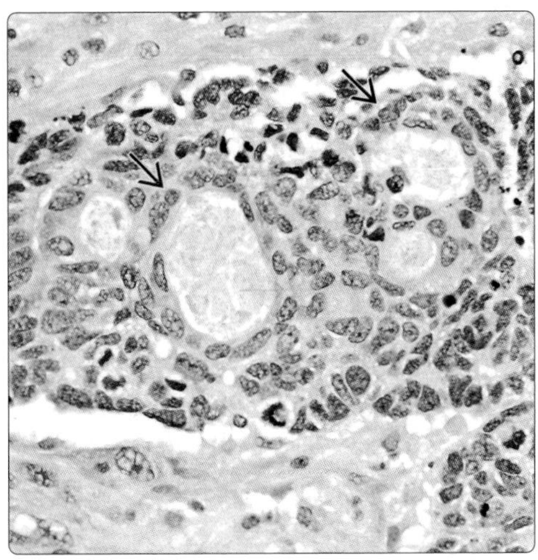

(Left) *Keratinizing squamous epithelium is a distinctive and rare form of epithelial metaplasia in GBM and gliosarcomas. It and other forms of epithelial metaplasia are more common in gliosarcomas.* **(Right)** *As seen here, discrete foci of compact, lumen-containing ➔ tissue represent rare glandular metaplasia.*

EMA in Epithelial Metaplasia

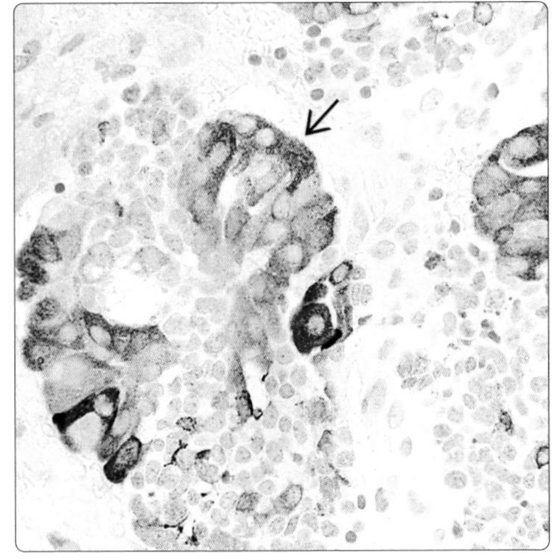

Lipidized Tumor Cells

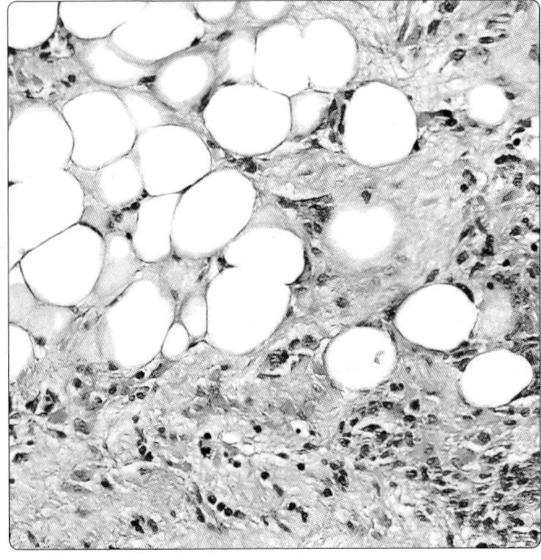

(Left) *Immunoreactivity for EMA helps define a component's epithelial nature ➔. Only a rare GBM of the epithelioid type is EMA positive in the absence of epithelial metaplasia.* **(Right)** *As with other CNS tumors, such as meningioma and neurocytoma, lipidized tumor cells in some GBMs bear a striking resemblance to adipocytes. Immunohistochemistry for GFAP will confirm their glial origin.*

Lipidized Tumor Cells Rimmed by GFAP

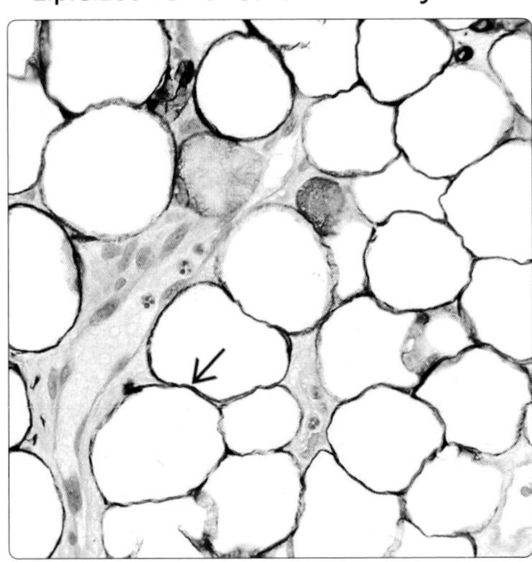

Oligodendroglial Component

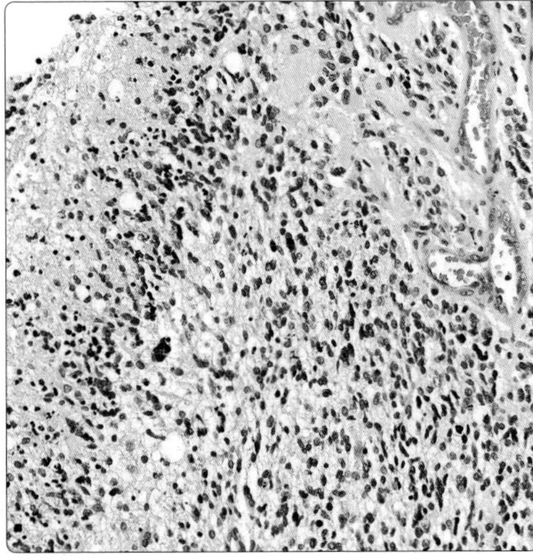

(Left) *The thin margins of compressed cytoplasm in lipid-laden, adipocyte-like cells are positive for GFAP ➔ in this lipidized GBM.* **(Right)** *Criteria for GBM with an oligodendroglioma component are fulfilled when an astrocytic lesion, such as this case with necrosis elsewhere, shows areas of classic oligodendroglioma.*

(Left) *A histologically classic oligodendroglioma element, in association with high-grade astrocytic tumor with necrosis, fulfills the diagnostic criteria for GBM with an oligodendroglioma component.* **(Right)** *A small percentage of GBMs often have well-defined areas of PNET-like tissue, in which cellularity is high and cells are generally round. As such, these areas lack the background fibrillarity of the parent lesion and its often dominant population of bi- or multipolar cells.*

Oligodendroglial Component

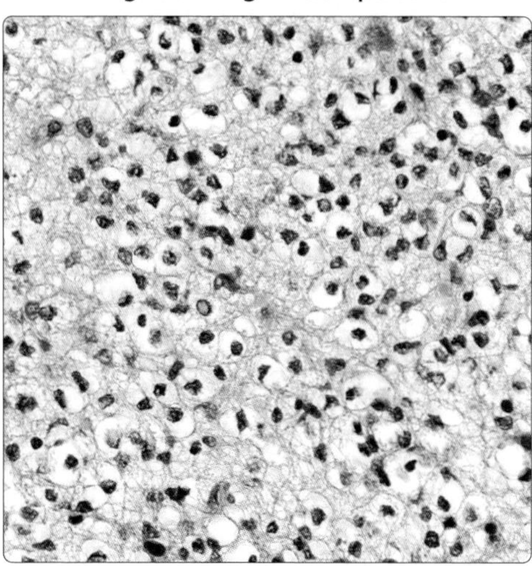

PNET-Like Component

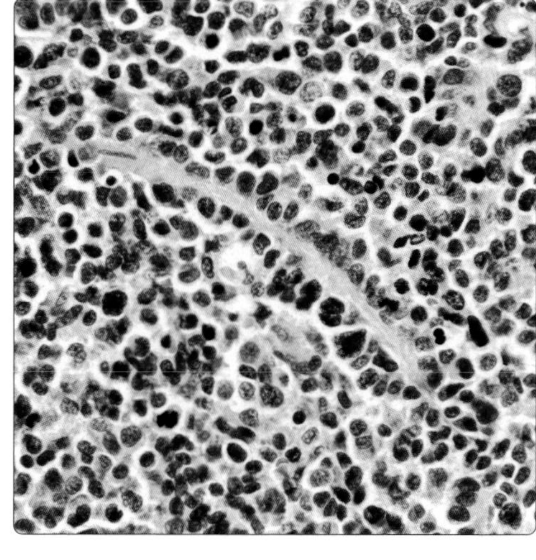

(Left) *PNET-like tissue in GBM may have Homer Wright (neuroblastic) rosettes ⇒ like those of medulloblastomas and neuroblastoma.* **(Right)** *PNET-like tissue in glioblastomas may have features of anaplasia, as seen in a minority of medulloblastomas. These qualities include large cell size, nuclear molding, cell-cell wrapping ⇒, and frequent apoptosis.*

Homer Wright Rosettes in PNET-Like Component

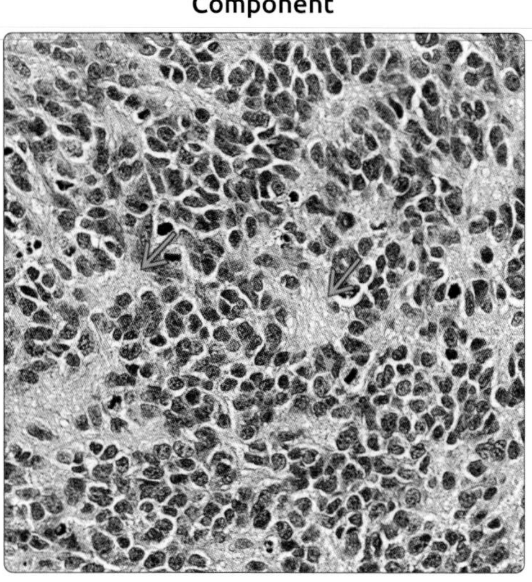

Anaplasia in PNET-Like Component

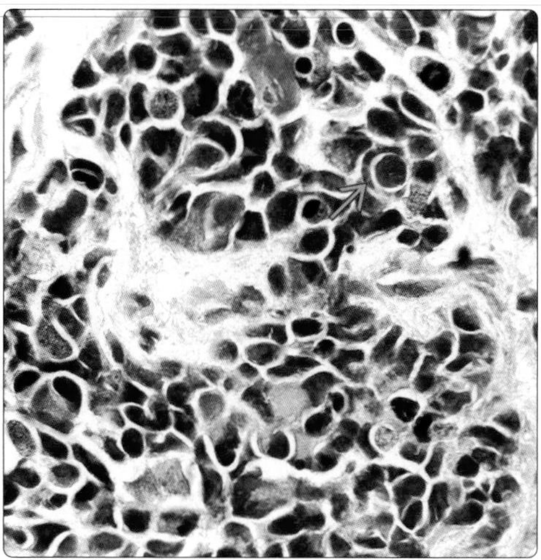

(Left) *In contrast to the glioma in which it arose, PNET-like tissue is immunoreactive for synaptophysin. The illustrated positivity is clearly that of the tumor, not merely background brain parenchyma.* **(Right)** *PNET-like tissue in glioblastomas has an especially high Ki-67 index.*

Synaptophysin in PNET-Like Component

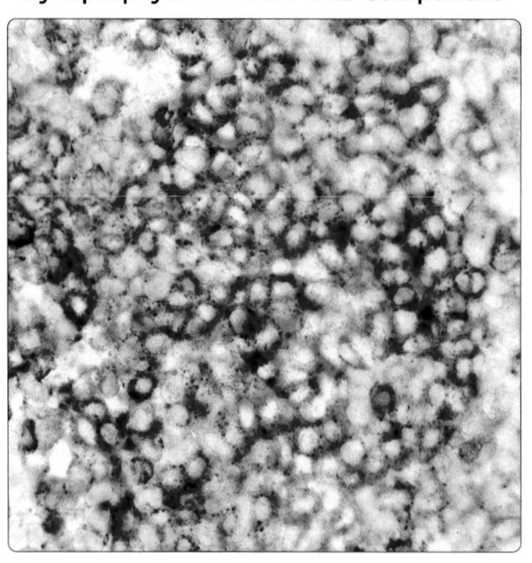

Extremely High Labeling Index

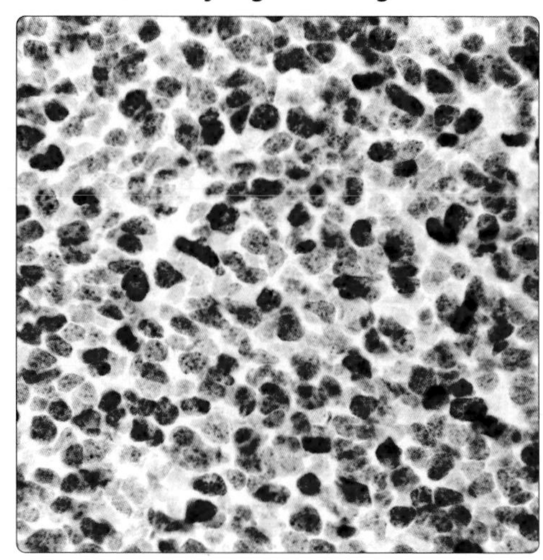

GFAP Focal, Giant Cell GBM

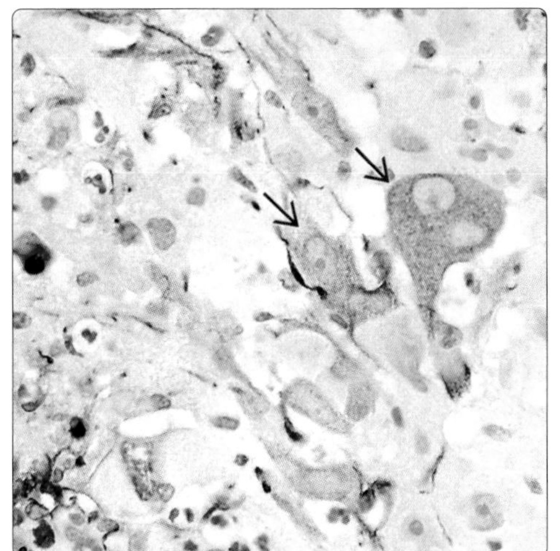

p53, Giant Cell GBM

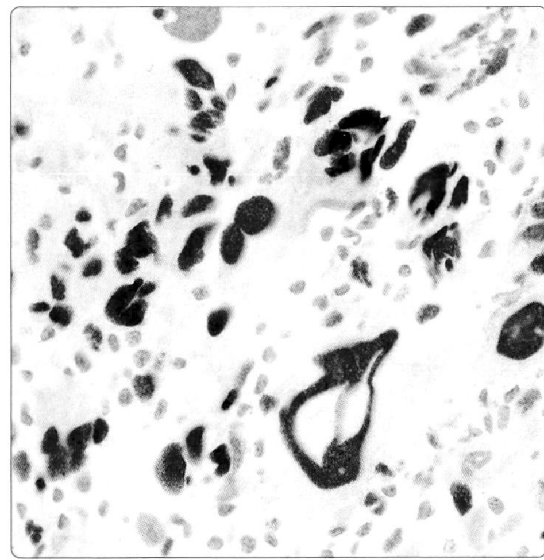

(Left) *GFAP staining* ⇨ *is often focal &/or faint in GBM of the giant cell type. The diagnosis, therefore, often rests more on histological features and exclusion of alternative diagnoses.* **(Right)** *Giant cell GBMs are often diffusely immunoreactive for p53.*

Synaptophysin, Giant Cell GBM

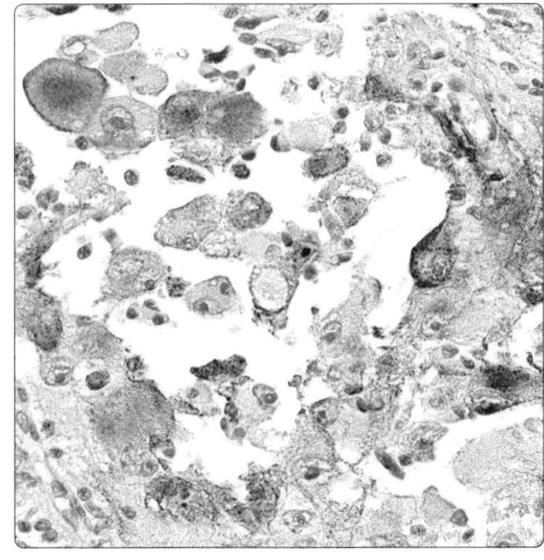

GFAP Variable

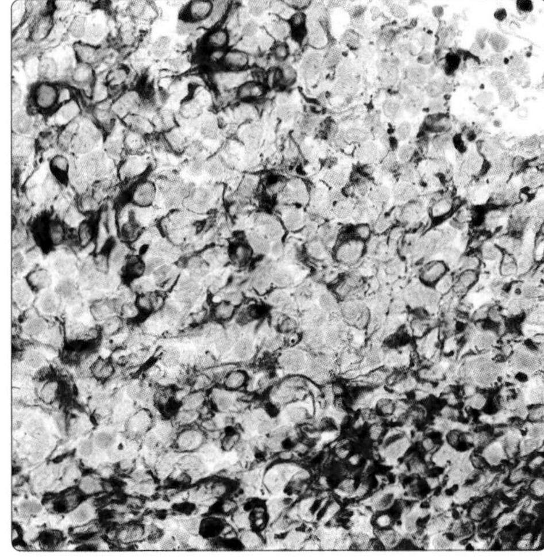

(Left) *Synaptophysin immunopositive cells are present in some GBMs, especially in the giant cell type. While such lesions are technically glioneuronal, this designation should, in general, be reserved for tumors in which neuronal differentiation is obvious in H&E sections.* **(Right)** *Some GBMs are extensively GFAP positive, whereas others are largely negative. Somewhat better differentiated regions, as seen in this case, are more likely to be positive than regions composed only of small, undifferentiated cells.*

Focal GFAP, Epithelioid GBM

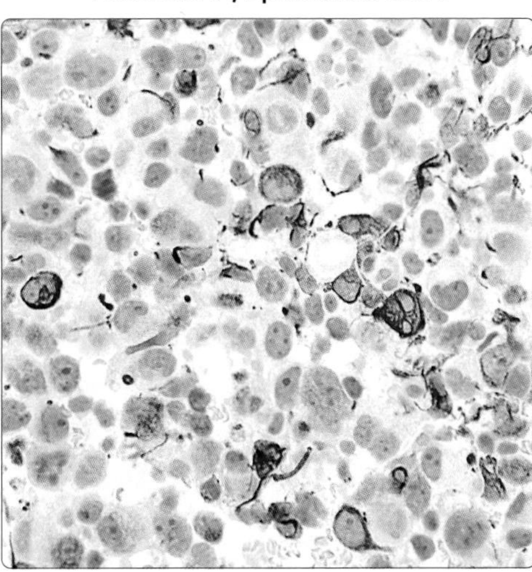

Ki-67(+) Elongate, Irregular Nuclei

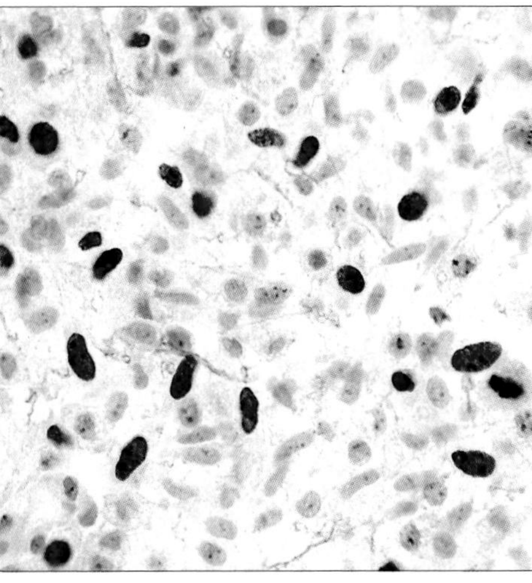

(Left) *GFAP positivity may be focal in epithelioid glioblastomas. It is convincing in this case, but can be so restricted as to be equivocal in others.* **(Right)** *While not a cancer-specific marker like IDH1, Ki-67 positivity helps identify small, elongated atypical tumor cells in a macrophage-rich infiltrate. Cytological features, such as atypia and increased nuclear size relative to that of phagocytes, remain critical diagnostic features, however.*

(Left) *Unlike secondary GBM that evolves from a lower grade precursor astrocytoma, primary glioblastomas, such as this mitotically active small cell example, are immunonegative for IDH1.* **(Right)** *Secondary glioblastomas that evolve from a lower grade precursor astrocytoma are often immunoreactive for IDH1. The considerably more common primary glioblastomas are not.*

Primary GBM, Negative for IDH1

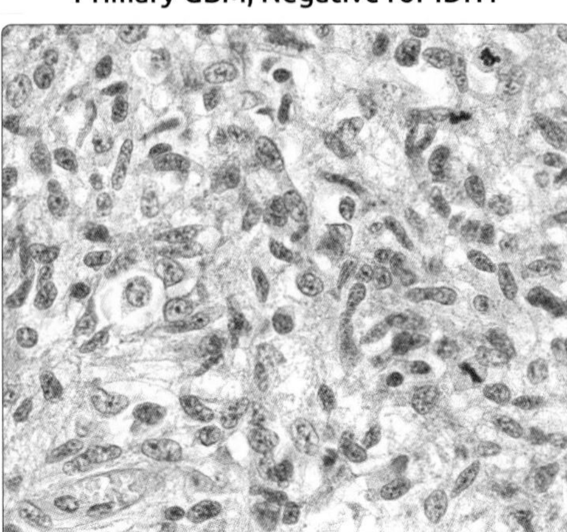

Secondary GBM, Positive for IDH1

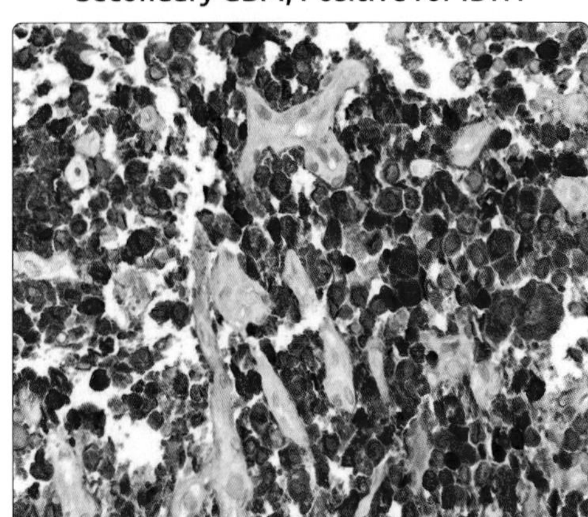

(Left) *GBMs infiltrate cortex and white matter as single cells and, in those secondary examples that express IDH1, individual tumor cells can be confidently identified.* **(Right)** *Most adult primary GBMs show retention of nuclear ATRX, as well as an absence of IDH1 IHC (+) (or IDH1/2 mutation). In contrast, adult secondary GBMs are more likely to demonstrate loss of nuclear ATRX and IDH1 IHC (+).*

IDH1 Cortical Infiltration

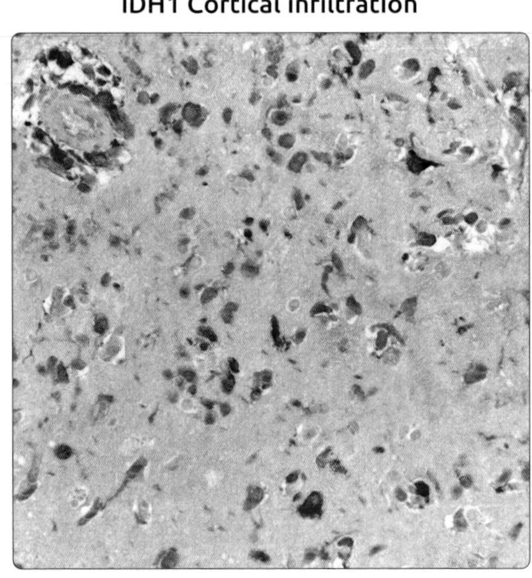

Adult GBM, Retained Nuclear ATRX

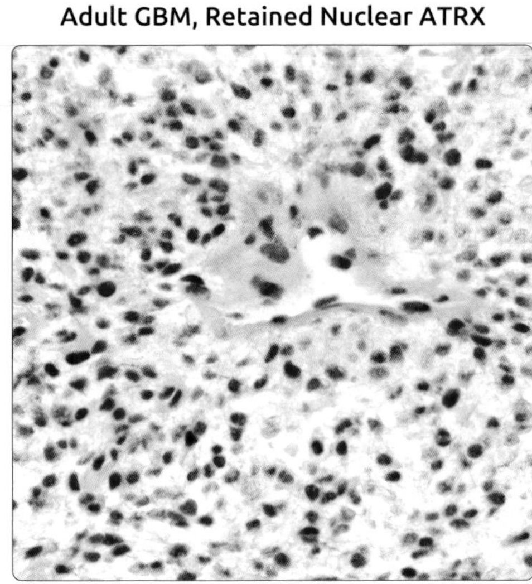

(Left) *CD68 positive macrophages ➡ may be numerous enough to partially obscure tumor cells ⇨. Long nuclei of the latter aid in identification.* **(Right)** *Small, elongate cells in a finely fibrillar matrix ⇨ are common in smear preparations of GBM. Nuclear size (small) and shape (elongate) help exclude oligodendroglioma and primary central system lymphoma. The fibrillar background, in particular, is alien to lymphoma, metastatic carcinoma, and melanoma.*

Admixed Macrophages

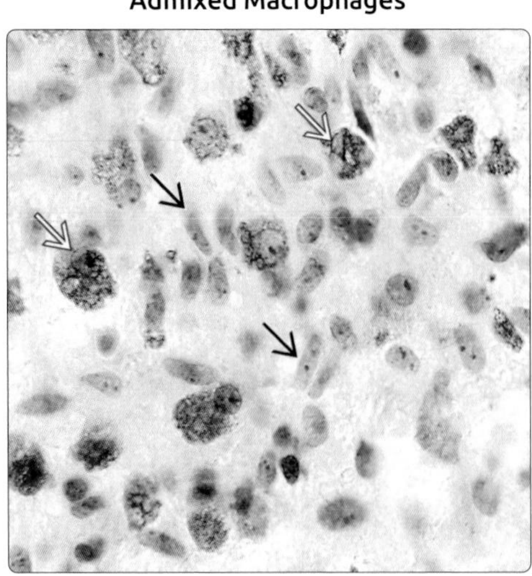

Smear, Small Elongate Cells

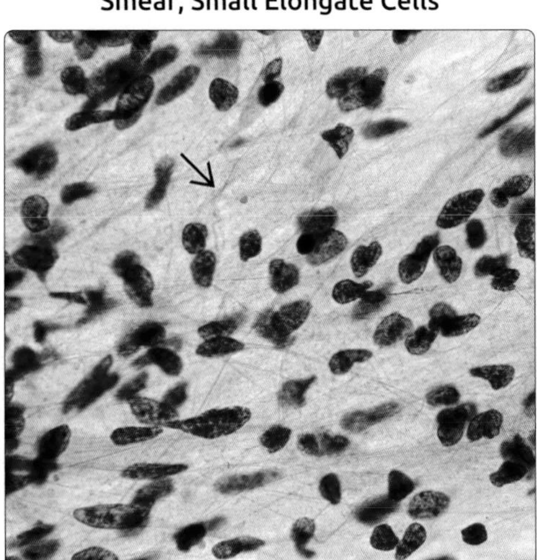

Smear: Giant Cell GBM

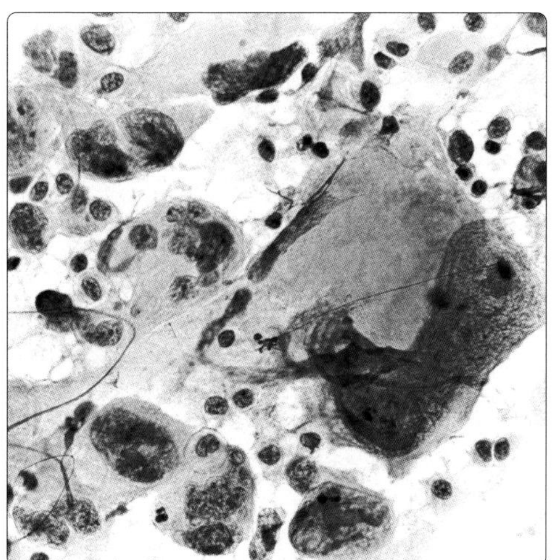

Smear: Necrotic Center

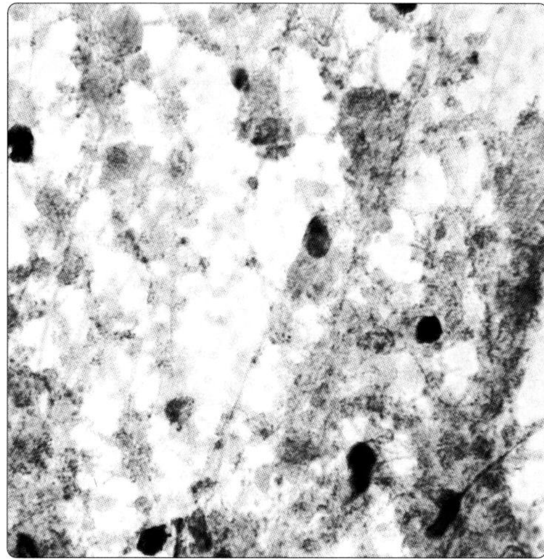

(Left) *Monstrous, pleomorphic nuclei characterize the giant cell variant of GBM in smear preparations.* **(Right)** *Cytological preparations of tissue from the nonenhancing center of a GBM will show little other than necrosis. Unlike infarcts and demyelinating disease, only smeared granular debris, not macrophages, are the result.*

Smear: Vascular Proliferation

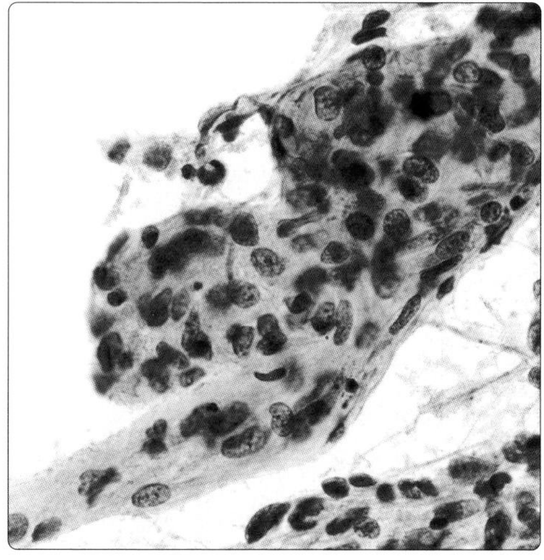

Smear: Post Treatment

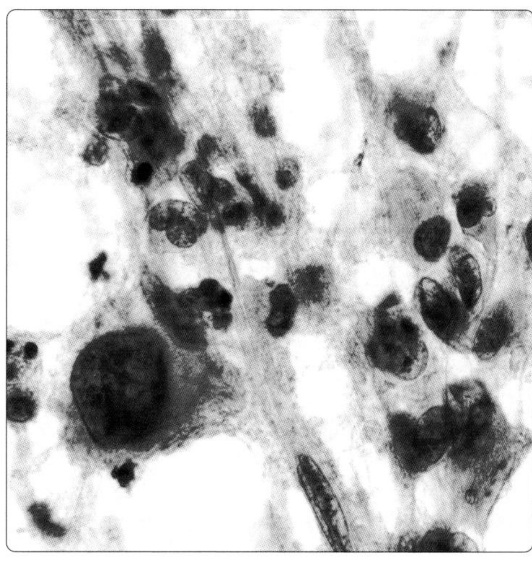

(Left) *Glomeruloid microvascular proliferation is prominent in smear preparations of many GBMs. It is not always easy to distinguish this proliferative response from vessels with merely hypertrophic endothelium.* **(Right)** *Considerable nuclear pleomorphism may be present in posttreatment glioblastomas, as illustrated here in a smear preparation. Intraoperatively, the degree of activity of a clinically recurrent lesion is better evaluated in frozen sections.*

***PTEN* Loss**

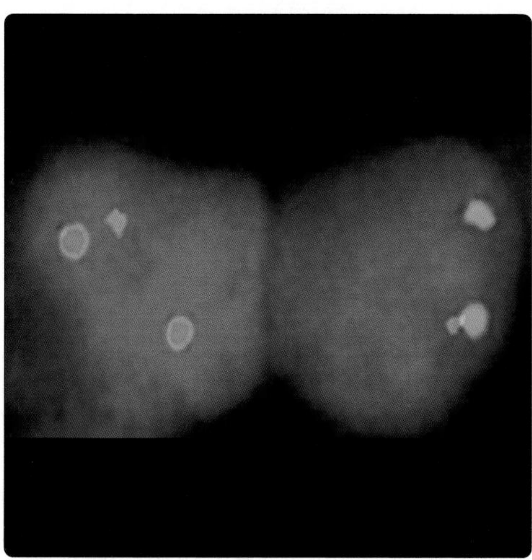

EGFR Amplification

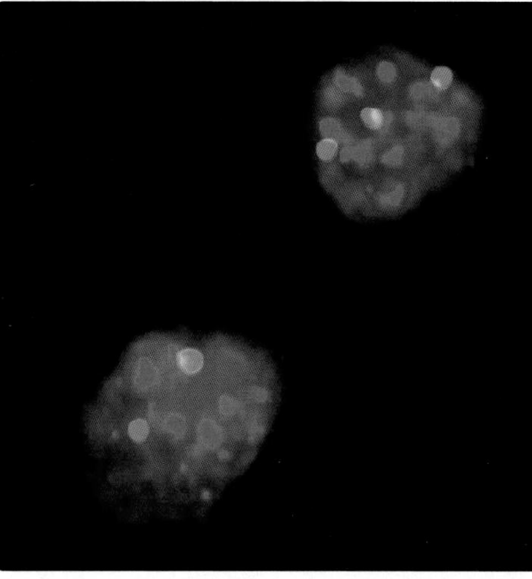

(Left) *The tumor suppressor gene PTEN (red signal) is lost along with much, if not all, of chromosome 10q in a significant percentage of glioblastomas. There is only 1 red signal per cell, but 2 green signals for the chromosome 10 centromere probe.* **(Right)** *Amplification of the EGFR receptor, common in primary GBM, is recognized by innumerable red FISH signals. One cell is trisomic, as indicated by 3 green signals for CEP7. (Courtesy M. Janawar, MD.)*

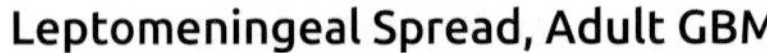

Leptomeningeal Spread, Adult GBM

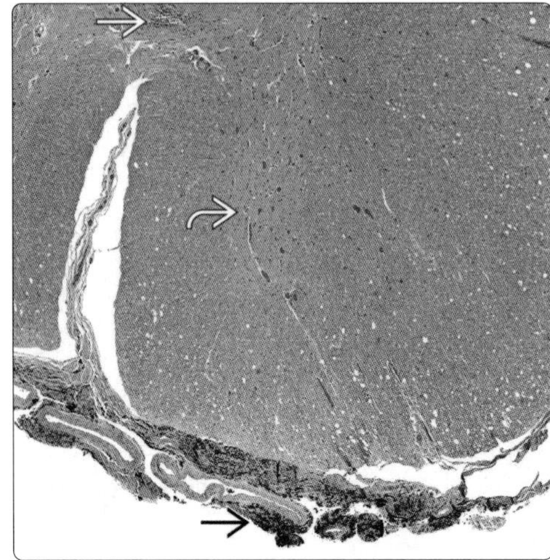

GBM With Leptomeningeal Spread

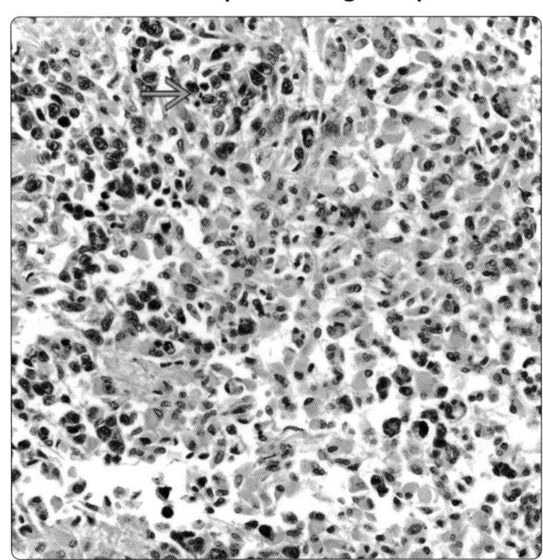

(Left) *While adult GBMs usually do not produce leptomeningeal spread, and then usually only at late stages of disease, it can occasionally be identified at autopsy, as in this patient. Tumor within ventral CSF spaces* ⇨ *can be readily seen; the anterior horn cell* ➦ *and central canal* ➡ *are highlighted for orientation.* **(Right)** *This adult GBM, spread to both leptomeninges and subventricular areas at autopsy, shows admixed poorly differentiated* ⇨ *and clearly astrocytic features.*

Axial MR: Pontine GBM

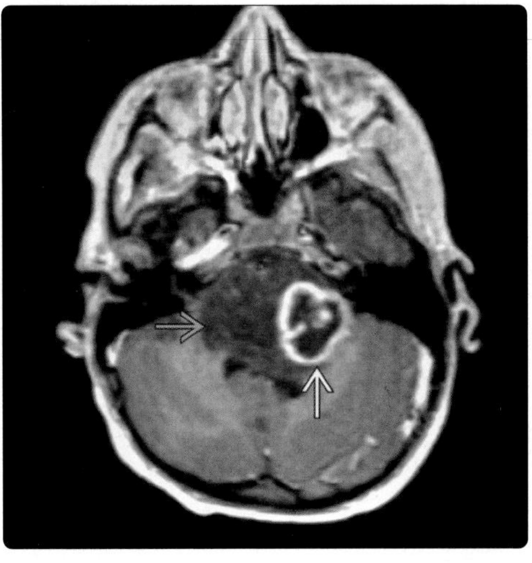

Spinal Cord Metastasis

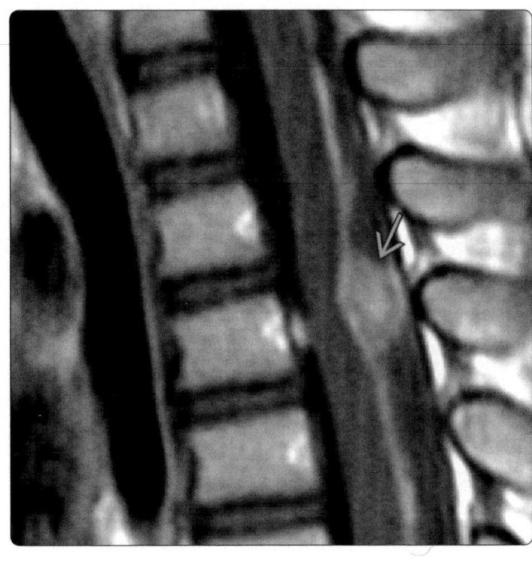

(Left) *On contrast-enhanced scans, this child with a diffuse intrinsic pontine glioma shows not only hypointensity that highlights the diffuse enlargement of the pons* ⇨*, but also a focus of rim-enhancing, centrally necrotic tumor* ➡*.* **(Right)** *This child with a diffuse intrinsic pontine glioma (DIPGs) was found to have a drop metastasis* ⇨ *in the spinal cord. DIPGs in children have a significant tendency to produce leptomeningeal spread.*

Diffuse Intrinsic Pontine Glioma

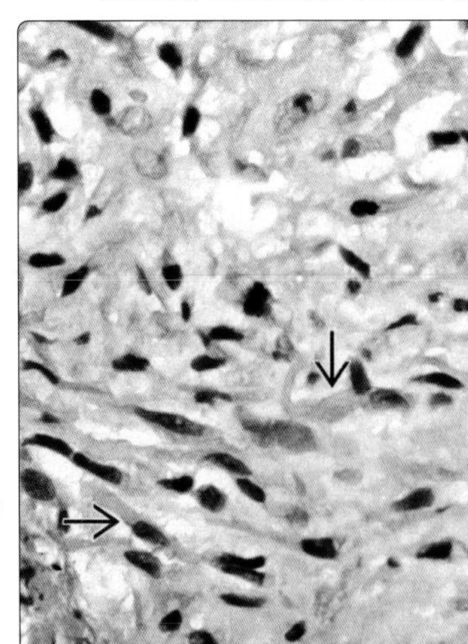

GFAP(+) Leptomeningeal Metastasis

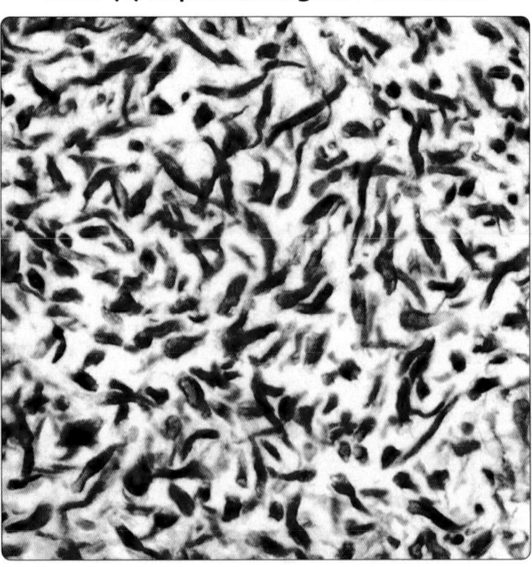

(Left) *This child with a DIPG presented early during her course of disease with leptomeningeal dissemination and the spinal cord drop metastasis was biopsied for diagnosis. Note the eosinophilic cytoplasm in only scattered cells* ⇨*.* **(Right)** *This child with a diffuse intrinsic pontine glioma presented early in her course of disease with a drop metastasis to the spinal cord, which proved on biopsy to be high-grade glioma with strong diffuse GFAP(+).*

Axial MR: Pseudoprogression

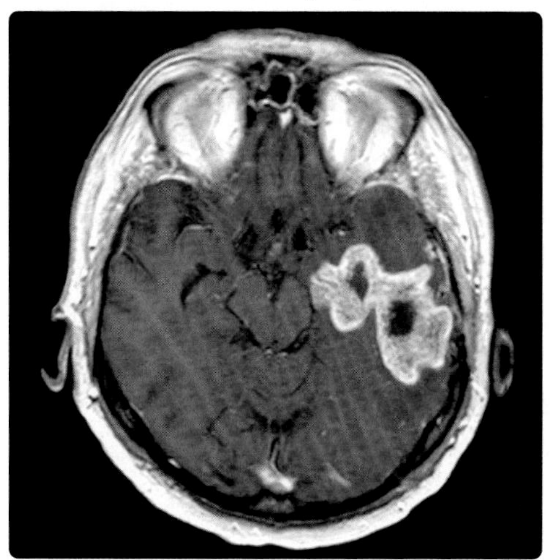

Post Treatment

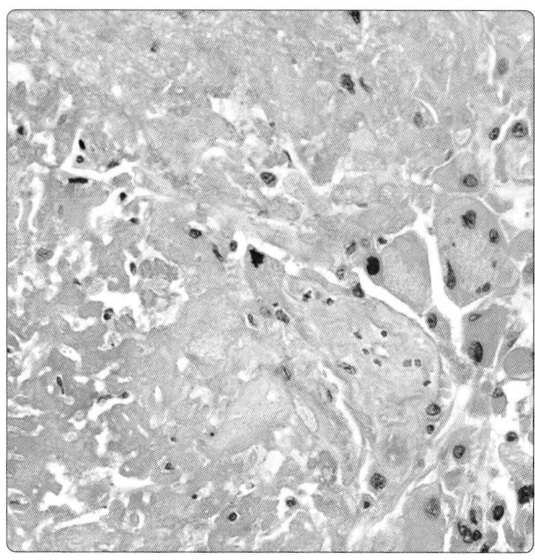

(Left) *An expansile, ring-enhancing GBM similar to a pretreatment lesion is, in some instances, due largely to treatment effects (pseudoprogression), rather than active tumor regrowth.* **(Right)** *Only coagulation necrosis and scattered cells, presumably neoplastic, are present in a patient after treatment with chemotherapy and radiation therapy. Other areas may contain highly cellular active tumor and tissue intermediate in composition between the 2 patterns.*

Posttreatment GBM

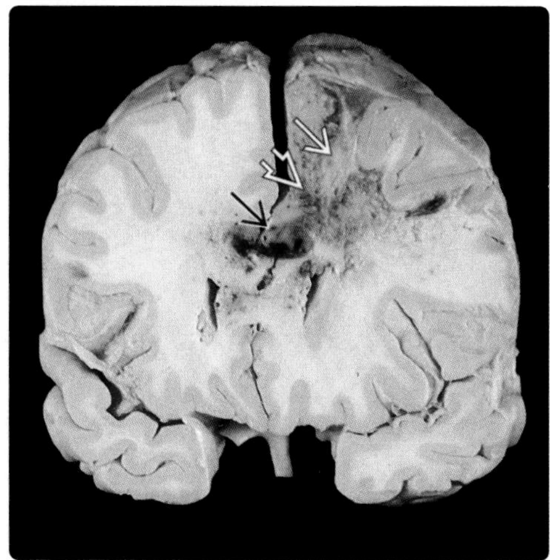

Posttreatment GBM

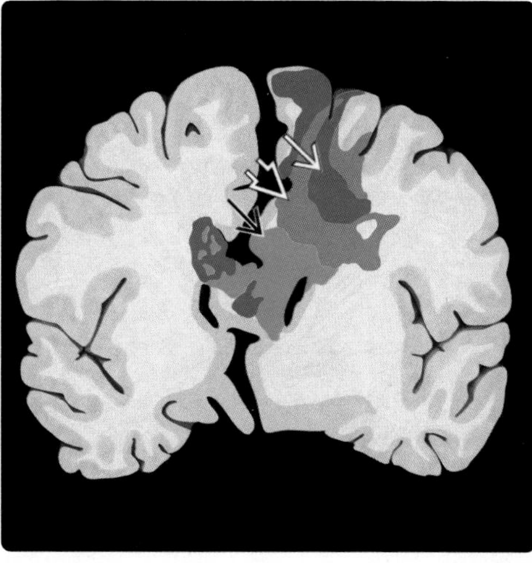

(Left) *Previously treated GBMs are often heterogeneous in composition. Active tumor is present ➙, as is radiation necrosis ➙, and tumor microscopically showing effects of prior treatment ➙.* **(Right)** *This graphic shows tissue types often seen post treatment. The green areas are active, recurrent tumor ➙. The blue regions are radionecrosis ➙. Areas of paucicellular neoplasm with cytological features of prior treatment are shown in purple ➙.*

Posttreatment, Thickened Vessels

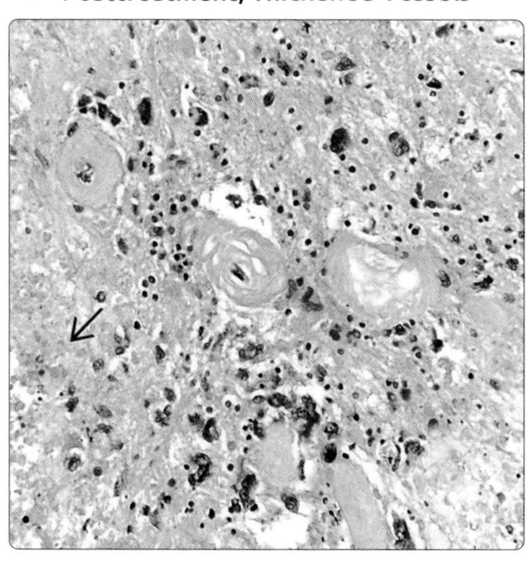

Admixed Necrosis and Paucicellular Tumor

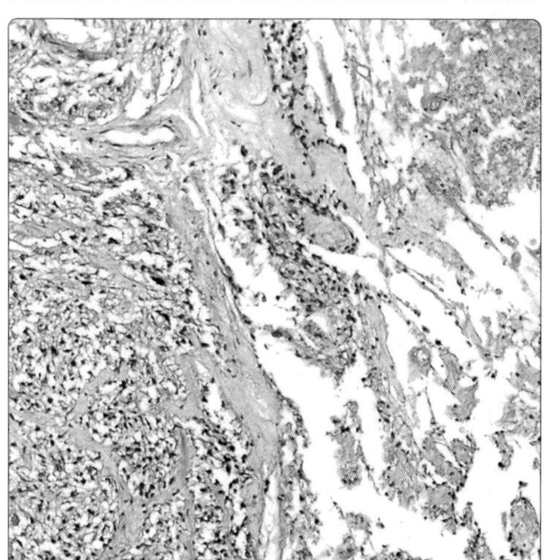

(Left) *While viable tumor is present, low cellularity and pleomorphism are consistent with persistent, but not actively recurrent, tumor. The thickened vessels reflect prior therapy. Necrosis ➙ as an irradiation effect is present as well.* **(Right)** *A mixture of necrosis and paucicellular tumor is not uncommon in GBM at recurrence or "pseudoprogression." The tissue is neoplastic, but not active high grade.*

KEY FACTS

TERMINOLOGY

- Typically variant of glioblastoma, but occasionally variant of oligodendroglioma, ependymoma, or subependymoma
- Mesenchymal metaplasia of glial cells, not true mixed glial/mesenchymal neoplasm

CLINICAL ISSUES

- Poor prognosis, akin to that of glioblastoma, ± mesenchymal differentiation

IMAGING

- Usually supratentorial and superficial; well demarcated; enhancing

MACROSCOPIC

- Variably discrete, intraoperatively may simulate metastasis or meningioma

MICROSCOPIC

- Bulk of lesion can have mesenchymal features
- Spread along vessels, mesenchymal component
- Tendency of mesenchymal component to mature into low-grade tumor or apparent reactive fibrosis
- Specific mesenchymal differentiation, some cases

ANCILLARY TESTS

- Abnormalities, e.g., *P53* mutations, identical in areas both of glial and mesenchymal differentiation (clonal neoplasm)
- Olig2(-) unlike typical glioblastoma
- CD34 often (+) in mesenchymal component, but not in infiltrating component
- p53(+), if present in both glial and mesenchymal tissue

DIAGNOSTIC CHECKLIST

- Consider gliosarcoma in any anaplastic fibroblastic process, even if glial component not obvious
- Reticulin and GFAP staining useful in distinguishing glial from mesenchymal component

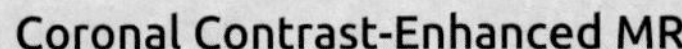
Coronal Contrast-Enhanced MR

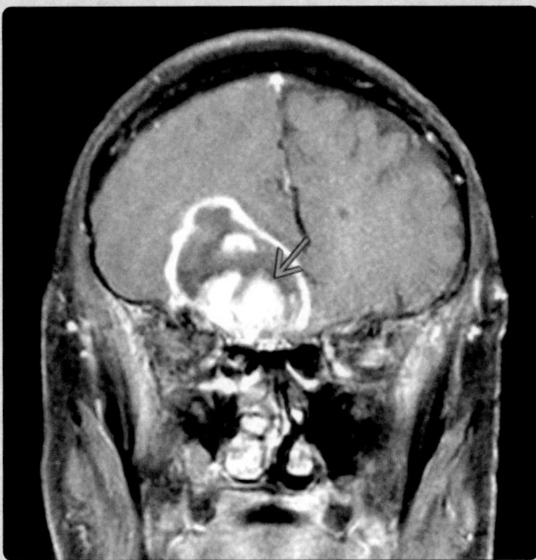

Discrete, Often Superficial

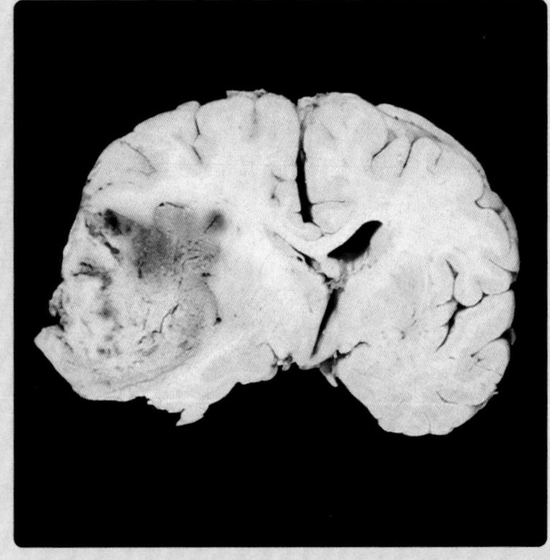

(Left) *Gliosarcomas often enhance with a rim profile typical of high-grade gliomas but also solidly and superficially, as seen here in a region of mesenchymal differentiation* →. **(Right)** *The firm, discrete, often superficial mass may be misinterpreted intraoperatively as meningioma or metastasis.*

Mesenchymal and Glial Features

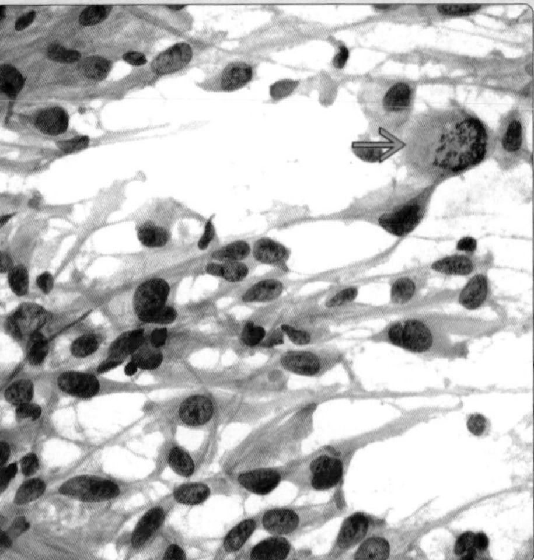

Mesenchymal and Glial Components

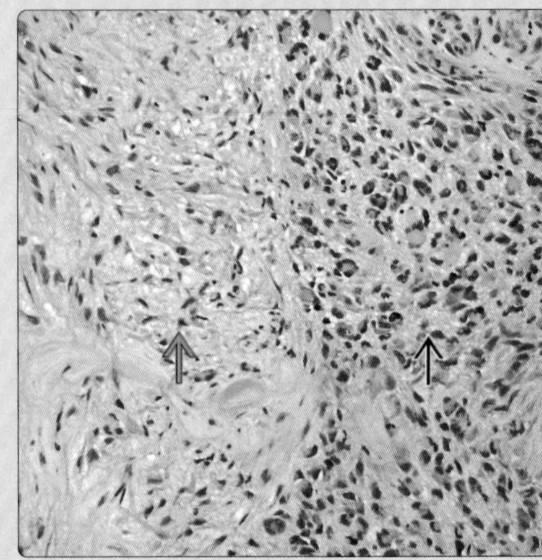

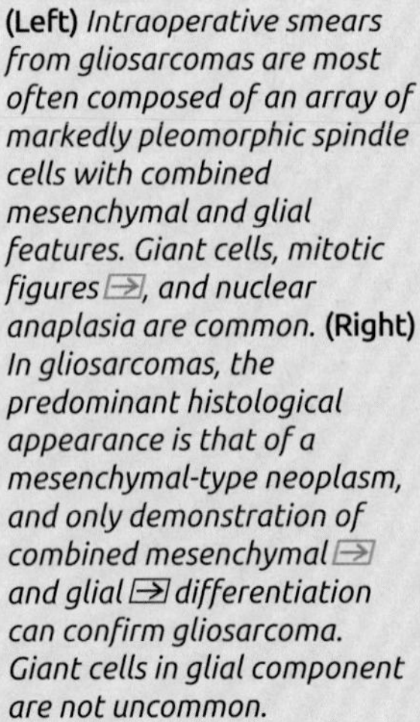
(Left) *Intraoperative smears from gliosarcomas are most often composed of an array of markedly pleomorphic spindle cells with combined mesenchymal and glial features. Giant cells, mitotic figures* →, *and nuclear anaplasia are common.* **(Right)** *In gliosarcomas, the predominant histological appearance is that of a mesenchymal-type neoplasm, and only demonstration of combined mesenchymal* → *and glial* → *differentiation can confirm gliosarcoma. Giant cells in glial component are not uncommon.*

TERMINOLOGY

Definitions

- Variant of glioblastoma, WHO grade IV
- Phenotypically mixed lesion with glial and mesenchymal differentiation
  - Evident at initial presentation (primary gliosarcoma)
  - Mesenchymal differentiation in preexisting malignant glioma, usually after treatment (secondary gliosarcoma)
- Occasionally variant of oligodendroglioma, ependymoma, subependymoma
- Mesenchymal differentiation of glial cells, not true mixed glial/mesenchymal neoplasm

ETIOLOGY/PATHOGENESIS

Environmental Exposure

- Past history of irradiation for CNS tumor in some cases

CLINICAL ISSUES

Epidemiology

- Age
  - Adults: Same age distribution as glioblastoma
    - Any age, but usually > 40 years
  - Children (rare)

Site

- Supratentorial, most cases
  - Temporal lobe classic, but not only site
- Posterior fossa associated with ependymoma, rare

Presentation

- Similar to glioblastoma
- Focal neurological deficit depending on site
- Headaches, seizures, cognitive dysfunction
- Macrocephaly, infants (rare)
- No prior history of glioma (primary gliosarcoma)
- Past history of glioma in some cases (secondary gliosarcoma)

Treatment

- Surgery, irradiation, and chemotherapy similar to glioblastoma

Prognosis

- Poor, similar to that of ordinary glioblastoma
  - Also poor for tumors arising in setting of oligodendroglioma (oligosarcoma) or ependymoma (ependymosarcoma)
- Skull penetration with extracranial extension in some cases
- Systemic metastases (exceptional)

IMAGING

MR Findings

- Usually supratentorial
- Typically superficial and well-demarcated
- Mass effect and peritumoral edema
- Contrast enhancing
  - Classic rim pattern of glioblastoma, some cases
  - Compact superficial mass, some cases

MACROSCOPIC

General Features

- Generally superficial location
- Variably discrete; intraoperatively often simulates metastasis or meningioma
- Firm
- Necrosis, some cases
- Skull penetration (rare)

MICROSCOPIC

Histologic Features

- Conventional astrocytic phenotype (glioblastoma variant)
  - Infiltrating glial component may be scant
  - Nests or lobules without reticulin, glial component
  - Spread along vessels, mesenchymal component
  - Dense, fascicular, sometimes herringbone pattern, reticulin-rich mesenchymal component
  - Tendency of mesenchymal component to mature into low-grade tumor or apparent reactive fibrosis
  - Often considerable atypia in vascular cells
  - Specific mesenchymal differentiation, some cases
    - Osteosarcoma
    - Chondrosarcoma
    - Rhabdomyosarcoma, rare
    - Angiosarcoma, rare
    - Liposarcoma or lipoma, rare
    - Leiomyosarcoma, rare
  - Epithelial differentiation, occasional cases
    - Glandular
    - Squamous
  - Foci of primitive neuroectodermal tumor (PNET)-like tissue, uncommon
    - Large round cells
    - High mitotic activity
    - Abundant apoptosis
    - Cell-cell wrapping
    - Nuclear molding
    - Small cells, some cases, occasionally with Homer Wright rosettes
- Oligosarcoma
  - Arising in setting of oligodendroglioma, WHO grade II or III
  - Dense fascicular reticulin-rich mesenchymal component
- Ependymosarcoma
  - Arising in setting of ependymoma, WHO grade II or III
  - Dense, fascicular, reticulin-rich mesenchymal component
- Subependymomasarcoma, exceedingly rare

ANCILLARY TESTS

Cytology

- Variable features of glioblastoma
- Bipolar malignant cells, sarcomatous component, may be scanty
- Variable mesenchymal differentiation, e.g., cartilaginous, lipoblasts, rhabdoid cells

Immunohistochemistry

- GFAP(+), often focal

- Nests or fields of glial component
- Some spindle cells within mesenchymal component
- Olig2(-) unlike typical glioblastoma
- CD34 often (+) in mesenchymal component, but not in infiltrating component
- Desmin (+) in lesions with myogenic differentiation
- p53(+), if present in both glial and mesenchymal tissue
- PNET-like tissue
  - Synaptophysin (+)
  - p53(+), often
  - Ki-67, very high index

Genetic Testing

- Abnormalities, e.g., *P53* mutations, identical in areas of both glial and mesenchymal differentiation (clonal neoplasm)
- Molecular profile similar to primary glioblastomas, but no *EGFR* overexpression or amplification

DIFFERENTIAL DIAGNOSIS

Glioblastoma in Meninges

- Distinction between gliosarcoma and glioblastoma with desmoplastic reaction often problematic
- Leptomeningeal tissue or location sometimes recognizable
- GFAP(+), Olig2(+) and more pronounced than gliosarcoma
- Often mesenchymal markers are negative, e.g., CD34
- Radiological image more typical of diffuse tumor as opposed to well-demarcated
- Prognostic relevance minimal, if any

Meningioma

- Rarely as high grade or fascicular
- No glial component
- Generally whorls &/or psammoma bodies
- Less reticulin, not pericellular
- EMA(+), SSTR2A(+), PR(+) some cases
- GFAP(-), S100(-) most cases

Metastatic Tumor

- No glial component
- Epithelial, melanocytic differentiation
- More necrosis, usually with perivascular sparing
- Little reticulin
- Neuroepithelial and glial markers are negative

Pleomorphic Xanthoastrocytoma

- No biphasic glial-mesenchymal architecture
- Less reticulin, generally not as pericellular
- No reticulin-rich anaplastic spindle cell component
- Eosinophilic granular bodies
- Xanthomatous (lipidized) cells
- Giant cells
- Less frequent mitoses, no vascular proliferation or palisading necrosis

Solitary Fibrous Tumor (SFT)/Hemangiopericytoma (HPC)

- Usually less anaplastic
- No glial component
- CD34(+) in classic SFT, but less staining in HPC
- Little reticulin in classic SFT, but usually abundant in HPC
- STAT6(+)
- BCL2(+), almost all cases

Fibrosarcoma and Undifferentiated Sarcoma

- Usually in children
- More fascicular
- No glial component
- Usually monomorphous
- Glial or neuroepithelial markers are negative

DIAGNOSTIC CHECKLIST

Clinically Relevant Pathologic Features

- Surgeon intraoperative impression often meningioma or metastasis
- Macroscopically often well circumscribed but behaves as malignant glioma
- Can penetrate skull

Pathologic Interpretation Pearls

- Consider lesion in any anaplastic fibroblastic process, even if glioma not initially apparent
- Reticulin staining useful in distinguishing glial from mesenchymal component
- GFAP staining often necessary to confirm presence of glial component
- Sarcomatous component typically Olig2(-) and often CD34(+)
- Sarcomatous component can occur in gliomas other than glioblastoma
- Spindle cell appearance occasionally seen in glioblastoma; do not diagnose sarcomatous component without interspersed reticulin

SELECTED REFERENCES

1. Joseph NM et al: Diagnostic implications of IDH1-R132H and OLIG2 expression patterns in rare and challenging glioblastoma variants. Mod Pathol. 26(3):315-26, 2013
2. Han SJ et al: Clinical characteristics and outcomes for a modern series of primary gliosarcoma patients. Cancer. 116(5):1358-66, 2010
3. Han SJ et al: Secondary gliosarcoma after diagnosis of glioblastoma: clinical experience with 30 consecutive patients. J Neurosurg. 112(5):990-6, 2010
4. Karremann M et al: Clinical and epidemiological characteristics of pediatric gliosarcomas. J Neurooncol. 97(2):257-65, 2010
5. Barut F et al: Gliosarcoma with chondroblastic osteosarcomatous differentation: report of two case with clinicopathologic and immunohistochemical features. Turk Neurosurg. 19(4):417-22, 2009
6. Han L et al: Magnetic resonance imaging of primary cerebral gliosarcoma: a report of 15 cases. Acta Radiol. 49(9):1058-67, 2008
7. Rodriguez FJ et al: Epithelial and pseudoepithelial differentiation in glioblastoma and gliosarcoma: a comparative morphologic and molecular genetic study. Cancer. 113(10):2779-89, 2008
8. Beaumont TL et al: Gliosarcoma with multiple extracranial metastases: case report and review of the literature. J Neurooncol. 83(1):39-46, 2007
9. Kaplan KJ et al: Gliosarcoma with primitive neuroectodermal differentiation: case report and review of the literature. J Neurooncol. 83(3):313-8, 2007
10. Rodriguez FJ et al: Gliosarcoma arising in oligodendroglial tumors ("oligosarcoma"): a clinicopathologic study. Am J Surg Pathol. 31(3):351-62, 2007
11. Vlodavsky E et al: Gliosarcoma with liposarcomatous differentiation: the new member of the lipid-containing brain tumors family. Arch Pathol Lab Med. 130(3):381-4, 2006
12. Boerman RH et al: The glial and mesenchymal elements of gliosarcomas share similar genetic alterations. J Neuropathol Exp Neurol. 55(9):973-81, 1996
13. Meis JM et al: Mixed glioblastoma multiforme and sarcoma. A clinicopathologic study of 26 radiation therapy oncology group cases. Cancer. 67(9):2342-9, 1991

Superficial Tumor, Mass Effect

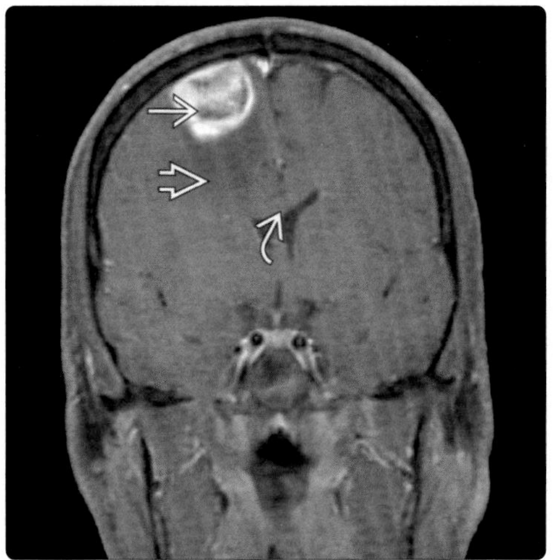

Vasculocentric Mesenchymal Component

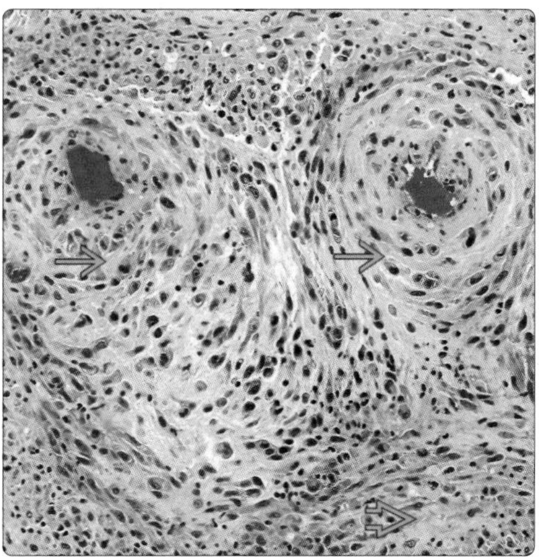

(Left) *Gliosarcomas are commonly superficial tumors, but otherwise show all the typical features of glioblastomas. Brisk enhancement with central hypointensity ➔, peritumoral edema ➔, and subfalcine herniation ➔ can be seen in this example.* **(Right)** *Many gliosarcomas demonstrate a brisk proliferation of atypical cells around the vessels ➔ imparting to the tumor an angiomatous appearance. The tumor cells around the vessels often show identical genetic aberrations as the surrounding glial component ➔.*

Cartilaginous Differentiation

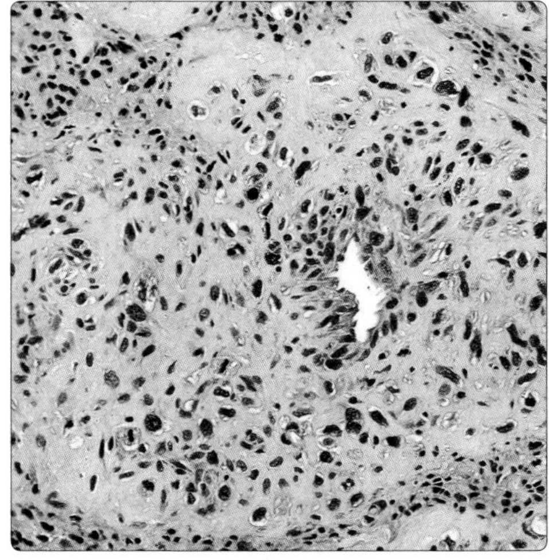

Myxoid Background + Vasculocentric Tumor

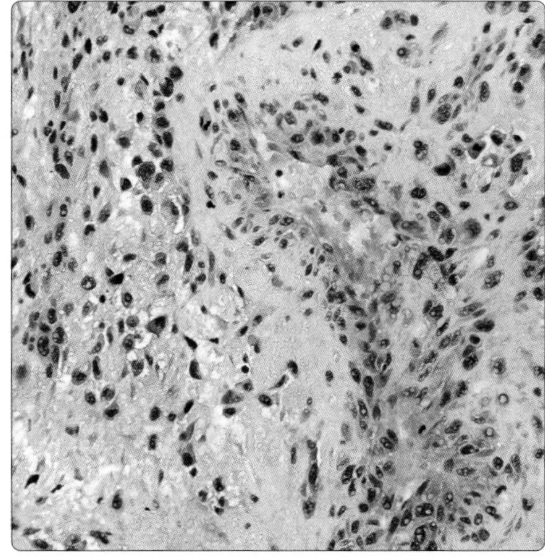

(Left) *The mesenchymal component that shows a vasculocentric arrangement can also demonstrate differentiation into other mesenchymal tissue types. Chondromatous or cartilaginous differentiation can be inferred from this image.* **(Right)** *The malignant cells in a background of rich myxoid matrix and those around the vascular structures constitute the mesenchymal component of this gliosarcoma. Some of the cells in both components are GFAP(+) but there was no Olig2 positivity in the section.*

Smear: Malignant Nuclei

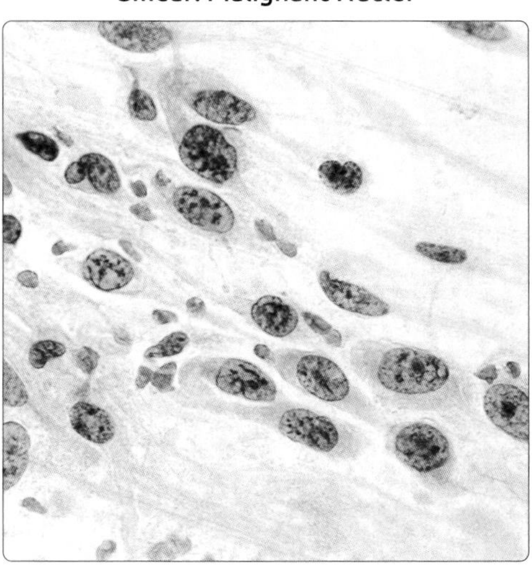

Smear: Mesenchymal Features

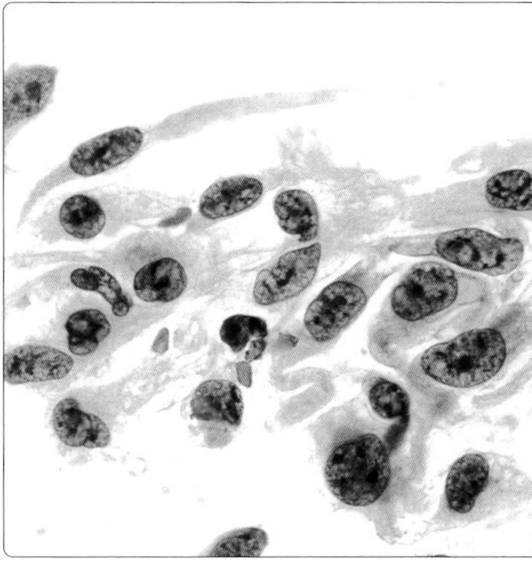

(Left) *Cells with large, irregular nuclei and coarse processes would help distinguish these cells as clearly malignant, but a clear distinction of glioblastoma from gliosarcoma at this cellular level is exceptionally difficult.* **(Right)** *Nuclei with malignant criteria reside in cells with thick, bipolar processes as seen in a smear preparation. Most cells in glioblastomas have smaller more delicate nuclei and finer processes.*

(Left) *Suggestively sarcomatous, microvascular proliferation may present as large, disorganized, tumefactive masses that are more exuberant in gliosarcoma than that expected of mere florid microvascular proliferation in glioblastoma.* **(Right)** *The distinction between the astrocytoma and the component with mesenchymal differentiation is not always as elementary as it is here, where a nest of astrocytes is surrounded by compact, histologically undifferentiated tumor.*

Vascular Proliferation

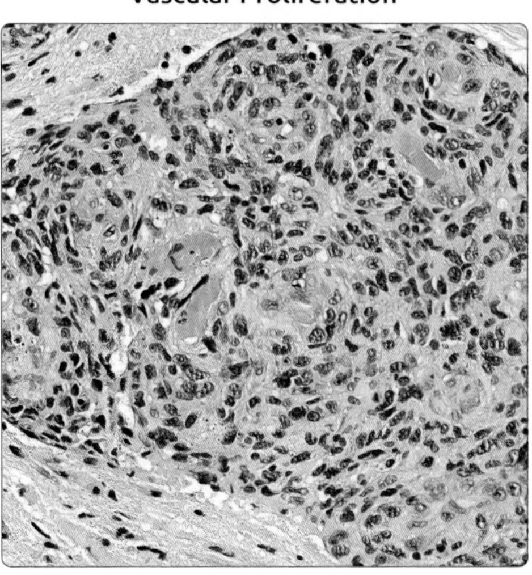

Evidence of Astrocytic Origin

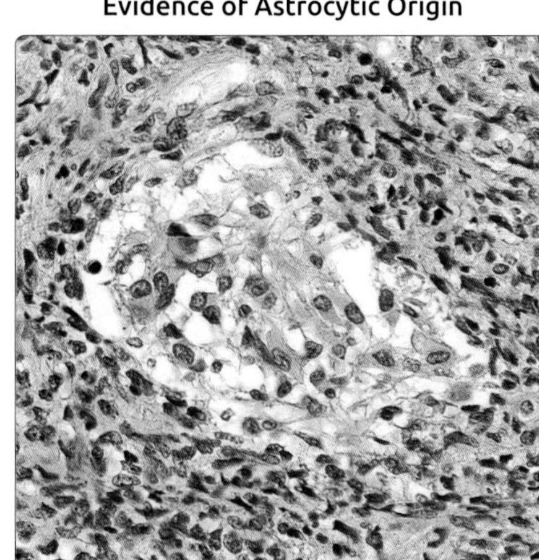

(Left) *Lobules of glioma with glassy "astrocytic" cytoplasm* ⇨ *sit in cellular spindle cell tissue with sarcomatous features. Reticulin staining aids in distinguishing the 2 components. Sarcomatous areas are reticulin-rich.* **(Right)** *While obvious glioblastoma such as this may be present, such inescapable evidence of grade IV astrocytoma may be difficult to find. Mesenchymal tissue predominates in many lesions, and staining for reticulin and GFAP may be required to identify the glioma in a lesion with dichotomous differentiation.*

Spindle Cells With Astrocytic Features

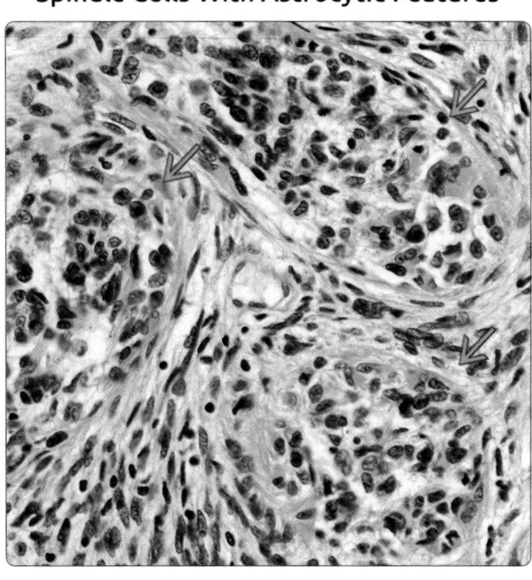

Palisading Necrosis in Glial Component

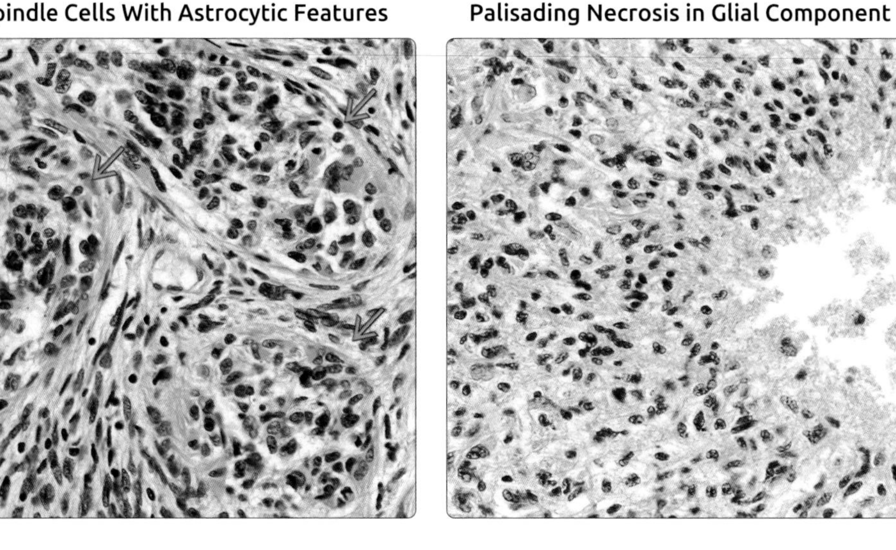

(Left) *The sarcomatous elements in gliosarcomas may be indistinguishable from conventional sarcomas of soft tissues. Typically, the sarcomatous component harbors multiple mitoses* ⇨ *and anaplastic nuclei akin to a high-grade sarcoma.* **(Right)** *Cellular mesenchymal tissue is clearly malignant in light of the cellular atypia and mitotic activity* ⇨*. The somewhat epithelioid, less spindled area of glial differentiation is on the right.*

Multiple Mitoses

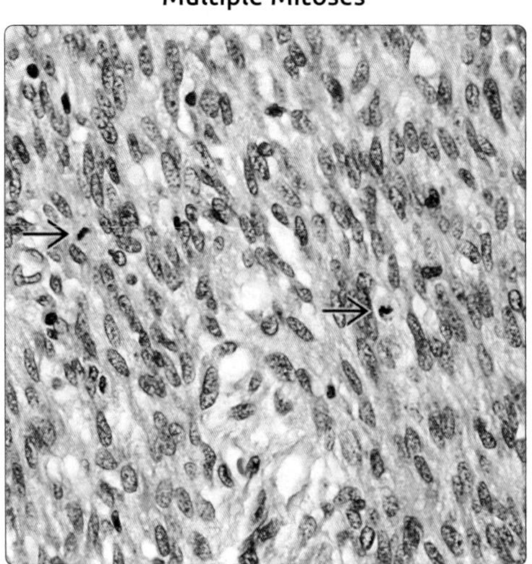

Mesenchymal and Glial Components

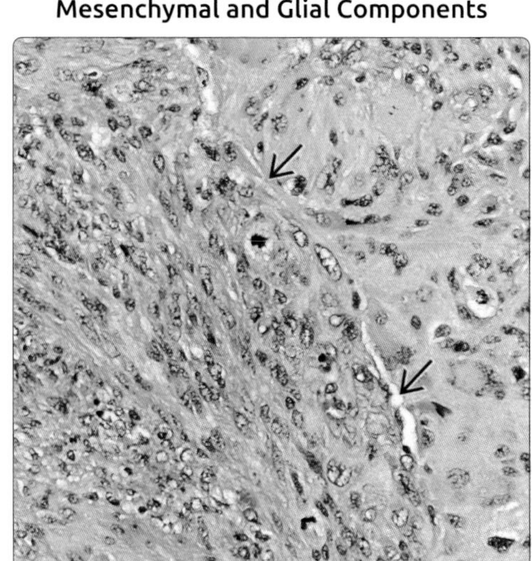

Mesenchymal and Glial Elements

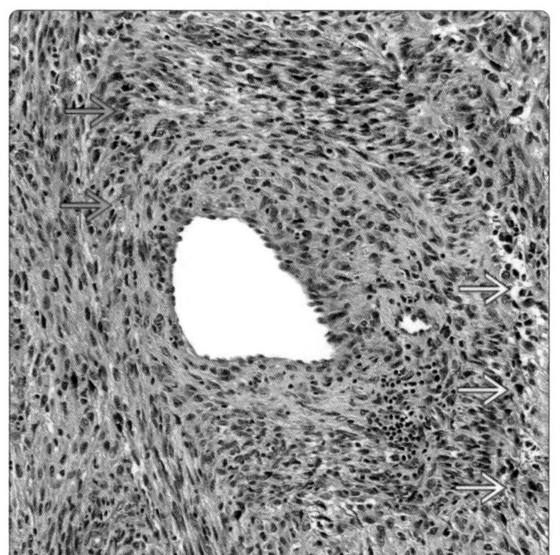

Reticulin-Rich Mesenchymal Component

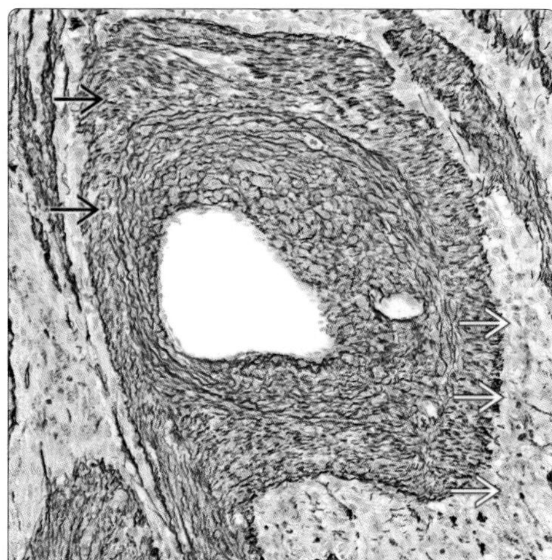

(Left) *The distinction between mesenchymal ⇨ and glial tissue is not always elementary but is simplified when adjacent sections are stained for H&E and reticulin. One suspects that the somewhat less cellular and more eosinophilic tissue ➡ shows glial differentiation.* **(Right)** *Reticulin that invests individual cells in perivascular mesenchymal tissue, but not the glial element, confirms the impression gleaned from the H&E section that this lesion has both glial ➡ and mesenchymal ⇨ differentiation.*

Mesenchymal Appearance

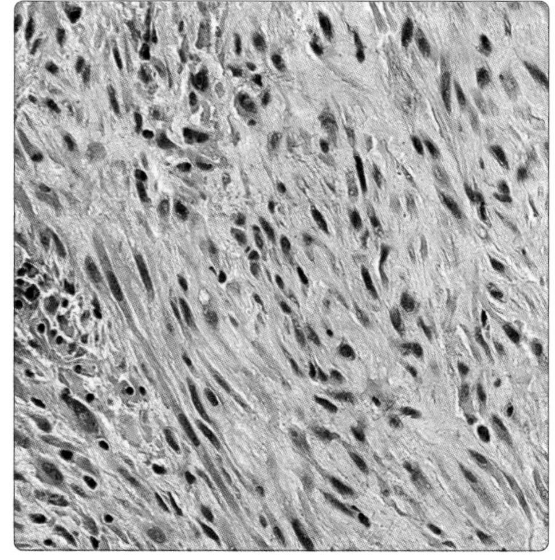

Osteoid Formation in Gliosarcoma

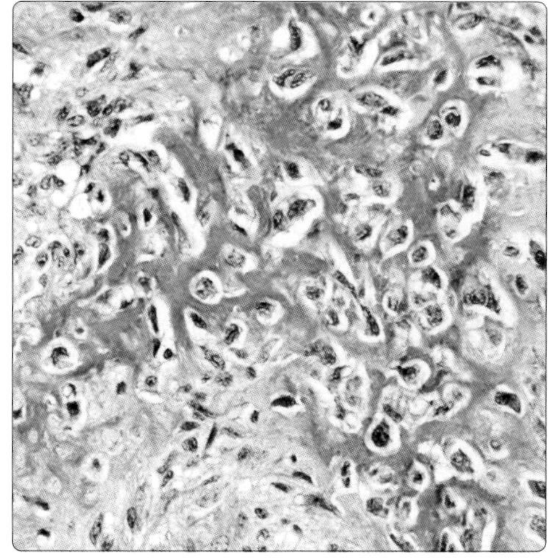

(Left) *Mesenchymal tissue sometimes appears to mature into low-grade sarcoma or even tissue that may appear more cicatricial than sarcomatous.* **(Right)** *Osteoid is less common than chondroid tissue in gliosarcomas. Rare primary or radiation-induced osteosarcomas should be excluded by virtue of demonstrating the glial component or derivation of this malignant neoplasm.*

Chondroid Differentiation

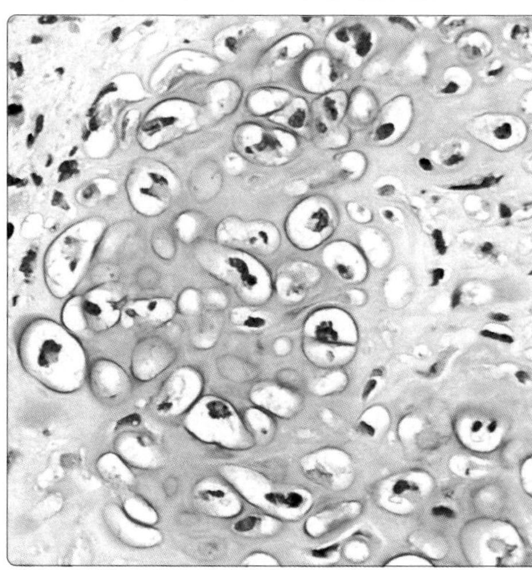

Severe Atypia in Mesenchymal Component

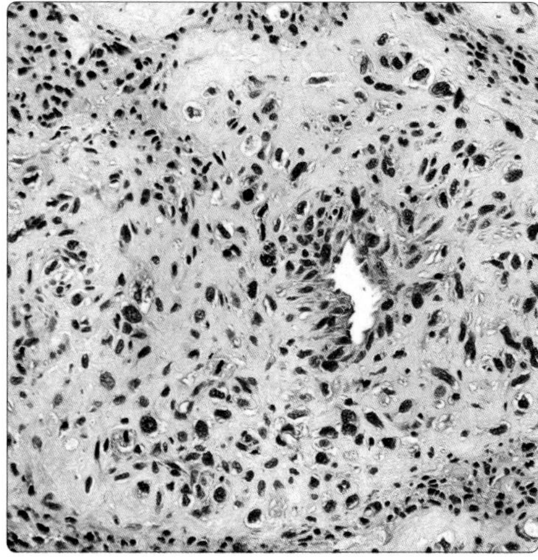

(Left) *Discrete islands of chondroid differentiation, usually only focal, are not uncommon in gliosarcomas. Other forms of mesenchymal differentiation, i.e., bone or muscle, are even less common. The possibility of teratoma comes to mind, but there is nothing else to support such an entity, and much to contradict it, i.e., the presence of a concomitant glioma.* **(Right)** *Severe atypia in the mesenchymal component surrounding the blood vessel leaves little doubt about the malignancy of the tumor in this case.*

(Left) *Liposarcomatous differentiation is rare gliosarcoma. Metaplasia to GFAP(+) "adipose tissue" also occurs in some glioblastomas. The illustrated cells of this gliosarcoma were GFAP(-).* **(Right)** *PNET-like tissue appears in some gliosarcomas, as with this "anaplastic" type with large cells, cell-cell wrapping ➔, frequent mitoses, and abundant apoptosis. Amplification of the c-myc oncogene is common in such cells. The cells are smaller and more conventionally neuroblastic in most other cases.*

Lipomatous Differentiation

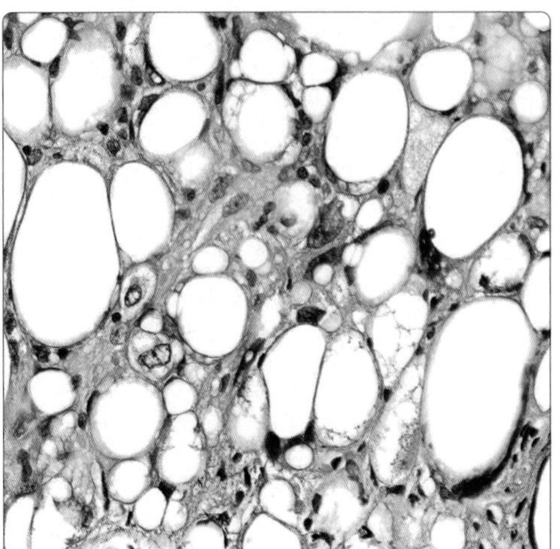

PNET-Like Component

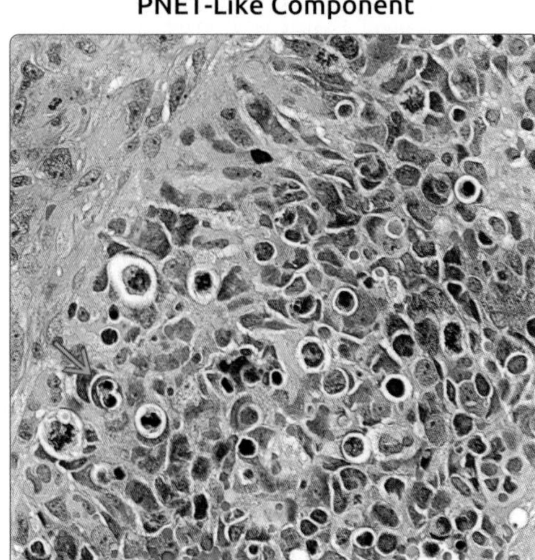

(Left) *Some ependymomas, grade II in this case, differentiate along mesenchymal lines (ependymosarcoma). A perivascular pseudorosette ➔ helps identify the ependymal component.* **(Right)** *Some gliosarcomas harbor cells with rhabdoid-like cytology suggestive of highly malignant neoplasm. Unlike the epithelioid glioblastoma, these cells are often devoid of GFAP positivity and may demonstrate markers such as desmin, reflecting their mesenchymal nature.*

Evidence of Ependymal Origin

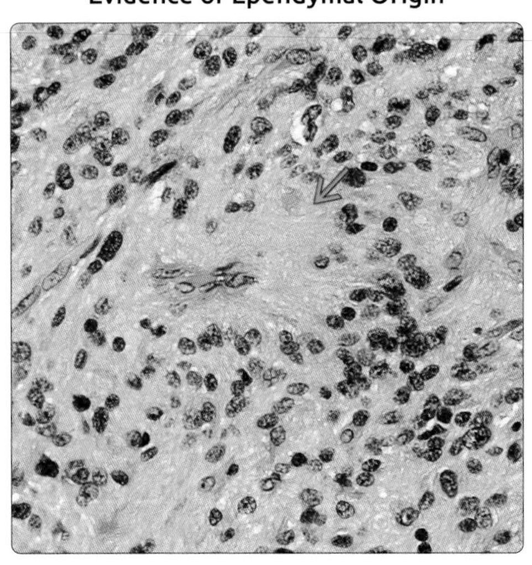

Rhabdoid-Like Sarcomatous Cells

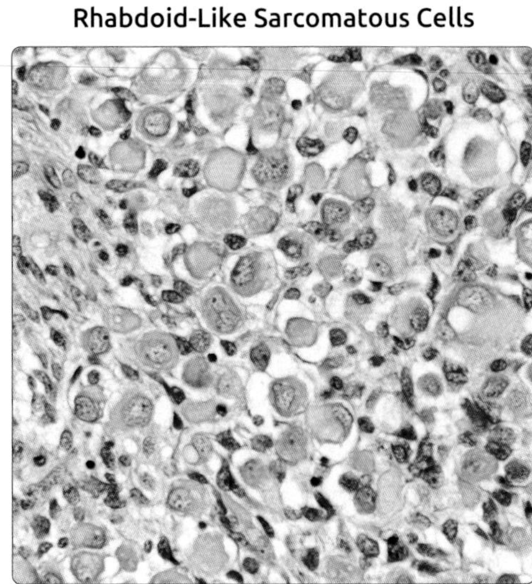

(Left) *In some mesenchymal components, the degree of anaplasia is severe enough to resemble an undifferentiated sarcoma or even carcinoma with highly pleomorphic nuclei and cell wrapping ➔.* **(Right)** *Some gliosarcomas have an intimate blending of glial and mesenchymal components. The mesenchymal component can display a herringbone type pattern ➔ reminiscent of other soft tissue sarcomas.*

Anaplasia and Cell Wrapping

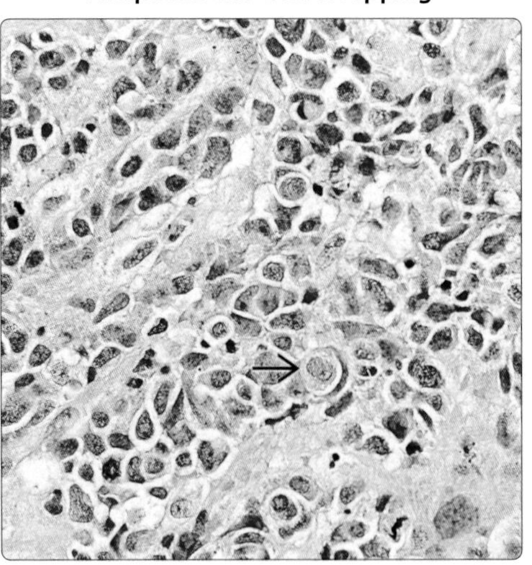

Herringbone Pattern

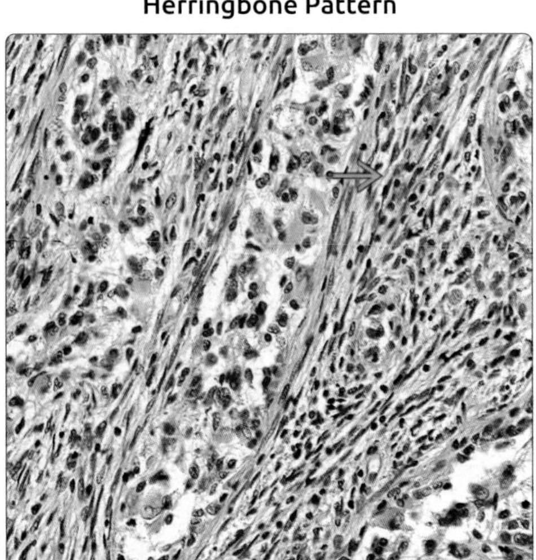

Rich Reticulin Staining

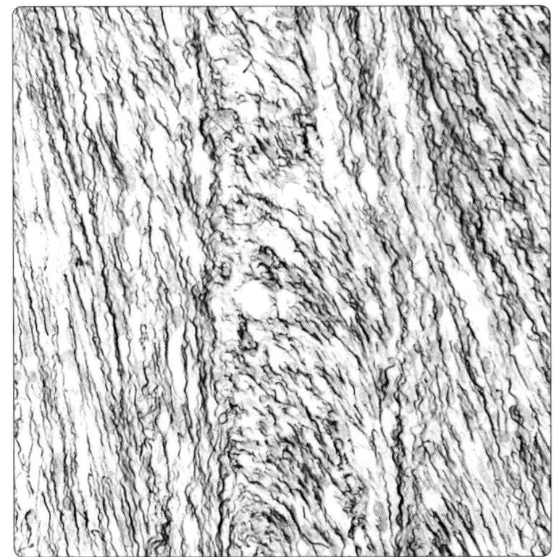

GFAP Staining of Mesenchymal Component

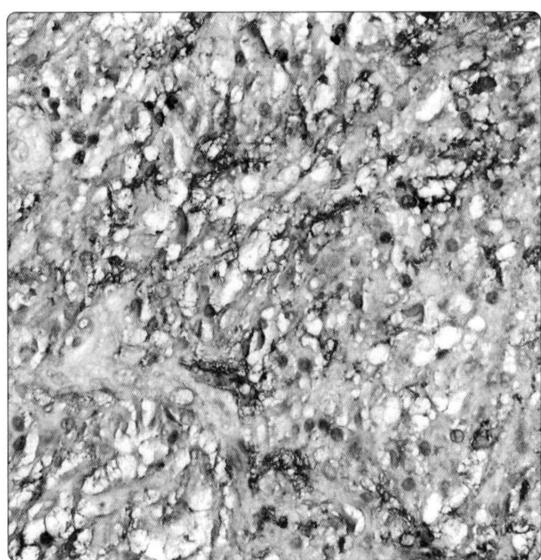

(Left) *Although not specific, the crisp, black reticulin fibers surrounding individual cells are strong evidence of mesenchymal differentiation. Reticulin fibers would be confined to vessels and their environs in the glial component.* **(Right)** *Foci of malignant cells with a glial phenotype of H&E are GFAP positive, as are scattered cells in a spindle cell tissue that is phenotypically mesenchymal.*

CD34(+) Mesenchymal Component

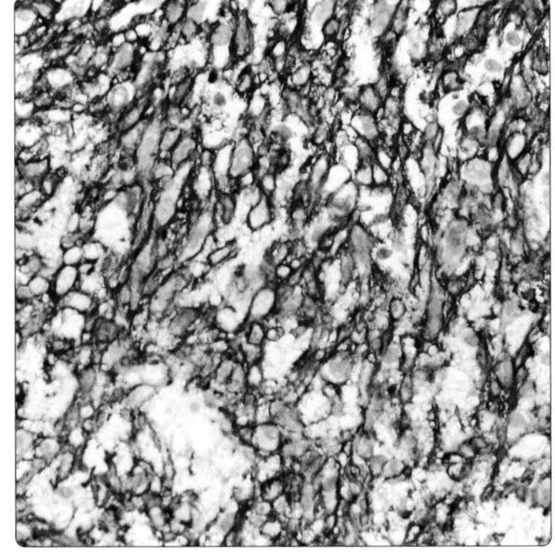

Desmin (+) Mesenchymal Cells

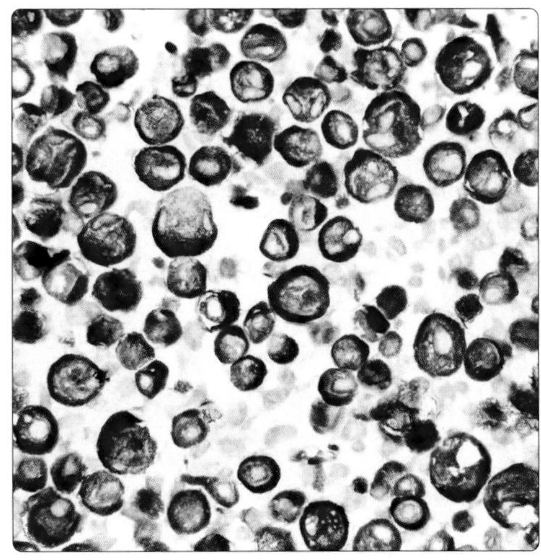

(Left) *The mesenchymal tumor component in gliosarcomas often demonstrates brisk positive staining with antibodies against CD34. The CD34 antibody highlights both the vascular network and the malignant mesenchymal component.* **(Right)** *Immunoreactivity for desmin helps identify the myoid nature of these globular cells and distinguish them from epithelioid astrocytes that populate occasional glioblastomas. The latter are usually GFAP(+).*

SMA(+) Tumor Cells

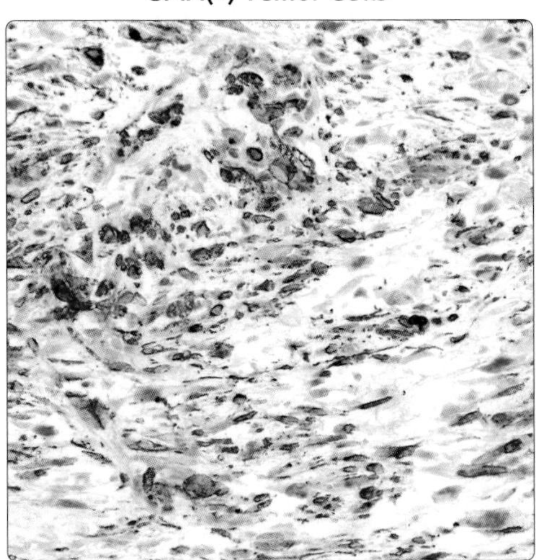

Olig2(-) Mesenchymal Component

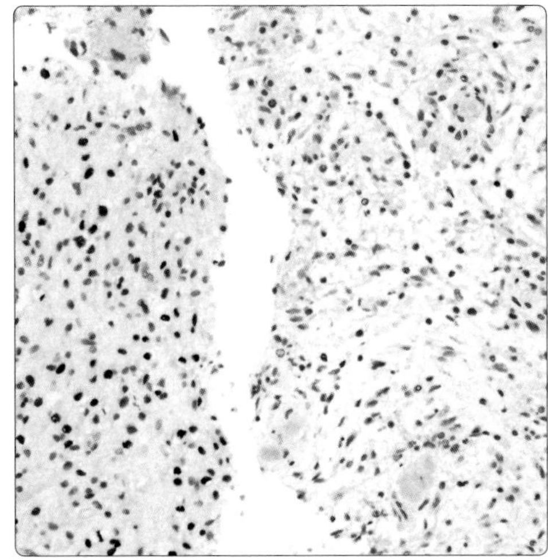

(Left) *In addition to desmin, and in addition to vascular structures in the sections, part of the mesenchymal component stains with muscular markers such as smooth muscle antigen (SMA).* **(Right)** *Typically, the glial component of gliosarcomas as well as the cells with astrocytic phenotype are positive with the antibodies for Olig2, while the mesenchymal component shows little or no staining, aiding in the diagnosis.*

Granular Cell Astrocytoma of the Cerebrum

KEY FACTS

TERMINOLOGY

- Infiltrating astrocytoma with dominant population of granular cells
- Unrelated to granular cell tumor of infundibulum or peripheral nerve

CLINICAL ISSUES

- Usually adults
- Poor prognosis
  - Usually behaves as high-grade astrocytoma

IMAGING

- Supratentorial expansile lesion
- Usually enhancing
  - Often with central area of necrosis (ring lesion)

MICROSCOPIC

- Resembles macrophage-rich lesion
- Bland nuclei with little nuclear pleomorphism belie aggressive nature of lesion
- Similar to gemistocytic astrocytoma in content of senescent cells, but clinically aggressive behavior

ANCILLARY TESTS

- CD68(+) but usually HAM56(-)
- Olig2 expression frequent
- S100(+), weak
- GFAP variable
- IDH1 (R132H) expression rare to absent

DIAGNOSTIC CHECKLIST

- Morphologically bland tumor with aggressive clinical behavior
- Can be misinterpreted as reactive, nonneoplastic, macrophage-rich process

Rim-Enhancing Profile

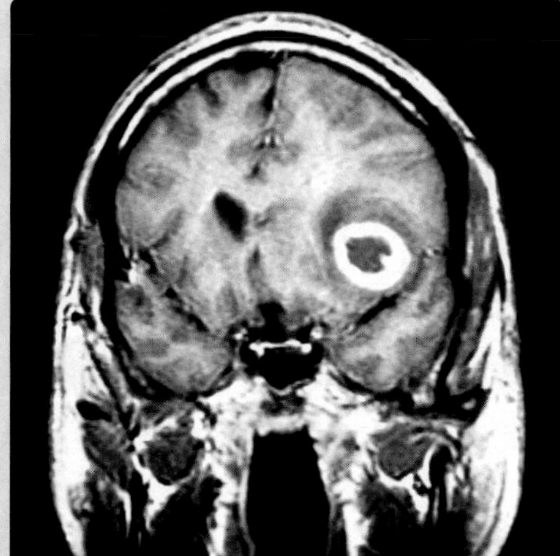

Tumor Cells Resembling Macrophages

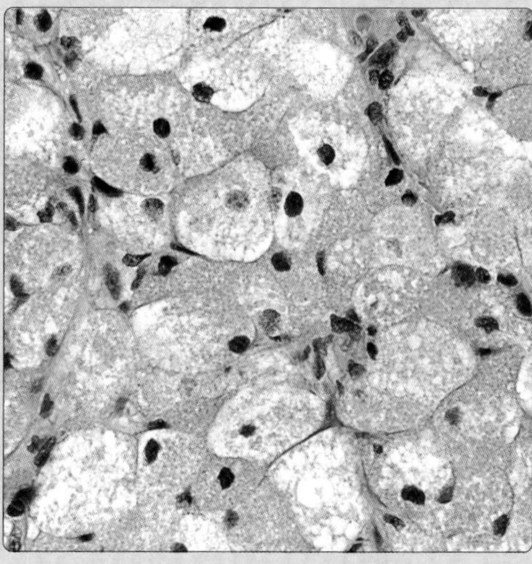

(Left) *A rim-enhancing, edema-generating profile similar to glioblastoma is the rule.* **(Right)** *Tumor cells resemble macrophages, but they are larger, more polygonal, and more granular than foamy.*

Granular Eosinophilic Cytoplasm

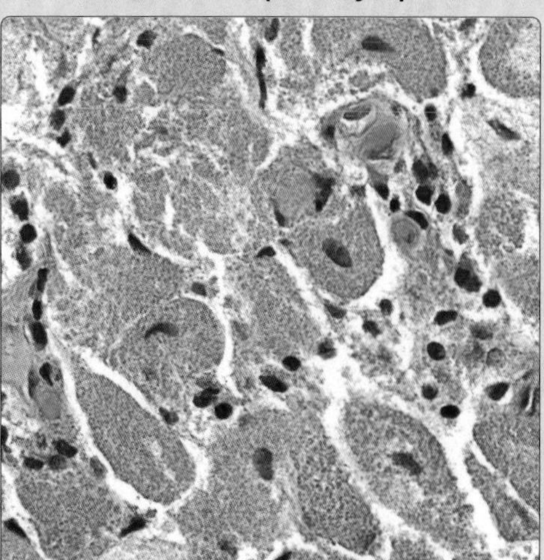

Variable GFAP Expression

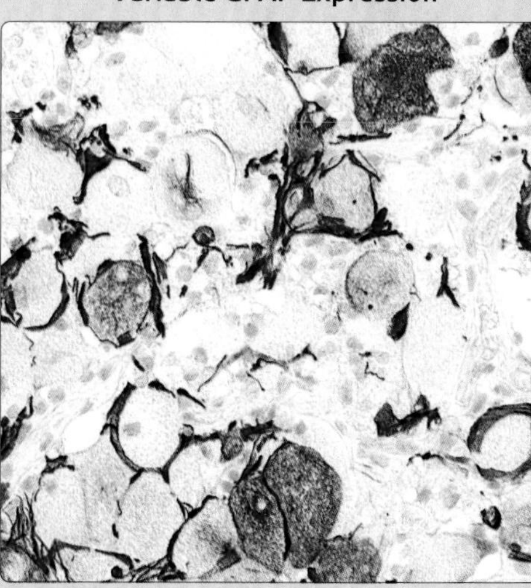

(Left) *Large cells with granular eosinophilic cytoplasm are the key diagnostic feature of granular cell astrocytoma.* **(Right)** *GFAP expression is variable in granular cell astrocytomas, being weak or negative in some cells and overtly positive in others.*

TERMINOLOGY

Definitions

- Infiltrating astrocytoma with abundant granular cells
- Unrelated to granular cell tumors of infundibulum and peripheral nerve
- Grading schemes likely to change
    - More aggressive behavior of grades II and III using traditional grading criteria

CLINICAL ISSUES

Presentation

- Usually adults
- Rare in children
- Neurological signs and symptoms dependent upon location
- Mass effects, seizures

Treatment

- Radiation and chemotherapy similar to other high-grade astrocytomas

Prognosis

- Poor; behavior similar to that of other high-grade astrocytomas
- Distinct histological appearance
- Median survival of 11 months in grade II and 9 months in grade III-IV in review of 59 cases
- Typically characterized by aggressive glioblastoma-like clinical behavior, even when histology satisfies criteria for only WHO grade II or III designation

IMAGING

MR Findings

- Supratentorial
- Usually enhancing
- Often central area of necrosis (ring lesion)
- Edema, mass effects

MICROSCOPIC

Histologic Features

- Infiltrating, but biopsied areas often compact sheets of granular cells
    - Transitions to conventional infiltrating astrocytoma, in some cases
- Tumor cells
    - Round to polygonal
    - Larger and somewhat more irregular than macrophages
    - Often back to back
    - Distinct cell borders
    - Fine cytoplasmic granulation
    - Cytologically bland nuclei
    - Rare mitoses
    - No perivascular accumulation
- Perivascular lymphocytes, in some cases
- Usually no vascular proliferation or necrosis
- Similar to gemistocytic astrocytoma in content of senescent cells, but aggressive behavior

ANCILLARY TESTS

Cytology

- Clumps of cells and individual cells
- Prominent granular cytoplasm with few short processes
- Bland nuclei with little nuclear pleomorphism (belies tumor's overall aggressive nature)

Histochemistry

- PAS-diastase
    - Reactivity: Positive with and without diastase
    - Staining pattern: Granular, lysosome-rich cytoplasm
- Reticulin
    - Variable amounts
    - Prominent, in minority of cases

Immunohistochemistry

- Macrophage markers
    - HAM56, CD163
        - Tumor cells (-)
        - Microglia (+)
    - CD68(+) (marker of lysosomes, not macrophages)
        - Tumor cells (+)
        - Microglia (+)
- GFAP
    - Diffuse blush (some cases)
    - Peripheral cytoplasm, intensely stained (some cases)
        - To be distinguished from displaced processes of neighboring reactive astrocytes
        - May be difficult to establish GFAP positivity of tumor cells
- Olig2 expression frequent
- S100(+), weak
- IDH1 (R132H) expression rare to absent
- Ki-67 index generally low

Genetic Testing

- Loss of heterozygosity at 1p, 9p, 10q, 17p, and 19q
    - Losses on 9p and 10q particularly frequent

Electron Microscopy

- Multiple granular lysosomes, membrane bound
- Few intermediate filaments

DIFFERENTIAL DIAGNOSIS

Macrophage-Rich Lesions

- Demyelinating disease
    - Smaller, rounder cells
    - Foamy rather than granular cells
    - Perivascular accumulation of macrophages
    - Multinucleated reactive astrocytes (Creutzfeldt cells)
    - HAM56(+) and CD163(+)
- Infarct
    - Small-sized macrophages
    - Foamy rather than granular cytoplasm
    - Perivascular accumulation of macrophages
    - Ischemic (red-dead) neurons
    - Hypertrophic and hyperplastic endothelial cells
    - Prominent cortical involvement
    - HAM56(+)

- Progressive multifocal leukoencephalopathy
  - Little contrast enhancement
    - Except in HAART-treated patients
  - Little mass effect
  - Less cellular
  - Multiple discrete foci of demyelination
  - Intranuclear, wine-red inclusions
    - Particularly in cells around demyelinated foci
  - Few perivascular lymphocytes
    - Except in HAART-treated patients
  - Immunoreactivity, with high index, for
    - p53 and Ki-67
  - JC virus identifiable through SV40 immunohistochemistry or in situ hybridization

Granular Cell Tumor

- Bland nuclei
- Essentially limited to neurohypophysis/sellar region in intracranial locations
- Low proliferative activity
- TTF-1(+)

Conventional Infiltrating Astrocytoma

- Areas of tissue infiltration by cells with glassy cytoplasm &/or those with little if any cytoplasm
- Multiple mitoses in grade III and IV examples
- High Ki-67 labeling index in grade III and IV examples
- No extravascular reticulin

DIAGNOSTIC CHECKLIST

Clinically Relevant Pathologic Features

- Seemingly bland tumor with aggressive clinical behavior
- Can be misinterpreted as reactive, nonneoplastic, macrophage-rich process

Pathologic Interpretation Pearls

- Do not accept CD68 immunoreactive granular cells as necessarily representing macrophages
- Search for more conventional high-grade glioma areas in biopsy/resection materials since these almost always coexist with granular cell astrocytoma
- No exact percentage of cells with granular cell features established for this diagnosis of granular cell astrocytoma

SELECTED REFERENCES

1. Campbell RN et al: Mistaken identity: granular cell astrocytoma masquerading as histiocytosis of the central nervous system. J Clin Neurosci. 21(8):1457-9, 2014
2. Wisell J et al: Sox10 nuclear immunostaining lacks diagnostic utility for CNS granular cell tumors. J Neuropathol Exp Neurol. 73(1):98-100, 2014
3. George AA et al: Unusual presentation of a granular cell astrocytoma. Histopathology. 63(6):883-5, 2013
4. Joo M et al: Cytogenetic and molecular genetic study on granular cell glioblastoma: a case report. Hum Pathol. 44(2):282-8, 2013
5. Joseph NM et al: Diagnostic implications of IDH1-R132H and OLIG2 expression patterns in rare and challenging glioblastoma variants. Mod Pathol. 26(3):315-26, 2013
6. Kang M et al: Crush cytologic findings of a cerebral granular cell astrocytoma. Acta Cytol. 56(5):571-5, 2012
7. Arvanitis LD et al: Cytologic features of granular cell astrocytoma in crush preparations. Diagn Cytopathol. 39(1):77-9, 2011
8. Schittenhelm J et al: Glioblastoma with granular cell astrocytoma features: a case report and literature review. Clin Neuropathol. 29(5):323-9, 2010
9. Shi Y et al: Granular cell astrocytoma. Arch Pathol Lab Med. 132(12):1946-50, 2008
10. Wierzba-Bobrowicz T et al: Granular cell astrocytoma. A case report with immunohistochemical and ultrastructural characterization. Folia Neuropathol. 46(4):286-93, 2008
11. Saad A et al: Granular cell astrocytoma of the cerebellum: report of the first case. Am J Clin Pathol. 126(4):602-7, 2006
12. Castellano-Sanchez AA et al: Granular cell astrocytomas show a high frequency of allelic loss but are not a genetically defined subset. Brain Pathol. 13(2):185-94, 2003
13. Brat DJ et al: Infiltrative astrocytomas with granular cell features (granular cell astrocytomas): a study of histopathologic features, grading, and outcome. Am J Surg Pathol. 26(6):750-7, 2002
14. Chorny JA et al: Cerebral granular cell astrocytomas: a Mib-1, bcl-2, and telomerase study. Clin Neuropathol. 19(4):170-9, 2000
15. Geddes JF et al: Granular cell change in astrocytic tumors. Am J Surg Pathol. 20(1):55-63, 1996

Pale Cells

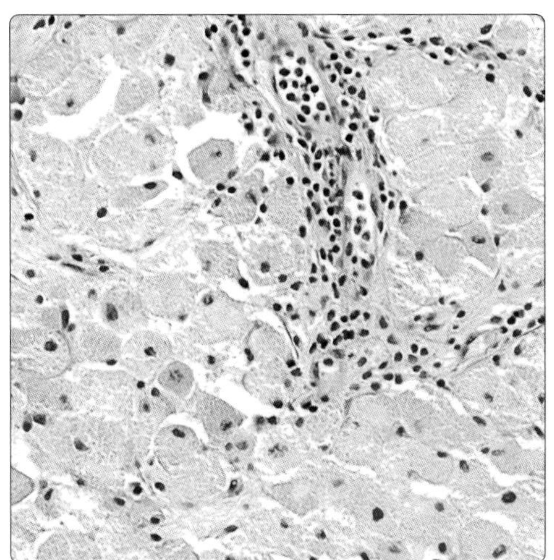

Chronic Inflammatory Cells

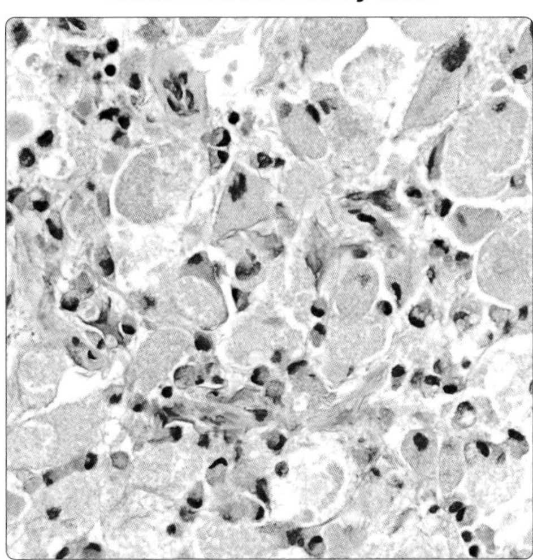

(Left) *In concert with perivascular lymphocytes, the pale cells in granular cell astrocytomas are easy to misinterpret as macrophages. Phagocytes are somewhat smaller, however, although this difference may be difficult to establish in individual cases.* **(Right)** *Intermingled chronic inflammatory cells may abet in a granular cell astrocytoma's simulation of an inflammatory process.*

Nuclear Angulation

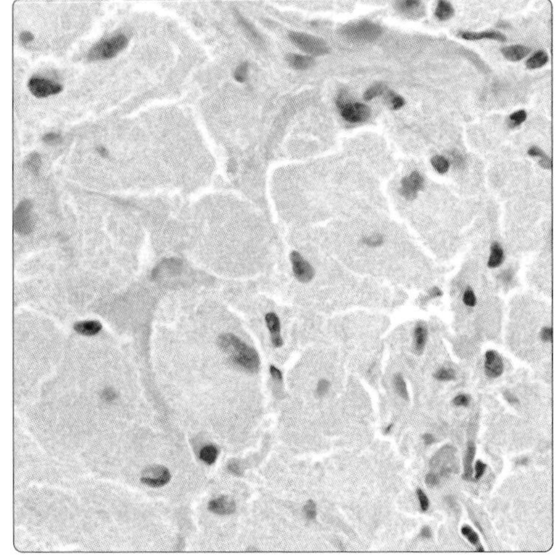

Cytoplasmic Granularity

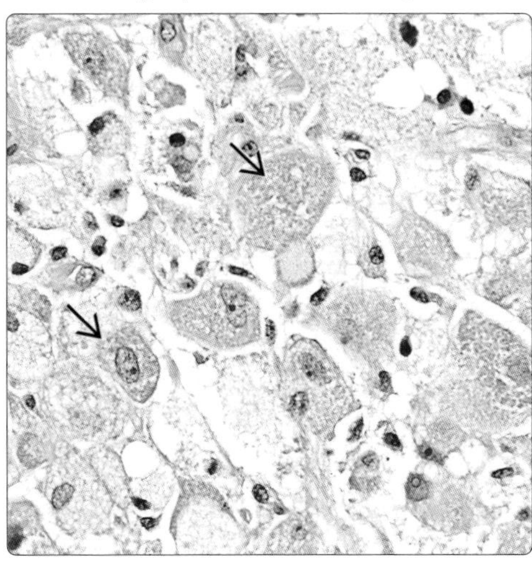

(Left) *The cells are considerably larger and more finely granular than those of a macrophage-rich lesion such as demyelinating disease. A degree of nuclear angulation here also aids in the distinction.* **(Right)** *Tumor cells are larger and more irregular than macrophages. Their nuclei are larger as well. Cytoplasmic granularity* ➙ *is especially apparent in this case.*

Nuclear Pleomorphism

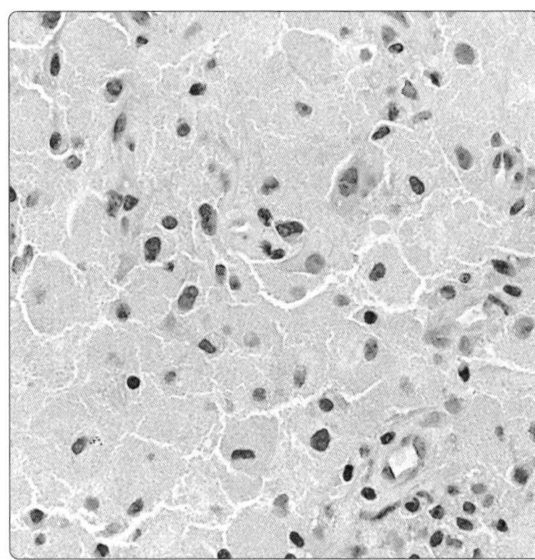

Granular Cytoplasm

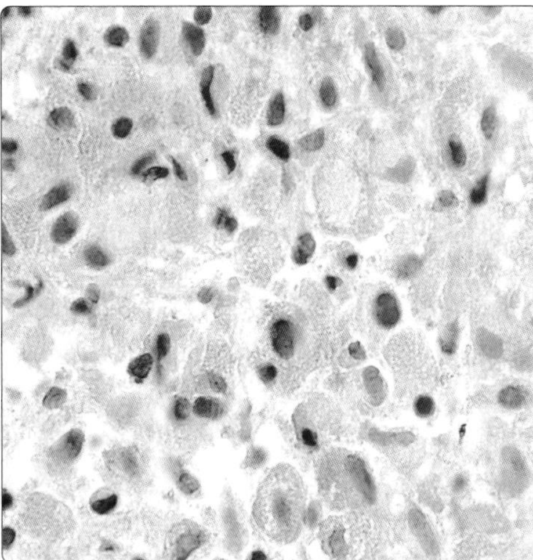

(Left) *The degree of nuclear pleomorphism helps identify granular cell astrocytes as neoplastic rather than phagocytic.* **(Right)** *This lesion combines prominent well-circumscribed macrophage-like cytoplasm and angulated pleomorphic nuclei typical of astrocytoma. The granular (as opposed to foamy) cytoplasm favors glioma over a reactive lesion.*

(Left) *The diagnosis of astrocytoma, grade III in light of the mitoses ⇨ is easy here because of transitions between granular cells and astrocytes with angulated naked nuclei common to many infiltrating astrocytomas.* **(Right)** *While there are some granular cells, the degrees of nuclear angulation and atypia are those of an infiltrating astrocytoma.*

Mitoses

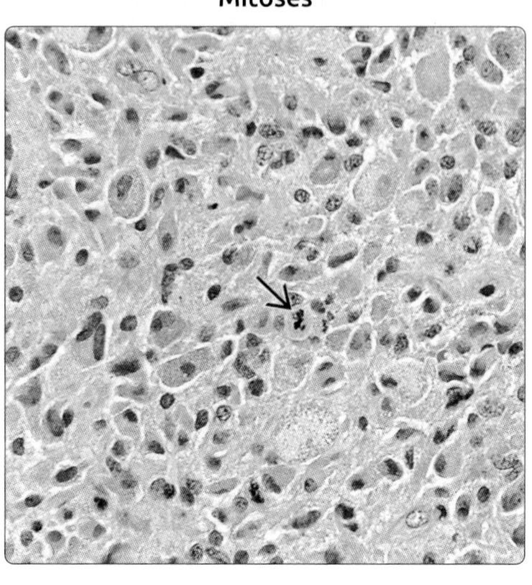

Nuclear Atypia

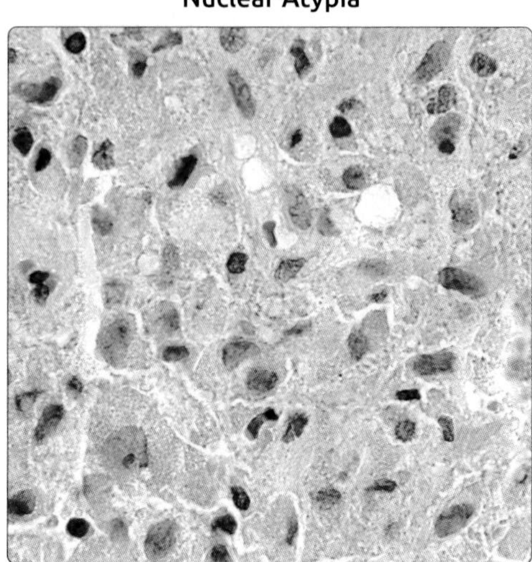

(Left) *The presence of microvascular proliferation supports a grade IV tumor designation in this case, although these tumors have a propensity for aggressive behavior regardless of grade.* **(Right)** *PAS positivity with and without diastase is a consistent feature of granular cell astrocytomas and supports lysosomes as the underlying morphologic basis for the cytoplasmic granules in these tumors.*

Microvascular Proliferation

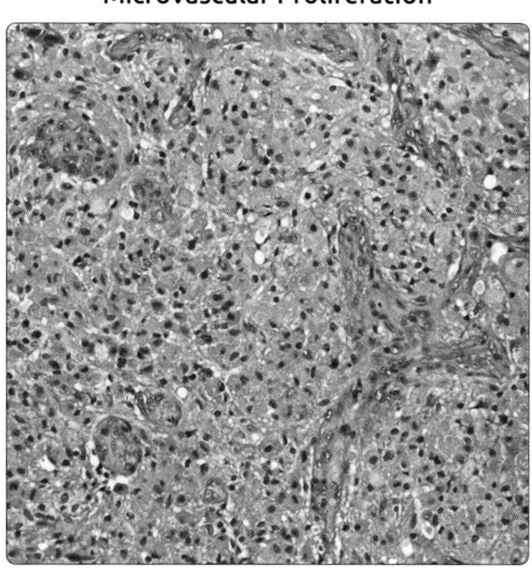

PAS Positivity

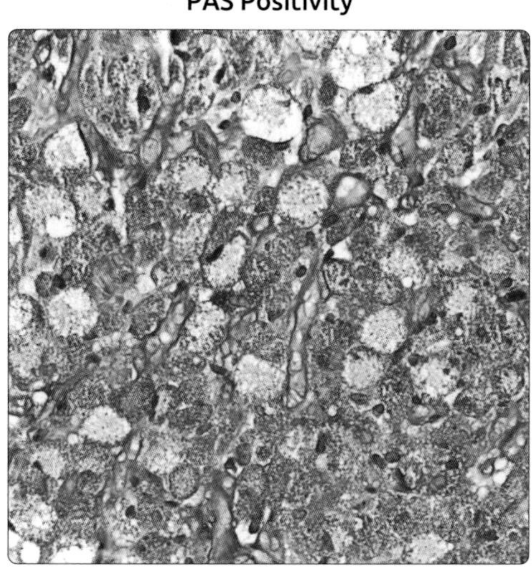

(Left) *Some cells may be peripherally immunoreactive for GFAP ⇨. Whether such staining is intrinsic to the granular cell or belongs to a passing process of a reactive astrocyte is frequently difficult to determine.* **(Right)** *The cells' fine granularity, round profiles, and short processes are obvious in a smear preparation. Although finely granular rather than coarsely granular or foamy, such cells can nevertheless be cytologically very similar to macrophages.*

Peripheral GFAP Immunoreactivity

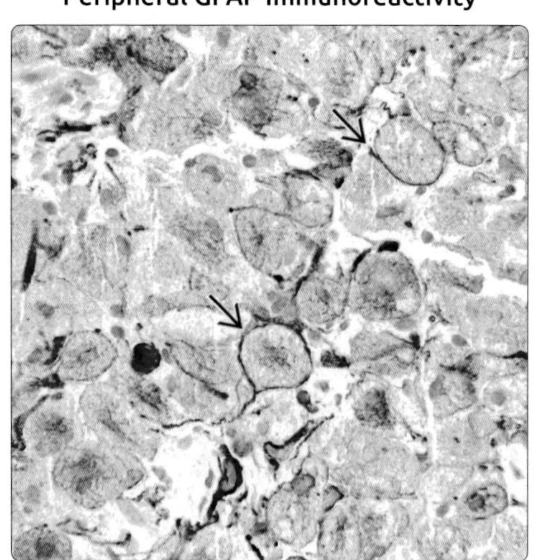

Fine Granularity

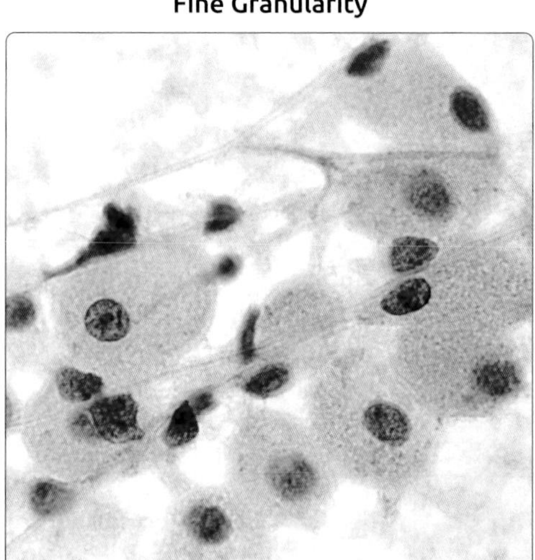

S100 Reactivity

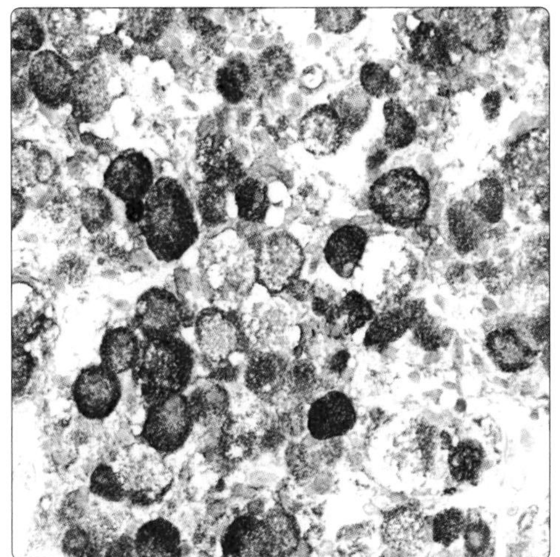

Olig2 Reactivity

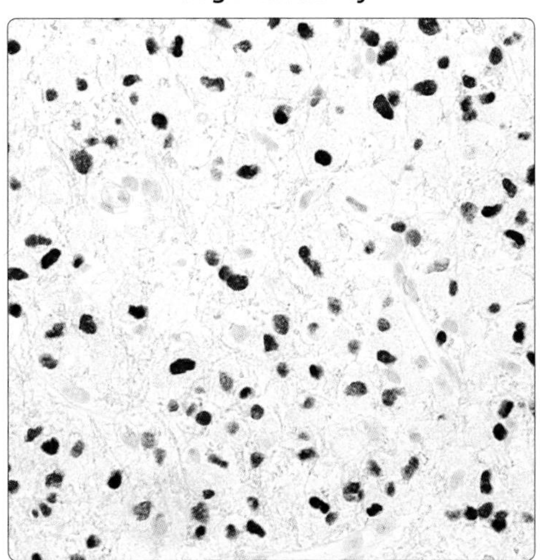

(Left) *Immunoreactivity for S100 is variable in granular cell astrocytomas but may be strong in individual cells.* **(Right)** *Olig2 expression, identifiable as a nuclear stain, is frequent in granular cell astrocytomas and diagnostically useful in separating the neoplastic cells from histiocytes.*

CD68 Reactivity

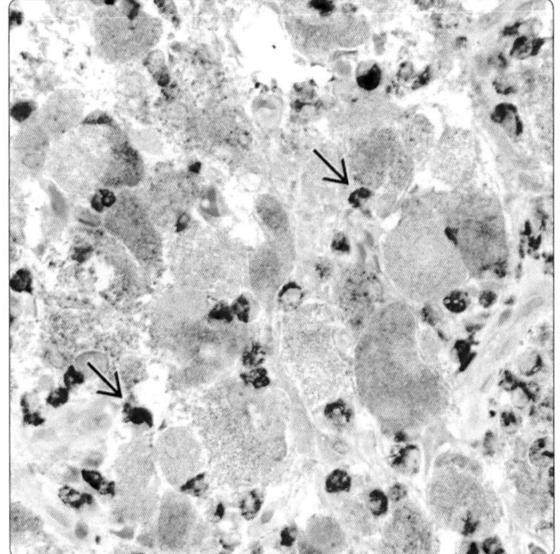

HAM56 Staining of Microglia

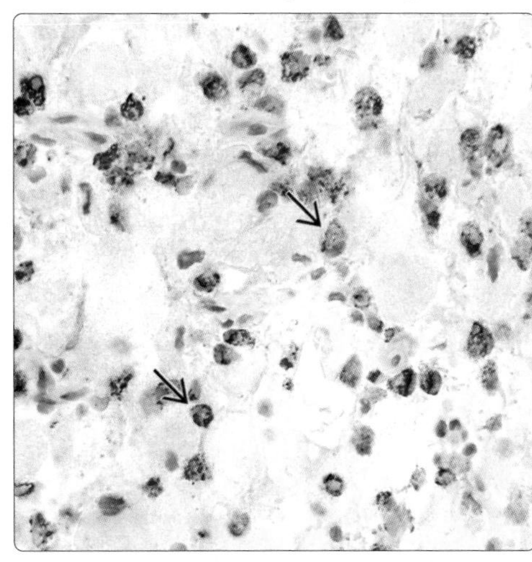

(Left) *Moderate to faint cytoplasmic reactivity for CD68 is typical of granular cell astrocytoma. Small nonneoplastic microglia are intensely stained ➔.* **(Right)** *A more specific maker than CD68 for macrophages, HAM56 usually stains only microglia ➔. Tumor cells are negative or only faintly positive.*

CD45 Immunoreactivity in Microglia

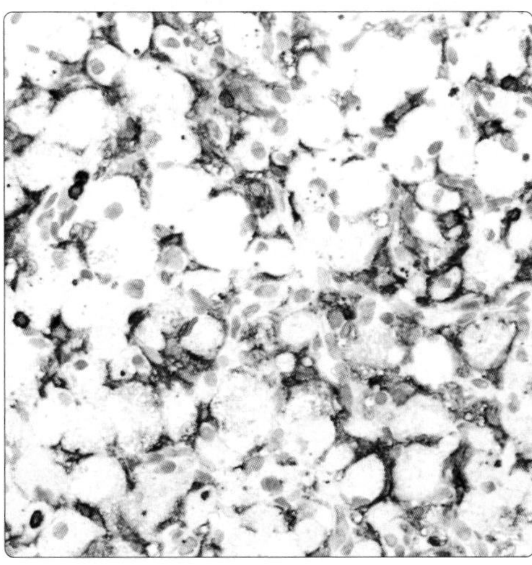

p53 Immunopositive Cells

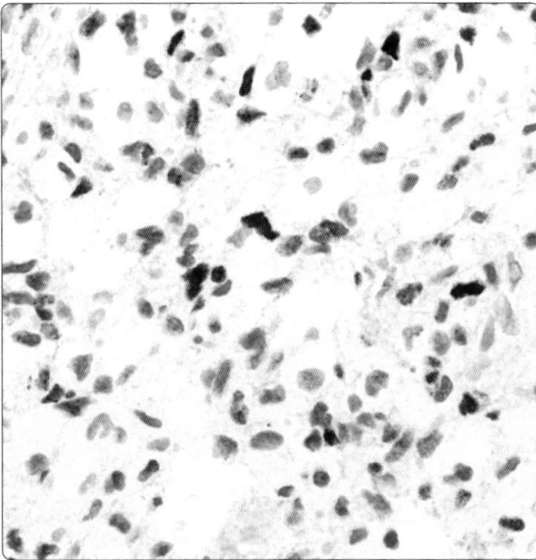

(Left) *CD45 is another marker that highlights microglia in granular cell astrocytomas, but is negative in neoplastic cells.* **(Right)** *p53 reactivity may be variable in granular cell astrocytomas and suggests that TP53 mutations may be present in a subset of cells.*

KEY FACTS

CLINICAL ISSUES

- Seizures, especially common given tumor's affinity for cerebral cortex
- Cerebral hemispheres
  - Most often frontal lobe
  - Uncommon in deep gray matter, basal ganglia, and thalamus
- Prognosis better than for astrocytoma grade II

IMAGING

- Almost always supratentorial
- Thickened cortex
- Calcifications, especially gyriform

MICROSCOPIC

- Infiltrating, with perineuronal satellitosis, perivascular and subpial accumulations
- Uniform cell distribution
- GFAP immunostaining in a subset of cells should not prompt diagnosis of mixed oligoastrocytoma
- Neuronal differentiation, uncommon
  - Neurocytes, sometimes delicate processes forming neuropil
  - Ganglion cells rarely tumoral, usually trapped neurons
- Mesenchymal differentiation (oligosarcoma) (rare)

ANCILLARY TESTS

- IDH-1(+) immunostaining and almost all adult cases show IHC(+) &/or *IDH1 IDH2* mutation
- 1p/19q codeletion
  - Increasingly used for histologic diagnosis and for directing treatment
  - Maintained by balanced translocation, der(1;19)(q10;p10)
- Retains nuclear ATRX; does not show strong nuclear p53 immunostaining

(Left) *Low-grade oligodendrogliomas are often relatively well-circumscribed areas of FLAIR hyperintensity of both white and gray matter. Affected cerebral cortex is usually thickened* ➡. **(Right)** *Best seen by CT, intracortical curvilinear, "gyriform" profiles* ➡ *are highly suggestive of the entity.*

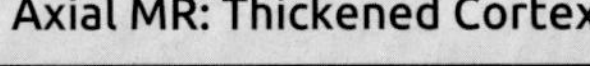

Axial MR: Thickened Cortex

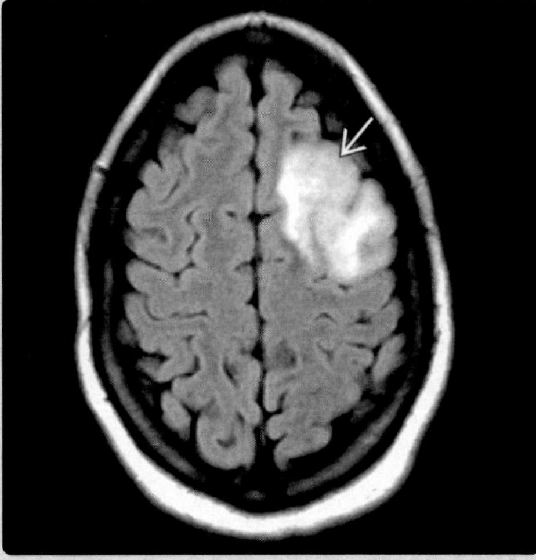

Axial CT: Curvilinear Calcification

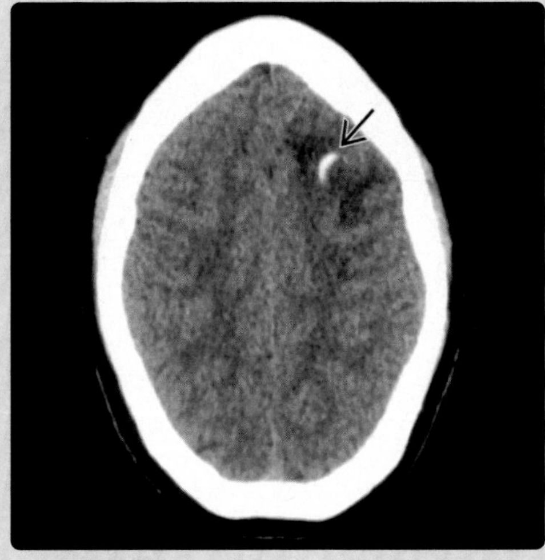

(Left) *Classic features of oligodendroglioma are those of a uniform population of tumor cells with round nuclei, scant cytoplasm, and an artifactual perinuclear halo. The latter can be absent in frozen sections and in very well-fixed small stereotactic biopsies. The diagnosis of oligodendroglioma does not rest solely on the presence of perinuclear halos.* **(Right)** *The Ki-67 index is low in grade II oligodendrogliomas.*

Classic Features

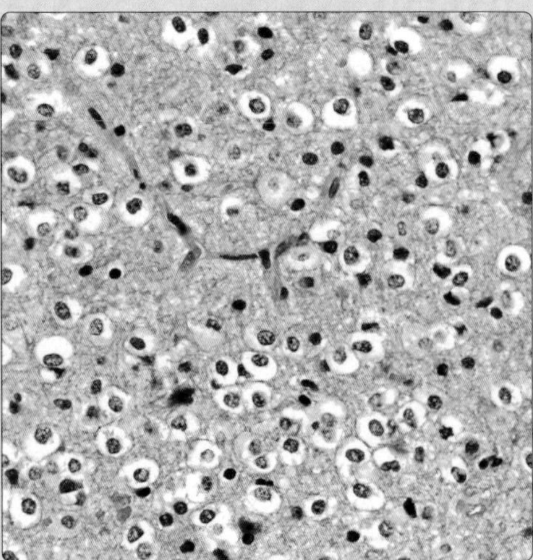

Low Ki-67

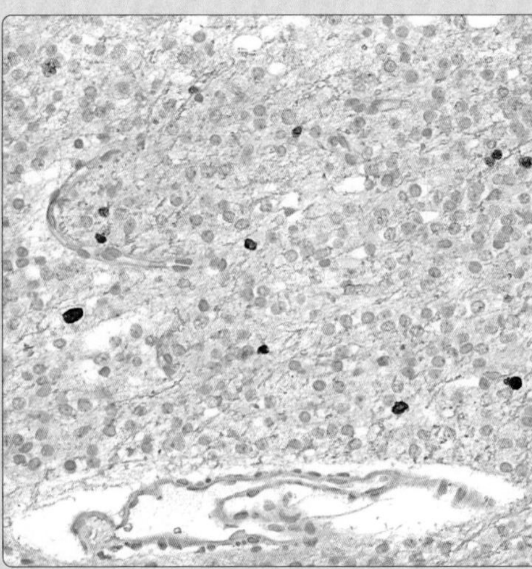

TERMINOLOGY

Definitions

- Infiltrating glioma with oligodendroglial features
- WHO grade II

CLINICAL ISSUES

Site

- Cerebral hemispheres
  - Most often frontal lobe
  - Uncommon in deep gray matter, basal ganglia, and thalamus
- Posterior fossa or spinal cord (rare)

Presentation

- Seizures; common given affinity of tumor for cerebral cortex
- Neurological deficit depending on site

Prognosis

- Variable, dependent in part on tumor grade, progression to anaplastic oligodendroglioma
- Years or decades with little growth (some cases)
- Better than for astrocytoma grade II
- Subarachnoid dissemination (uncommon)

IMAGING

MR Findings

- Bright on FLAIR; variable mass effect
- Thickened cortex
- Sometimes apparent circumscription

CT Findings

- Calcifications, especially gyriform

MACROSCOPIC

General Features

- Thickened cortex
- Ill-defined borders
- Fleshy and more circumscribed when grade III

MICROSCOPIC

Histologic Features

- Infiltrative of parenchyma
- Affinity for cerebral cortex
- Secondary structures: Perineuronal satellitosis, perivascular and subpial accumulation of tumor cells
- Microcysts
- Somewhat organoid architecture, more frequent in grade III
- Uniform cell distribution frequent
- Variable cellularity
  - Very low to high cellular tumor
  - Hypercellular tumor nodules with increased mitoses
- Cytoplasm
  - Water clear (fried egg appearance)
  - Sharp borders when cells back-to-back
  - Smooth-contoured wedge-shaped cells with apical hyaline or fibrillary inclusion (gliofibrillary oligodendrocytes)
  - Small gemistocyte-like cells with glassy, fibrillar cytoplasm and short processes (minigemistocytes)
  - Brightly eosinophilic intracytoplasmic granules (mainly in grade III lesions)
    - Ultrastructural features of Rosenthal fibers &/or lysosomes
  - Sharp cell borders, large round nuclei giving epithelioid appearance (more common in grade III)
- Vessels
  - Delicate angulated ("chicken-wire") capillaries
  - Vascular hypertrophy/proliferation, especially in grade III tumors
  - Glomeruloid vessels (uncommon)
- Calcification
  - Usually cortical
  - Dense undulating, gyriform pattern characteristic
- Neuronal differentiation (uncommon)
  - Neurocytes, sometimes delicate processes forming neuropil
  - Ganglion cells rarely tumoral, usually entrapped neurons
  - Synaptophysin immunopositivity in absence of histological neuronal differentiation (more common)
- Mesenchymal differentiation (oligosarcoma) (rare)
  - Spindle cell component with
    - Mitoses
    - Reticulin-rich matrix

ANCILLARY TESTS

Cytology

- Nuclei
  - Generally round, delicate chromatin, small nucleoli, monomorphous
  - Occasional overlap in degree of pleomorphism with astrocytomas of equivalent grade
- Cytoplasm
  - Usually scant with few processes
  - Little fibrillar background in tissue aggregates
  - Eosinophilic cytoplasm in minigemistocytes and gliofibrillary oligodendrocytes (more prominent in grade III lesions)
  - Intracytoplasmic, brightly eosinophilic, refractile bodies (more often in grade III)

Immunohistochemistry

- Mutant IDH-1(+): Nuclear and cytoplasmic staining, about 90% of adult cases, but generally (-) in pediatric cases
- Olig2(+)
- GFAP(+)
  - Variable
  - Cells with eosinophilic cytoplasm often (+)
    - Minigemistocytes and gliofibrillary oligodendroglia
  - Presence of GFAP(+) cells should not prompt diagnosis of mixed oligoastrocytoma, a diagnosis that has virtually disappeared
  - New genetic studies indicate that almost all mixed oligoastrocytomas either show genetic signature of astrocytic or oligodendroglial lineage, not both
- Synaptophysin (+)
  - In areas of neurocytic differentiation, especially neuropil

- Patchy to diffuse without histological evidence of neuronal differentiation (occasional)
- Unlike most IDH1(+) diffuse astrocytomas, does not show strong nuclear p53(+) &/or loss of nuclear ATRX

In Situ Hybridization

- Codeletion chromosomes 1p and 19q

Genetic Testing

- 1p/19q codeletion
  - Increasingly used to make histologic diagnosis and for directing treatment
  - Maintained by balanced translocation, der(1;19)(q10;p10)
  - Variable percentage of cases depending on histological stringency of diagnosis; higher incidence in association with classic histology
- *IDH1 IDH2* mutation
  - Almost all cases
- *CIC*, *FUBP1* mutations frequent: Loss of protein expression may have prognostic implications
- *TERT* promotor mutations frequent: Associated with increased expression of telomerase

DIFFERENTIAL DIAGNOSIS

Diffuse Astrocytoma, Grade II

- Irregular cell distribution, variably variable
- Greater nuclear pleomorphism, angulation
  - Hyperchromatic nuclei, inconspicuous nucleoli
- Fibrillar background (some cases)
- p53 immunostaining (+), diffuse nuclear (approximately 25% of cases)
- Nuclear ATRX (-) in tumor cells
- 1p/19q codeletion (-)

Dysembryoplastic Neuroepithelial Tumor

- Not always distinguishable, especially in small fragmented specimens
- Largely cortical with nodular architecture
- Floating neurons
- Internodular specific glioneuronal element
- Little or no perineuronal satellitosis
- Codeletion 1p/19q (-), but pediatric oligodendrogliomas almost always (-)
- IDH-1(-)

Clear Cell Ependymoma

- Compact architecture, no trapped brain elements except in the periphery
- Perivascular pseudorosettes
  - May be small and are GFAP(+_
- Grooved or clefted nuclei
- EMA(+) microlumina (some cases)
- Olig2(-), or only very focally (+); IDH-1(-)

Neurocytic Tumors

- Often intraventricular with little or no infiltration
- Finely fibrillar neuropil, sometimes in rosettes (only occasionally in oligodendrogliomas)
- Diffuse immunoreactivity for synaptophysin
- Olig2(-), or only very focally (+)
- IDH-1(-) and no 1p/19 co-deletion

Macrophage-Rich Lesions

- Demyelinating disease
  - Imaging, open ring pattern of enhancement
  - Sharp border
  - Perivascular chronic inflammation
  - Macrophages
    - Foamy or granular, non-water-clear cytoplasm
    - PAS(+), CD68(+), HAM65(+)
    - Olig2(-) and IDH1 (-)
  - Multinucleated astrocytes (Creutzfeldt cells)
- Infarct
  - Loss of axons
  - Macrophages
    - Foamy or granular, not water-clear
    - PAS(+), CD68(+), HAM56(+), IDH-1(-)
  - Ischemic red-dead neurons in acute phase
  - Endothelial cell hypertrophy and hyperplasia

DIAGNOSTIC CHECKLIST

Clinically Relevant Pathologic Features

- Seizures especially common given tumor's affinity for cerebral cortex

Pathologic Interpretation Pearls

- Do not interpret round cells with perinuclear halo necessarily as evidence of oligodendroglioma, or even as neoplasm
- Do not interpret GFAP (+) cells as indicative of mixed oligoastrocytoma; diagnosis of mixed glioma has virtually disappeared
- IDH-1 IHC (or *IDH1 IDH2* mutational testing), molecular studies for 1p/19q, frequently employed for diagnosis and prognosis

SELECTED REFERENCES

1. Appin CL et al: Molecular pathways in gliomagenesis and their relevance to neuropathologic diagnosis. Adv Anat Pathol. 22(1):50-8, 2015
2. Baumgarten P et al: Loss of FUBP1 expression in gliomas predicts FUBP1 mutation and is associated with oligodendroglial differentiation, IDH1 mutation and 1p/19q loss of heterozygosity. Neuropathol Appl Neurobiol. 40(2):205-16, 2014
3. Chan AK et al: Loss of CIC and FUBP1 expressions are potential markers of shorter time to recurrence in oligodendroglial tumors. Mod Pathol. 27(3):332-42, 2014
4. Sahebjam S et al: Emerging biomarkers in anaplastic oligodendroglioma: implications for clinical investigation and patient management. CNS Oncol. 2(4):351-8, 2013
5. Perry A et al: Oligodendroglial neoplasms with ganglioglioma-like maturation: a diagnostic pitfall. Acta Neuropathol. 120(2):237-52, 2010
6. Rossi S et al: Primary leptomeningeal oligodendroglioma with documented progression to anaplasia and t(1;19)(q10;p10) in a child. Acta Neuropathol. 118(4):575-7, 2009
7. Yan H et al: IDH1 and IDH2 mutations in gliomas. N Engl J Med. 360(8):765-73, 2009
8. Griffin CA et al: Identification of der(1;19)(q10;p10) in five oligodendrogliomas suggests mechanism of concurrent 1p and 19q loss. J Neuropathol Exp Neurol. 65(10):988-94, 2006
9. Jenkins RB et al: A t(1;19)(q10;p10) mediates the combined deletions of 1p and 19q and predicts a better prognosis of patients with oligodendroglioma. Cancer Res. 66(20):9852-61, 2006
10. Perry A et al: Oligodendrogliomas with neurocytic differentiation. A report of 4 cases with diagnostic and histogenetic implications. J Neuropathol Exp Neurol. 61(11):947-55, 2002
11. Burger PC et al: Losses of chromosomal arms 1p and 19q in the diagnosis of oligodendroglioma. A study of paraffin-embedded sections. Mod Pathol. 14(9):842-53, 2001

Infiltrative at Edge

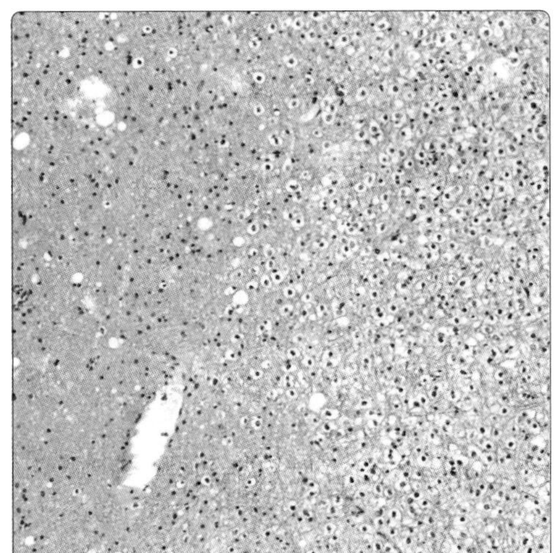

Perinuclear Halos

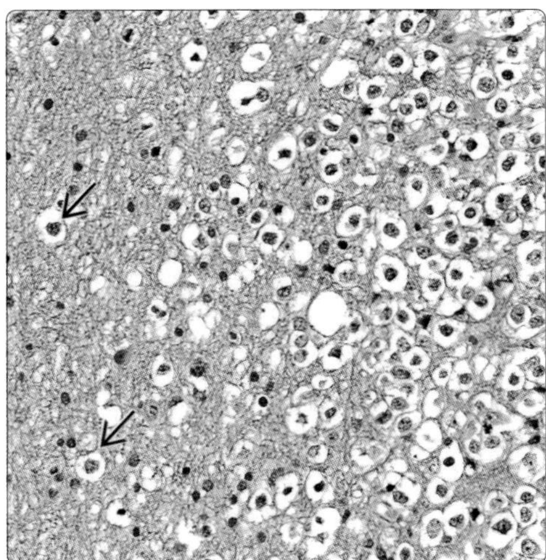

(Left) *The lesion's infiltrating quality is well-seen at the edge of a cellular region wherein tumor cells appear to move into less affected brain on the left.* **(Right)** *Individual tumor cells ➙ infiltrate into previously normal brain. Round uniform nuclei, nucleoli, and perinuclear halos are typical of oligodendrogliomas.*

Perineuronal Satellitosis

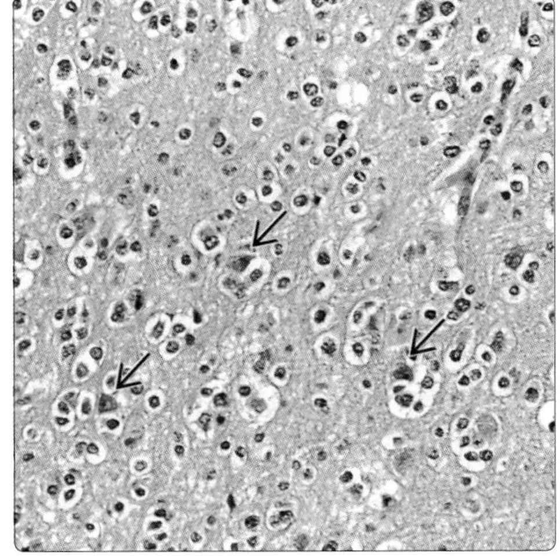

Surround Blood Vessels

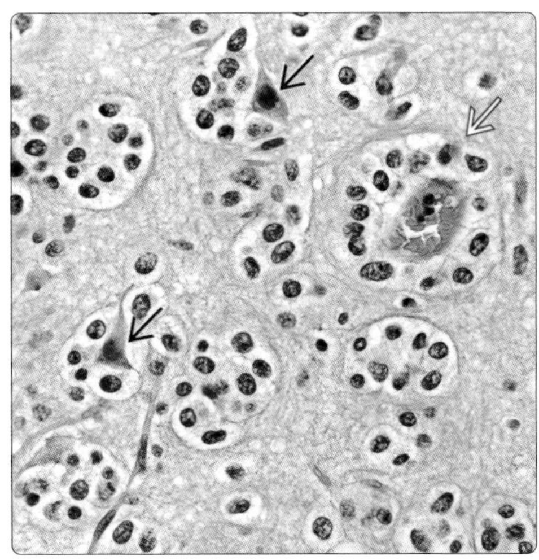

(Left) *The infiltrative qualities of oligodendrogliomas are well seen in gray matter, where perineuronal satellitosis ➙ is usually prominent. The latter is not as common, or pronounced, in diffuse astrocytomas.* **(Right)** *Uniform, round nuclei and prominent perinuclear halos are highly suggestive of oligodendroglioma. Surrounding ganglion cells ➙ and vessels ➡ are almost diagnostic thereof.*

Entrapped Axons

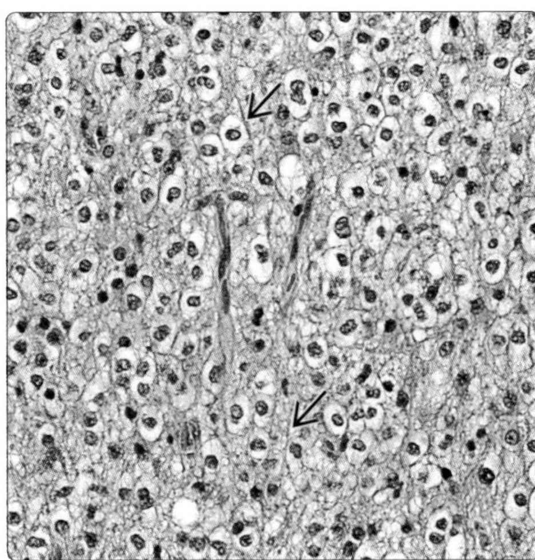

Conspicuous Entrapped Axons

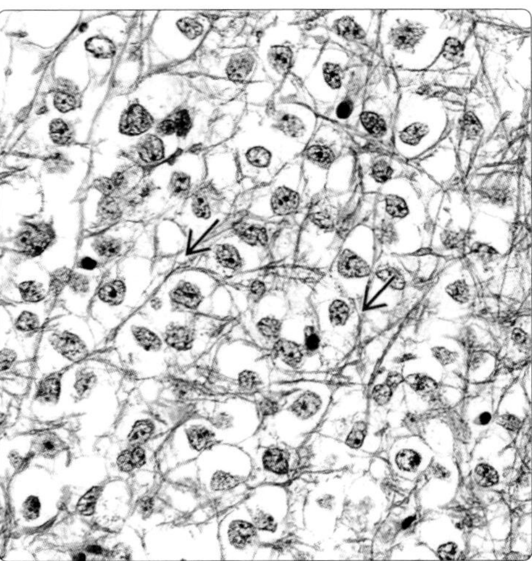

(Left) *Oligodendrogliomas, along with diffuse astrocytomas, are infiltrating neoplasms that creep into adjacent brain. As a consequence, fine, thread-like axons lie in the background of white matter ➙.* **(Right)** *Hyphae-like, axons trapped within the infiltrating lesion ➙ are often conspicuous in edematous white matter. Note open chromatin and prominent nucleoli typical of grade II oligodendrogliomas.*

(Left) *Monomorphisms in cell size, density, and distribution are cardinal qualities of oligodendrogliomas.* **(Right)** *Cells are more evenly distributed in oligodendrogliomas than in diffuse (infiltrative) astrocytomas.*

Monomorphic

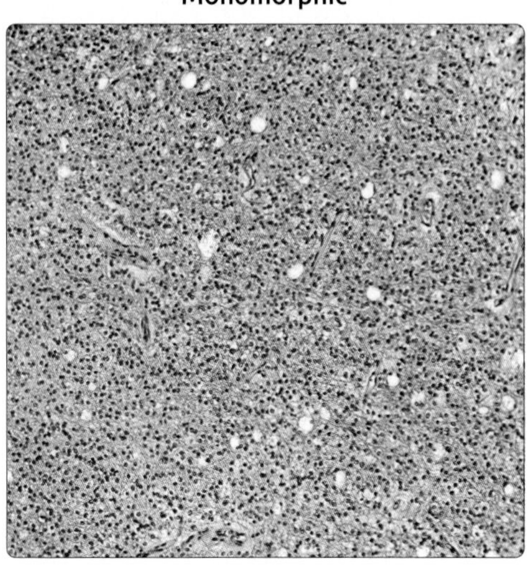

Even Cellular Distribution

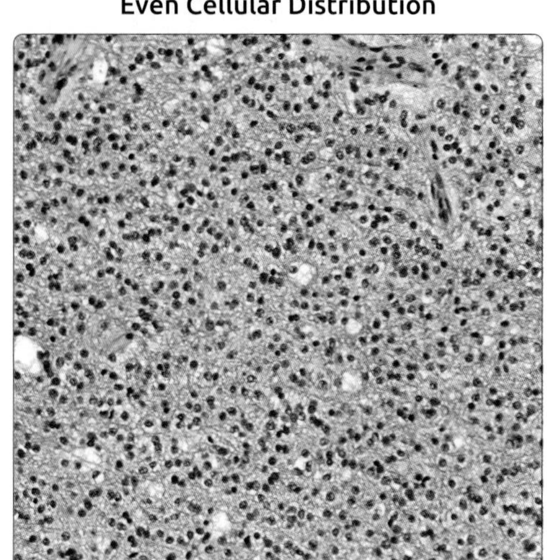

(Left) *Back-to-back cells with halos about uniform nuclei facilitate tumor typing. Given the seemingly compact architecture, a neurocytoma would be a possibility in this case.* **(Right)** *Quintessential oligodendrogliomas have monomorphism, round, back-to-back cells, and perinuclear halos.*

Back-to-Back Cells

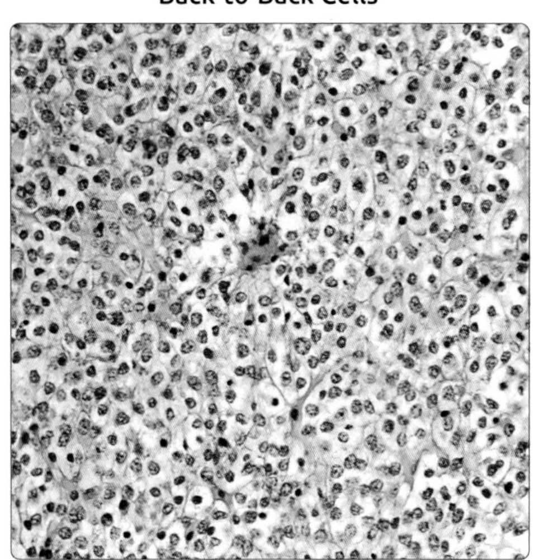

Classic Oligodendroglioma

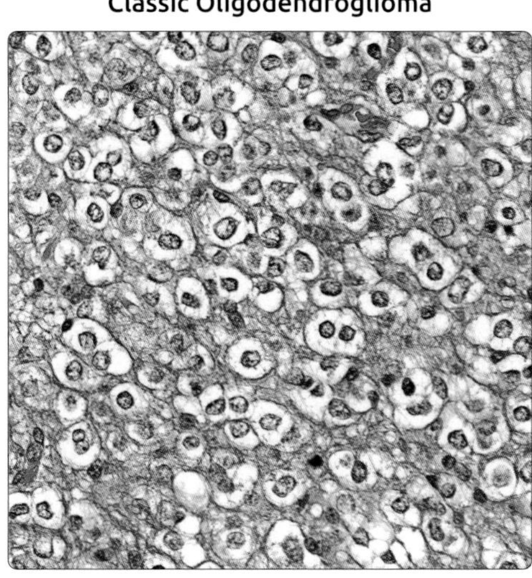

(Left) *Oligodendrogliomas with unevenly distributed cells may resemble diffuse astrocytomas. Round nuclei with distinct nucleoli, visible at even low magnification, are distinguishing features.* **(Right)** *Without perinuclear halos, oligodendrogliomas are not as distinctive, or visually appealing, as in textbook cases. Nevertheless, round nuclei and distinct nucleoli help distinguish such a lesion from diffuse astrocytoma. Halos are especially likely to be absent in frozen sections and well-fixed small biopsies.*

Uneven Cell Distribution

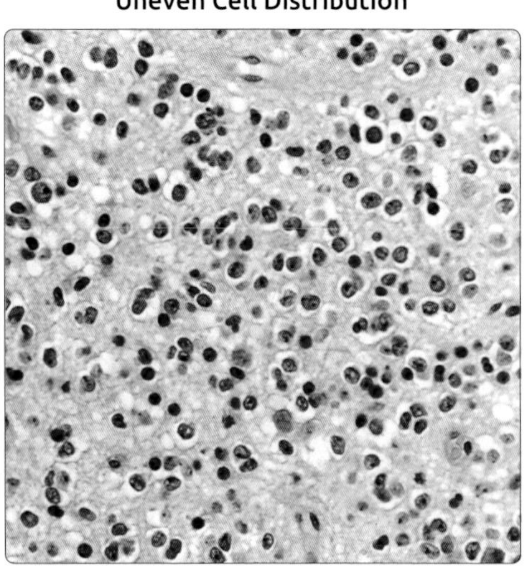

Without Perinuclear Halos

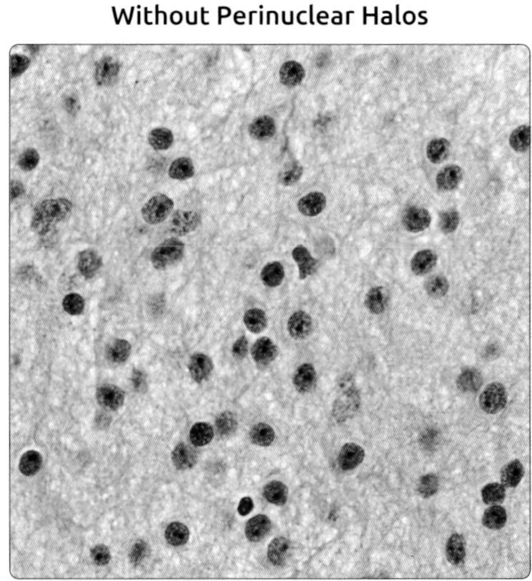

Gliofibrillary Oligodendrocytes

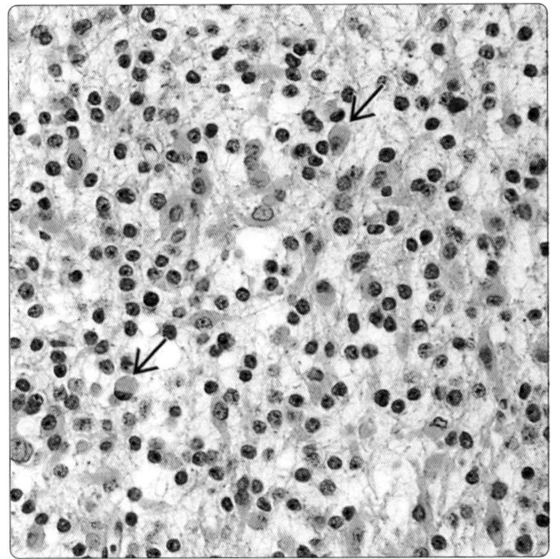

Minigemistocytes

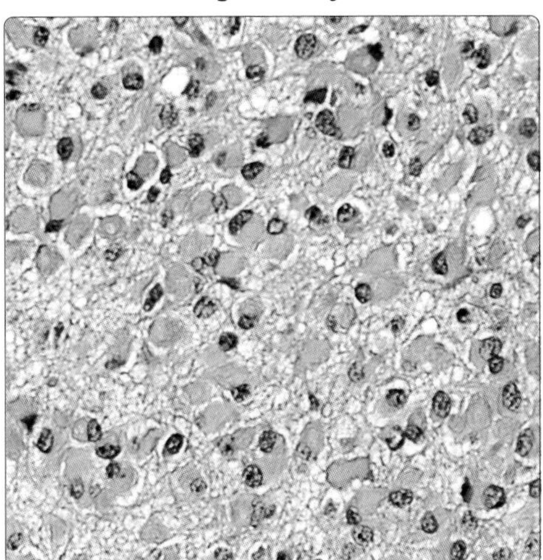

(Left) *Cells with features suggesting astrocytic differentiation* ⇨*, gliofibrillary oligodendrocytes in this case, are not uncommon in low-grade oligodendrogliomas, but are more frequent when grade III.* **(Right)** *As small versions of gemistocytes, the globular rather than polygonal mini version has hyaline cytoplasm and short processes. Such cells overlap with gliofibrillary oligodendrocytes, and the term minigemistocyte is often used for both. The cells will be GFAP(+).*

Cobweb Appearance

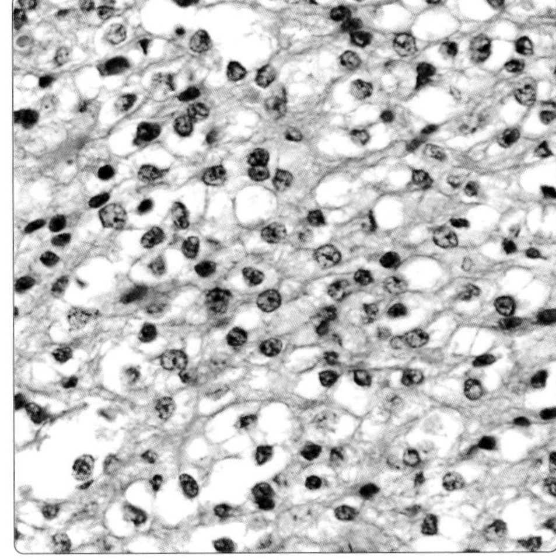

Minor Nuclear Pleomorphism

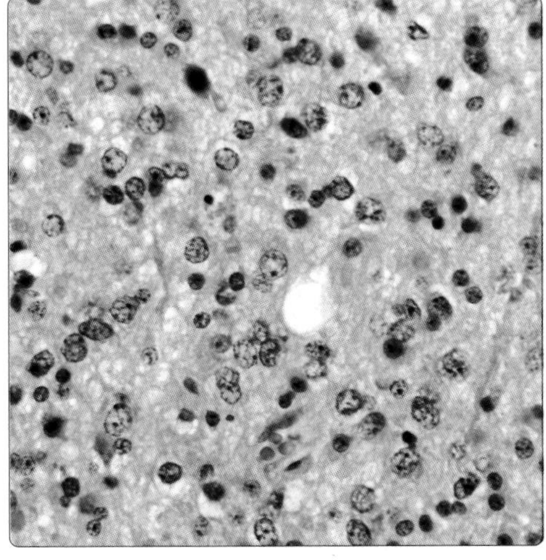

(Left) *In combination, perinuclear halos and parenchymal edema can produce a cobweb effect.* **(Right)** *The minor nuclear pleomorphism of this oligodendroglioma overlaps with that of diffuse astrocytoma. Nonetheless, it has the open nuclei and distinct nucleoli of oligodendroglioma. Molecular studies, 1p/19q, are often applied, even to classic lesions.*

Freezing Artifact

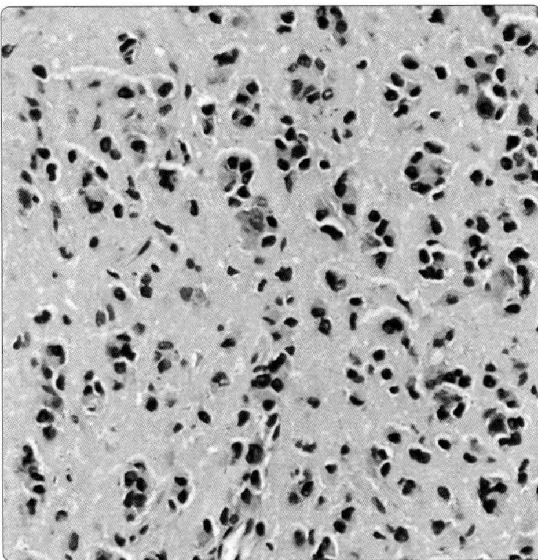

Freezing Artifact

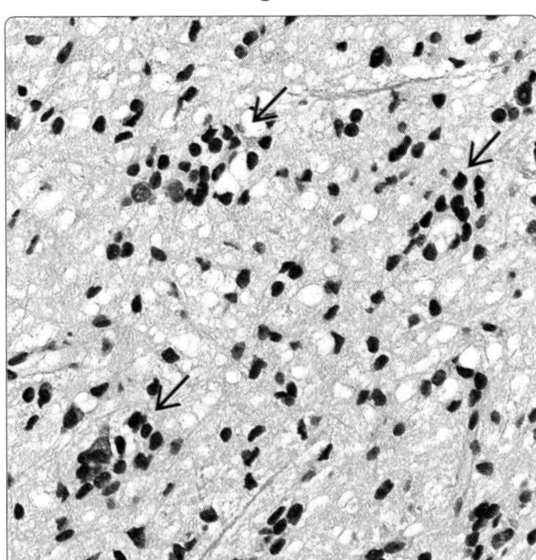

(Left) *Nuclear condensation and pleomorphism are consequences of prior freezing. The prominent perineuronal satellitosis is a clue as to the oligodendroglial nature of this infiltrating neoplasm.* **(Right)** *Nuclear angulation and hyperchromatism are artifacts of freezing. Oligodendrogliomas in frozen section controls often resemble astrocytomas. Perineuronal satellitosis* ⇨ *is more suggestive with oligodendroglioma.*

(Left) *Oligodendrogliomas are more prone to microcystic change than are infiltrating astrocytomas.* **(Right)** *Straight, curved, and angulated segments of capillaries create the classic chicken-wire vasculature → reflecting accentuated normal vessels, a soft clue to the diagnosis.*

Microcystic Change

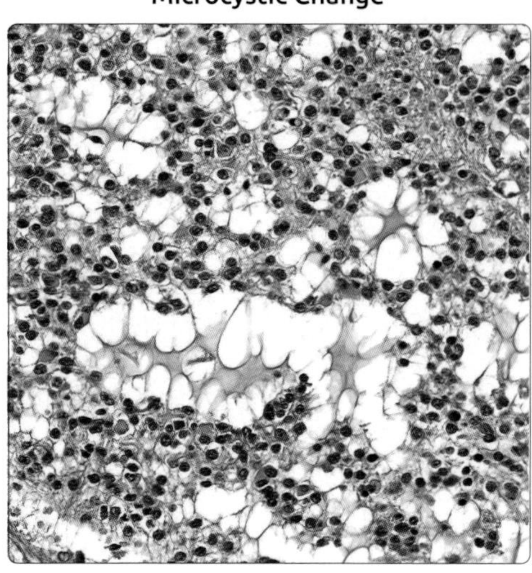

Chicken-Wire Vasculature

(Left) *Ribbons of cells are focal features in a minority of oligodendrogliomas. While this example is grade II, the phenomenon is more common in grade III examples.* **(Right)** *Calcospherites are common, but nonspecific, features of oligodendrogliomas. For example, small cell anaplastic astrocytoma, a WHO grade III tumor with poor prognosis, often shows small calcifications (as well as perinuclear halos).*

Ribbons of Cells

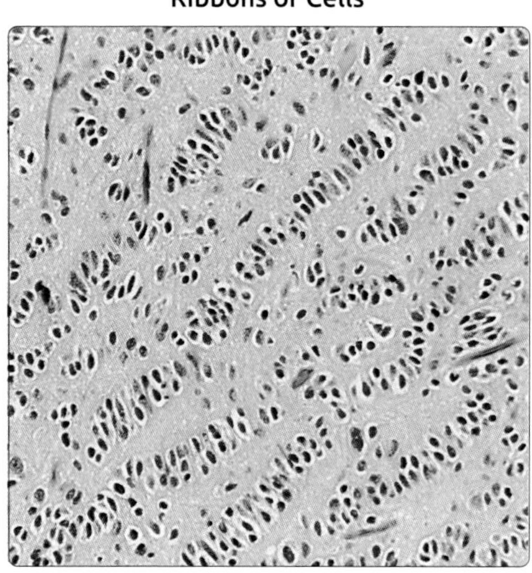

Calcospherites

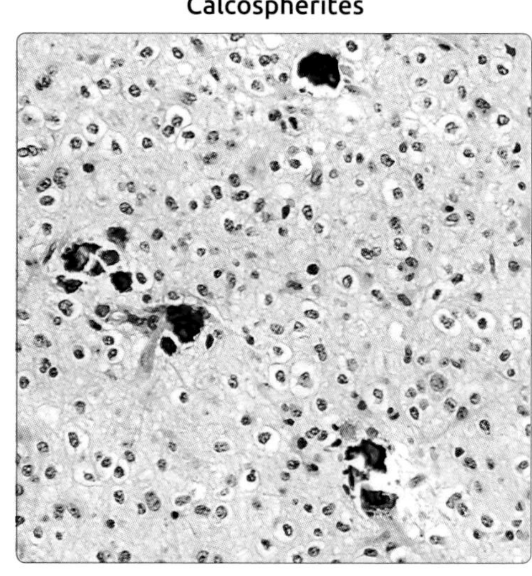

(Left) *Concentration of neoplastic cells beneath the pia is a frequent form of secondary structure in oligodendrogliomas →.* **(Right)** *Well-circumscribed cellular nodules → are not uncommon in oligodendrogliomas of either grade II or III. It is not always reflexly possible to assign their degree of atypia and mitotic activity grade III (anaplastic) oligodendroglioma. This example was grade II.*

Secondary Structures

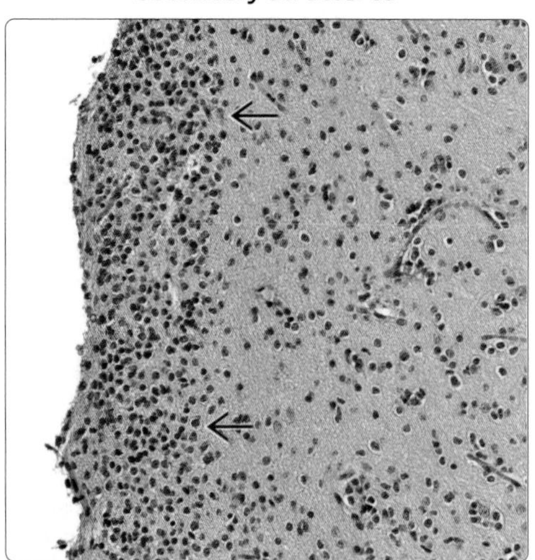

Hypercellular Tumor Nodules

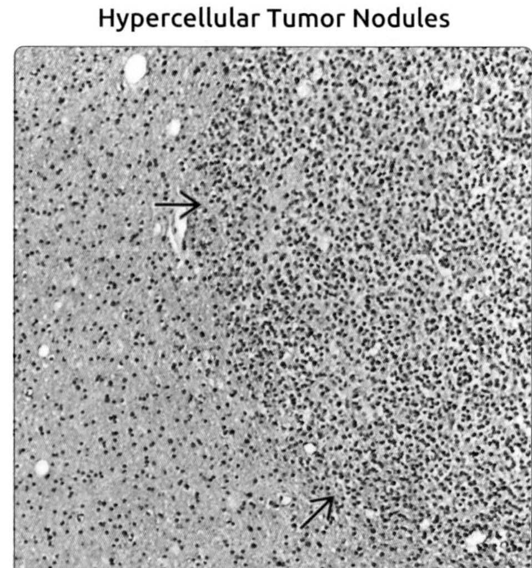

Smear, Round Nuclei

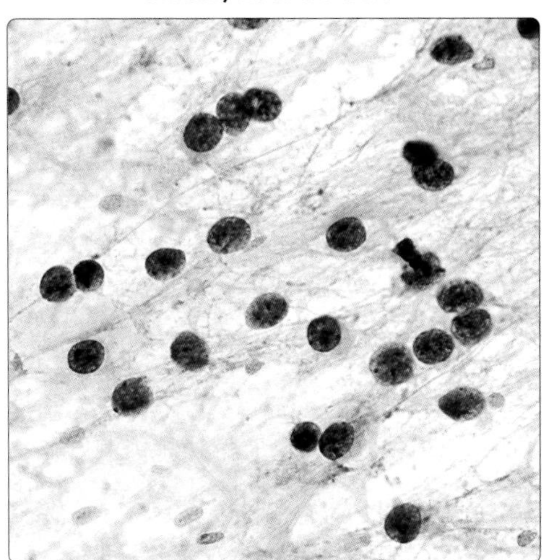

Smear, Minigemistocytes

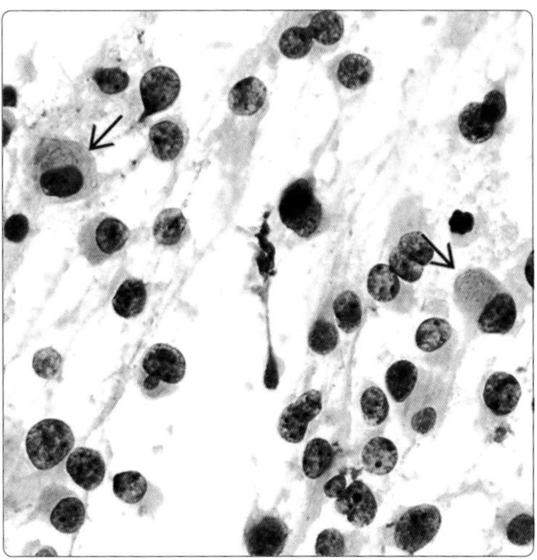

(Left) *Round nuclei, distinct nucleoli, scant cytoplasm, and little if any fibrillar background are cardinal features of oligodendroglioma in smear preparations.* **(Right)** *Astrocyte-like cells, minigemistocytic oligodendrocytes in this case ⮕, are helpful cytological features suggesting oligodendroglioma. The degree of nuclear atypia in this case suggests a grade III or borderline lesion.*

IDH-1(+)

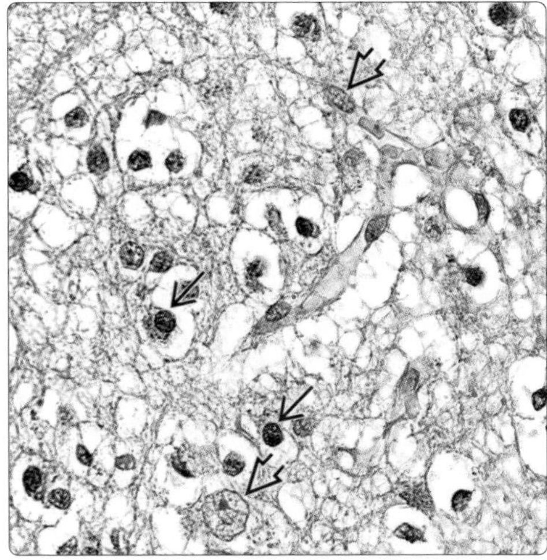

Reciprocal Translocation

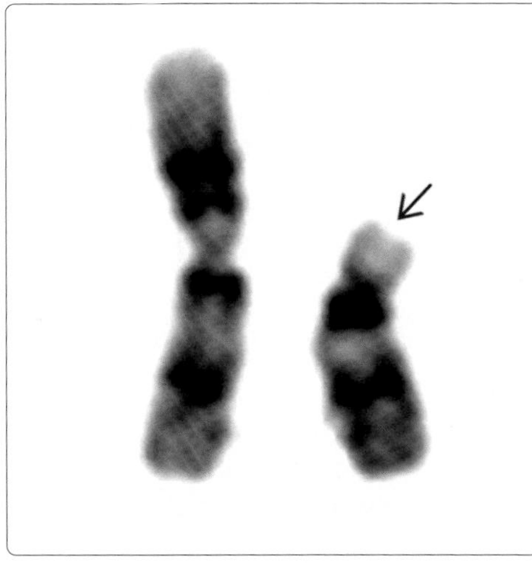

(Left) *Nuclei and cytoplasm of most oligodendrogliomas are immunoreactive for IDH-1 ⮕. Normal cells such as neurons and vessels are not immunoreactive ⮕. Reactive astrocytes would also be negative.* **(Right)** *As illustrated in an excerpt from a G-banded metaphase spread, the 1p/19q codeletion is maintained by a 19q-to-1 reciprocal translocation ⮕. The other derivative chromosome, composed of 1q and 19p, has been lost.*

FISH, Loss of 1p

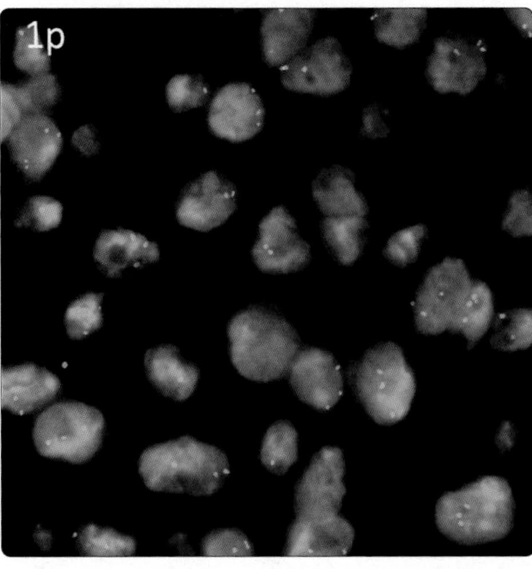

FISH, Loss of 19q

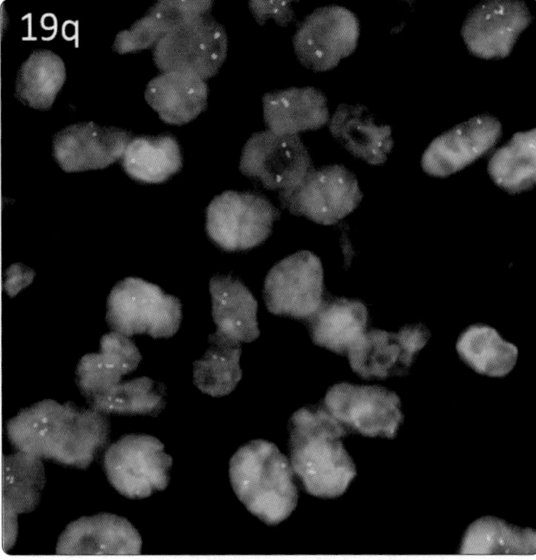

(Left) *Hybridization for a marker on chromosome 1p (red) and chromosomal enumeration probe 1 (CEP1) (green) found loss of the 1p locus, as inferred from the 2 signals for CEP1 and only 1 for the 1p. There was also loss of a marker on 19q.* **(Right)** *Hybridization for a marker on chromosome 19q (red) and chromosomal enumeration probe 19 (CEP19) (green) found loss of the 19q locus, as inferred from the 2 signals for CEP19 and only 1 for 1p. There was also loss of a marker on 1p.*

Anaplastic Oligodendroglioma

KEY FACTS

CLINICAL ISSUES

- Prognosis better than that of anaplastic astrocytoma (grade III)

IMAGING

- Enhancing, at least focally, in most cases

MICROSCOPIC

- Infiltrative, but sometimes focally compact with little or no infiltration
- Can have epithelioid, carcinoma-like appearance
- Occasional nodules with increased cytologic atypia
- Associated areas of grade II oligodendroglioma in some cases
- Astrocyte-like cells common: Minigemistocytes and gliofibrillary oligodendrocytes
  - Presence of GFAP(+) cells should not prompt diagnosis of "mixed anaplastic oligoastrocytoma," a category no longer recognized by new WHO classification
- Often with endothelial hypertrophy &/or proliferation
- More atypia, mitoses (> 5/10 HPF), and more frequent minigemistocytes, gliofibrillary oligodendrocytes than grade II oligodendroglioma

TOP DIFFERENTIAL DIAGNOSES

- Anaplastic astrocytoma (especially small cell astrocytoma, which is always *IDH1/2* wild type (ie., nonmutated)
- Glioblastoma (± *IDH1/2* mutation) (category of glioblastoma with oligodendroglioma component no longer recognized)
- Clear cell ependymoma (no LOH of 1p/19q)

DIAGNOSTIC CHECKLIST

- Molecular studies for 1p/19q codeletion required for diagnosis, important for prognosis
- IHC phenotype of IDH1 IHC(+) with nuclear ATRX retention, minimal nuclear p53(+) suggestive of oligodendroglial lineage

(Left) *Anaplastic oligodendrogliomas are typically bulky. As with grade II equivalents, the frontal lobe is a common site. (Courtesy K. Salzman, MD.)* **(Right)** *Anaplastic oligodendrogliomas are cellular and mitotically active →.*

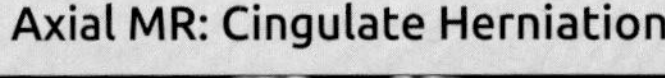

Axial MR: Cingulate Herniation

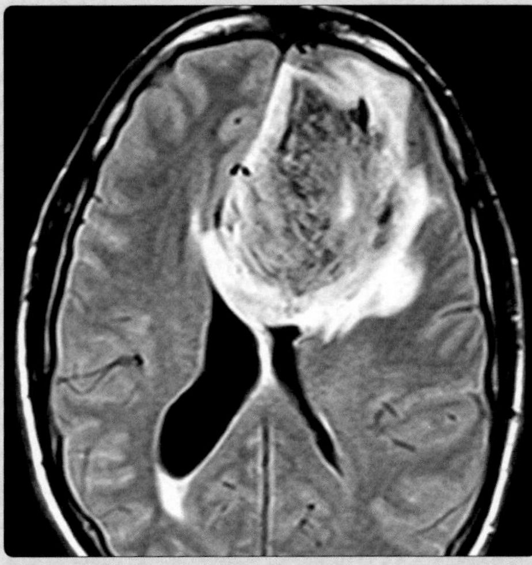

Hypercellular, Mitotically Active

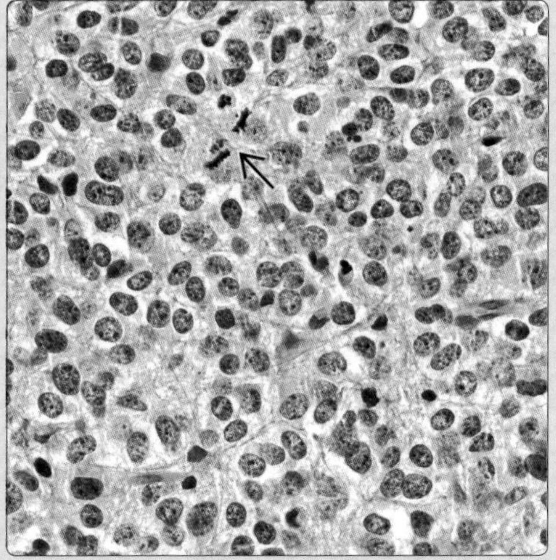

(Left) *Mucinous pools and prominent nucleoli are often found in anaplastic oligodendrogliomas; these features may prompt diagnostic consideration of metastatic carcinoma.* **(Right)** *Astrocyte-like cells in oligodendrogliomas, whether gliofibrillary oligodendrocyte, minigemistocyte, or cells intermediate between the 2, are often strongly immunoreactive for GFAP. The presence of these cells should not prompt diagnosis of oligoastrocytoma, a diagnosis that has virtually disappeared.*

Mucinous Pools

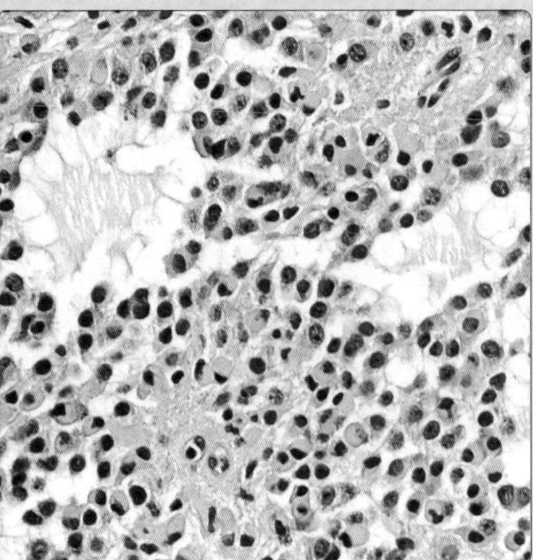

GFAP(+) Cells

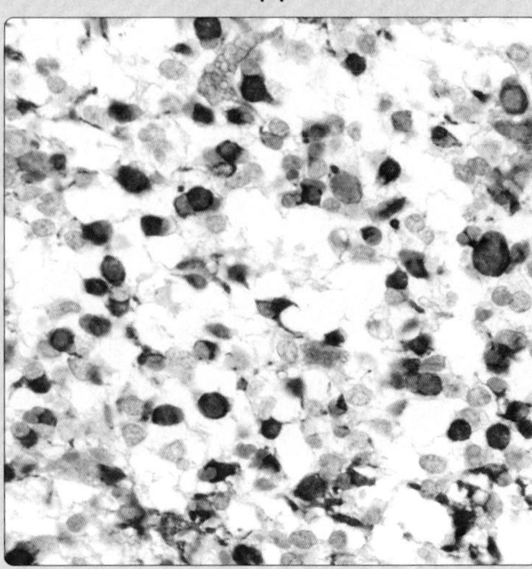

TERMINOLOGY

Definitions

- High-grade glioma with oligodendroglial features
  - WHO grade III
  - Presence of LOH 1p/19q required for diagnosis of anaplastic oligodendroglioma in new "integrated diagnosis" system

CLINICAL ISSUES

Treatment

- Adjuvant therapy
  - Standard approach: Temozolomide
- Radiation
  - Most cases

Prognosis

- Poor
  - Better than that for anaplastic (grade III) astrocytoma

IMAGING

MR Findings

- Often bulky
- Enhancing, at least focally, in ~ 1/2 of cases

CT Findings

- Calcifications
  - Common
  - May be cortical (gyriform)

MICROSCOPIC

Histologic Features

- Infiltrative but often partly compact with little intervening parenchyma
  - Perineuronal satellitosis
  - Perivascular and subpial accumulation
- High cellularity
  - Predominantly diffuse
  - Occasional nodules with increased cytologic atypia
- Associated areas of grade II oligodendroglioma in some cases
- Lobulated in some cases
- Cytologically monomorphous
- Epithelioid quality (some cases)
  - Round nuclei
  - Sharp cell borders
  - Cell dehiscence
- Astrocyte-like cells
  - Minigemistocytes
    - Glassy cytoplasm
    - Short processes
  - Gliofibrillary oligodendrocytes
    - Polygonal-triangular cells often with apical glial filaments
    - Few processes
  - Cells with eosinophilic granules (Rosenthal fibers or lysosomes)
  - Presence of GFAP(+) cells should not prompt diagnosis of mixed anaplastic oligoastrocytoma, diagnosis that has virtually disappeared
    - New genetic studies indicate that almost all mixed oligoastrocytomas either show genetic signature of astrocytic or oligodendroglial lineage, not both
- Artifactually dark, astrocytoma-like nuclei in frozen section controls
- Calcifications, often cortical (gyriform)
- Mitoses
  - WHO: High mitotic activity
    - "High" not defined
    - > 5/10 HPF or more in 1 study; others require fewer
- Endothelial hypertrophy &/or hyperplasia
- Necrosis
  - Seen in some cases
  - Usually little or no pseudopalisading
  - Presence or absence of necrosis does not significantly affect prognosis within anaplastic oligodendroglioma with LOH 1p/19q
- Neuronal differentiation, uncommon
  - Neurocytic, with islands of neuropil
  - Ganglion cells
- PNET-like component similar to that in glioblastomas (rare)
- Mesenchymal metaplasia (oligosarcoma) (rare)

ANCILLARY TESTS

Cytology

- Round nuclei
- Cytologic atypia
- Occasional astrocyte-like cells
- Mitoses but may be difficult to find

Immunohistochemistry

- GFAP often partly positive
- Mutant *IDH1* in most cases; rare oligodendrogliomas *IDH2*-mutated
  - IDH1 IHC(+), including neoplastic ganglion cells, if any
- Olig2(+)
- Synaptophysin often partly positive
  - With neurocytic or ganglion cell differentiation
- NeuN(+), neurocytes, some in neuropil islands
- Usually no strong nuclear p53(+) or loss of nuclear ATRX, unlike most IDH1(+) anaplastic astrocytomas, i.e., IDH1(+) + ATRX retention suggests oligodendroglial lineage

Genetic Testing

- 1p/19q codeletion (whole arm loss of both) used to classify tumors as oligodendroglial lineage
- *CIC*, *FUBP1* mutations frequent: Loss of protein expression may correlate with prognosis
- TERT promoter mutations frequent: Associated with increased expression of telomerase

SELECTED REFERENCES

1. Reuss DE et al: ATRX and IDH1-R132H immunohistochemistry with subsequent copy number analysis and IDH sequencing as a basis for an "integrated" diagnostic approach for adult astrocytoma, oligodendroglioma and glioblastoma. Acta Neuropathol. 129(1):133-46, 2015
2. Sahm F et al: Farewell to oligoastrocytoma: in situ molecular genetics favor classification as either oligodendroglioma or astrocytoma. Acta Neuropathol. 128(4):551-9, 2014

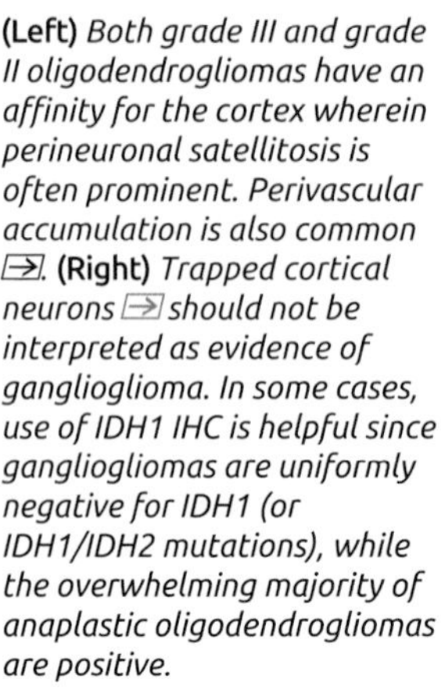

(Left) *Both grade III and grade II oligodendrogliomas have an affinity for the cortex wherein perineuronal satellitosis is often prominent. Perivascular accumulation is also common* ➙. **(Right)** *Trapped cortical neurons* ➙ *should not be interpreted as evidence of ganglioglioma. In some cases, use of IDH1 IHC is helpful since gangliogliomas are uniformly negative for IDH1 (or IDH1/IDH2 mutations), while the overwhelming majority of anaplastic oligodendrogliomas are positive.*

Affinity for Cortex

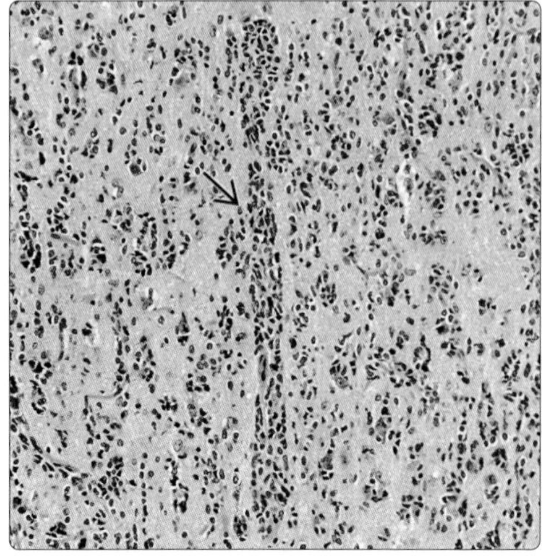

Entrapped Cortical Neurons

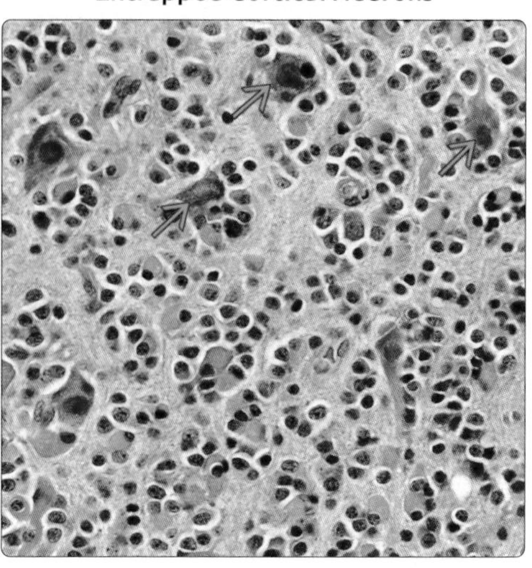

(Left) *Cytologically, many grade III oligodendrogliomas resemble primary CNS lymphoma, especially when there is little perineuronal satellitosis.* **(Right)** *Anaplastic oligodendrogliomas are sometimes histologically compact and cytologically epithelioid. This can simulate a metastasis.*

Simulating Lymphoma

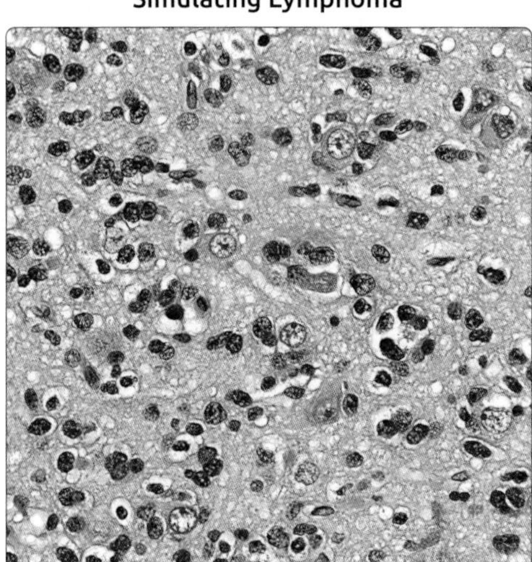

Simulating Metastasis

(Left) *Well-circumscribed "clonal" regions of increased cellularity* ➙ *are common in oligodendrogliomas, especially those that are grade III.* **(Right)** *A relatively sharp border demarcates pauci- and highly cellular regions.*

Hypercellular Nodules

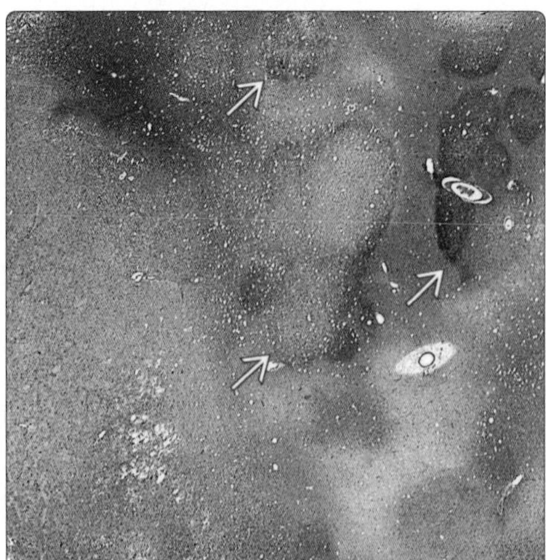

Contrast Between Hyper- and Hypocellular Areas

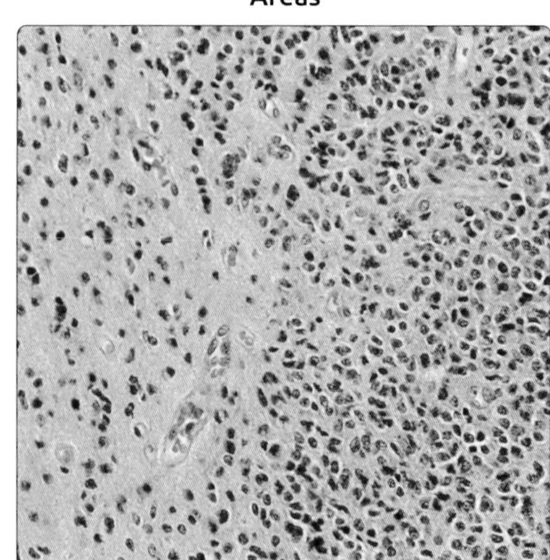

Cytological Monotony

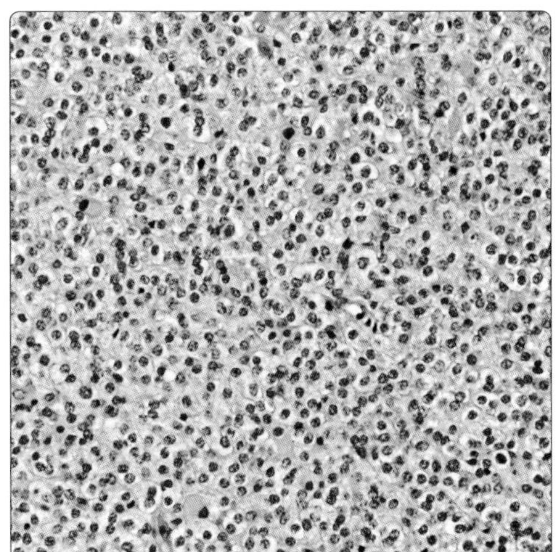

Infiltrative Tumor, Mitoses

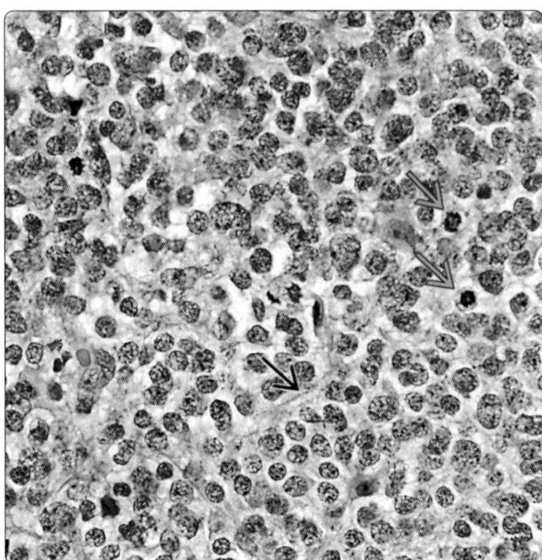

(Left) *Even distribution and cytological monotony are, in combination, highly suggestive of oligodendroglioma, either low or high grade.* **(Right)** *Monomorphous, round, and closely packed cells with mitoses ⇨ are typical features of grade III oligodendrogliomas. Small cell glioblastoma can have this same high cell density, but will not be composed exclusively of round cells. Axons course through this infiltrating lesion ⇨.*

Back-to-Back Cells

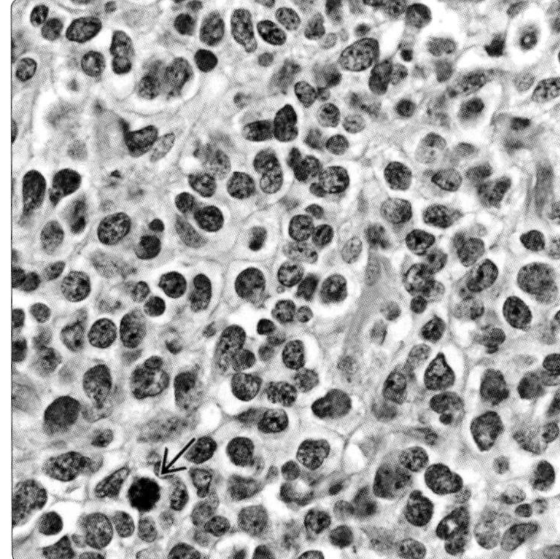

Eosinophilic Cytoplasm

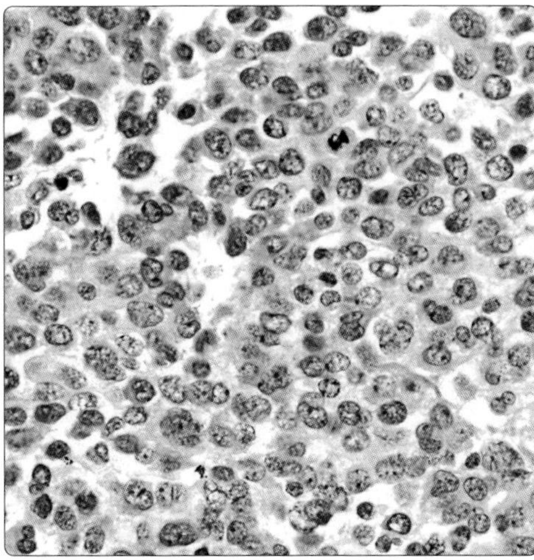

(Left) *Not as round as in the classic lesion, but rounder than in most high-grade astrocytic tumors, the cells of this cellular tumor are back-to-back, as is typical of oligodendrogliomas. A mitosis ⇨ and subtle perivascular halos are present.* **(Right)** *Anaplastic oligodendrogliomas are densely cellular, mitotically active tumors whose round cells help distinguish them from high-grade astrocytomas. A skirt of well-circumscribed pink cytoplasm is not unusual.*

Back-to-Back Cells

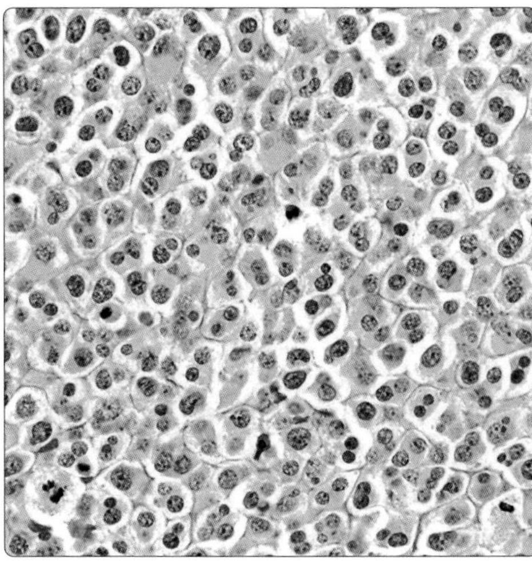

Simulating Astrocytoma

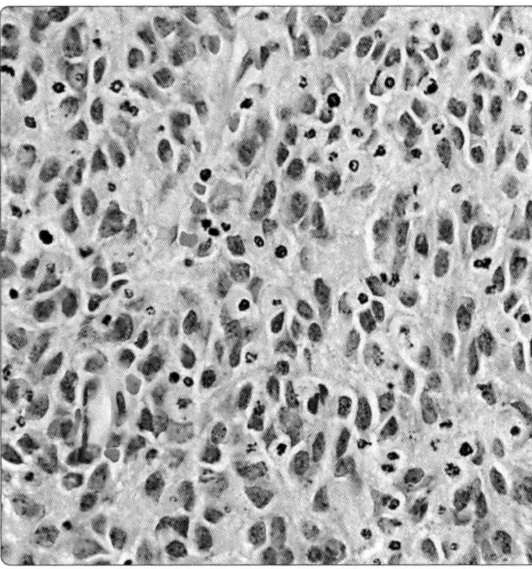

(Left) *Round, back-to-back cells are highly suspicious for those of oligodendroglioma, grade III.* **(Right)** *Nuclei can be somewhat irregular and even elongate so as to appear more "astrocytic." The diagnosis in such a setting depends on the presence of classic oligodendroglioma elsewhere in the specimen &/or molecular findings.*

(Left) *Nuclear elongation and pleomorphism give some high-grade oligodendrogliomas an astrocytic appearance. The dense, compact architecture is more consistent with the former. Calcifications also favor oligodendroglioma but are nonspecific.* **(Right)** *It can be difficult to distinguish anaplastic oligodendrogliomas with considerable nuclear pleomorphism, such as this, from anaplastic astrocytomas. The distinct cell borders favor the former. Classic low-grade oligodendroglioma will usually be present elsewhere in the specimen.*

Nonspecific Calcifications

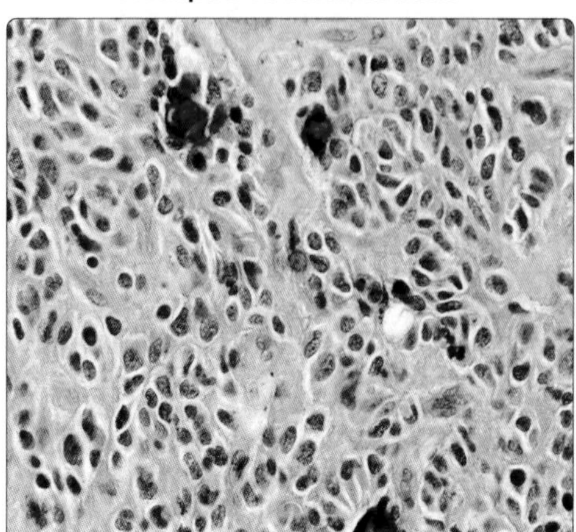

Nuclear Pleomorphism

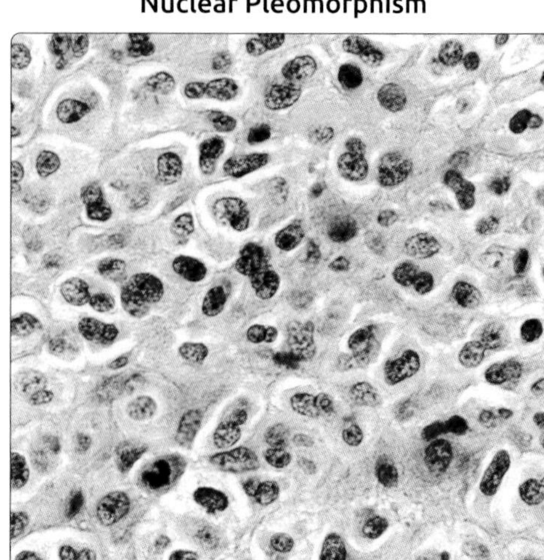

(Left) *Microcysts are prominent in some high- and, of course, low-grade oligodendrogliomas. Their presence or absence does not impact grading.* **(Right)** *Ribboning is an eye-catching feature of some oligodendrogliomas, usually of grade III.*

Microcysts

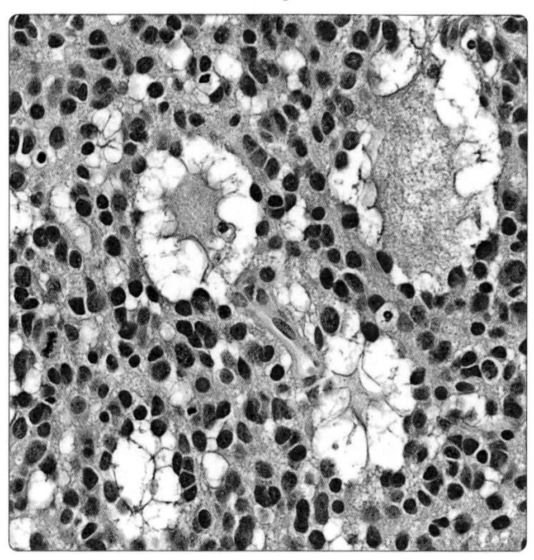

Ribbons of Cells

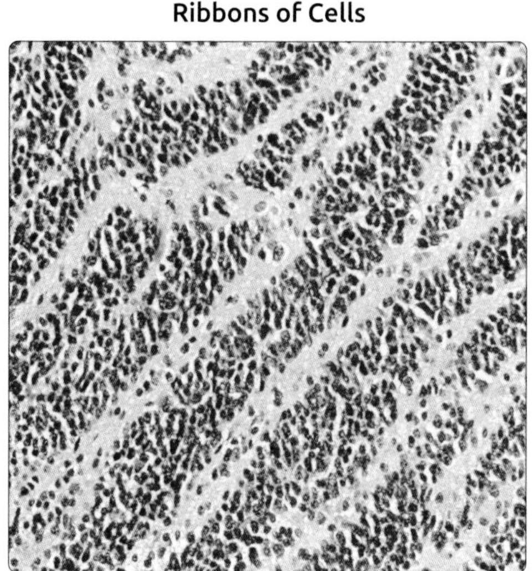

(Left) *Nuclear profiles can be intermediate in roundness between those of classic oligodendroglioma and astrocytoma. Focal or extensive pink cytoplasm is a feature of some high-grade oligodendrogliomas. As is typical of oligodendrogliomas, cells are back-to-back.* **(Right)** *Cells of grade III oligodendrogliomas may have the eosinophilic cytoplasm ⇒ more expected of astrocytes than oligodendrocytes. The sharp cell borders and round nuclei aid classification.*

Irregular Nuclei

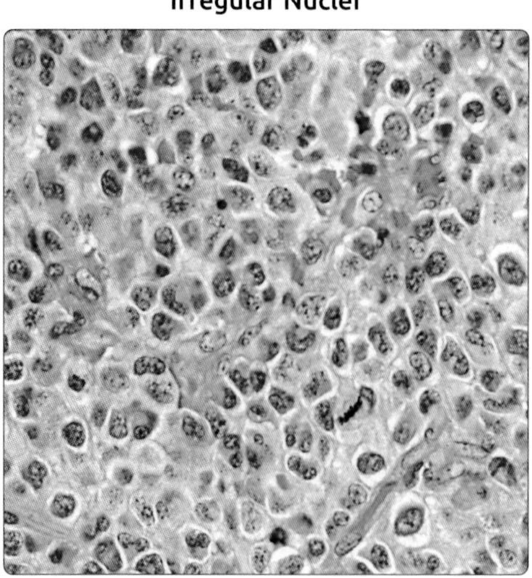

Rounded Cytoplasmic Profiles

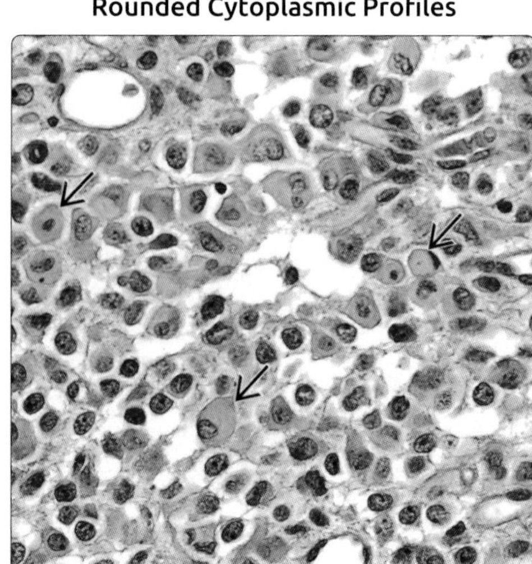

Minigemistocytes

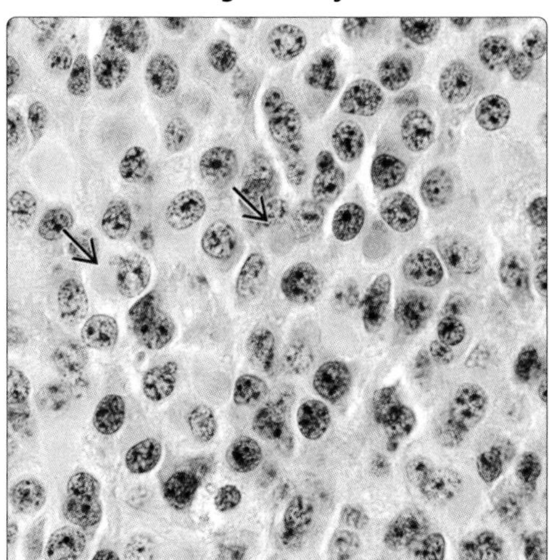

Heterogeneous Population

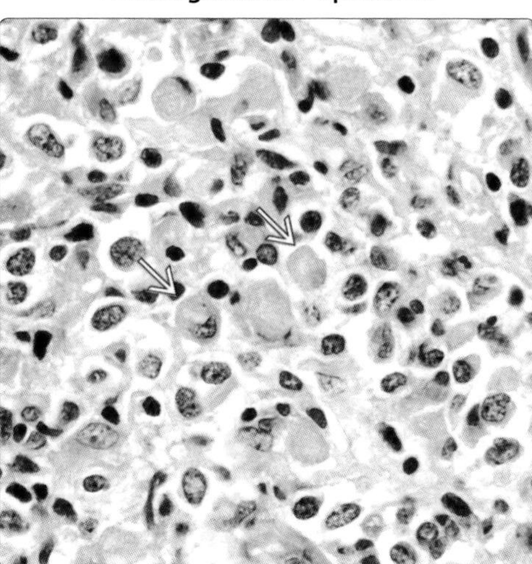

(Left) *Small intracytoplasmic pink bodies* ⇨ *are common in cells often referred to as minigemistocytes. The illustrated round nuclei are typical of oligodendrogliomas.* **(Right)** *Prominent pink cytoplasm* ➡, *whether circumferential or segregated as a small paranuclear mass, is common in oligodendrogliomas, especially those that are grade III. Note the heterogeneous population of tumor cells in this tumor.*

Triangular Gliofibrillary Oligodendrocytes

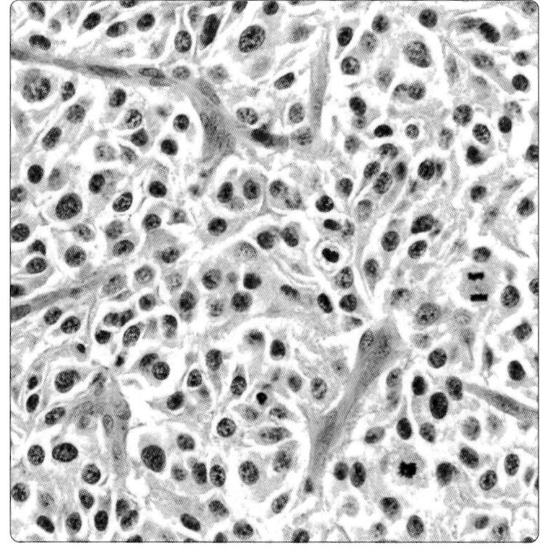

Fibrillar Background

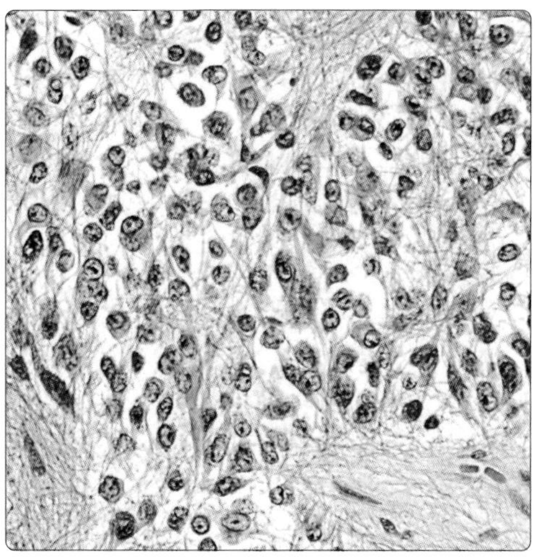

(Left) *Gliofibrillary oligodendrocytes with their polygonal to triangular apical cytoplasm and processes closely simulate the cells of astrocytoma. Endothelial cells are hypertrophic within the chicken-wire vessels.* **(Right)** *Astrocytoma-like tumor cell processes can focally aggregate to form an astrocytoma-like fibrillar background. All oligodendrogliomas now require genetic confirmation of LOH 1p/19q for an "integrated diagnosis."*

Gliofibrillary Oligodendroglioma

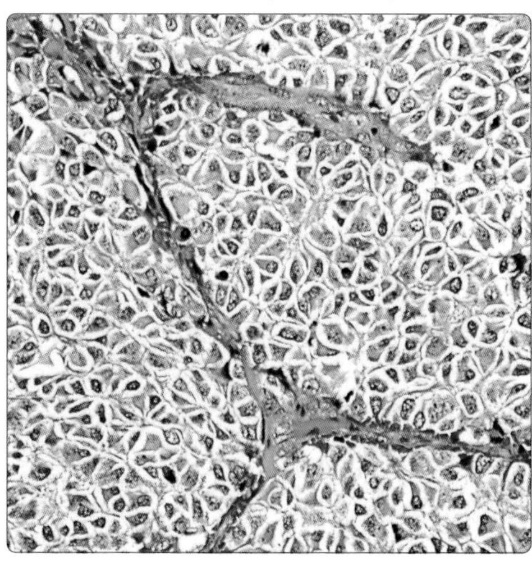

Angular-Shaped Cells

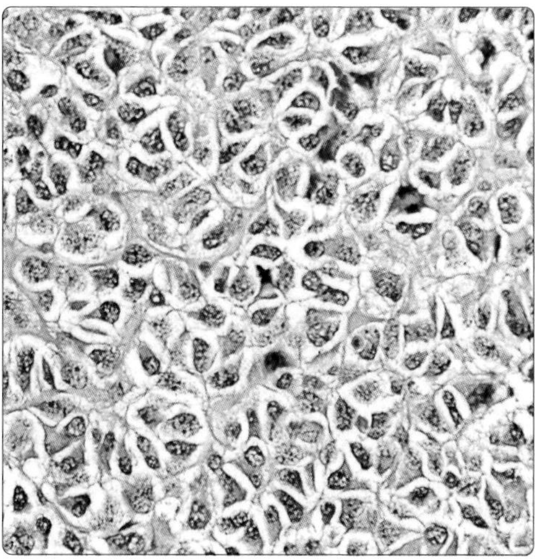

(Left) *Gliofibrillary oligodendrogliomas, especially when high grade, may be compact, lobulated masses with seemingly few overrun normal brain elements.* **(Right)** *Cells in gliofibrillary oligodendrogliomas, particularly grade III examples, can simultaneously appear epithelioid and glial. Note the angular profiles. Oligodendrogliomas require identification of LOH1p, 19q for an "integrated diagnosis."*

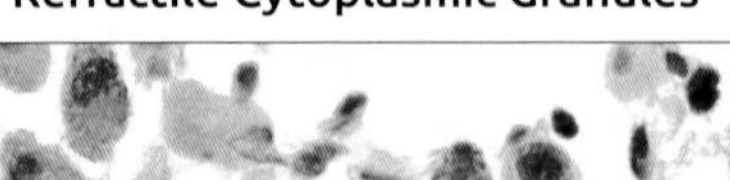

Refractile Cytoplasmic Granules

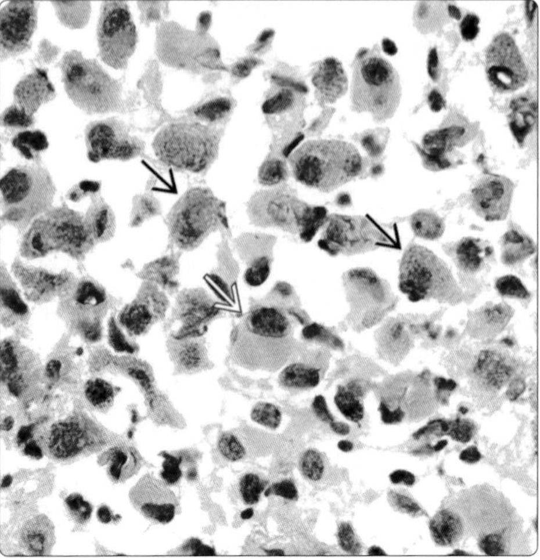

Prominent Nucleoli

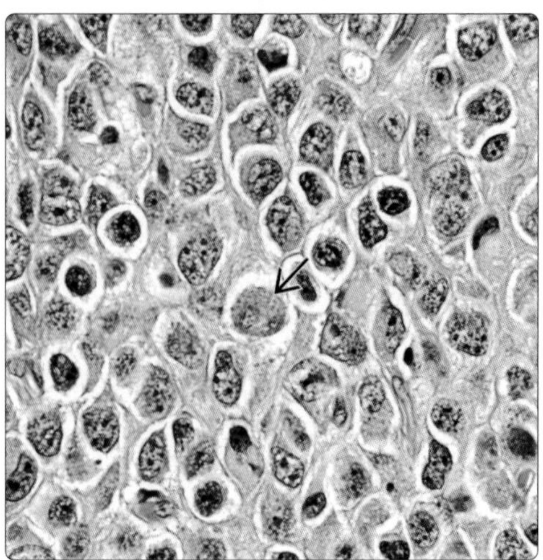

(Left) *Tumor cells stippled with fine, refractile, brightly eosinophilic granules → are almost diagnostic of high-grade oligodendroglioma. Small cells with hyaline cytoplasm → are common but nonspecific since they also occur in astrocytomas.* **(Right)** *Large round nuclei, prominent nucleoli, and sharp cell borders lend an epithelioid or lymphoma-like appearance to some anaplastic oligodendrogliomas. A granule-filled cell → is a clue to the diagnosis.*

Highly Refractile Granular Cells

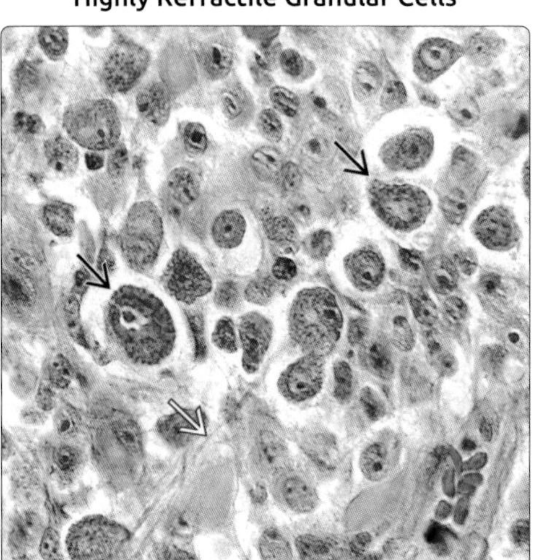

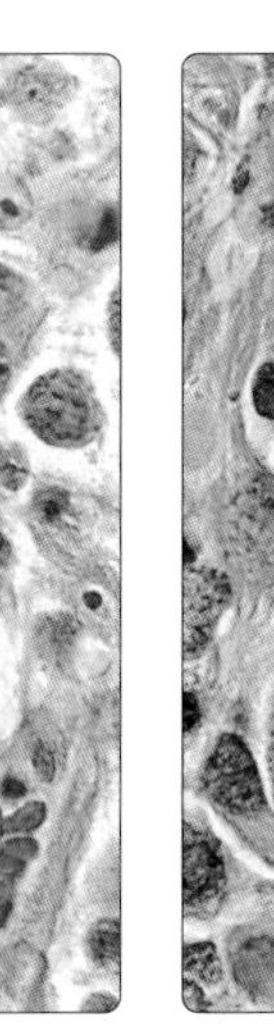

Prominent Eosinophilic Cytoplasm

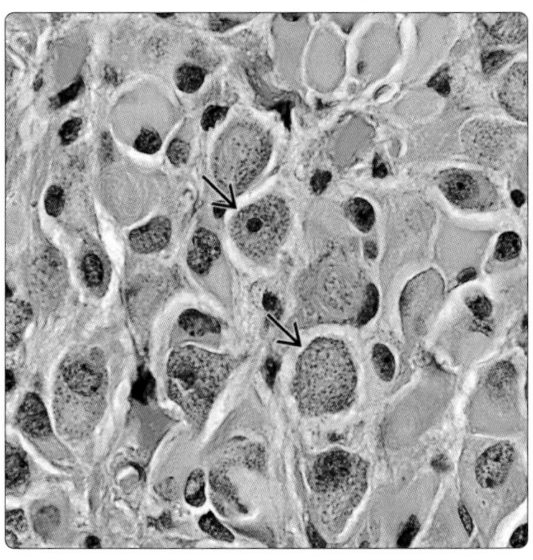

(Left) *Cells with refractile granules → are generally markers of oligodendroglioma, usually anaplastic. Nucleoli are more prominent in oligodendrogliomas than in astrocytomas. An axon traverses the lesion →.* **(Right)** *Regions of some grade III oligodendrogliomas are phenotypically very astrocytic, except for the telltale intracytoplasmic granules →, which are generally not features of astrocytomas.*

Simulating Gemistocytic Astrocytoma

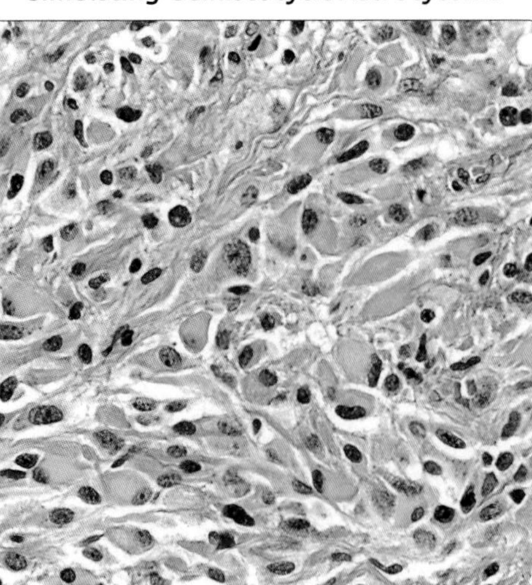

Simulating Fibrillary Astrocytoma

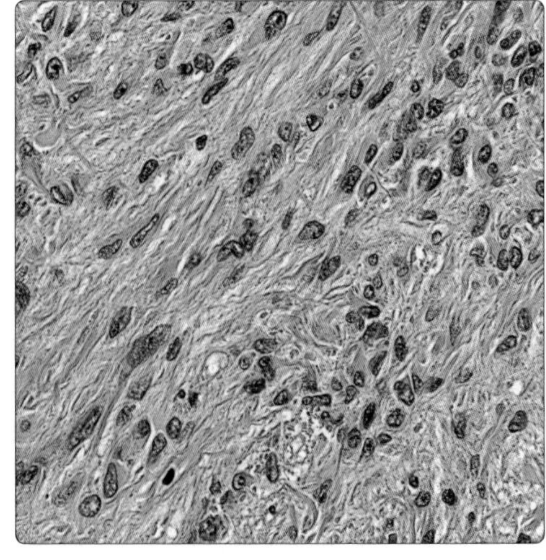

(Left) *Astrocytoma-like areas of grade III oligodendrogliomas somewhat resemble gemistocytic astrocytoma. As here, however, nuclei are less dense and nucleoli are more apparent. The finding of LOH 1p/19q is now required for an "integrated diagnosis" of oligodendroglioma.* **(Right)** *Compact fibrillar areas resembling astrocytoma are not uncommon in anaplastic oligodendrogliomas. Finding classic oligodendroglioma features elsewhere, and 1p/19q codeletion, is important in this setting.*

Bipolar Astrocyte-Like Cells

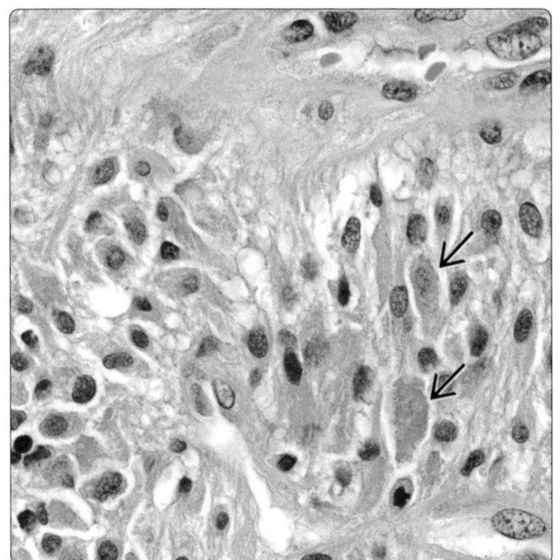

Intracytoplasmic Fibrillar Whorls

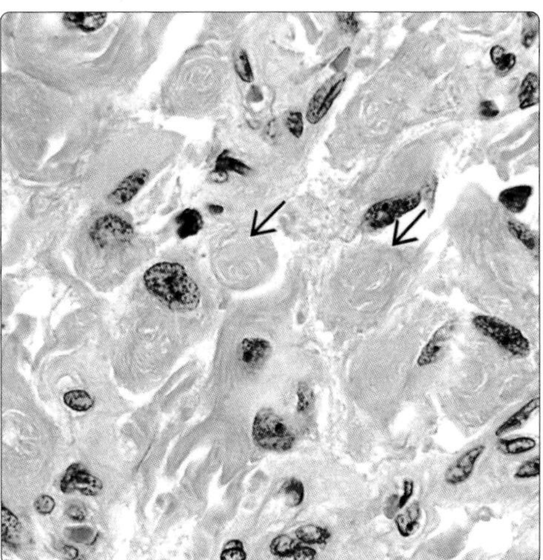

(Left) *Astrocyte-like cells in anaplastic oligodendroglioma assume many forms. Some are spherical, whereas others are bipolar. Intracytoplasmic granules ⇨ suggest oligodendroglioma.* **(Right)** *Phenotypically astrocytic cells are present in some grade III oligodendrogliomas. Intracytoplasmic fibrillar whorls ⇨, like those in more classic minigemistocytes, are characteristic of neoplastic oligodendrocytes in this context.*

Perinuclear Refractile Bands

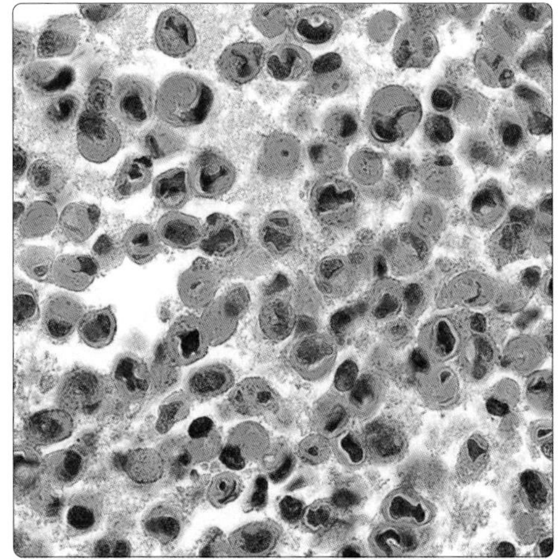

Linear Vascular Proliferation

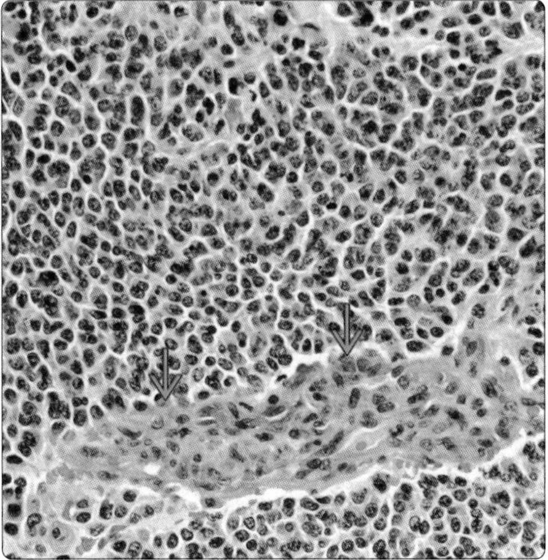

(Left) *Perinuclear, brightly eosinophilic bands appear to distort or "strangle" the nuclei of some grade III oligodendrogliomas.* **(Right)** *While not required for the designation of grade III, the presence of microvascular proliferation ⇨ simplifies the determination in cellular, mitotically active lesions such as this. Vascular proliferation is often more linear than the classic globose, "glomeruloid" masses seen in glioblastoma.*

Necrosis

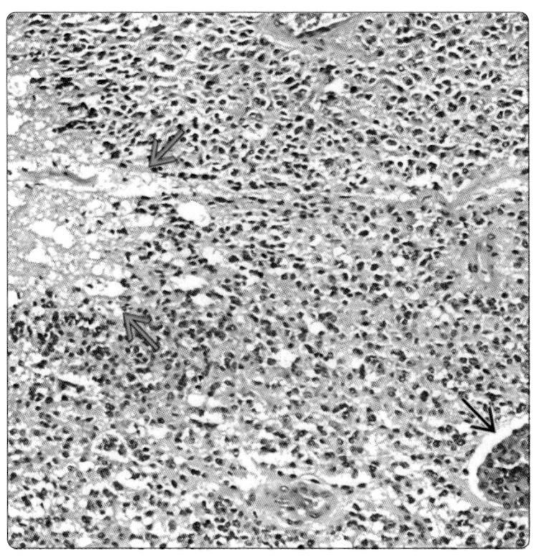

Pseudopalisading Necrosis

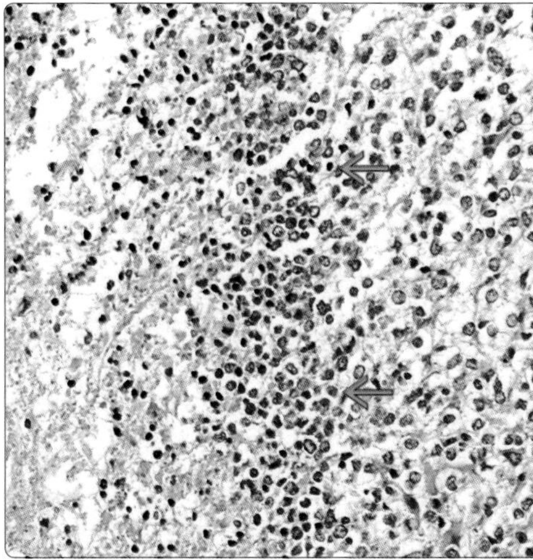

(Left) *Both vascular proliferation ⇨ and necrosis ⇨ are present in some grade III oligodendrogliomas. Small cell glioblastoma would be the principal differential diagnosis in such a case. The necrosis may show pseudopalisading.* **(Right)** *Necrosis in anaplastic oligodendrogliomas may have peripheral pseudopalisading ⇨ but may be only subtle, if present at all. In general, palisading is not as prominent as in glioblastoma.*

Uncommon Metaplastic Ganglion Cells

Metaplastic Ganglion Cells

(Left) *Neuronal differentiation, including metaplastic ganglion cells ⇒, is uncommon in oligodendrogliomas. Far more frequently, large intratumoral ganglion cells are trapped normal elements.* **(Right)** *Metaplastic ganglion cells that uncommonly occur in oligodendrogliomas are immunoreactive for synaptophysin.*

Smaller Sized Metaplastic Ganglion Cells

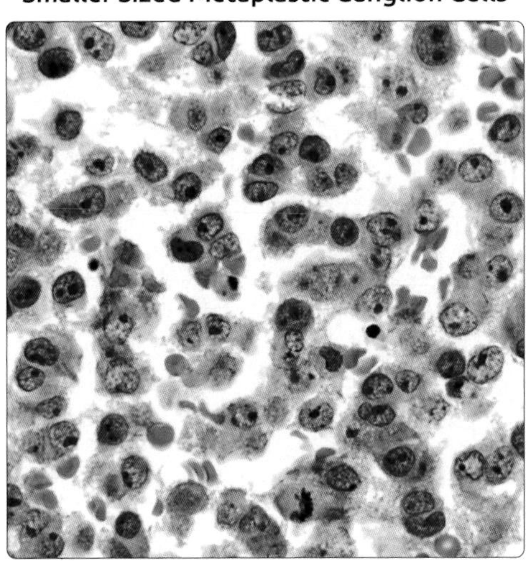

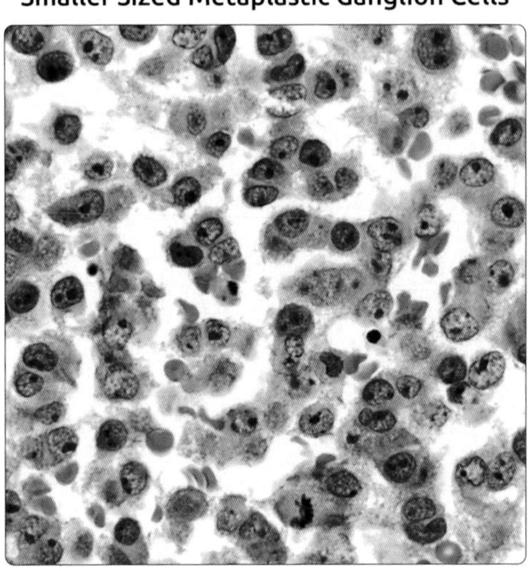

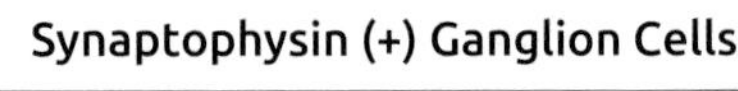

Synaptophysin (+) Ganglion Cells

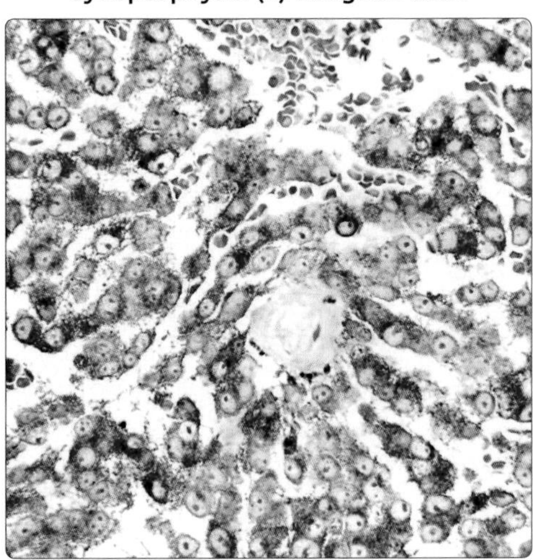

(Left) *Neuronal differentiation may result in cells intermediate between oligodendrocytes and ganglion cells.* **(Right)** *In oligodendrogliomas, tumor cells with neuronal differentiation are immunoreactive for synaptophysin. Cells in this case are smaller than ganglion cells but larger than classic neoplastic oligodendrocytes. Prominent nucleoli typical of large neurons are apparent, even at low magnification.*

Neuropil-Like Areas

Synaptophysin (+) Neuropil

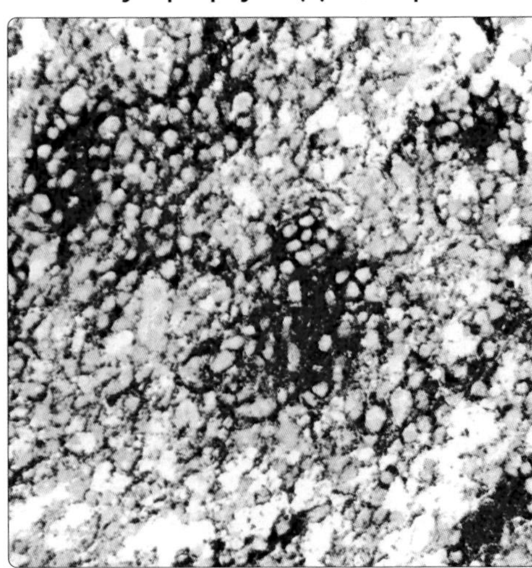

(Left) *Focal area of neuronal differentiation may occur in oligodendrogliomas of grades II or III. In either, such differentiation is expressed as islands of finely fibrillar neuropil ⇒ surrounded by cells whose neuronal nature is affirmed by immunohistochemistry.* **(Right)** *Islands of neuropil react strongly with antibodies to synaptophysin. Similar neuronal differentiation occurs also in infiltrating astrocytomas, usually of high grade.*

Smear: Uniform Round Nuclei

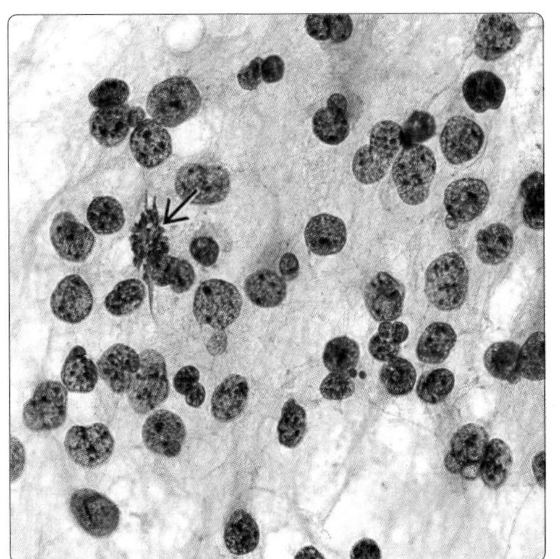

Smear: Gliofibrillary Oligodendrocytes

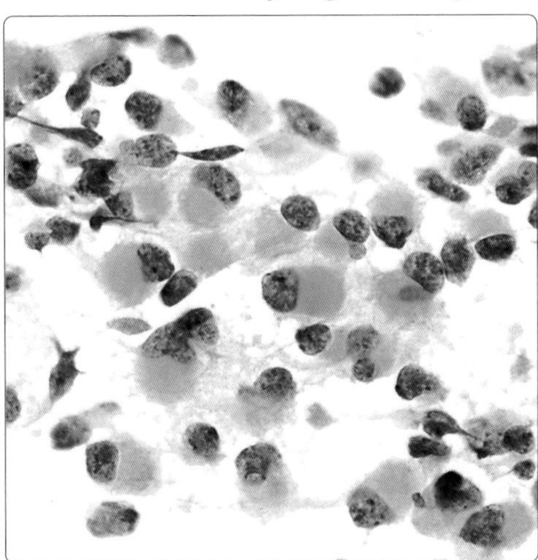

(Left) *Cells with generally round, uniform nuclei and scant cytoplasm are typical of oligodendroglioma. A mitosis is present ➡ in this grade III example.* **(Right)** *Gliofibrillary oligodendrocytes, common in grade III oligodendrogliomas, resemble gemistocytic astrocytes in smear preparations, although processes would be more prominent in the latter. Nuclei are also rounder and less dense than in neoplastic astrocytes.*

GFAP(+) Minigemistocytes

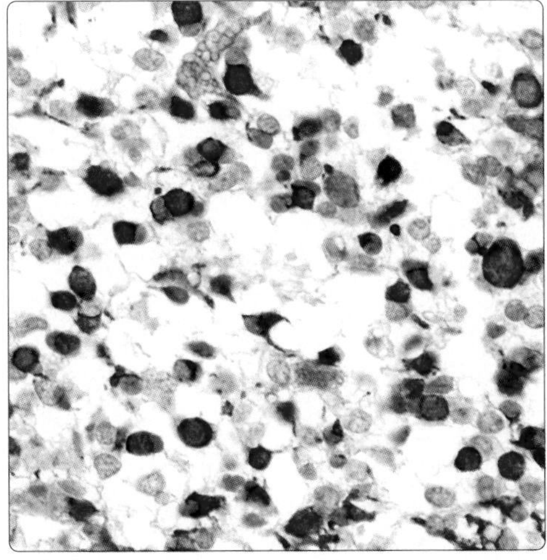

GFAP(+) Gliofibrillary Oligodendrocytes

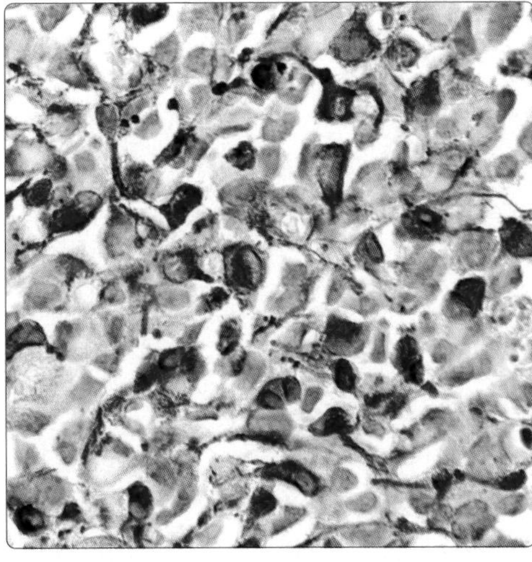

(Left) *Astrocyte-like cells in oligodendrogliomas, whether gliofibrillary, minigemistocyte, or intermediate between them, are often strongly immunoreactive for GFAP.* **(Right)** *GFAP(+) cells with processes are not unusual in oligodendrogliomas, particularly in gliofibrillary oligodendrocytes in grade III tumors. Such cells tend to occur in homogeneous sheets.*

Synaptophysin (+)

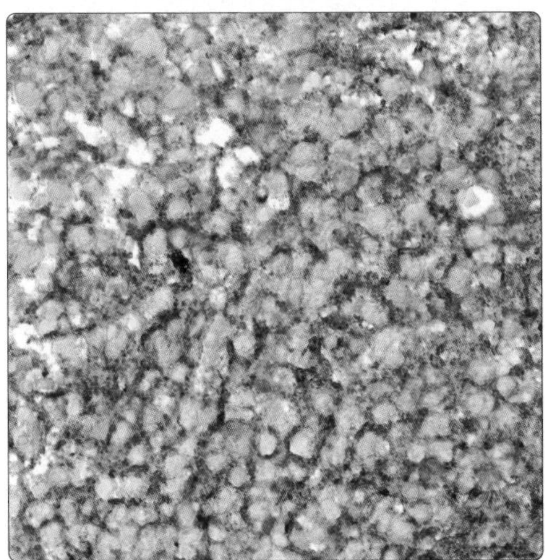

Brisk Ki-67

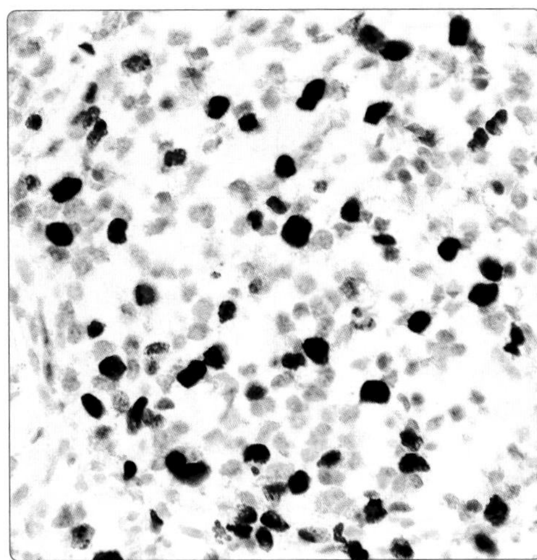

(Left) *Oligodendrogliomas may be immunoreactive for synaptophysin, even in the absence of histologically evident neuronal differentiation. This does not impact grading or prognosis. Such a tumor would be IDH1(+) (or have IDH1/IDH2 mutation) as well as LOH 1p/19q; a neurocytoma would have neither of these genetic features.* **(Right)** *The Ki-67 rate is brisk in grade III oligodendrogliomas, although no threshold index has been established to distinguish them from grade II tumors.*

Mixed Oligoastrocytoma

KEY FACTS

TERMINOLOGY

- Likely to be removed from WHO classification as specific entity
- Subjective, observer-dependent criteria for astrocytes, oligodendrocytes, and intermediate forms
- Molecular studies fail to define oligoastrocytoma (OA) genotype
- Defined by histological characteristics, not molecular features

MICROSCOPIC

- Tumors previously diagnosed as OA are diffuse gliomas of either astrocytic or oligodendroglial molecular subtypes

ANCILLARY TESTS

- Those with astrocytic molecular subtype are mostly IDH-1(+), ATRX(-) and p53(+)
- Those with oligodendroglial molecular subtype are mostly IDH-1(+) and 1p19q codeleted

DIAGNOSTIC CHECKLIST

- Particularly subjective in diagnosing common lesions without clearly defined, distinct areas of astrocytoma and oligodendroglioma
- No firm genetic definition, may be omitted from future WHO classifications
- Consider astrocytoma or oligodendroglioma, especially if IDH-1 immunopositive
- Use IDH-1, ATRX, and p53 immunostaining and FISH analysis for 1p/19q co-deletion
  - Astrocytic if IDH-1, ATRX mutated, ± p53 positivitiy
  - Oligodendroglial if IDH-1 mutated and 1p/19q co-deleted
  - Astrocytic if IDH-1, ATRX and p53 wild type; these tumors may be high grade despite histologic appearance
  - Without these markers, diagnosis should include term not otherwise specified (NOS)

Axial FLAIR MR

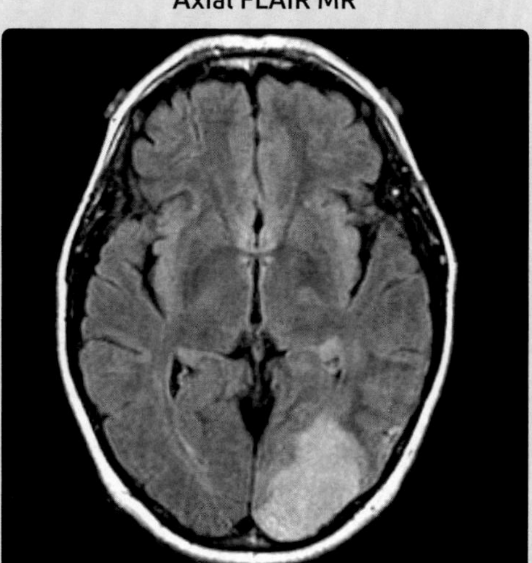

Axial T2WI MR

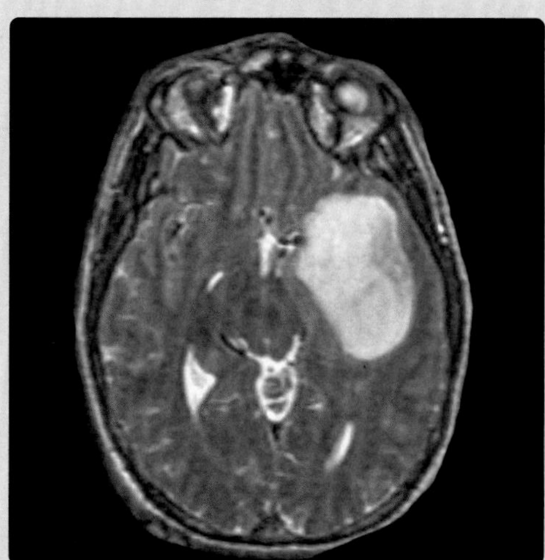

(Left) *This tumor originally reported as oligoastrocytoma with a prominent oligodendroglial component had an IDH1 mutation and 1p19q codeletion. Currently, it will be reported as oligodendroglioma.* **(Right)** *This tumor originally reported as oligoastrocytoma has IDH1 and TP53 mutations and loss of ATRX nuclear immunostaining. There is no 1p or 19q loss. Currently, it will be reported as diffuse astrocytoma.*

Ambiguity in Nuclear Morphology

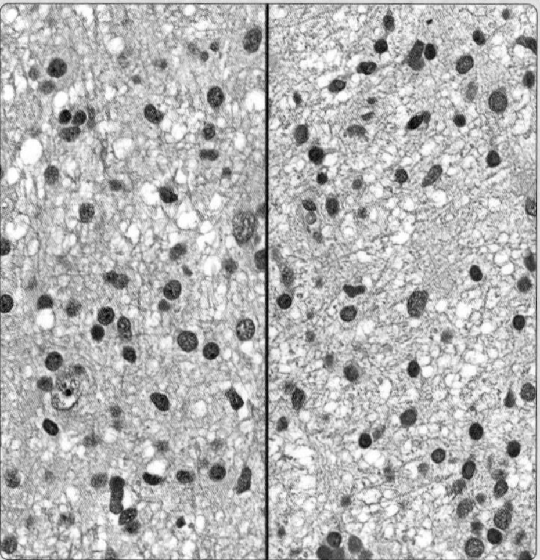

Difficulty in Grading Malignant Gliomas

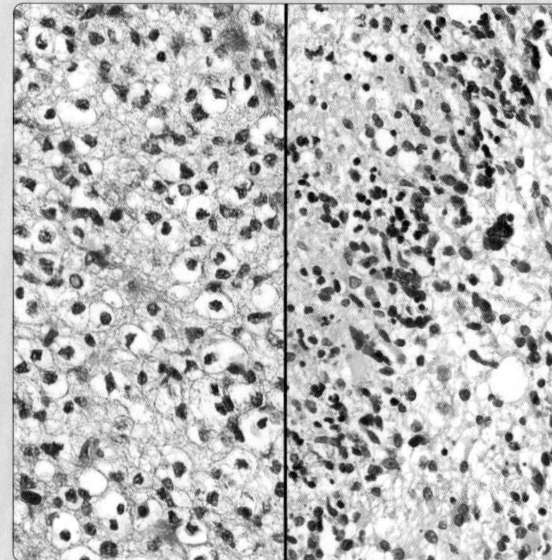

(Left) *One of the challenging issues in the diagnosis of infiltrating gliomas is the presence of variable nuclear size and shape that is interpreted as astrocytoma by some and oligodendroglioma or oligoastrocytoma by others.* **(Right)** *High-grade gliomas with areas of variable nuclear morphology and presence of necrosis were considered either glioblastoma with an oligodendroglioma component or anaplastic oligoastrocytoma, presenting a major dilemma in management.*

TERMINOLOGY

Abbreviations

- Mixed oligoastrocytoma (MOA)
- Oligoastrocytoma (OA)

Synonyms

- Mixed glioma

Definitions

- Subjective diagnosis
  - Varying observer-dependent criteria for what are astrocytes, oligodendrocytes, and intermediate forms
  - Ill-defined clinicopathologic entity
- Defined by histological characteristics, not molecular features
  - No molecular signature
  - Molecular classification of grade II infiltrating gliomas (*ATRX*, *TP53*, *IDH1*, or *IDH2* mutations and 1p/19q codeletion) help avoid ambiguity in diagnosis

CLINICAL ISSUES

Epidemiology

- Age
  - Adults

Site

- Supratentorial

Presentation

- Site-dependent neurological deficits
- Mass effects

Treatment

- Similar to other infiltrating gliomas of equal WHO grade

Prognosis

- Suggested to be better than astrocytoma and worse than oligodendroglioma of comparable WHO grade

MICROSCOPIC

Histologic Features

- No specific histologic feature defined and this tumor type is likely to be omitted from the WHO classification scheme

ANCILLARY TESTS

Immunohistochemistry

- Those with astrocytic molecular subtype are mostly p53(+), IDH-1(+), and ATRX(-)
- Those with oligodendroglial molecular subtype are mostly IDH-1(+) and 1p19q codeleted

Genetic Testing

- Current classification attempts failed to identify genetically unique disease under this diagnosis

DIFFERENTIAL DIAGNOSIS

Reactive Lesions

- Demyelinating disease
  - Sharp border relative to white matter
    - Little or no involvement of gray matter
  - HAM56(+), CD68(+) macrophages
  - Widely scattered multinucleated reactive cells, Creutzfeldt cells
  - Perivascular lymphocytes
- Infarct
  - Cortical necrosis, with ischemic "dead red" neurons
  - Macrophages, prominent
  - Hypertrophy and hyperplasia of small vessel endothelial cells

Astrocytoma

- No clearly defined oligodendroglioma features

Oligodendroglioma

- No astrocytic differentiation

DIAGNOSTIC CHECKLIST

Pathologic Interpretation Pearls

- Consider astrocytoma or oligodendroglioma, especially if IDH-1 immunopositive
- No genetic signature for OA recognized in recent TCGA studies
- Likely to be removed as a specific entity

SELECTED REFERENCES

1. Hartmann C et al: Molecular markers in low-grade gliomas: predictive or prognostic? Clin Cancer Res. 17(13):4588-99, 2011
2. Ohgaki H et al: Genetic profile of astrocytic and oligodendroglial gliomas. Brain Tumor Pathol. 28(3):177-83, 2011
3. Kim YH et al: Molecular classification of low-grade diffuse gliomas. Am J Pathol. 177(6):2708-14, 2010
4. Miller CR et al: Significance of necrosis in grading of oligodendroglial neoplasms: a clinicopathologic and genetic study of newly diagnosed high-grade gliomas. J Clin Oncol. 24(34):5419-26, 2006
5. van den Bent MJ et al: Adjuvant procarbazine, lomustine, and vincristine improves progression-free survival but not overall survival in newly diagnosed anaplastic oligodendrogliomas and oligoastrocytomas: a randomized European Organisation for Research and Treatment of Cancer phase III trial. J Clin Oncol. 24(18):2715-22, 2006
6. Perry A et al: Small cell astrocytoma: an aggressive variant that is clinicopathologically and genetically distinct from anaplastic oligodendroglioma. Cancer. 101(10):2318-26, 2004
7. Maintz D et al: Molecular genetic evidence for subtypes of oligoastrocytomas. J Neuropathol Exp Neurol. 56(10):1098-104, 1997
8. Hart MN et al: Mixed gliomas. Cancer. 33(1):134-40, 1974

Pilocytic Astrocytoma

KEY FACTS

TERMINOLOGY

- Low-grade, generally well-circumscribed tumor with biphasic pattern, WHO grade I
- Criteria for anaplasia or WHO grades higher than I not well established
- Increased mitotic rate ± palisading necrosis may imply more aggressive behavior
- Pilomyxoid astrocytoma (PMA) only recognized variant to date

CLINICAL ISSUES

- Extent of resection is most important prognostic factor
- Overall survival excellent, but residual tumor and neurological deficits may remain

IMAGING

- Cystic tumor with enhancing mural nodule
- Optic PA more solid and variable enhancement

MICROSCOPIC

- Generally well circumscribed
- Infiltration in some cases, especially cerebellum, optic nerve, chiasm, and tract
- Rosenthal fibers and less commonly eosinophilic granular bodies (EGBs)
- Compact fibrillar tissue, sometimes with spongy component (biphasic pattern)
- Vascular proliferation, usually glomeruloid microvascular proliferation common in cystic tumors
- Some tumors may have mixed PA and PMA features

ANCILLARY TESTS

- Activation of MAPK pathway
  - Mostly *KIAA1549-BRAF* fusion detectable, especially in posterior fossa tumors
  - Few tumors are BRAF V600E(+) or carry *NF1* mutations
- Immunohistochemical studies can help differentiate diffuse gliomas from PA

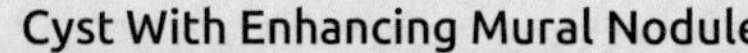

Cyst With Enhancing Mural Nodule

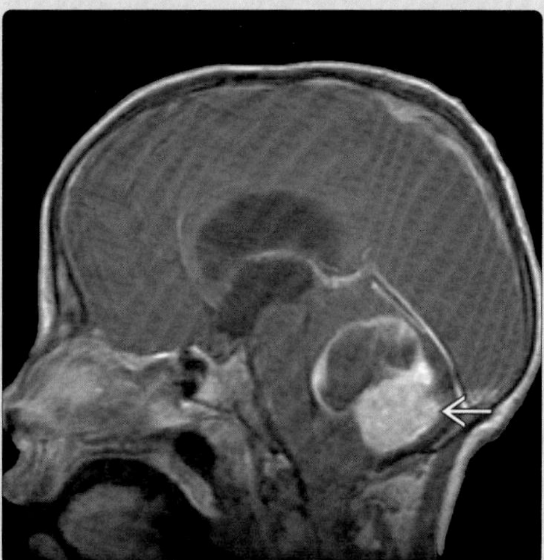

Biphasic, Focally Myxoid Tumor

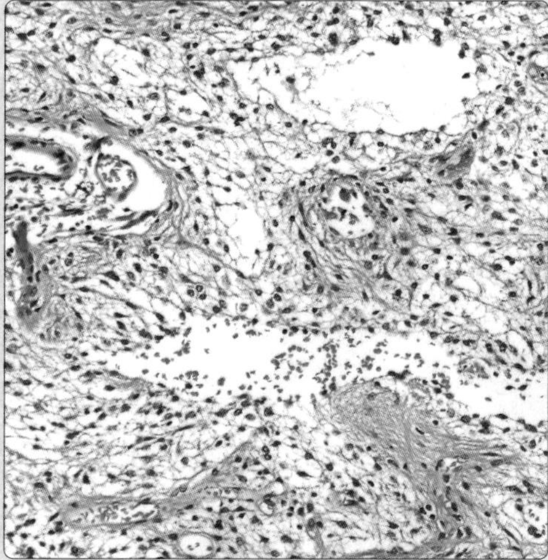

(Left) *Typically, pilocytic astrocytoma (PA) in the posterior fossa has a solid-cystic appearance with a diffusely enhancing solid component ➡. Despite the presence of hydrocephalus in most cases, there is limited mass effect or peritumoral edema.* **(Right)** *PAs often demonstrate biphasic pattern with loose, myxoid areas admixed with eosinophilic compact regions. The compact areas often harbor Rosenthal fibers.*

Rosenthal Fibers

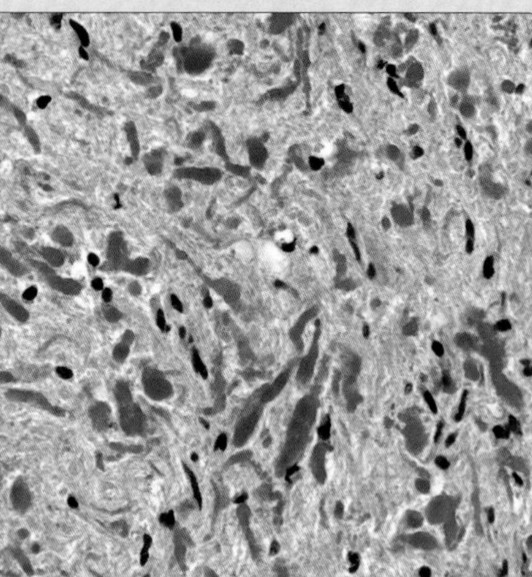

FISH for BRAF Fusion

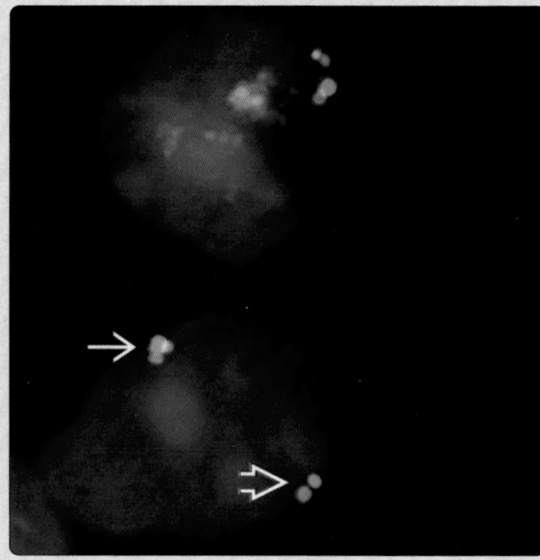

(Left) *Rosenthal fibers are eosinophilic irregular elongated "corkscrew" protein aggregates and when identified in tumor tissue, they help establish the diagnosis of PA.* **(Right)** *The KIAA1549-BRAF duplication can be detected using FISH. The duplicated gene segment can be visualized as 2 red spots ➡, in comparison with the normal chromosome 7 probes showing 1 signal each for the BRAF probe and the centromeric probe ➡.*

TERMINOLOGY

Abbreviations

- Pilocytic astrocytoma (PA)
- Juvenile pilocytic astrocytoma (JPA), obsolete term
- Pilomyxoid astrocytoma (PMA) variant of PA

Definitions

- Low-grade, generally well-circumscribed tumor with typical biphasic fibrillar piloid and hypofibrillar spongy patterns
- WHO grade I
- Tumors with anaplastic features described, but WHO grade is not assigned to these tumors
- Only 1 variant, pilomyxoid astrocytoma, described to date

ETIOLOGY/PATHOGENESIS

Neurofibromatosis 1 (NF1) Association

- Minority of cases
- Usually optic nerve PAs, typically bilateral, but may be seen anywhere in neuraxis

CLINICAL ISSUES

Presentation

- Variable presentation depending on location
  - Optic nerves: Proptosis, visual loss
  - Optic chiasm/hypothalamus: Visual loss, hypothalamic dysfunction, diencephalic syndrome (rare)
  - Cerebellum: Cerebellar dysfunction (ataxia), especially with vermian lesions, consequences of obstructive hydrocephalus
  - Spinal cord: Motor and sensory deficits depending on level affected
  - Intra- and paraventricular: Obstructive hydrocephalus
  - Peripheral cerebral hemispheres: Seizures, focal neurological deficits, mass effects

Treatment

- Surgical approaches
  - Extent of resection most important prognostic factor
  - Some tumors may remain dormant or even regress following partial resection
- Drugs
  - Usually considered for recurrent, multifocal, or progressive tumors
  - MAPK pathway inhibitors appear promising
- Radiation
  - Usually after recurrence or progression
  - Suggestion that early radiation may not be advisable
  - Rare examples of malignant progression years after radiation treatment

Prognosis

- Overall survival good, but residual tumor and neurological deficits may persist
- Most favorable for cerebellar, optic nerve, superficial cerebral, and spinal cord tumors
- Less favorable when central or hypothalamic
- Solid component often stable or slow growing
- Cyst recurrence or reformation is common especially for subtotally resected tumors
- Spontaneous regression, especially in optic nerve PAs in NF1 (rare)
- Dissemination in CSF pathways (rare) more common with the pilomyxoid variant
- Transformation to high-grade lesion (rare)
  - Radiation induced
    - Anaplastic transformation of primary tumor
    - Emergence of malignant infiltrating glioma in radiation field
  - Spontaneous
    - Some anaplastic PAs emerge de-novo without prior low-grade tumor, and nature of such tumors is controversial
    - Some typical PAs can progress to malignant gliomas in absence of prior radiation

IMAGING

MR Findings

- Discrete, usually with enhancing component
- Often macrocystic with enhancing nodule, especially in cerebellum, peripheral cerebral hemispheres, and spinal cord
- Often dorsally exophytic on brainstem or with cerebellopontine angle extension
- Usually little peritumoral edema
- More infiltrative in visual pathways
- Optic PA often solid without cystic component and variable enhancement
- Rare examples demonstrate leptomeningeal spread on contrast enhanced images
- Cyst wall occasionally enhances
- Rare examples with peripheral rim enhancement around cystic component

MACROSCOPIC

General Features

- Well circumscribed
- Often cystic with mural nodule in cerebellum, cerebrum, and spinal cord
- Occasional examples with hemorrhage

MICROSCOPIC

Histologic Features

- Borders/growth pattern
  - Generally well circumscribed
  - Infiltration in some cases, especially cerebellum and at tumor periphery
  - Leptomeningeal extension, especially in optic nerve and cerebellum, **not** sign of aggressive behavior
  - Filling of perivascular spaces
  - Astrocytic appearance, fibrillary background (majority)
  - Oligodendroglioma like, especially in cerebellum
  - Polar-spongioblastoma-like pattern (rare)
  - Diffuse infiltrative appearance (rare)
  - Focal areas with perivascular or angiocentric arrangement
- Cellular patterns
  - Compact fibrillar tissue with spongy component producing biphasic pattern

- Spongy tissue with myxoid appearance
- Degenerative nuclear atypia, more often in adult tumors
- Nuclear clustering or multinucleation, imparting pennies on a plate appearance
- Transitions to, or mixed features with PMA
- Myxoid background (variable and almost always focal if present)
- Rosenthal fibers in piloid or compact tissue
- Eosinophilic granular bodies, especially in spongy tissue
- Calcification in minority of cases, psammoma bodies exceptional
- Macrocyst, usually nonneoplastic wall
- Degenerative changes
  - Nuclear pleomorphism and smudgy chromatin
  - Multiple nuclei in large cells with ample cytoplasm
  - Angioma-like sclerotic vessels, especially cerebellar
  - Often seen in tumors from older patients
- Necrosis: Coagulative, usually no pseudopalisading
- Vascular proliferation
  - Intraparenchymal telangiectatic or glomeruloid in many cases
  - Cyst wall: Telangiectatic or glomeruloid in linear arrangement
  - Multilayered (true endothelial proliferation) in some anaplastic tumors
- Features of rare anaplastic examples
  - Histological criteria for anaplasia in PA not currently well established
  - Often adults and exceptionally children
  - Increased cellularity and infiltrative pattern
  - Increased rate of mitoses, more than just focal
    - Mitotic rate threshold for anaplastic examples not established
    - High Ki-67 index similar to high-grade gliomas, but cut-off value has not been established
  - Nuclear pleomorphism and cytological atypia reminiscent of malignant glioma beyond simple multinucleation or degenerative atypia
  - Palisading necrosis, (rare)

ANCILLARY TESTS

Cytology

- Bipolar, hair-like cells with long, narrow processes
- Round or ovoid, elongate nuclei
- Focal myxoid background
- Rosenthal fibers and eosinophilic granular bodies
- Bland nuclei with vesicular chromatin

Immunohistochemistry

- GFAP(+)
- Olig2(+), especially in oligodendroglioma-like and spongy areas
- Synaptophysin
  - Sometimes (+), especially in pilomyxoid variant
  - Not sign of neuronal differentiation
- Neurofilament often sparse positive, highlighting axonal structures at periphery
- Vimentin, SOX2, S100 protein, and MAP-2 (+), often diffuse and strong (all nonspecific)
- pERK(+) especially for tumors with BRAF duplication
- p16(+) often diffuse nuclear, negative p16 staining associated with worse outcome
- Ki-67
  - Tumors have low labeling (< 5%) but occasional tumor may be higher
  - Proliferating vessels, high
- IDH-1(-)

Genetic Testing

- Activation of MAPK pathway
  - Tandem duplication of *BRAF;* fusion with *KIAA1549*
    - Highest incidence in posterior fossa and optic pathways (60% or more); low in cerebral cortex
    - Often detected by FISH assay
  - Other fusion types have also been reported
  - *BRAF* mutation (V600E) in a small percentage of tumors
  - Other activating events include *SRGAP3-RAF1*
  - Mutations lead to MAPK pathway activation through increased pERK
- *NF1* mutation (rare)
- Molecular changes typical of diffuse astrocytomas are absent

DIFFERENTIAL DIAGNOSIS

Piloid Gliosis

- Accompanying tumors (e.g., craniopharyngioma, hemangioblastoma), cysts, and nonneoplastic lesions
- No loose, spongy component
- Low cellularity, variable amount of inflammatory cells
- Hemosiderin, e.g., around ependymoma
- Often MAP-2(-)

Pilomyxoid Astrocytoma

- Monomorphous, small bipolar cells
- Perivascular formations resemble pseudorosettes of ependymoma (angiocentric pattern), often prominent
- Prominent myxoid background
- No (or only few) eosinophilic granular bodies or Rosenthal fibers

Fibrillary (Diffuse) Astrocytoma

- Diffuse or infiltrating
- Secondary structures, e.g., subpial accumulation of cells or perineuronal satellitosis
- Generally no Rosenthal fibers or eosinophilic granular bodies
- Generally not macrocystic
- IDH-1(+); and no BRAF duplication in adults and adolescents
- Pediatric tumors ATRX loss &/or H3.3. K27M(+) on immunohistochemistry

Oligodendroglioma

- Diffusely infiltrating, predilection to cortex
  - Secondary structures: Perineuronal satellitosis, subpial spread
- 1p/19q codeletion but usually absent in pediatric tumors
- Unusual in cerebellum and spinal cord
- Almost always IDH-1(+) in adults
- Exceedingly rare in the posterior fossa

Ganglioglioma

- Overlap between ganglioglioma with pilocytic features and pilocytic astrocytoma with trapped or neoplastic ganglion cells
- Perivascular lymphocytes
- Eosinophilic granular bodies usually more prominent
- Generally higher ganglion cells:piloid tissue ratio
- BRAF V600E(+) and no *BRAF-KIAA1549* fusion
- CD34(+) in arachnoid pattern in neoplastic ganglion cells

Pleomorphic Xanthoastrocytoma

- Significant component in subarachnoid space
  - Compact rather than loose, spongy architecture
  - Giant cells
  - Pleomorphism
  - Eosinophilic granular bodies (EGBs); no significant Rosenthal fibers
  - Lipidized cells
  - Reticulin rich in leptomeningeal component
  - Perivascular lymphocytes
- Associated infiltrating cortical component

Dysembryoplastic Neuroepithelial Tumor

- Intracortical
- Well-circumscribed, patterned nodules with myxoid background [Alcian blue (+)]
- Almost exclusively uniform oligodendroglioma-like cells
  - Only minority with overtly glial appearing component
- Floating neurons, mostly between nodules
- Leptomeningeal involvement uncommon
- No biphasic pattern
- Surrounding cortical dysplasia in some cases
- As a rule, no Rosenthal fibers or granular bodies
- Little if any mass effect

Rosetted Glioneuronal Tumor (of 4th Ventricle)

- Glial component may be exactly like PA
- Neurocytic rosettes
- Synaptophysin(+) perivascular pseudorosettes
- More often in adults

Ependymoma

- Small biopsies of posterior fossa or spinal cord ependymomas may contain Rosenthal fibers in surrounding tissue (piloid gliosis)
- Perivascular pseudorosettes different than angiocentric pattern of PA
- Salt and pepper-type nuclear chromatin pattern and occasional true ependymal rosettes
- No *BRAF* mutation or duplication
- Olig2 often stains small percentage of tumor cells

DIAGNOSTIC CHECKLIST

Clinically Relevant Pathologic Features

- Stable, exceptional malignant transformation; typically chronic disease
- Spontaneous regression (uncommon), especially in neurofibromatosis 1
- Malignant progression ± prior radiation treatment (rare)

Pathologic Interpretation Pearls

- Do not exclude because of focal infiltrative pattern, especially in cerebellum
- Do not misinterpret vascular proliferation or necrosis as malignant glioma
- Molecular features are helpful in diagnosis
  - Almost all tumors IDH-1 immunonegative (no mutation)
  - RAS/RAF/MAPK pathway activation majority of tumors
  - FISH assay for BRAF duplication recommended

SELECTED REFERENCES

1. Kleinschmidt-DeMasters BK et al: Pilomyxoid Astrocytoma (PMA) Shows Significant Differences in Gene Expression vs. Pilocytic Astrocytoma (PA) and Variable Tendency Toward Maturation to PA. Brain Pathol. ePub, 2014
2. Tihan T et al: Pathologic characteristics of pediatric intracranial pilocytic astrocytomas and their impact on outcome in 3 countries: a multi-institutional study. Am J Surg Pathol. 36(1):43-55, 2012
3. Schindler G et al: Analysis of BRAF V600E mutation in 1,320 nervous system tumors reveals high mutation frequencies in pleomorphic xanthoastrocytoma, ganglioglioma and extra-cerebellar pilocytic astrocytoma. Acta Neuropathol. 121(3):397-405, 2011
4. Capper D et al: Characterization of R132H mutation-specific IDH1 antibody binding in brain tumors. Brain Pathol. 20(1):245-54, 2010
5. Horbinski C et al: Association of molecular alterations, including BRAF, with biology and outcome in pilocytic astrocytomas. Acta Neuropathol. 119(5):641-9, 2010
6. Horbinski C et al: Impact of morphology, MIB-1, p53 and MGMT on outcome in pilocytic astrocytomas. Brain Pathol. 20(3):581-8, 2010
7. Johnson MW et al: Spectrum of pilomyxoid astrocytomas: intermediate pilomyxoid tumors. Am J Surg Pathol. 34(12):1783-91, 2010
8. Riemenschneider MJ et al: Molecular diagnostics of gliomas: state of the art. Acta Neuropathol. 120(5):567-84, 2010
9. Rodriguez FJ et al: Anaplasia in pilocytic astrocytoma predicts aggressive behavior. Am J Surg Pathol. 34(2):147-60, 2010
10. Korshunov A et al: Combined molecular analysis of BRAF and IDH1 distinguishes pilocytic astrocytoma from diffuse astrocytoma. Acta Neuropathol. 118(3):401-5, 2009
11. Bar EE et al: Frequent gains at chromosome 7q34 involving BRAF in pilocytic astrocytoma. J Neuropathol Exp Neurol. 67(9):878-87, 2008
12. Ishizawa K et al: Olig2 and CD99 are useful negative markers for the diagnosis of brain tumors. Clin Neuropathol. 27(3):118-28, 2008
13. Tanaka Y et al: Diversity of glial cell components in pilocytic astrocytoma. Neuropathology. 28(4):399-407, 2008

(Left) *Solid components of PAs are often hyperintense on T2 and FLAIR and isointense on T1-weighted images when compared to gray matter. There is often limited mass effect and peritumoral edema.* **(Right)** *In most PAs, the contrast enhancement is seen in the solid component, but occasional PAs demonstrate enhancement around the cyst wall. This pattern may be mistaken for the rim enhancement of malignant gliomas. Note the limited amount of mass effect and peritumoral edema.*

Solid Tumor on FLAIR MR

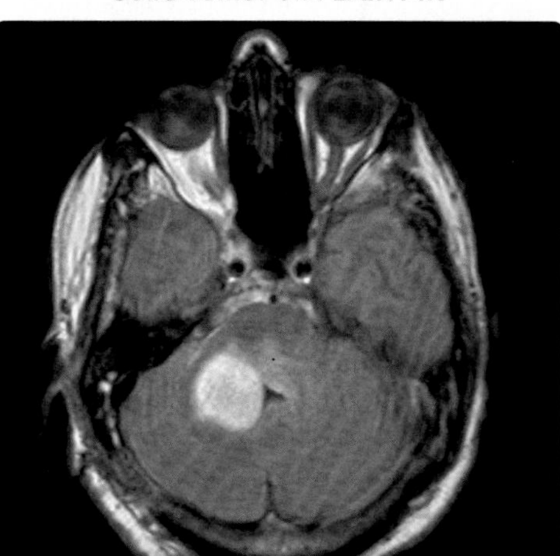

Cystic Contrast-Enhancing Mass

(Left) *Most PAs typically demonstrate loose, myxoid component and a more compact, eosinophilic component in which Rosenthal fibers are more commonly observed. This classical pattern is present in most, but not all, examples.* **(Right)** *Most PAs demonstrates a very elaborate fibrillary or hair-like (piloid), as well as variably myxoid, background on smear. Most tumor cells have bipolar processes and bland, oval, or round nuclei.*

Biphasic Architecture

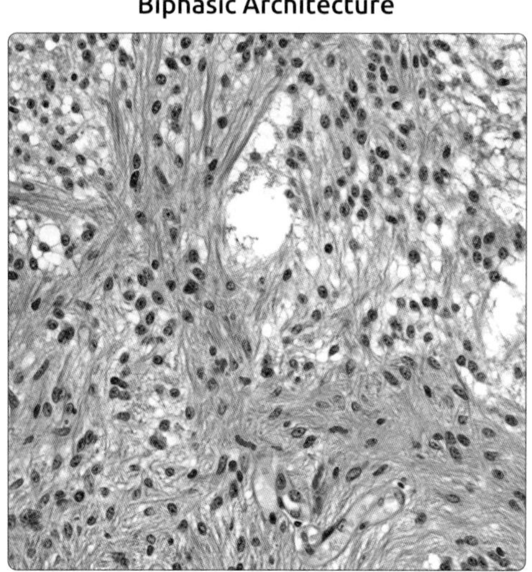

Piloid Background on Smear

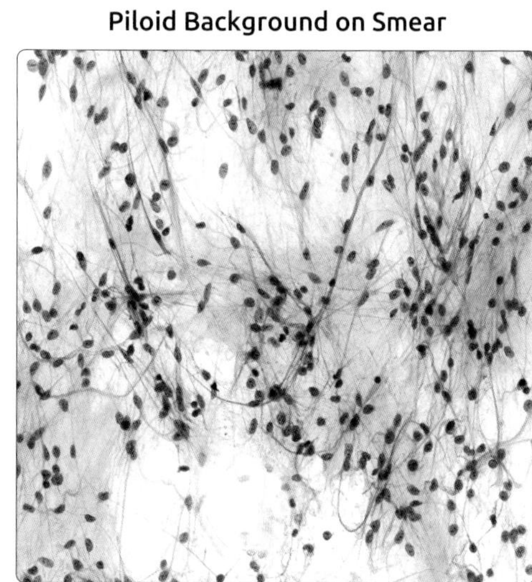

(Left) *The typical piloid or hair-like cells of PA often have conspicuous, but variable amount, of eosinophilic cytoplasm. In paraffin sections, the bipolar nature of the cells ⇒ may not be readily recognizable.* **(Right)** *Rosenthal fibers, while not specific for PA, are often present in the compact, cellular component of the tumor. It is critical to recognize these structures within the tumor tissue, since Rosenthal fibers are more commonly seen in the reactive parenchyma adjacent to many other pathological processes.*

Piloid Cells in Sections

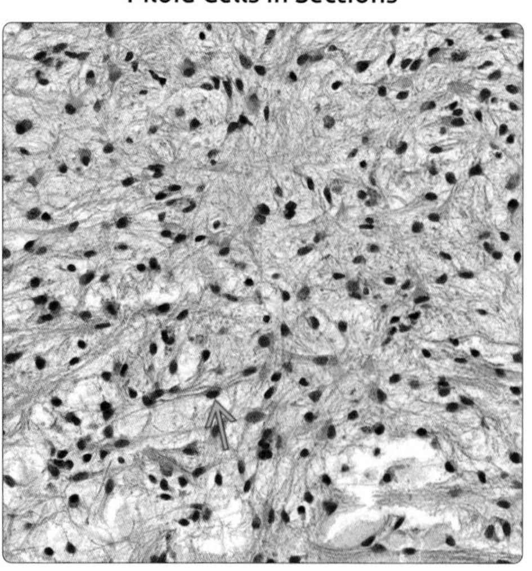

Rosenthal Fibers

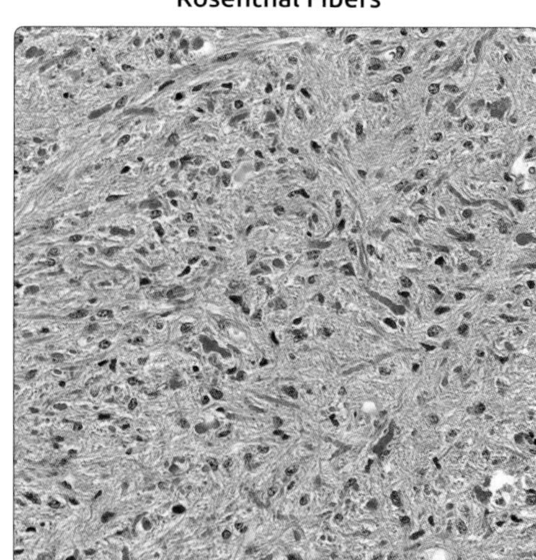

Microcystic Architecture

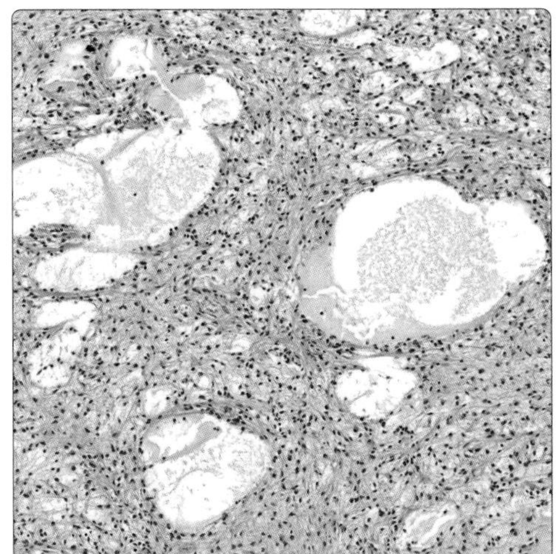

Rosenthal Fibers

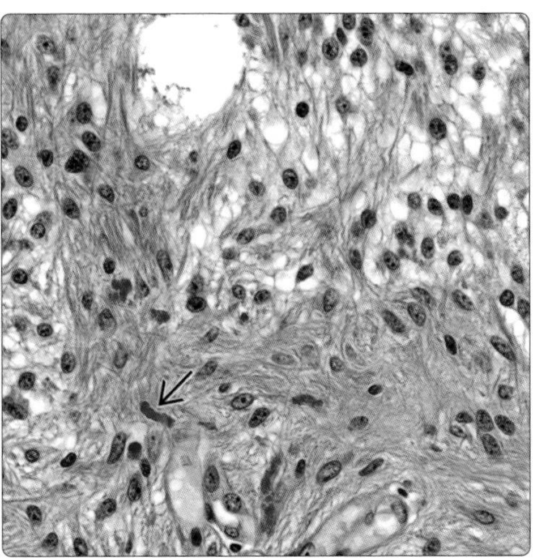

(Left) *Many PAs have numerous microscopic "cysts," which are in reality not true cysts but expansion of extracellular space that often contain myxoid material. This pattern may be confused with the so-called microcystic appearance of diffuse gliomas.* **(Right)** *The classic biphasic lesion has loose, spongy tissue and a densely fibrillar element, often with Rosenthal fibers ➙.*

Mural Nodule: Solid Component

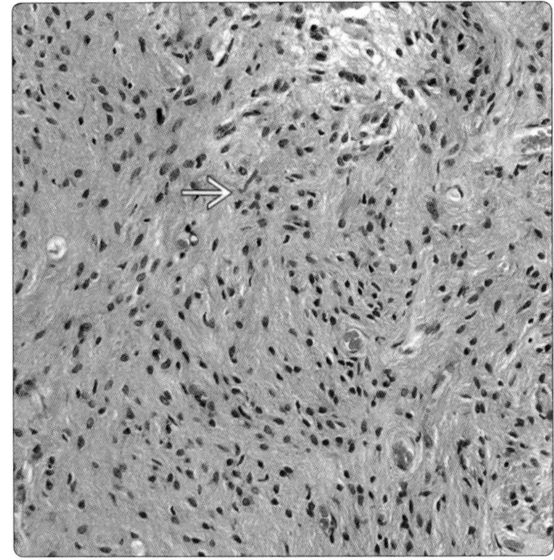

Hyalinized Vessels

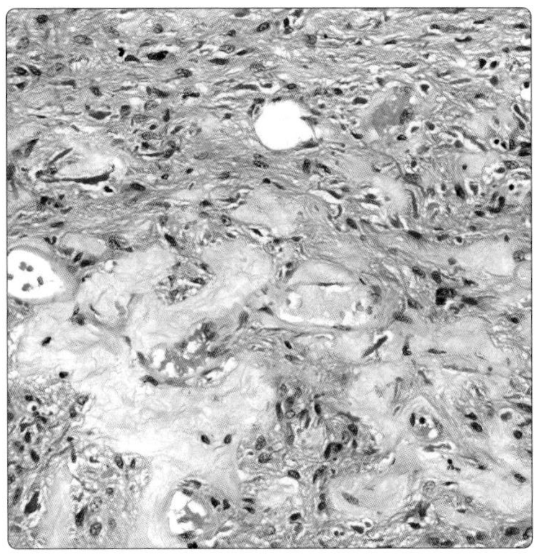

(Left) *The solid component of the tumor, or the tissue from the mural nodule, often demonstrates increased cellularity, a compact eosinophilic background, and Rosenthal fibers ➙. This appearance, along with the noninfiltrative nature of the tumor, is diagnostic of PA.* **(Right)** *In most PAs, the tumor vasculature as well as those in the surrounding tissues demonstrate mural hyalinization and thickening. Such vascular changes have been associated with an increased tendency for intratumoral bleeding.*

Pennies on a Plate

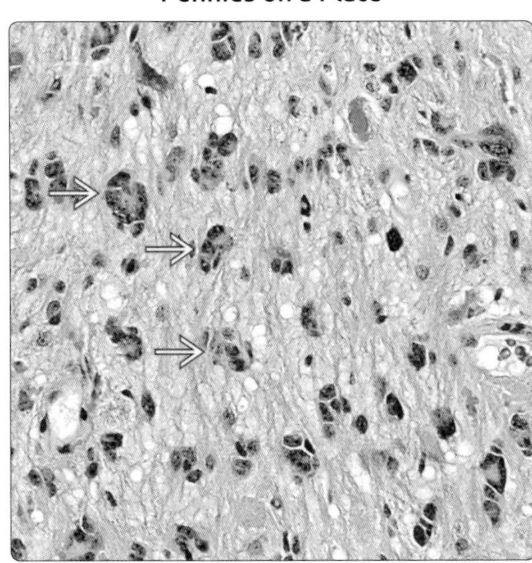

Hyalin Globules and EGBs

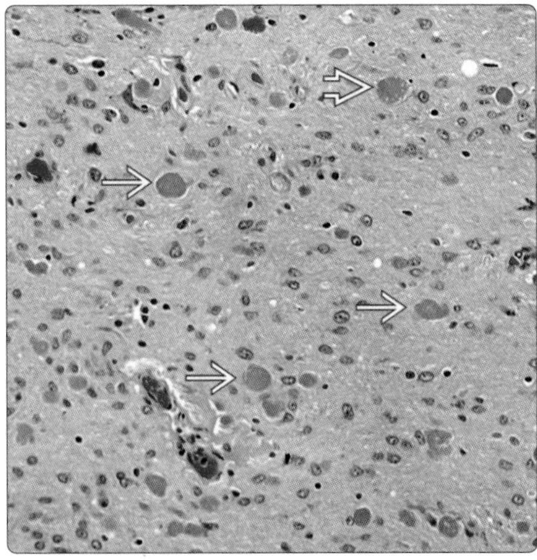

(Left) *Cells with a pennies on a plate ➙ distribution of their multiple nuclei are a common form of degenerative atypia. This is a very characteristic and helpful feature for the diagnosis of PA.* **(Right)** *Many PAs harbor eosinophilic structures that can either be classified as eosinophilic granular bodies (EGBs) ➙ or hyalin globules ➙. These structures often harbor an array of proteins. Such structures can also be encountered in ganglioglioma, a tumor in the differential diagnosis of PA.*

(Left) *A row of proliferating vessels* ➩ *often lies just outside a cyst lumen. This type of vascular proliferation, especially in a cyst wall, is generally a sign of a low-, rather than a high-grade, neoplasm.* **(Right)** *In some PAs, multinucleated cells along with bizarre nuclei in tumor cells with ample cytoplasm can evoke the appearance of a degenerative process. Such features have not been associated with aggressive behavior and are occasionally considered to represent ancient change.*

Granulation Tissue-Type Vascularity

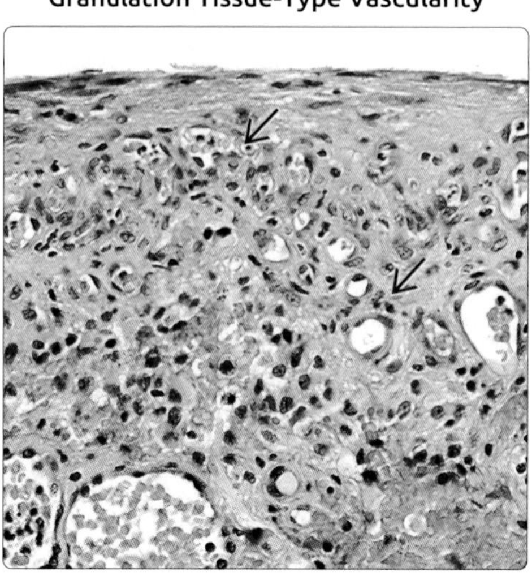

Degenerative Atypia

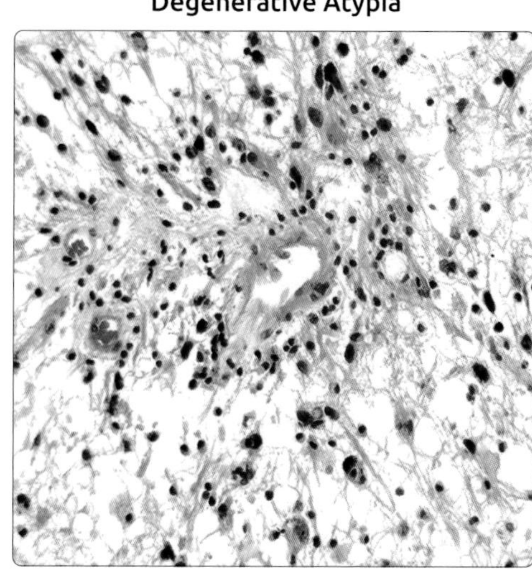

(Left) *The leptomeninges are seemingly conducive to tumor growth and expansion. The appearance of an extraaxial lesion can be created. As here, the leptomeningeal component typically has a sharp interface* ➩ *with the pial surface of the underlying brain.* **(Right)** *Nested cells may be the only decisive evidence of pilocytic astrocytoma in an example with predominantly infiltrative properties. Such tissue is most likely to be found in a leptomeningeal component.*

Leptomeningeal Growth

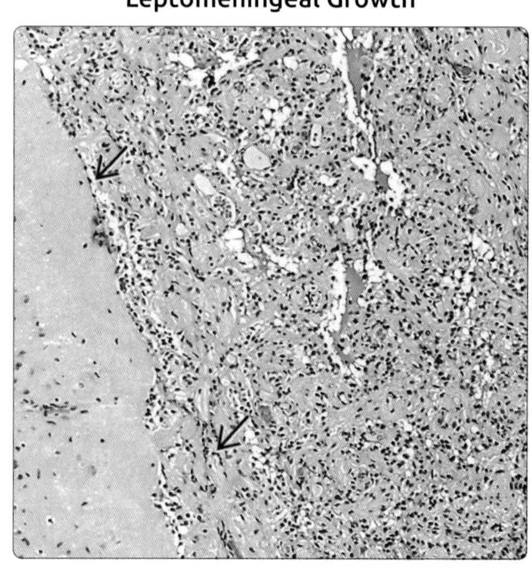

Leptomeningeal Component

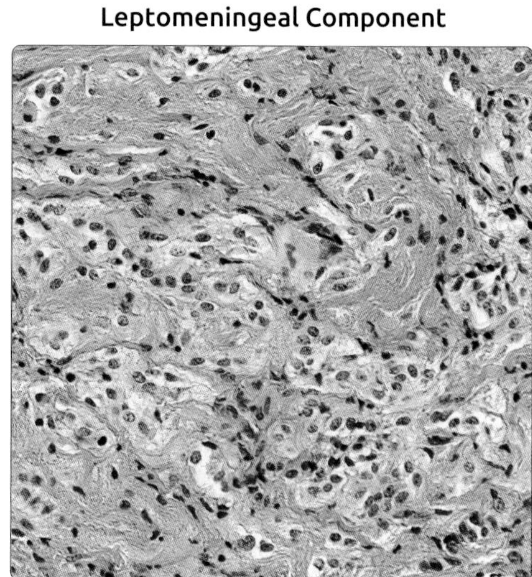

(Left) *Many pilocytic astrocytomas have loose, spongy tissue with microcysts with proteinaceous contents. The addition of encompassing condensed fibrillar tissue creates the classic biphasic pattern.* **(Right)** *Florid glomeruloid microvascular proliferation in linear arrays is not uncommon in PA. The proliferating vascular cells will have a high Ki-67 index. This should not be interpreted as sign of anaplasia.*

Microcystic Pattern

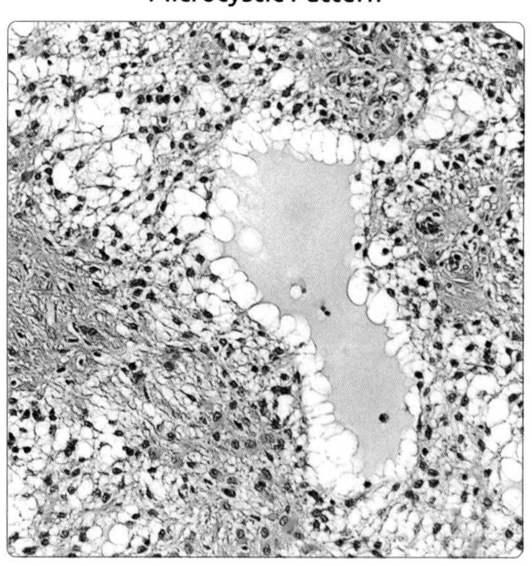

Microvascular Proliferation

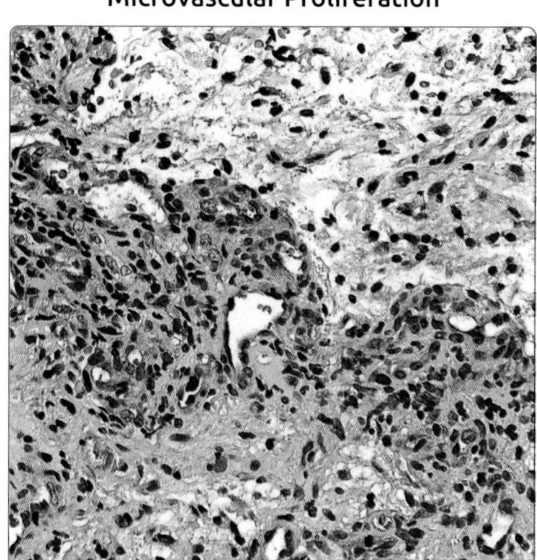

Gross Appearance: Hemorrhagic Tumor

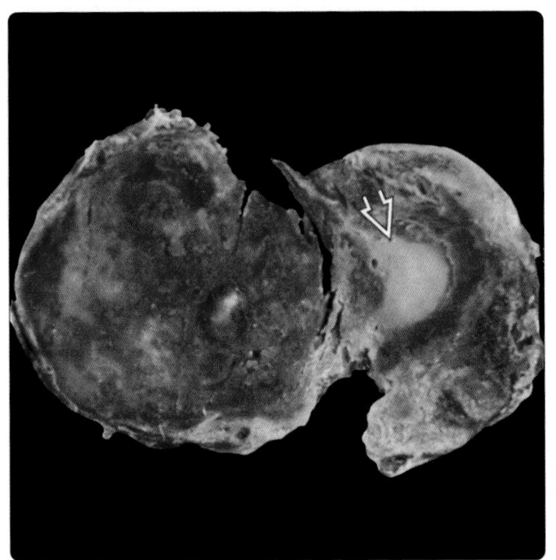

Hemorrhagic Tumor

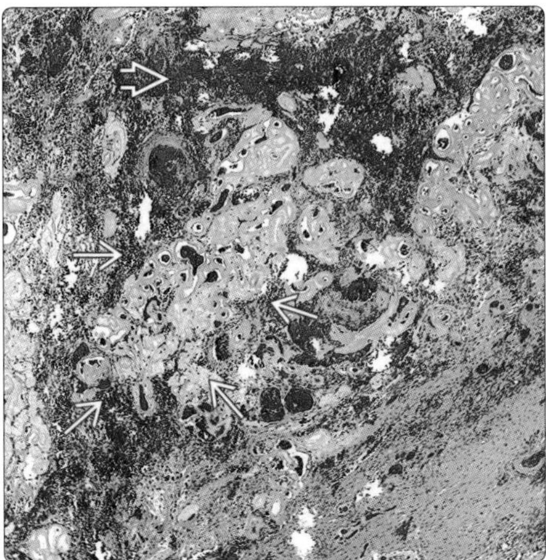

(Left) *Some PAs with vascular hyalinization in the posterior fossa are prone to hemorrhage and can come to the attention of the neurosurgeon as an emergency. In some of these cases intratumoral hemorrhage could obliterate both the cystic and solid components with only a small amount of viable tumor ➡.* **(Right)** *This PA presented with an acute picture and intratumoral hemorrhage. The presence of numerous hyalinized vessels ➡ and extravasated erythrocytes ➡ are consistent with this H&E.*

Oligodendroglioma-Like Pattern

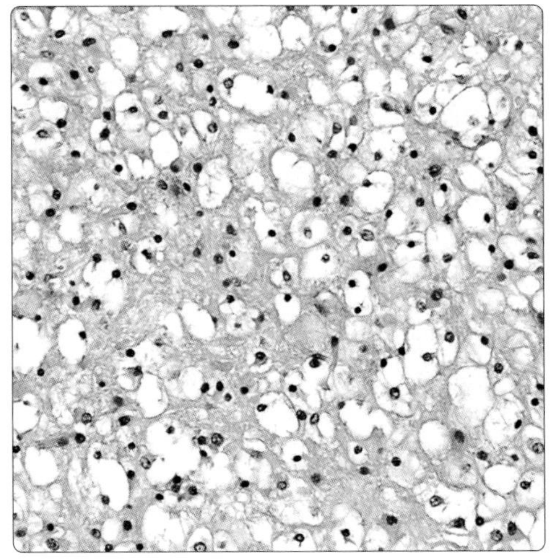

Psammomatous Calcifications

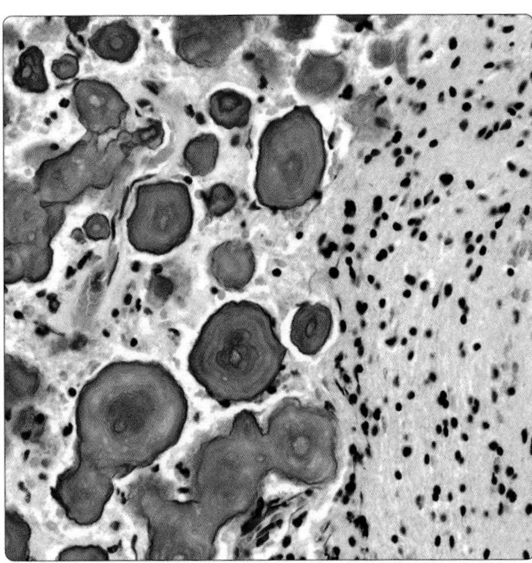

(Left) *Pilocytic astrocytomas may be remarkably similar to oligodendroglioma, even to the point of tissue infiltration. Such clear cells are especially prominent in pilocytic astrocytomas of the cerebellum.* **(Right)** *While calcifications are often seen in PAs, psammomatous calcifications are distinctly rare and evoke a differential diagnosis. Rare extensively calcified PAs harbor sufficient number of these structures to be confused with a meningioma.*

Nested or Organoid Pattern

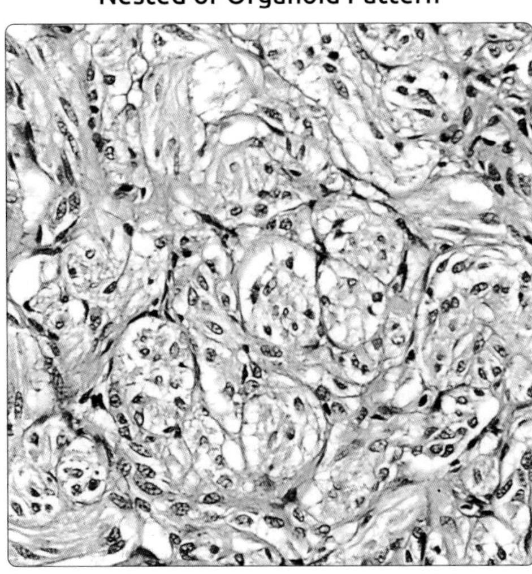

Eosinophilic Granular Body (EGB)

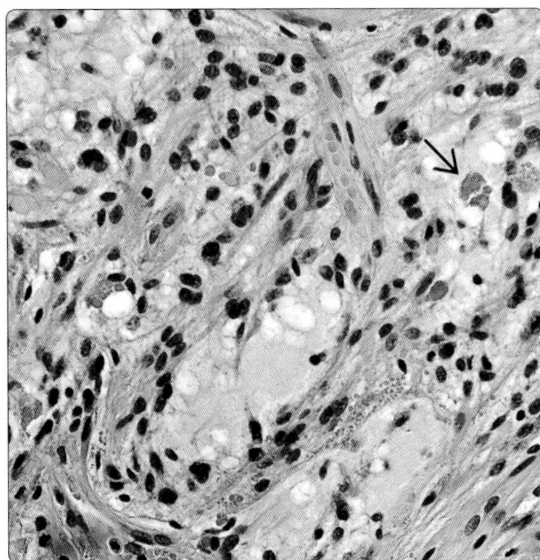

(Left) *Pilocytic astrocytomas in the leptomeninges often have a distinctive nested or organoid architecture that is not present in the intraparenchymal component.* **(Right)** *While the cellularity and nuclear hyperchromatism and pleomorphism may be concerning, the biphasic architecture is classic pilocytic astrocytoma. An eosinophilic granular body ➡ helps assure that this is pilocytic, not anaplastic, astrocytoma.*

(Left) *Piloid tissue and a myxoid background are easily overlooked in favor of the impressive, but prognostically insignificant, proliferating vessels ➩ in this smear preparation. Vascular proliferation, such as this, is common in PAs.* **(Right)** *Glomeruloid microvascular proliferation in a pilocytic astrocytoma is not evidence of anaplasia. On smear preparations, the interpretation of true vascular endothelial proliferation should be done with great caution.*

Intraoperative Smear

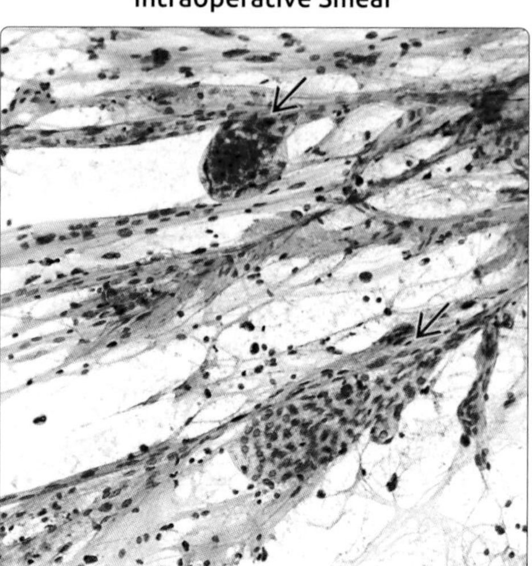

Vascular Changes on Smear

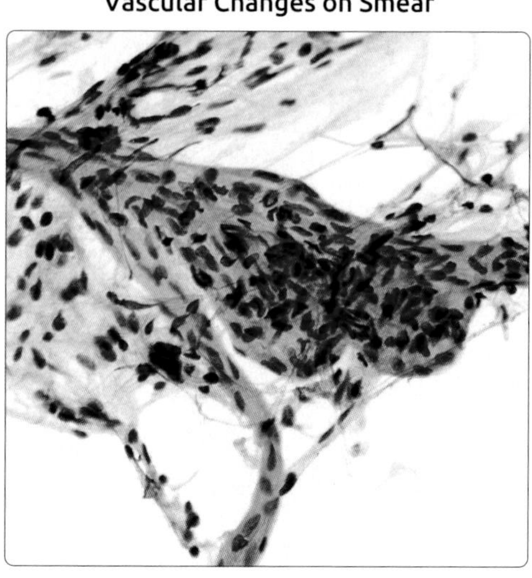

(Left) *Ribbons or palisaded arrangement of tumor cells impart an appearance of the so-called polar-spongioblastoma pattern, an arcane term that refers to a tissue pattern rather than a true entity. This pattern is not unique to PAs.* **(Right)** *Occasional ependymoma-like perivascular pseudorosettes can be seen in typical PA, but these are more common and abundant in the pilomyxoid variant. These rosette-like structures have fine processes interspersed with myxoid substance.*

Polar Spongioblastoma-Like Pattern

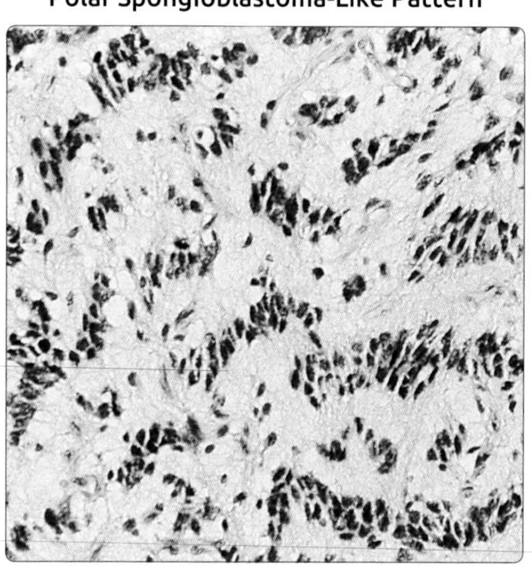

Focal Angiocentric Pattern

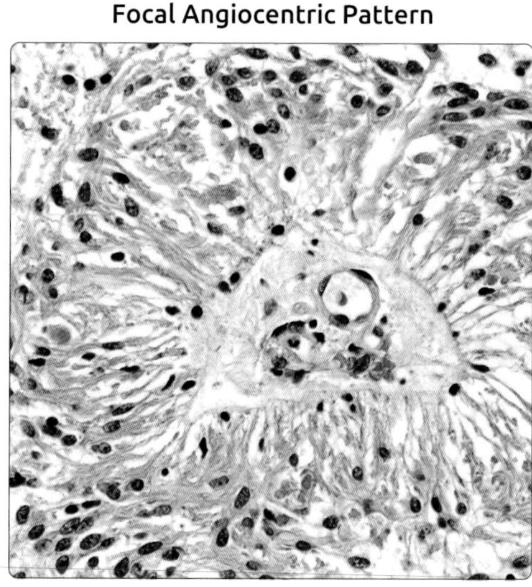

(Left) *PAs with neoplastic ganglion-like cells are difficult to classify as to whether they are ganglioglioma or pilocytic astrocytoma with bizarre ganglion-like cells.* **(Right)** *Glomeruloid microvascular proliferation is often present in PA, whereas the true vascular endothelial proliferation of the type seen in malignant gliomas is typically absent except for rare anaplastic examples.*

Neoplastic Ganglion Cells

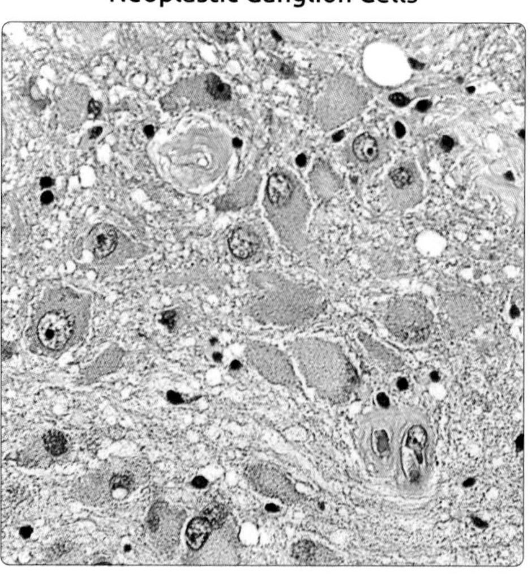

Glomeruloid Vascular Proliferation

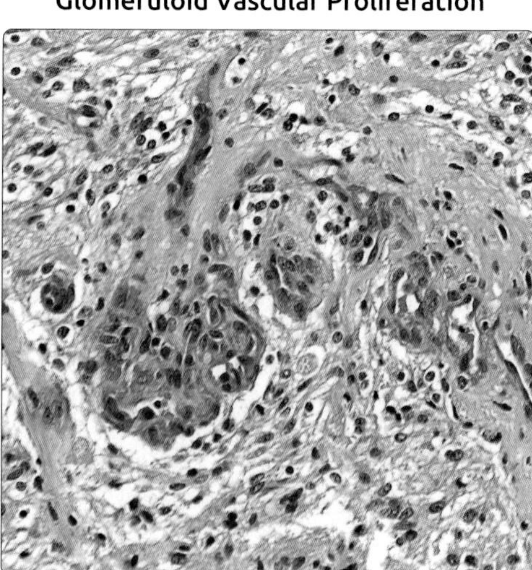

Anaplastic Features: Increased Mitoses

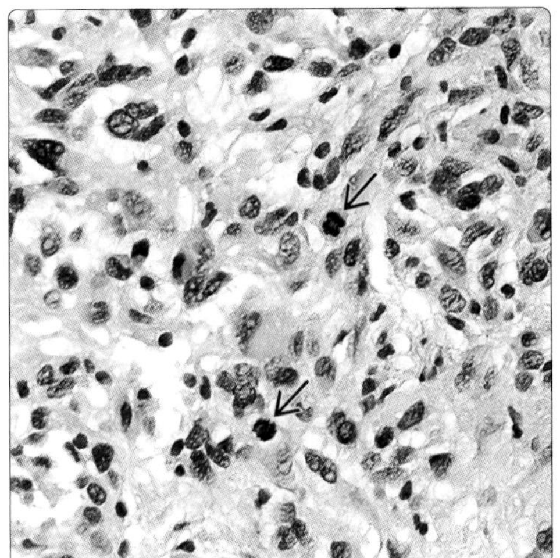

Low-Grade Area in Anaplastic Tumor

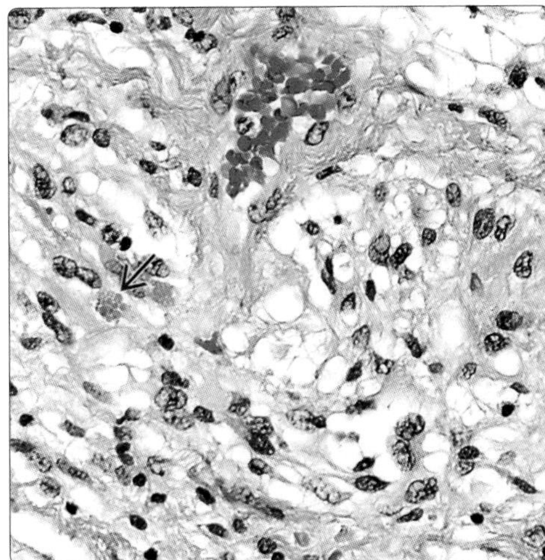

(Left) *Tissue, such as this, is clearly high grade in light of cellularity, atypia, and especially mitotic activity* →. *Elsewhere, there were classic features of pilocytic astrocytoma grade I.* **(Right)** *Only rarely do PAs undergo spontaneous anaplastic transformation. Low-grade elements, such as an EGB* →, *are present in this classically spongy lesion that had anaplastic features elsewhere.*

Multinucleated Cells and Mitoses

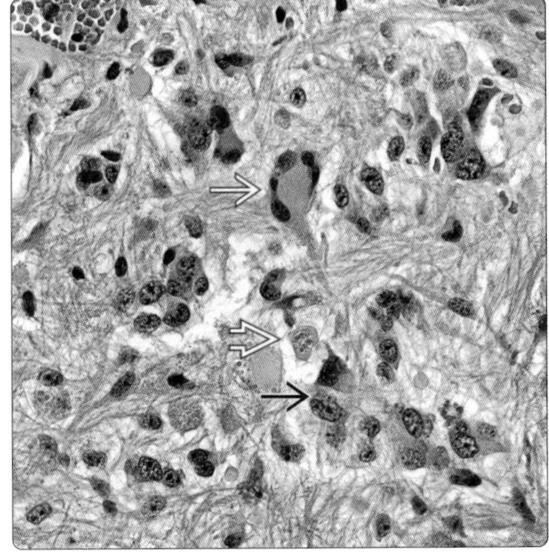

Infiltrative Appearance

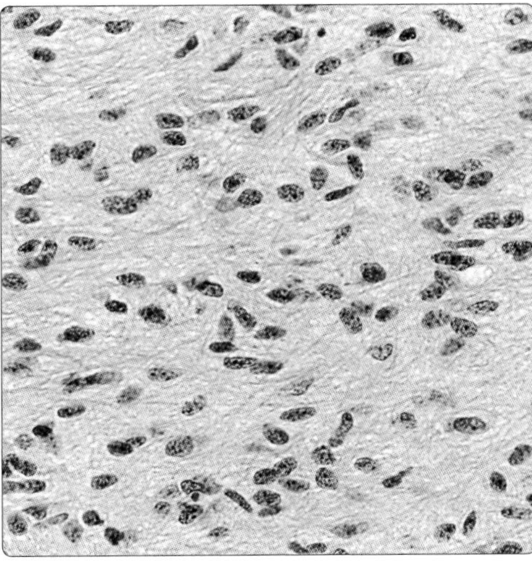

(Left) *Some PAs can harbor bizarre, multinucleated cells* ➡ *that appear to harbor evidence of degenerative change. This change is not worrisome, per se, unless accompanied by nuclear pleomorphism* →, *mitoses* ➡, *or other signs of anaplasia.* **(Right)** *The small cells in some PAs resemble those of infiltrating astrocytic neoplasms. Without additional typical features, the 2 lesions can be indistinguishable in small specimens. Small biopsies from PAs are often devoid of incorporated neuropil or axonal processes.*

Necrosis

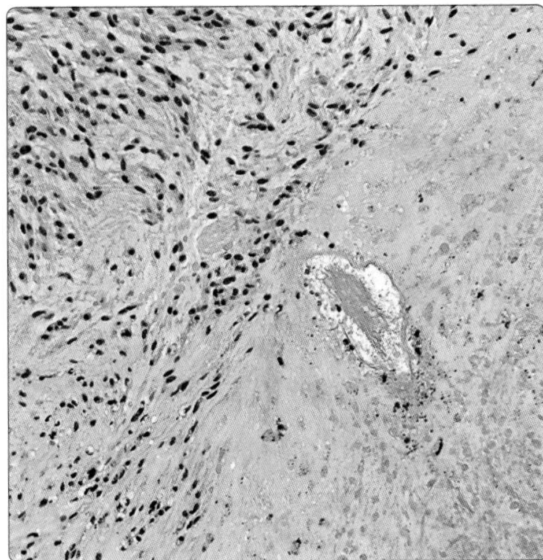

Increased Proliferation

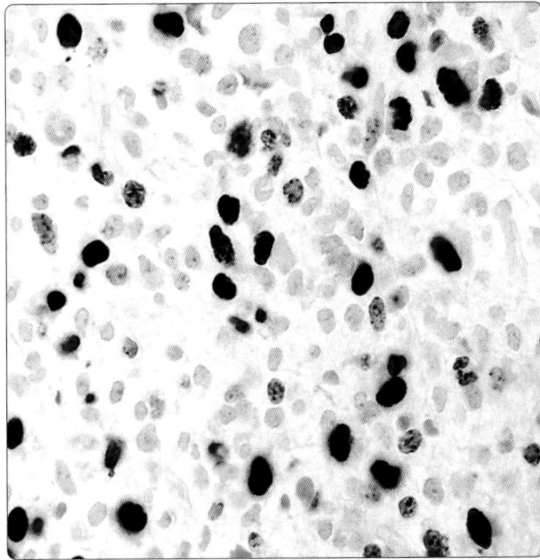

(Left) *Sharply defined areas of coagulation necrosis, involving both parenchyma and vasculature, are not uncommon in pilocytic astrocytomas. A suggestion of pseudopalisading is sometimes present. In the absence of increased mitoses, necrosis is not an indicator of anaplasia.* **(Right)** *While the Ki-67 index is sometimes somewhat higher than expected, this level is clearly exceptional and, in association with increased mitoses, helps establish the tumor as anaplastic.*

(Left) *Most optic gliomas, especially those in the setting of neurofibromatosis 1 (NF1), are PAs. The tumor often encases and expands the optic nerve and may extend caudally toward the optic chiasm.* (Right) *H&E shows the cross section of the optic nerve and the leptomeningeal spread of PA. Typically, PAs of the optic nerve proper appear much more infiltrative and expand the optic nerve.*

Sagittal MR: Optic Glioma

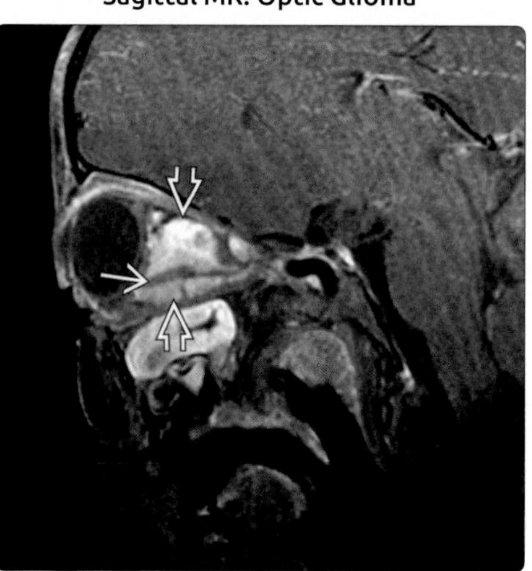

Optic Pilocytic Tumor

(Left) *The cross section of this tumor demonstrates an exaggerated nested structure of the optic nerve with intraneural tumor growth. There is limited distortion of the normal architecture at this level and the tumor infiltration is more conspicuous at the center.* (Right) *PA of the optic nerve infiltrate and expand compartments. In this section, the normal nested compartments of the optic nerve are expanded by tumor cells. The pial septa of the normal optic nerve are also thickened.*

Expanding Optic Nerve Proper

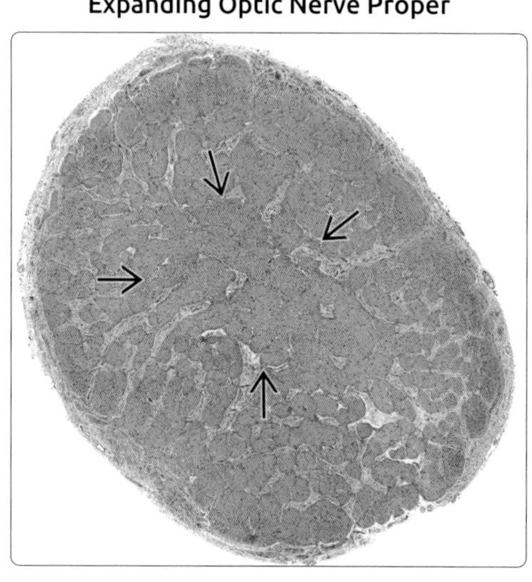

Expanding Optic Nerve Proper

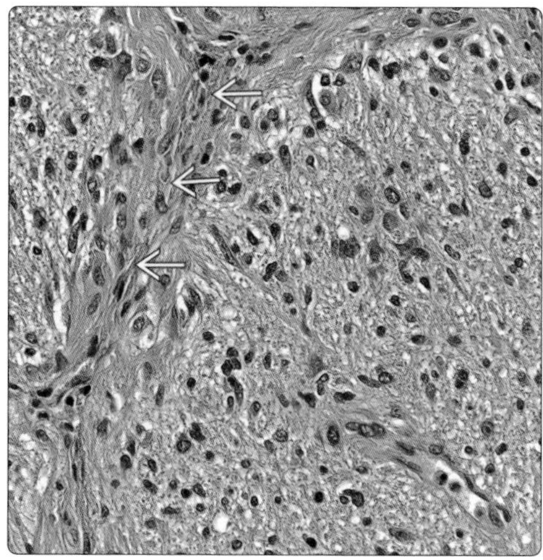

(Left) *Pilocytic astrocytomas of the optic nerves frequently broach the pia to reach and fill the subarachnoid space. These 2 components produce the classic radiologic bull's-eye appearance.* (Right) *PAs of the optic nerve typically fill the subarachnoid space and attach to the dura.*

Subarachnoid Involvement

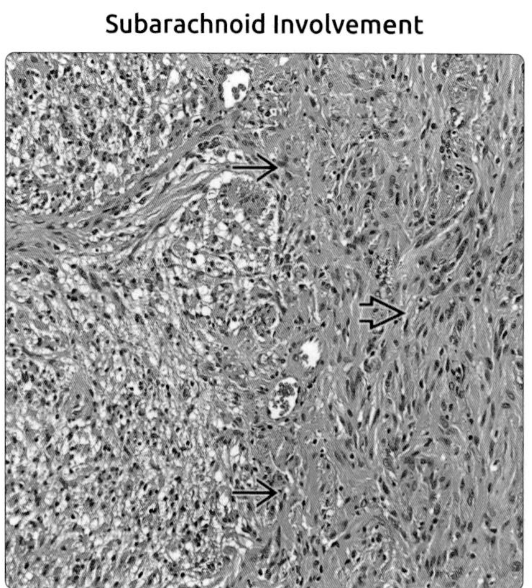

Optic Glioma Involving Dura Mater

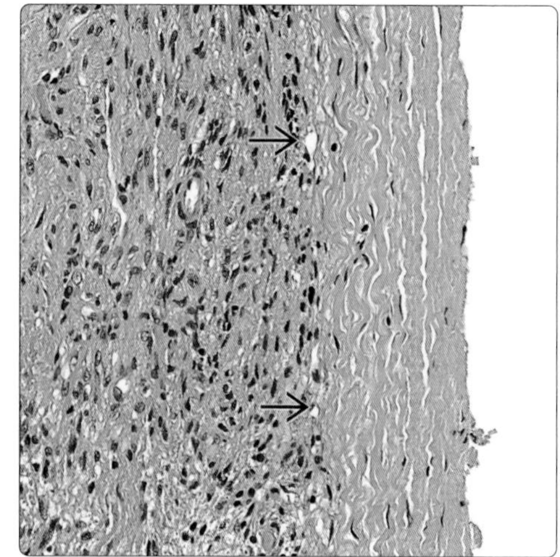

GFAP Positive

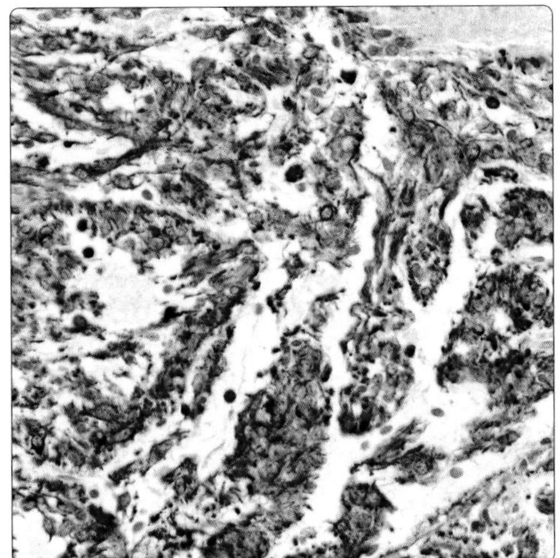

Olig2 Positive

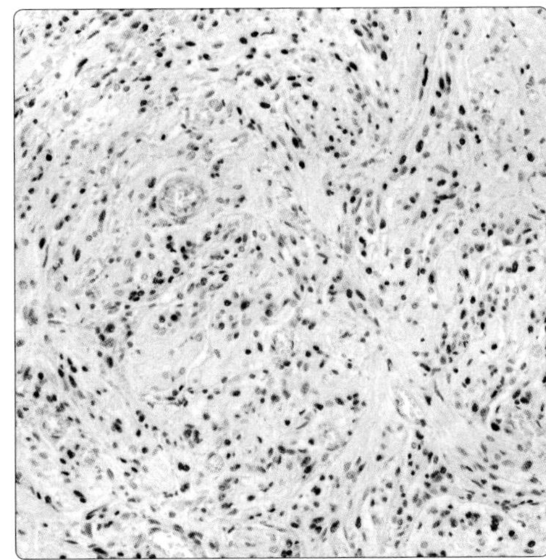

(Left) *PAs, especially their dense piloid component, are almost always immunoreactive with the GFAP antibodies.* **(Right)** *The glial marker Olig2 is a helpful adjunct to GFAP staining highlighting the majority of the tumor cells in PA. While there are some negative tumor cells, the ratio of these are much less compared to ependymal tumors in the same region.*

Synaptophysin Positive

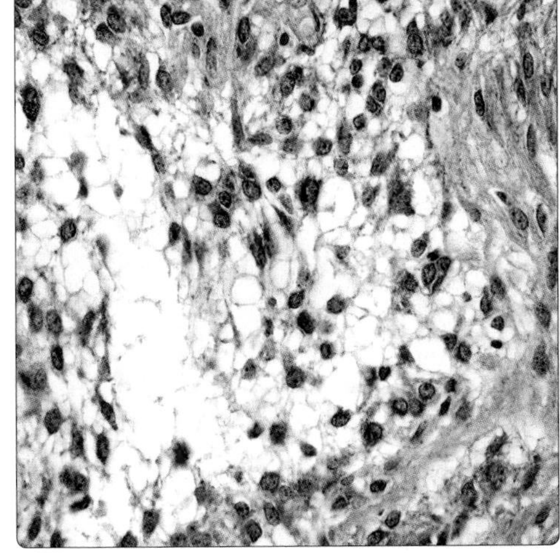

Neu-N Negative

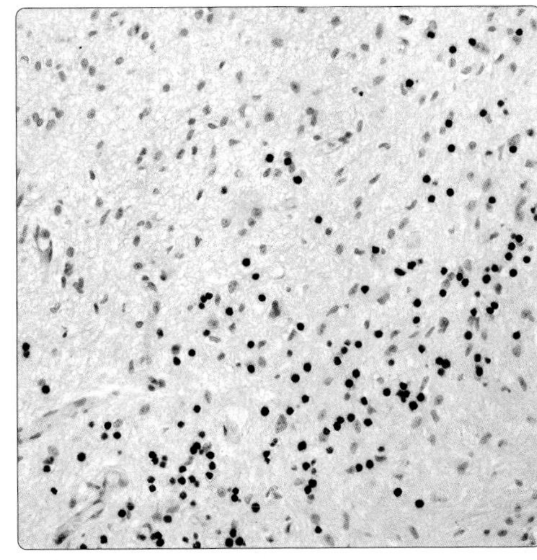

(Left) *Many PAs, as many as 40% in some studies, demonstrate significant positive staining with the synaptophysin antibodies. This staining should not be construed as a sign of neuronal differentiation.* **(Right)** *Some PAs in the posterior fossa can appear infiltrative, and the Neu-N staining highlighting the trapped internal granular layer neurons can highlight this pattern. An infiltrative pattern is more often seen at the tumor periphery.*

Neurofilament Staining

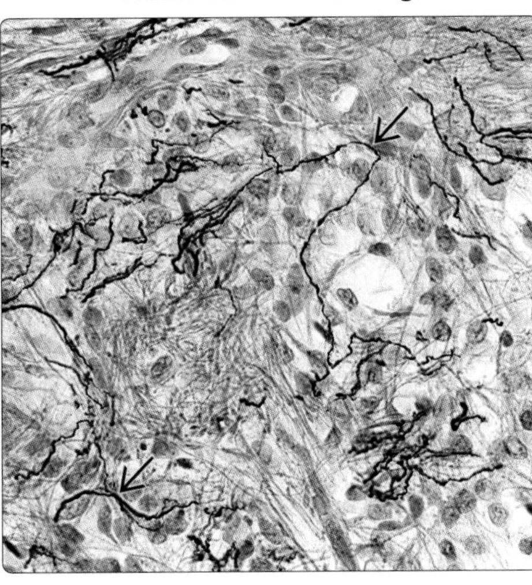

BRAF Duplication

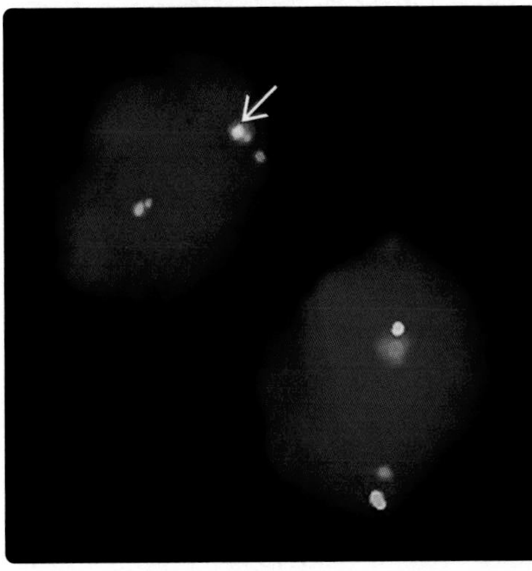

(Left) *Although macroscopically well circumscribed, PAs may contain axons ⇨. Such neuronal processes may be visualized by neurofilament immunohistochemistry even in the biphasic component.* **(Right)** *A tumor cell (top left) has 1 normal chromosome and 1 with a BRAF-KIAA fusion gene (red and green signals overlap so as to appear yellow ⇨). This genetic abnormality is common in cerebellar and optic pathway tumors but not in the cerebral cortex. (Courtesy V. P. Collins, MD.)*

Pilomyxoid Astrocytoma

KEY FACTS

TERMINOLOGY

- Variant of pilocytic astrocytoma with cytological monomorphism, small bipolar cells, myxoid background, and perivascular formations resembling ependymoma

CLINICAL ISSUES

- Almost always young children
- Many present with diencephalic syndrome

IMAGING

- Sites similar to pilocytic astrocytoma, but most hypothalamic/suprasellar
- Often bulky and solid when hypothalamic/suprasellar
- Often diffuse contrast enhancement

MICROSCOPIC

- Perivascular formations similar to ependymoma pseudorosettes
- Little, if any, compact fibrillar tissue
- Small, uniform, bipolar cells
- Rosenthal fibers essentially absent
- Glomeruloid vascular proliferation &/or necrosis in rare cases
- Occasional maturation to pilocytic astrocytoma

ANCILLARY TESTS

- GFAP(+)
- Synaptophysin (+) in some cases
- Olig2(+)
- *BRAF* abnormalities
  - Typical *KIAA1549-BRAF* fusion in 1/2 of cases
  - Rare tumors with *BRAF* V600E mutation

DIAGNOSTIC CHECKLIST

- Ependymoma-like but looser, more myxoid
- Occasional maturation to pilocytic astrocytoma
- Focal pilomyxoid pattern can be seen in typical pilocytic astrocytomas

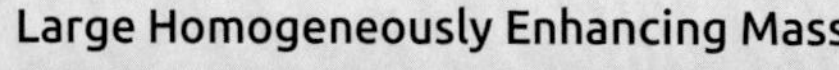

Large Homogeneously Enhancing Mass

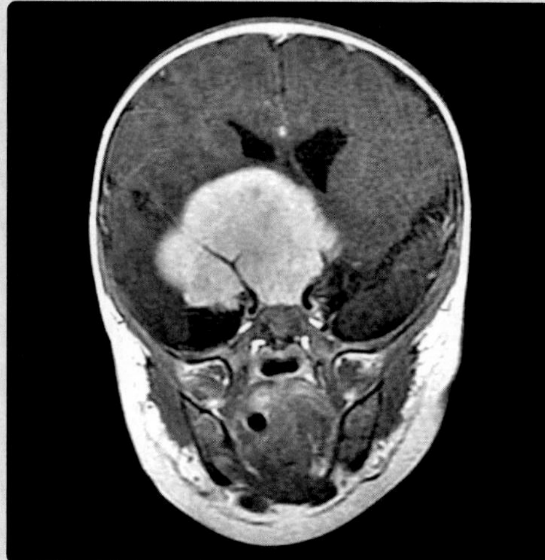

Bipolar Cells

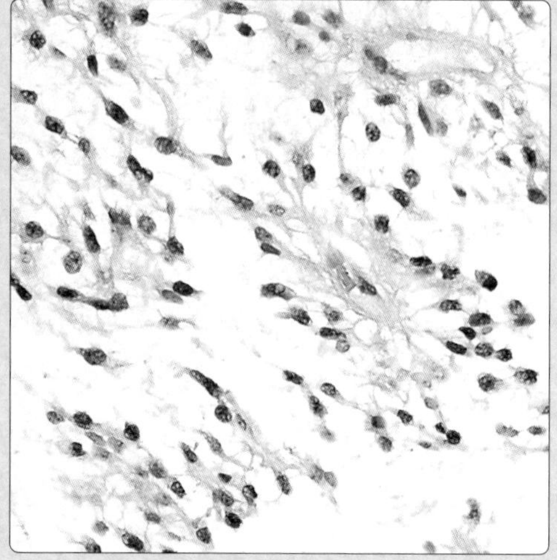

(Left) *Pilomyxoid astrocytomas in the frequently affected hypothalamic/suprasellar region are typically large. As elsewhere, most occur in infants and young children. They are often solid and homogeneously enhancing.* **(Right)** *PMA is characterized by monomorphous bipolar cells similar to those in PA, and the myxoid background often creates a loose texture that portends a dyscohesive nature to the tumor.*

Angiocentric Arrangement

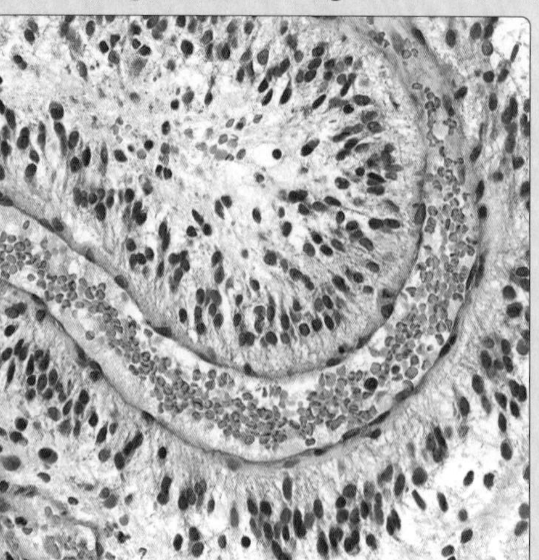

Myxoid Background

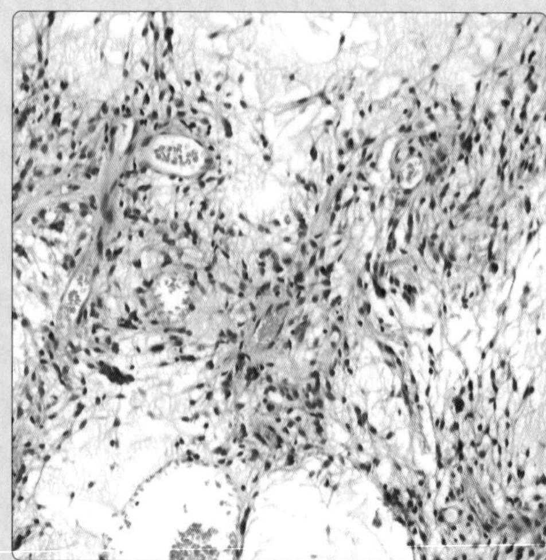

(Left) *The tumor cells in PMA demonstrate a striking perivascular or angiocentric arrangement in which the cells are aligned along the vascular tree in a perpendicular fashion. This arrangement, although slightly reminiscent of ependymomas, is distinct from the typical perivascular pseudorosettes of ependymal tumors.* **(Right)** *Paraffin sections highlight a prominent and often predominant myxoid background along with the monomorphous bipolar cells arranged in an angiocentric fashion, reminiscent of an ependymal tumor.*

TERMINOLOGY

Abbreviations

- Pilomyxoid astrocytoma (PMA)

Definitions

- Variant of pilocytic astrocytoma
  - Cytologic monomorphism
  - Small, hyperchromatic, bipolar tumor cells
  - Diffuse myxoid matrix
  - Angiocentric arrangement of tumor cells
    - Resemble ependymal pseudorosettes with some differences
- PMA implies aggressive behavior and more frequent CSF dissemination
  - Current WHO classification designates grade II for PMA
  - There is ambiguity in this designation and this may change in future iteration of classification scheme
- Classical pilocytic astrocytomas with focal changes are not considered in this category

ETIOLOGY/PATHOGENESIS

Associated Predisposing Conditions

- Neurofibromatosis type 1 in minority of cases

CLINICAL ISSUES

Site

- Similar to pilocytic astrocytoma, but more commonly suprasellar/hypothalamic/chiasmatic

Presentation

- Almost always young children, generally < 4 years
- Site-dependent symptomatology similar to that of pilocytic astrocytoma
- May have CSF dissemination at presentation
- Some present with diencephalic syndrome
  - Failure to thrive
  - Emaciation
  - Amnesia
  - Intense sleepiness
  - Unusual eye positions or blindness

Treatment

- Surgical approaches
  - Gross total resection is aim
  - Mostly biopsy or subtotal resection due to inaccessibility
- Drugs
  - Generally upon recurrence, vincristine, carboplatin
  - RAF and MEK inhibitors promising
- Radiation
  - Sometimes for recurrent tumors

Prognosis

- Generally favorable and better than diffuse astrocytomas
- More likely to progress and show CSF dissemination than conventional pilocytic astrocytoma
  - Some examples, especially if completely resected, have favorable prognoses
- Recurrent tumors may have more PA-like appearance, so-called maturation into PA
- Recurrence often in form of solid mass lesion

IMAGING

MR Findings

- Most often hypothalamic/suprasellar, but can occur anywhere along neuraxis
  - Solid iso- or hypointense on T1-weighted images
  - Hyperintense on T2-weighted and FLAIR images
  - Does not restrict on diffusion-weighted images
  - Solid component enhancing on contrast images
    - Most tumors are homogeneously enhancing
    - Some tumors have nonenhancing central components
    - Ring enhancement of some tumors (rare)
    - Basilar meninges or spinal enhancement in disseminated cases
- Often bulky when hypothalamic/suprasellar
- More likely solid than pilocytic astrocytoma
- Spinal seeding
  - At presentation, whole craniospinal imaging is advisable on diagnosis
  - Later during course of disease, or following surgical debulking

MICROSCOPIC

Histologic Features

- Overall solid and compact but may be partly infiltrative
- Often diffuse myxoid background matrix
- Perivascular or angiocentric arrangement of tumor cells similar to ependymoma pseudorosettes
- Little, if any, compact fibrillar tissue
- No biphasic (solid/microcystic) pattern
- Small uniform and bipolar cells
- Eosinophilic granular bodies distinctly rare
- Rosenthal fibers essentially absent
- Vascular proliferation in some cases
- Necrosis in some cases
- Occasional coexistence with, &/or transition to, pilocytic astrocytoma
- Focal angiocentric or myxoid pattern in an otherwise typical PA does not qualify for PMA
- Mitotic figures may be present, more often than in PA

ANCILLARY TESTS

Cytology

- Overall similar to pilocytic astrocytoma, but no Rosenthal fibers
- Delicate piloid cells with uniform, oval nuclei and bipolar processes
- Myxoid background

Immunohistochemistry

- GFAP(+)
- Olig2(+)
- Synaptophysin (+), approximately 1/2 of cases
- SOX2, Vim, S100 diffuse (+), nonspecific
- MAP-2(+)
- Rare cases positive with BRAF V600E stains
- p16 (+) in most tumor nuclei

- Negative p16 staining has been associated with more aggressive behavior

Genetic Testing

- Activation of RAS/BRAF pathway in at least 1/2 of cases
  - Tandem duplication of *BRAF* causing fusion with *KIAA1549* in some cases
  - *NF1* and RAS mutations exceptional
  - *BRAF* mutation (V600E), in minority of cases

DIFFERENTIAL DIAGNOSIS

Pilocytic Astrocytoma

- Radiologically more commonly cystic and solid
- Often biphasic tumor
- Rosenthal fibers
- Myxoid areas only focal
- Microcysts with eosinophilic granular bodies
- Few perivascular formations
- May have focal angiocentric pattern
- Clustered nuclei pennies on plate appearance

Ependymoma

- Cellular with epithelioid cells, no bipolar cells
- Little or no myxoid substance, except for myxopapillary type
- Well-developed, densely fibrillar perivascular pseudorosettes
- True, lumen-containing rosettes in some cases
- Most tumor cells Olig2(-) D2-40(+)

Angiocentric Glioma

- Corticocentric
- Perivascular linear ensheathment or radiating perivascular pseudorosettes
- Subpial perpendicular tumor cell layer
- Minimal to no myxoid background
- May resemble infiltrative areas of PMA
- EMA(+)

Malignant Glioma (Glioblastoma)

- Occasional malignant gliomas with angiocentric pattern misdiagnosed as PMA
- Infiltrative pattern, vascular endothelial proliferation, palisading necrosis
- Either EGRF amplification or IDH1/2 mutations
- None show BRAF tandem duplication
- Vascular endothelial proliferation or microvascular proliferation
- Palisading necrosis
- Marked nuclear pleomorphism and numerous mitoses

DIAGNOSTIC CHECKLIST

Clinically Relevant Pathologic Features

- Infiltrative properties, e.g., in hypothalamus and brainstem, may prevent total excision
- May mature into conventional pilocytic astrocytoma histology
- Somewhat more prone to CSF dissemination than pilocytic astrocytoma
- Typically more aggressive than PA even after accounting for location
- Solid, avidly enhancing tumor with little or no cystic component

Pathologic Interpretation Pearls

- Ependymoma-like but looser, more myxoid
- May be peripherally infiltrative and may be mistaken for diffuse astrocytoma
- No Rosenthal fibers, rare EGBs
- Diffuse myxoid background, monomorphous cells
- PA with focal PMA-like pattern not considered in this category
- Synaptophysin IHC does not exclude diagnosis

SELECTED REFERENCES

1. Alkonyi B et al: Differential imaging characteristics and dissemination potential of pilomyxoid astrocytomas versus pilocytic astrocytomas. Neuroradiology. 57(6):625-38, 2015
2. Kleinschmidt-DeMasters BK et al: Pilomyxoid Astrocytoma (PMA) Shows Significant Differences in Gene Expression vs. Pilocytic Astrocytoma (PA) and Variable Tendency Toward Maturation to PA. Brain Pathol. ePub, 2014
3. Lee IH et al: Imaging characteristics of pilomyxoid astrocytomas in comparison with pilocytic astrocytomas. Eur J Radiol. 79(2):311-6, 2011
4. Linscott LL et al: Pilomyxoid astrocytoma: expanding the imaging spectrum. AJNR Am J Neuroradiol. 29(10):1861-6, 2008
5. Rodriguez FJ et al: Gliomas in neurofibromatosis type 1: a clinicopathologic study of 100 patients. J Neuropathol Exp Neurol. 67(3):240-9, 2008
6. Ceppa EP et al: The pilomyxoid astrocytoma and its relationship to pilocytic astrocytoma: report of a case and a critical review of the entity. J Neurooncol. 81(2):191-6, 2007
7. Komakula ST et al: Pilomyxoid astrocytoma: neuroimaging with clinicopathologic correlates in 4 cases followed over time. J Pediatr Hematol Oncol. 29(7):465-70, 2007
8. Khanani MF et al: Pilomyxoid astrocytoma in a patient with neurofibromatosis. Pediatr Blood Cancer. 46(3):377-80, 2006
9. Komotar RJ et al: Pilocytic and pilomyxoid hypothalamic/chiasmatic astrocytomas. Neurosurgery. 54(1):72-9; discussion 79-80, 2004
10. Arslanoglu A et al: MR imaging characteristics of pilomyxoid astrocytomas. AJNR Am J Neuroradiol. 24(9):1906-8, 2003
11. Fernandez C et al: Pilocytic astrocytomas in children: prognostic factors--a retrospective study of 80 cases. Neurosurgery. 53(3):544-53; discussion 554-5, 2003
12. Tihan T et al: Pediatric astrocytomas with monomorphous pilomyxoid features and a less favorable outcome. J Neuropathol Exp Neurol. 58(10):1061-8, 1999

Central Necrosis

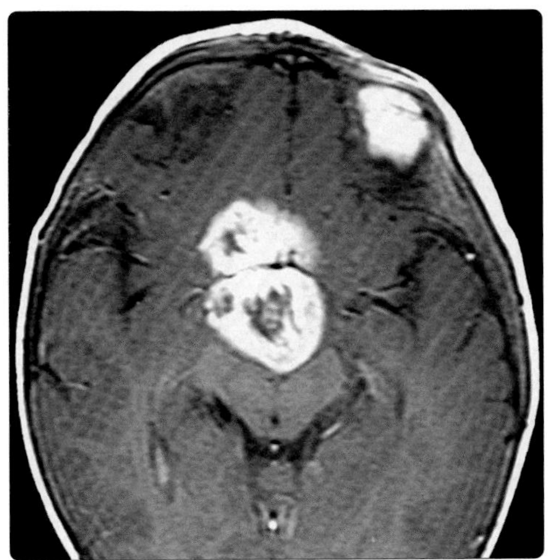

Intraoperative Smear, Bland Nuclei

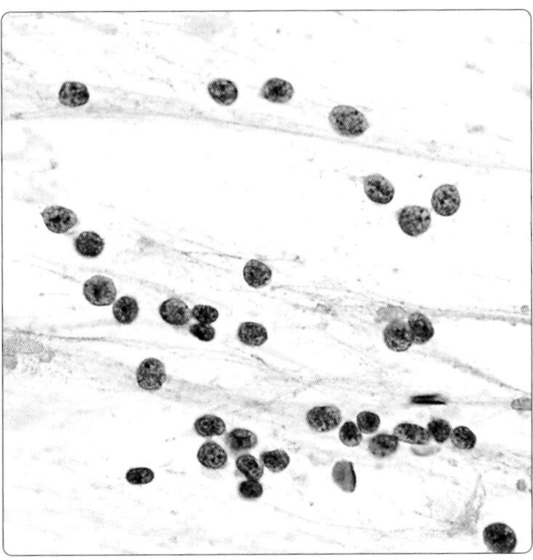

(Left) *While most PMAs have solid appearance on MR with little or no cystic component and enhance avidly, some demonstrate a hypointense central region that can sometimes correspond to the necrosis seen in the tumor tissue.* **(Right)** *In smears, cells have the same delicate piloid profiles and bland nuclei as those of pilocytic astrocytoma without clear bipolar processes. Rosenthal fibers are absent.*

Frozen Section, Monomorphic

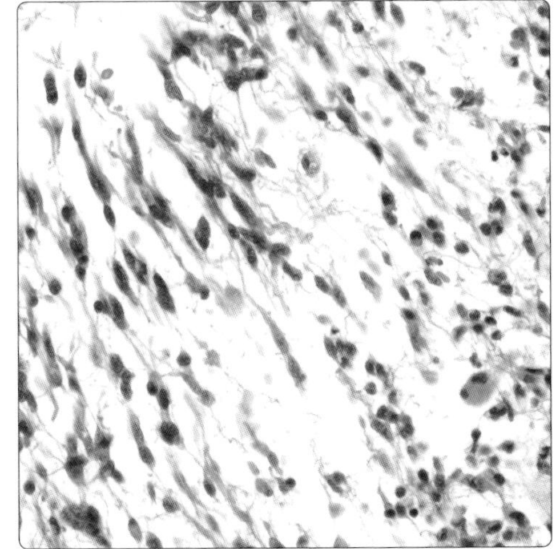

Bipolar Cells Myxoid Background

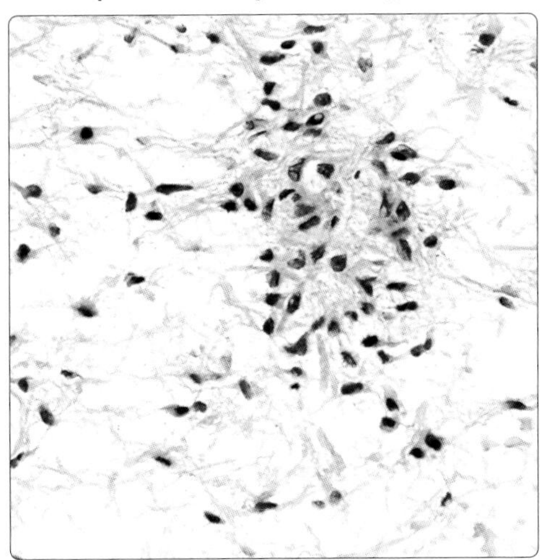

(Left) *The loose background in PMA may not be easily recognized as myxoid on frozen sections. The tumor cells are very similar to PA with their bipolar processes, but the extent of monomorphism may provide the clue to the diagnosis.* **(Right)** *When sparse, perivascular tumor cells can be dominated by a paucicellular myxoid background.*

Predominantly Myxoid Tumor

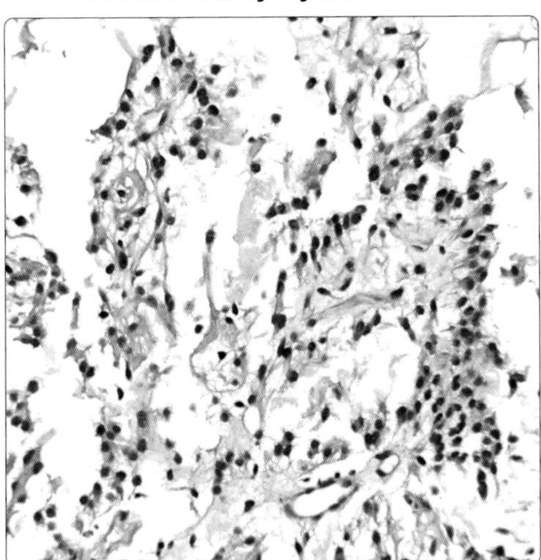

Angiocentric and Myxoid Tumor

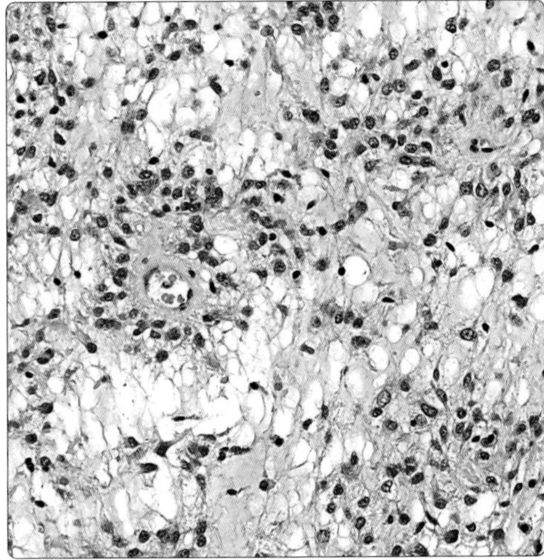

(Left) *The myxoid background is not specific to PMA and many PAs also demonstrate focal myxoid background and even microcysts with myxoid content. The distinctive feature of PMA is the presence of a myxoid background in the majority of the tumor tissue.* **(Right)** *Perivascular formations, small bland cells, and a rich myxoid background are a classic combination. The dense eosinophilic fibrillar tissue of pilocytic astrocytomas is missing.*

(Left) *PMAs are often solid neoplasms very similar to PA except in the periphery, where focal parenchymal infiltration may be observed. Samples from these regions may confuse the observer and mislead to a diagnosis of diffuse glioma.* **(Right)** *PMAs, like many other low-grade glial neoplasms, can demonstrate leptomeningeal spread* → *and many examples present with distant tumor spread along the leptomeninges. CSF or leptomeningeal spread can also occur after initial diagnosis.*

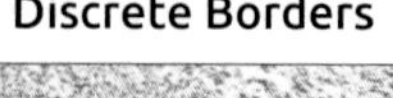

Discrete Borders

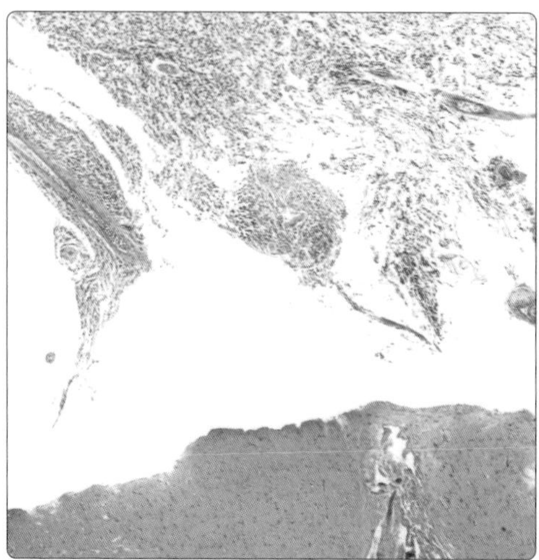

Leptomeningeal Spread

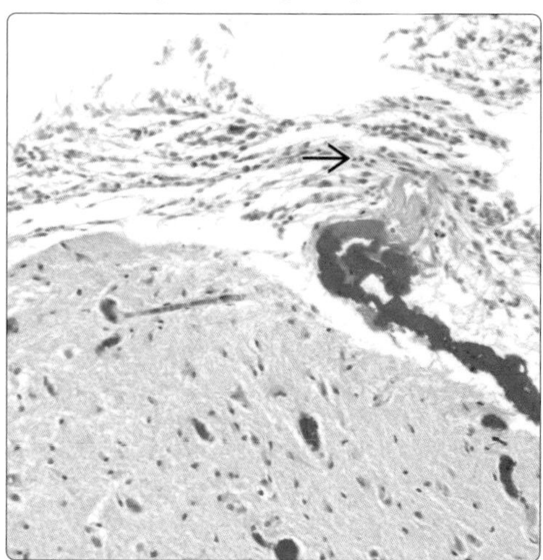

(Left) *The angiocentric pattern is another prominent feature of PMAs. However, many other CNS neoplasms, glial and otherwise, can demonstrate angiocentric arrangement of tumor cells, and this feature in isolation can mislead to an erroneous diagnosis of PMA.* **(Right)** *PMAs are often vascular neoplasms in which the tumor cells arrange in a striking angiocentric fashion. In many instances, this angiocentric arrangement may give the impression of an ependymal neoplasm.*

Perivascular Tumor Cells

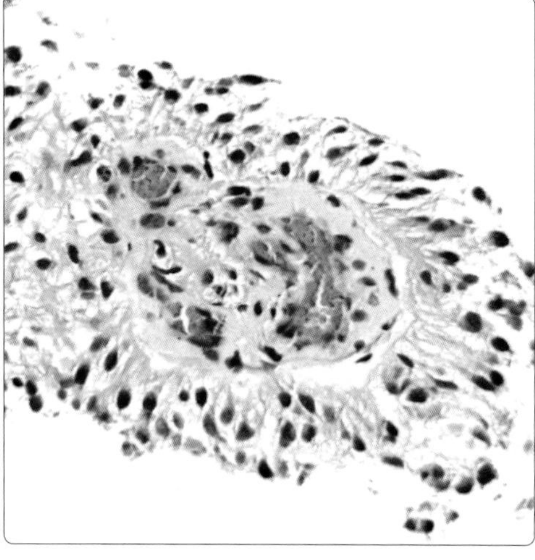

Highly Vascular Tumor

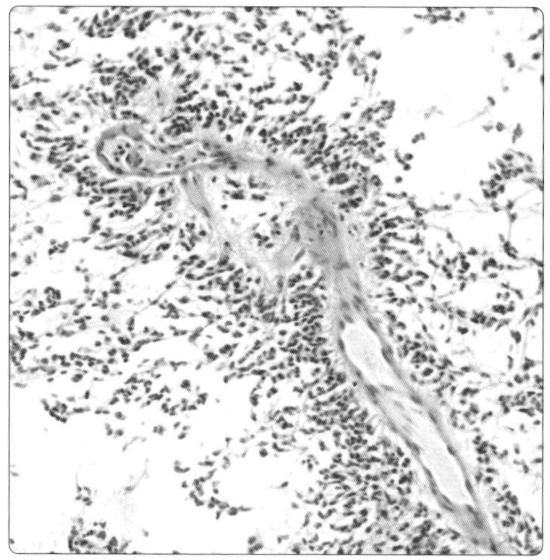

(Left) *Arcades of vascular proliferation seen in PMA are no different than those that occur in some cases of grade I pilocytic astrocytoma. The linear arrangement of these proliferative vessels is a clue to their reactive nature, and should not be misinterpreted as high grade.* **(Right)** *Mitoses* ⇒ *are encountered more commonly in PMA in comparison to PA. The combination of solid, noninfiltrative nature, angiocentric arrangement, myxoid background, and piloid cells distinguish PMA from a malignant glioma.*

Linear-Type Vascular Proliferation

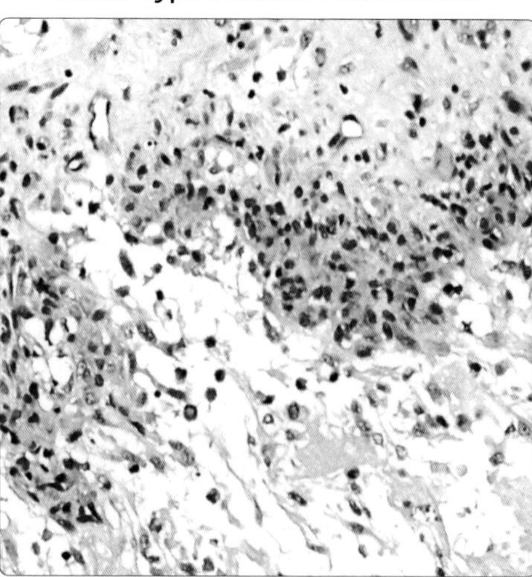

Angiocentric Tumor Cells and Mitoses

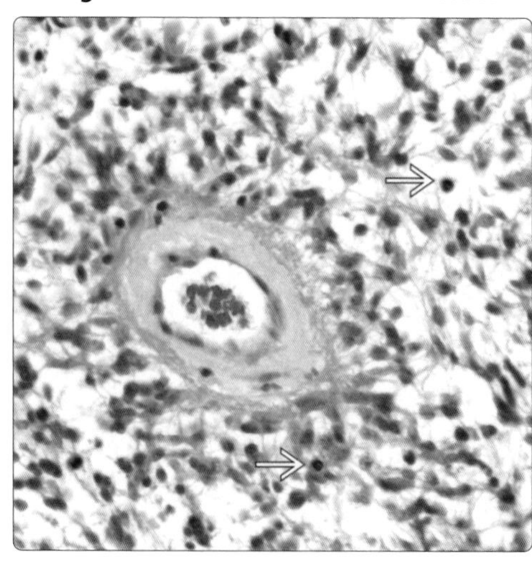

Necrosis

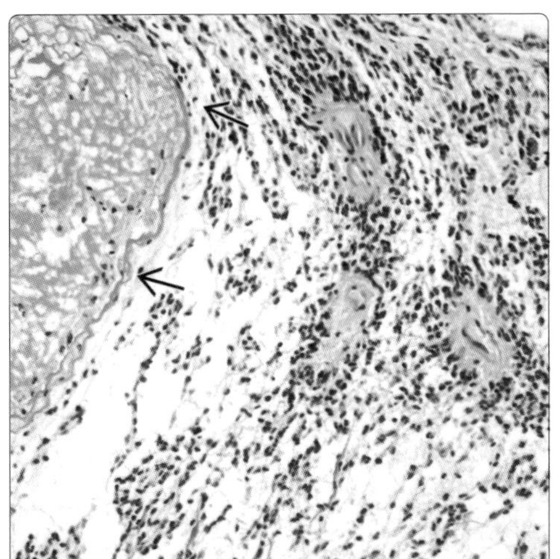

Diffuse Myxoid Background

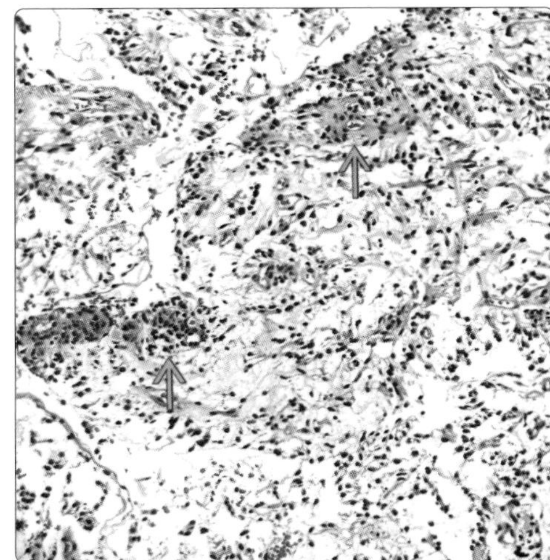

(Left) *While most PMAs do not demonstrate necrosis, some, especially those with central hypointense areas on contrast-enhanced images, can demonstrate geographic areas of necrosis* ➾. *However, palisading necrosis of the type seen in malignant gliomas is not encountered.* **(Right)** *PMA often demonstrates a diffuse prominent myxoid background and a population of monomorphous cells. Scattered angiocentric arrangement of tumor cells* ➾ *are also recognizable in this low-power magnification.*

GFAP, Strong

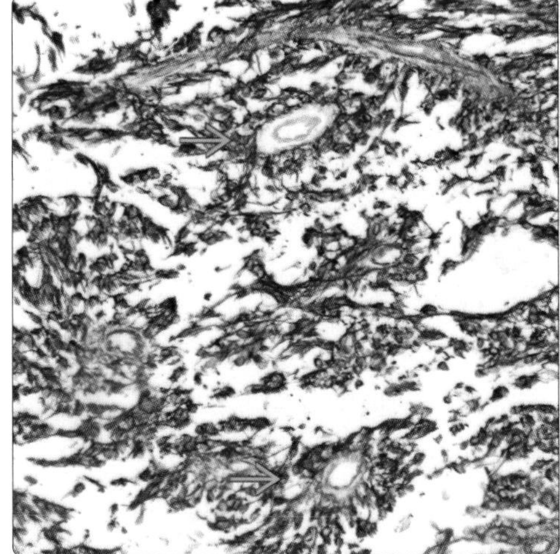

GFAP, Weaker

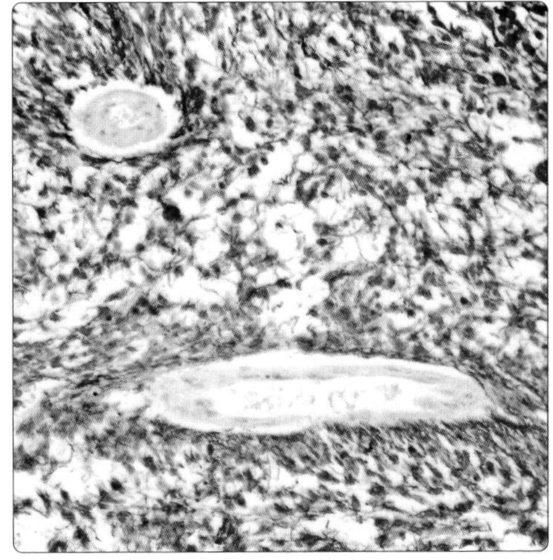

(Left) *Typically, PMAs are diffusely and strongly positive with antibodies against GFAP. In most instances, this immunostain highlights the angiocentric pattern of the tumor cells* ➾. **(Right)** *While diffuse, some tumors have weaker positivity with GFAP antibodies. Even in these cases, the perivascular arrangement of tumor cells can be readily identified.*

Synaptophysin

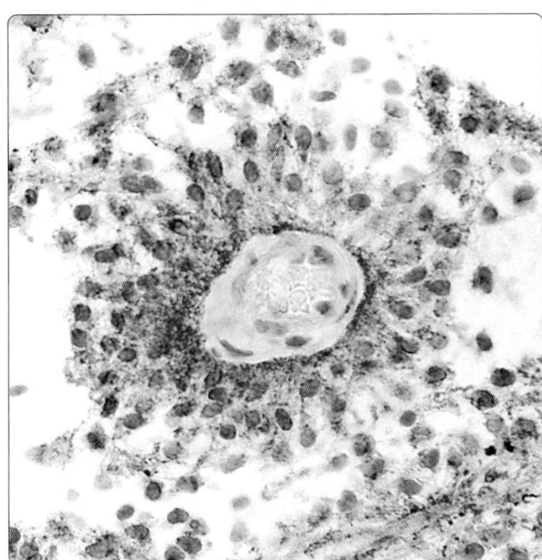

BRAF Fusion by FISH

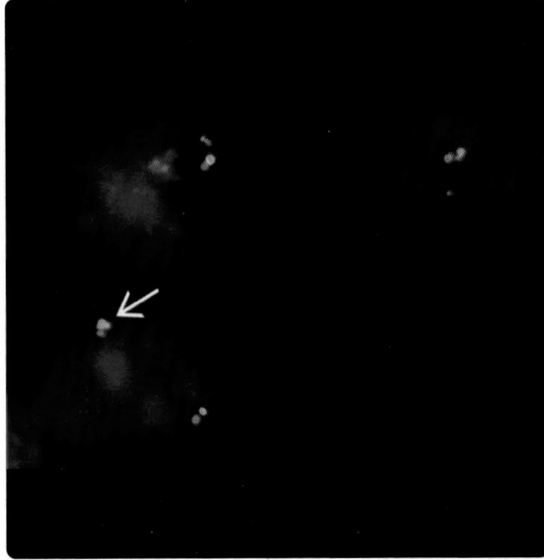

(Left) *Surprisingly, some pilomyxoid astrocytomas are immunoreactive for synaptophysin. A perivascular formation is stained in this case. This is, in a way, similar to many PAs that also demonstrate synaptophysin positivity.* **(Right)** *The duplication of the chromosome 7q34 region can be demonstrated by in situ hybridization using the probes against the BRAF gene* ➡. *This feature is seen is about half of the PMAs and the genetic alterations in the remaining tumors are still elusive.*

Pleomorphic Xanthoastrocytoma

KEY FACTS

TERMINOLOGY

- Superficial, pleomorphic, but generally low-grade astrocytoma

CLINICAL ISSUES

- Seen in children and young adults, often with seizures
- Generally good prognosis when superficial, cystic, and totally excised
- Less favorable prognosis with subtotal resection &/or features of anaplasia

IMAGING

- Usually superficial, discrete, enhancing, sometimes as mural nodule

MICROSCOPIC

- Solid component largely in subarachnoid space with
  - Pleomorphism and giant cells
  - Eosinophilic granular bodies
- Intracortical infiltrating component
- Anaplastic features, WHO grade III
  - Increased mitotic rate ≥ 5 per 10 HPF
  - Necrosis, rarely palisading type
  - Vascular endothelial proliferation
  - Occasionally, rhabdoid component

ANCILLARY TESTS

- PAS(+) eosinophilic granular bodies
- Reticulin around individual cells or small groups of cells
  - Collagen type IV immunohistochemistry can be also used to highlight same feature
- BRAF V600E mutation/(BRAF VE1 antibody staining) immunostaining positive in ~ 60% of cases

DIAGNOSTIC CHECKLIST

- Diagnose with caution in absence of eosinophilic granular bodies

(Left) *Pleomorphic xanthoastrocytoma (PXA) typically presents as a cystic lesion with an enhancing mural nodule ⇒ and are most commonly located in the temporal lobe.* **(Right)** *Giant cells with large, pleomorphic nuclei and abundant eosinophilic nuclei are one of the hallmarks of PXAs. While many such giant cells are mononuclear, others are multinucleated.*

Cystic Mass With Mural Nodule

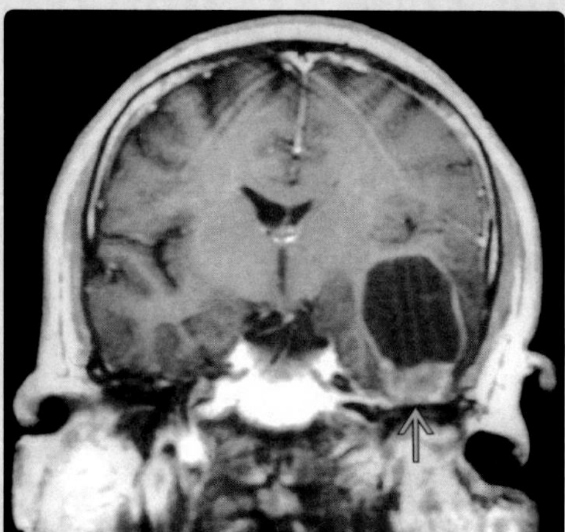

Pleomorphic Giant Cells

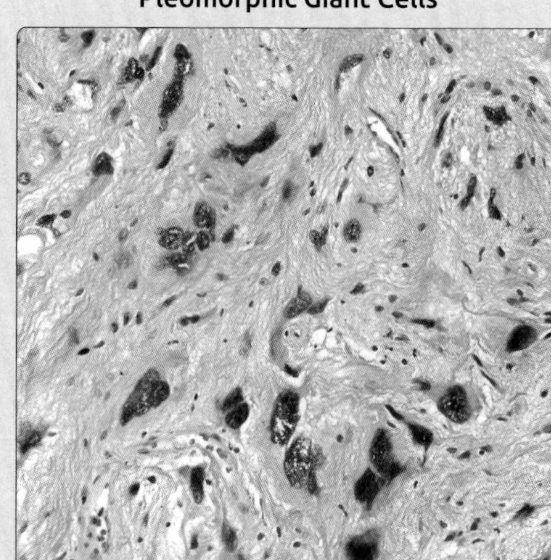

(Left) *One of the 3 most prominent features of PXAs is the presence of rich and delicate reticulin network that surrounds individual as well as small clusters of tumor cells.* **(Right)** *In this very high-power magnification, an eosinophilic granular body (EGB) appears as a cluster of small eosinophilic globules, often resembling a bunch of grapes ⇒. Notice the lipidized or xanthomatous cells in the background ⇒.*

Rich Reticulin Network

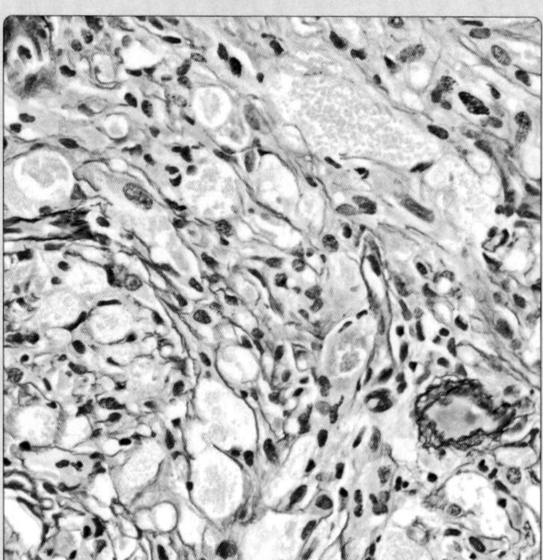

Eosinophilic Granular Body

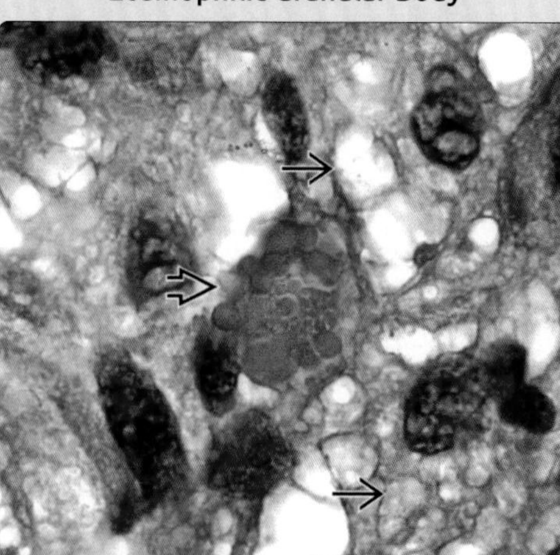

TERMINOLOGY

Abbreviations

- Pleomorphic xanthoastrocytoma (PXA)

Definitions

- Superficial, pleomorphic, but generally WHO grade II astrocytoma
  - PXA with anaplastic features now WHO grade III in new classification system
- Typically in children and young adults, relatively favorable prognosis compared to diffuse gliomas

CLINICAL ISSUES

Epidemiology

- Age
  - Children and young adults

Presentation

- Seizures
- Motor and sensory disturbance for spinal tumors

Treatment

- Surgical approaches
  - Gross total resection
  - Multiple resections
- Drugs
  - BRAF antagonists
  - e.g., vemurafenib used successfully
- Radiation
  - For cases with anaplastic features and unresectable, disseminated tumors

Prognosis

- Variable
  - Generally good when superficial, cystic, and totally excised WHO grade II
  - Less favorable when subtotally resected &/or showing anaplastic features
    - PXAs with anaplastic features are clinically aggressive
    - May warrant grade III designation
  - Gross total resection associated with longer recurrence free survival
  - No significant differences in recurrence-free survival and overall survival between children and adults
- BRAF V600E mutation status not significantly different between pediatric and adult groups with PXAs
  - More data required to know how BRAF V600E mutational status impacts prognosis
  - This mutation opens possibility of targeted drug therapy

IMAGING

MR Findings

- Generally in cerebral hemispheres
- Classically temporal
- Usually superficial
- Discrete, enhancing, sometimes as mural nodule
- Cystic in ~ 50% of cases
- PXA with anaplastic features still discrete but may be rim enhancing

MACROSCOPIC

General Features

- Generally discrete
  - Leptomeningeal component
- Cystic in ~ 50% of cases

MICROSCOPIC

Histologic Features

- Solid component often largely in subarachnoid space
  - Fascicular architecture
  - Nested architecture, some cases
  - Pleomorphism and giant cells
  - Large lipidized cells
    - They may be scanty or absent
  - Eosinophilic granular bodies (EGBs)
  - Intercellular reticulin around individual or clusters of cells
  - Leptomeningeal tumor spread
  - Perivascular lymphocytes
  - Ganglion cell component
    - Minority of cases
  - Melanotic tumor cells
    - Rare
  - May harbor epithelioid cells
  - Rosenthal fibers may be present but distinctly rare within tumor
- Intracortical component
  - Infiltrative
    - May be similar to diffuse astrocytoma
  - Calcifications
    - Some cases
- Anaplastic features
  - Grading criteria for higher grade (III, IV) not established, but high-grade lesions show
    - Higher cellularity
    - Less pleomorphism
    - Cells often more epithelioid and less elongated than classic grade II counterpart
    - Increased mitoses
      - $\geq$ 5 per 10 HPF
    - Vascular proliferation
      - Some cases
    - Necrosis
      - Some cases
    - Some tumors with epithelioid cell component

ANCILLARY TESTS

Cytology

- Tissue fragments and individual cells
- Eosinophilic glassy cytoplasm and large processes
- Nuclear pleomorphism
- Eosinophilic granular bodies
- Fibrillary, glial background

Histochemistry

- Reticulin around individual or small groups of cells
- PAS(+) eosinophilic granular bodies

Immunohistochemistry

- GFAP(+)
  - Usually some cells, but not all
- Synaptophysin
  - Neuronal component, if any
- Neurofilament typically (-)
  - Individual cells and rare clusters may be neurofilament (+)
- CD34(+)
  - Variable
- Ki-67
  - Variable index depending on degree of anaplasia
- (+) in ~ 60% of the cases
- Olig2(+) in small glial cells

Genetic Testing

- BRAF V600E mutations in 1/2-2/3 of tumors
  - PXA with anaplastic features have BRAF V600E mutation in < 50% of tumors
- Low incidence of *TP53* mutations
- Frequent loss of chromosome 9

DIFFERENTIAL DIAGNOSIS

Glioblastoma

- Giant cell and epithelioid glioblastoma confused often with PXA
- More infiltrative
  - Except for giant cell type
- Usually not compact
  - Except for giant cell type
- Usually not with fascicular architecture
- More pleomorphic (giant cell type)
- Few, if any, eosinophilic granular bodies
- Different genetic profiles
  - EGFR amplification or mutation
  - IDH 1/2 mutations
  - PXA harbors neither
- Epithelioid glioblastoma has more uniform smaller rounded cells
  - Less pleomorphism than WHO grade III PXA

Ganglion Cell Tumor

- Dysmorphic ganglion cells
- Nonpleomorphic glial component (ganglioglioma)
- Microcysts, some cases
- Lipidized, xanthomatous cells absent

Pilocytic Astrocytoma With Degenerative Atypia

- Microcystic component with myxoid matrix
- Compact component with bipolar cells
- Less pleomorphism
- Multinucleation (pennies on plate)
- More fibrillarity
- Rosenthal fibers
- Myxoid background
- Piloid cells with bipolar processes

DIAGNOSTIC CHECKLIST

Clinically Relevant Pathologic Features

- Discreteness facilitates complete resection, some cases
- Superficial, solid cystic with occasional mass effect
- Anaplastic change associated with poor prognosis
- Successful treatment using BRAF enzyme inhibitors in PXA with mutations

Pathologic Interpretation Pearls

- Minimal diagnostic features
  - Giant cells and pleomorphism
  - EGBs
  - Extensive reticulin network
- Diagnosis should be made with caution in absence of eosinophilic granular bodies
- Much of the tumor can be in subarachnoid space, with abundant reticulin
- Leptomeningeal component of tumor may look different
- The dilemma of anaplastic features
  - WHO 2007 does not have a grade III pleomorphic xanthoastrocytoma
  - Future versions may include higher-grade designations
  - Difficult to distinguish from giant cell glioblastoma
    - Similar histologic and molecular features except for EGBs
  - Threshold of 6 or more mitotic figures per 10 HPF accepted by most experts

SELECTED REFERENCES

1. Berghoff AS et al: BRAF alterations in brain tumours: molecular pathology and therapeutic opportunities. Curr Opin Neurol. 27(6):689-96, 2014
2. Ida CM et al: Pleomorphic Xanthoastrocytoma: Natural History and Long-Term Follow-Up. Brain Pathol. ePub, 2014
3. Koelsche C et al: BRAF-mutated pleomorphic xanthoastrocytoma is associated with temporal location, reticulin fiber deposition and CD34 expression. Brain Pathol. 24(3):221-9, 2014
4. Lee EQ et al: Successful Treatment of a Progressive BRAF V600E-Mutated Anaplastic Pleomorphic Xanthoastrocytoma With Vemurafenib Monotherapy. J Clin Oncol. ePub, 2014
5. Kahramancetin N et al: Aggressive behavior and anaplasia in pleomorphic xanthoastrocytoma: a plea for a revision of the current WHO classification. CNS Oncol. 2(6):523-30, 2013
6. Schmidt Y et al: Anaplastic PXA in adults: case series with clinicopathologic and molecular features. J Neurooncol. 111(1):59-69, 2013
7. Weber RG et al: Frequent loss of chromosome 9, homozygous CDKN2A/p14(ARF)/CDKN2B deletion and low TSC1 mRNA expression in pleomorphic xanthoastrocytomas. Oncogene. 26(7):1088-97, 2007
8. Martinez-Diaz H et al: Giant cell glioblastoma and pleomorphic xanthoastrocytoma show different immunohistochemical profiles for neuronal antigens and p53 but share reactivity for class III beta-tubulin. Arch Pathol Lab Med. 127(9):1187-91, 2003
9. Reifenberger G et al: Expression of the CD34 antigen in pleomorphic xanthoastrocytomas. Acta Neuropathol. 105(4):358-64, 2003
10. Giannini C et al: Immunophenotype of pleomorphic xanthoastrocytoma. Am J Surg Pathol. 26(4):479-85, 2002
11. Fouladi M et al: Pleomorphic xanthoastrocytoma: favorable outcome after complete surgical resection. Neuro Oncol. 3(3):184-92, 2001
12. Giannini C et al: Pleomorphic xanthoastrocytoma: what do we really know about it? Cancer. 85(9):2033-45, 1999
13. Perry A et al: Composite pleomorphic xanthoastrocytoma and ganglioglioma: report of four cases and review of the literature. Am J Surg Pathol. 21(7):763-71, 1997

Superficial Cerebral Tumor

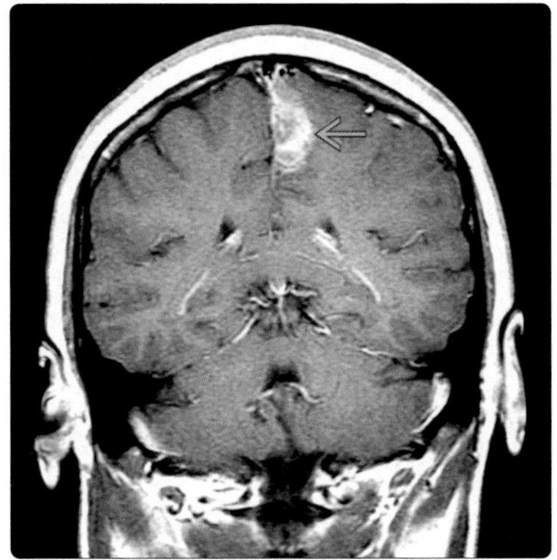

Enhancing Temporal Lobe Tumor Without Mass Effect

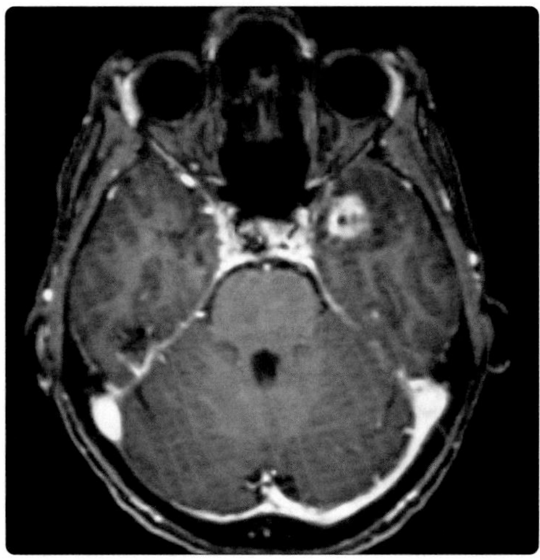

(Left) *PXAs are generally superficial, discrete, and enhancing ⇒. While often cystic, some are not, as in this example in a 23 year old. Cases such as this one could be mistaken on neuroimaging studies for meningioma.* **(Right)** *PXAs often have enhancing components and are often not associated with a significant degree of peritumoral edema or mass effect, as in this case.*

Giant Cells and Small Glial Cells

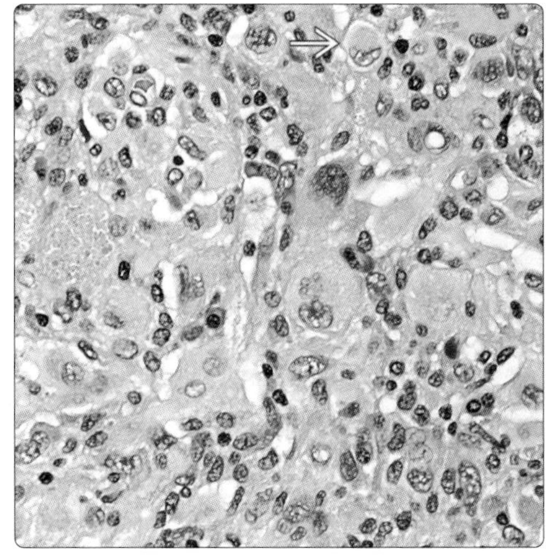

Pleomorphic Spindle Cell Tumor

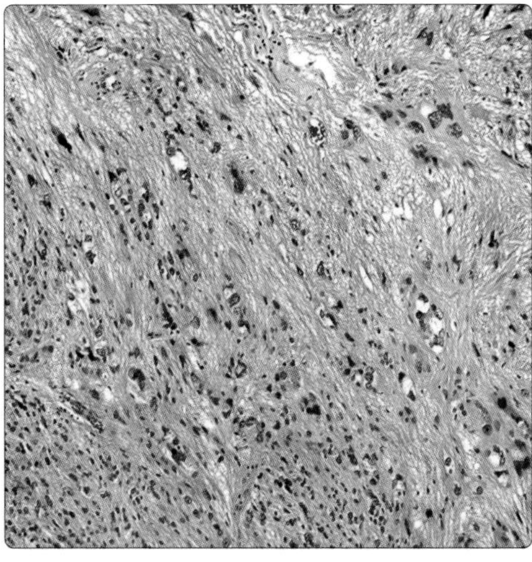

(Left) *The cytological composition is quite varied in PXA and often one can observe small glial or astrocytic cells next to pleomorphic cells with giant nuclei. In typical PXA, rare epithelioid-like cells can also be observed ➡. Unlike epithelioid glioblastoma, however, this tumor lacks other high-grade features or a relatively homogeneous population of epithelioid cells.* **(Right)** *Some PXAs can have areas with a spindle cell component simulating a mesenchymal tumor.*

Xanthomatous Cells

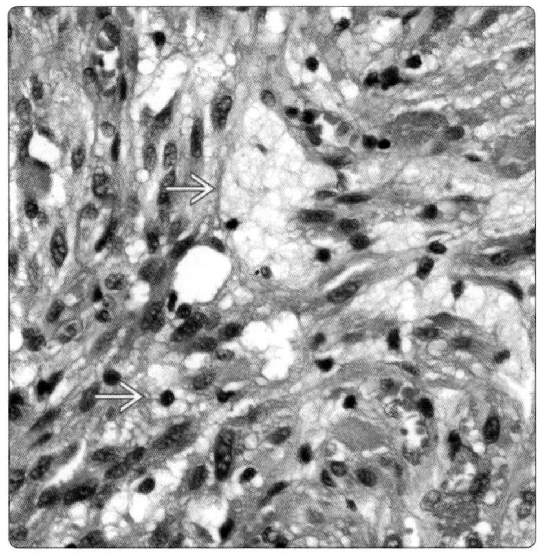

Compact Tumor, Perivascular Lymphocytes

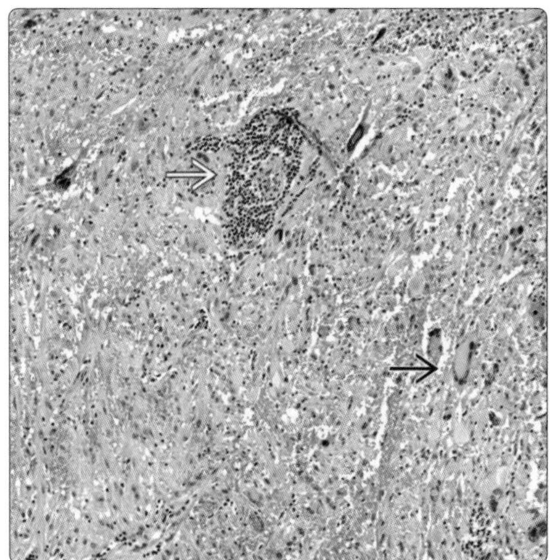

(Left) *Lipidized or xanthomatous cells ➡ may have a bubbly appearance. Such cells are often scarce and can greatly aid in the diagnosis. However, their absence does not negate the diagnosis of PXA.* **(Right)** *Low-power magnification in PXA demonstrates the compact nature of this pleomorphic spindle cell tumor with scattered giant cells ⇒ and perivascular lymphocytic infiltrates ➡.*

(Left) *The EGB is typical of low-grade neoplasms, such as PXA, ganglion cell tumor, or pilocytic astrocytoma. EGBs have been reported to react with antibodies against alpha B-crystallin, ubiquitin, and glial fibrillary acidic protein, although H&E is usually sufficient for recognition of these structures.* **(Right)** *Lipidized or xanthomatous cells often resemble lipoblasts but have been shown to be of glial origin, and the hypersegmented vacuolation is often not associated with lipid accumulation.*

Eosinophilic Granular Body

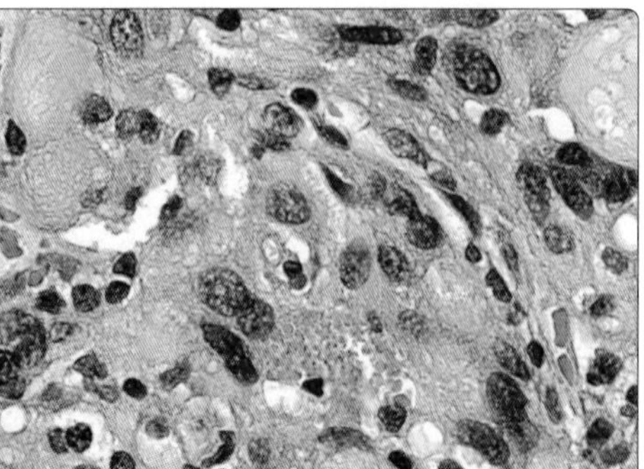

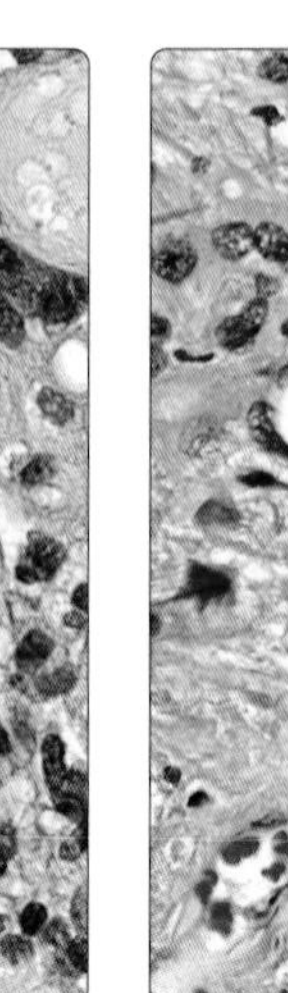

Xanthomatous Cells

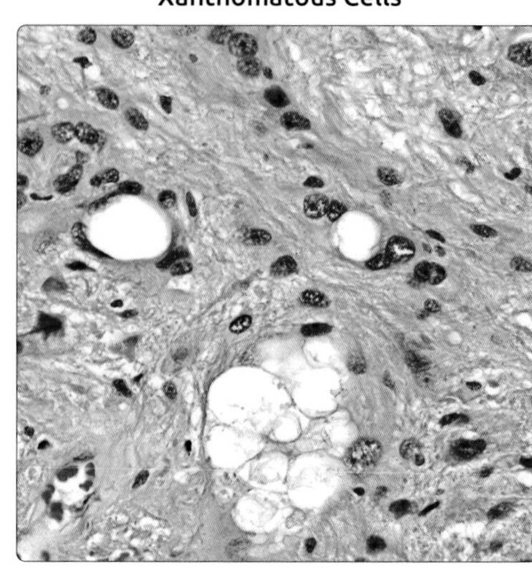

(Left) *While overall pleomorphic, PXAs generally lack the monstrous, multinucleated nuclei of giant cell glioblastoma. The presence of lipidized or xanthomatous cells* ➡ *helps establish the diagnosis.* **(Right)** *The tumor appears looser (and less PXA-like) when its pleomorphic cells are separated by artifact.*

Giant Cells of Pleomorphic Xanthoastrocytoma

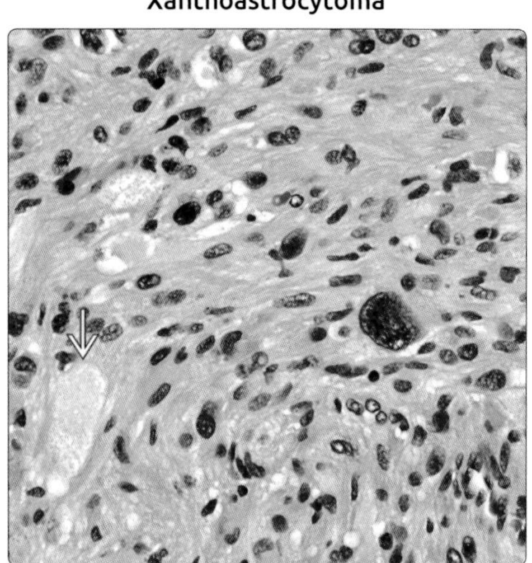

Loose, Pleomorphic Cells

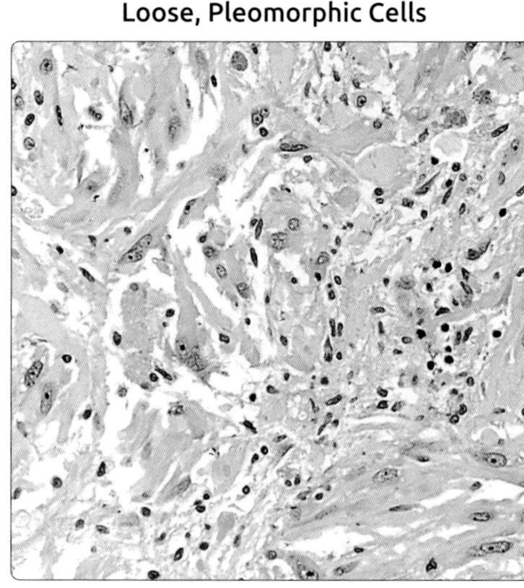

(Left) *Many PXAs harbor small cells, either admixed with the pleomorphic spindle cell component or in some foci as distinct clusters imparting the tumor a biphasic appearance.* **(Right)** *PXAs within the parenchyma or the cerebral cortex can often impart an appearance similar to that of infiltrating astrocytomas, and the degree of pleomorphism may mistakenly prompt a diagnosis of anaplastic astrocytoma or even glioblastoma.*

Small Cell Component

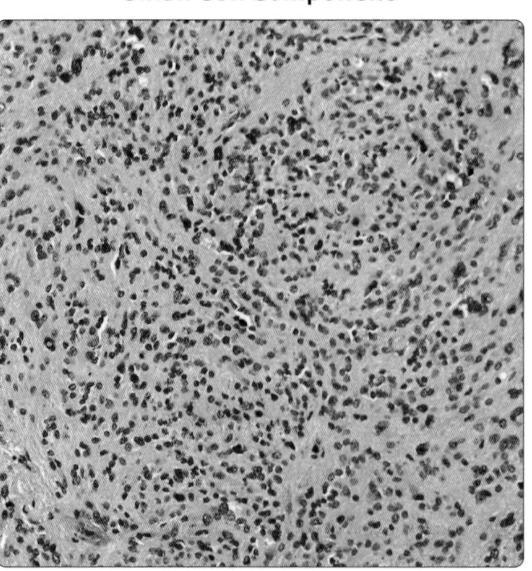

Infiltrative-Appearing Component

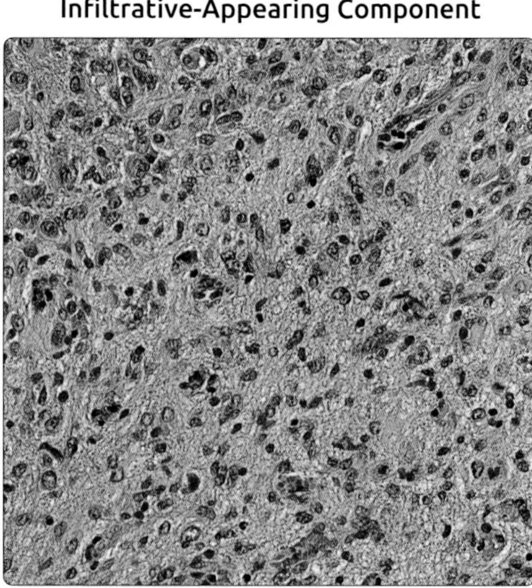

Pleomorphic Spindle Cells

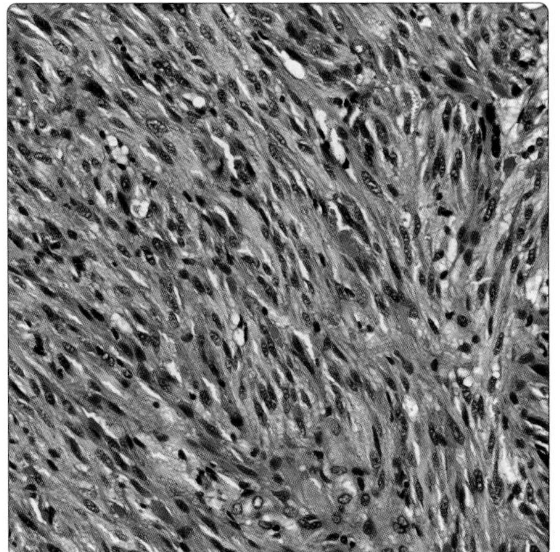

Rich Reticulin Network

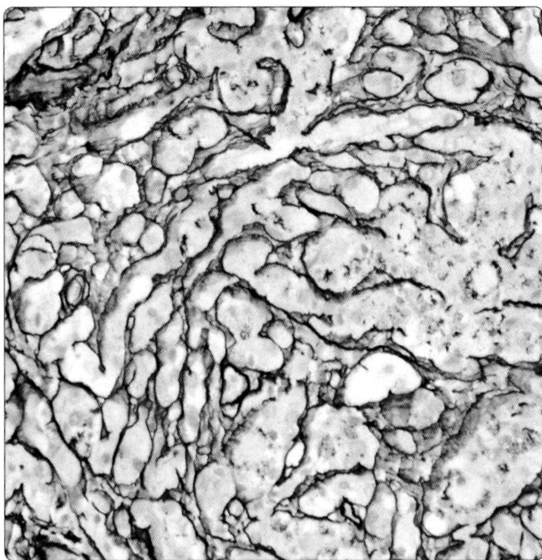

(Left) *The classic lesion has a somewhat fascicular architecture and spindle cells that, while pleomorphic, are not usually monstrous. The bulk of the lesion is compact and noninfiltrating.* **(Right)** *While not present in every specimen, reticulin is common in the leptomeningeal component. Reticulin fibers often surround small groups or individual cells.*

Leptomeningeal Spread

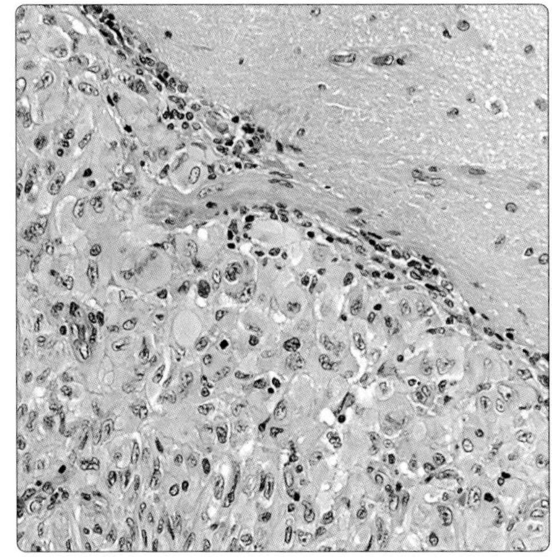

Leptomeningeal Tumor

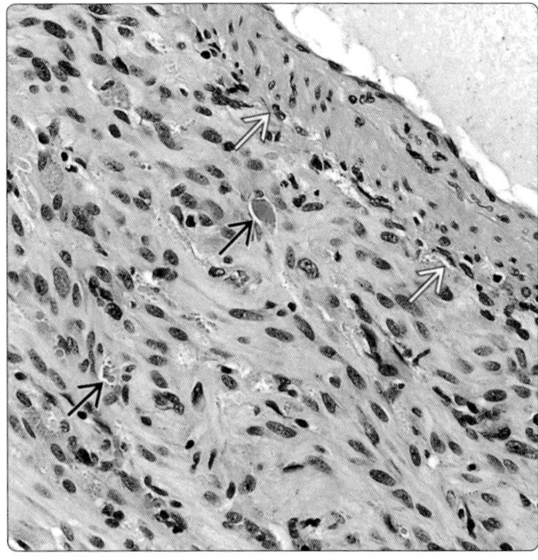

(Left) *Similar to other low-grade glial and glioneuronal tumors, PXAs are known to spread along the leptomeninges and Virchow-Robin spaces.* **(Right)** *An intratumoral artery with a clearly defined muscularis ➡ establishes the meningeal location of this compact tumor. There are multiple small EGBs ⇨. PXA, as well as pilocytic astrocytoma and ganglioglioma, can spread along the subarachnoid space. This does not impact grading or prognosis.*

Epithelioid Appearance

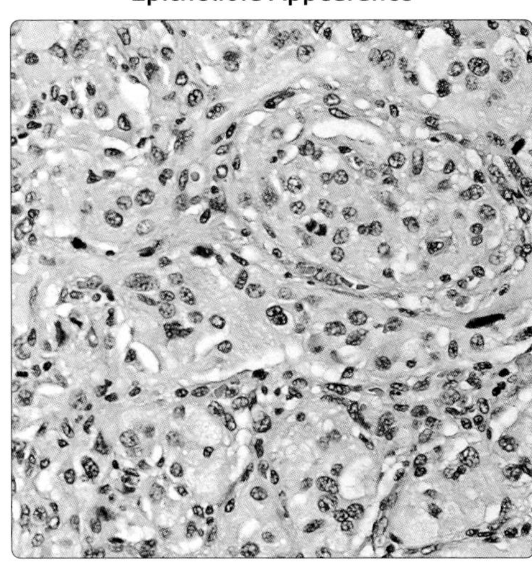

PAS-D(+) Eosinophilic Granular Body

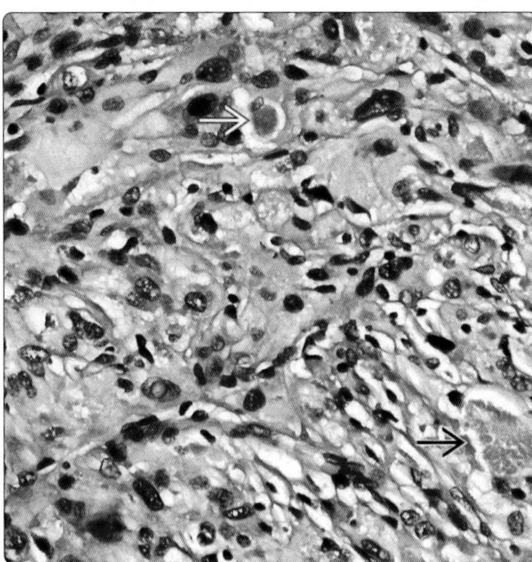

(Left) *In some areas, PXAs can appear whorled and epithelioid and may mimic other glial and nonglial neoplasms.* **(Right)** *EGBs can often be visualized using the PAS-D histochemical stain when they are few and not easily recognizable. While most EGBs stain strongly with the PAS-D stain ➡, some clusters are more inconspicuous ⇨.*

(Left) *Some PXAs may have unusual radiological features, such as a rim enhancement (this appearance may be accompanied by histological evidence of anaplasia). In this patient, the tumor presented as a rim-enhancing, albeit well-circumscribed mass. PXAs with anaplastic features are now officially graded as WHO grade III tumors.* **(Right)** *While not critical per se, increased cellular areas with mitotic figures are often seen in PXAs considered to have anaplastic features. PXAs with anaplastic features are now WHO grade III.*

Anaplastic PXA, WHO Grade III

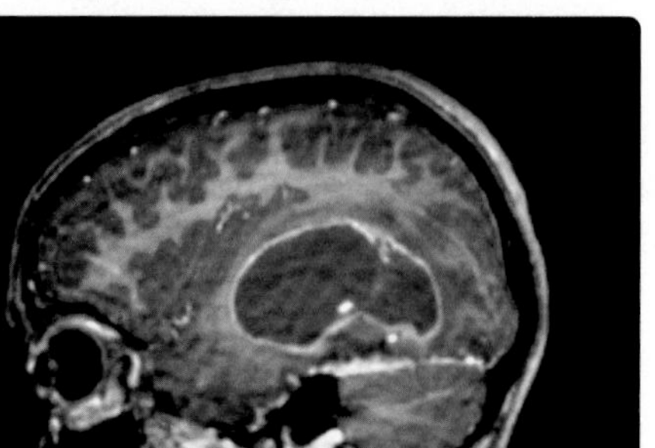

Anaplastic Features: Increased Cellularity

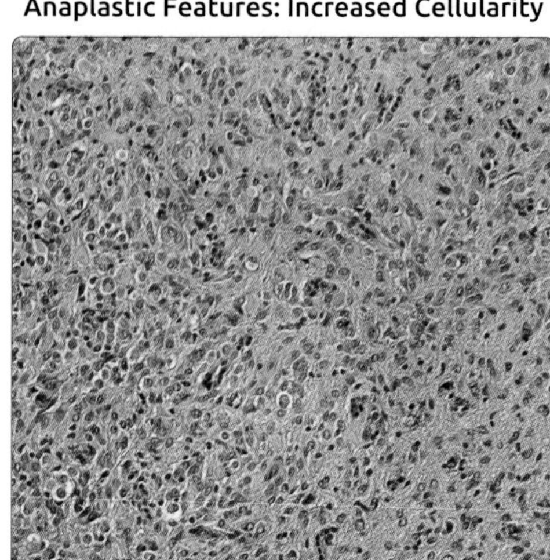

(Left) *Some PXAs may harbor rare epithelioid cells. In contrast to epithelioid glioblastomas, these are focally present in PXA, WHO grade III, and associated with other PXA features, such as EGBs and a pleomorphic population elsewhere in the tumor. Large numbers of such tumor cells, high-grade features, and absence of EGBs should prompt consideration of epithelioid GBM.* **(Right)** *Some PXAs harbor diffuse sheets of rhabdoid cells and palisading necrosis, which can be seen at presentation or in subsequent recurrences.*

Anaplastic Features: Epithelioid Cells

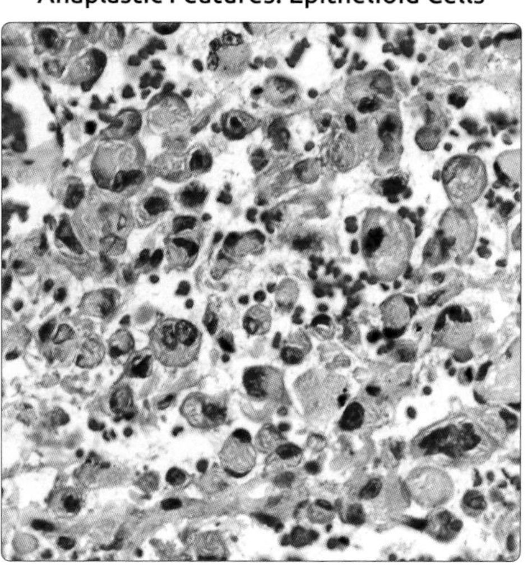

Rhabdoid Cells and Palisading Necrosis

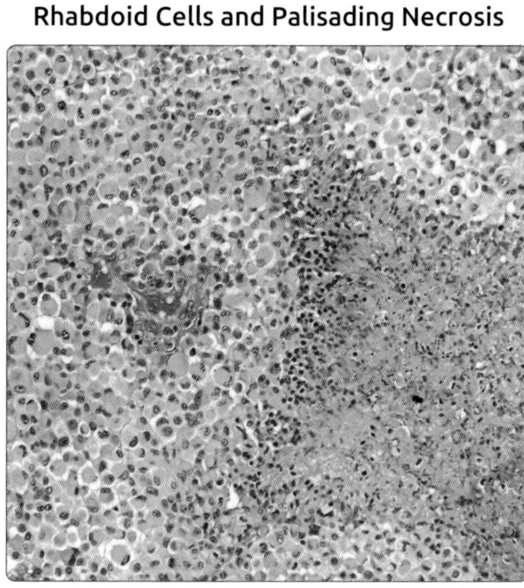

(Left) *Some PXAs have necrosis with pseudopalisading. These are not glioblastomas (WHO grade IV), but rather PXAs with anaplastic features, (WHO grade III), provided classic features of PXA were present historically or are present somewhere else in the current tumor.* **(Right)** *Even though distinctly rare, the presence of microvascular proliferation (vascular endothelial proliferation)* ➔ *distinct from the linear type reactive vascular proliferation may be a feature of PXA, WHO grade III.*

Anaplastic Features: Pseudopalisading

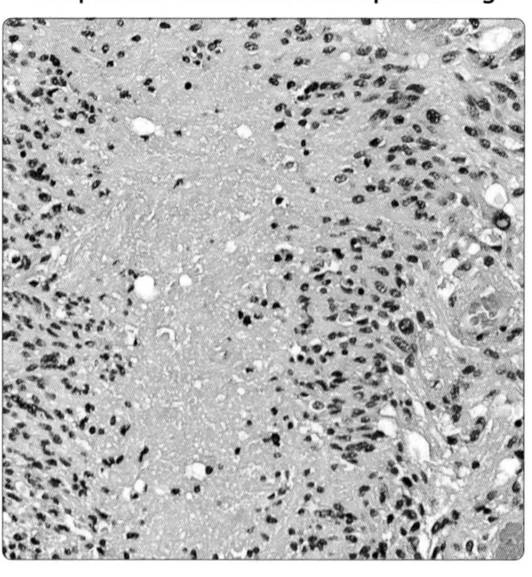

Anaplastic Features: Vascular Proliferation

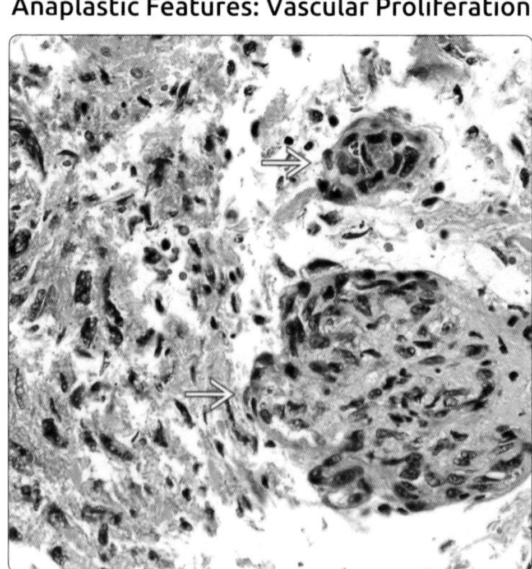

Glial Fibrillary Acidic Protein

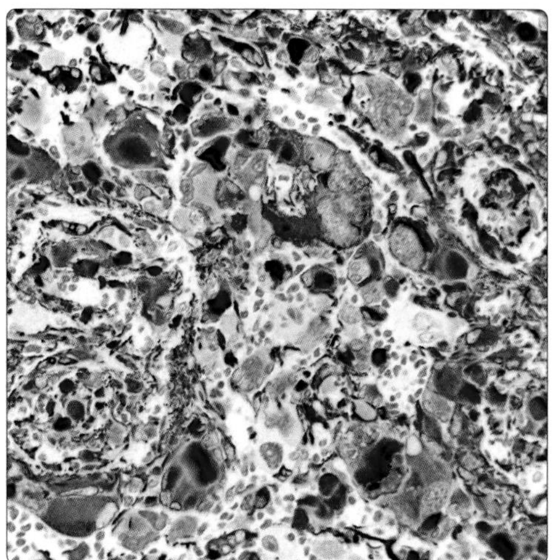

Glial Fibrillary Acidic Protein

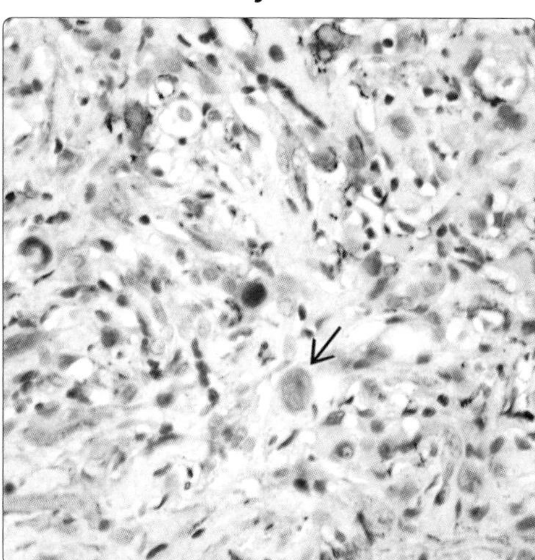

(Left) *Bundles of cells in the leptomeningeal component, as well as the parenchymal component, are GFAP(+). Both giant cells and small glial cells demonstrate GFAP staining.* **(Right)** *Not all cells of a PXA stain positively with the antibodies against GFAP. Here, some of the pleomorphic forms are negative* ➙.

Synaptophysin Staining

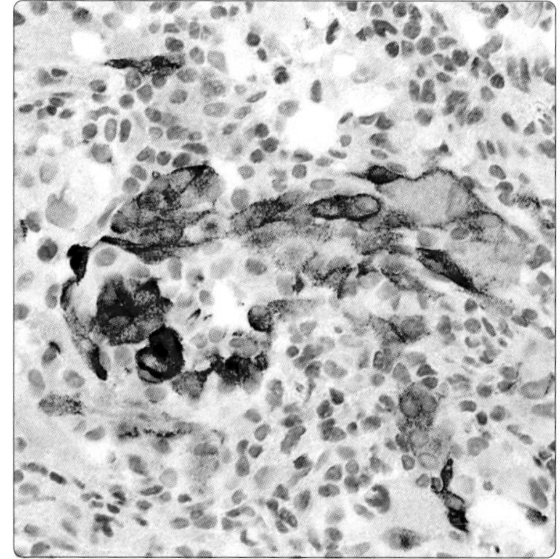

Olig2 Staining

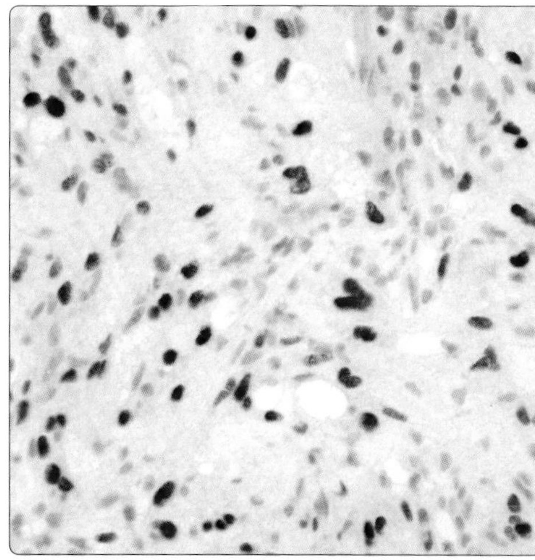

(Left) *A ganglion cell component will be immunoreactive for synaptophysin. This is a fairly frequent finding in PXAs.* **(Right)** *Olig2 immunostaining can be found in a subset of cells in PXAs but is far from specific for this entity, since it is identified in many types of diffuse astrocytic and oligodendroglial tumors.*

Neurofilament Staining

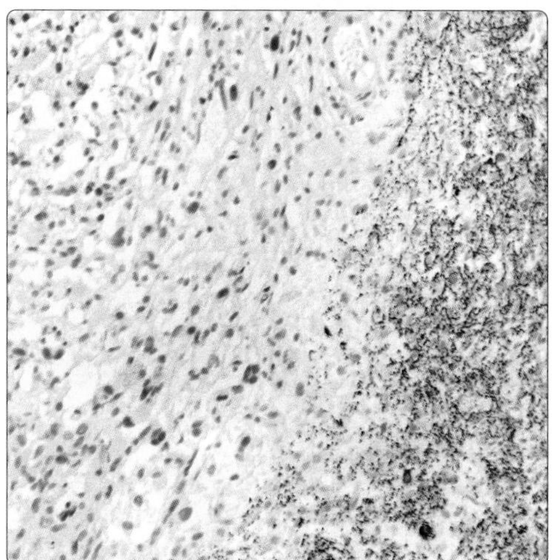

BRAF V600E Staining

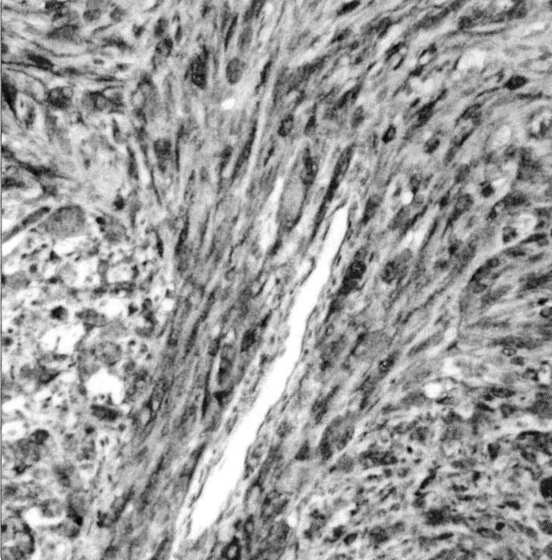

(Left) *The absence of immunoreactivity for neurofilament protein within the PXA on the left side of the image shows the cohesive rather than predominantly infiltrative nature of the tumor.* **(Right)** *Approximately 60% of PXAs and anaplastic PXAs harbor the BRAF V600E mutation, which can be recognized using the mutation-specific antibodies for BRAF VE1 on paraffin-embedded specimens. There is a good correlation between immunohistochemistry and BRAF sequencing, with rare exceptions.*

Subependymal Giant Cell Astrocytoma

KEY FACTS

TERMINOLOGY

- Neuroglial tumor composed of spindle to large cells occurring near foramen of Monro

ETIOLOGY/PATHOGENESIS

- Most cases in tuberous sclerosis complex

CLINICAL ISSUES

- Usually first 2 decades
- Intraventricular, near foramen of Monro
- Prognosis good, but subtotally resected lesions may regrow

MACROSCOPIC

- Well circumscribed

MICROSCOPIC

- Large (but not giant) cells resembling astrocytes &/or ganglion cells typical
- Fascicular architecture with spindle cells less common
- Mitoses infrequent

ANCILLARY TESTS

- Tumor cells show variable IHC(+) for
  - GFAP
  - S100
  - Neurofilament protein
  - Neuropeptides

TOP DIFFERENTIAL DIAGNOSES

- Ependymoma
- Ganglion cell tumor
- Gemistocytic astrocytoma
- Chordoid glioma of 3rd ventricle

DIAGNOSTIC CHECKLIST

- Large cells often with neuronal and astrocytic features
- Variable appearance, not always with classic large cells

(Left) *Subependymal giant cell astrocytomas (SEGAs) are brightly enhancing, discrete, exophytic masses near the foramen of Monro. Although usually unilateral, as in this case, bilaterality is not uncommon.* **(Right)** *SEGAs are discrete masses that lend themselves to complete or near-complete resection.*

Axial MR: Foramen of Monro Mass

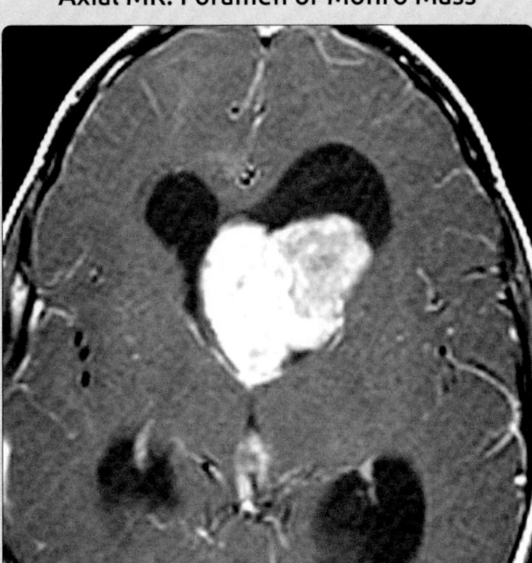

Resectable Discrete Mass

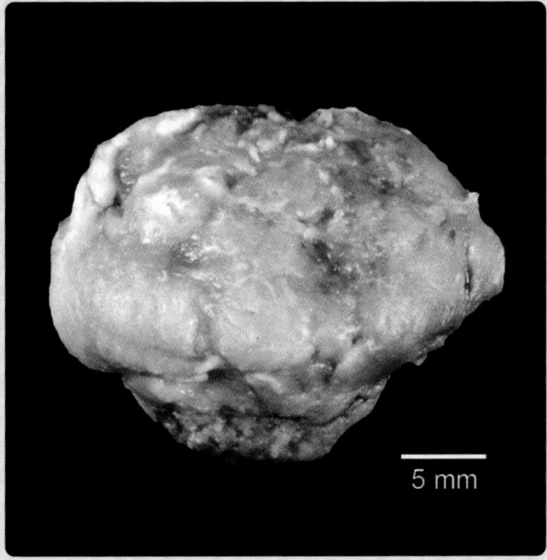

(Left) *SEGAs often contain large pleomorphic cells with abundant eosinophilic cytoplasm, large nuclei, and prominent nucleoli. Taken out of clinical and anatomical context, SEGAs can be easily mistaken for glioblastoma.* **(Right)** *Some SEGAs show bland cytological features and a more abundant fibrillary component.*

Pleomorphic Cells Simulating Glioblastoma

Fibrillar Background

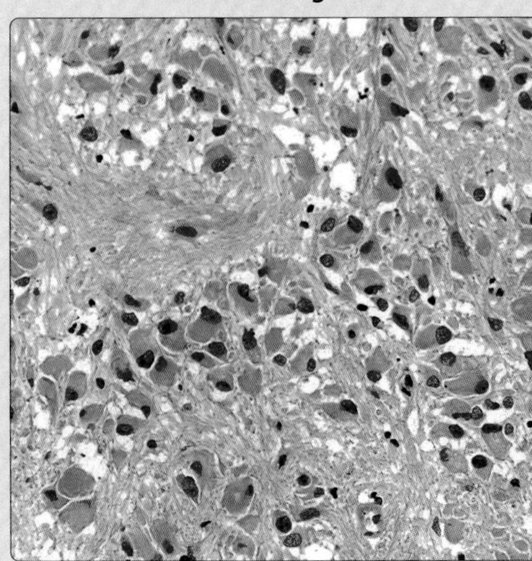

TERMINOLOGY

Abbreviations

- Subependymal giant cell astrocytoma (SEGA)

Definitions

- Neuroglial tumor composed of spindle to large epithelioid cells occurring near foramen of Monro

ETIOLOGY/PATHOGENESIS

Tuberous Sclerosis Complex

- Most cases of SEGA occur in tuberous sclerosis complex (TSC)
  - TSC due to *TSC1* (chromosome 9q34) or *TSC2* mutation (chromosome 16p13)
- SEGA is most common CNS neoplasm in tuberous sclerosis
- SEGA not seen in all TSC patients
  - Only occurs in minority of patients (~ 20% or less) with tuberous sclerosis
- Congenital SEGA develops in 2.2% of TSC patients
  - Patients with *TSC2* mutations, and especially with *TSC2/PKD1* mutations, are more prone to develop SEGA earlier in childhood; possibly should be screened for SEGA from birth

Sporadic

- Without other abnormalities of syndrome, occasional

CLINICAL ISSUES

Site

- Intraventricular, near foramen of Monro

Presentation

- Usually first 2 decades
- Clinical features of cerebrospinal fluid flow obstruction
- Seizures, associated with tuber(s)
- Symptoms precipitated by intratumoral/intraventricular hemorrhage (rare)
- Most SEGAs grow slowly
- SEGAs in patients with *PKD1/TSC2* mutations may grow more rapidly

Treatment

- Surgical approaches
  - Relief of obstruction, total excision if possible
- Drugs
  - Mammalian target of rapamycin signaling pathway inhibitor (everolimus)
  - Limited information on histologic features in SEGA following rapamycin therapy
    - In 1 report, rapamycin therapy did not change histopathological characteristics of subependymal giant cell astrocytoma
  - Everolimus demonstrates sustained effect on SEGA tumor reduction over ≥ 5 years of treatment

Prognosis

- Good
- Subtotally resected lesions may slowly regrow

IMAGING

MR Findings

- Discrete, intraventricular enhancing mass at foramen of Monro
- Sometimes bilateral
- Multiple, often calcified subependymal hamartomas (SEGA-like nodules) in walls of lateral ventricles
- Cortical tubers (most cases)
  - Thickened cortex
  - Linear areas of FLAIR or T2WI hyperintensity from lesion to subjacent ventricle

CT Findings

- Calcified tumor and subependymal hamartomas

MACROSCOPIC

General Features

- Well circumscribed, solid
- Intraventricular, near foramen of Monro

MICROSCOPIC

Histologic Features

- Well circumscribed, with interface with brain infrequently sampled
- Large (but not truly giant) cells resembling astrocytes &/or ganglion cells (typical)
- Fascicular architecture with spindle cells (less common)
- Fibrillar background
- Mitoses: Variable but often few
- Calcifications (some cases)
- Chronic inflammation (some cases)
- Mast cells in small number (common)
- Necrosis (infrequent)

ANCILLARY TESTS

Cytology

- Tissue fragments and large cells with
  - Well-circumscribed cytoplasm and processes
  - Large, round, usually eccentric nuclei with open chromatin and prominent nucleoli

Immunohistochemistry

- Tumor cells variably positive for
  - GFAP
  - Neurofilament protein, especially nonphosphorylated
  - Neuropeptides such as somatostatin, substance P
  - One study showed consistent nuclear expression of TTF-1 in subependymal giant cell astrocytomas
    - Study did not find TTF-1 immunoreactivity in cortical tuber or 2 renal angiomyolipomas resected from TSC patients
    - Intensity and number of IHC(+) cells depends on TTF-1 clone utilized
- Low Ki-67 index

Genetic Testing

- Mutation/deletion
  - *TSC1* or *TSC2*

DIFFERENTIAL DIAGNOSIS

Ependymoma

- More cellular
- More distinct perivascular pseudorosettes, occasional true rosettes
- Small, uniform cells
- EMA(+)
- Tumor cells show no neuronal immunohistochemistry (+) markers
  - Although variable in subependymal giant cell astrocytoma

Ganglion Cell Tumor

- More obvious ganglion cell differentiation
- Perivascular lymphocytes
- Eosinophilic granular bodies
- More cells immunoreactive for synaptophysin, neurofilament protein

Gemistocytic Astrocytoma

- Infiltrative growth pattern
- Smaller, more uniform cells
- Perivascular lymphocytes
- Tumor cells show no neuronal immunohistochemistry (+) markers
  - Although variable in subependymal giant cell astrocytoma
- Not confined in anatomic location to wall of lateral ventricles
  - More likely to be intraparenchymal

Chordoid Glioma of 3rd Ventricle

- Usually adults
- 3rd rather than lateral ventricle
- Chordoid architecture
- Cells smaller and more uniform
- No perivascular pseudorosettes
- IHC
  - GFAP more uniformly (+)
  - NFP(-)
  - CD34(+)
  - TTF-1(+)

DIAGNOSTIC CHECKLIST

Clinically Relevant Pathologic Features

- Discrete
- Large cells often with neuronal and astrocytic features
- Lend themselves to a complete resection or a near-complete resection

Pathologic Interpretation Pearls

- Variable appearance, not always with classic large cells
- Confined in anatomic location to the wall of the lateral ventricles
- Mixed glioneuronal phenotype leads some to prefer designation as subependymal giant cell tumor rather than astrocytoma

SELECTED REFERENCES

1. Beaumont TL et al: Subependymal giant cell astrocytoma in the absence of tuberous sclerosis complex: case report. J Neurosurg Pediatr. 1-4, 2015
2. Cheng S et al: Pathological findings of a subependymal giant cell astrocytoma following treatment with rapamycin. Pediatr Neurol. 53(3):238-242.e1, 2015
3. Franz DN et al: Everolimus for subependymal giant cell astrocytoma: 5-year final analysis. Ann Neurol. ePub, 2015
4. Hewer E et al: Consistent nuclear expression of thyroid transcription factor 1 in subependymal giant cell astrocytomas suggests lineage-restricted histogenesis. Clin Neuropathol. 34(3):128-31, 2015
5. Adriaensen ME et al: Natural history and CT scan follow-up of subependymal giant cell tumors in tuberous sclerosis complex patients. J Clin Neurosci. 21(6):939-41, 2014
6. Chatzopoulos K et al: Thyroid transcription factor-1 and epithelial membrane antigen expression in four cases of subependymal giant cell astrocytoma. Histopathology. 66(7):1035-6, 2014
7. Franz DN et al: Everolimus for subependymal giant cell astrocytoma in patients with tuberous sclerosis complex: 2-year open-label extension of the randomised EXIST-1 study. Lancet Oncol. 15(13):1513-20, 2014
8. Kotulska K et al: Congenital subependymal giant cell astrocytomas in patients with tuberous sclerosis complex. Childs Nerv Syst. 30(12):2037-42, 2014
9. Lee D et al: BRAF V600E mutations are frequent in dysembryoplastic neuroepithelial tumors and subependymal giant cell astrocytomas. J Surg Oncol. 111(3):359-64, 2014
10. Skalicky AM et al: The burden of subependymal giant cell astrocytomas associated with tuberous sclerosis complex: results of a patient and caregiver survey. J Child Neurol. 30(5):563-9, 2014
11. Campen CJ et al: Subependymal giant cell astrocytoma (SEGA) treatment update. Curr Treat Options Neurol. 13(4):380-5, 2011
12. Krueger DA et al: Everolimus for subependymal giant-cell astrocytomas in tuberous sclerosis. N Engl J Med. 363(19):1801-11, 2010
13. Buccoliero AM et al: Subependymal giant cell astrocytoma (SEGA): Is it an astrocytoma? Morphological, immunohistochemical and ultrastructural study. Neuropathology. 29(1):25-30, 2009
14. Takei H et al: Solitary subependymal giant cell astrocytoma incidentally found at autopsy in an elderly woman without tuberous sclerosis complex. Neuropathology. 29(2):181-6, 2009
15. Chan JA et al: Pathogenesis of tuberous sclerosis subependymal giant cell astrocytomas: biallelic inactivation of TSC1 or TSC2 leads to mTOR activation. J Neuropathol Exp Neurol. 63(12):1236-42, 2004
16. Sharma MC et al: Subependymal giant cell astrocytoma--a clinicopathological study of 23 cases with special emphasis on histogenesis. Pathol Oncol Res. 10(4):219-24, 2004
17. Kim SK et al: Biological behavior and tumorigenesis of subependymal giant cell astrocytomas. J Neurooncol. 52(3):217-25, 2001
18. Lopes MB et al: Immunohistochemical characterization of subependymal giant cell astrocytomas. Acta Neuropathol. 91(4):368-75, 1996

Compact Tumor

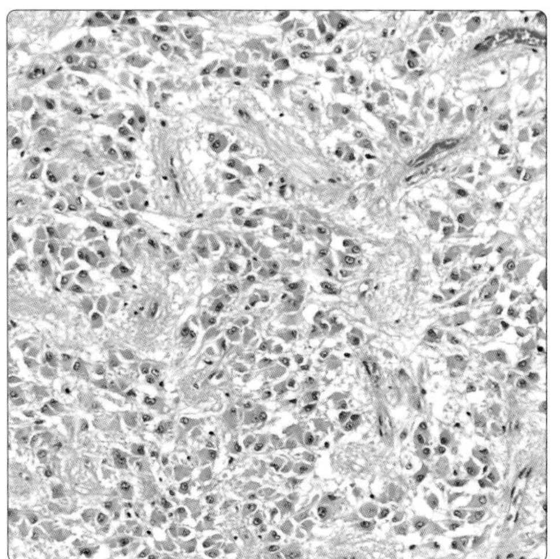

Perivascular Pseudorosettes

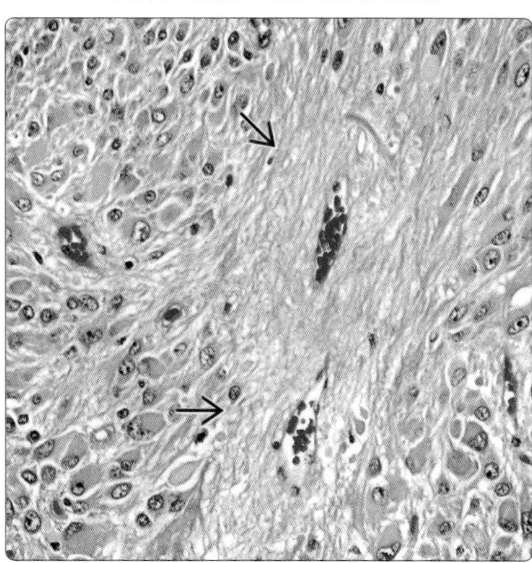

(Left) *SEGAs are compact, noninfiltrating tumors with perivascular fibrillar zones that resemble ependymoma pseudorosettes.* **(Right)** *Perivascular pseudorosettes ⇒ are especially prominent in lesions such as this, wherein aggregates of fine cytoplasmic process comprise much of the tissue. The neuronal overtones of the tumor are evident here, even at low magnification.*

Neuron-Like Cells

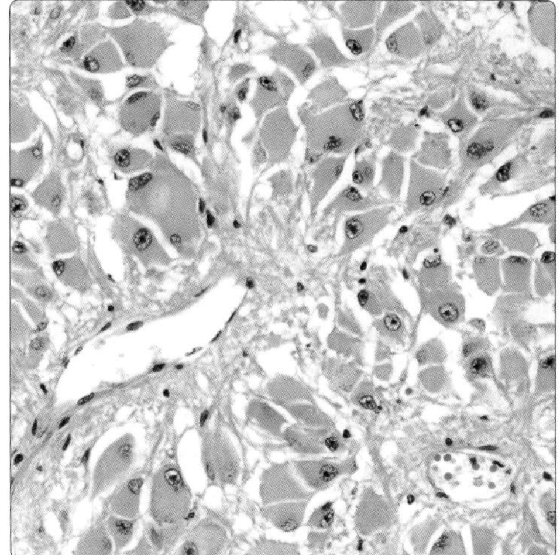

Peripherally Displaced Nuclei

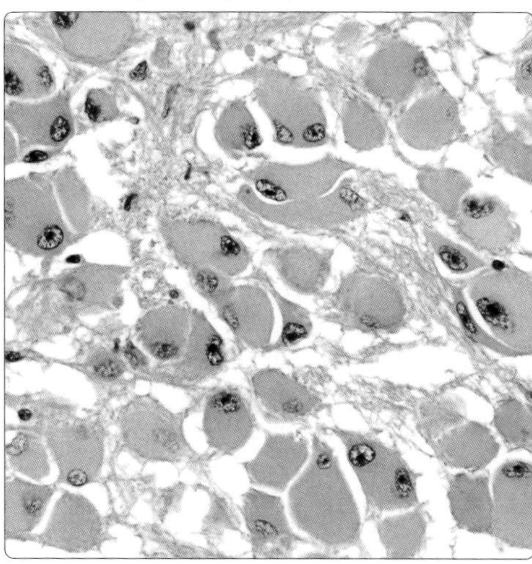

(Left) *Large, glassy, neuron-like cells and perivascular pseudorosettes are classic features.* **(Right)** *Large cells, with profiles that are simultaneously round and polygonal, resemble both ganglion cells and caricatures of gemistocytic astrocytes. Peripherally displaced nuclei are typical. While large, the cells are not typically giant.*

Nissl Substance

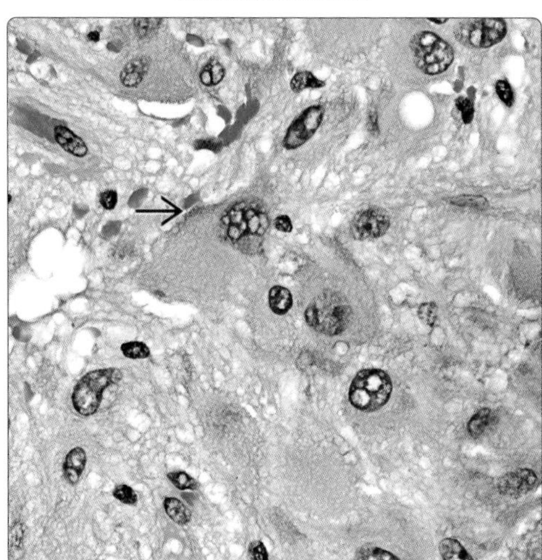

Calcospherites

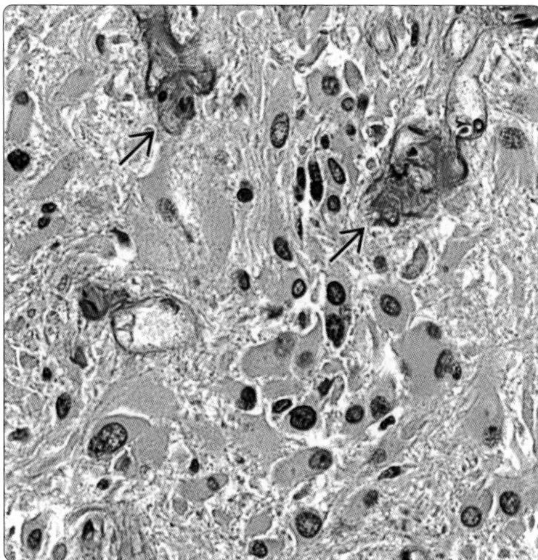

(Left) *Some cells within SEGAs have overt neuronal features, evidenced even on H&E by the presence of basophilic cytoplasmic Nissl substance ⇒. This material is identical to that seen in large nonneoplastic neurons in normal brain.* **(Right)** *SEGAs, or areas thereof, can be nondescript, with little other than an occasional large cell to intimate the diagnosis. Calcospherites help raise the possibility ⇒.*

(Left) *A common variant composed of spindle cells has a fascicular architecture.* **(Right)** *Reference to the clinical setting and location would be helpful to consider in the case of a seemingly nonspecific calcified SEGA such as this.*

Fascicular Architecture

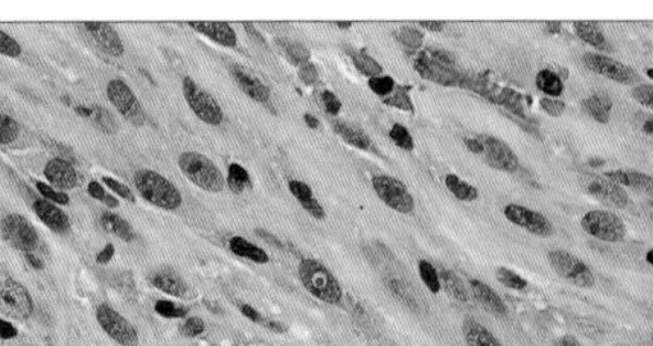

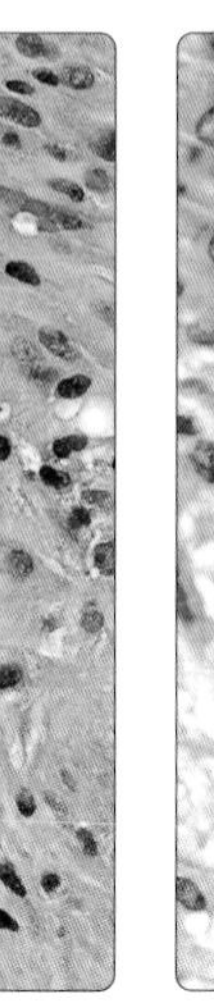

Less Classic SEGA

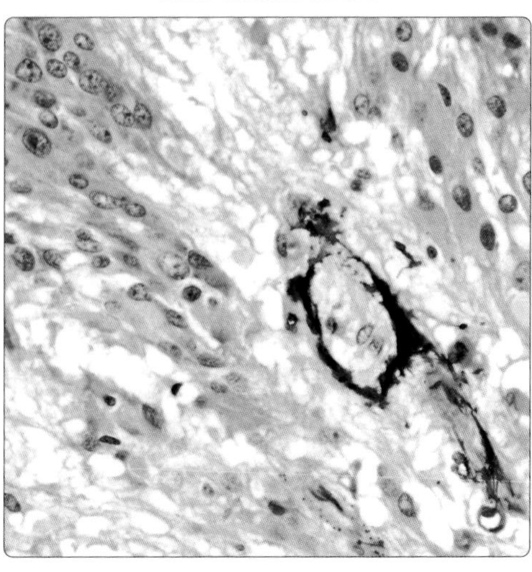

(Left) *SEGAs with smaller cells resemble gemistocytic astrocytes although the round, open nuclei with prominent nucleoli are more consistent with a tumor with neuronal qualities, such as SEGA.* **(Right)** *The similarity to ordinary astrocytomas may be marked in SEGAs such as this. The diagnosis depends on clinical context, site, lack of infiltration, presence of classic features elsewhere in the tumor, and immunohistochemistry.*

Simulating Gemistocytic Astrocytoma

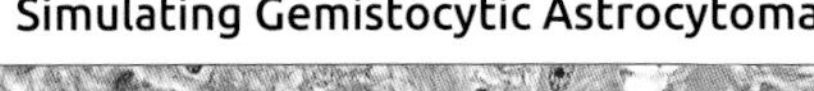

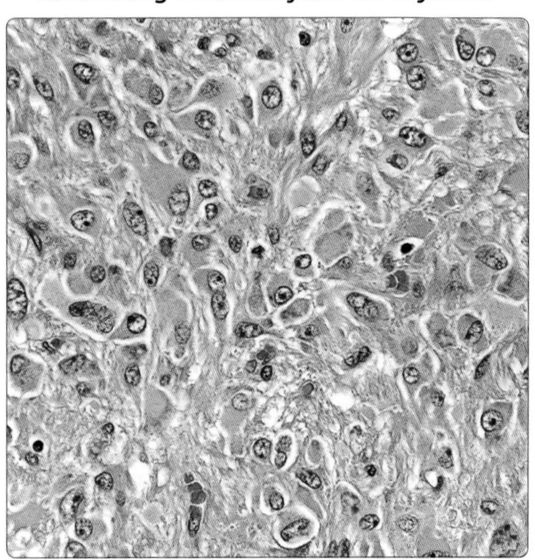

Simulating Ordinary Astrocytoma

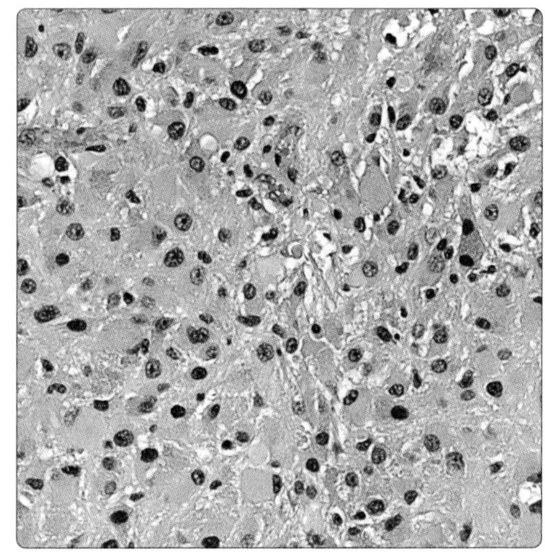

(Left) *Some, but not all, cells in SEGAs are GFAP immunopositive.* **(Right)** *Confirming suspicions from H&E sections, the tumors react for neuronal markers such as phosphorylated neurofilament protein (SM132). Immunostaining is typically focal and, even in regions of positivity, usually does not mark all cells.*

Subset of Cells, GFAP(+)

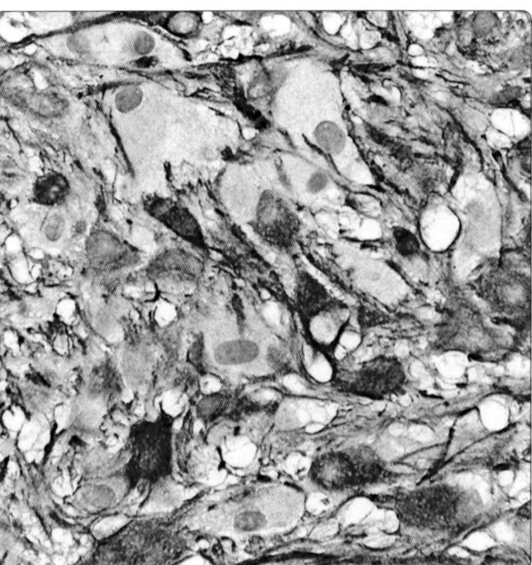

Subset of Cells, NFP(+)

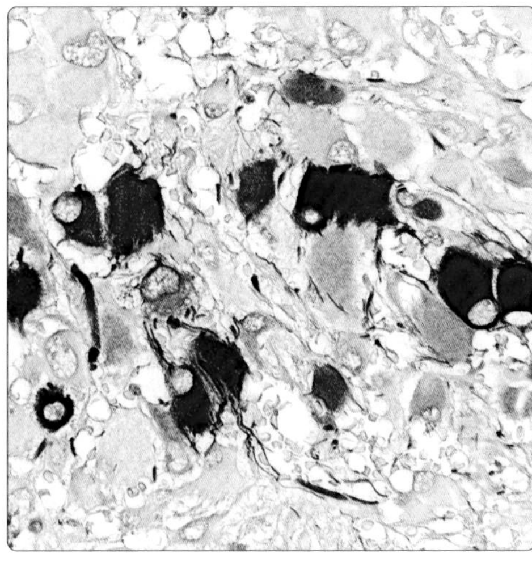

Axial MR: Candle Gutterings

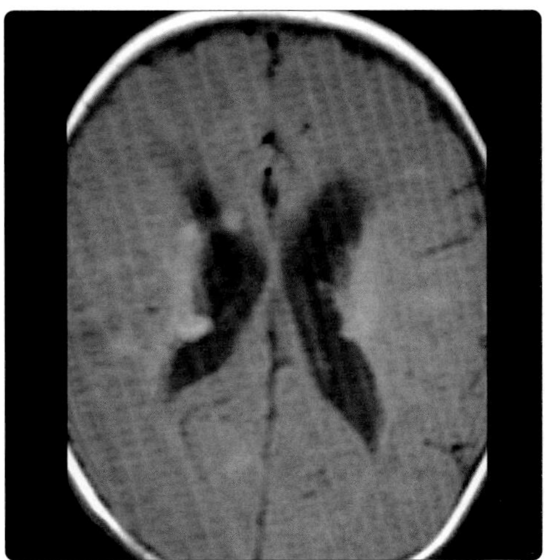

Coronal MR: TS

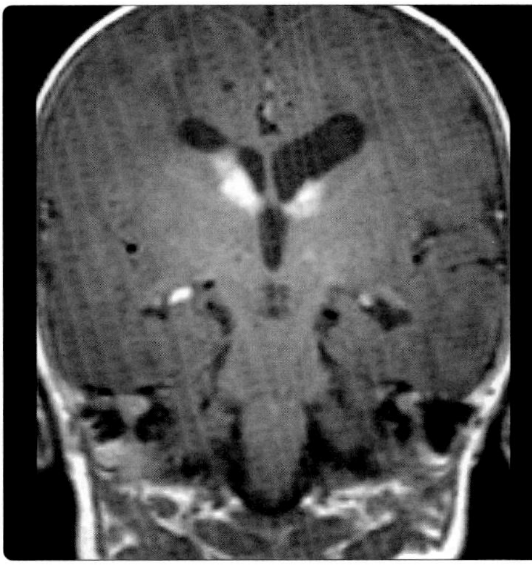

(Left) *This 3-month-old child with tuberous sclerosis has multiple nodules lining the bilateral ventricles, so-called candle guttering. By age 9, one of these had grown into a SEGA.* **(Right)** *This 3-month-old child with TS has bilateral masses in the walls of bilateral lateral ventricles; one of these grew to the extent that surgical resection was undertaken when the patient was 9 years old.*

Coronal MR: TS

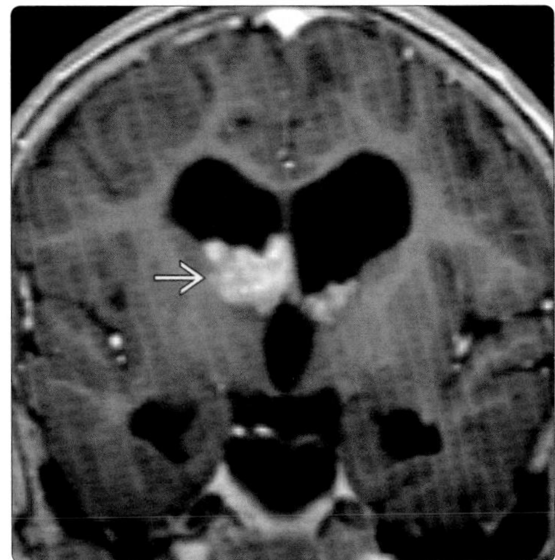

Mitosis

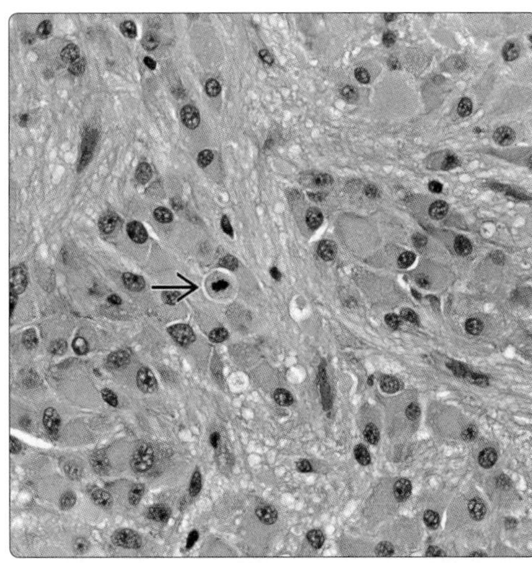

(Left) *This child had TS diagnosed very early in life and at 1st imaging study at age 3 months already was found to have bilateral lateral ventricular wall candle gutterings. One of these nodules showed growth ➡ and was removed when the patient was 9 years old; features were those of SEGA.* **(Right)** *SEGAs do grow and can have mitotic figures ➡, but these do not impact prognosis or grading; all SEGAs are WHO grade I.*

Focally Elevated Ki-67

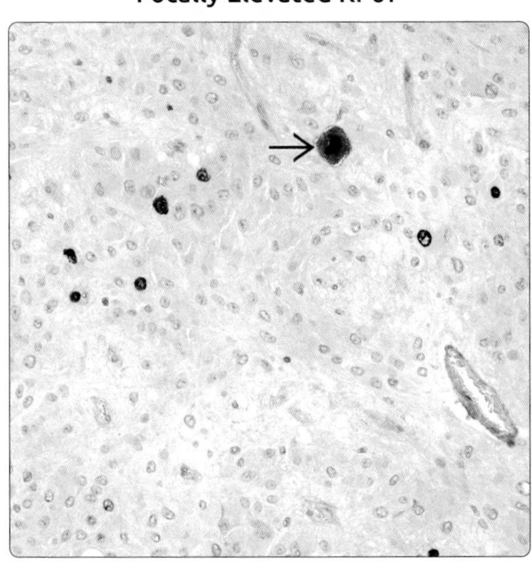

Smear: Prominent Nucleoli

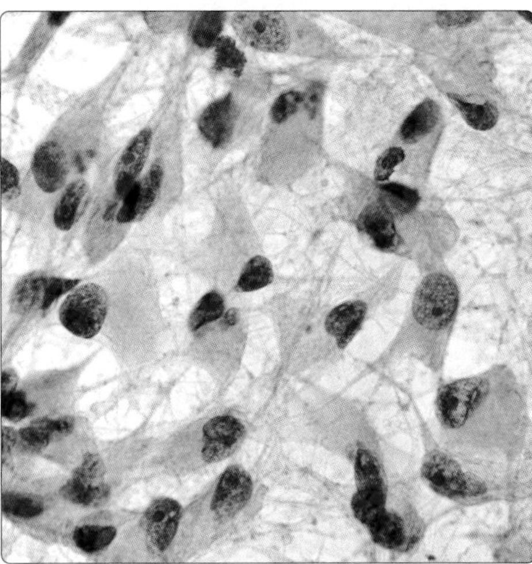

(Left) *SEGAs can show varying degrees of Ki-67 cell cycle labeling, and IHC can further highlight mitotic figures ➡.* *This parallels the fact that these tumors do grow over time, necessitating removal.* **(Right)** *The cells, with hybrid glial/neuronal qualities, typically have nuclei displaced to one pole. Prominent nucleoli contribute to the neuronal, ganglion cell quality.*

Ependymoma

KEY FACTS

TERMINOLOGY

- Generally well-circumscribed neoplasm with ependymal differentiation, WHO grade II

CLINICAL ISSUES

- Location
  - Adults: Mostly spinal cord; intracranial rare
  - Children: Most common posterior fossa, followed by supratentorial; spinal cord rare
- Prognosis
  - Adult and spinal cord: Excellent
  - Posterior fossa in children, fair prognosis, worse with high-grade and partial resection
  - Supratentorial, high-grade, partial resection associated with poor prognosis

IMAGING

- Spinal: Solid, cystic enhancing
- Supratentorial, solid and cystic, enhancing except for cortical ependymoma

MICROSCOPIC

- Variants
  - Classic cellular: Ependymoma, clear cell variant, papillary variant, tanycytic variant
- Histological patterns
  - Giant cell ependymoma, cortical ependymoma, mixed subependymoma/ependymoma, and myxopapillary ependymoma/ependymoma

ANCILLARY TESTS

- GFAP(+)
  - Perivascular pseudorosettes and fibrillar zones
- EMA(+)
  - Dot-like, highlighting microlumina and surfaces of true rosettes and epithelia
- C11orf95-RELA fusion with L1CAM positivity in some supratentorial tumors

Midline Cerebellar Tumor

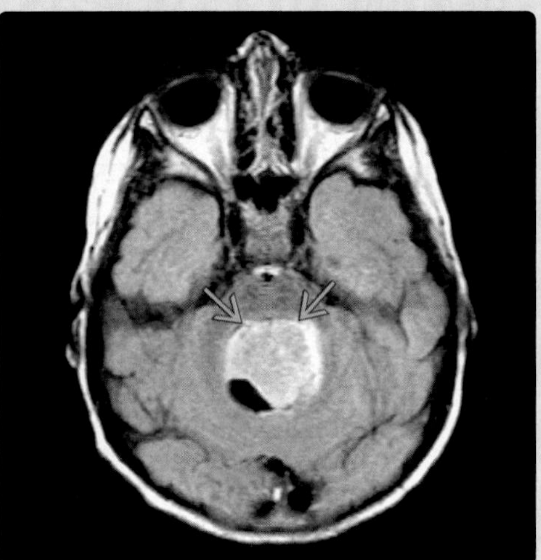

Intramedullary Enhancing Tumor

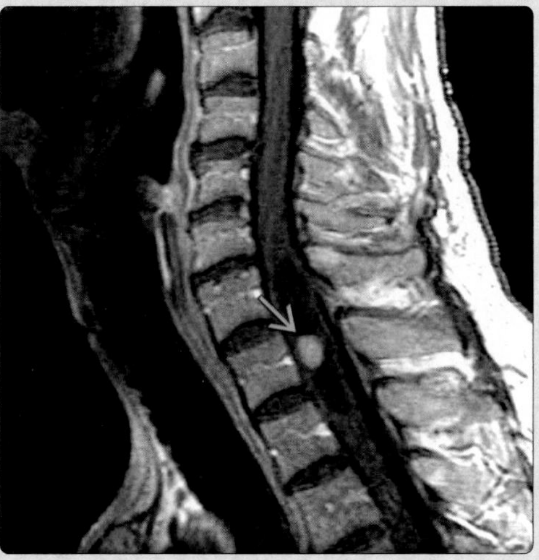

(Left) *This 4th ventricle tumor involves the vermis ➡ and the differential diagnoses include medulloblastoma, ependymoma, or pilocytic astrocytoma. The broad attachment to the ventricular floor favors ependymoma.* **(Right)** *Spinal ependymoma is often discrete and enhancing after gadolinium administration ➡. This cervical example is associated with cystic expansion of the cord both rostrally and caudally (syrinx).*

Intramedullary Spinal Cord Tumor

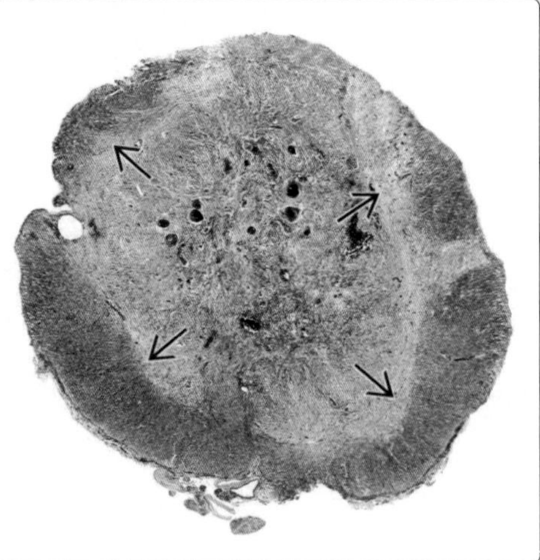

Perivascular Pseudorosette

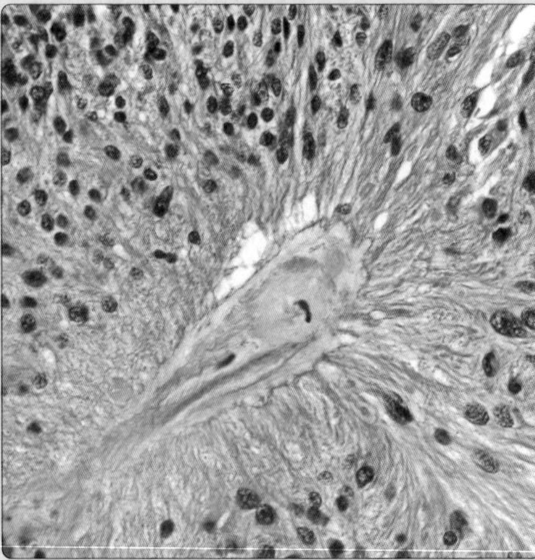

(Left) *As a result of a pushing rather than an infiltrative border ➡, an intraspinal ependymoma is usually cured by excision without the need for postoperative radio- or chemotherapy. This section is stained with H&E/Luxol fast blue.* **(Right)** *The typical perivascular arrangement of tumor cells in ependymoma and some other tumors with ependymal qualities is the diagnostic hallmark of this tumor, with rare exceptions.*

TERMINOLOGY

Definitions

- Generally well-circumscribed mass with ependymal differentiation
- WHO grade II

ETIOLOGY/PATHOGENESIS

Unknown Etiology

- Majority of tumors

Neurofibromatosis 2

- Minority of spinal cord tumors
- Often multiple

CLINICAL ISSUES

Epidemiology

- Age
  - Adults
    - Most commonly in spinal cord
    - Supratentorial and posterior fossa rare
  - Children
    - Most commonly in posterior fossa
    - Supratentorial location is less common, but anaplastic examples predominate in this location
    - Spinal is rare; may also be due to seeding from intracranial tumors

Site

- Spinal cord
  - Rostral, usually cervical; most common intramedullary tumor in adults
  - Conus medullaris and filum terminale, usually myxopapillary
  - Seeding of intracranial tumor should be considered in children
- Posterior fossa
  - Typically around 4th ventricle
  - Extension through foramina of Luschka and Magendie
- Supratentorial
  - Most often paraventricular with parenchymal component
  - Pure intraventricular tumor is rare
  - Most tumors are not directly connected to ventricles
    - Cortical ependymoma is rare, histologic features overlap with angiocentric glioma

Presentation

- Spinal
  - Pain
  - Neurological deficit, weakness, or sensory loss with level
  - Incontinence is rare
  - Signs and symptoms of neurofibromatosis 2 are rare
- Posterior fossa
  - Signs and symptoms of obstructive hydrocephalus
- Supratentorial
  - Features of mass effect, focal neurological deficit, seizures (uncommon)

Treatment

- Surgical approaches
  - Gross total resection is treatment of choice
  - Many posterior fossa tumors require shunting
- Drugs
  - Usually when subtotally resected, recurrent, or anaplastic
- Radiation
  - Standard for intracranial primary, except for some select supratentorial, grade II, totally resected tumors
  - Upon recurrence
  - Craniospinal for select patients, especially with CSF dissemination

Prognosis

- Spinal: Excellent
- Posterior fossa
  - Gross total resection is most critical prognostic factor
  - Patients younger than 3 years have poorer prognosis
  - WHO grade influences prognosis
- Supratentorial
  - Extent of resection, single most critical prognostic factor
  - L1CAM(+) tumors with C11orf95-RELA fusion have worse prognosis
  - WHO grade III and clear cell variant have worse prognosis

IMAGING

MR Findings

- Discrete with limited mass effect
- Mostly solid, cystic with rare enhancing mural nodule appearance
- Often hyper- or isointense on T2WI and hypointense on T1WI
- Extension into cisterna magna, posterior fossa tumors
- Enhancing nodules along spinal cord: CSF dissemination
- Hemorrhage or calcifications, low signal on T2
- Variable enhancement
  - Spinal cord tumors typically avid
  - Posterior fossa tumors, none to moderate
  - Cortical ependymomas, little or no enhancement
- Cystic component
  - Spinal intramedullary, more common
  - Supratentorial, extraventricular more common

MACROSCOPIC

General Features

- Well circumscribed
- May be cystic
- Hemorrhagic, cherry red appearance

MICROSCOPIC

Histologic Features

- Classic (cellular) ependymoma
  - Perivascular pseudorosettes
  - True rosettes, lumina, canals
  - Sheet-like growth pattern, hypercellular
  - Highly fibrillar areas, sometimes with few nuclei
  - Gemistocyte-like cells in fibrillar areas in some cases

- Necrosis common, especially in posterior fossa; not in itself indicator of anaplasia
- Tumor borders
  - Usually sharply circumscribed
  - Infiltrative occasionally, especially supratentorial and high grade
- Hypercellular nodules
  - Some in otherwise low-grade or typical ependymomas with only moderately increased mitotic rate
  - Some with increased atypia, high mitotic activity, and Ki-67 labeling, especially in posterior fossa
  - Some suggest presence of hypercellular nodules has limited effect on prognosis
- Presence of cystic structures and associated linear vascular proliferation
  - Some supratentorial and spinal intramedullary types
  - Telangiectatic vascular proliferation in wall
- Calcifications in some cases
- Hyalinized nodules in some intraspinal types
- Cytoplasmic vacuolization, sometimes lipidized-looking cells
- Epithelial surfaces less common than perivascular pseudorosettes; uncommon in intraspinal types
- Peritumoral piloid gliosis, especially spinal
- Bone &/or cartilage (rare)
- Neuronal differentiation, synaptophysin (+), nodules of neuronal differentiation (pale islands) similar to those of nodular/desmoplastic medulloblastoma (rare)

- Clear cell variant
  - Usually supratentorial
  - Especially sharp border with brain
  - Oligodendroglioma-like cytoplasmic clearing
  - Typical nuclei
    - Large relative to those of other ependymoma types
    - Round or polygonal, grooved, and clefted
  - Perivascular pseudorosettes may be inconspicuous
  - No true rosettes
- Papillary variant
  - Papillae with fibrovascular cores
  - Redundant columnar or cuboidal epithelium and round to oval nuclei
  - May be little fibrillar tissue
- Tanycytic variant
  - Fascicular architecture
  - Long, slender cells
  - Inconspicuous perivascular pseudorosettes
  - No true rosettes
  - Vacuolated cells
- Other histological patterns
  - Giant cell ependymoma
    - Degenerative atypia, usually in myxopapillary but rarely classic cellular ependymoma
    - Almost no perivascular pseudorosettes, epithelial cell
  - Cortical ependymoma
    - Supratentorial, not associated with ventricles
    - Predominantly spindle cells, tanycytic variant-like
    - Vacuolated cells, tubules
    - Occasional angiocentric glioma-like, infiltrative pattern
  - Ependymosarcoma
    - Malignant mesenchymal differentiation
  - Mixed ependymal tumors
    - Subependymoma/ependymoma
      - Foci of typical subependymoma in classical ependymoma
      - Prognostic significance not clear, but does not imply aggressive behavior
    - Myxopapillary/classic cellular ependymoma
      - Typically in spinal cord
      - Grading controversial
      - Prognostic significance not clear
  - Melanotic differentiation, often melanin-like lipochrome
- WHO grading criteria
  - Not clearly established
  - Mitotic rates < 5 per 10 high-power field (HPF) compatible with grade II ependymoma
    - Cutoff for anaplastic ependymoma unclear, 5/10 HPF and 10/10 HPF have been used
  - Vascular endothelial proliferation strong predictor of recurrence, not compatible with grade II
  - Palisading necrosis not compatible with grade II
  - No conspicuous pleomorphism or nuclear anaplasia in grade II ependymomas

ANCILLARY TESTS

Cytology

- Tissue fragments of cohesive cells
- Cell processes and fibrillar background
- Perivascular orientation (pseudorosettes)
- Small, oval nuclei in most types
- Larger, rounder nuclei with clefts and grooves in clear cell type
- Nuclear atypia in proportion to anaplasia
- Nuclear pleomorphism (degenerative atypia) not uncommon, particularly in giant cell type

Immunohistochemistry

- GFAP(+)
  - Processes more than cytoplasm
  - Well seen in perivascular pseudorosettes
- EMA(+)
  - Surfaces, especially true rosettes, canals, papilla
  - Dot-like staining of microlumina
- CD56(+), throughout tumor and microlumina
- D2-40(+), S100(+), both diffuse and strong, nonspecific
- Keratin (CAM5.2) focal, sometimes diffuse and strong
- Synaptophysin (+)
  - Classic ependymoma, focal, some cases
  - Neuronal differentiation, medulloblastoma-like pale islands (rare)
- L1CAM(+) in some supratentorial tumors
- Olig2 mostly (-) or rare (+) nuclei
- IDH-1(-)
- Ki-67 often high in pediatric and posterior fossa tumors

Genetic Testing

- Losses on chromosomes 1p, 3, 6q, 7, 9p, 10q, 13q, 16p, 17, 21, and 22q
  - Loss of 22q, site of *NF2* gene, especially relevant to spinal types, more often in adults

- Some neurofibromatosis 2 patients have solitary or multiple ependymomas
- Gains on 1q, 4q, 5, 7, 8, 9, 12q, and 20
- Recent studies suggest different genetic subgroups, but clear categorization based on molecular features are still elusive
- Supratentorial tumors with C11orf95-RELA fusion

Electron Microscopy

- Microlumina with microvilli
- Cilia and ciliary apparatus
- Runs of intermediate junctions, especially near microlumina

Gene Expression Profiling

- 3 types, possibly related to stem cell radial glia in all craniospinal compartments

DIFFERENTIAL DIAGNOSIS

DDx of Intraspinal Ependymoma

- Diffuse astrocytoma
  - Infiltrating (diffuse) growth pattern
    - Axons within tumor
  - No perivascular pseudorosettes
  - No EMA(+) dot-like profiles
- Pilocytic and pilomyxoid astrocytoma (PMA)
  - Loose, spongy architecture (pilocytic)
  - Piloid cells with Rosenthal fibers (pilocytic)
  - Eosinophilic granular bodies (pilocytic)
  - Perivascular rosettes (PMA)
  - Myxoid background (PMA)
- Schwannoma
  - Almost always extraaxial
  - More intensely and extensively S100(+) (including nuclei) than tanycytic ependymoma
  - Less intensely and diffusely GFAP(+)
  - Pericellular reticulin or collagen type IV
- Meningioma
  - Extraaxial
  - Whorls and psammoma bodies
  - EMA surface staining, S100 patchy (20%), GFAP(-)
- Hemangioblastoma
  - Lobular, sometimes vague, architecture
  - High vascularity
  - No perivascular pseudorosettes
  - Vacuolated (lipidized) tumor cells
  - Inhibin-α (+)

DDx of Intracranial Ependymoma

- Astroblastoma
  - Overlap with ependymoma in some cases
  - Perivascular thick; unipolar process more epithelioid
  - Vascular hyalinization
- Angiocentric glioma
  - Overlap with cortical ependymoma in some cases
  - Infiltrative growth pattern
  - Longitudinal as well as radial orientation of perivascular cells
  - Subpial vertical palisading
- Oligodendroglioma (vs. clear cell ependymoma)
  - Infiltrative, overruns normal brain elements
  - No large clefted and grooved nuclei
  - Codeletion of chromosomes 1p and 19q (adult cases)
- Medulloblastoma
  - Perivascular pseudorosettes less prominent
  - Neuroblastic (Homer Wright) rosettes (minority)
  - No true rosettes or epithelial surfaces
  - Nodules (pale islands) in nodular desmoplastic type
  - Synaptophysin (+)
- Neurocytoma
  - Cytologically monotonous
  - Finely fibrillar areas of neuropil
  - Synaptophysin diffusely (+)
- Pilocytic and pilomyxoid astrocytoma

DIAGNOSTIC CHECKLIST

Pathologic Interpretation Pearls

- Isolated perivascular pseudorosette formation in otherwise diffuse infiltrating glioma is not diagnostic for ependymoma
- EM may be necessary in problematic examples to establish ependymal lineage
- Grading is not affected by number or type of rosettes
- Grading is problematic in ependymomas, especially for mixed lesions and those with modest numbers of hypercellular nodules

SELECTED REFERENCES

1. Mack SC et al: Epigenomic alterations define lethal CIMP-positive ependymomas of infancy. Nature. 506(7489):445-50, 2014
2. Parker M et al: C11orf95-RELA fusions drive oncogenic NF-κB signalling in ependymoma. Nature. 2014 Feb 27;506(7489):451-5. Epub 2014 Feb 19. Erratum in: Nature. 508(7497):554, 2014
3. Tarapore PE et al: Pathology of spinal ependymomas: an institutional experience over 25 years in 134 patients. Neurosurgery. 73(2):247-55; discussion 255, 2013
4. Ellison DW et al: Histopathological grading of pediatric ependymoma: reproducibility and clinical relevance in European trial cohorts. J Negat Results Biomed. 10:7, 2011
5. Van Gompel JJ et al: Cortical ependymoma: an unusual epileptogenic lesion. J Neurosurg. 114(4):1187-94, 2011
6. Mack SC et al: The genetic and epigenetic basis of ependymoma. Childs Nerv Syst. 25(10):1195-201, 2009
7. Lehman NL: Patterns of brain infiltration and secondary structure formation in supratentorial ependymal tumors. J Neuropathol Exp Neurol. 67(9):900-10, 2008
8. Tihan T et al: The prognostic value of histological grading of posterior fossa ependymomas in children: a Children's Oncology Group study and a review of prognostic factors. Mod Pathol. 21(2):165-77, 2008
9. Taylor MD et al: Radial glia cells are candidate stem cells of ependymoma. Cancer Cell. 2005 Oct;8(4):323-35. Erratum in: Cancer Cell. 9(1):70, 2006
10. Fouladi M et al: Clear cell ependymoma: a clinicopathologic and radiographic analysis of 10 patients. Cancer. 98(10):2232-44, 2003
11. Ebert C et al: Molecular genetic analysis of ependymal tumors. NF2 mutations and chromosome 22q loss occur preferentially in intramedullary spinal ependymomas. Am J Pathol. 155(2):627-32, 1999
12. Min KW et al: Clear cell ependymoma: a mimic of oligodendroglioma: clinicopathologic and ultrastructural considerations. Am J Surg Pathol. 21(7):820-6, 1997

(Left) *Tumor cells often arrange themselves around vessels and their fibrillary processes extend to the vessel wall, creating a paucicellular area immediately surrounding the vascular wall, typically referred to as perivascular pseudorosette.* **(Right)** *Historical accounts of ependymomas refer to the perivascular radial formation of cells with nucleus-free mantles as pseudorosettes to distinguish them from neurocytic neuroblastic rosettes.*

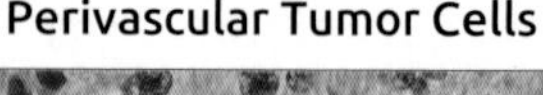

Perivascular Tumor Cells

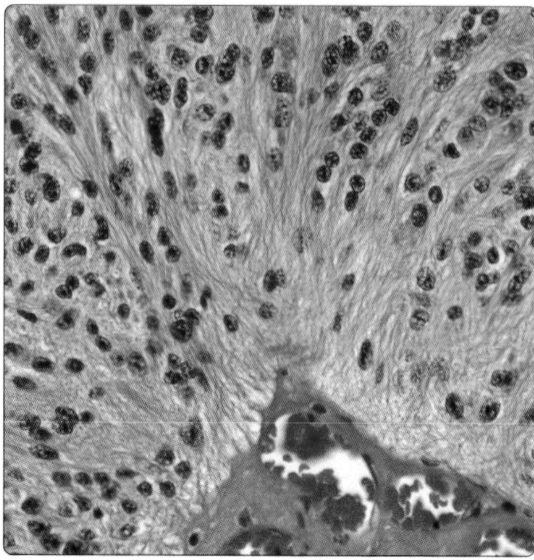

Perivascular Pseudorosettes

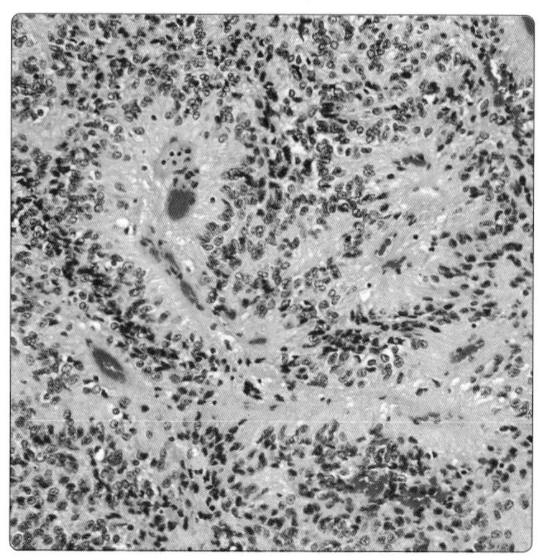

(Left) *The cuff-like, paucicellular areas around the vascular structures are not specific but are almost diagnostic of ependymal tumors. Identifying these structures impart a greater confidence to the diagnosis of ependymoma.* **(Right)** *In some tumors, perivascular pseudorosettes are sparse and may not be readily identifiable. In such cases, a more careful search may be aided by immunohistochemical stains that can expose the arrangement of the cells around vessels.*

Perivascular Pseudorosette

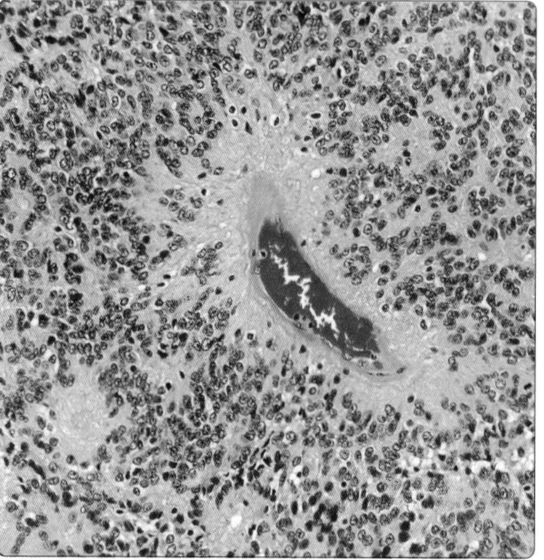

Incipient Perivascular Pseudorosette

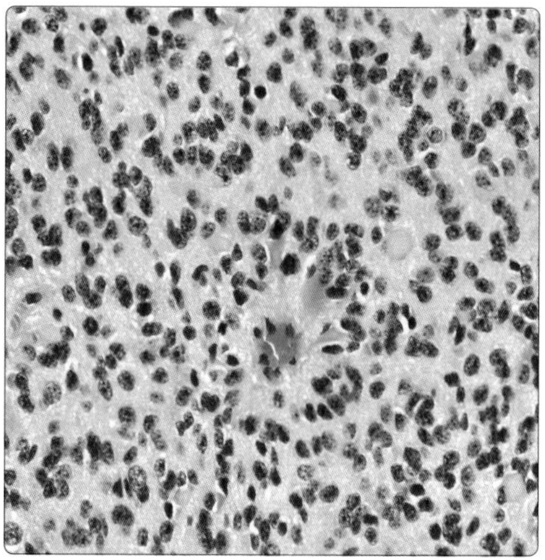

(Left) *In some sections, the perivascular pseudorosettes are not oriented in a plane to impart the classical appearance; rather, they show a network of vessels with nucleus-free mantles enabling the diagnosis.* **(Right)** *In some tumors, the presence of cytologically atypical or anaplastic-looking cells making up the perivascular pseudorosette may evoke the possibility of a higher grade neoplasm. While insufficient per se, such aggressive-looking pseudorosettes should prompt a more careful assessment of the tumor grade.*

Perivascular Pseudorosette

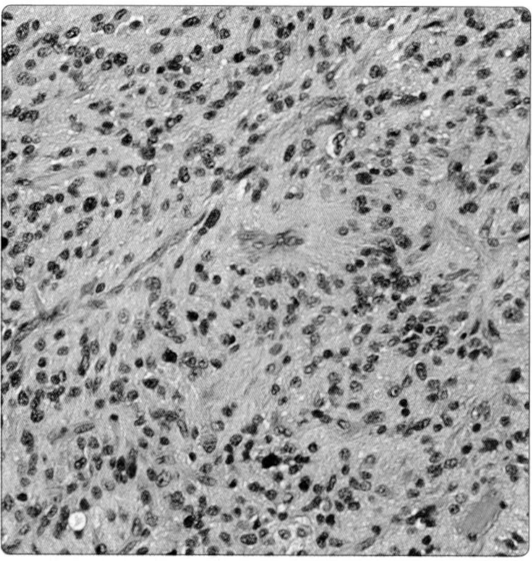

Perivascular Pseudorosette

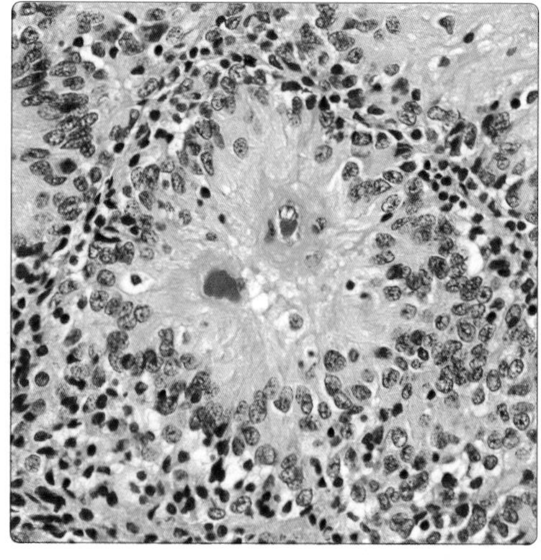

Pseudorosettes and True Rosettes

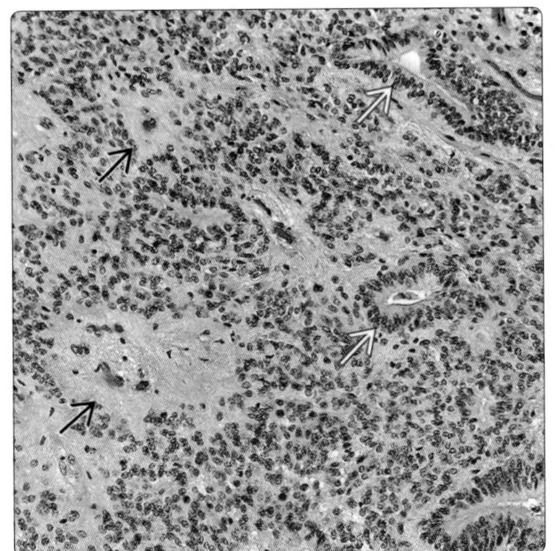

True Ependymal Rosettes

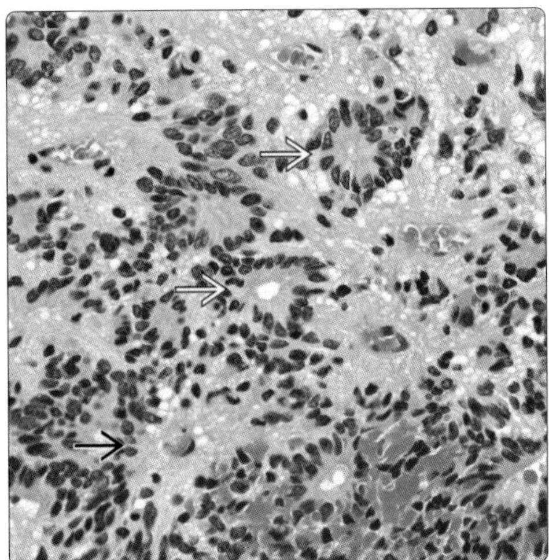

(Left) *Some ependymomas have both perivascular pseudorosettes ⇨ and true, ependymal rosettes ➡. Overall, as seen here, the former are more common. The term true is often used to identify lumen-containing structures without a central vessel.* **(Right)** *This type of rosettes with a central lumen suggests an abortive attempt to form a central canal. While these are suggested to be more common in the posterior fossa, any ependymal tumor can have a mixture of true ➡ and perivascular pseudo- ⇨ rosettes.*

True Rosettes and Tubules

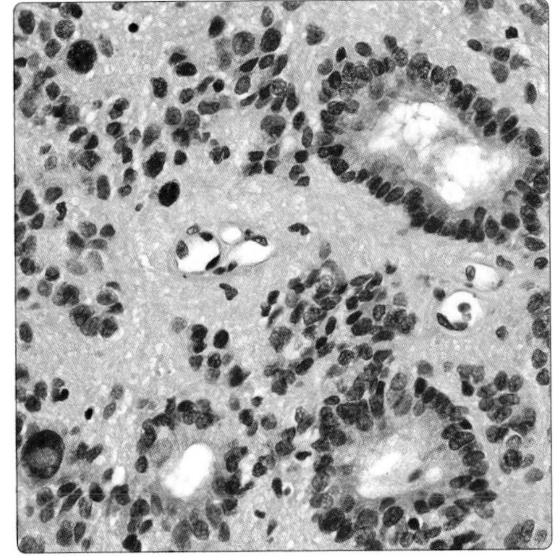

Pseudorosettes and Vacuolated Cells

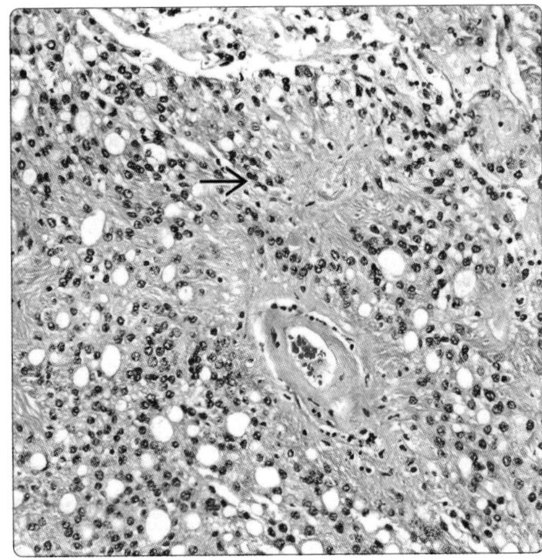

(Left) *Typical ultrastructural features attributed to ependymomas, such as ciliary formations, microvilli, and desmosome-like cell junctions are best appreciated in samples obtained from the true rosettes or some resembling tubules.* **(Right)** *Vacuolated cells can be encountered in any type of ependymoma and the extent of these cells can be quite varied. Some of these cells have a clear cell appearance, and the presence of perivascular pseudorosette ⇨ is reassuring of the diagnosis.*

Vacuolated Cells

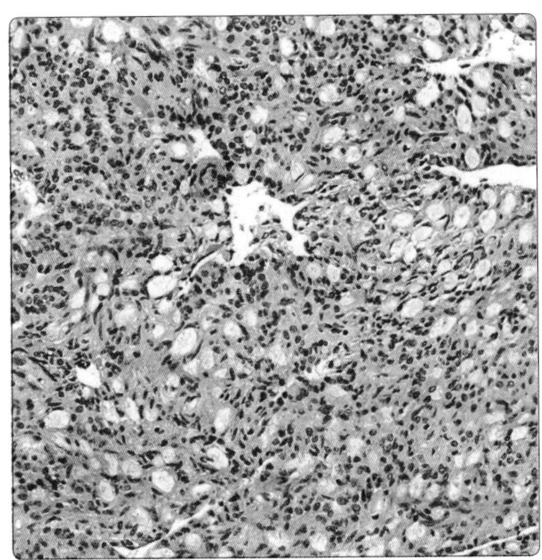

Vacuolated Signet Ring-Type Cells

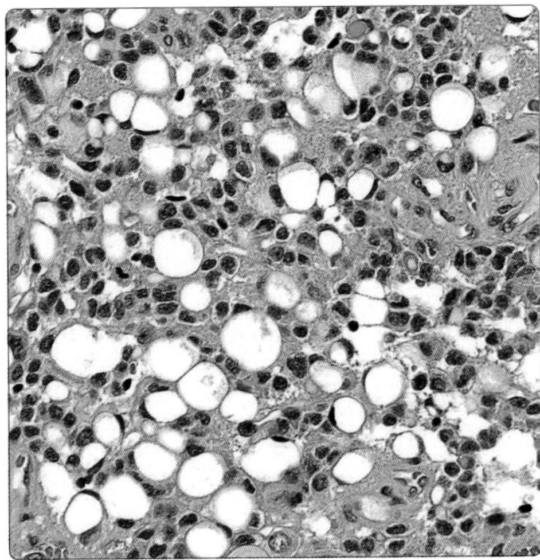

(Left) *Some ependymomas contain cells with single or multiple cytoplasmic vacuoles, compactly arranged and showing an oligodendroglioma-like appearance. In most other areas, the tumor had conspicuous perivascular pseudorosettes.* **(Right)** *While the designation of signet ring cells are of an ominous implication to the surgical pathologist in other tumor types, vacuolated cells with this appearance do not seem to portend any significance to the behavior of ependymomas.*

(Left) *In many ependymomas, the tumor cells can be observed in a linear or tubular arrangement, simulating normal ependyma lining the ventricles. In this section, the tumor had no direct association with the ventricles even though there was an ependymal lining-like area* ⇒. **(Right)** *Lesions, such as this epithelial ependymoma, overlap somewhat with choroid plexus papilloma, but the cells are less regimented and lack subepithelial basal lamina.*

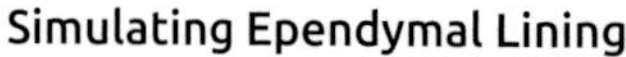

Simulating Ependymal Lining

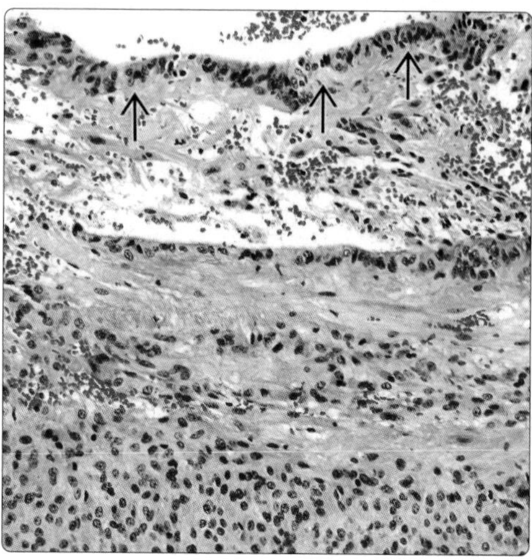

Epithelial Features

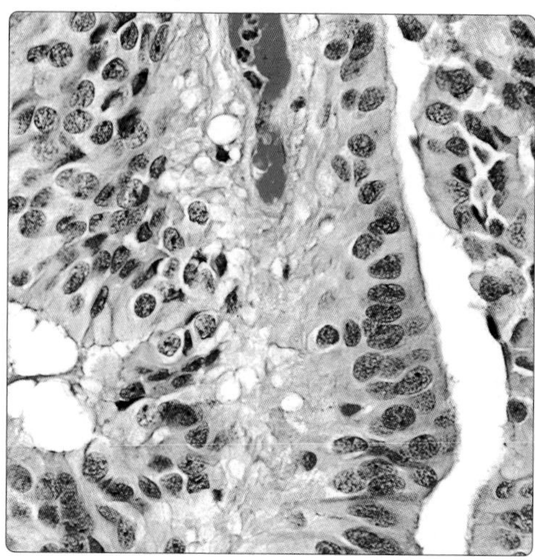

(Left) *Many ependymomas have a tendency to spread along the cerebrospinal space as well as along the leptomeninges. This can be seen following surgical resections but can also happen without any surgical manipulation of the tumor.* **(Right)** *Slit-like spaces lined by columnar cells are 1 form of epithelial differentiation. While this may suggest other entities, this feature is often focal within an otherwise typical ependymoma.*

Leptomeningeal Spread

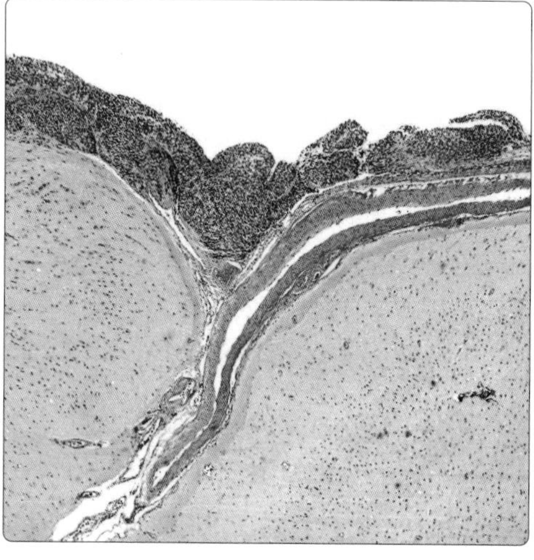

Epithelioid Slit-Like Spaces

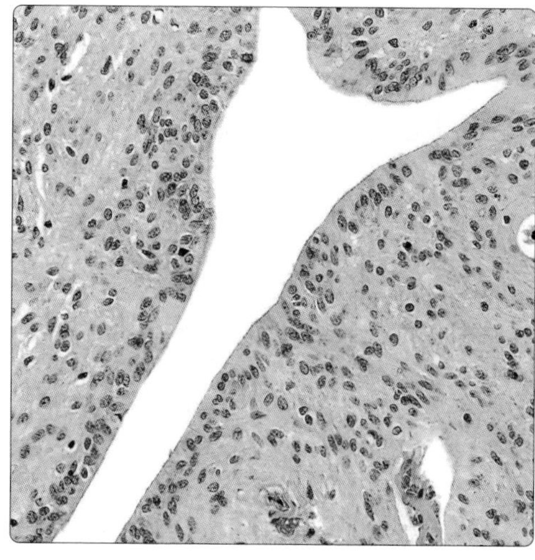

(Left) *Ependymomas generally have a sharp interface with the surrounding brain* ⇒. **(Right)** *While ependymomas are, overall, well circumscribed, a degree of tissue infiltration is not out of character, particularly in supratentorial types. In this case, tumor cells appear to move into the brain* ⇒ *from the cellular, more cohesive mass at the top.*

Well-Defined Borders

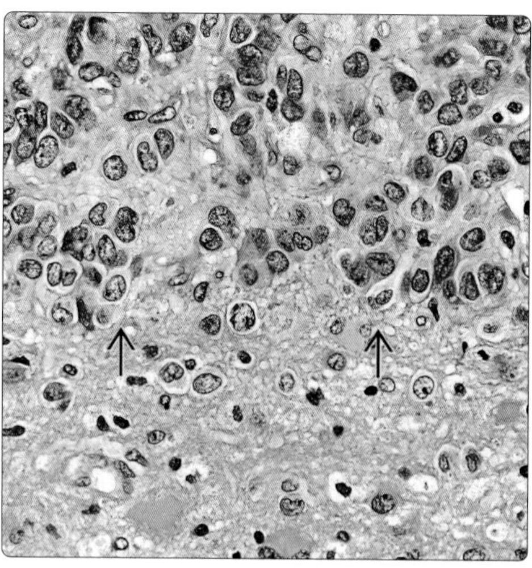

Focally Infiltrative Borders

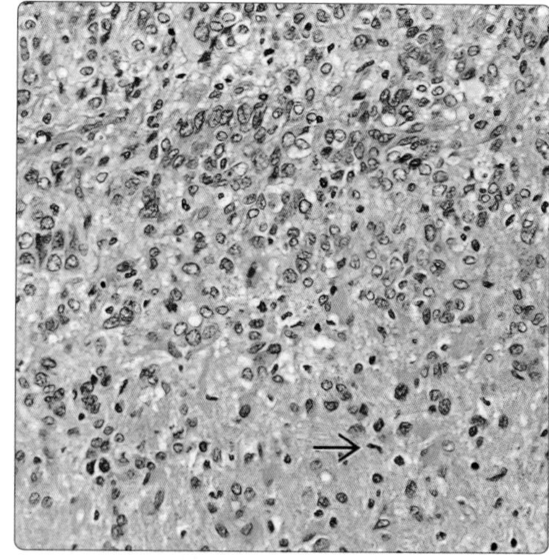

Hyalinized Vessels, Epithelioid Tumor

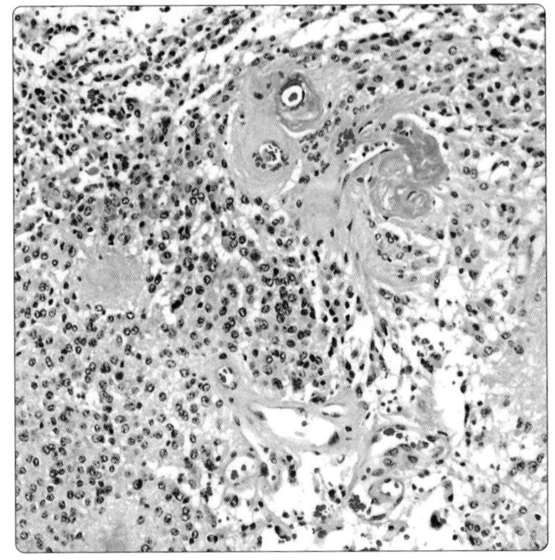

Vascular Proliferation in Cyst Wall

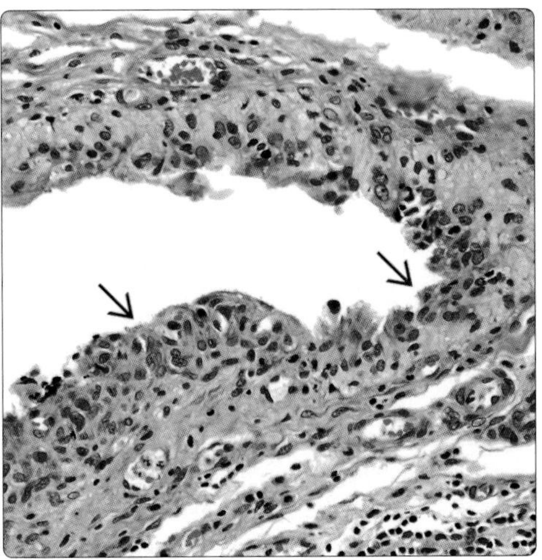

(Left) *The vascular changes in ependymomas can also be observed in other tumors, such as pilocytic astrocytoma. Focal vascular hyalinization is more common in spinal examples.* **(Right)** *Glomeruloid vascular proliferation in the cyst wall* ⇒ *should not be interpreted as evidence for grade III anaplastic ependymoma. Similar mural vascular change is common in other CNS tumors with a cystic component, such as pilocytic astrocytoma, ganglion cell tumor, and pleomorphic xanthoastrocytoma.*

Round Nuclei

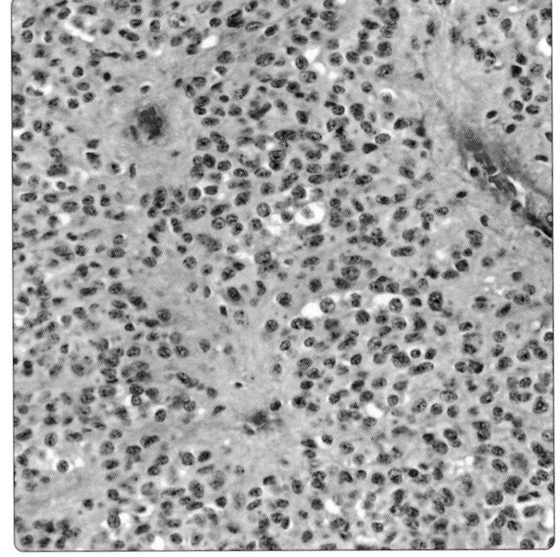

Dystrophic Calcifications

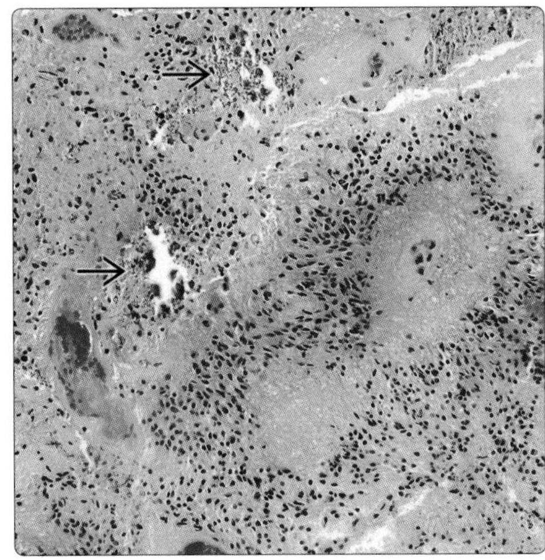

(Left) *Round nuclei lend an oligodendroglioma quality, but the dense cellularity, compact noninfiltrative architecture, and perivascular pseudorosettes reflect the lesion's ependymal nature. Ependymomas with even more pronounced oligodendroglial qualities (i.e., clear cell types) also exist.* **(Right)** *Many low-grade ependymomas demonstrate dystrophic calcifications* ⇒*. This feature can be prominent in resections following adjuvant therapy.*

Pseudorosettes and Calcifications

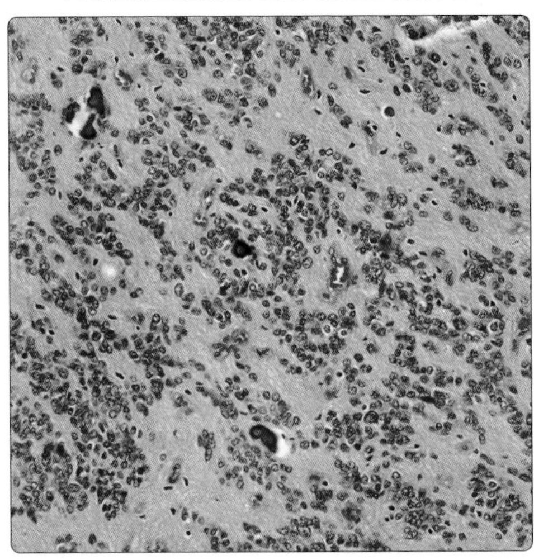

Psammomatous Calcifications

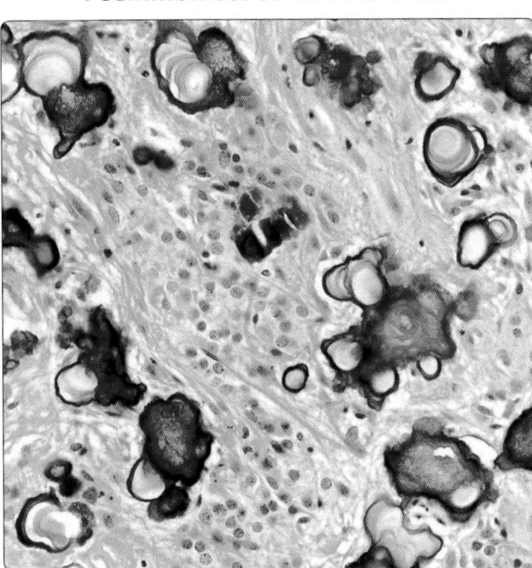

(Left) *Calcifications can be large and dystrophic or involve individual cells and may be in the form of psammoma bodies.* **(Right)** *Laminated calcospherites or "psammoma bodies" may be abundant in rare examples of ependymomas. They also can be only focal but are more often absent.*

(Left) *Some ependymomas, especially in the spinal cord, can harbor significantly large nuclei with dystrophic changes, mostly indicative of a degenerative process. When this is extensive, the term giant cell ependymoma is used.* **(Right)** *Overt nuclear pleomorphism characterizes the prognostically insignificant giant cell ependymoma. This form of degenerative atypia occurs both in cellular ependymomas, as seen here, and in myxopapillary types in the distal spinal cord.*

Bizarre Degenerated Cells

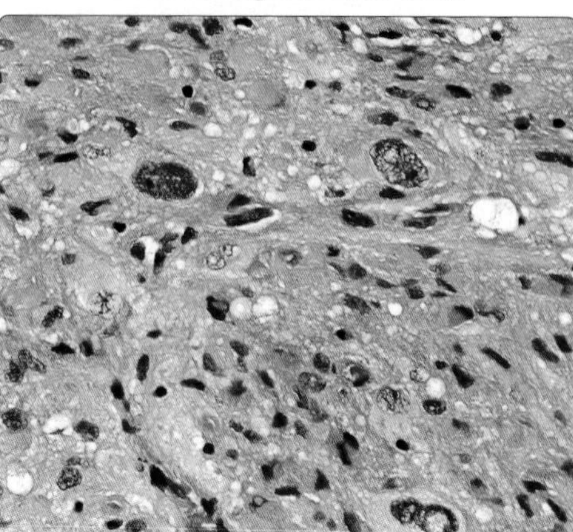

Nuclear Pleomorphism

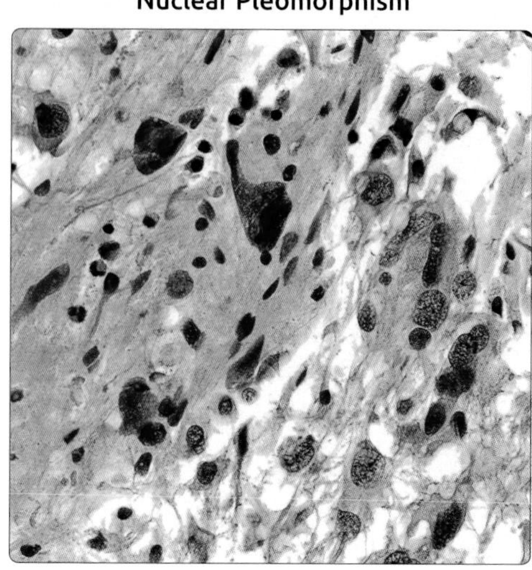

(Left) *Bone* ➡ *and hyaline cartilage* ⇨ *are uncommon metaplastic elements in ependymoma.* **(Right)** *The parenchymal tissue surrounding the ependymal tumors can demonstrate numerous Rosenthal fibers and gliosis. This is most typical in spinal cord tumors and may lead to a misdiagnosis if the real tumor tissue is overlooked.*

Metaplastic Elements

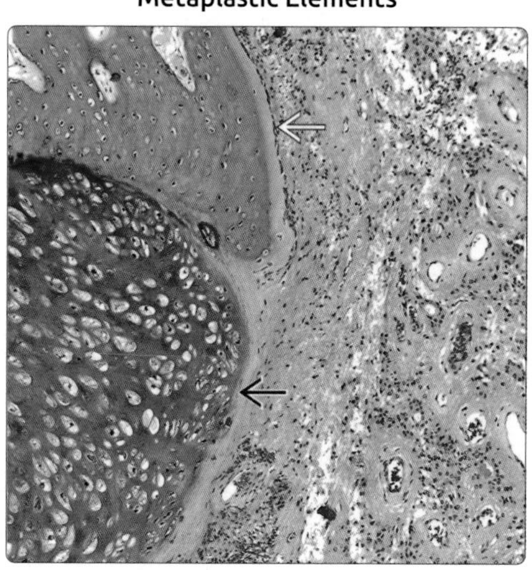

Rosenthal Fibers

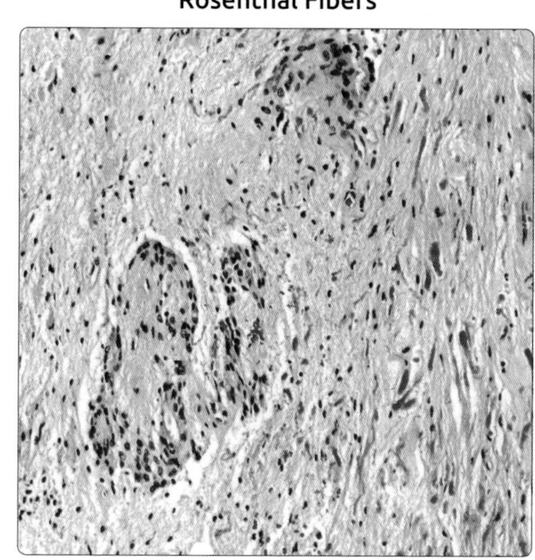

(Left) *Paucicellular regions of ependymomas can resemble an infiltrating glioma, either astrocytic with true gemistocytes or oligodendroglial with its mini gemistocytes.* **(Right)** *Small, gemistocyte-like cells are not uncommon in paucicellular areas of ependymomas* ➡*. The round nuclei of such cells create the appearance of oligodendroglioma with mini gemistocytes; although, oligodendroglioma would be most unusual as an exophytic pontine mass.*

Gemistocytes in Ependymoma

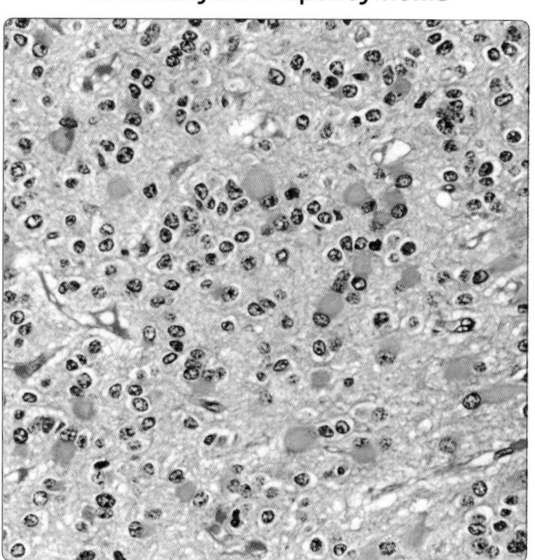

Gemistocytic Cells in Cerebellar Tumor

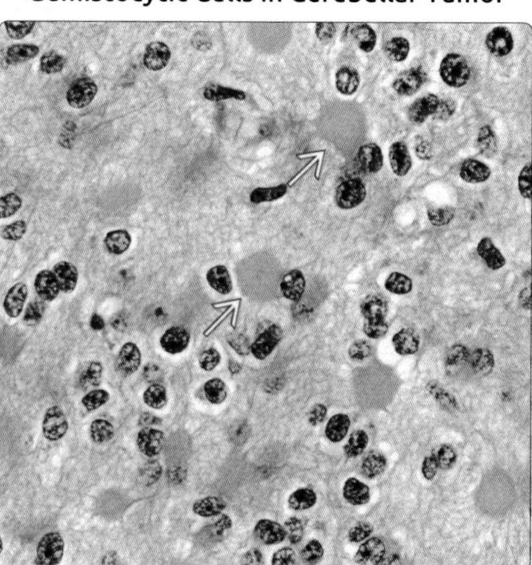

Hypercellular Nodules

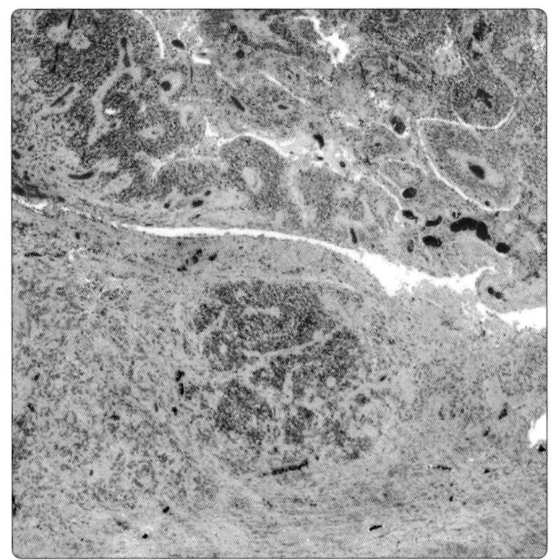

Hypercellular Nodule

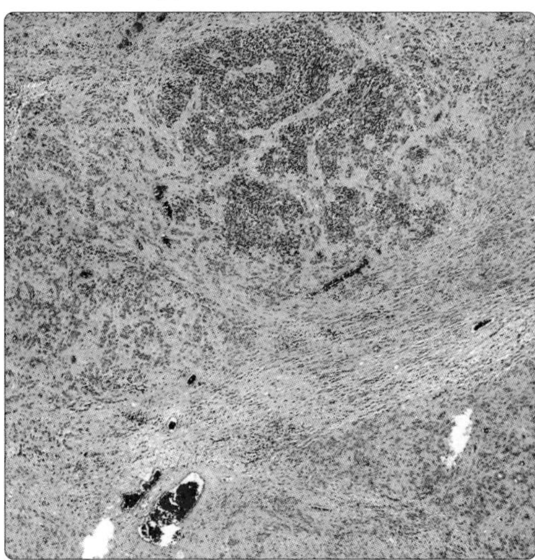

(Left) *Many ependymomas harbor foci of tumor cells with marked hypercellularity. Some of these nodules also demonstrate brisk mitoses. While these are more typical of the anaplastic variant, some low-grade ependymomas can also harbor such foci.* **(Right)** *The hypercellular nodule would typically have a higher mitotic count per high-power fields (HPF) compared to the low cellular areas. The significance of these nodules in grading and prognosis has not been established.*

Hypercellular Nodules

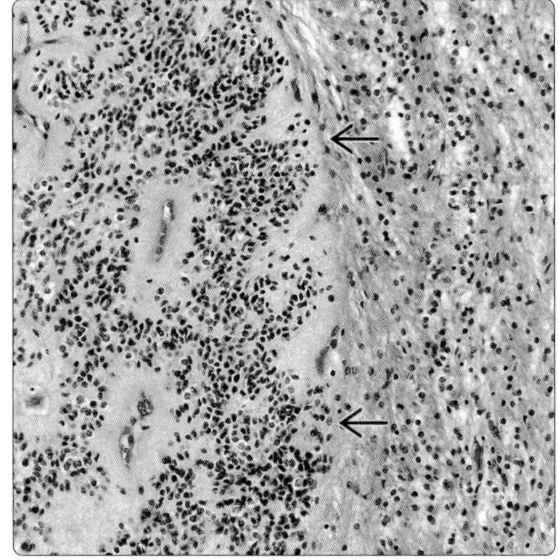

Hypercellular Nodule

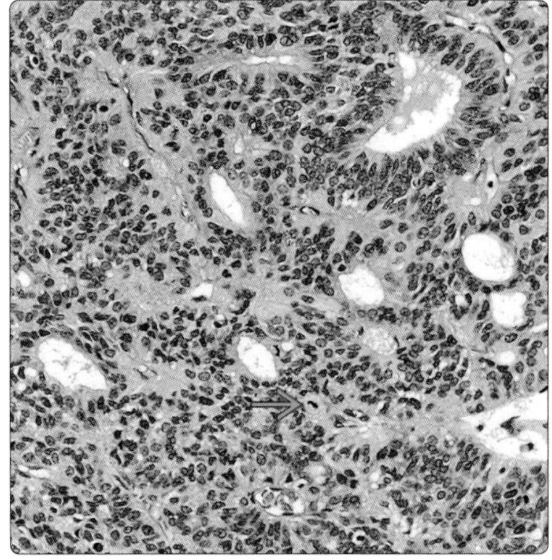

(Left) *Well-defined, generally spherical, seemingly clonal nodules of high cellularity and with a sharp border ➙ arise in some ependymomas, particularly those in the posterior fossa. Grading is complicated by the presence of these formations when they are more than very focal but less than numerous.* **(Right)** *Typically, there is a markedly increased cell density in the hypercellular nodules, and the mitotic figures are easier to find ➙. The conventional method of counting mitoses per 10 HPF may not be that accurate.*

Neuronal Differentiation

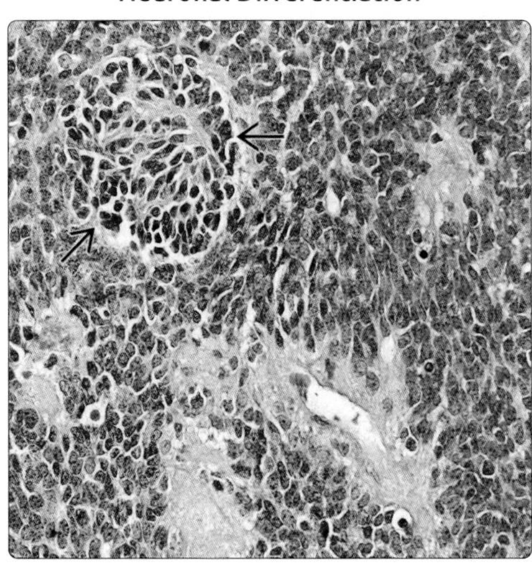

Neuronal Differentiation

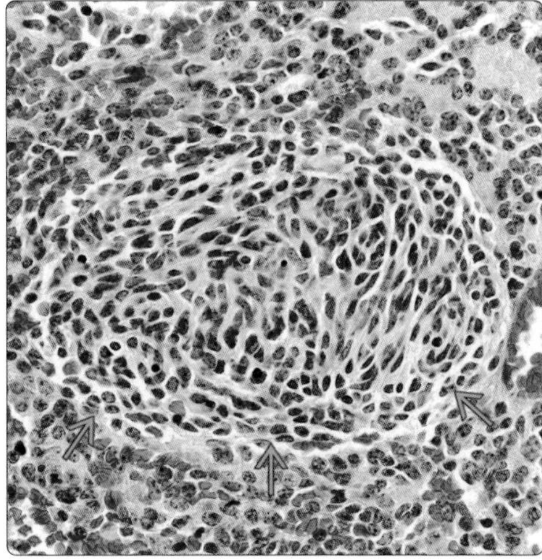

(Left) *Discrete nodules of neuronal differentiation ➙ similar to nodules in desmoplastic/nodular medulloblastoma are surprising findings in some ependymomas, grade III in this case. As in medulloblastomas, they are immunoreactive for synaptophysin.* **(Right)** *High-power magnification shows a nodule ➙ with neuronal differentiation in an otherwise typical ependymoma. These nodules can resemble medulloblastoma and are often strongly positive with neuronal antibodies.*

(Left) *A rare histopathological variant, papillary ependymoma has fronds of tumor without the overt epithelial features of a choroid plexus tumor. While some of these tumors predominantly appear papillary, many also have a classical pattern.* **(Right)** *In some papillary ependymomas, the pseudorosettes are replaced by frank papillary structures. Vacuolation ⇒, ribbon-like arrangement of tumor cells →, and a focal myxoid pattern ⇒ can aid in the diagnosis.*

Papillary Variant

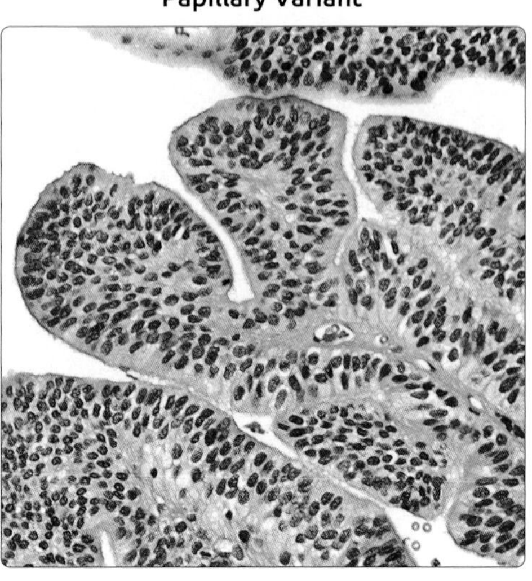

Papillary Variant: Ribbons

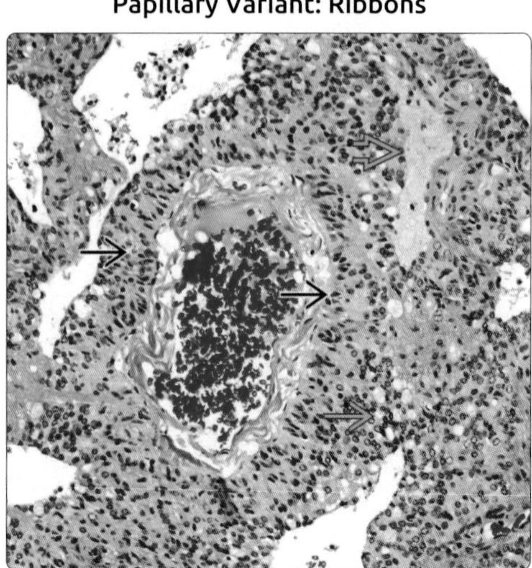

(Left) *This ependymoma's organization into compact sheets with thickened vessels and sharp borders helps identify this distinctive clear cell variant. Individually, its cells closely resemble those of oligodendroglioma.* **(Right)** *Clear cell ependymomas are not just ependymomas with perinuclear haloes. They are especially compact, i.e., noninfiltrative lesions with branching vessels and distinctive nuclei.*

Clear Cell Variant

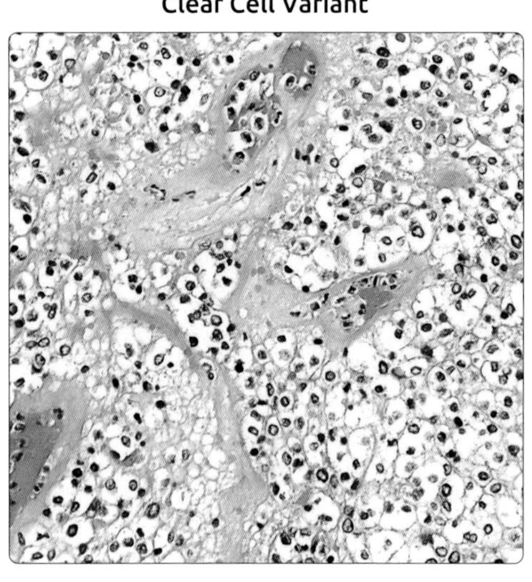

Clear Cell Variant

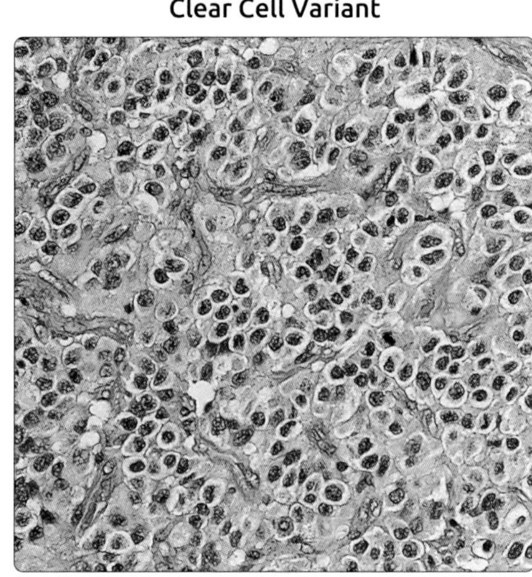

(Left) *A clear cell variant often resembles oligodendrogliomas and is more often seen as a supratentorial tumor in children. There is a suggestion that the clear cell variant follows a more aggressive clinical course, but this requires further validation.* **(Right)** *Some clear cell tumors have hypercellular foci with mitotic figures ⇒ and nuclear atypia. These tumors may qualify for the WHO grade III designation, and this complicates the significance of the clear cell variant in terms of prognosis.*

Clear Cell Variant

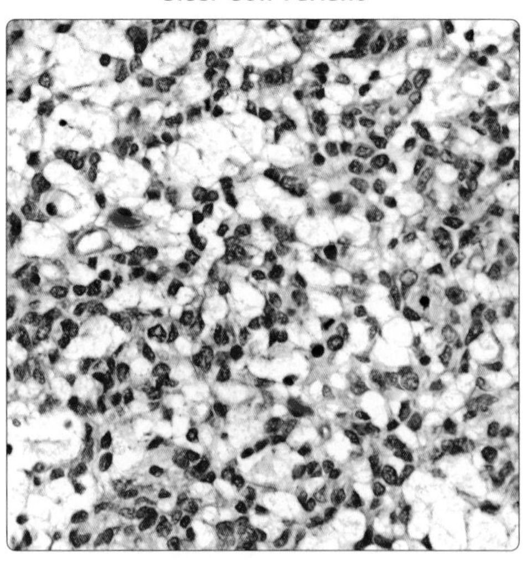

Clear Cell Variant

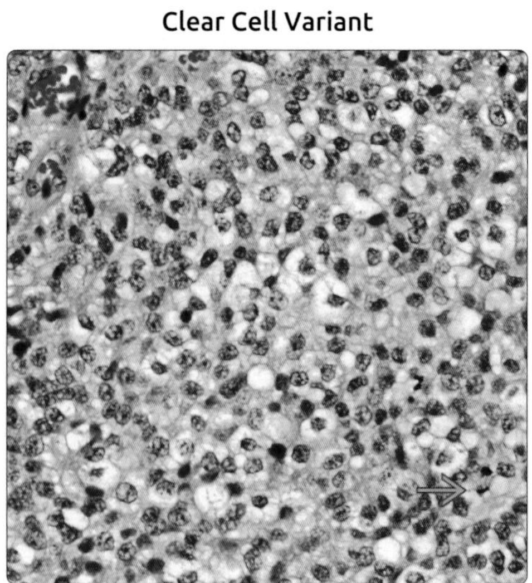

Tanycytic Variant: Bipolar Cells

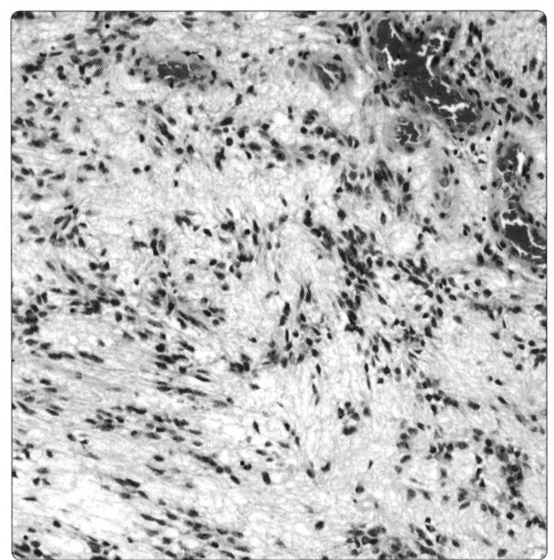

Tanycytic Variant: Piloid Cells

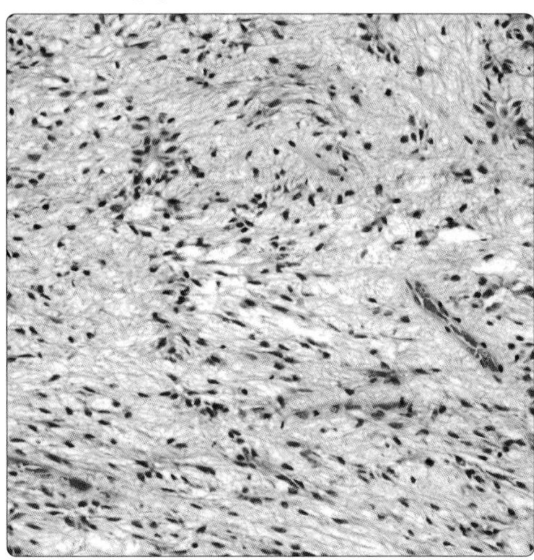

(Left) *Some ependymomas are predominantly composed of bipolar spindle cells with variable density from tumor to tumor. These tumors are more typical in the spinal cord but can also be seen intracranially.* **(Right)** *Some ependymomas may be mistaken for pilocytic astrocytoma by virtue of their myxoid background, piloid-appearing cells, and a compact glial background. This picture is often compounded by the lack of clear perivascular pseudorosettes. Immunostains are very helpful for the correct diagnosis.*

Tanycytic Variant

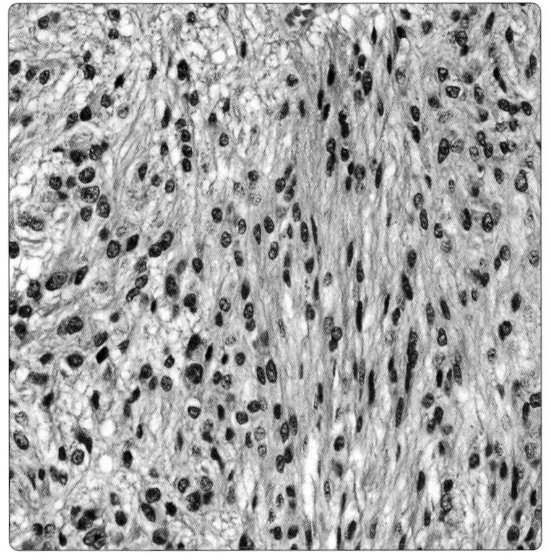

Subependymoma-Like Areas

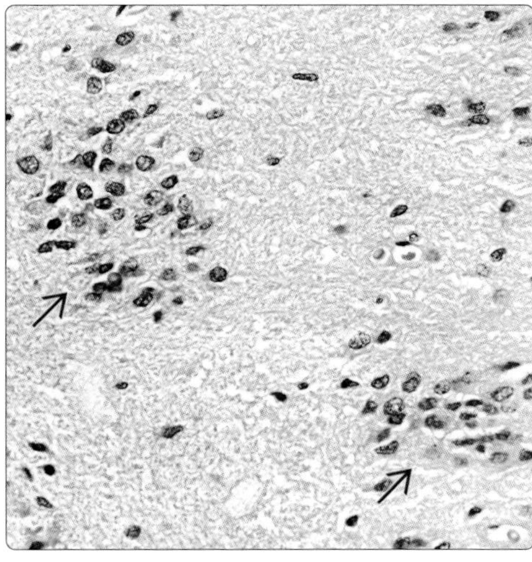

(Left) *This spinal cord tumor has a vaguely epithelioid appearance but has spindle, bipolar cells that were suggested to resemble tanycytes. Perivascular and true ependymal rosettes were distinctly absent, as is the case for most tanycytic ependymomas.* **(Right)** *This subependymoma-like area occurred in association with a typical WHO grade II posterior fossa ependymoma. The tumor's distinctive clustered nuclei ⇒ and fibrillar, process-rich, almost anuclear, background are classic features.*

Dense Collagenous Nodules

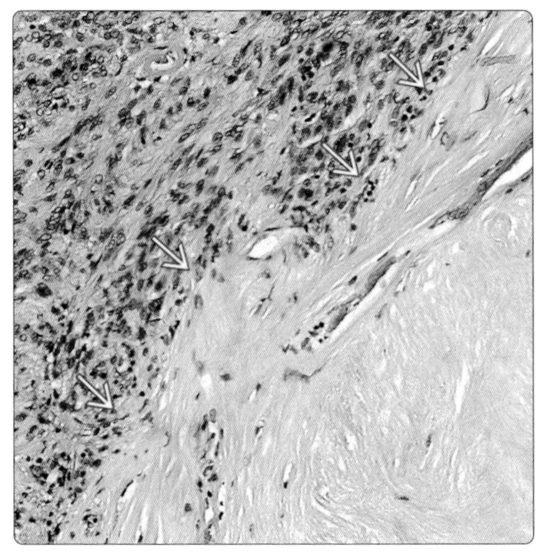

Dense Collagenous Nodules

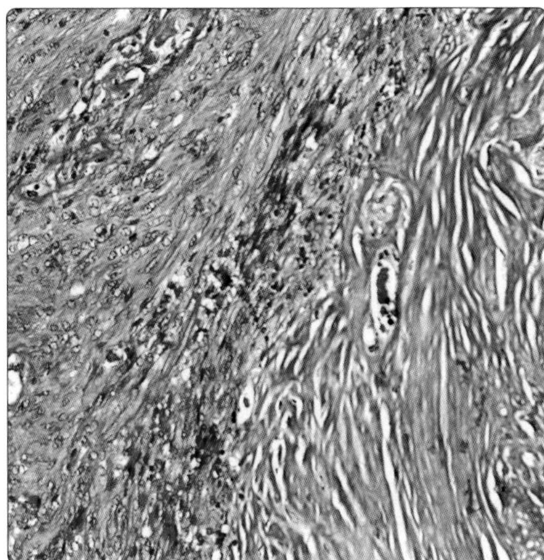

(Left) *Nodules of dense collagen ➡, highlighted here on the right side of the section, are distinctive features of some spinal ependymomas.* **(Right)** *Collagenous nodules in some spinal intramedullary ependymomas can be highlighted by a strong, positive trichrome staining.*

(Left) *While the so-called cortical ependymoma is not considered a variant, the radiological and histological appearance is quite unique. The tumor is often superficial with little connection to the ventricle and has a solid-cystic appearance and variably enhancing mural nodule ➡.* **(Right)** *Cortical ependymoma often demonstrates variable ependymal features with a prominent tanycytic pattern. Most tumors have significant spindle cell components as well as small, tubule-like rosettes ⇨.*

Cortical Ependymoma

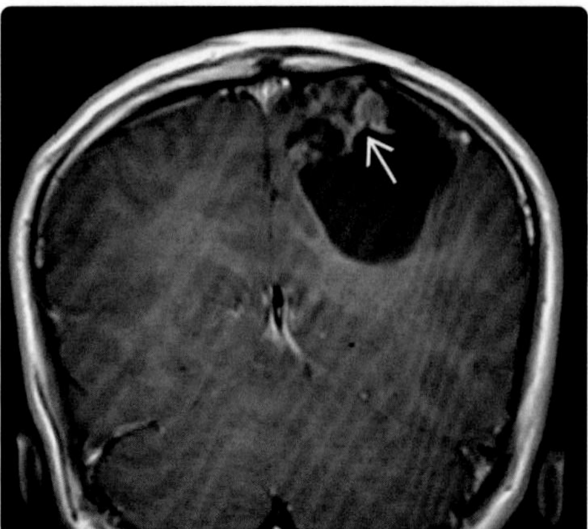

Cortical Ependymoma

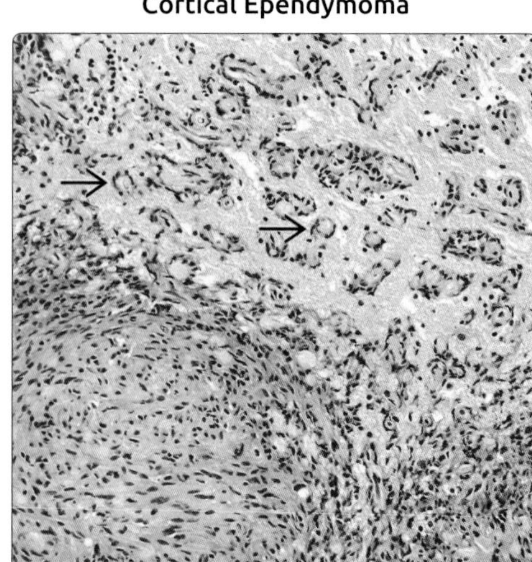

(Left) *The perivascular pseudorosettes and the tubule-like rosettes in cortical ependymomas are somewhat unique and appear more infiltrative into the cortical parenchyma. Nevertheless, histological, immunohistochemical, and ultrastructural features are typical of ependymomas.* **(Right)** *Cortical ependymomas, similar to tanycytic variant, harbor prominent spindle cell components as well as numerous vacuolated, or signet ring-like, cells.*

Cortical Ependymoma: Rosettes

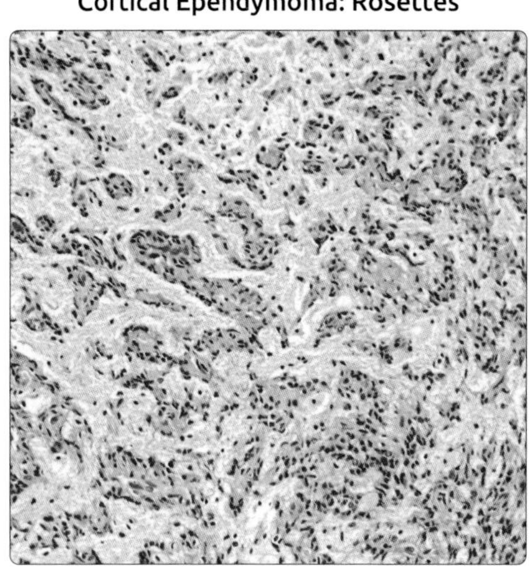

Cortical Ependymoma: Spindle Cells

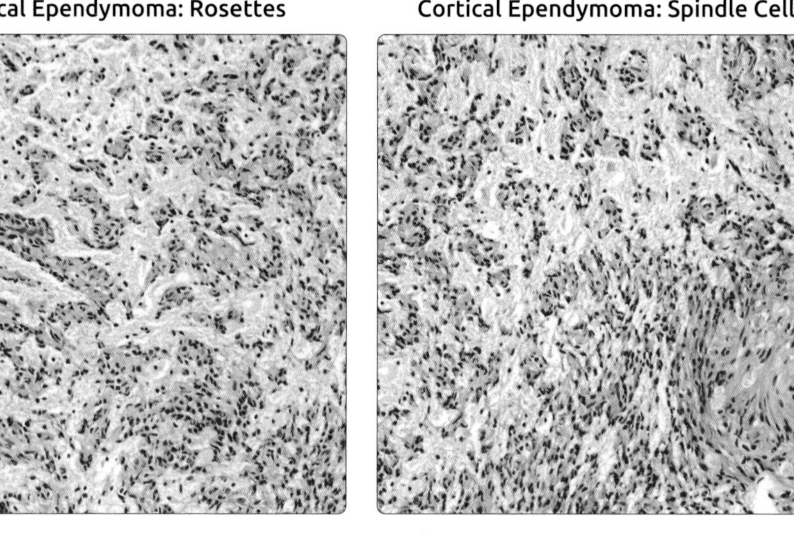

(Left) *Cortical ependymomas can have a number of unusual features: They may appear more papillary or pseudopapillary with epithelioid character, forming ribbons. Many other patterns have been associated with cortical ependymomas.* **(Right)** *Vacuolated, or signet ring-like, cells typical of any ependymoma can also be seen in cortical ependymomas.*

Cortical Ependymoma: Ribbons

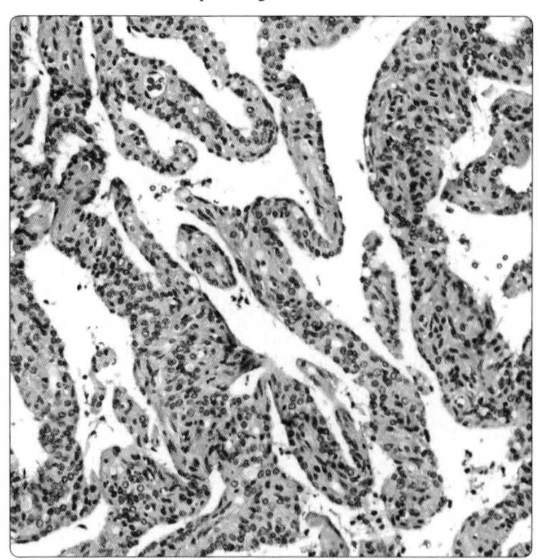

Cortical Ependymoma: Vacuolated Cells

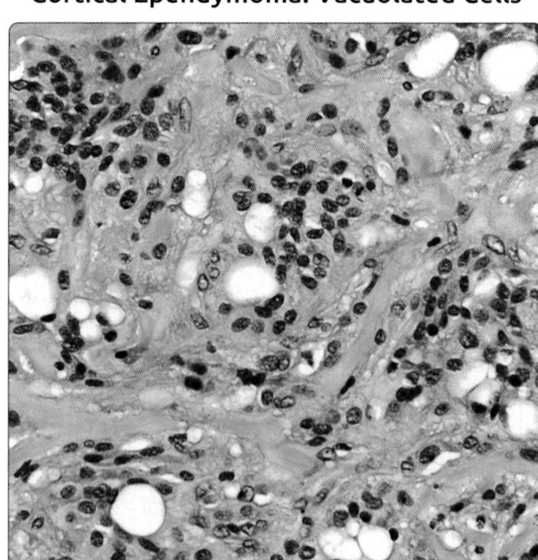

Vascular Proliferation

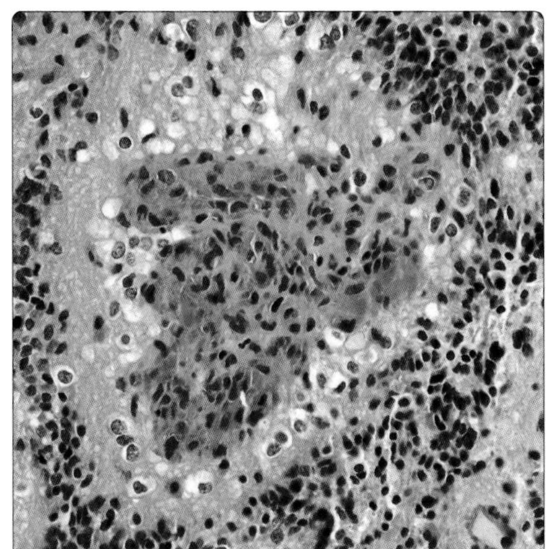

Vascular Proliferation

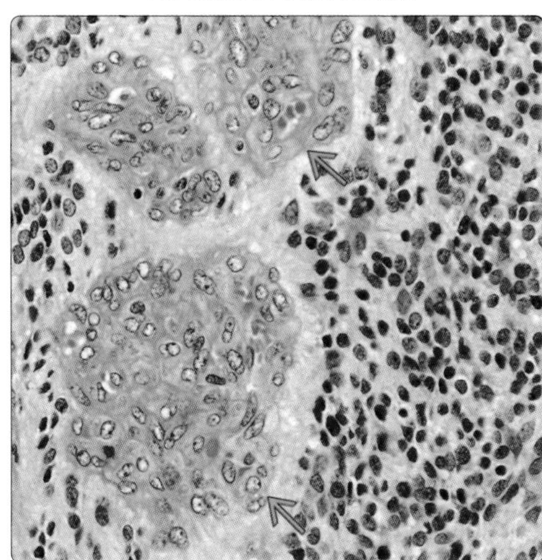

(Left) *The presence of bona fide vascular endothelial proliferation is indicative of a more aggressive tumor and is not compatible with a WHO grade II designation.* **(Right)** *Overt vascular proliferation ⇨ in a cellular, mitotically active ependymoma helps establish WHO grade III.*

Anaplasia and Increased Mitoses

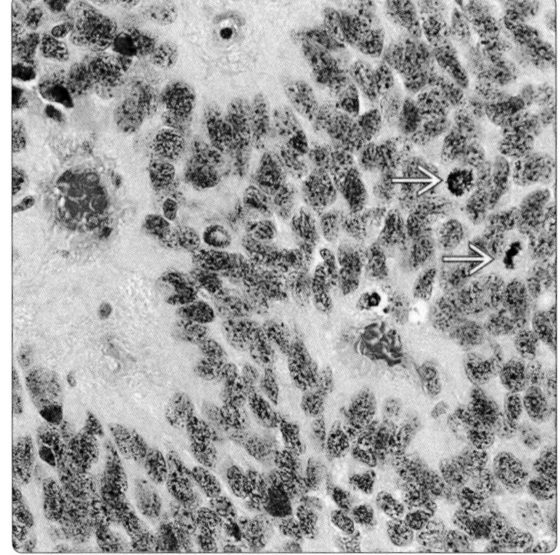

Atypical Mitoses

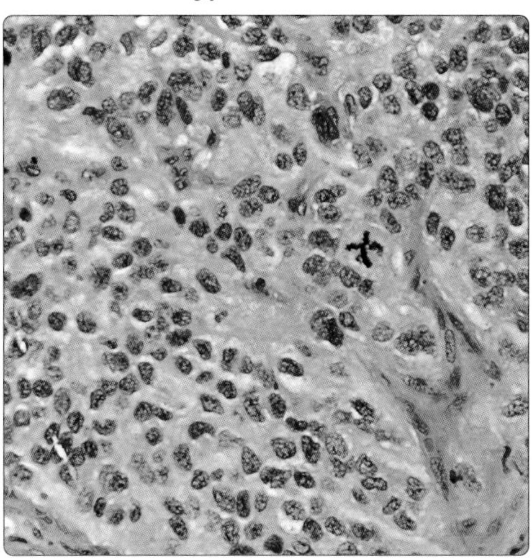

(Left) *Mitotic activity is the principal grading parameter. Given the degree of atypia and the number of mitoses ➔ in this high-power magnification, this ependymoma would be a WHO grade III neoplasm.* **(Right)** *While an atypical mitotic figure does not confer a high grade in ependymomas, the presence of such mitoses are more typical of WHO grade III neoplasms.*

Palisading Necrosis

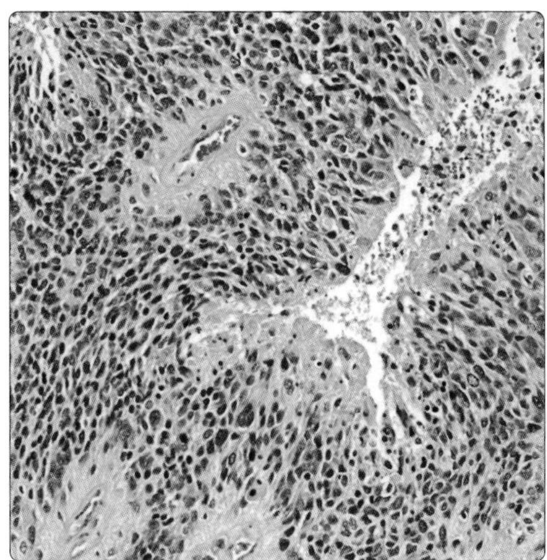

Incipient Perivascular Pseudorosette

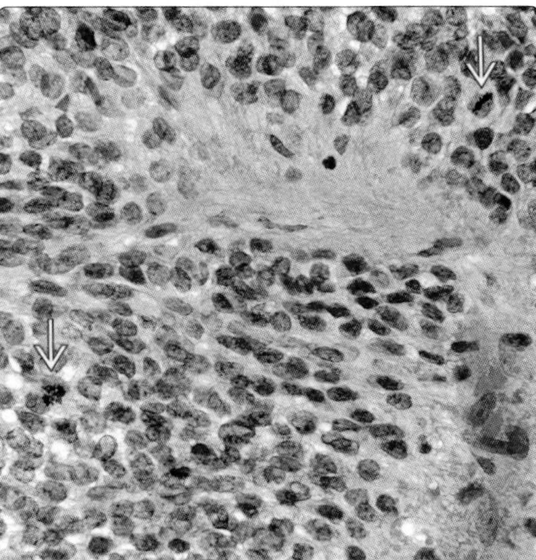

(Left) *While distinctly uncommon, the presence of palisading necrosis, unlike common coagulative necrosis, is more in keeping with an anaplastic tumor (WHO grade III).* **(Right)** *A perivascular pseudorosette, while poorly formed, is strong evidence that this cellular, cytologically anaplastic tumor with numerous mitoses ➔ is ependymoma grade III.*

(Left) *Smears from ependymomas can underscore the perivascular pseudorosettes in the tumor. Typically, most ependymomas smear well & can be easily recognized. However, grading of such tumors based on frozen section findings is not wise & should be deferred to final diagnosis.* **(Right)** *Intraoperative smears from ependymomas display a prominent fibrillary background suggestive of glial neoplasm, while the nuclei appear distinctly epithelial with "salt and pepper" chromatin and vacuoles* ➡.

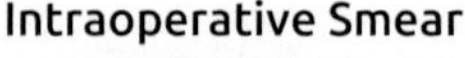

Intraoperative Smear

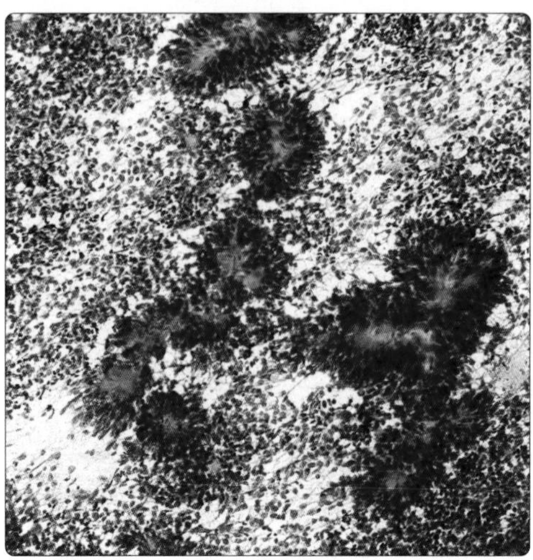

Fibrillary and Epithelial Features

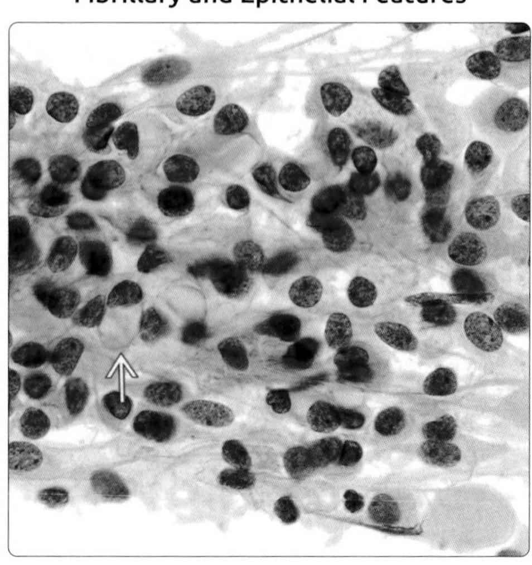

(Left) *Multiple long, dark, cell-cell, intermediate junctions* ⇨ *attach adjacent tumor cells as the latter abut one another about a microlumina* ⇨*. Microvilli and cilia fill the tiny space; the complex is responsible for the dot-like EMA staining typical of tumors with ependymal differentiation.* **(Right)** *Diffuse, intense staining for GFAP, and less avid reactivity for S100 (not shown), help distinguish tanycytic ependymoma from schwannoma.*

Ultrastructural Characteristics

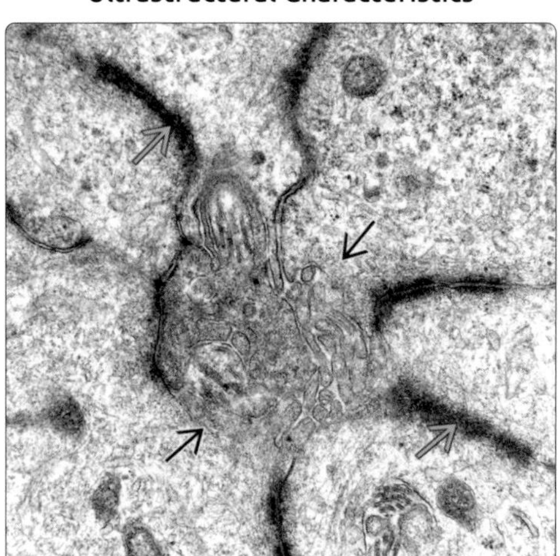

GFAP Positivity

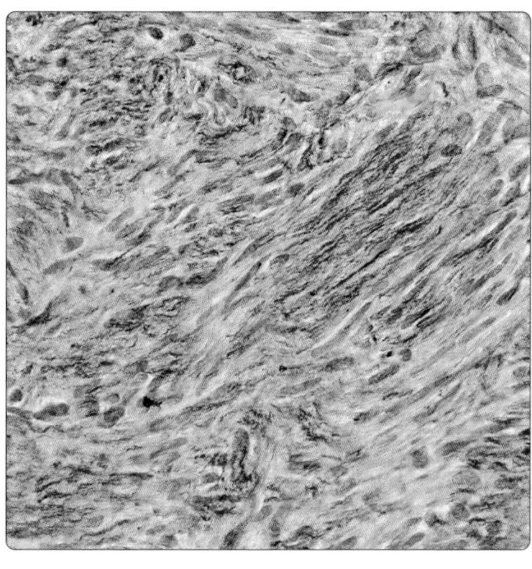

(Left) *While less common, some ependymomas have focal and sometimes weak GFAP staining. Even so, the perivascular staining suggests the diagnosis.* **(Right)** *There is variably positive staining with the GFAP antibodies in ependymomas and the tumor cells can be diffusely or focally positive. In all circumstances, the typical perivascular positivity is evident.*

GFAP Positivity

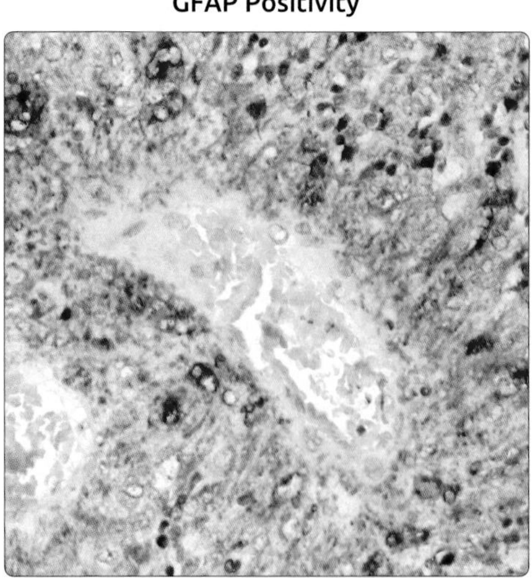

GFAP Positivity

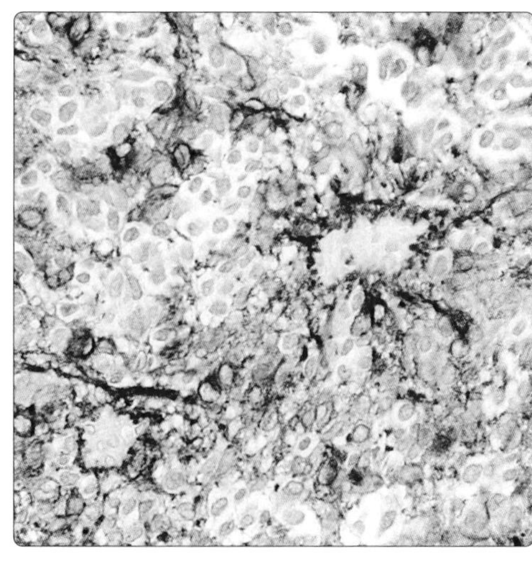

D2-40 Positivity

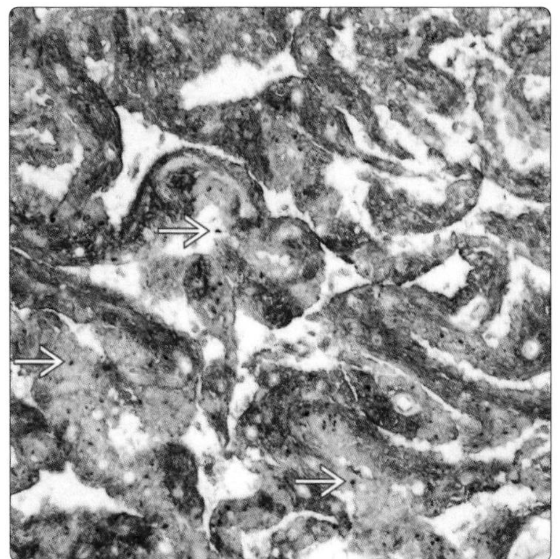

Cytokeratin Positivity

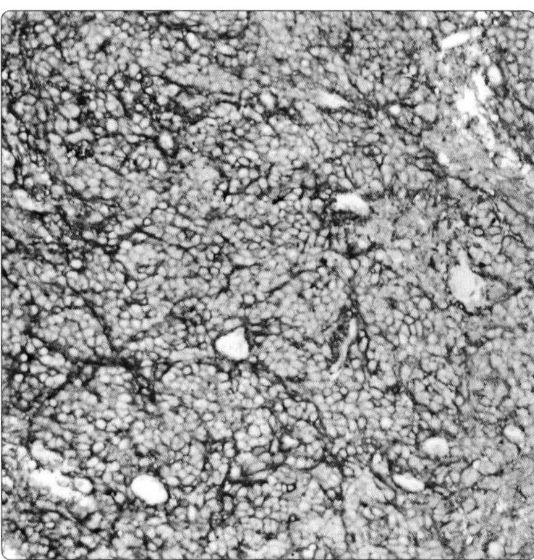

(Left) *The punctate positivity with D2-40 ➡ akin to positivity with EMA is often seen in ependymomas. In some cases, the positivity is very strong and diffuse, partially obscuring the punctate nature of the staining.* **(Right)** *Many ependymomas demonstrate strong membranous positivity with the antibodies against cytokeratin, low molecular weight (CAM 5.2) in this example.*

EMA Positivity

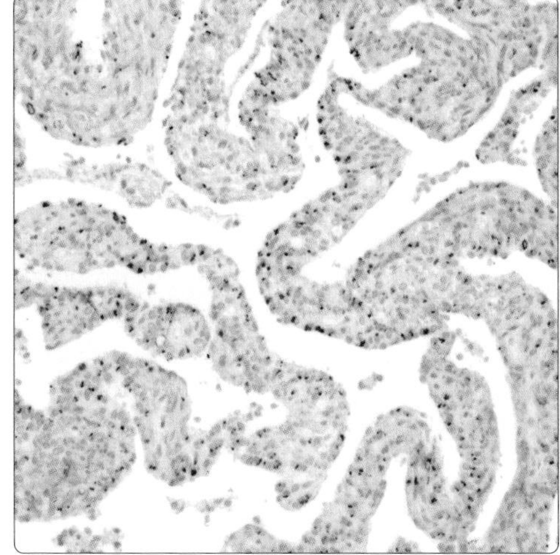

EMA Positivity

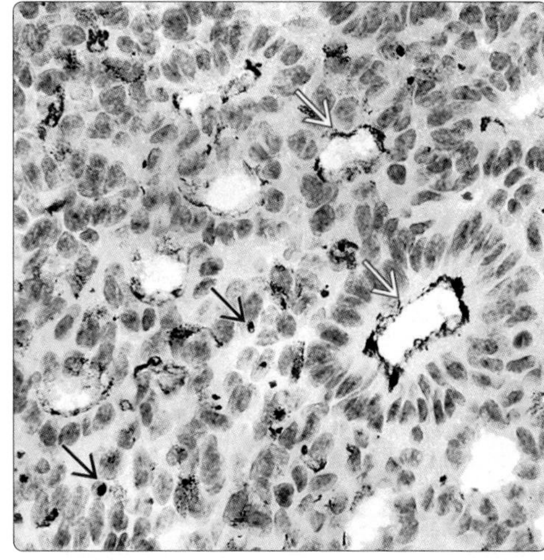

(Left) *Dot-like perinuclear positivity is especially pronounced in this cortical ependymoma. Most ependymoma variants are positive with EMA in the same fashion.* **(Right)** *Luminal surfaces of true ependymoma rosettes ➡ are EMA immunoreactive, as are microlumina ➡.*

Olig2(-) Tumor

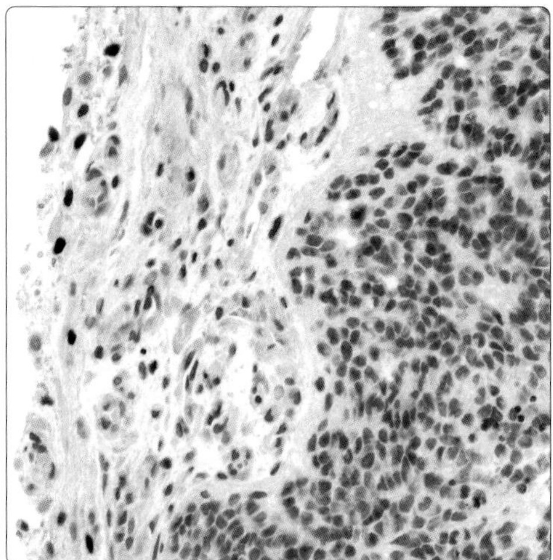

Proliferative Hypercellular Foci

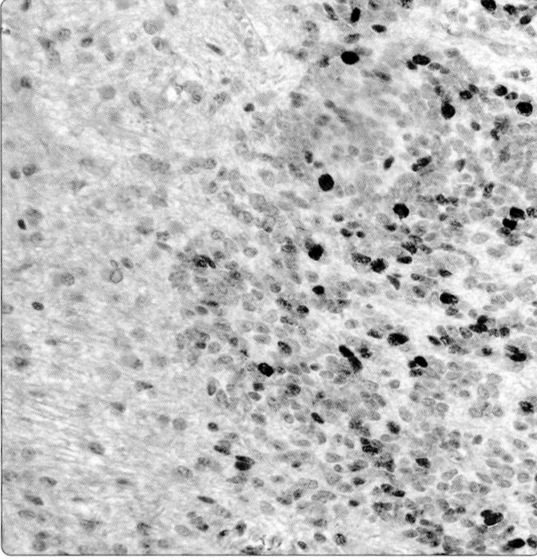

(Left) *Most ependymomas have only rare, scattered single positive cells or are negative with Olig2 antibodies. Rare tumors are focally but strongly positive, and the significance of the latter is not known.* **(Right)** *The Ki-67 index is considerably higher in the discrete cellular foci. It is unclear at what point such nodules are numerous enough to warrant diagnosis as grade III. The presence of widely scattered nodules, as illustrated here, is not sufficient for the diagnosis of grade III anaplastic ependymoma.*

Anaplastic Ependymoma

KEY FACTS

TERMINOLOGY

- WHO: Malignant glioma with ependymal differentiation, with high mitotic activity often accompanied by microvascular proliferation and pseudopalisading necrosis
- No consensus grading system
- ≥ 10 mitoses per 10 HPF, often with microvascular proliferation
- Molecular characterization may assist classification in future

CLINICAL ISSUES

- Rare in spinal cord
- Disease usually uncontrollable after initial recurrence

IMAGING

- Often bulky, discrete, and enhancing

MICROSCOPIC

- Diffuse high cellularity (some cases)
- Cellular nodular areas, especially in posterior fossa examples
- Mitotic activity increased over grade II
- May have infiltrative growth pattern

ANCILLARY TESTS

- GFAP(+), especially perivascular pseudorosettes
- EMA(+)
  - Surfaces, especially of true rosettes and other epithelial surfaces
  - Dot-like staining of microlumina
- L1CAM strongly (+) in most c11orf95-RELA fusion tumors

DIAGNOSTIC CHECKLIST

- Difficult, subjective distinction from grade II in many cases
- Medulloblastoma can mimic anaplastic ependymoma, especially on frozen sections
- Consider possibility with any compact, monomorphous, high-grade tumor, especially in young children

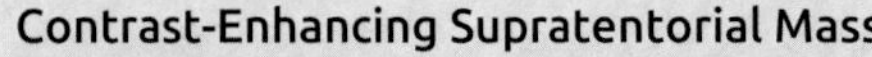

Contrast-Enhancing Supratentorial Mass

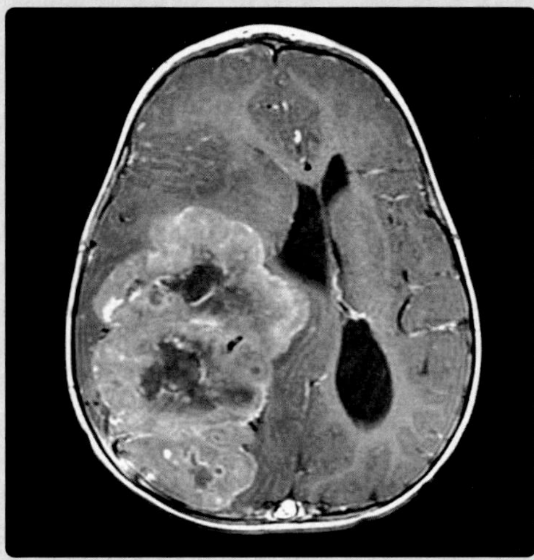

Vascular Proliferation

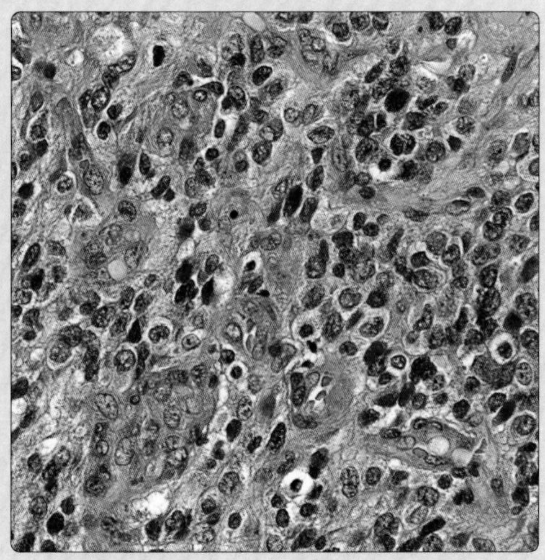

(Left) *High-grade ependymomas are often bulky masses. Children are principally affected. A supratentorial mass without obvious relationship to a ventricle does not preclude diagnosis of ependymoma.* **(Right)** *Even when grade III with vascular proliferation, ependymomas usually retain a compact architecture. Finding some feature of ependymal differentiation, whether histological or immunohistochemical, becomes important.*

Palisading Necrosis

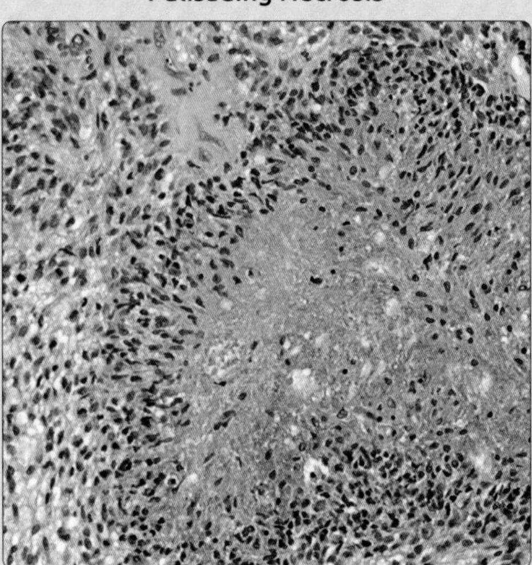

Clear Cell Variant

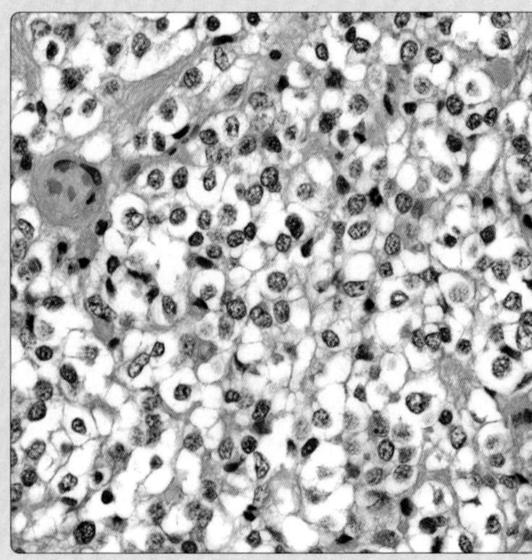

(Left) *Rare anaplastic ependymomas demonstrate palisading necrosis akin to those seen in classical glioblastomas.* **(Right)** *The clear cell variant of ependymomas, albeit not absolutely clear, have been associated with a more aggressive course. These neoplasms can be mistaken for many others such as oligodendroglioma, and have been considered anaplastic.*

TERMINOLOGY

Definitions

- WHO: Malignant glioma with ependymal differentiation, with high mitotic activity often accompanied by microvascular proliferation and pseudopalisading necrosis
- No consensus grading system
- WHO grade III

CLINICAL ISSUES

Site

- Supratentorial or infratentorial
- Spinal cord (uncommon)

Treatment

- Drugs
  - Often when supratentorial and subtotally resected
- Radiation
  - Standard for children older than 3 years

Prognosis

- Unfavorable
  - Local recurrence common
  - CNS dissemination can occur at presentation or later following local recurrence

IMAGING

MR Findings

- Often bulky and enhancing and cystic (some cases)

MICROSCOPIC

Histologic Features

- Discrete borders (some cases), especially clear cell variant
  - Infiltrative, but less compared to infiltrating gliomas
- High cellularity, often diffuse
  - Multiple nodules, especially common in posterior fossa tumors
    - Nodules contain cytologic atypia, high mitotic activity, and high Ki-67 index
- High mitotic activity but no precise cutoff for grade III
- Microvascular proliferation typical, but not present in all
- Necrosis
  - Nonpalisading type common in grade II ependymomas and not criterion for grade III
  - Pseudopalisading necrosis more closely associated with tumor aggressiveness
- Clear cell type, often, but not necessarily, grade III
- Mesenchymal differentiation (ependymosarcoma) rare

ANCILLARY TESTS

Cytology

- Cell processes and fibrillar background
- Generally more nuclear atypia than grade II

Immunohistochemistry

- GFAP(+), especially perivascular pseudorosettes
- EMA(+)
  - Epithelial surfaces, especially of true rosettes
  - Dot-like staining of microlumina
- Synaptophysin, neurofilament protein, both may be focal
- D2-40 often strong, either focal or diffuse, but nonspecific
- Olig2 staining is often negative in majority of tumor nuclei; exceptional examples are (+)
- L1CAM strongly (+) in most c11orf95-RELA fusion tumors

Genetic Testing

- C11orf95-RELA fusions in supratentorial tumors

DIFFERENTIAL DIAGNOSIS

Medulloblastoma

- Neuroblastic (Homer Wright rosettes) (some cases)
- Perivascular rosettes similar to ependymoma (some cases) but synaptophysin (+)
- Nodular/desmoplastic pattern (some cases)
  - Perinodular reticulin network
- Synaptophysin, diffusely (+) especially in nodules
- Nuclear (+) for β-catenin in Wnt type, and cytoplasmic (+) for GAB1 in SHH type

Embryonal Tumor With Multilayered Rosettes

- Finely fibrillar, synaptophysin (+) neuropil background
- Rosettes containing small round or slit-like lumina and anaplastic nuclei
- LIN28A(+)
- Chr 19q13.42 amplification

Glioblastoma

- Diffusely infiltrative
- More polymorphous, except for small cell type
- IDH-1 and p53 (+) with loss of ATRX in secondary glioblastoma, H3.3 K27M (+) in pediatric glioblastoma

Atypical Teratoid/Rhabdoid Tumor

- More often polymorphous
- Large rhabdoid or pale cells
- No fibrillar perivascular pseudorosettes
- Polyimmunophenotypic, e.g., EMA, cytokeratins, GFAP, synaptophysin, smooth muscle actin, desmin, etc.
- Loss of nuclear INI1 immunoreactivity

Choroid Plexus Carcinoma

- Often with focal papillary architecture and anaplasia
- Hyaline globules (some cases)
- No microvascular proliferation
- Cytokeratins stronger (+), no EMA (+) microlumina, weak GFAP

Astroblastoma

- Hyalinized vascular walls and perivascular cells with short stout processes
- Inconspicuous fibrillar matrix
- Radial papillary or ribboned profiles

SELECTED REFERENCES

1. Pajtler KW et al: Molecular classification of ependymal tumors across all CNS compartments, histopathological grades, and age groups. Cancer Cell. 27(5):728-43, 2015
2. Ellison DW et al: Histopathological grading of pediatric ependymoma: reproducibility and clinical relevance in European trial cohorts. J Negat Results Biomed. 10:7, 2011

Brisk Vascular Proliferation

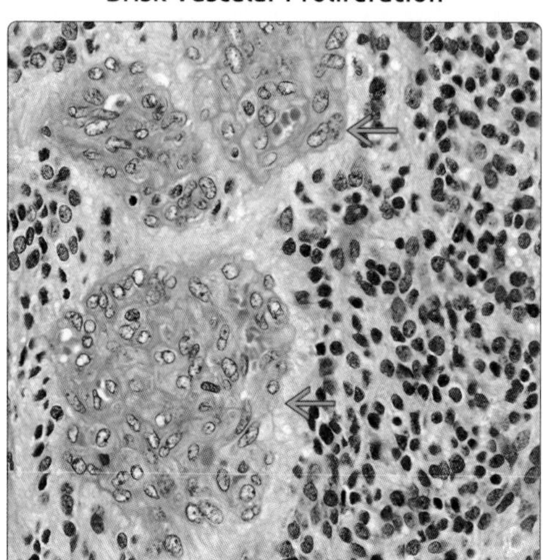

Geographic Necrosis

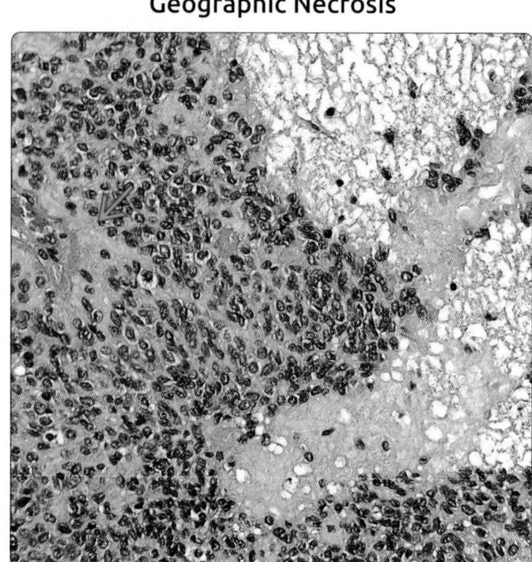

(Left) *The presence of microvascular proliferation ⇒ in a cellular lesion with mitoses simplifies the often thorny issue of grading an ependymoma.* **(Right)** *Sheet-like architecture and poorly formed perivascular pseudorosettes ⇒ help establish the diagnosis of ependymoma. While consistent with a grade III lesion, nonpalisading necrosis is not a grading parameter.*

Subtle Perivascular Pseudorosettes

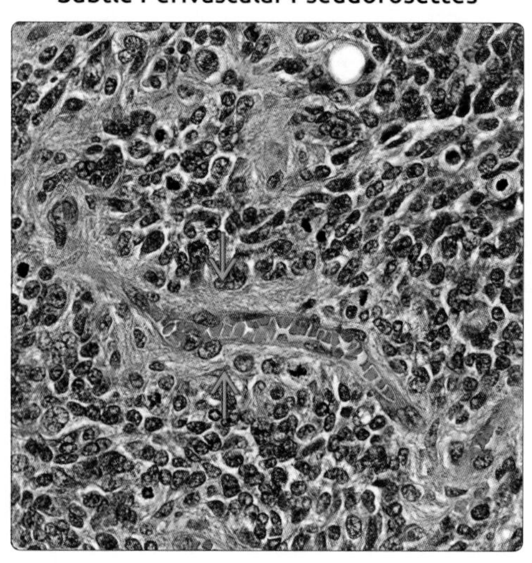

Numerous Mitoses

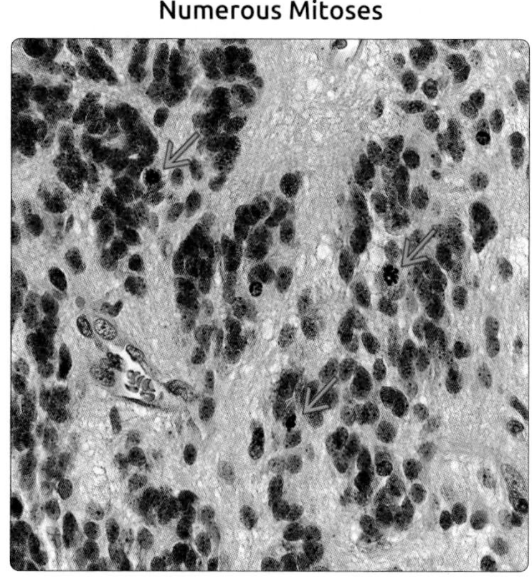

(Left) *Perivascular pseudorosettes ⇒ may be subtle and require immunohistochemistry for GFAP.* **(Right)** *Most anaplastic ependymomas have fibrillarity and perivascular pseudorosettes, at least to some degree. Assuming that the field is in any way representative, its 3 mitoses ⇒ leave little doubt that this tumor is grade III.*

Patternless Morphology

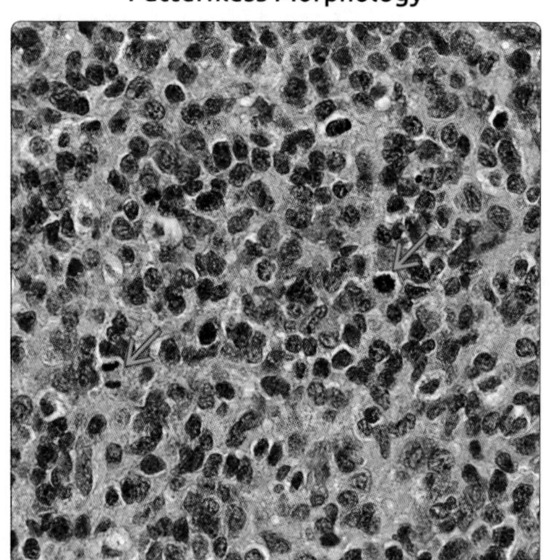

Primitive Rosettes

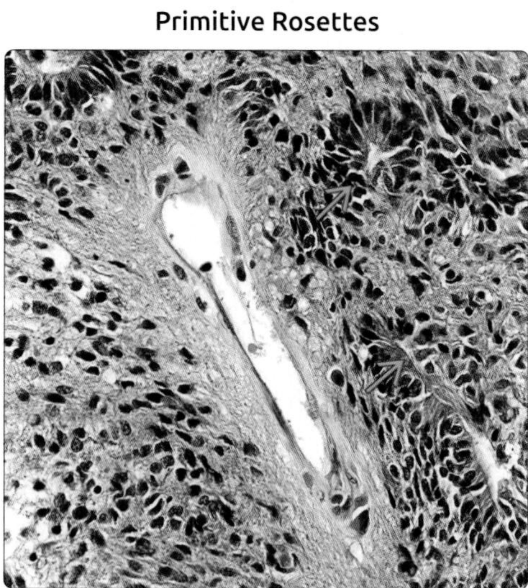

(Left) *Some anaplastic ependymomas lack perivascular pseudorosettes. A patternless lesion such as this with brisk mitotic activity ⇒ is clearly grade III.* **(Right)** *Round and slit-like, primitive, mitotically active rosettes ⇒ similar to those of embryonal tumor with multilayered rosettes appear in some grade III ependymomas. In ependymomas, such rosettes represent abortive ependymal canals.*

Mitoses but No Atypia

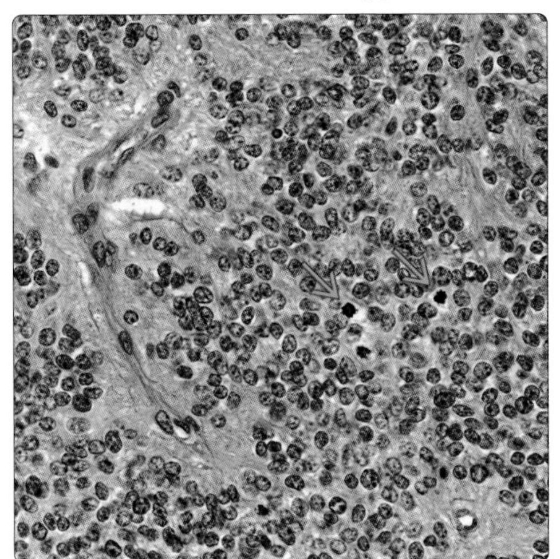

Atypia and Vascular Proliferation

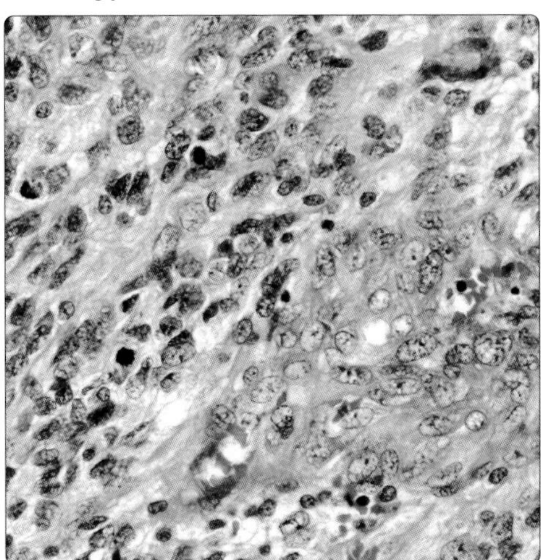

(Left) *Although a classic ependymoma with little atypia, there are too many mitoses for grade II* ⇨ *in this lesion that had multiple other similar nodules. Cellularity is higher than in grade II equivalents, and perivascular pseudorosettes are less prominent. There is considerable overlap, however, in cellularity and cytological features between ependymomas grades II and III.* **(Right)** *Marked cytological atypia, mitoses, and microvascular proliferation, in combination, are clear indicators of anaplasia.*

Necrosis and High Cellularity

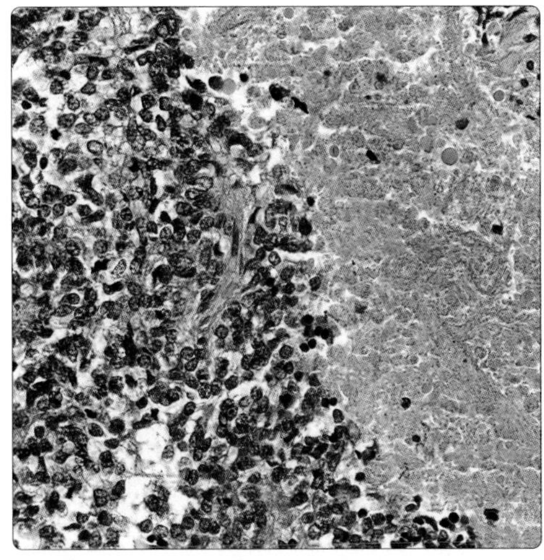

Low-Grade Area in Anaplastic Tumor

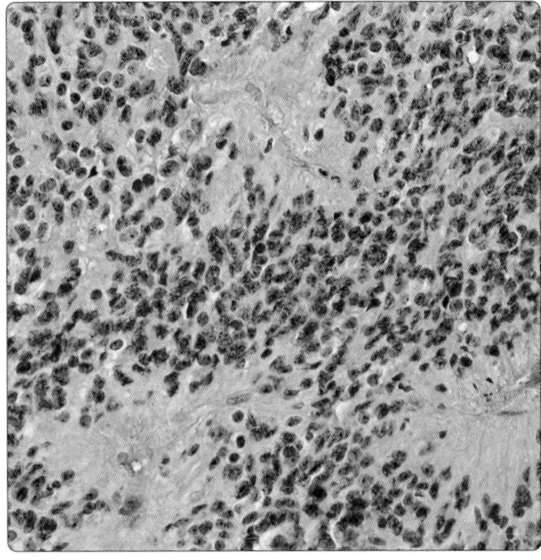

(Left) *Some ependymomas are so cellular and mitotically active that they are clearly anaplastic. Determining whether such tumors are ependymomas can be a more difficult issue.* **(Right)** *The degree of atypia suggests grade III, but confirmatory mitoses would be necessary for the designation of grade III. In many anaplastic ependymomas, foci that are indistinguishable from a low-grade tumor can be observed.*

Compact Architecture With Mitoses

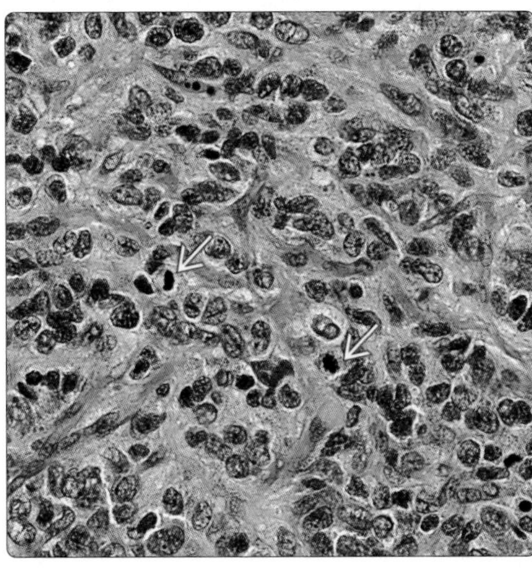

Cellular Anaplasia

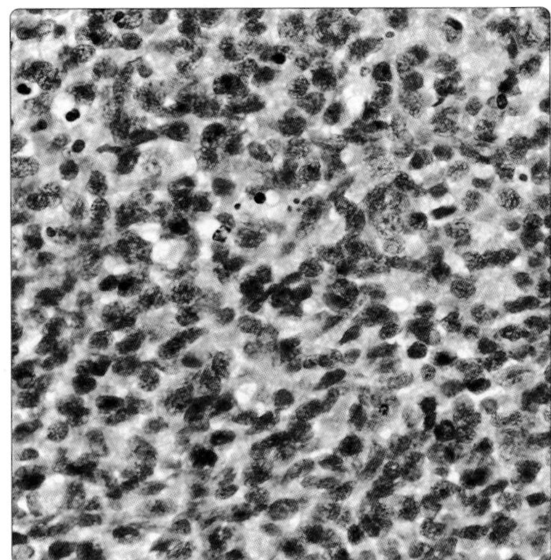

(Left) *Features suggesting ependymoma include compact architecture, vague perivascular pseudorosettes, and small, uniform, dark, oval nuclei. Mitoses, found here without difficulty* ➡*, are critical for the designation of grade III.* **(Right)** *In some anaplastic ependymomas, there is little to suggest ependymoma other than compact architecture and small, dark, uniform nuclei.*

(Left) *Particularly in the posterior fossa, ependymomas may have well-circumscribed nodules with varying cellularity, cytologic atypia, and mitotic activity. The one at the top is highly cellular, whereas that at bottom left is only marginally more cellular than the surrounding tumor. Mitoses were easy to find in the former. More than a few mitotically active nodules are required for grade III designation.* **(Right)** *Even if solitary, hypercellular nodules with cytologic atypia and mitotic activity suggest grade III.*

Hypercellular Nodules

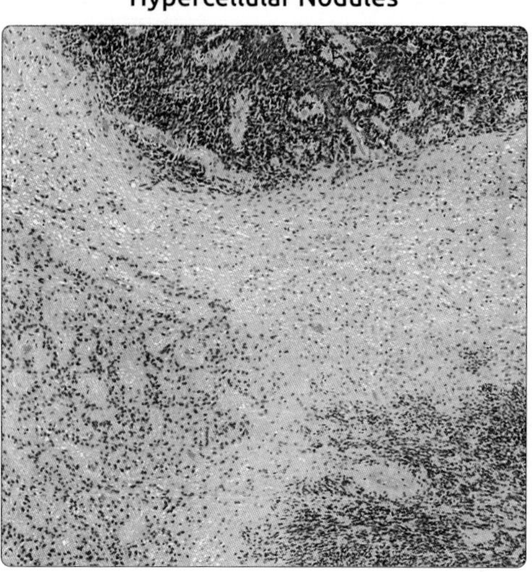

Hypercellular Nodule, Close-Up

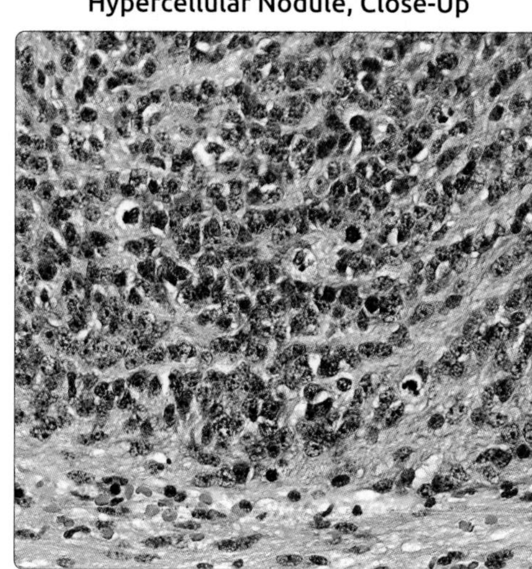

(Left) *Generally supratentorial and grade III, clear cell ependymomas have sharp borders. The clear cell variant can simulate either neurocytic tumors or oligodendrogliomas in some instances.* **(Right)** *Not all grade III clear cell ependymomas are particularly "clear cell." In such cases, the designation is based on architecture and pleomorphic nuclei. Mitoses are present* ⇨ *in this grade III example.*

Clear Cell Ependymoma

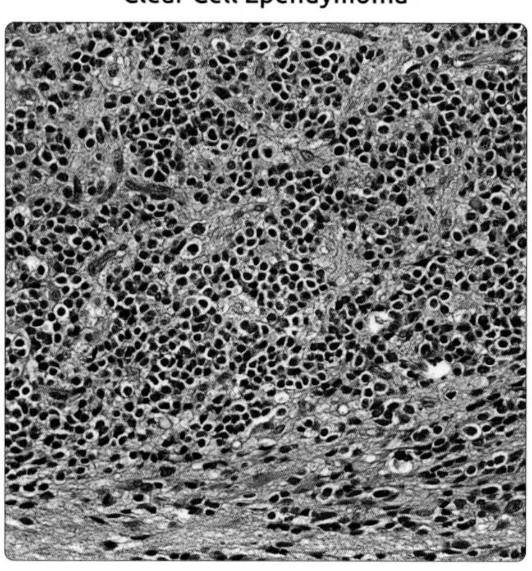

Clear Cell Ependymoma

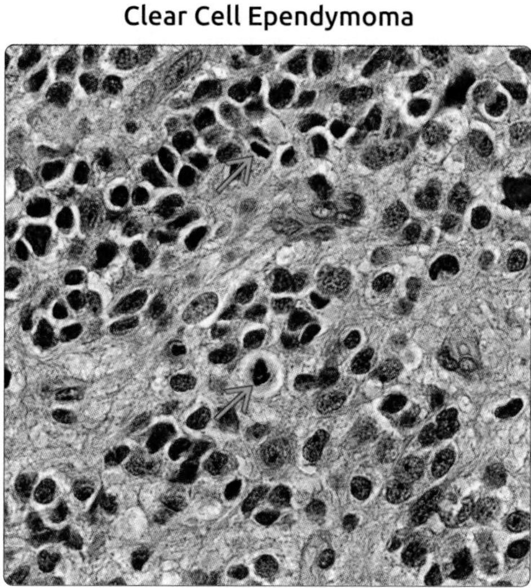

(Left) *Smear preparations often capture perivascular rosettes. Nuclei in grade III ependymomas are typically darker and cytologically more atypical than those of the grade II counterpart.* **(Right)** *Nuclei of clear cell ependymomas are larger and more clefted and grooved than those of other variants. A cell in prophase is about to divide* ⇨.

Pseudorosettes in Intraoperative Smear

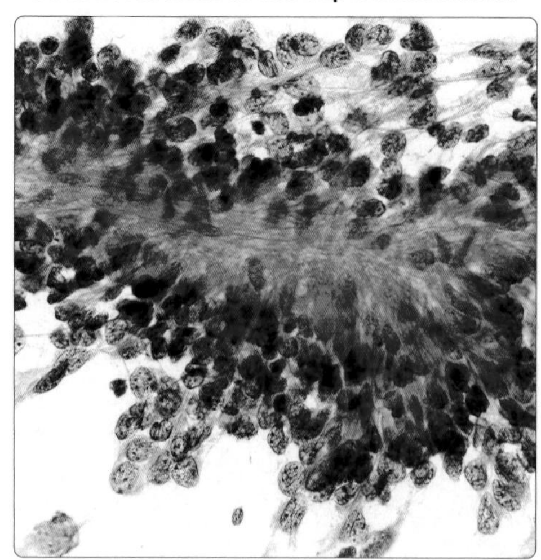

Intraoperative Smear Cytology, Prophase

GFAP, Strongly Positive

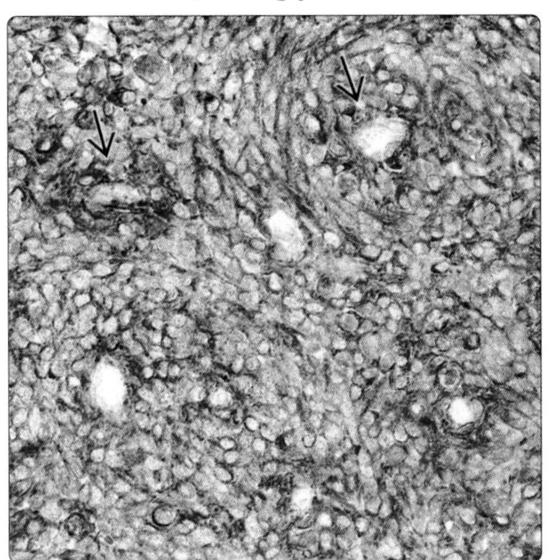

S100 Staining, Nuclear and Cytoplasmic

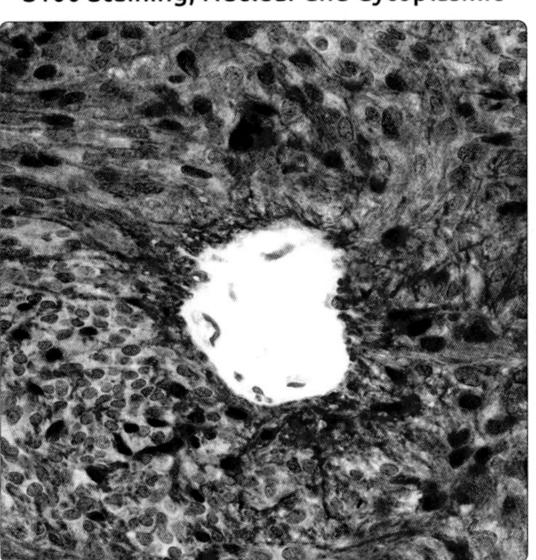

(Left) *GFAP is positive in some cases in both perivascular pseudorosettes* ➙ *and intervascular areas, but immunoreactivity may be restrained in other cases. GFAP IHC can assist in highlighting pseudorosettes.* **(Right)** *Ependymomas, as well as anaplastic ependymomas, are focally but strongly positive with S100 antibodies, and show both a nuclear and cytoplasmic staining pattern.*

Ki-67 in Hypercellular Nodules

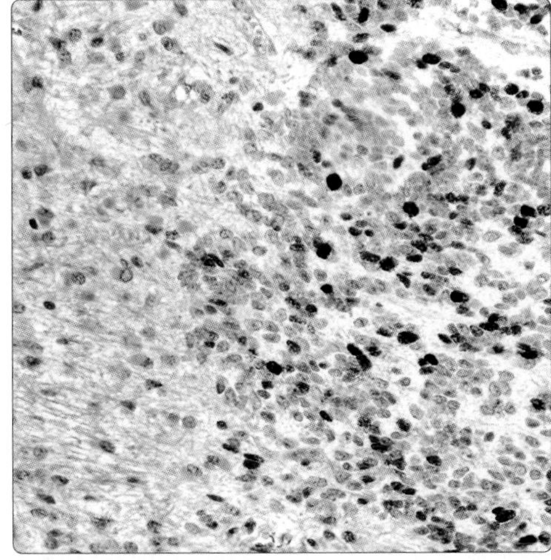

Epithelial Membrane Antigen

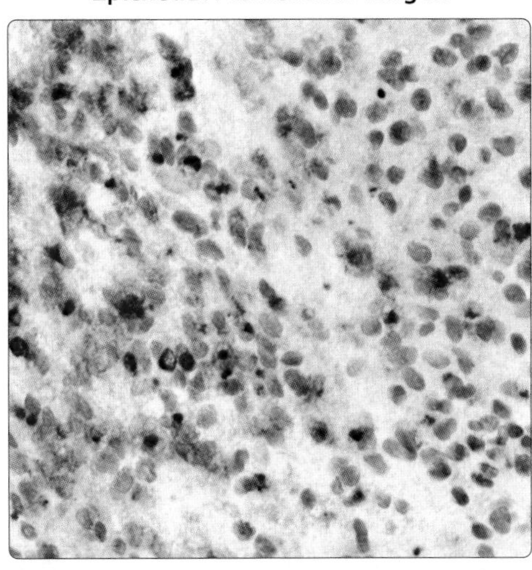

(Left) *The Ki-67 index is considerably higher within the hypercellular nodules in ependymomas.* **(Right)** *EMA demonstrates focal and scattered dot-like perinuclear immunopositivity in anaplastic ependymomas. While often less pronounced than grade II lesions, this staining is often helpful to recognize the tumor as an ependymal neoplasm.*

D2-40 Cytoplasmic Staining

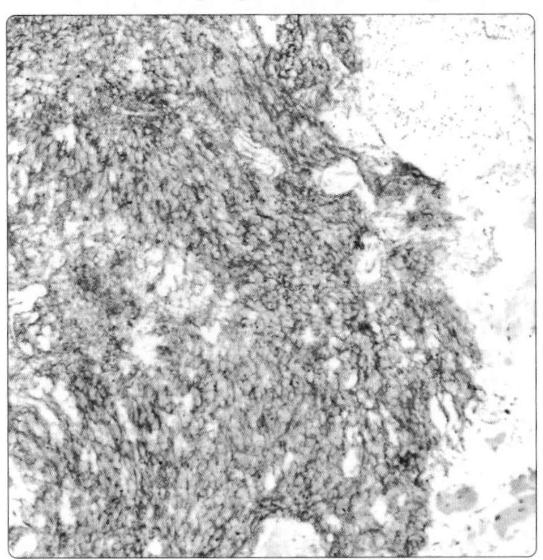

L1CAM Antibody Staining

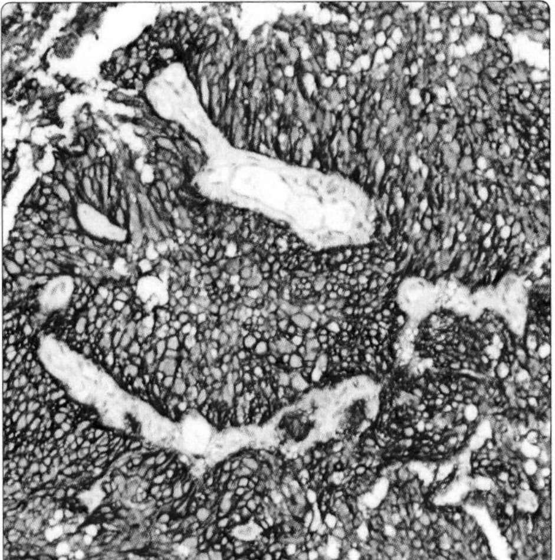

(Left) *While completely nonspecific, strong D2-40 staining (either focal or diffuse) supports the diagnosis of anaplastic ependymoma in lieu of more specific markers of ependymoma.* **(Right)** *Some anaplastic astrocytomas, especially those in the supratentorial region in children, demonstrate strong L1CAM positivity. Immunostaining for L1CAM often parallels the presence of C11orf95-RELA fusion.*

Myxopapillary Ependymoma

KEY FACTS

TERMINOLOGY

- Low-grade, mucin-rich ependymal neoplasm most commonly located in filum terminale, WHO grade I

CLINICAL ISSUES

- Distal spinal cord (filum terminale/conus medullaris)
- Extradural, pre- or postsacral or intraosseous (rare)
- Exceptionally above foramen magnum
- Generally good, but may seed neuraxis
- Recurrence related to extent of resection and intactness of capsule during removal
- Dissemination more likely in children
- Poor for rare pre- or postsacral lesions; potential for metastases

MACROSCOPIC

- Soft, sometimes myxoid "bag"

MICROSCOPIC

- Large, dark, pleomorphic without increased mitotic or Ki-67 rate (giant cell ependymoma) in rare cases
- Perivascular arrangement of epithelial cells around mucin
- Pseudopapillae, ribbons or strands of epithelial cells
- Fibrillar tumor similar to tanycytic ependymoma, but often with perivascular myxoid substance
- Dense sclerosis or infarction in some cases

ANCILLARY TESTS

- Alcian blue
- GFAP(+), S100(+) focal
- Dot-like pattern or focal surface staining

DIAGNOSTIC CHECKLIST

- Well-circumscribed filum terminale lesion amenable to complete resection in some cases
- Do not interpret nuclear pleomorphism in giant cell ependymoma as evidence of anaplasia

(Left) *Myxopapillary ependymoma is a sausage-shaped, homogeneously enhancing mass in the lower spinal cord and filum terminale* ➔*. Schwannoma and paraganglioma are principal differential diagnoses.* **(Right)** *A soft, bag-like myxoid mass arising from the filum terminale* ➔ *is almost certainly myxopapillary ependymoma.*

Sagittal Contrast-Enhanced MR

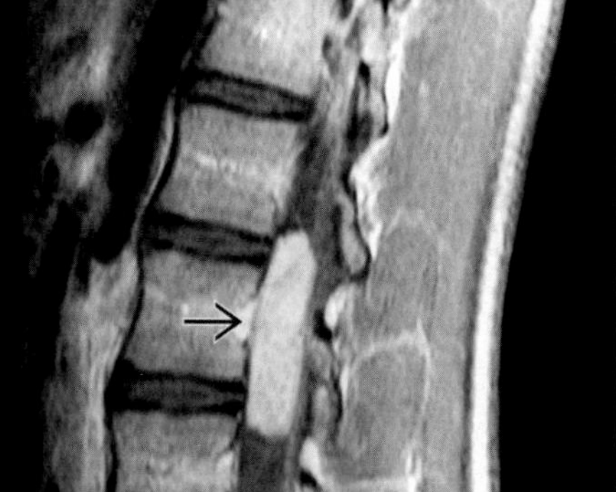

Bag-Like Myxoid Mass

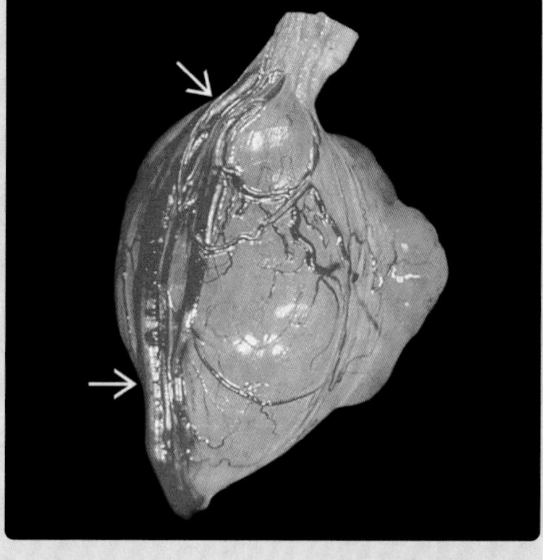

(Left) *Myxopapillary ependymomas have variable morphological characteristics and are composed of papillary structures with abundant mucin around the vascular lumina, with epithelial cells located around this mucinous matrix.* **(Right)** *Alcian blue (+) myxoid substance collars small vessels* ➔*.*

Mucinous With Papillary Architecture

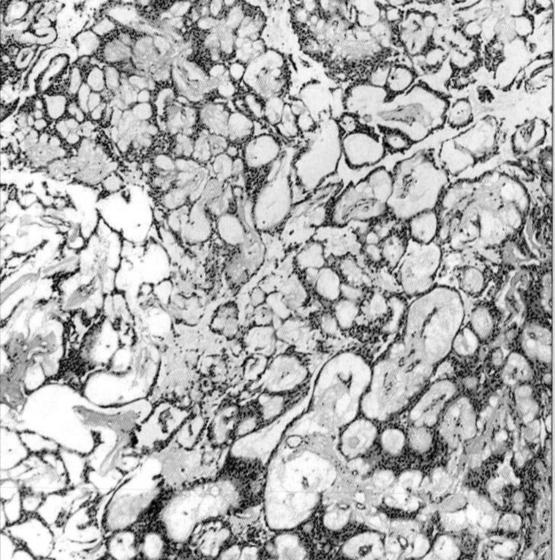

Abundant Mucin Around Vessels

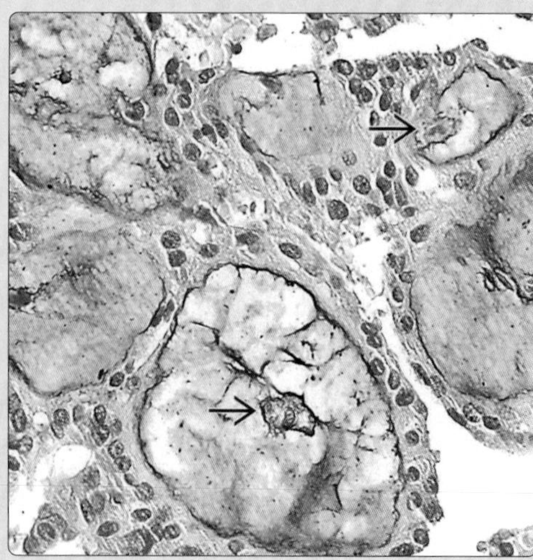

TERMINOLOGY

Abbreviations

- Myxopapillary ependymoma (MPE)

Definitions

- Low-grade, mucin-rich ependymal neoplasm most commonly located in filum terminale
- WHO grade I

CLINICAL ISSUES

Epidemiology

- Age
  - More common in adults, rare in children

Site

- Distal spinal cord (filum terminale/conus medullaris)
- Extradural, pre- or postsacral or intraosseous (rare)
- Exceptionally above the foramen magnum

Presentation

- Motor or sensory disturbance depending on location within spinal cord

Treatment

- Surgery
  - Total resection is treatment of choice
- Radiation
  - Reserved for subtotal resection, recurrence, or disseminated disease

Prognosis

- Generally good, but may seed neuraxis
- Recurrence related to extent of resection and intactness of capsule during removal
- Dissemination more likely in children
- Poor for rare pre- or postsacral lesions; potential for metastases

IMAGING

MR Findings

- Discrete, contrast enhancing

MACROSCOPIC

General Features

- Well circumscribed, encapsulated in some cases
- Spontaneous rupture with involvement of nerve roots or CSF dissemination possible
- Soft, sometimes mucinous "bag"

MICROSCOPIC

Histologic Features

- Perivascular arrangement of epithelial cells around mucin
- Pseudopapillae, ribbons or strands of epithelial cells
- Epithelial surfaces in some cases
- Fibrillar tumor similar to tanycytic ependymoma, but often with perivascular myxoid substance
- Microcysts
- Dense sclerosis or infarction in some cases, absence of interspersed reticulin fibers, unlike schwannoma
- Large, hyperchromatic pleomorphic nuclei without increased mitotic or Ki-67 rate (giant cell ependymoma) in occasional cases

ANCILLARY TESTS

Cytology

- Smears show fibrillar, mucinous background
- Epithelial cells with ependymal characteristics

Histochemistry

- Alcian blue
  - Perivascular, may be only focal

Immunohistochemistry

- Ki-67 low, usually < 2%
- GFAP(+), S100(+) focal
- EMA(+), D2-40(+)
  - Dot-like pattern or focal surface staining

Gene Expression Profiling

- DNA methylation profiling of ependymal tumors identifies 9 distinct molecular subgroups; MPE in its own subgroup and distinct from other spinal cord ependymomas
- Gene expression profiling for all ependymomas may better predict prognosis than histological features

DIFFERENTIAL DIAGNOSIS

Schwannoma

- Nerve root origin, rather than filum terminale
- Antoni A and B tissue, Verocay bodies, interspersed reticulin fibers, especially in Antoni A
- No epithelial features
- Diffuse rather than perivascular mucinous material in myxoid variants
- Diffuse and strong S100(+), SOX10(+) and GFAP(-) or focal

Paraganglioma

- Acinar architecture (zellballen)
- No (or only scant) myxoid background
- Chromogranin (+), S100(+) sustentacular cells &/or chief cells, cytokeratins (+) in some cases

DIAGNOSTIC CHECKLIST

Clinically Relevant Pathologic Features

- Well-circumscribed filum terminale lesion amenable to complete resection in some cases
- Disseminated or multifocal in some cases
- Exactly what amount of mucin needs to be present to diagnose MPE in filum terminale lesion unclear

Pathologic Interpretation Pearls

- May be only focally mucinous, typically around vessels
- Nuclear pleomorphism in giant cell ependymoma not to be interpreted necessarily as evidence of anaplasia

SELECTED REFERENCES

1. Pajtler KW et al: Molecular Classification of Ependymal Tumors across All CNS Compartments, Histopathological Grades, and Age Groups. Cancer Cell. 27(5):728-43, 2015
2. Barton VN et al: Unique molecular characteristics of pediatric myxopapillary ependymoma. Brain Pathol. 20(3):560-70, 2010

(Left) *Prominent fibrillary background with a conspicuous mucinous matrix and round to oval epithelioid cells with ependymal characteristics are helpful diagnostic features for MPE.* **(Right)** *On smear, MPEs retain the angiocentricity of ependymomas in general. Tumor cells extend processes to a small vessel ⇨ in the cytological equivalent of a perivascular pseudorosette. The cell cytoplasm, with fine processes, differs fundamentally from that of another local entity, paraganglioma.*

Smear, Oval Uniform Nuclei

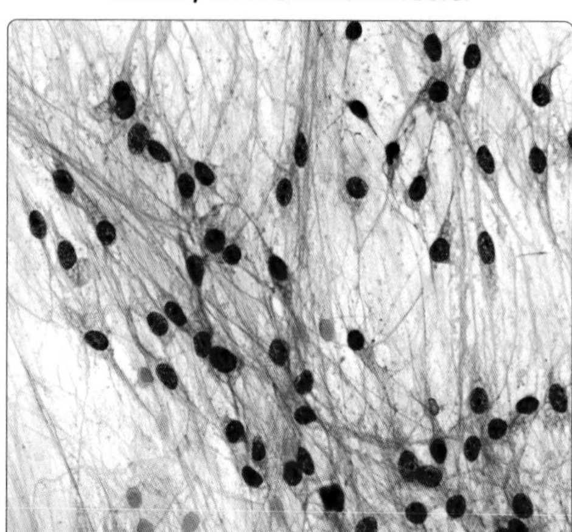

Smear, Angiocentricity

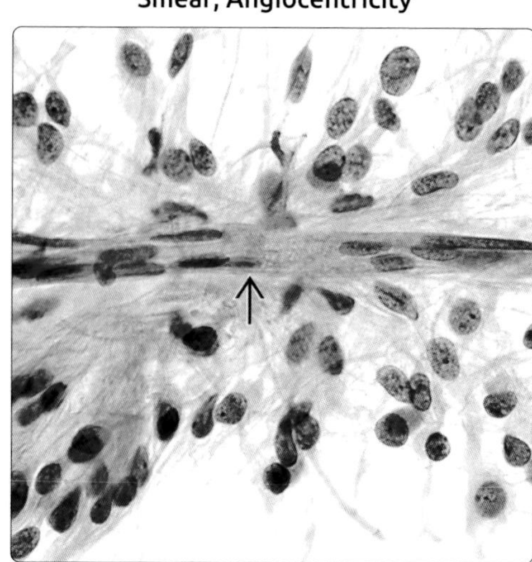

(Left) *Smears can highlight the perivascular arrangement of the fibrillary processes ➡ in myxopapillary ependymomas. The tumor cells seem to be connected to the vascular walls with these fibrillary processes, which imparts the appearance of perivascular pseudorosettes.* **(Right)** *The nuclei of myxopapillary ependymomas have the typical salt and pepper type punctate chromatin pattern and small but distinct nucleoli. While the mucinous matrix is not obvious, the fibrillary background suggests a glial neoplasm.*

Smear, Perivascular Glial Processes

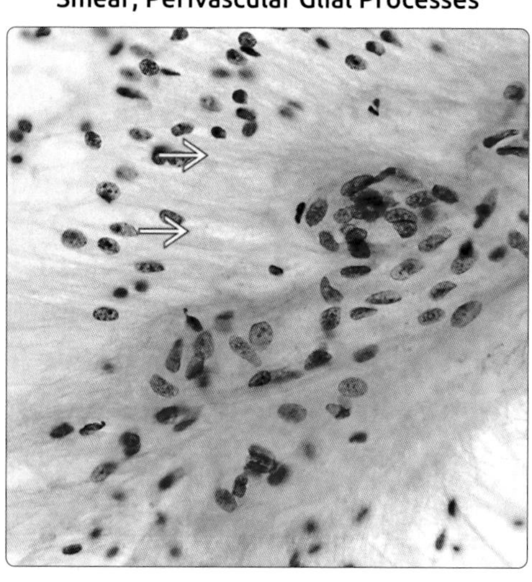

Ependymal Nuclei

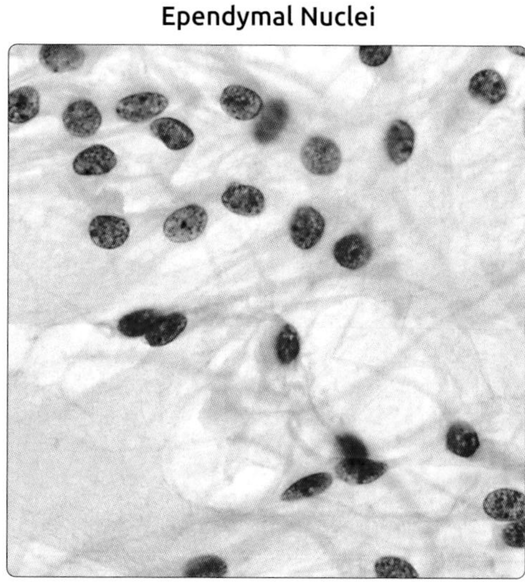

(Left) *Balls of epithelioid cells with myxoid cores are distinctive features in smear preparations.* **(Right)** *Whether obviously perivascular or not, circular profiles filled with myxoid substance are characteristic of myxopapillary ependymoma.*

Balls of Epithelioid Cells

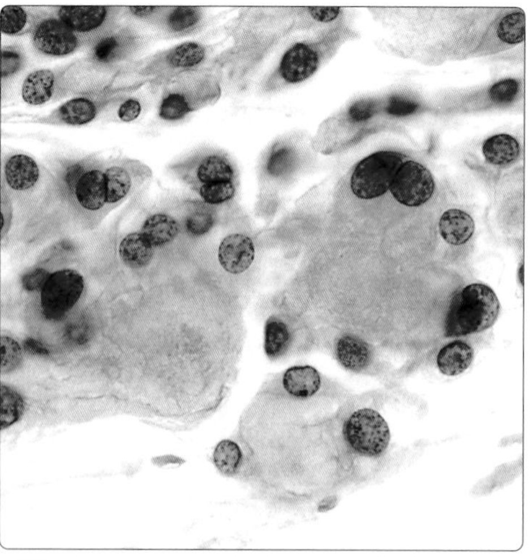

Frozen Section, Circular Mucin-Filled Areas

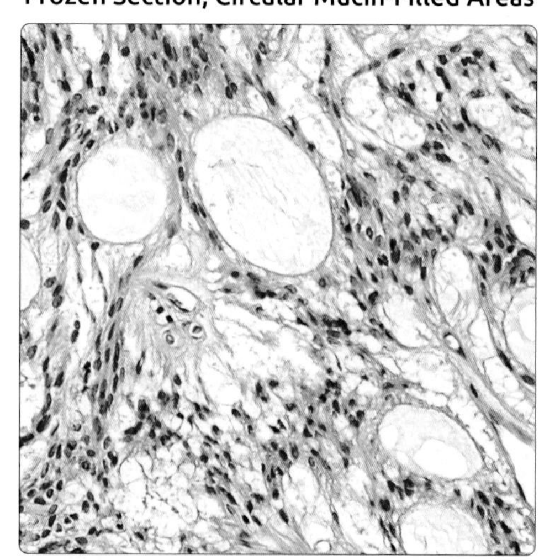

Attachment to Filum Terminale

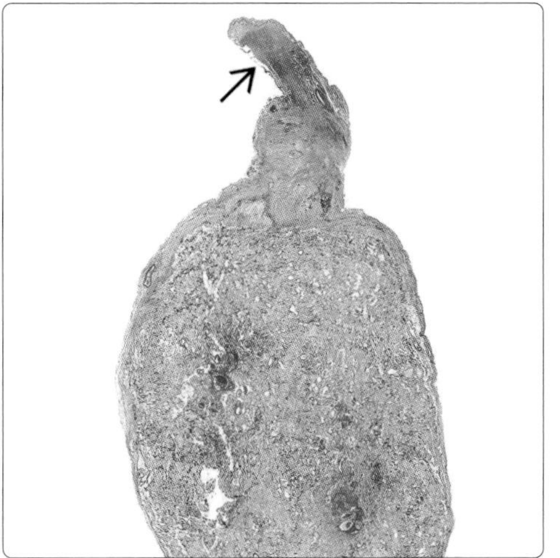

Connective Tissue Capsule

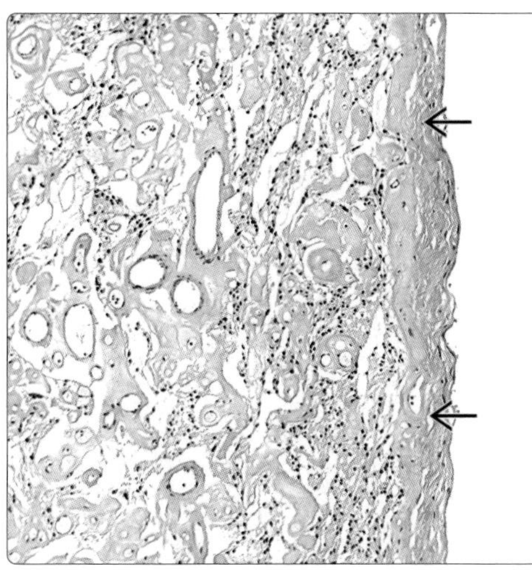

(Left) *Well-circumscribed MPE arises from the filum terminale ⇒. The lesion's faintly basophilic myxoid background is apparent here even at low magnification.* **(Right)** *A thin band of connective tissue ⇒ encapsulates the compact, noninvasive lesion that in this case has considerable perivascular sclerosis.*

Classic Mucinous Papillae

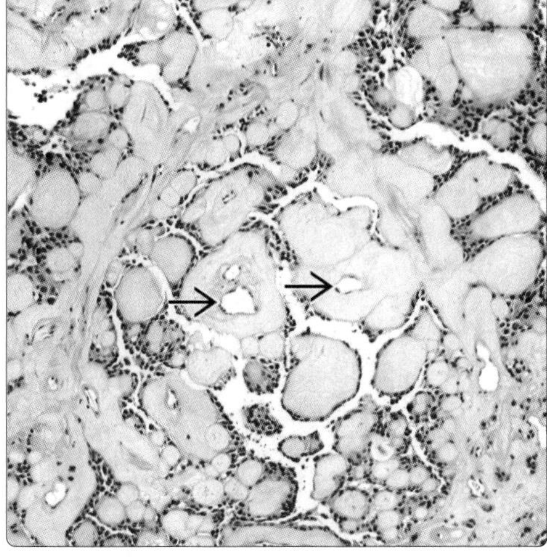

Tumor Lobules

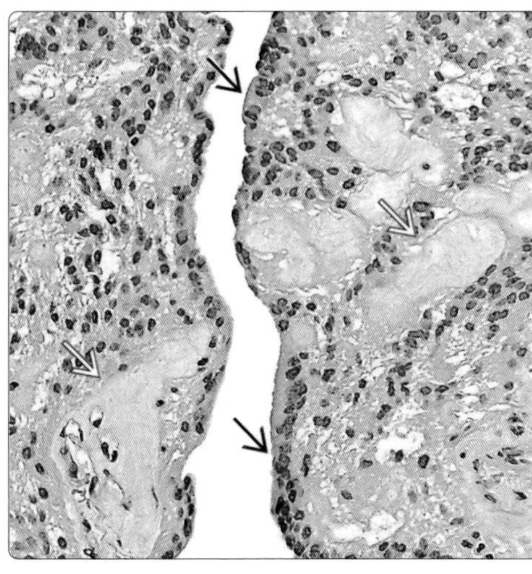

(Left) *The prominent mucinous appearance of the papillary structures and epithelioid cells lining the mucinous material are typical of myxopapillary ependymomas. The vascular structures ⇒ at the center of the mucinous material is clearly distinguishable.* **(Right)** *Neoplastic ependymal cells cover large lobules in some MPEs ⇒. Perivascular myxoid substance is also present ➡.*

Fibrillary, Tanycytic-Like Pattern

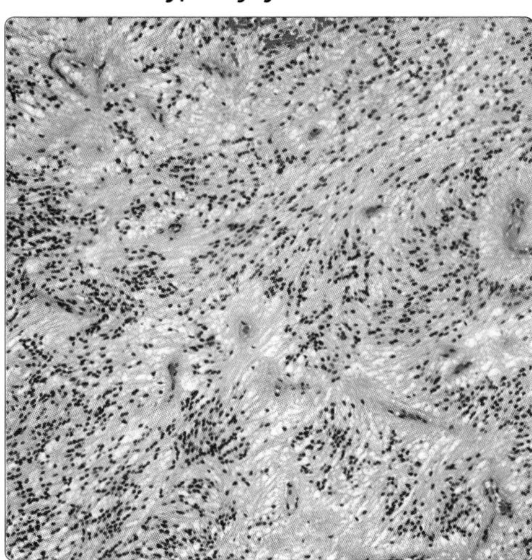

Fibrillary, Tanycytic-Like Pattern

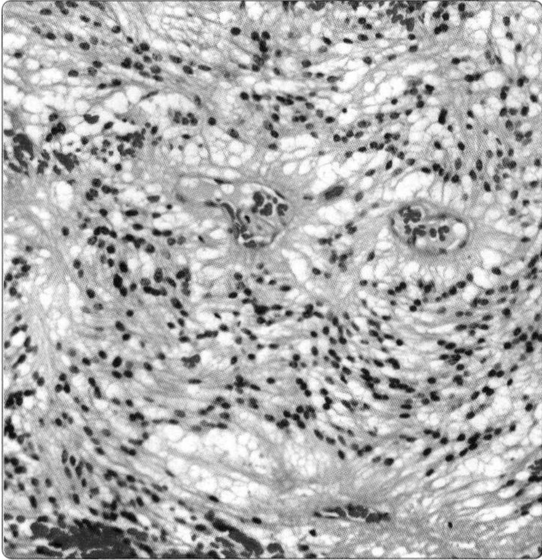

(Left) *Some myxopapillary ependymomas show a striking resemblance to tanycytic ependymomas with moderately cellular, highly fibrillary tumor with a fascicular architecture. The perivascular ependymal-type rosettes are also conspicuous.* **(Right)** *High magnification shows fibrillary areas with a fascicular pattern and conspicuous perivascular pseudorosettes. The mucinous background can be recognized in this section but an Alcian blue stain helps to underscore the extent of mucinous matrix.*

(Left) *Degenerative atypia akin to "ancient change" in schwannomas occasionally appears in MPEs.* **(Right)** *Glioblastoma would come to mind but for location and, usually, typical features of MPE elsewhere in the specimen. The absence of mitoses and a low Ki-67 index would be cautionary findings in such a giant cell ependymoma.*

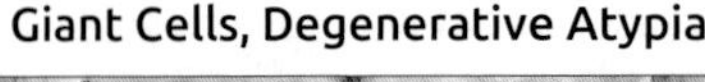

Giant Cells, Degenerative Atypia

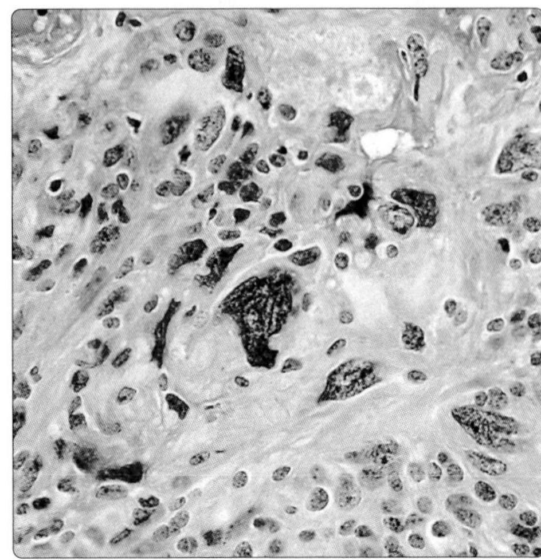

Cellular Atypia, Giant Cell Ependymoma

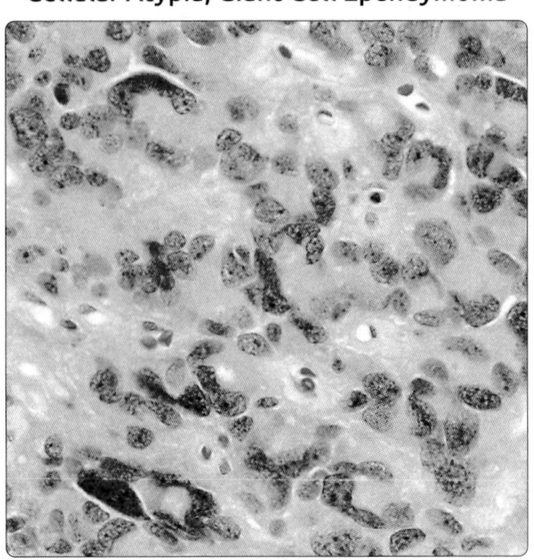

(Left) *Areas of zonal necrosis → are common in ependymomas from any anatomical site, but without surrounding pseudopalisading, necrosis in these areas is without prognostic or grading implications.* **(Right)** *Sclerosis crowds out tumor cells in some cases. Cyst-like spaces filled with myxoid substance → leave no doubt about the diagnosis.*

Necrosis Without Prognostic Implication

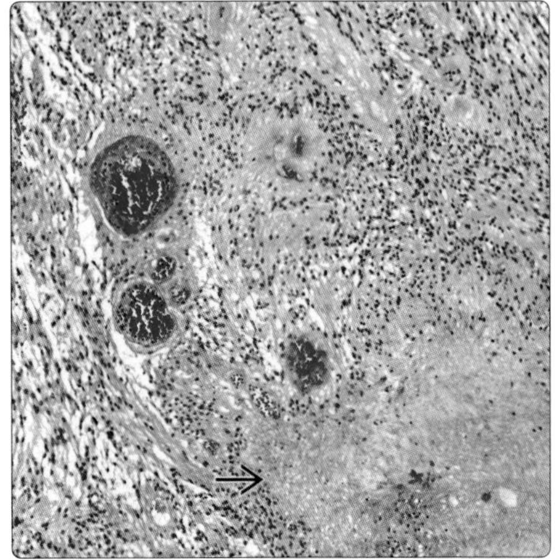

Sclerotic Tumor

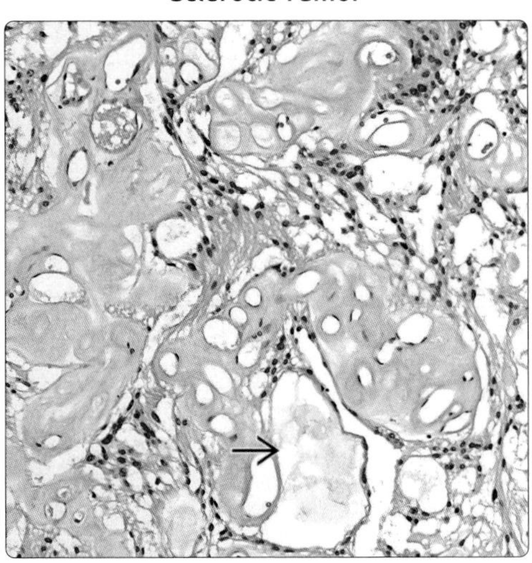

(Left) *Some tumors in spinal cord, especially within lumbosacral cord, demonstrate areas more typical of classical ependymoma, whereas in other foci the tumor possesses MPE morphology. Note the focal mucin between perivascular cells →.* **(Right)** *Some tumors have variable histological patterns focally resembling classical ependymoma and MPE. These tumors often have higher mitotic rates than typical MPE, but the prognostic significance of this hybrid morphology is not clear.*

Hybrid Ependymoma-MPE

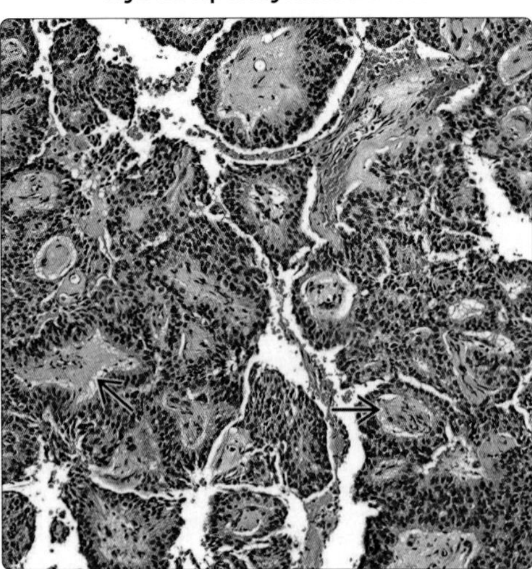

Hybrid Tumors: Classic MPE Area

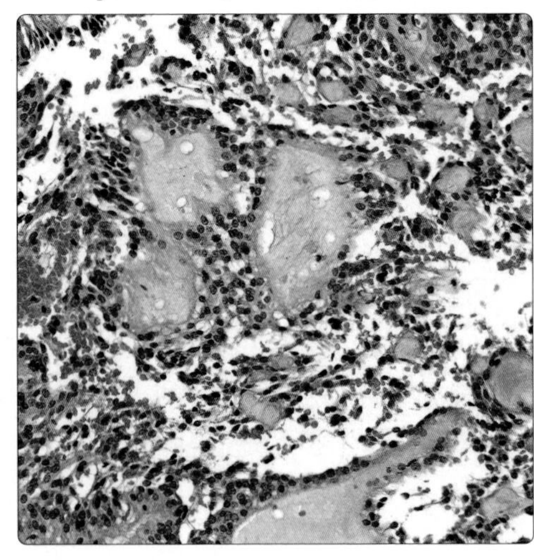

Mucinous Matrix With Alcian Blue

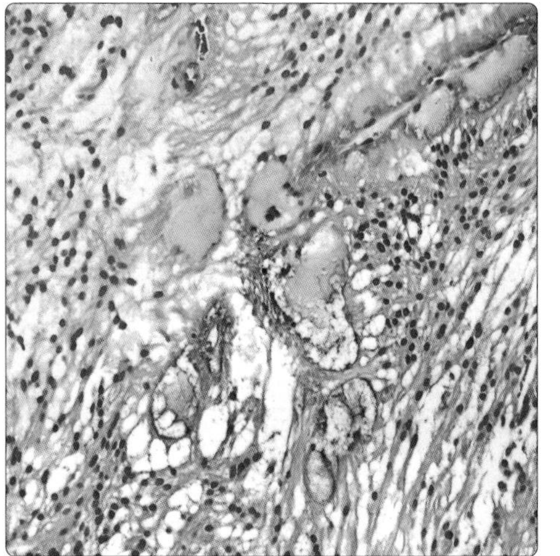

Trichrome (+) Vascular Structures

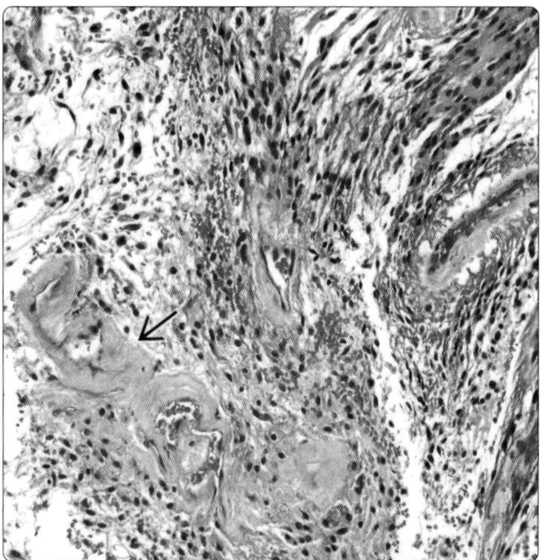

(Left) *A signature feature of MPE is the presence of Alcian blue (+) mucinous pools. In this area the perivascular ependymoma cell processes and central blood vessel have degenerated, leaving only the amorphous pools.* **(Right)** *The stains for collagen, like trichrome, highlight the prominent perivascular hyalinization and basal lamina ⇒ in MPE.*

GFAP(+) Highlighting Perivascular Pseudorosettes

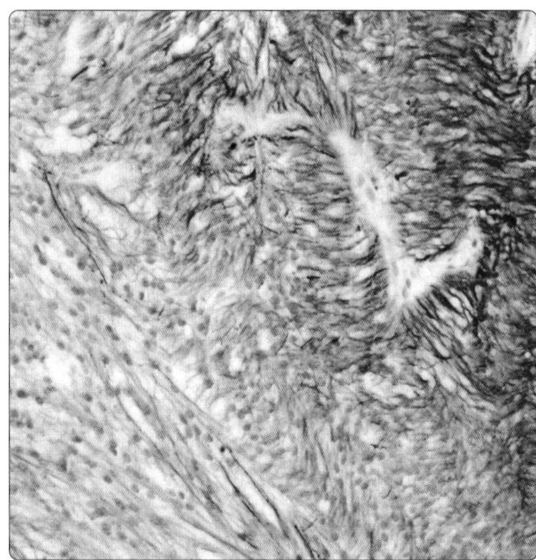

D2-40(+) Perivascular Pseudorosettes

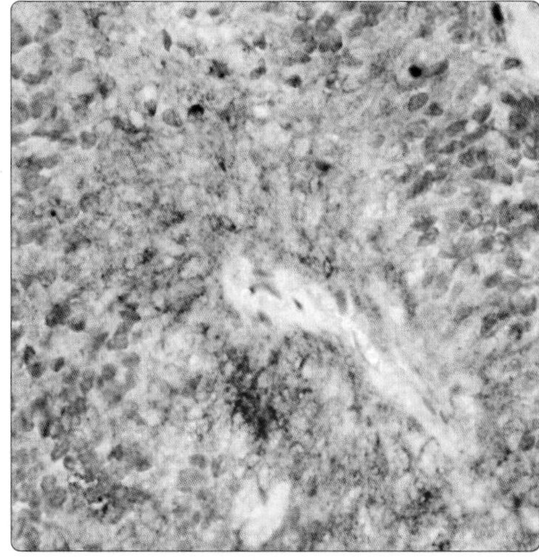

(Left) *Most MPEs are strongly positive for antibodies against GFAP. This positivity may be focal or diffuse, and is most noticeable around the vascular structures, similar to typical ependymomas.* **(Right)** *While entirely nonspecific, D2-40 highlights the perivascular structures in MPE and, similar to other ependymal neoplasms, is often diffusely positive. The staining may be weak or variable.*

EMA(+) Surface and Dot-Like Pattern

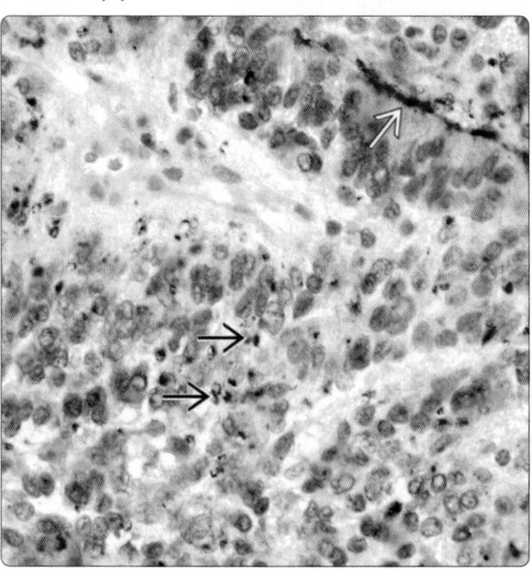

Low Proliferation Rate

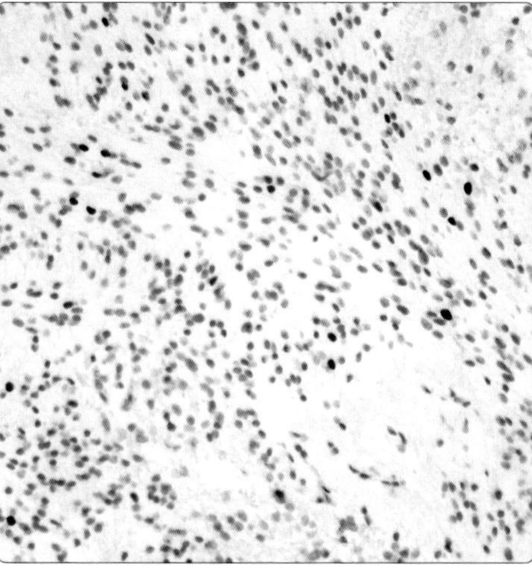

(Left) *EMA is positive in most ependymal tumors and MPEs are no exception. Two different staining patterns can be observed: (1) an epithelial surface staining ➡ and (2) dot-like perinuclear pattern ⇒. Both can be seen in this example. The dot-like pattern represents microlumina.* **(Right)** *Typically, MPEs demonstrate rare mitotic figures and the proliferation rate as measured with the Ki-67 antibody is low. Typically this index does not exceed 5%.*

Subependymoma

KEY FACTS

TERMINOLOGY

- Low-grade (WHO grade I), discrete tumor with ependymal differentiation and high ratio of fibrillar background to clustered nuclei

CLINICAL ISSUES

- More common in lateral & 4th ventricle; mostly middle-aged adults
- Well circumscribed; total excision possible in many cases
- Excellent prognosis

IMAGING

- Often little (if any) enhancement; exception to rule that discrete CNS tumors enhance

MICROSCOPIC

- Nuclear clustering, bland nuclei
- Densely fibrillar, paucicellular background
- Microcysts, especially when near foramen of Monro
- Subtle pseudorosettes, nodular architecture

ANCILLARY TESTS

- Smears poorly, often only tissue fragments, with fine processes
- Dot-like EMA(+) microlumina, some cases, GFAP(+)
- Ki-67 typically low but can be variable; significance of higher rate unclear

TOP DIFFERENTIAL DIAGNOSES

- Ependymoma
- Subependymal giant cell astrocytoma

DIAGNOSTIC CHECKLIST

- More microcysts in examples near foramen of Monro
- More clustering of nuclei in examples away from foramen of Monro
- Occasional examples with mixed subependymoma + ependymoma components; grade according to ependymoma component, but exact amount of latter in tumor necessary to be designated "mixed" is not specified

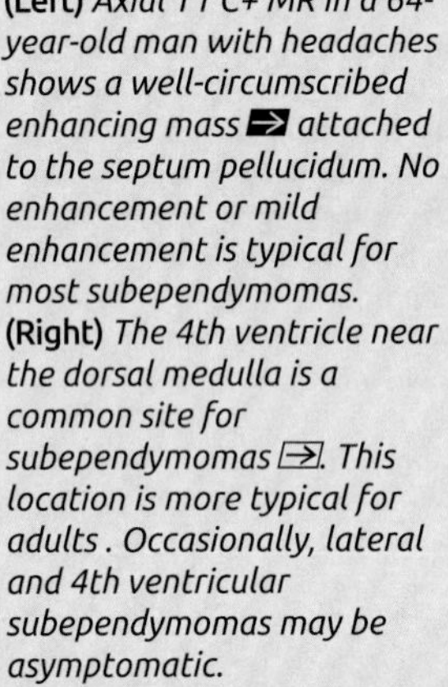

(Left) *Axial T1 C+ MR in a 64-year-old man with headaches shows a well-circumscribed enhancing mass ➡ attached to the septum pellucidum. No enhancement or mild enhancement is typical for most subependymomas.* **(Right)** *The 4th ventricle near the dorsal medulla is a common site for subependymomas ⇨. This location is more typical for adults . Occasionally, lateral and 4th ventricular subependymomas may be asymptomatic.*

Well-Circumscribed Enhancing Tumor

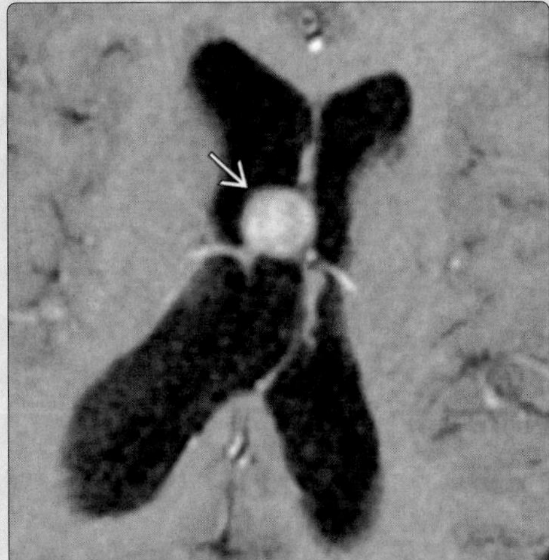

Intraventricular Location

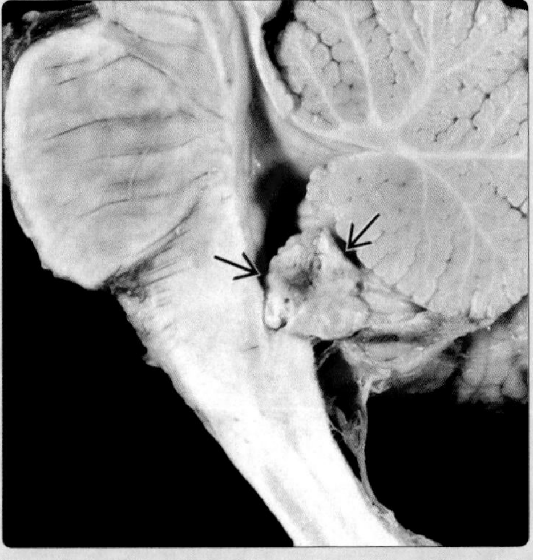

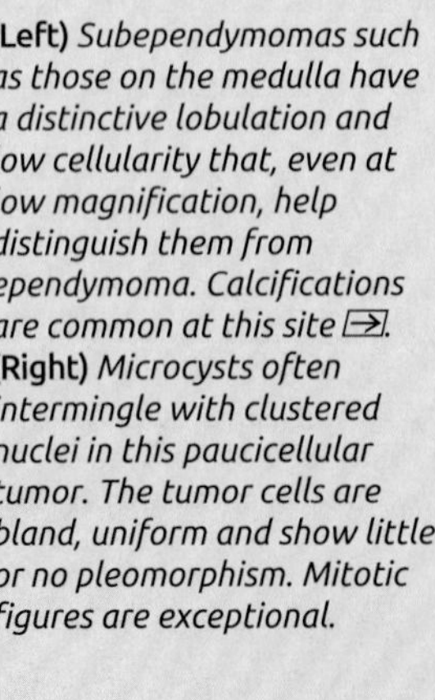

(Left) *Subependymomas such as those on the medulla have a distinctive lobulation and low cellularity that, even at low magnification, help distinguish them from ependymoma. Calcifications are common at this site ⇨.* **(Right)** *Microcysts often intermingle with clustered nuclei in this paucicellular tumor. The tumor cells are bland, uniform and show little or no pleomorphism. Mitotic figures are exceptional.*

Paucicellular, Lobulated Mass

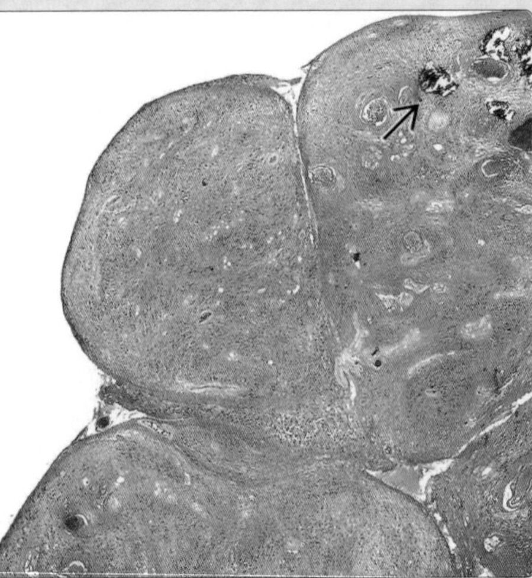

Microcysts and Clustered Nuclei

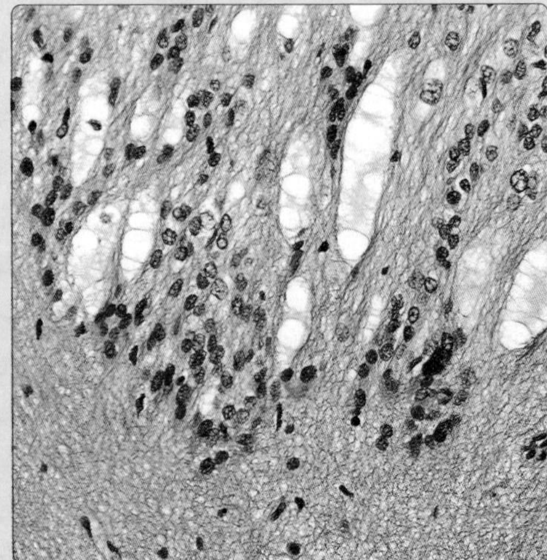

TERMINOLOGY

Definitions

- Discrete WHO grade I paucicellular neoplasm with clustered nuclei showing ependymal differentiation

CLINICAL ISSUES

Epidemiology

- Age
  - Mostly middle-aged adults, rare in children

Site

- Intraventricular
  - Lateral and 4th ventricle more common
- Intraparenchymal
  - Spinal cord; cerebral hemisphere, sometimes superficial and remote from ventricles

Presentation

- Obstructive hydrocephalus with lesions at foramen of Monro or 4th ventricle
- Other expressions, including seizures with supratentorial intraparenchymal lesions
- Acute deficit, some cases, precipitated by intraventricular hemorrhage in large tumor near foramen of Monro

Treatment

- Surgical approaches
  - Well circumscribed; total excision possible in many cases

Prognosis

- Good; mixed subependymoma/ependymoma presumably less favorable; amount of latter component necessary to diagnose mixed lesion not specified in WHO

IMAGING

Radiographic Findings

- Any location, but most often on medulla, near foramen of Monro, or in spinal cord
- Well circumscribed
- Bright in T2W and FLAIR images
- Often little, if any, enhancement; exception to rule is discrete CNS tumor enhancement
- May be calcified, especially on medulla

MACROSCOPIC

General Features

- Well circumscribed
- Lobular, especially on medulla
- Gritty when densely calcified

MICROSCOPIC

Histologic Features

- At foramen of Monro
  - Finely fibrillar, paucicellular background
  - Small, uniform, cytologically bland nuclei
  - Microcysts
  - Nuclear clustering, variable
  - Subtle or no perivascular pseudorosettes
- Other sites, e.g., medulla, spinal cord
  - Nuclear clustering, more prominent
  - Few microcysts, if any
  - Subtle pseudorosettes
  - Calcifications more common
  - Rarely ependymoma component, usually 4th ventricle

ANCILLARY TESTS

Cytology

- Smears poorly, often only tissue fragments, with fine processes
- Finely fibrillar background & bland, ependymoma-like nuclei

Immunohistochemistry

- Diffusely GFAP (+)
- Dot-like EMA (+) microlumina, some cases
- Ki-67, variable; significance of higher rate unclear
- Neurofilament protein (axons) (-); no overrun parenchyma

DIFFERENTIAL DIAGNOSIS

Ependymoma

- Uniform medium to high cellularity
- Perivascular pseudorosettes
- True rosettes, some cases
- Few microcysts, if any
- No nuclear clustering, except for combined ependymoma-subependymoma (usually 4th ventricular)
- Tanycytic type more fascicular than clustered

Subependymal Giant Cell Astrocytoma

- More cellular, compact, back-to-back large gemistocyte-like cells
- Large astrocytes and ganglion-like cells
- Immunostaining for GFAP, neurofilament protein, & synaptophysin
- Some patients with tuberous sclerosis complex

Pilocytic Astrocytoma

- Smears readily (pilocytes)
- More spongy, less fibrillar tissue with eosinophilic granular bodies
- Piloid tissue, usually with Rosenthal fibers

Central Neurocytoma

- Uniform high cellularity
- Synaptophysin (+), GFAP(-)
- Smears well; many markedly uniform cells with little cytoplasm
- Oligodendroglioma-like, neuropil background

Infiltrating (Diffuse) Astrocytoma

- Infiltrating growth pattern
- Little nuclear clustering
- No pseudorosettes
- EMA(-), isocitrate dehydrogenase 1 (+), p53(+), loss of nuclear X-linked α-thalassemia mental retardation staining

SELECTED REFERENCES

1. Rushing EJ et al: Subependymoma revisited: clinicopathological evaluation of 83 cases. J Neurooncol. 85(3):297-305, 2007

(Left) *FLAIR MR demonstrates that subependymomas near the foramen of Monro may attain considerable size. Large subependymomas are associated with periventricular hyperintensities on FLAIR images, suggesting impaired fluid dynamics and hydrocephalus.* **(Right)** *Most subependymomas near the foramen of Monro are small nubbins discovered incidentally postmortem. Only rarely are they massive intraventricular lesions such as this, in which massive hemorrhage may ensue.*

Intraventricular Tumor

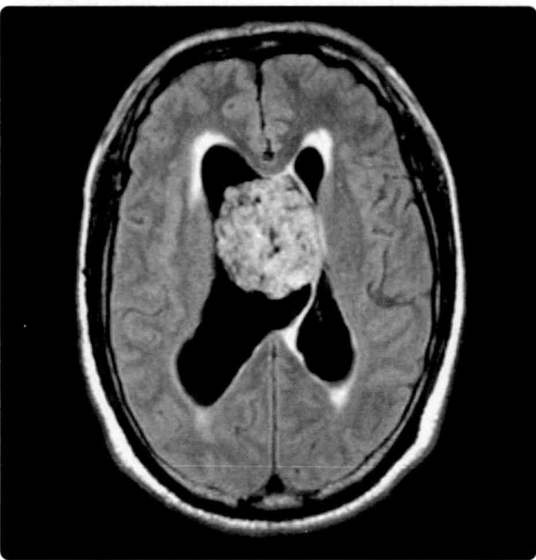

Large Tumor With Hydrocephalus

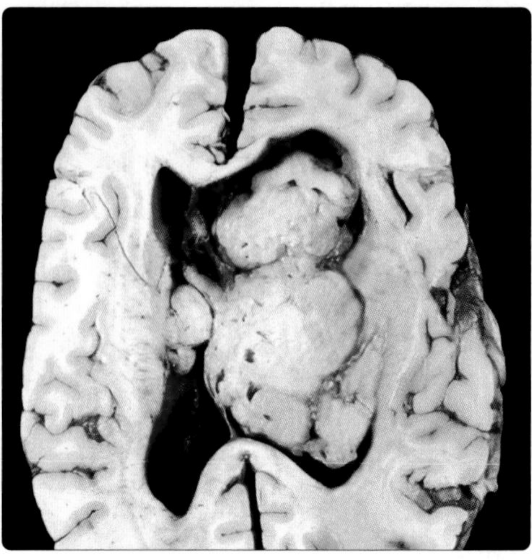

(Left) *On cross section, subependymomas have a brain-like appearance on fresh specimens. Lobulated appearance is often recognizable. Notice the well-circumscribed nature of the tumor. Foci of intratumoral hemorrhage are not uncommon* ⇒. **(Right)** *In this whole-mount preparation, the lobulated appearance is much more pronounced compared with the gross specimen. Even in this magnification, the tumor appears paucicellular.*

Solid Tumor and Hemorrhagic Foci

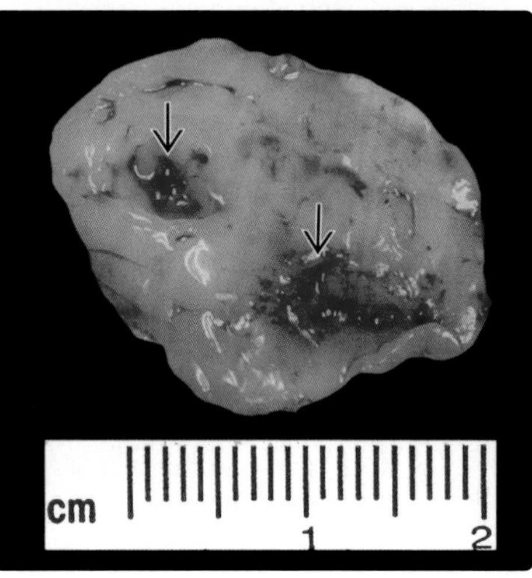

Lobulated Lateral Ventricle Tumor

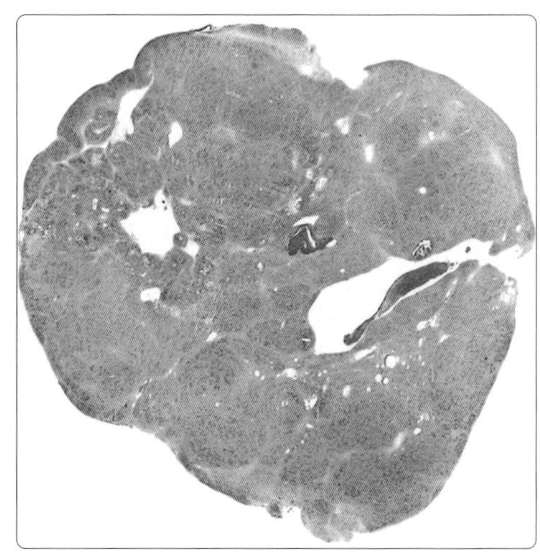

(Left) *In this example, lobulation can be appreciated at low magnification. Hyalinized vessels* ⇒ *are also commonly encountered at the periphery or the parenchyma of the tumors.* **(Right)** *Subependymomas often portend a markedly lobulated architecture with variably sized clusters of tumor cells embedded in a richly fibrillary matrix. The tumor often appears paucicellular at this magnification.*

Hyalinized Vessels

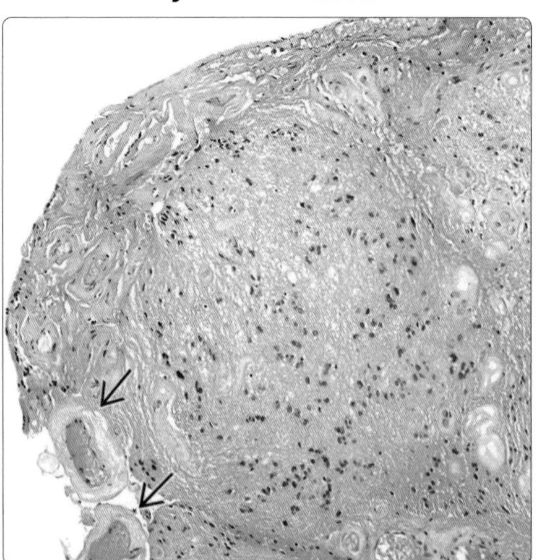

Clustered Nuclei

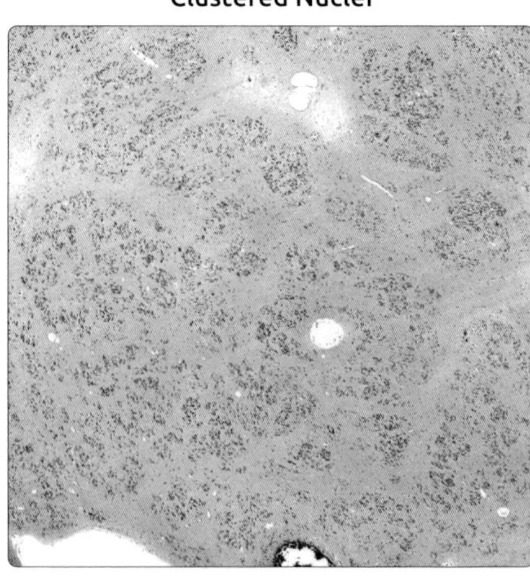

Microcysts

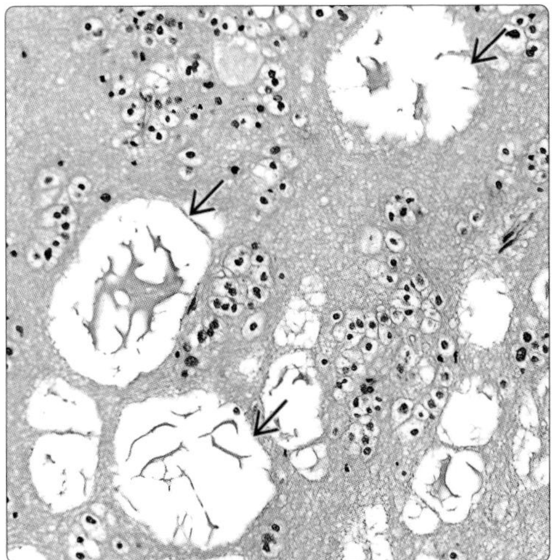

Lobulated Paucicellular Tumor

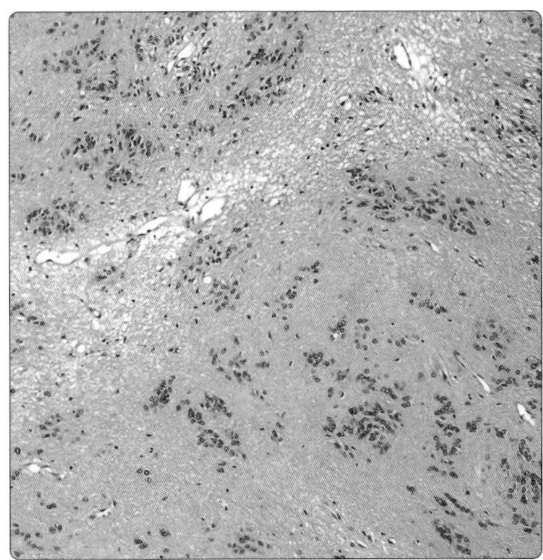

(Left) *Microcysts filled with basophilic myxoid substance* ➙*, subtle clustering of nuclei, and finely fibrillar background are essential features of subependymomas, as they occur near the foramen of Monro. Microcysts are uncommon in subependymomas at other sites.* **(Right)** *Low-power magnification of subependymoma demonstrates the richly fibrillary lobules separated often by a loose matrix and clusters of cells embedded in the fibrillary matrix.*

Fibrillary Matrix

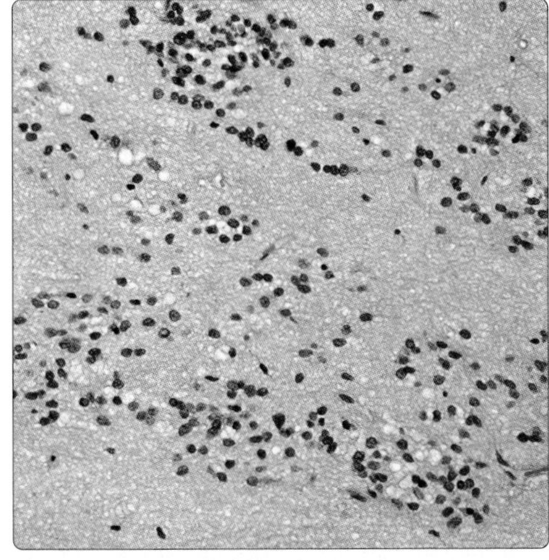

Bland Ependymal Cells

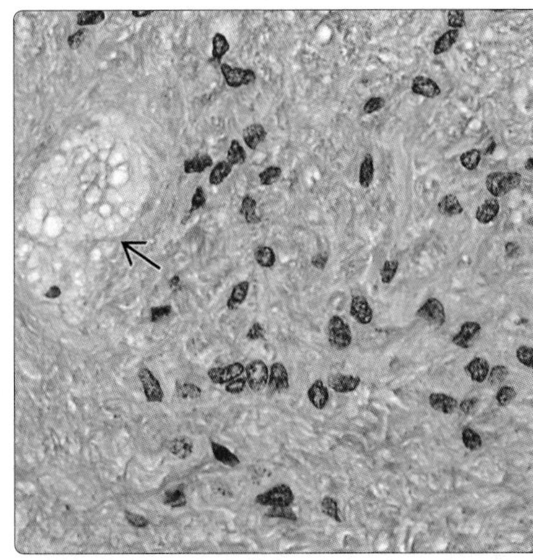

(Left) *High-power magnification of subependymoma demonstrates the richly fibrillary matrix and small ependymal type cells often in variably sized clusters. There is little or no nuclear pleomorphism or hyperchromasia and often no mitotic figures.* **(Right)** *Subependymomas often harbor cells with bland nuclei without pleomorphism, inconspicuous nucleoli, and the rich glial fibrillary matrix is often prominent. Small microcysts with mucoid matrix are often present* ➙*.*

Smear, Low Magnification

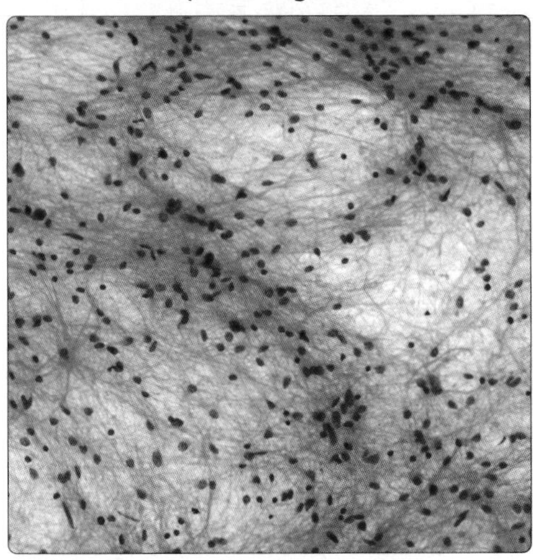

Smear, High Magnification

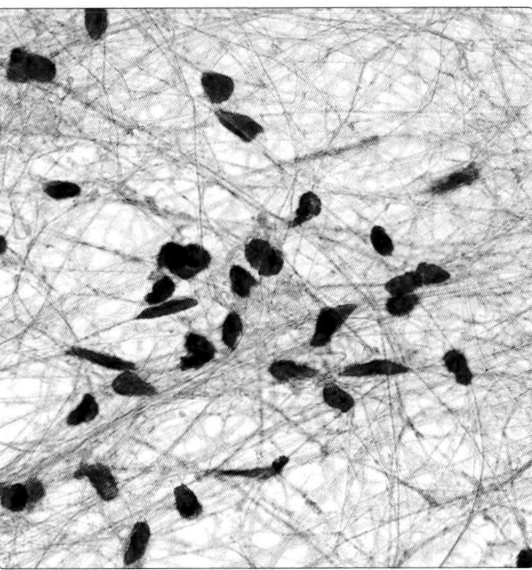

(Left) *Subependymomas do not readily smear, but the poorly spread tumor tissue highlights the marked fibrillary background and small, bland tumor cells with elaborate processes.* **(Right)** *The fibrillar background seen in histological sections is best resolved in smear preparations wherein the feltwork of delicate cell processes is well seen. Subependymomas typically do not smear out well.*

Astroblastoma

KEY FACTS

TERMINOLOGY

- Relationship and overlap with ependymoma not clear
- Compact tumor with perivascular pseudorosettes and, often, marked sclerosis

CLINICAL ISSUES

- Age: Children and young adults
- Treatment: Surgical excision potentially curative in low-grade examples
- Prognosis
    - Good: Low-grade examples
    - Poor: High-grade examples

IMAGING

- Discrete, usually superficial mass
- Sometimes cystic
- Dark signal of dense collagen in some cases (FLAIR and T2-weighted images)

MICROSCOPIC

- Perivascular pseudorosettes, may be narrow
- Cells larger, plumper than in ependymoma
- Overall less fibrillar

ANCILLARY TESTS

- GFAP
    - Irregularly alternating (+) and (-) cells
    - Some cases largely, if not entirely (-)
- EMA
    - Surface (+), limited
    - Dot-like staining of microlumina, focal

DIAGNOSTIC CHECKLIST

- Compact architecture, potentially cured by excision

Axial MR: Discrete Superficial Mass

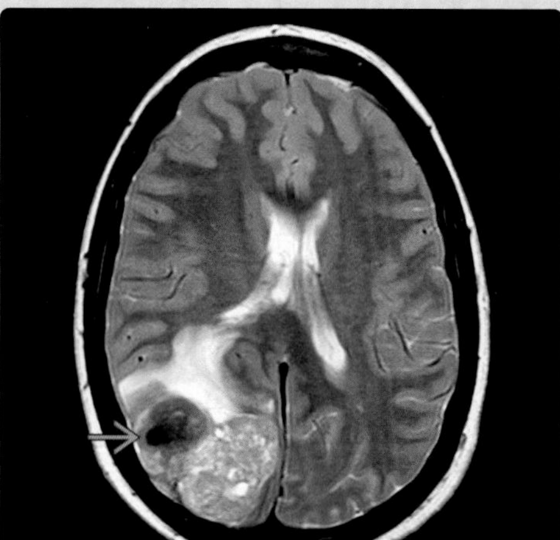

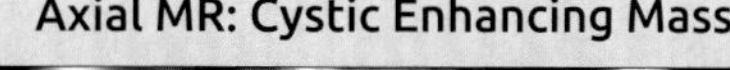

Axial MR: Cystic Enhancing Mass

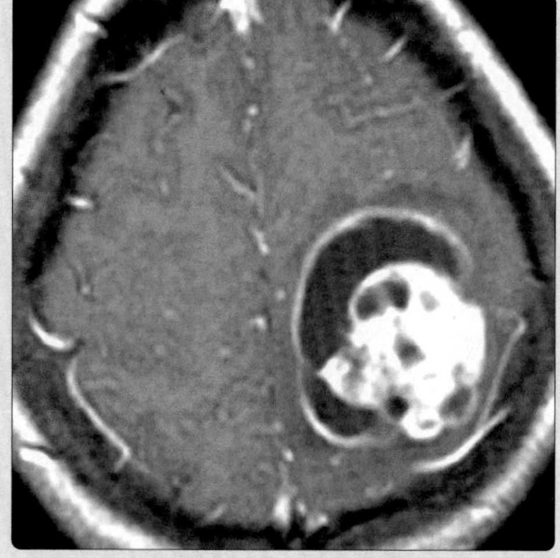

(Left) *Astroblastomas are discrete, superficial masses, often with dark regions ⇨ in T2W images that reflect dense sclerosis and in some cases calcification.* **(Right)** *Astroblastomas are superficial, often cystic, enhancing masses. Children and young adults are the usual hosts.*

Prominent Sclerosis

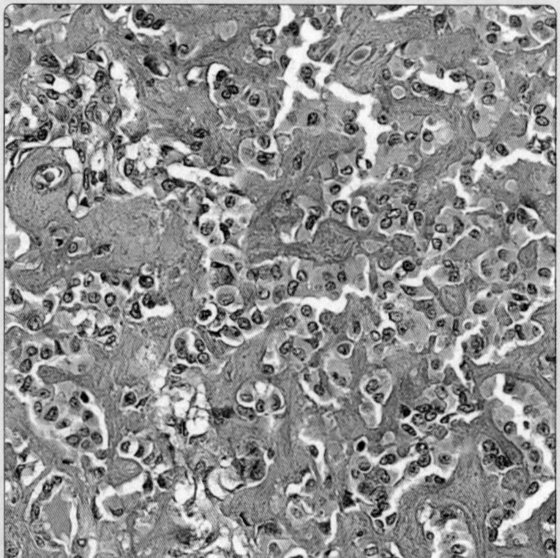

Plump Cells

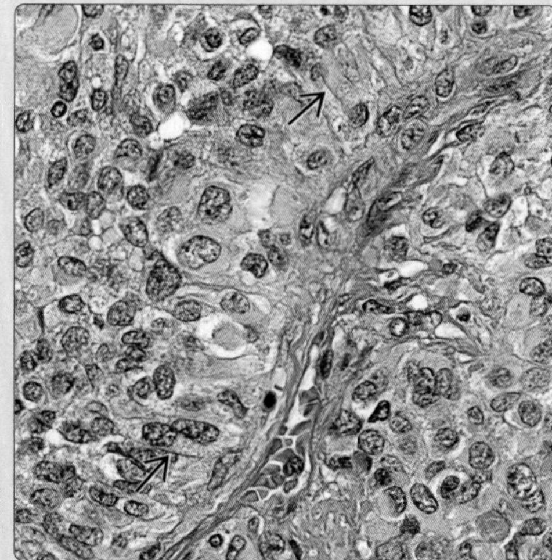

(Left) *Sclerosis is one of the most distinctive features of astroblastoma but is not invariably present.* **(Right)** *Plump cells with sharply defined cell borders ⇨ help distinguish this lesion from ependymoma with its more perivascular, finely fibrillar zones.*

TERMINOLOGY

Definitions

- Compact tumor with perivascular pseudorosettes and, often, marked sclerosis
- Distinction from ependymoma not clear
- No WHO grades assigned for astroblastoma or anaplastic astroblastoma

CLINICAL ISSUES

Epidemiology

- Age
  - Children and young adults

Presentation

- Seizures
- Expression of mass effect
- Neurological deficit depending on site

Treatment

- Surgical approaches
  - Surgical excision potentially curative in low-grade examples

Prognosis

- Good: Low-grade examples
- Poor: High-grade examples

IMAGING

General Features

- Location
  - Cerebral hemispheres
  - Often superficial
- Morphology
  - Discrete
  - Contrast enhancing, heterogeneously in some cases
  - Often cystic
  - Dark signal of dense collagen and calcium in some cases (FLAIR and T2W images)
  - Peritumoral edema in some cases, especially when high grade

MACROSCOPIC

General Features

- Mass lesion
- Often cystic
- Firm

MICROSCOPIC

Histologic Features

- Discrete, "pushing" borders
- Potentially infiltrative when high grade
- High cellularity
- Perivascular pseudorosettes
  - May be narrow
  - Component cells plumper and somewhat more pleomorphic than in ependymoma
  - Processes thicker than in ependymoma
  - Nuclei larger, rounder than in ependymoma
- Little fibrillar background
- Vascular sclerosis and hyalinization, often prominent
- Calcification, especially in tumors with abundant sclerosis
- Mitoses, necrosis (sometimes with pseudopalisading), vascular proliferation in high-grade examples

ANCILLARY TESTS

Cytology

- Tissue fragments and individual cells
- Plump, sometimes bipolar cells
- Nuclei somewhat larger and rounder than in ependymoma

Immunohistochemistry

- GFAP
  - Irregularly alternating (+) and (-) cells
  - Some cases largely, if not entirely, (-)
- EMA
  - Surface (+), limited
  - Dot-like staining of microlumina, focal

Genetic Testing

- Gains of chromosomes 20q and 19 in some cases

Electron Microscopy

- Small lumina with
  - Microvilli, cilia
- Intermediate junctions
  - Multiple, especially numerous near microlumina

DIFFERENTIAL DIAGNOSIS

Ependymoma

- More widely distributed in CNS
- More fibrillarity in
  - Background
  - Perivascular pseudorosettes
- Nuclei smaller, less pleomorphic, and less epithelioid
- Rosettes or canals in some cases
- Less sclerosis

Pleomorphic Xanthoastrocytoma

- Prominent leptomeningeal component in most cases
- Fascicular architecture
- Pleomorphism
- Perivascular chronic inflammation
- Eosinophilic granular bodies (hyaline droplets)
- Lipidization

Pilocytic Astrocytoma

- Less cellular
- Microcysts
- Myxoid background
- Fibrillar tissue with Rosenthal fibers
- Eosinophilic granular bodies (hyaline droplets)
- Less sclerosis

Papillary Meningioma

- More often dural-based than intraparenchymal
- More common meningioma patterns may be co-existent with papillary pattern
- Many are brain invasive, unlike sharp demarcation of astroblastoma

- IHC(+) for SSTR2A
- IHC(-) for GFAP
- No dot-like IHC(+) for EMA

DIAGNOSTIC CHECKLIST

Clinically Relevant Pathologic Features

- Compact architecture, potentially cured by excision
- Often cystic
- May be very sclerotic

Pathologic Interpretation Pearls

- Compact architecture
- Ependymoma-like, but
  - Narrower perivascular pseudorosettes
  - More uniformly and highly cellular without fibrillar zones
  - More sclerosis
  - Cells rounder, more epithelioid

SELECTED REFERENCES

1. Sabharwal P et al: Intraventricular Astroblastoma in an Infant: A Case Report and Review of the Literature. Pediatr Neurosurg. ePub, 2015
2. Singla N et al: Hemorrhage in astroblastoma: An unusual manifestation of an extremely rare entity. J Clin Neurosci. ePub, 2015
3. de la Garma VH et al: High-grade astroblastoma in a child: Report of one case and review of literature. Surg Neurol Int. 5:111, 2014
4. Salvati M et al: Cerebral astroblastoma: analysis of six cases and critical review of treatment options. J Neurooncol. 93(3):369-78, 2009
5. Lehman NL: Central nervous system tumors with ependymal features: a broadened spectrum of primarily ependymal differentiation? J Neuropathol Exp Neurol. 67(3):177-88, 2008
6. Lehman NL: Patterns of brain infiltration and secondary structure formation in supratentorial ependymal tumors. J Neuropathol Exp Neurol. 67(9):900-10, 2008
7. Port JD et al: Astroblastoma: radiologic-pathologic correlation and distinction from ependymoma. AJNR Am J Neuroradiol. 23(2):243-7, 2002
8. Brat DJ et al: Astroblastoma: clinicopathologic features and chromosomal abnormalities defined by comparative genomic hybridization. Brain Pathol. 10(3):342-52, 2000
9. Bonnin JM et al: Astroblastomas: a pathological study of 23 tumors, with a postoperative follow-up in 13 patients. Neurosurgery. 25(1):6-13, 1989
10. Rubinstein LJ et al: The astroblastoma and its possible cytogenic relationship to the tanycyte. An electron microscopic, immunohistochemical, tissue- and organ-culture study. Acta Neuropathol. 78(5):472-83, 1989

Sharp Border

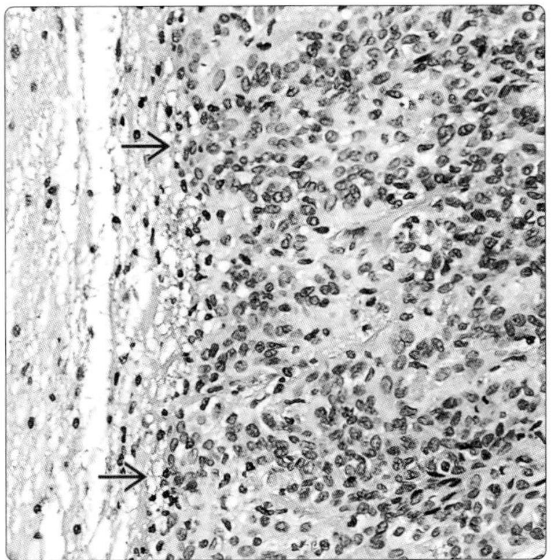

More Pleomorphic Than Ependymoma

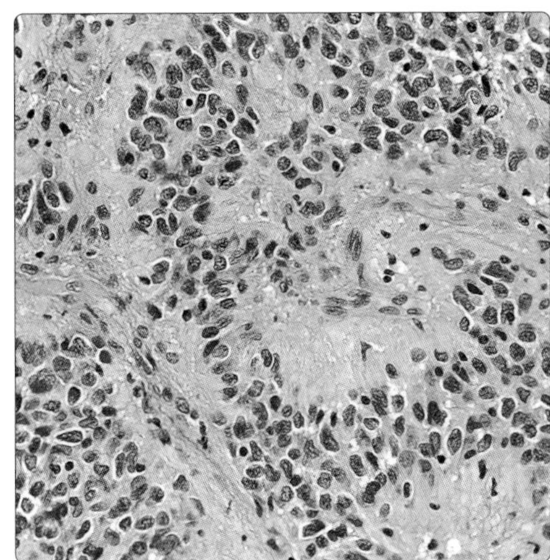

(Left) *Low-grade astroblastomas have an especially sharp border ⮕. Even at low magnification, tumor cells have a plumper, more epithelioid quality than those in ependymoma.* **(Right)** *Cells in astroblastoma perivascular pseudorosettes are rounder and somewhat more pleomorphic than those in ependymoma.*

Coarse Perivascular Cell Processes

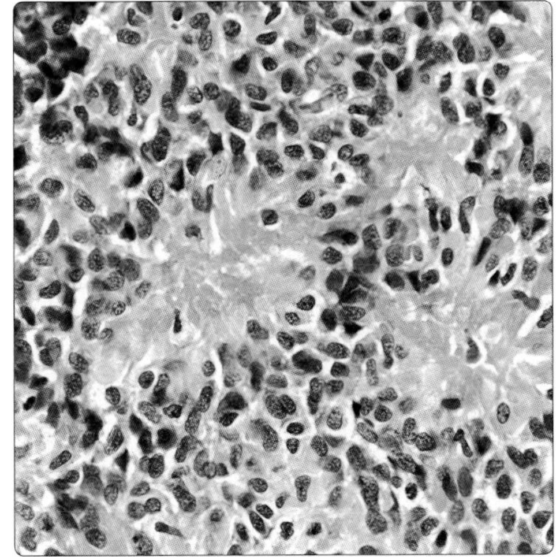

Short Perivascular Cell Processes

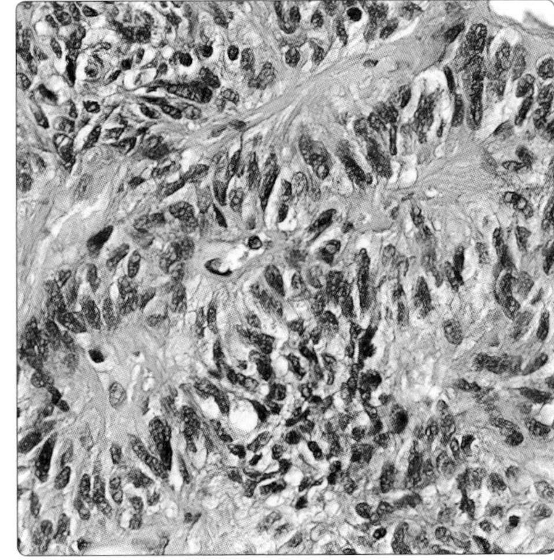

(Left) *Coarse processes of plump cells converge on vessels to form perivascular pseudorosettes. Cells are somewhat larger and more pleomorphic than those in ependymomas. There is also less fibrillarity.* **(Right)** *Perivascular cell processes are shorter, stouter, and less tapering and fibrillar in astroblastoma than in ependymoma.*

Osteoid-Like Sclerosis

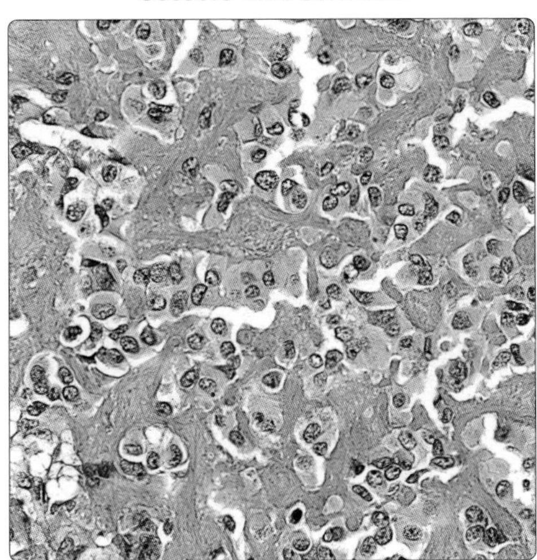

Advanced Sclerosis, Calcification

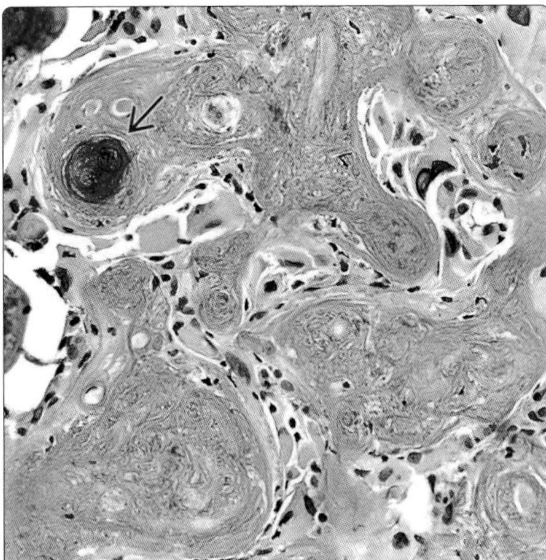

(Left) *Osteoid-like sclerotic tissue is present in most astroblastomas, at least focally.* **(Right)** *Advanced sclerosis, in which calcifications ⮕ are common, crowds out tumor cells in astroblastomas. Such hyalinization is not a feature of classic ependymomas. The distinction, or relationship, between the 2 tumors remains a subject of discussion, however.*

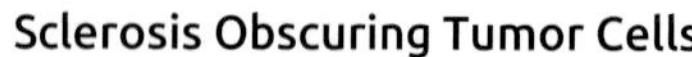

Sclerosis Obscuring Tumor Cells

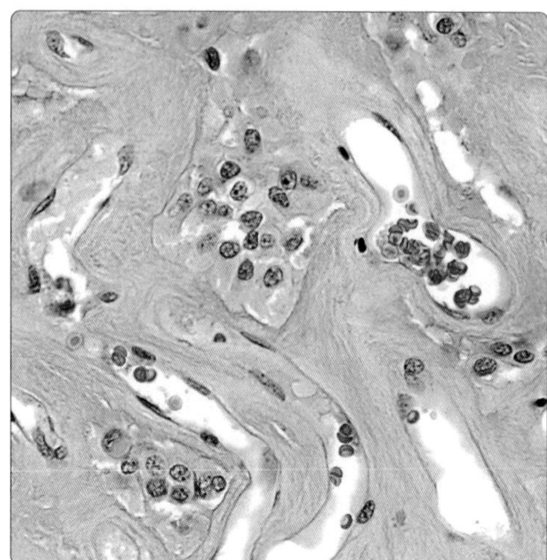

Pseudopapillary Appearance

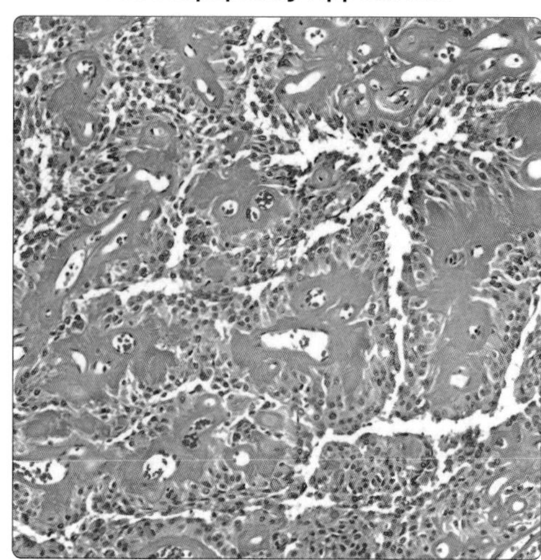

(Left) *Sclerosis in some areas may be so abundant that tumor cells are relatively obscured.* **(Right)** *Astroblastomas may have a pseudopapillary appearance with prominent perivascular cell arrangement.*

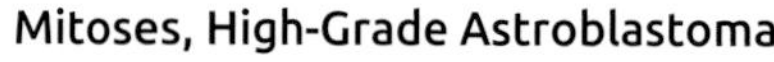

Mitoses, High-Grade Astroblastoma

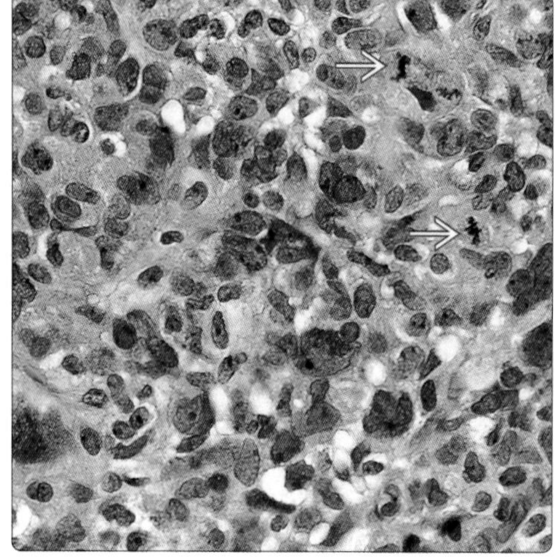

Necrosis, High-Grade Astroblastoma

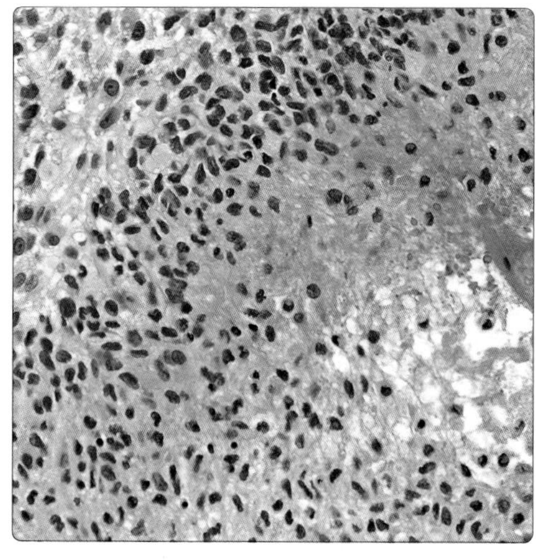

(Left) *Higher cellularity and multiple mitoses* ➡ *characterize high-grade examples as well. While there is nothing diagnostic of astroblastoma in this section, the plump, somewhat epithelioid cells are nevertheless typical.* **(Right)** *Necrosis with pseudopalisading is present in some high-grade astroblastomas. Precise grading criteria remain to be defined.*

Subset Cells, GFAP(+)

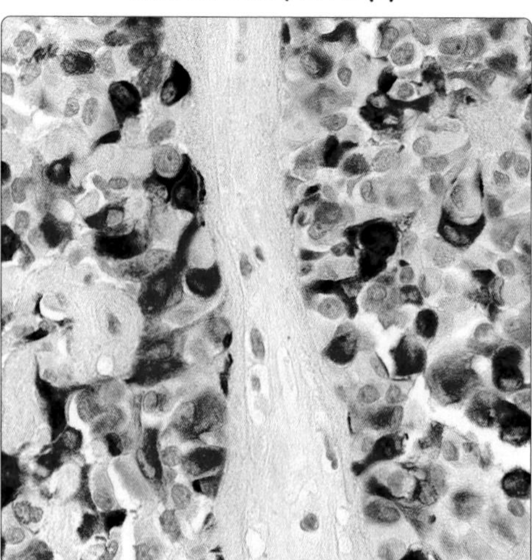

EMA, Membranous Pattern

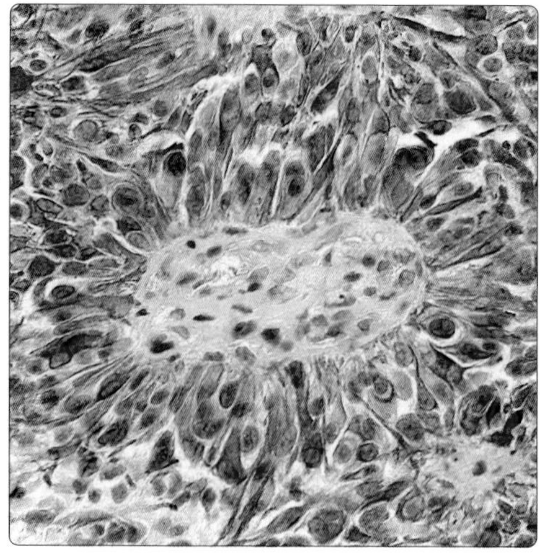

(Left) *In astroblastomas, plump perivascular cells that are strongly GFAP(+) alternate with those that fail to react. Cells in ependymoma perivascular pseudorosettes are typically more delicate and more uniformly positive for GFAP.* **(Right)** *Some astroblastomas will manifest cell membrane immunostaining for EMA, but this is often only present focally.*

EMA: Cell Surface and Dot-Like

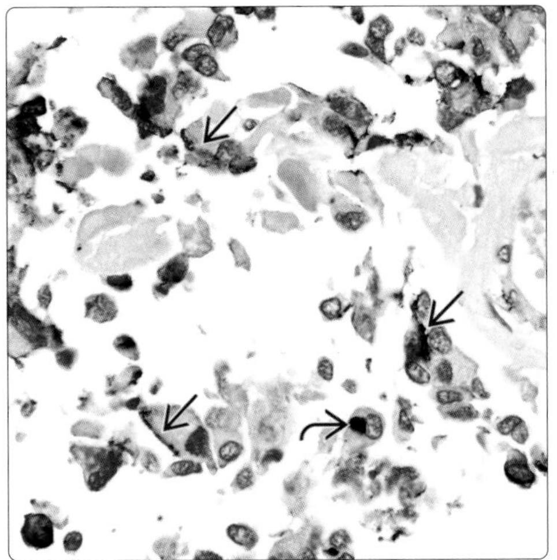

EMA: Dot-Like Microlumina

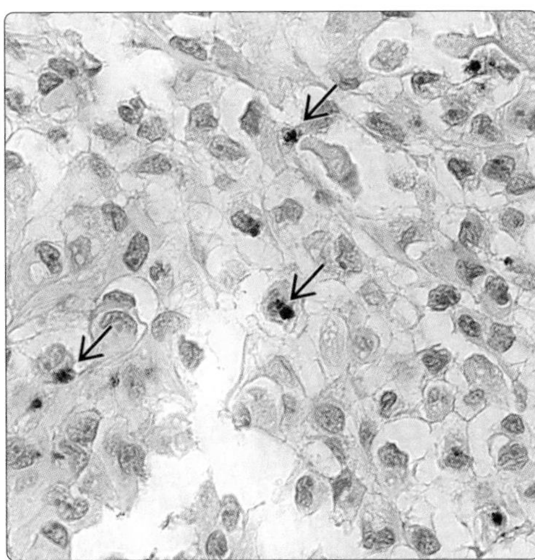

(Left) *As with other tumors with ependymal differentiation, there may be surface staining for EMA ⇒ and focal dot-like profiles of microlumina ⇒. Both may be only focal or even absent.* **(Right)** *The presence of dot-like lumina ⇒ on EMA immunostaining is consistent with probable ependymal differentiation in astroblastoma.*

Sagittal MR: Simulating Meningioma

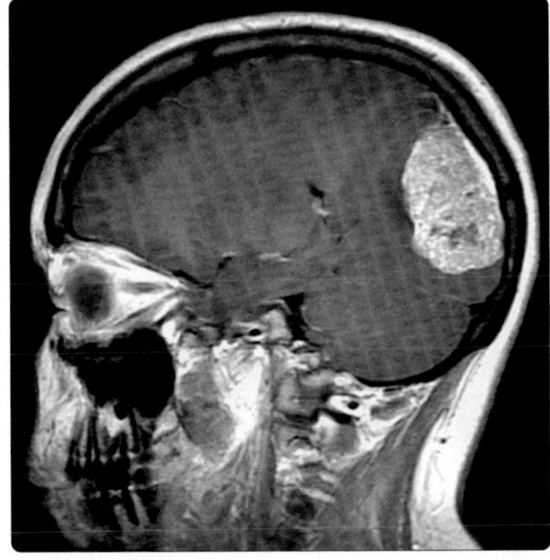

Focally Calcified

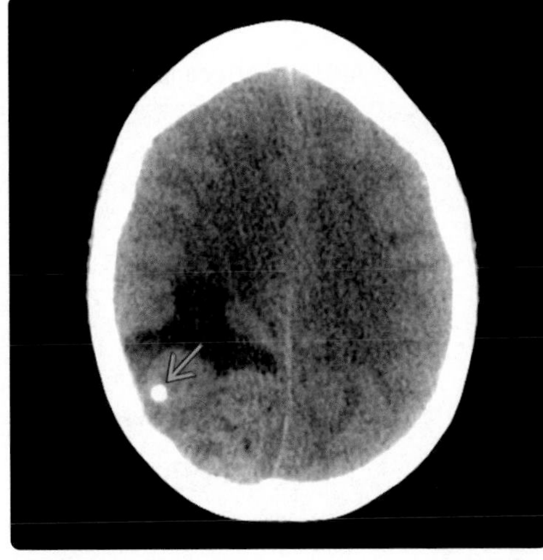

(Left) *Some astroblastomas secondarily attach to dura and simulate meningiomas, as did this high-grade example.* **(Right)** *As best seen by CT, astroblastomas may be focally calcified ⇒.*

Smear: Tissue Fragments

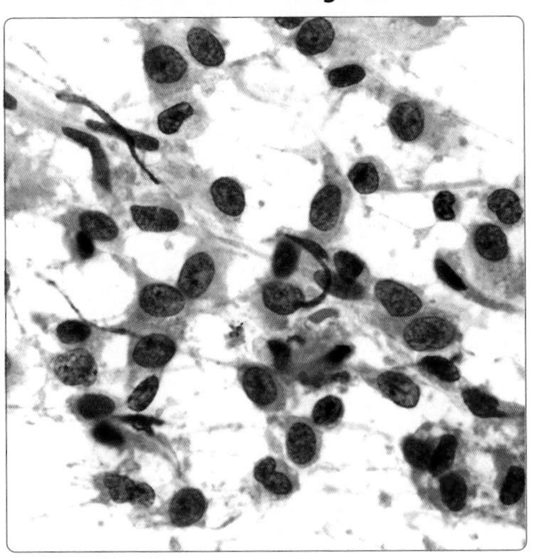

Smear: Epithelioid Cells

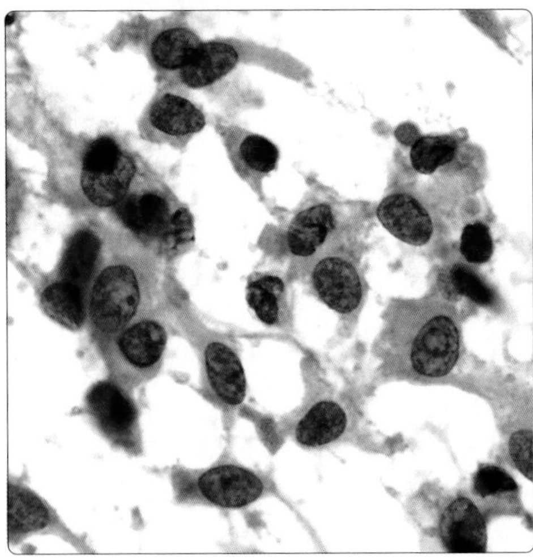

(Left) *Smear preparations from astroblastoma generate tissue fragments as they do with other tumors with ependymal differentiation.* **(Right)** *The round, mildly pleomorphic, epithelioid cells are typical of astroblastoma. Those of ependymoma are generally smaller and more uniform. The degree of background fibrillarity is often greater in ependymomas as well.*

Angiocentric Glioma

KEY FACTS

TERMINOLOGY

- Overlap with and relationship to intracortical ependymoma unclear
- Definition and incidence of anaplastic types unknown

CLINICAL ISSUES

- Children and young adults
- Seizures
- Prognosis generally favorable
  - Long-term stability
  - Only rarely aggressive or recurrent

IMAGING

- Cortically based
- Little if any contrast enhancement

MICROSCOPIC

- Neoplasm combining features of infiltrating glioma and schwannoma- and ependymoma-like areas
- Distinctive subpial palisading
- Infiltration, but little perineuronal satellitosis
- Both radial (ependymoma-like) and longitudinal orientation to vessels
- Compact areas resembling schwannoma &/or ependymoma
- Multiphenotypic "hybrid" tumors with glioneuronal, ependymal features with angiocentric pattern reported in literature

ANCILLARY TESTS

- Dot-like EMA staining of microlumina
- Focal surface EMA staining, especially in perivascular formations

DIAGNOSTIC CHECKLIST

- Distinctive subpial palisading
- Save tissue for immunohistochemistry and electron microscopy

(Left) *This gray matter-based lesion is bright on FLAIR imaging →. As is typical, there is little mass effect and there was no contrast enhancement.* **(Right)** *Angiocentric gliomas are often superficial parenchymal tumors that are hyperintense on T2-weighted images and hypo-/isointense on T1-weighted images. There is limited or no enhancement or mass effect.*

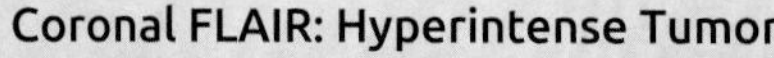

Coronal FLAIR: Hyperintense Tumor

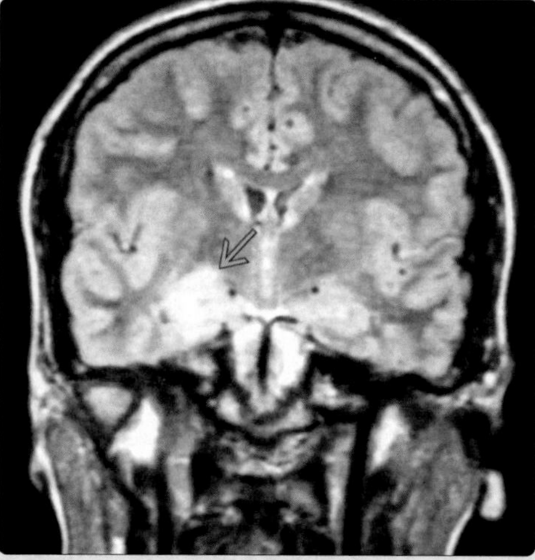

Intracortical FLAIR: Bright Lesion

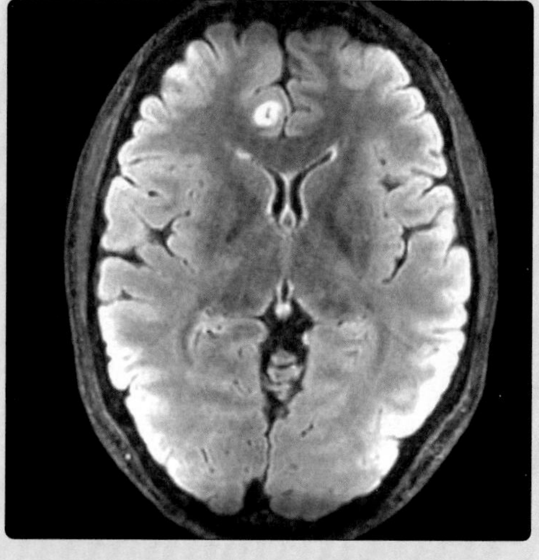

(Left) *The tumor cells in angiocentric glioma appear to infiltrate the parenchyma and arrange themselves in a linear fashion around the vascular structures, even though some tumor cells appear to have little connection with the vasculature.* **(Right)** *Distinctively aligned to the pial surface, tumor cells find repose near the surface of the brain →. Equivalent subpial cells in oligodendrogliomas and astrocytomas lack the perpendicular polarity illustrated here.*

Angiocentric Arrangement of Tumor Cells

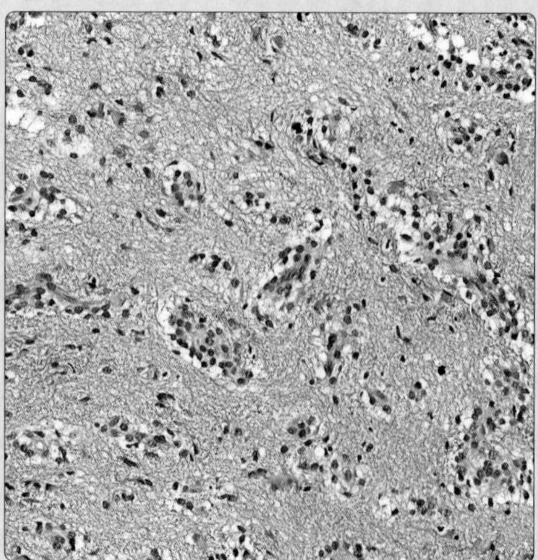

Subpial Cells Perpendicular to Surface

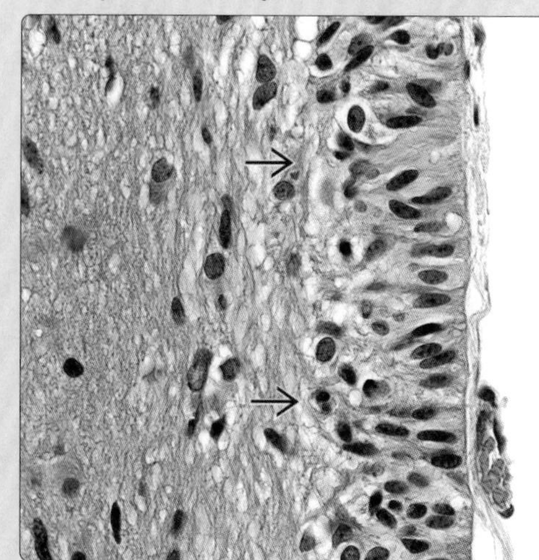

TERMINOLOGY

Definitions

- Neoplasm combining features of infiltrating glioma and ependymoma, WHO grade I
- Distinction from other tumors with ependymal differentiation not clear

CLINICAL ISSUES

Epidemiology

- Age
  - Children and young adults

Presentation

- Seizures

Treatment

- Surgical approaches
  - Gross total resection is treatment of choice

Prognosis

- Generally favorable
- Only rarely recurrent or aggressive

IMAGING

General Features

- Morphology
  - Ill defined, occasionally cystic

MR Findings

- Cerebral hemispheres, particularly cortical
- Extension to underlying ventricle in some cases
- Little or no mass effect, often ill defined
- Some cases have hypodense center or cysts

MACROSCOPIC

General Features

- Ill-defined mass, cystic in some cases, firm in others

MICROSCOPIC

Histological Features

- Infiltrative appearance, but little perineuronal satellitosis
- Both radial (ependymoma-like) and longitudinal orientation of cells to vessels
- Subpial palisading
- Compact areas resembling schwannoma or ependymoma
- Myxoid background in some cases
- Calcifications and cysts in rare cases
- Trapped neurons with neurofibrillary change in some cases
- Mitoses absent or occasional
- High cellularity, rare
- Minute, dark, intracytoplasmic microlumina are uncommon (immunohistochemistry for EMA usually required for detection)

ANCILLARY TESTS

Cytology

- Tissue fragments with few individual cells
- Bipolar cells with long nuclei with speckled chromatin

Immunohistochemistry

- EMA(+), focal punctate, perivascular
- GFAP(+) in some tumor cells and background

Electron Microscopy

- Small lumina with microvilli and cilia
- Multiple intermediate junctions joining cells and forming microlumina

DIFFERENTIAL DIAGNOSIS

Ependymoma

- Solid, generally enhancing mass
- Mostly solid, noninfiltrating except boundaries
- Transitional cases occur (cortical ependymoma)

Subependymoma

- Discrete, noninfiltrating
- Nodular architecture without angiocentric arrangement

Infiltrating Astrocytoma

- No perivascular pseudorosettes or subpial, perpendicular orientation of columnar cells
- IDH1(+) in most cases, ATRX loss in some cases

Astroblastoma

- Largely solid, noninfiltrating
- Perivascular pseudorosettes composed of epithelioid cells with plump processes
- Dense vascular sclerosis

Pilocytic Astrocytoma

- Solid, enhancing mass
- Biphasic architecture with eosinophilic granular bodies and Rosenthal fibers

Ganglion Cell Tumor

- Usually enhancing
- Cytologically abnormal ganglion cells
- Perivascular inflammation

DIAGNOSTIC CHECKLIST

Pathologic Interpretation Pearls

- Distinctive combination of infiltration, perivascular pseudorosettes, and subpial aggregation
- Ependymal features but diffuse infiltration
- Distinctive subpial palisading

SELECTED REFERENCES

1. Ni HC et al: Angiocentric glioma: a report of nine new cases, including four with atypical histological features. Neuropathol Appl Neurobiol. 41(3):333-46, 2015
2. Lellouch-Tubiana A et al: Angiocentric neuroepithelial tumor (ANET): a new epilepsy-related clinicopathological entity with distinctive MRI. Brain Pathol. 15(4):281-6, 2005
3. Wang M et al: Monomorphous angiocentric glioma: a distinctive epileptogenic neoplasm with features of infiltrating astrocytoma and ependymoma. J Neuropathol Exp Neurol. 64(10):875-81, 2005

(Left) *The typical appearance of angiocentric glioma is that of an infiltrating tumor with a peculiar predilection to perivascular spaces creating a distinctive, angiocentric distribution.* **(Right)** *Compact Antoni A-like tissue sometimes arise abruptly in the infiltrating component. Verocay bodies are not expected.*

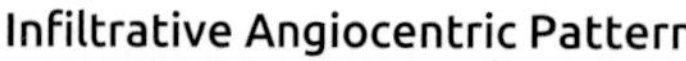

Infiltrative Angiocentric Pattern

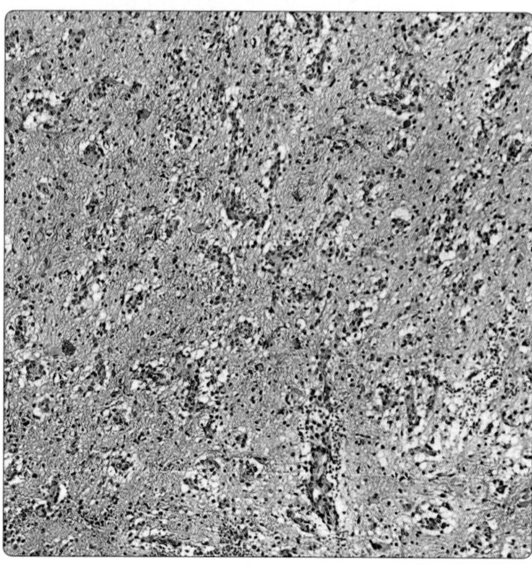

Compact Areas

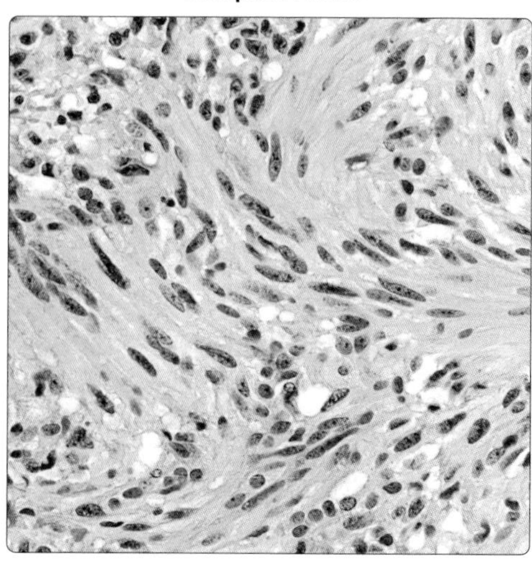

(Left) *Some angiocentric gliomas have solid, sheet-like growth. Note that cytologically, the cells have oval-round nuclei and small amounts of eosinophilic cytoplasm, similar to ependymomas.* **(Right)** *Perivascular pseudorosettes sometimes have an especially prominent anuclear zone immediately surrounding the vessel. Nuclei are more elongated than in ependymomas. The speckled chromatin is another distinguishing feature.*

Ependymoma-Like Cells

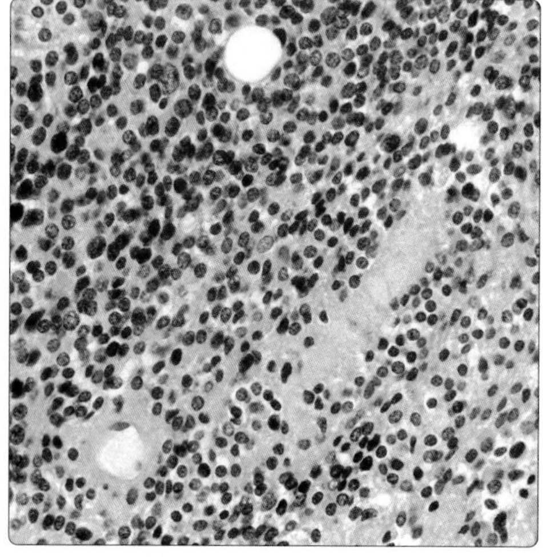

More Elongated Nuclei Than Ependymoma

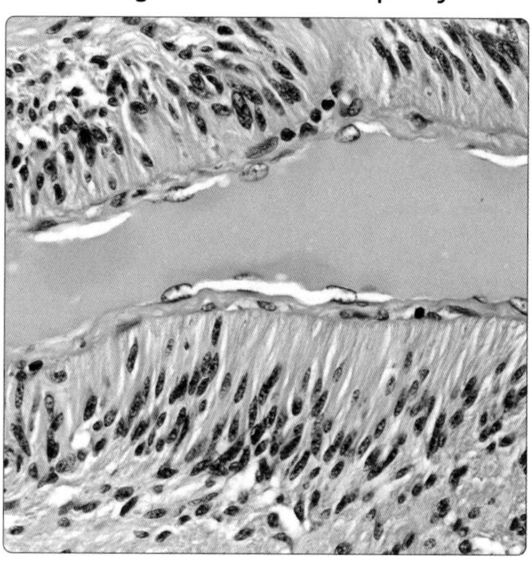

(Left) *Some tumors have densely cellular compact areas, and there is little evidence of the angiocentric pattern typical of this tumor in this region.* **(Right)** *Histological appearance of some of the tissue sections in angiocentric glioma, such as this one, raises the possibility of glioma, mesenchymal tumor, or schwannoma.*

Hypercellular Regions

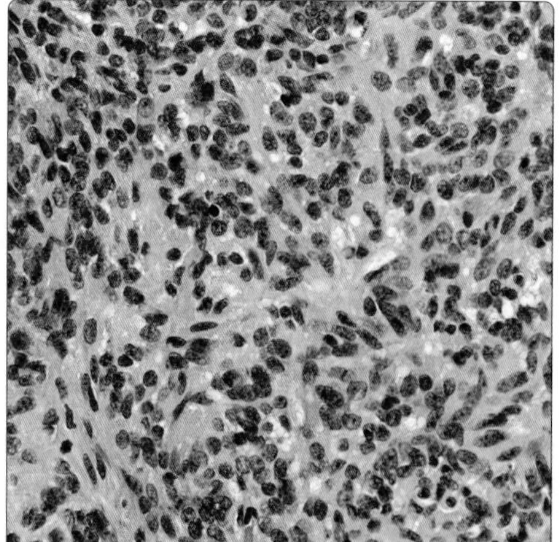

Bipolar Spindle Cells

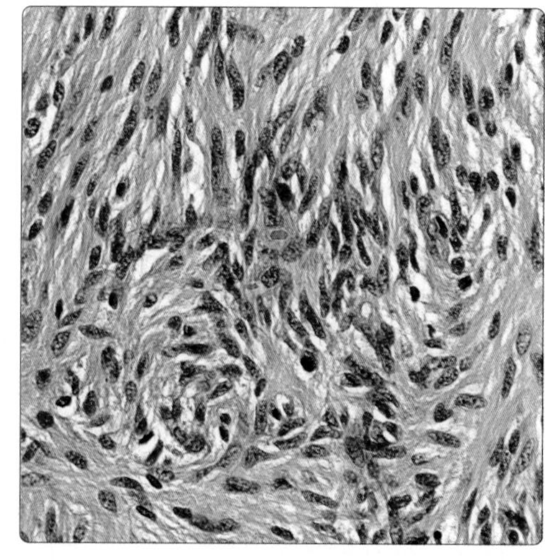

Subpial Arrangement of Tumor Cells

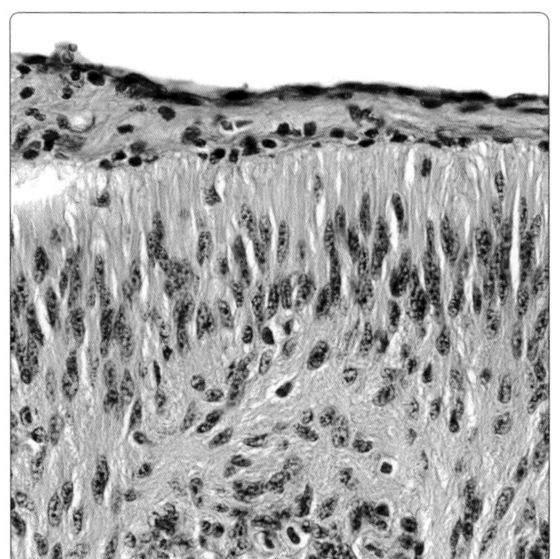

Perivascular, Subpial Tumor Cells

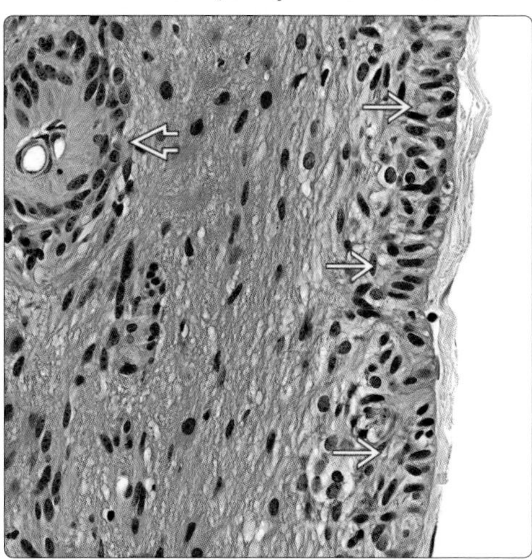

(Left) *The tumor cells in angiocentric glioma have a peculiar tendency to arrange themselves perpendicular to the pia mater just below the leptomeningeal space. This arrangement is almost unique to angiocentric glioma.* **(Right)** *The tumor cells arranged below the pia mater and perpendicular to it ➔ also coexist with the angiocentric or perivascular architecture ➔ more typical of the entity.*

Fascicular Pattern

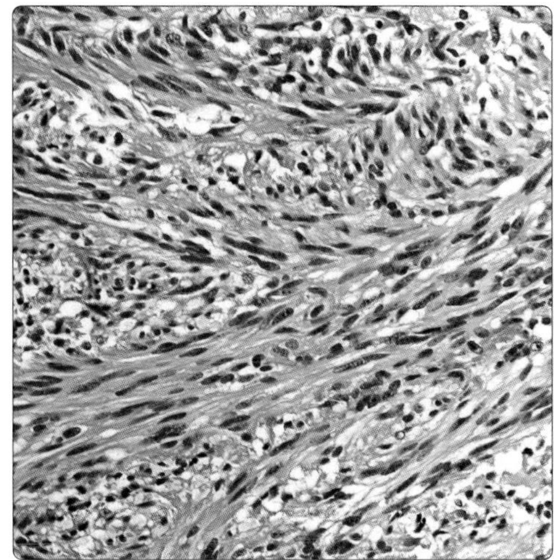

Predominant Angiocentric Pattern

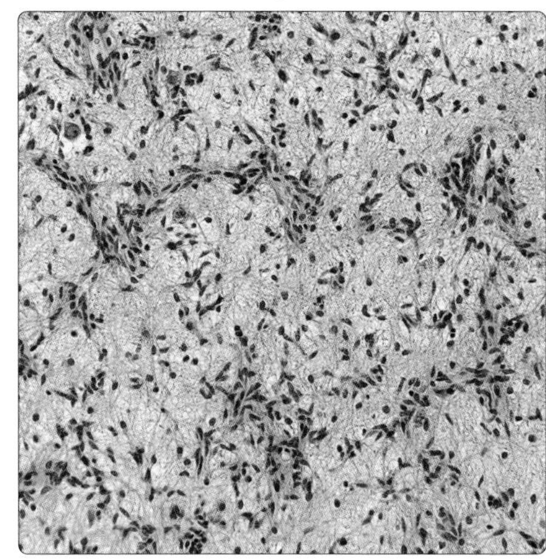

(Left) *Interwoven fascicles in angiocentric glioma may simulate those of a mesenchymal tumor, such as fibrosarcoma. This pattern is also reminiscent of other spindle cell tumors, such as schwannoma.* **(Right)** *The combination of polar tumor cells, here radiating from vessels, and a basophilic background lends a myxomatous quality similar to that of pilocytic astrocytoma, particularly its pilomyxoid variant.*

Perivascular Tumor Cells

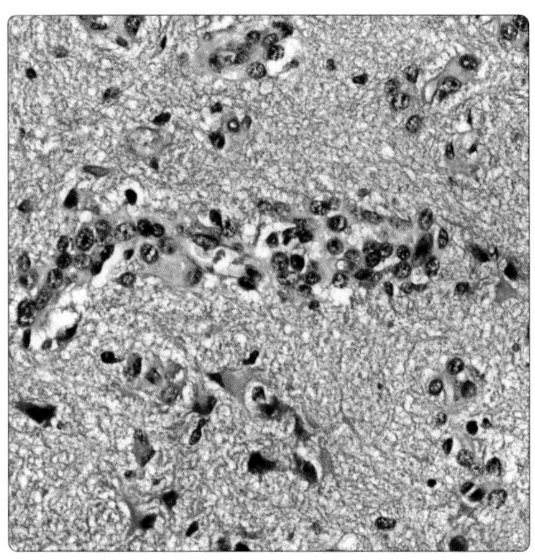

Perivascular Tumor Cells

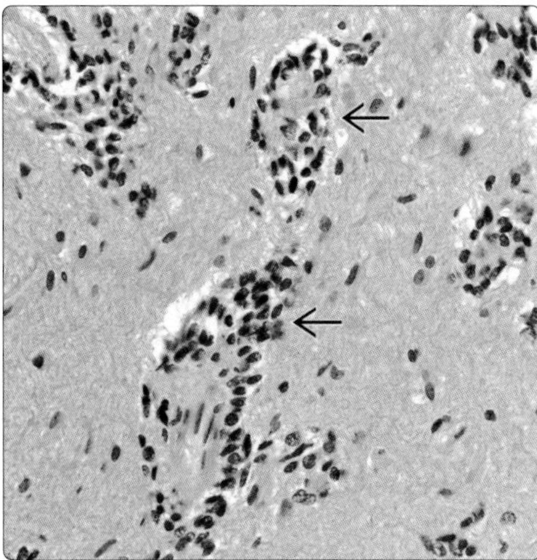

(Left) *The tumor cells appear glial in nature and are often arranged along the vascular channels. The cells typically have small bland nuclei, with virtually no pleomorphism or high-grade features.* **(Right)** *Perivascular tumor cells ➔ occur here in a lesion that, elsewhere, was classic ependymoma. It remains unclear whether such lesions should be considered angiocentric glioma with prominent ependymoma features or ependymoma with perivascular extension.*

(Left) *A smear preparation captures the tumor's angiocentricity and long, thin nuclei. Perivascular cells align longitudinally in this case* ➡. **(Right)** *Tumor cells distributed around a small vessel create a loose, poorly structured perivascular pseudorosette. Tumor cells in this entity are typically small and have glial character. The smear background is typically glial and entrapped ganglion cells can be observed.*

Intraoperative Smear: Elongated Nuclei

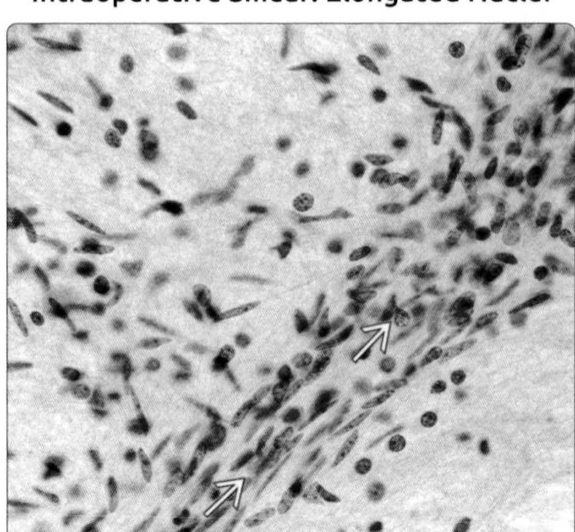

Angiocentric Arrangement of Cells

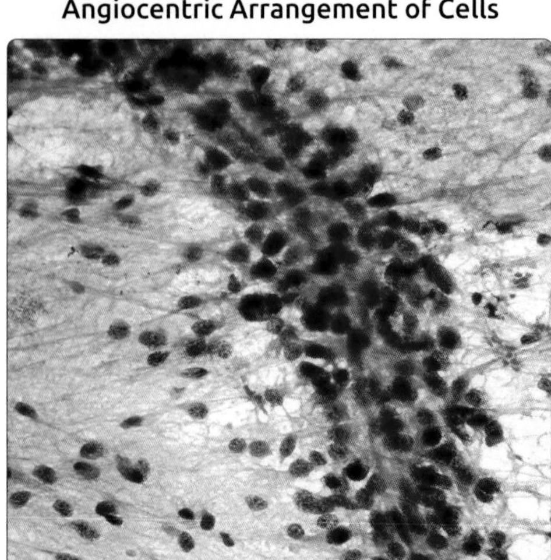

(Left) *The tumor cells, especially those in schwannoma-like areas, have pilocytic morphology with marked fibrillary processes and elongated nuclei.* **(Right)** *Myxoid background, cytological bipolarity, and a perivascular formation create a resemblance to pilomyxoid glioma.*

Bipolar Cells

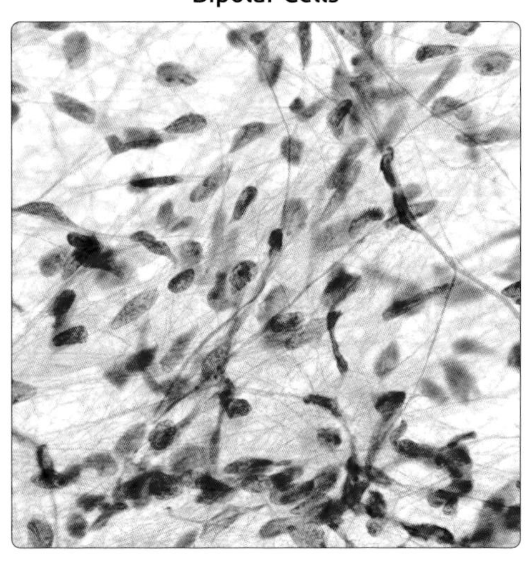

Myxoid Background

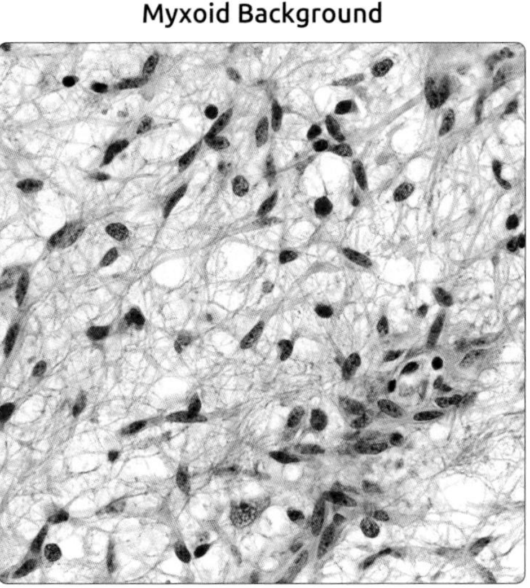

(Left) *Trapping neurons* ➡ *and other preexisting elements, this lesion can closely resemble infiltrating astrocytoma.* **(Right)** *Entrapped, cytologically normal ganglion cells with Nissl substance reflect the infiltrating nature of the lesion. Small bipolar cells are typical of angiocentric glioma but may not be distinguished individually from those of an infiltrating astrocytoma.*

Infiltrative Appearance

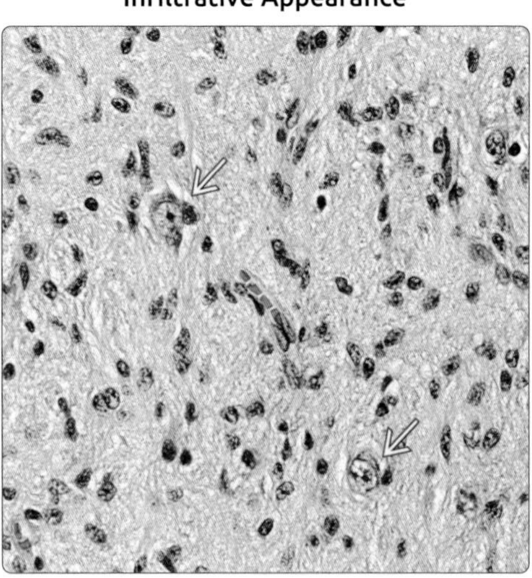

Trapped Neuronal Cells

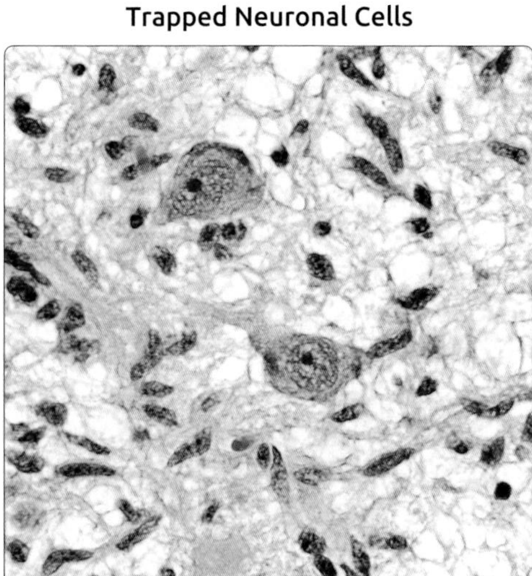

Microvilli, Ependymal Features

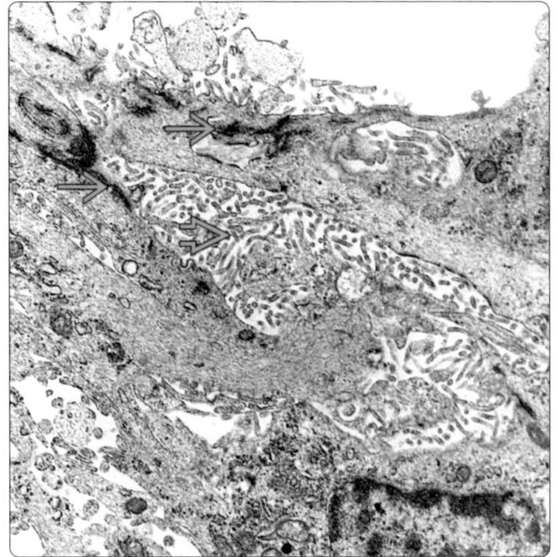

GFAP Staining Background

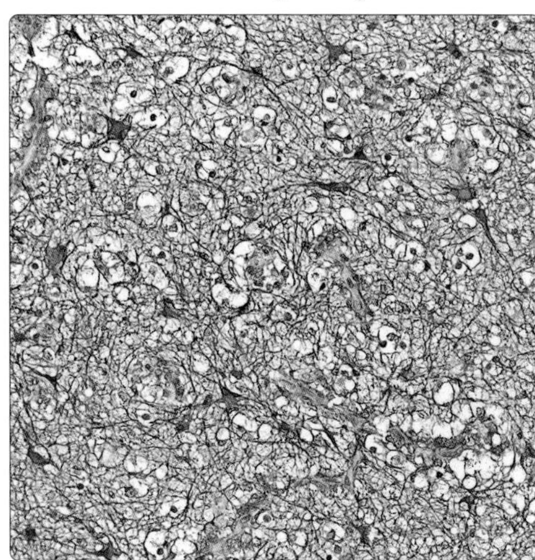

(Left) *Microvilli ⇨ fill small lumina between cells joined by multiple intermediate junctions ⇨. Cilia often complete the ultrastructural picture of ependymal differentiation.* **(Right)** *The tumor cells are only faintly positive for GFAP or other glial markers, but the background neuropil demonstrates significant staining, complicating the interpretation.*

EMA Positivity

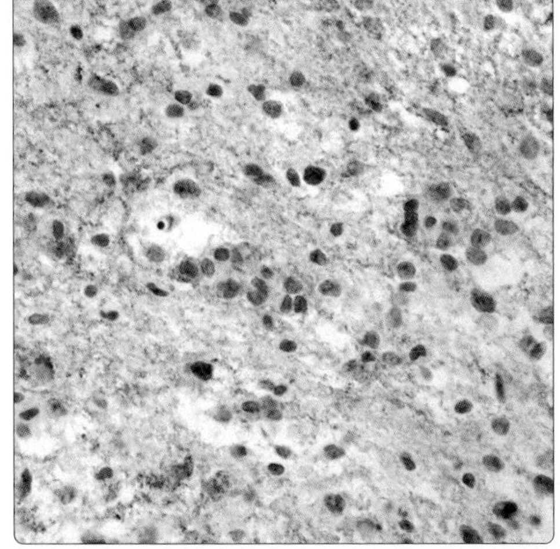

EMA Positivity

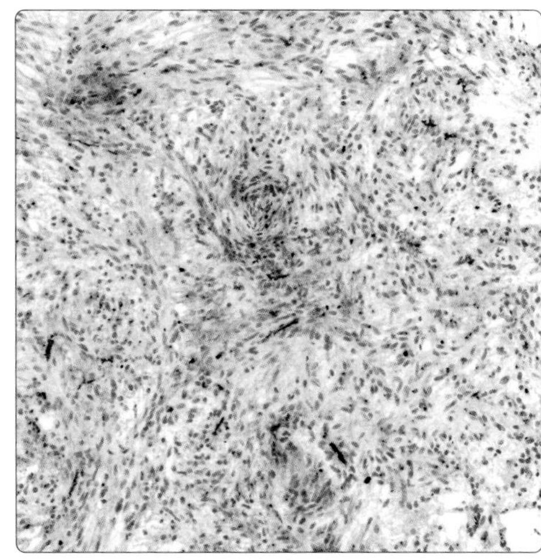

(Left) *The tumor cells of angiocentric glioma often demonstrate faint or weak positivity for EMA in a dot-like pattern reminiscent of ependymal tumors.* **(Right)** *Occasionally, the staining pattern of EMA is not typical for this tumor or ependymomas, and in addition to the dot-like staining, demonstrates membrane or cytoplasmic diffuse staining.*

Ki-67 Staining: Low Labeling Index

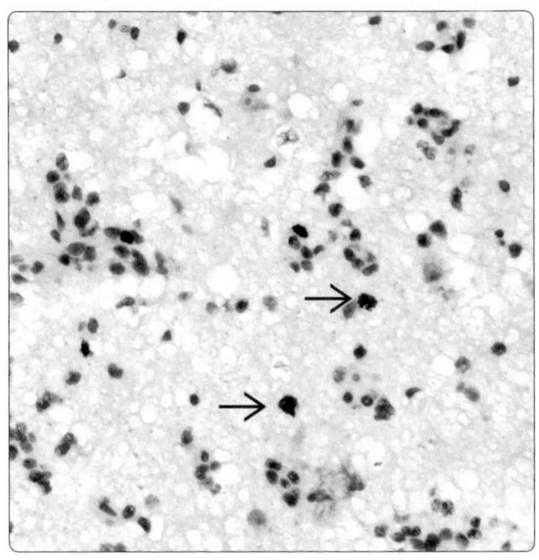

Neu-N Positive Neurons

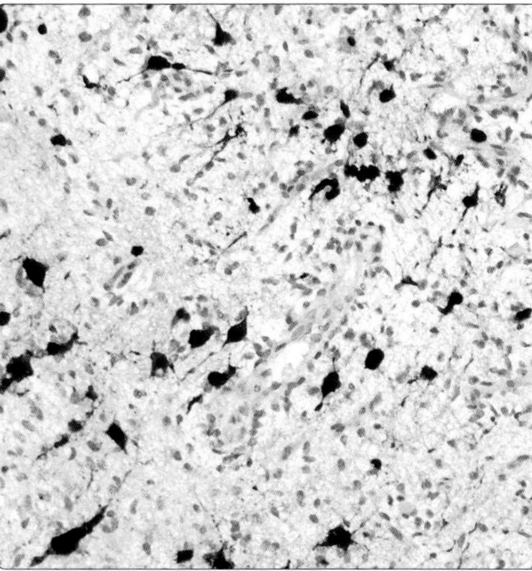

(Left) *Only rare tumor cells are highlighted by the MIB1 antibody (Ki-67) emphasizing the slow-growing nature of the tumor. Presence of individual positive cells ⇨ in the parenchyma suggests that tumor cells are not only around the vessels but also occur as single cells within brain tissue.* **(Right)** *The trapped neurons of angiocentric glioma are readily demonstrable with neuronal stains, such as Neu-N.*

Chordoid Glioma of 3rd Ventricle

KEY FACTS

CLINICAL ISSUES

- Adults
- Obstructive hydrocephalus
- Psychiatric and memory changes
- Hypothalamic and pituitary dysfunction
- Excision: Total removal usually impossible without neurological deficits

IMAGING

- 3rd ventricle
- Well circumscribed
- Ovoid
- Intensely and homogeneously enhancing

MACROSCOPIC

- Pushing, noninfiltrative borders
- Fills 3rd ventricle

MICROSCOPIC

- Chordoid architecture
- Myxoid background
- Prominent lymphoplasmacytic infiltrate with Russell bodies
- Sharp border with, and dense adherence to, walls of 3rd ventricle

ANCILLARY TESTS

- GFAP(+)
- CD34(+)
- TTF-1(+) nuclear immunostaining
- EMA and cytokeratins (+), focal in some cases

DIAGNOSTIC CHECKLIST

- Chordoid architecture
- Lymphoplasmacytic infiltrates
- TTF-1(+)
- Densely adherent to walls of 3rd ventricle

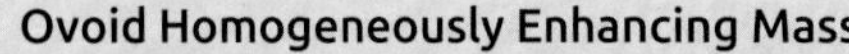

(Left) *Chordoid gliomas are ovoid, homogeneously enhancing masses that fill the 3rd ventricle, as seen here on sagittal MR.* **(Right)** *The firm, well-circumscribed lesion fills the 3rd ventricle and adheres to its walls.*

Ovoid Homogeneously Enhancing Mass

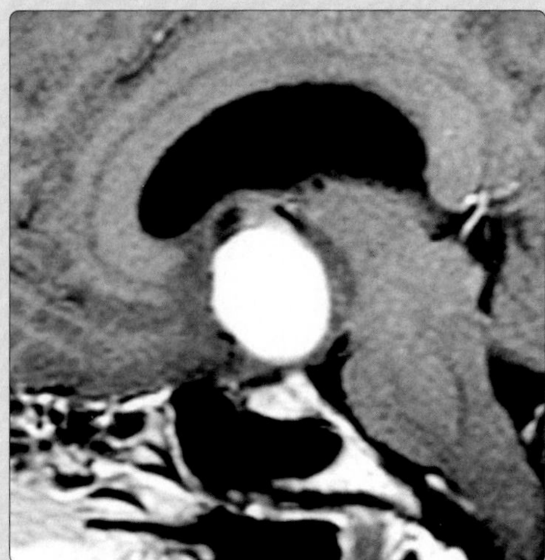

3rd Ventricle Mass

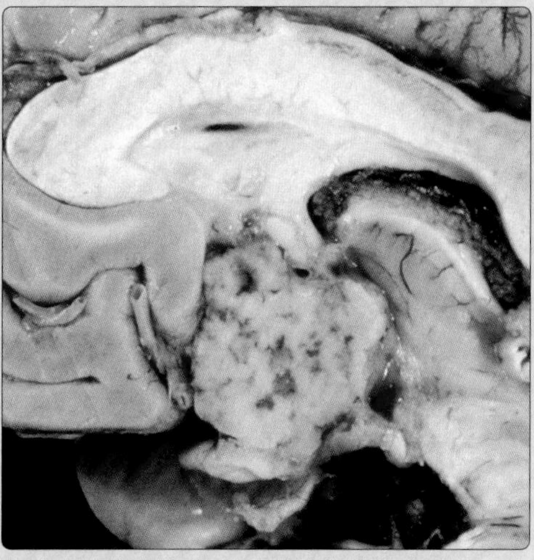

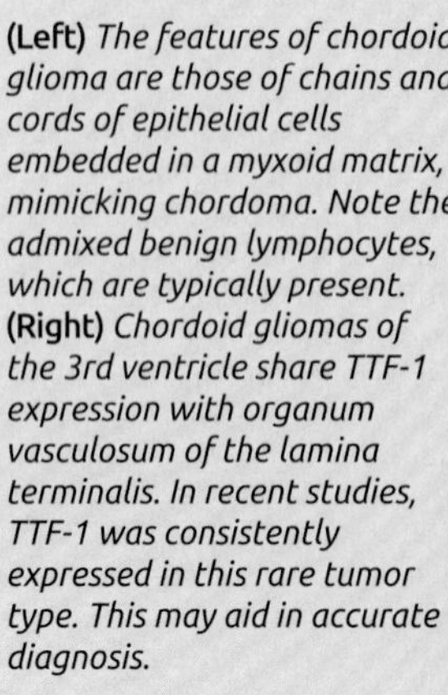

(Left) *The features of chordoid glioma are those of chains and cords of epithelial cells embedded in a myxoid matrix, mimicking chordoma. Note the admixed benign lymphocytes, which are typically present.* **(Right)** *Chordoid gliomas of the 3rd ventricle share TTF-1 expression with organum vasculosum of the lamina terminalis. In recent studies, TTF-1 was consistently expressed in this rare tumor type. This may aid in accurate diagnosis.*

Classic Example Mimics Chordoma

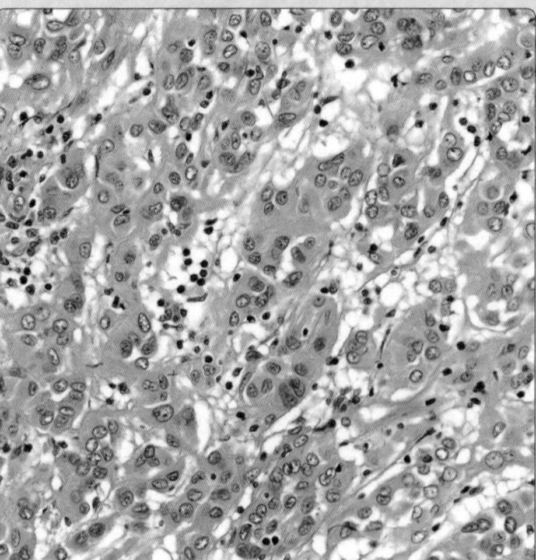

TTF-1(+), Distinctive Feature

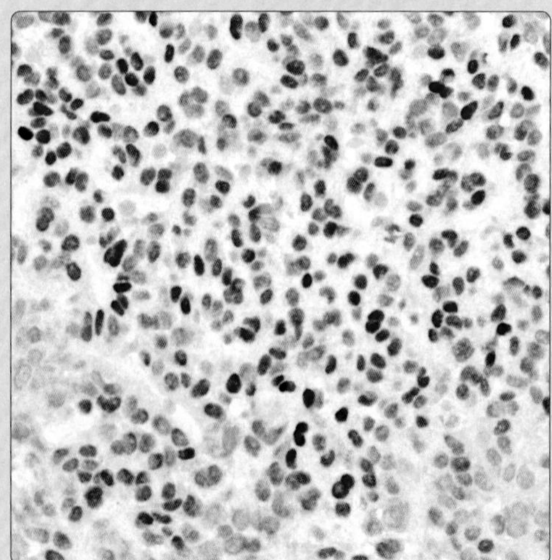

TERMINOLOGY

Definitions

- Discrete 3rd ventricular tumor with chordoid architecture

CLINICAL ISSUES

Epidemiology

- Age
  - Adults
- Sex
  - More often women

Presentation

- Obstructive hydrocephalus, acute or chronic
- Psychiatric and memory changes
- Hypothalamic and pituitary dysfunction

Treatment

- Surgical approaches
  - Excision, but total removal usually impossible without neurological deficits

Prognosis

- Slowly growing
- Details of long-term prognosis unclear

IMAGING

General Features

- Location
  - 3rd ventricle
- Morphology
  - Well circumscribed
  - Intensely and homogeneously enhancing
  - Ovoid

MACROSCOPIC

General Features

- Well circumscribed, firm
- Pushing, noninfiltrative border
- Dense adherence to walls of 3rd ventricle

MICROSCOPIC

Histological Features

- Sharp border with dense adherence to walls of ventricle
- Chordoid architecture with myxoid background
- Lymphoplasmacytic infiltrate with Russell bodies
- Round to oval bland nuclei
- Small distinct nucleoli
- Chondroid differentiation (rare)
- Peritumoral piloid gliosis

ANCILLARY TESTS

Cytology

- Clumps and individual cells
- Myxoid background
- Polygonal or elongated cells
- Binucleation
- Lymphocytes and plasma cells

Immunohistochemistry

- GFAP(+)
- CD34(+)
- EMA and cytokeratins (+), focal in some cases
- TTF-1 nuclear immunostaining

DIFFERENTIAL DIAGNOSIS

Pilocytic Astrocytoma

- Piloid cells in smear preparation
- Spongy microcystic tissue alternating with compact component
- Rosenthal fibers in tumor cells, eosinophilic granular bodies
- Little chronic inflammation

Ependymoma

- Prominent glial processes in smears
- Perivascular pseudorosettes &/or lumen-containing "true" rosettes
- No chronic inflammation

Chordoma

- Skull base (not intraventricular) tumor
- Vacuolated (physaliphorous) tumor cells
- More myxoid; little chronic inflammation
- Brachyury (+), GFAP(-)

Germinoma

- More suprasellar than 3rd ventricular
- No chordoid architecture or myxoid matrix
- OCT4(+), CD117(+), PLAP(+)
- Granulomas, some cases

Yolk Sac Tumor

- Vitelline pattern more delicate and lacy than chordoid architecture
- Hyaline droplets
- α-fetoprotein (+)

Meningioma (Lymphoplasmacytic and Chordoid Subtypes)

- Intraventricular types usually lateral rather than 3rd ventricle
- Little inflammation in chordoid subtype
- Usually some areas of conventional meningioma
- Whorls
- Psammoma bodies

Pineal Parenchymal Tumor

- Rosettes or sheet-like architecture
- Little if any inflammation
- Synaptophysin (+)
- Posterior 3rd ventricle

SELECTED REFERENCES

1. Bielle F et al: Chordoid gliomas of the third ventricle share TTF-1 expression with organum vasculosum of the lamina terminalis. Am J Surg Pathol. ePub, 2015
2. Michotte A et al: Expression of thyroid transcription factor 1 in a chordoid glioma. J Neurol Sci. 346(1-2):362-3, 2014

(Left) *This lesion is densely adherent along a sharp interface with the walls of the 3rd ventricle* ➡. *As a result, aggressive attempts at resection may damage the hypothalamus.* **(Right)** *Cords of cells in a myxoid background create the distinctive chordoid appearance. Nuclei are bland in this low-grade, slowly growing lesion with only rare mitoses.*

Sharp Interface

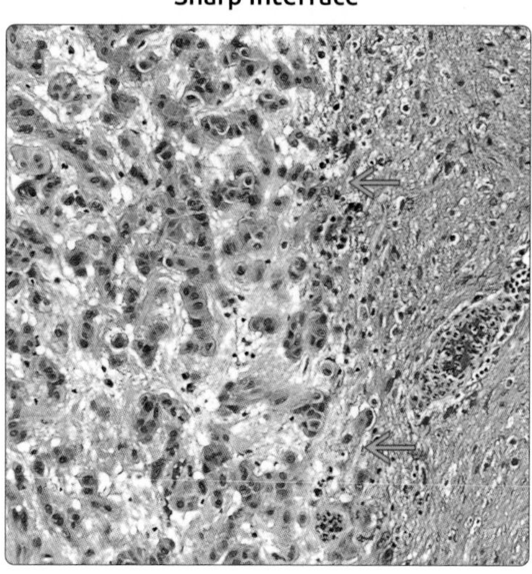

Bland Nuclei, Scant Mitoses

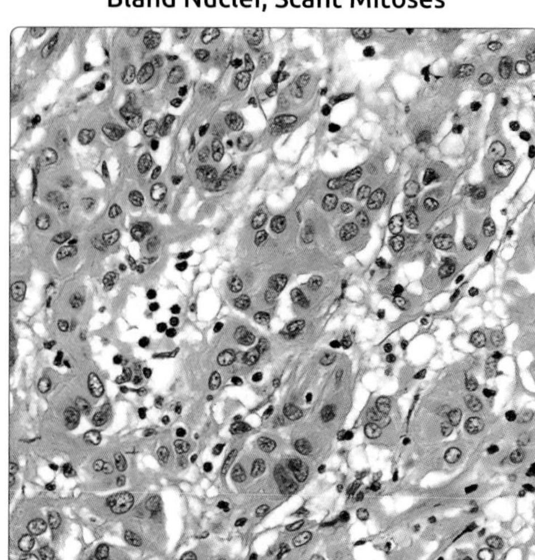

(Left) *Some examples are less chordoid than others, but a basophilic myxoid matrix remains as a diagnostic clue.* **(Right)** *Chronic inflammation is a common feature in a lesion that otherwise can resemble meningioma.*

Less Abundant Myxoid Matrix

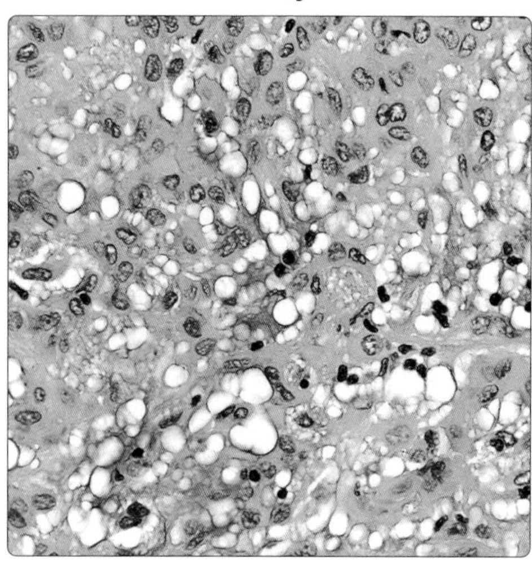

Frequent Chronic Inflammation

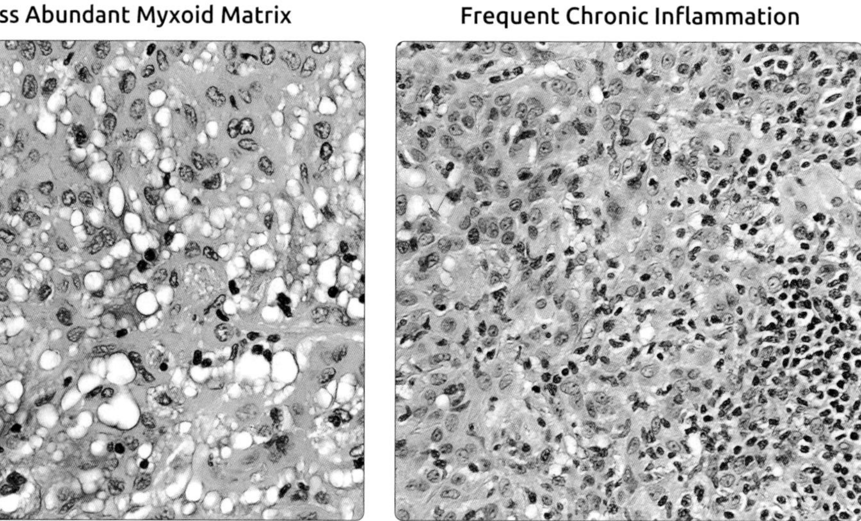

(Left) *Large numbers of plasma cells intermingle with tumor cells.* **(Right)** *While nonspecific, plasma cells with Russell bodies* ➡ *are highly suggestive of the entity.*

Admixed Plasma Cells

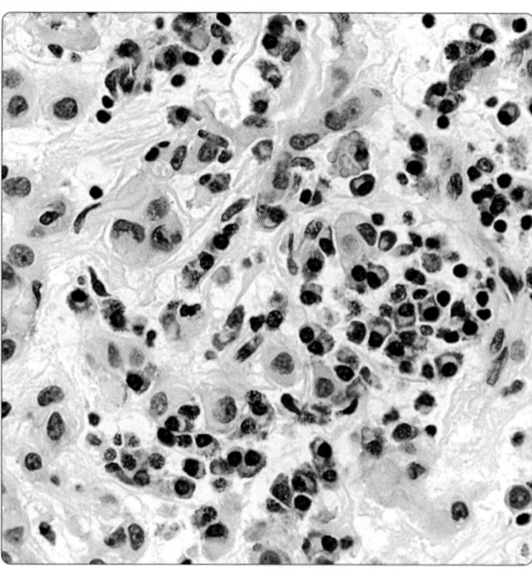

Russell Bodies

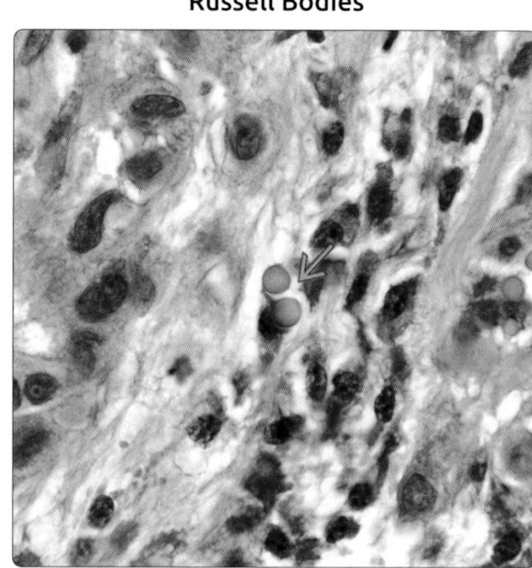

Vacuoles

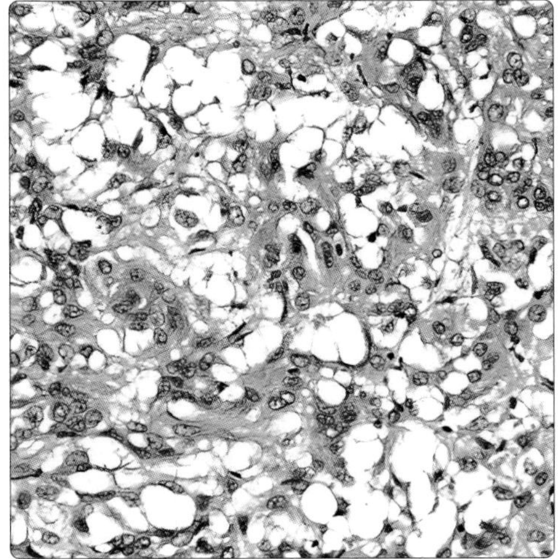

Piloid Gliosis

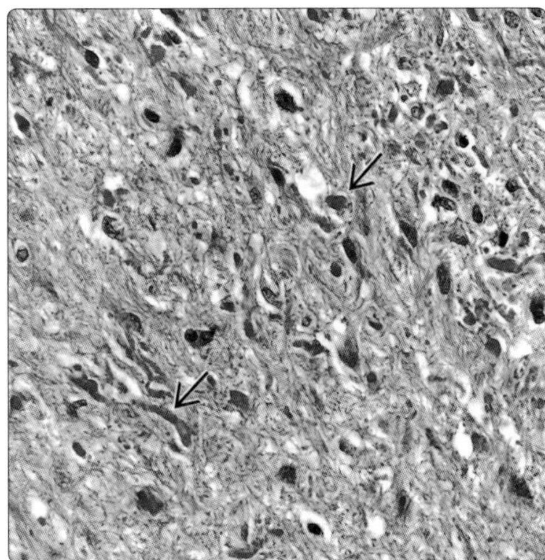

(Left) *Vacuoles and artifact can obscure the tumor's chordoid architecture.* **(Right)** *This tumor typically incites piloid gliosis with Rosenthal fibers in 3rd ventricular walls ➙. Lacking is the microcystic or spongy tissue of most pilocytic astrocytomas.*

GFAP Highlights Chordoid Architecture

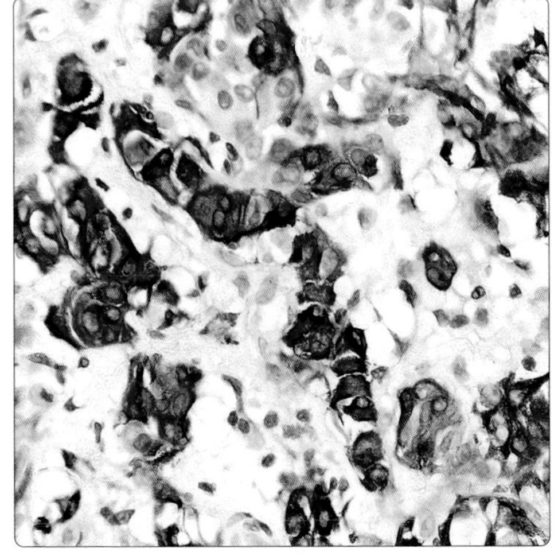

CD34 Highlights Epithelioid Features

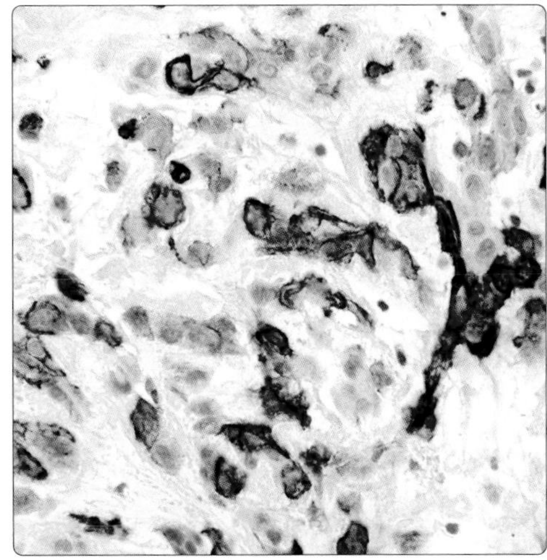

(Left) *GFAP staining emphasizes the tumor's chordoid architecture.* **(Right)** *Chordoid gliomas are often immunoreactive for CD34.*

Smear: Cell-Cell Cohesion

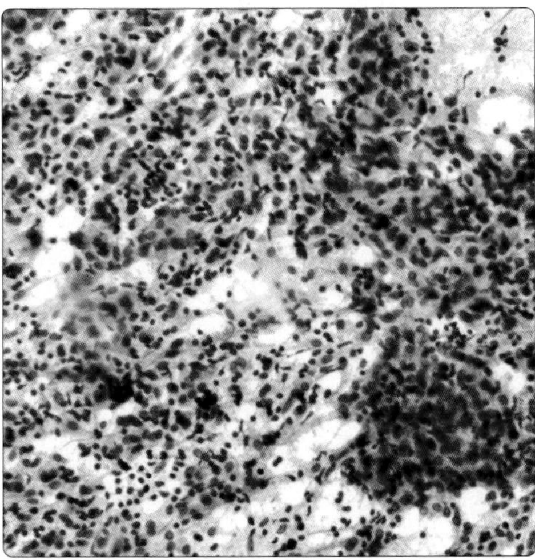

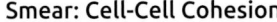

Smear: Mixed Epithelial/Glial Features

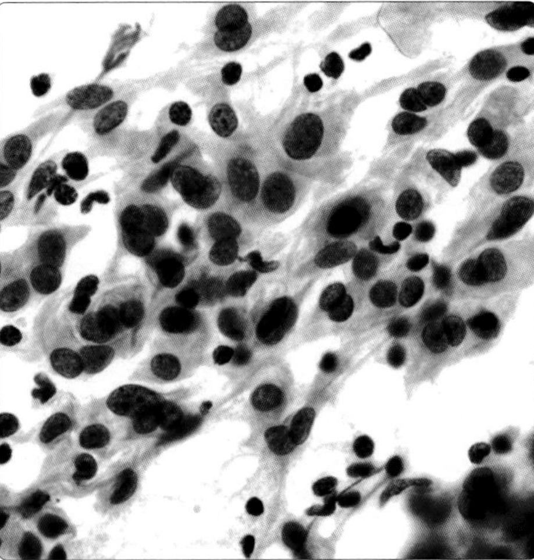

(Left) *Cell-cell cohesion results in large tissue fragments and clumps in smear preparations. (Courtesy A. Adesina, MD.)* **(Right)** *Both epithelial and glial features are present. Among the former are sharp cell borders and large round nuclei. Scattered cytoplasmic processes reflect the tumor's glial heritage. Note the lymphocytes that are common in this distinctive 3rd ventricular lesion. (Courtesy A. Adesina, MD.)*

KEY FACTS

TERMINOLOGY

- Papillary neoplasms arising from choroid plexus epithelium

CLINICAL ISSUES

- Children
  - Lateral or 3rd ventricle
- Adults
  - 4th ventricle or cerebellopontine angle
- Total excision most important prognostic factor
- Prognosis excellent
  - Malignant progression rare
  - Cerebrospinal fluid (CSF) dissemination uncommon
  - Chance of recurrence greater with atypical papilloma

MICROSCOPIC

- More complex papillary architecture than normal plexus
- Surface of epithelium flat rather than normal cobblestone
- Atypical papilloma: ≥ 2 mitoses per 10 HPF (suggested)

ANCILLARY TESTS

- Cytokeratins, usually CK7(+) and CK20(-)
- GFAP(+) in some cases, especially cells with long bipolar processes (glial differentiation)
- EMA(+), membranous in some cases, S100(+), Kir7.1(+)
- Synaptophysin (+) diffuse in many cases, neuropil islands (rare)
- Transthyretin (+) in most cases

TOP DIFFERENTIAL DIAGNOSES

- Papilloma vs.
  - Normal choroid plexus
  - Atypical papilloma
- Atypical papilloma vs.
  - Carcinoma
- Papillary ependymoma
- Papillary endolymphatic sac tumor
  - At cerebellopontine angle

Papilloma With Pedicle

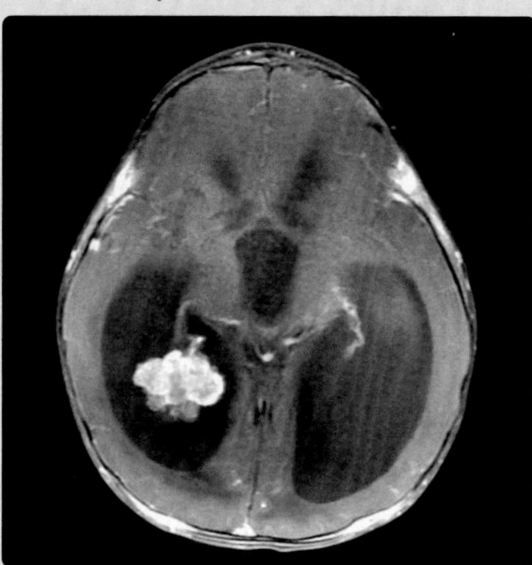

Papilloma Villi

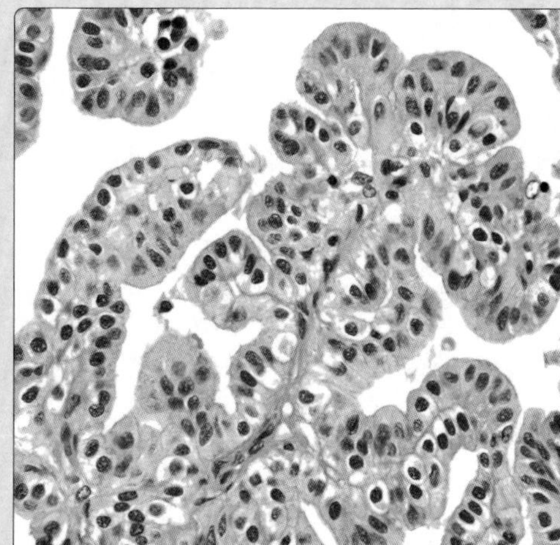

(Left) *Postcontrast T1WI MR shows a papilloma dangling from its pedicle in a ventricular system massively dilated from the tumor's secretion of cerebrospinal fluid (CSF).* **(Right)** *The redundancy and flat surface of the papilloma villi distinguish tumor from normal choroid plexus.*

Solid Areas

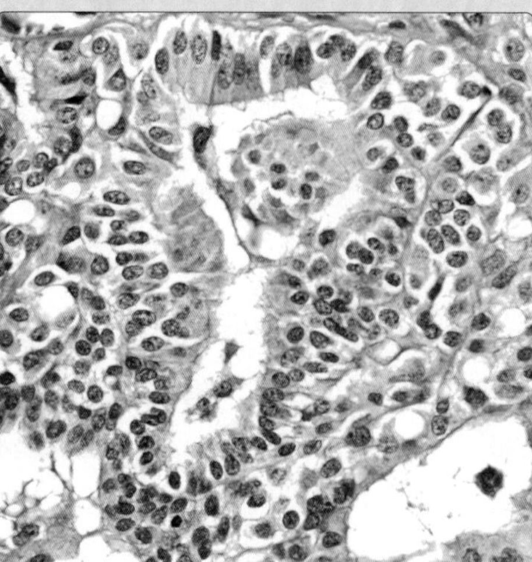

Compact Architecture

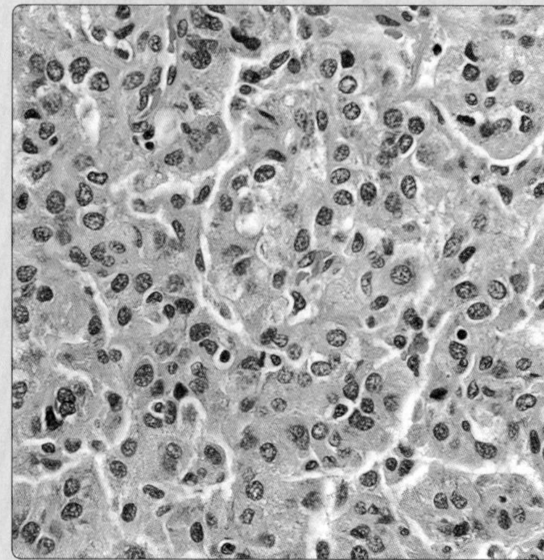

(Left) *Solid area and focal pseudostratification help distinguish this papilloma from normal choroid plexus.* **(Right)** *Some choroid plexus tumors are more compact than papillary. Higher grade choroid plexus tumors, atypical and carcinoma, need to be excluded.*

Choroid Plexus Papilloma and Atypical Papilloma

TERMINOLOGY

Definitions

- Papillary neoplasms arising from choroid plexus epithelium
- Papilloma: WHO grade I; atypical papilloma: WHO grade II

ETIOLOGY/PATHOGENESIS

Inherited Tumor Syndromes

- Germline *TP53* mutation, e.g., Li-Fraumeni (uncommon)
- Aicardi (rare)

CLINICAL ISSUES

Site

- Lateral or 3rd ventricle (children), 4th ventricle or cerebellopontine angle (adults)

Presentation

- Symptoms of increased intracranial pressure, craniosynostosis resulting in premature suture (before 2 years of age)

Prognosis

- Papilloma, excellent
- Atypical papilloma: Good, but higher rate of recurrence and cerebrospinal fluid spread

IMAGING

MR Findings

- Intraventricular or cerebellopontine angle, intensely enhancing
- Irregular, lobulated, if not overtly papillary
- Diffuse ventriculomegaly in some cases

MACROSCOPIC

General Features

- Discrete, often papillary, intraoperative bleeding (occasionally)

MICROSCOPIC

Histologic Features

- Papilloma
  - Transition to normal choroid plexus common
  - Variably complex papillary architecture, surface epithelium flat, not cobblestone
  - Limited (usually no) extension into brain
  - Variably pseudostratified, unlike simple epithelium of normal plexus
  - Foci with elongate, bipolar tumor cells (glial differentiation)
  - Acinar rather than papillary architecture (rare)
  - Prominent vascular hyalinization in some cases
  - Variable intratumoral cytological atypia, pleomorphic nuclei (unusual)
  - Mitoses, necrosis (uncommon)
  - Calcifications in some cases, bone or cartilage (rare)
  - Focal lipofuscin pigmentation epithelium (uncommon)
  - Oncocytic change, focal (occasional)
  - Neuropil islands, synaptophysin (+) (rare)
- Atypical papilloma
  - Same features as papilloma, but also
    - More crowding, cytological atypia, pseudostratification (usually)
    - Solid, nonpapillary areas, necrosis in some cases
  - ≥ 2 mitoses per 10 HPF is suggested threshold

ANCILLARY TESTS

Cytology

- Tissue fragments with smooth epithelial surfaces; individual, nonciliated columnar cells

Immunohistochemistry

- Immunophenotype of normal choroid plexus
  - GFAP(+) in some cases, especially cells with long bipolar cells (glial differentiation)
  - EMA(+), membranous in some cases, S100(+), Kir7.1(+)
  - Synaptophysin (+) diffuse in many cases, neuropil islands (rare)
  - Transthyretin (+) in most cases
  - Cytokeratins, usually CK7(+) and CK20(-)
- Ki-67 labeling index ~ 1-2%
- p53(+), papilloma rare; atypical papilloma ~ 10%

Genetic Testing

- No specific molecular features separating papilloma from atypical papilloma
- Frequent chromosome-wide gains in papilloma and atypical papilloma, but few losses

DIFFERENTIAL DIAGNOSIS

Normal Choroid Plexus

- Simple papillary architecture without pseudostratification or cytologic atypia
- Cobblestone cell surfaces
- Calcifications deeply situated in stroma, not peripherally in papillae
- No mitoses
- Thicker vessels

Choroid Plexus Carcinoma

- More mitoses; number distinguishing atypical papilloma from carcinoma generally ≥ 5-10 per 10 HPF, but no consensus number; often ≥ 5 in presence of solid architecture, necrosis, etc.
- Greater atypia, but overlap with atypical papilloma
- Solid, nonpapillary architecture in some cases
- Overt anaplasia in some cases
- Necrosis, but also in some atypical papillomas and rare papillomas

Papillary Ependymoma

- Less papillary, fibrillated, glial cytologic features
- EMA(+) microlumina in some cases

SELECTED REFERENCES

1. Japp AS et al: High-resolution genomic analysis does not qualify atypical plexus papilloma as a separate entity among choroid plexus tumors. J Neuropathol Exp Neurol. 74(2):110-20, 2015

(Left) *The epithelium of papillomas such as this is more complex than that of normal choroid plexus.* **(Right)** *The flat-surfaced epithelium of a choroid plexus papilloma ➙ is to be distinguished from an undulating (or cobblestone) profile of normal choroid plexus. Papillae of the tumor are also more irregular and complex.*

Complex Epithelium

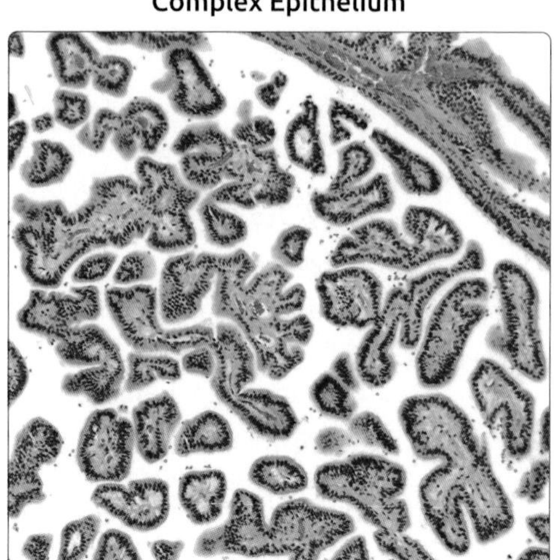

Flat-Surfaced Epithelium

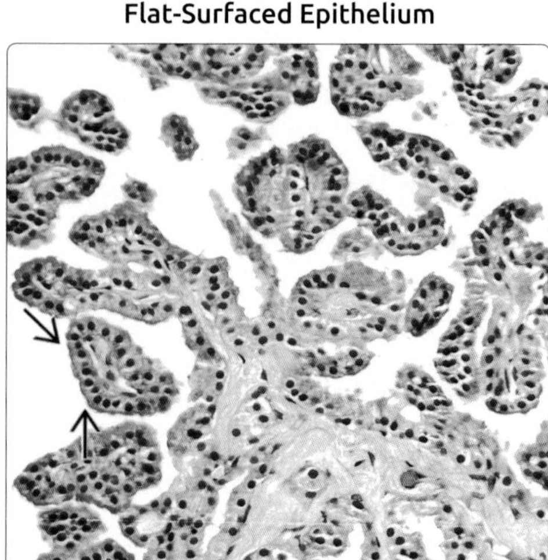

(Left) *Crowding of papillae, subtle pseudostratification, and increased nuclear:cytoplasmic ratio of a papilloma can overlap with those of atypical papilloma. Mitoses were rare in this papilloma, however.* **(Right)** *Concretions in a papilloma often lie within the small papillations. Mineralizations in normal choroid plexus are larger and arise deeper within the substance of the tissue.*

Crowding of Papillae

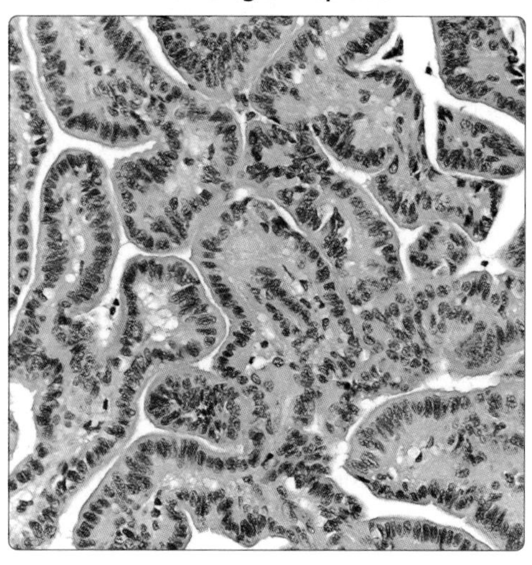

Concretions

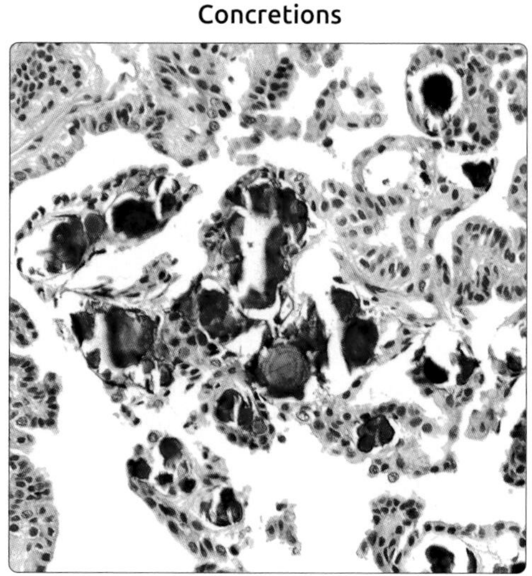

(Left) *Even very well-differentiated papillomas are easy to identify when their epithelium is as flat as it is here. Papillae, in addition, are not well formed.* **(Right)** *The epithelium of normal choroid plexus such as this is simpler, more cuboidal, and more cobblestoned than that of a papilloma.*

Flat Epithelium

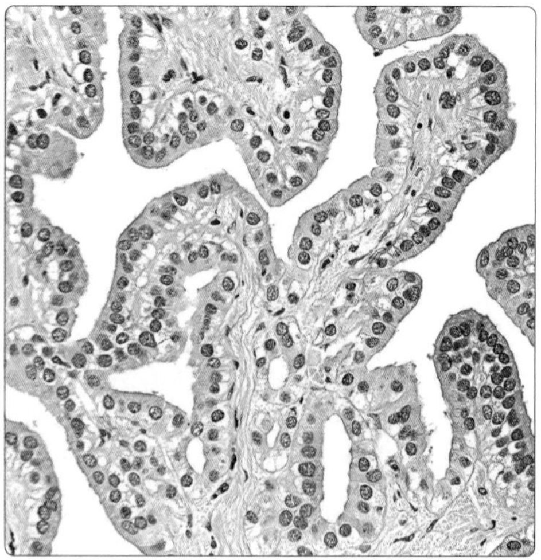

Simple, Cuboidal Epithelium

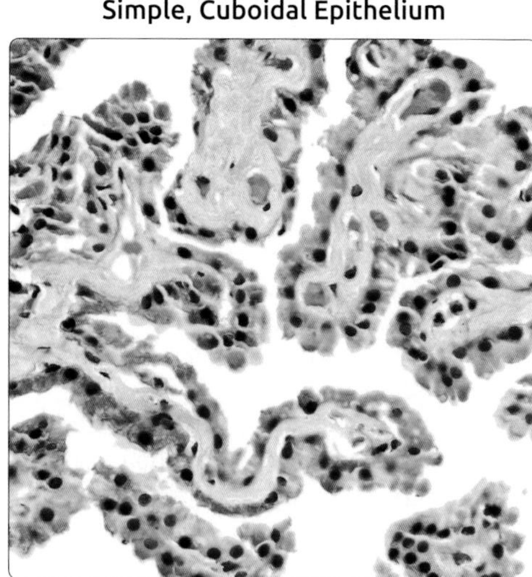

Architectural Disarray

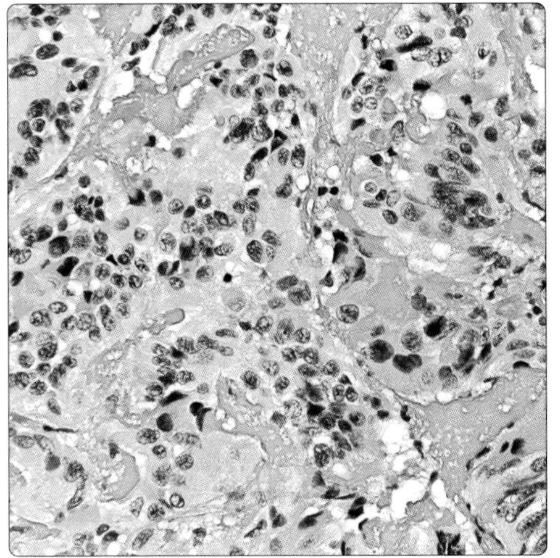

Stromal Hyalinization

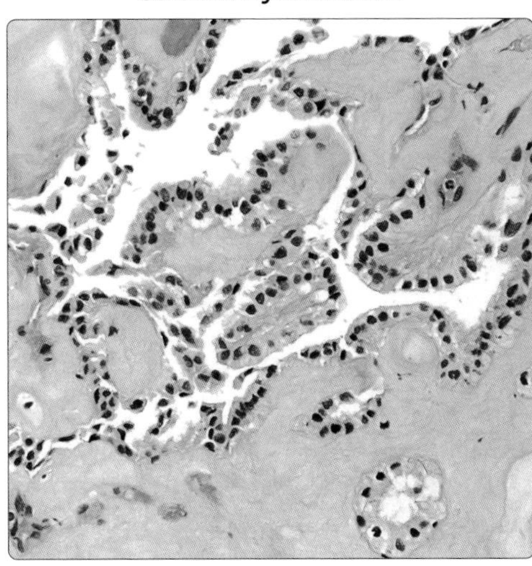

(Left) *While worrisome, architectural disarray and nuclear atypia are not, in themselves, evidence of anaplasia in choroid plexus papillomas. Substantial mitotic activity, missing in this case, is required.* **(Right)** *Stromal hyalinization is prominent in some choroid plexus papillomas with chronic changes.*

Mitotic Activity

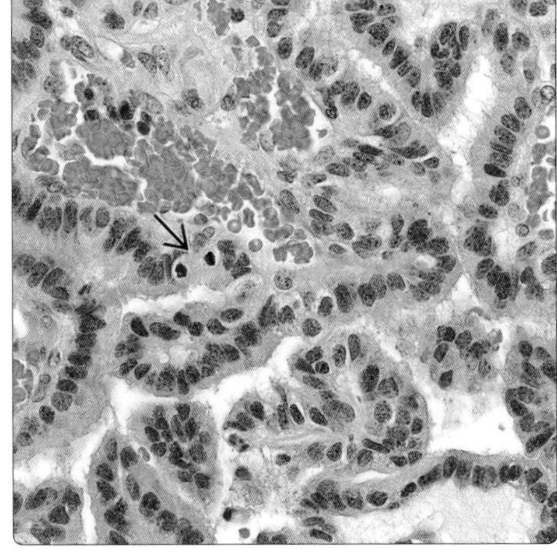

Mitoses

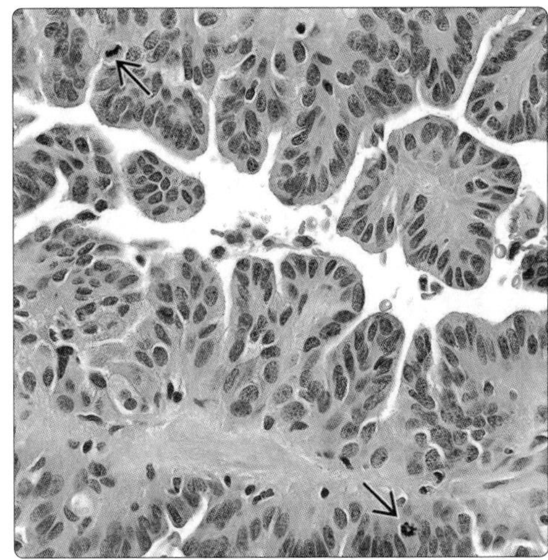

(Left) *Overtly papillary choroid plexus tumors such as this are diagnosed as atypical on the basis of mitotic activity* ➔ *that is higher than those of grade I papillomas. A threshold of 2 or more mitoses per 10 HPF has been suggested.* **(Right)** *Two mitoses in 1 HPF* ➔ *are evidence that a lesion is at least atypical papilloma. There were other mitoses in this case, but fewer than in a carcinoma.*

Juxtaposed Papilloma and Choroid Plexus

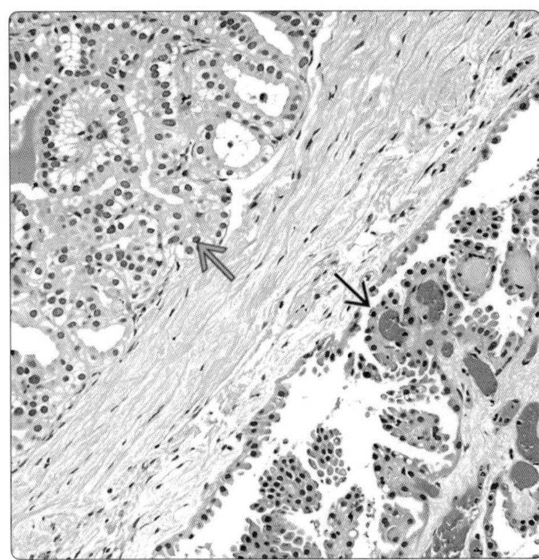

Hobnail Surface

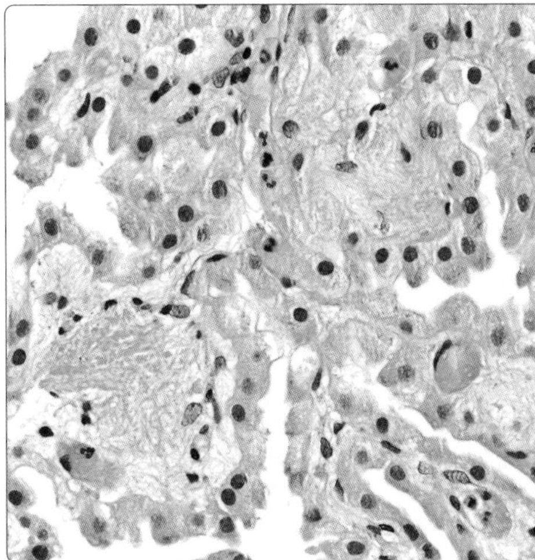

(Left) *Juxtaposed papilloma* ➔ *and normal choroid plexus* ➔ *emphasize the differences in the 2 epithelia: The former simple and cobblestone in surface profile, the latter flat-surfaced and overall more complex.* **(Right)** *Normal choroid plexus has an undulating cobblestone or hobnail surface profile as opposed to the flat surfaces in papillomas and atypical papillomas.*

(Left) *This degree of atypia is worrisome for atypical papilloma, or even well-differentiated carcinoma, but in the absence of mitoses papilloma is the diagnosis. The cells are more columnar and the nuclei more atypical than those of normal choroid plexus. The surface is especially flat ⇒ in this case.* **(Right)** *The epithelium of a choroid papilloma may, focally, be ribbon-like rather than papillary.*

Atypia

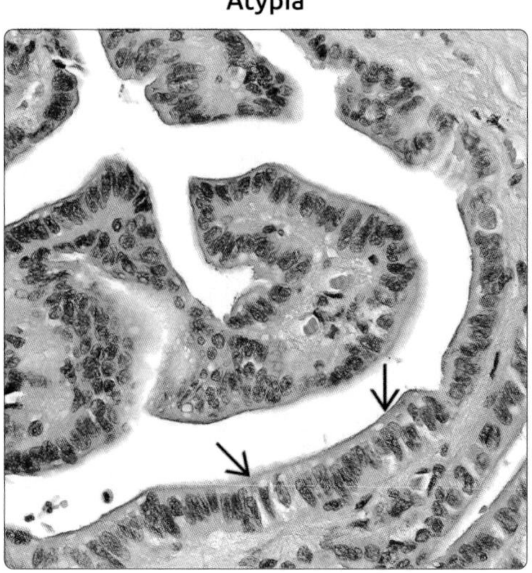

Ribbon-Like Epithelium

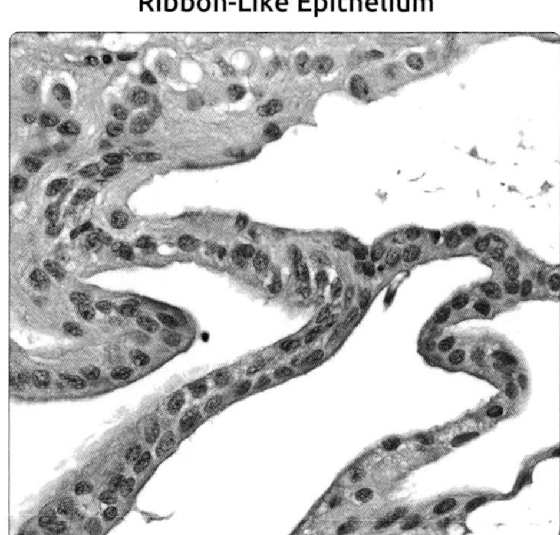

(Left) *Rare choroid plexus tumors are more acinar than papillary. The possibility of adenoma or adenocarcinoma may come to mind.* **(Right)** *Glial differentiation in choroid plexus tumors takes the form of ependymoma-like perivascular pseudorosettes produced by long cytoplasmic processes ⇒ inserting into vessel walls.*

Acinar Architecture

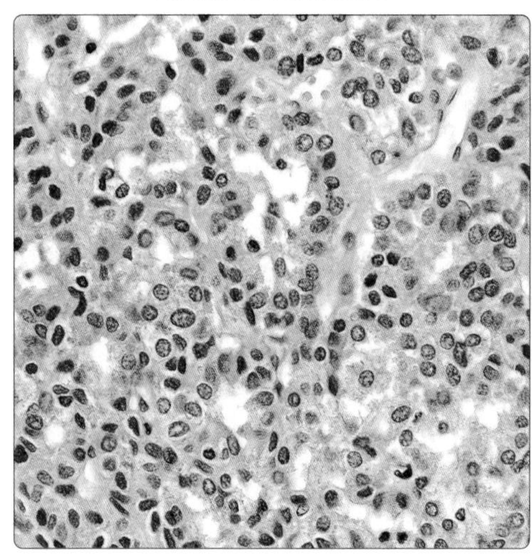

Glial Differentiation

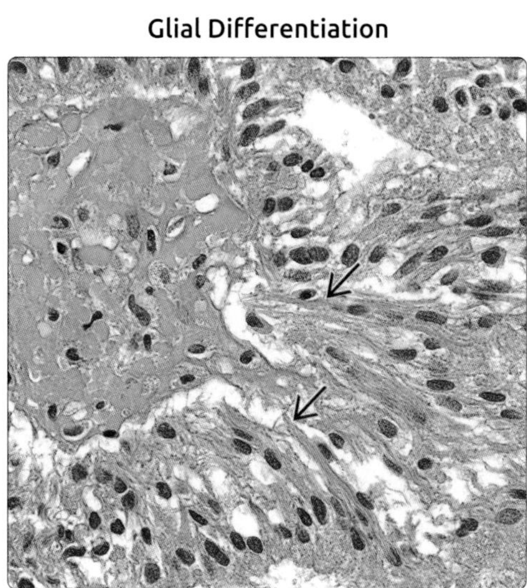

(Left) *Tumor cell cytoplasm occasionally has a finely granular, mitochondria-rich oncocytic quality. This prognostically neutral change is usually focal.* **(Right)** *As a rule, it is lipofuscin ⇒, not true melanin, that stipples the epithelium of melanotic choroid plexus papillomas.*

Oncocytic Cytoplasm

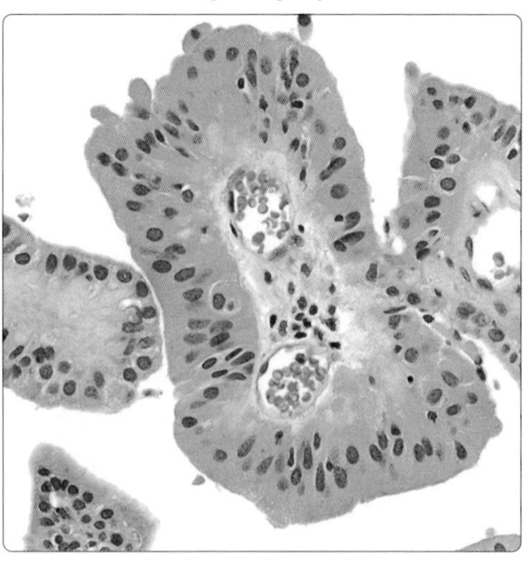

Lipofuscin

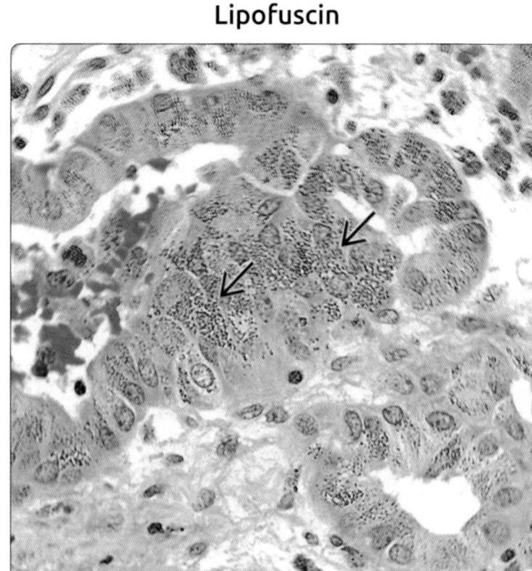

Cohesive Tissue Fragments

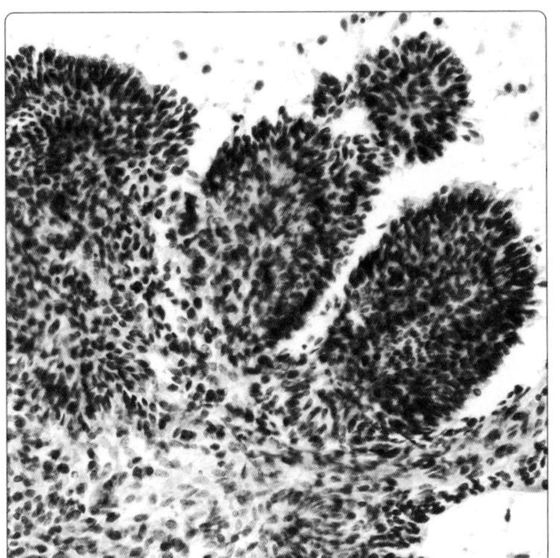

Columnar Cells

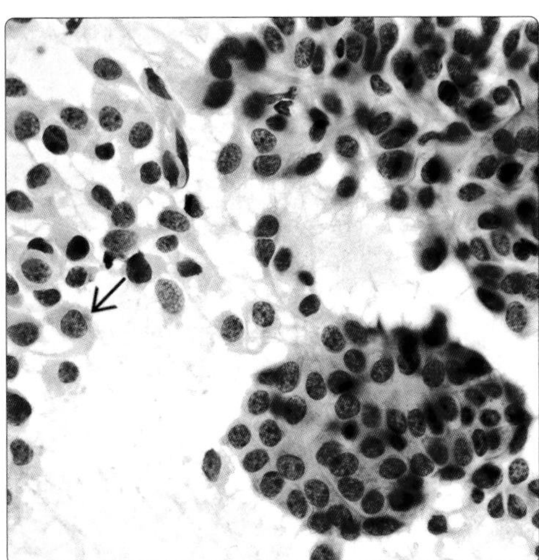

(Left) *In smear preparations, cohesive tissue fragments of crowded cells with a columnar surface epithelium help establish the diagnosis of papilloma.* **(Right)** *Tissue fragments with sharp borders, as well as individual columnar cells ⇒, are clear evidence of an epithelial lesion.*

GFAP(+) Processes

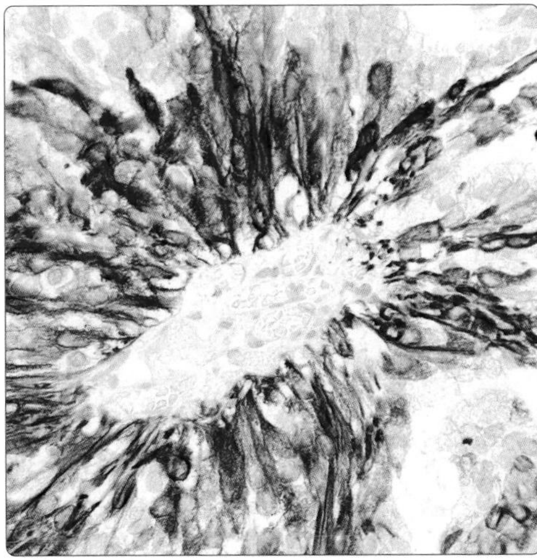

GFAP Immunoreactive Cells

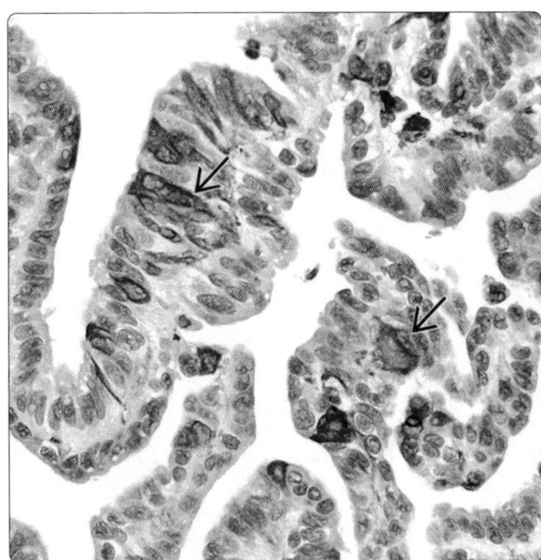

(Left) *Radiating perivascular, GFAP-positive processes indicate glial differentiation in some choroid plexus tumors. It is usually only focal.* **(Right)** *Scattered cells immunoreactive for GFAP ⇒ are occasionally present in choroid plexus papillomas; however, most are immunonegative throughout.*

Synaptophysin Immunoreactivity

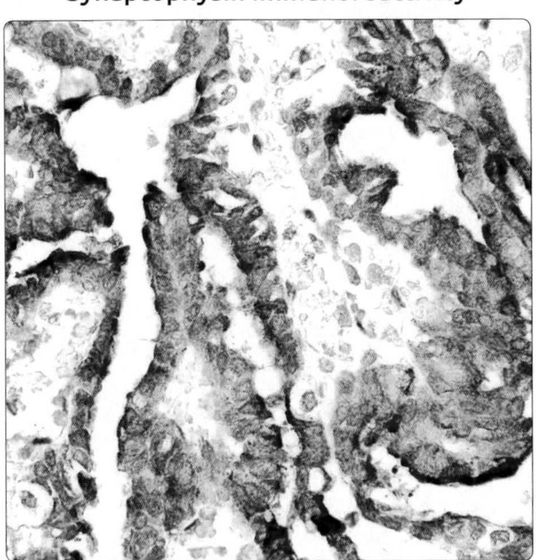

CK7 Immunoreactivity

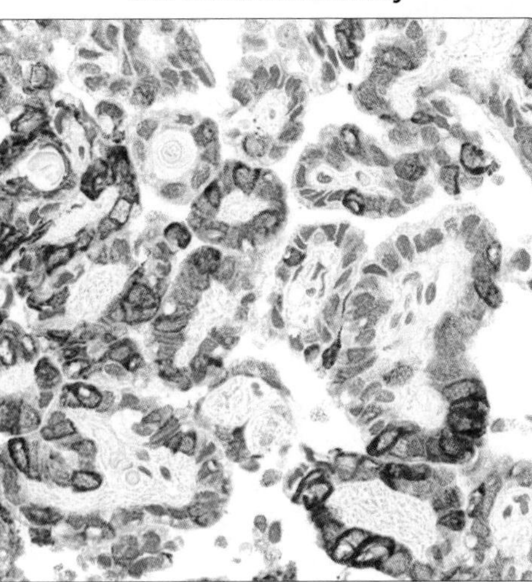

(Left) *Many, but not all, papillomas are diffusely immunoreactive for synaptophysin.* **(Right)** *Most papillomas are immunoreactive, at least in part, for CK7. As is often the case, staining was negative for CK20.*

Choroid Plexus Carcinoma

KEY FACTS

TERMINOLOGY

- Anaplastic epithelial neoplasm of choroid plexus

ETIOLOGY/PATHOGENESIS

- Rare cases syndromic
  - Germline *TP53* mutation, e.g., Li-Fraumeni
  - Aicardi

CLINICAL ISSUES

- Lateral ventricle (most cases)
- 4th ventricle (rare)
- Usual age < 3 years
- Prognosis
  - Excellent for well-differentiated examples after gross total resection
  - Poor in highly anaplastic types

MICROSCOPIC

- More cellular than papilloma
- Considerable inter- and intratumoral variation in degree of anaplasia
- Mitotically, no precise cutoff from atypical papilloma, but carcinoma generally ≥ 5-10 per 10 HPF; often ≥ 5 per 10 HPF in presence of solid areas, hypercellularity, and necrosis
- Solid, nonpapillary areas (most cases)

ANCILLARY TESTS

- *TP53* mutations; ~ 50% of cases
- Chromosomal instability frequent in choroid plexus carcinoma
- Cytokeratins, generally CK7(+) and CK20(-)
- BER-EP4(-) and S100(+) in most cases

TOP DIFFERENTIAL DIAGNOSES

- Atypical papilloma
- Atypical teratoid/rhabdoid tumor
- Metastatic carcinoma
- Anaplastic ependymoma and astroblastoma

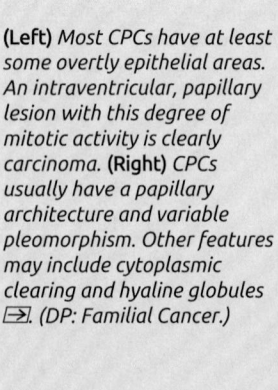

(Left) *Choroid plexus carcinomas (CPCs) are highly malignant neoplasms and may form huge, fleshy masses with associated edema and mass effect.* **(Right)** *CPCs are malignant neoplasms that almost always develop in young children and demonstrate variable contrast enhancement. (DP: Familial Cancer.)*

Huge Fleshy Mass

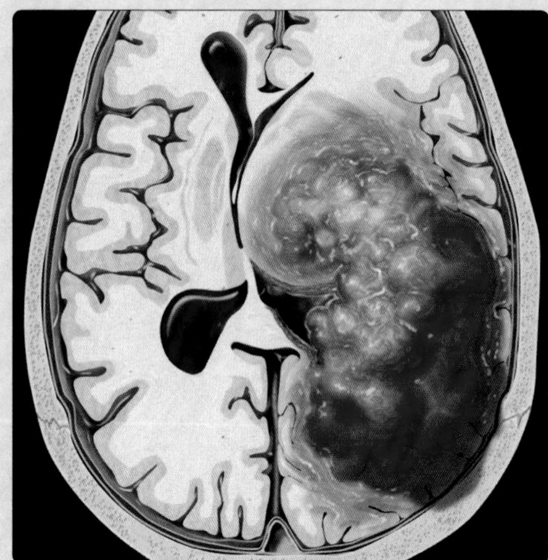

Variable Contrast Enhancement

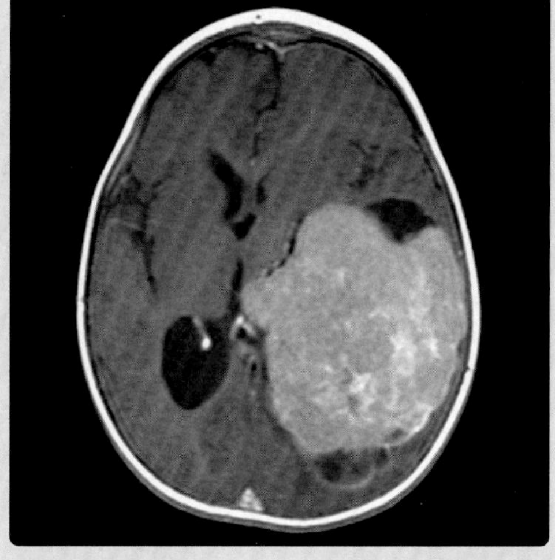

(Left) *Most CPCs have at least some overtly epithelial areas. An intraventricular, papillary lesion with this degree of mitotic activity is clearly carcinoma.* **(Right)** *CPCs usually have a papillary architecture and variable pleomorphism. Other features may include cytoplasmic clearing and hyaline globules* ➔*. (DP: Familial Cancer.)*

Overt Epithelial Areas

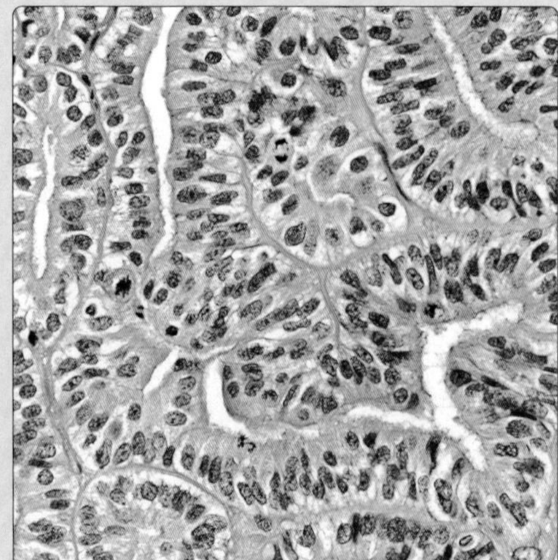

Papillary Architecture

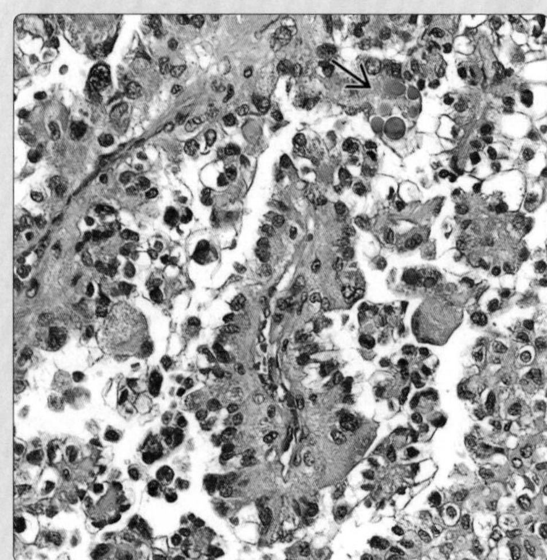

TERMINOLOGY

Abbreviations

- Choroid plexus carcinoma (CPC)

Definitions

- Anaplastic neoplasm originating in choroid plexus epithelium (WHO grade III)

ETIOLOGY/PATHOGENESIS

Inherited Tumor Syndromes

- Germline *TP53* mutation, e.g., Li-Fraumeni (uncommon)
- Aicardi (rare)

CLINICAL ISSUES

Site

- Lateral (most cases)
- 4th ventricle (rare)

Presentation

- Pediatric tumor
- Usually in patients < 3 years

Natural History

- Evolution from papilloma, rarely evident

Treatment

- Irradiation and chemotherapy, depending on age
- Observation alone in some centers if totally resected and well differentiated

Prognosis

- Excellent for well-differentiated examples after gross total resection
- Poor for anaplastic types and with p53 diffuse staining/mutation
- Risk of cerebrospinal fluid dissemination, especially anaplastic types

IMAGING

MR Findings

- Generally large
  - Lobular; papillary (in some cases)
- Enhancing
- Diffuse dilation of ventricular system (in some cases)

MACROSCOPIC

General Features

- Fleshy
- Hemorrhage and necrosis mainly in anaplastic types
- Invasive in some cases
- Intraoperative bleeding in some cases

MICROSCOPIC

Histologic Features

- More cellular and cytologically more atypical than papilloma
- Separate areas of &/or transitional areas to regions of lower grade tumor (frequent)
- Invasion of adjacent brain in some cases, but may be seen in papillomas
- Variable differentiation
  - Overtly papillary
  - Papillary and focal solid growth patterns
  - Predominantly solid with sometimes conspicuous nuclear pleomorphism
  - Solid, undifferentiated
- Calcifications (occasional)
- Eosinophilic globules
  - Usually in areas with marked nuclear pleomorphism and prominent cytoplasm
- Necrosis (frequent)
- Oncocytic change (uncommon)
- Mitoses
  - Generally ≥ 5-10 per 10 HPF
  - No precise cutoff from atypical papilloma, but
    - Often ≥ 5 mitoses per 10 HPF in presence of solid areas, hypercellularity, and necrosis

Cytologic Features

- Tissue fragments
- Individual columnar cells
- Nuclear atypia, mitoses

ANCILLARY TESTS

Immunohistochemistry

- Cytokeratins, generally CK7(+) and CK20(-)
- BER-EP4(-) and S100(+) in most cases
- Kir7.1(+)
- Ki-67
  - Inter- and intratumoral variability
  - Usually > 10% in large areas

Genetic Testing

- *TP53* mutations; ~ 50% of cases
- *TP53* alterations associated with poorer prognosis in choroid plexus tumors in some studies
- Notch pathway activation induces choroid plexus tumors in mice and is present in subset of human choroid plexus tumors
- Chromosomal instability frequent in CPC
- Increased number of *TP53* mutant copies associated with worse survival in CPC
- *TAF12*, *NFYC*, and *RAD54L* putative oncogenes concurrently gained

DIFFERENTIAL DIAGNOSIS

Atypical Choroid Plexus Papilloma, Grade II

- Fewer mitoses
  - No consensus on distinction by mitotic count
  - Atypical papilloma ≥ 2 and generally ≤ 5-10 per 10 HPF
  - In carcinoma, often ≥ 2 and < 5 per 10 HPF in presence of solid areas, increased cellularity, pleomorphism, necrosis
- Usually less cellular, more papillary, little, if any, solid tissue and necrosis

Atypical Teratoid/Rhabdoid Tumor

- Jumbled, nonpapillary architecture
- Rhabdoid cells, in most cases

- Polyimmunophenotypic
- Nuclear INI1 loss in neoplastic cells
- Difficult to distinguish in some cases

Metastatic Carcinoma

- Usually intraparenchymal
- Near cerebral cortical gray-white junction or cerebellum
- More epithelial markers (+), e.g., EMA, BER-EP4, TTF-1
- Almost always limited to adults, while CPC usually limited to young children

Glioblastoma

- Epicenter in brain parenchyma
- Diffusely infiltrative, nonpapillary
- Generally smaller cells
- Necrosis with pseudopalisading &/or microvascular proliferation
- Often GFAP(+)
- Epithelial markers (-), except for those with epithelial metaplasia

Anaplastic Ependymoma and Astroblastoma

- Paraventricular location
- Perivascular pseudorosettes; no true papillae
- Prominent hyalinization in astroblastoma
- GFAP(+) in most cases
- EMA(+), especially of microlumina

Embryonal Neoplasms

- Small cell, nonpapillary neoplasms
- No epithelial differentiation
- Synaptophysin (+)

Cribriform Neuroepithelial Tumor

- Very rare, low-grade intraventricular neoplasm
- Cribriform/trabecular architecture
- Surface EMA staining, INI1 loss

Papillary Tumor of Pineal Region

- Similar morphologic and immunophenotypic features
- Pineal gland location not feature of choroid plexus tumors
- Cell pleomorphism and mitotic activity less pronounced

DIAGNOSTIC CHECKLIST

Pathologic Interpretation Pearls

- CPC extremely rare in adults
  - Consider metastatic adenocarcinoma 1st in adults rather than CPC

SELECTED REFERENCES

1. Merino DM et al: Molecular characterization of choroid plexus tumors reveals novel clinically relevant subgroups. Clin Cancer Res. 21(1):184-92, 2015
2. Tong Y et al: Cross-species genomics identifies TAF12, NFYC, and RAD54L as choroid plexus carcinoma oncogenes. Cancer Cell. 27(5):712-27, 2015
3. Ruland V et al: Choroid plexus carcinomas are characterized by complex chromosomal alterations related to patient age and prognosis. Genes Chromosomes Cancer. 53(5):373-80, 2014
4. Gozali AE et al: Choroid plexus tumors; management, outcome, and association with the Li-Fraumeni syndrome: the Children's Hospital Los Angeles (CHLA) experience, 1991-2010. Pediatr Blood Cancer. 58(6):905-9, 2012
5. Schittenhelm J et al: Atypical teratoid/rhabdoid tumors may show morphological and immunohistochemical features seen in choroid plexus tumors. Neuropathology. 31(5):461-7, 2011
6. Tabori U et al: TP53 alterations determine clinical subgroups and survival of patients with choroid plexus tumors. J Clin Oncol. 28(12):1995-2001, 2010
7. Wrede B et al: Atypical choroid plexus papilloma: clinical experience in the CPT-SIOP-2000 study. J Neurooncol. Epub ahead of print, 2009
8. Jeibmann A et al: Malignant progression in choroid plexus papillomas. J Neurosurg. 107(3 Suppl):199-202, 2007
9. Dang L et al: Notch3 signaling initiates choroid plexus tumor formation. Oncogene. 25(3):487-91, 2006
10. Jeibmann A et al: Prognostic implications of atypical histologic features in choroid plexus papilloma. J Neuropathol Exp Neurol. 65(11):1069-73, 2006
11. Judkins AR et al: INI1 protein expression distinguishes atypical teratoid/rhabdoid tumor from choroid plexus carcinoma. J Neuropathol Exp Neurol. 64(5):391-7, 2005
12. Ang LC et al: An immunohistochemical study of papillary tumors in the central nervous system. Cancer. 65(12):2712-9, 1990

Crowding, Atypia, and Mitotic Activity

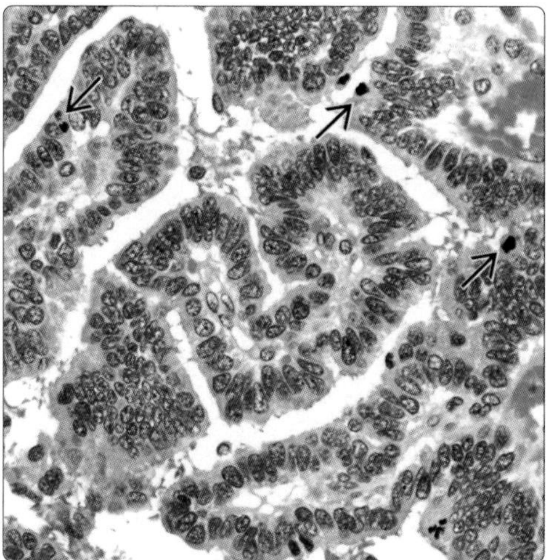

Pseudostratified Columnar Epithelium

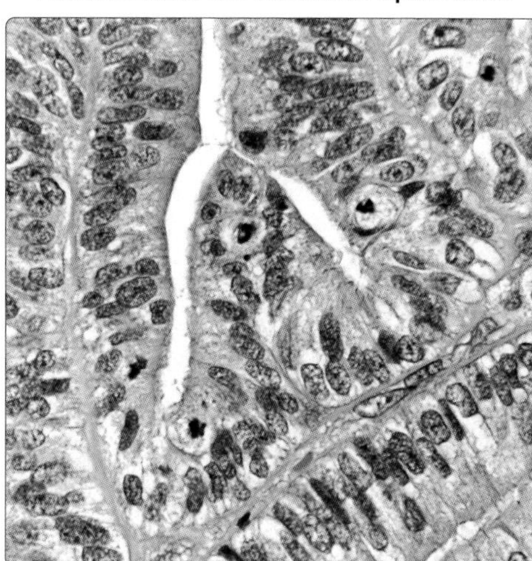

(Left) *This degree of crowding, atypia, and mitotic activity* ➔ *establishes the diagnosis of CPC.* **(Right)** *The pseudostratified, distinctly columnar epithelium is too mitotically active for atypical papilloma.*

Necrosis

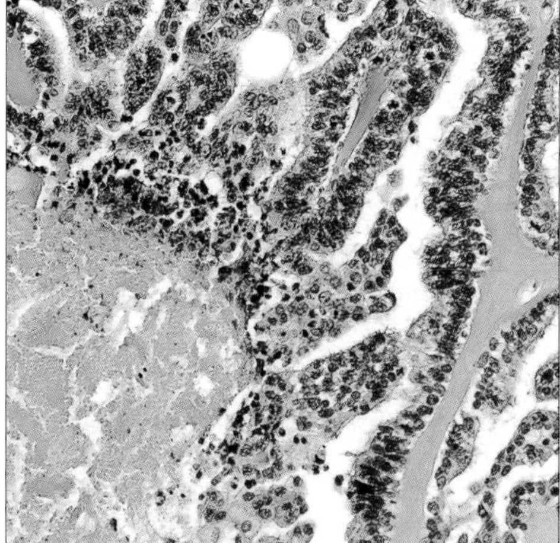

Atypia

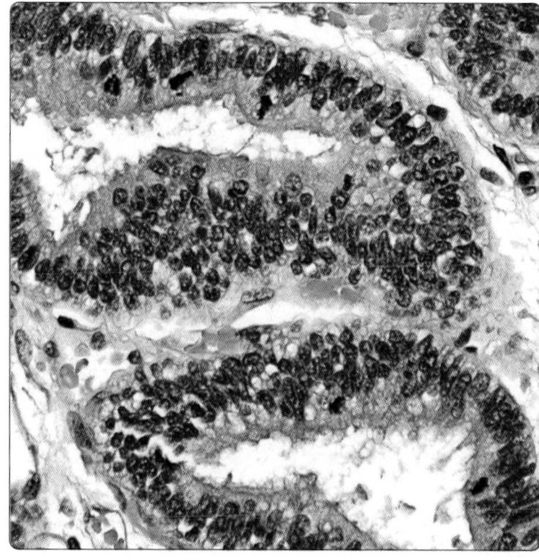

(Left) *While common in CPCs, even ones such as this with well-formed papillae, necrosis is not diagnostic since it occurs in atypical papillomas and even rarely in papillomas.* **(Right)** *This degree of atypia occurs in atypical papillomas, but mitotic activity to this extent requires the diagnosis of carcinoma.*

Extensive Necrosis

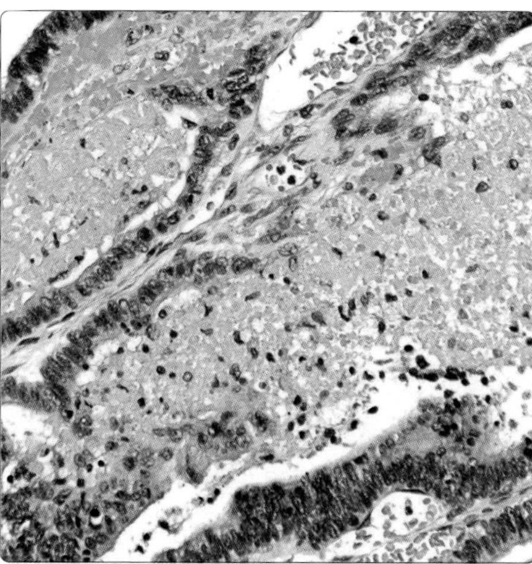

Epithelial Differentiation

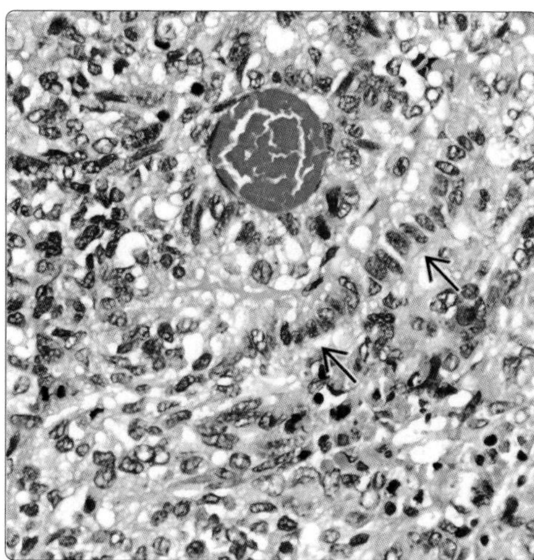

(Left) *Necrosis is extensive in some plexus carcinomas. Only linear fragments of epithelium remain in this case.* **(Right)** *Epithelial differentiation* ➔ *in anaplastic CPCs may be subtle and focal.*

(Left) *Crude papillae and solid, nonpapillary architecture are distinctive features of some plexus carcinomas.* **(Right)** *Epithelial formations ➡, even when subtle, help establish the diagnosis of carcinomas largely undifferentiated. Even this minor degree of epithelial differentiation helps exclude atypical teratoid/rhabdoid tumor.*

Solid Architecture

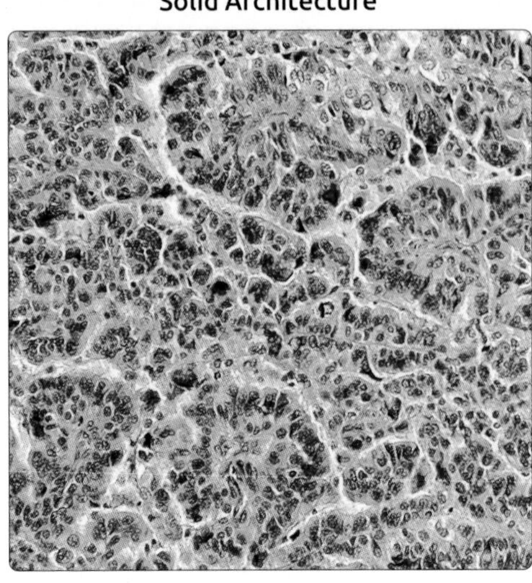

Epithelial Formations

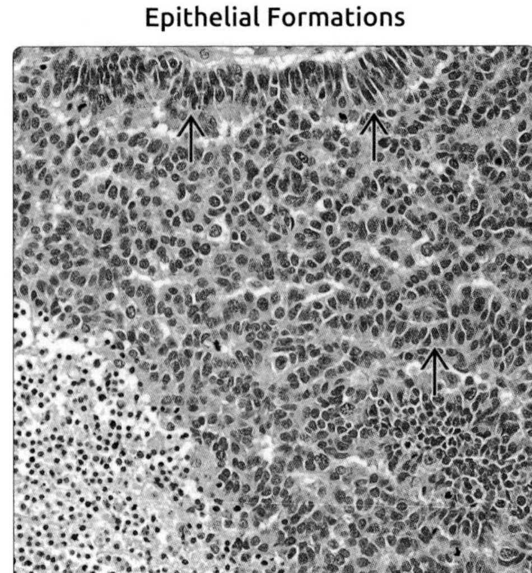

(Left) *Perivascular cell arrangement, while resembling that of ependymoma, is more consistent with an epithelial lesion, such as CPC.* **(Right)** *Focal parallel alignment of tumor cells along a basement membrane ➡ is a clue to the plexus origin of this otherwise undifferentiated tumor.*

Perivascular Cell Arrangement

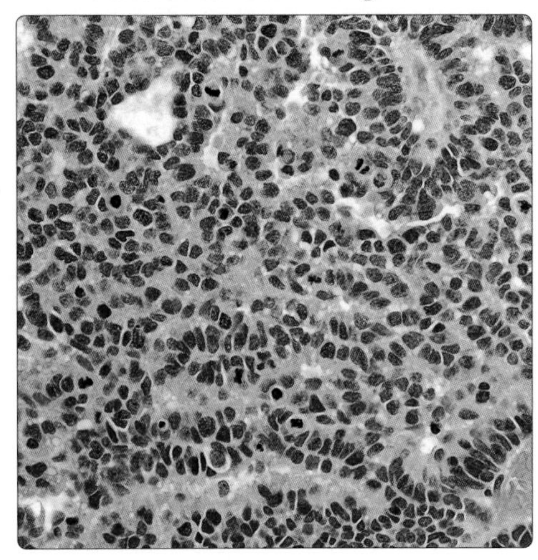

Basement Membrane

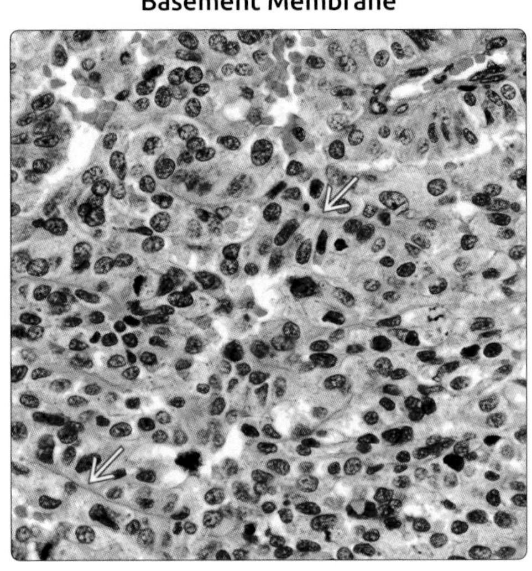

(Left) *The compact, vaguely epithelial architecture is highly suggestive of CPC. A calcospherite ➡ aids somewhat in its identification, but the diagnosis depends largely on epithelial features, subtle in this case. Immunopositivity for appropriate markers is also important.* **(Right)** *In combination, poorly formed papillae, cytological atypia, and mitoses leave no doubt about the diagnosis of CPC.*

Calcospherite

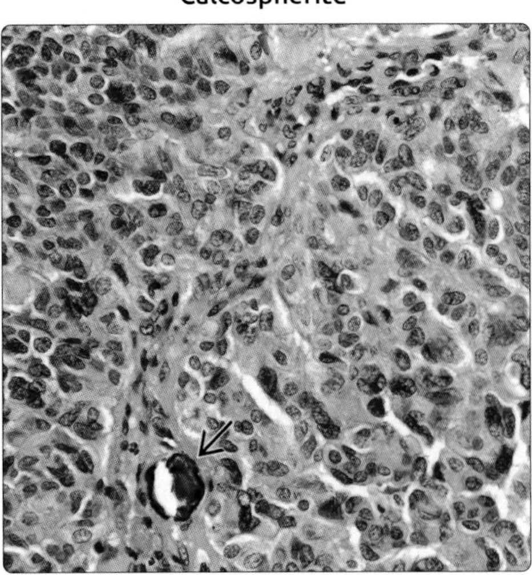

Poorly Formed Papillae

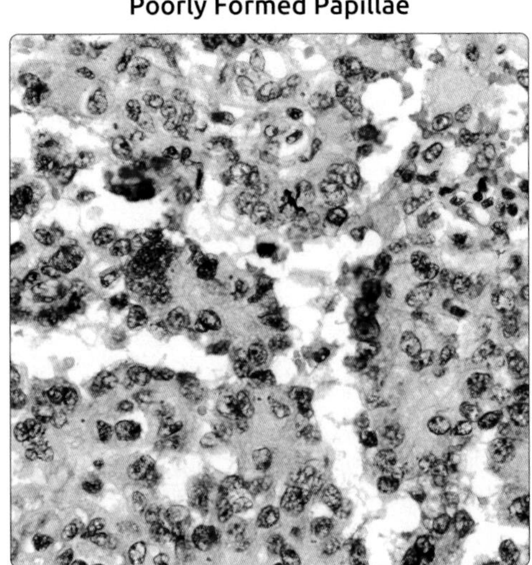

Noninfiltrative Growth

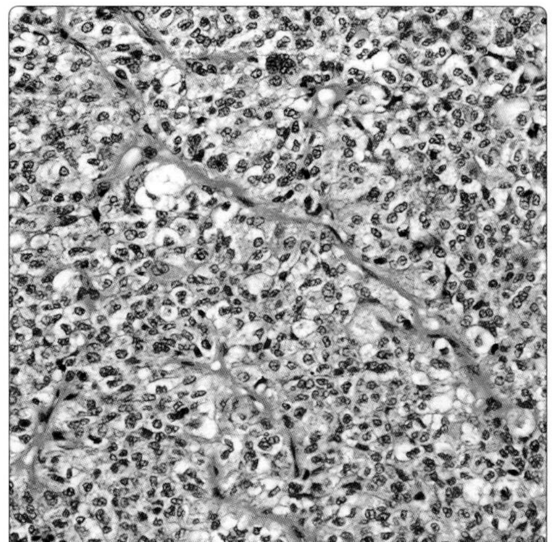

Compact Lesion

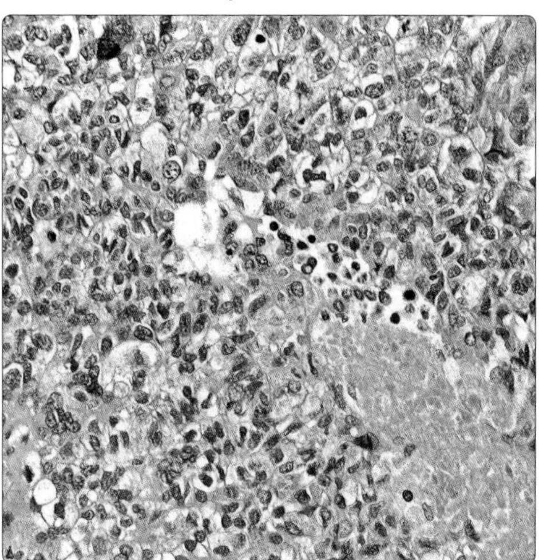

(Left) *Compact, noninfiltrative growth is more consistent with CPC than infiltrating glioma, such as glioblastoma.* **(Right)** *CPC should be high on the list of differential diagnoses in compact intraventricular lesions such as this. Atypical teratoid/rhabdoid tumor would be another possibility. Nuclear staining for INI1/BAF47 would be retained in the carcinoma.*

Solid Sheets of Cells

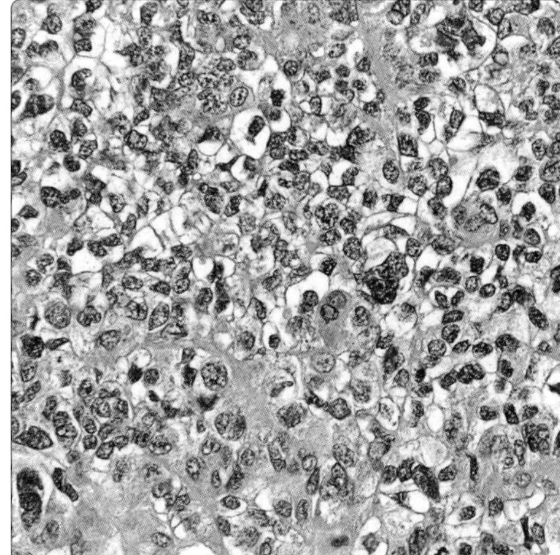

Bizarre Mitoses

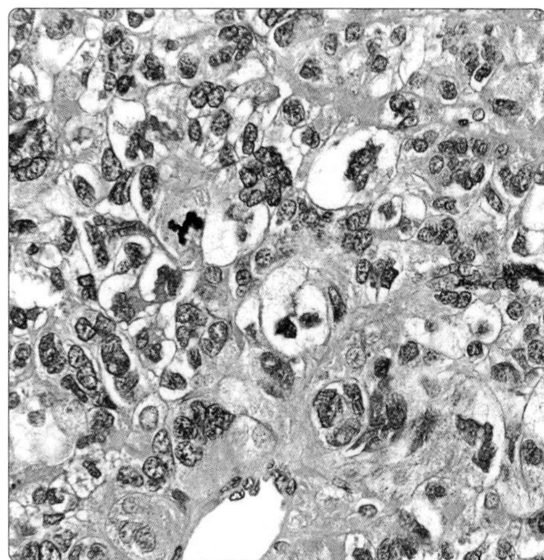

(Left) *Solid sheets of cells lend a vague oligodendroglial appearance to some plexus carcinomas. Atypical teratoid/rhabdoid tumor would also come to mind.* **(Right)** *Bizarre mitoses in a pleomorphic tumor with vague epithelial features occur in some CPCs. This tumor has more multinucleation than most atypical teratoid/rhabdoid tumors.*

Microcysts

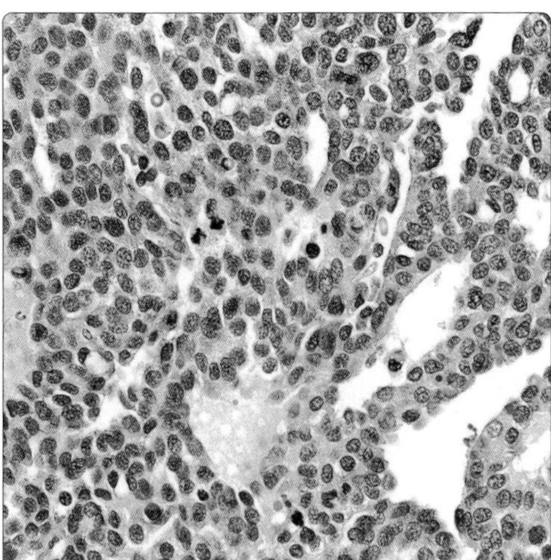

Solid Architecture

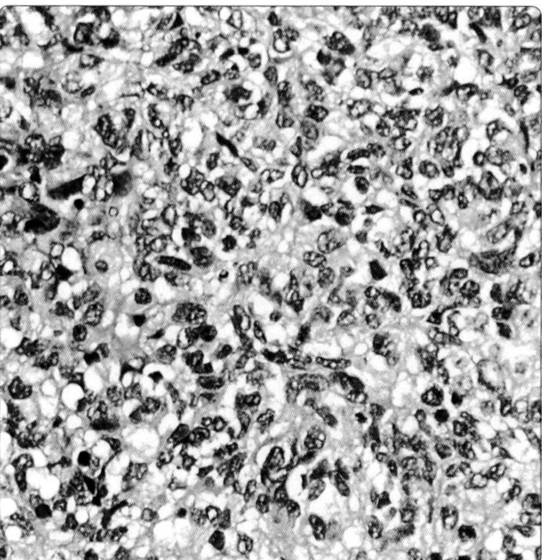

(Left) *Microcysts unassociated with epithelial features are present in some CPCs.* **(Right)** *A definitive diagnosis of CPC depends on the presence of papillary architecture &/or immunopositivity for appropriate markers. A descriptive designation may need to suffice when neither is evident.*

(Left) *CPCs like this with sheet-like growth patterns may resemble atypical teratoid/rhabdoid tumor.* **(Right)** *A rhabdoid quality is present in some CPCs. The distinction between atypical teratoid/rhabdoid tumor (AT/RT) and CPC is made immunohistochemically with antibodies to INI1/BAF47. Both neoplasms favor the very young, but especially AT/RT.*

Sheet-Like Growth

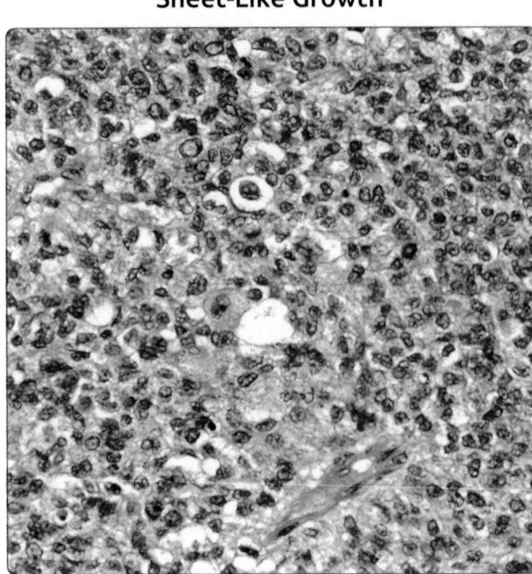

Rhabdoid Quality

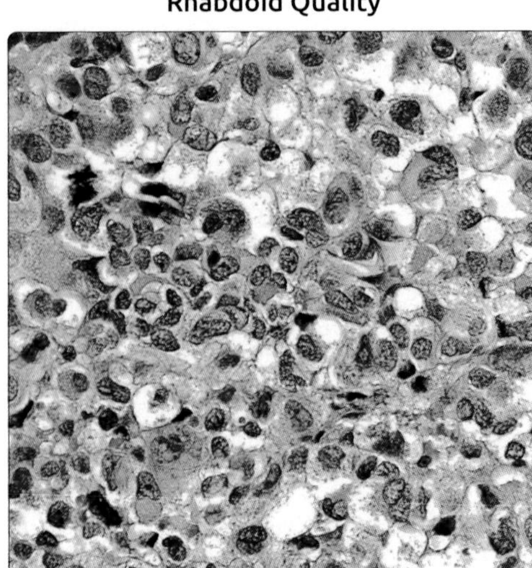

(Left) *Immunohistochemistry &/or the presence of papillary features elsewhere in the specimen would be necessary to establish the nature of undifferentiated lesions such as this.* **(Right)** *Hyaline globules ➙ are present in pleomorphic, cytoplasm-rich areas of some CPCs.*

Undifferentiated Lesion

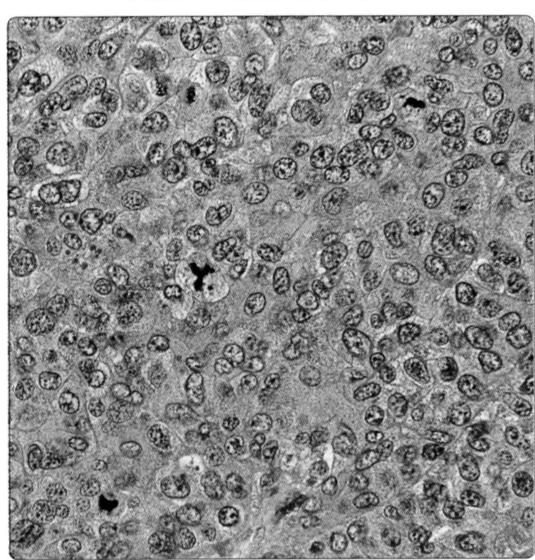

Hyaline Globules

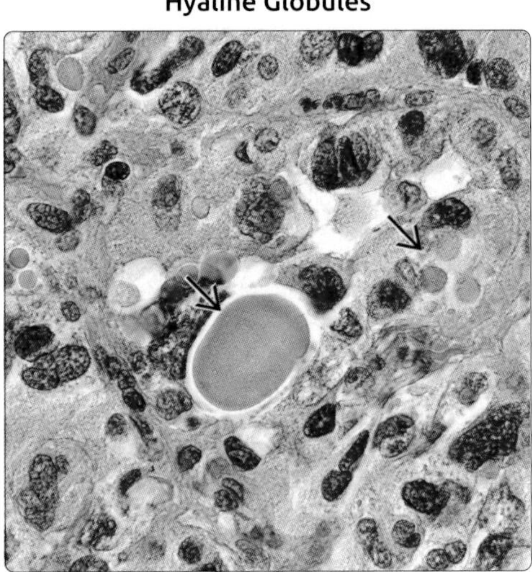

(Left) *Dyscohesive tumor fragments composed of cells with little cytoplasm are consistent with CPC but leave open the possibility of alternative diagnoses.* **(Right)** *Prominent cytoplasm and sharp cell borders suggest an epithelial neoplasm.*

Dyscohesive Tumor Fragments

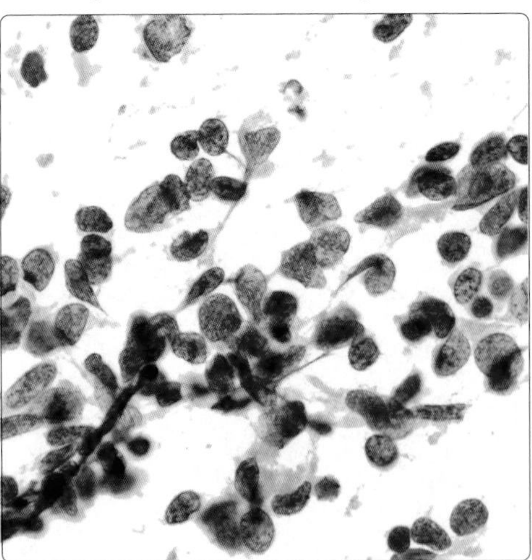

Prominent Cytoplasm

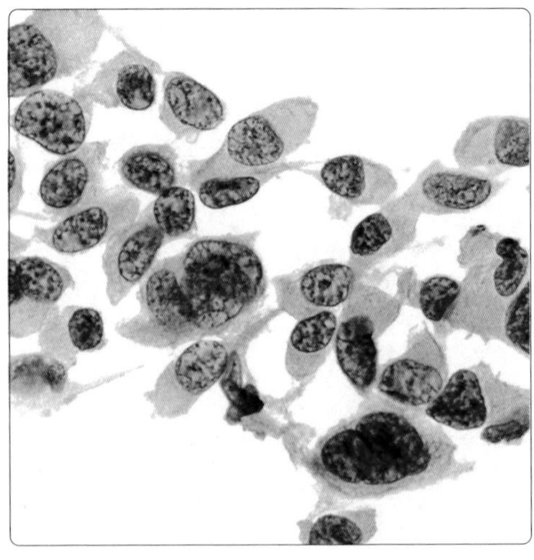

Cytokeratin Expression

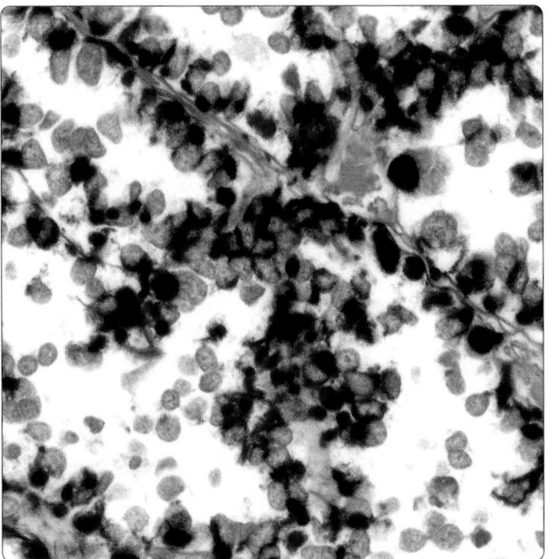

EMA Immunoreactivity

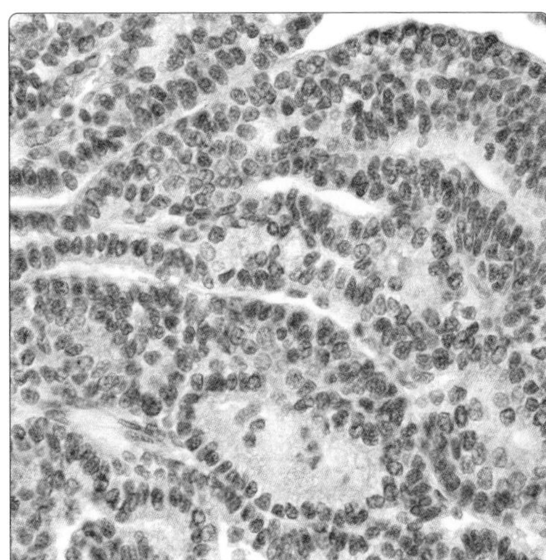

(Left) *Cytokeratin expression is a consistent feature of CPC, which attests to its epithelial nature.* **(Right)** *EMA immunoreactivity is more variable than keratins in choroid plexus neoplasms. Although frequent in carcinomas, it may be weak or altogether negative as in this example.*

S100 Expression

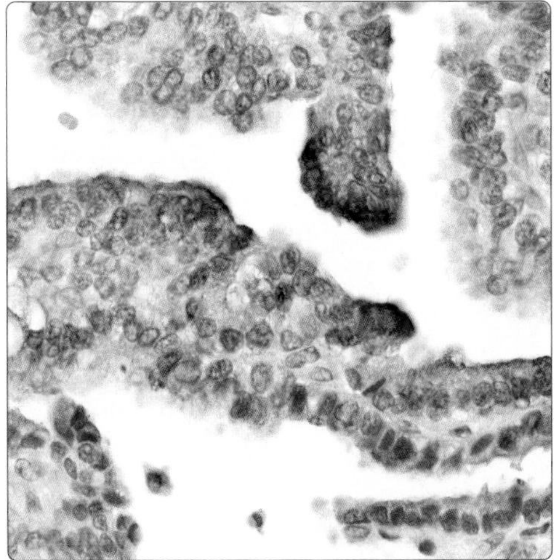

Strong S100 Expression

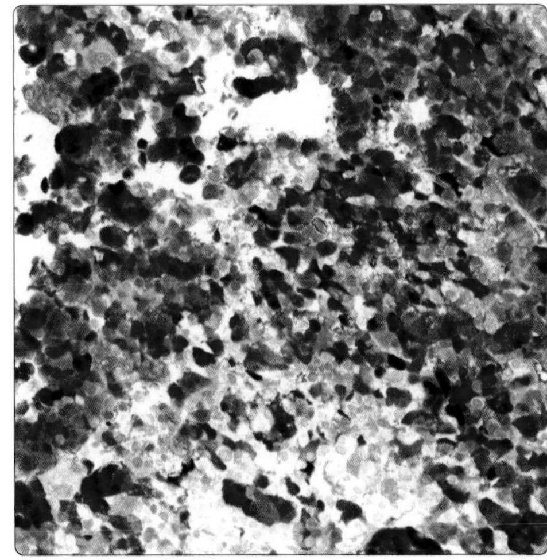

(Left) *S100 expression in CPC is variable but usually present, at least focally.* **(Right)** *S100 expression may be strong in a subset of CPCs.*

Ki-67 Labeling Index

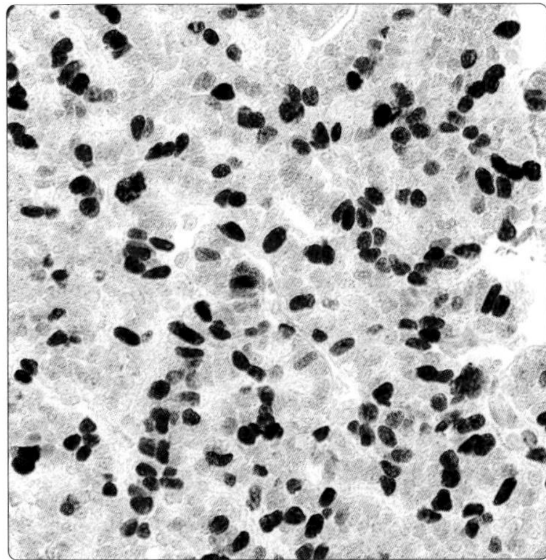

Retained INI1 Expression

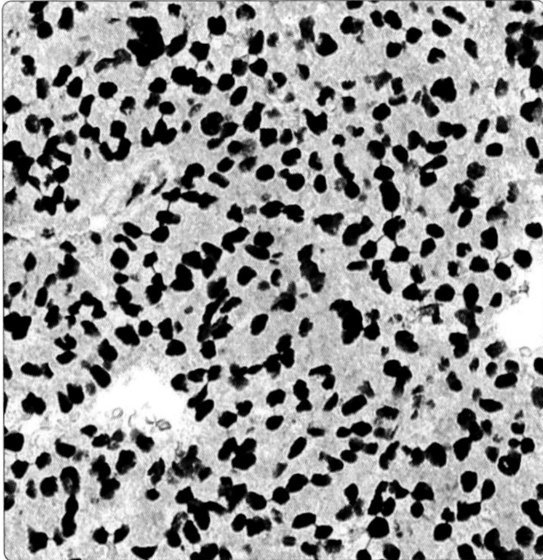

(Left) *A high proliferation rate, represented by a high mitotic rate or Ki-67 labeling index is a consistent feature of CPCs and a main requirement to separate them from atypical or conventional papillomas.* **(Right)** *One of the main differential diagnoses of CPCs is atypical teratoid rhabdoid tumor. The distinction in practical terms can be made by the recognition of INI1 retention in CPCs.*

Ganglion Cell Tumors

KEY FACTS

TERMINOLOGY

- Benign, well-differentiated tumors with dysplastic ganglion cells, either alone (gangliocytoma) or with neoplastic glial component (ganglioglioma)

CLINICAL ISSUES

- Slow growing, indolent
- Frequent history of seizures
- Cyst with enhancing mural nodule, many cases
- Resectable, excellent prognosis, rarely fatal

MICROSCOPIC

- Compact (not infiltrative) with dysplastic neurons
  - Large pleomorphic vesicular hyperchromatic nuclei
  - Irregular apical dendrites, coarse peripheral Nissl
- Pure ganglion cell composition (gangliocytoma) or additional neoplastic glial component, often pilocytic-appearing (ganglioglioma)
- Eosinophilic granular bodies, lymphocytes

ANCILLARY TESTS

- Neoplastic neurons: Positive, granular/surface synaptophysin, neurofilament protein, NeuN
- Glial component and intermediate cells: S100, GFAP positive
- Ki-67 labeling low (< 3%) in glial component

TOP DIFFERENTIAL DIAGNOSES

- Infiltrating glioma with trapped normal neurons
- Pilocytic astrocytoma
- Pleomorphic xanthoastrocytoma

Cyst Mural Nodule

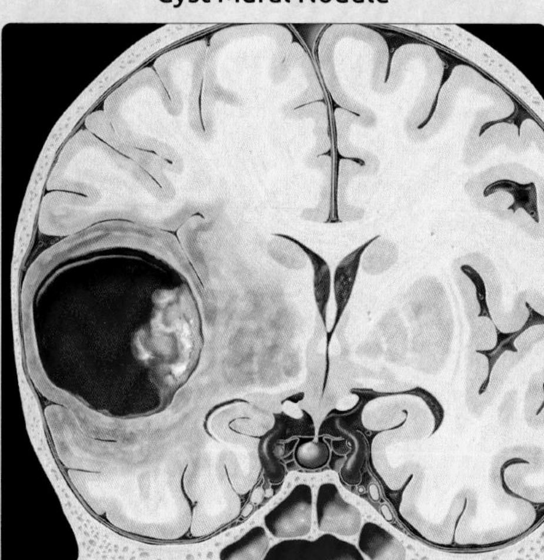

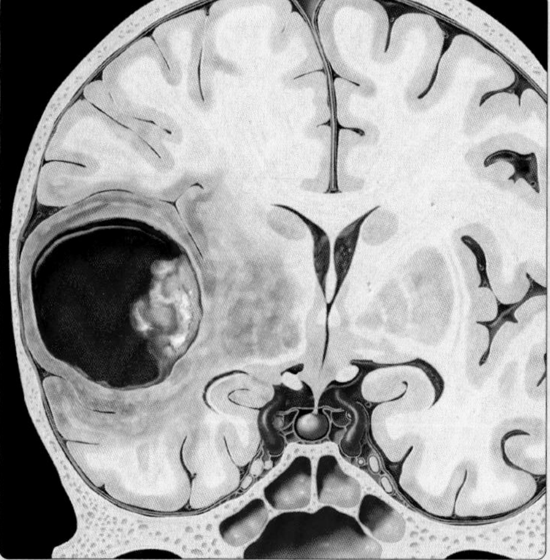

Cystic and Enhancing Components

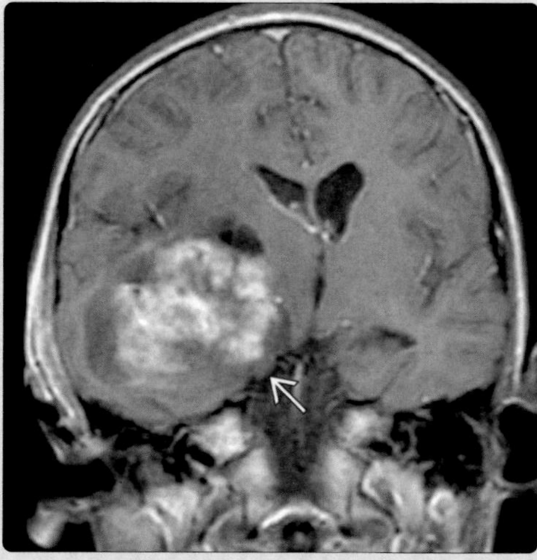

(Left) *Cyst mural nodule architecture typifies ganglion cell tumors (GCTs).* **(Right)** *Coronal T1WI C+ MR shows a large, heterogeneous right temporal mass with cystic and enhancing solid components ➡. Note there is no significant surrounding edema.*

Multinucleated Ganglion Cells

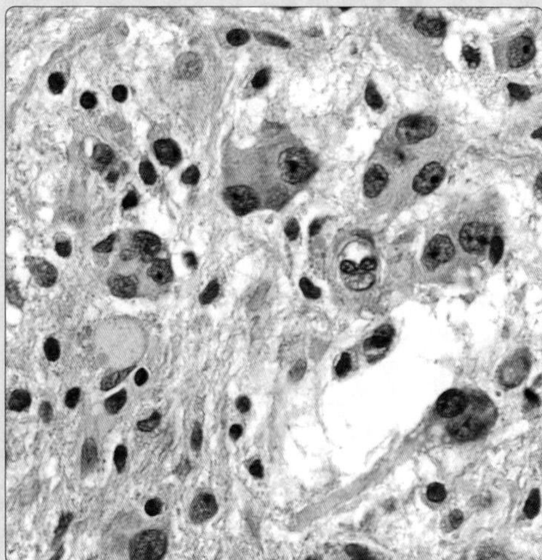

Mutant *BRAF* (V600E) in Ganglion Cells

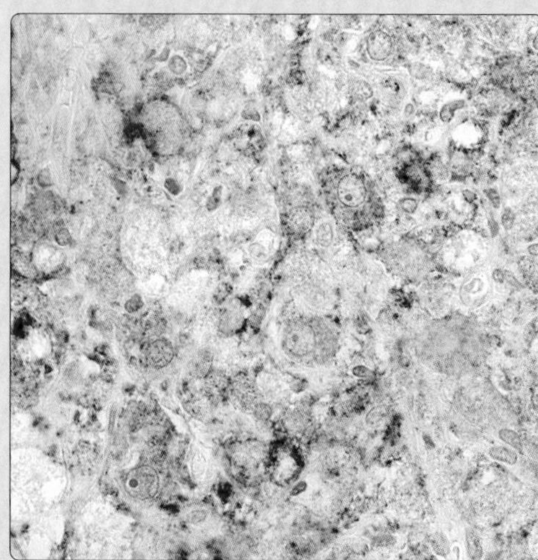

(Left) *Bi- and multinucleated ganglion cells establish the diagnosis of a neuronal neoplasm.* **(Right)** *A subset of gangliogliomas have a BRAF (V600E) mutation that may be detected with antibodies specific against the mutant protein, particularly in the neoplastic ganglion cell component.*

TERMINOLOGY

Abbreviations

- Ganglion cell tumors (GCT)

Definitions

- Well-differentiated tumors composed mainly of large, mature neurons
  - Exclusive ganglion cell composition (gangliocytoma) or mixed ganglion cell and glial elements (ganglioglioma): WHO grade I
    - Diagnostic criteria for WHO grade II ganglion cell tumors not established
  - Anaplastic ganglioglioma: WHO grade III
    - No consensus on grading criteria
    - Substantial mitotic activity
    - Microvascular proliferation in some cases
    - Necrosis in some cases; grade IV designation not applied to GCTs

ETIOLOGY/PATHOGENESIS

Histogenesis

- Gangliocytomas may appear more malformative (hamartomatous) than neoplastic
- Gangliocytomas may be associated with developmental lesions
  - Adjacent cortical dysplasia
- Presumed origin of ganglioglioma from pluripotential progenitor cells showing divergent differentiation to glial and neuronal cells
- Presence of less mature neurons (ganglioid cells) suggests stepwise transformation to larger neurons

CLINICAL ISSUES

Epidemiology

- Incidence
  - Low, < 2% of all brain tumors
- Age
  - All ages but usually children or young adults

Site

- Most supratentorial; predilection for temporal lobe
  - Also cerebellum, optic nerve, brainstem, pineal region, spinal cord, neurohypophysis (rare)

Presentation

- Symptoms may precede diagnosis by several years
  - Seizures
  - Obstructive hydrocephalus, increased intracranial pressure, headaches
  - Site-dependent neurologic deficits

Natural History

- Slowly growing or stable
- Involvement of subarachnoid space not indicative of malignancy
- Aggressive upon rare anaplastic transformation

Treatment

- Surgical approaches
  - Simple, even partial, resection may suffice

Prognosis

- Excellent long-term prognosis
- Infrequent recurrence
- Poor with rare anaplastic transformation
  - Usually of glial component

IMAGING

MR Findings

- Hypointense on T1WI, hyperintense on T2WI
- Cyst with contrast-enhancing mural nodule in classic ganglioglioma
- Solid, nodular, or rim-like enhancement, occasional ganglioglioma
- Solid, noncystic appearance frequent in gangliocytoma
- No enhancement in some gangliocytomas

CT Findings

- Iso- or hypodense, heterogeneous
- Frequent calcification
- Scalloped calvaria in superficial examples

MACROSCOPIC

General Features

- Superficial, corticocentric, &/or subarachnoid location
- Solid or cystic with little mass effect, except for cyst
- Well-circumscribed nodule, often in cyst wall
- Sometimes calcified (gritty)

Sections to Be Submitted

- Entire mural nodule (if small), portion of cyst wall

MICROSCOPIC

Gangliocytoma

- Compact, noninfiltrative growth pattern
  - Cellularity similar to or less than normal gray matter
  - Architecturally disorganized
  - No small neurons, perineuronal oligodendroglia, reactive astrocytes, or microglia
- Neuropil-rich background (neuritic processes)
- Cytologically dysmorphic, multipolar neurons
  - Poorly formed, irregularly arranged apical dendrites
    - Disorganized architecture, not oriented toward pial surface
  - Large, pleomorphic vesicular or hyperchromatic nuclei
    - Bi- or multinucleated, with prominent nucleoli
    - Intranuclear cytoplasmic inclusions
  - Nissl substance
    - Coarse, irregular, peripherally misplaced
    - Absent in many cases
- Ganglioid cells: Less mature, intermediate-sized neurons
- No mitotically active neuroblasts
- Neurodegenerative pathology
  - Related to age
    - Absent in patients < 30 years of age
    - No effect of *APOE* genotypes
  - Granulovacuolar degeneration (cytoplasmic vacuoles with basophilic granules)
  - Tau-related changes

    - Neurofibrillary cytoplasmic, fibrillar and basophilic tangles; argyrophilic, tau protein, and ubiquitin (+)
  - Neuropil threads
  - α-synuclein pathology, minority of cases
- Glomeruloid vasculature in some cases
  - In cyst wall
    - Linear, more telangiectatic than actively proliferating
    - Often associated with hemosiderin
  - May be more glomeruloid in parenchyma
  - No prognostic significance in grade I and II types
  - Microvascular proliferation &/or necrosis in anaplastic transformation
- Reticulin fibers, often perivascular
- Perivascular lymphocytes
  - Common, variable numbers
- Calcifications
  - Scattered small calcospherites, common
  - Dense, confluent ("brain stone")
    - Not specific for GCTs

Ganglioglioma

- Compact growth pattern, overall
- Extension into nearby subarachnoid space
  - Common, not indicative of anaplasia
- Neuronal component
  - Vesicular, often multiple nuclei, prominent nucleoli
  - Variable Nissl substance
  - Neuronal component sometimes inconspicuous, requiring immunohistochemistry for neuronal markers
  - 2 patterns: Compact nodules or dispersed individual neoplastic ganglion cells
- Glial component, mixed or geographically separate
  - Astrocytic; pilocytic or fibrillary-like
  - Often lobular architecture
    - Nests of neoplastic cells, trapped or encircled
    - Reticulin-, collagen-rich interlobular stroma, ± lymphocytes
  - Microcyst-rich pattern
    - Smaller ganglion cells and piloid glia
    - May mimic pilocytic astrocytoma
  - Mixed ganglion cells, astrocytes in fibrillar stroma
- Eosinophilic granular bodies
- Desmoplasia
  - Especially with tumors involving subarachnoid space
    - Trichrome positive, reticulin-rich

Histologic Variants

- Anaplastic ganglioglioma, WHO grade III
  - Anaplastic component usually glial, GFAP(+)
    - Frequent mitoses, necrosis; may resemble conventional anaplastic astrocytoma or glioblastoma
    - Aggressive, like malignant gliomas; tend to recur
    - Diagnose only when clear neuronal component present; infiltrating gliomas with trapped normal neurons far more frequent
  - Anaplastic neuronal component
    - Rare
    - Overlaps practically and conceptually with ganglioneuroblastoma and primitive neuroectodermal tumor (PNET); criteria unclear
  - Sarcomatous change in anaplastic ganglioglioma, rare

ANCILLARY TESTS

Cytology

- Ganglion cells better preserved than in frozen sections
  - Larger, rounder than normal ganglion cells
  - Ample cytoplasm
  - Nuclei
    - Open chromatin
    - Prominent nucleoli
    - Nissl substance coarse and peripheral
- Fibrillar background of glial cell processes
- Eosinophilic granular bodies
- Lymphocytes

Histochemistry

- Trichrome and reticulin
  - Reactivity: Positive in desmoplastic areas

Immunohistochemistry

- Synaptophysin
  - Fine granular surface staining of ganglion cells, but not specific for neoplastic neurons
- Chromogranin: Punctate cytoplasmic staining in ganglion cells
- NeuN
  - Best stains for nonneoplastic neurons
  - Nuclei positive in some cases, but may be negative
  - Negative result of little diagnostic significance
- GFAP(+) glial component, intermediate cells, and reactive astrocytes
- Some tumor cells positive for both neuronal and glial markers
- S100(+) in glial and variable in neuronal cells
- CD34
  - Tumor cells positive, variable percentage colabel with S100 or neuronal (NeuN) markers
  - Large protoplasmic astrocytes in surrounding cortex positive
- Neuropeptides: Vasoactive intestinal peptide, enkephalins, dopamine, tyrosine hydroxylase, serotonin, β-hydroxylase, somatostatin, and substance-P may be positive
- Collagen IV and laminin positive in desmoplastic tumors
- Ki-67: Very low index in glial component and negative in neuronal component
- BRAF V600E immunopositivity in mutant cases
  - Stronger in neuronal component
  - Negative prognosticator in pediatric ganglioglioma in 1 study

Genetic Testing

- MAPK pathway activation
  - *BRAF* (V600E) point mutation, in up to 50% of cases
    - *KIAA1549:BRAF* fusion rare (unlike pilocytic astrocytoma)
- Abnormalities of tuberous sclerosis genes (*TSC1* and *TSC2*) may play role
- Gains of chromosomes 5, 7, 8, and 12; loss of chromosomes 9, 10, and 22 most common
- Pediatric posterior fossa and spinal cord gangliogliomas separated into 2 clinicopathologic and molecular subgroups in recent study

- Group I (classic gangliogliomas): *BRAF* (V600E) mutation in subset, lack of *KIAA1549:BRAF*
- Group II (pilocytic astrocytoma with foci of gangliocytic differentiation): Frequent *KIAA1549:BRAF*
- Possible relation of *BRAF* (V600E) mutation with prognosis in gangliogliomas controversial

Electron Microscopy

- Dense core granules in ganglion cells
  - Inconspicuous in normal CNS neurons
- Synaptic junctions, neurosecretory vesicles
- Intermediate filaments and basal lamina in astrocytes

DIFFERENTIAL DIAGNOSIS

Normal Brain

- Ordered, organized complexity
- Layered cortical architecture, with apical dendrites directed to cortical surface, but
  - No layering in normal deep gray matter (basal ganglia and thalamus)
- Cytologically normal neurons only rarely binucleate
- Perineuronal ("satellite") oligodendroglia
- No calcifications

Infiltrating Glioma With Trapped Normal Neurons

- Consider in cases of suspected anaplastic ganglioglioma
- Much more common than GCT
- Especially oligodendroglioma, but also diffuse astrocytoma
- Normal cortical neurons
  - Polar cytoplasm, apical dendrites oriented toward pial surface
  - Size variation not present to extent seen in GCT
  - Cytologically atypical (neoplastic) perineuronal "satellite" glial cells
  - Trapped native neurons within tumors may acquire cytologic abnormalities but no abnormal clustering or binucleation
- Reactive, "activated" microglia; CD68, CD45, HAM56(+)
- *IDH1*/*IDH2* mutations characteristic of infiltrating glioma

Meningioangiomatosis With Trapped Cortical Ganglion Cells

- Plaque-like intracortical lesion; not round or cystic mass
- Perivascular fibroblastic or meningothelial cells deep into cortex
  - EMA(+), some cases
- Laminated psammoma bodies, not nondescript calcospherites
- Associated meningioma, some cases

Cortical Dysplasia and Tubers

- No cyst or compact architecture
  - Abnormal neurons in cortex, subcortical white matter
  - Large, glassy cells (balloon cells); PAS, S100(+)
- No perivascular lymphocytes
- Hyperintensity, T2W and FLAIR MR, in underlying white matter

Hypothalamic Hamartoma

- Nonneoplastic malformative lesion with classic location
- Solid, little or no mass effect
- Essentially identical to nonneoplastic gray matter, little dysmorphism
- No enhancement on MR

Dysplastic Cerebellar Gangliocytoma (Lhermitte-Duclos Disease)

- Site specific; cerebellum
- Association with Cowden syndrome
- Pathognomonic radiological appearance
- Differentiation of internal granule cells to large ganglion cells
- Myelinated axons in abnormal molecular layer

Desmoplastic Infantile Ganglioglioma

- Solid, dura-attached, superficial mass with surrounding cyst
- Markedly desmoplastic
- GFAP(+) glia
- Neurons smaller than conventional ganglion cells (ganglioid cells)
  - Overlap in size and shape with neoplastic astrocytes
- Highly cellular, mitotically active PNET-like area, some cases

Neurocytic Tumors With Ganglion Cell Component

- Predominant population of small neurocytes
  - Monotonous, oligodendroglioma-like
- Ganglion cell and glial component, some cases (ganglioglioneurocytoma)

Dysembryoplastic Neuroepithelial Tumor

- Cortical lesion
  - Normal background of cortical cells, including ganglion cells
- Usually solid, not cystic
- Patterned, nodular architecture
- Prominent component of oligodendroglia-like cells
- Large neurons "floating" in micropools of mucin
  - Little dysmorphism, clustering, or atypia
- Axons ensheathed by oligodendroglioma-like cells in "specific glioneuronal element"
  - May be difficult to find
  - Appropriate plane of section needed for its detection
- Mucoid background, Alcian blue positive
  - Nodules especially positive
- No desmoplasia
- Few, if any, eosinophilic granular bodies (EGB)s in nodules
- No chronic inflammation

Pleomorphic Xanthoastrocytoma (PXA)

- Large, pleomorphic, spindle to epithelioid astrocytes, some lipidized
- Coarse and delicate granular bodies
- Minor infiltration of cortex and white matter
- Trapped nonneoplastic neurons
- Anaplastic features in pleomorphic xanthoastrocytoma component (~ 15% of cases)
- Composite pleomorphic xanthoastrocytoma-ganglioglioma far less common
  - Difficult practical and conceptual distinction between GCT and PXA with ganglion cell component

Pilocytic Astrocytoma

- Classic lesion without neoplastic ganglion cells

- May contain some synaptophysin (+) cells
- Pilocytic astrocytoma with neuronal component
  - Difficult practical and conceptual distinction from GCT
  - Glial component of ganglioglioma often pilocytic

Subependymal Giant Cell Astrocytoma (Tuberous Sclerosis)

- Tuberous sclerosis complex association in most cases
- Site specific; near foramen of Monro
- Mixed glioneuronal immunophenotype
- Large cells, some with ganglion cell features, but usually not full ganglion cell phenotype
- No chronic inflammation, but mast cells frequent

Embryonal Tumors With Ganglion Cell Differentiation

- Medulloblastoma
  - Predominant small round blue cell component except in highly differentiated nodular/desmoplastic examples
  - Posttreatment maturation and small cell depletion, some cases
- Ganglioneuroblastoma
  - Concomitant, ganglion cell and small round blue cell component
  - Lesions with more equal ratios of differentiated to undifferentiated cells
  - Practical and conceptual overlap with GCT with only focal immature neurons or neuroblasts

Ganglion Cell Metaplasia

- Pituitary adenoma
  - Site specific: Sella
  - Varying population of adenoma cells, often GH or ACTH producing
- Gliomas, especially oligodendroglioma
  - Focal phenomenon in otherwise typical infiltrating oligodendroglioma
  - Synaptophysin (+) in 20%
  - 1p/19q codeletion, including ganglion cells of oligodendrogliomas
- Paraganglioma
  - Site specific: Filum terminale
  - Dominant population of chief cells
- ATRT
  - Extremely rare

Multinodular and Vacuolating Neuronal Tumors of Cerebrum

- Recently described neuronal tumors occurring in cerebrum of adults
- Low grade, excellent prognosis
- Nodular architecture
- Cell component varies from overtly neuronal to cytologically ambiguous
- Nuclear reactivity for HuC/HuD neuronal markers
- Variable reactivity for conventional neuronal markers (synaptophysin, chromogranin, neurofilament protein)

DIAGNOSTIC CHECKLIST

Pathologic Interpretation Pearls

- Perivascular sprinkling of lymphocytes often clue to presence of GCT
- Rule out infiltrating glioma with entrapped neurons

SELECTED REFERENCES

1. Donson AM et al: Pediatric brainstem gangliogliomas show BRAF(V600E) mutation in a high percentage of cases. Brain Pathol. 24(2):173-83, 2014
2. Gupta K et al: Posterior fossa and spinal gangliogliomas form two distinct clinicopathologic and molecular subgroups. Acta Neuropathol Commun. 2:18, 2014
3. Krishnan C et al: Atypical teratoid/rhabdoid tumor with ganglioglioma-like differentiation: case report and review of the literature. Hum Pathol. 45(1):185-8, 2014
4. Lummus SC et al: Massive dissemination from spinal cord gangliogliomas negative for BRAF V600E: report of two rare adult cases. Am J Clin Pathol. 142(2):254-60, 2014
5. Yust-Katz S et al: Clinical and prognostic features of adult patients with gangliogliomas. Neuro Oncol. 16(3):409-13, 2014
6. Dahiya S et al: BRAF(V600E) mutation is a negative prognosticator in pediatric ganglioglioma. Acta Neuropathol. 125(6):901-10, 2013
7. Huse JT et al: Multinodular and vacuolating neuronal tumors of the cerebrum: 10 cases of a distinctive seizure-associated lesion. Brain Pathol. 23(5):515-24, 2013
8. Koelsche C et al: Mutant BRAF V600E protein in ganglioglioma is predominantly expressed by neuronal tumor cells. Acta Neuropathol. 125(6):891-900, 2013
9. Horbinski C et al: Isocitrate dehydrogenase 1 analysis differentiates gangliogliomas from infiltrative gliomas. Brain Pathol. 21(5):564-74, 2011
10. Perry A et al: Oligodendroglial neoplasms with ganglioglioma-like maturation: a diagnostic pitfall. Acta Neuropathol. 120(2):237-52, 2010
11. Piao YS et al: Neuropathological findings in intractable epilepsy: 435 Chinese cases. Brain Pathol. 20(5):902-8, 2010
12. Luyken C et al: Supratentorial gangliogliomas: histopathologic grading and tumor recurrence in 184 patients with a median follow-up of 8 years. Cancer. 101(1):146-55, 2004
13. Yin XL et al: Genome-wide survey for chromosomal imbalances in ganglioglioma using comparative genomic hybridization. Cancer Genet Cytogenet. 134(1):71-6, 2002
14. Becker AJ et al: Mutational analysis of TSC1 and TSC2 genes in gangliogliomas. Neuropathol Appl Neurobiol. 27(2):105-14, 2001
15. Brat DJ et al: Tau-associated neuropathology in ganglion cell tumours increases with patient age but appears unrelated to ApoE genotype. Neuropathol Appl Neurobiol. 27(3):197-205, 2001
16. Raghavan R et al: Alpha-synuclein expression in central nervous system tumors showing neuronal or mixed neuronal/glial differentiation. J Neuropathol Exp Neurol. 59(6):490-4, 2000
17. Blümcke I et al: The CD34 epitope is expressed in neoplastic and malformative lesions associated with chronic, focal epilepsies. Acta Neuropathol. 97(5):481-90, 1999
18. Lindboe CF et al: Epiperikaryal synaptophysin reactivity in the normal human central nervous system. Clin Neuropathol. 17(5):237-40, 1998
19. Quinn B: Synaptophysin staining in normal brain: importance for diagnosis of ganglioglioma. Am J Surg Pathol. 22(5):550-6, 1998
20. Hirose T et al: Ganglioglioma: an ultrastructural and immunohistochemical study. Cancer. 79(5):989-1003, 1997
21. Perry A et al: Composite pleomorphic xanthoastrocytoma and ganglioglioma: report of four cases and review of the literature. Am J Surg Pathol. 21(7):763-71, 1997
22. Zhang PJ et al: Synaptophysin expression in the human spinal cord. Diagnostic implications of an immunohistochemical study. Am J Surg Pathol. 20(3):273-6, 1996
23. Prayson RA et al: Cortical architectural abnormalities and MIB1 immunoreactivity in gangliogliomas: a study of 60 patients with intracranial tumors. J Neuropathol Exp Neurol. 54(4):513-20, 1995
24. Wolf HK et al: Ganglioglioma: a detailed histopathological and immunohistochemical analysis of 61 cases. Acta Neuropathol. 88(2):166-73, 1994

Binucleate Ganglion Cell

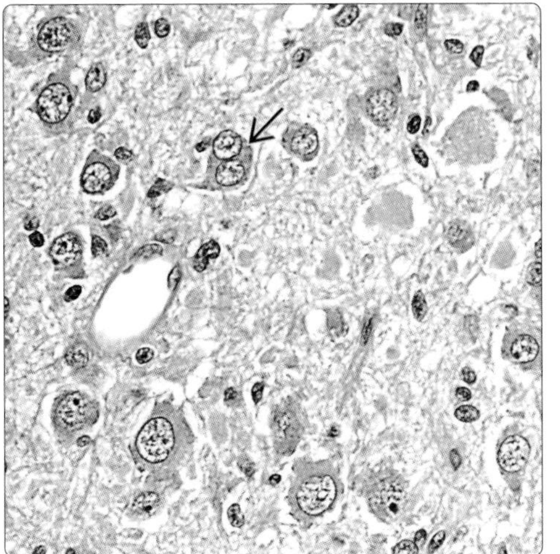

Closely Packed Cells

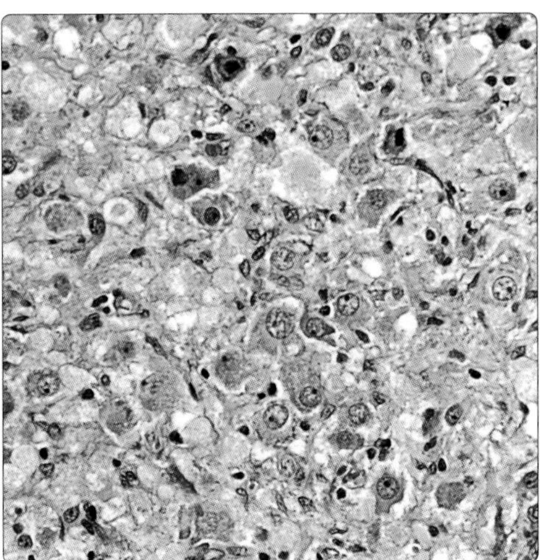

(Left) *Gangliocytomas include paucicellular lesions that are more hamartomatous than neoplastic. While such lesions may resemble normal brain, their disorganized and abnormally juxtaposed neurons are clearly abnormal; some are even binucleate ➙.* **(Right)** *Gangliocytomas vary in cellularity and ratio of nuclei to anucleate fibrillar background. Nuclei are closely packed in this gangliocytoma with little intervening neuropil.*

Binucleate Ganglion Cell

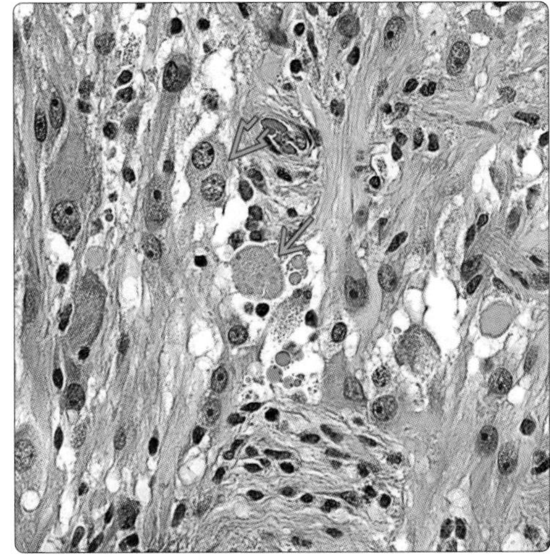

Eosinophilic Granular Body

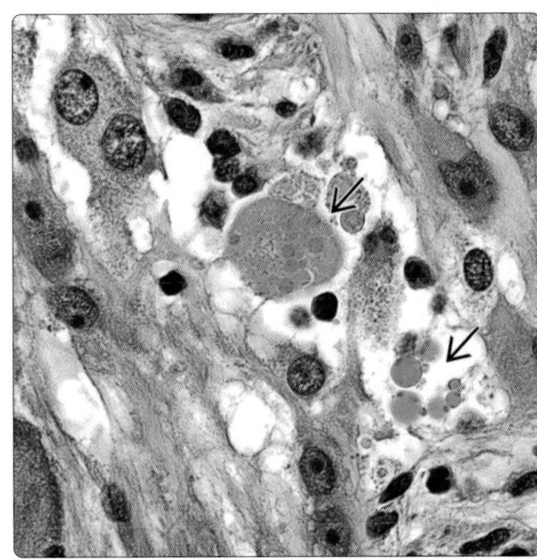

(Left) *Ganglion cells have copious cytoplasm, round nuclei, and prominent nucleoli. A binucleate example ➙ and an eosinophilic granular body (EGB) are present ➙.* **(Right)** *EGBs are packaged accumulations of hyaline droplets ➙ common in longstanding neuronal tumors. They also populate other low-grade, circumscribed tumors, such as pleomorphic xanthoastrocytoma and pilocytic astrocytoma.*

Lymphoid Aggregates

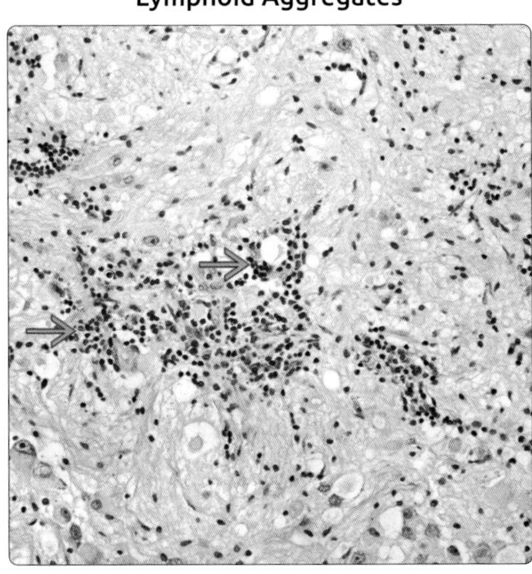

Abnormal Ganglion Cells

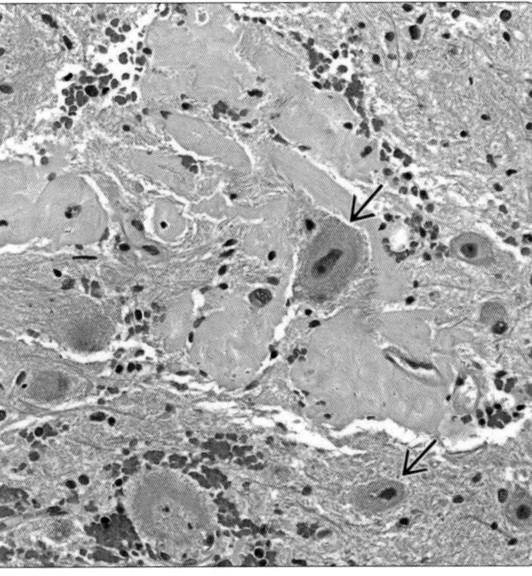

(Left) *Hematoxylin and eosin shows a medium-power view of a ganglioglioma with prominent lymphoid aggregates, most of which are perivascular ➙. Perivascular lymphocytes are characteristic of, but not exclusive to, GCTs and should prompt consideration of the diagnosis.* **(Right)** *Hyalinized vessels and large abnormal ganglion cells ➙ indicate this is a gangliocytoma, not normal gray matter. The distinction is not always easy, however, especially in small, fragmented specimens.*

(Left) *Microcalcifications (calcospherites) in a gangliocytoma may be more conspicuous than the ganglion cells* →. **(Right)** *Lamellated, geode-like mineralization may be seen in longstanding GCTs. While distinctive, it is in no way diagnostic of a neuronal tumor; it occurs in other lesions, such as low-grade gliomas. Calcification to this degree is a marker of chronicity, whatever the host lesion.*

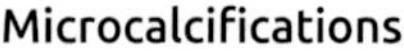

Microcalcifications

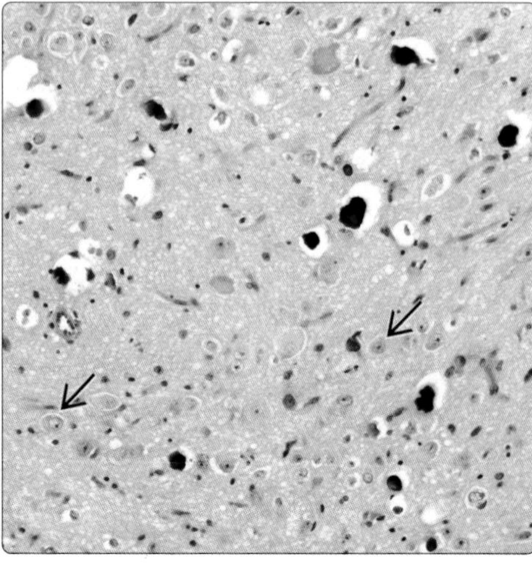

Lamellated, Geode-Like Mineralization

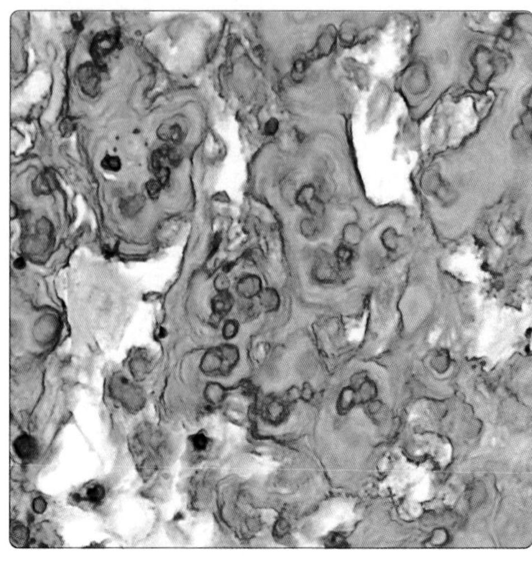

(Left) *Perivascular lymphocytes in a CNS tumor should suggest the possibility of a GCT. Prominent nucleoli and binucleation* → *distinguish this GCT from pleomorphic glioma.* **(Right)** *Fine neuronal processes create a coarse neuropil between cytologically abnormal ganglion cells. An eosinophilic granular body* → *is a helpful finding.*

Perivascular Lymphocytes and Binucleation

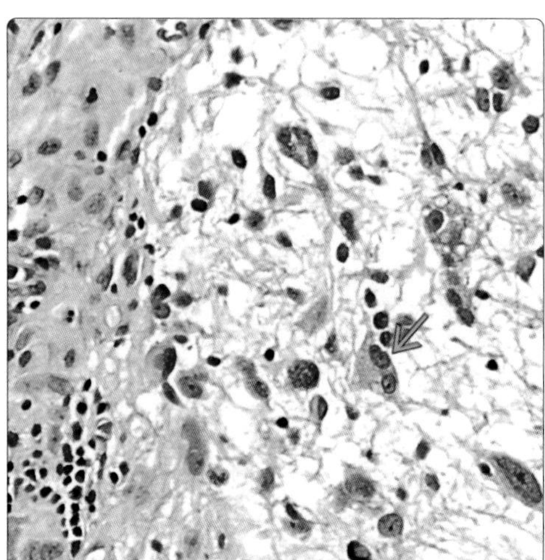

Coarse Neuropil

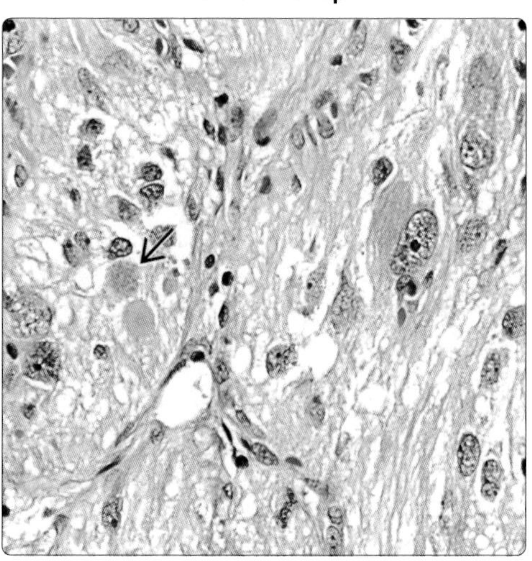

(Left) *Ganglion cells varying in size and pleomorphism may suggest astrocytoma rather than ganglioglioma. Prominent nucleoli, at least in some cells, are clues to the tumor's neuronal nature. Immunostaining may resolve the issue in cellular, pleomorphic lesions, such as this.* **(Right)** *Both neurofibrillary change* → *and granulovacuolar degeneration* ➡ *are present in some longstanding GCTs.*

Pleomorphism

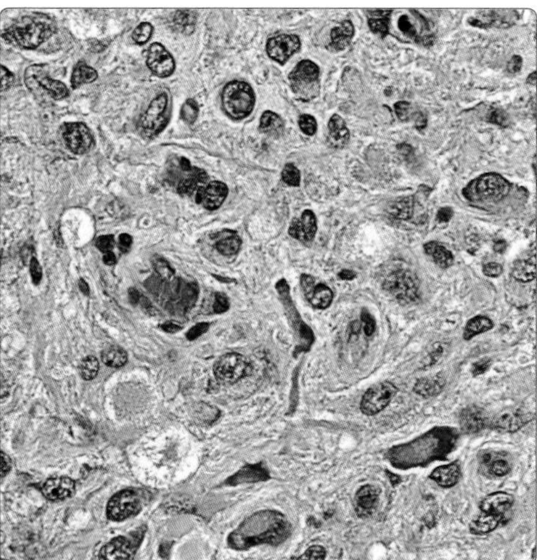

Neurofibrillary Change and Granulovacuolar Degeneration

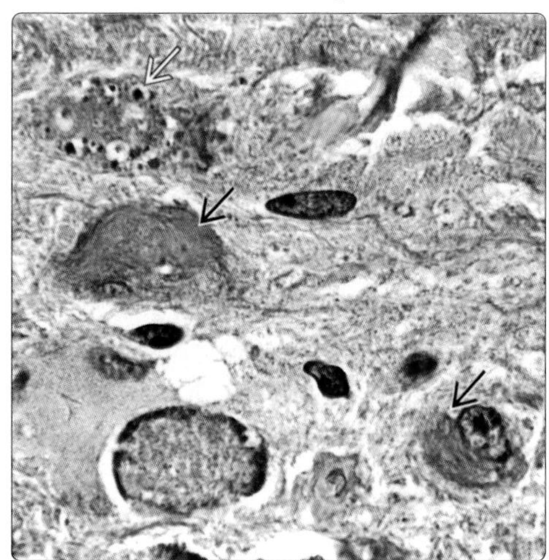

Perivascular Chronic Inflammation

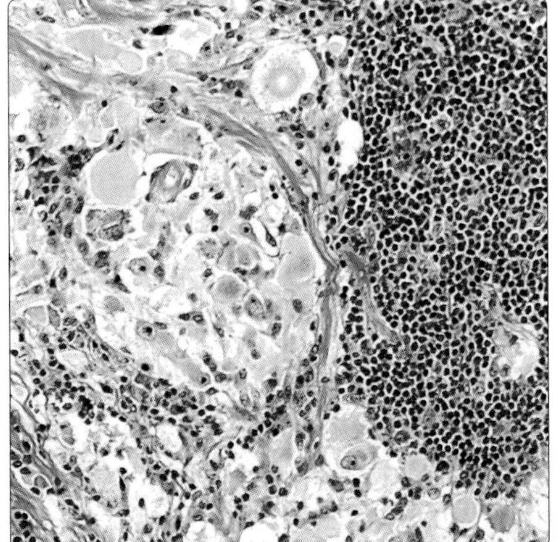

Prominent Nucleoli

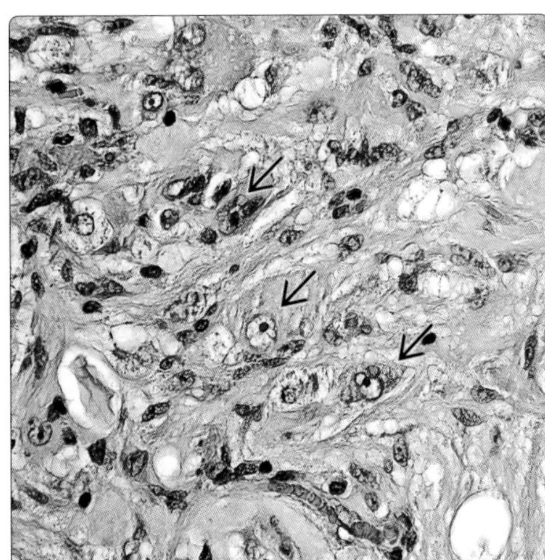

(Left) *Perivascular chronic inflammation, common in GCTs, may be very prominent. At low magnification, the large tumor cell-lymphocyte combination might even prompt consideration of germinoma.* **(Right)** *Prominent nucleoli are giveaway features in GCTs, such as this ganglioglioma, wherein ganglion cells ⇒ blend in with the background and resemble astrocytes.*

Intratumoral Lymphocytes

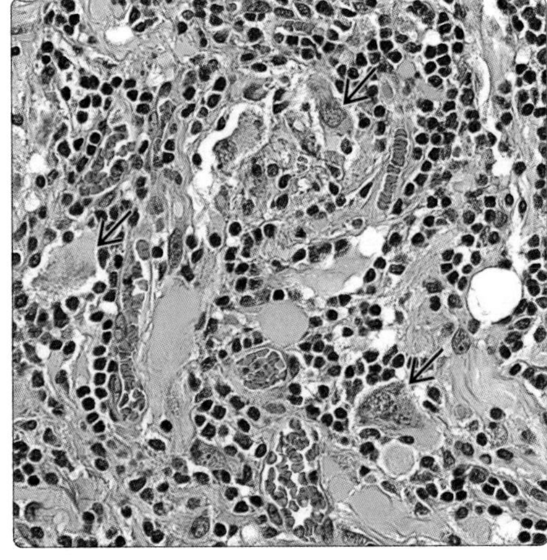

Perivascular Inflammation

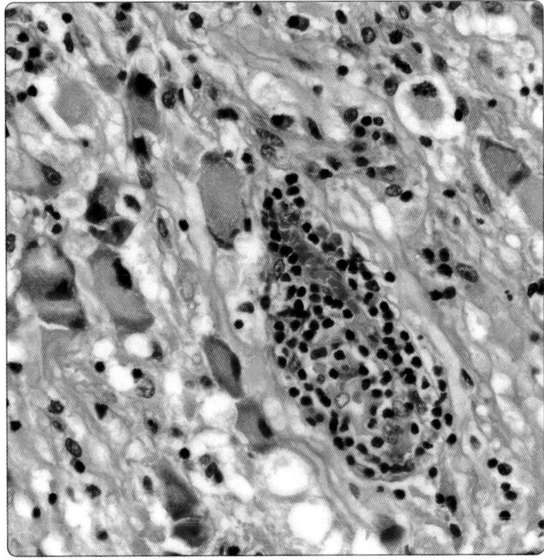

(Left) *Intratumoral lymphocytes are often clues as to the diagnosis of a GCT. Here, ganglion cells ⇒ hide, germinoma-like, in a dominant lymphoid infiltrate.* **(Right)** *Chronic inflammatory changes are commonly present in gangliogliomas. Perivascular inflammation may raise the possibility of an inflammatory disorder, but the aggregates of large, abnormal ganglion cells are diagnostic of a neoplasm.*

Organoid Architecture

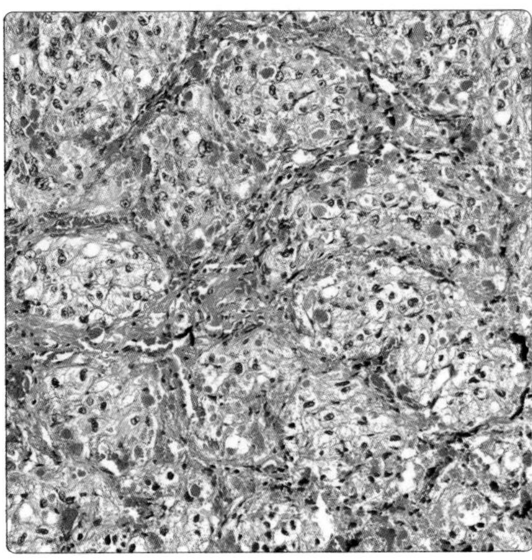

Perivascular Lymphocytes

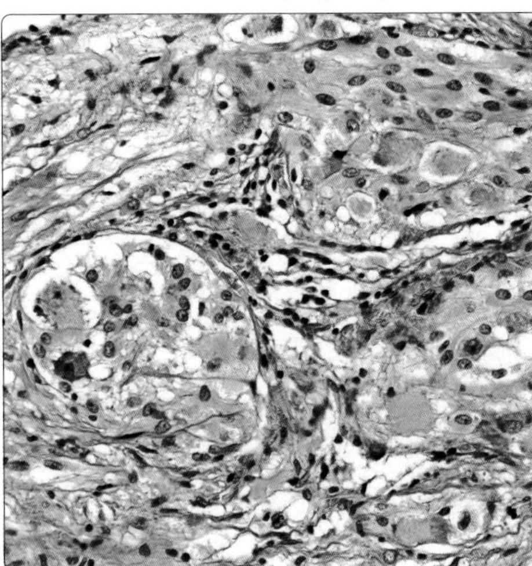

(Left) *Some gangliogliomas have an organoid or nested architecture.* **(Right)** *As in this ganglioglioma, the difference between neuronal and glial components may be subtle; some cells having neither clearly defined neuronal nor glial features. While nonspecific, perivascular lymphocytes, even in small numbers, are consistent with GCT.*

(Left) *Conventional gangliogliomas such as this may overlap with desmoplastic infantile ganglioglioma (DIG) in the degree of desmoplasia. Small ganglion cells interspersed in the stroma* ⇒ *are difficult to identify, just as they are in DIG.* **(Right)** *Here, ganglioid cells* ⇒ *hide in the Masson trichrome positive stroma of a noninfantile desmoplastic ganglioglioma. Immunohistochemistry for synaptophysin and GFAP may be necessary to identify neuronal and glial components, respectively.*

Desmoplasia

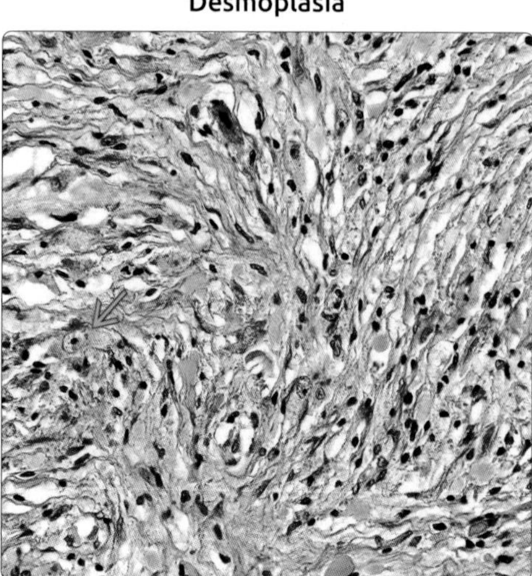

Masson Trichrome Positive Stroma

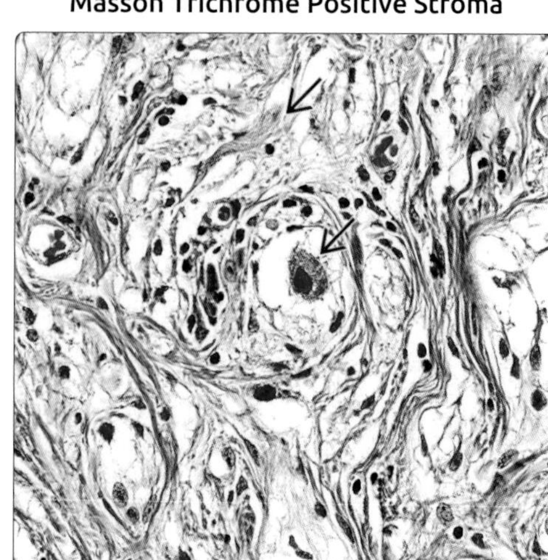

(Left) *GCTs composed entirely of mature, or largely mature, ganglion cells are termed gangliocytomas. Calcifications* ⇒ *are common. This tumor was elsewhere neurocytoma, in a composite lesion known as ganglioneurocytoma.* **(Right)** *Neurocytomas with ganglion cell differentiation are known as ganglioneurocytomas. Here, in the neurocytoma component, small, round neurocytes sit in a delicate neuropil background. A gangliocytoma component was present elsewhere.*

Microcalcifications

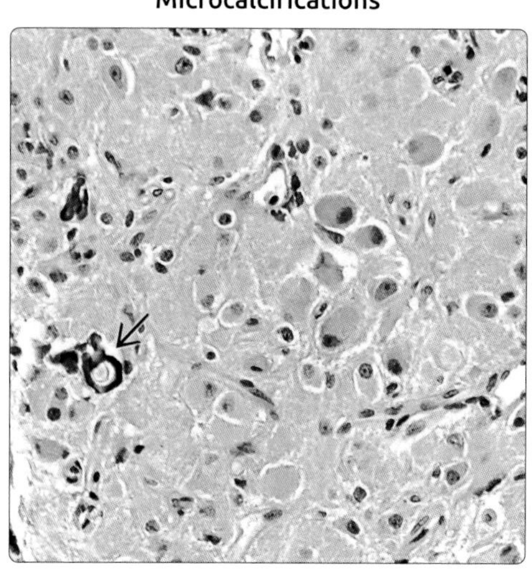

Neurocytoma Component

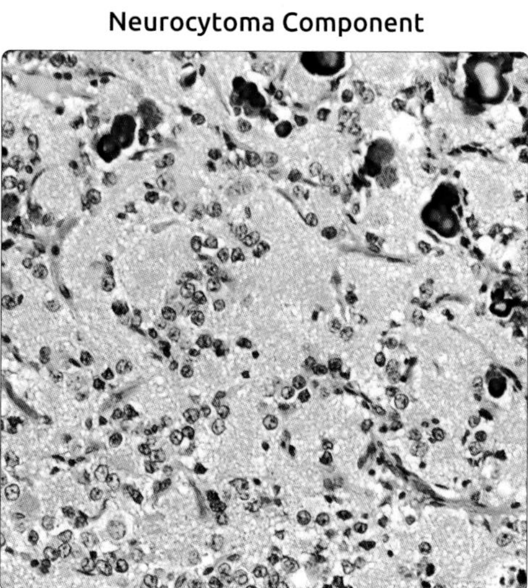

(Left) *Only rare gangliogliomas undergo anaplastic transformation. This lesion with large ganglion cells* ⇒ *had a mitotically active glial component elsewhere in the specimen.* **(Right)** *Multiple mitoses* ⇒ *in the cellular spindle cell element are clear evidence of anaplastic transformation of the glial component. Low-grade ganglioglioma was present elsewhere. Criteria for grading such neoplasms, and the prognostic significance of anaplastic changes, are unclear.*

Anaplastic Transformation

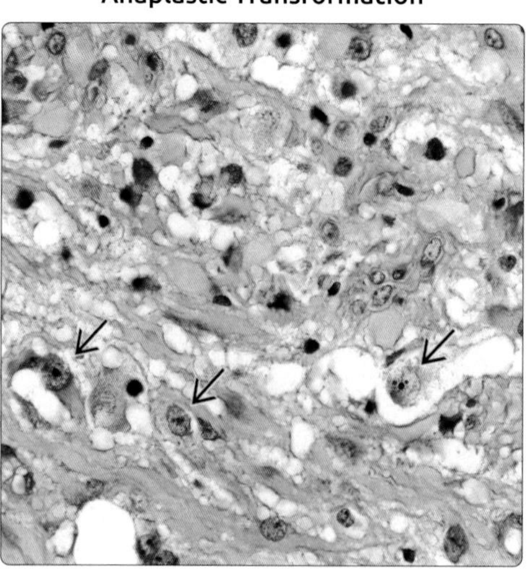

Mitotic Activity

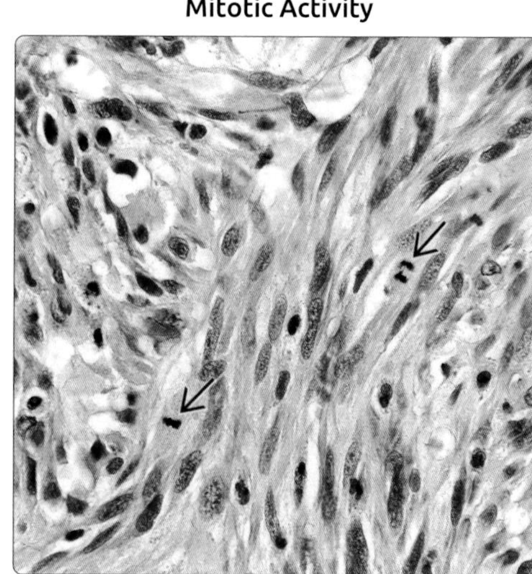

Ganglion Cells With Macronucleoli

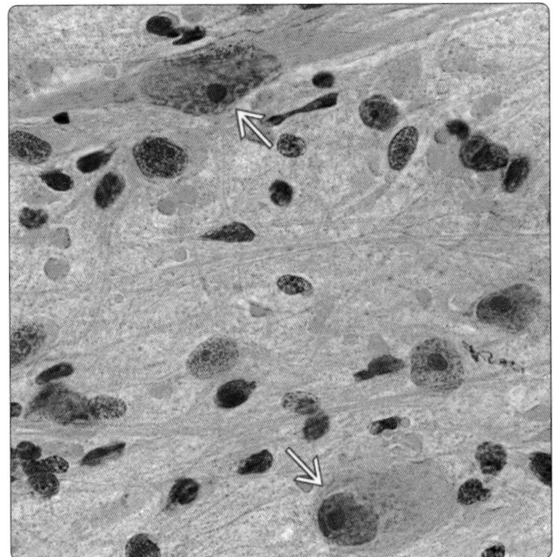

Binucleated Ganglion Cells

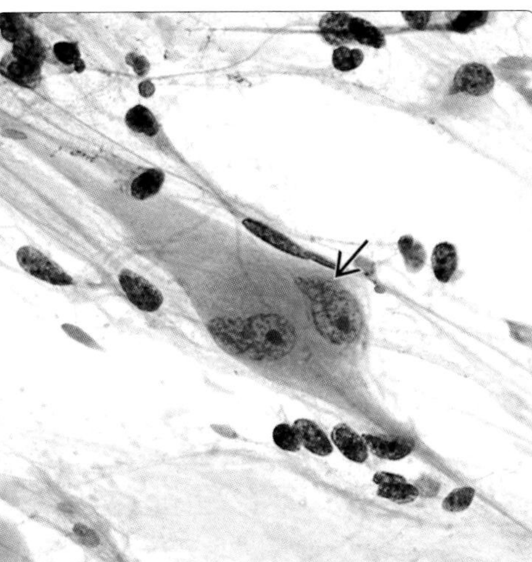

(Left) *Ganglion cells with large nuclei, ample basophilic cytoplasm, and macronucleoli ➡ may be conspicuous in smear preparations of GCTs, gangliocytoma in this case.* **(Right)** *Gangliocytoma's large, cytologically atypical, binucleated ganglion cells ➡, as illustrated in a smear preparation, strongly support the diagnosis.*

Synaptophysin Immunoreactivity

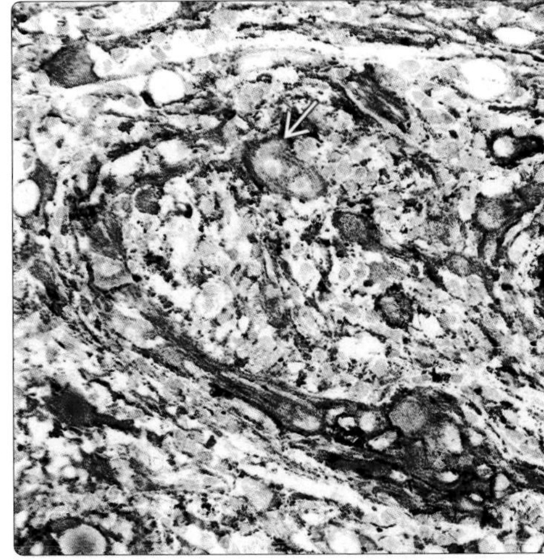

Membranous Synaptophysin Immunoreactivity

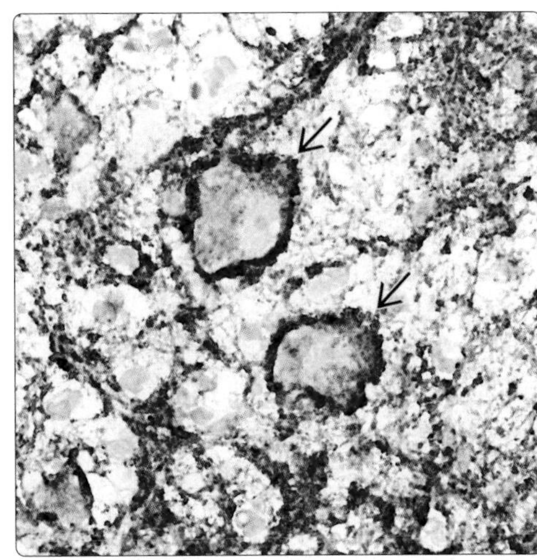

(Left) *Almost by definition, ganglion cells are immunoreactive for synaptophysin in patterns either cytoplasmic or membranous. A binucleate form is present ➡ in this ganglioglioma.* **(Right)** *Ganglion cells' immunoreactivity for synaptophysin is often heavily membranous ➡. Such a pattern suggests a neoplastic cell in the cerebral cortex but not in many other CNS sites, wherein normal ganglion cells also have this distinctive dense positivity.*

Chromogranin Immunoreactivity

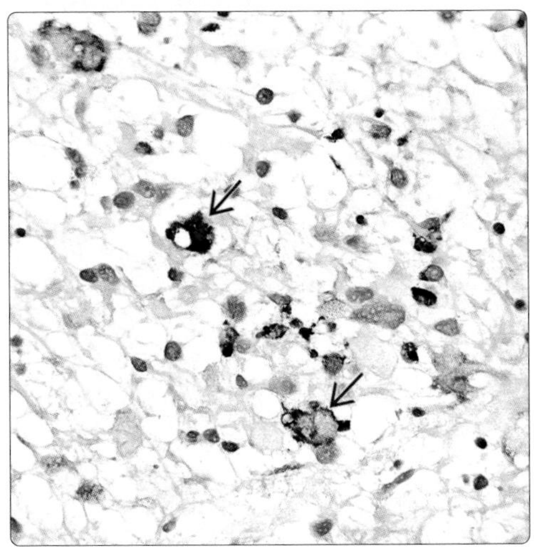

CD34 Immunoreactivity

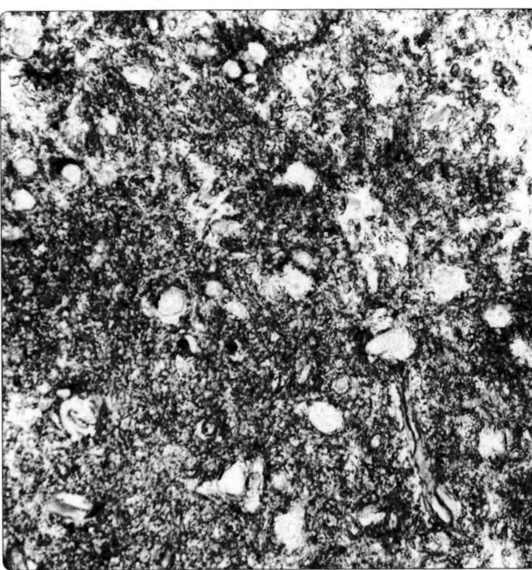

(Left) *Finely granular cytoplasmic immunoreactivity for chromogranin ➡ is clear evidence of neuronal differentiation, either in normal or neoplastic cells. These are neoplastic in a gangliocytoma.* **(Right)** *Immunoreactivity for CD34 is common in GCTs, both in the tumor, as here, and in surrounding cortex. Positivity is also frequent in pleomorphic xanthoastrocytoma, an entity in the differential diagnosis.*

KEY FACTS

TERMINOLOGY

- Glioneuronal tumor with spindle cell glial component, prominent collagenous stroma, and small ganglion cells

CLINICAL ISSUES

- Infants < 1 year
- Macrocephaly, seizures
- Generally favorable outcome; regression after subtotal resection (some cases)

IMAGING

- Large, cystic lesion over cerebral convexities
- ↓ T2 signal in desmoplastic areas
- Focal contrast enhancement in mural nodule

MACROSCOPIC

- Sharp demarcation from brain
- May be dura-attached

MICROSCOPIC

- Spindle astrocytic cells in desmoplastic stroma
- Small ganglion cells difficult to identify, solitary or clustered
- Conventional ganglion cell component with eosinophilic granular bodies in some cases
- Tumors without ganglion cell component termed desmoplastic infantile astrocytoma (DIA)
- Small cell component in some cases

ANCILLARY TESTS

- Spindle cells GFAP, S100(+)
- Ganglion and small cells: Synaptophysin, chromogranin (+), NeuN(+/-)
- Low Ki-67 labeling indices (< 5%)
- *BRAF* (*V600E*) mutation in minority
- Similar molecular profile of DIG and DIA suggests histologic spectrum of same entity

(Left) *Massive, cystic, and cerebral hemispheric, desmoplastic infantile gangliogliomas (DIGs) typically have a contrast-enhancing mural nodule ➔.* **(Right)** *Like many other ganglion cell tumors, DIGs may assume a cyst-mural nodule ➔ configuration.*

Large Cyst With Enhancing Mural Nodule

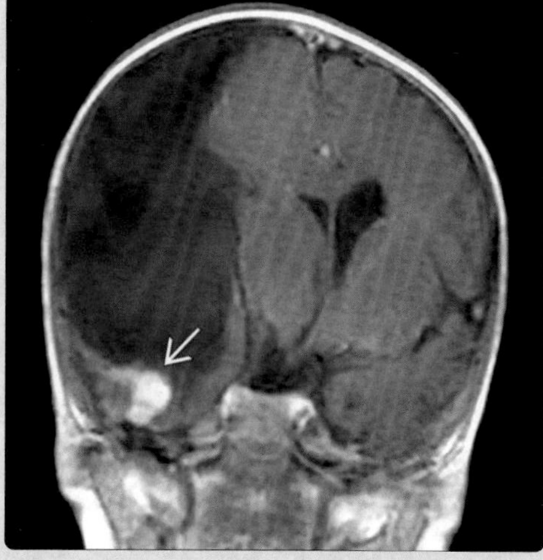

Cyst With Mural Nodule

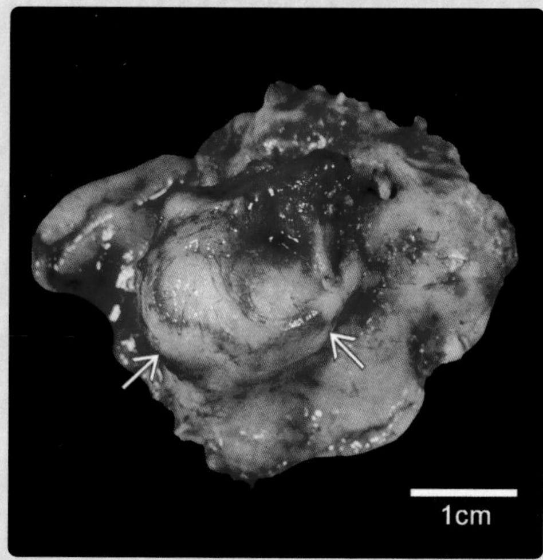

(Left) *A dominant bland spindle cell component in a desmoplastic stroma is the hallmark of DIG. A storiform pattern is common.* **(Right)** *GFAP is strongly expressed in many cells of DIG and highlights their spindle, tapering cytoplasm.*

Desmoplasia

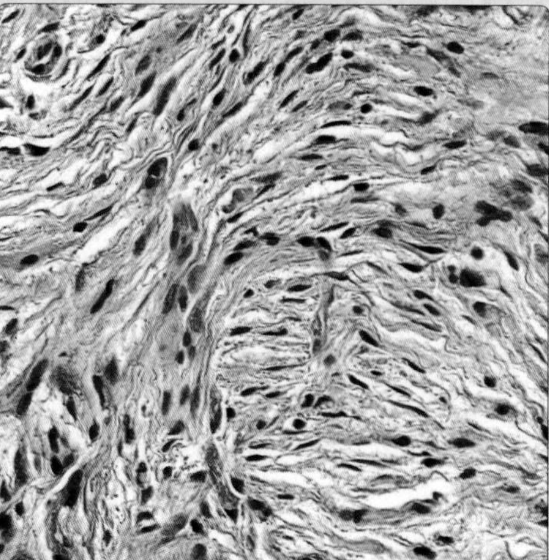

GFAP Expression

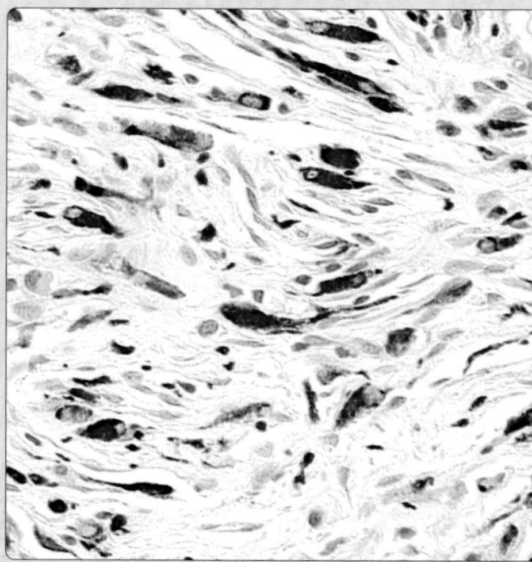

TERMINOLOGY

Abbreviations

- Desmoplastic infantile astrocytoma (DIA)

Definitions

- Glioneuronal tumor with prominent collagen-rich stroma and small ganglion cells (WHO grade I)

CLINICAL ISSUES

Presentation

- Typically in infants; rare outside pediatric population
- Macrocephaly, seizures

Treatment

- Excision
  - Complete removal often difficult
  - Stabilization or cure usually results

Prognosis

- Generally favorable; some regress after subtotal resection
- No prognostic difference between tumors with astrocytic or ganglion cell predominance
- Rare aggressive examples
- Prognostic significance of cellular, mitotically active small cell component unclear
  - Not necessarily predictive of aggressive behavior
  - Possibly unfavorable prognosis when dominant

IMAGING

General Features

- Location
  - Supratentorial

MR Findings

- Large, often massive
- ↓ T2 signal in desmoplastic areas
- Contrast enhancement of cyst wall and solid areas/mural nodule

MACROSCOPIC

General Features

- Massive
- Sharp demarcation from brain
- Macrocyst
- Firm to hard
- May incorporate regional vessels
- May be dura-attached

MICROSCOPIC

Histologic Features

- Sharp demarcation from brain
- Leptomeningeal involvement; spread into Virchow-Robin spaces
- Spindle glial cells in desmoplastic stroma
- Plump astrocytes with glassy cytoplasm/gemistocytes
- Small ganglion cells singly distributed or in small clusters
  - Often difficult to identify and distinguish from plump astrocytes
- Conventional ganglion cell component with eosinophilic granular bodies in some cases
- Tumors without ganglion cell component termed desmoplastic infantile astrocytoma (DIA)
  - Not equated with other astrocytomas with desmoplasia
- Small cell component in some cases
  - Mitotically active
  - Microvascular proliferation and even necrosis

ANCILLARY TESTS

Immunohistochemistry

- Spindle cells GFAP, S100(+)
- Ganglion cells and small cell component: Synaptophysin, chromogranin (+)
- Low Ki-67 labeling indices (< 5%)
  - Moderate to high in small cell components

Genetic Testing

- Low genetic instability
- Common alterations of gliomas not present
- *BRAF* (*V600E*) mutation in minority
- Similar molecular profile of DIG and DIA suggests histologic spectrum of same entity

DIFFERENTIAL DIAGNOSIS

Ganglioglioma (Conventional)

- Older patients, smaller tumors
- Large ganglion cells and eosinophilic granular bodies
- Perivascular lymphocytes

Meningioma

- Rare in infants
- Fibrous subtype potential mimic, but generally not cystic
- EMA(+)

Primitive Neuroectodermal Tumor

- No macrocyst or desmoplastic glial component

Pleomorphic Xanthoastrocytoma

- Desmoplasia less pronounced
- Pleomorphism
- Xanthic tumor cells (most cases)

Meningeal Sarcoma

- Malignant pleomorphic spindle cells, reticulin-rich
  - GFAP(-), S100(-)

Pilocytic Astrocytoma

- Spongy, microcystic component, little desmoplasia
- Rosenthal fibers, eosinophilic granular bodies

SELECTED REFERENCES

1. Koelsche C et al: BRAF V600E expression and distribution in desmoplastic infantile astrocytoma/ganglioglioma. Neuropathol Appl Neurobiol. 40(3):337-44, 2014
2. Gessi M et al: Genome-wide DNA copy number analysis of desmoplastic infantile astrocytomas and desmoplastic infantile gangliogliomas. J Neuropathol Exp Neurol. 72(9):807-15, 2013
3. VandenBerg SR et al: Desmoplastic supratentorial neuroepithelial tumors of infancy with divergent differentiation potential ("desmoplastic infantile gangliogliomas"). Report on 11 cases of a distinctive embryonal tumor with favorable prognosis. J Neurosurg. 66(1):58-71, 1987

(Left) *Principally leptomeningeal, DIGs involve the brain more by extension along perivascular spaces* → *than by diffuse, single-cell infiltration.* **(Right)** *There may be limited infiltration into adjacent brain parenchyma* →*.*

Perivascular Space Extension

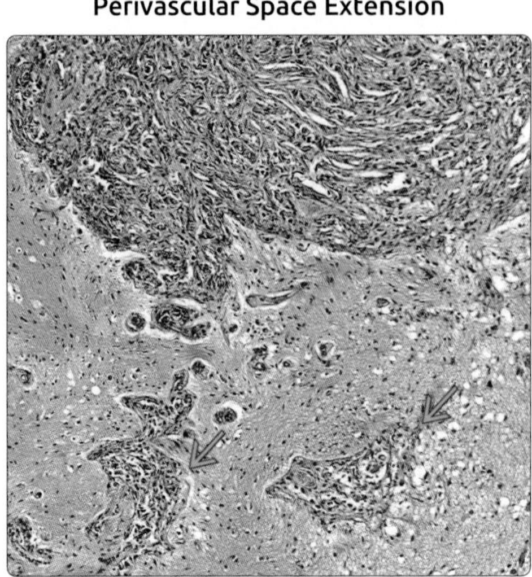

Brain Infiltration

(Left) *Incorporation of leptomeningeal vessels* → *in DIGs reflects the superficial position of the entity. As is typical, the tumor itself may be nonspecific in appearance.* **(Right)** *Delicate spindle cells in a desmoplastic stroma typical of DIG should prompt GFAP staining. A surprising number of positive cells will be present in what appears to be a mesenchymal tumor.*

Leptomeningeal Vessels

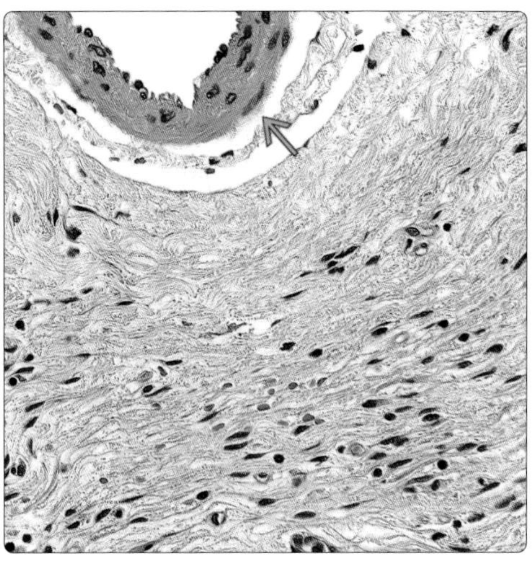

Spindle Cells

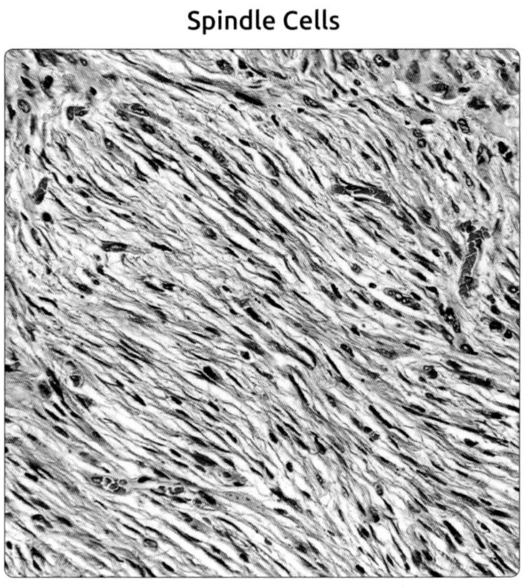

(Left) *Positive trichrome staining can resolve doubts as to the nature of the paucicellular stroma in DIGs. Such areas generate diagnostically helpful dark signal in T2W and FLAIR images.* **(Right)** *Pericellular reticulin staining in desmoplastic areas is characteristic of DIG.*

Positive Trichrome Stain

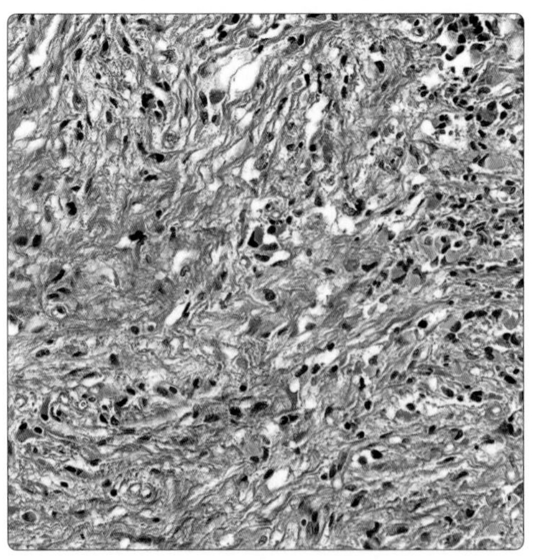

Pericellular Reticulin

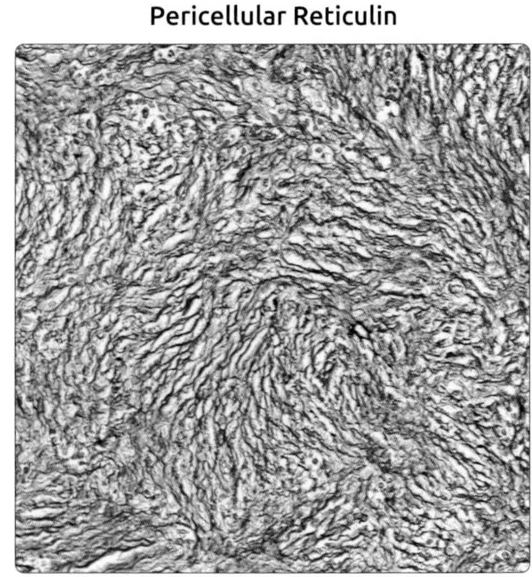

Stroma-Rich Tumor

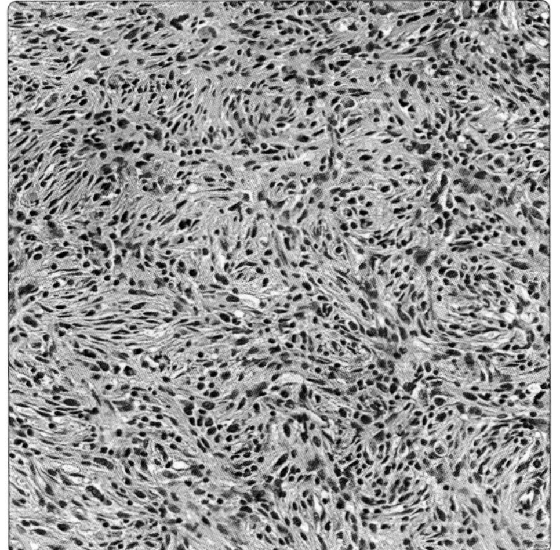

Spindle Neoplastic Glia

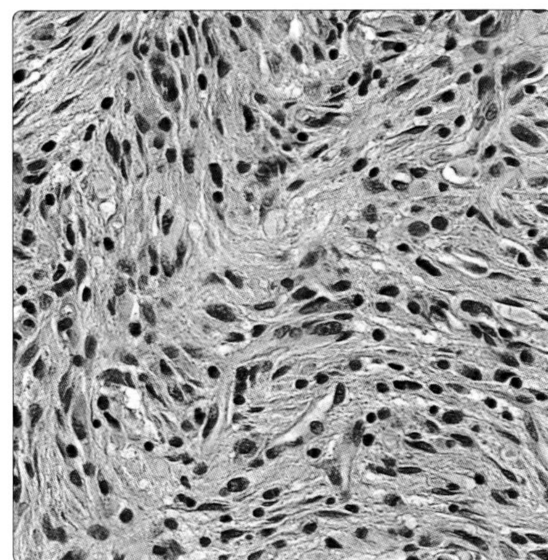

(Left) *DIG is a stroma-rich tumor with variable cellularity. Some areas are moderately cellular and not very fibrotic.* **(Right)** *The predominant cellular component of DIG is spindle neoplastic glia in a collagen-rich stroma.*

Pleomorphic Glial Tissue

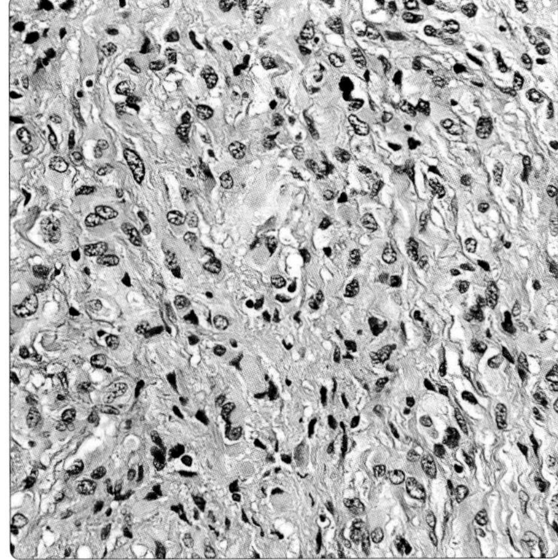

Compact Pleomorphic Cell Areas

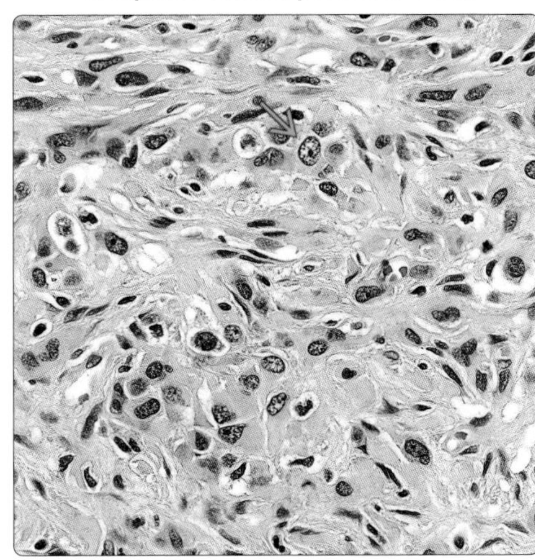

(Left) *Out of clinical/radiological context, pleomorphic glial tissue in desmoplastic infantile gangliogliomas may be misinterpreted as an infiltrating glioma or sarcoma.* **(Right)** *Compact areas of cells with pleomorphic nuclei and glassy cytoplasm suggest astrocytic differentiation. Only an occasional cell may appear ganglionic ⇒.*

Eccentric Hyaline Cytoplasm

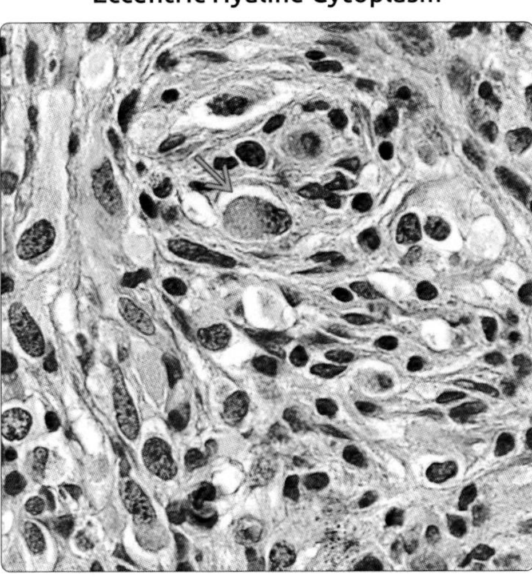

Compact Tissue

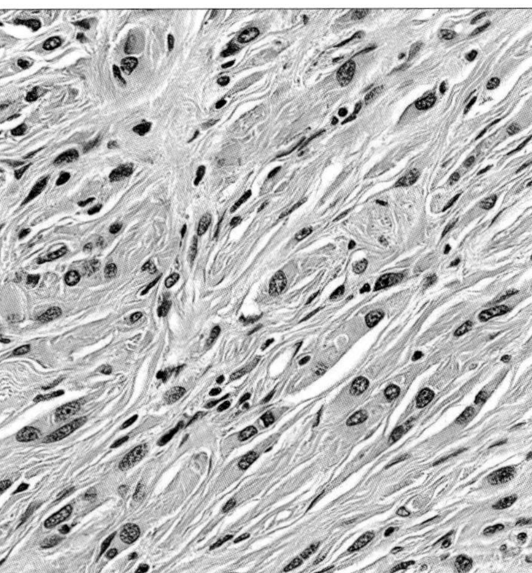

(Left) *Small, round cells with eccentric hyaline cytoplasm ⇒ common in DIGs have features intermediate between ganglion cells and astrocytes.* **(Right)** *Elongated astrocytes form compact tissue in some regions of many DIGs.*

(Left) *Only in some instances are ganglion cells ⇒ identified on the basis of their features in H&E sections alone. Immunohistochemistry for synaptophysin and chromogranin are helpful.* **(Right)** *Polymorphous tissue in DIGs contains neoplastic glia and neurons ⇒. An index of suspicion, prompted by typical patient age and imaging characteristics, aids in the identification of the neuronal component.*

Ganglion Cells

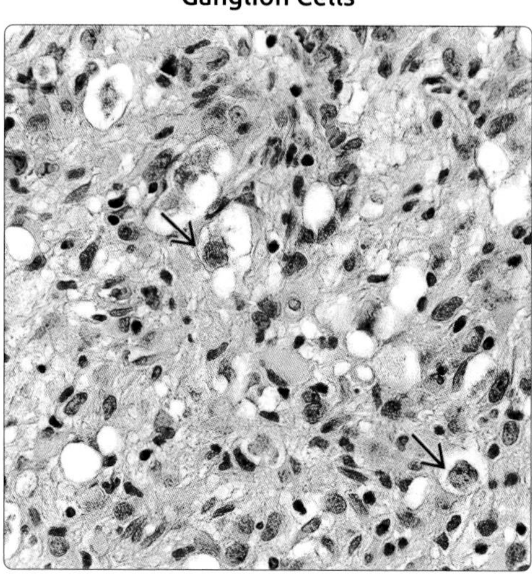

Polymorphous Tissue

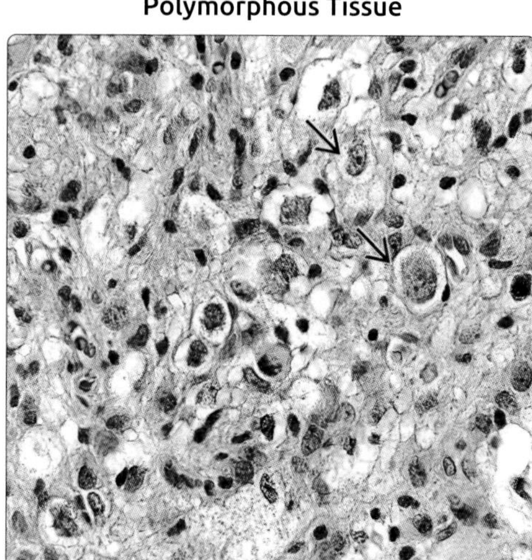

(Left) *Ganglion cells in desmoplastic infantile gangliogliomas are typically small and somewhat round ⇒, with prominent nucleoli that aid in identification.* **(Right)** *Although known for their desmoplasia, cells in DIGs may be arranged in a back-to-back manner. These often have H&E features of both neurons and glia.*

Ganglion Cells

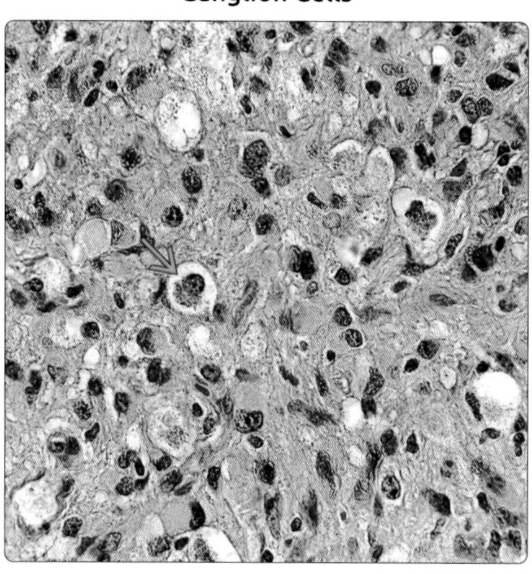

Back-to-Back Arrangement

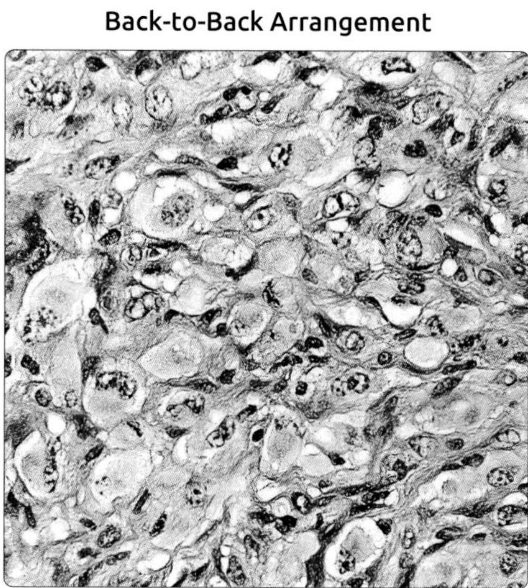

(Left) *Areas closely resembling conventional ganglion cell tumors are present focally in some DIGs. Large ganglion cells ⇒ stand out among other cell components.* **(Right)** *Large cells with prominent nucleoli ⇒ simplify the diagnosis of a neuronal tumor. However, smaller, less obviously neuronal cells are the rule in DIGs.*

Large Ganglion Cells

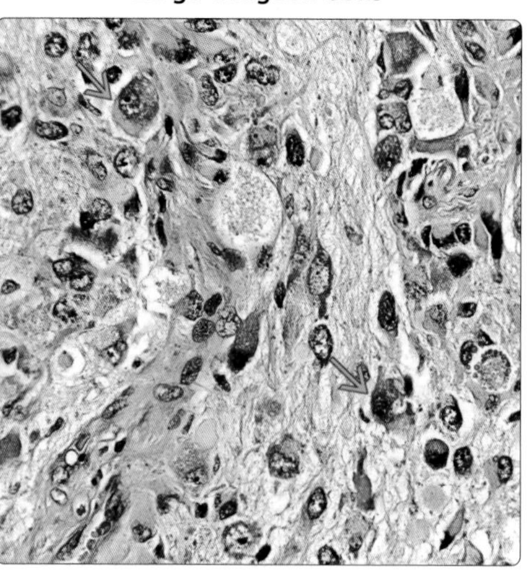

Large Ganglion Cells

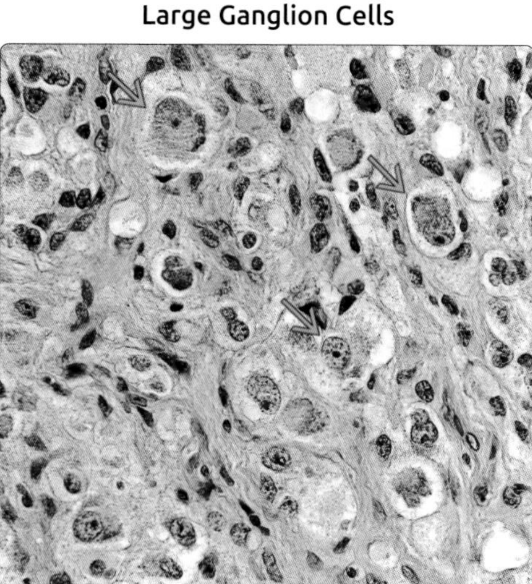

Necrosis

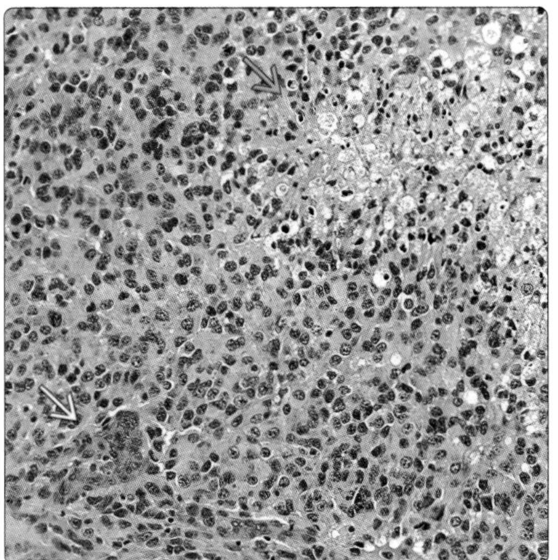

Small Cell Component

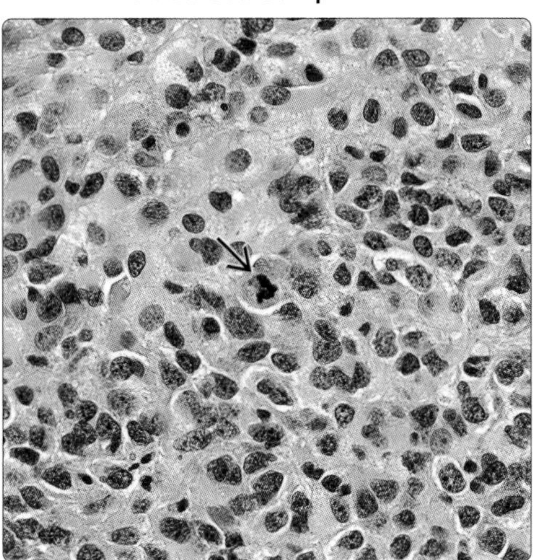

(Left) *DIGs sometimes contain small cell, mitotically active tissue with microvascular proliferation* ➡ *and necrosis* ⇨ *that fulfill criteria of PNET or glioblastoma. The prognosis is not always adversely affected by such anaplastic components.* **(Right)** *The small cell component of a DIG may have all of the cytological features and mitotic activity* ⇨ *of a high-grade tumor, either PNET or glioblastoma.*

GFAP-Positive Areas

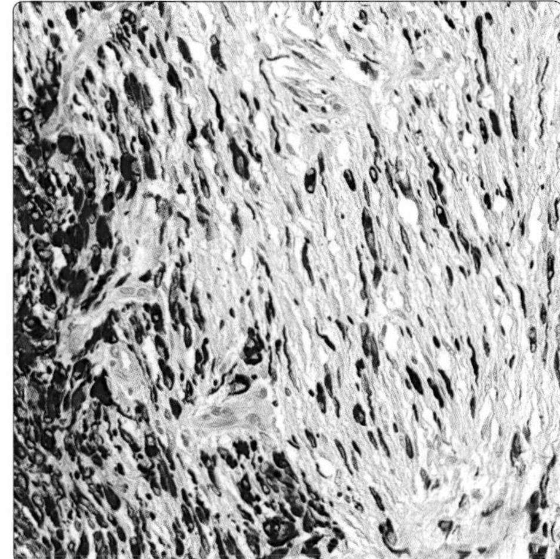

GFAP Immunostaining

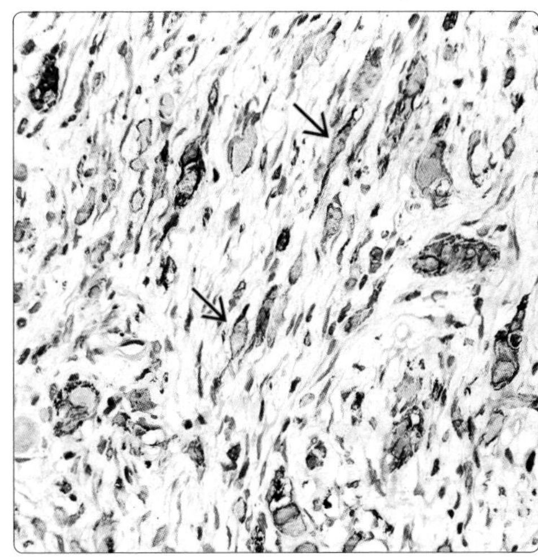

(Left) *The density of GFAP-positive areas is high where tumor cells are more polygonal, and low in desmoplastic areas wherein cells are spindle-shaped.* **(Right)** *Immunostaining of DIGs for GFAP usually discloses more positive cells* ⇨ *than would be expected on the basis of findings in H&E sections alone.*

Synaptophysin Positivity

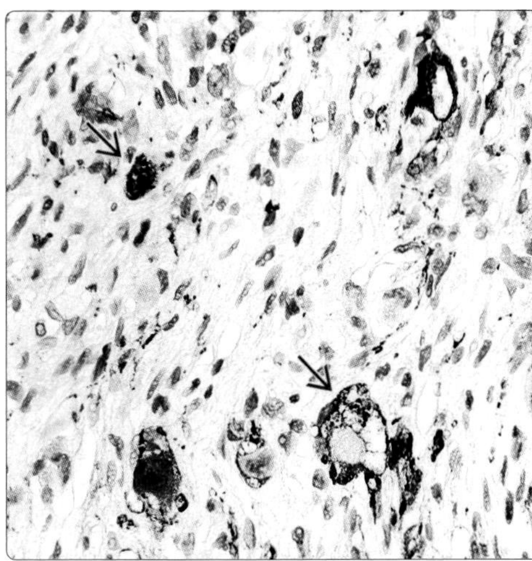

Chromogranin Immunoreactivity

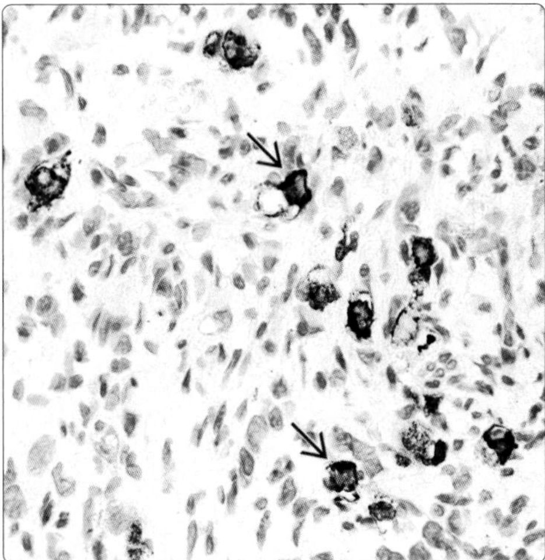

(Left) *Ganglion cells in desmoplastic infantile gangliogliomas are best identified by immunohistochemistry for synaptophysin* ⇨. **(Right)** *Immunoreactivity for chromogranin is also used to confirm the presence of a neuronal component* ⇨.

Dysplastic Cerebellar Gangliocytoma (Lhermitte-Duclos Disease)

KEY FACTS

TERMINOLOGY

- Hamartomatous lesion of cerebellum characterized by thickened folia and replacement of internal granular layer by abnormal ganglion cells

CLINICAL ISSUES

- Usually component of Cowden syndrome
- Headaches, ataxia, visual disturbance
- Mass effect, CSF obstruction
- Good prognosis, but may recur (25%) requiring reexcision

IMAGING

- Unilateral, cerebellar lesion
- Striped appearance on FLAIR and T2W MR images is highly suggestive of entity

MICROSCOPIC

- Replacement of normal internal granular layer by small to large ganglion cells
- Myelinated processes in molecular layer extending to pial surface
- Clear spaces (vacuolation) in white matter and molecular layer

ANCILLARY TESTS

- Germline *PTEN* mutations in most patients
- Synaptophysin (+) ganglion cells
- Neurofilament protein (+) neuronal processes
- NeuN variably (+)
- Phospho-AKT and phospho-S6 (+) in large ganglion cells; reflects AKT/mTOR pathway activation

(Left) *On T2WI MR, the focal, striped appearance → is almost diagnostic of Lhermitte-Duclos disease (LDD).* **(Right)** *Foliar expansion of LDD is best appreciated at low magnification, wherein the thickness of the affected cerebellar cortex → and loss of darkly staining internal granule cells are most apparent.*

Striped Appearance

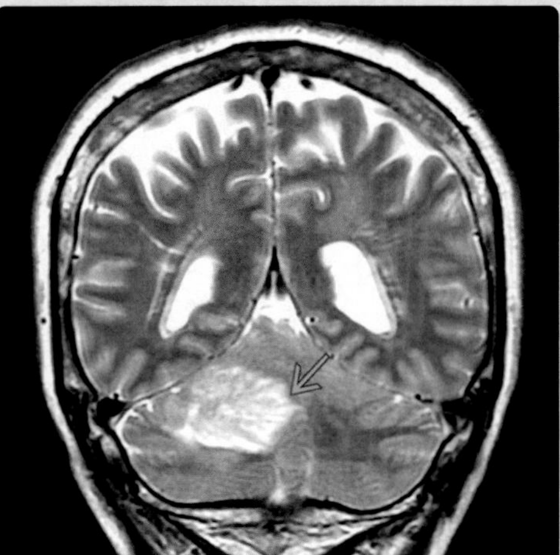

Foliar Expansion

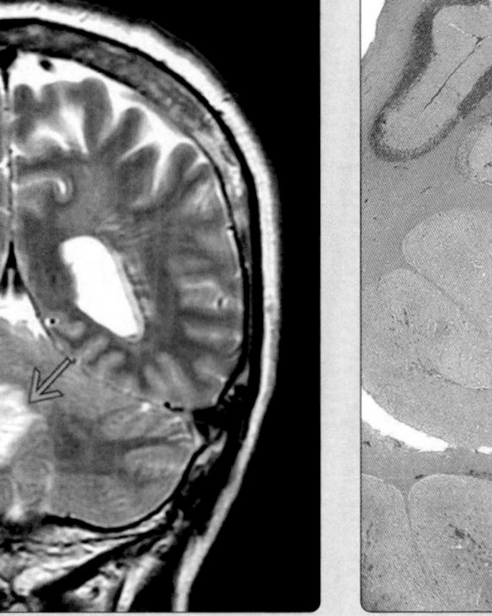

(Left) *Replacement of the internal granular layer in areas may be near complete →. Only rare, isolated granule cells may be present.* **(Right)** *Dysplastic ganglion cells in LDD are immunoreactive for synaptophysin.*

Internal Granular Layer Replacement

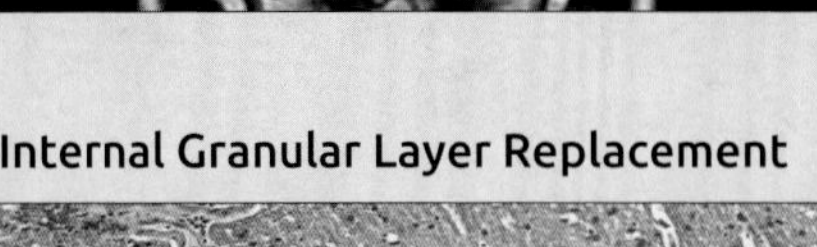

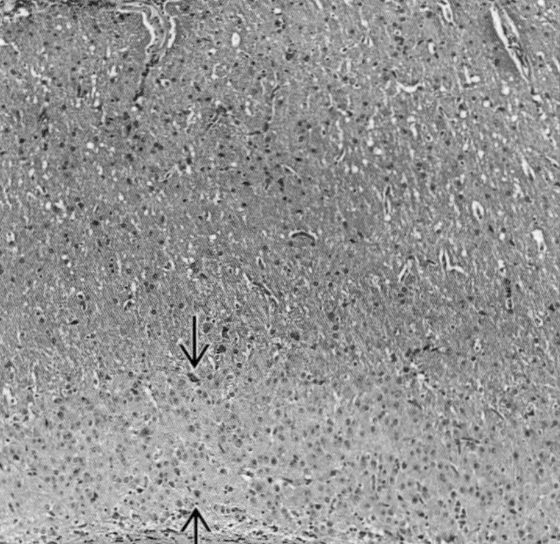

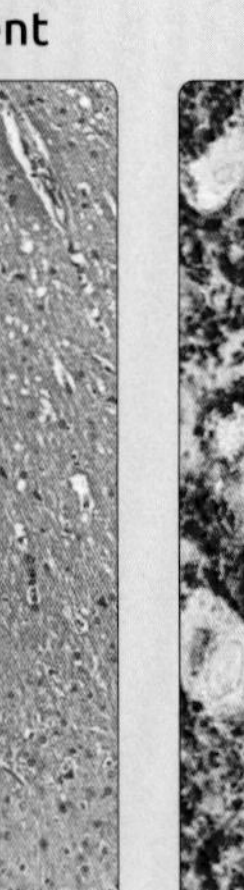

Synaptophysin Immunoreactivity

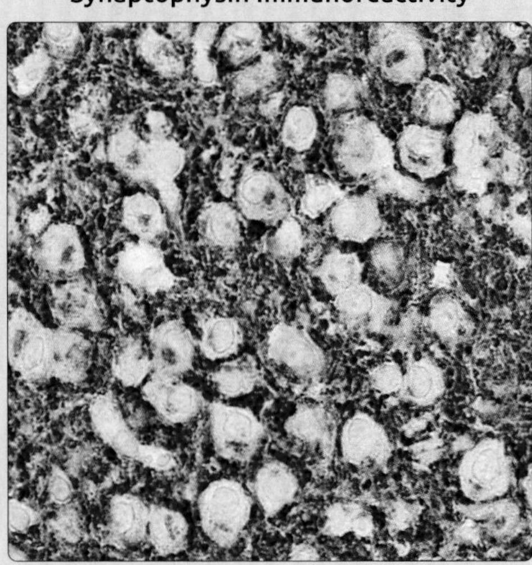

TERMINOLOGY

Synonyms

- Lhermitte-Duclos disease (LDD)

Definitions

- Hamartomatous lesion of cerebellum characterized by thickened folia and replacement of internal granular layer by abnormal ganglion cells
- WHO grade I

ETIOLOGY/PATHOGENESIS

Tumor Predisposition Syndrome

- Cowden syndrome (germline *PTEN* mutation)

CLINICAL ISSUES

Presentation

- Young adults, occasionally children
- Headaches, ataxia, mass effect, obstruction

Natural History

- Slow enlargement of lesion

Treatment

- Surgical approaches
  - Resection if symptomatic

Prognosis

- Good but may recur (25%), requiring 2nd surgery
- No malignant potential

IMAGING

MR Findings

- Unilateral, cerebellar
- Striped appearance on FLAIR and T2W images
- Contrast enhancement secondary to prominent draining veins in minority of cases

MACROSCOPIC

General Features

- Enlarged folia

MICROSCOPIC

Histologic Features

- Replacement of normal internal granular layer by small to large ganglion cells
  - Transformation accentuated in superficial portion of internal granular layer
- Haphazard arrangement of neurons compared to single layer of Purkinje cells
- Myelinated axons extending through molecular layer to pial surface
- Clear spaces (vacuolation) in white matter and molecular layer
- Calcifications in some chronic cases

ANCILLARY TESTS

Histochemistry

- Hematoxylin and eosin/Luxol fast blue
  - Reactivity: Myelin sheaths in molecular layer

Immunohistochemistry

- Synaptophysin (+) ganglion cells
- Neurofilament protein (+) neuronal processes
- NeuN variably (+)
- Phospho-AKT and phospho-S6 (+) in large ganglion cells; reflects AKT/mTOR pathway activation

Genetic Testing

- Germline *PTEN* mutations in most, but not all cases
- Activation of mTOR pathway
- Phenotypic features of Lhermitte-Duclos modeled in mice with *PTEN* loss

Electron Microscopy

- Ganglion cells with neuronal features, including microtubules, synapses, clear vesicles

DIFFERENTIAL DIAGNOSIS

Conventional Ganglion Cell Tumor

- Gangliocytoma
  - Not centered on internal granular cell layer
    - Mass; no respect of local architecture
  - Eosinophilic granular bodies
  - Perivascular chronic inflammation
- Ganglioglioma
  - Complex architecture, cyst/mural nodule
  - GFAP(+) glial component
  - Eosinophilic, PAS-positive granular bodies

Infiltrating Glioma With Trapped Purkinje Cells

- Hypercellularity in molecular layer, internal granular cell layer, and white matter
- Single cell layer of overrun ganglion cells (Purkinje cell layer)
- Atypical glia, often with mitoses

DIAGNOSTIC CHECKLIST

Pathologic Interpretation Pearls

- Neuroimaging highly suggestive of diagnosis
- Broad bands of ganglion cells not seen in other lesions

SELECTED REFERENCES

1. Abel TW et al: Lhermitte-Duclos disease: a report of 31 cases with immunohistochemical analysis of the PTEN/AKT/mTOR pathway. J Neuropathol Exp Neurol. 64(4):341-9, 2005
2. Capone Mori A et al: Lhermitte-Duclos disease in 3 children: a clinical long-term observation. Neuropediatrics. 34(1):30-5, 2003
3. Zhou XP et al: Germline inactivation of PTEN and dysregulation of the phosphoinositol-3-kinase/Akt pathway cause human Lhermitte-Duclos disease in adults. Am J Hum Genet. 73(5):1191-8, 2003
4. Kwon CH et al: Pten regulates neuronal soma size: a mouse model of Lhermitte-Duclos disease. Nat Genet. 29(4):404-11, 2001
5. Yachnis AT et al: Expression of neurofilament proteins in the hypertrophic granule cells of Lhermitte-Duclos disease: an explanation for the mass effect and the myelination of parallel fibers in the disease state. J Neuropathol Exp Neurol. 47(3):206-16, 1988

(Left) *LDD is a hamartomatous, layered process rather than a discrete mass, as small neurons in the internal granular layer are replaced by ganglion cells → of varying sizes.* **(Right)** *A thin layer of residual small internal granular cells persists adjacent to the white matter → in an area where transformation is less than complete.*

Replacement by Ganglion Cells

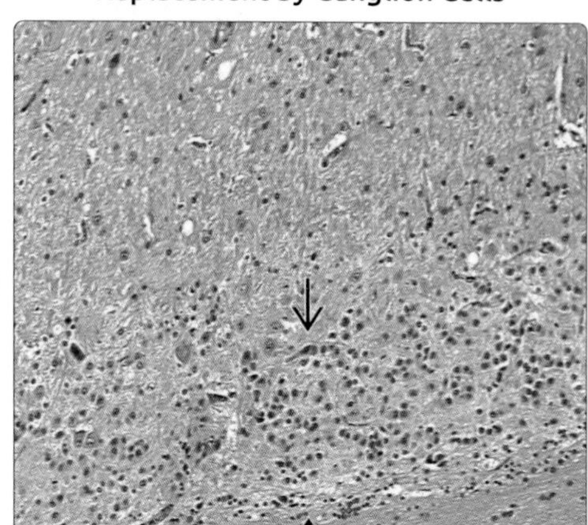

Residual Internal Granular Cells

(Left) *Medium to large ganglion cells with mild cytologic abnormalities fill the internal granular layer in LDD.* **(Right)** *Out of context at high magnification where the laminar nature of the process may not be apparent, abnormal neurons of Lhermitte-Duclos disease may be misinterpreted as those of gangliocytoma.*

Medium to Large Ganglion Cells

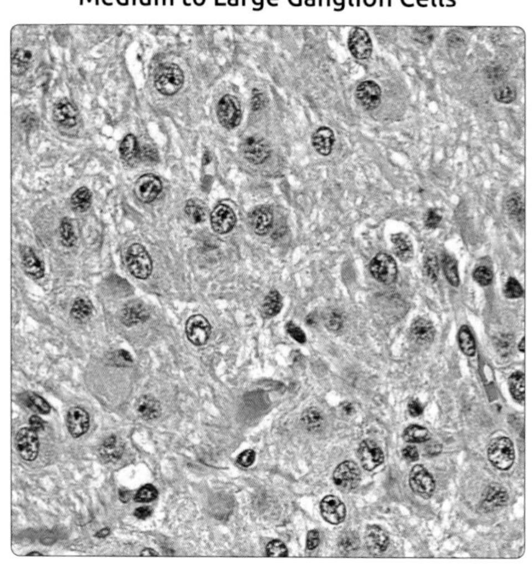

Abnormal Neurons

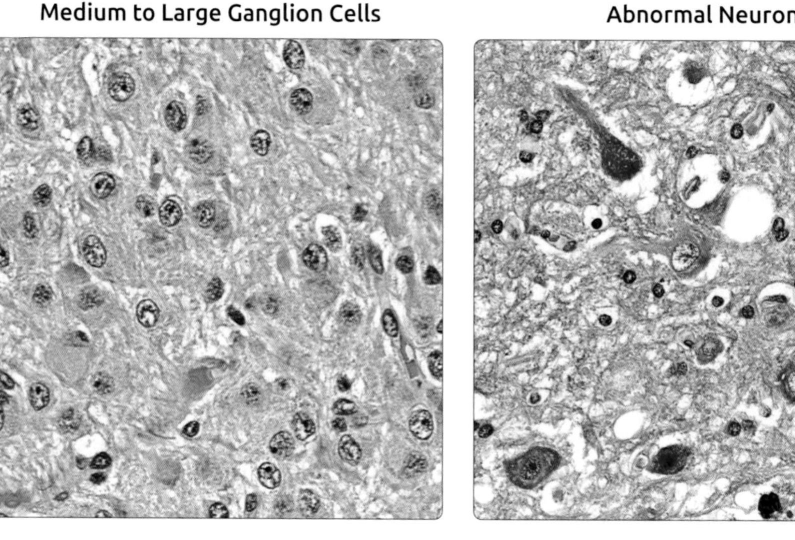

(Left) *The superficial internal granular layer contains only abnormal ganglion cells and smaller ganglioid cells →, whereas the deeper portion features a normal complement of small neurons →. A Purkinje cell is present →.* **(Right)** *Internal granular cells are replaced by small ganglion cells or "ganglioid" cells in the internal granular cell layer →. Larger ganglion cells would be present in maximally affected areas. Purkinje cells are unaffected →.*

Internal Granular Layer

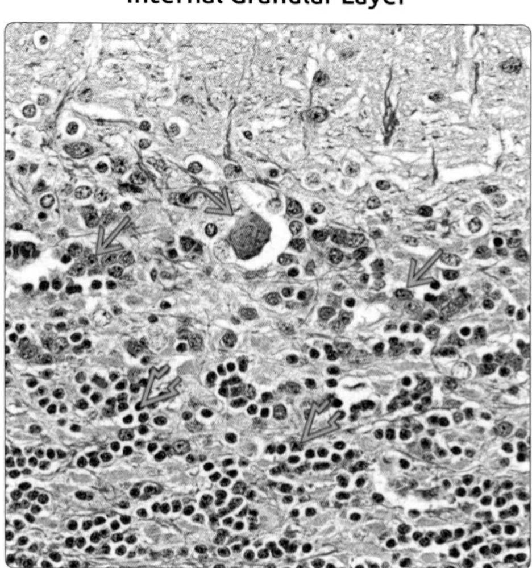

Ganglion and Ganglioid Cells

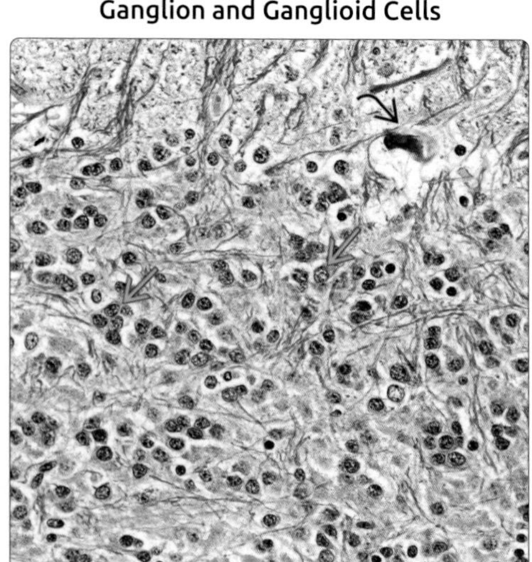

Myelinated Fibers

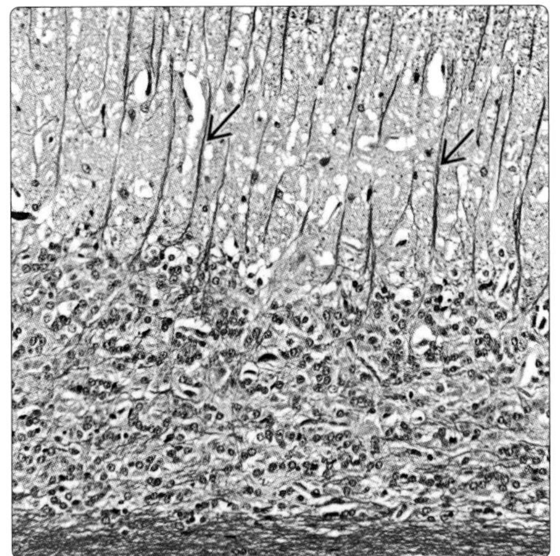

Myelinated Fibers

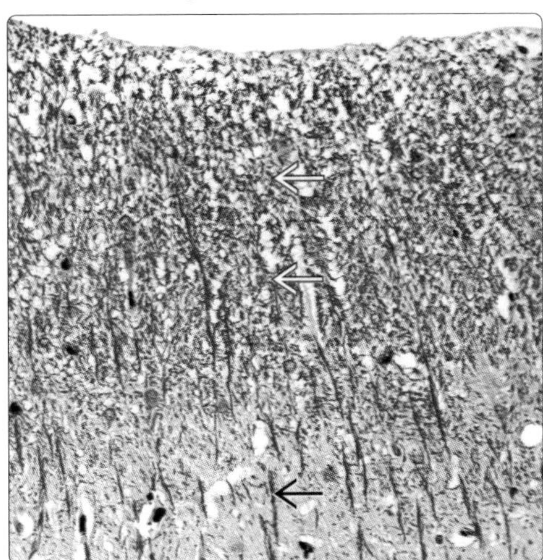

(Left) *Bundles of myelinated fibers ⇨ course vertically to the leptomeningeal surface within the normally myelin-free molecular layer.* **(Right)** *A zone of fine myelinated fibers ➡ lies beneath the pial surface in a Luxol fast blue stain. Bundles of larger, more heavily myelinated fibers ⇨ are also present.*

Clear Spaces

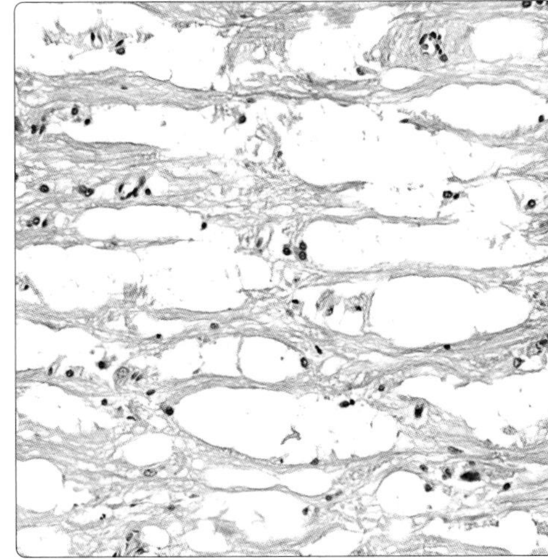

Coarse Calcifications

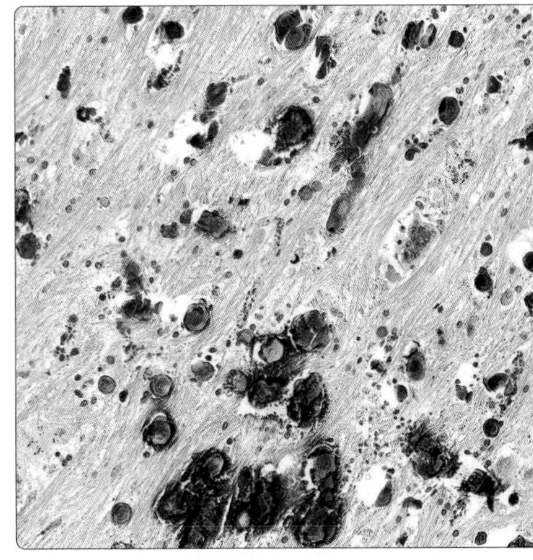

(Left) *Clear spaces and clefts are distinctive in white matter. The spaces are not to be confused with intratumoral microcysts common in ganglion cell tumors, infiltrating gliomas, and pilocytic astrocytoma.* **(Right)** *Coarse calcifications are conspicuous in some chronic examples of dysplastic cerebellar gangliocytoma.*

NeuN Labeling

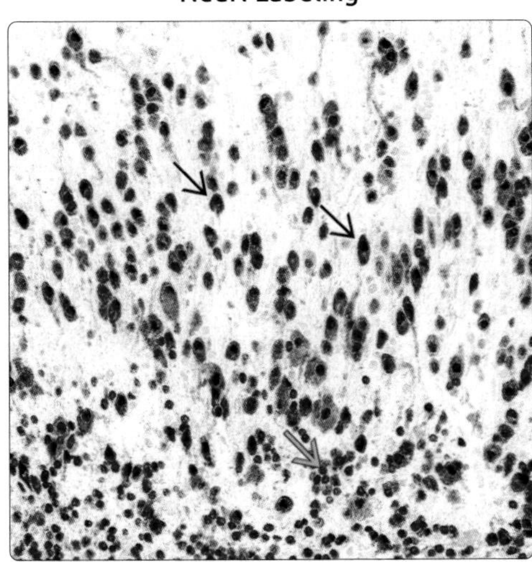

Phospho-S6 Immunostaining

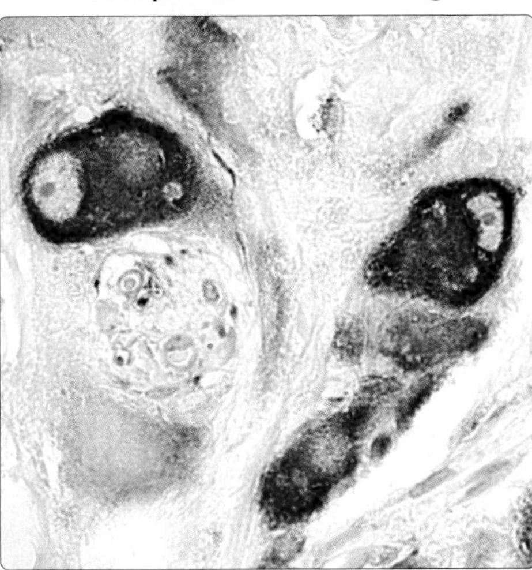

(Left) *Nuclear and cytoplasmic labeling with NeuN antibody confirms the neuronal nature of the large cells in the external granule cell layer. Affected cells ⇨ are considerably larger than residual granule cells ⇨.* **(Right)** *Aberrant mTOR pathway activation, reflected by increased phospho-s6 immunostaining, may explain many of the cytomorphologic features, particularly cytomegaly. (Courtesy T. Abel, MD, PhD.)*

Central Neurocytoma

KEY FACTS

TERMINOLOGY

- Well-differentiated intraventricular neoplasm with neurocytic differentiation near foramen of Monro

CLINICAL ISSUES

- Signs of increased intracranial pressure
- Favorable prognosis
- Extent of resection most important prognostic factor

MICROSCOPIC

- Cytologic monomorphism
- Resembles oligodendroglioma
- Perivascular, ependymoma-like neuropil rosettes, in most cases
- Microcalcifications frequent
- Atypical neurocytoma defined by Ki-67 labeling indices
  - > 2% in 1 study and > 3% in another

ANCILLARY TESTS

- Synaptophysin positive in neurocytes and neuropil
- Loss of heterozygosity in 1p and 19q frequent
- Whole chromosomal arm 1p/19q codeletion typical of oligodendroglial tumors usually absent

TOP DIFFERENTIAL DIAGNOSES

- Oligodendroglioma
- Ependymoma
- Dysembryoplastic neuroepithelial tumor-like neoplasm of septum pellucidum
- Pineocytoma
- Primitive neuroectodermal tumor
- Subependymal giant cell astrocytoma (tuberous sclerosis)

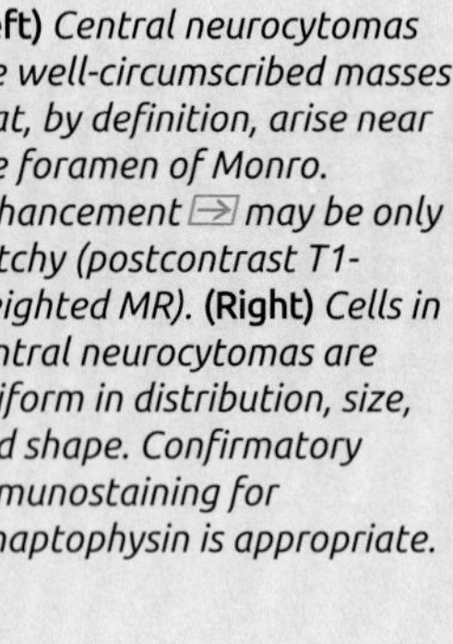

(Left) *Central neurocytomas are well-circumscribed masses that, by definition, arise near the foramen of Monro. Enhancement* ➡ *may be only patchy (postcontrast T1-weighted MR).* **(Right)** *Cells in central neurocytomas are uniform in distribution, size, and shape. Confirmatory immunostaining for synaptophysin is appropriate.*

Intraventricular Mass Near Foramen of Monro

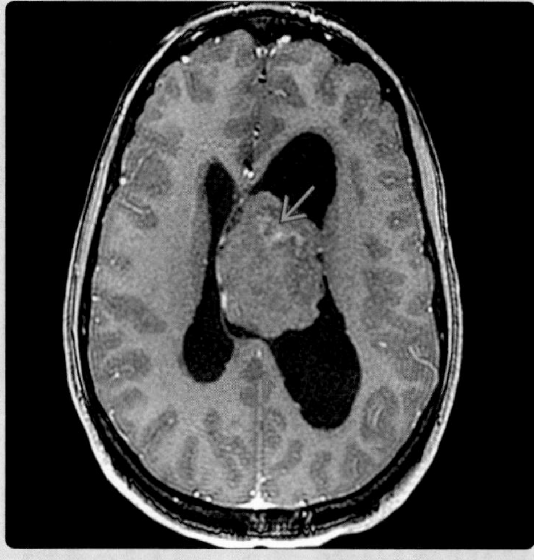

Cellular Uniformity

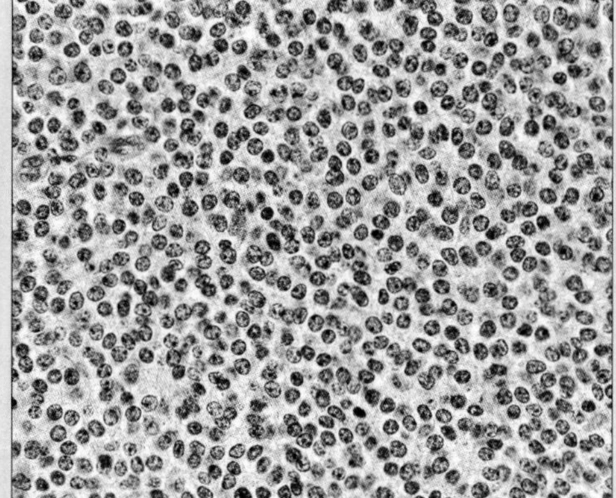

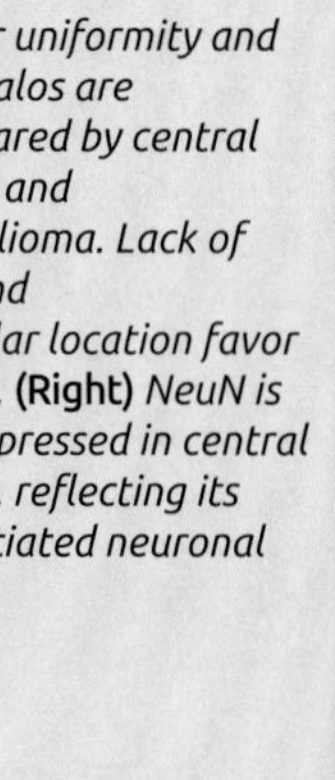

(Left) *Nuclear uniformity and perinuclear halos are properties shared by central neurocytoma and oligodendroglioma. Lack of infiltration and intraventricular location favor neurocytoma.* **(Right)** *NeuN is frequently expressed in central neurocytoma, reflecting its well-differentiated neuronal nature.*

Oligodendroglial Mimic

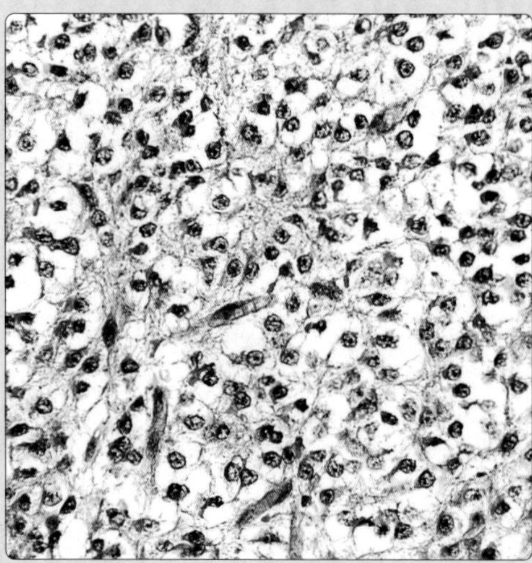

NeuN Expression

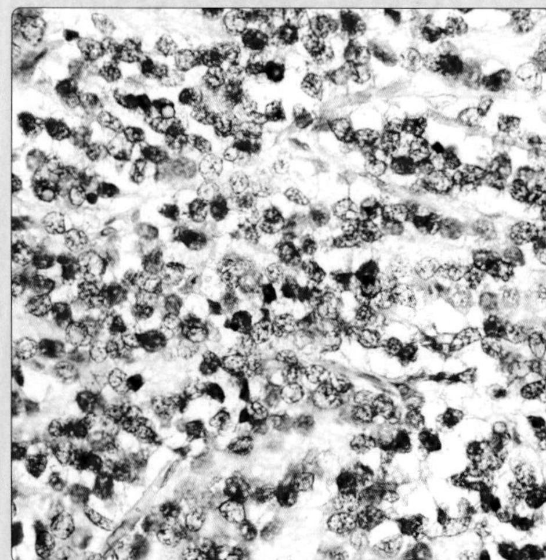

TERMINOLOGY

Definitions

- Well-differentiated intraventricular tumor of neurocytes arising near foramen of Monro
- WHO grade II
- Numerical grading for "atypical" category not developed

CLINICAL ISSUES

Presentation

- Signs of increased intracranial pressure
- Intraventricular hemorrhage, minority of cases

Prognosis

- Favorable
- Extent of resection most important factor
  - Only independent prognostic factor in recent multiinstitutional study
- Recurrence rate greater for "atypical" examples

IMAGING

MR Findings

- Often large mass
- Heterogeneous contrast enhancement, often patchy
- Attached to ependymal surface and septum pellucidum near foramen of Monro
- Obstructive hydrocephalus
- Hemorrhage occasional

CT Findings

- Calcifications, frequent

MICROSCOPIC

Histologic Features

- Cells in sheets or large lobules
- Remarkable cytological uniformity
- Artifactual perinuclear halos lend oligodendroglioma-like appearance, sometimes striking
- Ependymoma-like perivascular pseudorosette-like, nucleus-free zones &/or larger patches of neuropil
- Microcalcifications, frequent
- Delicate vessels, with little surrounding stroma
- Differentiation to ganglion cells, uncommon
- Lipidization, rare
- Atypical neurocytoma defined by Ki-67 labeling indices > 2 or 3%
  - Increased mitoses (usually ≥ 3 per 10 HPF)
  - Atypia, often minor
  - Microvascular proliferation, some cases
  - Necrosis, some cases
  - Ki-67 labeling index not uniform prognostic factor in all studies

ANCILLARY TESTS

Cytology

- Round, uniform nuclei with delicate chromatin and small nucleoli
- Little cytoplasm
- Delicate vessels

Immunohistochemistry

- Synaptophysin (+) neurocytes, perivascular pseudorosette-like and larger neuropil zones
- NeuN, variably (+)
- Chromogranin-A (-), except in neoplastic or entrapped normal ganglion cells

Genetic Testing

- Loss of heterozygosity in 1p and 19q frequent
- Whole chromosomal arm 1p/19q codeletion typical of oligodendroglial tumors usually absent
- Frequent gains of 2p, 10q, 11q, and 18q
- Frequent losses of 1p, 6q, 12q, 17p, 17q, and 20p
- Whole gains of chromosome 7 but without *EGFR* amplification

DIFFERENTIAL DIAGNOSIS

Oligodendroglioma

- Not a midline intraventricular mass
- Diffuse infiltration with "secondary structures"
- 1p/19q codeletion

Dysembryoplastic Neuroepithelial Tumor-Like Neoplasm of Septum Pellucidum

- Low cellularity
- Myxoid background
- Largely synaptophysin (-)
- Floating neurons and "specific glioneuronal element," some cases

Subependymal Giant Cell Astrocytoma (Tuberous Sclerosis)

- Exclusively large, spindle to epithelioid cells

Ependymoma (Especially Clear Cell Type)

- Para- not intraventricular when supratentorial
- Clefted, lobulated nuclei in clear cell type
- Not as cytologically monomorphous
- Coarser processes in perivascular pseudorosettes
- GFAP(+) perivascular pseudorosettes
- EMA(+) paranuclear dot-like microlumina

Pineocytoma

- Site specific, large pineocytomatous rosettes, less cytologically monomorphic

Primitive Neuroectodermal Tumor

- High cellularity
- Cytologically malignant
- Brisk mitotic index activity; high Ki-67 labeling index

SELECTED REFERENCES

1. Vasiljevic A et al: Prognostic factors in central neurocytomas: a multicenter study of 71 cases. Am J Surg Pathol. 36(2):220-7, 2012
2. Kobayashi TK et al: Cytologic diagnosis of central neurocytoma in intraoperative squash preparations: a report of 2 cases. Acta Cytol. 54(2):209-13, 2010
3. Korshunov A et al: Recurrent cytogenetic aberrations in central neurocytomas and their biological relevance. Acta Neuropathol. 113(3):303-12, 2007

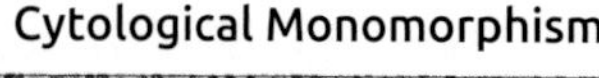

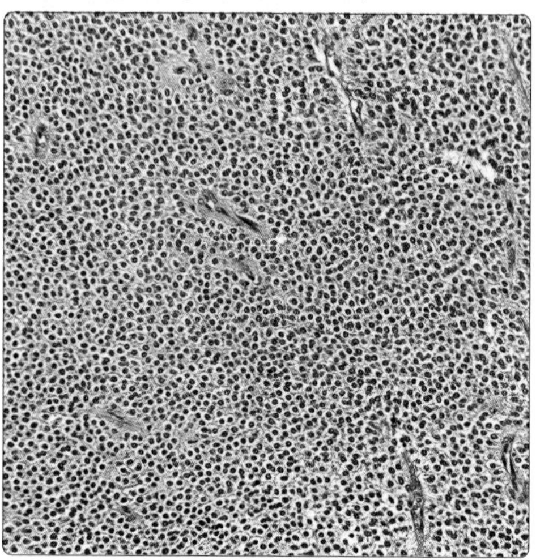

Cytological Monomorphism

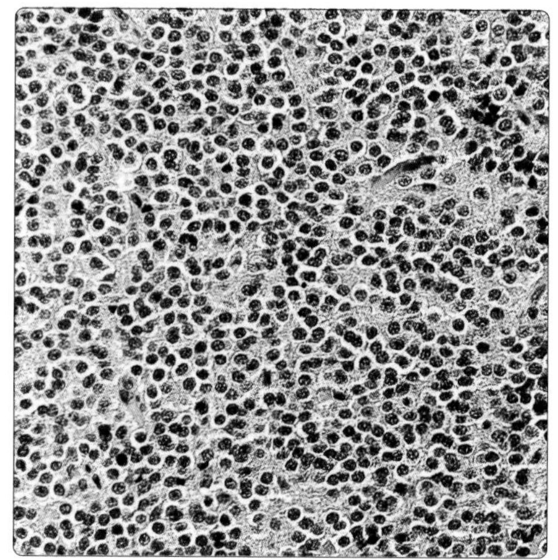

(Left) *Central neurocytomas are compact, noninvasive, and cytologically more monomorphous than other CNS tumors. Vessels are characteristically delicate. These features, in a lesion near the foramen of Monro, leave few diagnostic alternatives.* **(Right)** *Cytological monomorphism of this degree is typical of central neurocytoma. Note the delicate intercellular neuropil.*

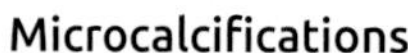

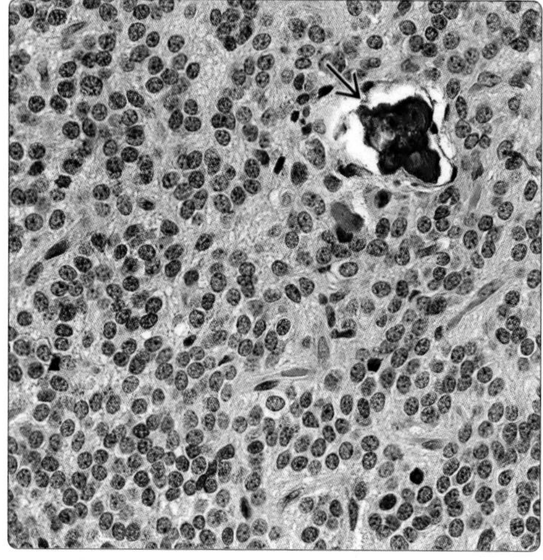

Dense Microcalcifications

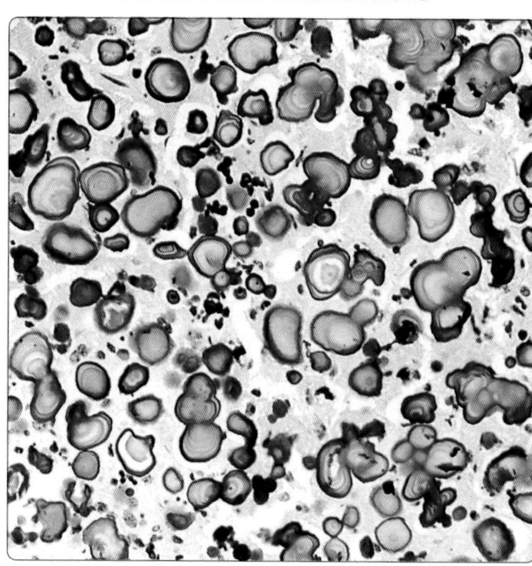

(Left) *Central neurocytomas share compact architecture, high cellularity, and calcifications* → *with ependymoma but are cytologically more monomorphous. The distinction, nevertheless, often rests largely upon immunohistochemistry for synaptophysin positivity and GFAP negativity.* **(Right)** *Some central neurocytomas are so densely calcified as to be a "brain stone."*

Neuropil Zones

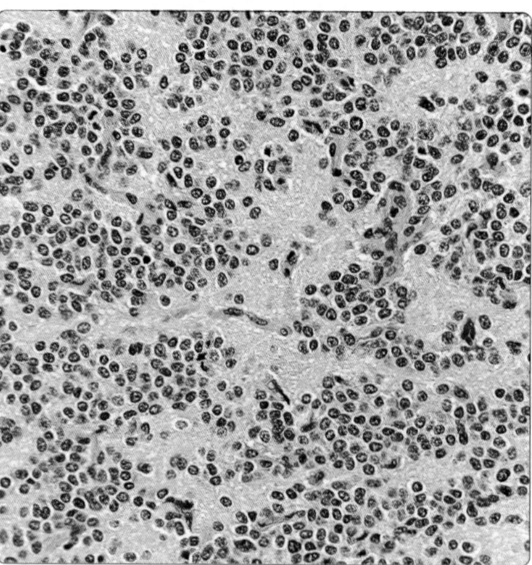

Perivascular Neuropil Zones

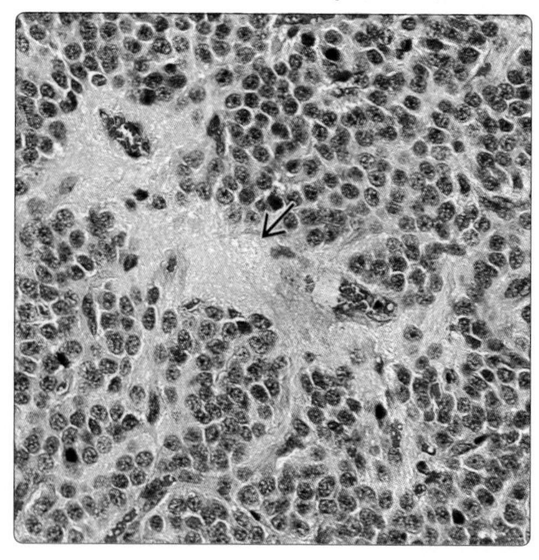

(Left) *Round or stellate often perivascular neuropil zones interrupt the sheet-like architecture of some neurocytomas, producing a resemblance to ependymoma. Immunohistochemistry, synaptophysin positivity and GFAP negativity, makes the distinction.* **(Right)** *Perivascular fibrillar zones* → *in central neurocytomas mimic perivascular pseudorosettes of ependymoma.*

Cellular Monomorphism

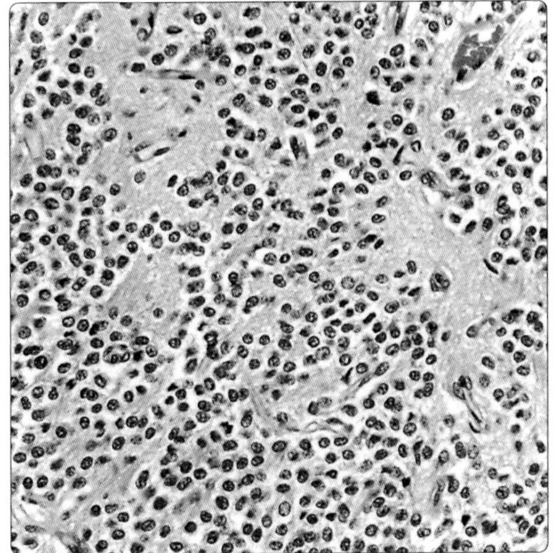

Perivascular Pseudorosette-Like Structures

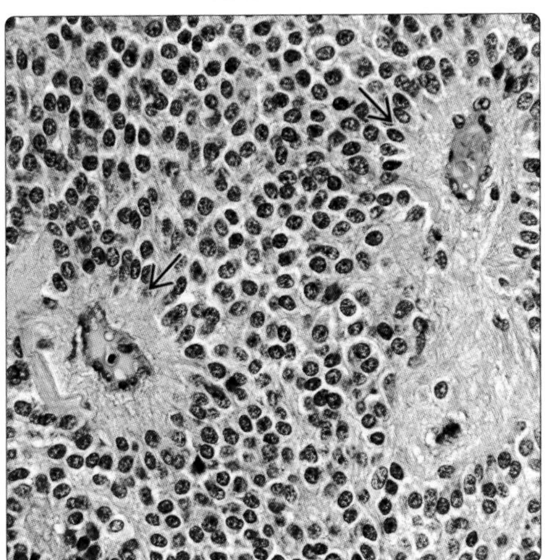

(Left) *Monomorphism and neuroendocrine qualities of neurocytomas facilitate the diagnosis. Oligodendroglioma is a reasonable alternative but lacks compact, noninfiltrative architecture and central localization near the foramen of Monro.* **(Right)** *Given the pseudorosette-like structures of perivascular formations ➙, ependymoma of the foramen of Monro was an early designation for central neurocytoma.*

Neuropil Zones

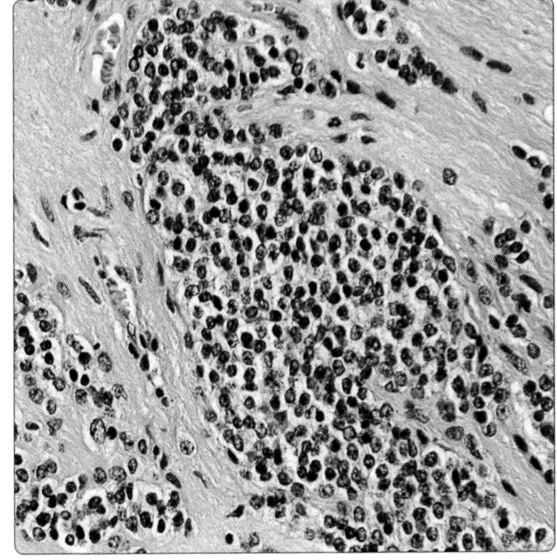

Ganglioid and Ganglion Cells

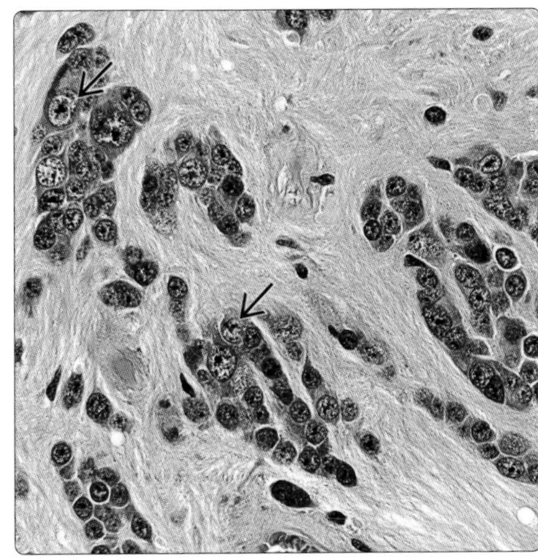

(Left) *Densely cellular islands of neurocytes alternate with eosinophilic, almost acellular, neuropil that will immunolabel for synaptophysin. Only intratumoral reactive astrocytes will react for GFAP.* **(Right)** *Ganglioid cells and even ganglion cells ➙ appear in some central neurocytomas. Processes of such cells contribute the more robust processes within neuropil, here seen to separate clusters of cell bodies.*

Ganglion Cell Differentiation

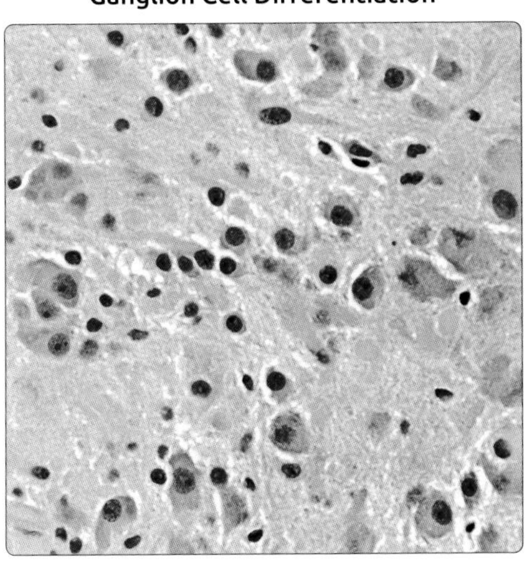

Ganglioid Cells

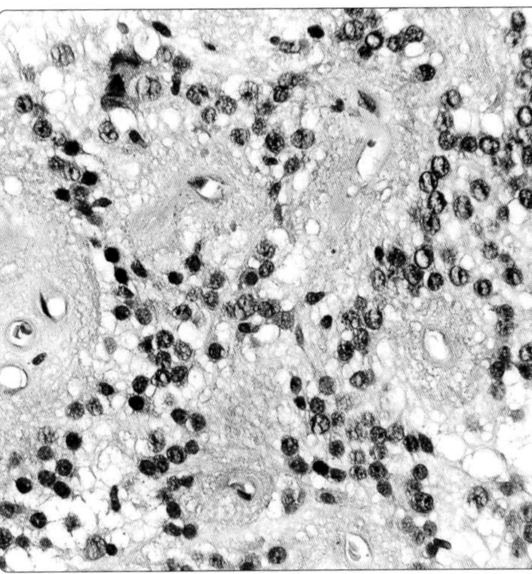

(Left) *In some central neurocytomas, advanced ganglion cell differentiation mimics the appearance of a conventional gangliocytoma.* **(Right)** *Neurocytes and small ganglioid cells form perivascular arrays in some neurocytomas, particularly in extraventricular examples.*

(Left) *Nuclear roundness, clear halos, and "chicken-wire" vasculature in many neurocytomas mimic oligodendroglioma. The intraventricular location of neurocytoma and compact, noninfiltrative architecture resolve the issue.* **(Right)** *Perinuclear halos produce a close mimic of oligodendroglioma.*

Oligodendroglial-Like Appearance

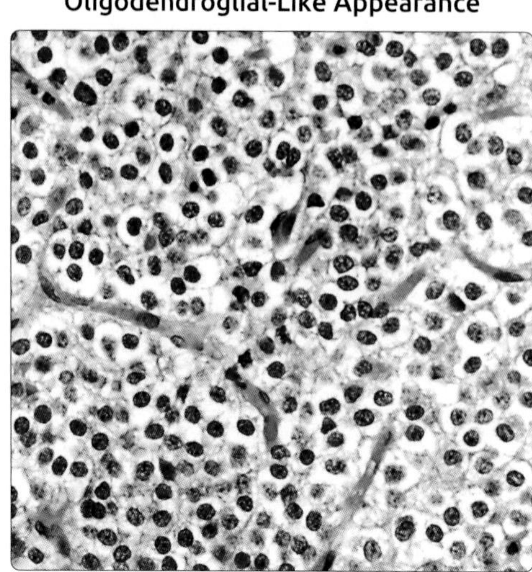

Perinuclear Halos

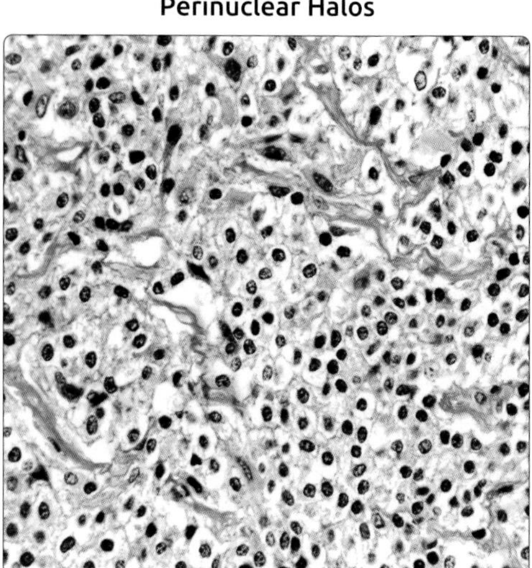

(Left) *Uniform nuclear roundness, in concert with particularly prominent halos, creates the appearance of oligodendroglioma. Not surprisingly, central neurocytomas were once considered intraventricular oligodendroglioma.* **(Right)** *Occasional neurocytomas contain islands of lipidized neurocytes resembling adipocytes. Lipidized neurocytomas are usually cerebellar rather than central.*

Oligodendroglial-Like Appearance

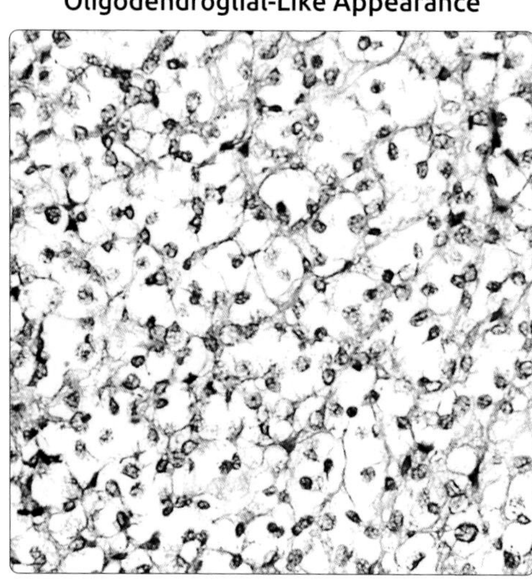

Lipidized Central Neurocytoma

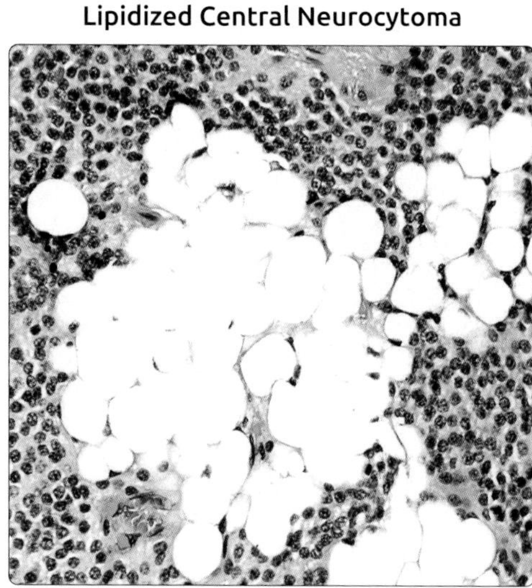

(Left) *While defined mainly by Ki-67 labeling indices, mitoses ⇨ are present in most atypical central neurocytomas. Other features in some cases include nuclear atypia and microvascular proliferation. Mitoses are rare in the classic neurocytoma.* **(Right)** *A significant degree of nuclear pleomorphism occurs in some mitotically active ⇨ atypical neurocytomas. Still, a Ki-67 index > 2 or 3% defines atypical neurocytomas.*

Atypical Neurocytoma

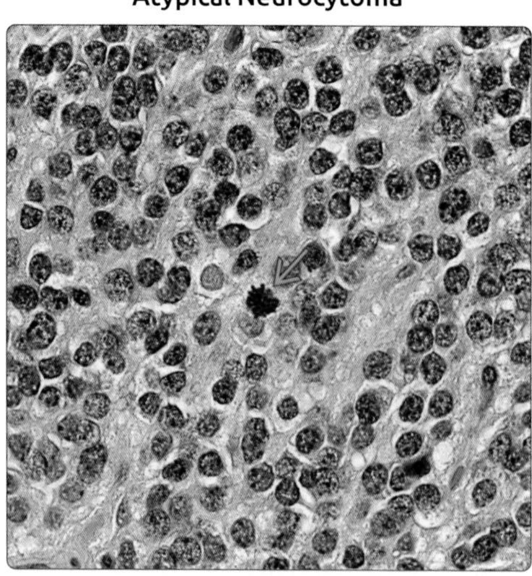

Atypical Neurocytoma

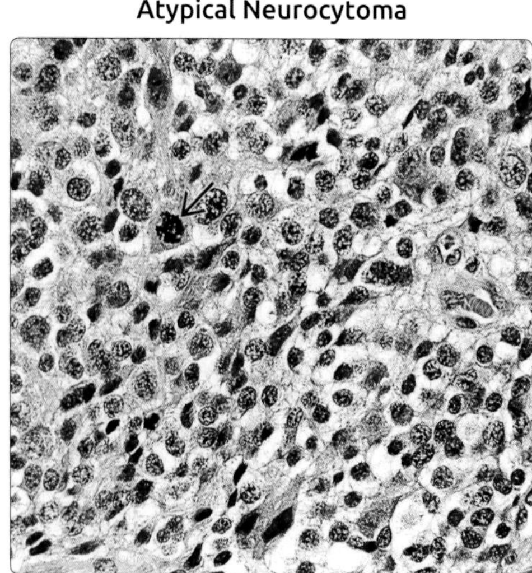

Nuclear Uniformity

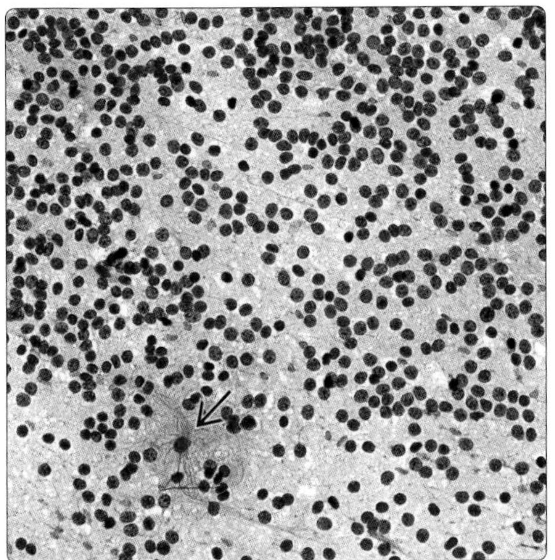

"Salt and Pepper" Chromatin

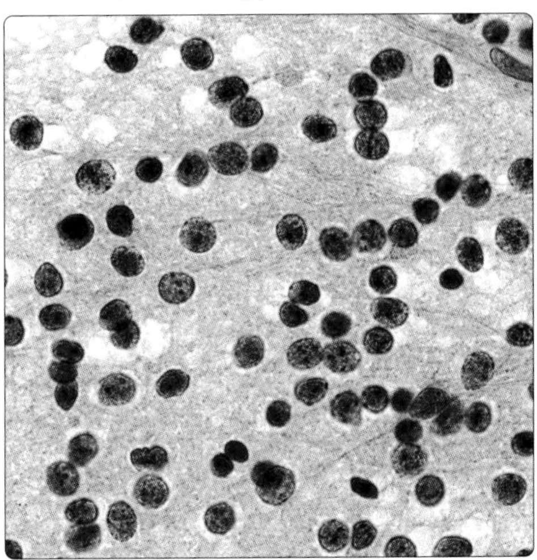

(Left) *Uniformity of nuclear size and shape and absence of axons make central neurocytoma a consideration in this smear preparation of an intraventricular tumor. Note a reactive astrocyte* ⇒. **(Right)** *Dispersed in a monolayer, the cells of central neurocytoma show nuclear uniformity and bland "salt and pepper" chromatin. Unlike ependymoma, there are few cytoplasmic processes.*

Synaptophysin Expression

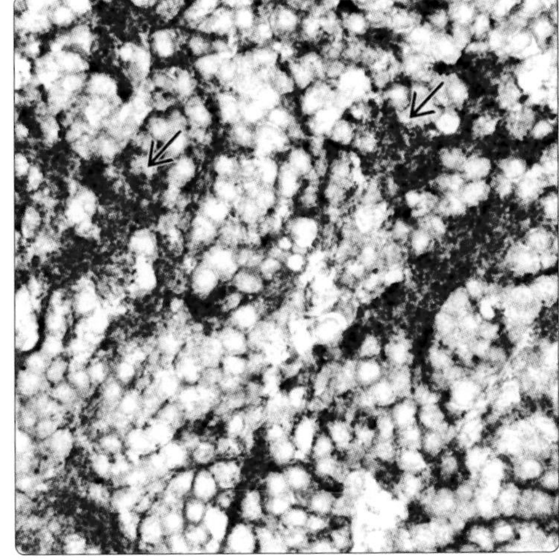

Reactive Astrocytes

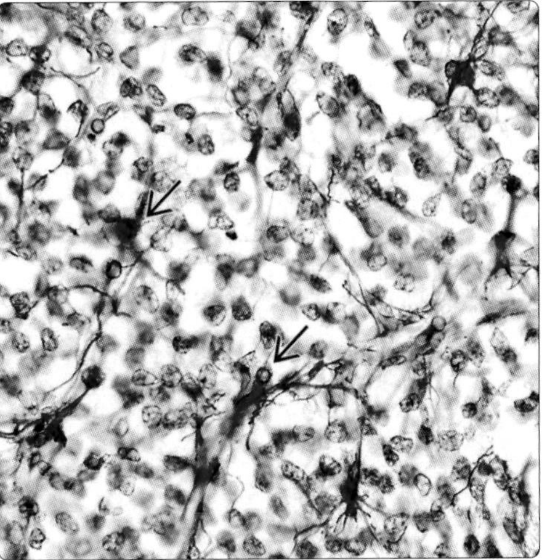

(Left) *The most useful immunomarker of central neurocytoma is synaptophysin, here strongly expressed in neurocytes and neuropil islands* ⇒. *Similar areas in ependymomas are GFAP immunoreactive, rather than synaptophysin immunoreactive.* **(Right)** *Trapped GFAP(+) reactive astrocytes* ⇒ *with long processes are common around small vessels in central neurocytoma. Glial differentiation is not a feature.*

Ki-67 Labeling Index in Neurocytoma

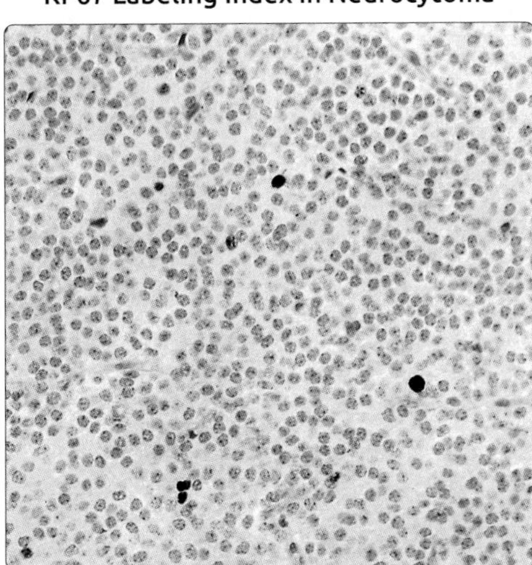

Ki-67 Labeling Index in Atypical Neurocytoma

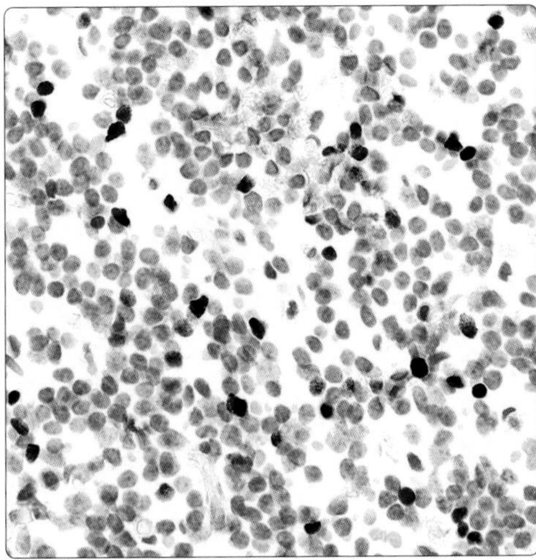

(Left) *The Ki-67 labeling index is low (≤ 1%) in typical central neurocytomas.* **(Right)** *Atypical neurocytomas are defined mainly by increased (> 2-3%) Ki-67 labeling. It is ~ 10% in this case. Such lesions often have mitoses and even microvascular proliferation.*

KEY FACTS

IMAGING

- Well circumscribed
- Variable contrast enhancement
- "Cyst with mural nodule" architecture, in some cases

MACROSCOPIC

- Gross circumscription is rule
- Unlike ill-defined borders seen in oligodendroglioma

MICROSCOPIC

- Sharp interface with nonneoplastic brain
- Sheets of round cells with stippled "salt and pepper" chromatin
- Large neuropil islands or Homer Wright rosettes
- Frequent ganglion cell differentiation in ~ 2/3 of cases
- Frequently calcified

ANCILLARY TESTS

- Neuronal proteins
    - Synaptophysin uniformly expressed
- GFAP immunoreactive cells present in > 50% of cases

TOP DIFFERENTIAL DIAGNOSES

- Oligodendroglioma
    - Infiltrating growth pattern
    - Secondary structures, e.g., perineuronal satellitosis, subpial accumulation of tumor cells
    - Microcysts frequent
    - 1p/19q codeletion in most cases
- Dysembryoplastic neuroepithelial tumor
- Infiltrating astrocytoma
    - Infiltrating growth pattern
- Ganglioglioma
    - Conspicuous ganglion cell and glial component not feature of pure extraventricular neurocytoma
- Papillary glioneuronal tumor

(Left) *Extraventricular neurocytoma (EVN) ➔ is a well-circumscribed neoplasm, often with a cyst-mural nodule architecture. A differential diagnostic possibility, grade II oligodendroglioma, does not enhance.* **(Right)** *EVN is characterized by prominent neurocytic differentiation, including the presence of well-developed rosettes with delicate neuropil cores in some cases.*

Cyst-Mural Nodule Architecture

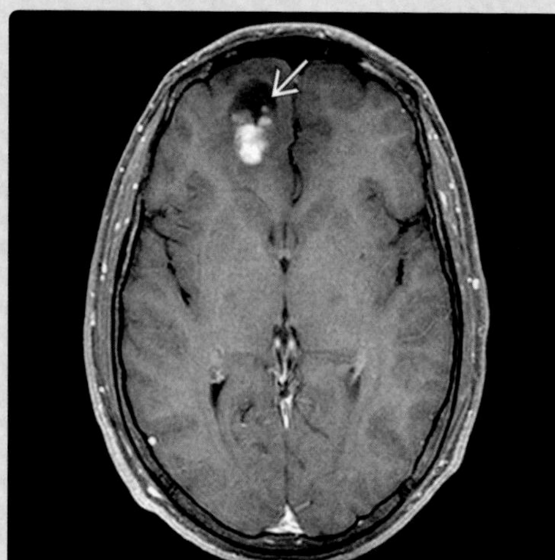

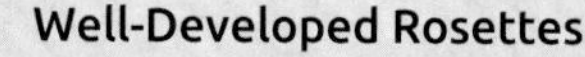

Well-Developed Rosettes

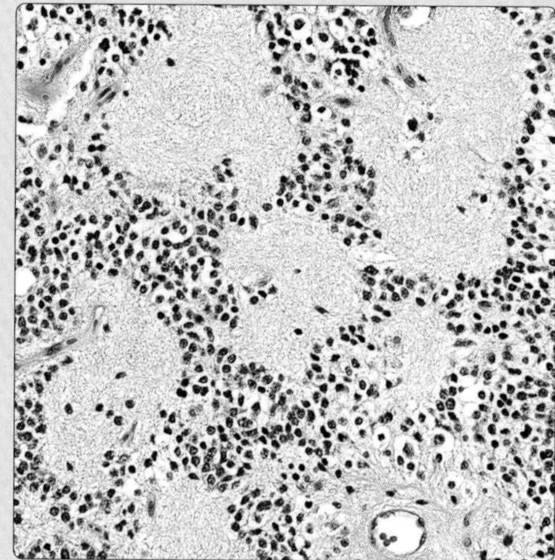

(Left) *Microcalcifications are not uncommon in EVN, as shown in this example.* **(Right)** *All EVNs strongly express synaptophysin. This example demonstrates sharp circumscription with adjacent gliotic brain.*

Microcalcifications

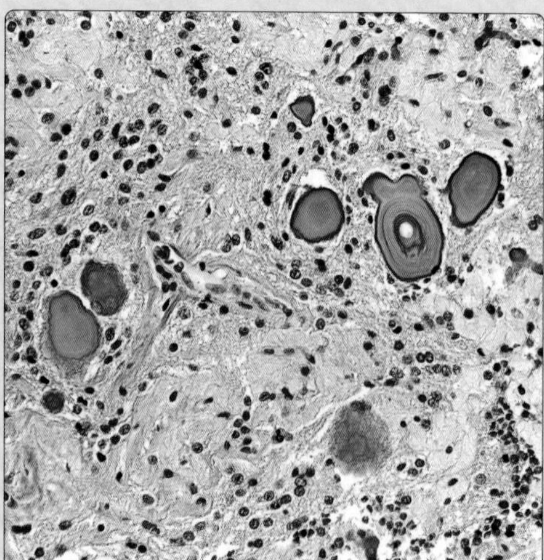

Synaptophysin Expression

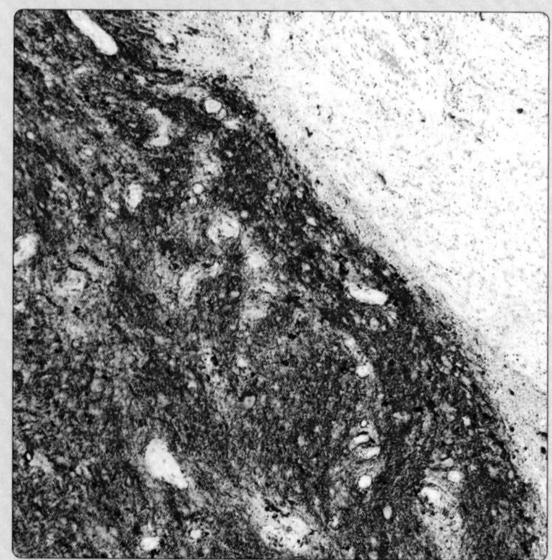

TERMINOLOGY

Abbreviations

- Extraventricular neurocytoma (EVN)

Definitions

- Well-differentiated neurocytic neoplasm arising outside lateral ventricles and septum pellucidum, usually in cerebral hemispheres
- No WHO grade assigned but probably grade II

CLINICAL ISSUES

Treatment

- Complete resection optimal
- Radiation therapy for subtotally resected tumors

Prognosis

- Usually favorable after gross total resection
- Recurrence associated with subtotal resection &/or atypical histologic features

IMAGING

General Features

- Location
  - Supratentorial brain or spinal cord

MR Findings

- Well circumscribed
- Contrast enhancement variable
- Cyst with mural nodule (some cases)

CT Findings

- Calcifications common

MACROSCOPIC

General Features

- Gross circumscription is rule
- Unlike ill-defined borders seen in oligodendroglioma

MICROSCOPIC

Histologic Features

- Sharp interface with surrounding brain
- Sheets of round cells with "salt and pepper" chromatin
  - Similar in cellularity to central neurocytoma in some cases, but often lower
  - Oligodendroglioma quality in cytology and pattern
- Large neuropil islands or Homer Wright rosettes
- Ganglion cell differentiation (majority of cases)
- Frequently calcified
  - Extensive calcification ("brain stone") uncommon
- Hyalinized vessels
- Mitoses low level

Grading Criteria

- Not well established
- Atypical designation appropriate in subset with necrosis, vascular proliferation, mitoses > 3 per 10 HPF

ANCILLARY TESTS

Cytology

- Monotonous cells with stippled chromatin

Immunohistochemistry

- Neuronal proteins
  - Synaptophysin (+)
    - Neurocytes, rosettes, and ganglion cells
  - Chromogranin (+), more often in ganglion cells
  - NeuN expression often positive
    - Negative result does not exclude EVN
- GFAP
  - Tumor cells (+), > 50%
    - Positive cells in central form of neurocytoma are reactive astrocytes

DIFFERENTIAL DIAGNOSIS

Oligodendroglioma

- Infiltrating growth pattern
  - Secondary structures, e.g., perineuronal satellitosis, subpial accumulation of tumor cells
- Microcysts frequent
- 1p/19q codeletion, in most cases
  - Some extraventricular neurocytomas reported as codeleted and containing t(1;19)
- *IDH1/2* mutations present in most cases but usually lacking in extraventricular neurocytoma

Dysembryoplastic Neuroepithelial Tumor

- Overruns normal cortex
  - Not discrete mass; nodular architecture
  - Floating neurons
- Low cellularity; no cellular sheets of neurocytes
- No hyalinized vessels

Infiltrating Astrocytoma

- No contrast enhancement in grade II and some grade III
- Infiltrating growth pattern
  - Secondary structures and nuclear pleomorphism
  - Nuclear irregularity

Ganglioglioma

- Conspicuous ganglion cell and glial component, not features of pure extraventricular neurocytoma
- If neurocytic component in ganglioglioma is extensive or predominates, best to place it in EVN category

Papillary Glioneuronal Tumor

- Papillary or pseudopapillary architecture
  - Perivascular small astrocytes
  - Interpapillary neurocytes ± ganglion cells

SELECTED REFERENCES

1. Rodriguez FJ et al: Interphase cytogenetics for 1p19q and t(1;19)(q10;p10) may distinguish prognostically relevant subgroups in extraventricular neurocytoma. Brain Pathol. 19(4):623-9, 2009
2. Brat DJ et al: Extraventricular neurocytomas: pathologic features and clinical outcome. Am J Surg Pathol. 25(10):1252-60, 2001

Rosettes

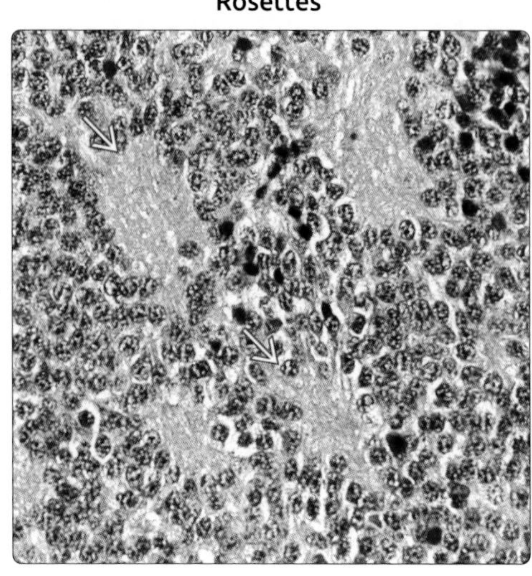

Finely Fibrillar Tissue

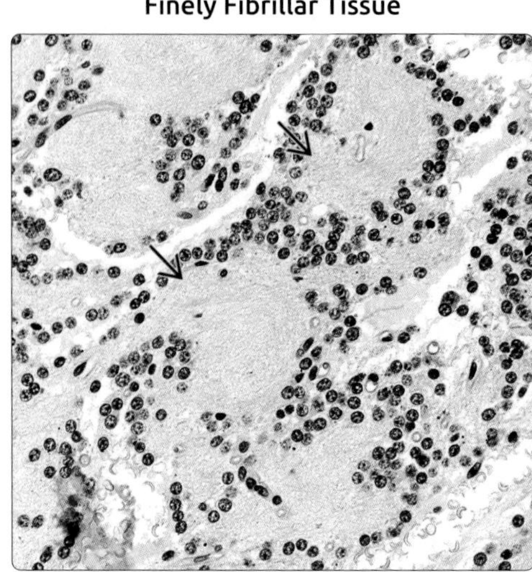

(Left) *Some extraventricular neurocytomas are indistinguishable in terms of cellularity from their central counterparts near the foramen of Monro. Rosettes with finely fibrillar neuropil cores ➡ are common in both lesions.* **(Right)** *Finely fibrillar tissue ➡ may be the dominant tissue when neurocytic rosettes are numerous and large. The cellularity of these largely anuclear cores is considerably less than that of normal gray matter.*

Compact Nests

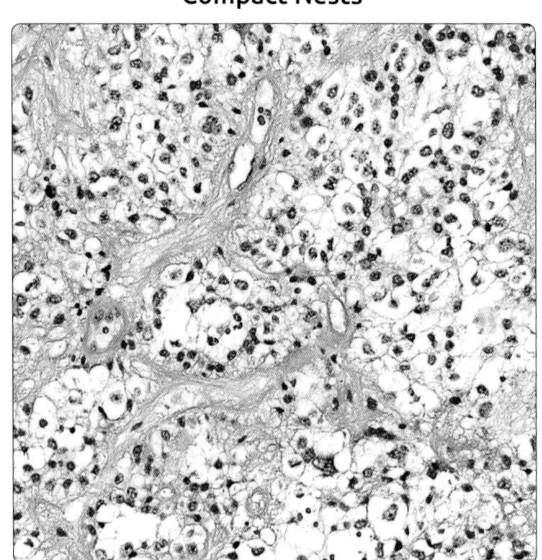

Cellular Monotony

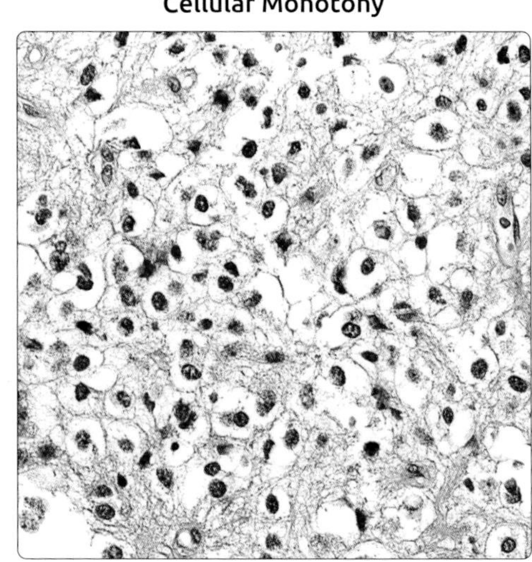

(Left) *Compact nests of tumor cells in a fibrillary background are present in some EVNs, particularly those with glial differentiation.* **(Right)** *Although cellular monotony is an important diagnostic feature of EVN, a degree of pleomorphism is compatible with the diagnosis. The illustrated tumor is also entirely consistent with oligodendroglioma, although the latter is an infiltrating and generally synaptophysin negative tumor.*

Round Nuclei and Perinuclear Clearing

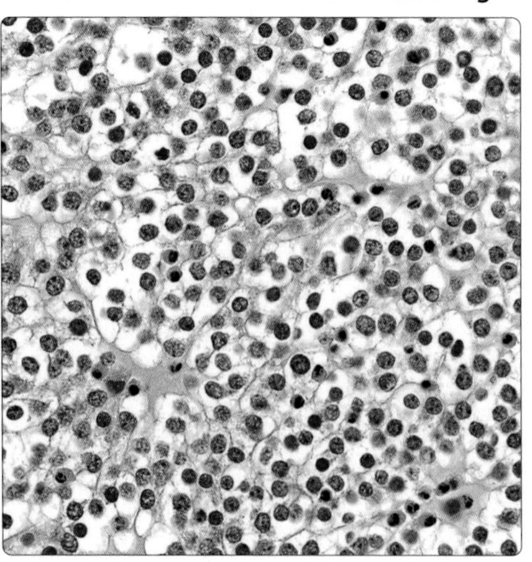

Eosinophilic Cytoplasm

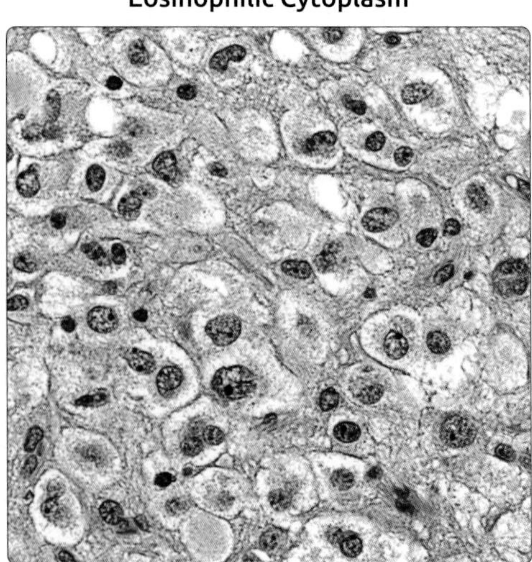

(Left) *Round nuclei with perinuclear clearing are cytologic features that overlap with those of oligodendroglioma. The latter are infiltrating tumors, however, whereas neurocytomas are discrete masses.* **(Right)** *Perinuclear clearing is not a universal feature of EVN. In this example, eosinophilic cytoplasm lacks the prominent clear cell artifact that gives some neurocytomas their oligodendroglioma appearance.*

Vascular Hyalinization and Microcalcifications

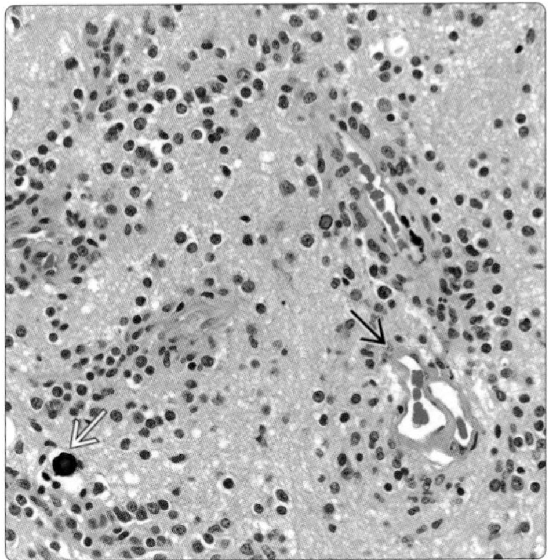

Rows of Neurocytes

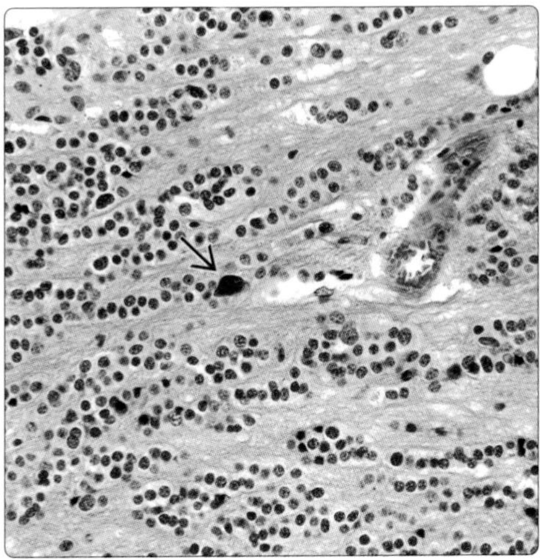

(Left) *Subtle features of chronicity in some EVN include vascular hyalinization ⇨ and focal microcalcifications ➡.* **(Right)** *Straight rows of monotonous neurocytes suggest neurocytic differentiation in low-grade CNS neoplasms. EVNs may contain occasional pleomorphic cells ⇨, a finding without prognostic significance.*

Discrete Tumor Margin

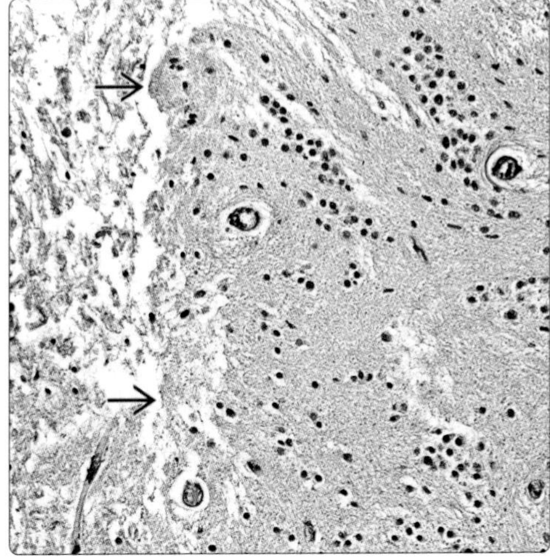

Large Calcifications

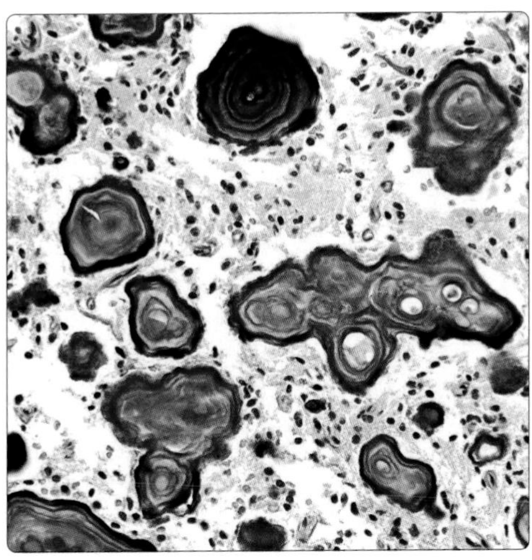

(Left) *Areas of EVN may be markedly hypocellular and difficult to distinguish from nonneoplastic brain. A discrete margin between them ⇨, however, is a clue as to the nature of the lesion. It at least raises the possibility that the tumor is not infiltrating glioma.* **(Right)** *Large, concentric, coalescing calcifications are a conspicuous feature of some EVNs. Microcalcifications may rarely be so extensive and closely packed as to produce a "brain stone."*

Ganglion Cell Differentiation

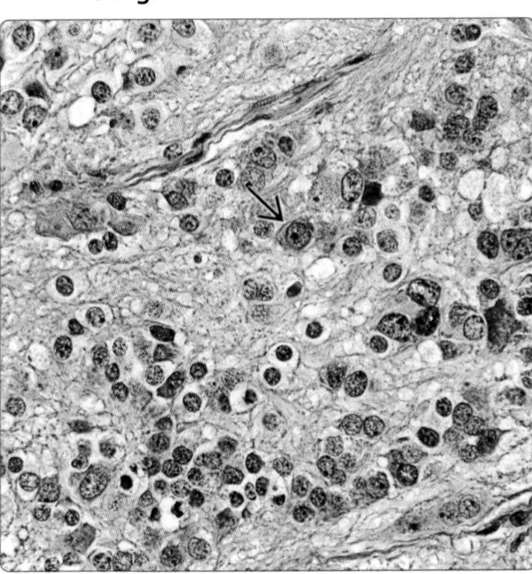

Large Ganglion Cells

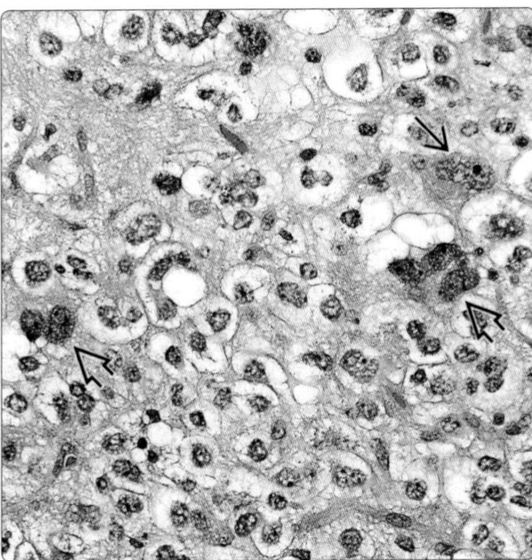

(Left) *Ganglion cell differentiation is more frequent in EVN than in its central counterpart. Small ganglioid cells ⇨ are suggested by the subtle increase in cytoplasm and a large central nucleolus.* **(Right)** *Larger ganglion cells are present in some EVNs ⇨, as are pleomorphic cells ⇨ that are difficult to assign to glial or neuronal lineage based on morphology alone.*

(Left) *Oligodendroglioma-like cells in a compact, noninfiltrative mass are entirely consistent with neurocytoma, whether extraventricular as here, or when centrally situated at the foramen of Monro.* **(Right)** *Glial differentiation is more frequent in EVNs than in central neurocytomas. Here, it takes the form of bundled elongated cells with cytoplasmic processes ⇒.*

Oligodendroglioma-Like Cells

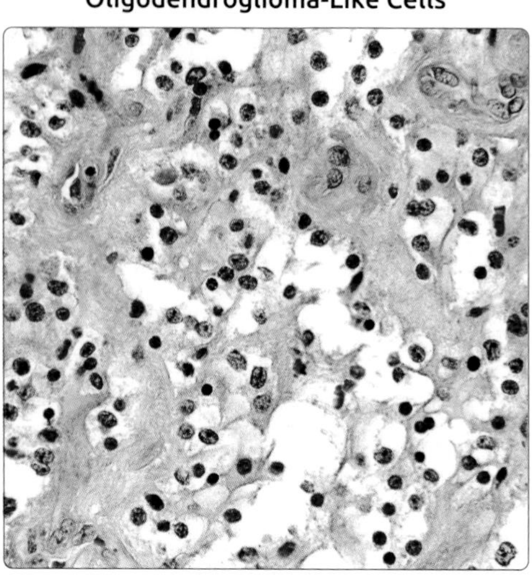

Glial Differentiation

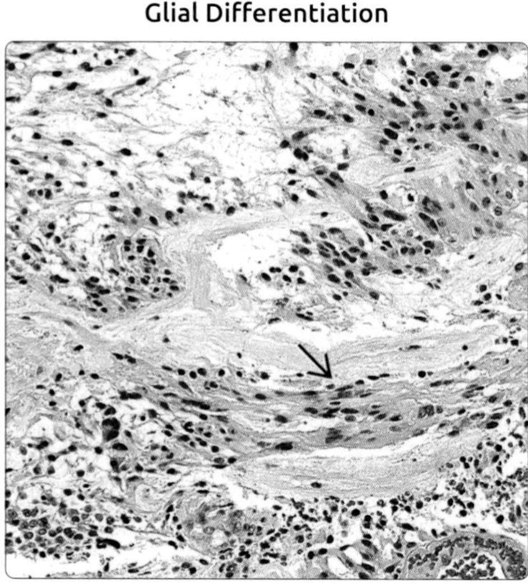

(Left) *In contrast to ependymomas, the finely fibrillar background in EVNs consists of neuropil that would be immunoreactive for synaptophysin rather than GFAP. The degree of fibrillarity is consistent with either entity.* **(Right)** *Areas of high cellularity among a fibrillar background are common in both EVNs and ependymoma. While there may be distinguishing histological features, relative immunoreactivities for synaptophysin and GFAP often make the distinction.*

Neuropil

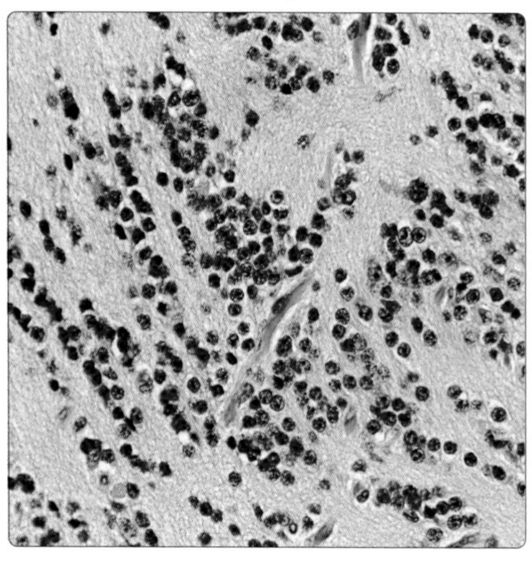

High Cellularity

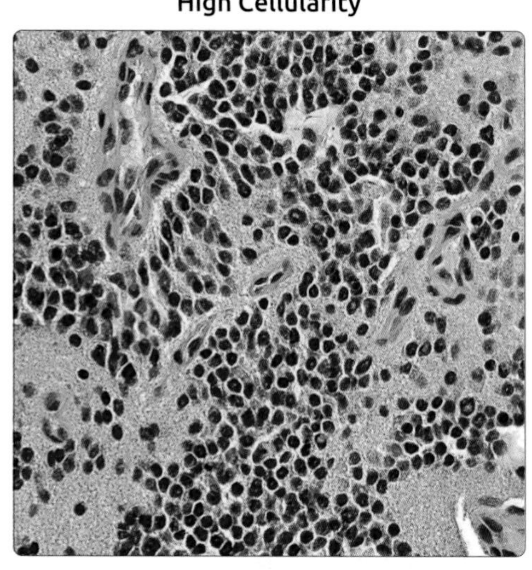

(Left) *Increased cellularity in EVNs is a worrisome finding that should prompt a search for other atypical features, such as increased mitotic activity and microvascular proliferation. Grading criteria for EVNs are not well formulated, however.* **(Right)** *Necrosis is a worrisome finding in EVNs, and it helped place this particular tumor in the atypical category. Necrosis suggests the potential for more aggressive behavior than in conventional EVNs.*

Increased Cellularity

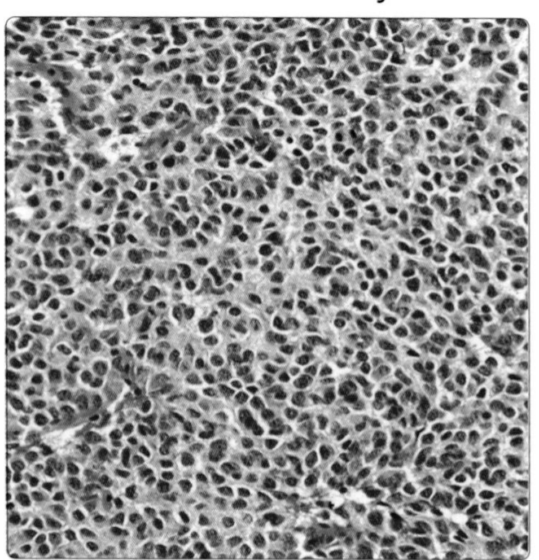

Necrosis

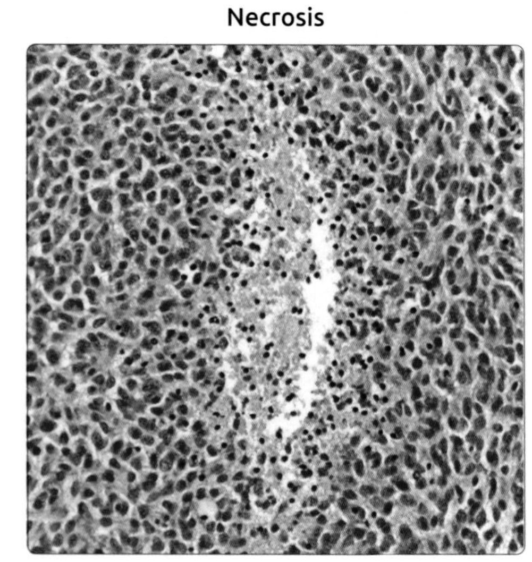

Diffuse Synaptophysin Staining

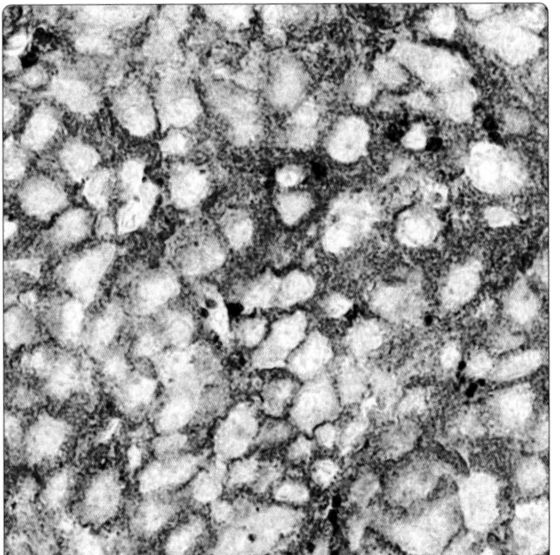

Chromogranin Labeling

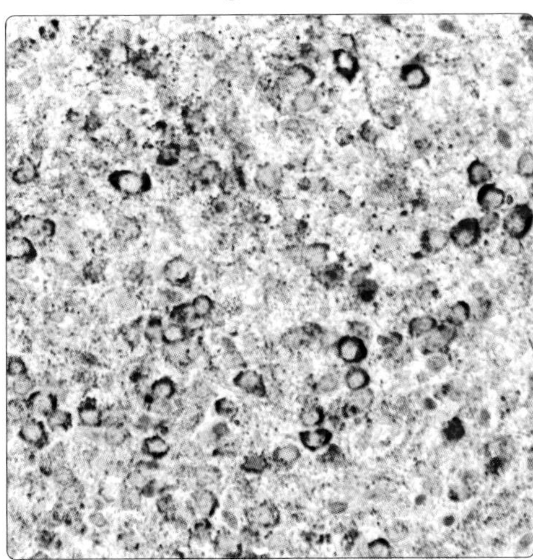

(Left) *Strong, diffuse synaptophysin staining of membranes, cytoplasm, and neuropil helps distinguish EVN from morphologic mimics.* **(Right)** *Chromogranin labeling in some EVNs confirms neuronal differentiation. Immunopositivity to this degree is more commonly seen for synaptophysin, however.*

Glial Differentiation

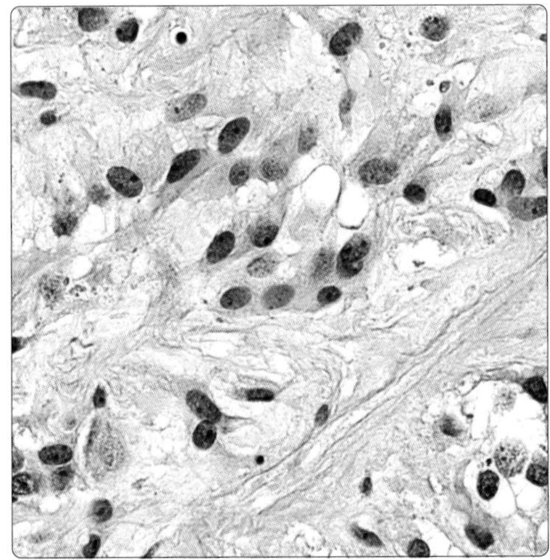

GFAP Immunoreactivity

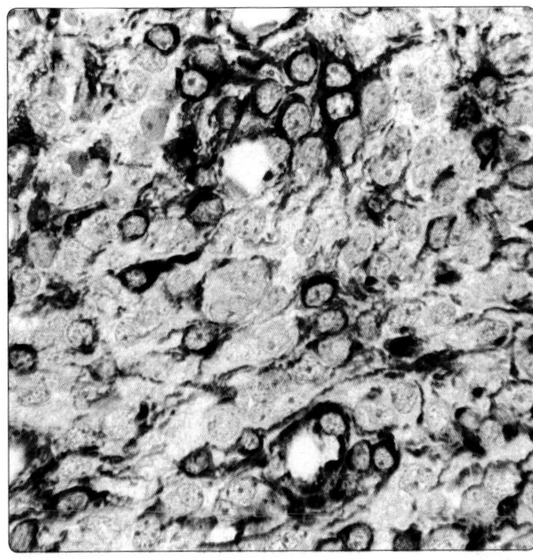

(Left) *Focal glial differentiation is conspicuous in this EVN containing elongated cells with oval nuclei and eosinophilic cell processes in a coarse fibrillary background.* **(Right)** *Immunoreactivity for GFAP in cytologically abnormal cells confirms glial differentiation, which may be only focal.*

Neurosecretory Granules

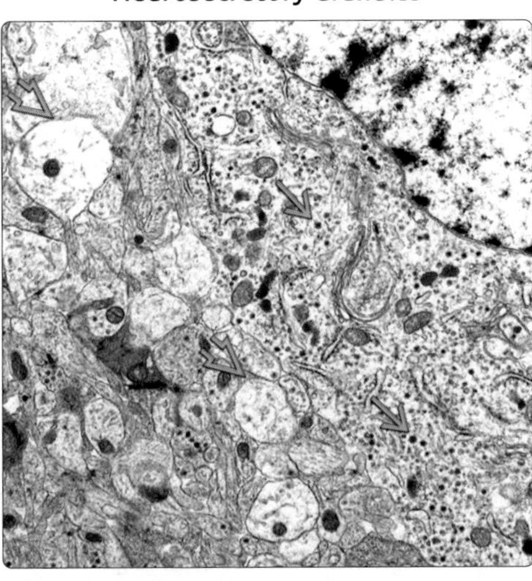

t(1;19) Translocation

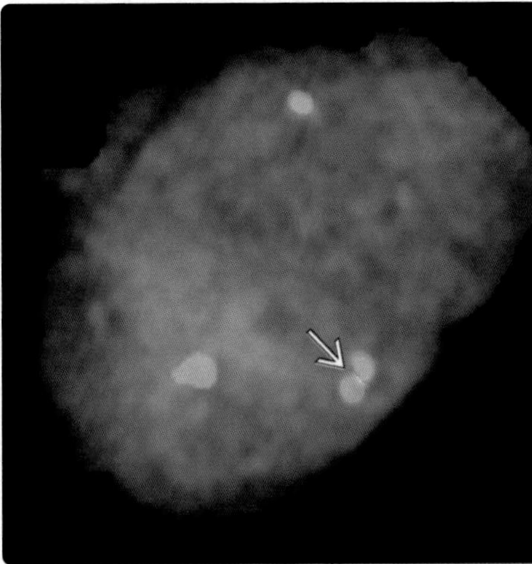

(Left) *Numerous small neurosecretory granules are shown ⇨ in the cytoplasm of an EVN cell at the ultrastructural level. Note numerous neuronal processes ⇨ that, in aggregate, form neuropil.* **(Right)** *FISH study demonstrates juxtaposition of centromere 1 (red) and 19p12 (green) reflecting t(1;19) ➡, a feature in ~ 25% of EVN. Its significance is unclear but supports a biologic overlap with oligodendroglioma.*

Cerebellar Liponeurocytoma

KEY FACTS

TERMINOLOGY

- WHO grade II, largely on basis of relatively frequent recurrence

CLINICAL ISSUES

- Headache, obstructive hydrocephalus
- Good overall survival, but relatively frequent (~ 50%) recurrence

MICROSCOPIC

- Round, monotonous cells with scant cytoplasm and stippled chromatin (neurocytes)
- Large lipid vacuoles in subset of cells resembling mature adipocytes
- Infiltrating glial component (some cases)
- Myoid cells (rare)
- Mitotic figures rare to absent

ANCILLARY TESTS

- Diffusely (+) for neuronal antigens (synaptophysin, MAP2)
- Focal GFAP(+) in some cases
- *TP53* mutations in 20%
- Gene expression profiles similar to central neurocytoma but different from medulloblastoma

TOP DIFFERENTIAL DIAGNOSES

- Lipoma
- Clear cell ependymoma
- Teratoma
- Oligodendroglioma

DIAGNOSTIC CHECKLIST

- Low proliferation reflects better prognosis and distinguishes it from medulloblastoma
- Consider cerebellar liponeurocytoma for neoplasm with uniform, round, adipocyte-like cells and low proliferation rate

T1 Hyperintensity

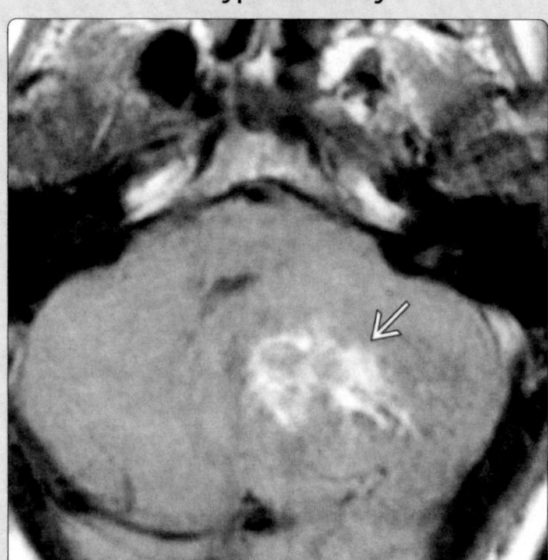

Neurocytes and Lipidized Cells

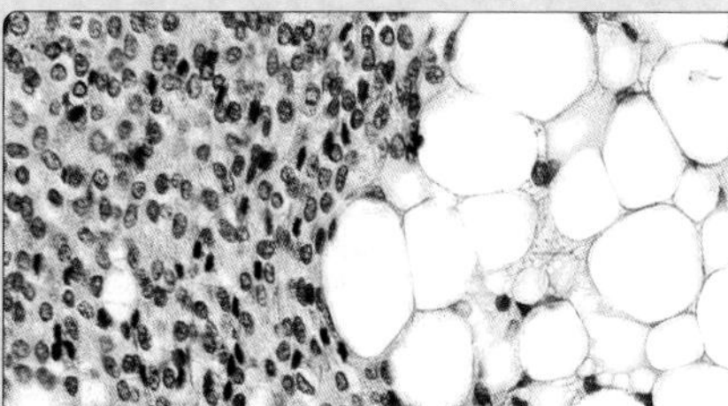

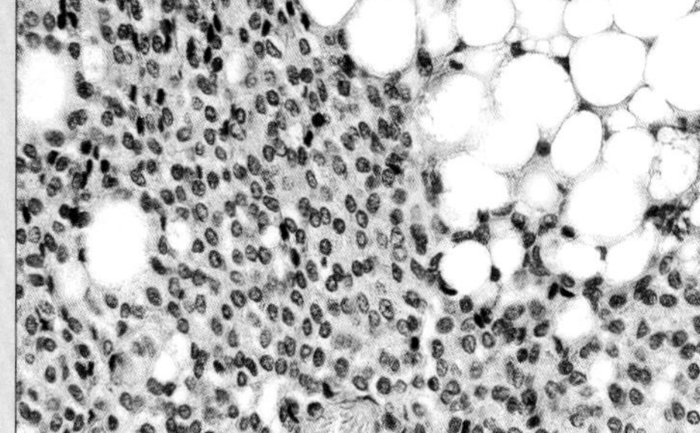

(Left) *Cerebellar liponeurocytomas are generally well circumscribed and, due to their lipid content, hyperintense on T1-weighted precontrast MR images ➡.* **(Right)** *The principal components of cerebellar liponeurocytoma include classic neurocytes and distinctive, variably lipidized cells resembling adipose tissue.*

Synaptophysin Expression

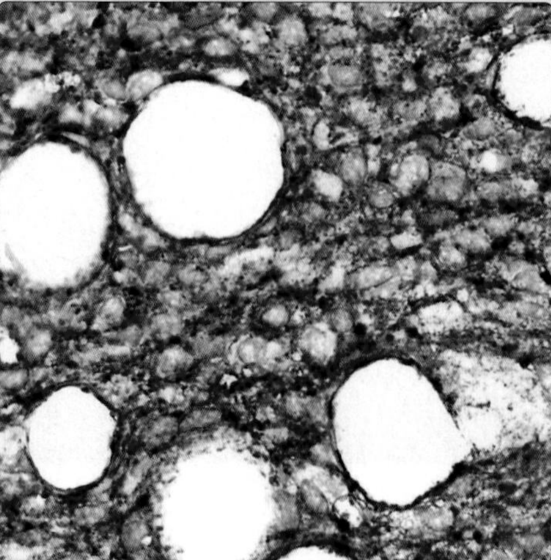

GFAP(+) Component

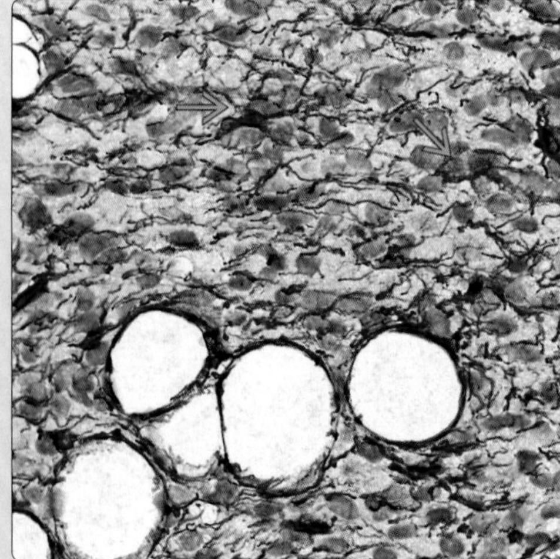

(Left) *As it is typical of well-differentiated neurocytic neoplasms, cerebellar liponeurocytomas are intensely immunoreactive for synaptophysin.* **(Right)** *A GFAP(+) component may be present in cerebellar liponeurocytomas, but more often only reactive astrocytes ➡ are positive.*

TERMINOLOGY

Synonyms

- Medullocytoma
- Lipomatous glioneurocytoma
- Liponeurocytoma
- Lipidized mature neuroectodermal tumor of cerebellum

Definitions

- Well-differentiated neurocytic neoplasm with adipocyte-like cells
- WHO grade II, largely on basis of relatively frequent recurrence

CLINICAL ISSUES

Epidemiology

- Age
  - Adults, mean age: 50 years

Presentation

- Headache, obstructive hydrocephalus, focal neurologic deficits

Prognosis

- Good overall survival, but relatively frequent (~ 50%) recurrence rate

IMAGING

General Features

- Location
  - Cerebellum
    - Mainly hemispheric

MR Findings

- Well circumscribed
- Variable T1 and T2 hyperintensity
- Heterogeneous enhancement
- Little or no peritumoral edema

MICROSCOPIC

Histologic Features

- Round, monotonous cells with scant cytoplasm and stippled chromatin typical of neurocytes
- Large lipid vacuoles in subset of cells resembling mature adipocytes
- Mitotic figures rare to absent
- Well-differentiated glial, infiltrative component (some cases)
- Myoid differentiation (rare)

ANCILLARY TESTS

Immunohistochemistry

- Diffusely (+) for neuronal antigens (synaptophysin, MAP2)
- Focal GFAP(+) in some cases
- Desmin (+) myoid components (rare)

Genetic Testing

- *TP53* mutations in 20%
- Gene expression profiles similar to central neurocytoma but different from medulloblastoma
- Absent *PTCH*, *APC*, or *β-catenin* mutations
  - Absent isodicentric 17q
  - Absent monosomy 6

Electron Microscopy

- Microtubule-containing processes
- Neurosecretory granules
- Nonmembrane bound lipid

DIFFERENTIAL DIAGNOSIS

Lipoma

- Only adipose tissue, no neurocytoma

Clear Cell Ependymoma

- Rare in posterior fossa
- Well-formed GFAP(+) pseudorosettes, at least focally
- Grooved/clefted nuclei
- Scant to absent immunoreactivity for neuronal markers
- EMA(+) dots or microlumina in most cases

Teratoma

- Other tissue types or germ cell tumor constituents
- No neurocytic component

Oligodendroglioma

- Rare in posterior fossa
- 1p19q codeletion and *IDH1/2* mutations

DIAGNOSTIC CHECKLIST

Clinically Relevant Pathologic Features

- Low proliferation reflects better prognosis and distinguishes it from medulloblastoma

Pathologic Interpretation Pearls

- Consider cerebellar liponeurocytoma for neoplasm with uniform, round, adipocyte-like cells and low proliferation rate

SELECTED REFERENCES

1. Chakraborti S et al: Supratentorial and cerebellar liponeurocytomas: report of four cases with review of literature. J Neurooncol. 103(1):121-7, 2011
2. Hortobágyi T et al: Adult cerebellar liponeurocytoma with predominant pilocytic pattern and myoid differentiation. Neuropathol Appl Neurobiol. 33(1):121-5, 2007
3. Kuchelmeister K et al: Liponeurocytoma of the left lateral ventricle–case report and review of the literature. Clin Neuropathol. 25(2):86-94, 2006
4. Aker FV et al: Cerebellar liponeurocytoma/lipidized medulloblastoma. J Neurooncol. 71(1):53-9, 2005
5. Horstmann S et al: Genetic and expression profiles of cerebellar liponeurocytomas. Brain Pathol. 14(3):281-9, 2004
6. Giordana MT et al: Medulloblastoma with lipidized cells versus lipomatous medulloblastoma. Clin Neuropathol. 19(6):273-7, 2000
7. González-Cámpora R et al: Lipidized mature neuroectodermal tumour of the cerebellum with myoid differentiation. Neuropathol Appl Neurobiol. 24(5):397-402, 1998
8. Giangaspero F et al: Medullocytoma (lipidized medulloblastoma). A cerebellar neoplasm of adults with favorable prognosis. Am J Surg Pathol. 20(6):656-64, 1996

Dysembryoplastic Neuroepithelial Tumor

KEY FACTS

TERMINOLOGY

- Dysembryoplastic neuroepithelial tumor (DNET, DNT)

CLINICAL ISSUES

- Site
    - Cerebral cortex; temporal lobe (including mesial structures) most frequently affected
- Prognosis
    - Limited growth potential; stabilization even after subtotal resections is rule

IMAGING

- Multiple T2-hyperintense nodules limited to cerebral cortex, no edema, little mass effect
- Lack of enhancement in majority of cases

MICROSCOPIC

- Round, small, monotonous cells (oligodendroglial-like) forming well-distinct macronodules
- Pyramidal neurons in pools of mucin ("floating" neurons) lacking satellitosis highly characteristic
- Specific glioneuronal element
- Cortical dysplasia of adjacent cortex in some cases
- Microcysts [Alcian blue (+)]

ANCILLARY TESTS

- 1p/19q codeletion typical of oligodendroglioma is not feature

TOP DIFFERENTIAL DIAGNOSES

- Oligodendroglioma
    - Often difficult to exclude
- Pilocytic astrocytoma
- Ganglioglioma
- Extraventricular neurocytoma
- Rosette-forming glioneuronal tumor

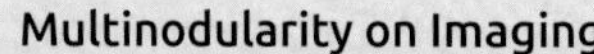

Multinodularity on Imaging

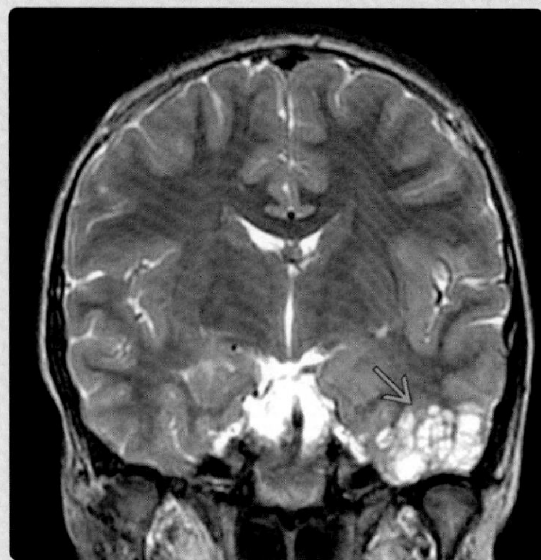

Cortical-Based Nodules

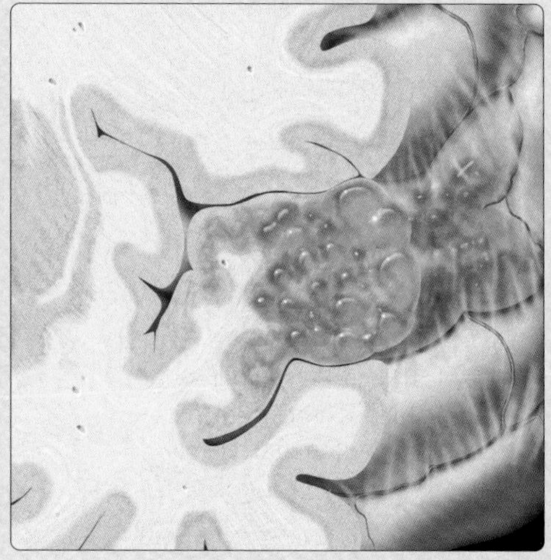

(Left) *A multinodular, T2W hyperintense, corticocentric abnormality ⇒ with little mass effect is characteristic of dysembryoplastic neuroepithelial tumor (DNET).* **(Right)** *Clusters of cortical-based nodules are a key diagnostic feature of DNET. The temporal lobe is a common, but not exclusive, site.*

Oligodendroglial-Like Morphology

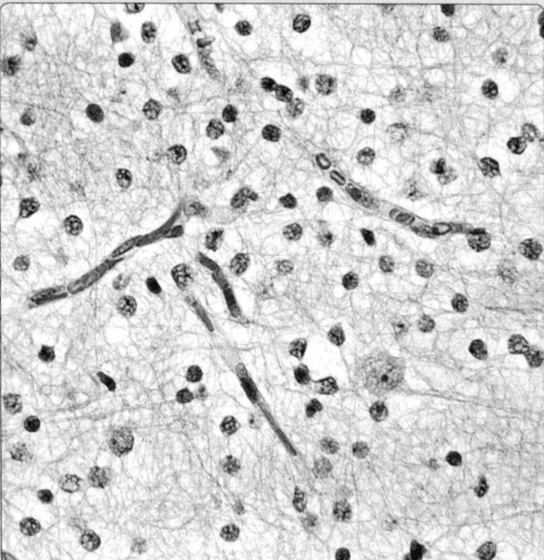

"Floating" Neurons

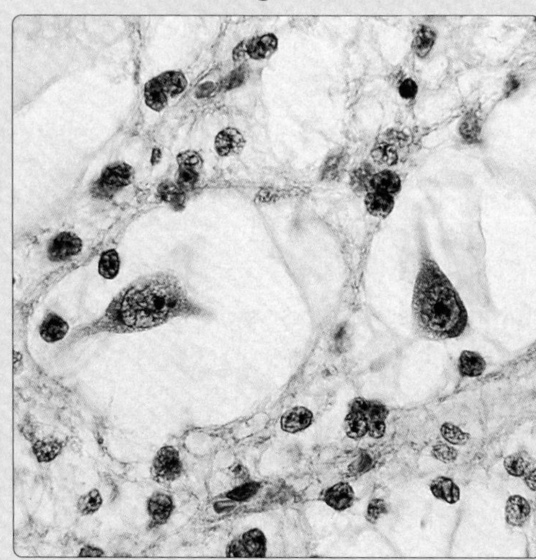

(Left) *Round uniform cells resembling those found in oligodendrogliomas represent the key cellular component of DNET.* **(Right)** *Large ganglion cells suspended in small pools of mucin ("floating" neurons) are very helpful diagnostic features of DNET.*

TERMINOLOGY

Abbreviations

- Dysembryoplastic neuroepithelial tumor (DNET, DNT)

Definitions

- Cortical-based multinodular lesion associated with chronic seizures
- WHO grade I

CLINICAL ISSUES

Site

- Cerebral cortex, particularly mesial temporal lobe (common)
- Septum pellucidum, caudate (uncommon)
- Brainstem and cerebellum (rare)

Presentation

- Children and young adults
- Chronic seizures, partial complex type
- Obstructive hydrocephalus with septum pellucidum lesions

Natural History

- Slow growth or long-term stability in most cases
  - Morphologic changes over time

Treatment

- Resection in symptomatic cases

Prognosis

- Limited growth potential; stabilization even after subtotal resection
- Excellent seizure control, even after subtotal resection
- Occasional recurrence with filling of surgical defect
- Anaplastic transformation to high-grade glioma (rare)
  - Spontaneous (extremely rare)
  - Post irradiation

IMAGING

MR Findings

- Typically small, complex masses, up to 7 cm
- T1 hypointensity, sometimes multinodular
- Multiple T2-hyperintense nodules largely limited to cerebral cortex
- Large hemispheric lesion (uncommon)
  - Gray and limited white matter involvement
  - Extension to lateral ventricle
- Little or no mass effect or perilesional edema
- Lack of enhancement in most cases
  - Small punctate or ring enhancement in some cases
    - May slowly enlarge over time

CT Findings

- Hypodense, cortical-based
- Comprehensive "scalloping" of overlying calvaria

MACROSCOPIC

General Features

- Intracortical nodules
- Focal elevations, "blisters" on cortical surface

MICROSCOPIC

Histologic Features

- Cortical-based; white matter also affected (some cases)
  - Large variant examples, usually temporal lobe, extend to lateral ventricle
  - Variant involves septum pellucidum
- Round, small, monotonous cells (oligodendroglial-like)
  - In well-defined, patterned (ring-like) nodules
    - Nodules can be composed of pilocytic or nonspecific astrocytes
  - Diffuse, intracortical oligodendrocyte-like cells
  - Vertically oriented axons ensheathed by granular oligodendrocyte-like cells
- Pyramidal neurons
  - Preexisting cortical neurons in pools of mucin ("floating" neurons)
  - No perineuronal satellitosis
- Microcysts
- Internodular specific glioneuronal element
- Diffuse basophilic mucoid matrix
- Extension to subpial zone or into leptomeninges (some cases)
- Glomeruloid vascular changes
  - Usually in recurrent cases
  - Semicircular arcades
  - Associated radiologically with small rings of intense contrast enhancement on MR
    - Eosinophilic granular bodies in some cases
- Cortical dysplasia of adjacent cortex in some cases
- Mitoses (rare)
- Associated tumors (uncommon)
  - Ganglioglioma
  - Pleomorphic xanthoastrocytoma
- Anaplastic transformation (exquisitely rare)

Histologic Subtypes

- Simple DNT
  - Classic form with nodular areas and specific glioneuronal element
- Complex DNT
  - Additional features, including cortical dysplasia
- Nonspecific DNT
  - Controversial, lacks diagnostic histologic features of DNET and overlaps with other glial and glioneuronal tumors
  - Diagnosis based predominantly on clinicoradiologic features (stable cortically based, well-circumscribed lesion; history of chronic seizures)
  - Not histopathological entity
- DNET incorporated into recent proposals for classification of long-term epilepsy-associated tumors (LEATs)

ANCILLARY TESTS

Cytology

- Trapped cortical ganglion cells
- Oligodendrocyte-like cells
  - Monomorphous, round, delicate nuclei
  - Little cytoplasm
- Myxoid background

- Delicate capillaries

Histochemistry

- Alcian blue
  - Reactivity: Microcysts and background matrix

Immunohistochemistry

- S100(+) oligodendroglial-like cells
- Oligodendrocyte markers (e.g., myelin oligodendrocyte glycoprotein) also (+)
- Olig2(+)
- Glial (GFAP) and neuronal markers (synaptophysin, neurofilament, tubulin, NeuN) variably (+)
- MIB1 labeling index low except in some nonspecific DNETs
- Overexpression of multidrug transporters (P-gp, MRP2, MRP5, BCRP), and BDNF-TrkB pathway components
  - May explain intrinsic epileptogenicity and resistance to antiepileptic drugs

In Situ Hybridization

- Expression of proteolipid protein gene (myelin associated)

Genetic Testing

- No 1p/19q codeletion
  - Codeletion usually lacking in pediatric oligodendrogliomas
- *BRAF V600E* mutation reported in minority of cases, in both specific and nonspecific forms

Electron Microscopy

- Oligodendroglial-like cells sometimes with glial/oligodendroglial features (pericellular lamination, intermediate filaments) or neuronal features (dense core granules, synapses)

DIFFERENTIAL DIAGNOSIS

Oligodendroglioma

- Diffuse infiltration, white and gray matter
- Perineuronal satellitosis
- Nonpatterned nodules in some cases
- Calcifications, uncommon in DNETs
- 1p/19 codeletion
  - In adults, but rare in children
- Distinction from DNET sometimes impossible in small, fragmented specimens

Pilocytic Astrocytoma

- Contrast enhancement on MR
- Biphasic pattern (compact and microcystic) in most cases
- Fibrillar, GFAP(+) tissue
- Rosenthal fibers
- Eosinophilic granular bodies
  - Occasionally seen in DNET

Ganglioglioma

- Obviously dysmorphic ganglion cells and usually lack of oligodendroglial-like cells
- Rosenthal fibers
- Eosinophilic granular bodies
  - Occasionally present in DNET
- Perivascular lymphocytes
- Occasional reticulin-rich stroma

Extraventricular Neurocytoma

- Mass, intracortical expansion with trapped preexisting elements
- Usually more cellular
- Well-formed rosettes
- Ganglion cell differentiation, many cases
- Diffuse staining for neuronal markers

Rosette-Forming Glioneuronal Tumor of 4th Ventricle

- Well-formed, compact rosettes
  - Synaptophysin(+)
- Pilocytic astrocytoma-like component
- Not always related to 4th ventricle

Angiocentric Glioma

- Ependymal rather than oligodendroglial qualities
  - Perivascular pseudorosettes
- Subpial perpendicular palisading
- Nodules of schwannoma-like tissue
- GFAP(+)
- EMA(+) microlumina

DIAGNOSTIC CHECKLIST

Pathologic Interpretation Pearls

- Consider DNET when evaluating bland intracortical oligodendroglioma-like lesion
- Small fragmented specimens may preclude definitive diagnosis
  - Diagnosis of low-grade oligodendroglioma-like lesion may be appropriate

SELECTED REFERENCES

1. Blumcke I et al: A neuropathology-based approach to epilepsy surgery in brain tumors and proposal for a new terminology use for long-term epilepsy-associated brain tumors. Acta Neuropathol. 128(1):39-54, 2014
2. Chappé C et al: Dysembryoplastic neuroepithelial tumors share with pleomorphic xanthoastrocytomas and gangliogliomas BRAF(V600E) mutation and expression. Brain Pathol. 23(5):574-83, 2013
3. Komori T et al: Dysembryoplastic neuroepithelial tumor, a pure glial tumor? Immunohistochemical and morphometric studies. Neuropathology. 33(4):459-68, 2013
4. Chang EF et al: Seizure control outcomes after resection of dysembryoplastic neuroepithelial tumor in 50 patients. J Neurosurg Pediatr. 5(1):123-30, 2010
5. Ray WZ et al: Clinicopathologic features of recurrent dysembryoplastic neuroepithelial tumor and rare malignant transformation: a report of 5 cases and review of the literature. J Neurooncol. 94(2):283-92, 2009
6. Fujisawa H et al: Genetic differences between neurocytoma and dysembryoplastic neuroepithelial tumor and oligodendroglial tumors. J Neurosurg. 97(6):1350-5, 2002
7. Baisden BL et al: Dysembryoplastic neuroepithelial tumor-like neoplasm of the septum pellucidum: a lesion often misdiagnosed as glioma: report of 10 cases. Am J Surg Pathol. 25(4):494-9, 2001
8. Stanescu Cosson R et al: Dysembryoplastic neuroepithelial tumors: CT, MR findings and imaging follow-up: a study of 53 cases. J Neuroradiol. 28(4):230-40, 2001
9. Daumas-Duport C et al: Dysembryoplastic neuroepithelial tumors: nonspecific histological forms – a study of 40 cases. J Neurooncol. 41(3):267-80, 1999
10. Prayson RA: Composite ganglioglioma and dysembryoplastic neuroepithelial tumor. Arch Pathol Lab Med. 123(3):247-50, 1999
11. Hirose T et al: Dysembryoplastic neuroeptihelial tumor (DNT): an immunohistochemical and ultrastructural study. J Neuropathol Exp Neurol. 53(2):184-95, 1994
12. Daumas-Duport C et al: Dysembryoplastic neuroepithelial tumor: a surgically curable tumor of young patients with intractable partial seizures. Report of thirty-nine cases. Neurosurgery. 23(5):545-56, 1988

Intracortical Nodules

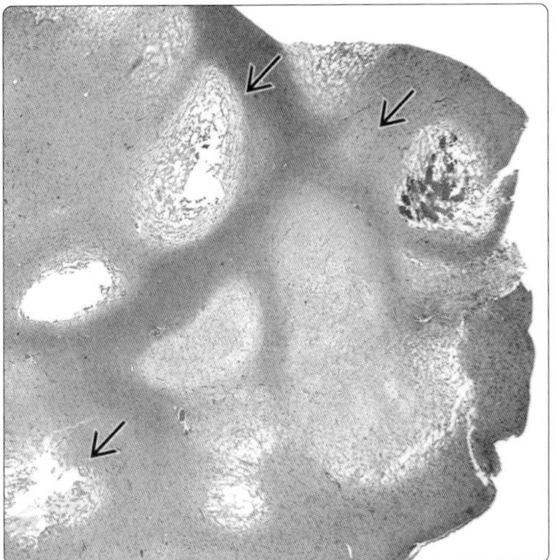

Intracortical Nodules

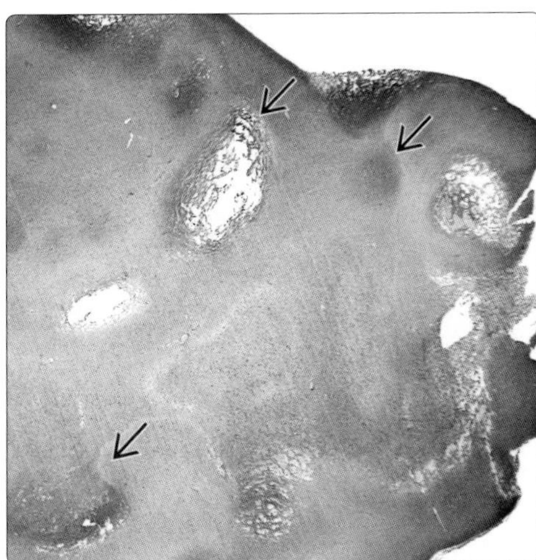

(Left) *In DNET, intracortical nodules ⇨ are best seen in largely intact specimens.* **(Right)** *Given their content of acid mucopolysaccharide, intracortical nodules of DNET ⇨ are well seen after staining with Alcian blue.*

Intracortical Nodule

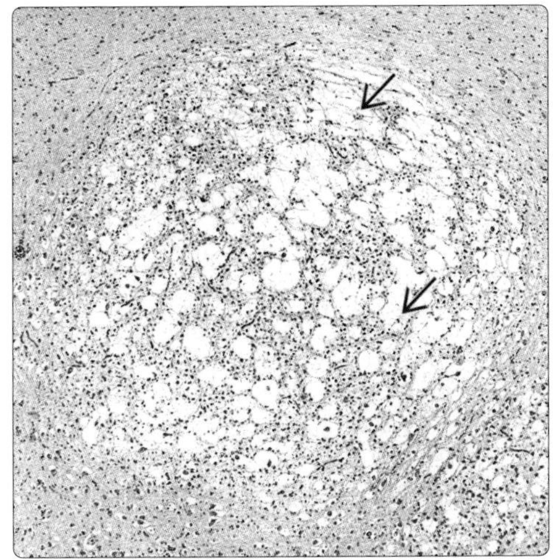

Intracortical Nodule

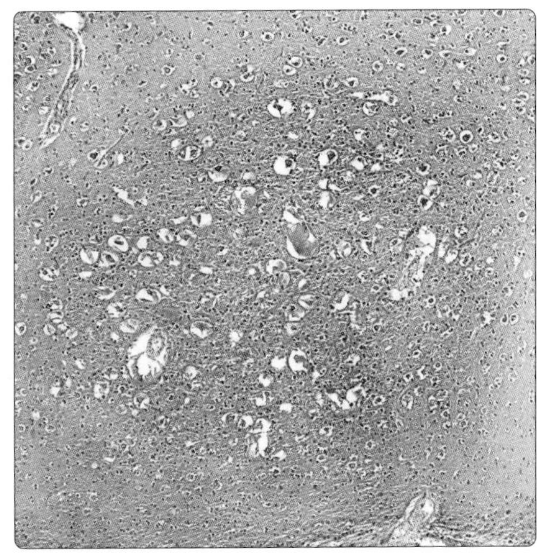

(Left) *Intracortical nodules in DNETs consist of oligodendroglial-like cells in a vacuolated, microcystic background. Neurons sit, or "float," in clear spaces ⇨. Lack of significant white matter involvement is the norm.* **(Right)** *Acid mucopolysaccharide gives the stroma of nodules and contents of microcysts their reactivity for Alcian blue. Ill-defined, nonnodular foci are often positive as well.*

Leptomeningeal Extension

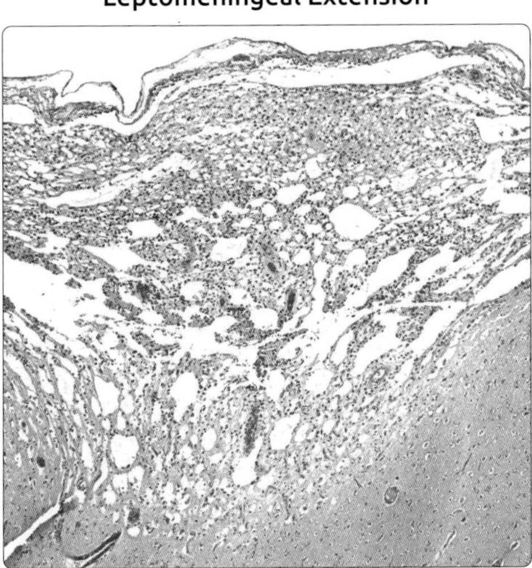

Microcysts

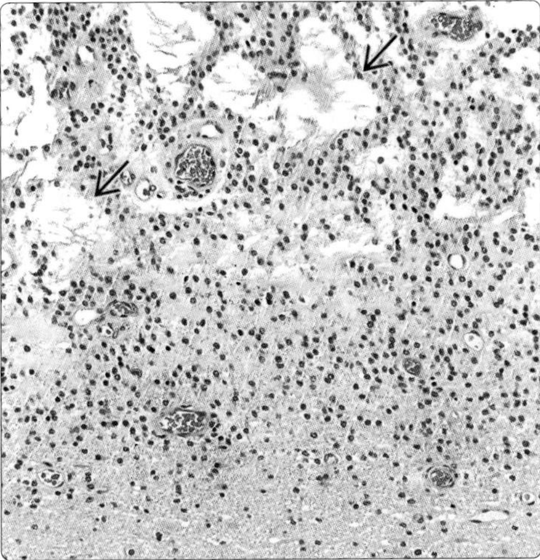

(Left) *DNETs may extend into adjacent leptomeninges wherein microcysts may be plentiful. Ganglion cell tumors, pilocytic astrocytoma, and pleomorphic xanthoastrocytoma are other low-grade tumors prone to similar extensions.* **(Right)** *Microcysts ⇨ are often prominent in the leptomeningeal component. Immediately below this microcyst-rich region, the intracortical element may closely resemble oligodendroglioma.*

(Left) *The specific glioneuronal component, often difficult to visualize, consists of parallel rows of axons ➡ oriented perpendicular to the pial surface. Each is ensheathed by oligodendroglial-like cells. Cortical neurons ⇨ lie interspersed.* **(Right)** *Often within mucus, such "floating" neurons are eye-catching features of DNET. Parallel bundles of axons, the specific glioneuronal element ➡, course vertically through the field.*

Specific Glioneuronal Component

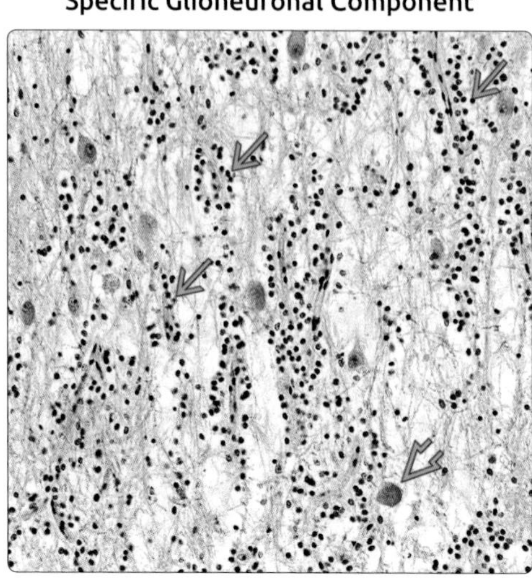

"Floating" Neurons

(Left) *Axons ➡ within the specific glioneuronal element are neurofilament protein immunoreactive.* **(Right)** *Nodular architecture and neurons seemingly suspended, "floating," in mucus ➡ are the 2 most distinctive features of DNET. The diagnosis is, nevertheless, often not elementary.*

Axons Within Specific Glioneuronal Component

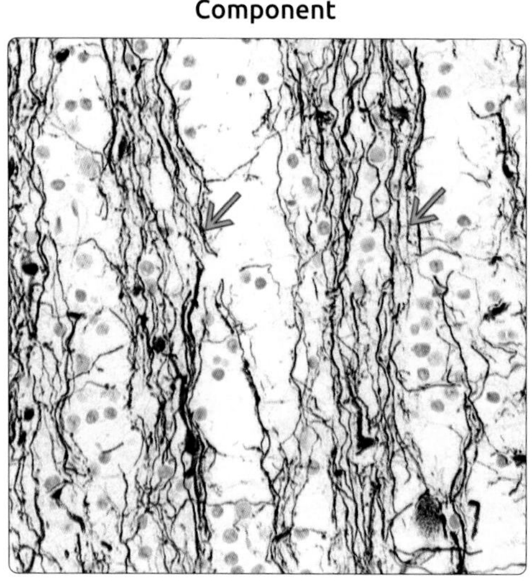

Nodules and "Floating" Neurons

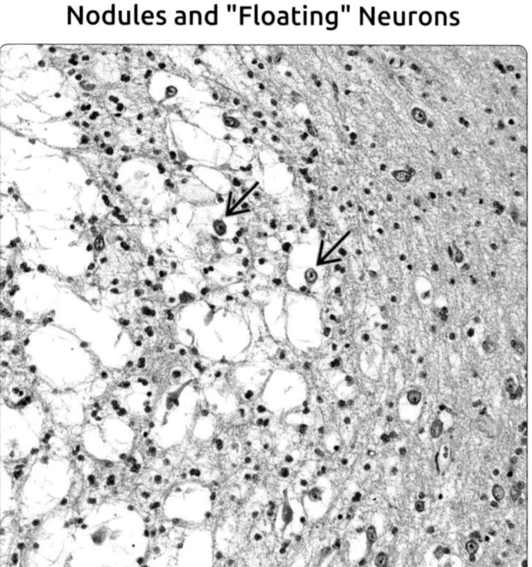

(Left) *Microcysts sometimes elongate in profile and are common in DNET. Oligodendroglioma would also be a plausible diagnostic possibility.* **(Right)** *Microcysts lined by small uniform cells are present in many DNETs. Such architecture is shared by low-grade gliomas, both astrocytic and oligodendroglial.*

Microcysts

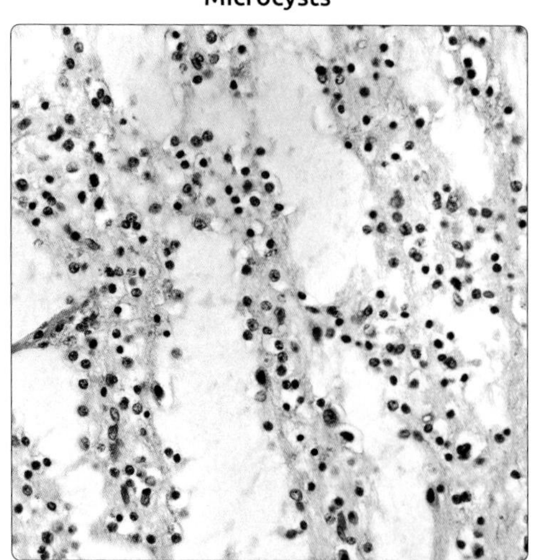

Microcysts

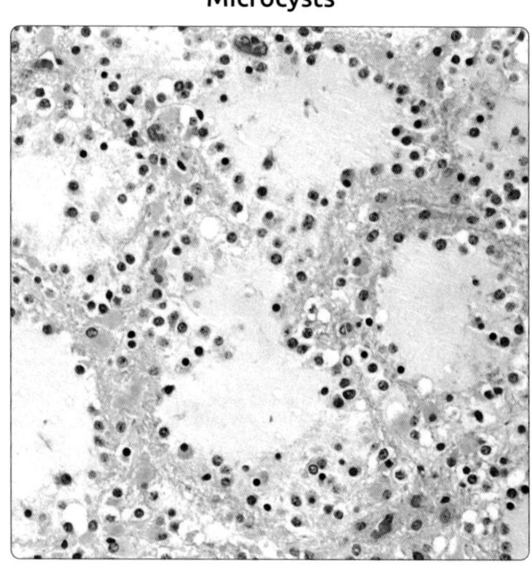

Ribboning and Cytological Uniformity

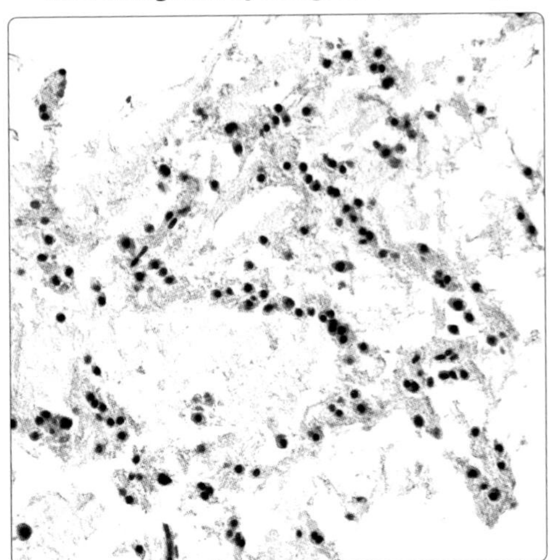

"Floating" Neurons

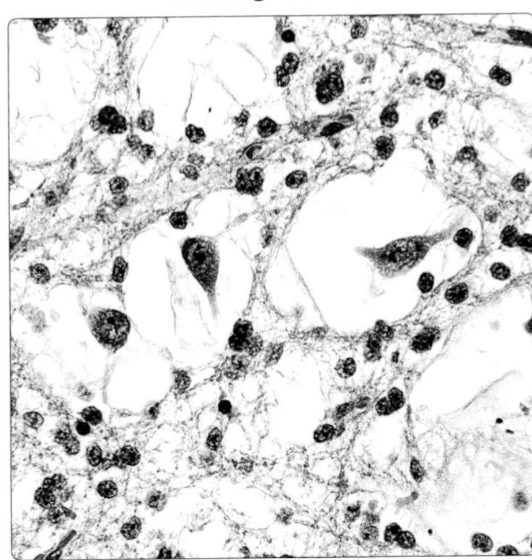

(Left) *A specific diagnosis of DNET may not be possible when architectural features are distorted in small fragmented specimens. The ribboning and cytological uniformity here are suggestive, but not diagnostic of DNET.* **(Right)** *So-called "floating" neurons are an important diagnostic feature usually not found in oligodendrogliomas.*

"Floating" Neuron

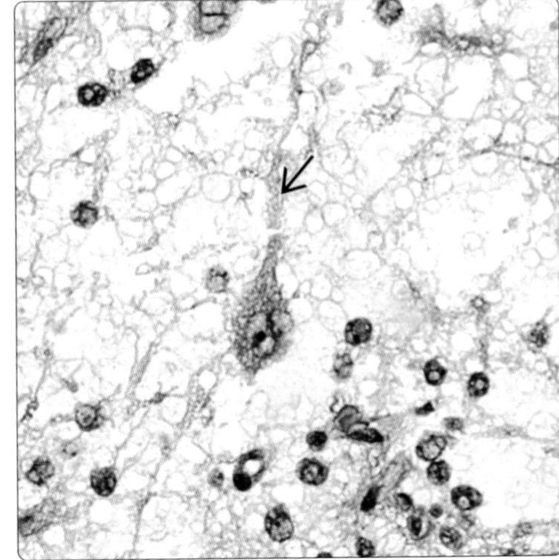

"Floating" Neuron

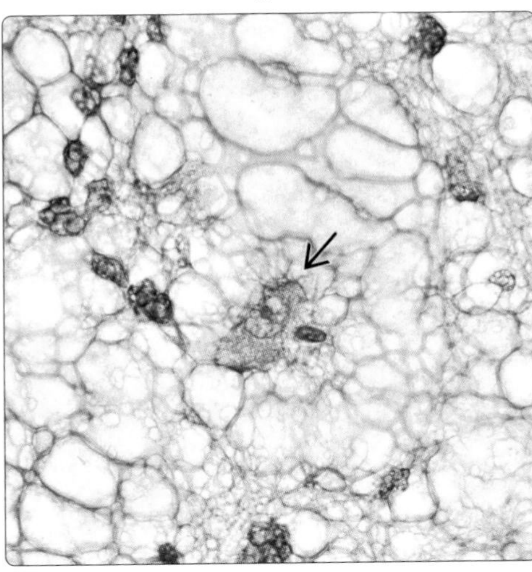

(Left) *A feature almost unique to DNETs, and rare in oligodendrogliomas, is large pyramidal neurons ➙ "floating" in pools of mucin. They and the absence of perineuronal satellitosis help distinguish DNET from infiltrative glioma.* **(Right)** *Alcian blue staining colorfully identifies the mucopolysaccharide pools around large, "floating" neurons ➙.*

Nuclear Roundness

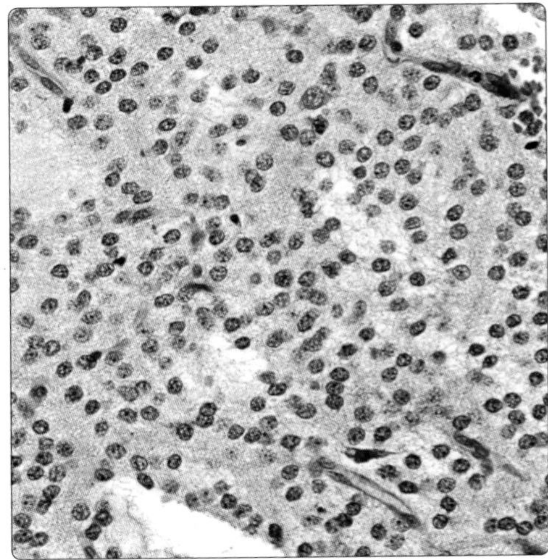

Chicken-Wire Vasculature

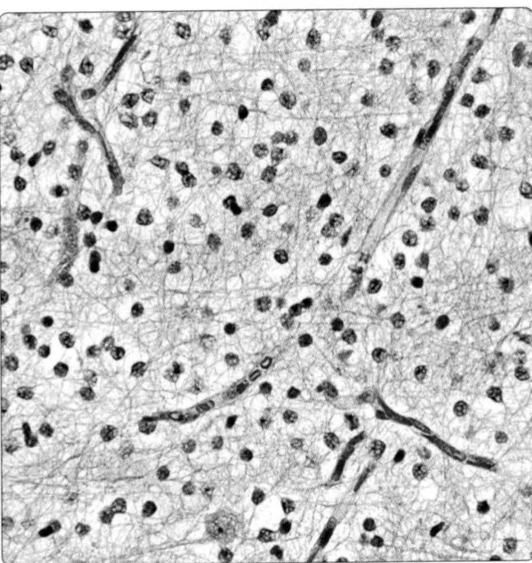

(Left) *In combination, the illustrated degree of cellularity and nuclear roundness in this DNET make oligodendroglioma a strong differential diagnosis. Other features would be required to make the distinction.* **(Right)** *Even the chicken-wire vasculature of an oligodendroglioma may be present in a DNET. A diagnosis of oligodendroglial-like lesion may be appropriate if no additional specific features of DNET are found.*

(Left) *Dysembryoplastic neuroepithelial tumors may have a loose, histologically nonspecific cobweb architecture similar to that of infiltrating gliomas.* **(Right)** *Cytologically bland cells with round nuclei, intercalated between axons* → *create a picture indistinguishable from low-grade oligodendroglioma.*

Cobweb Architecture

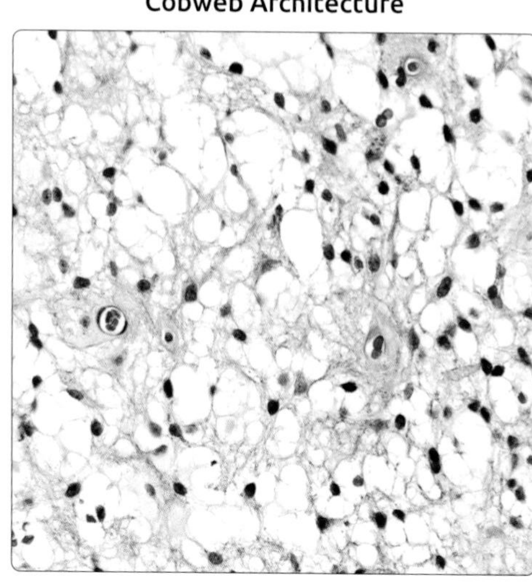

Round Nuclei

(Left) *Widely scattered oligodendroglioma-like cells create a slight hypercellularity which, alone, cannot be distinguished from that of oligodendroglioma.* **(Right)** *Conspicuous nuclear pleomorphism in some DNETs should not raise concern for an astrocytic tumor as long as other pathologic characteristics of DNET are present.*

Slight Hypercellularity

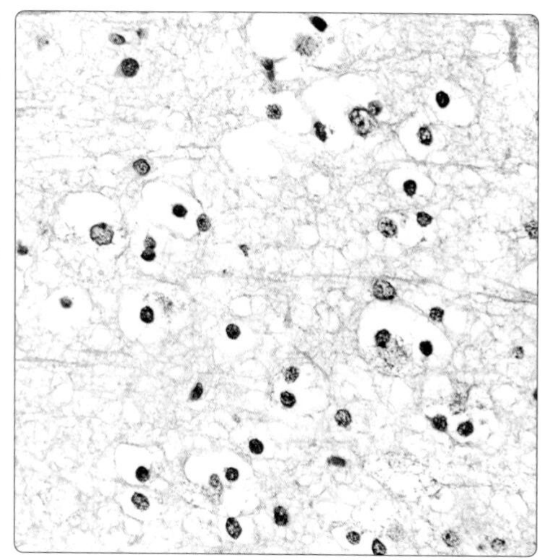

Nuclear Pleomorphism

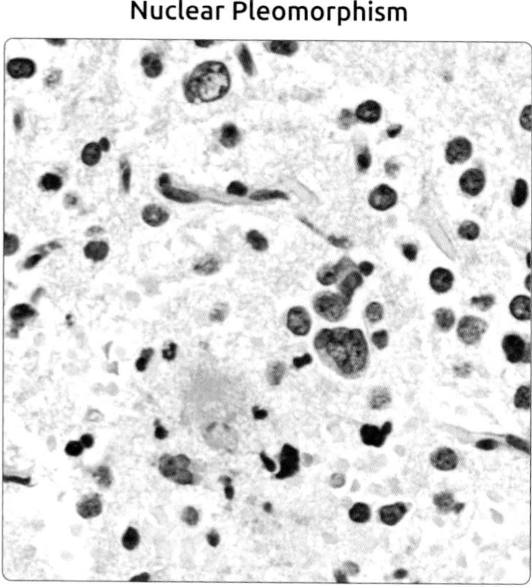

(Left) *T1-weighted coronal MR image shows small areas of intense ring enhancement* → *present in some DNETs, particularly recurrent lesions. Due to arcades of microvascular proliferation, the phenomenon may be misinterpreted both radiologically and pathologically as evidence of anaplasia.* **(Right)** *Areas of ring enhancement in DNET correspond histologically to arcades of loose glomeruloid vessels* →.

Ring Enhancement

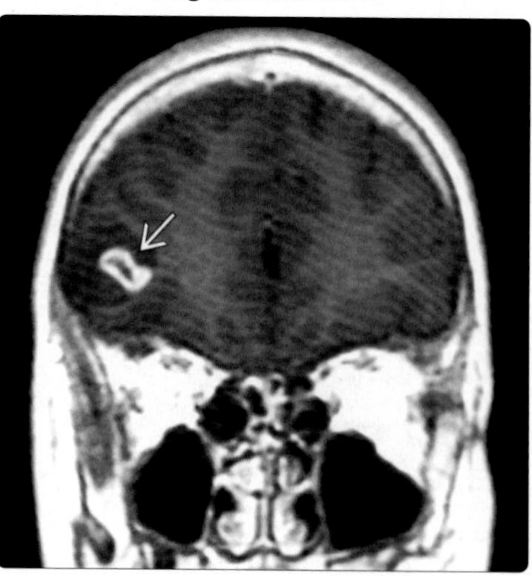

Arcades of Glomeruloid Vessels

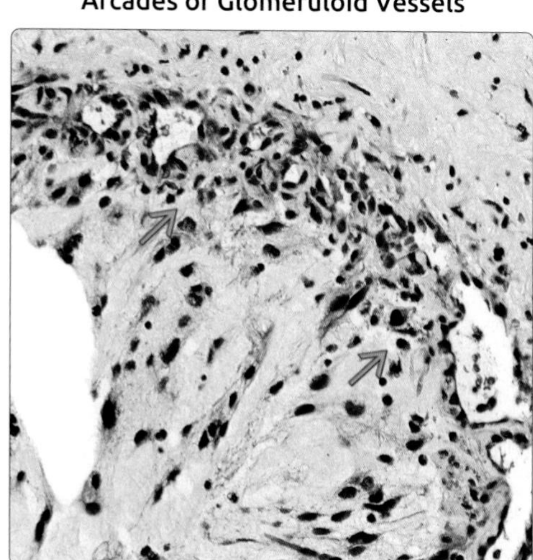

Microvascular Proliferation

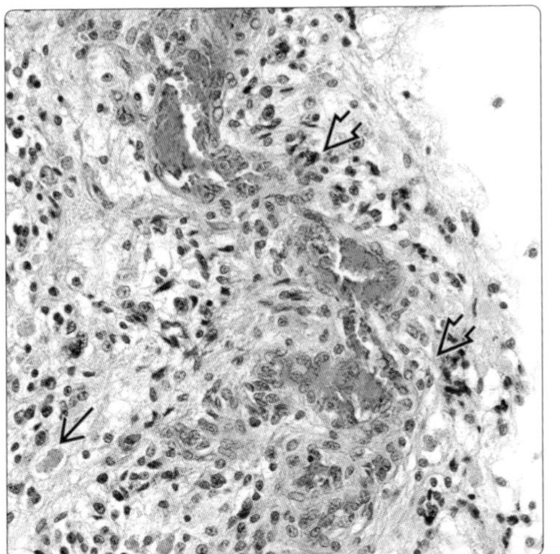

Myxoid Background

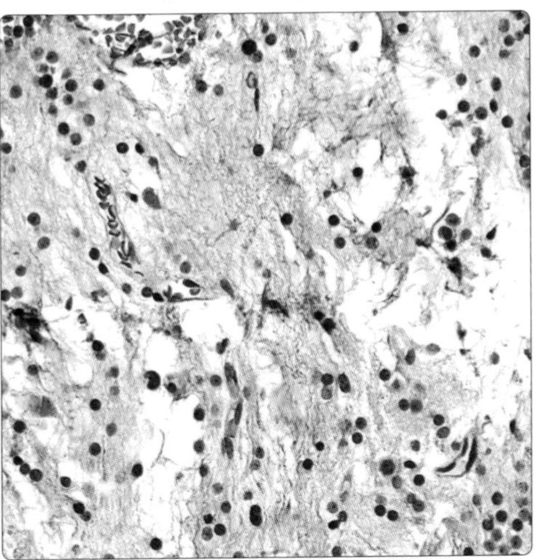

(Left) *Loose, almost telangiectatic microvascular proliferation, generally in circular arcades ⮚, is common in DNETs. Although more a feature of low-grade gliomas, eosinophilic granular bodies → may be present.* **(Right)** *A basophilic myxoid background is a common, although nonspecific, feature of DNT. Tissue such as this is consistent with, but not diagnostic of, DNET.*

Ribbon-Like Palisades

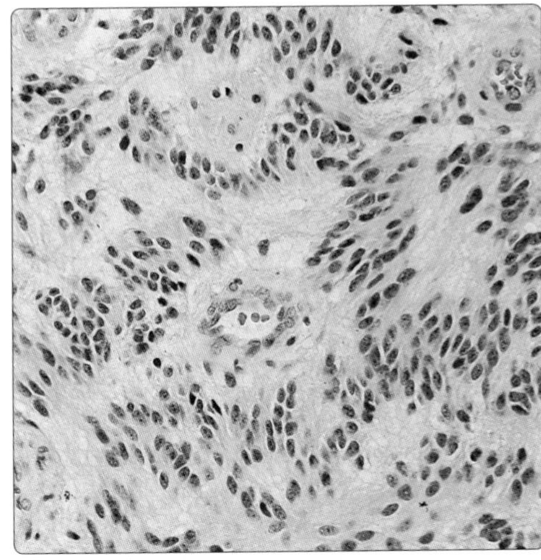

Oligodendroglial-Like Cells and Trapped Neurons

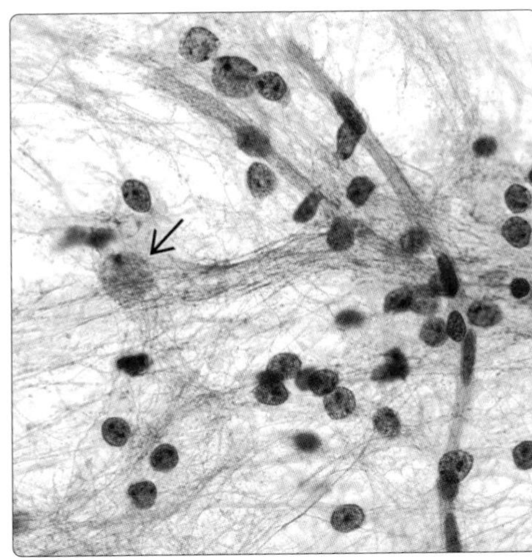

(Left) *Complex ribbon-like palisades are distinctive features of some DNTs. Similar ribboning occurs in oligodendrogliomas, usually of high grade.* **(Right)** *Cytologically bland oligodendroglial-like cells, trapped neurons →, myxoid background, and delicate capillaries are essential features of DNETs in smear preparations.*

Septum Pellucidum DNET

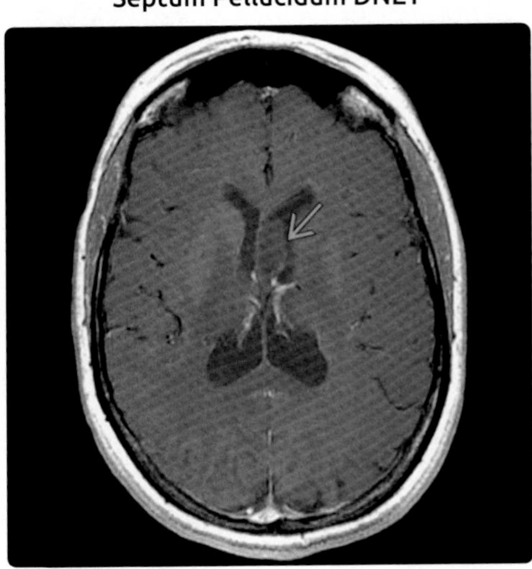

Septum Pellucidum DNET

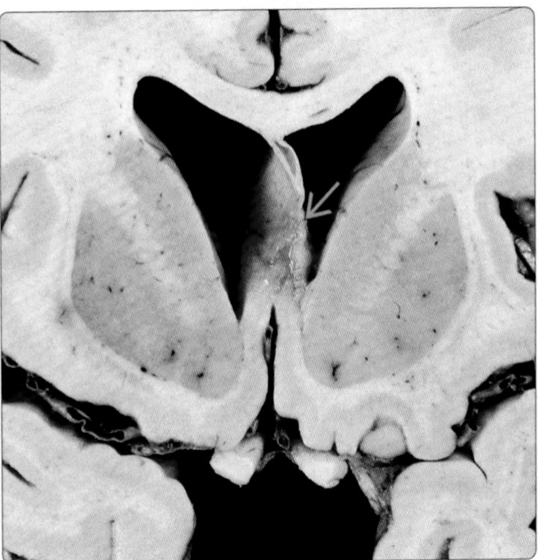

(Left) *On T1W postcontrast MR images, dysembryoplastic neuroepithelial tumors, or close mimics thereof, occasionally appear as nonenhancing masses in the septum pellucidum and anterior lateral ventricles →.* **(Right)** *At this unusual site, DNETs may appear as a gelatinous growth along the septum pellucidum →.*

Rosette-Forming Glioneuronal Tumor of 4th Ventricle

KEY FACTS

TERMINOLOGY

- Low-grade glioneuronal neoplasm arising in the posterior fossa with neurocytes, distinctive rosettes, and associated glial component
- Rosette-forming glioneuronal tumor (RGNT)

CLINICAL ISSUES

- Usually involves cerebellum (vermis) and 4th ventricle
  - But not always related to cerebellum or 4th ventricle
- Favorable prognosis, curable with gross total resection

IMAGING

- Well circumscribed and solid, or cystic and solid, midline
- T2-hyperintense, heterogeneous contrast enhancement

MICROSCOPIC

- Small neurocytic rosettes with eosinophilic neuropil core or perivascular arrangement
- Low-grade glial component resembling pilocytic astrocytoma
- Linear arrangements of oligodendroglia-like cells and mucin pools reminiscent of dysembryoplastic neuroepithelial tumor, in some cases

ANCILLARY TESTS

- Synaptophysin most useful immunohistochemical target, highlights rosettes
- *PIK3CA* and *FGFR1* mutations reported in RFGT
- Lack of *BRAF* alterations

TOP DIFFERENTIAL DIAGNOSES

- Pilocytic astrocytoma
- Dysembryoplastic neuroepithelial tumor
- Oligodendroglioma
- Ependymoma
- Cerebellar liponeurocytoma

DIAGNOSTIC CHECKLIST

- Rosettes distinctive but may be focal

(Left) *RFGTs are usually, but not always, located in the 4th ventricle. Imaging studies may demonstrate a small lesion with circles of intense contrast enhancement ➡. **(Right)** Bland round neurocytes around an eosinophilic neuropil core ➡ are a diagnostic feature of this tumor.*

4th Ventricle Mass

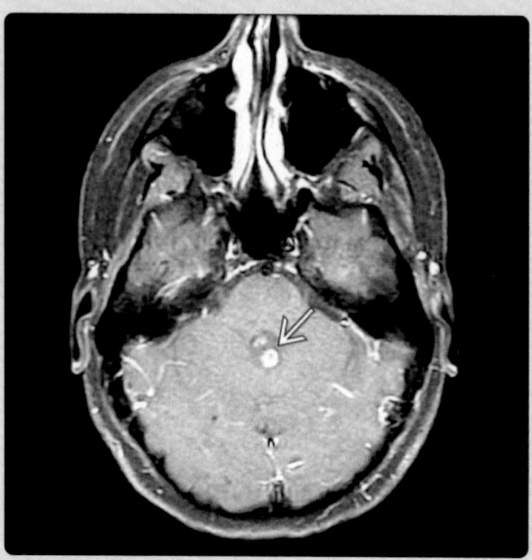

Neuropil Cores

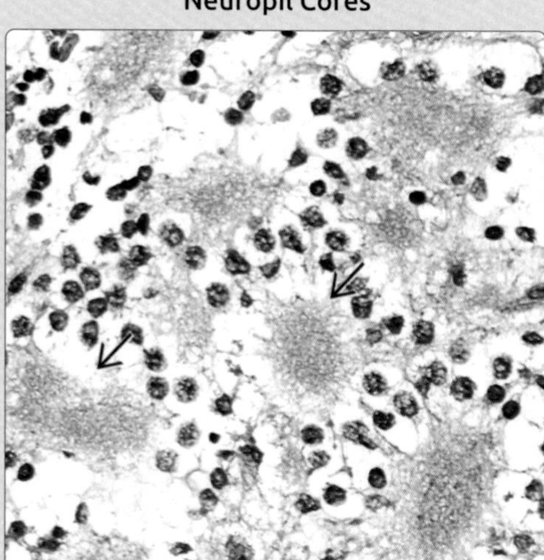

(Left) *Although slightly distorted by the smearing process, rosettes with delicate fibrillary cores are still evident on smears. **(Right)** The glial component of rosette-forming glioneuronal tumor may be nondescript, as seen here, or similar to pilocytic astrocytoma. In either case, it is often inconspicuous.*

Rosettes

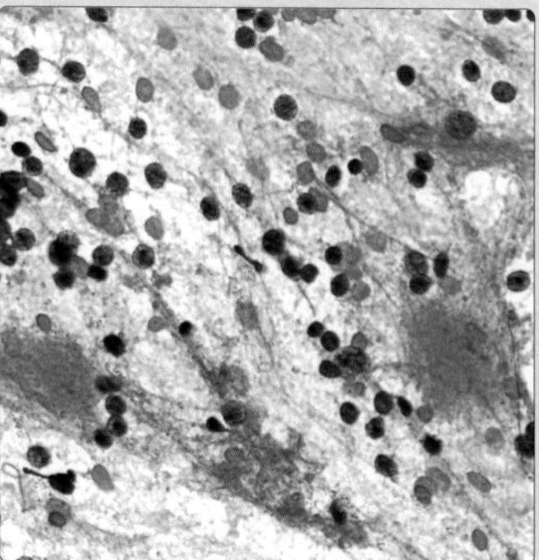

Glial Component

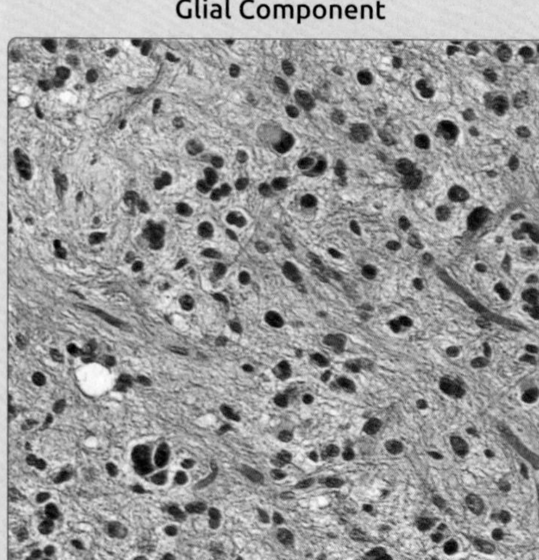

TERMINOLOGY

Definitions

- Low-grade glioneuronal neoplasm arising in posterior fossa with neurocytes, distinctive rosettes, and associated glial component

ETIOLOGY/PATHOGENESIS

Genetic

- Rare case in NF1 or Noonan syndrome

CLINICAL ISSUES

Site

- Usually involves cerebellum and 4th ventricle
- Pineal gland/tectal region, hypothalamus/optic chiasm, and spinal cord (minority of cases)
- Multifocal or intraventricular dissemination, rare

Presentation

- Headache, obstructive hydrocephalus
- Intratumoral hemorrhage, occasionally

Prognosis

- Favorable; curable with gross total resection

IMAGING

MR Findings

- Well circumscribed and solid or cystic and solid midline
- T2-hyperintense, heterogeneous contrast enhancement

MICROSCOPIC

Histologic Features

- Loose, mucoid matrix &/or microcysts
- Small uniform neurocytes
  - Round nuclei with fine stippled chromatin
- Small perivascular rosettes (neurocytic) with eosinophilic core
- Linear arrangements of oligodendroglia-like cells and mucin pools reminiscent of dysembryoplastic neuroepithelial tumor, in some cases
- Low-grade glial component resembling pilocytic astrocytoma
  - Compact, without microcysts and sponginess of classic pilocytic astrocytoma
  - Bipolar astrocytes
  - Eosinophilic granular bodies and Rosenthal fibers
  - Microcalcifications
  - Glomeruloid vasculature and hyalinized vessels with hemosiderin deposition
- Purkinje cells floating in myxoid substance, in some cases
- Mitoses: Usually none; necrosis: None

ANCILLARY TESTS

Cytology

- Uniform, round nuclei with delicate chromatin

Immunohistochemistry

- Synaptophysin (+) rosettes but Neu-N usually (-)
- Other markers of neuronal differentiation (e.g., MAP2) also (+) in rosettes
- GFAP and S100(+) in glial component
- Ki-67 index low

Genetic Testing

- *PIK3CA* and *FGFR1* mutations reported in RGNT
- Lack of *BRAF* alterations

Electron Microscopy

- Aligned microtubules, dense core granules, and mature synapses (rare)
- Dense glial filaments in glial component

DIFFERENTIAL DIAGNOSIS

Pilocytic Astrocytoma

- No neurocytic rosettes

Dysembryoplastic Neuroepithelial Tumor

- Almost always supratentorial, but
  - Occasionally in posterior fossa where features (e.g., floating neurons) overlap
- Lacks well-formed rosettes, but overlaps in some cases with RGNT

Oligodendroglioma

- Rare in posterior fossa
- Infiltrative growth pattern, no rosettes
- 1p/19q codeletion in adults

Ependymoma

- Highly cellular, most cases
- Perivascular pseudorosettes
  - GFAP(+) and often Olig2 and synaptophysin (-)

Cerebellar Liponeurocytoma

- High cellularity, low Ki-67 index
- Lipidized tumor cells without rosette formation
- Diffusely synaptophysin (+)

DIAGNOSTIC CHECKLIST

Pathologic Interpretation Pearls

- Rosettes distinctive but may be focal
- Not always in or around 4th ventricle

SELECTED REFERENCES

1. Gessi M et al: FGFR1 mutations in Rosette-forming glioneuronal tumors of the fourth ventricle. J Neuropathol Exp Neurol. 73(6):580-4, 2014
2. Schlamann A et al: An individual patient data meta-analysis on characteristics and outcome of patients with papillary glioneuronal tumor, rosette glioneuronal tumor with neuropil-like islands and rosette forming glioneuronal tumor of the fourth ventricle. PLoS One. 9(7):e101211, 2014
3. Ellezam B et al: Recurrent PIK3CA mutations in rosette-forming glioneuronal tumor. Acta Neuropathol. 123(2):285-7, 2012
4. Scheithauer BW et al: Rosette-forming glioneuronal tumor: report of a chiasmal-optic nerve example in neurofibromatosis type 1: special pathology report. Neurosurgery. 64(4):E771-2; discussion E772, 2009
5. Preusser M et al: Rosette-forming glioneuronal tumor of the fourth ventricle. Acta Neuropathol. 106(5):506-8, 2003
6. Komori T et al: A rosette-forming glioneuronal tumor of the fourth ventricle: infratentorial form of dysembryoplastic neuroepithelial tumor? Am J Surg Pathol. 26(5):582-91, 2002

(Left) *Individual and coalescing microcysts are nonspecific features, but multiple neurocytic rosettes → are specific. An index of suspicion facilitates identification of diagnostic rosettes with their fibrillar cores.* **(Right)** *The diagnostic feature of the rosette-forming glioneuronal tumor is a small rosette with either a fibrillar core → or a centrally placed vessel. In either case, the fibrillar tissue, composed of neuritic processes, will be immunoreactive for synaptophysin.*

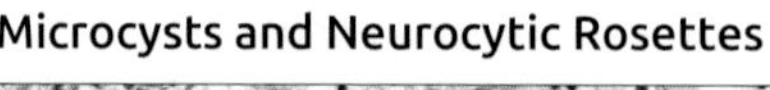

Microcysts and Neurocytic Rosettes

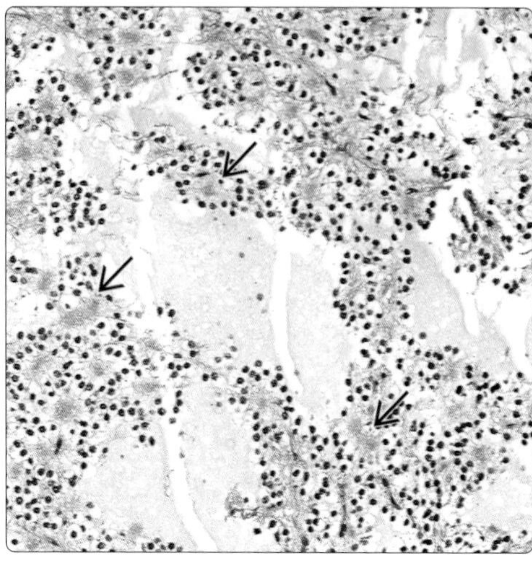

Small Rosettes

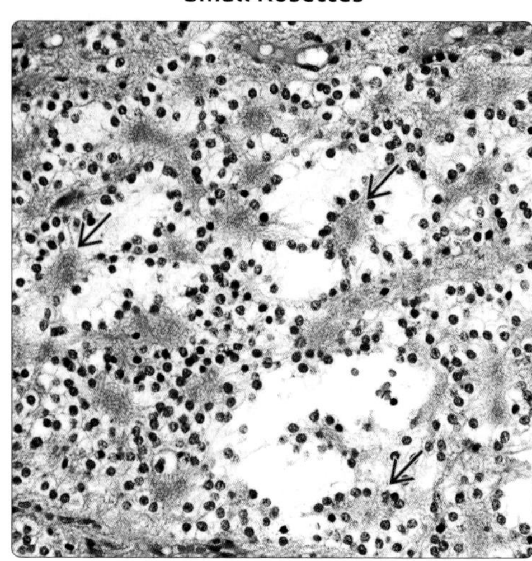

(Left) *It may be easy to overlook the small rosettes → and focus on the oligodendroglioma-like cells, which may mislead to the diagnosis of oligodendroglioma and pilocytic astrocytoma. Location and pattern of contrast enhancement bring the correct entity into the differential list.* **(Right)** *Rosettes in rosette-forming glioneuronal tumors have finely fibrillar cores → similar to those of neuroblastic (or Homer Wright) rosettes, which occur in neuroblastomas and some medulloblastomas.*

Small Rosettes

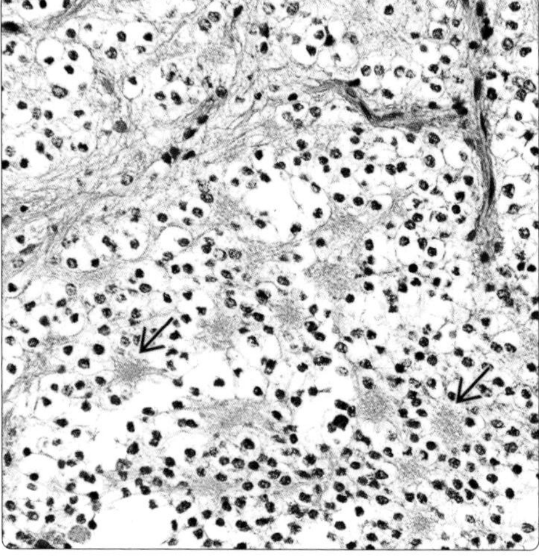

Rosettes

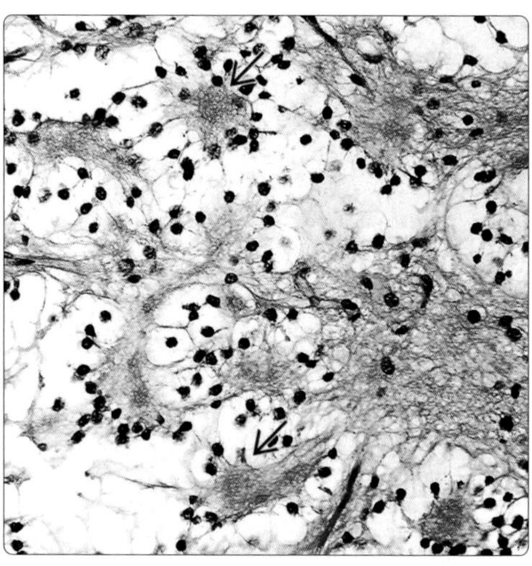

(Left) *Pale-staining neurocytic rosettes →, however focal and difficult to find, are critical features in the diagnosis of rosette-forming glioneuronal tumor. In spite of its name, the tumor does not always occur in the 4th ventricle.* **(Right)** *The finely fibrillar neuropil core of the rosettes may be inconspicuous, and only clusters of small uniform cells → are present to introduce the possibility of the entity.*

Neurocytic Rosettes

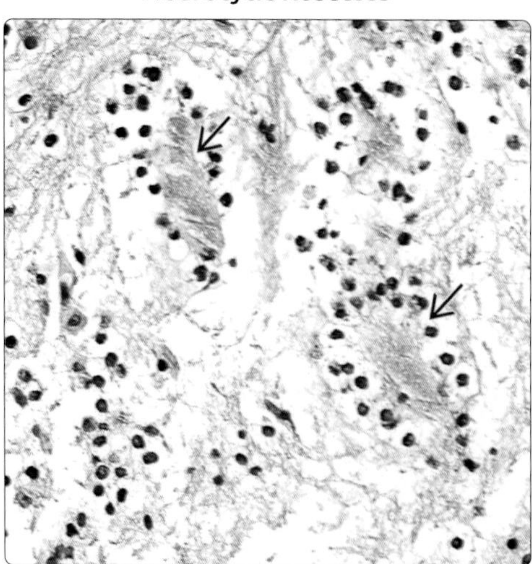

Clusters of Small Uniform Cells

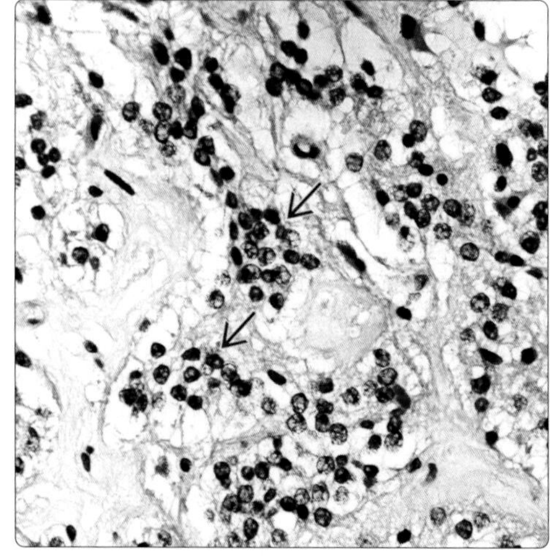

Oligodendroglioma-Like Cells

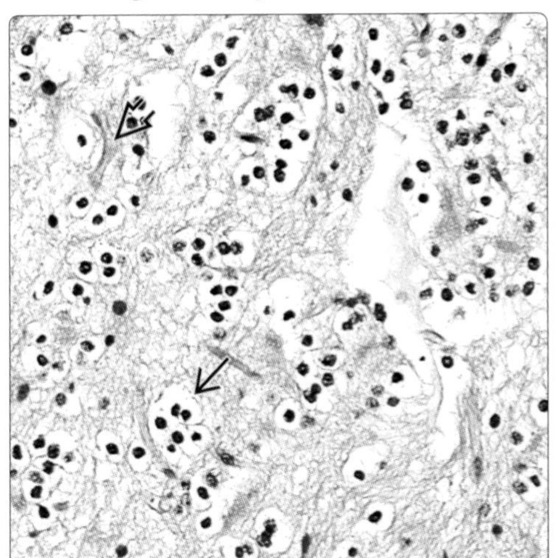

Perivascular Rosettes

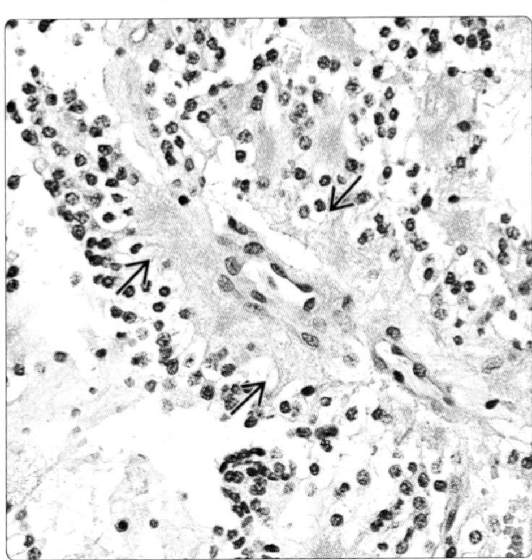

(Left) *There are only clusters of oligodendroglioma-like cells* ⮕ *in some cases to hint at the nature of the lesion. The suggestively perivascular orientation of some* ⮕ *helps raise the possibility of RFGT.* **(Right)** *Rosettes in rosette-forming glioneuronal tumors are frequently perivascular* ⮕*. In contrast to ependymoma, the anuclear component is composed of fine neuropil rather than coarser glial processes. As such, it is synaptophysin (+) rather than GFAP(+).*

Pilocytic Component

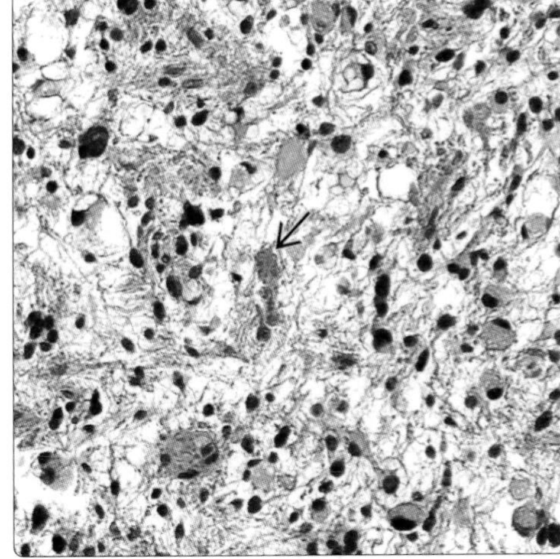

Rosenthal Fibers

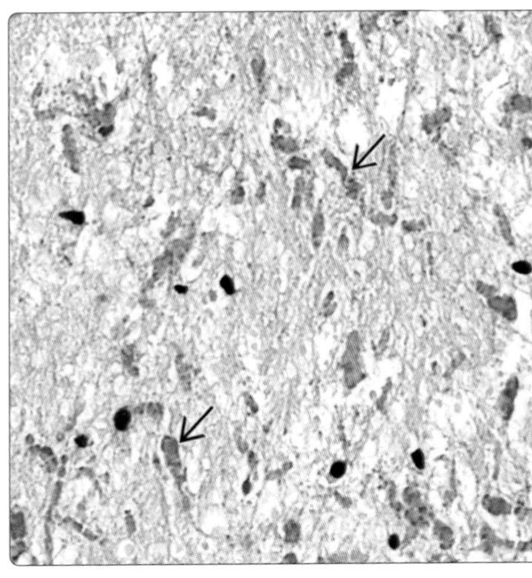

(Left) *A well-differentiated, glial, pilocytic component is almost always present in rosette-forming glioneuronal tumors. This example is loose, myxomatous tissue with Rosenthal fibers* ⮕*.* **(Right)** *In the absence of loose, spongy tissue, the piloid tissue, with Rosenthal fibers* ⮕*, could represent piloid gliosis rather than the glial component of RFGT.*

Rosettes

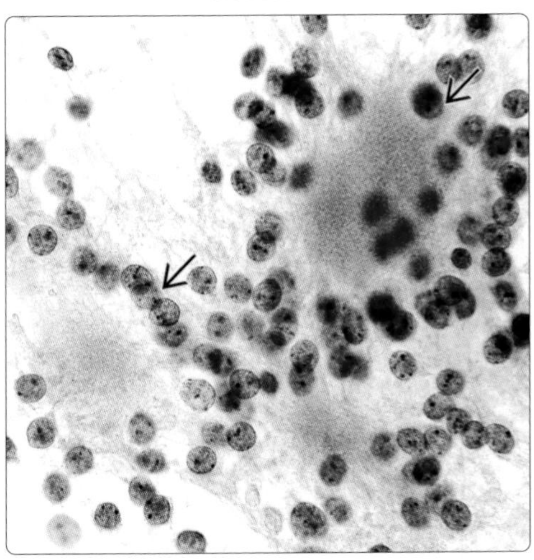

Synaptophysin (+) Rosettes

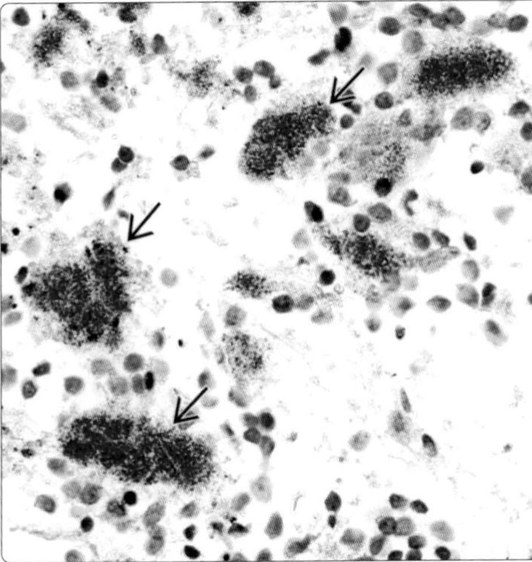

(Left) *Smear preparations capture the lesion's distinctive rosettes* ⮕*. (Courtesy E. Stopa, MD.)* **(Right)** *The fibrillar, neuropil core neurocytic rosettes* ⮕ *have a delicate, granular immunopositivity for synaptophysin.*

Papillary Glioneuronal Tumor

KEY FACTS

CLINICAL ISSUES

- Throughout CNS
  - Predilection for temporal lobe
- Young adults
- Headaches and seizures
- Favorable prognosis with gross total resection

IMAGING

- Supratentorial, well circumscribed, often cystic
- Cyst with mural nodule (some cases)

MICROSCOPIC

- Hyalinized vessels form pseudopapillae surrounded by single layer of small, cuboidal cells
- Neurocytes in interpapillary space
  - Large ganglion cells and smaller ganglioid cells more common

ANCILLARY TESTS

- Perivascular astrocytes GFAP(+) and Olig2(+)
- Neurocytic interpapillary component
  - Synaptophysin (+)
- Ganglioid/ganglion cells neurofilament protein (+)
- Low Ki-67 indices
- Novel *SLC44A1-PRKCA* fusion

TOP DIFFERENTIAL DIAGNOSES

- Oligodendroglial tumors
- Extraventricular neurocytoma
- Dysembryoplastic neuroepithelial tumor
- Choroid plexus papilloma
- Pilocytic astrocytoma
- Rosette-forming glioneuronal tumor
- Clear cell ependymoma

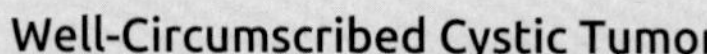

Well-Circumscribed Cystic Tumor

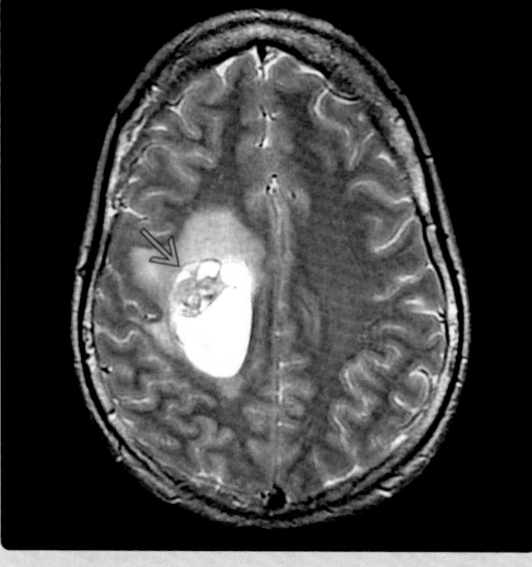

Dual Population of Cells

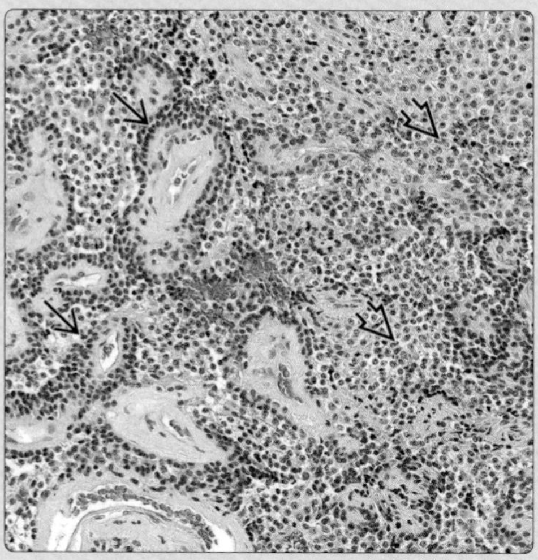

(Left) *Papillary glioneuronal tumors (PGNTs) are well circumscribed, often cystic tumors with a mural nodule ⇨ and a configuration that suggests a favorable surgically curable lesion.* **(Right)** *The defining feature of PNGT is a dual population of cells, including a glial perivascular layer ⇨ and usually predominant round interpapillary neurocytes ⇨.*

Pseudopapillae

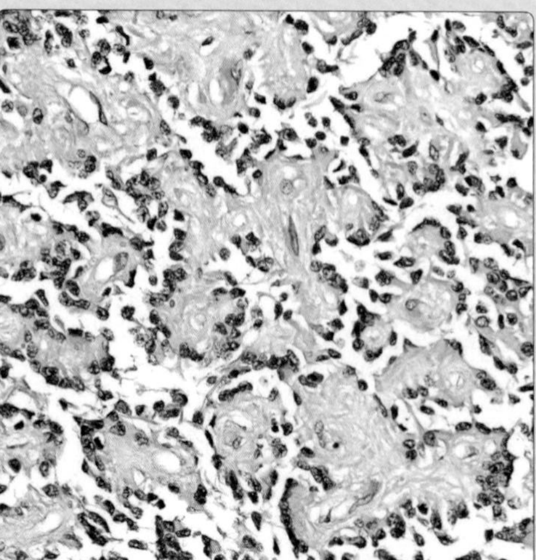

Hyalinization of Vessels

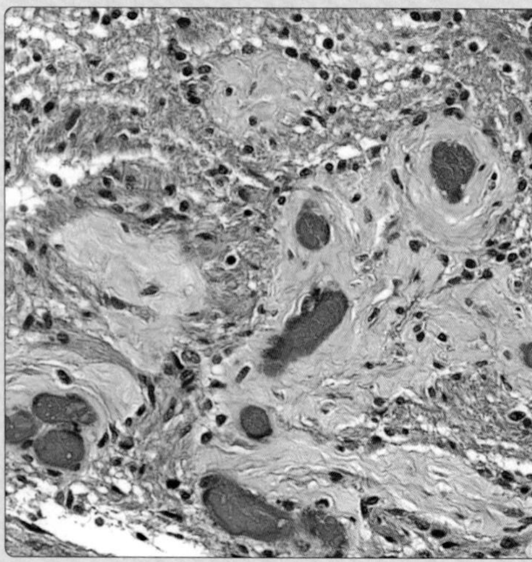

(Left) *As the result of tissue dehiscence, pseudopapillae are prominent in some examples. As is often the case, the biphasic neuronal/glial composition may not be apparent in H&E sections alone.* **(Right)** *Hyalinization of vessels may be present in some examples with an associated gliotic response. Hyalinization of vessels is a feature of slowly growing neoplasms.*

TERMINOLOGY

Abbreviations

- Primary glioneuronal tumor (PGNT)

Definitions

- Low-grade pseudopapillary neoplasm with small perivascular astrocytes and interpapillary neurocytes (WHO grade I)

CLINICAL ISSUES

Epidemiology

- Age
  - Young adults

Site

- Throughout CNS; predilection for temporal lobe

Presentation

- Headaches and seizures

Treatment

- Complete resection optimal

Prognosis

- Favorable with gross total resection
- Possible local recurrence with subtotal resection

IMAGING

MR Findings

- Well circumscribed, often cystic
- Cyst with mural nodule architecture (some)

MACROSCOPIC

General Features

- Cystic or occasionally solid

MICROSCOPIC

Histologic Features

- Pseudopapillae composed of hyalinized vessels covered by single layer of small, somewhat cuboidal cells
- Well-differentiated neurocytes
  - Filling interpapillary space
  - Uniform, round
  - Perinuclear halos similar to oligodendroglioma (some cases)
- Large ganglion cells, as well as smaller ganglioid forms; less common in interpapillary zones
- Mitoses (rare)
- Peritumoral reactive gliosis

ANCILLARY TESTS

Cytology

- Nonspecific; may feature uniform cellularity and vague papillary structures in smears

Immunohistochemistry

- Perivascular glial cells
  - GFAP(+)
  - Olig2(+)
- Neurocytes, ganglion, and ganglioid cells
  - Synaptophysin (+), NeuN(+/-)
- Ki-67 index very low
  - Neurofilament protein (+) in larger neuronal cells

Genetic Testing

- Novel *SLC44A1-PRKCA* fusion
- Cytogenetic hallmarks of diffuse gliomas absent
  - 1p/19q codeletion absent
  - Chromosome 7 gains, without *EGFR* amplification in 1 case

DIFFERENTIAL DIAGNOSIS

Oligodendroglioma

- Diffuse infiltration, with secondary structures
  - Perineuronal satellitosis, subpial and perivascular aggregation
- Frequent 1p/19q deletion

Extraventricular Neurocytoma

- No perivascular GFAP(+) neoplastic astrocytic component
  - Only scattered processes of reactive astrocytes

Dysembryoplastic Neuroepithelial Tumor

- Intracortical lesion
- Nondiscrete mass
- Myxoid background
- Distinctive nodular architecture
- Perineuronal myxoid material ("floating neurons")

Choroid Plexus Papilloma

- Intraventricular
- True, rather than pseudopapillae
- Epithelial markers, especially cytokeratins, (+)

Pilocytic Astrocytoma

- Biphasic compact/loose-textured pattern with microcysts
- Rosenthal fibers and eosinophilic granular bodies
- Vague oligodendroglioma pattern, in some cases
- Extensively GFAP(+)

Rosette-Forming Glioneuronal Tumor

- Synaptophysin (+) perivascular neuropil
- Small Homer Wright rosettes with synaptophysin (+) cores
- Predilection for 4th ventricular region

Clear Cell Ependymoma

- Perivascular pseudorosettes
- Extensively GFAP(+)
- EMA(+) cytoplasmic dots, &/or microlumina

DIAGNOSTIC CHECKLIST

Clinically Relevant Pathologic Features

- Discreteness often permits curative total excision

Pathologic Interpretation Pearls

- Consider PGNT in presence of hemispheric tumor with low-grade appearance and pseudopapillary architecture

SELECTED REFERENCES

1. Komori T et al: Papillary glioneuronal tumor: a new variant of mixed neuronal-glial neoplasm. Am J Surg Pathol. 22(10):1171-83, 1998

Perivascular Glia and Interpapillary Neurocytes

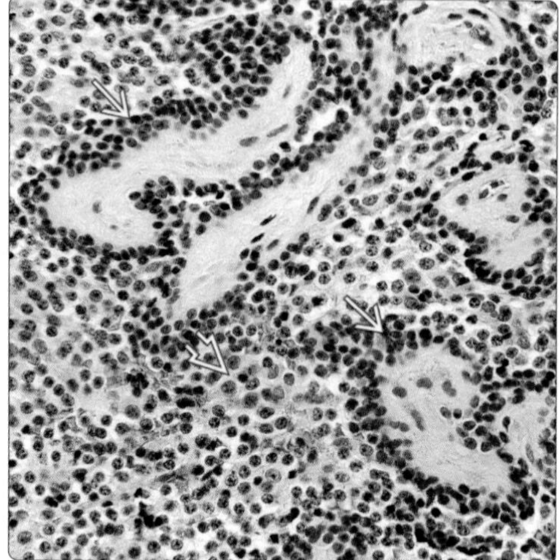

Dual Cell Population

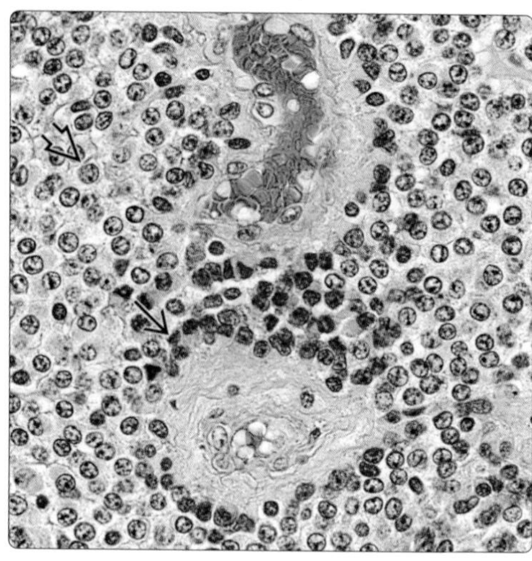

(Left) *The dichotomous nature of the lesion is apparent in most cases; perivascular glia ➡ are being readily distinguishable from the pale interpapillary neurocytes ➡.* **(Right)** *The dual population of PGNT includes a single layer of perivascular glial cells ➡ and the numerically predominant, somewhat oligodendroglioma-like, neurocytes ➡. Awareness of PGNT aids considerably in identifying these 2 components in H&E sections.*

Sheets of Neurocytes

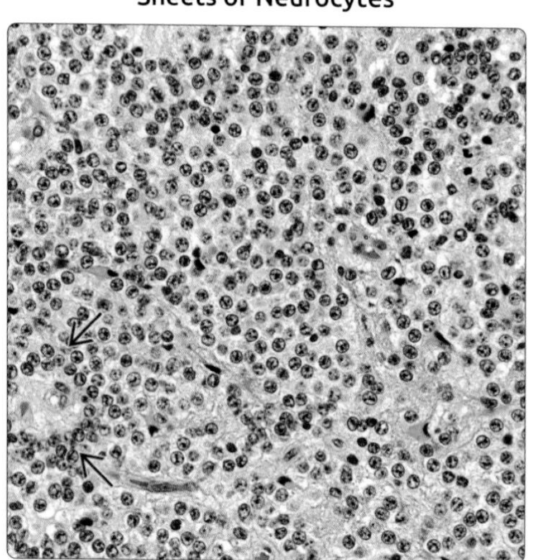

Glial and Neurocytic Components

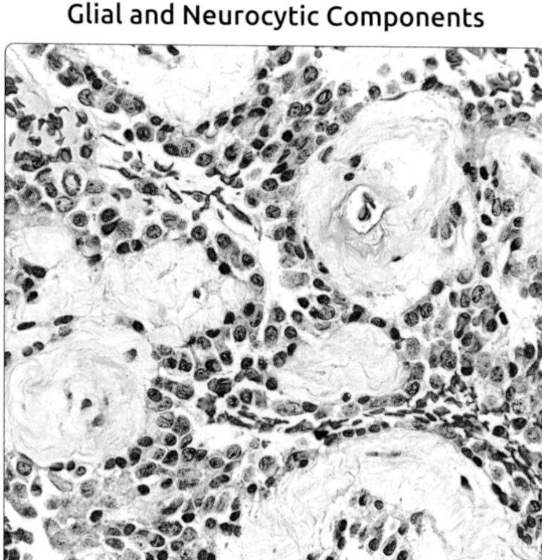

(Left) *Sheets of neurocytes may engender a broad differential diagnosis, including oligodendroglioma, extraventricular neurocytoma, and pilocytic astrocytoma. Only focal perivascular layering of glial cells ➡ suggests PGNT.* **(Right)** *In some cases, there is no apparent distinction in H&E sections between glial and neurocytic components.*

Neurocytic Component

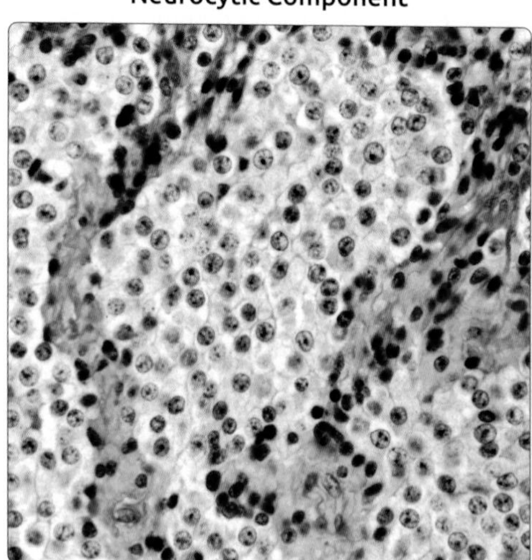

Thickened Vessels

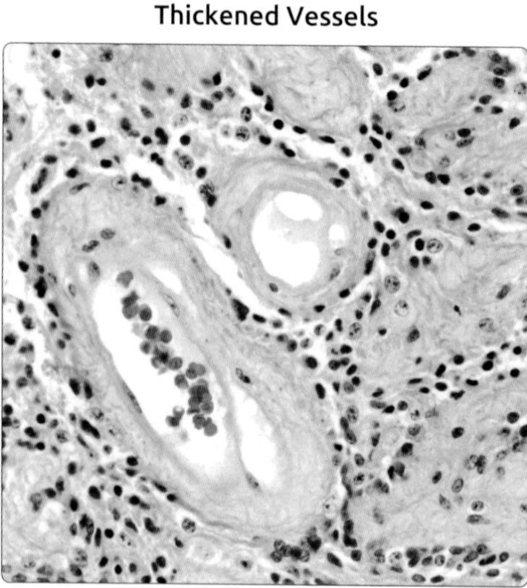

(Left) *The neurocytic component may assume a more lobular or nested pattern in tumors that have less well-developed pseudopapillae.* **(Right)** *Thickened vessels and scant intervening tumor cells suggest a compact, noninfiltrating tumor but do little to suggest PGNT.*

Perivascular Glial Component

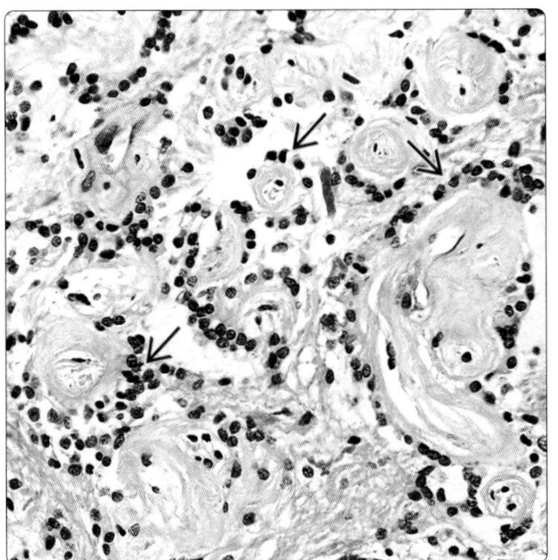

Tissue Dehiscence

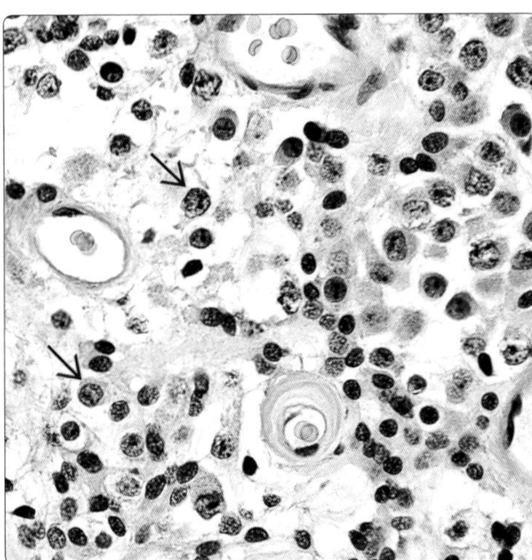

(Left) *The perivascular glial component ⮕ in some PGNTs is more apparent than the neurocytic element.* **(Right)** *Tissue dehiscence creates a generic, compact tumor with little architectural specificity; however, the pale uniform nuclei ⮕ suggest a neurocytic tumor. Immunostaining for GFAP and synaptophysin is necessary to show the tumor's biphasic composition.*

Ganglion Cell Differentiation

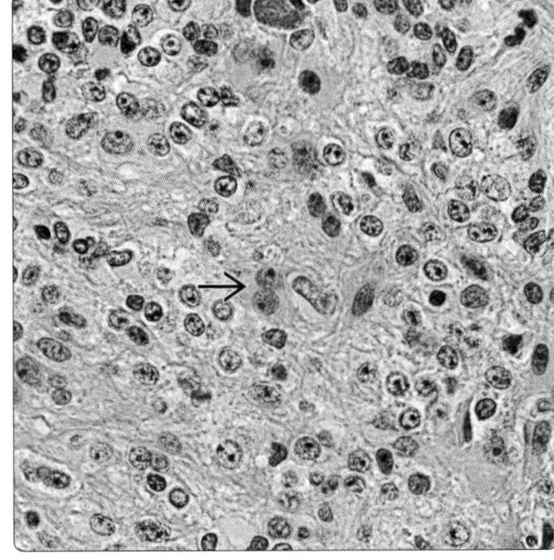

Neurocytic Component

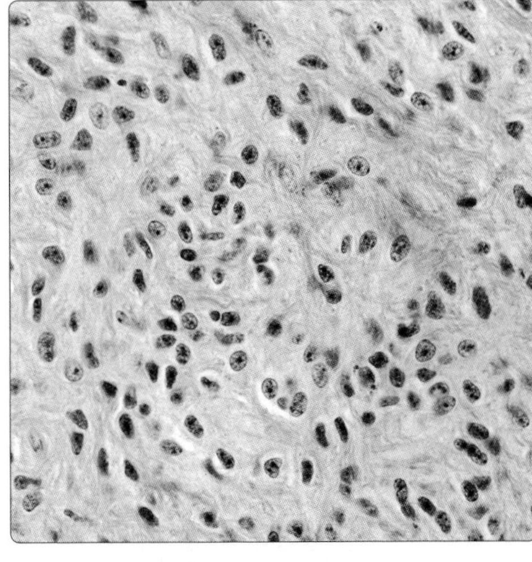

(Left) *Early ganglion cell differentiation, including binucleate forms ⮕, is a frequent focal finding. Neurocytes resembling oligodendroglia populate the background.* **(Right)** *The neurocytic component occasionally resembles infiltrating glioma. Immunostaining is necessary to identify such PGNTs.*

GFAP-Positive Glial Component

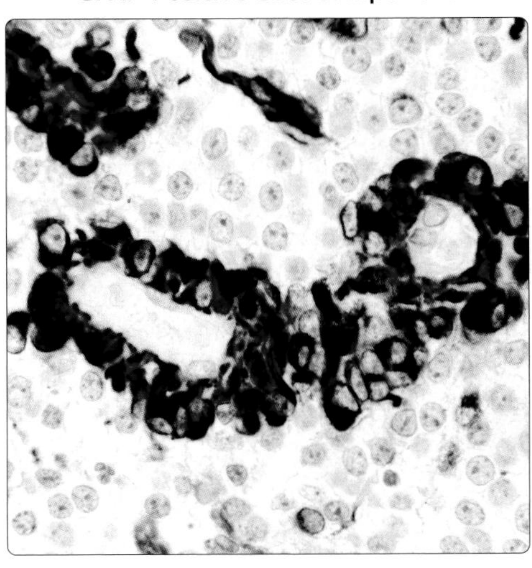

Synaptophysin-Positive Neurocytic Component

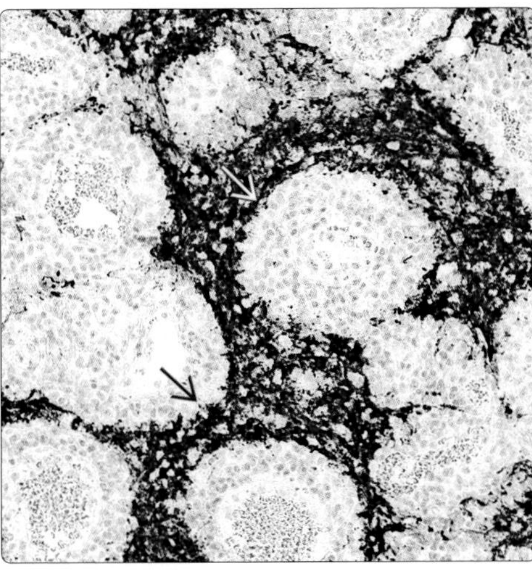

(Left) *The perivascular glial component is immunoreactive for GFAP, sometimes strikingly so.* **(Right)** *The interpapillary neurocytic component ⮕ strongly labels with synaptophysin, while the perivascular glial layer ➡ is negative.*

Paraganglioma of Filum Terminale

KEY FACTS

CLINICAL ISSUES

- Often not considered preoperatively

IMAGING

- Discrete contrast-enhancing mass in cauda equina (filum terminale)

MACROSCOPIC

- Smooth surface
- Attached to filum terminale

MICROSCOPIC

- May resemble ependymoma
- Perivascular formations less pronounced and less fibrillar than in ependymoma
- Ganglion cell metaplasia, ~ 25%

ANCILLARY TESTS

- Smear preparations helpful in excluding ependymoma and schwannoma
- Synaptophysin, diffusely (+)
- Chromogranin: Some (but usually not all) cells (+)
- Cytokeratins (CAM5.2, AE1/AE3), especially CAM5.2, may be extensively (+)
- S100(+) sustentacular cells, inconstant, sometimes only focal

TOP DIFFERENTIAL DIAGNOSES

- Ependymoma
- Schwannoma

DIAGNOSTIC CHECKLIST

- Discreteness and location (filum terminale) facilitate total resection
- Consider possibility of paraganglioma for any filum terminale mass; rarely clinical or radiological diagnosis

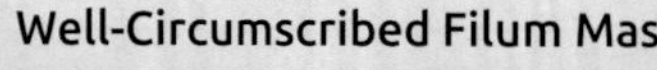

Well-Circumscribed Filum Mass

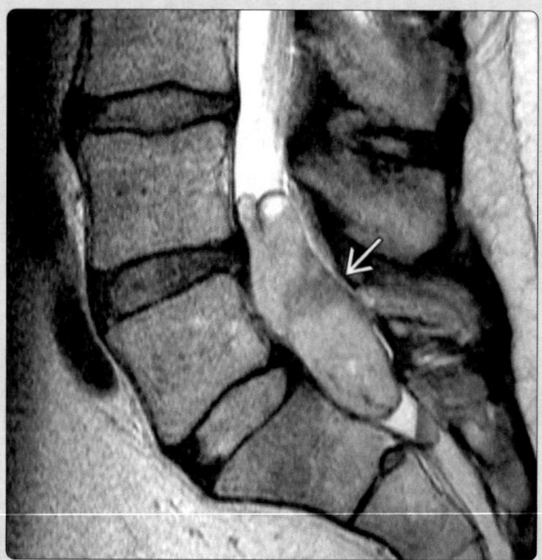

Discrete Mass

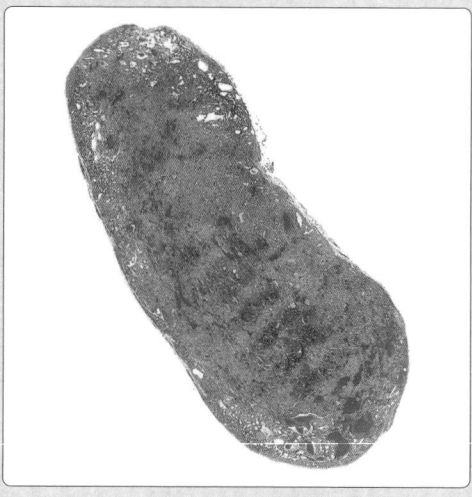

(Left) *As seen in a T2WI MR, paragangliomas of the filum terminale ➔ are well-circumscribed masses amenable to total resection. Myxopapillary ependymoma and schwannoma are the usual preoperative suspects.* **(Right)** *A whole-mount histological section underscores the lesion's discreteness and ease of surgical excision. Another local lesion, myxopapillary ependymoma, is similarly well circumscribed.*

Round to Oval Nuclei

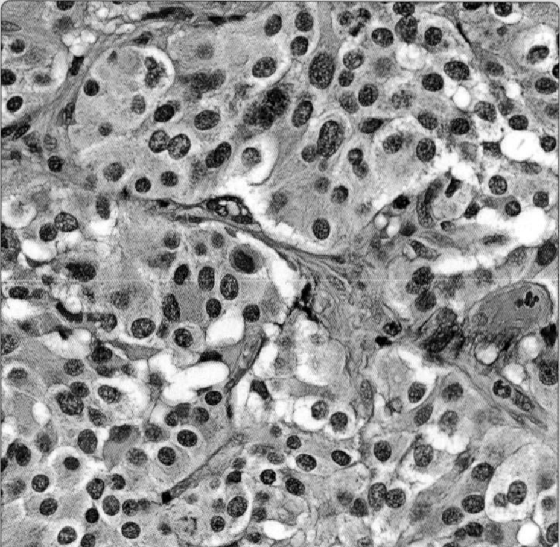

Perivascular Formations

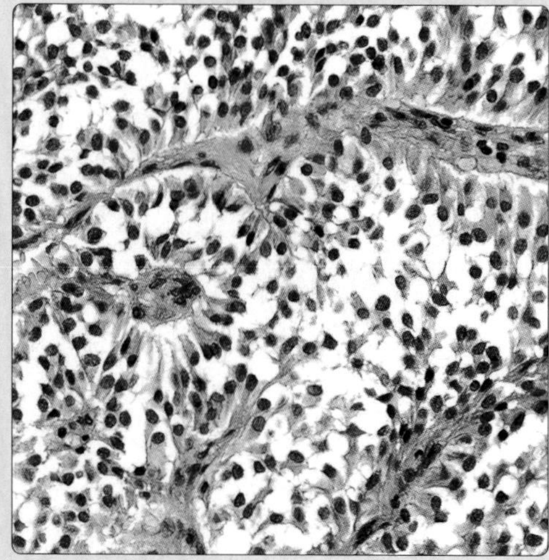

(Left) *The round to oval nuclei are cytologically bland. Sharp cell borders are sometimes apparent.* **(Right)** *Perivascular formations and artifactual dehiscence combine to create an ependymoma-like appearance.*

TERMINOLOGY

Definitions

- Low-grade, well-circumscribed neuroendocrine tumor of filum terminale
- Paragangliomas are WHO grade I

CLINICAL ISSUES

Epidemiology

- Age
  - Adults; children (rare)

Presentation

- Pain, sensorimotor deficits (less common)

Treatment

- Surgical approaches
  - Surgical excision curative

Prognosis

- Excellent
- Cerebrospinal fluid dissemination (rare)

IMAGING

MR Findings

- Cauda equina (filum terminale), discrete, homogeneously enhancing

MACROSCOPIC

General Features

- Attached to filum terminale
- Smooth surface
- Delicate capsule
- Soft, red
- Bleeds freely

MICROSCOPIC

Histologic Features

- Capsule, sometimes calcified
- Organoid architecture (zellballen)
- Rich vascularity
- Perivascular formations: Similar to but less pronounced and less fibrillar than in ependymoma
- Ribbons, some cases
- Sharp cell borders, particularly around vessels
- Sustentacular cells: Perilobular, inconspicuous, need immunohistochemistry, S100, for identification
- Ganglion cell metaplasia, ~ 25%
  - Ganglion cells
  - Schwann cell component (ganglioneuroma) in some cases
- Oncocytic change (occasional)
- Melanotic cells (rare)
- Extensive fibrosis (some cases)

Cytologic Features

- Dyscohesive uniform round cells
- Sharp cell borders (no fibrillar processes)
- Bland, "salt and pepper" nuclei

ANCILLARY TESTS

Immunohistochemistry

- Synaptophysin diffusely (+)
- Chromogranin: Some (but usually not all) cells (+)
- Cytokeratins (CAM5.2, AE1/AE3), especially CAM5.2, may be extensively (+)
- S100(+), sustentacular cells, inconstant, sometimes focally
- Somatostatin (+), some cases

DIFFERENTIAL DIAGNOSIS

Ependymoma

- Myxopapillary
  - Pseudopapillae rather than nested (zellballen) architecture
  - Perivascular myxoid material
  - Fibrillar background in some cases
  - Little reticulin
  - Fibrillar processes and smaller, darker nuclei in smears
  - GFAP(+) and sometimes EMA(+), dot-like microlumina
  - Tissue fragments and cells with processes in smears
- Cellular
  - No capsule
  - Perivascular pseudorosettes
  - Little reticulin
  - Fibrillar processes and smaller darker nuclei in smears
  - GFAP(+) and sometimes EMA(+) dot-like microlumina
  - Tissue fragments and fibrillated cells in smears
- Tanycytic
  - No capsule
  - Fascicular architecture
  - Elongated cells
  - Little reticulin
  - Perivascular pseudorosettes, but may be inconspicuous
  - Prominent fibrillar, GFAP(+) background
  - Tissue fragments and fibrillated cells in smears

Schwannoma

- Variable fascicular (Antoni A) and loose, spongy (Antoni B) tissue
- Tissue fragments and few individual cells in smears, spindle cells
- Strongly and diffusely S100(+), SOX10(+)
- Synaptophysin and chromogranin (-)
- Pericellular reticulin and collagen IV staining

DIAGNOSTIC CHECKLIST

Clinically Relevant Pathologic Features

- Discreteness and location (filum terminale) facilitate total resection

Pathologic Interpretation Pearls

- Consider possibility of paraganglioma for any filum terminale mass; is rarely clinical or radiological diagnosis
- Stain suspicious cases for synaptophysin and chromogranin

SELECTED REFERENCES

1. Sonneland PR et al: Paraganglioma of the cauda equina region. Clinicopathologic study of 31 cases with special reference to immunocytology and ultrastructure. Cancer. 58(8):1720-35, 1986

(Left) *Paragangliomas have a delicate, sometimes mineralized, capsule* ⇨. **(Right)** *Closely packed small lobules (zellballen) are the tumor's classic feature. Delicate nuclei have a "salt and pepper" quality that helps identify the entity, although the overall appearance raises the possibility of ependymoma, a far more common tumor than paraganglioma.*

Mineralized Capsule

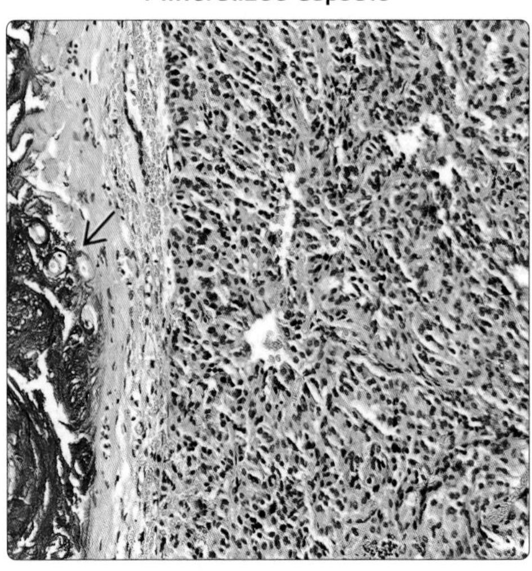

Zellballen

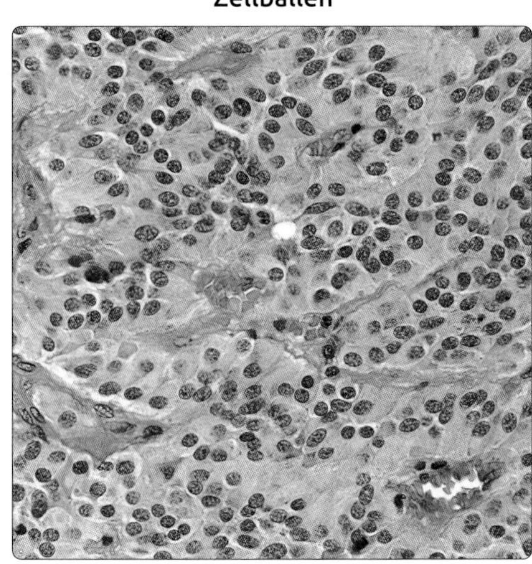

(Left) *The cells have a vague epithelioid quality due to distinct cell borders, especially in perivascular formations that resemble ependymoma pseudorosettes. The delicate, ovoid, speckled nuclei are typical of neuroendocrine tumors, paraganglioma included.* **(Right)** *Microcysts with myxoid material create a similarity to myxopapillary ependymoma. Immunopositivity for neuronal markers would resolve the issue.*

Vague Epithelioid Quality

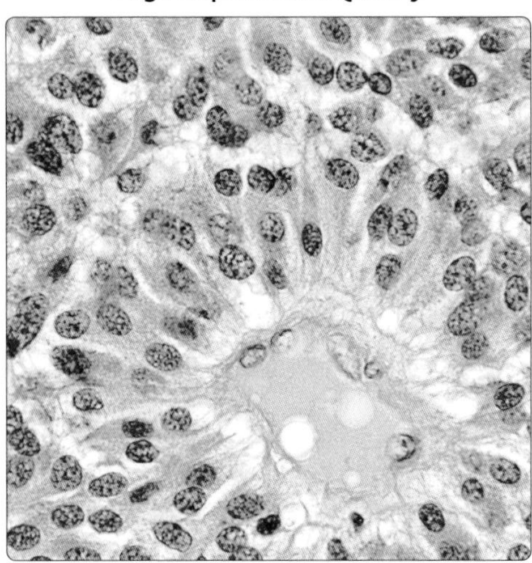

Microcysts

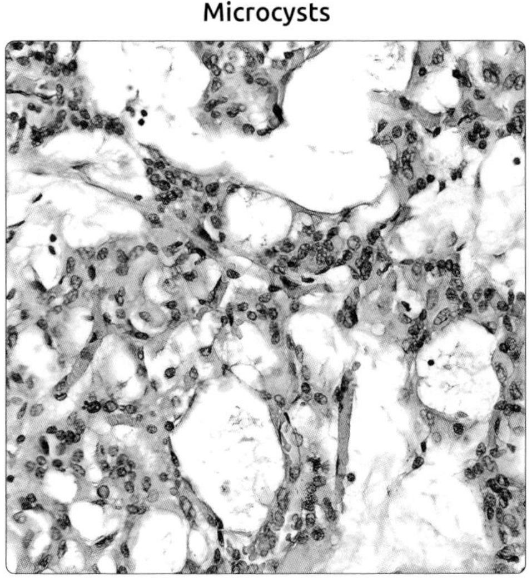

(Left) *Anastomosing cords of cells create a distinctive feature in a minority of paragangliomas.* **(Right)** *Ganglion cell metaplasia enlivens a minority of cases. The presence of Nissl substance* ➡ *facilitates identification of the large cells with prominent nucleoli. A Schwann cell component will also be present in some cases.*

Anastomosing Cords

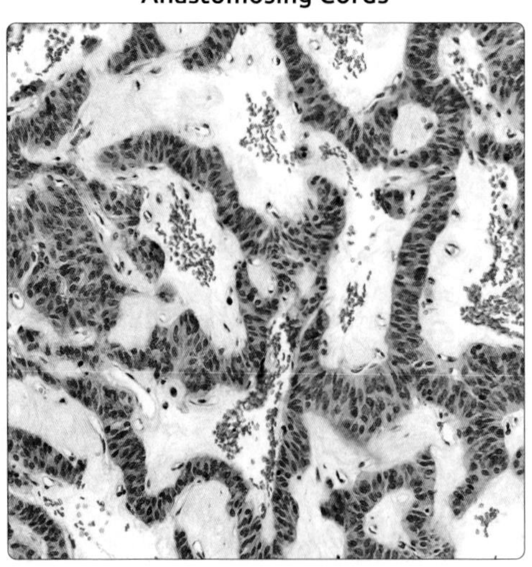

Ganglion Cell Metaplasia

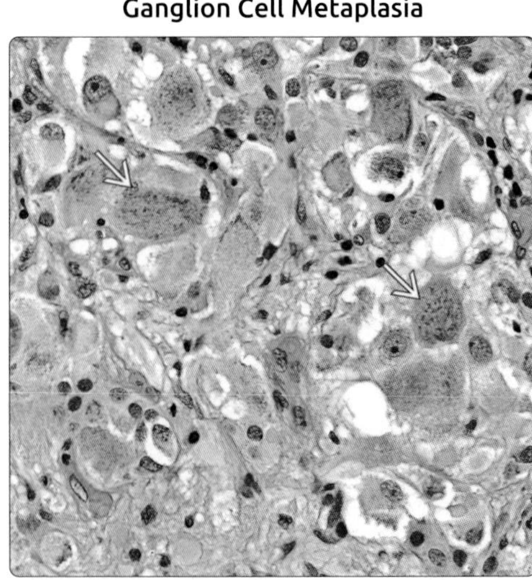

"Salt and Pepper" Nuclei

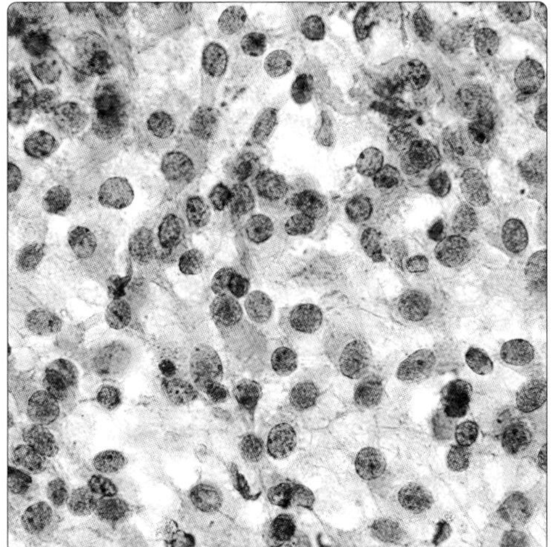

Small Lobules

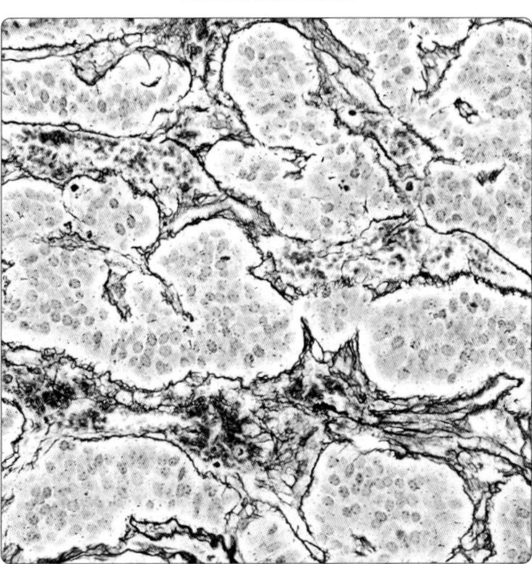

(Left) *Uniform, cytologically bland nuclei with the "salt and pepper" quality of a neuroendocrine neoplasm are best seen in smear preparations.* **(Right)** *Reticulin circumscribes small lobules. Tumor and stroma would not be so segregated in ependymoma, nor would such a lobular architecture be present.*

Diffuse Synaptophysin Positivity

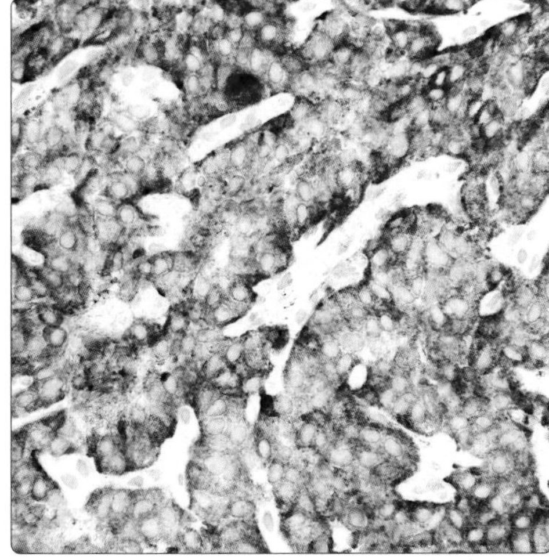

Chromogranin Immunoreactivity

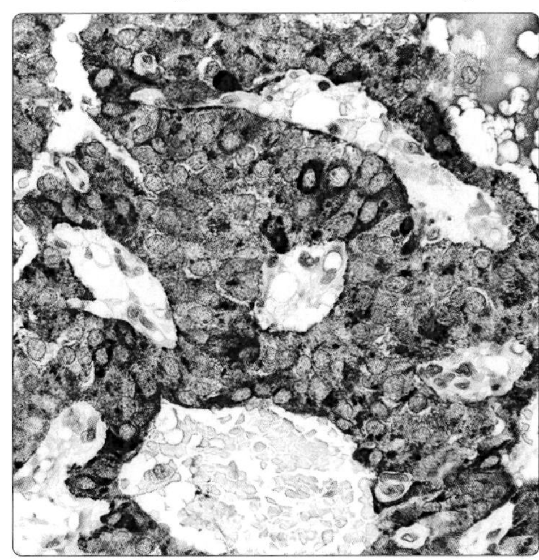

(Left) *Diffuse positivity for synaptophysin is typical of paraganglioma. This finely granular cytoplasmic staining, in concert with minimal if any GFAP staining, helps confirm the diagnosis.* **(Right)** *Cells vary over a broad range in the degree of immunoreactivity for chromogranin. Some are negative, others strongly positive, and many are intermediate.*

Cytokeratin Immunoreactivity

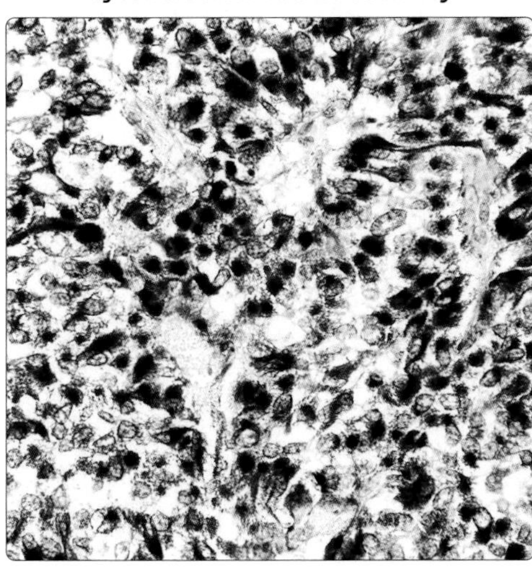

Sustentacular Cells

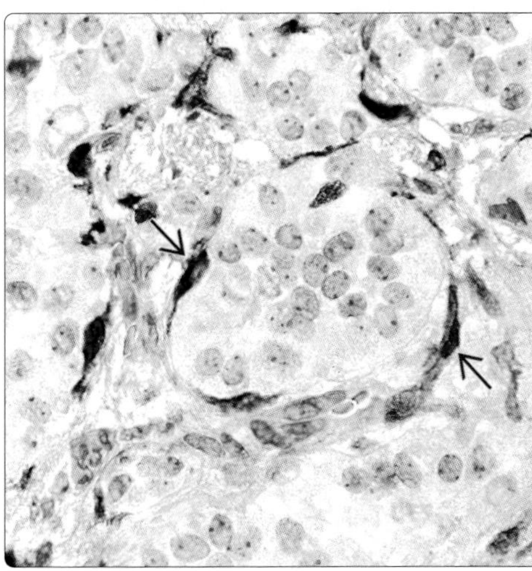

(Left) *Immunoreactivity for cytokeratins (CAM5.2) should not be a surprise in paragangliomas of the filum terminale.* **(Right)** *S100-positive sustentacular cells* ⇒ *delimit zellballen in some paragangliomas. The delicate cells are usually not as obvious as in this immunohistochemical preparation, and almost invisible in H&E sections.*

Malignant Glioneuronal Tumors

KEY FACTS

TERMINOLOGY

- Heterogeneous group of malignant tumors with differentiation along both neuronal and glial lines
  - Poorly characterized
  - No consensus grading criteria
- Anaplastic gangliogliomas prototypic but rare
- Designation best applied to tumors not fitting into specified WHO categories

CLINICAL ISSUES

- Prognosis unfavorable to poor, but details unclear given uncertainties in classification

MICROSCOPIC

- Anaplastic ganglioglioma
- Anaplastic ganglioglioneurocytoma
- Anaplastic glioma with focal neuronal differentiation or immunotype

ANCILLARY TESTS

- Neuronal component, including neuropil islands: Synaptophysin (+), NeuN(+/-)
  - Neurofilament protein (+) in ganglion cells, if any
- Glial component: GFAP and S100 protein (+)

TOP DIFFERENTIAL DIAGNOSES

- High-grade infiltrating glioma with trapped neurons
  - Much more common than malignant glioneuronal tumor
- Embryonal tumors
  - Overlap as category with high-grade glioneuronal tumors
  - Embryonal tumor designation applied predominantly to small, round blue cell tumors/undifferentiated tumors with minor glial differentiation
- Atypical teratoid/rhabdoid tumor

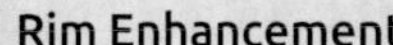

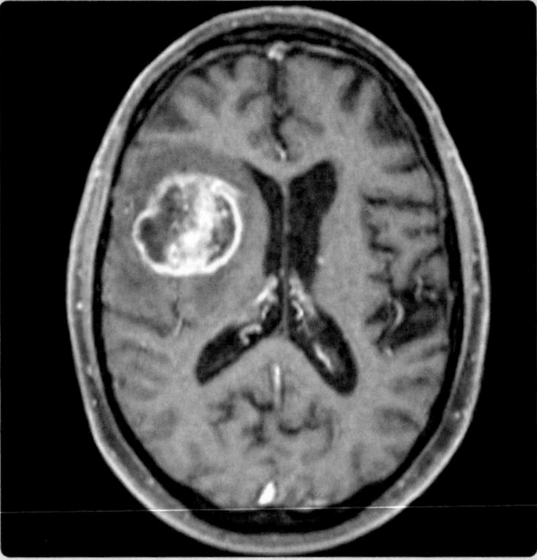

Epithelioid Cells

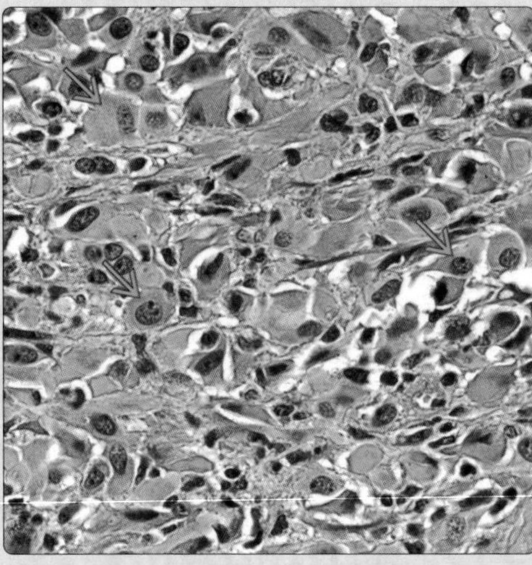

(Left) *Some malignant glioneuronal tumors (MGNTs) share the radiologic features of glioblastoma including rim enhancement, mass effect, and edema.* **(Right)** *MGNTs may contain epithelioid cells; some with macronucleoli appear neuronal →, but others do not. Staining with neuronal and glial markers is usually required.*

Heterogeneous Cell Components

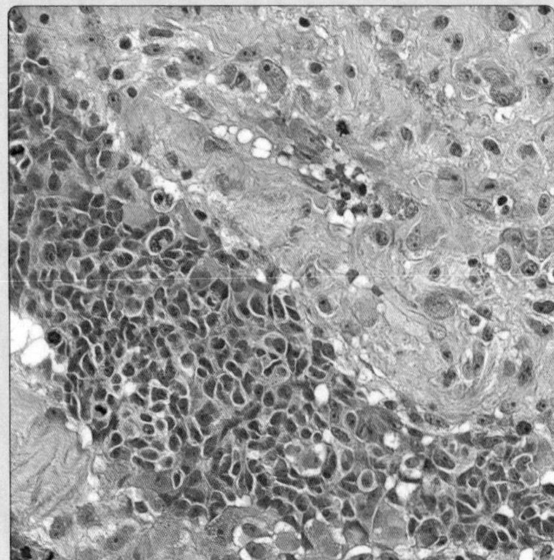

Ambiguous Lineage

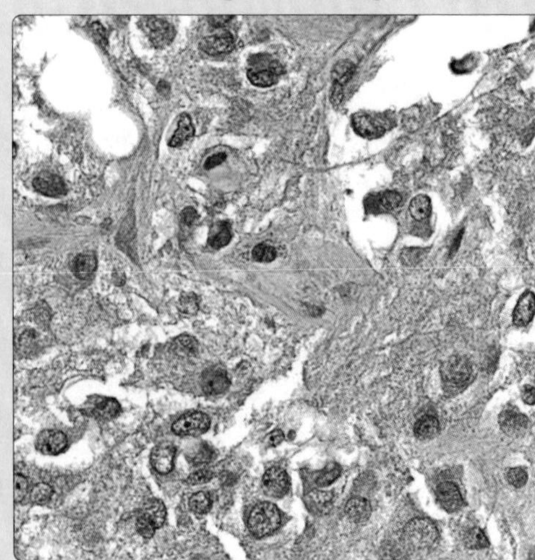

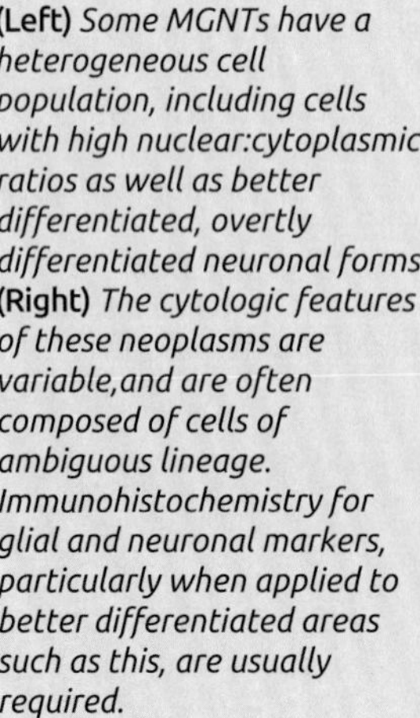

(Left) *Some MGNTs have a heterogeneous cell population, including cells with high nuclear:cytoplasmic ratios as well as better differentiated, overtly differentiated neuronal forms.* **(Right)** *The cytologic features of these neoplasms are variable,and are often composed of cells of ambiguous lineage. Immunohistochemistry for glial and neuronal markers, particularly when applied to better differentiated areas such as this, are usually required.*

TERMINOLOGY

Abbreviations

- Malignant glioneuronal tumor (MGNT)

Definitions

- Heterogeneous group of malignant tumors with differentiation along both neuronal and glial lines
  - Poorly characterized group
  - No consensus regarding grading criteria
  - Designation best applied to tumors not fitting into specified WHO categories

CLINICAL ISSUES

Presentation

- May affect any age group, including children and elderly

Treatment

- Surgery plus radiation therapy
- Chemotherapy may be tailored to dominant component, glial or neuronal, if distinction can be made

Prognosis

- Unfavorable, but details unclear given unsettled classification and nomenclature

MICROSCOPIC

Anaplastic Ganglioglioma

- Equates with WHO grade III
- Demarcated
- Neuronal component
  - Ganglion cells, often with smaller ganglioid cells
  - Usually low grade but cellular, pleomorphic, and mitotically active in rare cases
- Anaplastic glial component
  - Astrocytic; rarely oligodendroglial
    - Variably epithelioid, giant cell, fibrillary
  - Variable architectural patterns
    - Ribbons, pseudopapillae, cohesive nests, pseudorosettes
  - Eosinophilic granular bodies
  - Perivascular lymphocytes

Anaplastic Ganglioglioneurocytoma

- Ill-defined entity
- Ganglion cells &/or smaller ganglioid cells
- Neurocytes resembling oligodendrocytes
- Anaplastic glial component

Anaplastic Glioma With Partial Neuronal Differentiation

- Pleomorphic xanthoastrocytoma
  - Mitotically active, ± microvascular proliferation, necrosis
  - Neuronal differentiation, ganglion cells
    - No prognostic significance
- Oligodendroglioma, grade III or II with
  - Neuronal differentiation
    - Ganglion cells and ganglioid cells
    - Neuropil rosettes
    - No known prognostic significance
- Glioblastoma
  - Immunoexpression of neuronal proteins
    - Not infrequent, especially in giant cell type
    - No definite prognostic significance
  - Embryonal tumor component
    - Islands, nodules, or sheets of primitive cells
    - Anaplasia as seen in some medulloblastomas
    - Very high mitotic and Ki-67 rate
    - Immunopositive for synaptophysin and often p53
    - Therapy for embryonal tumors possibly efficacious
- Glioma with neuropil islands
  - Glioma usually anaplastic, distinctive pale regions of fine neuropil surrounded by round neurocytes
    - Astrocytoma grade III or IV (typical)
    - Oligodendroglioma (uncommon)
    - Ependymoma (rare)
  - Neuronal element often neurocytic; ganglion cells few
  - Low (Ki-67) indices
  - Histologic pattern rather than specific entity
  - No prognostic significance

ANCILLARY TESTS

Immunohistochemistry

- Neuronal component, including neuropil islands
  - Synaptophysin (+)
  - Neurofilament protein (+) in ganglion cells, if any
  - NeuN(+/-)
- Glial component
  - GFAP and S100 protein (+)

DIFFERENTIAL DIAGNOSIS

High-Grade Infiltrating Glioma With Trapped Neurons

- Much more common than malignant glioneuronal tumor
- Overrun cortical neurons with aligned apical dendrites directed to cortical surface
- Trapped, overrun neurons may appear atypical, but changes usually minor; binucleation rare

Embryonal Tumors

- Overlap as category with high-grade glioneuronal tumors
- Embryonal tumor designation applied predominantly to small, round blue cell tumors/undifferentiated tumors with minor glial differentiation

Atypical Teratoid/Rhabdoid Tumor

- No ganglion cell morphology
- Additional immunoreactivities: EMA, keratin, smooth muscle actin, desmin, etc.
- Loss of nuclear immunoreactivity for INI1

DIAGNOSTIC CHECKLIST

Pathologic Interpretation Pearls

- Infiltrative gliomas with trapped ganglion cells much more common than malignant glioneuronal tumors

SELECTED REFERENCES

1. Donev K et al: Expression of diagnostic neuronal markers and outcome in glioblastoma. Neuropathol Appl Neurobiol. 36(5):411-21, 2010

(Left) *A biphasic, mitotically active ⇒ MGNT has both a small cell glial component ⇒ and a ganglion cell element ⇒.* **(Right)** *Complex architectural patterns, including pseudopapillae or ependymoma-like perivascular pseudorosettes, engender a broad differential diagnosis that usually requires immunohistochemistry for resolution.*

Biphasic Tumor

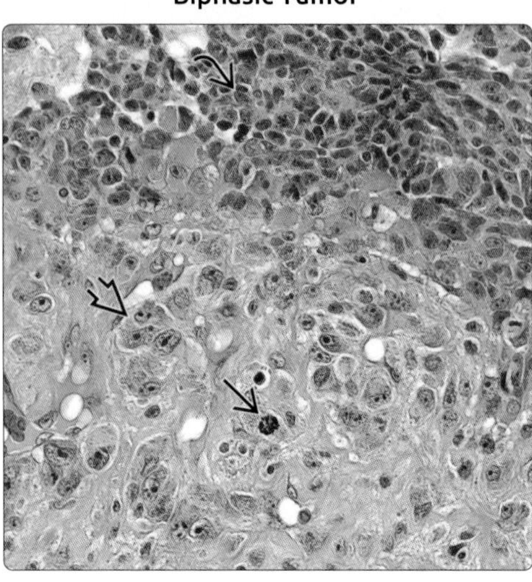

Pseudopapillae

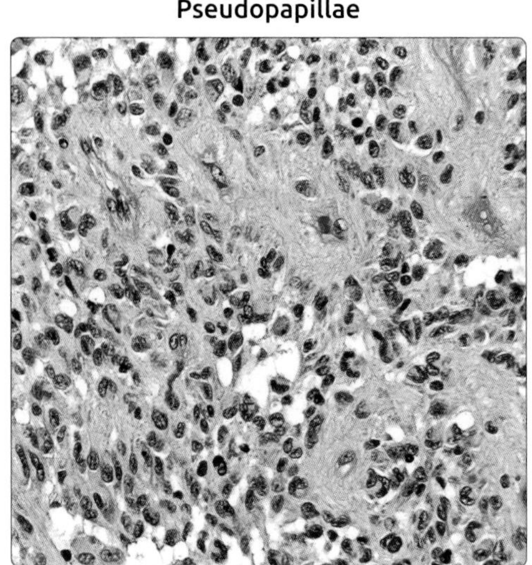

(Left) *This MGNT contained a moderately cellular, somewhat monotonous neuronal component with mitotic activity ⇒. There were ganglion cells, neurocytes, and neuropil in other regions.* **(Right)** *Neuronal differentiation is focally present in the form of ganglion cells ⇒ with Nissl substance and macronucleoli. This tumor was mitotically active elsewhere. Delicate neuropil and oligodendroglioma-like neurocytes are present as well.*

Mitotic Activity

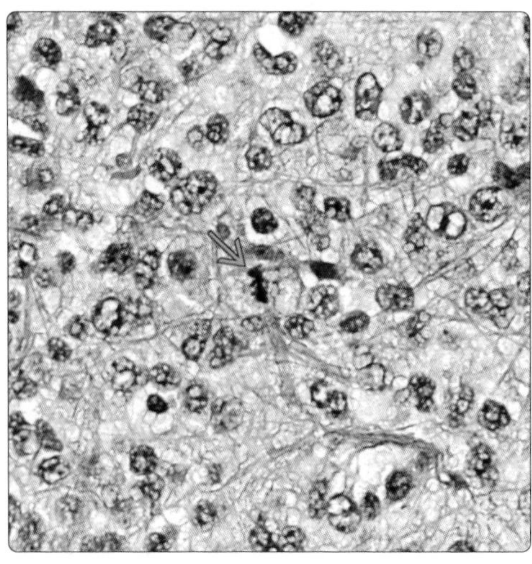

Neuronal Differentiation

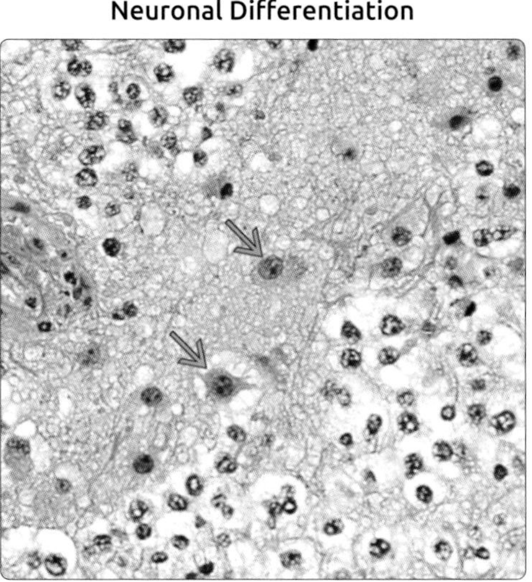

(Left) *Some MGNTs may contain pleomorphic cells with bizarre hyperchromatic nuclei or intranuclear inclusions. Pleomorphism, in itself, is insufficient for a diagnosis of anaplasia. Mitoses were present elsewhere.* **(Right)** *High cellularity, mitoses, and microvascular proliferation ⇒ are features of anaplasia in glioneuronal tumors. A high Ki-67 index was also present.*

Pleomorphic Cells

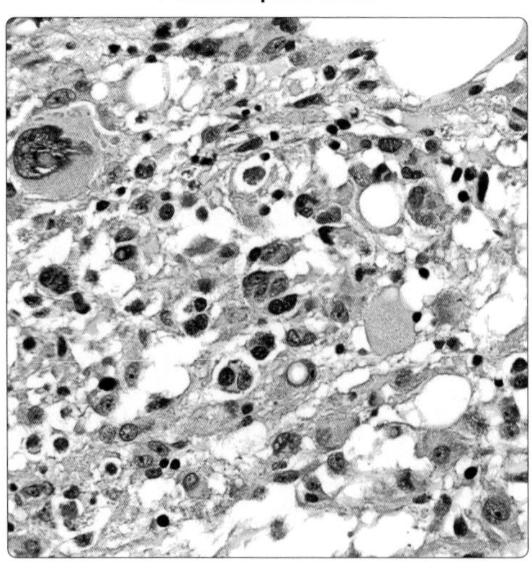

Microvascular Proliferation

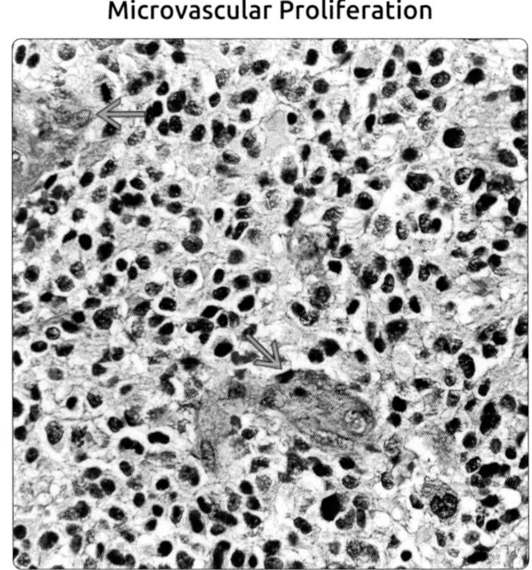

Neuronal Component

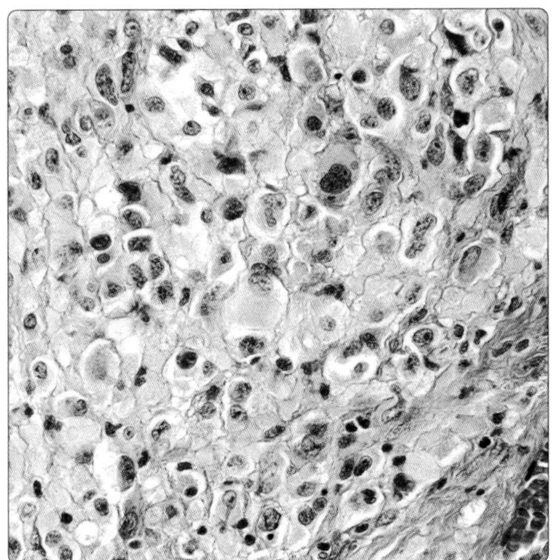

Synaptophysin Immunoreactivity

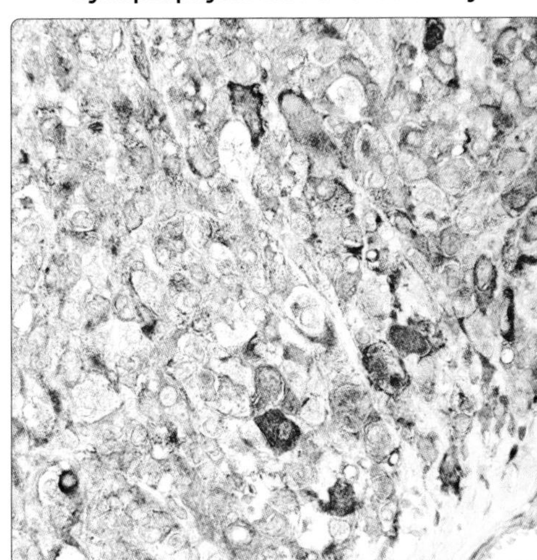

(Left) *The neuronal component may appear malignant in rare gangliogliomas. The suggestive ganglion cell differentiation was confirmed by diffuse immunoreactivity for synaptophysin. Mitoses and a high Ki-67 labeling index were present.* **(Right)** *Immunostaining for synaptophysin may be critical in confirming a neuronal element when histological features are suggestive but not diagnostic of ganglion cells.*

GFAP Staining

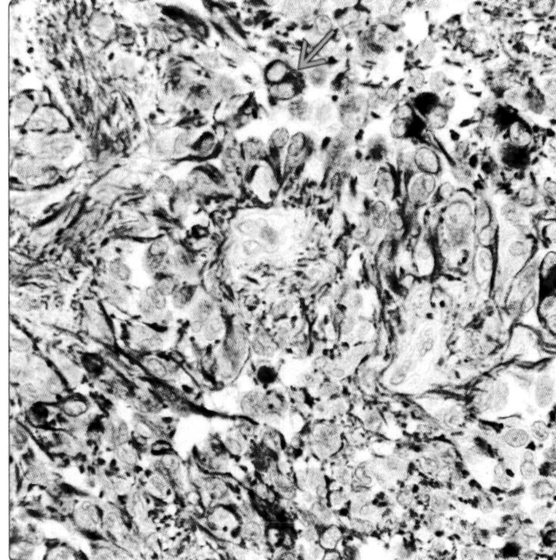

Chromogranin Immunopositivity

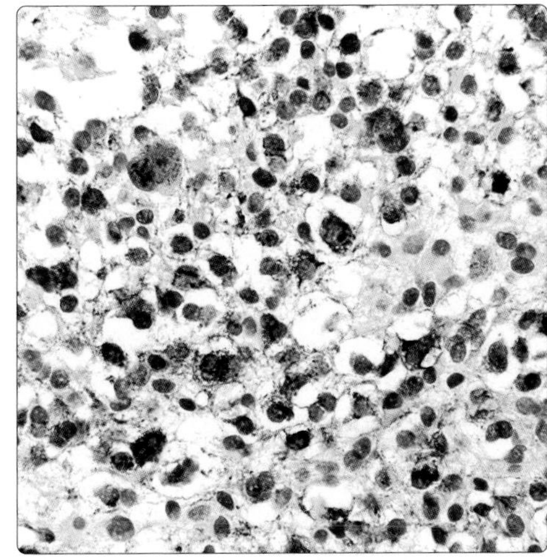

(Left) *Partial staining for GFAP is usually required to establish the diagnosis of a glial component in malignant glioneuronal tumors. Some* ⇒ *but not all cells are positive in this case.* **(Right)** *Chromogranin immunopositivity also supports the presence of a neoplastic neuronal component. Focal weak staining for a single neuronal marker is not sufficient to diagnose MGNT.*

Neuropil Islands

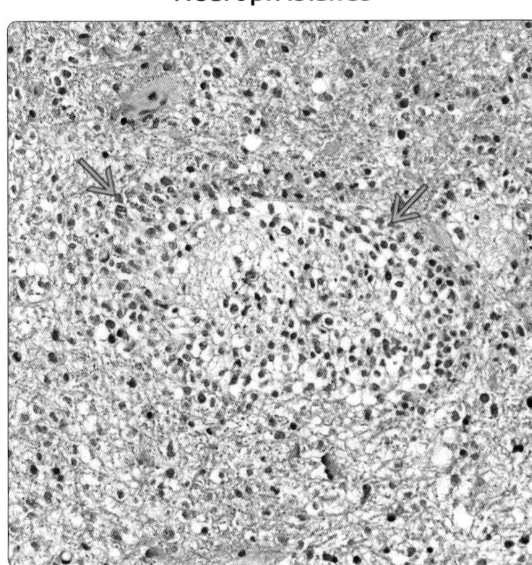

Rosetted Islands

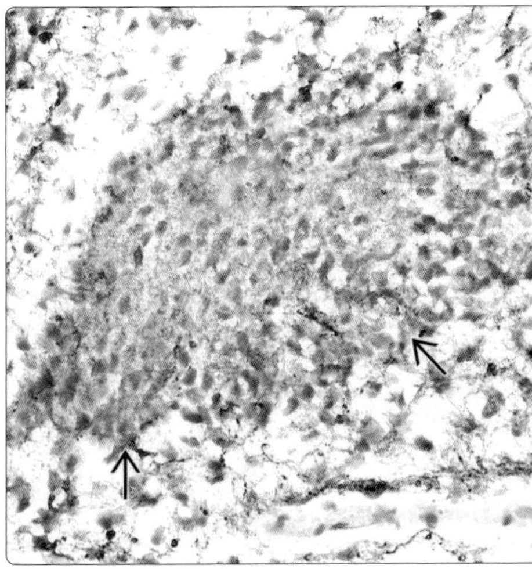

(Left) *Anaplastic glioma with neuropil islands represents a variant of infiltrating glioma with sharply demarcated areas of neurocytes and neuropils* ⇒*. The latter are a morphologic reflection of neuronal differentiation. The glial element is typically anaplastic astrocytoma.* **(Right)** *Rosetted islands in infiltrating gliomas such as this anaplastic astrocytoma are immunopositive for synaptophysin. Most staining lies in the fibrillar, neuropil core. Neurocytes* ⇒ *delineate the focus.*

Diffuse Leptomeningeal Glioneuronal Tumor

KEY FACTS

TERMINOLOGY

- Indolent neoplasm characterized by oligodendroglioma-like cytology, usually affecting children and demonstrating extensive leptomeningeal and superficial parenchymal CNS spread

CLINICAL ISSUES

- Indolent neoplasm characterized by periods of stabilization and slow progression

IMAGING

- Superficial cyst-like/nodular T2 hyperintense lesions throughout CNS
- Diffuse leptomeningeal enhancement
- Small, enhancing, discrete intraparenchymal masses, particularly in spinal cord

MICROSCOPIC

- Bland round cells with perinuclear halos with associated leptomeningeal desmoplasia
- Rare to absent mitotic activity
- Overt neuronal/ganglion cell differentiation in subset of cases

ANCILLARY TESTS

- Olig2 and S100 expression consistent
- GFAP and synaptophysin variable
- IDH1 (R132H) (-)
- Concurrent *BRAF-KIAA1549* fusion and 1p loss most frequent molecular alteration

TOP DIFFERENTIAL DIAGNOSES

- Macrophage-rich inflammatory lesions
- Oligodendroglioma
- Desmoplastic infantile ganglioglioma/astrocytoma
- Pilocytic astrocytoma
- Embryonal tumors

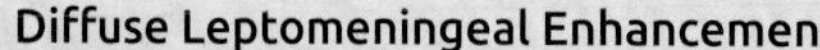

Diffuse Leptomeningeal Enhancement

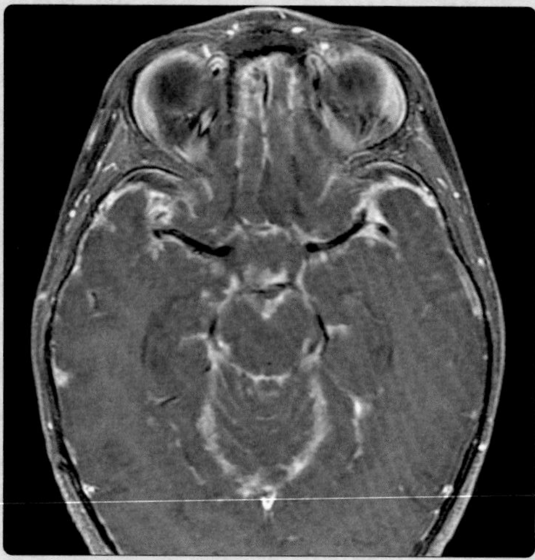

Nerve Root Involvement

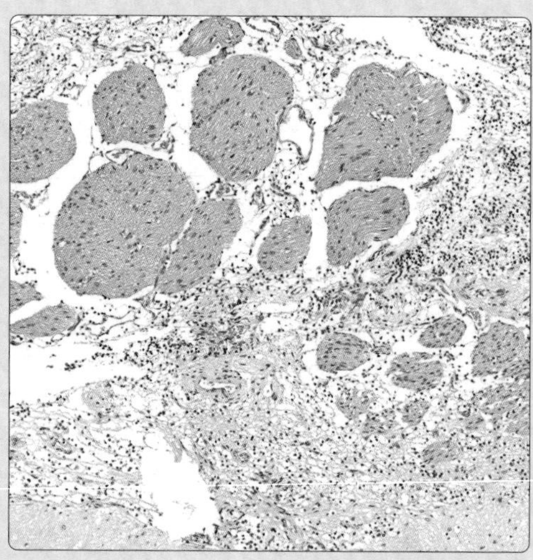

(Left) *The hallmark of disseminated leptomeningeal glioneuronal tumors (DLGNT) is extensive involvement of intracranial and spinal leptomeninges, as demonstrated by extensive superficial enhancement in this T1-weighted postcontrast MR.* **(Right)** *Extensive dissemination in leptomeninges by DLGNT may lead to infiltration and entrapment of nerve roots in the spine.*

Leptomeningeal Desmoplasia

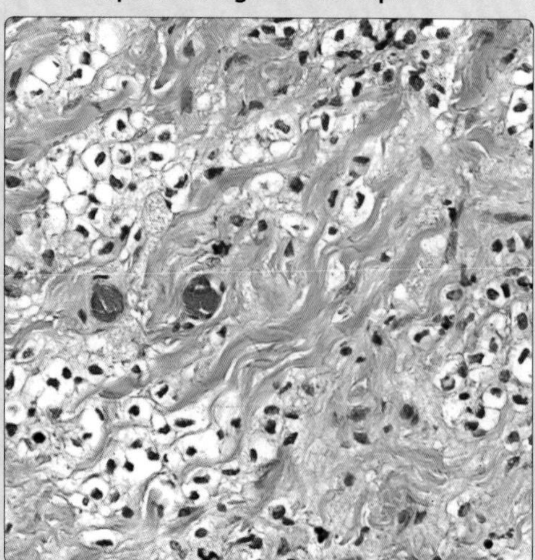

Ganglion Cell Differentiation

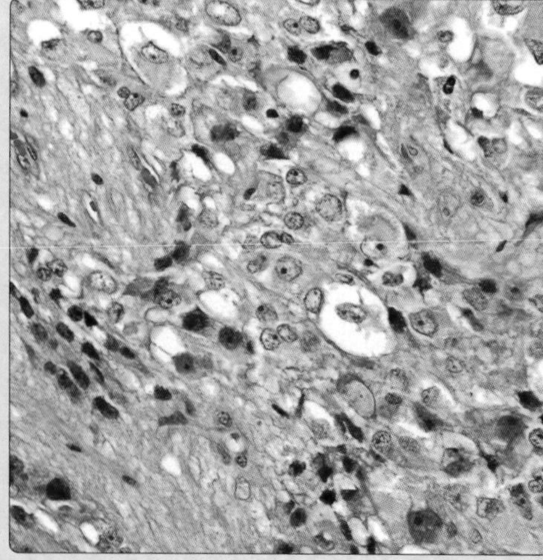

(Left) *When present in small leptomeningeal biopsies, DLGNT elicits a characteristic desmoplastic response. Cellularity is often low and the main differential diagnosis in these cases is an inflammatory/macrophage-rich process.* **(Right)** *A subset of DLGNT demonstrates overt neuronal differentiation in the form of ganglion cells, which may form significant aggregates.*

TERMINOLOGY

Abbreviations

- Diffuse leptomeningeal glioneuronal tumor (DLGNT)

Synonyms

- Disseminated oligodendroglial-like neoplasm
- Disseminated oligodendroglioma-like neoplasm
- Primary leptomeningeal oligodendrogliomatosis

Definitions

- Indolent neoplasm characterized by oligodendroglioma-like cytology, usually affecting children and demonstrating extensive leptomeningeal and superficial parenchymal CNS spread, out of proportion to putative intraparenchymal primary lesions

CLINICAL ISSUES

Presentation

- Signs secondary to increased intracranial pressure
- Meningeal signs, cranial and spinal nerve deficits, spinal cord compression in subset

Prognosis

- Indolent neoplasm characterized by periods of stabilization and slow progression
- Morbidity often significant

IMAGING

MR Findings

- Superficial cyst-like/nodular T2 hyperintense lesions throughout CNS
- Diffuse leptomeningeal enhancement on postcontrast T1-weighted sequences
- Small enhancing discrete intraparenchymal masses, particularly in spinal cord

MICROSCOPIC

Histologic Features

- Bland round cells with perinuclear halos with associated leptomeningeal desmoplasia
- Rare to absent mitotic activity
- Overt neuronal/ganglion cell differentiation in subset of cases
- Anaplastic transformation rare

Cytologic Features

- CSF samples usually negative

ANCILLARY TESTS

Immunohistochemistry

- Olig2 and S100 expression consistent
- GFAP and synaptophysin expression variable
- IDH1 (R132H) (-)

Genetic Testing

- Concurrent *BRAF-KIAA1549* fusion and 1p loss most frequent molecular alteration

DIFFERENTIAL DIAGNOSIS

Macrophage-Rich Inflammatory Lesions

- Larger cells with oval nuclei and foamy cytoplasm
- CD68(+)
- Olig2 and S100(-)

Oligodendroglioma

- Pathologic and molecular overlap in subset of cases
- Leptomeningeal dissemination and *BRAF-KIAA1549* fusion rare

Desmoplastic Infantile Ganglioglioma/Astrocytoma

- Discrete, cystic cerebral mass, rather than leptomeningeal dissemination
- Astrocytic rather than oligodendroglial-like morphology

Pilocytic Astrocytoma

- Oligodendroglioma-like regions present in subset of cases
- Pilocytic morphology present at least focally (piloid areas, eosinophilic granular bodies, Rosenthal fibers)

Embryonal Tumors

- More cellular and high proliferative activity

DIAGNOSTIC CHECKLIST

Clinically Relevant Pathologic Features

- Suspect diagnosis of leptomeningeal glioneuronal tumor in presence of diffuse leptomeningeal enhancement in pediatric patient

Pathologic Interpretation Pearls

- Think of DLGNT when encountering small leptomeningeal biopsies with subtle increase in cellularity

SELECTED REFERENCES

1. Rodriguez FJ et al: High rate of concurrent BRAF-KIAA1549 gene fusion and 1p deletion in disseminated oligodendroglioma-like leptomeningeal neoplasms (DOLN). Acta Neuropathol. 129(4):609-10, 2015
2. Schniederjan MJ et al: Diffuse leptomeningeal neuroepithelial tumor: 9 pediatric cases with chromosome 1p/19q deletion status and IDH1 (R132H) immunohistochemistry. Am J Surg Pathol. 37(5):763-71, 2013
3. Agamanolis DP et al: An unusual form of superficially disseminated glioma in children: report of 3 cases. J Child Neurol. 27(6):727-33, 2012
4. Rodriguez FJ et al: Disseminated oligodendroglial-like leptomeningeal tumor of childhood: a distinctive clinicopathologic entity. Acta Neuropathol. 124(5):627-41, 2012
5. Perilongo G et al: Spinal low-grade neoplasms with extensive leptomeningeal dissemination in children. Childs Nerv Syst. 18(9-10):505-12, 2002

KEY FACTS

TERMINOLOGY

- Non-germ cell, nonteratomatous tumor of pineal region derived from pineal parenchymal cells

CLINICAL ISSUES

- Clinical presentation nearly identical for different types of pineal parenchymal tumors, germinomas, teratomas

IMAGING

- Pineocytomas and PPTIDs well circumscribed
- Pineocytomas noninvasive
- Homogeneous enhancement with contrast
- Tumor size for pineocytomas, PPTIDs usually 2-5 cm
- Pineoblastomas more likely poorly demarcated, noncalcified

MICROSCOPIC

- Isomorphic cells with scant cytoplasm
- Pineocytomatous rosettes in pineocytoma, variably present in PPTID, absent in pineoblastoma
- Grading based on mitotic activity, presence or absence of immunostaining with neurofilaments
- Pineocytomas, some PPTID may contain ganglion cells, pleomorphic cells

ANCILLARY TESTS

- Immunohistochemistry positive for synaptophysin, neurofilament protein
- Ki-67 helpful in distinguishing types of PPTs

TOP DIFFERENTIAL DIAGNOSES

- Germinoma
- Metastatic carcinoma

Axial NECT: Pineocytoma Calcification, No Hydrocephalus

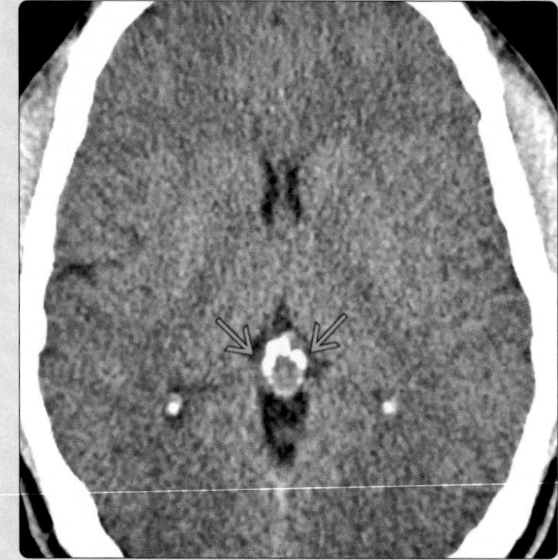

Pineocytomatous Rosettes

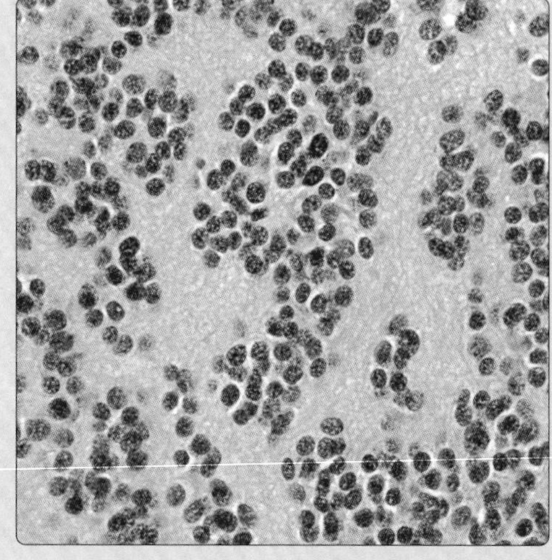

(Left) *Axial NECT shows a classic example of pineocytoma with exploded peripheral calcification ⇒. This small mass, just over 1 cm in size, produces no hydrocephalus.* **(Right)** *Broad rosettes formed by neuritic processes, resulting in anuclear fibrillar eosinophilic areas unassociated with blood vessels, are a signature feature of pineocytoma.*

Pineocytomatous Rosettes, Synaptophysin

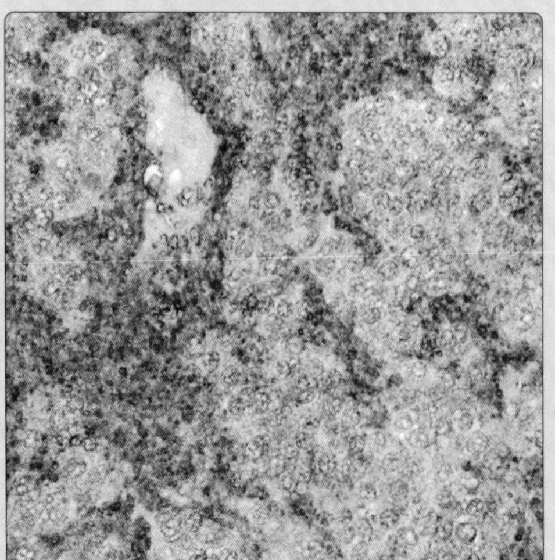

Pineocytoma, Absent Cell Cycling

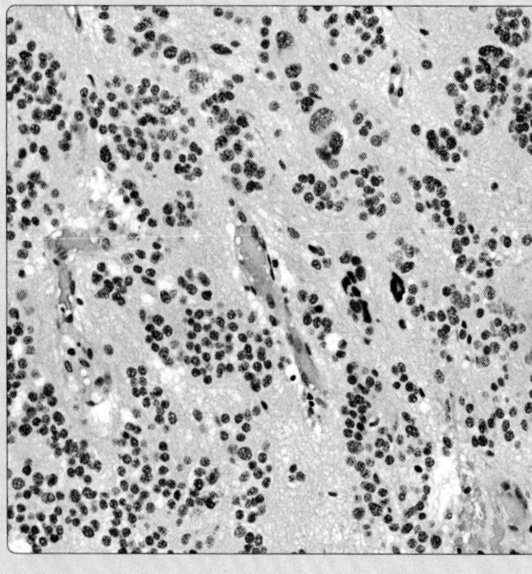

(Left) *Synaptophysin highlights the broad pineocytoma rosettes. This degree of immunoreactivity for synaptophysin serves to distinguish this type of rosette from perivascular rosettes in ependymoma; the latter would be GFAP (+).* **(Right)** *Cell cycle labeling should be nearly absent in a pineocytoma, WHO grade I, as illustrated in this image.*

TERMINOLOGY

Abbreviations

- Pineal parenchymal tumor (PPT)
- Pineal parenchymal tumor of indeterminate differentiation (PPTID)

Definitions

- Non-germ cell, nonteratomatous tumors of pineal gland originating from pineal parenchymal cells

ETIOLOGY/PATHOGENESIS

Unknown for Most PPTs

- Pineoblastomas may be associated with germline *RB1* (retinoblastoma 1 gene, chromosome 13) mutation
- Pineoblastomas described as occurring in *DICER1* mutation (pleuropulmonary blastoma familial tumor predisposition syndrome)

CLINICAL ISSUES

Epidemiology

- Incidence
  - Rare, account for < 1% of all brain tumors
  - PPTs account for only 30% of all pineal region tumors
    - Germinomas, teratomas, cysts more prevalent
- Age
  - Pineocytoma, WHO grade I; PPTIDs, grade II-II
    - Average age: 38 years
  - Pineoblastoma, WHO grade IV
    - Average age: 18 years

Presentation

- Indistinguishable from other pineal region masses
  - Symptoms referable to hydrocephalus
  - Compression of tectal plate and paralysis of upward gaze

Treatment

- Resection for pineocytomas
- Adjuvant chemotherapy, radiotherapy for higher grade PPTs

Prognosis

- Excellent, with resection only, for pineocytoma
- Outcome based on grading

IMAGING

General Features

- Pineocytomas, PPTIDs often well circumscribed
- Usually homogeneous, may show peripheral calcification or occasional cystic change
- Pineoblastomas more likely poorly demarcated, noncalcified
- Some clues, but neuroimaging features cannot reliably distinguish grade

MICROSCOPIC

Grading Criteria

- Pineocytoma, WHO grade I
  - Lobular or diffuse patterns
  - Varying size and numbers of pineocytomatous rosettes
    - Large, irregular, pineocytomatous rosettes typical of pineocytoma
    - May also see Homer Wright smaller, more circular rosettes
  - Rosettes contain neuritic processes, absence of nuclei
  - Cells isomorphic
    - Round nuclei, stippled chromatin, scant cytoplasm
  - Large ganglion cells or multinucleated cells with bizarre appearance in some cases
  - No mitotic activity
- Pineal parenchymal tumor of intermediate differentiation, WHO grades II-III
  - Dense lobular arrangement
  - Diffuse proliferation mimicking neurocytoma
  - Transitional forms with areas of intermediate differentiation combined with pineocytomatous rosettes
  - Biphasic pattern with pineocytoma admixed with pineoblastoma
    - Rarest form
  - Cells isomorphic
    - Round nuclei, stippled chromatin, scant cytoplasm
  - Criteria for grade II
    - < 6 mitoses/10 HPF
    - Positive immunoreactivity for neurofilament protein
  - Criteria for grade III
    - ≥ 6 mitoses/10 HPF **or**
    - < 6 mitoses, but absence of immunoreactivity for neurofilament protein
- Pineoblastoma, WHO grade IV
  - Monotonous sheet-like appearance
  - Absence of large pineocytomatous rosettes
    - May show Homer Wright rosettes, Flexner-Wintersteiner rosettes
  - Small blue cells, cytological features similar to other primitive neuroectodermal tumors
  - Brisk mitotic activity
  - High Ki-67 labeling index

ANCILLARY TESTS

Immunohistochemistry

- Pineocytomatous rosettes synaptophysin (+)
- Cell cytoplasm synaptophysin, NSE (+)
- Neurofilament (+) labels in filament pattern; can also highlight ganglionic differentiation in pineocytoma, PPTID
- Neurofilament (+) cells in PPTID prognostically favorable
- Ki-67 rate
  - 3-7% for PPTID grade II
  - High for pineoblastoma

DIFFERENTIAL DIAGNOSIS

Papillary Tumor of Pineal Region

- Vague epithelial features
- Cytoplasmic vacuoles
- Immunophenotype
  - Diffusely (+) for CK8
  - Diffusely (+) 18 (CAM5.2), especially CK18 alone

Germinoma

- Germ cells with large prominent nucleoli, vacuolated cytoplasm
- Immunophenotype:
  - CD117 (C-kit) (+)
  - Placental alkaline phosphatase (+)
  - OCT4(+)
  - SALL4(+)
- Usually accompanied by nonneoplastic CD45(+) lymphocytes

Metastatic Carcinoma

- Usually immunoreactive for keratins, epithelial membrane antigen
- May have gland formation, more necrosis

Pineal Cyst

- Glial cyst wall without ependymal or epithelial lining
- Gliotic, often with Rosenthal fibers
- Nonneoplastic condition
- Often biopsies contain accompanying normal pineal gland
  - Normal pineal gland lobular
  - Normal gland intensely synaptophysin IHC(+)
  - Normal gland with interspersed GFAP(+) inter- and intralobular astrocytes
  - Ki-67 labeling low

DIAGNOSTIC CHECKLIST

Pathologic Interpretation Pearls

- Rule out papillary tumor of pineal region
- Do not mistake PPTs with large ganglion cells for germinoma
- Neurocytomas and pineocytomas nearly identical histologically; differentiate by location
- Do not mistake pleomorphism in PPTs for metastatic carcinoma

SELECTED REFERENCES

1. Edson MA et al: Outcomes After Surgery and Radiotherapy for Papillary Tumor of the Pineal Region. World Neurosurg. ePub, 2015
2. Gener MA et al: Clinical, Pathological, and Surgical Outcomes for Adult Pineoblastomas. World Neurosurg. ePub, 2015
3. Heim S et al: Papillary Tumor of the Pineal Region: A Distinct Molecular Entity. Brain Pathol. ePub, 2015
4. Kang YJ et al: Integrated genomic characterization of a pineal parenchymal tumor of intermediate differentiation. World Neurosurg. ePub, 2015
5. Maiti TK et al: Rare pathologies in the posterior third ventricular region in children: case series and review. Pediatr Neurosurg. 50(1):42-7, 2015
6. Sandip S et al: Leptomeningeal metastases in pineoblastoma. BMJ Case Rep. 2015, 2015
7. Szathmari A et al: Anatomical, molecular and pathological consideration of the circumventricular organs. Neurochirurgie. 61(2-3):90-100, 2015
8. Yu T et al: Twenty-seven cases of pineal parenchymal tumours of intermediate differentiation: mitotic count, Ki-67 labelling index and extent of resection predict prognosis. J Neurol Neurosurg Psychiatry. ePub, 2015
9. Bielle F et al: Late dural relapse of a resected and irradiated pineal parenchymal tumor of intermediate differentiation. Clin Neuropathol. 33(6):424-427, 2014
10. de Kock L et al: Germ-line and somatic DICER1 mutations in pineoblastoma. Acta Neuropathol. 128(4):583-95, 2014
11. Farnia B et al: Clinical Outcomes and Patterns of Failure in Pineoblastoma: A 30-Year, Single-Institution Retrospective Review. World Neurosurg. 82(6):1232-1241, 2014
12. Goschzik T et al: PTEN mutations and activation of the PI3K/Akt/mTOR signaling pathway in papillary tumors of the pineal region. J Neuropathol Exp Neurol. 73(8):747-51, 2014
13. Ito T et al: Clinicopathologic study of pineal parenchymal tumors of intermediate differentiation. World Neurosurg. 81(5-6):783-9, 2014
14. Jouvet A et al: Pineal parenchymal tumours and pineal cysts. Neurochirurgie. ePub, 2014
15. Murro D et al: Cytologic features of the normal pineal gland on squash preparations. Diagn Cytopathol. 42(11):939-43, 2014
16. Sasani M et al: An unusual location for a choroid plexus papilloma: the pineal region. Childs Nerv Syst. 30(7):1307-11, 2014
17. Watanabe T et al: Pineal parenchymal tumor of intermediate differentiation: Treatment outcomes of five cases. Mol Clin Oncol. 2(2):197-202, 2014
18. Sabbaghian N et al: Germline DICER1 mutation and associated loss of heterozygosity in a pineoblastoma. J Med Genet. 49(7):417-9, 2012
19. Han SJ et al: Pathology of pineal parenchymal tumors. Neurosurg Clin N Am. 22(3):335-40, vii, 2011
20. Dahiya S et al: Pineal tumors. Adv Anat Pathol. 17(6):419-27, 2010
21. Fèvre-Montange M et al: Histopathology of tumors of the pineal region. Future Oncol. 6(5):791-809, 2010
22. Fèvre-Montange M et al: Pineocytoma and pineal parenchymal tumors of intermediate differentiation presenting cytologic pleomorphism: a multicenter study. Brain Pathol. 18(3):354-9, 2008
23. Jouvet A et al: Pineal parenchymal tumors: a correlation of histological features with prognosis in 66 cases. Brain Pathol. 10(1):49-60, 2000
24. Oller-Daurella L et al: Partial epilepsy with seizures appearing in the first three years of life. Epilepsia. 30(6):820-6, 1989

Rosettes Lack Central Vessel

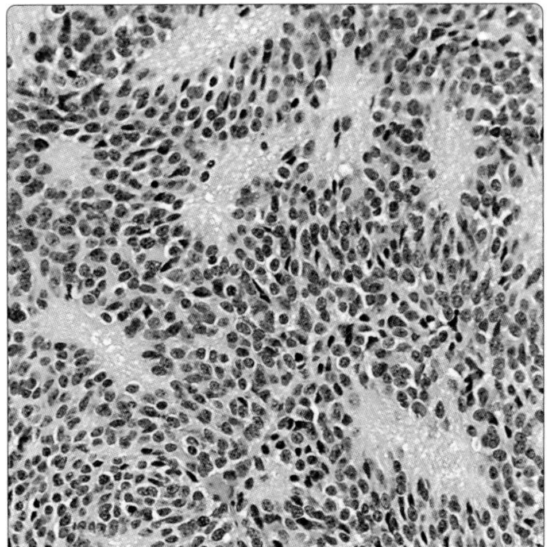

Rosettes, Homer Wright-Like

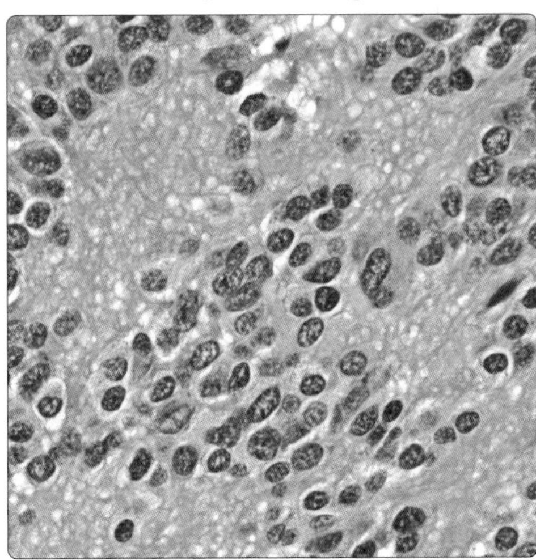

(Left) *Pineocytomatous rosettes are often large, round to oval, and finely fibrillar. Unlike perivascular pseudorosettes in lesions such as ependymoma, there is no centrally placed vessel.* **(Right)** *Rosettes in pineocytoma may approach the smaller size of the Homer Wright type (the latter being typical of neuroblastic tumors, including pineoblastoma).*

Pineocytoma, Lobularity

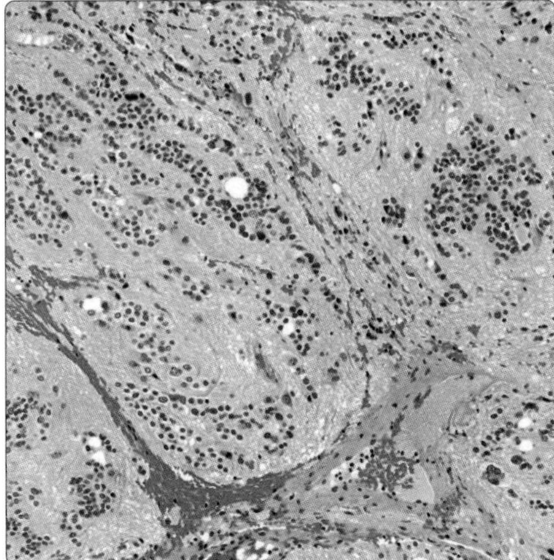

Pineocytoma, Neuronal Differentiation

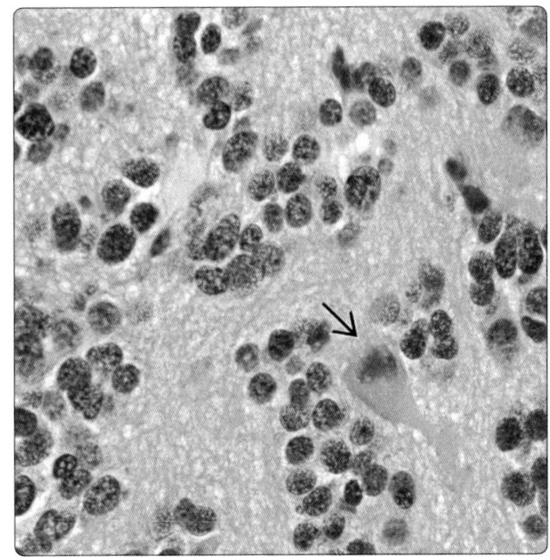

(Left) *Some pineocytomas are lobulated. Note the extensive neurocytic differentiation with abundant eosinophilic anuclear areas. These are immunoreactive for synaptophysin, and, unlike ependymoma, negative for GFAP.* **(Right)** *Pineocytomas are composed of a monotonous population of cells with stippled nuclear chromatin, scant cytoplasm, and near absent mitotic activity. Pineocytomas may contain prognostically insignificant neurons ➙ with varying degrees of maturation.*

Prognostically Insignificant Pleomorphism

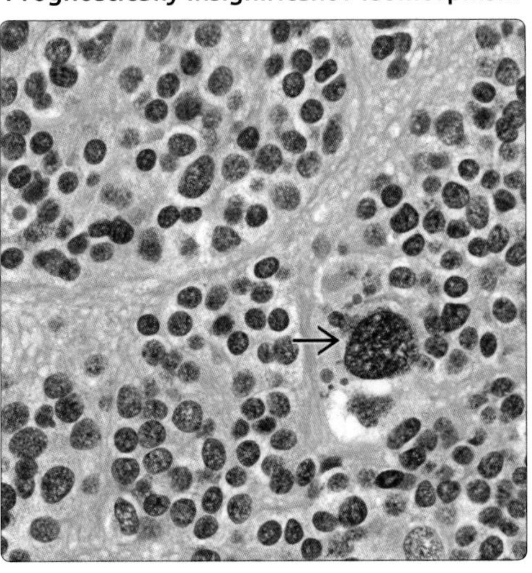

Concentric Calcification

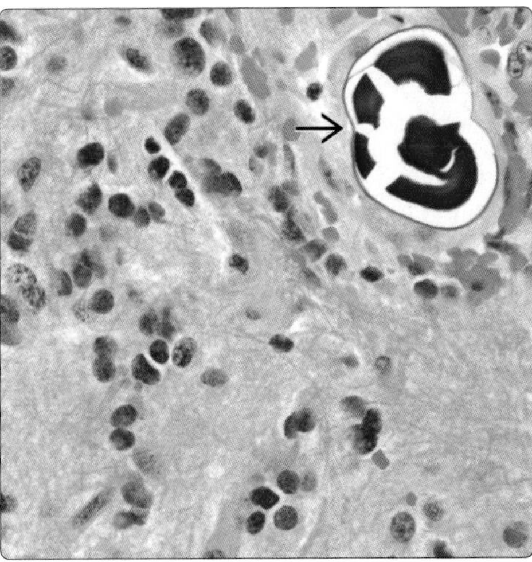

(Left) *Nuclear enlargement and pleomorphism ➙ in rosette-forming pineocytomas should not be misconstrued as evidence of anaplasia. Prognosis is not affected by this feature in either pineocytoma or PPTID.* **(Right)** *Pineocytomas may contain calcifications ➙, either microscopically or on neuroimaging. This does not affect prognosis.*

(Left) *Pineocytomas (as well as PPTIDs) are diffusely and intensely immunoreactive for synaptophysin, both within rosettes and individual cell cytoplasm. As is typical, immunoreactivity is granular.* **(Right)** *Antineurofilament protein immunostain labels in a filament-like pattern are shown. There is nonimmunoreactivity of the paranuclear cell cytoplasm. Note the large immunoreactive neuron ⇨.*

Granular Synaptophysin

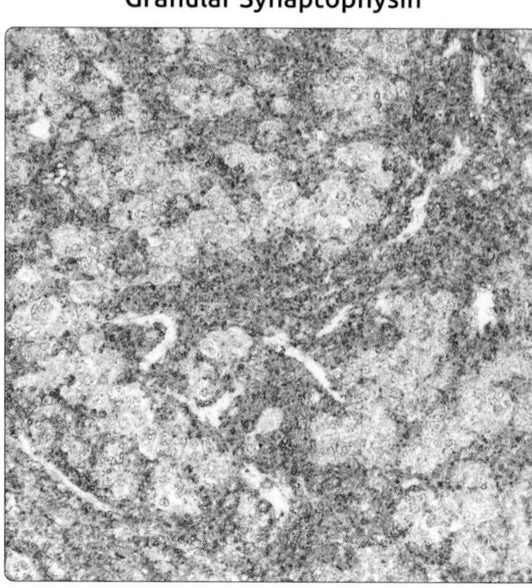

Neuronal Differentiation, Neurofilament Protein

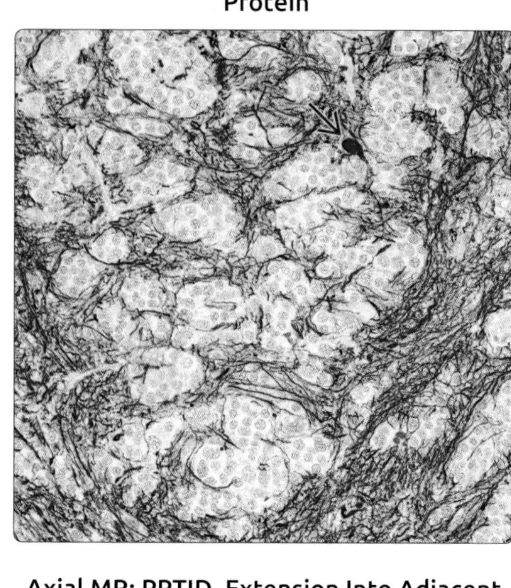

(Left) *Pineocytomas are GFAP(-) but may show reactive GFAP(+) reactive astrocytic cell processes at their perimeter.* **(Right)** *Axial T2WI MR of a PPTID in a 57-year-old woman shows an inhomogeneous, iso-/mildly hyperintense pineal mass ⇨ that contains some cystic foci. The mass appears relatively well demarcated but focally invades the right thalamus ⇨. Extension into adjacent structures is more typical of PPTID than pineocytoma.*

Reactive Astrocytes at Periphery

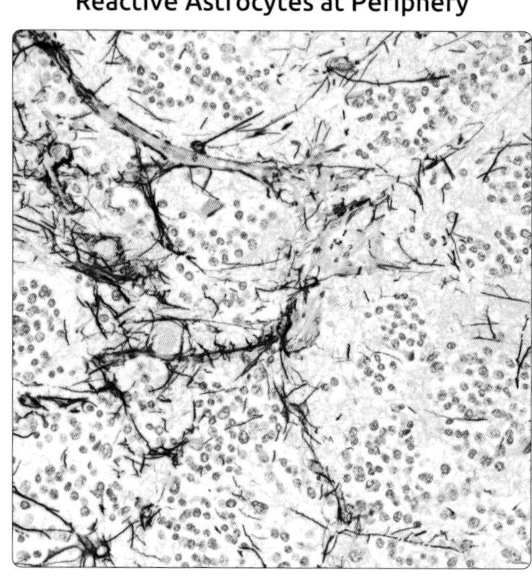

Axial MR: PPTID, Extension Into Adjacent Structures

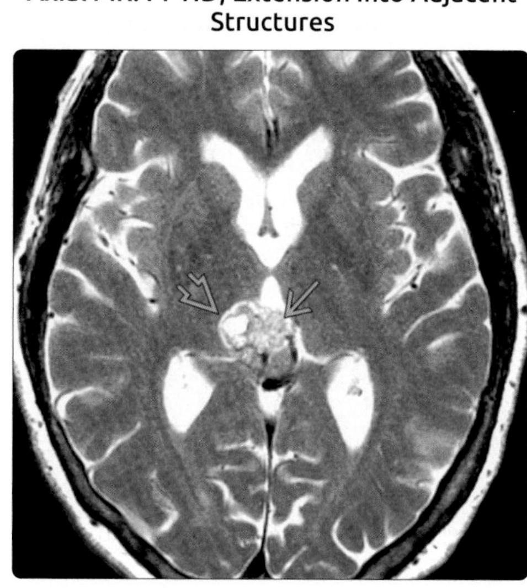

(Left) *Sagittal MR, with contrast, shows a pineal region mass ➡ that proved to be a PPTID. Neuroimaging features cannot confidently distinguish the type, or even grade, of a pineal region tumor.* **(Right)** *PPTID with a diffuse architectural pattern shows patternless sheets of monotonous, medium-sized cells. Note the absence of pineocytomatous rosettes.*

Sagittal MR: PPTID

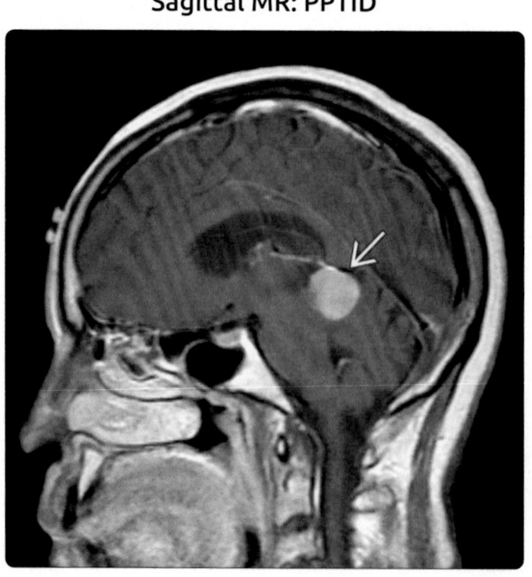

PPTID, Diffuse Architecture

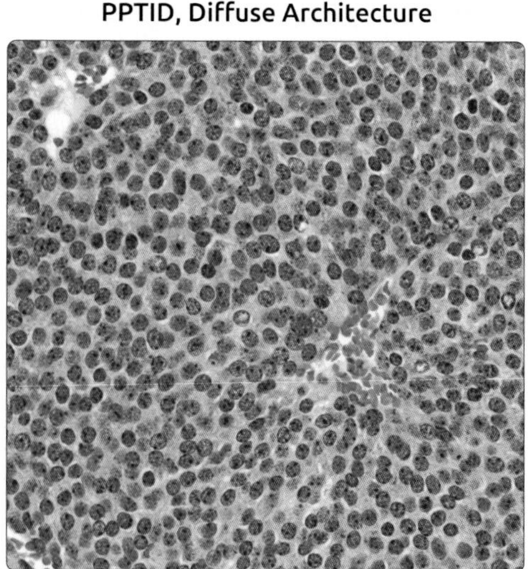

PPTID, Lobular Architecture

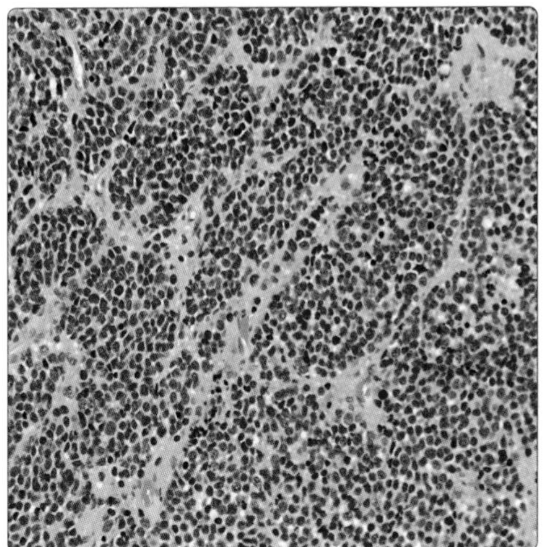

PPTID, Mitoses

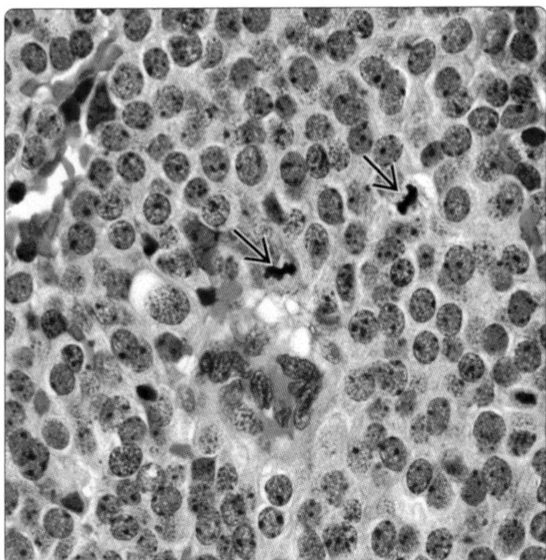

(Left) *PPTIDs show several patterns, including lobular architecture, as in this case. Note the moderate to high cellularity and absence of pineocytomatous rosettes.* **(Right)** *This PPTID with a diffuse pattern shows mitotic figures ⇒ in numbers > 6 per 10 HPF. The PPTID showed scattered cells with immunoreactivity to neurofilament protein, but with this degree of mitotic activity, the neoplasm met criteria for grade III.*

PPTID, Pleomorphism

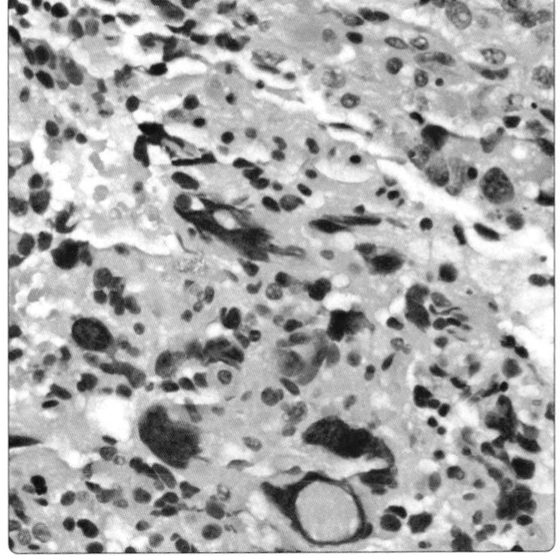

PPTID, NFP

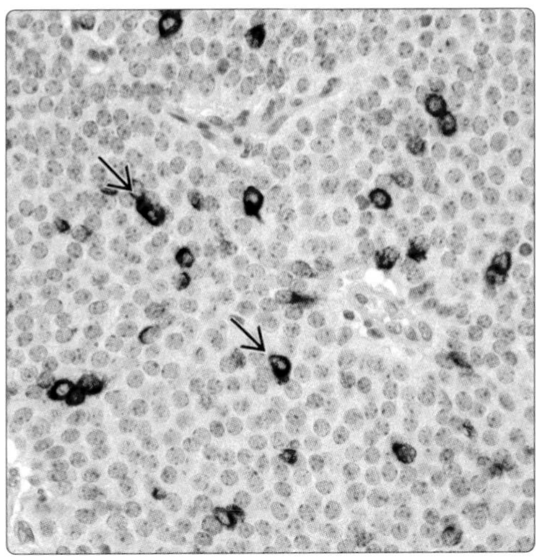

(Left) *This PPTID showed extreme cytological atypia but very little mitotic activity, diffuse architecture, and low Ki-67 labeling. The pleomorphism does not impart a higher grade to PPTID and does not adversely affect prognosis.* **(Right)** *PPTID with diffuse architectural pattern shows scattered smaller-sized cells with antineurofilament immunoreactivity ⇒ but also had significantly increased mitotic activity. It met criteria for grade III.*

PPTID, Ganglionic Differentiation

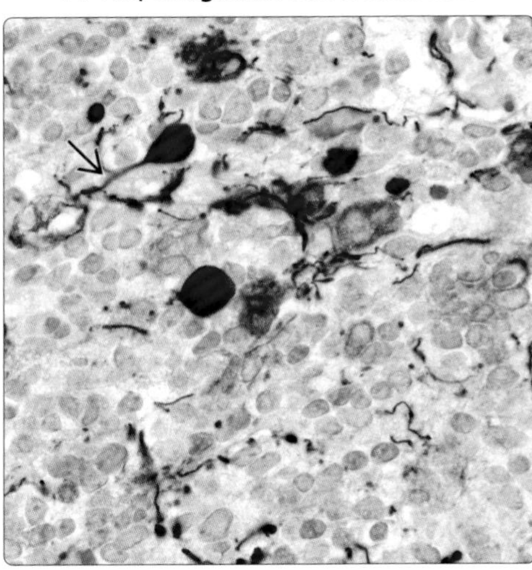

PPTID, NSE

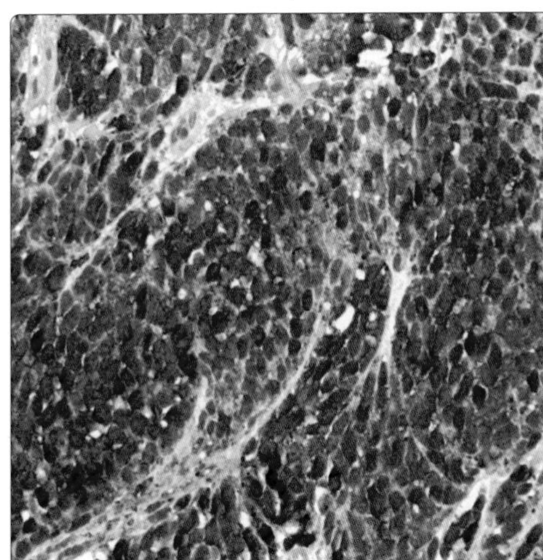

(Left) *This PPTID shows extensive ganglionic differentiation by antineurofilament protein immunostaining, with well-developed cell processes ⇒.* **(Right)** *PPTID show strong diffuse cytoplasmic immunoreactivity for neuron-specific enolase.*

(Left) *Note the negatively immunostained blood vessels in this synaptophysin-immunopositive PPTID.* **(Right)** *This PPTID manifests the least frequent pattern, with biphasic, admixed better differentiated pineal parenchymal tumor cells ⇨ and pineoblastoma ➡.*

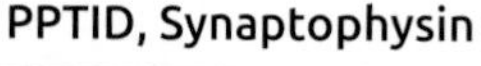

PPTID, Synaptophysin

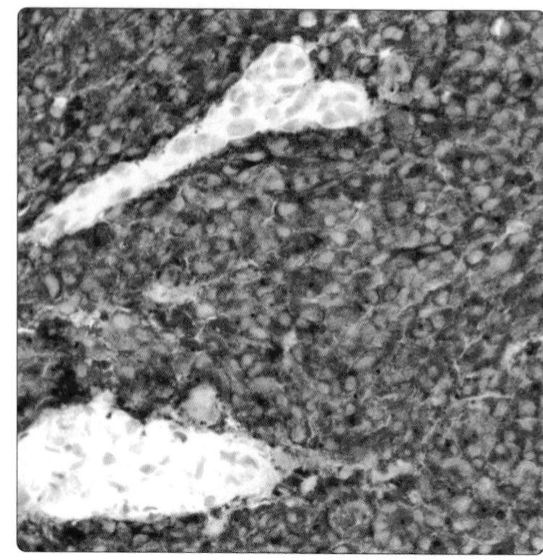

Biphasic Pattern

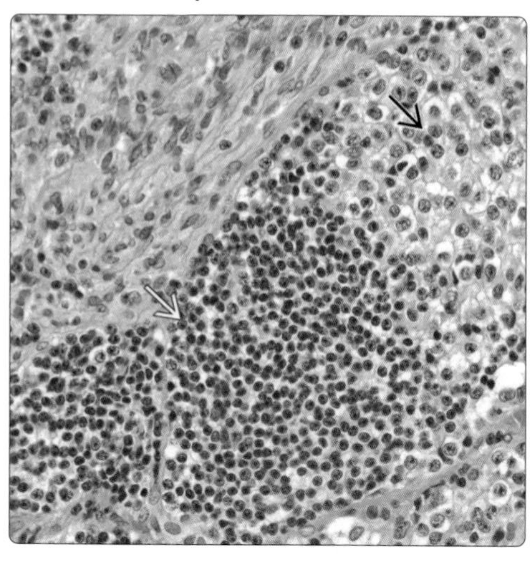

(Left) *Sagittal graphic shows a large, heterogeneous pineal mass with areas of hemorrhage and necrosis. Note the compression of adjacent structures, hydrocephalus, and diffuse CSF seeding ⇨, all typical of pineoblastoma.* **(Right)** *Sagittal T1WI MR of a pineoblastoma ⇨ shows its position underneath the splenium, elevation of the internal cerebral veins, and compression of the tectal plate. Note the moderate hydrocephalus.*

Pineoblastoma With CSF Seeding

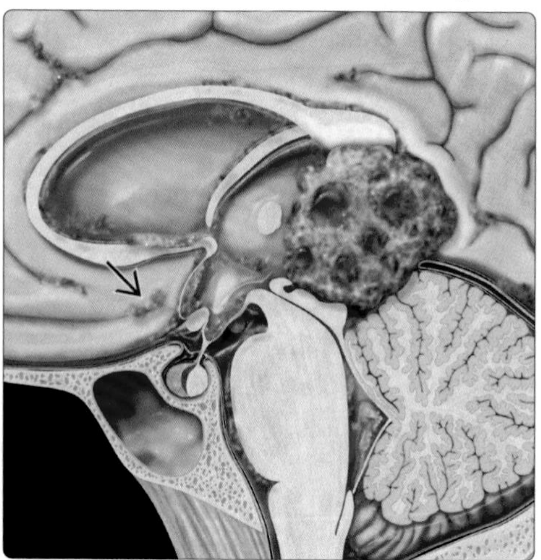

Sagittal MR: Pineoblastoma, Hydrocephalus

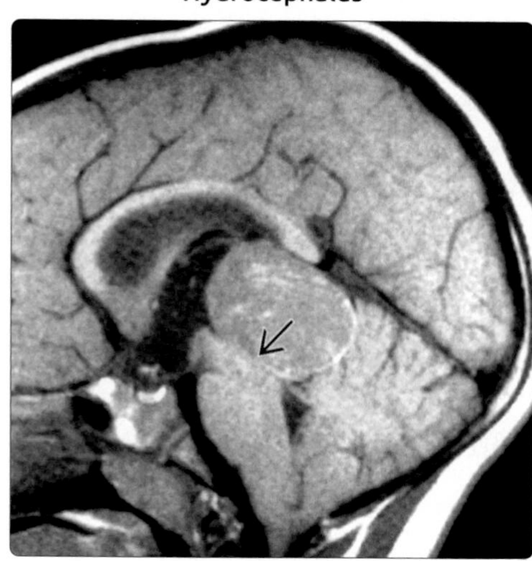

(Left) *Pineoblastoma shows small round blue cell appearance and scattered mitotic figures ⇨. As is typical with small round blue cell tumors, while mitotic activity is brisk, often the number of mitotic figures that can be confidently identified on H&E is less than the number of cells revealed to be in cell cycle by Ki-67. Note the Homer Wright rosettes ➡.* **(Right)** *Pineoblastoma consists of a monotonous population of densely packed cells with round to mildly irregular nuclei, stippled chromatin, and scant cytoplasm.*

Homer Wright Rosettes

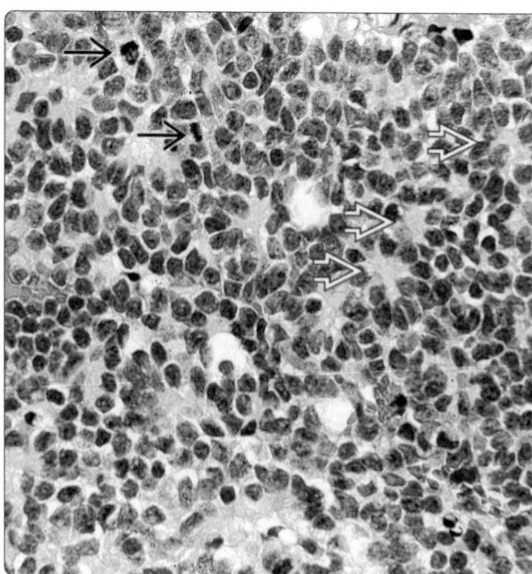

Pineoblastoma, Stippled Chromatin

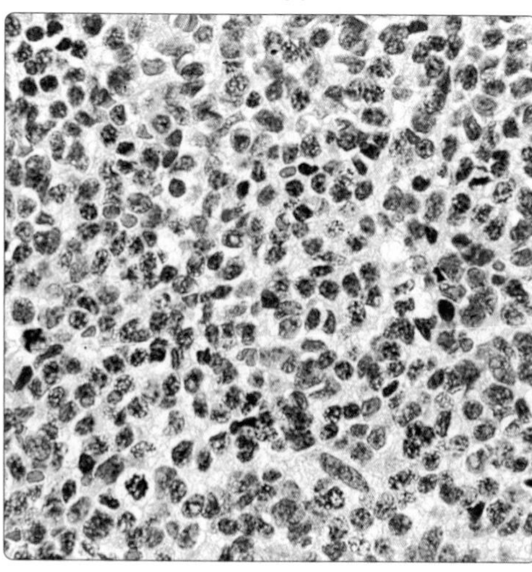

Pineoblastoma, Anaplasia

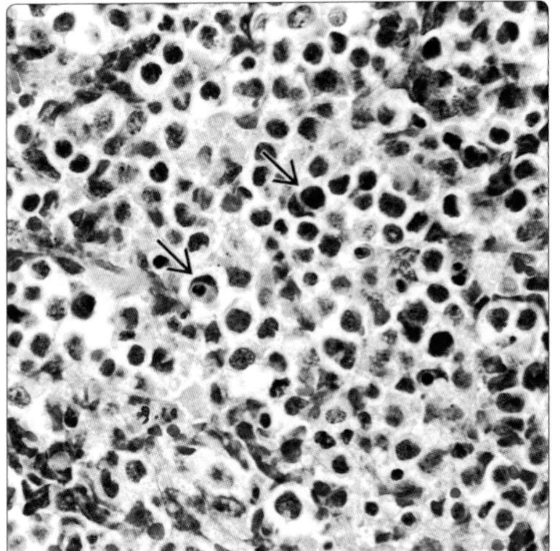

Apoptotic Cells

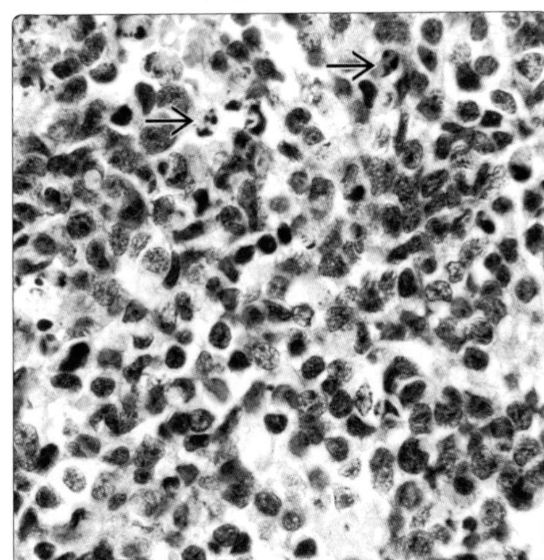

(Left) *Pineoblastomas occasionally have features of anaplasia, similar to medulloblastoma. These include large cell size, cell-cell wrapping ➙, and frequent apoptosis. Nuclear molding is also common.* **(Right)** *Pineoblastoma with anaplastic features similar to those seen in medulloblastoma, including apoptotic cells ➙, is shown.*

Pineoblastoma, High Ki-67

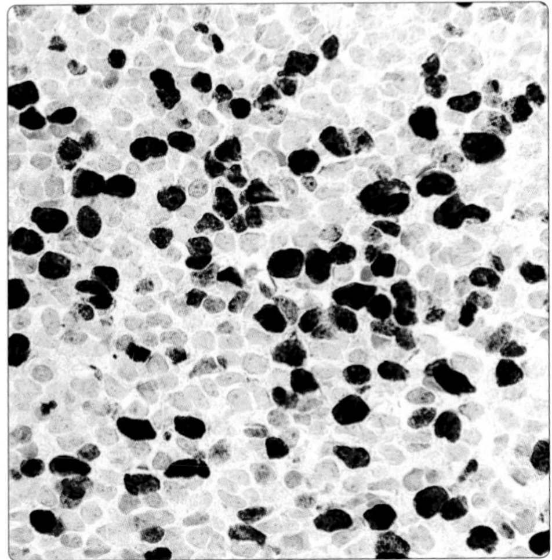

Smear, Pineoblastoma

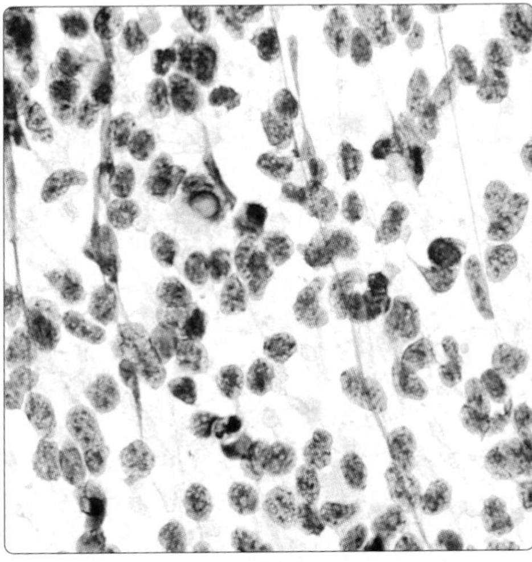

(Left) *Pineoblastomas (similar to all small, blue, undifferentiated tumors) have a high cell cycle labeling rate, as shown here on Ki-67 immunostaining.* **(Right)** *Smear of hypercellular, cytologically monotonous pineoblastoma is shown.*

Smear, Pineoblastoma

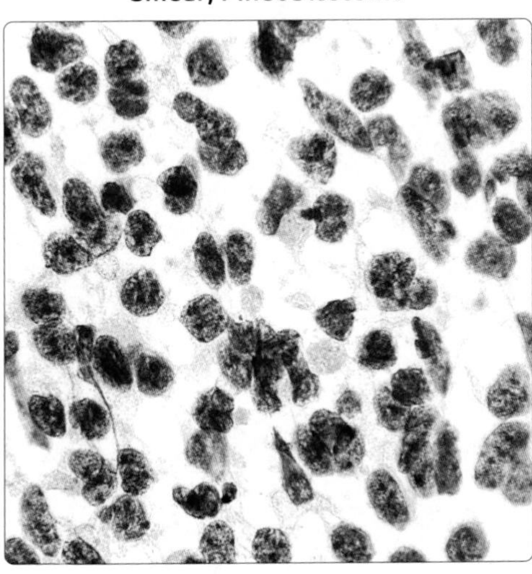

MR Does Not Distinguish Pineal Tumor Types

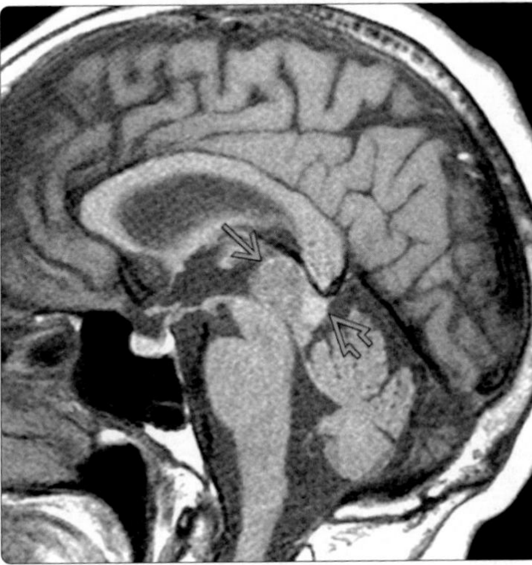

(Left) *Intraoperative smear preparation of a pineoblastoma illustrates the nuclear monotony, scant cytoplasm, and stippled chromatin pattern typical of this high-grade tumor.* **(Right)** *Sagittal T1WI MR in a 57-year-old woman with headaches and visual problems and an outside MR interpreted as germinoma is shown. Repeat imaging shows a slightly hypointense pineal mass ➙ that compresses and invades the tectal plate ➙.*

Papillary Tumor of the Pineal Region

KEY FACTS

TERMINOLOGY

- Subtly epithelial neoplasm of pineal region

CLINICAL ISSUES

- Signs and symptoms of CSF flow obstruction
- Prognosis guarded
- Frequent local recurrence &/or cerebrospinal fluid dissemination

IMAGING

- Heterogeneously enhancing mass in pineal region

MICROSCOPIC

- Epithelial surfaces, e.g., tubules
- Perivascular rosettes with distinct cell border
- Pseudopapillae
- Mitoses, scant to moderate
- Necrosis in some cases
- Intracytoplasmic vacuoles

ANCILLARY TESTS

- CAM5.2 (CK8/18) (+)
- CK18 more positive when done alone
- Losses: Chromosomes 3, 10, and 22q
- Gains: Chromosomes 4, 5, 8p, 9, and 12
- 2 global methylation subgroups: Group 1 (better progression-free survival) and group 2 (higher overall methylation)

TOP DIFFERENTIAL DIAGNOSES

- Normal pineal
- Ependymoma
- Choroid plexus papilloma
- Pineal parenchymal tumors
- Metastatic carcinoma and melanoma
- Germinoma

(Left) *The brightly enhancing, well-circumscribed lesion with an epicenter in the pineal region* ➙ *is prone to obstruct the flow of cerebrospinal fluid and produce hydrocephalus.* **(Right)** *Subtle epithelial features help distinguish the lesion from pineal parenchymal tumors.*

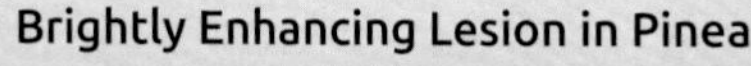
Brightly Enhancing Lesion in Pineal

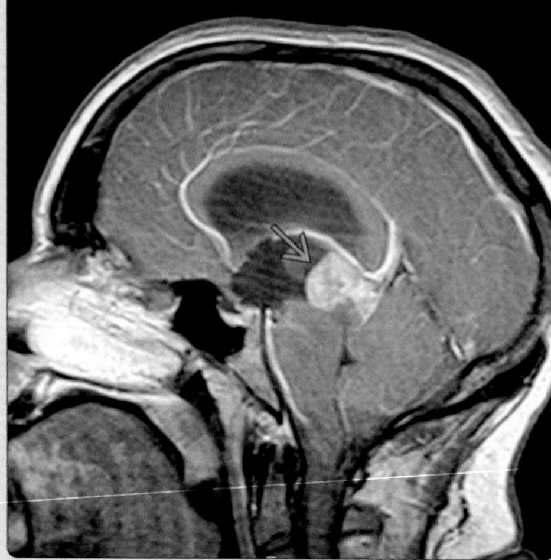

Subtle Epithelial Features

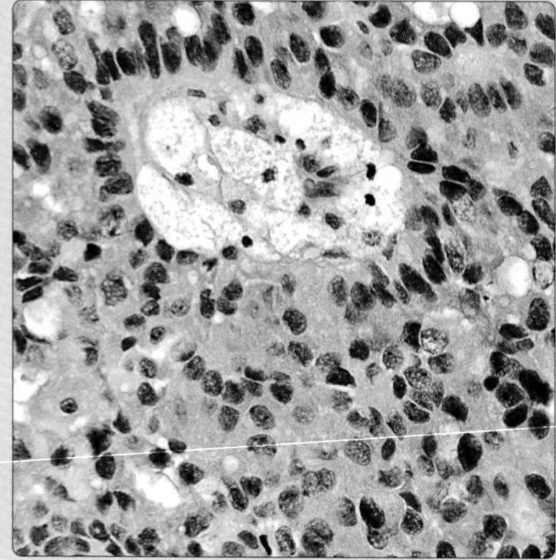

(Left) *Compact architecture and sharp cell borders are diagnostic clues in pineal region tumors.* **(Right)** *Small canals or tubules are not uncommon.*

Compact Architecture

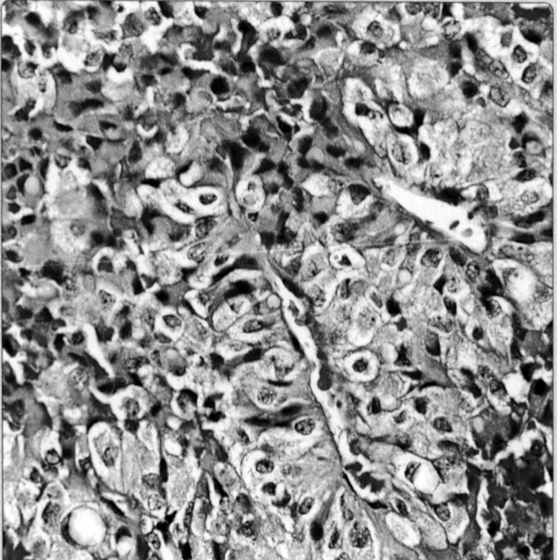

Small Tubule

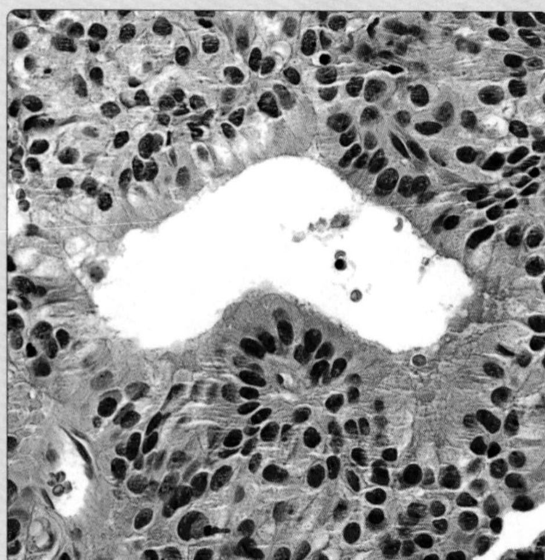

TERMINOLOGY

Definitions

- Subtly epithelial neoplasm of pineal region; grading criteria not well defined

ETIOLOGY/PATHOGENESIS

Cytogenesis

- Proposed origin from subcommissural organ in posterior wall of 3rd ventricle

CLINICAL ISSUES

Epidemiology

- Age
  - Adults, rarely children

Presentation

- Results of cerebrospinal fluid (CSF) obstruction
  - Headaches, gait instability, loss of recent memory
- Impairment of upward gaze (Parinaud syndrome)

Treatment

- Surgical approaches
  - Gross total excision key prognostic factor
- Adjuvant therapy
  - Role of chemotherapy unclear
- Radiation
  - Commonly employed

Prognosis

- Guarded
- Local recurrence frequent
- CSF dissemination uncommon

IMAGING

MR Findings

- Pineal region, especially near posterior commissure
- Avid heterogeneous enhancement
- Intrinsic T1 hyperintensity in some cases

MICROSCOPIC

Histologic Features

- Solid, compact architecture
- Subtly epithelial with pseudopapillae, perivascular rosettes with distinct cell borders, epithelial surfaces
- Intracytoplasmic vacuoles
- Mitoses, scant to moderate
- Hyalinized vessels and necrosis in some cases

ANCILLARY TESTS

Cytology

- Tissue fragments and few individual cells
- Plump oval nuclei
- Cytoplasm with short, thick processes
- Nuclear grooves in some cells

Immunohistochemistry

- CAM5.2 (CK8/18) (+)
  - CK18 more positive when done alone than when part of CAM5.2
- S100(+)
- GFAP(-)
- Synaptophysin, EMA (+/-)

Genetic Testing

- Losses: Chromosomes 3, 10, and 22q
- Gains: Chromosomes 4, 5, 8p, 9, and 12
- 2 global methylation subgroups: Group 1 (better progression-free survival) and group 2 (higher overall methylation)
- *SPDEF* (known to be expressed in rodent subcommissural organ) ↑

Electron Microscopy

- Epithelial features
  - Microvilli, small lumina
  - Zipper-like intermediate junctions (zonulae adherences)
  - Dense core granules, scant

DIFFERENTIAL DIAGNOSIS

Normal Pineal

- Lobular architecture, less epithelial cytology, no mitoses, calcifications (brain sand)
- Synaptophysin diffusely (+), GFAP(+) in scant intralobular cells
- CAM5.2(-)
- Very low Ki-67 index

Ependymoma

- Prominent fibrillated perivascular pseudorosettes
- GFAP(+), EMA(+) in microlumina (dot-like, luminal) or membrane pattern

Choroid Plexus Papilloma

- Overtly epithelial with true papillae
- Keratin (+), synaptophysin [(+) in most cases]
- Calcifications (occasional)

Pineal Parenchymal Tumors

- No epithelial differentiation
- Large, pineocytomatous rosettes (pineocytoma)
- Synaptophysin diffusely (+)

Metastatic Carcinoma and Melanoma

- Carcinoma
  - Generally older patients, more anaplastic
  - Often EMA(+)
- Melanoma
  - SOX10, HMB-45, Melan-A, and tyrosinase all (+)

Germinoma

- Large, dyscohesive cells with prominent nucleoli

SELECTED REFERENCES

1. Heim S et al: Papillary tumor of the pineal region: a distinct molecular entity. Brain Pathol. ePub, 2015
2. Fèvre-Montange M et al: Prognosis and histopathologic features in papillary tumors of the pineal region: a retrospective multicenter study of 31 cases. J Neuropathol Exp Neurol. 65(10):1004-11, 2006
3. Jouvet A et al: Papillary tumor of the pineal region. Am J Surg Pathol. 27(4):505-12, 2003

Overt Epithelial Features

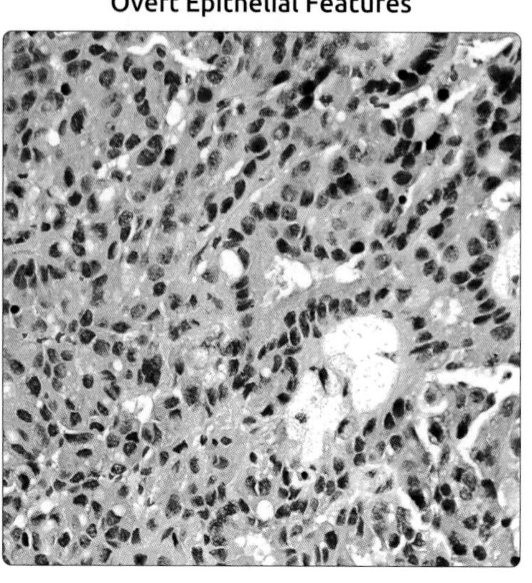

Pseudopapillae

(Left) *Some tumors of the pineal region are overtly epithelial, at least focally.* **(Right)** *Tissue dehiscence produces pseudopapillae; the latter being overall more common than those of the true type.*

Intracytoplasmic Vacuoles

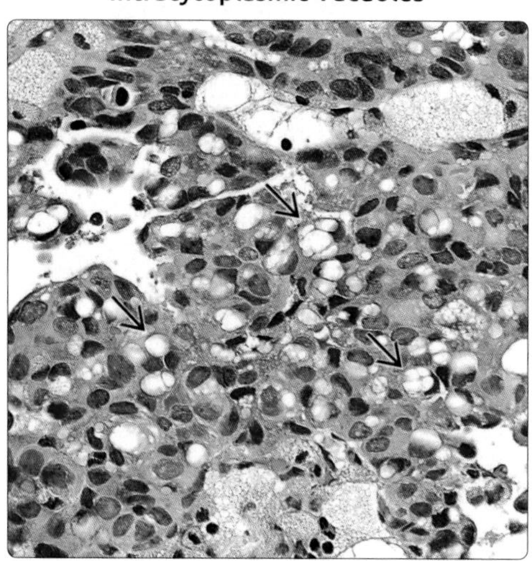

Columnar Perivascular Cells

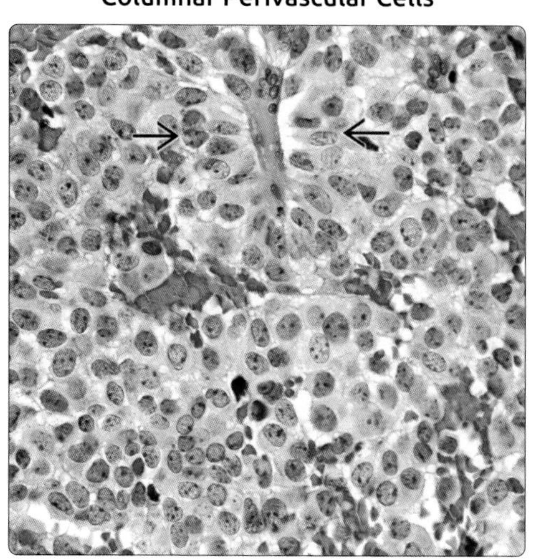

(Left) *Intracytoplasmic vacuoles* → *are common in this neoplasm with vague epithelial features.* **(Right)** *Only a hint of epithelial differentiation may be present, usually in the form of short, columnar perivascular cells with distinct cell borders* →.

Vaguely Lobular Architecture

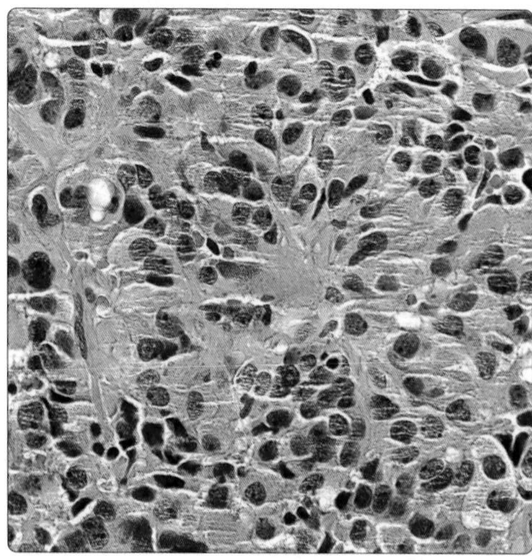

Solid Areas

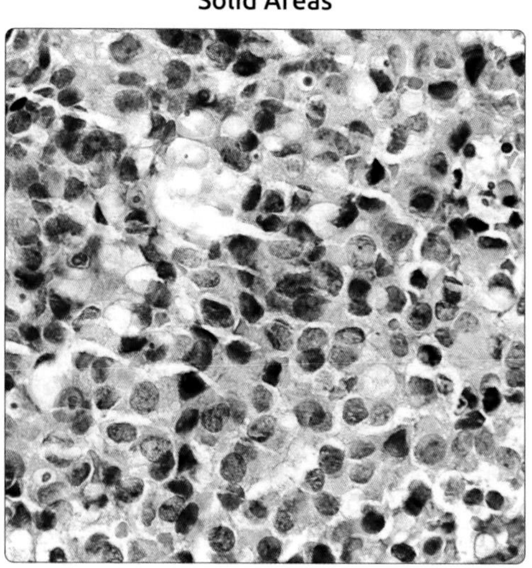

(Left) *A vaguely lobular architecture creates a similarity to normal pineal gland.* **(Right)** *Solid areas may resemble germinoma, normal pineal, pineal parenchymal tumors, and even metastatic carcinoma or melanoma.*

Distinct Cell Borders

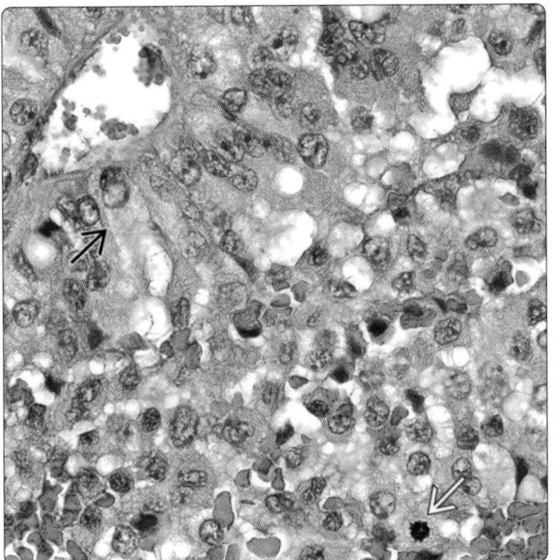

Necrosis

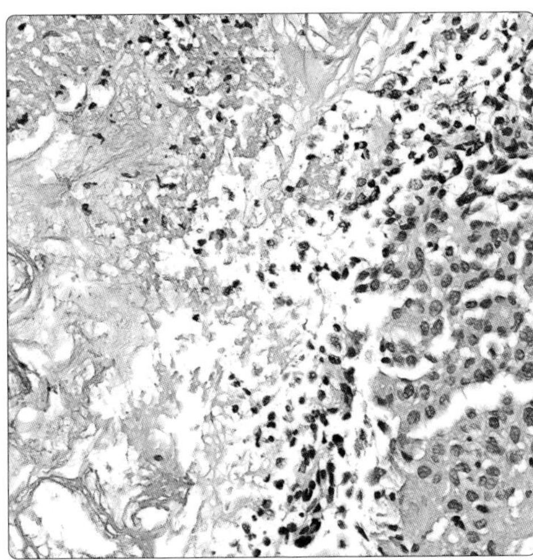

(Left) *Distinct cell borders* ⇨*, especially in perivascular formations, lend a distinctive, yet often subtle, epithelial quality. Mitoses may be present* ➡. **(Right)** *Necrosis is not uncommon in papillary tumors of the pineal region.*

Orientation to Vessel

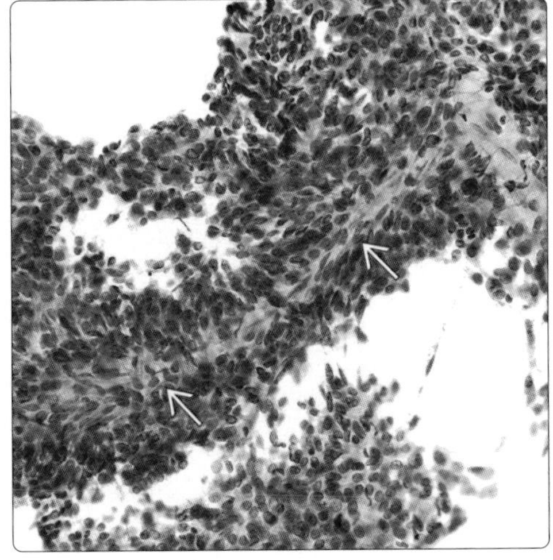

Plump Nuclei

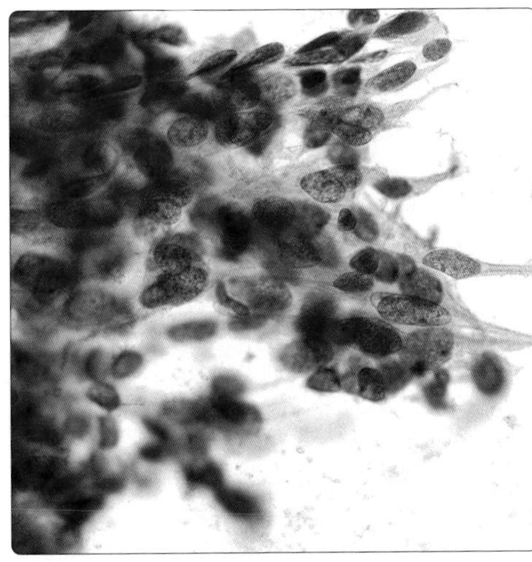

(Left) *Orientation to a vessel* ➡ *creates a cytological equivalent to the perivascular formations seen in tissue sections.* **(Right)** *Plump nuclei are somewhat elongated. Cytoplasm is extended into processes that are shorter and thicker than those of ependymoma.*

CAM5.2 Immunopositivity

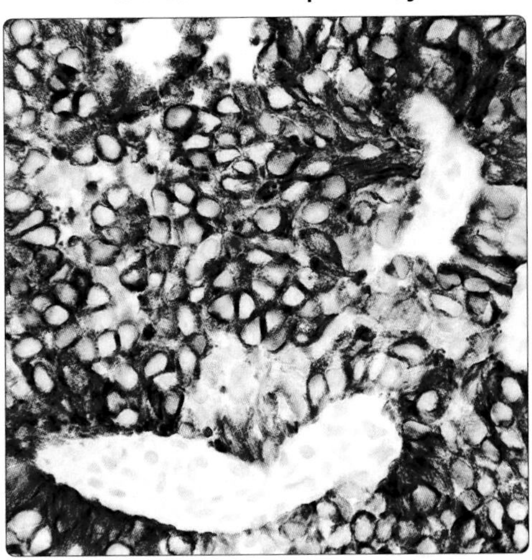

Ki-67 Labeling Index

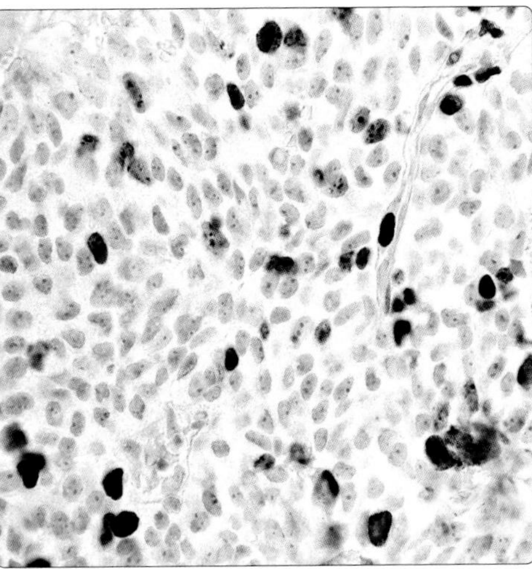

(Left) *Papillary tumors of the pineal region are diffusely immunopositive for CAM5.2 (CK8/18), and even more so when CK18 is used alone.* **(Right)** *While sometimes giving the impression of a low-grade "benign" tumor, the Ki-67 rate is often brisk.*

Pineal Anlage Tumor

KEY FACTS

TERMINOLOGY
- Malignant pineal region tumor with both neuroepithelial and ectomesenchymal differentiation
- Overlap in terminology with melanotic neurectodermal tumor of infancy (melanotic progonoma)

CLINICAL ISSUES
- Very rare
- Mostly children, usually infants
- Aggressive, but full understanding of biologic behavior and appropriate treatment is incomplete due to rarity of lesion

IMAGING
- Solid and cystic
- Contrast enhancing
- Obstructive hydrocephalus

MACROSCOPIC
- Firm, often cystic, focally black

MICROSCOPIC
- Neuroepithelial differentiation
- Epithelium, often pigmented
- Small cell tissue potentially with Homer Wright or Flexner-Wintersteiner rosettes
- Ectomesenchymal differentiation
  - Cartilage, striated muscle, etc.

TOP DIFFERENTIAL DIAGNOSES
- Teratoma
- Medulloblastoma with myoblastic &/or melanotic differentiation
- Pineal parenchymal tumor
- Melanotic neurectodermal tumor of infancy (melanotic progonoma)

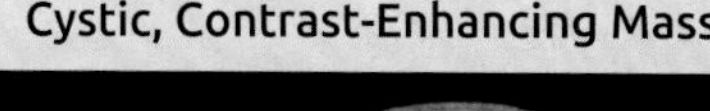

Cystic, Contrast-Enhancing Mass

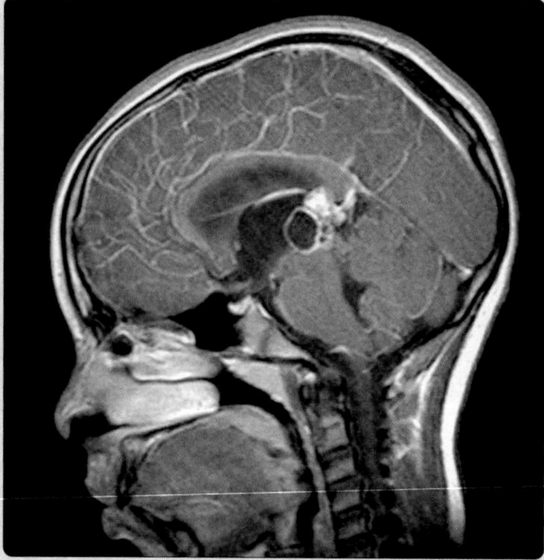

Mesenchymal Differentiation

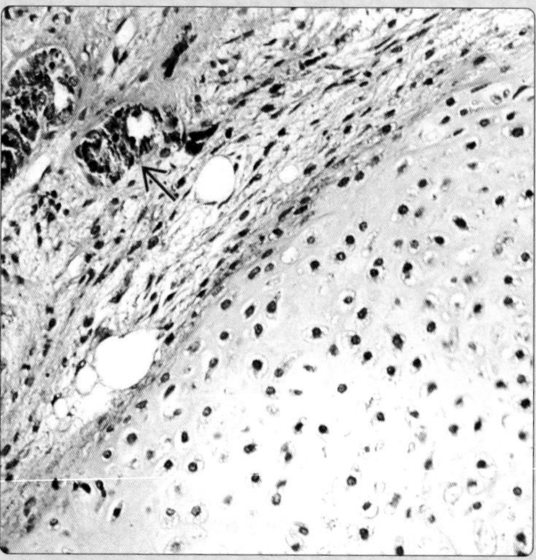

(Left) *Pineal anlage tumors are cystic, contrast-enhancing masses positioned so as to impede the flow of cerebrospinal fluid. Patients are usually infants.* **(Right)** *Mesenchymal differentiation, cartilage in this case, in combination with pigmented epithelium →, introduces the possibilities of pineal anlage tumor and teratoma.*

Multinodularity

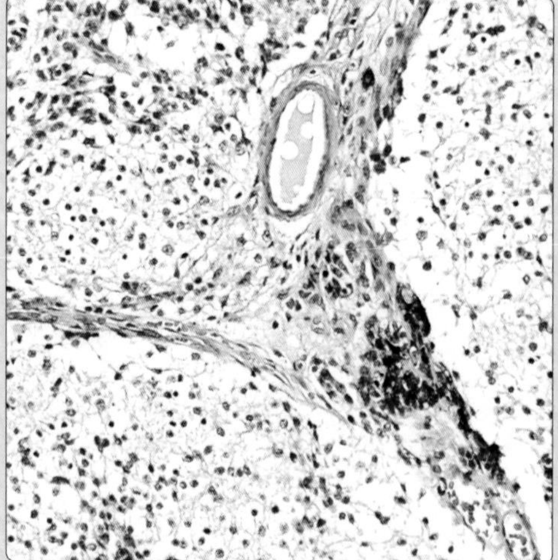

Circumscribed Areas of Neuropil

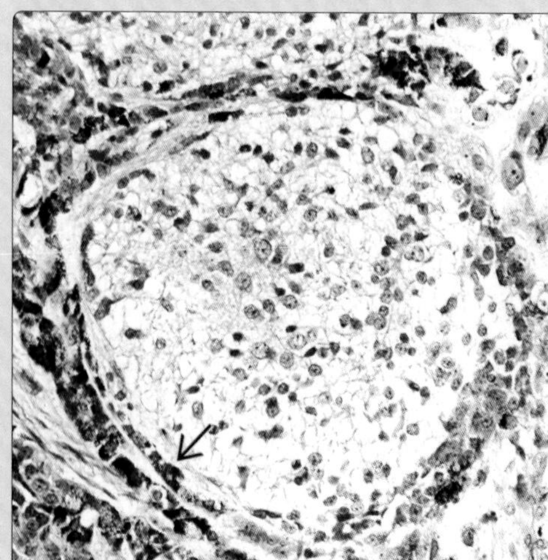

(Left) *Multinodularity may be present in a subset of pineal anlage tumors.* **(Right)** *Distinctive features of pineal anlage tumors are well-circumscribed areas of neuropil, ± small ganglion cells. Pigment epithelium → often delineates the nodules, at least in part.*

TERMINOLOGY

Definitions

- Malignant pineal region tumor with both neuroepithelial and ectomesenchymal differentiation
  - Ectomesenchyme is neural crest-derived mesoderm
- Overlap in terminology with melanotic neuroectodermal tumor of infancy (melanotic progonoma)

CLINICAL ISSUES

Epidemiology

- Incidence
  - Very rare
- Age
  - Mostly children, usually infants

Site

- Pineal region

Presentation

- Consequences of obstructive hydrocephalus
  - Macrocephaly, vomiting, obtundation, papilledema, Parinaud sign

Treatment

- No consensus given rarity of disease

Prognosis

- Poor
- Rapid local recurrence, potential for cerebrospinal fluid dissemination
- Full understanding of biologic behavior is incomplete due to rarity of this lesion

IMAGING

MR and CT Findings

- Solid and cystic
- Contrast enhancing
- Obstructive hydrocephalus

MACROSCOPIC

General Features

- Firm, often cystic, focally black

MICROSCOPIC

Histologic Features

- Neuroepithelial differentiation
  - Mature or immature CNS tissue
    - Discrete islands, ganglion cells, glia
  - Epithelium
    - Tubules, cords
    - Variably pigmented, often extensively
    - Often partially around islands of neuroblasts or more mature CNS tissue
  - Small cell component, potentially with
    - Homer Wright (neuroblastic) rosettes
    - Flexner-Wintersteiner (retinoblastomatous) rosettes
    - Mitoses
- Ectomesenchymal differentiation
  - Cartilage, striated muscle, fibrous tissue, adipose tissue
- No endodermal or cutaneous derivatives, e.g., lung, gastrointestinal tract, or skin/adnexa
- Conceptually similar in scope to normal fetal pineal gland, some species

ANCILLARY TESTS

Immunohistochemistry

- Synaptophysin (+)
  - Neuronal tissue
- GFAP(+)
  - Glial tissue
- Muscle markers
  - Desmin (+), myogenin (+)
- Ki-67
  - High in densely cellular areas, low in differentiated components
- INI1 (BAF47), retained

Electron Microscopy

- True melanosomes (i.e., not lipochrome-like neuromelanin) within pigmented epithelium

DIFFERENTIAL DIAGNOSIS

Teratoma

- Endodermal tissues, e.g., lung, gastrointestinal tract
- Choroid plexus, common
- Ependyma, medullary epithelium, and germinal matrix common
- Generally less pigmented epithelium

Medulloblastoma With Myogenic &/or Melanotic Differentiation

- Largely small cell undifferentiated tumor
- Fewer pigmented tubules, no cartilage
- No pigmented cells surrounding islands of neuroglial tissue

Pineal Parenchymal Tumor

- Monomorphous small cell lesion
- Pineocytomatous rosettes in pineocytoma

Melanotic Neurectodermal Tumor of Infancy (Melanotic Progonoma)

- Typically in bone, especially maxilla, but reported in brain, including pineal region
- No mesodermal derivatives, e.g., cartilage, muscle
- Generally benign, with low-level proliferative activity
- Overlap in terminology with pineal anlage tumor

SELECTED REFERENCES

1. Olaya JE et al: Pineal anlage tumor in a 5-month-old boy. J Neurosurg Pediatr. 5(6):636-40, 2010
2. Berns S et al: Review of pineal anlage tumor with divergent histology. Arch Pathol Lab Med. 130(8):1233-5, 2006
3. Rickert CH et al: Melanotic progonoma of the brain: a case report and review. Childs Nerv Syst. 14(8):389-93, 1998
4. Raisanen J et al: Primitive pineal tumor with retinoblastomatous and retinal/ciliary epithelial differentiation: an immunohistochemical study. J Neurooncol. 9(2):165-70, 1990
5. Schmidbauer M et al: Neuroepithelial and ectomesenchymal differentiation in a primitive pineal tumor ("pineal anlage tumor"). Clin Neuropathol. 8(1):7-10, 1989

(Left) *Areas of neuronal differentiation reminiscent of medulloblastoma nodules are delineated by cellular, tubule-forming, focally pigmented epithelium* ⇒. **(Right)** *Well-circumscribed areas of CNS tissue surrounded by tubules of pigment epithelium are distinctive features of the rare pineal anlage tumor.*

Neuronal Differentiation

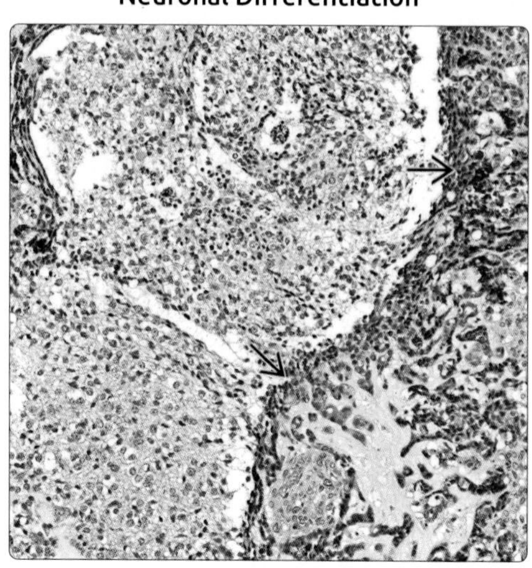

CNS Tissue

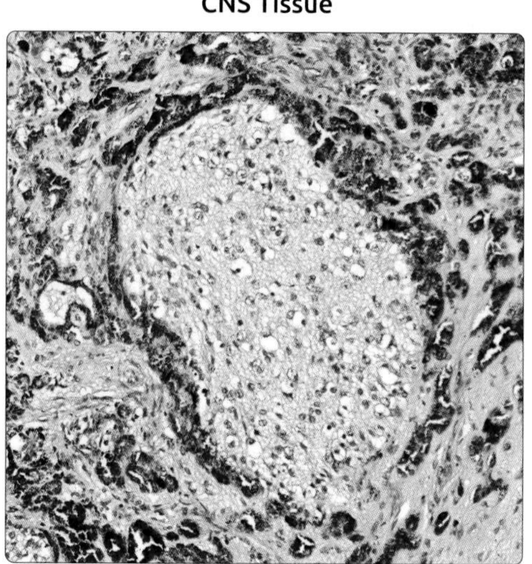

(Left) *Anastomosing cords and tubules are a distinctive feature not present in the histologically similar teratomas that frequent this region. The epithelium of the anlage tumor is variably pigmented. Little pigment is present in this area* ⇒. **(Right)** *Variably pigmented epithelium forms multiple tubules and anastomosing strands.*

Anastomosing Cords and Tubules

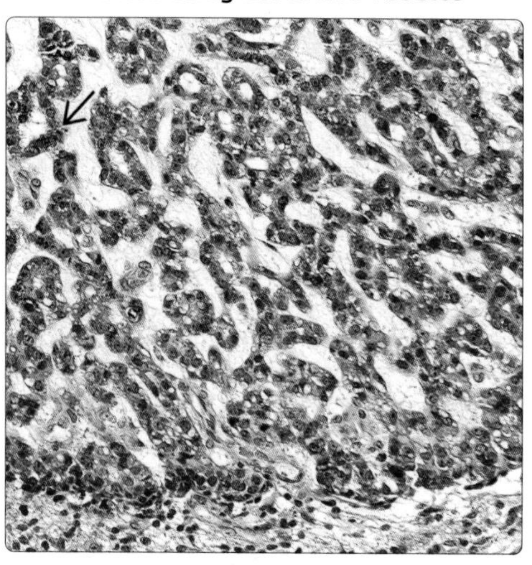

Pigmented Epithelium

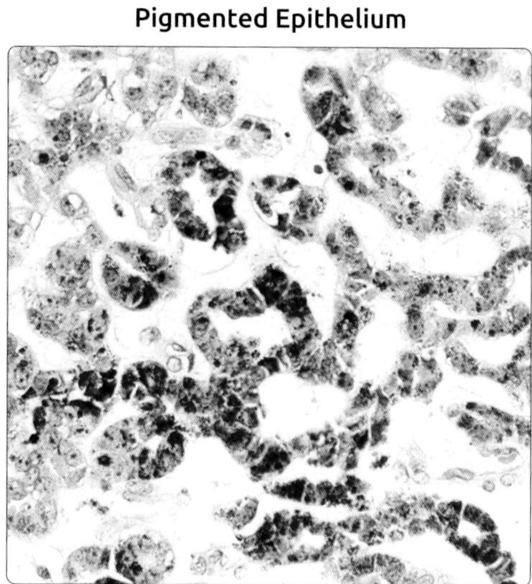

(Left) *The neuroglial element may be nondescript glioma-like tissue with only a hint of neuronal differentiation.* **(Right)** *Small ganglion cells* ⇒ *with prominent nucleoli may be present in neuroglial areas.*

Neuroglial Element

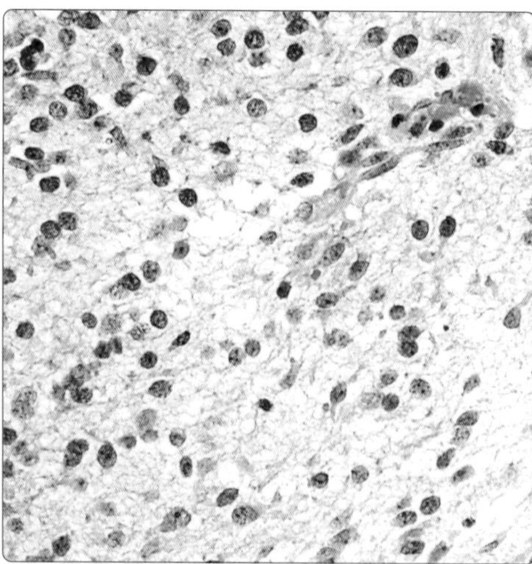

Small Ganglion Cells

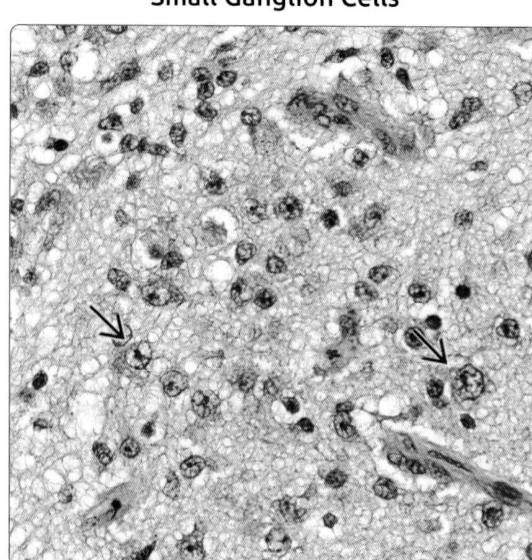

Strap-Shaped Myocytes

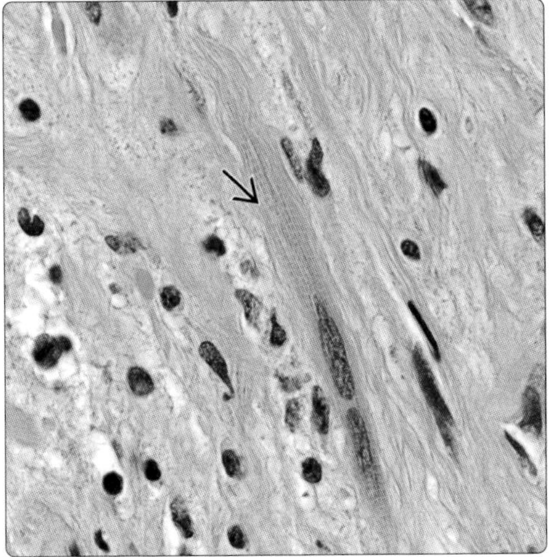

Muscle Fibers

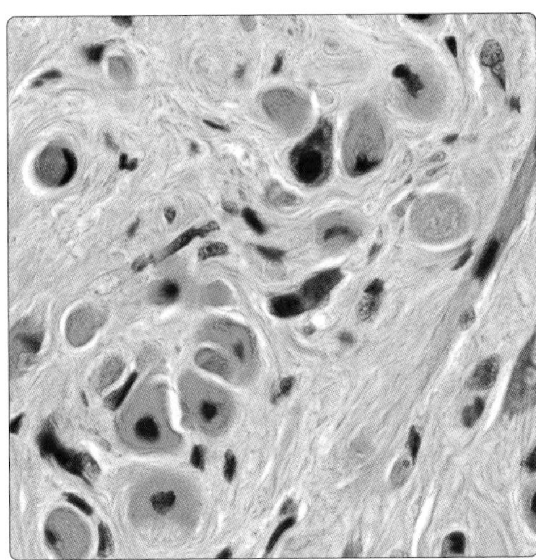

(Left) *The presence of strap-shaped myocytes with cross striations ➙ narrows the differential to teratoma and medulloblastoma with myogenic differentiation. The former is more likely to have abundant CNS tissue with embryonal components, ependyma, endodermal derivatives, and skin.* **(Right)** *Muscle fibers may not be as apparent when cut in cross section as they are when sectioned longitudinally.*

Mesenchymal Differentiation

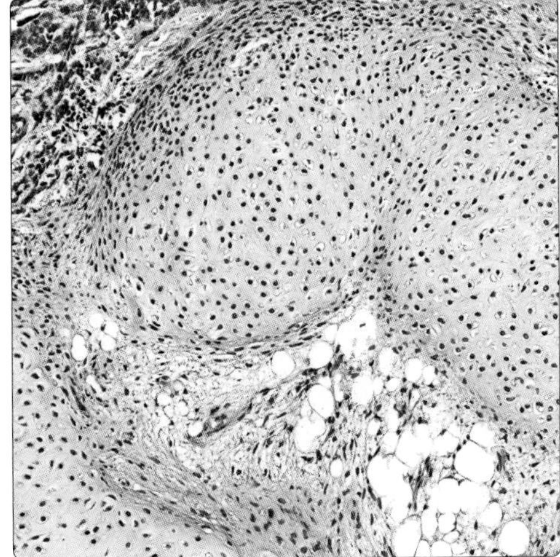

Cellular Areas

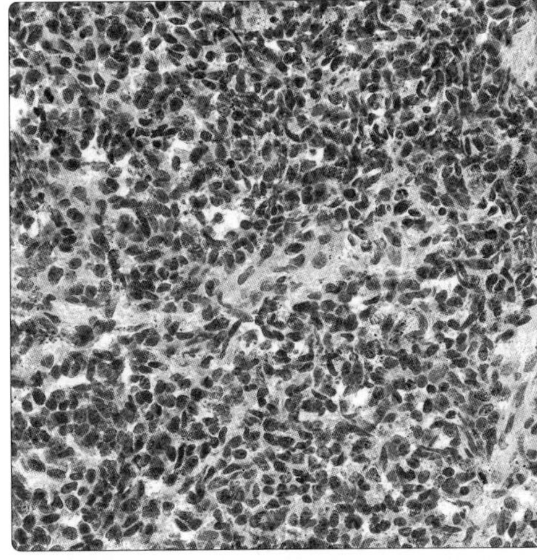

(Left) *Cartilage, and even adipose tissue in this case, are patent evidence of mesenchymal differentiation. While definitional issues remain unresolved, the presence of mesenchymal tissue has, in general, distinguished pineal anlage tumor from melanotic neurectodermal tumor of infancy (melanotic progonoma).* **(Right)** *Densely cellular embryonal-like areas are variably present.*

Islands of Neuroglial Tissue

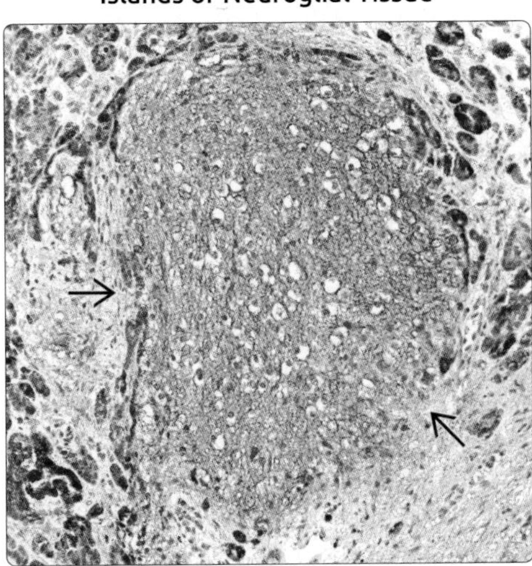

Desmin Staining

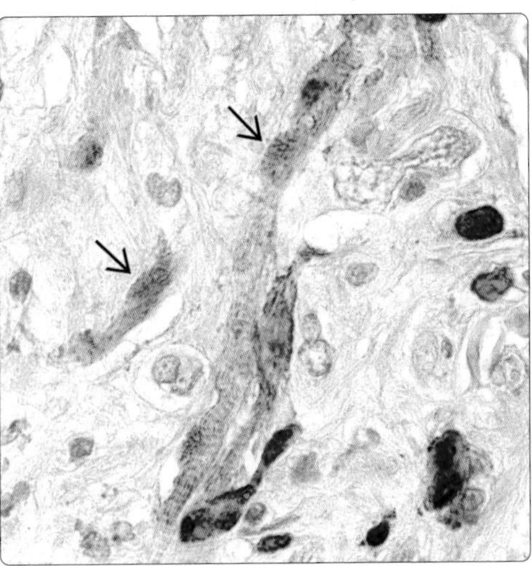

(Left) *Islands of neuroglial tissue are immunoreactive for synaptophysin ➙.* **(Right)** *Immunostaining for muscle markers such as desmin helps confirm the presence of myoid differentiation ➙.*

Medulloblastoma

KEY FACTS

TERMINOLOGY

- Small cell anaplastic embryonal tumor of cerebellum
- Unrelated to other embryonal tumors
- Unrelated to peripheral PNET (Ewing sarcoma)

ETIOLOGY/PATHOGENESIS

- Gorlin: Nodular/desmoplastic type (rare)
- Turcot type 2, APC: Classic (nonnodular) (rare)

CLINICAL ISSUES

- Prognosis overall favorable, but dependent on stage and subtype
- Overall, most favorable type is WNT subtype, which is recognized by nuclear β-catenin and monosomy 6
- Most WNT pathway subtypes of medulloblastoma are classic medulloblastomas, but most classic medulloblastomas are not WNT pathway
  - WNT is rarest molecular type and most classic medulloblastomas are not WNT but group 3 or 4

MICROSCOPIC

- Classic: ~ 70%
- Nodular/desmoplastic: ~ 15-20%
- Large cell/anaplastic: Required degree of anaplasia and percent of tumor cross-sectional area unclear, but generally severe anaplasia &/or large cell type over 50% or more of tumor area

ANCILLARY TESTS

- Pathway: Classic (nonnodular) and biphasic
- Sonic hedgehog pathway: Nodular/desmoplastic

DIAGNOSTIC CHECKLIST

- Identification of molecular pathways (e.g., WNT, Shh) increasingly used in classification
- Separating groups 3 and 4 (lumped under non-Shh/non-WNT) is not as important for practical purposes, currently difficult to do with immunohistochemistry

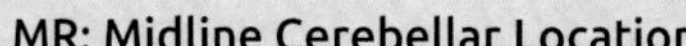

MR: Midline Cerebellar Location

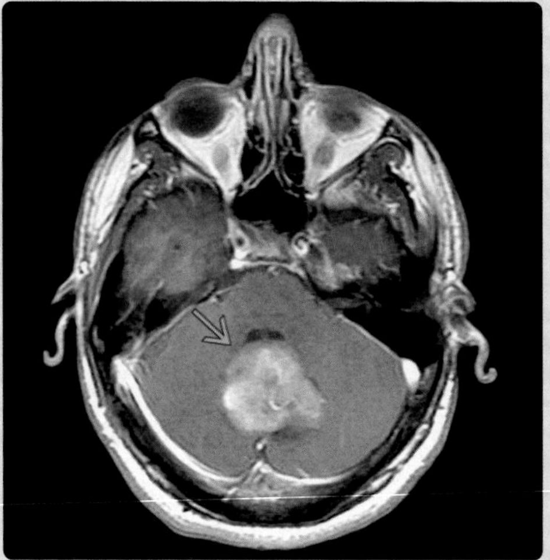

Intranodular Neurocytes

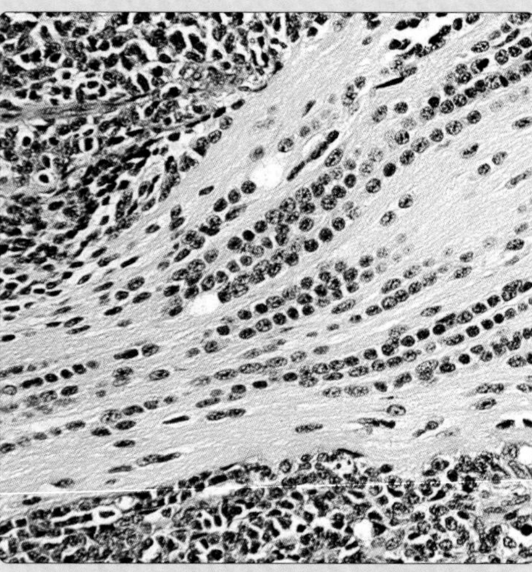

(Left) *Medulloblastomas are variably enhancing cerebellar masses, either vermian →, as seen here, or hemispheric.* **(Right)** *This case shows files of cytologically bland intranodular neurocytes contrast with the chaotic jumble of cytologically more atypical cells in surrounding extranodular areas.*

MR: Leptomeningeal Spread

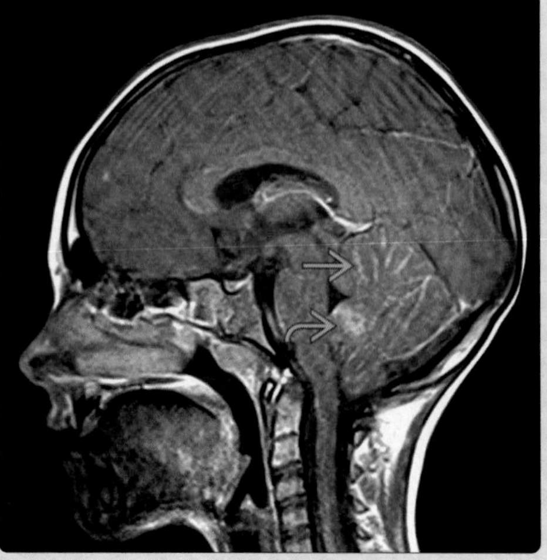

MR: Spinal Cord CSF Spread

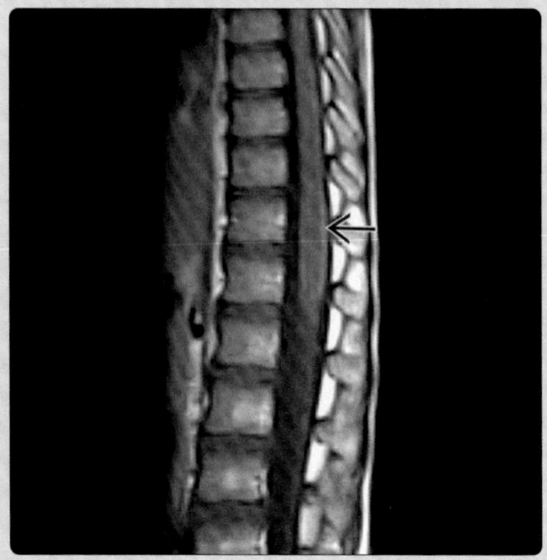

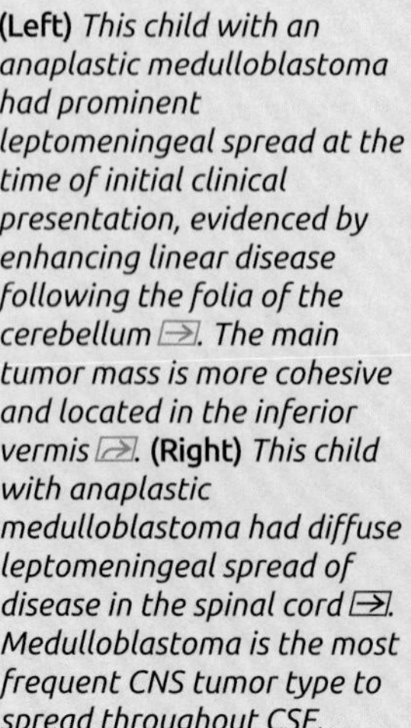

(Left) *This child with an anaplastic medulloblastoma had prominent leptomeningeal spread at the time of initial clinical presentation, evidenced by enhancing linear disease following the folia of the cerebellum →. The main tumor mass is more cohesive and located in the inferior vermis ↗.* **(Right)** *This child with anaplastic medulloblastoma had diffuse leptomeningeal spread of disease in the spinal cord →. Medulloblastoma is the most frequent CNS tumor type to spread throughout CSF.*

TERMINOLOGY

Synonyms

- None: Only medulloblastoma utilized

Definitions

- Small cell anaplastic embryonal tumor of cerebellum
- Unrelated to other embryonal tumors
- Unrelated to peripheral PNET (Ewing sarcoma)
- WHO grade IV

ETIOLOGY/PATHOGENESIS

Predisposing Cancer Syndromes

- Gorlin: Nodular/desmoplastic type (rare)
- Turcot type 2, APC: Classic (nonnodular) (rare)

2 Principal Pathways, Proposed

- External granule neuron precursor cells (nodular/desmoplastic type): Activation of sonic hedgehog (Shh) pathway
- Derivatives of ventricular matrix zone: Classic type: Activation of wingless (WNT) pathway medulloblastoma
  - Most WNT pathway subtypes of medulloblastoma are classic medulloblastomas, but most classic medulloblastomas are not WNT pathway since WNT pathway tumors are rare

CLINICAL ISSUES

Site

- Cerebellum
  - Vermis: Typically classic (nonnodular/desmoplastic) type
  - Hemisphere: Typically nodular/desmoplastic type

Presentation

- Expressions of obstructive hydrocephalus
- Cerebellar dysfunction
- Cranial nerve signs

Natural History

- Prone to CSF dissemination, especially as spinal drop metastases

Treatment

- Adjuvant therapy
  - Multiple course, combination therapy
  - Chemotherapy alone in nodular/desmoplastic and less than 3 years of age
- Radiation
  - Tumor plus neuraxis, standard except for very young patients
  - Role evolving for very favorable tumor subsets, especially in young patients

Prognosis

- Overall favorable with therapy, but dependent on stage and subtype
  - Very favorable, (80% survival), for WNT pathway/classic types and nodular desmoplastic types in children, both with total resection
  - Favorable (~ 70% overall survival) for sonic hedgehog nodular desmoplastic type
  - Less favorable for partially resected or metastatic disease
  - Unfavorable for large cell/anaplastic types
    - Especially unfavorable when associated with *MYC* amplification
- Overall, most favorable type is WNT subtype, which is recognized by nuclear beta catenin and monosomy 6
  - Most WNT pathway subtypes of medulloblastoma are classic medulloblastomas, but not all classic medulloblastomas are WNT pathway
- Late metastasis to bones, lymph nodes, lungs, uncommon
- Peritoneal implants through shunt, uncommon
- Radiation-induced 2nd primary, usually glioblastoma, is uncommon
  - Posterior cerebral hemispheres
  - Cerebellum, differential includes glial differentiation in original medulloblastoma
  - 5-10 years post irradiation

IMAGING

MR Findings

- Large
- Variable contrast enhancement, often only slight
- Striking nodularity (bunch of grapes) in extensively nodular type
- Metastatic leptomeningeal disease at presentation, intracranial or intraspinal, rare, any type but especially large cell/anaplastic

MACROSCOPIC

General Features

- Generally large
- Fleshy
- Involvement of subarachnoid space
- Firm, nodular in nodular/desmoplastic type
- Necrosis, especially when large cell/anaplastic

MICROSCOPIC

Histologic Features

- Patterns of spread
  - Infiltrates cerebellum and choroid plexus
  - Extension into subarachnoid space, common
  - Reenters brain as columns of cells in molecular layer
  - CSF dissemination, usually spinal drop metastases, especially in large cell/anaplastic types; subfrontal metastases also common
  - Potential for peritoneal implants with ventriculoperitoneal shunt
  - Late systemic metastases (uncommon)
- Classic (~ 70% of medulloblastomas)
  - Highly cellular sheets and lobules
  - Neuroblastic (Homer Wright) rosettes with fibrillar core
  - Stacked linear arrays
  - Perivascular pseudorosettes and stellate zones of finely fibrillar neuropil
  - WNT pathway medulloblastomas are classic type but WNT is rarest molecular type
    - Thus, majority classic medulloblastomas are not WNT but group 3 or 4

- Nodular/desmoplastic (~ 15-20%)
  - Conventional
    - Circumscribed pale areas (pale islands): Vary in size from small and identifiable only with reticulin staining to large and dominant
    - Intranodular neurocytic differentiation: Round, bland cells; finely fibrillar neuropil; cell streaming; few mitoses; often apoptotic cells
    - Extranodular tissue more cellular, cytologically atypical, mitotically active; higher Ki-67 index
  - Extensively nodular
    - Predominantly nodular tissue, but no established precise percentage
- Biphasic (~ 10%)
  - Nodules similar to, but often somewhat less well defined than, those in nodular/desmoplastic type
  - No perinodular reticulin
  - No GFAP(+) intranodular astrocytes as there is in nodular/desmoplastic type
- Large cell/anaplastic: Required degree of anaplasia and percent of tumor cross-sectional area unclear, but generally severe anaplasia &/or large cell type are over 50% of tumor area
  - Anaplastic (~ 10% of medulloblastomas)
    - Large cells, ≥ 2x as large over conventional small cells of medulloblastoma
    - Nuclear molding
    - Cell-cell wrapping, around apoptotic or viable cell
    - Nuclear pleomorphism
    - High mitotic activity
    - Abundant apoptosis
  - Large cell (~ 1%)
    - Sheets &/or lobules of monomorphous, large round cells with prominent nucleoli; abundant apoptosis
    - Often associated with severely anaplastic tissue
- Miscellaneous
  - Desmoplasia
    - Common in all types with leptomeningeal extension; without nodules, not diagnostic of nodular/desmoplastic type
    - Abundant reticulin
  - Apoptosis
    - Prominent overall
    - Especially prominent, sometimes as large areas (apoptotic lakes), in large cell/anaplastic type
    - In nodules of nodular desmoplastic type
  - Necrosis
    - Usually without pseudopalisading
    - Less common than apoptosis
  - Mitoses
    - Variable, from rare to many
  - Calcification
    - Generally uncommon
    - Dystrophic in necrotic or apoptotic areas
  - Maturation to gangliocytoma, especially in nodular/desmoplastic type (uncommon)
- With myogenic differentiation (medullomyoblastoma) (rare)
  - Striated muscle
- With melanocytic differentiation (melanotic medulloblastoma) (rare)
  - Pigmented epithelium, usually tubules
- With combined myoid and melanocytic differentiation (rare)

ANCILLARY TESTS

Cytology

- Conventional type: Small uniform cells with varying degrees of atypia, sometimes very slight
- Anaplastic type: Large angulated cells
- Large cell type: Large round cells with prominent nucleoli
- Few cell processes and little fibrillar background, as opposed to ependymoma

Immunohistochemistry

- Synaptophysin
  - Overall (+), but weak, equivocal, or even (-) in some cases
  - Especially (+) in
    - Nodules in nodular/desmoplastic type
    - Perivascular pseudorosettes and neuropil
    - Individual cells in large cell type
- GFAP
  - Extranodular cells in nodular/desmoplastic type, in some cases
  - Bipolar or stellate cells in nodules, often concentrated at periphery
  - Scattered foci, individual cells, in other types, in some cases
- Muscle markers
  - Medulloblastoma with myogenic differentiation
- Melanocytic markers
  - Medulloblastoma with melanotic differentiation
- Neurofilament protein
  - Variable, depending on antibody
  - Neuropil (+)
  - Pale islands (+)
- β-catenin (+) in both cytoplasm and nucleus (nuclear translocation) in tumors with pathway activation (histologically classic medulloblastomas)
- GAB1, filamin A, and YAP1, in nodular desmoplastic type

Genetic Testing

- Pathway: Classic (nonnodular) and biphasic lesions
  - Monosomy chromosome 6
  - Mutation in *CTNNB1* (β-catenin), *APC*, *AXIN1/2*
- Sonic hedgehog pathway: Nodular/desmoplastic lesions
  - *PTCH1* (95%)
  - Others (5%): *SMO*, *GLI*, *SUFU*
- Non-Shh/non-WNT
  - Recognition of WNT and Shh groups is important, but separating groups 3 and 4 (lumped under non-Shh/non-WNT) is not as important for practical purposes, currently difficult to do with immunohistochemistry
- Other
  - *c-MYC* and *N-MYC* amplifications, especially *c-MYC*, and especially in large cell/anaplastic types
    - Prognostically unfavorable
  - Inactivating mutations *MLL2* or *MLL3*, especially in large cell anaplastic type

- Adult tumors: 10q loss, and 17q gain unfavorable prognostic factors
  - Unlike in children, β-catenin activation and chromosome 6 loss not as favorable
- i(17)q
  - Usually with classic type
  - Prognostic significance debated, isolated 17p loss may be unfavorable
  - Copy number changes principally in non-Shh/non-WNT tumors
- Monosomy 6, marker of pathway activation
  - Classic and biphasic types
  - Prognostically favorable

Gene Expression Profiling

- Subgroups
  - Pathway activation
  - Shh pathway activation
  - 2-4 other groups, depending on reporting laboratory
    - Less favorable features (e.g., *MYC* amplification, chromosome 17 copy number changes) concentrated in these

DIFFERENTIAL DIAGNOSIS

Atypical Teratoid/Rhabdoid Tumor

- Common in posterior fossa; mimics medulloblastoma
- Generally more nuclear pleomorphism and more cytoplasm, but occasional medulloblastoma-like small cell architecture
- Polyimmunophenotypic
  - EMA
  - GFAP
  - Cytokeratins
  - Synaptophysin
  - Actin
- Loss of nuclear immunostaining for INI1(BAF47)
  - Defining feature in majority of cases (which show *SMARCB1* mutation); small minority have *SMARCA4* mutation

Embryonal Tumor With Multilayered True Rosettes (ETMR)

- Formerly, embryonal tumor with abundant neuropil and true rosettes (ETANTR)
- Defined by presence of genetic features
  - Any CNS embryonal tumor with C19MC amplification or fusion given ETMR designation, including those without rosettes
  - Tumors formerly designated ependymoblastoma, medulloepithelioma now recognized to share same genetic features; now incorporated into ETMR designation
- Prominent neuropil
  - Not in discrete islands as in nodular/desmoplastic medulloblastoma
- True (lumen-containing) rosettes
  - Sometimes arising in neuropil areas
  - Distinctive, granular subapical band

Anaplastic Glioma and Glioblastoma

- May be radiation-induced 2nd primary
- Microvascular proliferation and necrosis with pseudopalisading more common
- Synaptophysin (-), except for trapped brain
- GFAP(+), in some cases

Ependymoma

- Generally sharper tumor-cerebellum interface
- Less involvement of subarachnoid space
- More prominent perivascular pseudorosettes
- Nodules of higher cellularity in less cellular background tumor (common)
- True (lumen-containing) rosettes, in some cases
- Microvascular proliferation, rare in medulloblastoma
- GFAP(+), especially perivascular pseudorosettes
- Synaptophysin usually (-), but can be focally (+)
- EMA(+) microlumina, common but not required

DIAGNOSTIC CHECKLIST

Clinically Relevant Pathologic Features

- Propensity for CSF dissemination generally dictates neuraxis irradiation in most cases

Pathologic Interpretation Pearls

- Consider possibility of atypical teratoid/rhabdoid tumor, especially in patients < 2 years old: Immunostain for INI1(BAF47)
- Identification of molecular pathways (e.g., Shh) increasingly used in classification
- WNT is rarest molecular type and most classic medulloblastomas are not WNT but group 3 or 4

SELECTED REFERENCES

1. Remke M et al: Medulloblastoma molecular dissection: the way toward targeted therapy. Curr Opin Oncol. 25(6):674-81, 2013
2. Northcott PA et al: Rapid, reliable, and reproducible molecular sub-grouping of clinical medulloblastoma samples. Acta Neuropathol. 123(4):615-26, 2012
3. Ellison DW et al: Definition of disease-risk stratification groups in childhood medulloblastoma using combined clinical, pathologic, and molecular variables. J Clin Oncol. 29(11):1400-7, 2011
4. Ellison DW et al: Medulloblastoma: clinicopathological correlates of SHH, WNT, and non-SHH/WNT molecular subgroups. Acta Neuropathol. 121(3):381-96, 2011
5. Fellay CN et al: Medulloblastomas in adults: prognostic factors and lessons from paediatrics. Curr Opin Neurol. 24(6):626-32, 2011
6. McCabe MG et al: Chromosome 17 alterations identify good-risk and poor-risk tumors independently of clinical factors in medulloblastoma. Neuro Oncol. 13(4):376-83, 2011
7. Northcott PA et al: Medulloblastoma comprises four distinct molecular variants. J Clin Oncol. 29(11):1408-14, 2011
8. Northcott PA et al: Pediatric and adult sonic hedgehog medulloblastomas are clinically and molecularly distinct. Acta Neuropathol. 122(2):231-40, 2011
9. Parsons DW et al: The genetic landscape of the childhood cancer medulloblastoma. Science. 331(6016):435-9, 2011
10. Schwalbe EC et al: Rapid diagnosis of medulloblastoma molecular subgroups. Clin Cancer Res. 17(7):1883-94, 2011
11. Ellison DW: Childhood medulloblastoma: novel approaches to the classification of a heterogeneous disease. Acta Neuropathol. 120(3):305-16, 2010
12. Gibson P et al: Subtypes of medulloblastoma have distinct developmental origins. Nature. 468(7327):1095-9, 2010
13. Gilbertson RJ et al: The origins of medulloblastoma subtypes. Annu Rev Pathol. 3:341-65, 2008
14. Kool M et al: Integrated genomics identifies five medulloblastoma subtypes with distinct genetic profiles, pathway signatures and clinicopathological features. PLoS One. 3(8):e3088, 2008
15. McManamy CS et al: Nodule formation and desmoplasia in medulloblastomas-defining the nodular/desmoplastic variant and its biological behavior. Brain Pathol. 17(2):151-64, 2007

(Left) *As seen here, a sheet-like, nonnodular growth pattern is that of the predominant, classic medulloblastoma. While WNT pathway medulloblastomas display classic pattern, this is a rare subtype and thus most classic medulloblastomas are subgroup 3 or 4.* **(Right)** *Classic medulloblastomas may be composed of sheets of cells that are uniform in cytological features and distribution. Although highly cellular, there may be little nuclear pleomorphism and mitotic activity.*

Sheet-Like Growth, Classic Type

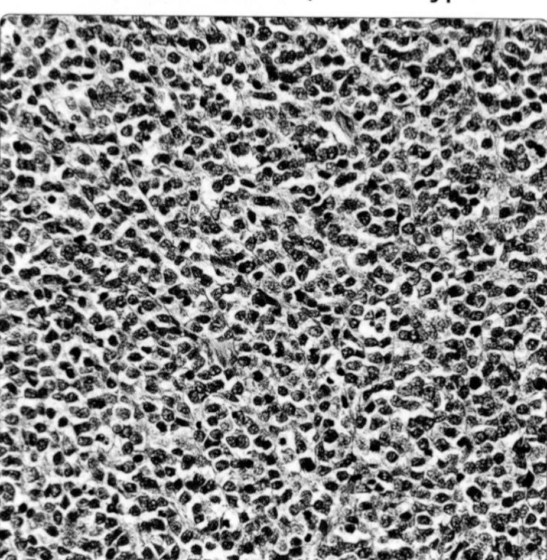

Uniform Cells, Classic Type

(Left) *Given the complex infoldings created by the cerebellum's foliar architecture, it is not surprising that medulloblastomas often reach, and fill, the subarachnoid space. Tumor cells may then invade the underlying molecular layer.* **(Right)** *Medulloblastomas in the subarachnoid space appear to descend along cell processes as they reenter the parenchyma. This downward spread recreates migration of external granular cells during embryonic development.*

Tumor in Subarachnoid Space, Classic Type

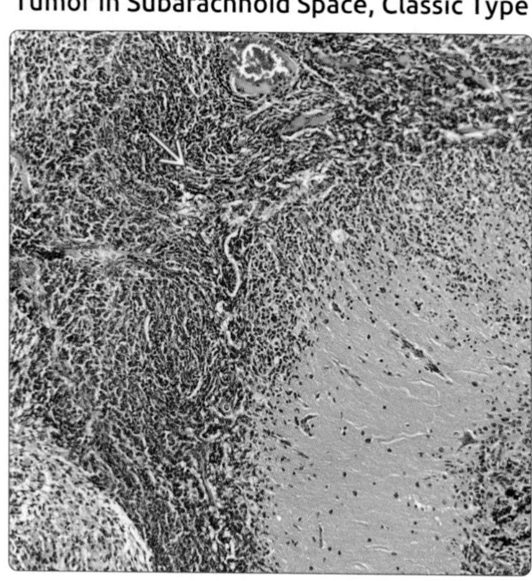

Reentry From Subarachnoid Space Along Cell Processes

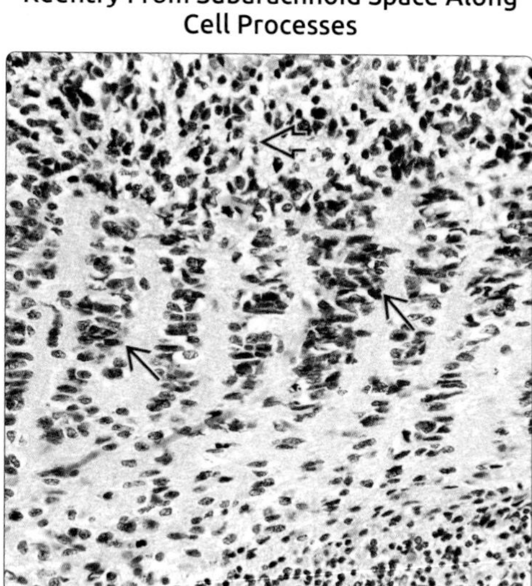

(Left) *Having reached the subarachnoid space, medulloblastomas often reenter the brain along perivascular spaces.* **(Right)** *Medulloblastomas often have an angiocentric pattern as they follow the course of intraparenchymal vessels, but the tumor is also capable of single cell, diffuse parenchymal infiltration.*

Extension Along Virchow-Robin Spaces

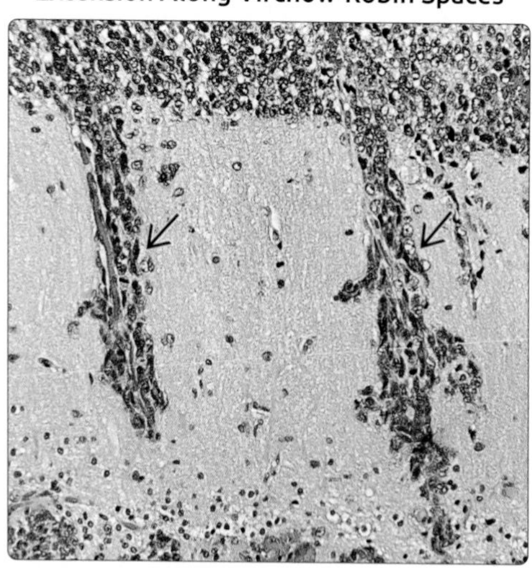

Perivascular Tumor, Classic Type

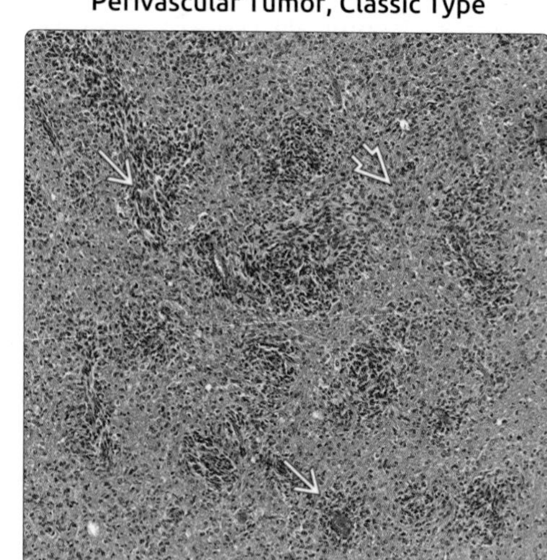

Densely Cellular, Classic Type

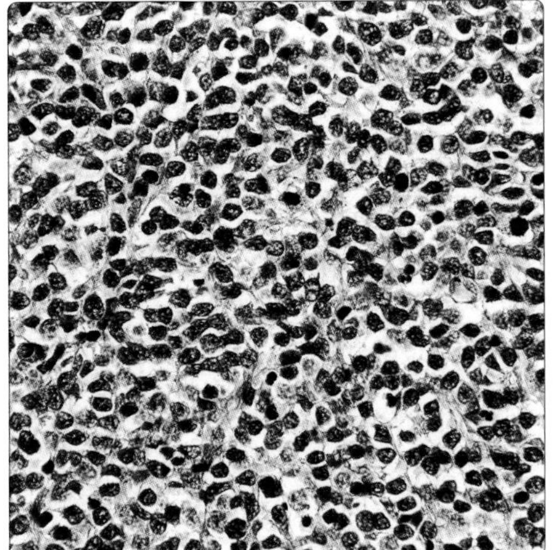

More Dispersed Tumor Cells, Classic Type

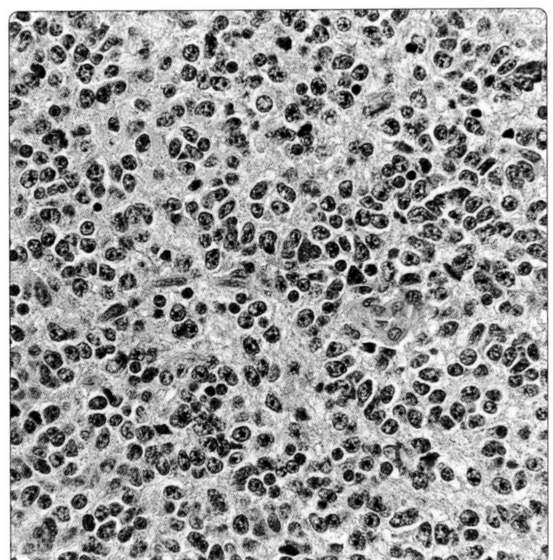

(Left) *Medulloblastomas are densely cellular grade IV tumors, but when favorable as to stage and molecular subtype have a cure rate of over 80%.* **(Right)** *When not back-to-back, tumor cells leave a glioma-like fibrillar background, as seen here.*

Variation in Cell Density, Classic Type

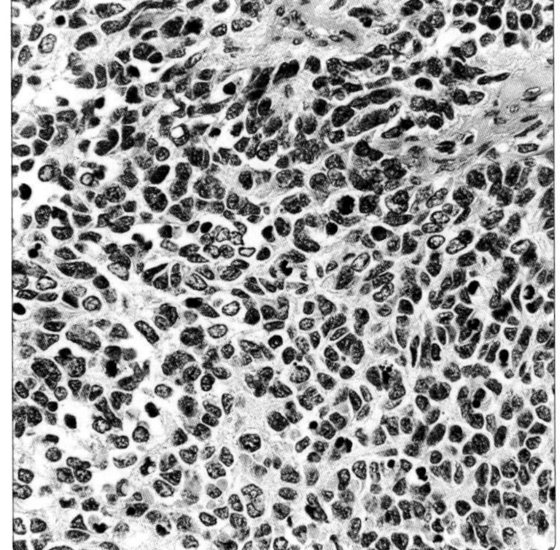

Elongate Nuclei, Classic Type

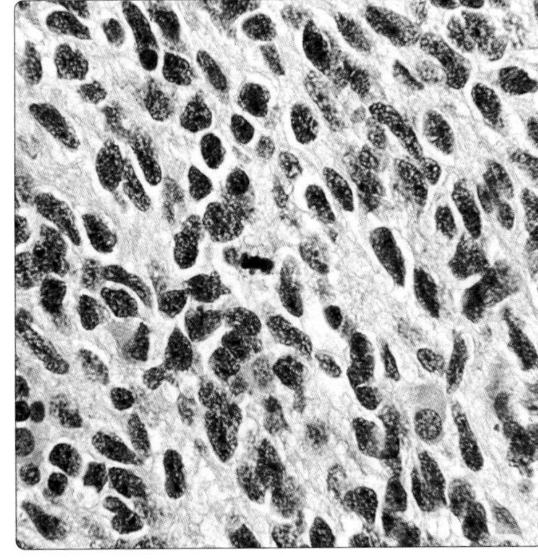

(Left) *Variation in cell density to the degree seen here is common in medulloblastomas, and not evidence of anaplasia.* **(Right)** *Moderately cellular areas with elongated nuclei may closely simulate high-grade astrocytoma. The degree of nuclear atypia and hyperchromatism seen here is that of moderate-degree anaplasia.*

Mild Anaplasia, Classic Type

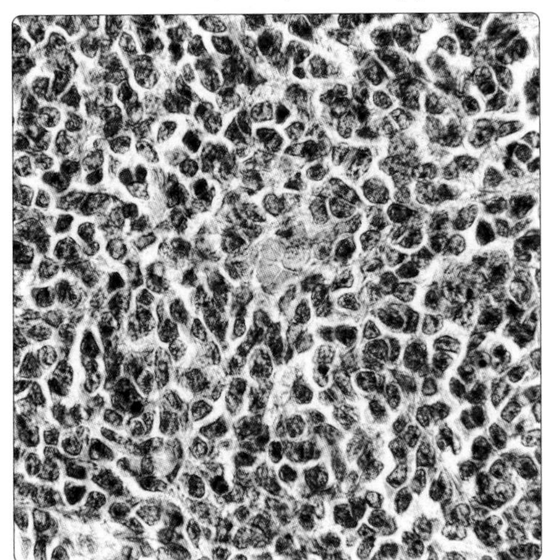

Mild Anaplasia, Classic Type

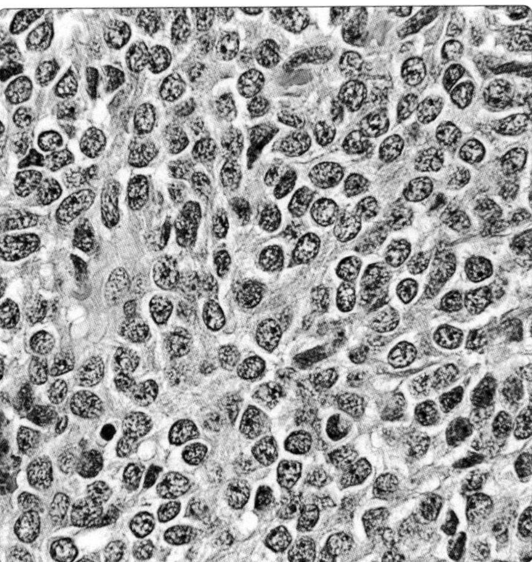

(Left) *Mild anaplasia is expressed as a restrained degree of nuclear pleomorphism and atypia. While highly cellular, this tumor is only slightly to moderately anaplastic.* **(Right)** *Only a mild degree of anaplasia is present in this case with minimal nuclear pleomorphism. The somewhat open nuclei raise the issue of atypical teratoid/rhabdoid tumor. Small blue cell tumors should be assessed by INI1 immunohistochemistry. AT/RTs show nuclear INI1 loss; medulloblastomas show retention.*

(Left) *Neuroblastic Homer Wright rosettes are uncommon features of classic (nonnodular) medulloblastomas. They are not perivascular and, unlike true rosettes, have no lumina.* **(Right)** *Uniform columns, as rosettes viewed longitudinally, are striking and diagnostic. These structurings are sometimes termed "en filade" to recall rows of marching soldiers.*

Homer Wright Rosettes, Classic Type

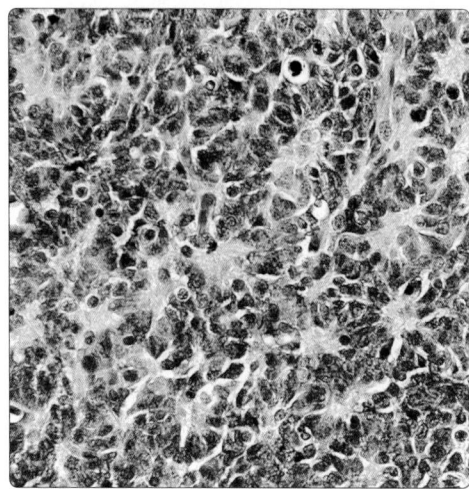

Rows of Tumor Cells, Classic Type

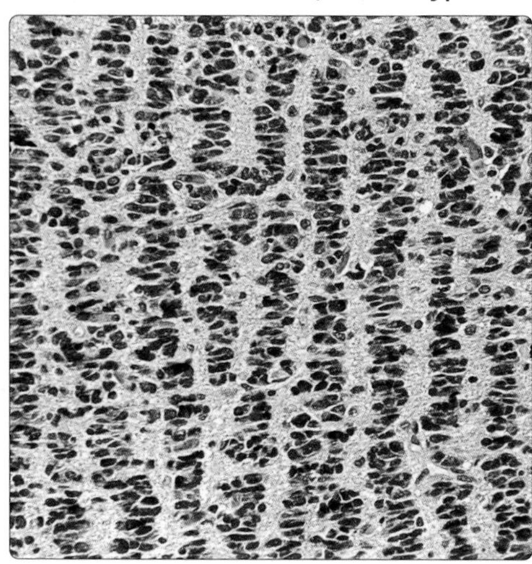

(Left) *Finely fibrillar neuropil, often somewhat perivascular, creates a decided resemblance to ependymoma. Since these areas are created by neuritic process, they would be immunoreactive for synaptophysin. Similar zones in ependymoma would be positive for GFAP.* **(Right)** *Perivascular pseudorosettes in some medulloblastomas, such as those seen here, create close facsimiles to those in ependymoma. Immunohistochemistry for GFAP, EMA, and synaptophysin are appropriate in the face of such formations.*

Finely Fibrillar Background

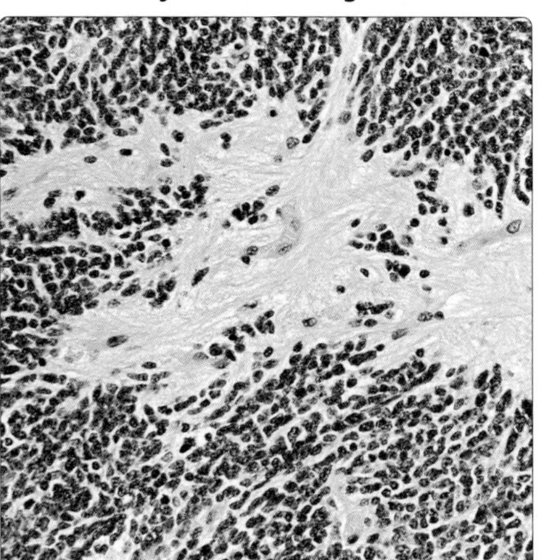

Simulating Ependymoma

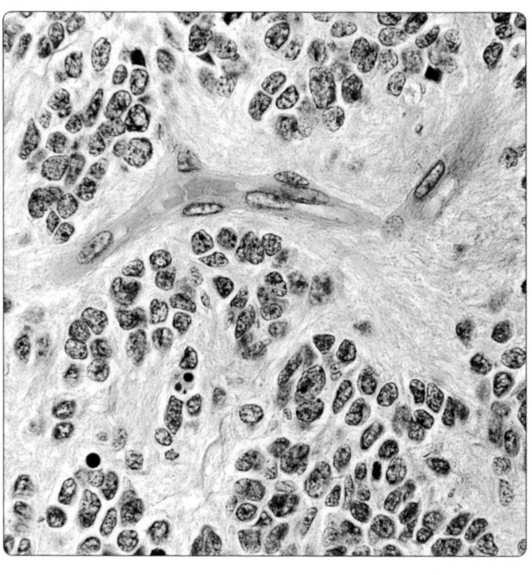

(Left) *Nodular/desmoplastic tumors may have a distinctive fine nodularity similar to that of a cirrhotic liver.* **(Right)** *Lightly stained nodules, or pale islands, stand out against the darker, less differentiated background of extranodular tissue in the nodular/desmoplastic medulloblastoma type. Nodules of this type would be delineated by reticulin fibers.*

Nodular/Desmoplastic Medulloblastoma

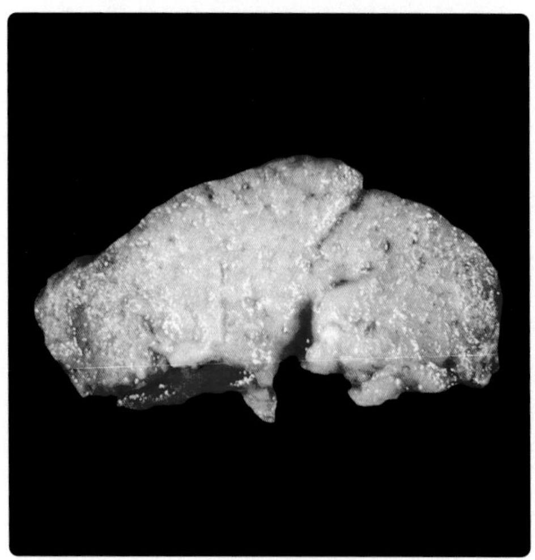

Pale Islands in Nodular/Desmoplastic Type

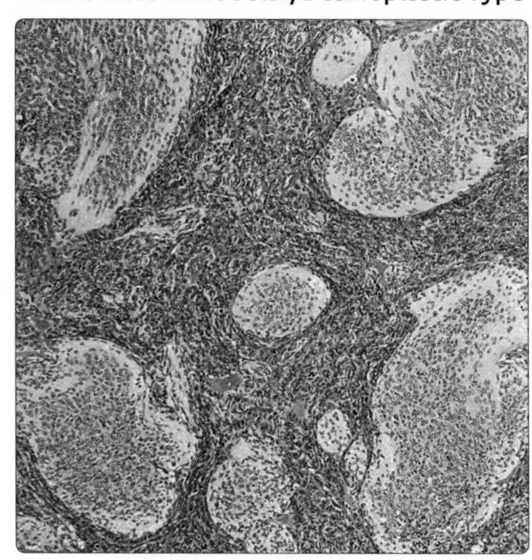

Nodular/Desmoplastic Type

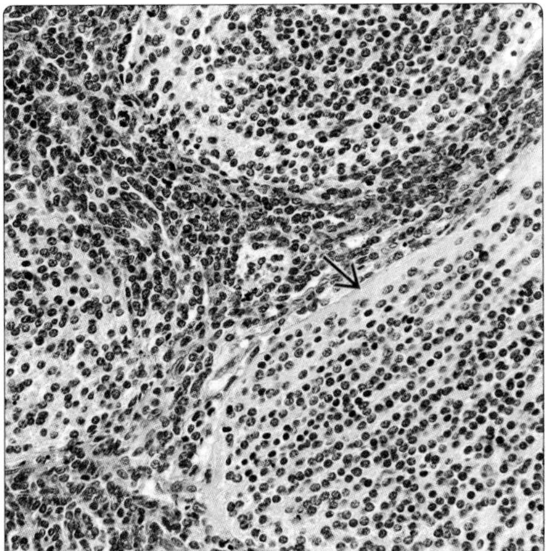

Paucinodular Variant, Nodular/Desmoplastic Type

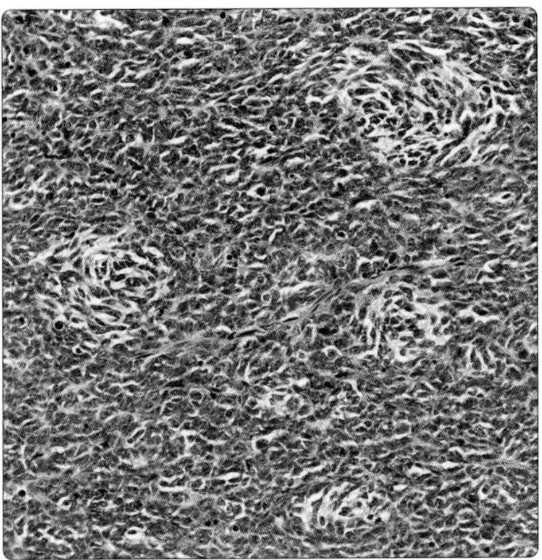

(Left) *There is considerable intra- and intertumoral variability among nodular/desmoplastic medulloblastomas in the amount of intranodular neuropil. The latter is sparse in this case, and most apparent at the periphery of the nodule* ➙*.* **(Right)** *Nodules of neurocytic differentiation may be small and poorly formed. Reticulin staining of the highly cellular, ostensibly anodular, tissue would find many incipient nodules in the form of small clusters. This is still a nodular/desmoplastic medulloblastoma.*

Apoptosis, Nodular/Desmoplastic Type

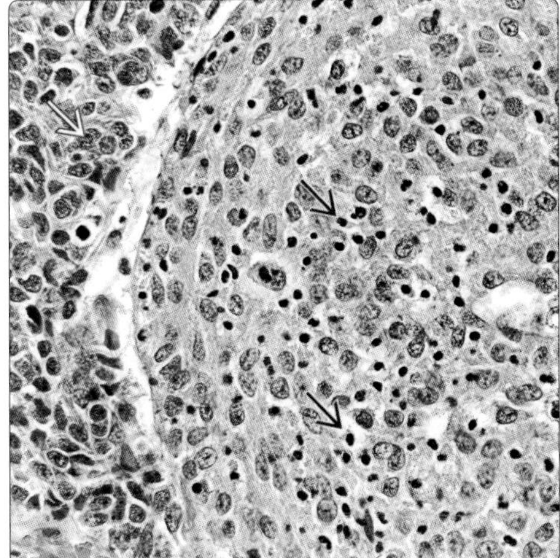

Medulloblastoma With Extensive Nodularity

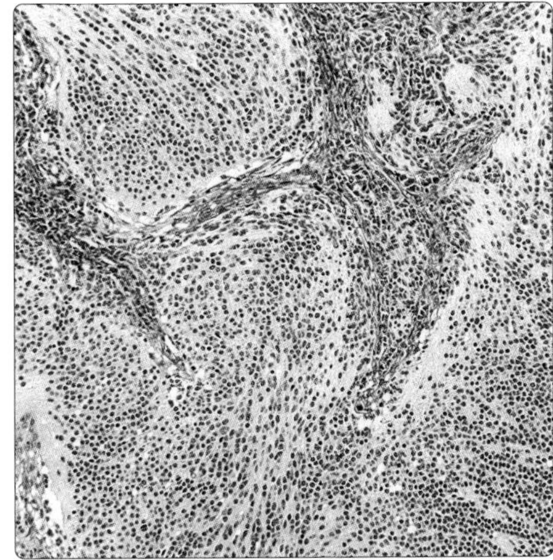

(Left) *Lymphocyte-like apoptotic cells* ➙ *are numerous in some developing nodules. Cellularity and cytological atypia are relatively increased in extranodular areas* ➙*.* **(Right)** *Nodules dominate the prognostically favorable lesion of infants, known as medulloblastoma with extensive nodularity (MBEN). Such lesions are part of the nodular/desmoplastic group, with no precise cutoff in terms of percentage of section area from ordinary nodular/desmoplastic lesions with prominent nodularity.*

Ill-Defined Nodules

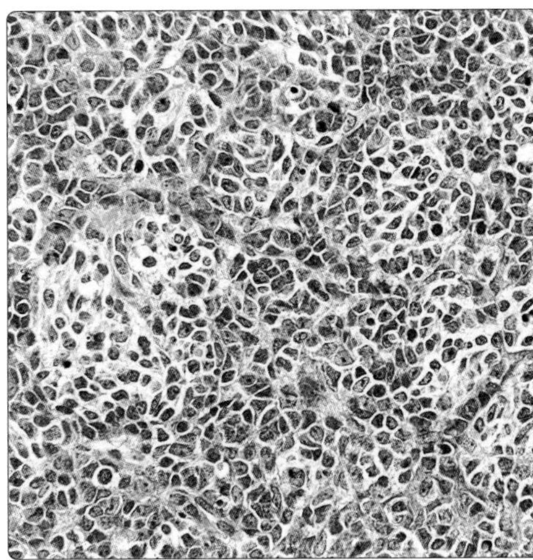

Reticulin, Nodular/Desmoplastic Type

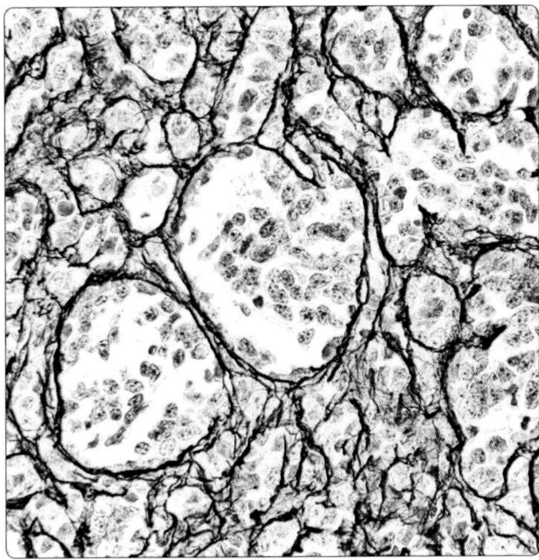

(Left) *Ill-defined nodules may await reticulin staining for confirmation. If reticulin surrounds the nodules then this is a nodular/desmoplastic type; if not, this is a biphasic classic type.* **(Right)** *Almost all of the apparently extranodular compartment is formed of small nodules or individual cells. Often, as seen here, tissue outside of the obvious nodules is actually multi- and micronodular.*

(Left) *As seen here, long cords or single cell rows of tumor sit in densely desmoplastic stroma. Without the requisite nodules, neither the cells nor connective tissue establish the presence of a nodular/desmoplastic medulloblastoma.* **(Right)** *Columns and narrow lobules of cells stream though reticulin-rich desmoplastic tissue in a nodular/desmoplastic lesion. Desmoplasia in itself is not a sufficient criterion for this medulloblastoma subtype. Reticulin-bound nodules are required.*

Desmoplasia Alone Not Nodular/Desmoplastic Subtype

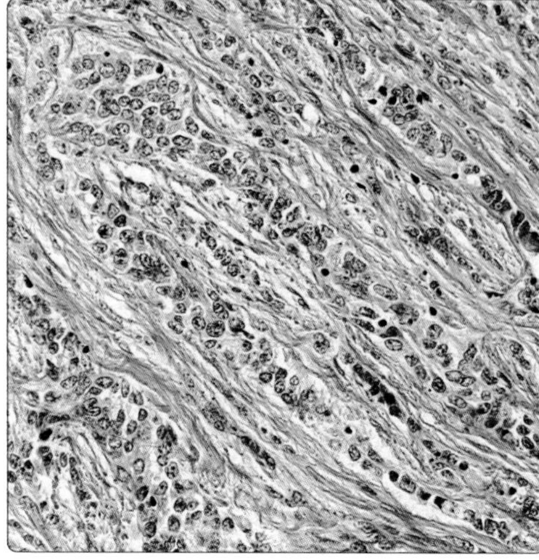

Desmoplasia Alone, Outlined by Reticulin

(Left) *The differentiating propensity inherent in the formation of nodules is carried to the extreme in some cases, as seen here.* **(Right)** *Occasional nodular/desmoplastic lesions differentiate into paucicellular, neuropil-rich tissue containing small ganglion cells →. Even the typically highly-cellular internodular component ⇒ has matured in this case.*

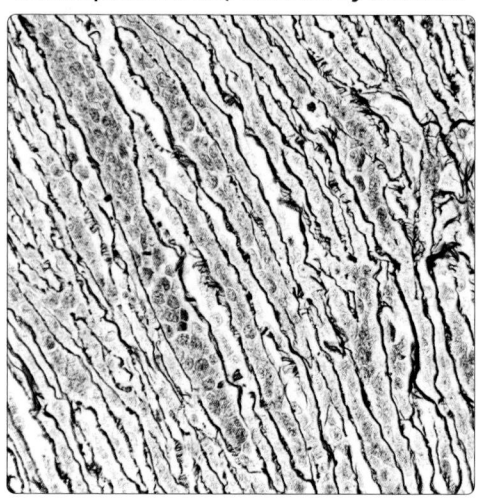

Extreme Nodularity and Differentiation

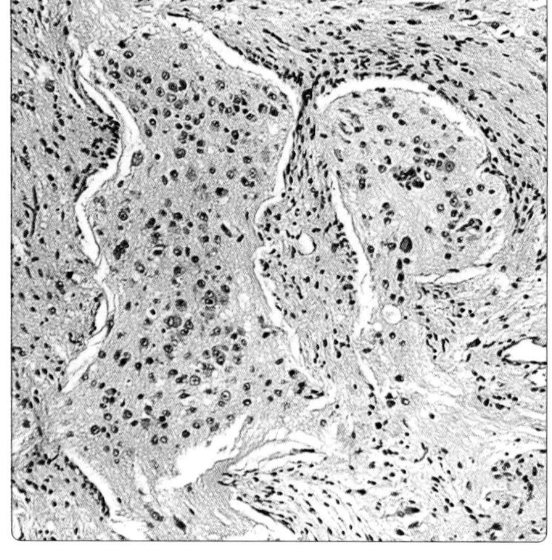

Occasional Ganglion Cells, Nodular/Desmoplastic Type

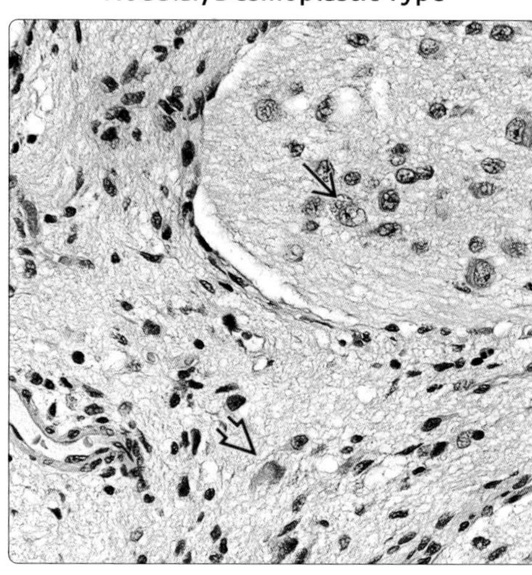

(Left) *Some classic medulloblastomas are nodular, yet not desmoplastic. There would be no perinodular reticulin, unlike nodules in nodular/desmoplastic tumors. This pattern in a classic medulloblastoma is designated biphasic.* **(Right)** *A reticulin stain demonstrates the absence of perinodular reticulin in the nodule in biphasic classic medulloblastomas.*

Ill-Defined Nodules, Biphasic Classic Type

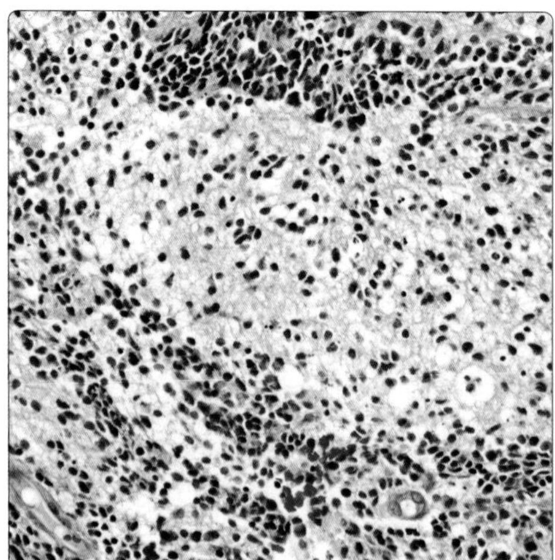

Absence of Reticulin, Biphasic Classic Type

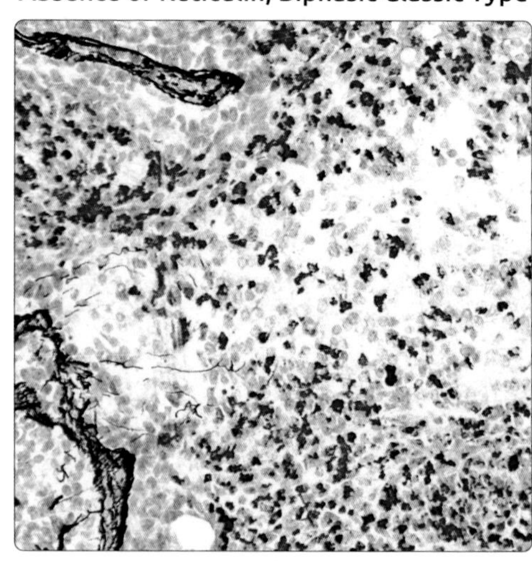

Rhabdomyoblasts

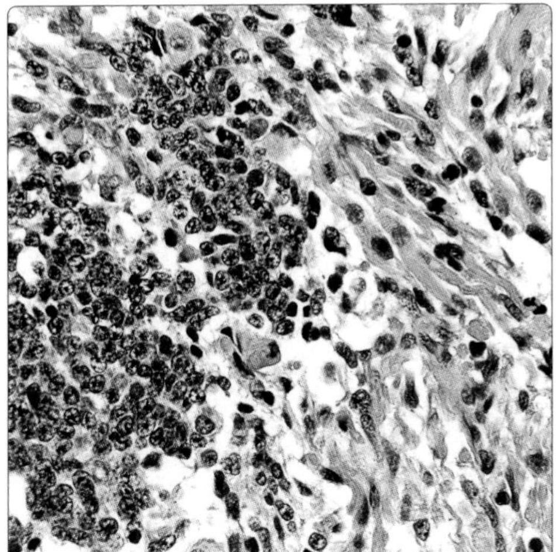

Striated Muscle Cells

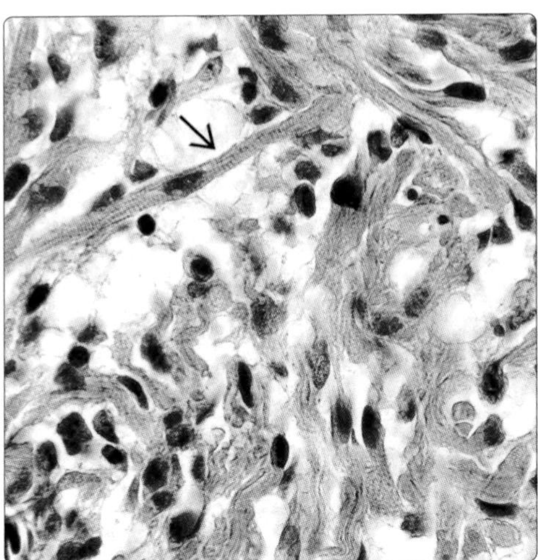

(Left) *Rare medulloblastomas contain eosinophilic strap cells, rhabdomyoblasts, in the tumor known as medulloblastoma with myogenic differentiation. An earlier designation was medullomyoblastoma.* **(Right)** *Striated muscle cells ⇒ are striking findings in rare medulloblastomas, known officially as medulloblastoma with myogenic differentiation. Medullomyoblastoma is a simpler, but older, term.*

Melanotic Differentiation

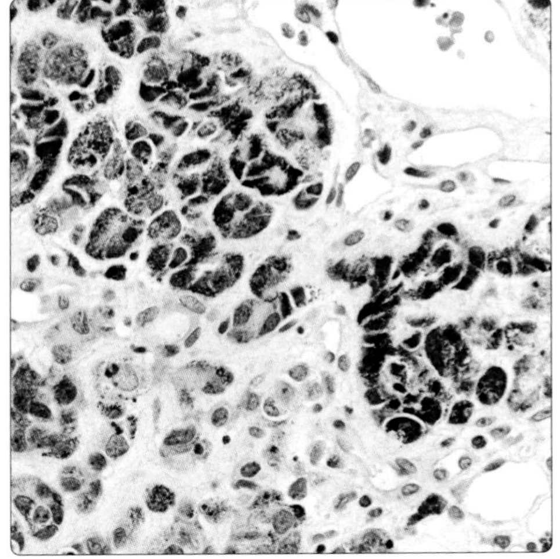

Rare Pigment-Laden Tubules

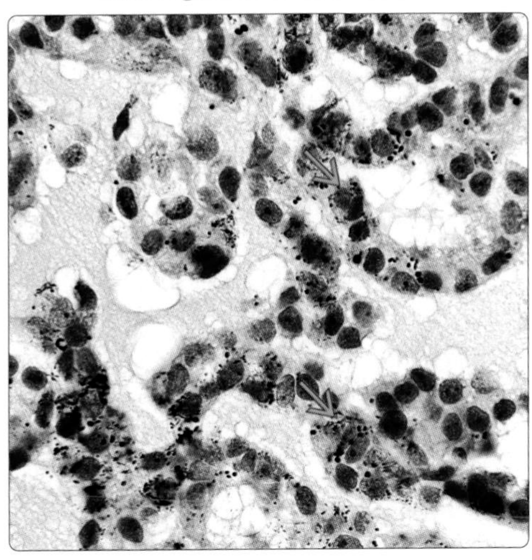

(Left) *Variably pigmented tubules are focal or widespread features of the rare medulloblastoma with melanocytic differentiation, melanotic medulloblastoma.* **(Right)** *Pigment-laden tubules ⇒ add interest to some medulloblastomas known as medulloblastoma with melanotic differentiation. Rare examples that also have a myoid component are even more interesting visually.*

Neuronal Differentiation

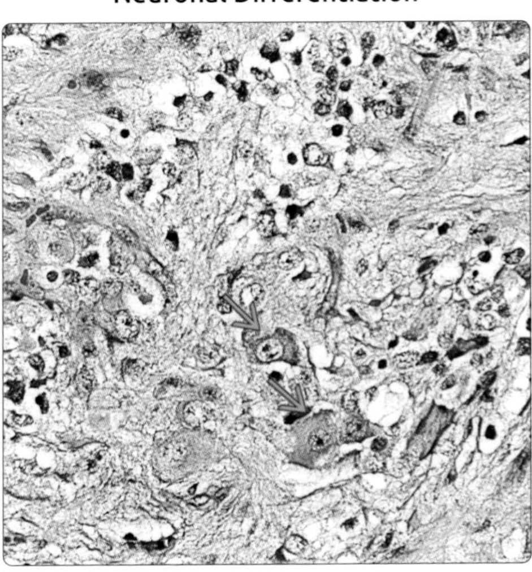

Ganglion Cells

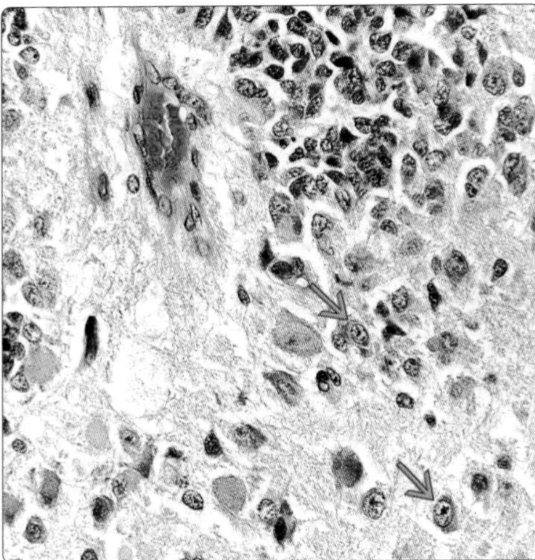

(Left) *Neuronal differentiation in medulloblastomas presents immunohistochemically as positivity for neuronal markers, or histologically as Homer Wright rosettes, neurocytes in nodular lesions, &/or, rarely, ganglion cells ⇒.* **(Right)** *Ganglion cell differentiation ⇒ is uncommon in medulloblastomas and often occurs in finely fibrillar areas of neuropil created by tumor cell processes.*

(Left) *Classic medulloblastomas are formed of sheets of small, uniform cells with little nuclear pleomorphism. Compared with large cell and severely anaplastic counterparts, anaplasia is not pronounced in this case. Although grade IV, mitoses may be few.* **(Right)** *There is a degree of nuclear pleomorphism in this slightly anaplastic tumor, but not the coarse, hard chromatin, nuclear angulation, and molding that characterizes severely anaplastic tissue.*

Classic Medulloblastoma

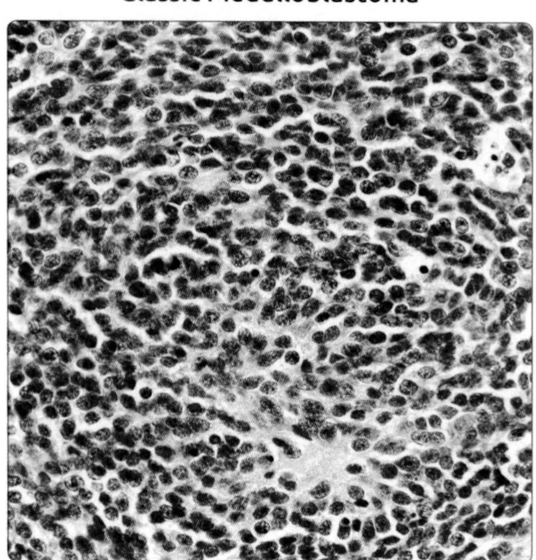

Mild Anaplasia

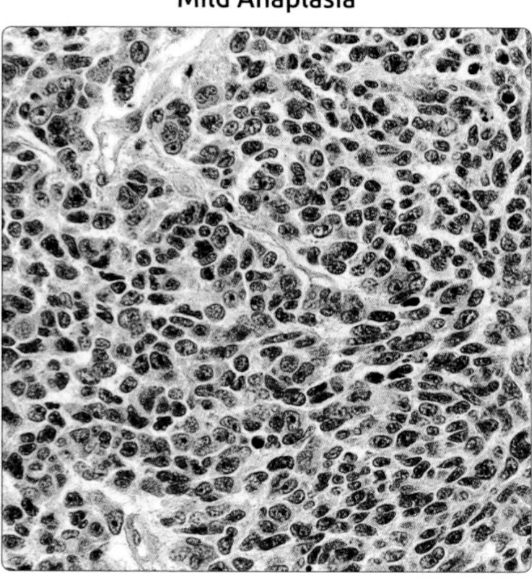

(Left) *Moderate anaplasia lacks the overt molding and cell-cell wrapping of anaplasia in its severe form. There are no absolute criteria to distinguish them, and there is often considerable intratumoral heterogeneity in the degree of anaplasia.* **(Right)** *Large pleomorphic cells with nuclear molding are typical of severe anaplasia. Nuclei in large cell medulloblastoma, in contrast, would be uniformly round and have prominent nucleoli. Molding would be minimal.*

Moderate Anaplasia

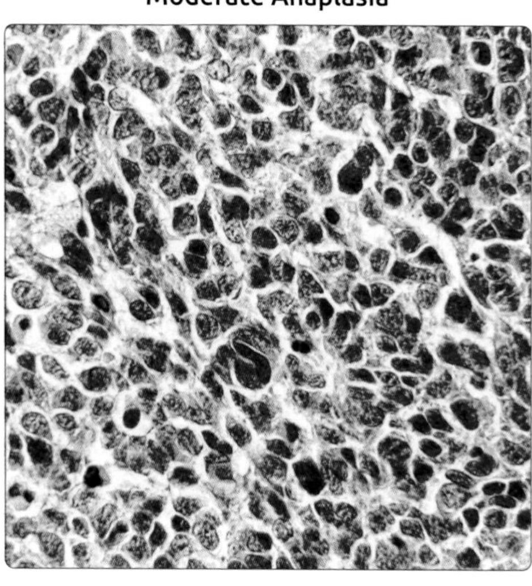

Severe Anaplasia, Anaplastic Type

(Left) *Severe anaplasia is characterized by large cells with irregular, molded nuclei. Nucleoli are less prominent than in large cell medulloblastoma. Both severely anaplastic and large cell medulloblastomas may resemble atypical teratoid/rhabdoid tumor.* **(Right)** *As demonstrated here, wrapping of one cell about another → is common in severely anaplastic tissue. As is typical, both apoptosis and mitoses are common.*

Severe Anaplasia, Anaplastic Type

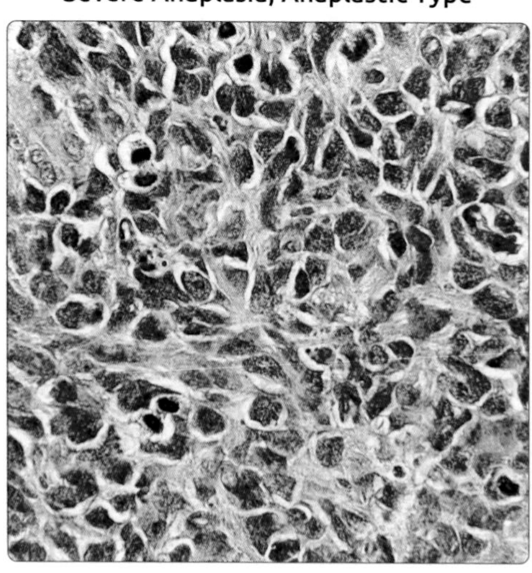

Cell Enwrapment, Anaplastic Type

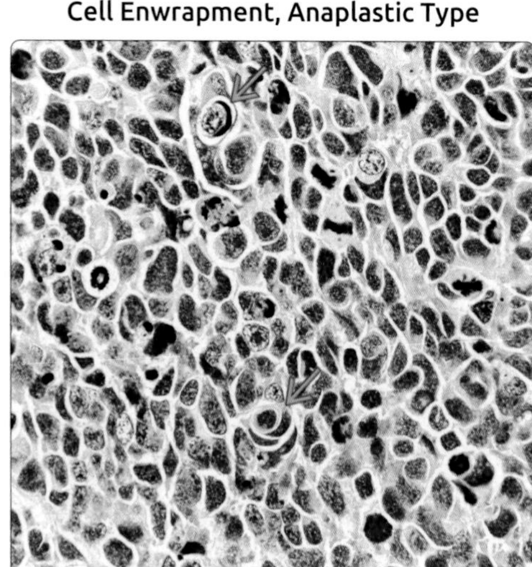

Large Cell Type

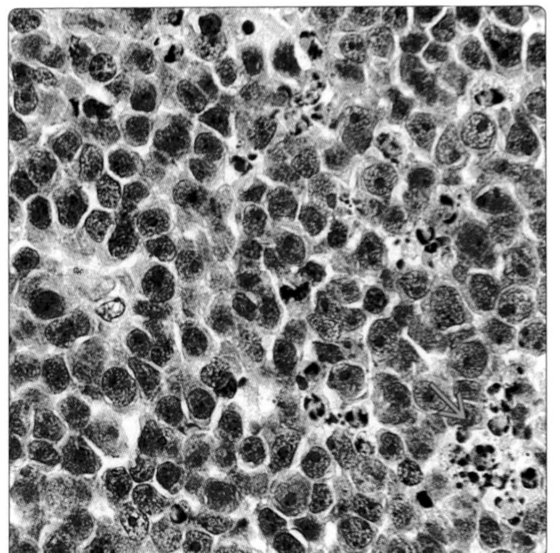

Prominent Apoptosis, Large Cell Type

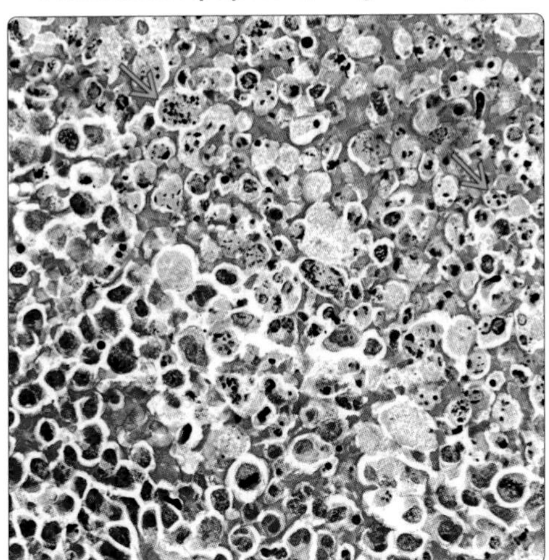

(Left) *Large cell medulloblastomas have sheets of cells with large, round nuclei with prominent nucleoli. Apoptosis ⇒ is prominent.* **(Right)** *Apoptosis ⇒ is prominent in large cell/anaplastic medulloblastoma. As seen here, there may be large confluent areas of self-destroying cells. This tumor has some features of the large cell type with round nuclei with prominent nucleoli, but has some angulation, as is typical of severe anaplasia.*

Severe Anaplasia, Anaplastic Type

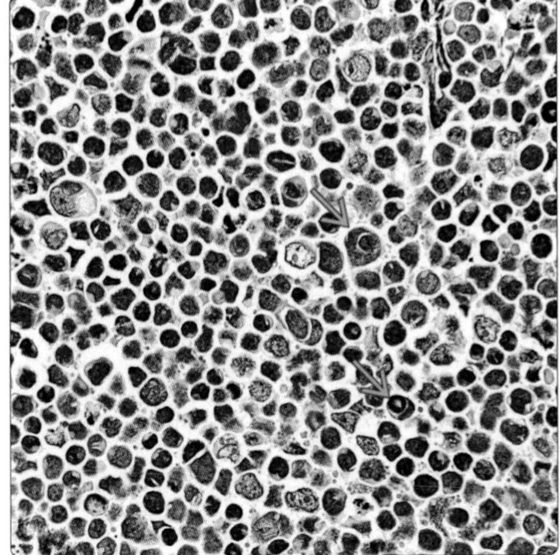

Large Cell Type

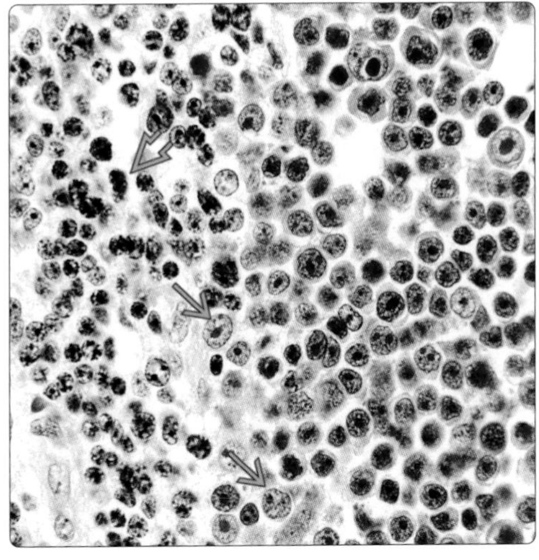

(Left) *Large cell tissue typically forms homogeneous lobules or sheets. Wrapping of one cell around another ⇒ is common, as it is seen in medulloblastomas with severe anaplasia.* **(Right)** *Sheets of large, round cells with prominent nucleoli ⇒ are defining features of large cell medulloblastoma. As is common, the lesion is not exclusively large cell, but also has cells with lesser degrees of anaplasia ⇒.*

Anaplastic Type With Homer Wright Rosettes

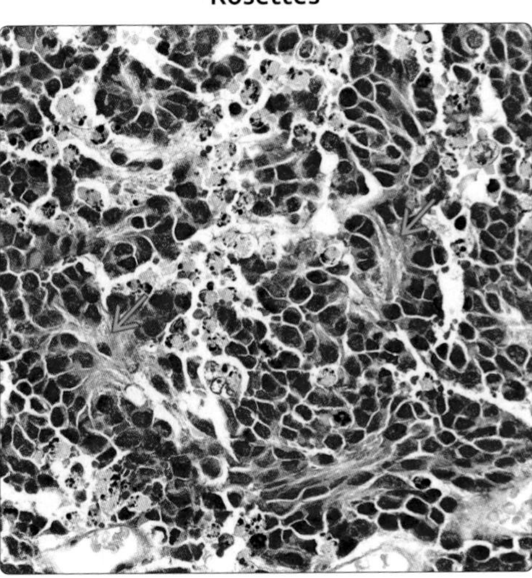

Severe Anaplasia in Nodular/Desmoplastic Type

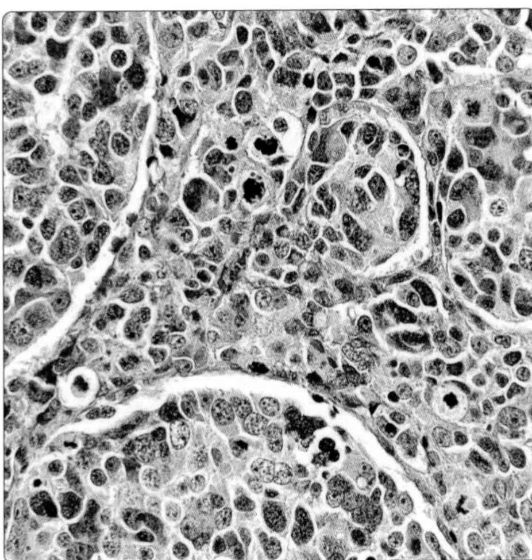

(Left) *Severe anaplasia does not necessarily preclude formation of Homer Wright rosettes ⇒. Severe anaplasia is evident in nuclear features of size, molding, and coarse chromatin. Abundant apoptosis is common.* **(Right)** *Severe anaplasia sometimes occurs in nodular/desmoplastic types. Note the marked atypia, mitoses, and abundant apoptosis that is present here.*

(Left) *The most common form of medulloblastoma is composed of small uniform cells with little cytoplasm that spread individually in smear preparations. In spite of the grade IV nature, mitoses may be difficult to find. Cells and tissue fragments, respectively, lack processes and fibrillar background that are typical of ependymoma.* **(Right)** *The large size, prominent nucleoli, and cell-cell wrapping ⇨ stand out in smear preparations of large cell/anaplastic medulloblastomas, as seen here.*

Smear, Small Uniform Cells, Classic Type

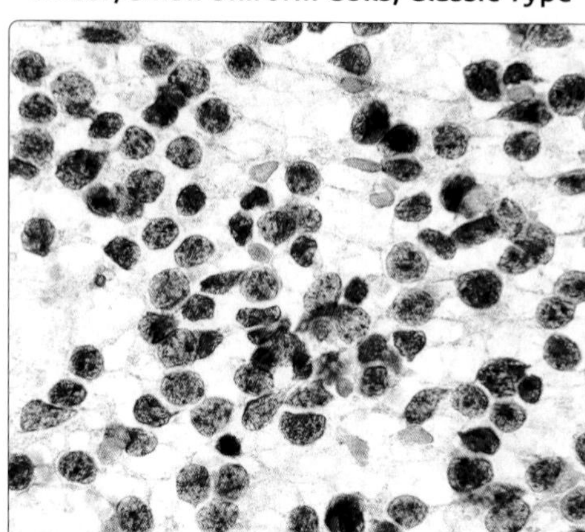

Smear, Large Anaplastic Cells

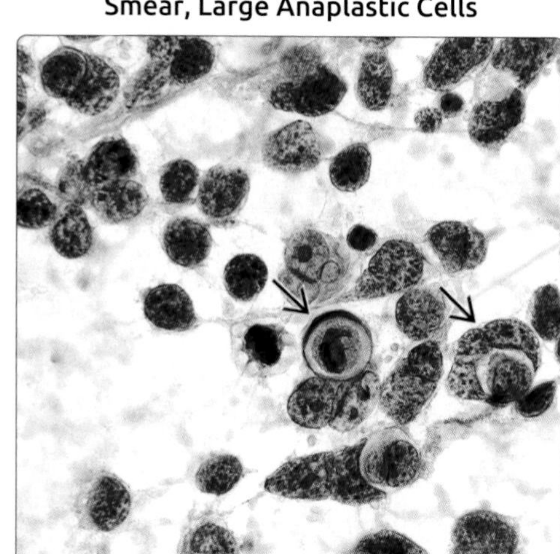

(Left) *Tumor cells are often diffusely positive for synaptophysin, although not always as robustly as seen here. Immunopositivity may even be slight, equivocal, or absent.* **(Right)** *Large nodules with advanced neurocytic differentiation are strongly immunoreactive for synaptophysin. A smaller nodule ⇨ is less positive. Extranodular cells are negative in this case.*

Synaptophysin Variable

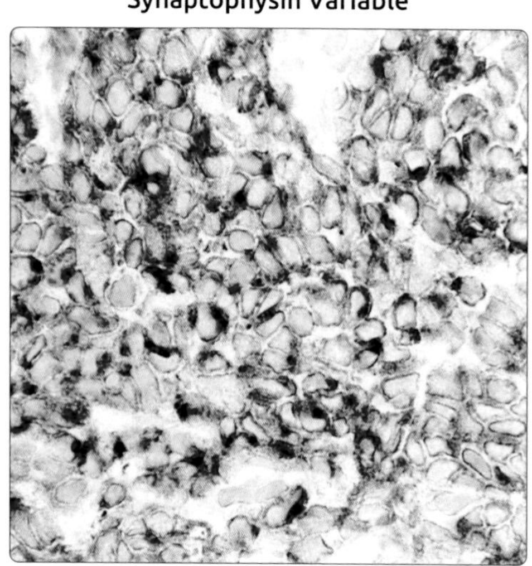

Nodules Strongly Synaptophysin (+)

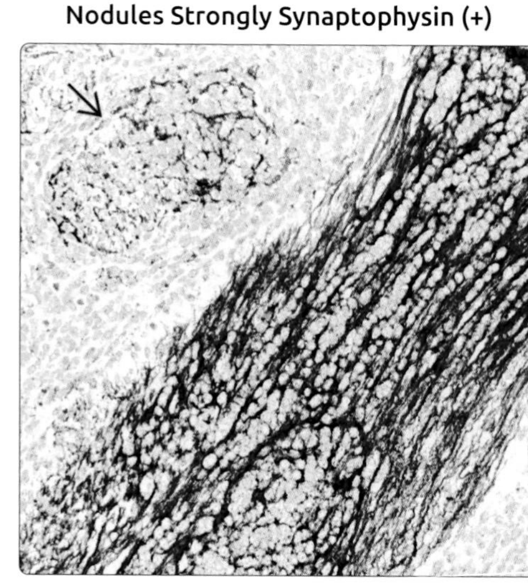

(Left) *Widespread immunoreactivity for GFAP is present in some medulloblastomas, especially in extranodular cells of the nodular/desmoplastic variant. More often, only trapped perivascular reactive astrocytes are positive.* **(Right)** *Long GFAP positive processes that are common in nodular/desmoplastic lesions are usually concentrated at the periphery of the nodules ⇨.*

Widespread GFAP, Nodular/Desmoplastic Type

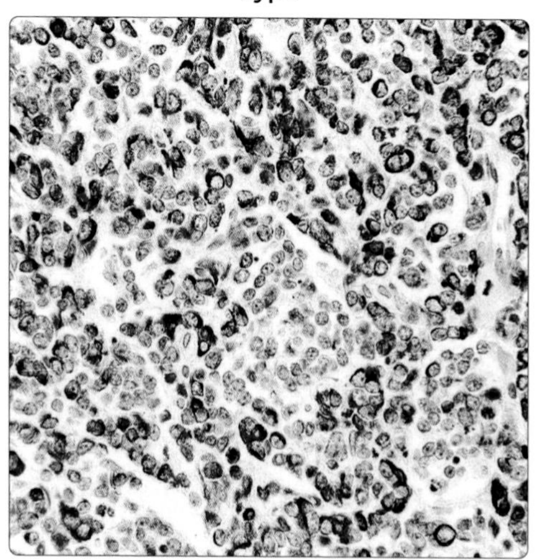

GFAP at Periphery of Nodules

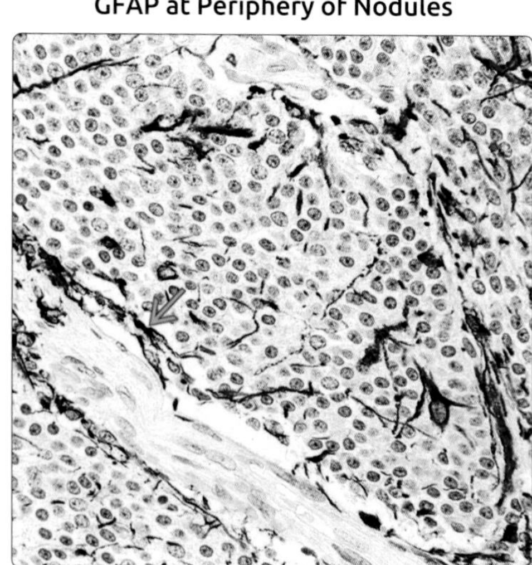

GAB1 IHC

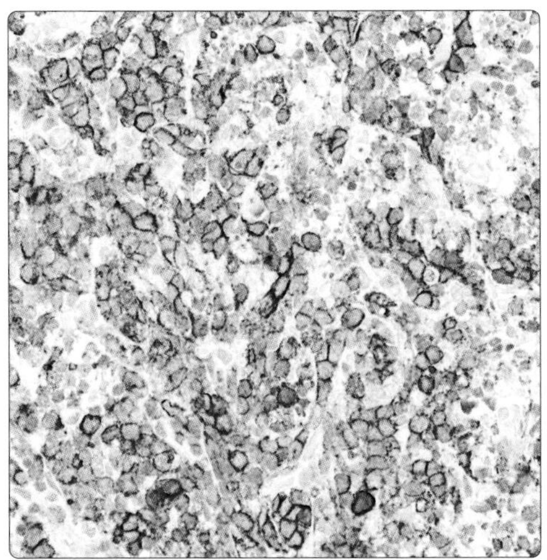

Nuclear β-Catenin Prognostically Favorable

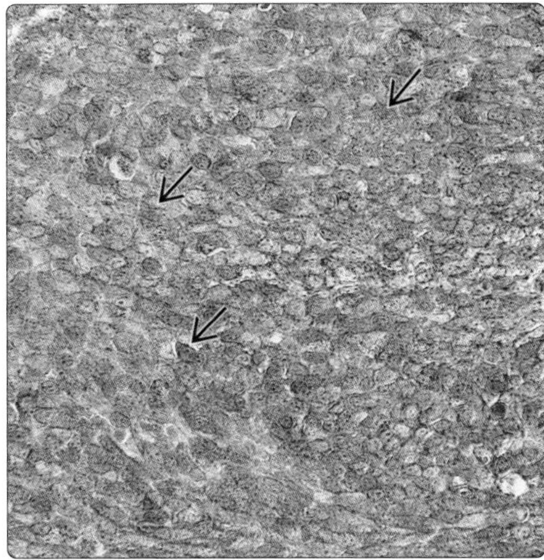

(Left) *Immunostaining, here positive, for a marker of sonic hedgehog (Shh) pathway activation, GAB1, can be used in subclassification. The other principal group, with activation of the WNT pathway, can be assessed using FISH for monosomy 6, or immunohistochemistry for nuclear β-catenin. (Courtesy D. Ellison, MD, PhD.)* **(Right)** *Nuclear ⇨ as well as cytoplasmic staining for β-catenin is an index of WNT pathway activation, and a prognostically favorable medulloblastoma subtype.*

Monosomy Chromosome 6, Favorable Prognosis

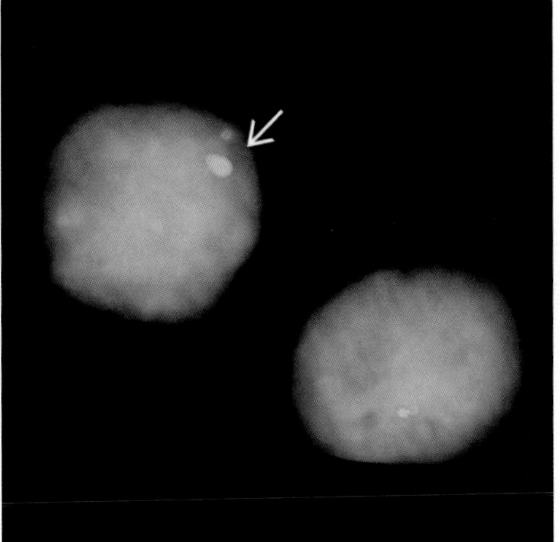

C-MYC Amplification, Unfavorable Prognosis

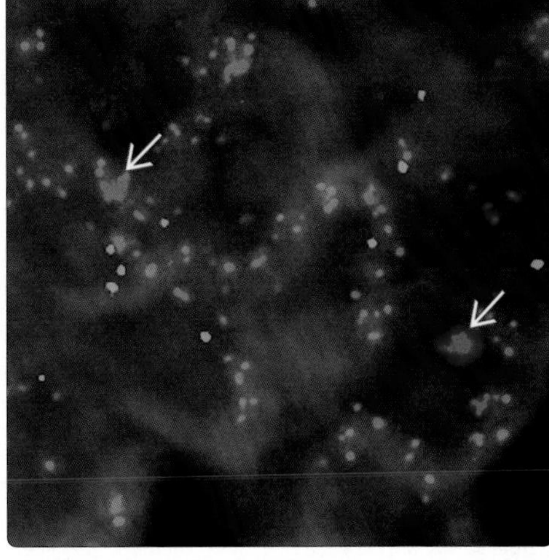

(Left) *Cells from a WNT pathway activated tumor are monosomic for chromosome 6. There is just 1 signal each ➡ for probes to 6p and 6q. (Courtesy D. Ellison, MD, PhD.)* **(Right)** *Innumerable red signals ➡ for C-MYC indicate amplification in this anaplastic medulloblastoma. Green signals are from a probe for chromosome 8p. (Courtesy D. Ellison, MD, PhD.)*

Systemic Spread via Ventriculoperitoneal Shunt

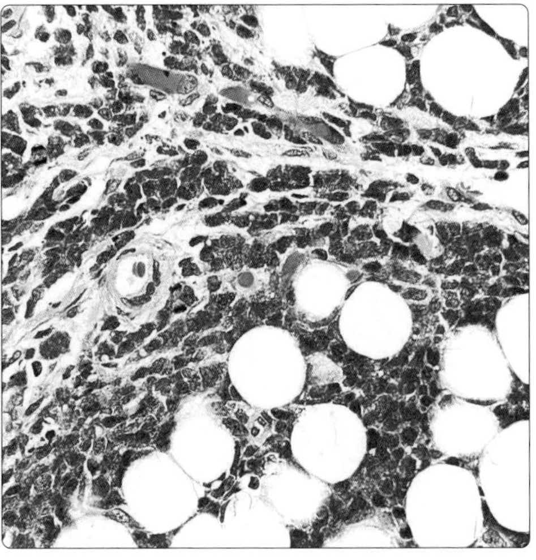

Bone Marrow Metastases

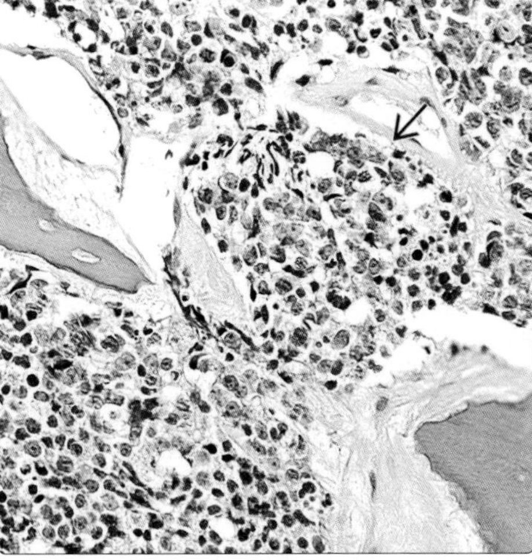

(Left) *Medulloblastomas may implant on the peritoneal surface after reaching the abdominal cavity through a ventriculoperitoneal shunt.* **(Right)** *Medulloblastomas occasionally disseminate systemically, with bone marrow being the most common secondary site ⇨.*

CNS Embryonal Neoplasms

KEY FACTS

TERMINOLOGY

- Heterogeneous group of embryonal neoplasms composed of poorly differentiated cells that may express neuronal and glial markers

CLINICAL ISSUES

- Predominantly tumors of children, but may present in adults
- Cerebral hemispheres are most frequent location
- Occasional cases in suprasellar region, brainstem, and spinal cord
- Embryonal neoplasms are highly aggressive neoplasms with propensity for CSF dissemination and metastasis outside CNS
- Worse prognosis as group than medulloblastoma
  - Not all embryonal neoplasms are equivalent

MICROSCOPIC

- Hypercellularity, round to oval, crowded nuclei with stippled chromatin
- Elevated mitotic activity and frequent apoptotic bodies
- Presence of severe anaplasia at increased frequency (~ 50% of CNS embryonal tumors) compared with medulloblastoma
- Relatively circumscribed, but may infiltrate adjacent brain tissue in some cases

ANCILLARY TESTS

- Synaptophysin expression most common
- Also may express neurofilament protein, chromogranin-A, NeuN
- GFAP expression variable

Enhancing Mass

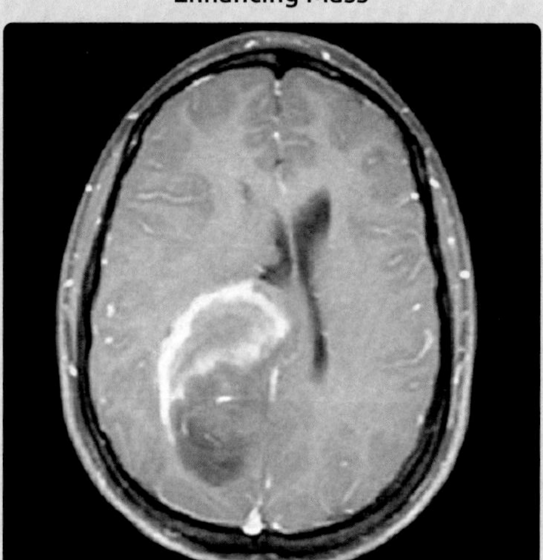

Hypercellularity

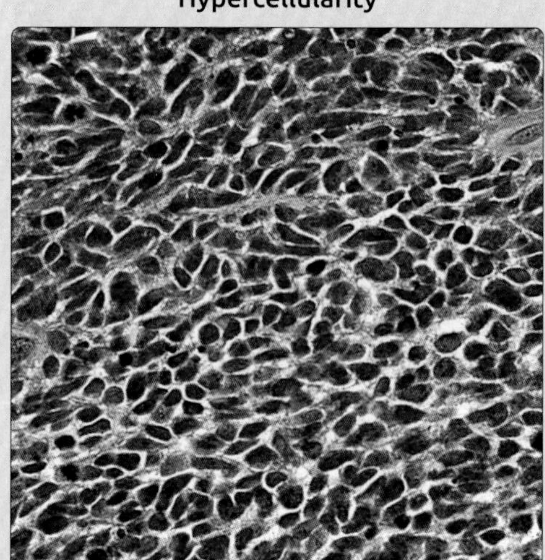

(Left) *CNS embryonal neoplasms may be large, enhancing masses. This lesion has a rim pattern; others are solidly enhancing, and some have surprisingly little enhancement given the overt histological abnormality.* **(Right)** *CNS embryonal neoplasms are highly cellular neoplasms whose diagnosis in undifferentiated cases rests largely on immunohistochemical findings (and even then can be difficult).*

Apoptotic Bodies

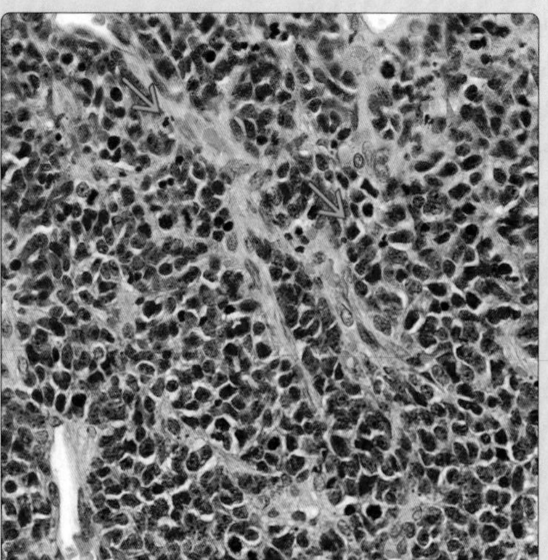

Synaptophysin Immunoreactivity

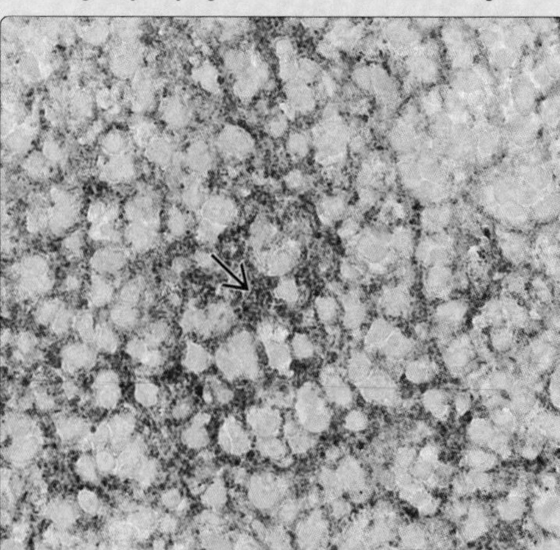

(Left) *In this cellular CNS embryonal neoplasm, conspicuous accumulation of apoptotic bodies is an important feature ⇒. Hypertrophic stromal vessels also impart a vague lobular pattern.* **(Right)** *Synaptophysin immunoreactivity is uniform in cerebral neuroblastoma and highly supportive of the diagnosis. The pattern of reactivity includes labeling of an individual cell or group of cells, as well as background neuropil ⇒.*

TERMINOLOGY

Synonyms

- Embryonal tumor with abundant neuropil and true rosettes (ETANTR)
- Embryonal tumor with multilayered rosettes (ETMR)

Definitions

- Heterogeneous group of embryonal neoplasms composed of poorly differentiated cells that may express neuronal and glial markers
- To be distinguished from primitive neuroectodermal tumor (PNET)-like tissue in some malignant gliomas (e.g., glioblastoma)
- Unrelated to peripheral "PNET" (Ewing sarcoma)
- WHO grade IV

CLINICAL ISSUES

Epidemiology

- Age
  - Predominantly in children (rarely in adults)

Site

- Cerebral hemispheres most frequent
- Near ventricular system in many cases
- Occasionally suprasellar, brainstem, and spinal cord

Presentation

- Symptoms secondary to mass effect, hydrocephalus

Treatment

- Craniospinal irradiation and multimodality chemotherapy

Prognosis

- Highly aggressive with propensity for CSF dissemination
- Overall worse prognosis than medulloblastoma
- May vary by age (children vs. adults)

IMAGING

MR Findings

- Relatively circumscribed compared to infiltrating gliomas
- Variable contrast enhancement
- Spinal MR required in most cases to exclude leptomeningeal dissemination

CT Findings

- Hyperdensity secondary to high cellularity
- Minority may calcify

MICROSCOPIC

Histologic Features

- Hypercellularity, round to oval crowded nuclei with stippled chromatin
- Elevated mitotic activity and frequent apoptotic bodies
- Relatively circumscribed, but may infiltrate
- Variable neuronal and glial differentiation
  - Immunohistochemistry for confirmation
  - Distinction from small cell malignant gliomas problematic, especially in cases with glial differentiation

Cerebral Neuroblastoma

- Applied to types with exclusive primitive neuronal (neuroblastic) differentiation
- Variable patterns, including sheets, rosettes, and palisades
- Fine, fibrillar neuropil in many regions
- Variable desmoplasia
- Mitoses scant to abundant
- Small, ganglioid cells (in some instances)

Ganglioneuroblastoma

- Neuroblastic differentiation, but also containing mature ganglion cells
- Significance of only a few neuroblasts unclear, but treatment similar to PNET

Medulloepithelioma

- Rare subtype predominantly in very young children
- Less frequent stereotypical locations include ciliary body, retina, and optic nerve, but may be separate entities
- Supra- or infratentorial
- Luminal mitoses
- Ribbons with obvious epithelial features, but primitive pseudostratified cells and external, PAS positive, limiting membrane
- Epithelioid ribbons have morphologic overlap with embryonic neural tube

Ependymoblastoma

- Ill-defined category, existence challenged
- Traditionally defined by presence of ependymoblastic or multilayered rosettes in otherwise conventional embryonal neoplasm
- Rosettes mitotically active
- Many ependymoblastomas fall into other more specific embryonal neoplasm categories, usually either ETANTR or medulloepithelioma

Embryonal Tumor With Abundant Neuropil and True Rosettes

- Rare aggressive tumor, usually of first 2 years
- Large, often well-circumscribed mass with little contrast enhancement
- Highly cellular undifferentiated tissue, prominent neuropil and distinctive rosettes with sharply defined lumina
- Neurocytes and small ganglion cells in neuropil areas
- Genetically distinct with frequent amplification at chromosome 19q13.41 microRNA polycistron

Undifferentiated Small Cell Embryonal Tumors

- Subset of tumors, particularly in children, may not demonstrate specific line of differentiation by morphology or immunohistochemistry
- Frequent difficulty arises in categorizing such lesions as high-grade glioma, or undifferentiated primary CNS tumor

Nodular Subtype

- Incompletely characterized
- Similar in part to nodular/desmoplastic medulloblastoma
  - Synaptophysin (+) nodules but no perinodular reticulin

ANCILLARY TESTS

Cytology

- Stippled chromatin similar to neuroendocrine neoplasms; loosely arranged clusters

Immunohistochemistry

- Should express at least 1 marker reflecting neuronal differentiation
  - Synaptophysin expression most common
  - Also may express neurofilament protein, chromogranin-A, NeuN
- GFAP expression variable
  - Difficult to distinguish from high-grade glioma when GFAP(+) and synaptophysin (-)
- Nuclear INI1 labeling uniformly present
- LIN28A immunoreactivity characteristic of ETANTR

Genetic Testing

- Alterations include *RASSIF1A* promoter methylation, *CDKN2A* deletions
- Gain of *PCDHGA3* and *FAM129A*
- High frequency of *TP53* mutations in CNS embryonal neoplasms of adults
- *IDH1* mutations in minority of adult cases suggests overlap with infiltrating gliomas
- Amplification at chromosome 19q13.41 microRNA cluster in subset of CNS embryonal neoplasms, including ETANTR
  - Associated with aggressive biologic behavior
- Presence of i(17q) very rare, as opposed to 30-50% occurrence in medulloblastoma
- 19p, 2p, and 1q gains
- 3 molecular subgroups of CNS embryonal neoplasms in recent study
  - Group 1 (primitive neural): LIN28 expression; shortest overall survival
  - Group 2 (oligoneural): Olig2 expression
  - Group 3 (mesenchymal lineage): LIN28/Olig2 negative
- Molecular signatures and 19q13.41 amplification shared by ETANTR, medulloepithelioma, and ependymoblastoma (grouped under ETMR)

DIFFERENTIAL DIAGNOSIS

Ewing Sarcoma

- Tendency for extradural or intradural extension from bone rather than CNS origin
- Frequent strong CD99 expression, but nonspecific
- Characterized at genetic level by somatic *EWS* rearrangements leading to various fusion transcripts
- Unrelated to CNS embryonal neoplasms

High-Grade Astrocytoma With PNET-Like Tissue Component

- Malignant neoplasm with high-grade infiltrating glioma and sharply circumscribed embryonal neoplasm areas
- GFAP(+) glioma and synaptophysin (+) embryonal neoplasm
- Incomplete sampling of glial component may account for some embryonal neoplasms in adults

High-Grade Astrocytoma

- More conspicuous infiltration at tumor-parenchymal interface
- Predominant expression of GFAP over neuronal markers favors infiltrating astrocytoma
- Difficult to distinguish from undifferentiated primary CNS tumor without expression of synaptophysin or GFAP

Anaplastic Ependymoma

- Overlaps practically with ependymoblastoma
- Well-developed pseudorosettes (at least focally)
- GFAP(+) (particularly in perivascular areas)
- EMA(+) dot-like or surface immunoreactivity in some, but not all, cases
- Little, if any, synaptophysin (+) neuropil

Anaplastic Oligodendroglioma

- Classic low-grade oligodendroglioma often present
- Often GFAP(+) (at least focally)
- Codeletion of 1p and 19q

Metastatic Small Cell Carcinoma

- Must be excluded always in adults
- Frequently cytokeratin and TTF-1(+), regardless of site of origin

Neurocytoma

- Low cellularity, more uniform cytologically, low Ki-67

Olfactory Neuroblastoma (Esthesioneuroblastoma)

- Must be excluded in adults (usually not diagnostic consideration in children)
- Clinical manifestations include epistaxis &/or nasal obstruction
- Cribriform plate involvement
- Involvement of CNS by direct extension (frontal lobes in particular)
  - Intradural, extraparenchymal involvement rather than intraparenchymal (as with CNS embryonal neoplasms)
- Lobular architecture and delicate vascular stroma

DIAGNOSTIC CHECKLIST

Pathologic Interpretation Pearls

- Consider supratentorial embryonal neoplasm in high-grade, relatively circumscribed cellular neoplasms in children
- Distinguishing embryonal neoplasm from anaplastic small cell gliomas is therapeutically relevant, but often difficult
- When considering embryonal neoplasm in adults think of high-grade astrocytoma with PNET component

SELECTED REFERENCES

1. Korshunov A et al: Embryonal tumor with abundant neuropil and true rosettes (ETANTR), ependymoblastoma, and medulloepithelioma share molecular similarity and comprise a single clinicopathological entity. Acta Neuropathol. 128(2):279-89, 2014
2. Judkins AR et al: Ependymoblastoma: dear, damned, distracting diagnosis, farewell*!. Brain Pathol. 20(1):133-9, 2010
3. Gessi M et al: Embryonal tumors with abundant neuropil and true rosettes: a distinctive CNS primitive neuroectodermal tumor. Am J Surg Pathol. 33(2):211-7, 2009
4. Li M et al: Frequent amplification of a chr19q13.41 microRNA polycistron in aggressive primitive neuroectodermal brain tumors. Cancer Cell. 16(6):533-46, 2009

Homer Wright Rosettes

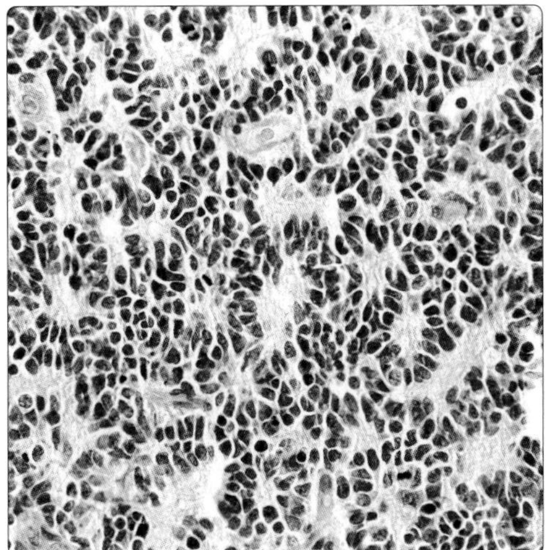

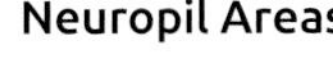

Neuropil Areas

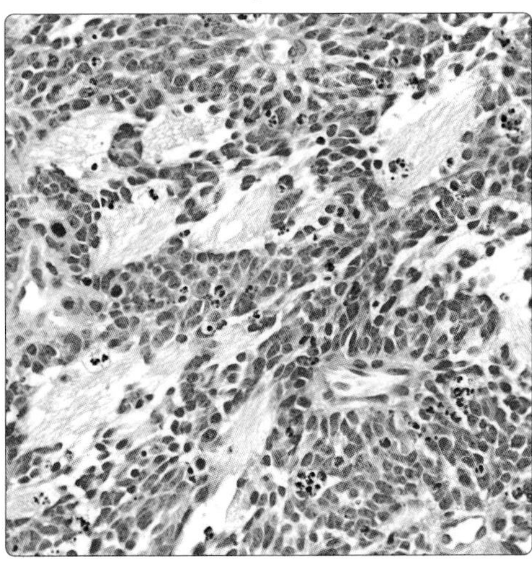

(Left) *Classic neuroblastic Homer Wright rosettes establish an unequivocal neuroblastic nature, and a clear place within the embryonal neoplasm group. Such lesions are rare, like other CNS embryonal neoplasms.* **(Right)** *Somewhat larger than neuroblastic Homer Wright rosettes, pale areas of neuropil are equally specific for neuroblastic differentiation. Both of these structures, and the cores of neuroblastic rosettes, would be immunoreactive for synaptophysin.*

Mixed Ganglion Cell and Neuroblastic Differentiation

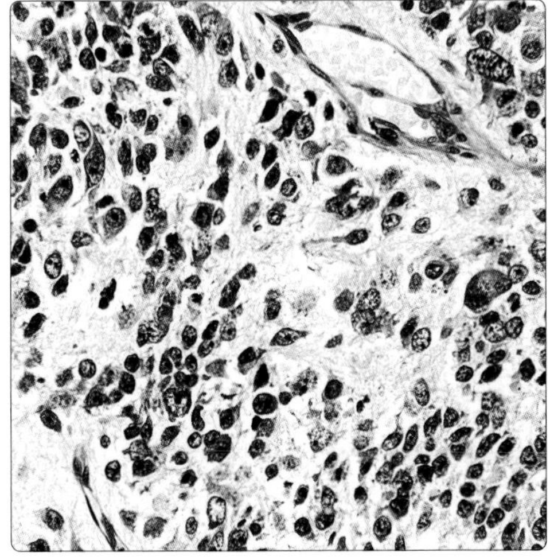

Ganglioneuroblastoma

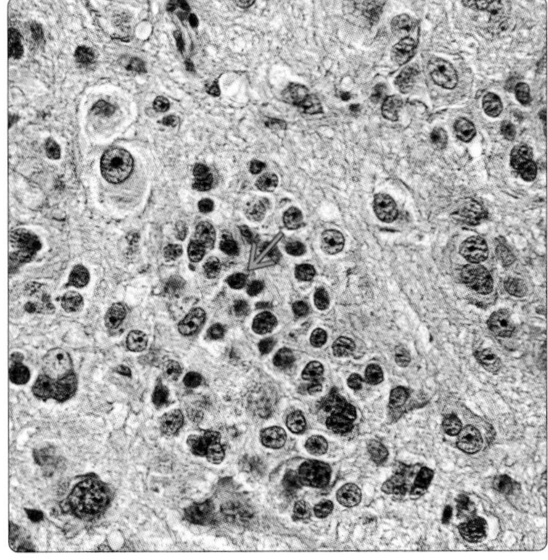

(Left) *Tumors with mixed ganglion cell and neuroblastic differentiation are difficult to classify as dedifferentiated ganglion cell tumors or differentiating neuroblastomas.* **(Right)** *Lesions with both ganglion cells, smaller gangliod cells, and small neuroblasts* → *are known as either ganglioneuroblastoma or dedifferentiating ganglion cell tumors. There is no consensus on terminology, grading, or treatment of these borderline lesions.*

Well-Defined Epithelial Surfaces

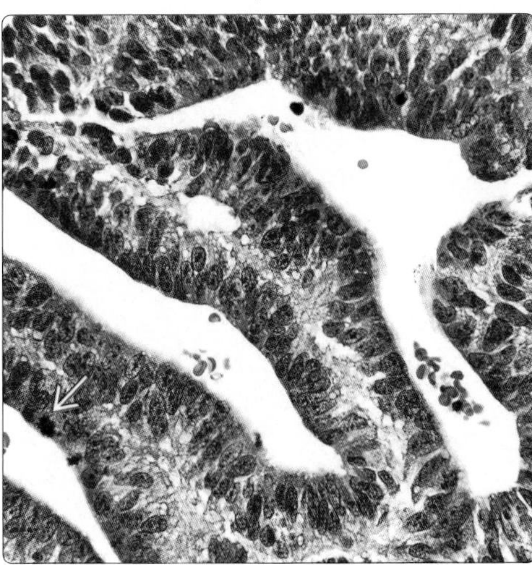

Luminal Mitoses

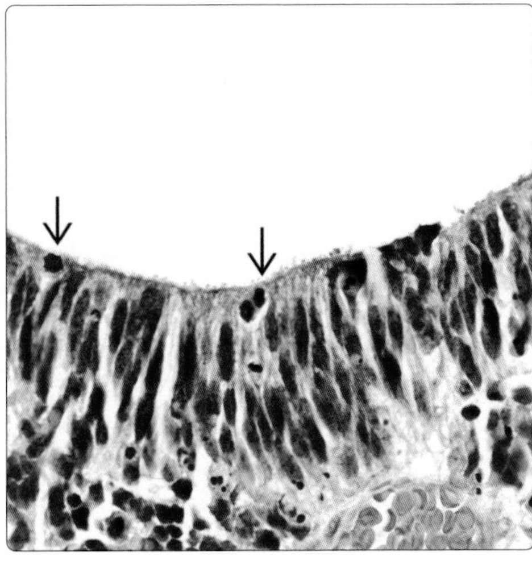

(Left) *Well-defined epithelial surfaces define the rare medulloepithelioma neoplasm that recapitulates the embryonic neural tube. Mitoses* ➡ *are characteristically located superficially, near the lumen side of the epithelium.* **(Right)** *Mitoses* → *in medulloepitheliomas are characteristically concentrated just below the lumen.*

(Left) *The defining property of ependymoblastoma, ependymoblastic rosettes* ➡, *represent epithelial, lumen-containing structures that resemble true rosettes of ependymoma but have the small cell primitive background of embryonal neoplasms. Existence of the entity has been challenged.* **(Right)** *Ependymoblastoma is a controversial embryonal neoplasm subtype. Most neoplasms interpreted as ependymoblastomas are nonspecific, highly cellular, primitive, and mitotically active over most of the tumor.*

Ependymoblastic Rosettes

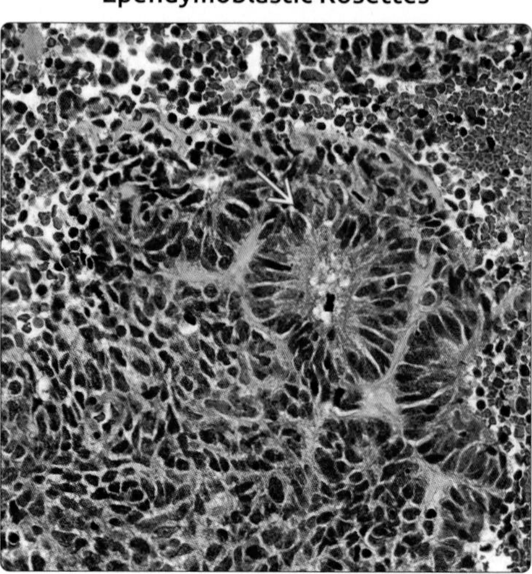

Ependymoblastoma

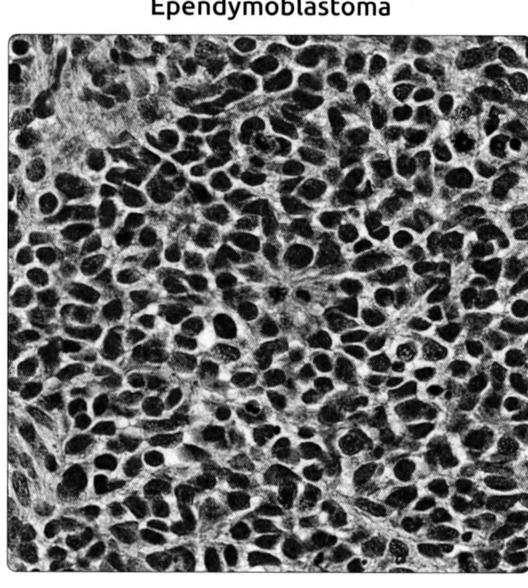

(Left) *Embryonal tumors with abundant neuropil and true rosettes (ETANTR) are crisscrossed by bands of prominent, finely fibrillar neuropil* ➡*. The tumor's relationship to ependymoblastoma is controversial.* **(Right)** *Neurite-rich neuropil areas* ➡ *in ETANTRs are appropriately immunoreactive for neurofilament protein. The same areas would also be strongly positive for synaptophysin.*

ETANTR

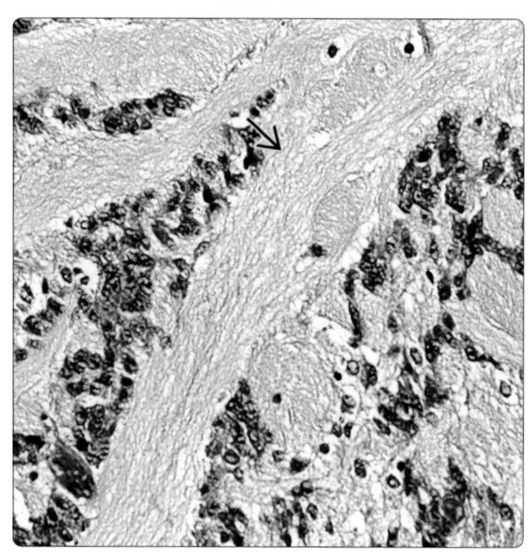

Neurite-Rich Neuropil Areas

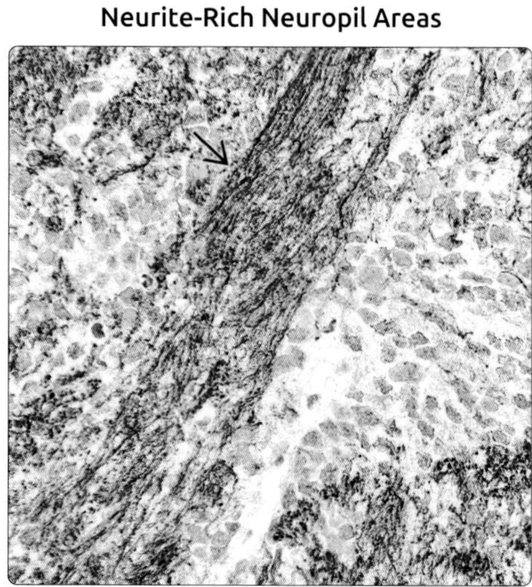

(Left) *Focal, densely cellular aggregates forming lumen-containing rosettes sit in a finely fibrillar, paucicellular tumor background, the latter somewhat resembling normal gray matter.* **(Right)** *Rosettes in ETANTRs have well-defined lumina* ➡*, although, some up-and-down focusing may be necessary for identification. Apoptosis is prominent in this case. This rare tumor has what appears to be a defining molecular signature (i.e., amplification at chromosome 19q13.41 microRNA polycistron).*

Lumen-Containing Rosettes

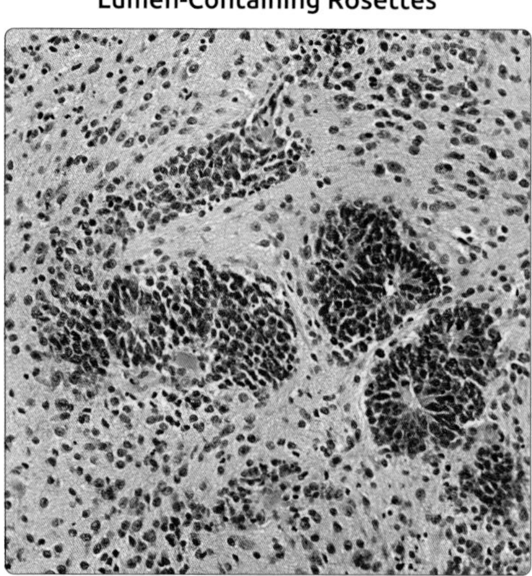

Rosettes With Well-Defined Lumina

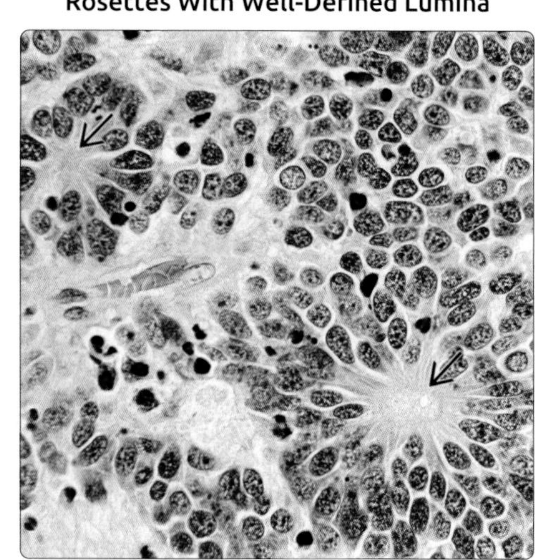

Medulloblastoma-Like Nodule

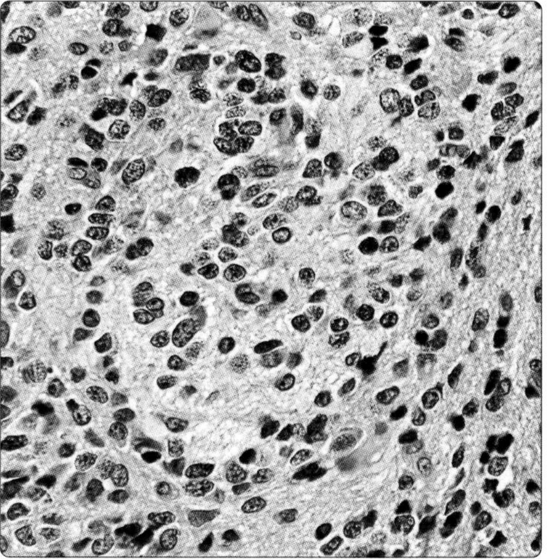

Medulloblastoma-Like Nodule

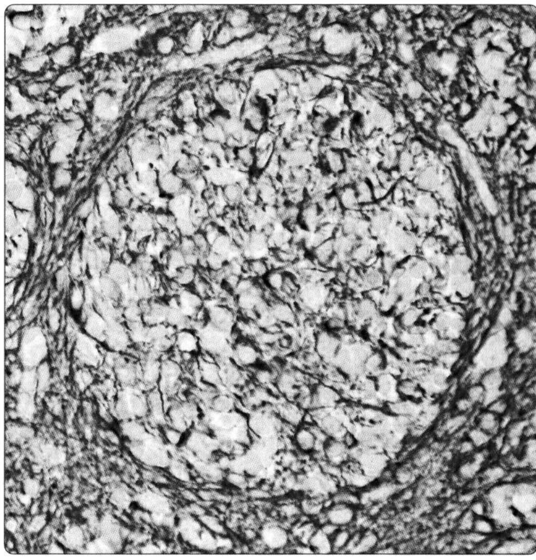

(Left) *A variant of CNS embryonal neoplasms (supratentorial, in this case) contains medulloblastoma-like nodules, but without the surrounding reticulin.* **(Right)** *Well-defined nodules in CNS embryonal neoplasms are characterized by strong immunoreactivity for synaptophysin, both in the nodule and surrounding tissue. In part, this CNS embryonal neoplasm variant resembles nodular/desmoplastic medulloblastoma. Unlike the latter tumor, nodules in this rare supratentorial lesion are not reticulin bound.*

CNS Embryonal Neoplasms in Familial Adenomatous Polyposis

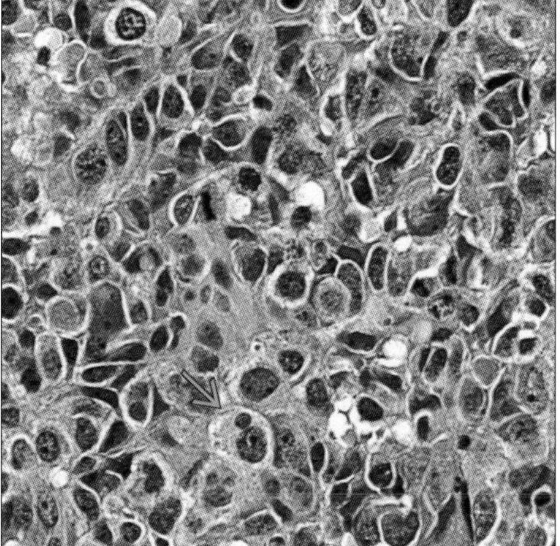

Nuclear β-Catenin Staining

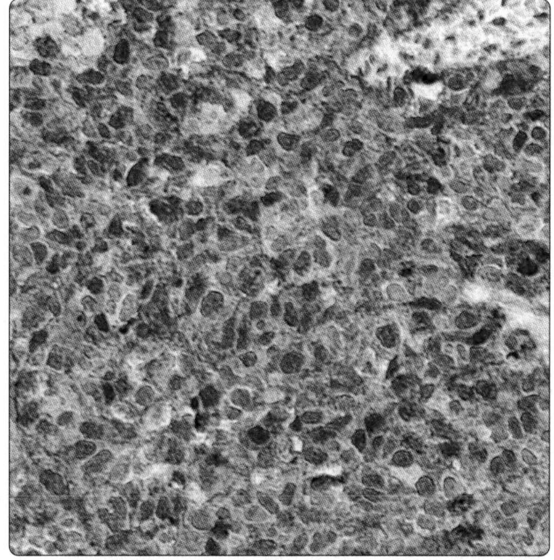

(Left) *Supratentorial CNS embryonal neoplasms can arise in familial adenomatous polyposis (FAP) syndrome. This example has considerable nuclear variability and large cells with a ganglioid appearance* ⇨*.* **(Right)** *Nuclear β-catenin staining (seen in this CNS embryonal neoplasm patient with FAP), reflects activation of the Wnt signaling pathway; this pathway is also operational in a subset of medulloblastomas.*

Synaptophysin Reactivity in PNET Component

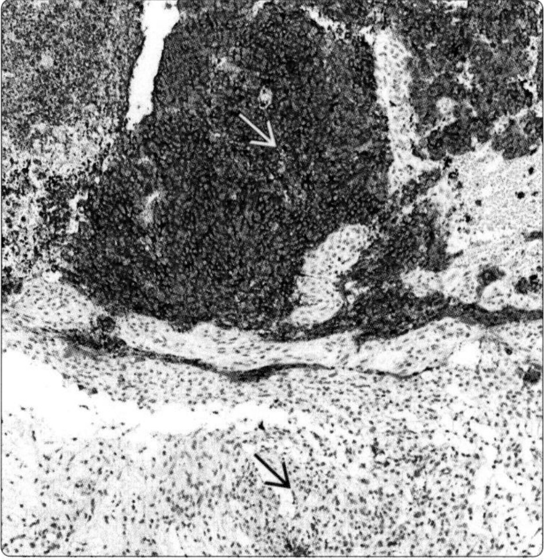

GFAP Immunoreactivity in Glial Component

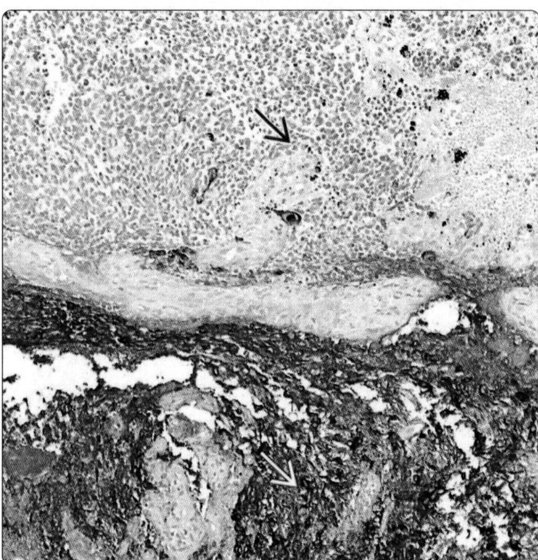

(Left) *Strong immunoreactivity for synaptophysin* ➡ *highlights embryonal tissue in this high-grade astrocytoma with a PNET component. The glial component* ⇨ *is negative.* **(Right)** *Strong immunoreactivity for GFAP* ➡ *highlights glioma tissue in this high-grade astrocytoma with a PNET component. The embryonal component* ⇨ *is negative.*

KEY FACTS

TERMINOLOGY

- Ependymoblastoma, medulloepithelioma now recognized to be same entity, fused into ETMR classification
- Any CNS embryonal tumor with C19MC amplification or fusion given ETMR designation, including those without distinctive histopathological features (such as true rosettes)

CLINICAL ISSUES

- Usually < 3 years
- Intracranial, supratentorial more common than cerebellum, brainstem
- Leptomeningeal dissemination, even extraneural metastases seen in later phases of disease
- Poor prognosis; highly aggressive

MICROSCOPIC

- Highly cellular unstructured primitive areas
- Paucicellular finely fibrillar neuropil
- True rosettes
- Focal differentiation, in neuropil areas, to neurocytes and ganglion cells in some cases
- Rosette lumina delineated by zone composed of cell-cell junctions
- Features of anaplasia similar to anaplastic medulloblastoma in some cases

ANCILLARY TESTS

- Synaptophysin (+), especially neuropil areas
- Amplification 19q13.42
- LIN28A(+)

DIAGNOSTIC CHECKLIST

- Abundant neuropil highly suggestive of entity
- Rosettes may be inconspicuous
- Rosettes possess true lumen, not of Homer Wright type

(Left) *As in this T2WI of a cerebellar example, the lesion is often well circumscribed and massive in size. Embryonal tumors with multilayered true rosettes (ETMRs) are more common in the cerebrum but also occur in brain stem and cerebellum.* **(Right)** *ETMR has a propensity to metastasize to the cerebrospinal fluid. Note the multifocal opacification of basilar meninges ➡, including near the optic chiasm.*

Often Well Circumscribed

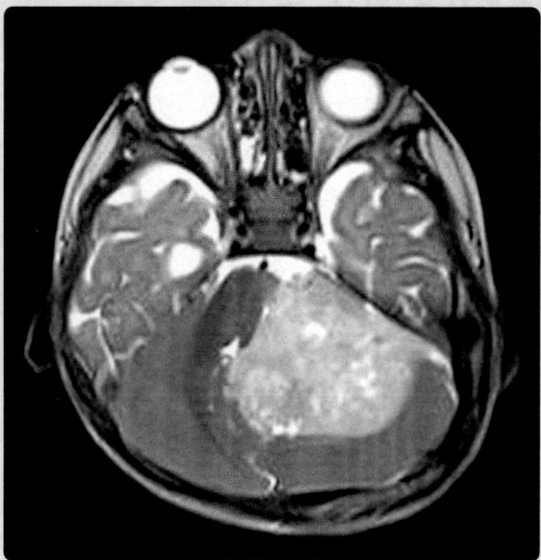

Leptomeningeal Metastases

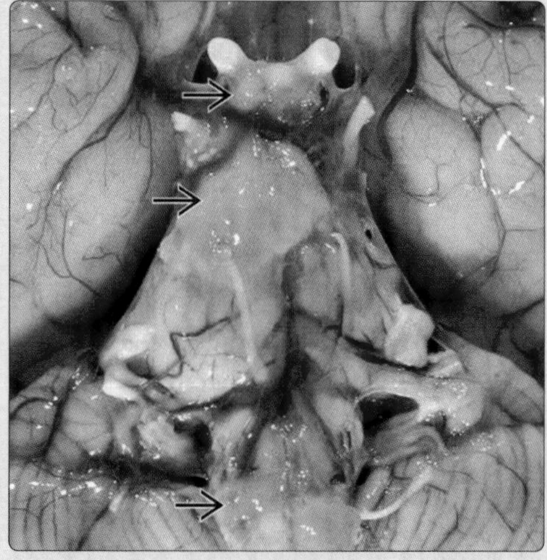

(Left) *Distinctively, the tumor combines finely fibrillar neuropil ➡ and true, lumen-containing rosettes ➡.* **(Right)** *LIN28A is usually strongly positive in the small cell component of ETMR and negative in medulloblastoma, which might enter the differential diagnosis. However, LIN28A immunoreactivity is also seen in germ cell tumors and hence is not completely specific to ETMR.*

Neuropil With True Rosettes

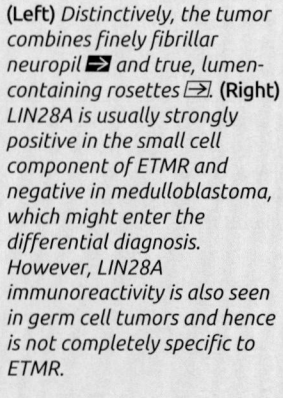

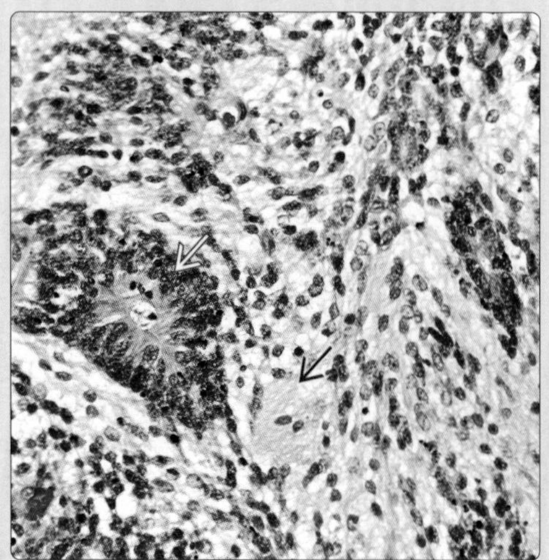

LIN28A

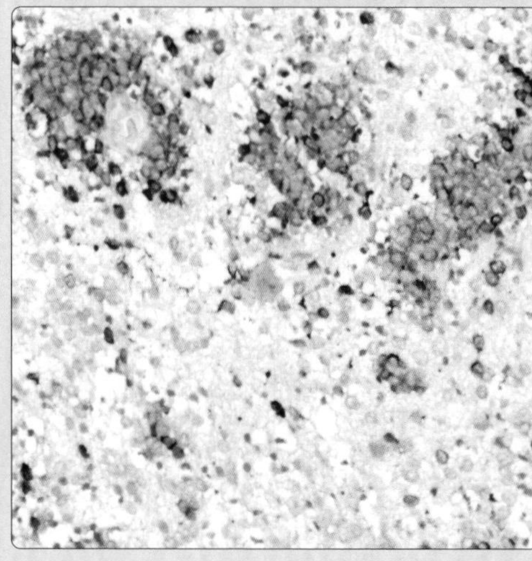

TERMINOLOGY

Abbreviations

- Embryonal tumor with multilayered true rosettes (ETMR), C19MC altered

Synonyms

- Includes embryonal tumor with abundant neuropil and true rosettes (ETANTR)

Definitions

- Now defined by alterations in C19MC locus at 19q13.42 (amplification and fusions)
- ETMR, ependymoblastoma, and subset of medulloepithelioma now recognized as single entity
- Embryonal tumor formed of finely fibrillar neuropil and lumen-containing, true rosettes
  - Any CNS embryonal tumor with C19MC amplification or fusion given ETMR designation, including those without distinctive histopathological features

CLINICAL ISSUES

Epidemiology

- Age
  - Usually < 3 years
- Sex
  - F > M

Site

- Intracranial, both supra- and infratentorial

Presentation

- Signs of increased intracranial pressure

Treatment

- Surgical approaches
  - Resection
- Adjuvant therapy
  - Chemotherapy
- Radiation
  - In some cases, despite patient age

Prognosis

- Poor, highly aggressive
  - Most die within 36 months; median survival: ~ 9 months
- Potential for cerebrospinal fluid (CSF) seeding, even extraneural metastases in late stages of disease

IMAGING

MR Findings

- Large, may be well circumscribed

MACROSCOPIC

General Features

- Fleshy, reddish-gray; may cause widespread CSF metastases

Size

- ≤ 10 cm

MICROSCOPIC

Histologic Features

- Highly cellular, unstructured primitive areas
- Paucicellular, finely fibrillar neuropil
- True rosettes
  - In highly cellular areas or arising abruptly in areas of neuropil
  - May be focal and inconspicuous
  - Lumen small and round or large and slit-like
  - Sharply defined luminal surface
  - Intraluminal granular debris
  - Lumina delineated by zone composed of cell-cell junctions
- Neurocytes and ganglion cells in neuropil areas in some cases
- Perivascular formations uncommon
- Features of anaplasia in some cases
  - Large cell size
  - Nuclear molding, cell-cell wrapping
  - Abundant apoptosis and mitoses

ANCILLARY TESTS

Immunohistochemistry

- Synaptophysin (+), especially neuropil areas; GFAP only focally if at all (+); LIN28A(+)

Genetic Testing

- Amplification 19q13.42 (now definitional of entity)

Electron Microscopy

- Microtubule-containing neurites
- Cell-cell junctions around rosette lumina

DIFFERENTIAL DIAGNOSIS

Medulloblastoma

- Sparse if any neuropil, except in nodular types
- Neuroblastic, Homer Wright-type rosettes, rather than true, lumen-containing rosettes

Anaplastic Ependymoma

- Fibrillar perivascular pseudorosettes; GFAP(+); EMA(+): Dot-like pattern of microlumina; surface staining, focal

Other Embryonal Tumors

- Lack amplification 19q13.42, usually not LIN28a(+); little, if any, neuropil; rosettes, if any, of Homer Wright type

DIAGNOSTIC CHECKLIST

Pathologic Interpretation Pearls

- Histological features highly variable; entity now defined by genetic signature
- Abundant neuropil highly suggestive of entity; rosettes may be focal and inconspicuous
- LIN28A protein expression not exclusive to ETANTR: Seen in most germ cell tumors

SELECTED REFERENCES

1. Edmonson CA et al: Embryonal tumor with multilayered rosettes of the fourth ventricle: case report. J Neurosurg Pediatr. 1-5, 2015

(Left) *The biphasic tumor contains finely fibrillar neuropil ⇨ and multiple true, lumen-containing rosettes ➡. Many examples lack such abundant rosettes, making genetic testing/LIN28A IHC mandatory.* **(Right)** *Strands of highly cellular tissue stream through neuropil that is not as abundant in this case as it is in most examples. Any doubts as to the presence of neuropil can be resolved by the component's strong immunopositivity for synaptophysin and negative reaction for GFAP. The tumor should be LIN28A(+).*

Multiple Rosettes

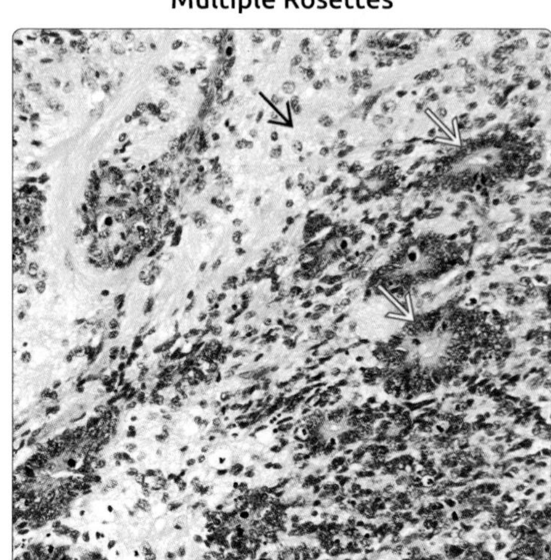

Less Typical Appearance

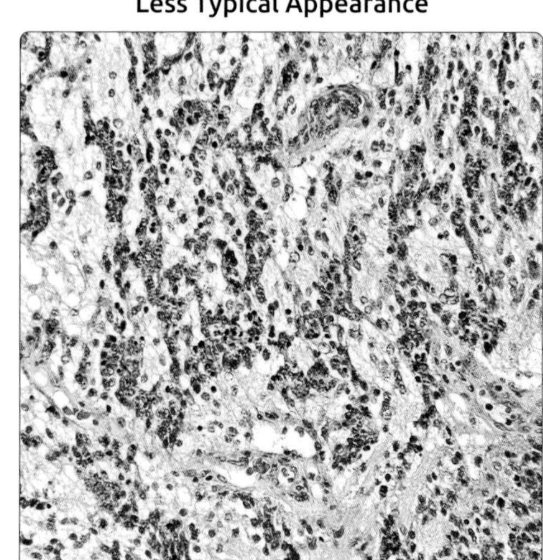

(Left) *Finely fibrillar, almost anuclear bands of neuropil ⇨ are 1 of the lesion's 2 signature features. Rosettes, the other, are not present here. However, any CNS embryonal tumor with C19MC amplification or fusion is to be given EMTR diagnosis, including those without distinctive histopathological features.* **(Right)** *Neuropil may dominate areas of the lesion, leaving only focal, highly cellular areas ⇨. Careful up-and-down focusing sometimes reveals small round lumina in such ostensibly undifferentiated areas.*

Area Lacking Rosettes

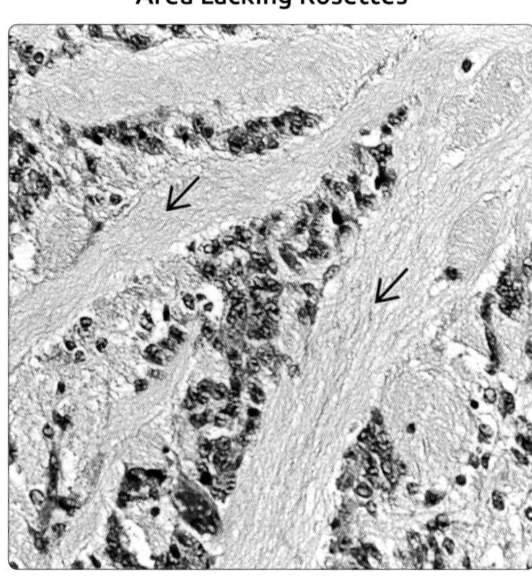

Only Focal Hypercellular Areas

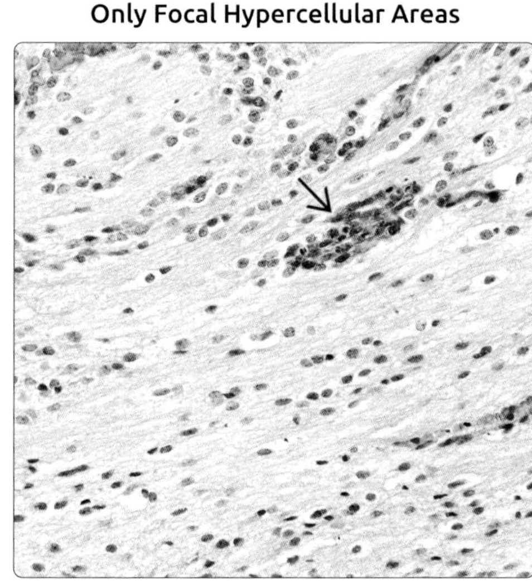

(Left) *Differentiation to neurocytes and small ganglion cells ⇨ occurs in some cases. Diagnosis by definition requires C19MC amplification or fusion and testing can be especially important in examples with unusual histological features.* **(Right)** *Diagnostically important small lumina ⇨ may be inconspicuous in highly cellular areas. The presence of abundant neuropil elsewhere in the tumor should encourage a search for such structures. The sharp eosinophilic border to the microlumina is a helpful diagnostic feature.*

Differentiation to Small Ganglion Cells

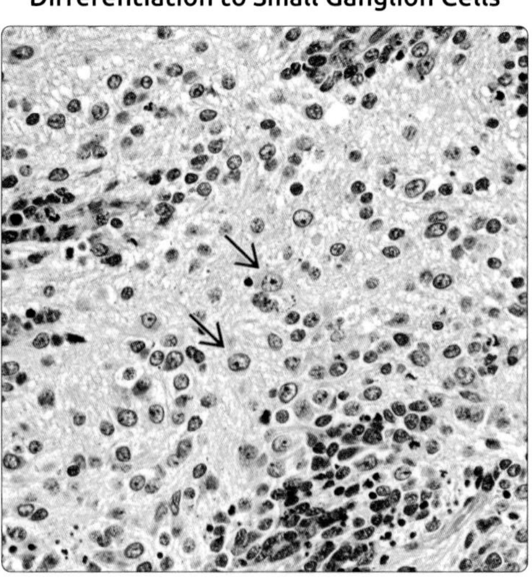

Small Lumina With Sharp Borders

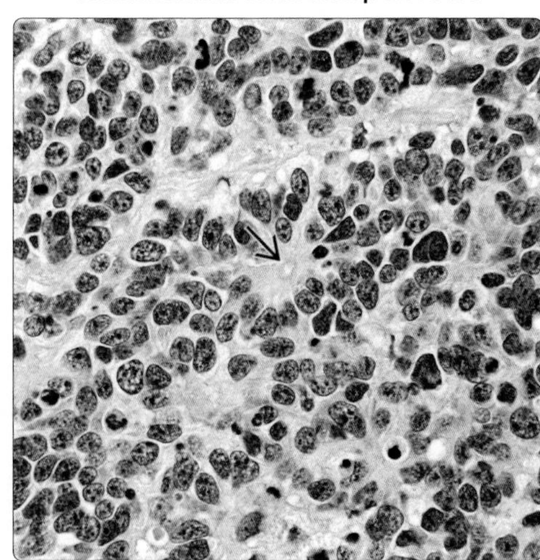

Intraluminal Granular Debris

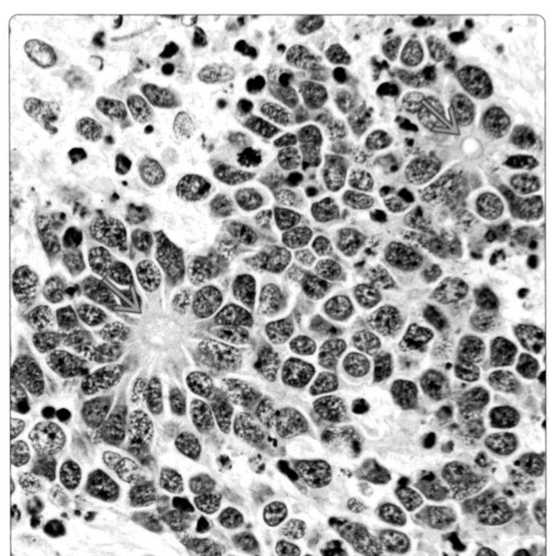

Subapical Granular Band Unlike Ependymoma

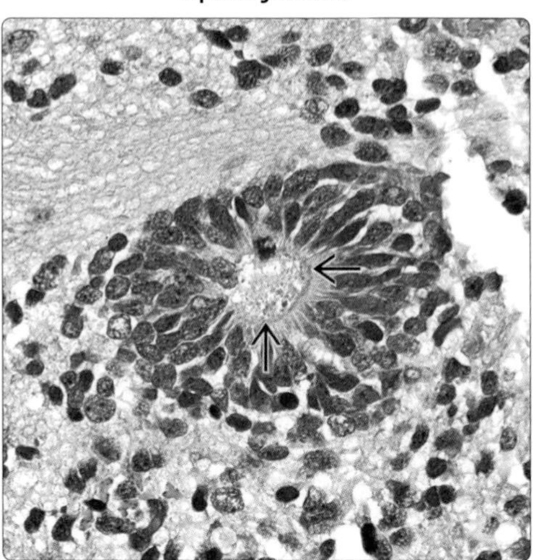

(Left) *Rosette lumina are often circular, as here, or sometimes slit-like. In aggregate, cell-cell connections near the lumen form a circular zone* ➡*, typical of the entity. Note the scant amount of intraluminal granular eosinophilic debris that can sometimes be seen within the lumina.* **(Right)** *Characteristic of the lesion is a subapical, darkly eosinophilic, granular band* ➡ *not present in ependymomas. CNS embryonal tumors with C19MC amplification or fusion should be given EMTR diagnosis.*

Simulating Ependymoma

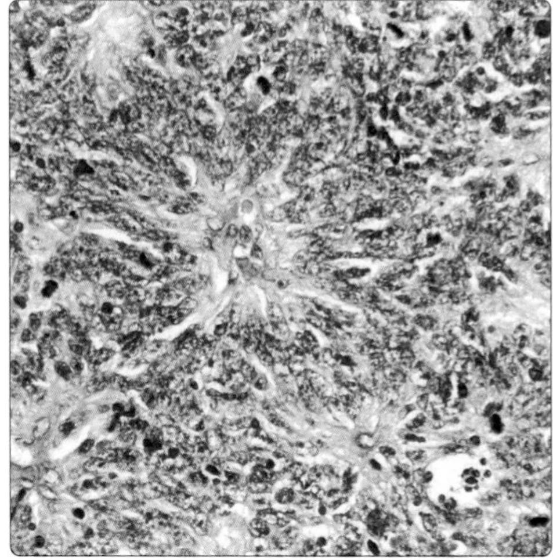

Anaplasia

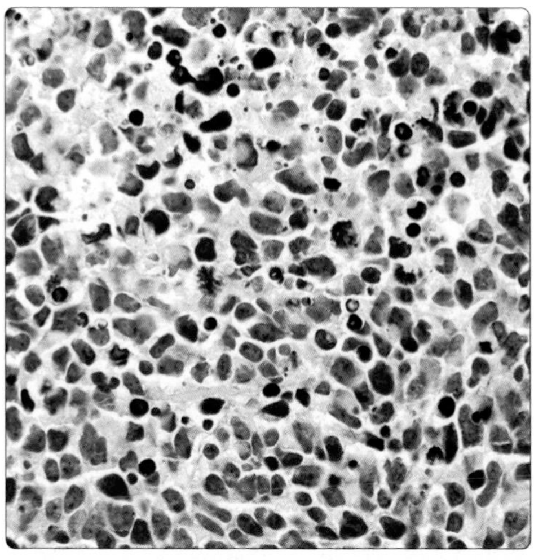

(Left) *Crude perivascular pseudorosettes are focal findings. The lesion, however, is a neuroblastic (not a glial) tumor. GFAP staining in ETMR is usually confined to scattered reactive astrocytes, unlike ependymoma where GFAP often highlights perivascular pseudorosettes. Ependymoma is further negative for LIN28A.* **(Right)** *Anaplasia, as occurs in some medulloblastomas, is present in some ETMRs. It is characterized by larger cell size, nuclear molding, and abundant mitotic activity and apoptosis.*

Synaptophysin (+) Neuropil

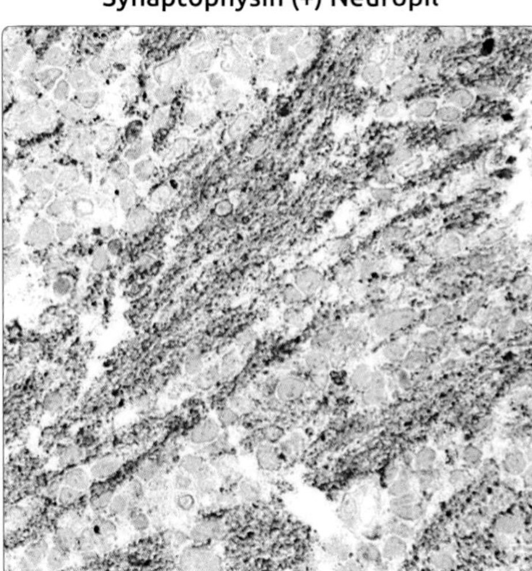

Neurofilament (+) Neuropil

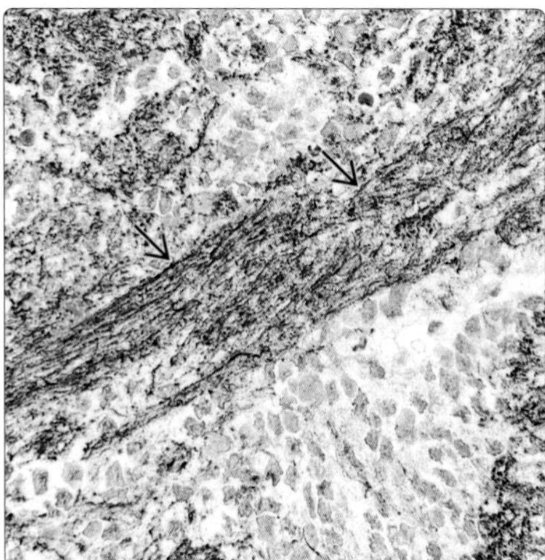

(Left) *Paucicellular regions of neuropil are strongly immunoreactive for synaptophysin. Those ETMRs without neuropil often fall into what was formerly called ependymoblastoma, a tumor now recognized to be ETMR.* **(Right)** *In aggregate, neurofilament protein-positive axons* ➡ *form neuropil. Cellular areas are usually negative. Some medulloblastomas also have neuropil but are confined to nodules in the nodular/desmoplastic type, especially the extensively nodular subtype.*

KEY FACTS

TERMINOLOGY

- Unrelated to intraparenchymal CNS embryonal tumors

ETIOLOGY/PATHOGENESIS

- Somatic rearrangements in *EWSR1* gene result in fusion transcripts with aberrant transcriptional, protumorigenic activity

CLINICAL ISSUES

- In CNS, secondary extension from epidural space, skull bones, or metastases to spine most common
- Primary dural locations intracranially or in spine (extraaxial)
- Aggressive neoplasms but long-term survival in patients with localized disease in recent years

MICROSCOPIC

- Sheets or lobules of cells with round to oval nuclei and variable cytoplasm
- Highly cellular, lack of significant stroma
- May infiltrate adjacent structures (e.g., nerve roots)
- High mitotic rate and necrosis (frequent)
- Homer Wright rosettes (rare)

ANCILLARY TESTS

- Cytology
  - Fine, delicate chromatin and small nucleoli
  - Scant amphophilic to clear cytoplasm
- Periodic acid-Schiff positivity
- Various fusion transcripts, usually involving *EWSR1* gene, by RT-PCR or FISH are almost definitional
- CD99(+), membranous pattern in majority of cases

TOP DIFFERENTIAL DIAGNOSES

- Medulloblastoma/CNS embryonal tumors
- Pediatric round blue cell tumors
- Small cell glioblastoma
- Lymphoma

(Left) *Ewing sarcoma affecting the central nervous system usually presents as an extraaxial, dural-based mass, or, as in this example ⇒, from adjacent bone (postcontrast T1WI MR).* **(Right)** *The cells of Ewing sarcoma are characterized by cytologic monotony and round to oval nuclei with fine chromatin. Variable amounts of clear cytoplasm and vague lobularity are typical.*

Extraaxial Mass

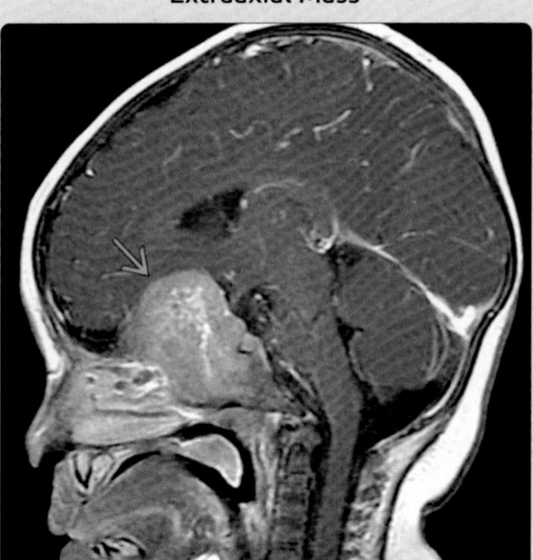

Cytologic Monotony

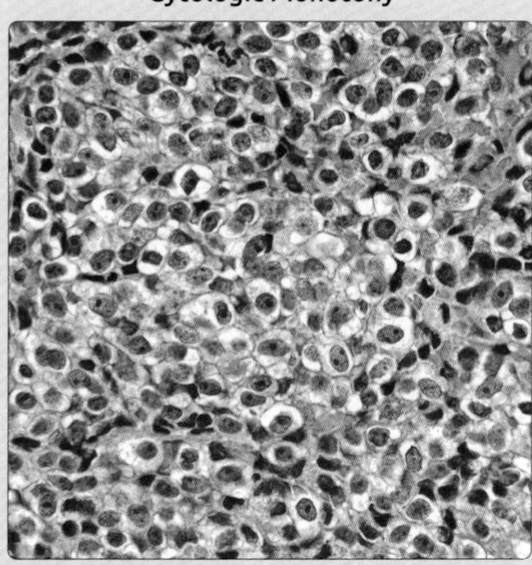

(Left) *Increased cytoplasmic glycogen is a frequent feature of Ewing sarcoma, may be highlighted by PAS without diastase, and is responsible for cytoplasmic clearing at the H&E level.* **(Right)** *Strong membranous CD99 immunoreactivity is present in almost all Ewing sarcomas. However, immunopositivity is not specific and is frequent in other round blue cell tumors in the differential diagnosis.*

Cytoplasmic Glycogen

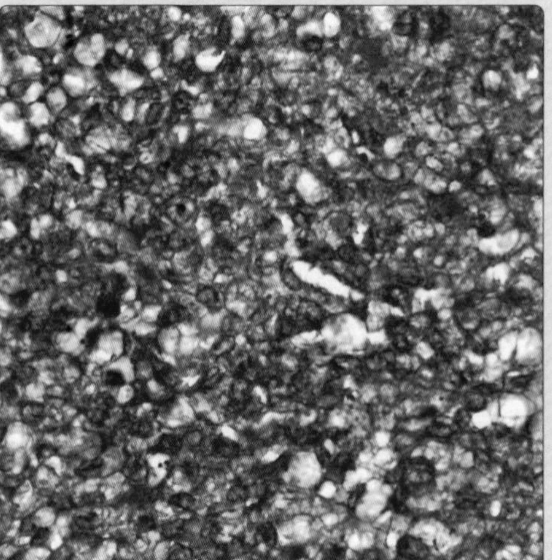

Membranous CD99

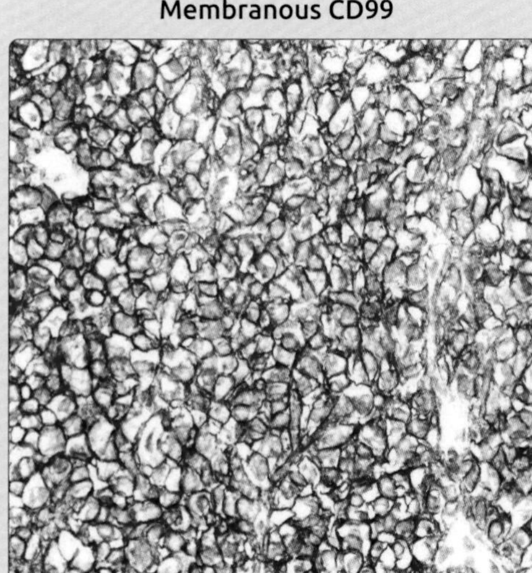

TERMINOLOGY

Definitions

- Malignant small round blue cell tumor with rearrangements in *EWSR1* gene
- Unrelated to intraparenchymal CNS round blue cell/embryonal tumors

ETIOLOGY/PATHOGENESIS

Genetic

- Somatic rearrangements in *EWSR1* gene result in fusion transcripts with aberrant transcriptional, protumorigenic activity

CLINICAL ISSUES

Site

- Favors lower extremities and chest wall in children and teenagers
- In CNS, secondary extension from epidural space, skull bones, or metastases to spine most common
- Primary locations include
  - Cauda equina/filum terminale
  - Intracranial or intraspinal dura (extraaxial)
  - Peripheral nerve

Treatment

- Irradiation and multiagent chemotherapy

Prognosis

- Aggressive neoplasms but long-term survival in patients with localized disease in recent years
- Some primary intraspinal examples recur with disseminated leptomeningeal disease

IMAGING

MR Findings

- Enhancing masses with dural tails may mimic meningioma intracranially

CT Findings

- Best demonstrates bone destruction

MICROSCOPIC

Histologic Features

- Sheets or lobules of cells with round to oval nuclei and variable cytoplasm
- Highly cellular, lack of significant stroma
- May infiltrate adjacent structures (e.g., nerve roots)
- High mitotic rate and necrosis (frequent)
- Homer Wright rosettes (rare)

ANCILLARY TESTS

Cytology

- Fine, delicate chromatin and small nucleoli
- Scant amphophilic to clear cytoplasm

Histochemistry

- Periodic acid-Schiff
  - Reactivity: Variable staining without diastase, reflecting glycogen
  - Staining pattern: Cytoplasmic

Immunohistochemistry

- CD99(+), membranous pattern in majority of cases
  - Also (+) in variety of morphologic mimics but usually (-) in CNS embryonal tumors
- Nuclear FLI-1 immunoreactivity in majority
- Neural markers (synaptophysin, chromogranin) variably (+)
- Cytokeratins (+) in minority of cases, usually isolated cells

Genetic Testing

- Various fusion transcripts, usually involving *EWSR1* gene, by RT-PCR or FISH are almost definitional
  - *EWSR1-FLI1* fusion transcript most common
  - *EWSR1-ERG* in minority of cases
  - Less commonly, *EWSR1* fusions to *ETV1*, *ETV4*, or *FEV*
- t(11;22)(q24;q12) resulting in *EWSR1-FLI1* fusion in majority of cases (80-90%)
- t(21;22) in others

DIFFERENTIAL DIAGNOSIS

Medulloblastoma/Central Nervous System Embryonal Tumors

- Principal differential diagnosis in CNS
- Intraparenchymal
- CD99 expression absent to weak
- Lack *EWSR1* rearrangements

Pediatric Round Blue Cell Tumors

- Includes neuroblastoma, alveolar rhabdomyosarcoma, poorly differentiated synovial sarcoma, desmoplastic round blue cell tumor, mesenchymal chondrosarcoma, and unclassifiable tumors
- Distinction rests on immunohistochemical and molecular features

Small Cell Glioblastoma

- Intraparenchymal location and radiologic characteristics of high-grade glioma (e.g., ring enhancement)
- Microvascular proliferation
- GFAP(+), in substantial subset

Lymphoma

- Dyscohesive architecture
- Lymphoid markers (+)

DIAGNOSTIC CHECKLIST

Clinically Relevant Pathologic Features

- Usually extraaxial compared with CNS embryonal tumors

Pathologic Interpretation Pearls

- CD99 also (+) in variety of morphologic mimics, but usually (-) in CNS embryonal tumors

SELECTED REFERENCES

1. Karikari IO et al: Primary intradural extraosseous Ewing sarcoma of the spine: case report and literature review. Neurosurgery. 69(4):E995-9, 2011
2. Mateen FJ et al: Spinal intradural extraosseous Ewing's sarcoma. Rare Tumors. 3(1):e7, 2011

(Left) *Ewing sarcomas are highly cellular tumors and prototypical of round blue cell tumors common in children. Sheets of monotonous cells with high nuclear:cytoplasmic ratios are typical.* **(Right)** *The presence of variable amounts of clear cytoplasm suggests the diagnosis of Ewing sarcoma in a round blue tumor. Cytoplasmic clearing is, in part, the result of glycogen accumulation.*

Prototypical Round Blue Cell Tumor

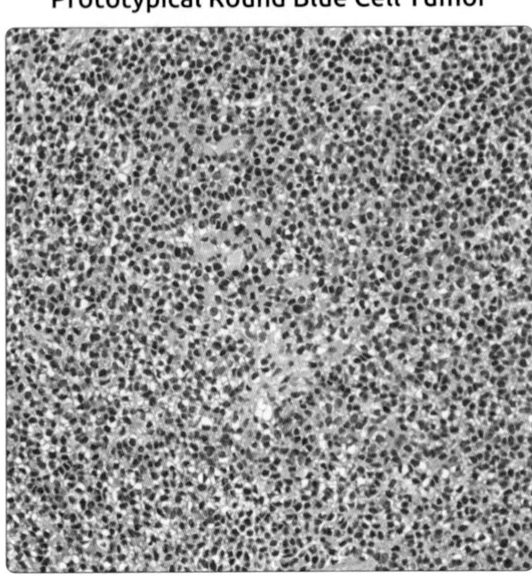

Clear Cytoplasm

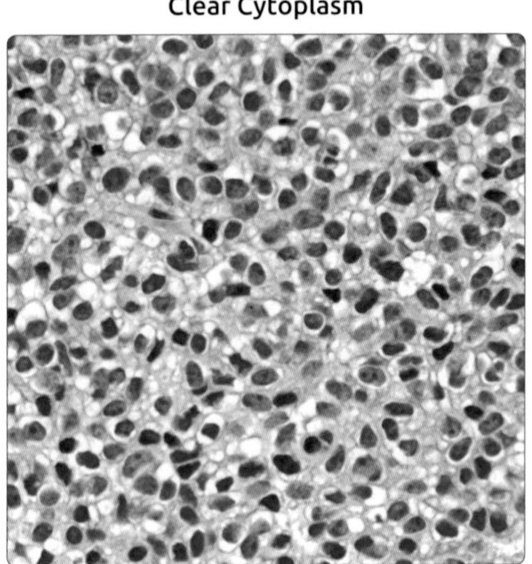

(Left) *Some Ewing sarcomas have somewhat more eosinophilic cytoplasm and larger nucleoli. Nuclei are, nevertheless, cytologically rather bland.* **(Right)** *A subset of Ewing sarcoma contains well-developed Homer Wright-type rosettes. Despite this feature of overt neuroblastic differentiation, such tumors are considered within the morphologic spectrum of the same entity.*

Eosinophilic Cytoplasm and Nucleoli

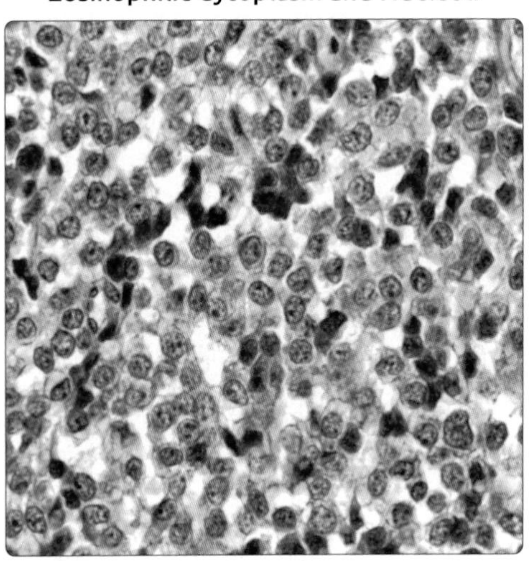

Homer Wright-Type Rosettes

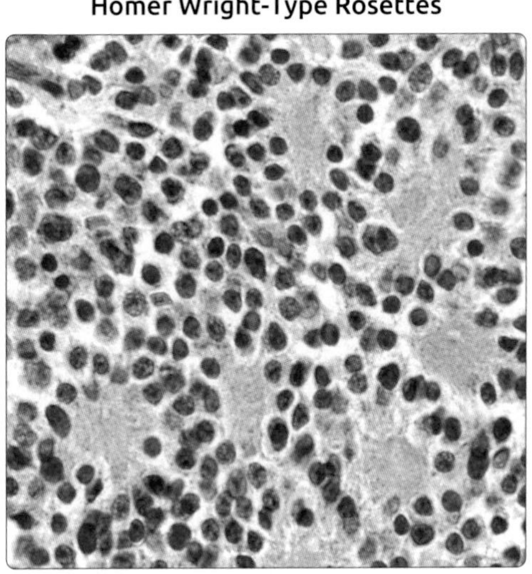

(Left) *Prominent infiltration of nerve roots may be a feature in some Ewing sarcomas, particularly those of the spine. Such involvement may represent secondary extension from vertebral bones, while, in others, it is the result of a true intradural primary, typically of the filum terminale/cauda equina.* **(Right)** *In smears, Ewing sarcomas appear as highly cellular neoplasms arranged in loose clusters composed of cells with high nuclear:cytoplasmic ratios.*

Nerve Root Infiltration

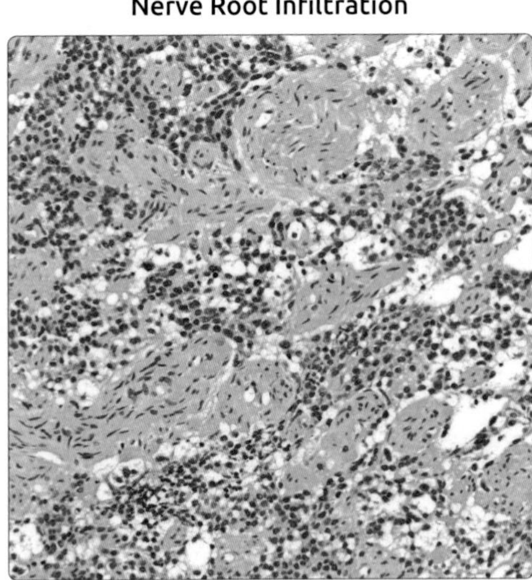

Loose Clusters

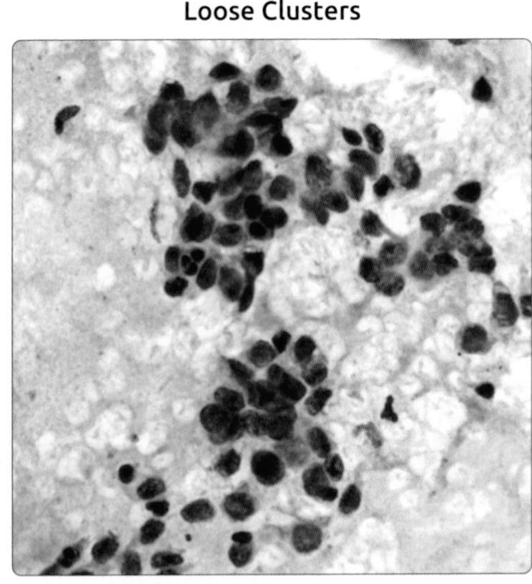

Calvarial Neoplasm

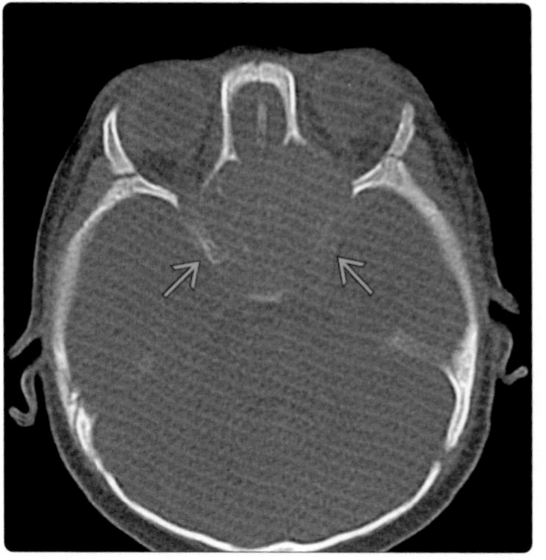

Filling of Intertrabecular Spaces

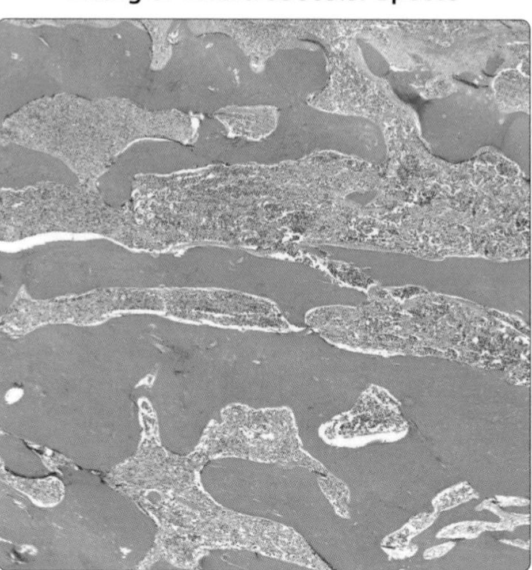

(Left) *Ewing sarcoma may present as a calvarial neoplasm that involves the CNS by direct extension. This axial CT with bone windows highlights a large osseodestructive tumor at the base of the skull ➡.* **(Right)** *Aggregates of small to medium-sized round cells fill the intertrabecular spaces. Direct extension from overlying bone represents the most frequent scenario of CNS involvement of Ewing sarcoma. (Courtesy A. Rosenberg, MD.)*

Intracranial Rhabdomyosarcoma

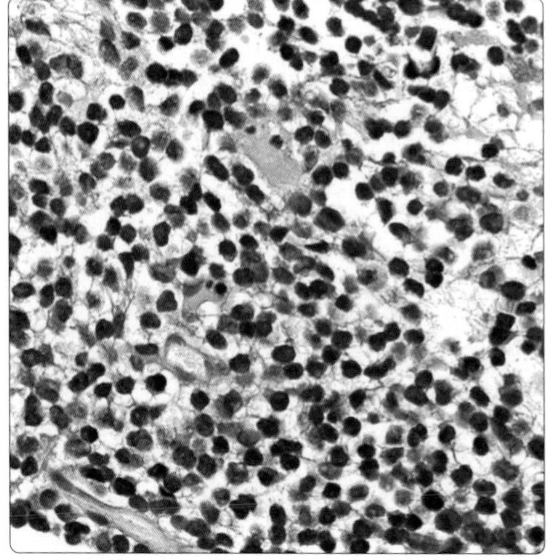

Myogenin Expression

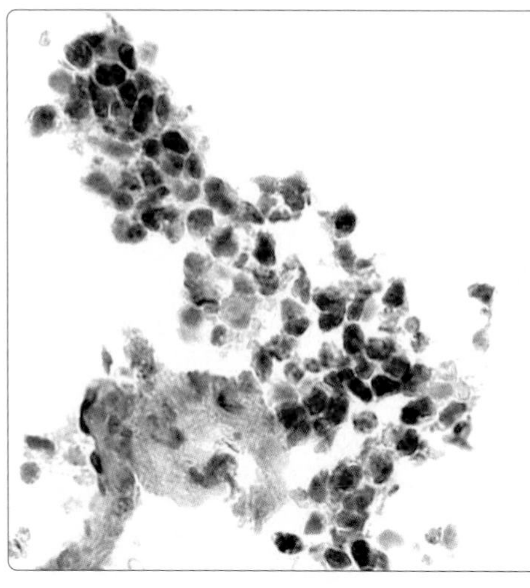

(Left) *Many round blue cell tumors enter into the differential diagnosis of Ewing sarcoma. In this example of an intracranial rhabdomyosarcoma, cells are more hyperchromatic than those typical of Ewing sarcoma. Immunohistochemical confirmation of myogenic differentiation was required, however.* **(Right)** *Strong, uniform nuclear expression of myogenin in this small round blue cell tumor supports a diagnosis of rhabdomyosarcoma and helps exclude Ewing sarcoma.*

Membranous CD99 Staining

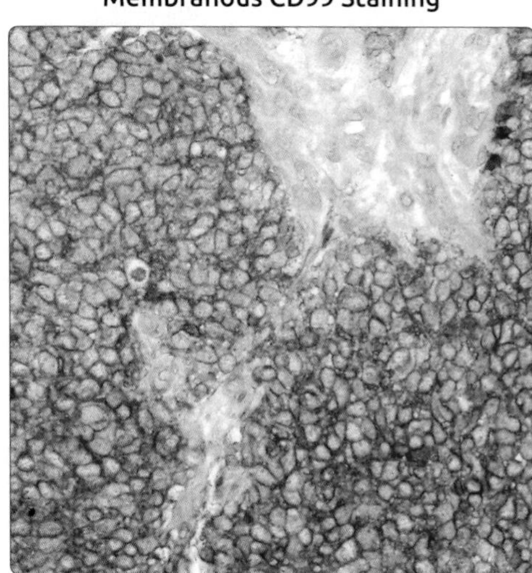

EWSR1-ERG Fusion

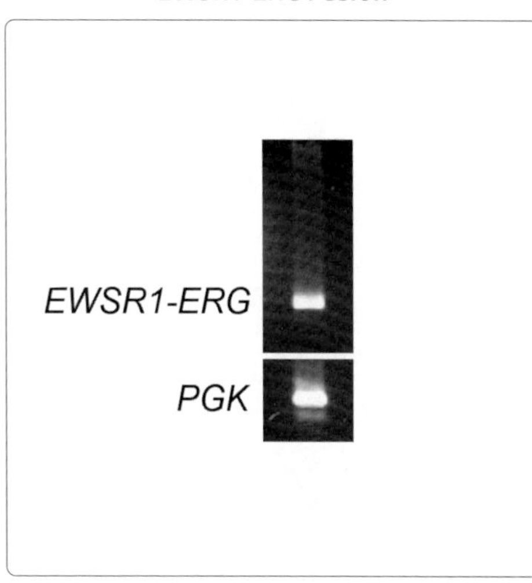

(Left) *Strong, membranous CD99 staining is present in the majority of Ewing sarcoma. It is not specific, however. (Courtesy A. Polydorides, MD, PhD.)* **(Right)** *Given the wide differential diagnosis and relative lack of specific IHC markers, molecular confirmation is almost always required. RT-PCR in formalin-fixed tissues represents a frequent approach. In this example, demonstration of an EWSR1-ERG fusion transcript confirmed the diagnosis. PGK (PGK1) (housekeeping gene) serves as an internal control for the PCR reaction.*

Atypical Teratoid/Rhabdoid Tumor

KEY FACTS

TERMINOLOGY

- Highly malignant CNS neoplasm similar to renal and extrarenal rhabdoid tumors occurring in infants and young children

ETIOLOGY/PATHOGENESIS

- Germline *INI1* mutations in ~ 1/3

CLINICAL ISSUES

- Rare: 1-2% of pediatric primary CNS tumors
- Generally first 2 years of life
- Nearly all intracranial; intraspinal rare
- Prognosis poor

MACROSCOPIC

- Large, soft, fleshy, and necrotic

MICROSCOPIC

- Distinctive, yet nondescript, large pale cells
- Rhabdoid cells
- Undifferentiated cells, sometimes simulating medulloblastoma
- Glands, rosettes, or chondroid matrix (uncommon)

ANCILLARY TESTS

- Polyimmunophenotypic, with variable positivity, often in individual cells or small groups
  - EMA, cytokeratins, GFAP, S100 protein, synaptophysin, neurofilament protein, chromogranin, smooth muscle actin, desmin
- Loss of nuclear immunoreactivity for INI1/BAF47 essentially diagnostic and required
- Deletions, mutations in *INI1/hSNF5/SMARCB1/BAF47* gene in almost all cases

TOP DIFFERENTIAL DIAGNOSES

- Medulloblastoma, choroid plexus carcinoma, embryonal tumors (formerly supratentorial PNET)

Axial MR: Massive Size

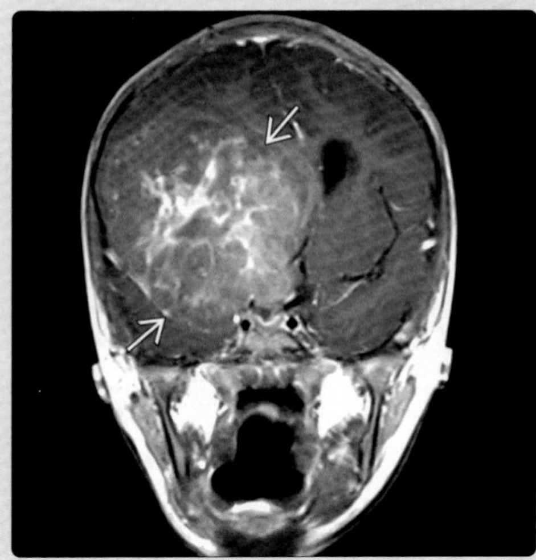

Large Jumbled Cells

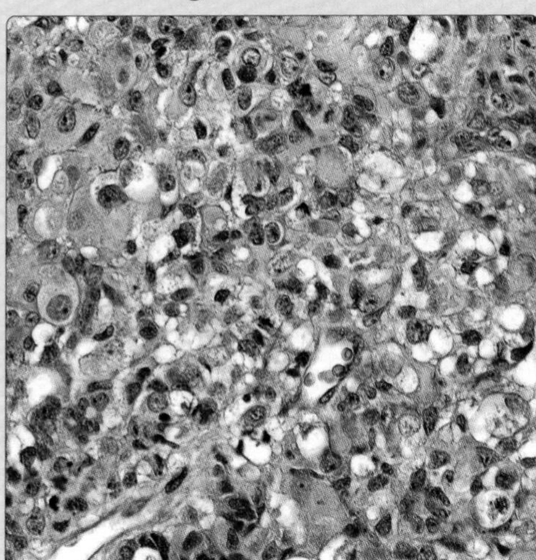

(Left) *Atypical teratoid/rhabdoid tumors (AT/RTs) are usually large, if not massive, tumors ➡ with variable degrees of contrast enhancement.* **(Right)** *In spite of the lesion's name, most examples are not overtly rhabdoid, if at all. Large, pale, jumbled cells are more characteristic.*

Brisk Cell Cycling

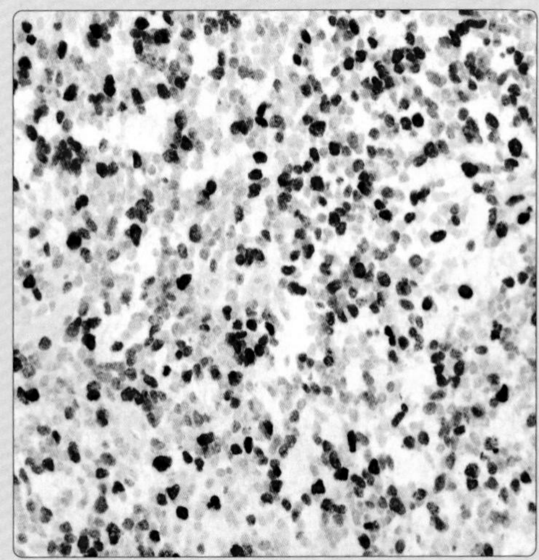

Loss of INI1

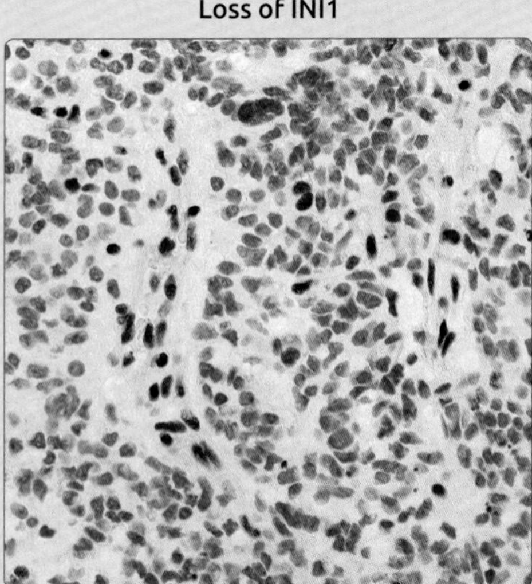

(Left) *AT/RTs are highly malignant tumors with brisk cell cycling rates.* **(Right)** *Loss of nuclear INI1 expression is the signature IHC feature of almost all AT/RTs. Evaluation of this immunostain should only be performed in areas of the slide in which the small blood vessel endothelial cells retain the nuclear expression and serve as internal controls for fidelity of technique/tissue fixation.*

TERMINOLOGY

Abbreviations

- Atypical teratoid/rhabdoid tumor (AT/RT)

Synonyms

- Rhabdoid tumor of CNS

Definitions

- Highly malignant early pediatric CNS neoplasm similar to renal and extrarenal rhabdoid tumor
- WHO grade IV

ETIOLOGY/PATHOGENESIS

Genetics

- Germline *INI1* mutations in ~ 1/3 of cases

CLINICAL ISSUES

Epidemiology

- Incidence
  - Rare: 1-2% of primary pediatric CNS tumors
- Age
  - Generally first 2 years of life
  - Rare in adults
    - Occasionally suprasellar
- Sex
  - Males > females (3:2)

Site

- Nearly all intracranial
  - 50-60% infratentorial
    - Often cerebellopontine angle
  - 40-50% supratentorial
    - Intracerebral
    - Suprasellar, especially in adults
- Rare intraspinal
- May show cerebrospinal fluid dissemination (i.e., drop metastases)

Presentation

- Variable
  - Site-dependent neurological deficits
  - Macrocephaly
  - Signs of increased intracranial pressure

Treatment

- Surgical approaches
  - Gross total resection optimal
    - Often not possible
- Adjuvant therapy
  - Chemotherapy; often sarcoma-like regimen
- Radiation
  - Standard
    - Despite young age of patients

Prognosis

- Poor
  - CSF dissemination common

IMAGING

MR Findings

- Large mass
- Variably enhancing
- Frequent hemorrhage and necrosis
- May show cerebrospinal fluid dissemination

MACROSCOPIC

General Features

- Large
- Soft, fleshy, hemorrhagic, and necrotic

MICROSCOPIC

Histologic Features

- Heterogeneous, variably textured, disordered, complex architecture
- Distinctive, yet nondescript, large pale cells
- Rhabdoid cells
  - Round eccentric nuclei
    - Open chromatin pattern
  - Prominent nucleoli
  - Eosinophilic cytoplasmic inclusion (sometimes)
    - Fibrillary or homogeneous
- Cords of cells
  - In basophilic mucoid matrix
  - Resemble chordoma or trabecular pattern of renal rhabdoid tumors
- Undifferentiated, embryonal-like cells
  - Flexner-Wintersteiner or Homer Wright rosettes
  - Totally undifferentiated, small cell
- Other patterns of differentiation (rare)
  - Epithelial patterns
    - Few small, gland-like spaces or nests or flat epithelial surfaces
    - Primitive squamous differentiation
    - Ependymal canals or neural tube-like structures
  - Chondroid matrix
  - Ganglioglioma-like differentiation
- Mitoses (frequent)
- Apoptosis (prominent)
- Necrosis (common)
  - Often with dystrophic calcification
- Fibrovascular septa

ANCILLARY TESTS

Cytology

- Large pale cells
- Rhabdoid cells
- Small primitive cells
- Abundant apoptosis, mitoses

Immunohistochemistry

- Polyimmunophenotypic, with variable positivity, often in individual cells or small groups
  - EMA
  - Cytokeratins
  - Smooth muscle actin (SMA), desmin

- GFAP
- S100 protein
- Synaptophysin
- Neurofilament protein
- Chromogranin
- Vimentin
  - Widespread IHC(+), little diagnostic value
  - May highlight cytoplasmic ball-like inclusions
- Most cases have vimentin, EMA, SMA IHC(+); other IHCs more variable
- True germ cell markers [CD117 (C-kit), OCT4, PLAP] negative
- Claudin-6
  - Role of strong expression in prognosis uncertain
  - In some studies found to be expressed in variety of other pediatric CNS and soft tissue tumors
- Loss of nuclear reactivity for INI1/BAF47 essentially diagnostic, and near-required
- High Ki-67 labeling index, often over 50%
- P53 protein expression often found
  - Usually no *TP53* mutation
  - May be due to deregulation of p16(INK4A) and p14(ARF) pathway

Genetic Testing

- Deletions, mutations in *INI1/hSNF5/SMARCB1/BAF47* gene in almost all cases
- Mutation in *SMARCA4/BRG1* gene (rare)
  - Retained nuclear INI1 immunostaining in rare AT/RTs with *SMARCA4/BRG1* mutation
- Loss of all (monosomy) or part (deletion) of chromosome 22 by FISH in almost all cases

Electron Microscopy

- Rhabdoid cell cytoplasm
  - Spherical, paranuclear, cytoplasmic inclusions
    - Tight, compact, whorled intermediate filaments
    - Ultrastructural variation with other cell types

DIFFERENTIAL DIAGNOSIS

Medulloblastoma

- Especially anaplastic/large cell variant
- More cell-cell wrapping, nuclear molding
- Coarser, more atypical, hyperchromatic nuclei
- Diffusely synaptophysin (+)
- Reticulin-defined nodules in desmoplastic/nodular variant
- Retained nuclear INI1 immunostaining

Embryonal Tumors

- Formerly supratentorial PNET
- More monomorphous histology; no rhabdoid cells
- Nodular architecture in 1 type
- Diffusely synaptophysin (+)
- Retained nuclear INI1 immunostaining

Malignant Glioma

- GFAP(+) but may be focal
- Retained nuclear INI1 immunostaining

Choroid Plexus Carcinoma

- EMA(-) or focal
- Retained INI1 staining
  - But some cases difficult to distinguish
- Trapped choroid plexus, especially in cerebellum

Rhabdoid Meningioma

- Very rare in infants
- Retained nuclear INI1 immunostaining

Germinoma

- Pineal and suprasellar locations most frequent
- More uniform large cells
- No rhabdoid inclusions
- Occasional noncaseating granulomas
- Glycogen-rich cells
- Immunoreactivity for CD117 (C-kit), OCT4, PLAP
- Retained INI1 nuclear immunostaining

DIAGNOSTIC CHECKLIST

Pathologic Interpretation Pearls

- Consider possibility of AT/RT in any hypercellular, poorly differentiated tumor in infants, including embryonal (formerly PNETs), medulloblastomas, choroid plexus carcinomas
  - Employ immunostaining for INI1
    - Many AT/RTs show paucity of rhabdoid cells
    - Test all CNS pediatric small blue cell/embryonal tumors for loss of INI1
  - AT/RTs show diffuse loss of INI1 immunostaining in all tumor cells
    - Do not incorrectly interpret entrapped nontumor cells that retain INI1
  - Check fidelity of immunostaining
    - Entrapped blood vessels with positive nuclear INI1 in endothelial cells are internal control
- Small subset of AT/RTs do not show loss of nuclear INI1 due to mutation in *SMARCA4/BRG1* gene
  - Most patients have inherited, germline mutations
  - Worse prognosis than with INI1 loss/mutation in *INI1/hSNF5/SMARCB1/BAF47* gene
- Not all tumors with INI1 loss/mutation in *INI1/hSNF5/SMARCB1/BAF47* gene are automatically atypical teratoid/rhabdoid tumors
  - Other rare CNS tumors have diffuse loss of INI1 immunostaining: Cribriform neuroepithelial tumor of ventricle
    - Rare tumors can develop subset of cells with loss of INI1
      - Pleomorphic astrocytomas
      - Gangliogliomas
      - Diffuse gliomas/glioblastomas
      - Likely clones of tumor cells with *SMARCB1* mutations evolve as late mutational event
  - Numerous nonglial tumors now recognized to have *INI1* mutations, i.e., *SMARCB1* mutated tumors
    - Highly variable percentage of cells show rhabdoid cells in these tumors
    - In children
      - Renal/extrarenal malignant rhabdoid tumors (MRT)
      - Renal medullary carcinoma

- ▫ Poorly differentiated chordomas; typical chordomas maintain strong nuclear INI1 immunoreactivity
- – Subsets of
  - ▫ Epithelioid sarcomas
  - ▫ Extraskeletal myxoid chondrosarcomas
  - ▫ Epithelioid malignant peripheral nervous system tumors
  - ▫ Rare rhabdoid carcinomas of gastroenteropancreatic, sinonasal, genitourinary tract
- Not all non-AT/RT tumors with *INI1* mutations follow highly aggressive clinical course
  - Transcriptional analyses have identified atypical teratoid rhabdoid tumor subgroups
    - Different gene expression patterns
    - Involvement of ASCL1, regulator of NOTCH signaling
    - ASCL1 expression, correlated with clinical prognostic factors, shows differences in survival between subgroups
- Rare examples of AT/RTs without INI1 protein loss or mutation in *SMARCA4/BRG1* gene
  - Diagnosis should be made with caution
  - Requires extensive additional testing, often by research methodologies

SELECTED REFERENCES

1. Dhir A et al: Lumbar spinal atypical teratoid rhabdoid tumor. J Clin Neurosci. ePub, 2015
2. Sredni ST et al: Rhabdoid tumor predisposition syndrome. Pediatr Dev Pathol. 18(1):49-58, 2015
3. Agaimy A: The expanding family of SMARCB1(INI1)-deficient neoplasia: implications of phenotypic, biological, and molecular heterogeneity. Adv Anat Pathol. 21(6):394-410, 2014
4. Bourdeaut F et al: Rhabdoid tumors: integrating biological insights with clinical success: A report from the SMARCB1 and Rhabdoid Tumor Symposium, Paris, December 12-14, 2013. Cancer Genet. 207(9):346-351, 2014
5. Hasselblatt M et al: SMARCA4-mutated atypical teratoid/rhabdoid tumors are associated with inherited germline alterations and poor prognosis. Acta Neuropathol. 128(3):453-6, 2014
6. Jeong JY et al: Atypical teratoid/rhabdoid tumor arising in pleomorphic xanthoastrocytoma: a case report. Neuropathology. 34(4):398-405, 2014
7. Krishnan C et al: Atypical teratoid/rhabdoid tumor with ganglioglioma-like differentiation: case report and review of the literature. Hum Pathol. 45(1):185-8, 2014
8. Margol AS et al: Pathology and diagnosis of SMARCB1-deficient tumors. Cancer Genet. ePub, 2014
9. Dufour C et al: Clinicopathologic prognostic factors in childhood atypical teratoid and rhabdoid tumor of the central nervous system: A multicenter study. Cancer. 118(15):3812-21, 2012
10. Bruggers CS et al: Clinicopathologic comparison of familial versus sporadic atypical teratoid/rhabdoid tumors (AT/RT) of the central nervous system. Pediatr Blood Cancer. 56(7):1026-31, 2011
11. Hasselblatt M et al: Nonsense mutation and inactivation of SMARCA4 (BRG1) in an atypical teratoid/rhabdoid tumor showing retained SMARCB1 (INI1) expression. Am J Surg Pathol. 35(6):933-5, 2011
12. Kleinschmidt-DeMasters BK et al: Atypical teratoid/rhabdoid tumor arising in a ganglioglioma: genetic characterization. Am J Surg Pathol. 35(12):1894-901, 2011
13. Birks DK et al: Claudin 6 is a positive marker for atypical teratoid/rhabdoid tumors. Brain Pathol. 20(1):140-50, 2010
14. Mobley BC et al: Loss of SMARCB1/INI1 expression in poorly differentiated chordomas. Acta Neuropathol. 120(6):745-53, 2010
15. Athale UH et al: Childhood atypical teratoid rhabdoid tumor of the central nervous system: a meta-analysis of observational studies. J Pediatr Hematol Oncol. 31(9):651-63, 2009
16. Biswas A et al: Atypical teratoid rhabdoid tumor of the brain: case series and review of literature. Childs Nerv Syst. 25(11):1495-500, 2009
17. de León-Bojorge B et al: Atypical teratoid/rhabdoid tumor of the central nervous system. Childs Nerv Syst. 25(11):1387; author reply 1389, 2009
18. Ertan Y et al: Atypical teratoid/rhabdoid tumor of the central nervous system: clinicopathologic and immunohistochemical features of four cases. Childs Nerv Syst. 25(6):707-11, 2009
19. Edgar MA et al: The differential diagnosis of central nervous system tumors: a critical examination of some recent immunohistochemical applications. Arch Pathol Lab Med. 132(3):500-9, 2008
20. Seno T et al: An immunohistochemical and electron microscopic study of atypical teratoid/rhabdoid tumor. Brain Tumor Pathol. 25(2):79-83, 2008
21. Warmuth-Metz M et al: CT and MR imaging in atypical teratoid/rhabdoid tumors of the central nervous system. Neuroradiology. 50(5):447-52, 2008
22. Zarovnaya EL et al: Atypical teratoid/rhabdoid tumor of the spine in an adult: case report and review of the literature. J Neurooncol. 84(1):49-55, 2007
23. Allen JC et al: Atypical teratoid/rhabdoid tumor evolving from an optic pathway ganglioglioma: case study. Neuro Oncol. 8(1):79-82, 2006
24. Biegel JA: Molecular genetics of atypical teratoid/rhabdoid tumor. Neurosurg Focus. 20(1):E11, 2006
25. Haberler C et al: Immunohistochemical analysis of INI1 protein in malignant pediatric CNS tumors: Lack of INI1 in atypical teratoid/rhabdoid tumors and in a fraction of primitive neuroectodermal tumors without rhabdoid phenotype. Am J Surg Pathol. 30(11):1462-8, 2006
26. Chen ML et al: Atypical teratoid/rhabdoid tumors of the central nervous system: management and outcomes. Neurosurg Focus. 18(6A):E8, 2005
27. Judkins AR et al: INI1 protein expression distinguishes atypical teratoid/rhabdoid tumor from choroid plexus carcinoma. J Neuropathol Exp Neurol. 64(5):391-7, 2005
28. Parwani AV et al: Atypical teratoid/rhabdoid tumor of the brain: cytopathologic characteristics and differential diagnosis. Cancer. 105(2):65-70, 2005
29. Raisanen J et al: Chromosome 22q deletions in atypical teratoid/rhabdoid tumors in adults. Brain Pathol. 15(1):23-8, 2005
30. Reddy AT: Atypical teratoid/rhabdoid tumors of the central nervous system. J Neurooncol. 75(3):309-13, 2005
31. Strother D: Atypical teratoid rhabdoid tumors of childhood: diagnosis, treatment and challenges. Expert Rev Anticancer Ther. 5(5):907-15, 2005
32. Judkins AR et al: Immunohistochemical analysis of hSNF5/INI1 in pediatric CNS neoplasms. Am J Surg Pathol. 28(5):644-50, 2004
33. Dang T et al: Atypical teratoid/rhabdoid tumors. Childs Nerv Syst. 19(4):244-8, 2003
34. Bambakidis NC et al: Atypical teratoid/rhabdoid tumors of the central nervous system: clinical, radiographic and pathologic features. Pediatr Neurosurg. 37(2):64-70, 2002
35. Biegel JA et al: Alterations of the hSNF5/INI1 gene in central nervous system atypical teratoid/rhabdoid tumors and renal and extrarenal rhabdoid tumors. Clin Cancer Res. 8(11):3461-7, 2002
36. Biegel JA et al: The role of INI1 and the SWI/SNF complex in the development of rhabdoid tumors: meeting summary from the workshop on childhood atypical teratoid/rhabdoid tumors. Cancer Res. 62(1):323-8, 2002
37. Kleihues P et al: The WHO classification of tumors of the nervous system. J Neuropathol Exp Neurol. 61(3):215-25; discussion 226-9, 2002
38. Lee MC et al: Atypical teratoid/rhabdoid tumor of the central nervous system: clinico-pathological study. Neuropathology. 22(4):252-60, 2002
39. Packer RJ et al: Atypical teratoid/rhabdoid tumor of the central nervous system: report on workshop. J Pediatr Hematol Oncol. 24(5):337-42, 2002
40. Oka H et al: Clinicopathological characteristics of atypical teratoid/rhabdoid tumor. Neurol Med Chir (Tokyo). 39(7):510-7; discussion 517-8, 1999
41. Burger PC et al: Atypical teratoid/rhabdoid tumor of the central nervous system: a highly malignant tumor of infancy and childhood frequently mistaken for medulloblastoma: a Pediatric Oncology Group study. Am J Surg Pathol. 22(9):1083-92, 1998
42. Rorke LB et al: Central nervous system atypical teratoid/rhabdoid tumors of infancy and childhood: definition of an entity. J Neurosurg. 85(1):56-65, 1996

Vacuolated Cells

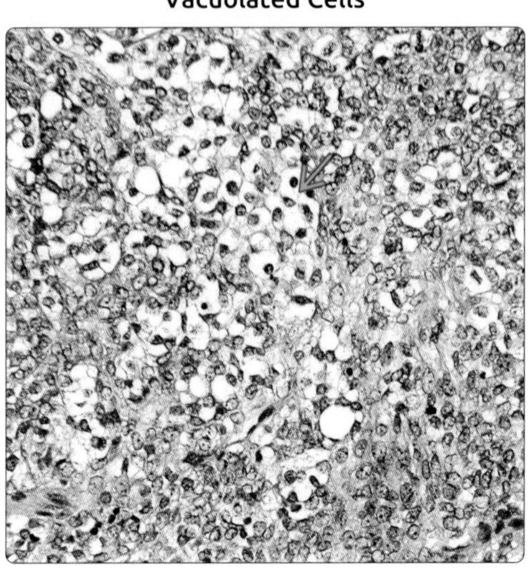

Large Pale Cells

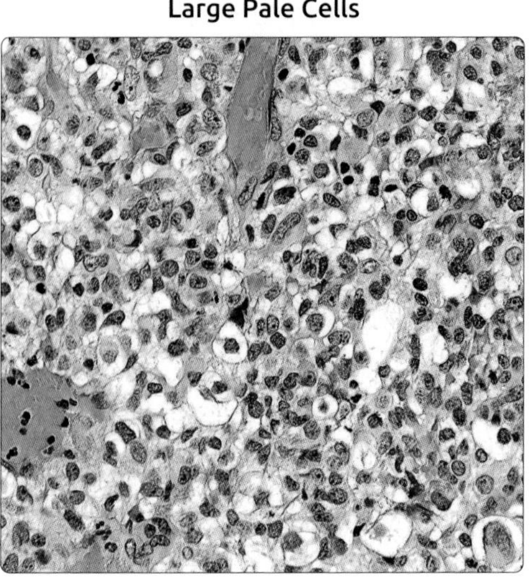

(Left) *While not a specific pattern, a disorganized mixture of vacuolated cells* ➩ *and smaller cells with a moderate amount of cytoplasm is common in AT/RTs.* **(Right)** *Large, jumbled, pale cells comprise a pattern that, while not diagnostic, is highly suggestive of AT/RT. Undifferentiated choroid plexus carcinoma would be a prime differential diagnostic entity, to be distinguished largely by immunohistochemistry.*

Extensive Vacuolation

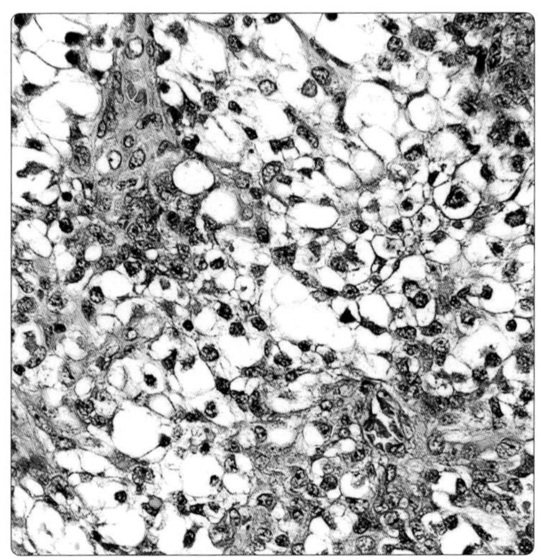

Patternless Architecture

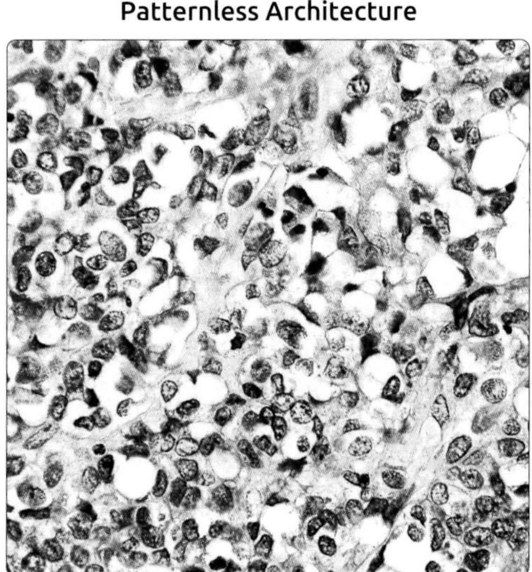

(Left) *AT/RTs are sometimes extensively vacuolated. Similar cells occur in a differential diagnostic entity: Choroid plexus carcinoma.* **(Right)** *Cells of AT/RT often include epithelioid cells in a disorganized structureless pattern. There is usually more cytoplasm than expected of medulloblastoma. While unstructured, the pattern is highly suggestive of atypical teratoid/rhabdoid tumor.*

Epithelioid Cells

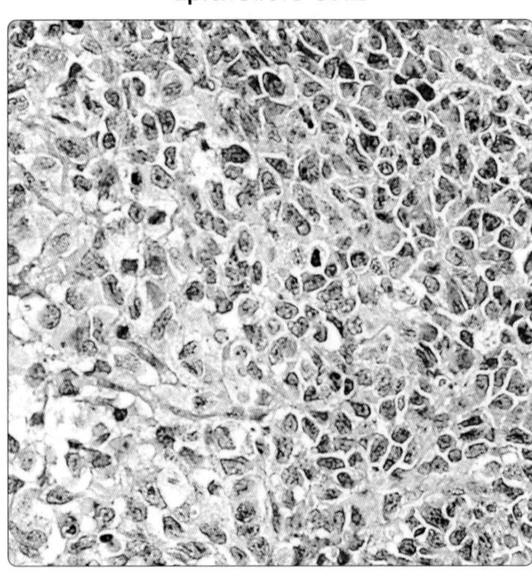

Simulating Glioma

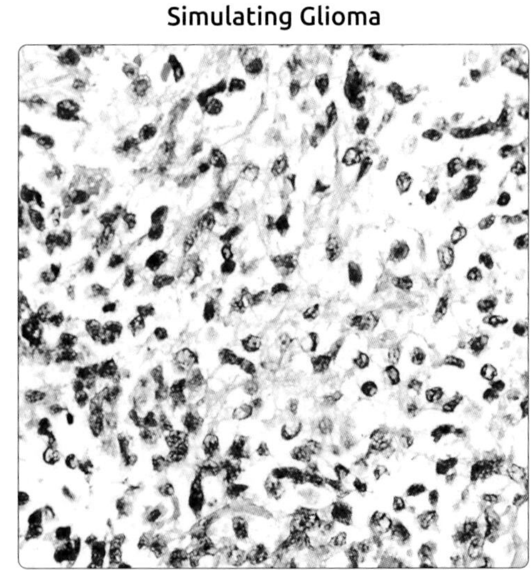

(Left) *Sheets of cytologically malignant, epithelioid cells comprise this AT/RT. While the degree of cellularity approaches, or equals, that of medulloblastoma or other embryonal tumors, AT/RTs generally have more nuclear pleomorphism and cytoplasm.* **(Right)** *Especially at higher magnification, disorganized tissue can have a glioma-like cellular randomness. AT/RTs are not diffusely infiltrating tumors, although they trap choroid plexus in some cases.*

Prominent Nucleoli

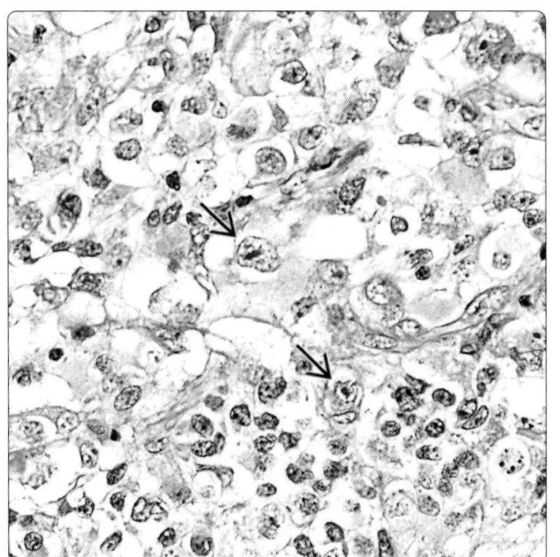

Rounded Nuclei

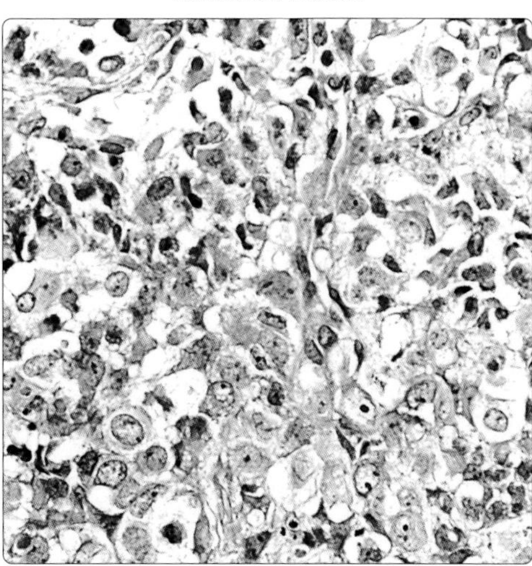

(Left) *Large pale cells with prominent nucleoli ➡ may mimic those of ganglion cell tumor or even germinoma. Loss of nuclear staining for INI1 would quickly resolve the issue in favor of AT/RT.* **(Right)** *Large round nuclei with prominent nucleoli are at least a focal feature of most AT/RTs. Such iconic cells are not present in all cases, however.*

Minimal Hyperchromatism

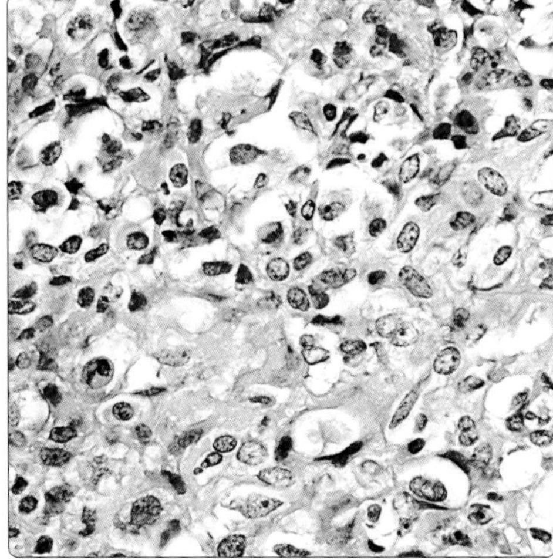

Simulating Germinoma

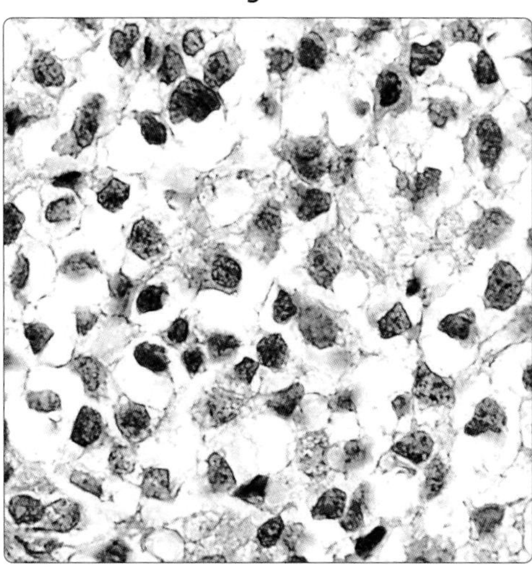

(Left) *Although moderately pleomorphic, AT/RT cells are often not especially hyperchromatic and can even be rather cytologically bland.* **(Right)** *Sheets of large round cells with prominent nucleoli and pale cytoplasm somewhat resemble those in germinomas. Unlike the latter neoplasm, however, AT/RTs feature inconspicuous lymphocytes. Immunostaining for INI1 and germ cell markers would readily resolve the issue.*

Rhabdoid Cell Inclusions

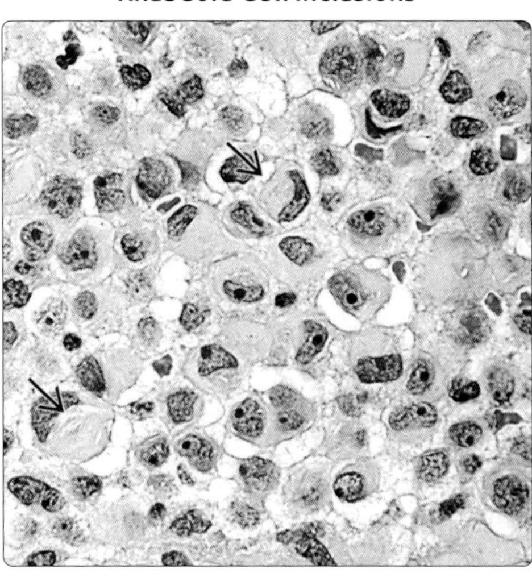

Paranuclear Filamentous Inclusions

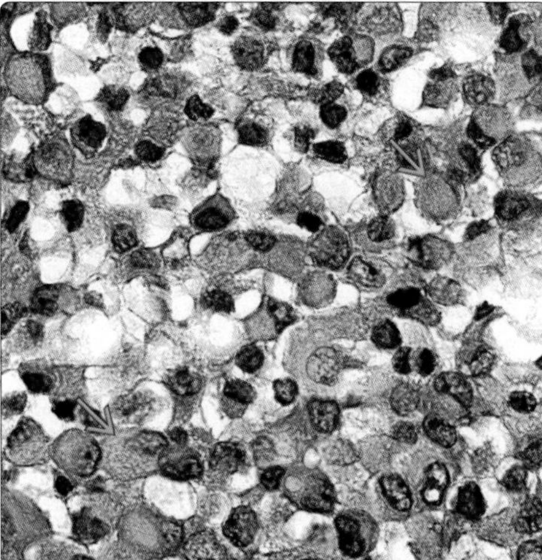

(Left) *Cytoplasmic inclusions, some fibrillar ➡, in combination with large nuclei containing prominent nucleoli, create the classic rhabdoid appearance. Most AT/RTs are not, however, overtly rhabdoid.* **(Right)** *Classic rhabdoid tissue may be a focal, but less often the dominant, tumor element. Large cell medulloblastomas are similar, to a degree, but lack the paranuclear, filamentous inclusions ➡ typical of rhabdoid cells.*

(Left) *Uniform high cellularity in an AT/RT suggests the possibility of an embryonal tumor or medulloblastoma. Immunostaining for INI1 is a sensible precaution in such lesions, especially those that occur in the very young.* **(Right)** *There is little, in a limited sample such as this, to firmly exclude medulloblastoma or an embryonal tumor. Tumor cells in both would be diffusely immunoreactive for synaptophysin and would retain nuclear INI1.*

Simulating Medulloblastoma

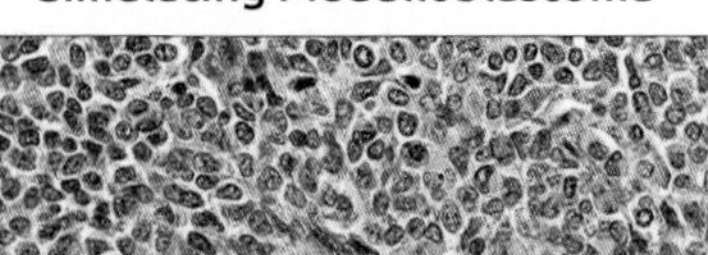

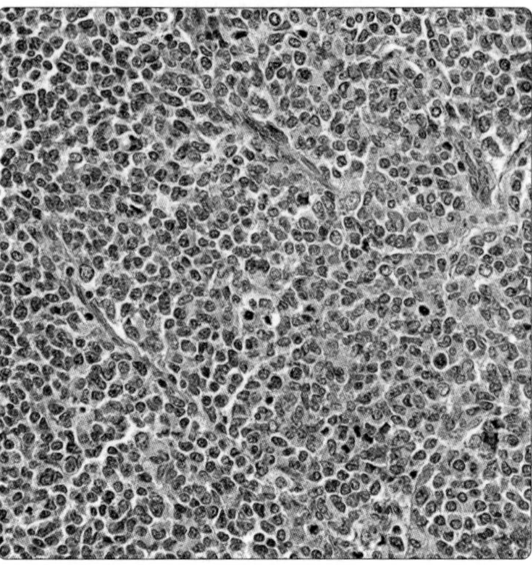

Small Blue Cell Areas

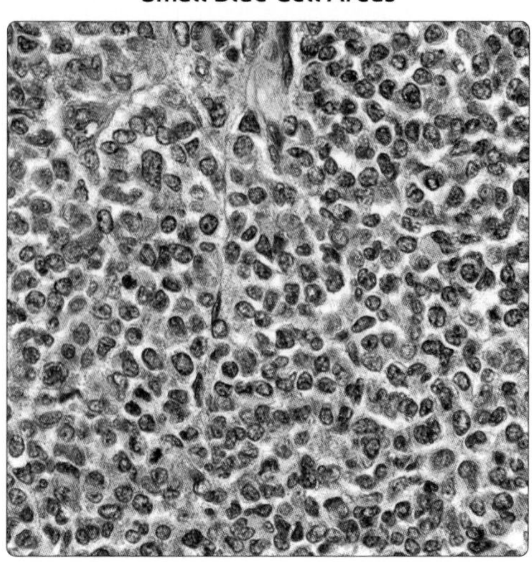

(Left) *Strands and cords of tumor cells in a myxoid matrix can mimic chordoma or the trabecular pattern of renal rhabdoid tumors. Such structures would be most unusual in medulloblastoma.* **(Right)** *Fine anastomosing strands of cells in basophilic, mucoid matrix resemble chondrosarcoma and chordoma, neoplasms that are extra- rather than intraaxial.*

Simulating Chordoma

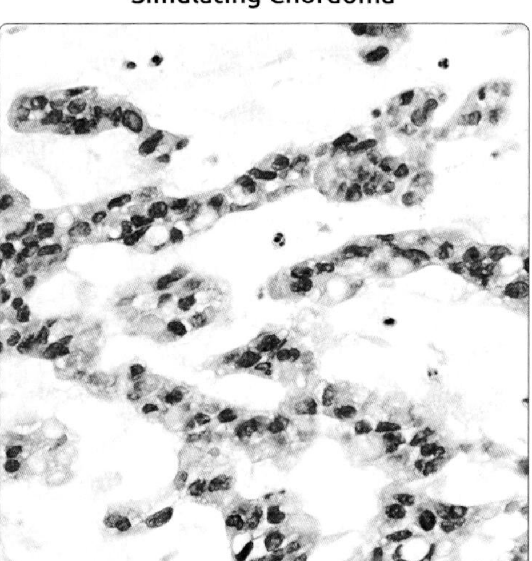

Simulating Myxoid Tumor

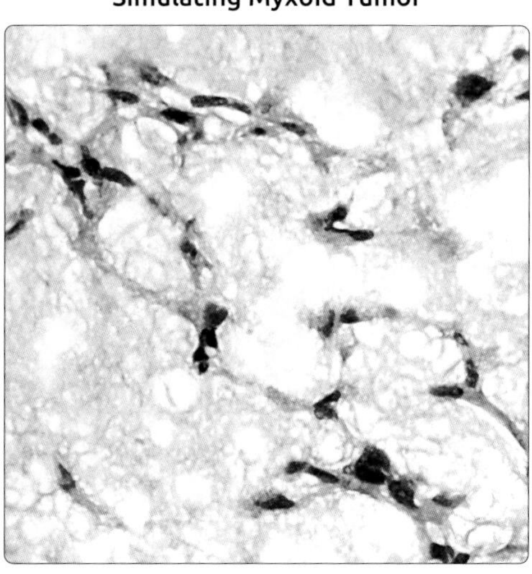

(Left) *Necrosis is a hallmark of the microscopic, macroscopic, and radiologic appearance of AT/RT. Microvascular proliferation is typically missing.* **(Right)** *Necrosis is often extensive in AT/RTs. A few large cells ⇨ with epithelioid qualities at the margin with viable tissue suggest the possibility of AT/RT. It would be prudent to stain such lesions for INI1.*

Necrosis Without Microvascular Proliferation

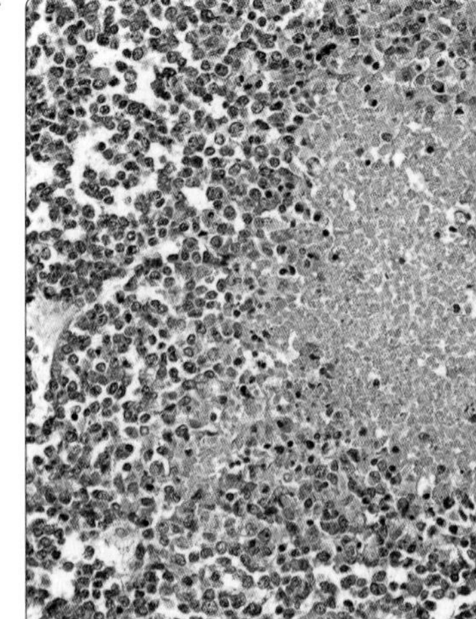

Rare Rhabdoid Cells

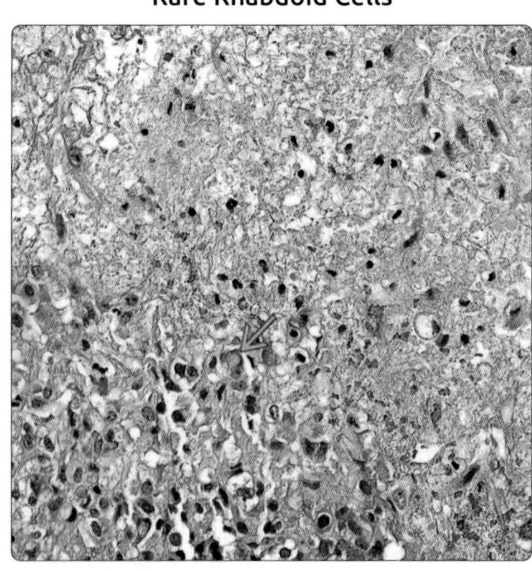

Simulating Ependymoma

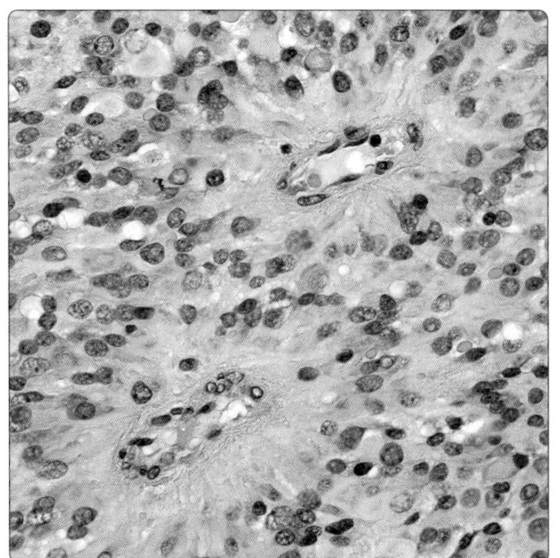

Simulating Sarcoma

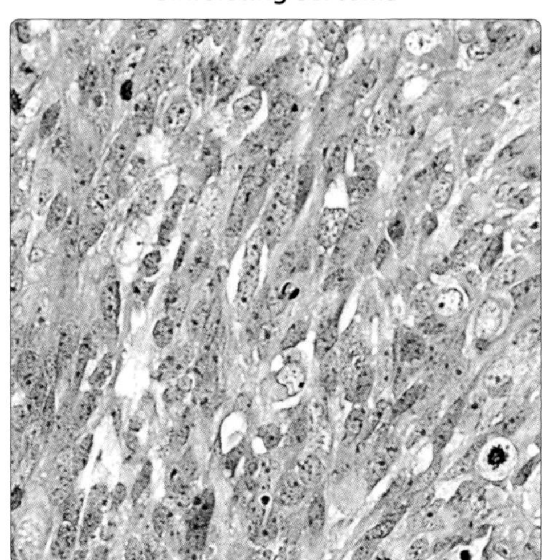

(Left) *Perivascular arrangement of cells lends an ependymoma-like quality to some AT/RTs. However, such formations are GFAP(-) in the AT/RT.* **(Right)** *Sheets of elongate cells are just 1 of the many expressions of AT/RT. Although not a specific pattern, they lend a mesenchymal appearance. Like the other components, such tissue would be nonspecifically immunopositive for vimentin.*

Simulating Carcinoma

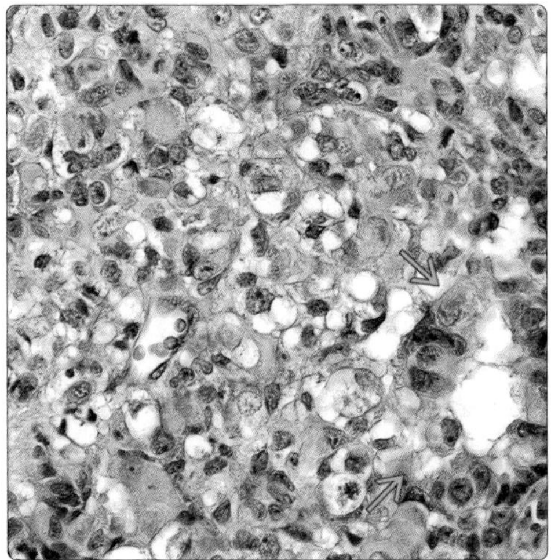

Epithelial Differentiation

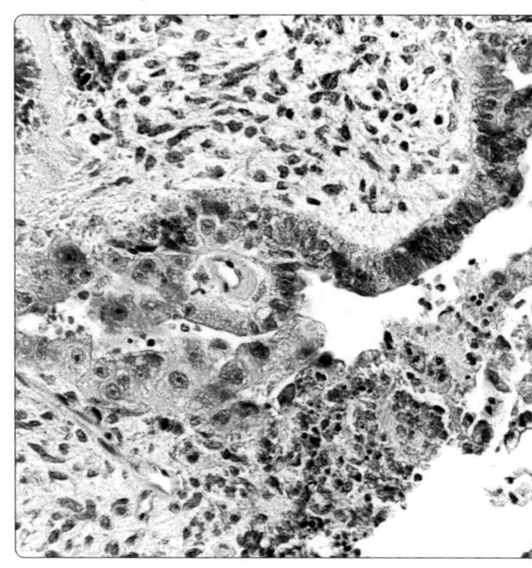

(Left) *Poorly formed glands ⇒ or epithelial surfaces are evidence of epithelial differentiation in AT/RT. Even these abortive structures are usually lacking.* **(Right)** *Occasional AT/RTs make attempts at epithelial differentiation, here in the form of a crude but unequivocal epithelial surface.*

Rosette-Like Structures

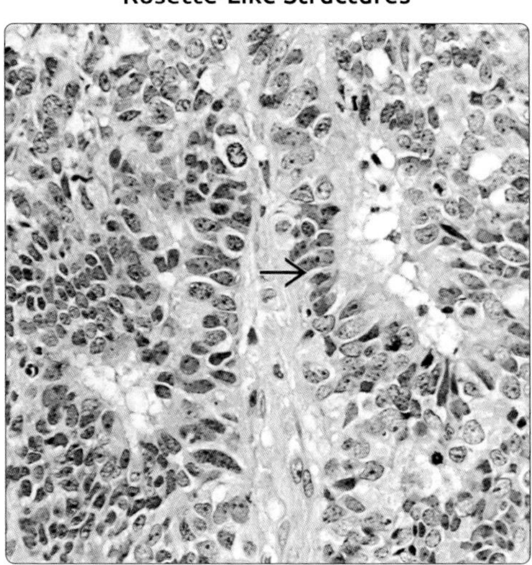

Epithelial Differentiation

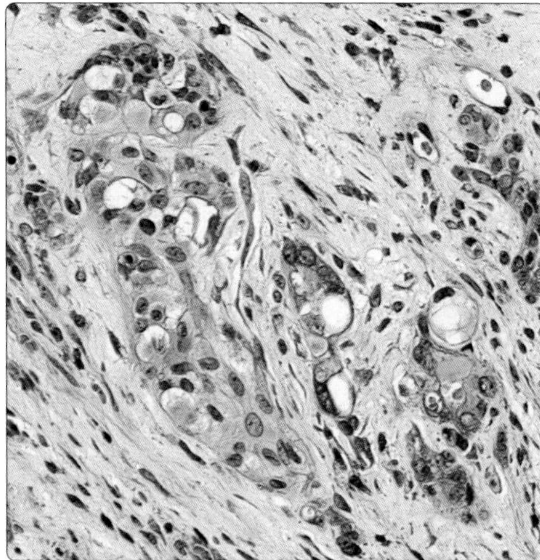

(Left) *Rare AT/RTs contain gland-like ⇒ or rosette-like structures with lumina. Remaining areas of such tumors have more typical AT/RT histological features and cells show loss of nuclear INI1 immunostaining, both providing for confident diagnosis.* **(Right)** *Occasionally AT/RTs show considerable epithelial differentiation.*

(Left) *Smear preparations reveal the AT/RT's polymorphous large cells with open chromatin and nucleoli. Although not illustrated here, intracytoplasmic inclusions are often present.* **(Right)** *Monomorphous, round, sharply defined cells with prominent nucleoli and intracytoplasmic inclusions ⇒ are the classic rhabdoid cells for which the lesion is named.*

Smear: Polymorphous Cells

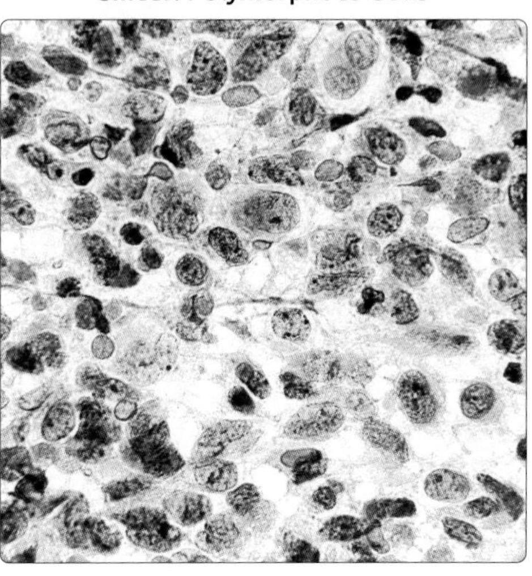

Smear: Rhabdoid Cells

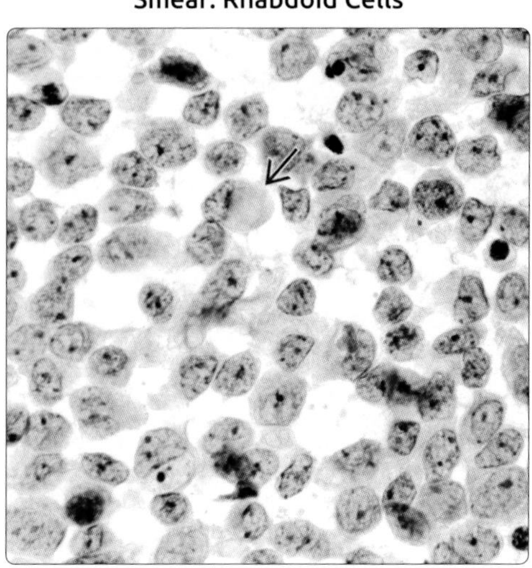

(Left) *AT/RTs are usually focally immunoreactive for cytokeratins, AE1/AE3 in this case. Medulloblastomas and supratentorial embryonal tumors would be negative. As here, not all cells in AT/RT are reactive for any 1 of the multiple antigens expressed by those tumors.* **(Right)** *Cells immunoreactive for EMA are common in AT/RT. An important differential diagnosis option, choroid plexus carcinoma, while often reactive for cytokeratins, is only uncommonly EMA positive.*

AE1/AE3

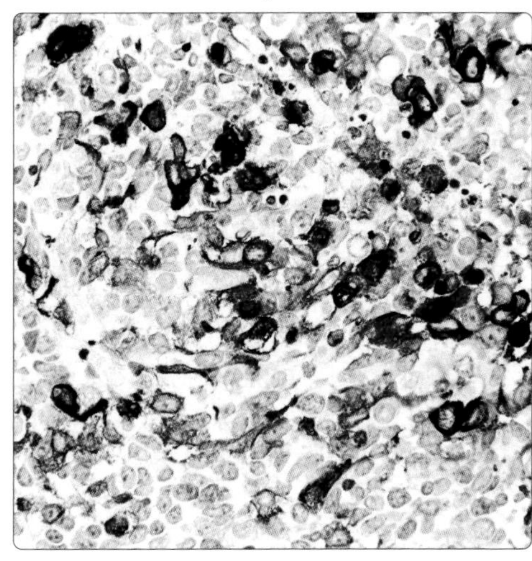

EMA

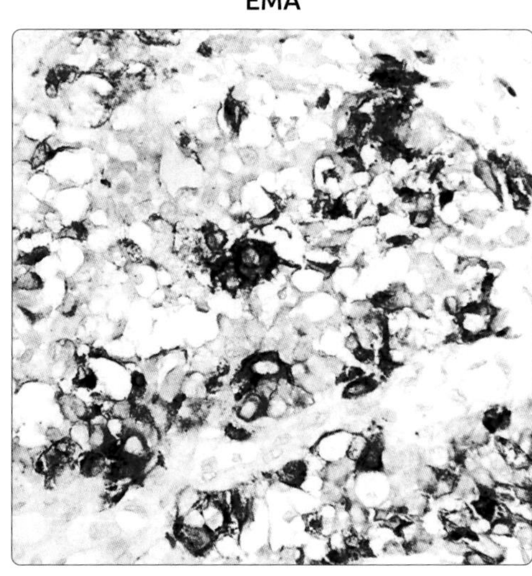

(Left) *GFAP immunostaining is part of the AT/RT immunophenotype, which includes variable reactivity for neuronal, glial, epithelial, and mesenchymal markers. Immunopositivity is patchy for most. Only staining for vimentin is diffuse.* **(Right)** *The hallmark and essential diagnostic feature of AT/RT is loss of nuclear staining for INI1. Normal vessels and stroma serve as positive internal controls with retained nuclear reactivity ⇒.*

GFAP

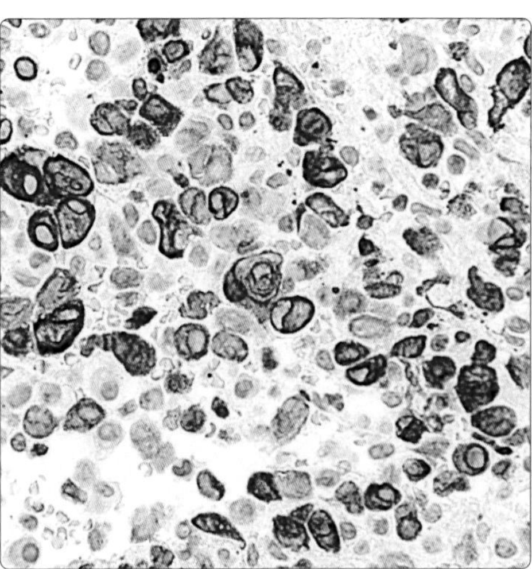

INI1

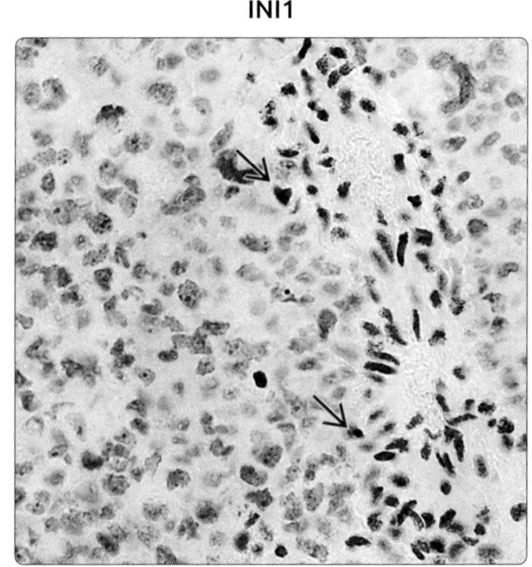

Posterior Fossa AT/RT

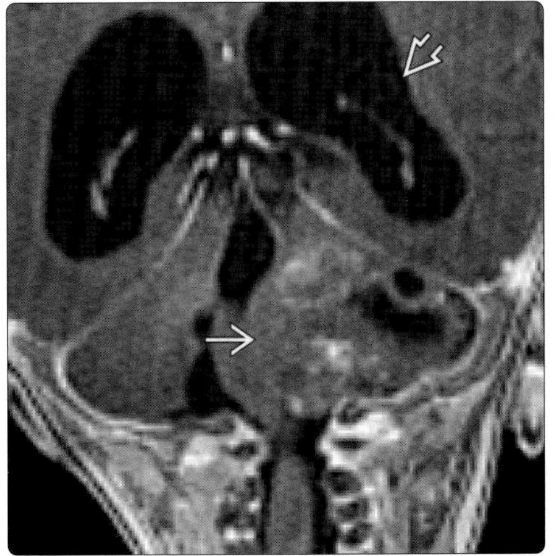

CSF Dissemination

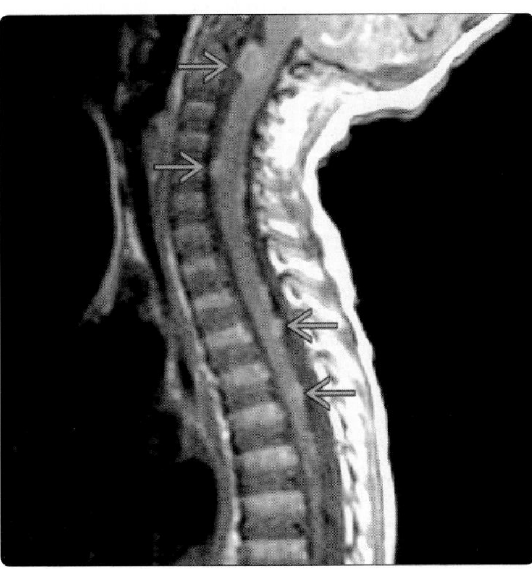

(Left) *When occurring in the posterior fossa, AT/RTs have a predilection for involvement of the cerebellopontine angle ➡. There is severe obstructive hydrocephalus with massive dilation of the lateral ventricles ➡.* **(Right)** *Sagittal T1WI MR with contrast shows multiple enhancing "drop mets" ➡ along the ventral and dorsal surfaces of the cervical and thoracic chord from a posterior fossa AT/RT. AT/RTs have a propensity for CSF dissemination.*

Touch Imprint AT/RT

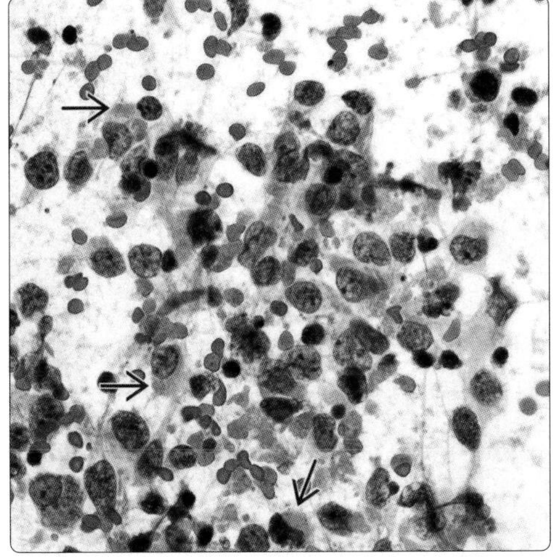

Rare Rhabdoid Cells

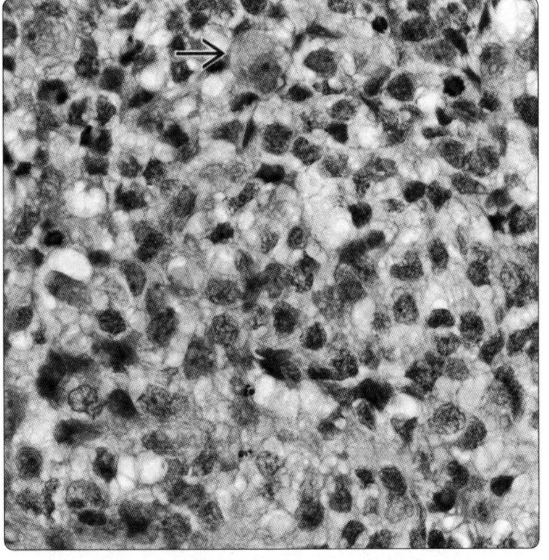

(Left) *Rhabdoid cells may be infrequent in AT/RTs. Perfect rhabdoid cells are lacking in this touch imprint, although a few tumor cells show dense eosinophilic cytoplasmic ball-like inclusions ➡.* **(Right)** *Permanent sections of AT/RTs have highly variable numbers of classic rhabdoid cells and in some tumors, such cells with large vesicular nuclei, prominent nucleoli, and eccentrically placed cytoplasmic showing rounded contours and ball-like inclusions, may be few and far between ➡.*

AT/RT With *SMARCA4* Mutation

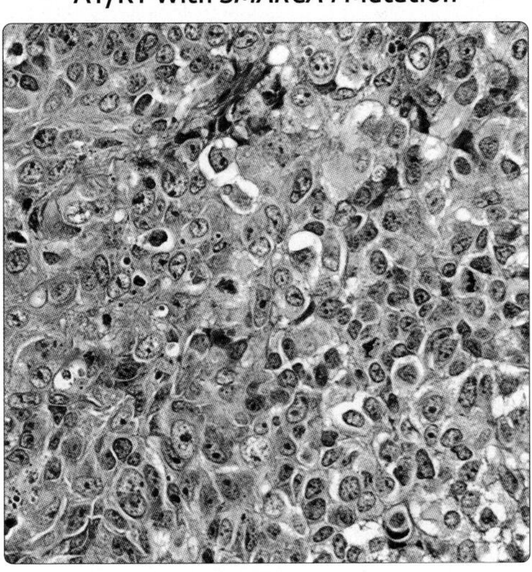

Retained INI1 in AT/RT With *SMARCA4* Mutation

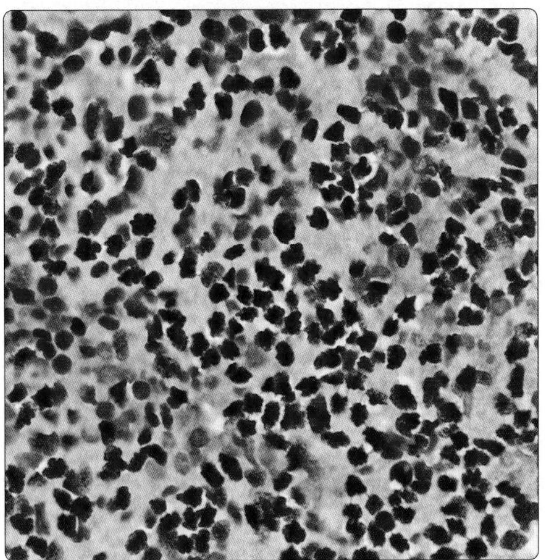

(Left) *Rarely, AT/RT may lack INI1 mutations and instead have mutations in associated proteins, such as SMARCA4. As this example demonstrates, histologic and other immunophenotypic findings are identical to INI1-mutant tumors. (Courtesy C. Giannini, MD.)* **(Right)** *Retained INI1 (SMARCB1) in an AT/RT containing SMARCA4 mutation is shown, although this tumor demonstrated classic histologic and immunohistochemical features of AT/RT. (Courtesy C. Giannini, MD.)*

Germinoma

KEY FACTS

CLINICAL ISSUES

- Predilection to midline structures: Pineal, pituitary, and suprasellar regions
- Paralysis of upward gaze and convergence (Parinaud syndrome) and diabetes insipidus
- Highly radiosensitive: Pure germinomas have > 90% 5-year survival rate
- Several-year history of symptoms, e.g., pituitary insufficiency, not inconsistent with germinoma
- Peak age incidence: 15-20 years

IMAGING

- Strong homogeneous enhancement
  - Pituitary or pineal location, occasionally both
- Occasionally enhancement along ventricular lining

ANCILLARY TESTS

- OCT4(+), SALL4(+), LIN28A(+)
- CD117 or c-kit(+)
- PLAP(+), but less reliable than other markers

TOP DIFFERENTIAL DIAGNOSES

- Teratomas or nonseminomatous germ cell tumor
- Granulomatous diseases (e.g., sarcoidosis)
- Langerhans cell histiocytosis
- Pineal parenchymal tumors
- Malignant lymphoma

DIAGNOSTIC CHECKLIST

- Crush artifact, sometimes severe, can distort tumor cells and obscure diagnosis
- Immunohistochemistry may be necessary for tumor detection
- Exclude other, nongerminomatous, components, e.g., yolk sac tumor, choriocarcinoma, especially in presence of positive serum or CSF markers

(Left) *Germinomas are typically midline tumors that enhance avidly upon contrast administration. This sagittal T1WI contrast-enhanced MR demonstrates a sellar tumor with suprasellar extension.* **(Right)** *Some germinomas synchronously affect pineal and sellar regions. This axial postcontrast T1WI MR demonstrates enhancing masses in both locations.*

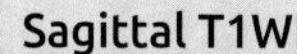

Sagittal T1WI

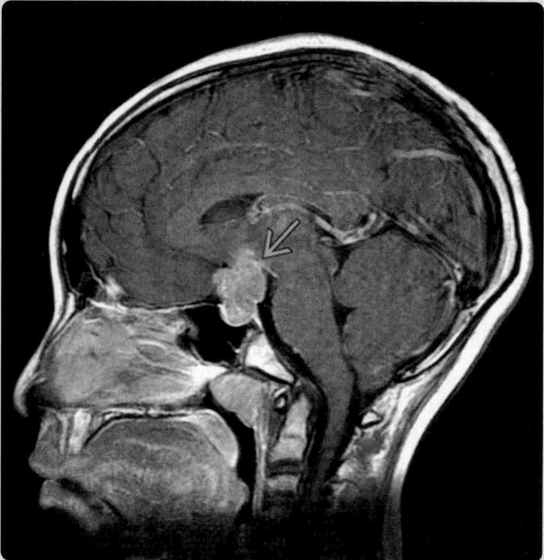

Pineal and Pituitary Involvement

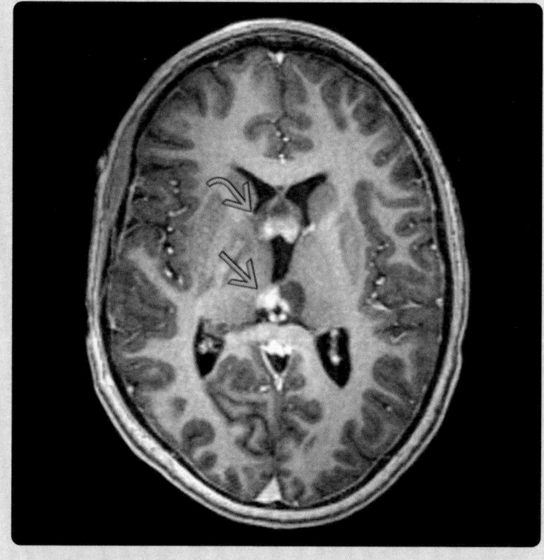

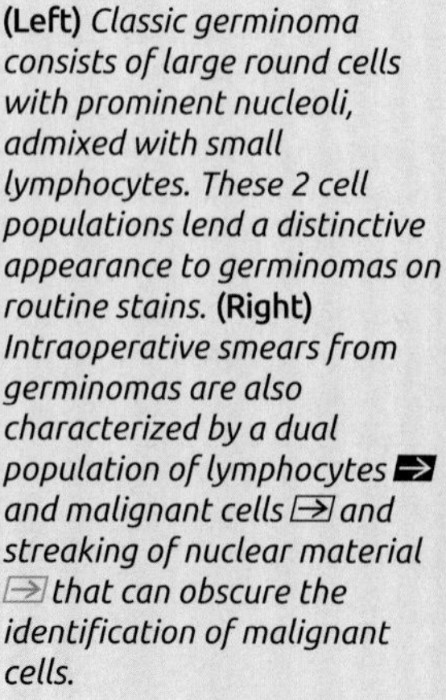

(Left) *Classic germinoma consists of large round cells with prominent nucleoli, admixed with small lymphocytes. These 2 cell populations lend a distinctive appearance to germinomas on routine stains.* **(Right)** *Intraoperative smears from germinomas are also characterized by a dual population of lymphocytes and malignant cells and streaking of nuclear material that can obscure the identification of malignant cells.*

Malignant Cells and Lymphocytes

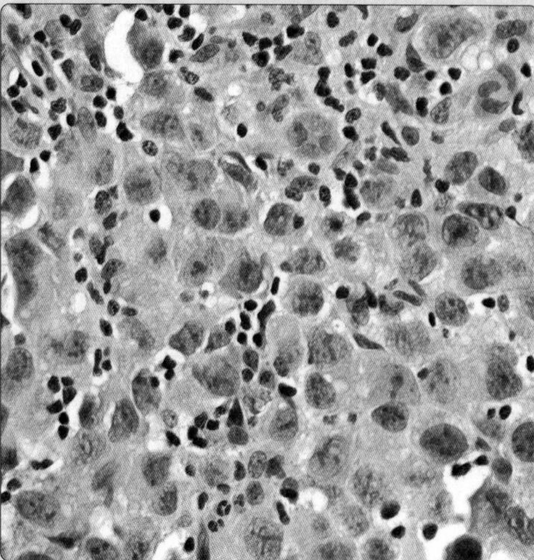

Intraoperative Smear

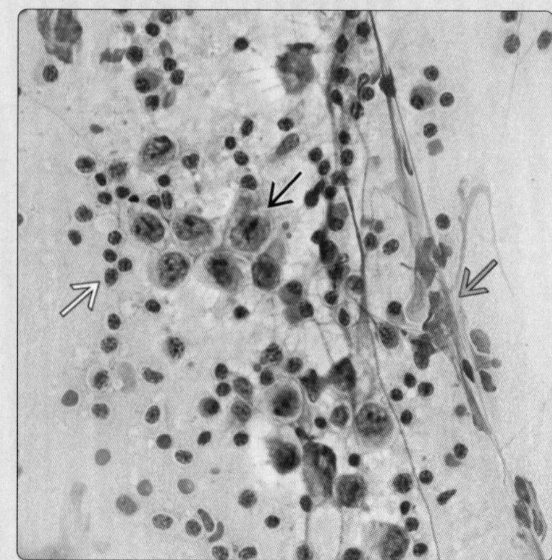

TERMINOLOGY

Definitions

- Morphologic and immunophenotypic counterpart of gonadal or extragonadal seminoma and dysgerminoma

CLINICAL ISSUES

Epidemiology

- Incidence
  - 2/3 of all intracranial germ cell tumors
  - Incidence varies geographically
    - Higher incidence in Japan
- Age
  - Principally in first 3 decades
  - Peak age incidence: 15-20 year
- Sex
  - Male predominance in pineal region
  - Slight female predominance in sellar/suprasellar tumors

Site

- Predilection for midline structures
  - Pineal, most common
  - Sellar/suprasellar
  - Synchronous pineal/suprasellar, rare
- Basal ganglia, uni- or bilateral, rare
- Other intracranial sites, rare
- Diffuse subependymal seeding, especially frontal horns of lateral ventricles, rare

Presentation

- Pineal
  - Paralysis of upward gaze and convergence (Parinaud syndrome)
  - Hydrocephalus
- Suprasellar/sellar
  - Visual disturbance, mostly field defects
  - Hypopituitarism
  - Diabetes insipidus
- Basal ganglia and thalamus
  - Hemiparesis
- Some tumors associated with precocious puberty, regardless of site
- Protracted (several years) pituitary insufficiency, rare

Treatment

- Highly radiosensitive
- Chemotherapy, timing relative to radiotherapy debated
- Surgical resection beyond biopsy provides no advantage in survival

Prognosis

- Pure germinomas: > 90% 5-year survival rate
  - Somewhat less favorable prognosis for tumors with syncytiotrophoblastic component
  - Some suggest deleterious effect of gross total resection on prognosis
- Risk of secondary tumor following radiation necessitates long-term follow-up

IMAGING

MR Findings

- Solid pineal tumor with occasional cystic component
- Isointense or hyperintense to gray matter on T1WI
- Hyperintense on FLAIR and T2WI
- Strong homogeneous enhancement
- Occasionally enhancing tumor along ventricular walls
  - Periventricular and subependymal spread can be seen in pineal and pituitary germinomas

MACROSCOPIC

General Features

- Affected sites difficult to access surgically
  - Specimens often small
- Tough consistency due to fibrous tissue, in some cases

MICROSCOPIC

Histologic Features

- Specimens often show crush artifact
- Homogeneous sheets, lobules, or individual cells
- Tumor cells
  - Large, round, dyscohesive cells
  - Prominent, irregular, bar-shaped nucleoli
  - Pale cytoplasm
  - Mitoses, common
  - Apoptosis, common
- Isolated multinucleated syncytiotrophoblasts, uncommon
- Inflammatory cell component
  - Always lymphocytic, sometimes dense
  - Germinal centers, some cases
  - Can obscure tumor cells
  - Often minimal or absent in areas of parenchymal infiltration
  - Noncaseating granulomas, variable
- Apoptosis, common
- Necrosis, uncommon
- Calcifications, usually overrun normal pineal corpora arenacea ("brain sand")
- Brain parenchymal infiltration, mimic other tumors, such as malignant glioma

ANCILLARY TESTS

Cytology

- Smear
  - Tumor cells
    - Large nuclei with central macronucleoli
    - Discrete cell membranes
    - Clear or vacuolated cytoplasm
  - Small lymphocytes
    - Variable number, mature T cells
  - Often significant nuclear "streaking" and crush artifact on smears
- CSF cytology: Rarely (+) for tumor cells

Histochemistry

- PAS diastase
  - Reactivity: (+), diastase labile

- Staining pattern: Highlights cytoplasmic glycogen in tumor cells

Immunohistochemistry

- PLAP(+)
  - Less reliable than other antibodies
  - Prone to background staining false-positives, and false-negatives
- OCT4(+)
- CD117 (c-kit)(+)
- D2-40(+)
- Cytokeratin (+), occasional
- Isolated syncytiotrophoblasts HCG-β(+)
- SALL4(+)
- LIN28A(+)
- Ki-67, high labeling index

Serologic Testing

- HCG-β(+) in CSF and serum in cases with syncytiotrophoblasts

DIFFERENTIAL DIAGNOSIS

Pineal Parenchymal Tumors

- Cohesive tumor architecture
- Absent or scant lymphocytic infiltrate
- Synaptophysin (+)
- OCT4(+) and CD117(-)

Granulomatous Lesions

- Sarcoidosis
  - Potentially confused with germinomas with abundant granulomatous reaction
  - No malignant cells
  - OCT4(-) and PLAP(-)
  - Common at base of brain, rare in pineal region
- Granulomatous hypophysitis/giant cell granuloma
  - Limited to pituitary
  - No atypical cells
  - Giant cells, mixed inflammatory infiltrates in some cases
  - OCT4(-) and PLAP(-)
- Tuberculosis
  - Necrosis
  - Acid-fast bacilli
  - No tumor cells

Langerhans Cell Histiocytosis

- Langerhans cells
  - Folded, clefted nuclei
  - May appear as dyscohesive as germinoma but may have focal clusters
- Eosinophils and mixed inflammatory cells
- CD1a(+)
- OCT4(-) and PLAP(-)
- Many BRAF VE1 IHC(+) (mutated for *BRAF V600E*)

Malignant Lymphoma

- Most common in older adults or immunocompromised individuals
- Periventricular dissemination, rare
- Typically CD20(+), CD79-a(+), and MUM1(+)
- SALL4(-), LIN28A(-), OCT4(-), and CD117(-)

Teratomas and Other Germ Cell Tumors

- Limited biopsies of mixed germ cell tumors may miss nongerminomatous component(s)
  - Increased serum or CSF α-fetoprotein levels
  - α-fetoprotein (+) on biopsy suggests yolk sac component
    - Carcinoma-like histologic features or Schiller-Duval bodies
  - CD30 positivity in biopsy suggests embryonal carcinoma component
- Midline tumor with cyst and MR signal characteristics of fat &/or calcification suggests teratomatous component

DIAGNOSTIC CHECKLIST

Clinically Relevant Pathologic Features

- More likely to produce diabetes insipidus than other tumors
- Compatible with year-long preoperative history in spite of brisk mitotic activity

Pathologic Interpretation Pearls

- Crush artifact, sometimes severe, can obscure tumor cells
- Immunohistochemistry (CD117 and OCT4) may be necessary for detection of rare tumor cells
- Exclude other, nongerminomatous, components, (e.g., yolk sac tumor and choriocarcinoma) in presence of positive serum/CSF markers

SELECTED REFERENCES

1. Acharya S et al: Long-term outcomes and late effects for childhood and young adulthood intracranial germinomas. Neuro Oncol. 17(5):741-6, 2015
2. Tan C et al: Expression of Kit and Etv1 in restricted brain regions supports a brain-cell progenitor as an origin for cranial germinomas. Cancer Genet. 208(3):55-61, 2015
3. Martens T et al: Long-term follow-up and quality of life in patients with intracranial germinoma. Neurosurg Rev. 37(3):445-50; discussion 451, 2014
4. Ono H et al: Spontaneous regression of germinoma in the pineal region before endoscopic surgery: a pitfall of modern strategy for pineal germ cell tumors. J Neurooncol. 103(3):755-8, 2011
5. Alapetite C et al: Pattern of relapse and outcome of non-metastatic germinoma patients treated with chemotherapy and limited field radiation: the SFOP experience. Neuro Oncol. 12(12):1318-25, 2010
6. Cuccia V et al: Suprasellar/pineal bifocal germ cell tumors. Childs Nerv Syst. 26(8):1043-9, 2010
7. Khatua S et al: Treatment of primary CNS germinomatous germ cell tumors with chemotherapy prior to reduced dose whole ventricular and local boost irradiation. Pediatr Blood Cancer. 55(1):42-6, 2010
8. Lee D et al: Histologically confirmed intracranial germ cell tumors; an analysis of 62 patients in a single institute. Virchows Arch. 457(3):347-57, 2010
9. Phi JH et al: Germinomas in the basal ganglia: magnetic resonance imaging classification and the prognosis. J Neurooncol. 99(2):227-36, 2010
10. Wang Y et al: Intracranial germinoma: clinical and MRI findings in 56 patients. Childs Nerv Syst. 26(12):1773-7, 2010
11. Wong JM et al: Germinoma with malignant transformation to nongerminomatous germ cell tumor. J Neurosurg Pediatr. 6(3):295-8, 2010
12. Yonezawa H et al: Germinoma with syncytiotrophoblastic giant cells arising in the corpus callosum. Neurol Med Chir (Tokyo). 50(7):588-91, 2010
13. Goodwin TL et al: Incidence patterns of central nervous system germ cell tumors: a SEER Study. J Pediatr Hematol Oncol. 31(8):541-4, 2009
14. Rivarola et al: Precocious puberty in children with tumours of the suprasellar and pineal areas: organic central precocious puberty. Acta Paediatr. 90(7):751-6, 2001
15. Matsutani M et al: Primary intracranial germ cell tumors: a clinical analysis of 153 histologically verified cases. J Neurosurg. 86(3):446-55, 1997

Coronal Contrast-Enhanced MR

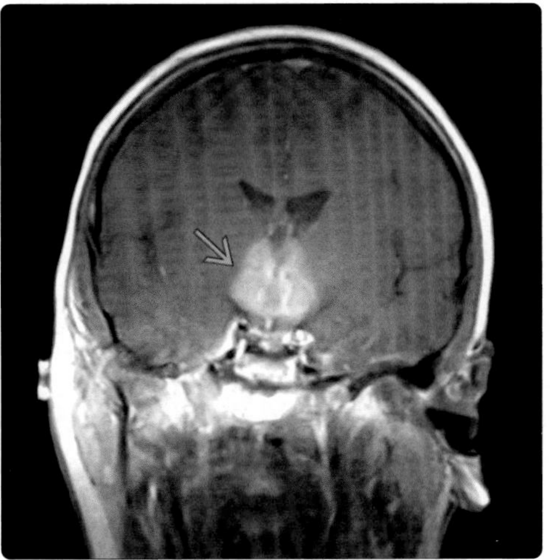

Involvement of Mammillary Body

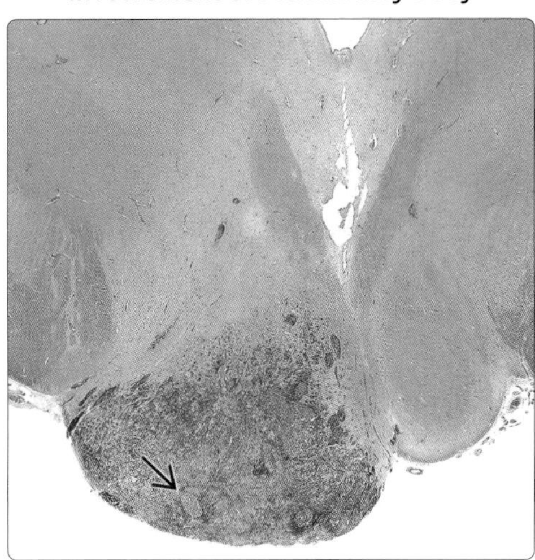

(Left) *Emphasizing the midline position of most germinomas, this coronal contrast-enhanced T1WI MR demonstrates a homogeneously enhancing hypothalamic mass ⇒ that extends along the periventricular space of the 3rd ventricle.* **(Right)** *As in this lesion centered on a mammillary body, germinoma should be suspected, even at low magnification, in the face of a dense lymphoid infiltrate with germinal centers ⇒. The suprasellar/hypothalamic region is a favored site, as is the pineal area.*

Intraoperative Smear

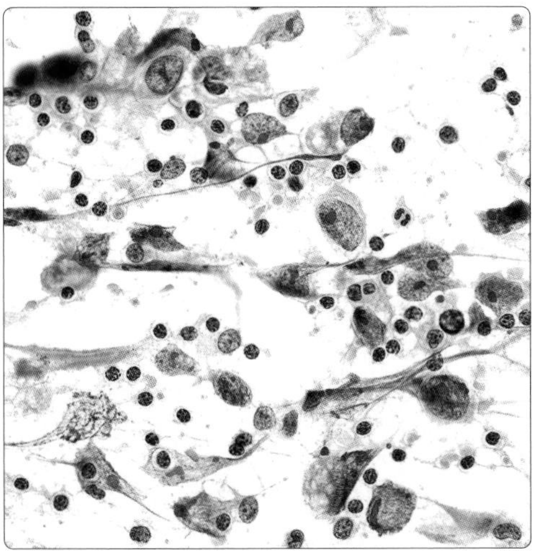

Intraoperative Smear

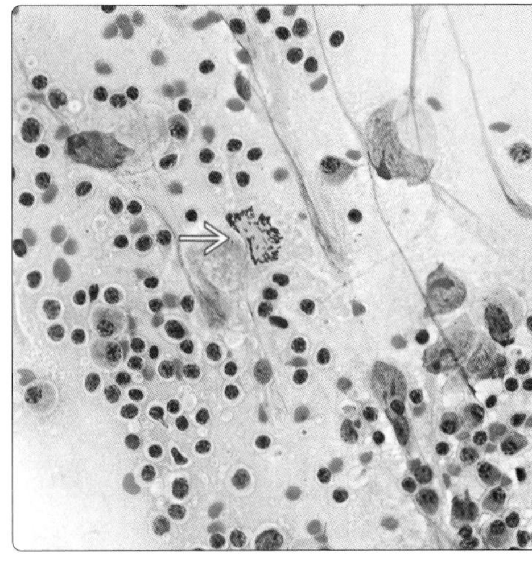

(Left) *An intraoperative diagnosis is often easier on smears than on frozen sections. Large tumor cells with prominent nucleoli, intermixed with small lymphocytes, leave few other diagnostic possibilities, especially in a lesion from the pineal or suprasellar region.* **(Right)** *Mitotic figures and large nuclei with macronucleoli on a background of lymphocytes and plasma cells are typical of germinomas. Mitotic figures ➡ also help identify the neoplastic cell population.*

Frozen Section

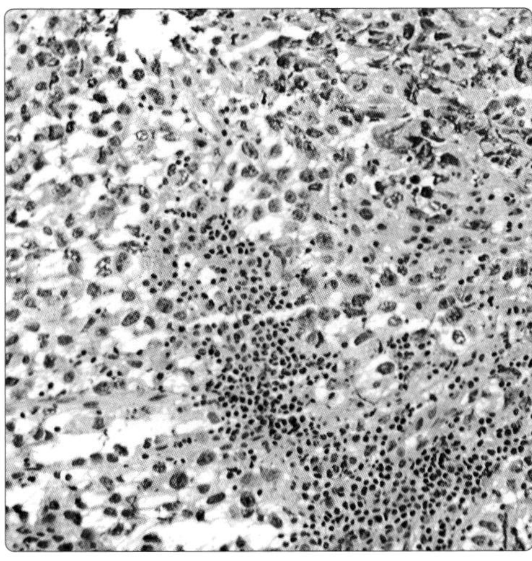

Crush Artifact in Biopsies

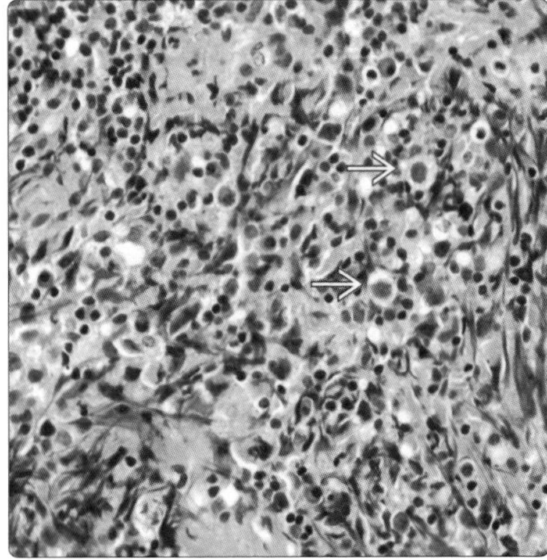

(Left) *Frozen sections from germinomas are often limited and demonstrate artifactual changes. Recognition of the malignant cells admixed with small, mature lymphocytes greatly aid in the diagnosis. Many tumor cells in frozen sections also appear fragmented.* **(Right)** *In many biopsies, despite the streaking of nuclear material and the crush artifact, the presence of noncrushed, large anaplastic cells with prominent nuclei ➡ can help make the diagnosis of germinoma.*

(Left) *Well-developed granulomas ⇒ are not uncommon in germinomas at any body site, including the CNS. However, large anaplastic tumor cells ⇒ can be recognized in these instances.* **(Right)** *Germinomas may have not only granulomas but multinucleated giant cells containing asteroid bodies ⇒. Tumor cells can be difficult to find in small biopsies wherein inflammation is more abundant than in this case. No tumor cells are detected in some cases that later prove to be germinoma.*

Granulomas in Germinoma

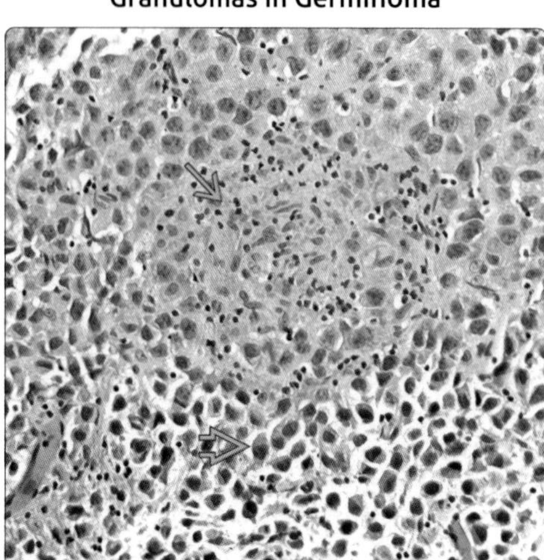

Granulomas and Asteroid Bodies

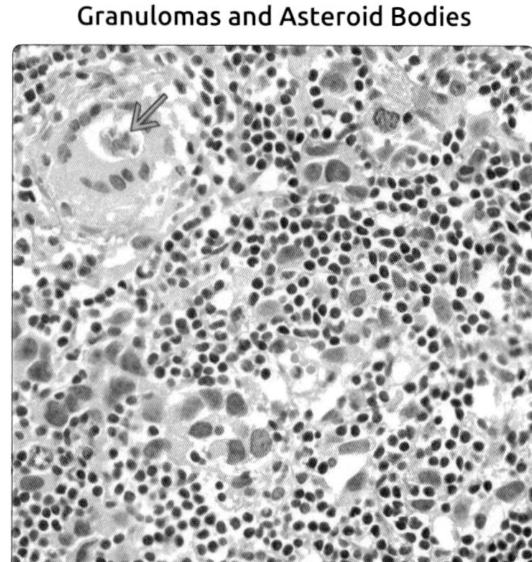

(Left) *Germinomas often show radiologic or histologic evidence of a subependymal spread. Tumor cells ⇒ aggregate beneath the ependyma ⇒ in this case.* **(Right)** *Abundant lymphocytes, as well as occasional plasma cells, constitute the background in germinomas. The neoplastic cells are often large with hyperchromatic nuclei and prominent nucleoli ⇒. This biphasic pattern is virtually diagnostic of germinomas.*

Subependymal Spread

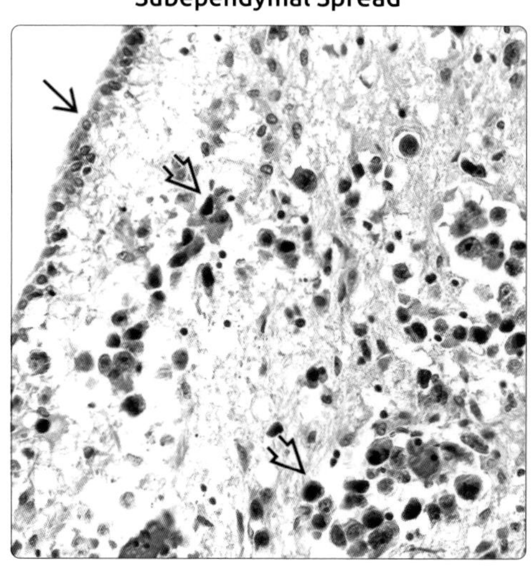

2 Populations of Cells

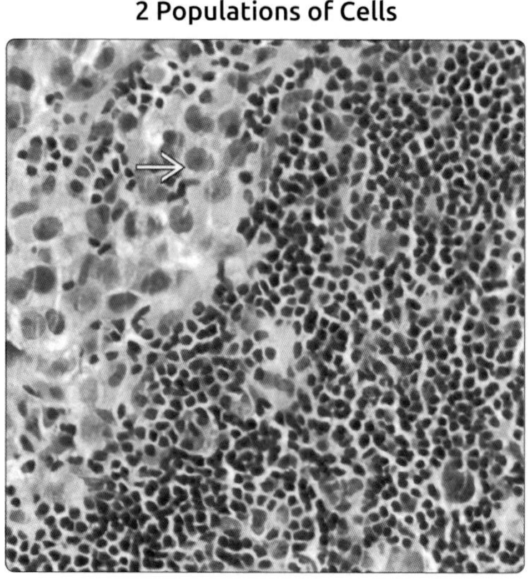

(Left) *Germinomas typically have variable ratios of large, anaplastic, polygonal cells to small lymphocytes. The latter is sparse here but may be so dominant that tumor cells may be difficult, or even impossible, to find in some cases. Mitoses are frequent ⇒.* **(Right)** *One of the typical histological appearances of germinomas is the so-called clear cell change that is reminiscent of an anaplastic oligodendroglioma.*

Anaplastic Tumor Cells With Mitoses

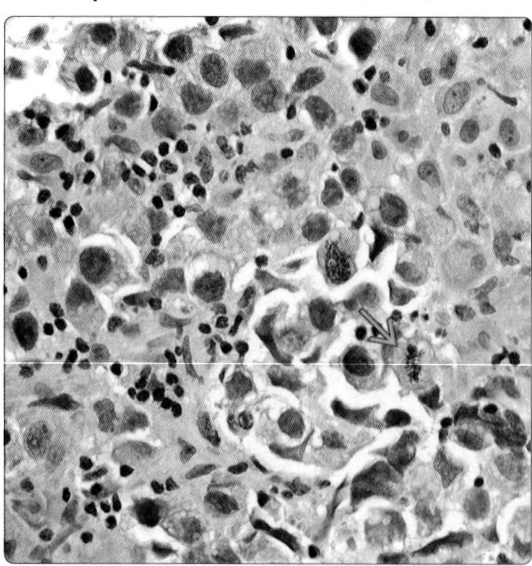

Clear Cell Tumor

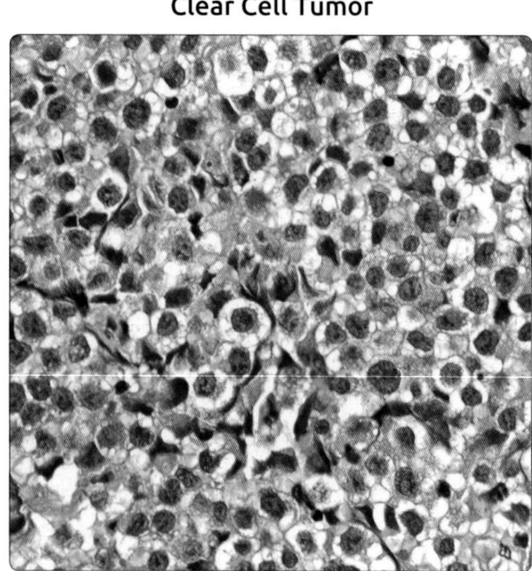

CD117 (C-kit) Positivity

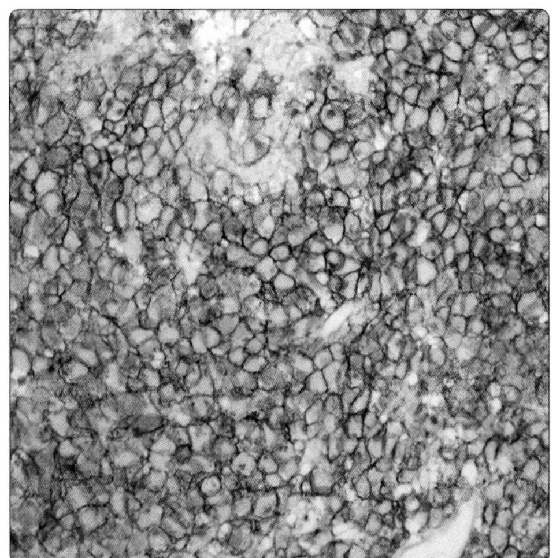

CD117 Positivity

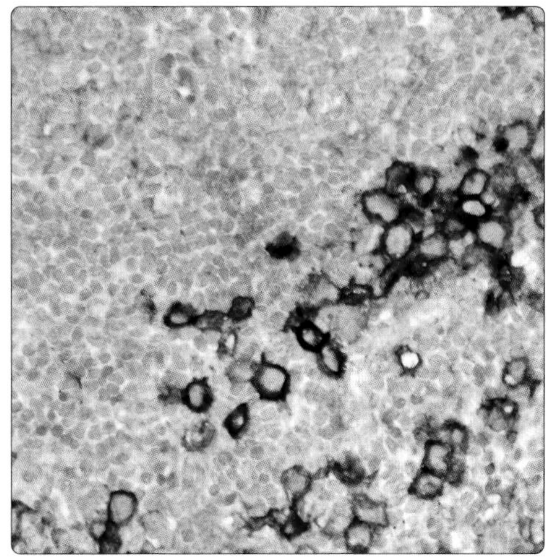

(Left) *Most of the neoplastic cells demonstrate strong membranous staining with antibodies against CD117 (c-kit).* **(Right)** *The scattered malignant cells in a background of inflammatory cells can be highlighted both with nuclear and cytoplasmic stains for diagnosis. In this image, the CD117(+) tumor cells with membranous staining can be seen in a background of abundant lymphocytes.*

Human Chorionic Gonadotrophin Positivity

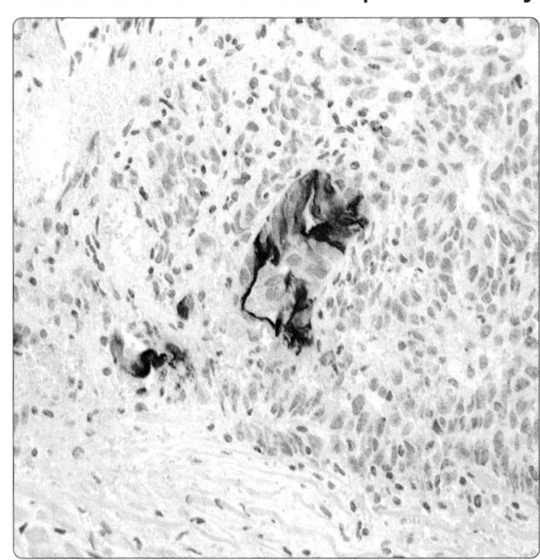

PLAP Positivity

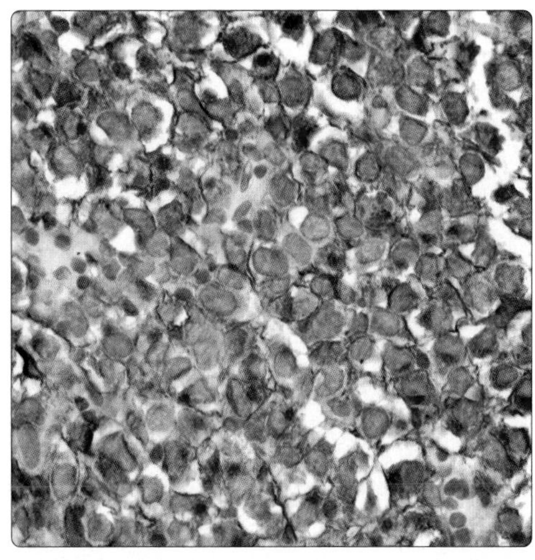

(Left) *Some germinomas harbor large cells that demonstrate immunopositivity with the antibodies against human chorionic gonadotrophin.* **(Right)** *PLAP is 1 of the most commonly used stains for the diagnosis of germinomas. While this stain is not as reliable as some of the newer markers, it is still positive in the overwhelming majority of germinomas.*

SALL4 Nuclear Positivity

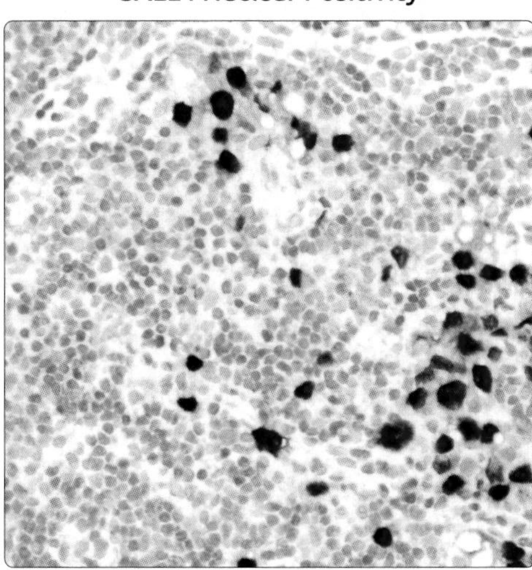

OCT-4 Nuclear Positivity

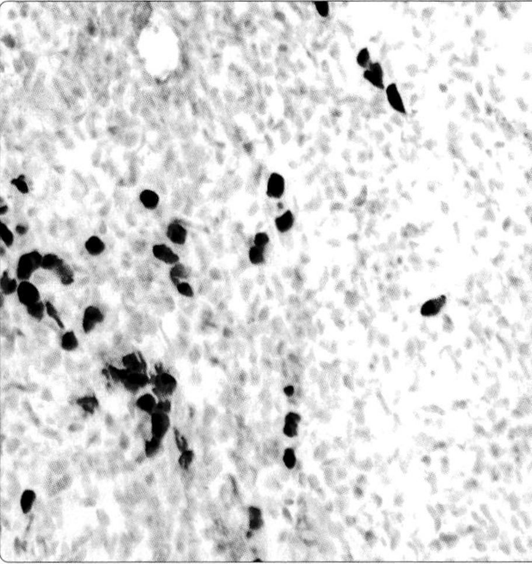

(Left) *SALL4 is a nuclear stain that is positive in most germ cell tumors and can identify tumor cells in a majority of germinomas.* **(Right)** *Octamer binding transcription factor-4 (OCT-4) antibody is directed against this homeodomain transcription factor and is strongly positive in almost all germinomas. This nuclear stain is suggested to be a critical factor in the self-renewal of undifferentiated embryonic stem cells.*

Teratomas

KEY FACTS

TERMINOLOGY

- Nonseminomatous germ cell tumors with tissue components resembling normal derivatives of all 3 germ layers

CLINICAL ISSUES

- Total excision treatment of choice for mature teratomas
- Teratomas harboring immature or malignant germ cell tumor elements may require multimodal therapy
- Prognosis depends on presence of other germ cell elements, especially embryonal carcinoma, yolk sac tumor, or choriocarcinoma

IMAGING

- Complex, heterogeneous, solid-cystic mass

MICROSCOPIC

- Haphazard arrangement of tissue types from all germ layers, including mesenchyme, epithelium, and neuroectoderm
- Unlike mature types, immature teratomas often have mitotic figures and apoptosis
- Associated other germ cell tumor(s) may be focal and require immunohistochemistry for detection and classification

ANCILLARY TESTS

- Epithelial elements positive for cytokeratins, including CK7, CK20, and AE1/AE3
- Mesenchymal elements positive for vimentin, muscle-specific actin, and desmin
- Germ cell markers in malignant germ cell tumor elements

TOP DIFFERENTIAL DIAGNOSES

- Dermoid cyst
- Craniopharyngioma
- Intraspinal endodermal (bronchogenic) cyst

(Left) *Teratomas are often bulky midline masses that contain calcifications and varying signal intensity. The solid components often have high signal intensity on FLAIR images and show variable enhancement.* **(Right)** *Some congenital teratomas, by occupying much of the intracranial compartment, displace the brain ➡ to the periphery.*

Large Midline Mass

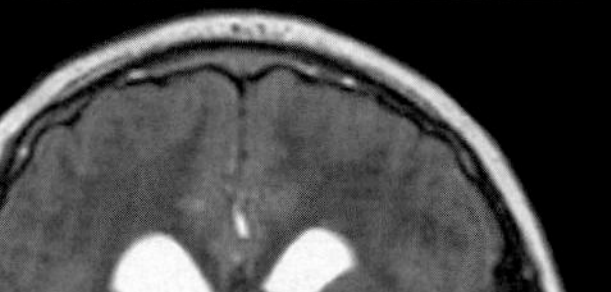

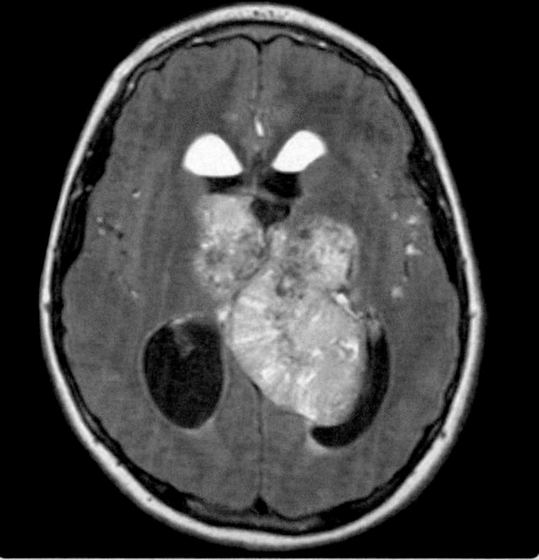

Massive Congenital Teratoma

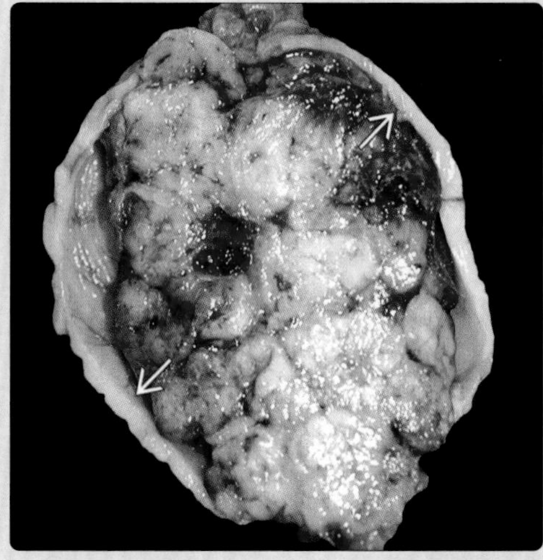

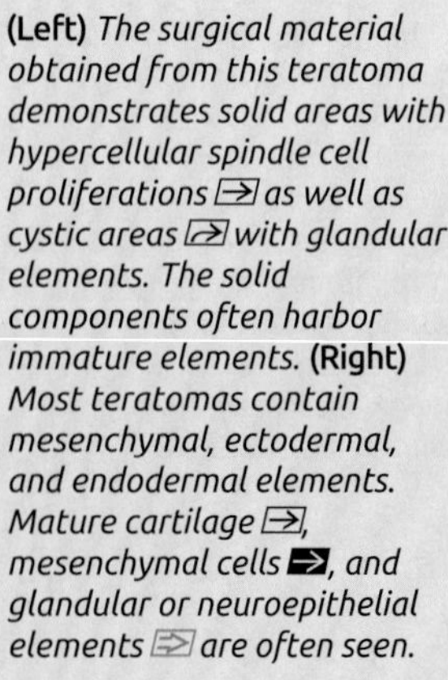

(Left) *The surgical material obtained from this teratoma demonstrates solid areas with hypercellular spindle cell proliferations ➡ as well as cystic areas ➡ with glandular elements. The solid components often harbor immature elements.* **(Right)** *Most teratomas contain mesenchymal, ectodermal, and endodermal elements. Mature cartilage ➡, mesenchymal cells ➡, and glandular or neuroepithelial elements ➡ are often seen.*

Complex Solid-Cystic Architecture

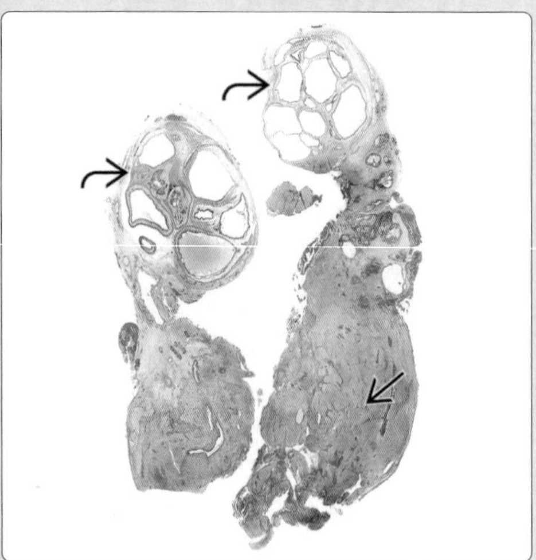

Tissues From All 3 Germ Layers

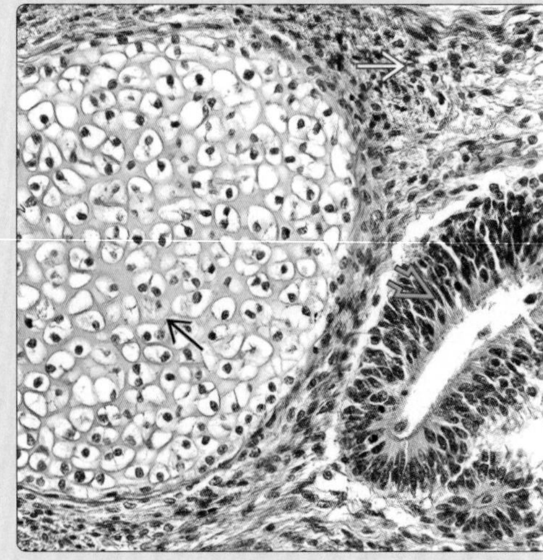

TERMINOLOGY

Definitions

- Nonseminomatous germ cell tumors with tissue components resembling normal derivatives of all 3 germ layers
- 3 subtypes recognized
  - Mature teratoma composed of fully differentiated (adult) tissue types
  - Immature teratoma with tissues resembling those of embryos
  - Teratoma with malignant transformation (rare)
    - Includes elements of somatic malignant tumors, such as carcinoma, sarcoma, or primitive neuroectodermal tumor (PNET)

CLINICAL ISSUES

Presentation

- Congenital immature teratomas
  - Present in early age with macrocephaly and hydrocephaly
  - May be massive and cause fetal demise
  - Can be diagnosed prenatally, but majority is unresectable
- Mature/immature teratomas
  - Most common in 1st and 2nd decades of life
  - Most commonly affect pineal region
  - Often coexist with other germ cell elements (e.g., germinoma, yolk sac tumor, embryonal carcinoma)

Treatment

- Total excision treatment of choice for mature teratoma
- Immature or malignant components require multimodal therapy

Prognosis

- Depends on presence of other germ cell elements, especially embryonal carcinoma, yolk sac tumor, or choriocarcinoma
- Excellent for mature teratomas with gross total excision
- Dismal for teratomas with malignant transformation
- Pure teratomas may recur as nonteratomatous tumors
- Congenital teratomas are often lethal

IMAGING

MR Findings

- Complex, heterogeneous, solid-cystic mass
- Cystic midline mass containing calcium, fat, soft tissue
- Variable signal on T1- and T2-weighted and contrast-enhanced images

MICROSCOPIC

Histologic Features

- Haphazard arrangement of tissue types from all germ layers, including mesenchyme, epithelium, and neuroectoderm
- Mature teratomas
  - Composed of mature epidermal, dermal tissues with adnexa
  - Calcifications (common)
  - Epithelial elements, including squamous and glandular (enteric or respiratory) components
  - Neuroectodermal elements include neurons, choroid plexus, ependymal tissue
- Immature teratomas
  - Unlike mature types, immature teratomas often have mitotic figures and apoptosis
  - Blastema-like stroma is most common immature element
- Teratomas with malignant component
  - Carcinoma or sarcoma-like foci without obvious differentiation
  - High-grade neuroepithelial component resembles PNET or medulloblastoma
- Associated other germ cell tumor(s)
  - May be focal and require immunohistochemistry
  - Germinoma most common
  - Yolk sac tumor (endodermal sinus tumor), embryonal carcinoma, &/or choriocarcinoma
  - Malignant nonteratomatous elements may escape detection on initial or subsequent specimens

ANCILLARY TESTS

Immunohistochemistry

- Epithelial elements positive for cytokeratins, including CK7, CK20, and AE1/AE3
  - Focally chromogranin or synaptophysin (+)
- Vimentin, muscle-specific actin, and desmin (+); mesenchymal elements
- Germ cell markers in malignant germ cell elements; CD117, OCT4, HCG-β, α-fetoprotein (+)

DIFFERENTIAL DIAGNOSIS

Dermoid/Epidermoid Cyst

- Only squamous epithelium and adnexa represented
  - Some consider this lesion monodermal form of mature cystic teratoma
- Excellent prognosis
- Most occur in posterior fossa

Neurenteric Intraspinal Cyst (Endodermal, Bronchogenic)

- Predominant ciliated, mucus-producing epithelium
- Sometimes with bronchial cartilage

Craniopharyngioma

- Palisaded epithelium and stellate reticulum
- Wet keratin
- No mesenchymal or neuroectodermal elements

SELECTED REFERENCES

1. Goyal N et al: Intracranial teratomas in children: a clinicopathological study. Childs Nerv Syst. 29(11):2035-42, 2013
2. Agrawal M et al: Teratomas in central nervous system: a clinico-morphological study with review of literature. Neurol India. 58(6):841-6, 2010
3. Bare JB et al: Congenital immature teratoma of the central nervous system: three case reports with literature review. Fetal Pediatr Pathol. 26(3):109-18, 2007
4. Phi JH et al: Immature teratomas of the central nervous system: is adjuvant therapy mandatory? J Neurosurg. 103(6 Suppl):524-30, 2005

(Left) *Mature squamous epithelium with abundant keratinization* → *is 1 of the most common components of mature teratomas. Unlike epidermoid cysts, teratomas harbor other germ layer elements, which are not illustrated in this image.* **(Right)** *Common mesenchymal elements in mature teratomas are cartilage* →*, smooth muscle, and fibrous tissue* ⇨*.*

Mature Squamous Epithelium

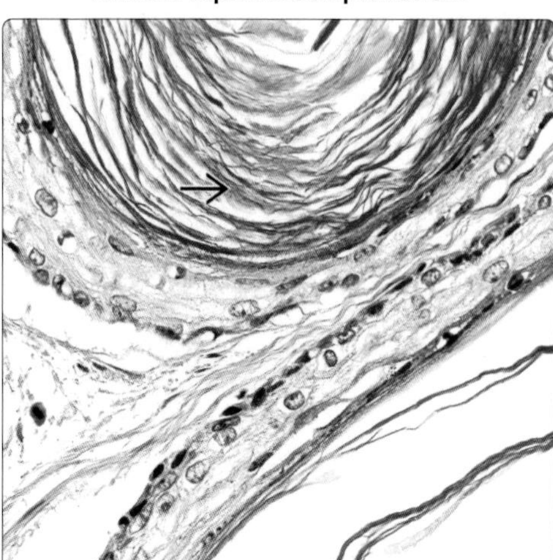

Cartilage and Smooth Muscle

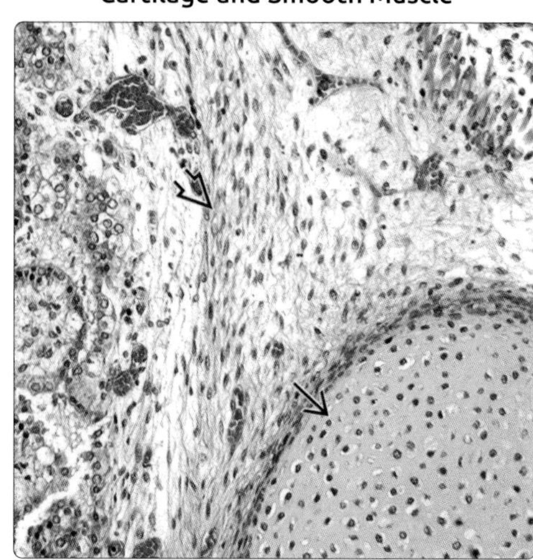

(Left) *In mature teratoma, epithelial elements* → *often occur with mesenchymal tissue, such as smooth muscle* ⇨*. Adipose tissue and skeletal muscle is also common.* **(Right)** *Glandular cells may demonstrate mucin production by goblet cells* →*. The glands can be of any type but are more commonly adnexal, intestinal, or gastric.*

Mesenchymal Elements

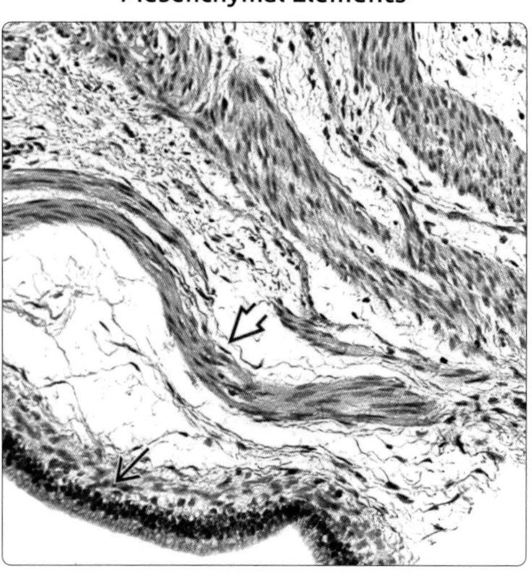

Various Glandular Structures

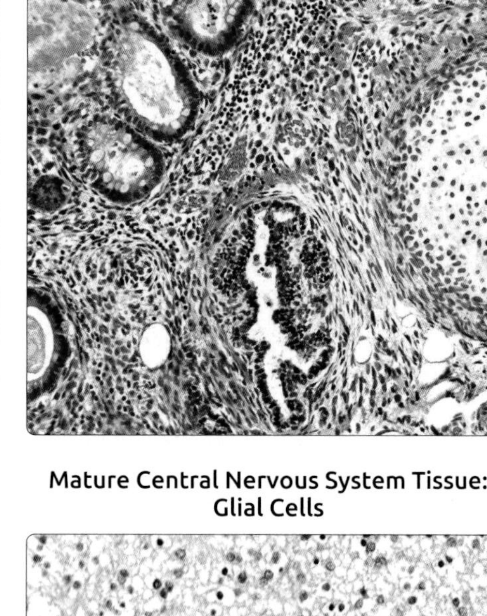

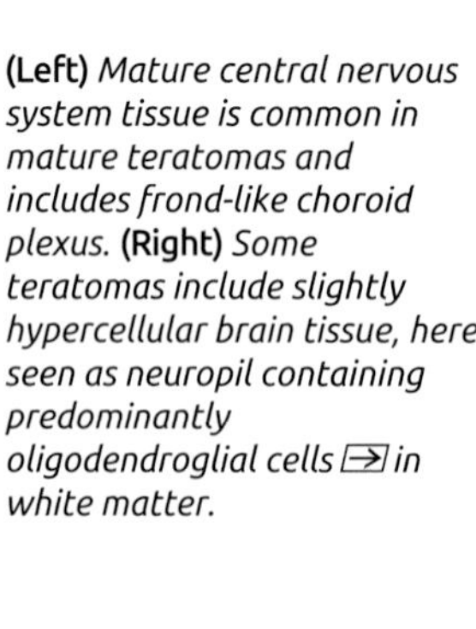

(Left) *Mature central nervous system tissue is common in mature teratomas and includes frond-like choroid plexus.* **(Right)** *Some teratomas include slightly hypercellular brain tissue, here seen as neuropil containing predominantly oligodendroglial cells* → *in white matter.*

Mature Central Nervous System Tissue: Choroid Plexus

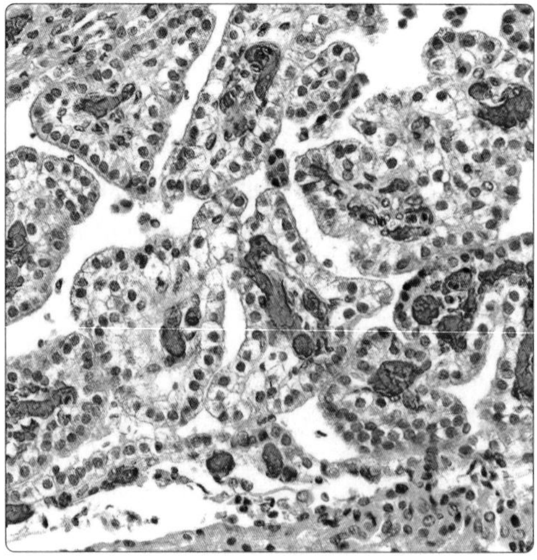

Mature Central Nervous System Tissue: Glial Cells

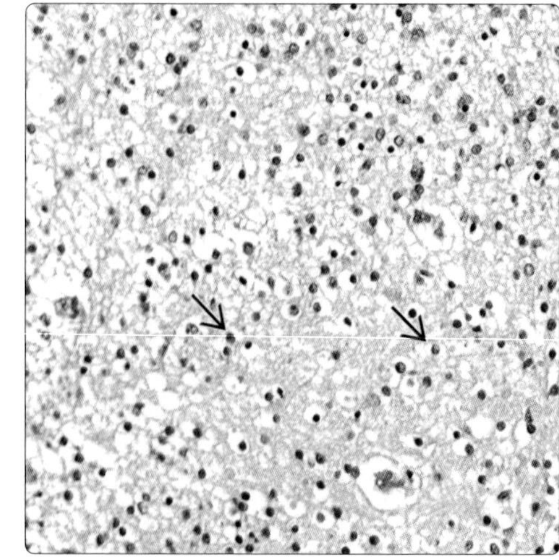

Immature Elements

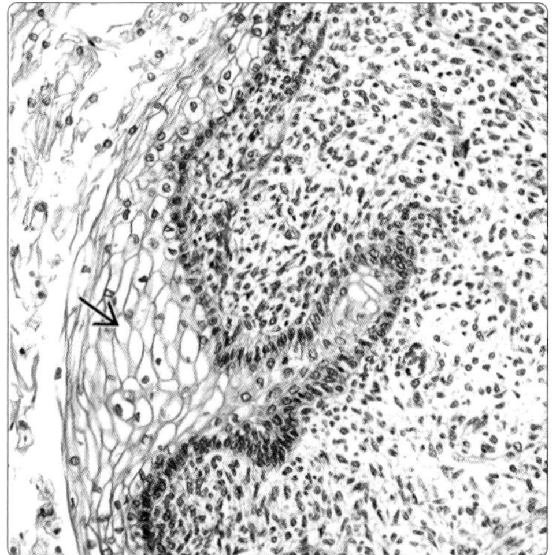

Immature Elements

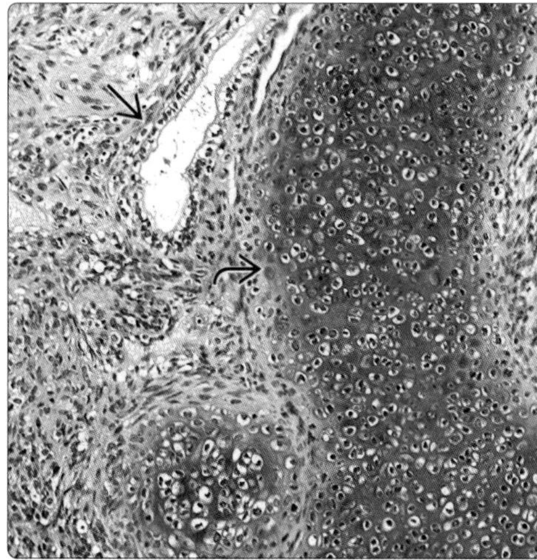

(Left) *Hypercellular, immature squamous epithelium ➡ with clear cytoplasm due to glycogenization is common in teratomas.* **(Right)** *Tissue disorganization and lack of maturation are well seen in this example that combines cartilage ↪ with very basophilic matrix and glandular epithelium ➡.*

Atypical Glandular Proliferations

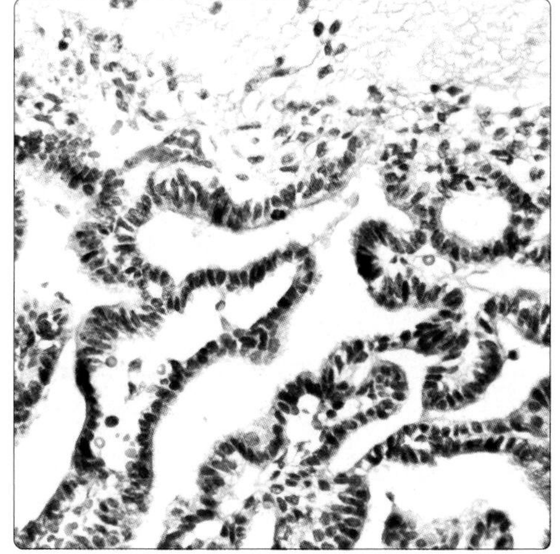

Embryonic Neuroepithelium

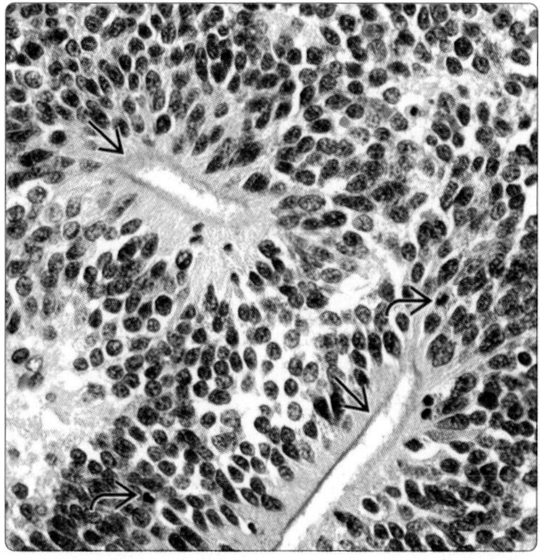

(Left) *Disordered glandular elements with hyperchromasia raise the possibility of a malignant germ cell component, such as a yolk sac tumor. Immunohistochemistry for a-fetoprotein can resolve the issue.* **(Right)** *Immature teratoma often consists largely of embryonic neuroepithelial elements. Note the increased cellularity and mitotic figures ↪. Slit-like lumina indicate immature neural tube/rudimentary ependymal differentiation ➡.*

Neuroepithelial Rosettes

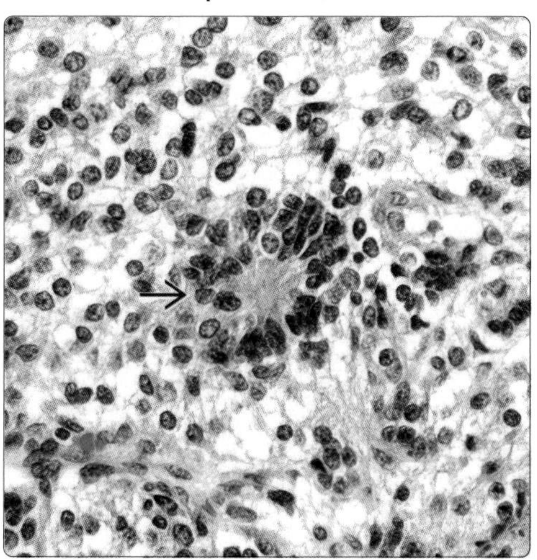

Immature Bone

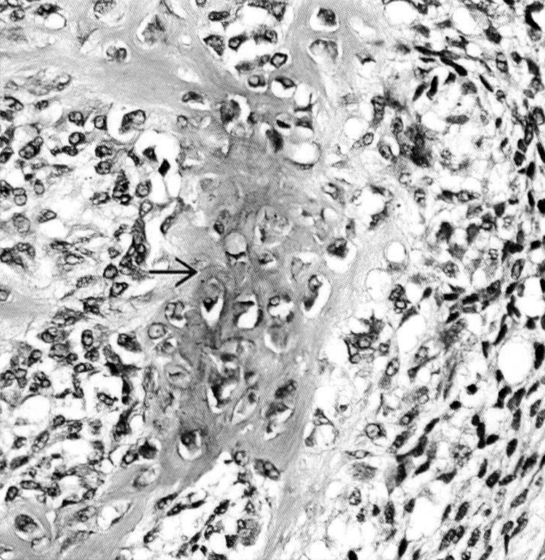

(Left) *Immature neuroepithelium may either include rosettes of the Homer Wright type or immature neuroepithelium with a central lumen; in this case, the presence of a central lumen is indefinite ➡. These immature elements are often immunoreactive for 1 or more neural markers, particularly synaptophysin.* **(Right)** *Immature bone ➡, as well as undifferentiated mesenchymal tissue, can have enough nuclear hyperchromasia and pleomorphism to suggest, falsely, the impression of sarcoma.*

Other Germ Cell Tumors

KEY FACTS

CLINICAL ISSUES

- Nongerminomatous cell tumors less radiosensitive than germinomas
- Pure embryonal carcinomas or endodermal sinus tumors behave more aggressive than mixed germ cell tumors
- Nongerminomatous germ cell tumors clinically separated into
  - Secreting tumors
    - Present with CSF α-fetoprotein level > 10 ng/mL &/or beta HCG > 50 IU/L
  - Nonsecreting tumors
    - Low α-fetoprotein &/or beta HCG levels
- Visual abnormalities and somnolence in about 1/2 of cases
- Diabetes insipidus with sellar region tumors

MICROSCOPIC

- Yolk sac tumor
  - Delicate fibrovascular projections forming distinct papillae (Schiller-Duval bodies)
- Embryonal carcinoma
  - Large anaplastic cells with epithelial features and abundant mitoses
- Choriocarcinoma
  - Mixture of cells resembling cyto- or syncytiotrophoblasts
  - Syncytiotrophoblasts line large angular blood-filled channels

ANCILLARY TESTS

- Some tumors with isochromosome 12p
- SALL4(+) LIN28A(+)
- OCT 3/OCT4 (+)
- AFP positive in yolk sac component and sometimes embryonal carcinoma component
- Cytokeratins diffuse and strong (+) in embryonal carcinoma component
- HCG(+) in choriocarcinomatous component

Mixed Germ Cell Tumor, Hydrocephalus

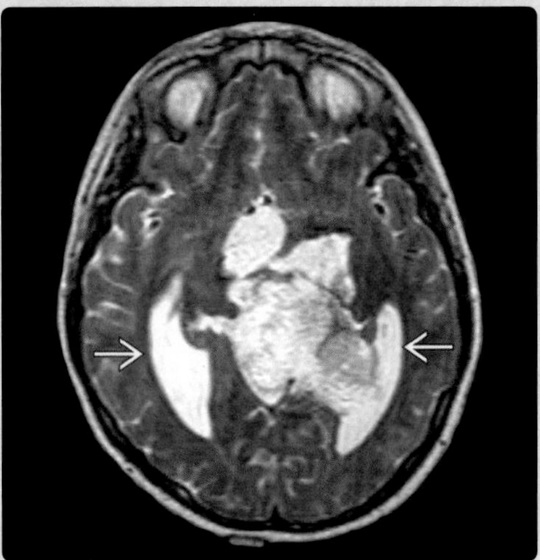

Embryonal Carcinoma

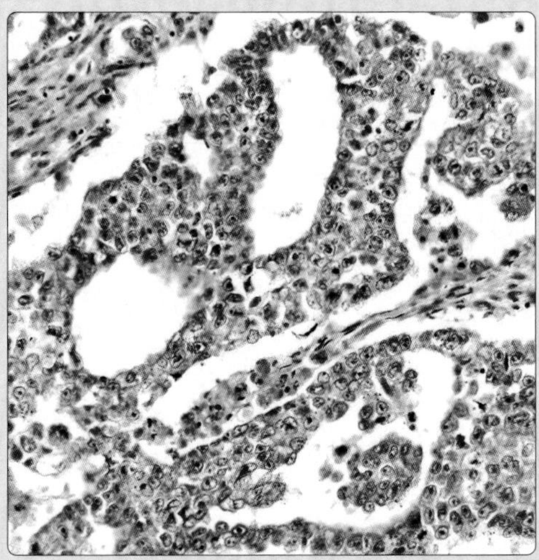

(Left) *Mixed germ cell tumors with or without germinomatous component are heterogeneous masses with iso- and hyperintense areas on T2-weighted images. They are often accompanied by hydrocephalus →.* **(Right)** *Rarely, even as a component of a mixed germ cell tumor, embryonal carcinoma forms thick bands composed of epithelioid cells with prominent nucleoli.*

Yolk Sac Endodermal Sinus Tumor

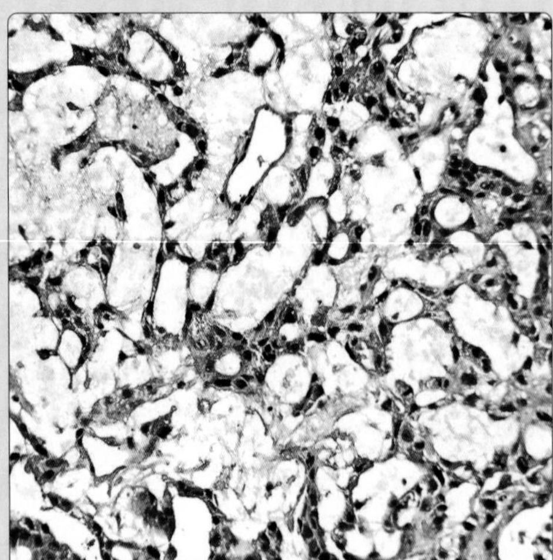

Choriocarcinoma

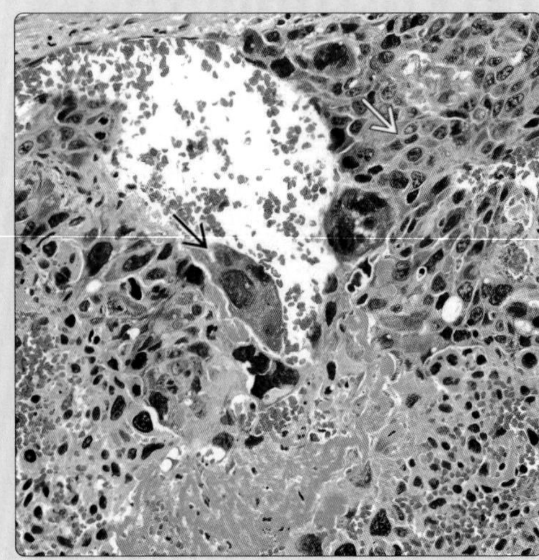

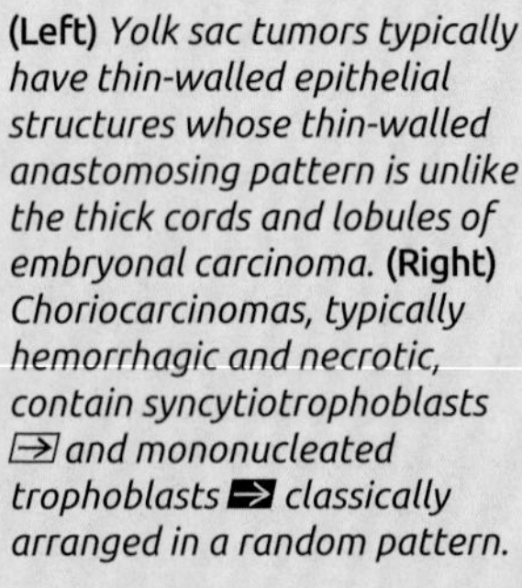

(Left) *Yolk sac tumors typically have thin-walled epithelial structures whose thin-walled anastomosing pattern is unlike the thick cords and lobules of embryonal carcinoma.* **(Right)** *Choriocarcinomas, typically hemorrhagic and necrotic, contain syncytiotrophoblasts → and mononucleated trophoblasts → classically arranged in a random pattern.*

TERMINOLOGY

Definitions

- Yolk sac tumor (endodermal sinus tumor)
  - Epithelial malignant neoplasm generally consisting of variety of loose patterns
- Embryonal carcinoma
  - Malignant tumor of epithelioid cells variably in sheets, cords, and cysts
- Choriocarcinoma
  - Malignant neoplasm composed of cytotrophoblasts and syncytiotrophoblasts
- Mixed germ cell tumor
  - Combination of any of the above
    - Most common combination is teratoma and germinoma
    - Often contain germinomatous component
    - More common than any pure lesion except for germinoma

CLINICAL ISSUES

Epidemiology

- Age
  - Median
    - ~ 10 years, similar to germinoma
  - Patients with metastatic germ cell tumors older

Site

- Similar to germinomas
  - Pineal and sellar/suprasellar regions most common
- Primary CNS choriocarcinomas rare
- Metastasis should always be considered
  - Other sites include
    - Testes
    - Lung
    - Mediastinum
  - Multiple and most commonly cerebral location
  - Majority of patients with cerebral metastases also have lung metastases
- Rare examples of metachronous testicular and CNS mixed germ cell tumors reported

Presentation

- Signs of increased intracranial pressure
- Visual abnormalities and somnolence in ~ 1/2 of cases
- Diabetes insipidus with sellar region tumors
  - Mixed germ cell tumors less commonly associated with diabetes insipidus
- Depends on site and multifocality
- Some present with extracranial metastases years after initial primary tumor

Laboratory Tests

- Nongerminomatous germ cell tumors clinically separated into tumors that are
  - Secreting and present with CSF α-fetoprotein levels > 10 ng/mL &/or beta HCG > 50 IU/L
    - AFP slightly more common than HCG
    - High levels seen in disseminated and metastatic tumors
    - Increased levels in recurrence or dissemination
  - Nonsecreting
- HCG expression reported in all types of germ cell tumors

Prognosis

- Nongerminomatous tumors less radiosensitive than germinomas
- 5-year overall survival rates much lower than germinomas: 30-50%
- Pure choriocarcinomas are metastatic and especially prone to CSF dissemination
- Pure embryonal carcinomas or endodermal sinus tumors more aggressive than mixed germ cell tumors
- Metastatic tumors have dismal prognoses
  - Some metastatic tumors successfully treated with chemotherapy
  - Long-term survival probability low despite chemo- and radiotherapy
- Patients who relapse early after radiotherapy have worse prognosis

IMAGING

MR Findings

- Hypo- to isointense on T1, and hyper- to isointense on T2-weighted images
- Heterogeneous enhancement
- Evidence of CSF spread

MICROSCOPIC

Histologic Features

- Yolk sac tumor
  - Endodermal sinus tumor
  - Primitive epithelial cells in loose and myxoid matrix
  - Epithelial cells, with mitoses, in reticular pattern or sinusoidal channels
  - Delicate fibrovascular projections forming distinct papillae
    - Schiller-Duval bodies, or endodermal sinuses
  - Solid, glandular, and microcystic patterns
  - PAS(+) proteinaceous globules
- Embryonal carcinoma
  - Large anaplastic cells with epithelial features, macronucleoli, and abundant mitoses
  - Cohesive nests, cords, and sheets
  - Rare clear glandular structures
- Choriocarcinoma
  - Sheets and clusters of trophoblasts
  - Marked hemorrhage, necrosis, and cytologic atypia
  - Mixture of cells resembling cyto- or syncytiotrophoblasts
  - Syncytiotrophoblasts line large angular blood-filled channels
  - Numerous mitoses, lymphocytic infiltrates, and multinucleated cells
- Mixed malignant germ cell tumor
  - Combination of any of the above, ± germinoma
    - More common than pure yolk sac tumor, embryonal carcinoma, or choriocarcinoma

ANCILLARY TESTS

Immunohistochemistry

- Yolk sac tumor
  - AFP(+)
    - Can be patchy
  - Antitrypsin (+)
  - Antichymotrypsin (+)
  - Cytokeratins (+)
  - SALL4(+)
  - LIN28A(+)
  - Glypican-3 (+)
- Embryonal carcinoma
  - Keratins
    - Including CK19(+)
  - CD30(+)
  - SALL4(+)
  - LIN28A(+)
  - May also be AFP(+), but C-Kit(-) or weak
  - OCT 3/OCT4(+)
- Choriocarcinoma
  - HCG(+)
  - LIN28A(+) diffuse, strong
- Mixed germ cell tumors
  - Most with germinomatous component, hence germinoma markers positive
  - Most SALL4(+), LIN28A(+) regardless of individual components

Genetic Testing

- Genomic alterations in CNS germ cell tumors indistinguishable from non-CNS germ cell tumors
  - Multiple chromosomal imbalances
  - Gain of 12p (common)
  - Isochromosome 12p (rare)

DIFFERENTIAL DIAGNOSIS

Pineoblastoma

- Small blue round cell tumors with rosettes
- May resemble embryonal carcinoma, solid pattern
  - But cells smaller and less epithelioid
- Synaptophysin (+)
- Neurofilament protein (+)
- Retinal S antigen (+)
- Cytokeratin (-)
- OCT4(-)

Papillary Tumor of Pineal Region

- Largely unstructured architecture
- CK8/18 (CAM5.2) (+)
  - Especially CK18 alone (+)
- Germ cell tumor markers (-)

Metastatic Carcinoma

- May resemble embryonal carcinoma
- Often older patients
- More often multifocal
- Most SALL4(-) and LIN28A(-)

DIAGNOSTIC CHECKLIST

Pathologic Interpretation Pearls

- Small biopsies may not include all components
- Immunostaining critical in most cases

SELECTED REFERENCES

1. Lai IC et al: Treatment results and prognostic factors for intracranial nongerminomatous germ cell tumors: single institute experience. Childs Nerv Syst. 31(5):683-91, 2015
2. Takami H et al: Human chorionic gonadotropin is expressed virtually in all intracranial germ cell tumors. J Neurooncol. ePub, 2015
3. Sukov WR et al: Isochromosome 12p and polysomy 12 in primary central nervous system germ cell tumors: frequency and association with clinicopathologic features. Hum Pathol. 41(2):232-8, 2010
4. Goodwin TL et al: Incidence patterns of central nervous system germ cell tumors: a SEER Study. J Pediatr Hematol Oncol. 31(8):541-4, 2009
5. Mei K et al: Diagnostic utility of SALL4 in primary germ cell tumors of the central nervous system: a study of 77 cases. Mod Pathol. 22(12):1628-36, 2009
6. Ngan KW et al: Immunohistochemical expression of OCT4 in primary central nervous system germ cell tumours. J Clin Neurosci. 15(2):149-52, 2008
7. Oechsle K et al: Cerebral metastases in non-seminomatous germ cell tumour patients undergoing primary high-dose chemotherapy. Eur J Cancer. 44(12):1663-9, 2008
8. Schneider DT et al: Molecular genetic analysis of central nervous system germ cell tumors with comparative genomic hybridization. Mod Pathol. 19(6):864-73, 2006
9. Sawamura Y et al: Germ cell tumours of the central nervous system: treatment consideration based on 111 cases and their long-term clinical outcomes. Eur J Cancer. 34(1):104-10, 1998
10. Calaminus G et al: Secreting germ cell tumors of the central nervous system (CNS). First results of the cooperative German/Italian pilot study (CNS sGCT). Klin Padiatr. 209(4):222-7, 1997

Yolk Sac Tumor Component

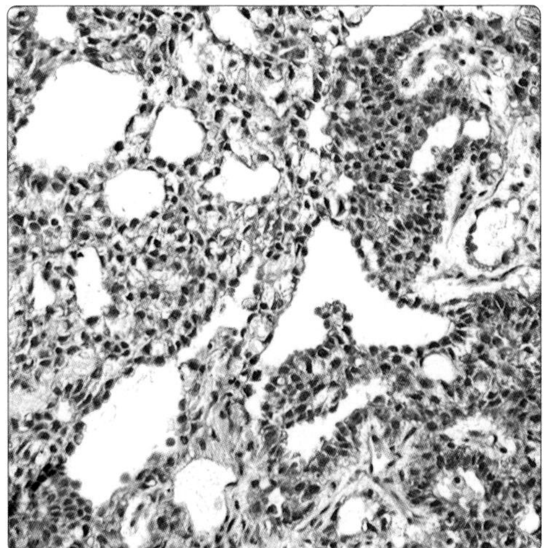

Yolk Sac Tumor Component

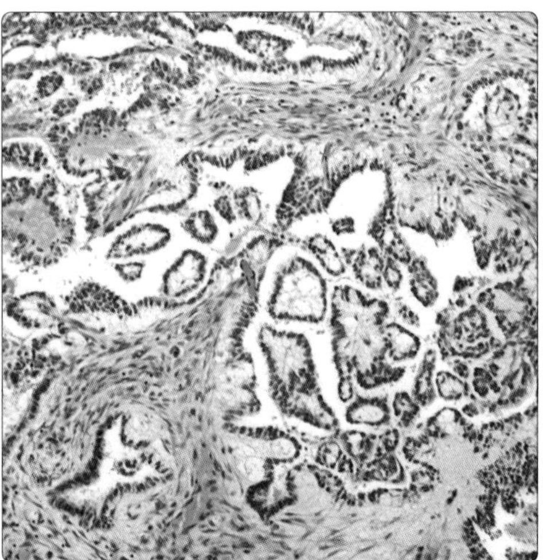

(Left) *Yolk sac tumors can have microcystic architecture with both scattered thin cords and focal solid nests. This glandular pattern often has alveolar-like cystic spaces in a variably myxoid stroma.* **(Right)** *Yolk sac tumors can have papillae embedded in a cellular stroma. Choroid plexus neoplasia would come to mind, but for the fibrous stroma and expected immunoreactivity for a-fetoprotein.*

Yolk Sac Endodermal Sinus Tumor

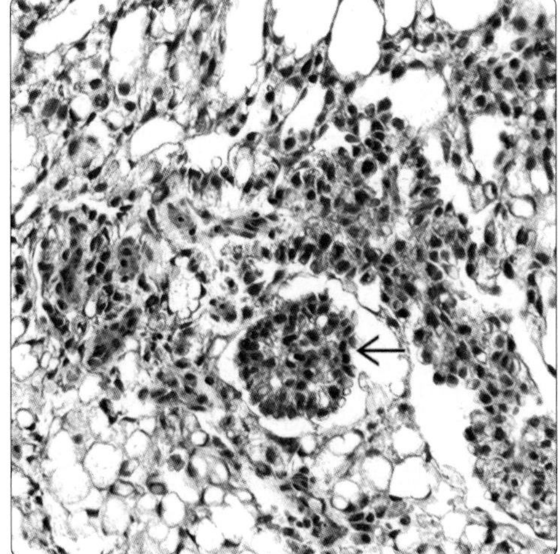

Embryonal Carcinoma

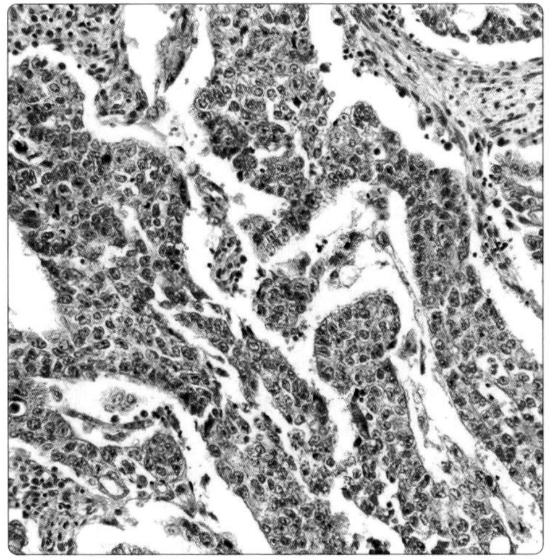

(Left) *Endodermal sinus tumors often show cystic or vacuolated pattern with clear cells and small glandular structures ➙. This microcystic pattern often intermingles with other patterns including macrocystic and reticular patterns.* **(Right)** *Embryonal carcinomas are formed of undifferentiated plump epithelioid cells forming large thick cords or lobules, not the usual delicate lacy pattern of yolk sac tumor.*

Embryonal Carcinoma

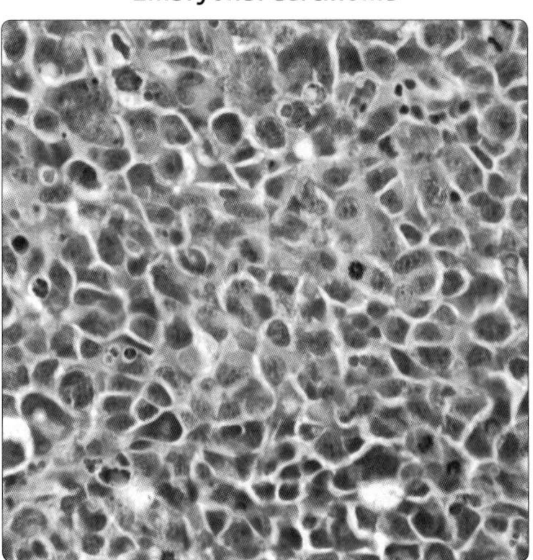

Embryonal Carcinoma

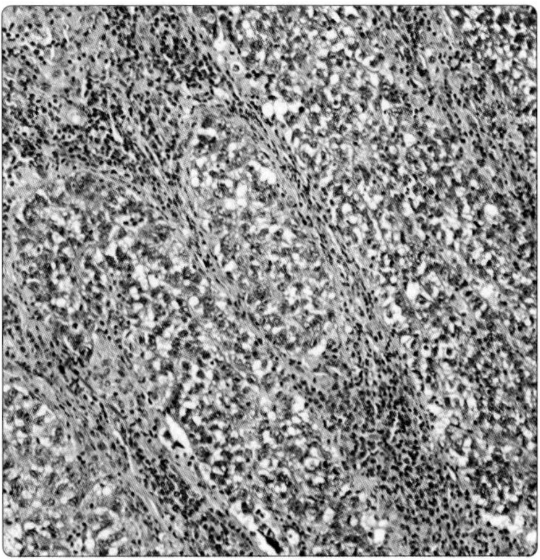

(Left) *Except for the highly basophilic cytoplasm, there is little evidence for a germ cell neoplasm for this embryonal carcinoma with the appearance similar to many high-grade malignancies such as metastatic carcinoma.* **(Right)** *In combination, lobules of large round cells, fibrous bands, and lymphocytes might suggest germinoma. Embryonal carcinomas are immunoreactive for cytokeratins, germinomas are not. Both are positive for OCT4.*

(Left) *Diffuse CD30 staining occurs in the overwhelming majority of embryonal carcinomas, highlighting the plasma membranes. This immunostain is typically negative in germinomas.* **(Right)** *Scattered HCG-positive syncytiotrophoblasts are sometimes present in germinomas. Diffuse strong positivity ➩ is expected only in choriocarcinoma.*

CD30 Positivity

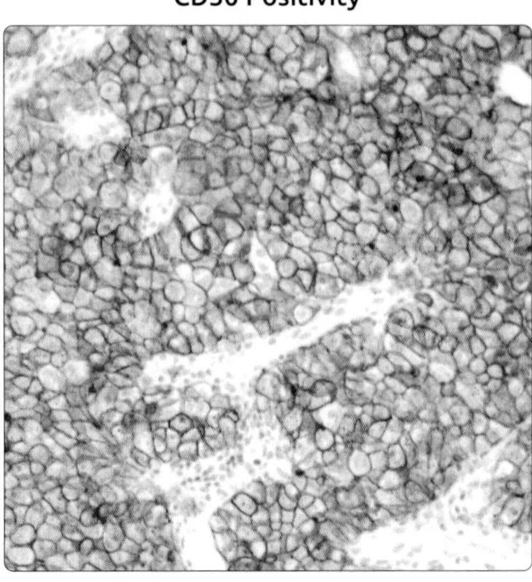

HCG Positivity

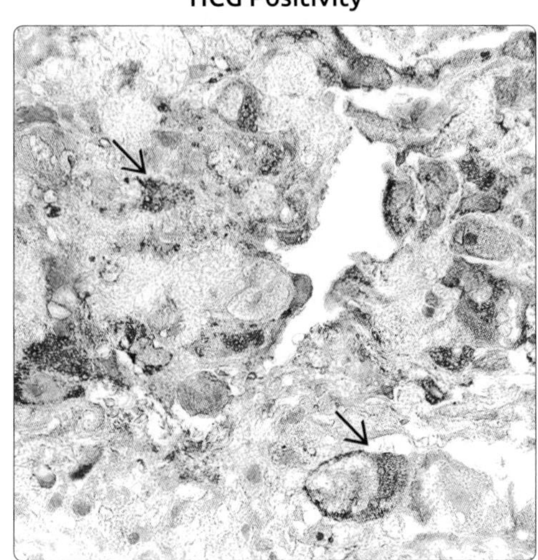

(Left) *Epithelial structures ➩ in yolk sac tumors are immunoreactive for a-fetoprotein. As in this case, reactivity is usually patchy and may be very focal.* **(Right)** *The transcription factor OCT4 is typically positive in embryonal carcinomas such as this, as well as in germinomas. Immunostaining is nuclear in both cases.*

AFP and Yolk Sac Tumor

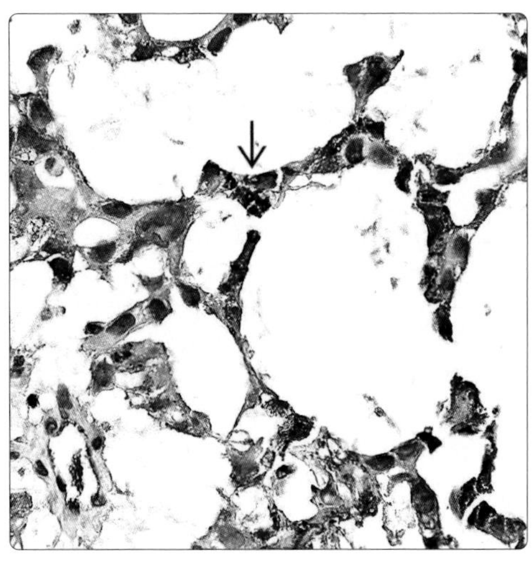

OCT4 Positivity

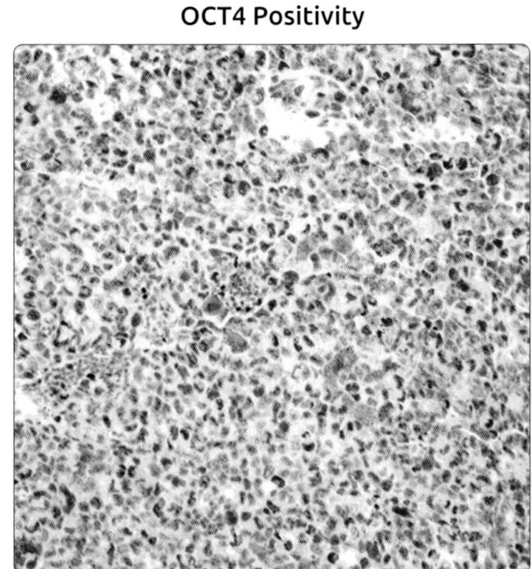

(Left) *CD30 antibodies preferentially identify embryonal carcinoma, a neoplasm with epithelioid qualities.* **(Right)** *Immunohistochemistry for cytokeratins is typically positive in embryonal carcinoma. Germinomas are negative.*

CD30 Positivity

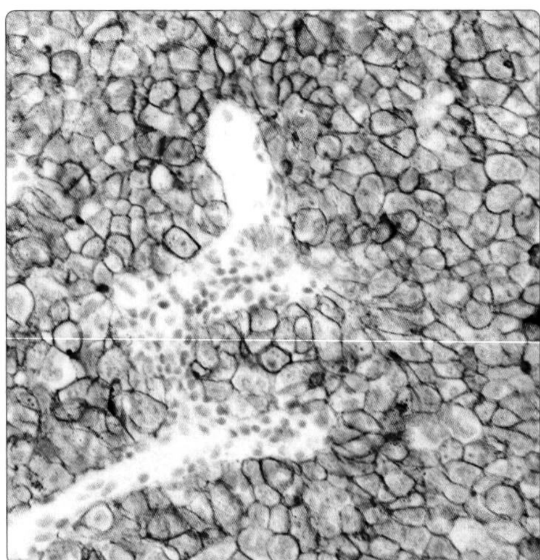

Cytokeratin Positivity

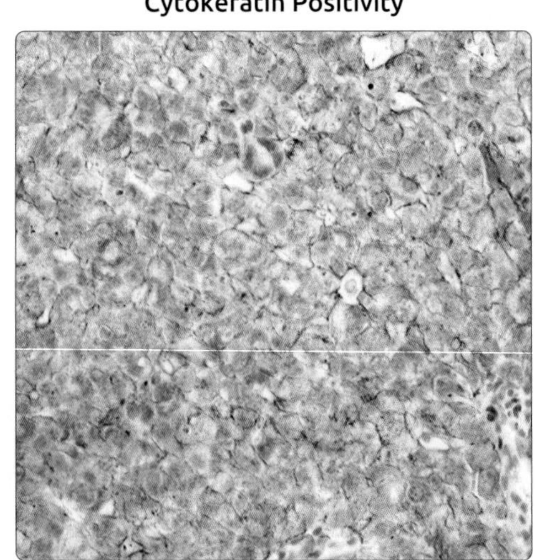

Contrast-Enhanced T1-Weighted MR

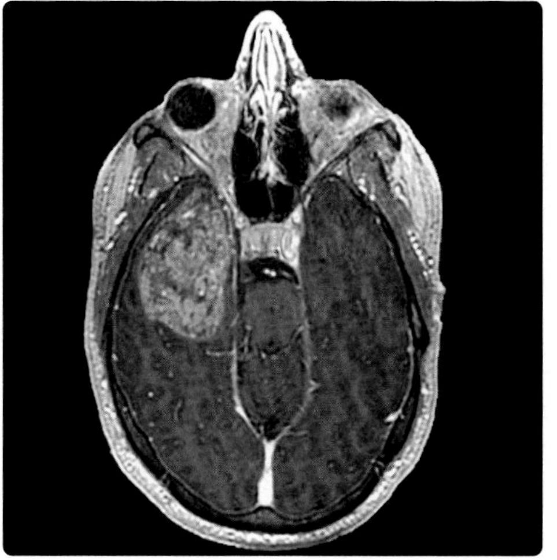

Embryonal Carcinoma

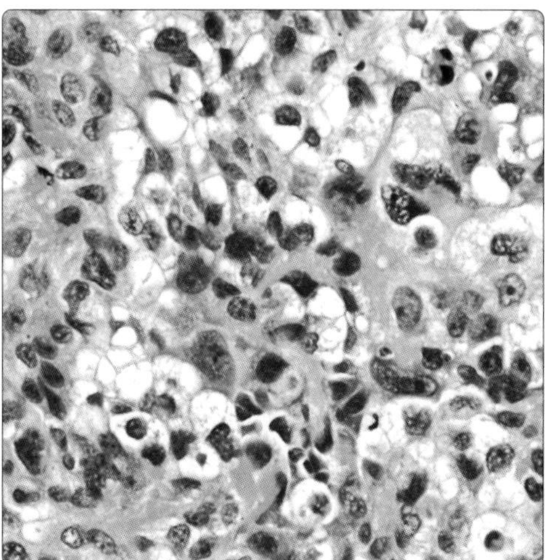

(Left) *This large tumor in a 33-year-old man demonstrates heterogeneous enhancement. The patient had a testicular tumor resected 3 years earlier and also has mediastinal masses. The patient's age is a good indication of this tumor being a metastatic mixed germ cell tumor.* **(Right)** *Embryonal carcinomas can attain a variety of forms, yet scattered cells with prominent nucleoli, and markedly pleomorphic, anaplastic nuclei with occasional clear cytoplasm are common. Most anaplastic cells have basophilic cytoplasm with indistinct borders.*

Cytokeratin Cocktail

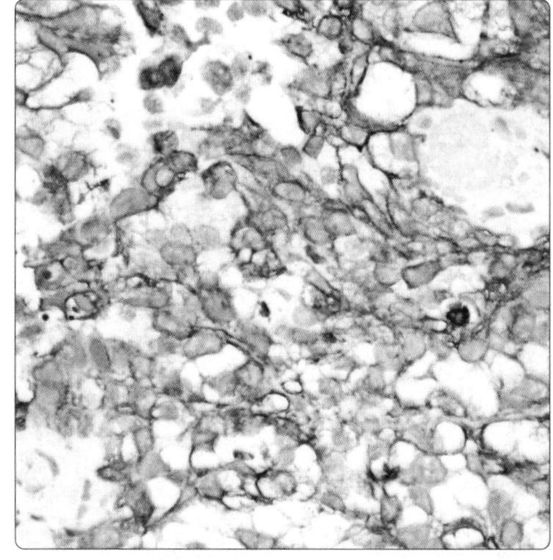

SALL4 Positivity

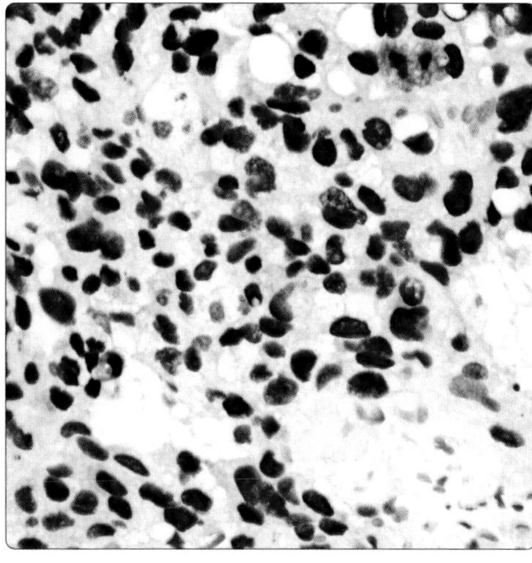

(Left) *Embryonal carcinomas are mostly strongly and diffusely positive with antibodies against cytokeratins (AE1/AE3 and CAM5.2).* **(Right)** *SALL4 (a nuclear transcription factor) is positive in most germ cell tumors, and also demonstrates strong diffuse nuclear staining in embryonal carcinomas.*

LIN28A Positivity

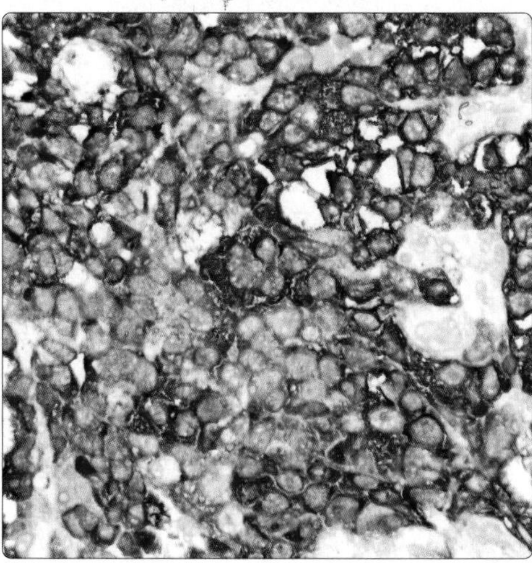

α-Fetoprotein

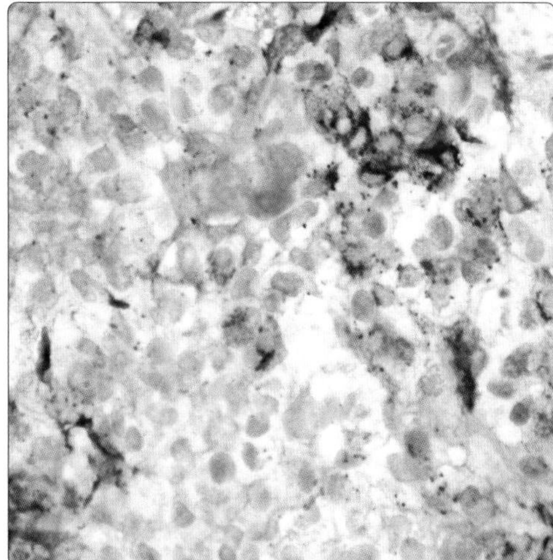

(Left) *Similar to SALL4, LIN28A is diffusely and strongly positive in all germ cell tumors, including embryonal carcinoma.* **(Right)** *While typical for yolk sac (endodermal sinus) tumor components, more than half of embryonal carcinomas are positive with the antibodies against α-fetoprotein.*

Hemangioblastoma

KEY FACTS

TERMINOLOGY

- Well-circumscribed, highly vascular, lipid-rich, low-grade neoplasm of uncertain histogenesis, WHO grade I

ETIOLOGY/PATHOGENESIS

- von Hippel-Lindau disease (germline mutation in *VHL* gene) in approximately 10% of patients
- Most sporadic tumors also have inactivated *VHL* gene

MACROSCOPIC

- Well circumscribed
- Yellow, due to lipid content
- Small mural nodules can escape detection at surgery

MICROSCOPIC

- Heterogeneous in ratio of vasculature to tumor cells
  - High ratio, reticular
  - Low ratio, cellular
- Nuclear pleomorphism and hyperchromasia: Scattered large dark nuclei
- Vacuolated tumor cells

ANCILLARY TESTS

- Smears poorly
- Stromal cells variably lipid laden, oil red O staining
- Inhibin-α (+) in stromal or interstitial cells, may be focal
- GLUT-1(+)
- Vascular markers (+), e.g., CD31, CD34, FXIIIA, in endothelial cells

DIAGNOSTIC CHECKLIST

- Can resemble astrocytoma, particularly in frozen sections
- Can closely resemble metastatic renal cell carcinoma
- Rare supratentorially: Microcystic meningioma more likely option

(Left) *Hemangioblastomas are cystic tumors with avidly enhancing nodules ➡ after gadolinium administration on T-1 weighted images, as seen here in the cerebellum, the tumor's most common location. Note the dark, medially located cystic component ➡.* **(Right)** *Macroscopic appearance of hemangioblastomas can be variable. In aggregate, lipid-laden stromal cells give some hemangioblastomas a bright yellow hue, while others appear more vascular and hemorrhagic.*

Cystic Tumor With Enhancing Nodule

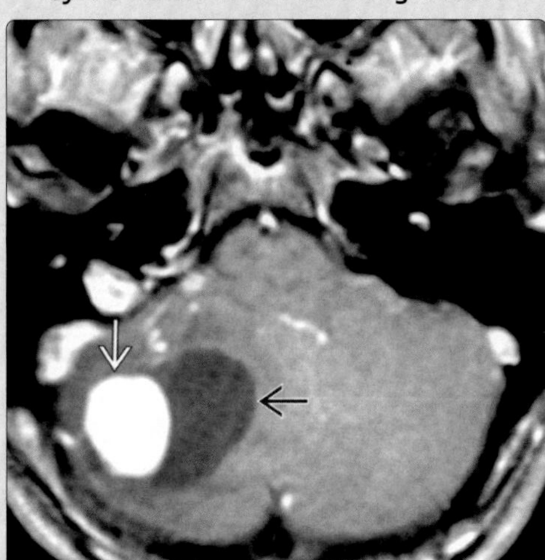

Gross Appearance

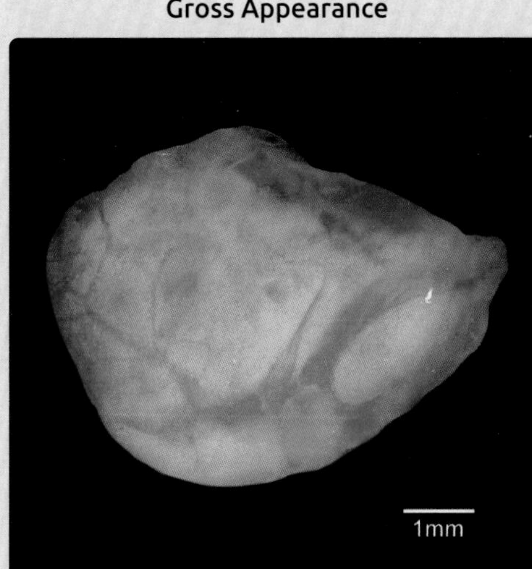

(Left) *Scattered large hyperchromatic nuclei ➡, vacuolated cells, and multiple capillaries are classic features of the cellular type of hemangioblastoma.* **(Right)** *Microscopic composition of hemangioblastoma is that of a highly vascular and vacuolated or lipid-rich cells. The degree of vacuolization, i.e., the clear cell appearance, varies significantly from tumor to tumor.*

Vascular Tumor With Vacuolated Cells

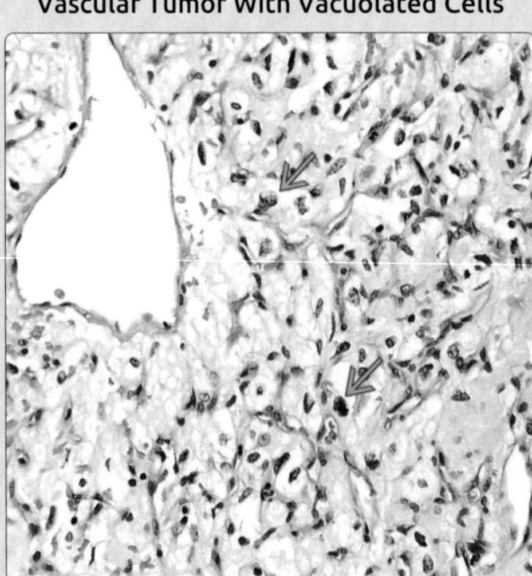

Vacuolated Stromal Cells

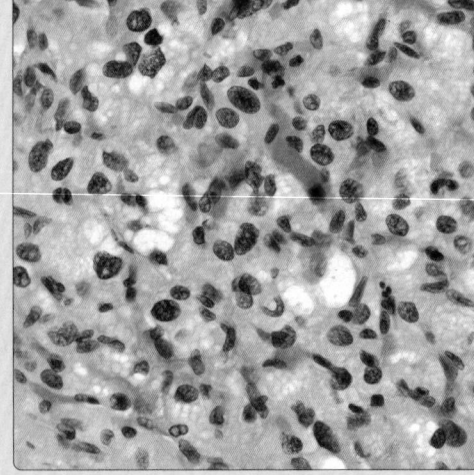

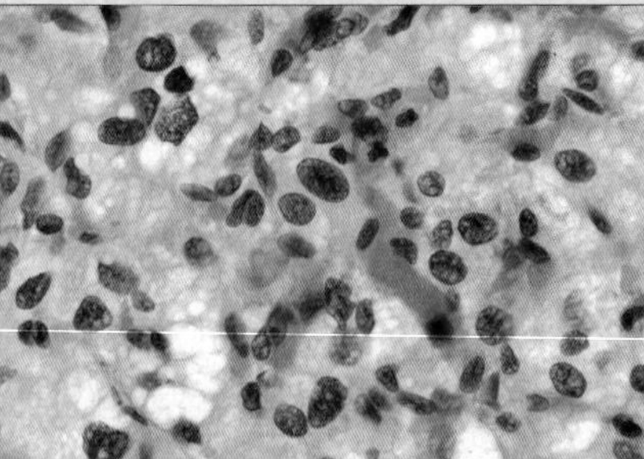

TERMINOLOGY

Definitions

- Well-circumscribed, highly vascular, lipid-rich, low-grade neoplasm of uncertain histogenesis, WHO grade I

ETIOLOGY/PATHOGENESIS

Sporadic

- Unknown etiology
- In most sporadic hemangioblastomas there is activation of *VHL* gene

Syndromic von Hippel-Lindau Disease

- Germline mutation in *VHL* gene in approximately 10% of patients
  - Hemangioblastoma, sometimes multiple
  - Endolymphatic sac tumor
  - Other findings of VHL disease: Renal cell carcinoma, renal cysts
  - Adrenal, pancreatic, &/or epididymal tumors

CLINICAL ISSUES

Site

- Cerebellum (most common) and brainstem
- Spinal cord, usually dorsal
- Retina
- Supratentorial, rare
- Multiple in von Hippel-Lindau disease

Presentation

- Dependent on location
  - Local mass effect
  - Obstructive hydrocephalus
- Polycythemia (rare)
- Acute symptoms due to hemorrhage (rare)

Treatment

- Surgical approaches
  - Total excision usually possible
- Drugs
  - Antiangiogenic therapy (bevacizumab) used successfully if tumor(s) not resectable

Prognosis

- Excellent in most sporadic cases
- Less favorable in von Hippel-Lindau disease because of comorbid tumors
- Disseminated or multifocal tumors, less certain

IMAGING

Radiographic Findings

- Angiography: Highly vascular, discrete

MR Findings

- Discrete, intensely enhancing
- Flow voids in T2WI and T1WI in some cases
- Often cystic with mural nodule
- Little surrounding edema
- Hemangioblastomatosis
  - Term used for disseminated hemangioblastoma or multifocal disease: Rare form

MACROSCOPIC

General Features

- Well circumscribed
- Superficial, centered on pial surface
- Bloody, dark red, or focally yellow due to lipid content

MICROSCOPIC

Histologic Features

- Discrete borders
- Piloid gliosis with Rosenthal fibers in surrounding parenchyma
- Highly vascular, often many large, thin-walled vessels
- Heterogeneous in ratio of vasculature to tumor cells
  - High ratio, reticular type
    - Highly cellular
    - Small nests of extravascular tumor cells (stromal or interstitial cells)
    - Vacuolated cytoplasm
    - Abundant reticulin
  - Low ratio, cellular type
    - Large lobules of cells
    - More cytoplasm than reticular type
    - Less cytoplasmic vacuolation
    - Glioma-like fibrillar areas, some cases
    - Vascular proliferation, perilobular
    - Less reticulin, little of it pericellular
- General features
  - Mitoses (absent or rare)
  - Scattered large dark nuclei
  - Hyaline globules, minority of cases
  - Extramedullary hematopoiesis (rare)
    - Microscopic foci with high Ki-67 staining
  - Cyst-like spaces
  - Dense sclerosis
  - Mast cells
  - Necrosis (rare)
- Cyst wall
  - Piloid gliosis with Rosenthal fibers
  - Vascular proliferation, telangiectatic
- Metastatic renal cell carcinoma to hemangioblastoma (rare)

ANCILLARY TESTS

Cytology

- Smears poorly
  - Tissue fragments only in most cases
  - Few individual cells
    - Vacuolated, with pleomorphic and hyperchromatic nuclei

Histochemistry

- Reticulin
  - Staining pattern: Around small groups of cells in reticular type
- PAS(+) globules, occasional
- Oil red O

- Stromal cells variably (+)

Immunohistochemistry

- Inhibin-α (+)
  - Variable in extent, may be focal
  - Stromal or interstitial cells positive
- EMA(-)
  - Usually negative
  - Occasionally focally positive, surface staining
- MIB-1
  - Generally low, but higher in cellular type
- GFAP(+)
  - Sometimes positive, especially in cellular type
- Vascular markers (+), e.g., CD31, CD34, FXIIIA
  - Endothelial cells positive but not stromal cells
- GLUT-1(+)
  - Often diffuse but weak
- Brachyury (-)
  - Only weak and cytoplasmic positivity, i.e., negative (not nuclear as in chordoma)

DIFFERENTIAL DIAGNOSIS

Metastatic Carcinoma, Especially Renal Cell Carcinoma

- Both occur in von Hippel-Lindau syndrome
- More mitoses, higher Ki-67 index
- Cytokeratins (+), EMA(+), CD10(+), pax-8(+)
- Inhibin-α, usually, but not always negative
- Imaging of kidneys reasonable when in doubt

Capillary Angioma

- Often intraspinal, extramedullary
- No interstitial cells
- Inhibin-α (-)
- Little or no neutral fat (oil red O)

Meningioma, Especially Microcystic Variant

- Thickened vessels
- Whorls and psammoma bodies, both may not be seen
- Little reticulin
- Smears out well, many individual cells
  - Uniform, bland nuclei with intranuclear inclusions and grooves
- EMA(+), inhibin-α (-) in some but (+) in others
- More likely diagnosis than hemangioblastoma if lesion is supratentorial

Pilocytic Astrocytoma

- Long, bipolar hair cells in smear preparation
- Spongy, microcystic component with eosinophilic granular bodies
- Dense piloid tissue with Rosenthal fibers
- Generally not exclusively piloid tissue without microcysts
- GFAP(+), inhibin-α (-)

Infiltrating, Diffuse Astrocytoma

- More similar to hemangioblastoma in frozen compared to permanent sections
- Infiltrating, not well circumscribed
  - Overrun axons and neuron cell bodies
- No lobular architecture
- Not highly vascular
- Little if any neutral fat
- Reticulin confined to vessels
- Inhibin-α (-) in some cases, (+) in others
- IDH-1(+) and Olig2(+)
- GFAP widely positive

Ependymoma

- Perivascular pseudorosettes
- Epithelial surfaces/true rosettes in some cases
- Fewer vessels
- Reticulin confined to vessels
- GFAP(+)
- EMA(+)
  - Surface
  - Dot-like microlumina
- Inhibin-α (-)

DIAGNOSTIC CHECKLIST

Clinically Relevant Pathologic Features

- Well circumscribed, usually amenable to complete excision
- Small mural nodule may not be apparent at surgery
- Highly vascular spinal cord examples potentially misinterpreted intraoperatively as arteriovenous malformations

Pathologic Interpretation Pearls

- Sharply defined
- Surrounding dense piloid gliosis
- May be histologically nondescript and similar to astrocytoma, especially in frozen sections
- Can closely resemble metastatic renal cell carcinoma
- Variable in histological appearance
  - Closely packed, highly vascular: Reticular type
  - Large, sometimes paucicellular lobules: Cellular type
- Fat stain on frozen section helpful in diagnosis
- Consider possibility in face of intensely enhancing discrete tumor in adult, especially in cerebellum, medulla, and spinal cord
- Scan kidneys to rule out renal cell primary in ambiguous cases
- Most cerebellar; supratentorial location rare

SELECTED REFERENCES

1. Barresi V et al: Brachyury: a diagnostic marker for the differential diagnosis of chordoma and hemangioblastoma versus neoplastic histological mimickers. Dis Markers. 2014:514753, 2014
2. Shankar GM et al: Sporadic hemangioblastomas are characterized by cryptic VHL inactivation. Acta Neuropathol Commun. 2:167, 2014
3. Barresi V et al: Expression of brachyury in hemangioblastoma: potential use in differential diagnosis. Am J Surg Pathol. 36(7):1052-7, 2012
4. Ramachandran R et al: Intradural extramedullary leptomeningeal hemangioblastomatosis and paraneoplastic limbic encephalitis diagnosed at autopsy: an unlikely pair. Arch Pathol Lab Med. 132(1):104-8, 2008
5. Woodward ER et al: VHL mutation analysis in patients with isolated central nervous system haemangioblastoma. Brain. 130(Pt 3):836-42, 2007
6. Gläsker S et al: Risk of hemorrhage in hemangioblastomas of the central nervous system. Neurosurgery. 57(1):71-6; discussion 71-6, 2005
7. Hasselblatt M et al: Cellular and reticular variants of haemangioblastoma revisited: a clinicopathologic study of 88 cases. Neuropathol Appl Neurobiol. 31(6):618-22, 2005
8. Jung SM et al: Immunoreactivity of CD10 and inhibin alpha in differentiating hemangioblastoma of central nervous system from metastatic clear cell renal cell carcinoma. Mod Pathol. 18(6):788-94, 2005

Solid-Cystic Cerebellar Tumor

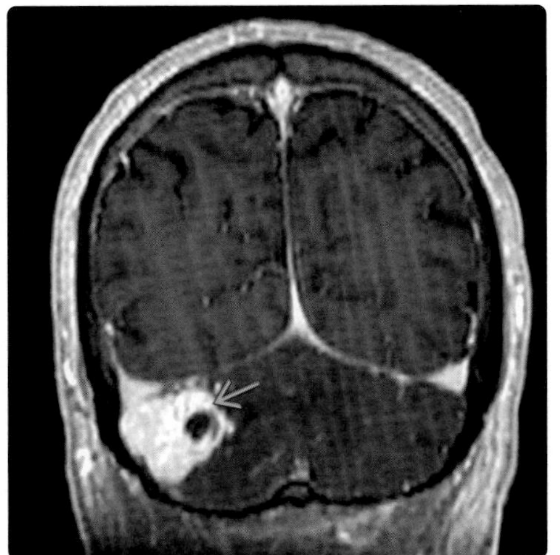

Solid Cerebellar Tumor

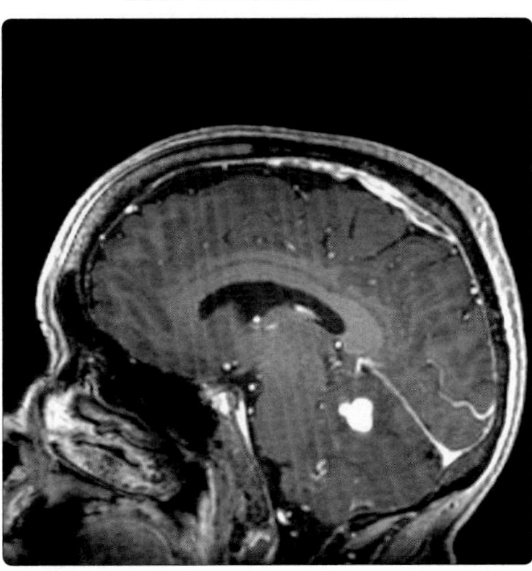

(Left) *This coronal contrast-enhanced T1WI MR demonstrates a predominantly solid neoplasm with a central hypointense cystic component ➔ with almost no mass effect.* **(Right)** *This small hemangioblastoma is entirely solid without a cystic component and demonstrates little mass effect or peritumoral edema.*

Temporal Lobe Tumor in VHL

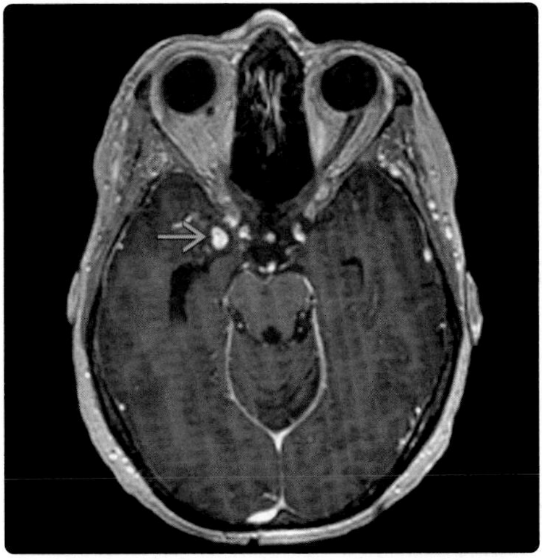

Thoracic Tumor

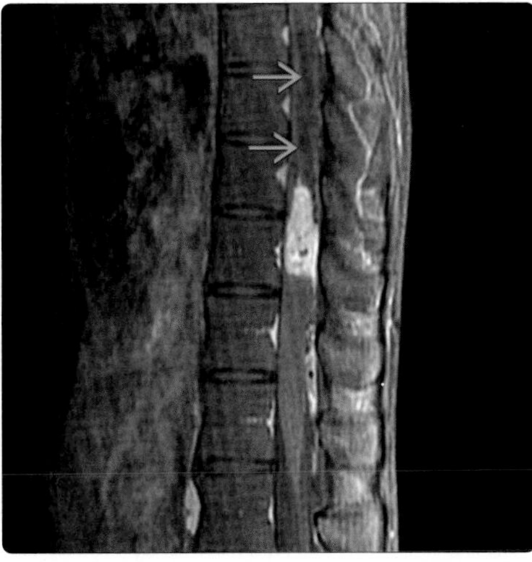

(Left) *This patient with von Hippel-Lindau disease had multiple hemangioblastomas, including a small tumor in the right temporal lobe ➔. This axial, contrast-enhanced T1WI MR demonstrates a small, predominantly solid tumor.* **(Right)** *In this patient without VHL, the tumor appears as a solid, markedly enhancing tumor on sagittal contrast-enhanced T1WI MR. Note the suggestion of syrinx ➔ formation rostral to the mass.*

Intradural Extramedullary Tumor

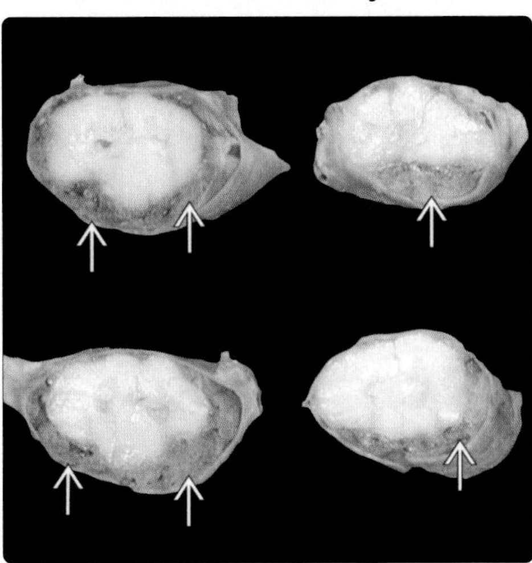

Extramedullary Intradural Tumor

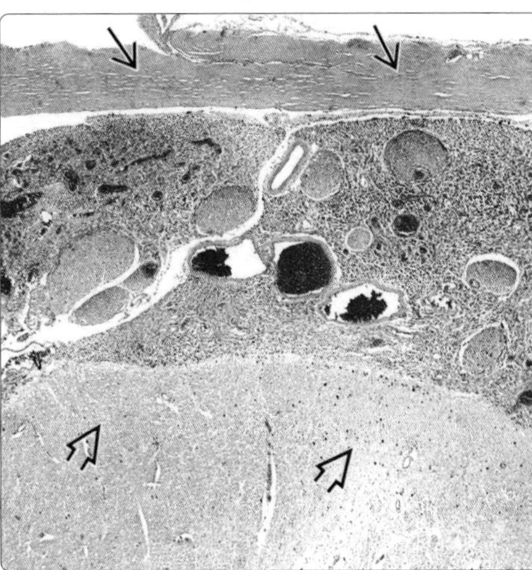

(Left) *In these axial sections of the thoracic spinal cord from an autopsy of a patient with disseminated hemangioblastoma (hemangioblastomatosis), the tumor is seen primarily as an extramedullary mass coating the surface of the spinal cord ➔.* **(Right)** *Histological sections from autopsy case with disseminated hemangioblastoma (hemangioblastomatosis) are shown. Tumor is seen filling the intradural space encasing nerve roots. The dura ➔ and the spinal cord parenchyma ➔ appear uninvolved.*

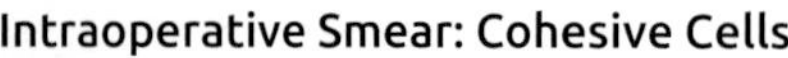

Intraoperative Smear: Cohesive Cells

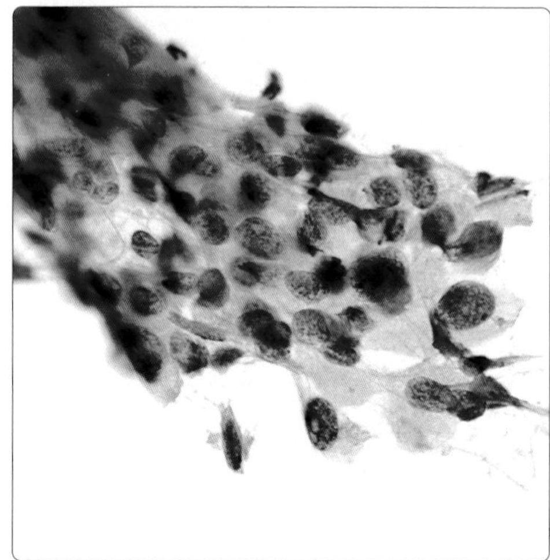

Vacuolated Cells in Smear

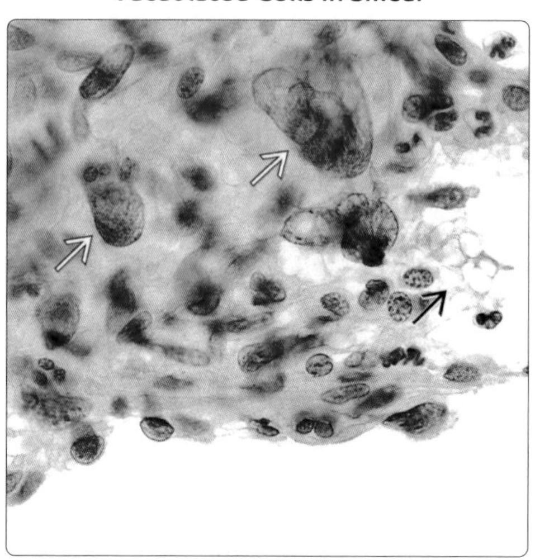

(Left) *In the absence of vacuolated cells, nuclear pleomorphism and high cellularity might suggest an anaplastic tumor. Smears from hemangioblastomas often do not contain single cells, which may be helpful.* **(Right)** *Hemangioblastomas generally do not smear out, remaining instead as tissue fragments in which vacuolated cells ⇨ may be present. Nuclear pleomorphism ➡ is common but is not an index of anaplasia.*

Frozen Section Mimicking Glioma

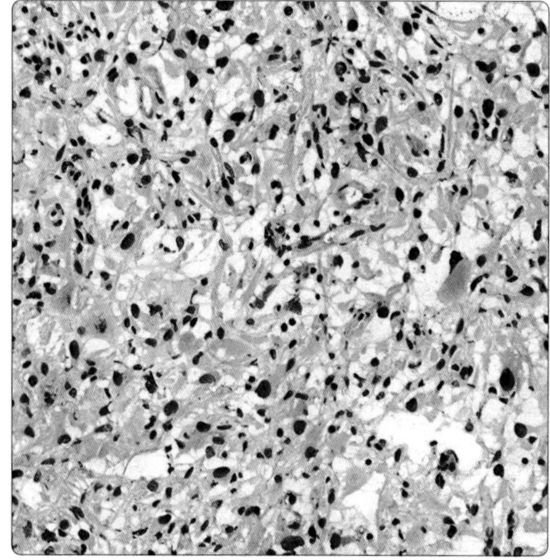

Paraffin Section: Post Frozen

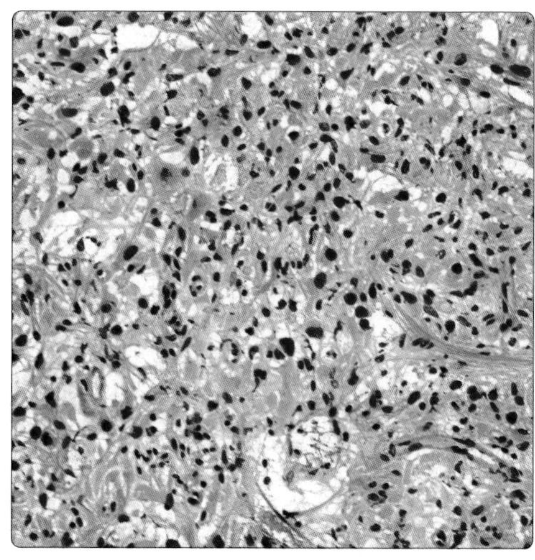

(Left) *Hemangioblastomas appear markedly pleomorphic in frozen sections. In the absence of relevant clinical and radiological information, they can easily be misdiagnosed as malignant glioma.* **(Right)** *Tissue samples subjected to frozen section will still pose a significant challenge the next day after paraffin processing. While this is only slightly easier, the chance of misdiagnosis is still present. An unfrozen sample must be retained to avoid a mistake in diagnosis.*

Frozen Section: Sharp Borders

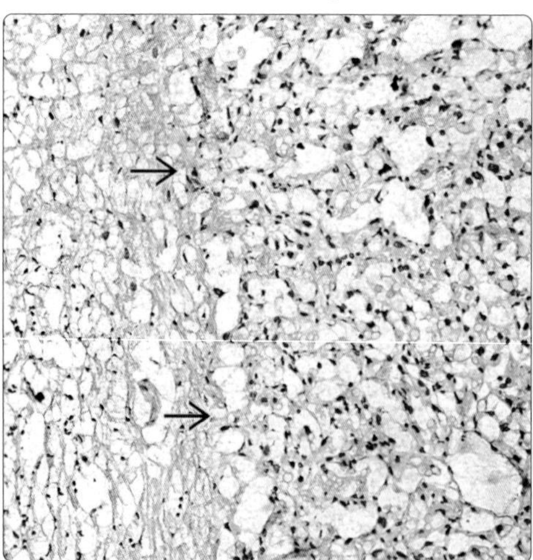

Frozen Section: Vacuolated Cells

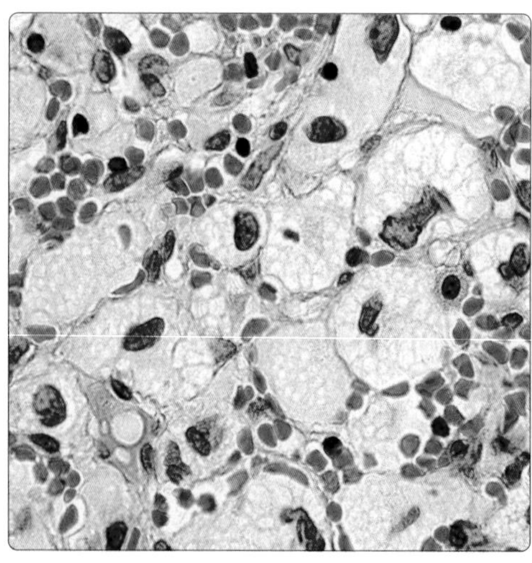

(Left) *The sharp border ⇨ helps distinguish a hemangioblastoma from an infiltrating glioma. Both the tumor and the surrounding gliotic parenchyma can resemble astrocytoma. In most frozen sections, it may not be possible to observe this sharp boundary.* **(Right)** *In frozen sections, it is cells such as these that stain prominently with oil red O. Cells with such vacuolated cytoplasm would be unusual in renal cell carcinoma. Supratentorial, dural-based masses with cells such as these are usually microcystic meningiomas.*

Whole Mount: Discrete Mass

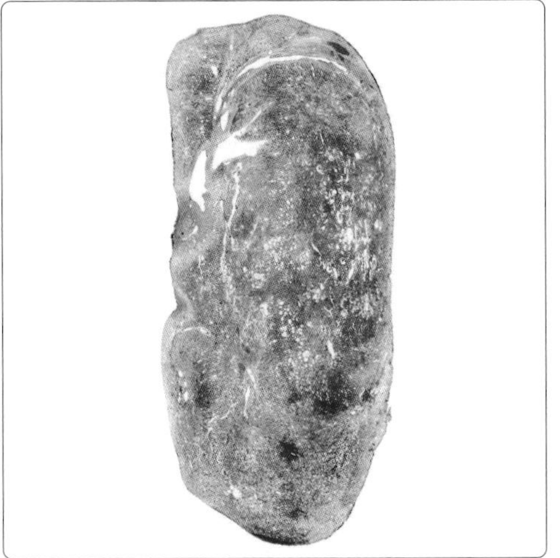

Whole Mount: Solid Circumscribed Tumor

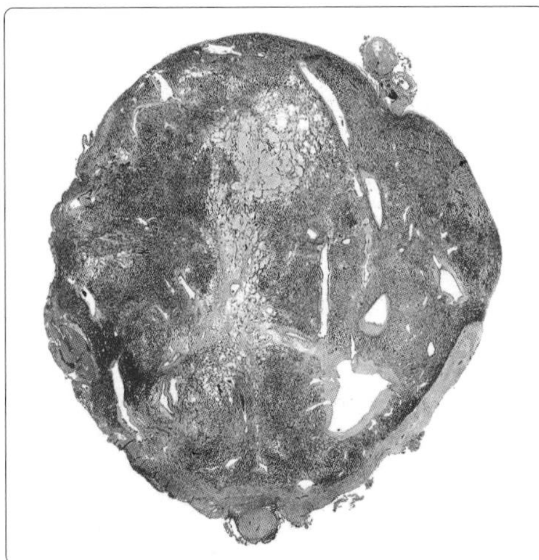

(Left) *Intermingled regions of high and low cellularity, gaping vessels, and cystic change give hemangioblastomas their typical variegated appearance. As is apparent in this whole-mount section, the lesion is a discrete mass that lends itself to surgical resection.* **(Right)** *The enhancing component is a well-circumscribed cellular nodule, as shown here in a whole-mount section. The varying degrees of cell density with loose and denser areas is typical.*

Well-Defined Cerebellar Tumor

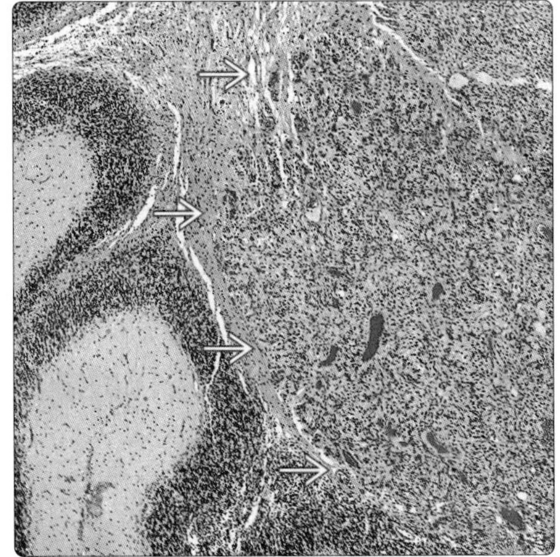

Vascular Mural Nodule

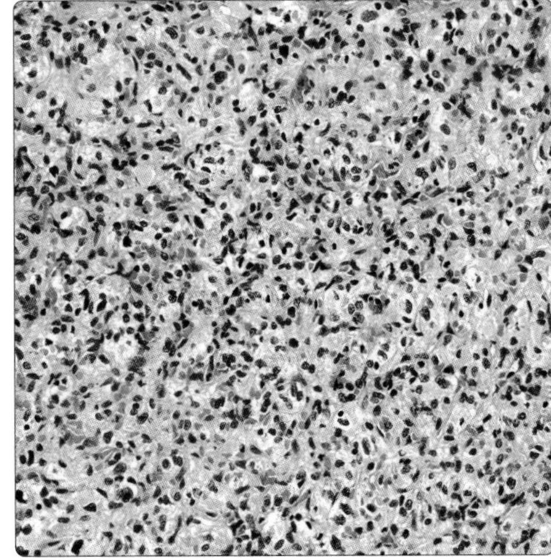

(Left) *In this low magnification, hemangioblastoma appears as an intraaxial mass with well-defined borders* ➔. **(Right)** *In the solid component of the tumors, as in this section from a mural nodule, the highly vascular nature as well as the vacuolated cells are quite conspicuous.*

Retinal Hemangioblastoma

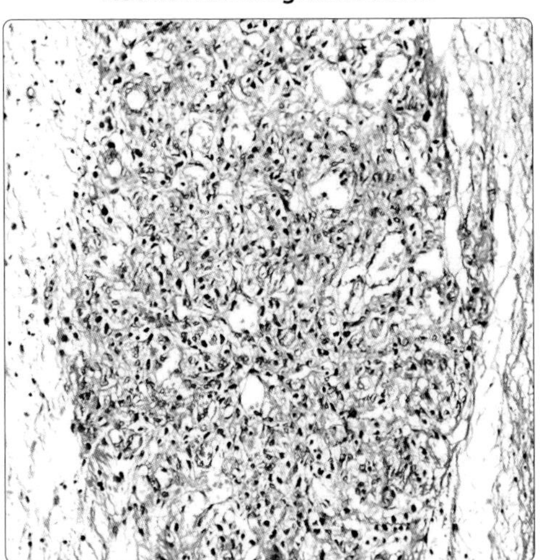

Organoid Architecture

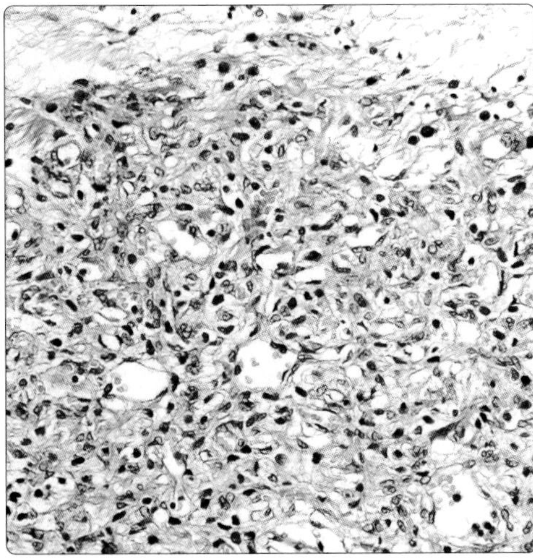

(Left) *The tumor's discreteness is especially apparent in small examples, such as this one in the retina. Histological features of tumors in the retina are essentially identical to spinal or cerebellar tumors.* **(Right)** *The tumor often has a vague organoid architecture imparted by the elaborate vascular network and the surrounding vacuolated cells with occasional bizarre nuclei.*

Stromal Cells in Hemangioblastoma

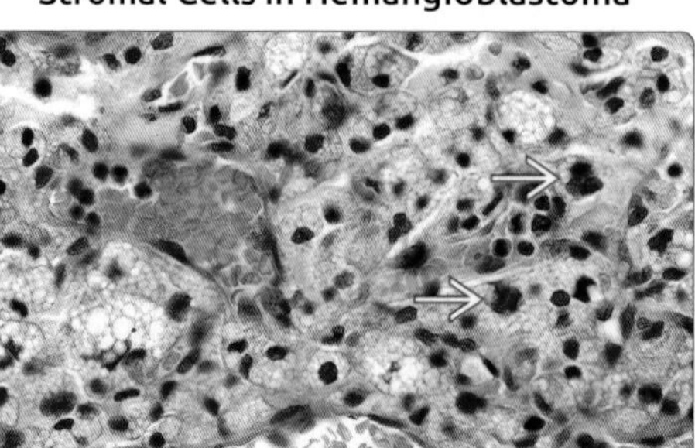

Clear Cells in Hemangioblastoma

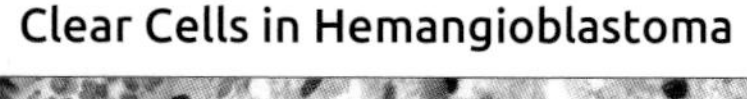

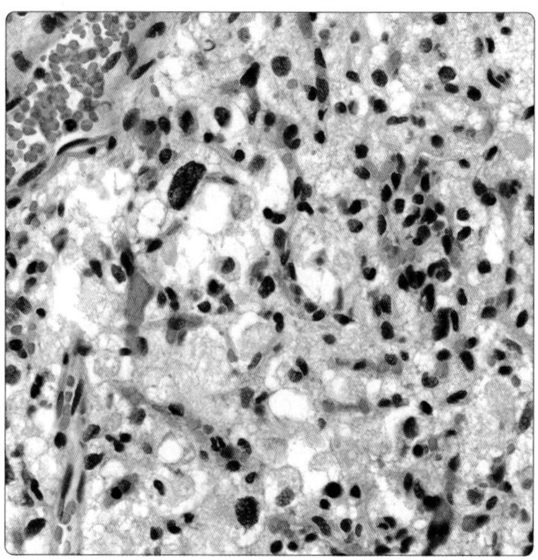

(Left) *The rich vascular network and the bubbly vacuolated cells define the high-magnification appearance of hemangioblastomas. Scattered atypical cells with bizarre nuclei* ➔ *are often present in most sections.* **(Right)** *The clear cytoplasm in hemangioblastomas are almost always vacuolated or contain some eosinophilic material, unlike the optically clear cytoplasm of renal cell carcinoma; however, the distinction can prove difficult on histology alone.*

Extramedullary Hematopoiesis

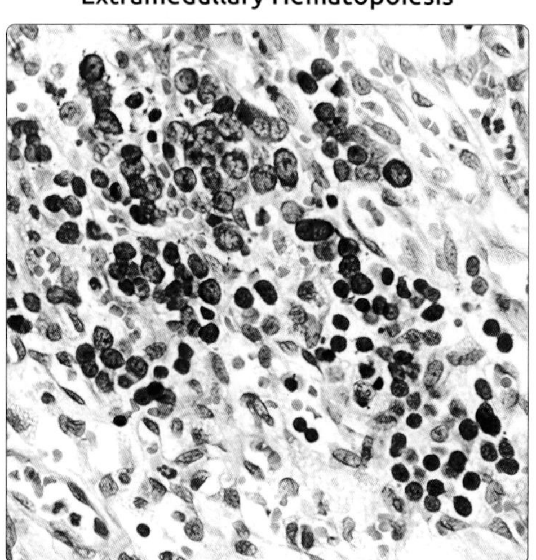

Hyaline Globules

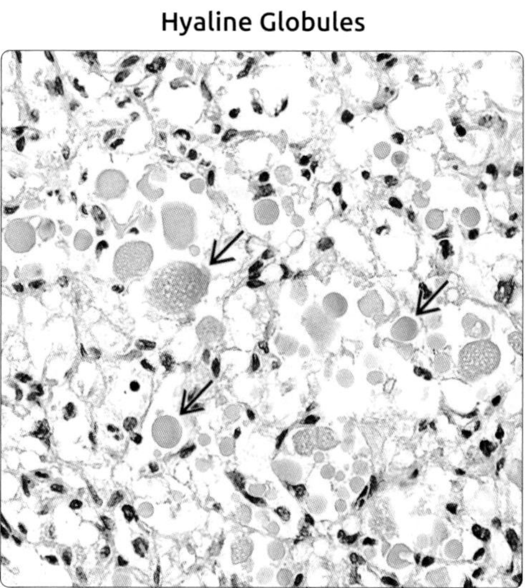

(Left) *Aggregated blue cells with high nuclear:cytoplasmic ratios cluster in a focus of extramedullary hematopoiesis. In such foci, Ki-67 labeling index may be very high, but this is not related to tumor proliferation rate.* **(Right)** *Hyaline globules* ➔ *are focal findings in some hemangioblastomas. While nonspecific, they are found in only a few other CNS tumors, e.g., choroid plexus carcinoma, yolk sac tumor, and secretory meningioma.*

Adjacent Reactive Tissue

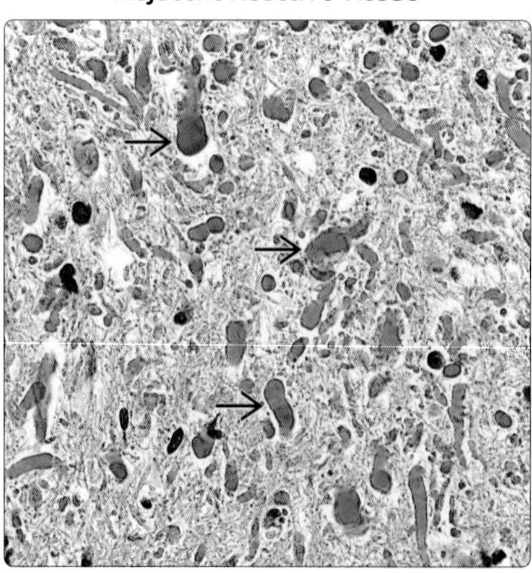

Dense Hyalinization

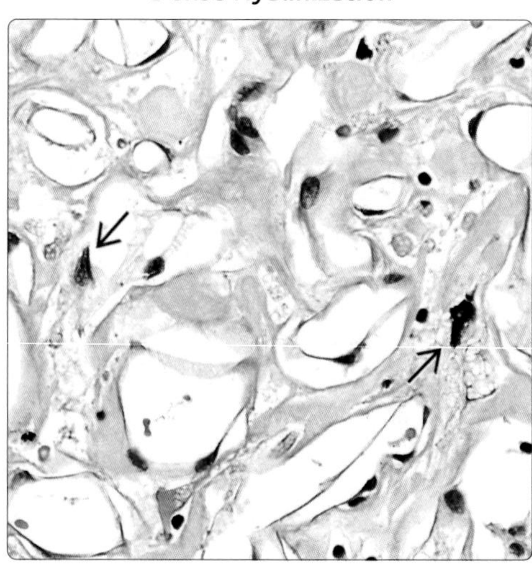

(Left) *Peritumoral fibrillar tissue with Rosenthal fibers* ➔*, i.e., piloid gliosis, may be mistaken for pilocytic astrocytoma. The illustrated reactive tissue lacks the myxoid background &/or microcysts that are present in most pilocytic astrocytomas.* **(Right)** *Few tumor cells* ➔ *remain in densely hyalinized areas. Other entities such as vascular malformations and sclerotic gliomas would have to be considered. Immunohistochemistry for inhibin-a would be especially important.*

Reticulin-Rich Tumor

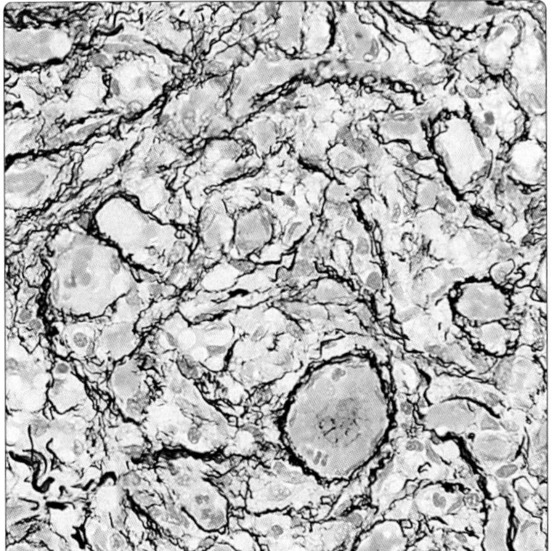

GLUT-1(+) Staining

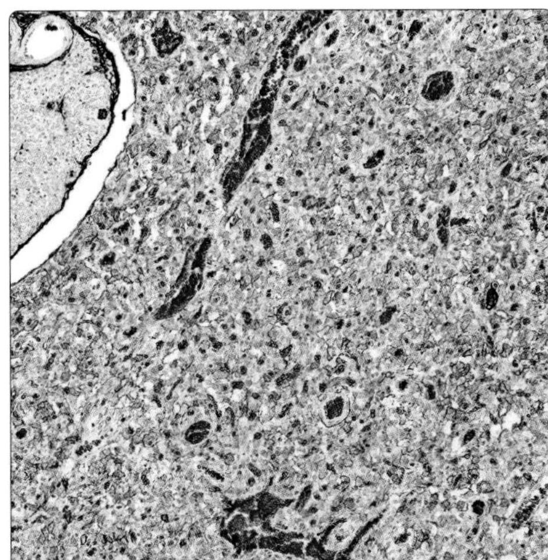

(Left) *Reticulin surrounds small groups of cells or individual cells in the reticular type. Reticulin in this abundance would be highly unlikely in other cerebellar or spinal intramedullary neoplasms. Extraaxial tumors such as capillary angioma and hemangiopericytoma/solitary fibrous tumor are, however, rich in reticulin fibers.* **(Right)** *Most hemangioblastomas, central and peripheral, demonstrate GLUT-1 positivity, which is often diffuse but weak.*

Inhibin-α Positivity

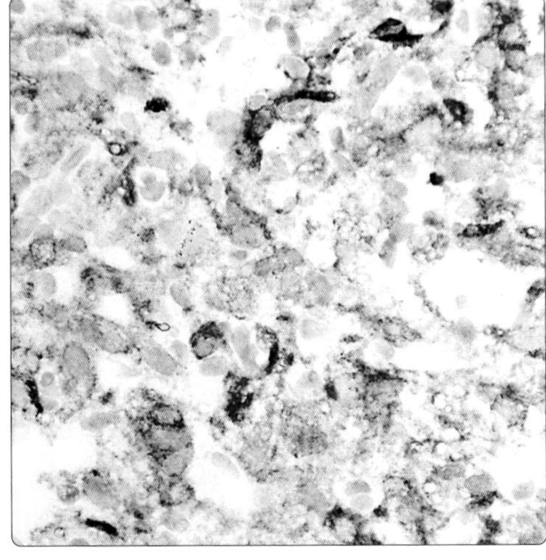

GFAP(+) Cells

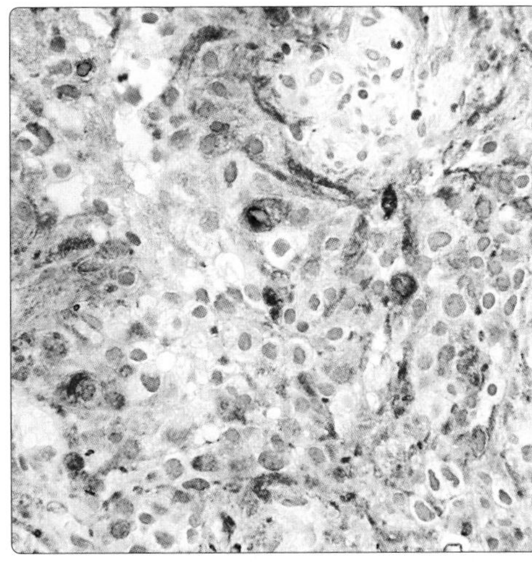

(Left) *Inhibin-a staining is finely granular and varies in intensity from cell to cell. Cells may be strongly positive, weakly reactive, or negative. Diffuse, strong positivity is unusual.* **(Right)** *Some stromal cells may be immunoreactive for GFAP, especially in the lobular, cellular type.*

CD34 Highlights Vasculature

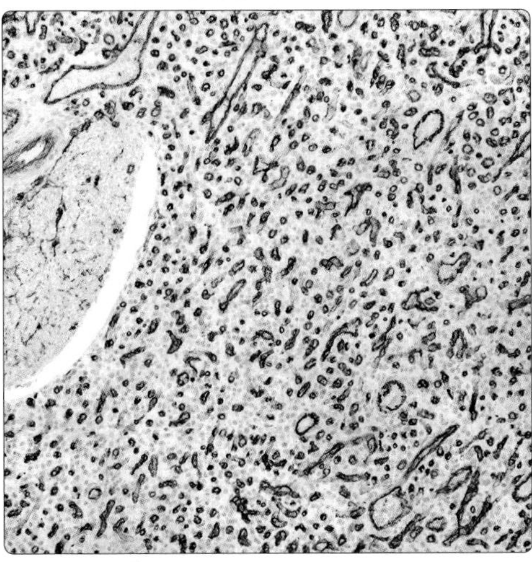

S100 Protein Positive

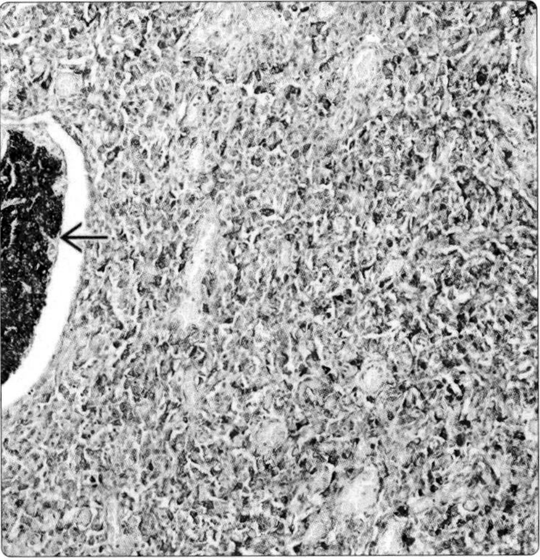

(Left) *Hemangioblastomas are highly vascular neoplasms, and endothelial stains such as CD34 or CD31 underscore the extent of vascularity in the neoplasm. Note that the stromal cells are immunonegative for CD31 or CD34.* **(Right)** *Hemangioblastomas are often strongly and diffusely positive with antibodies against S100 protein. The trapped nerve root ⇒ in this intradural extramedullary tumor serves as a positive control.*

KEY FACTS

CLINICAL ISSUES

- Median age at presentation
  - 60-65 years in immunocompetent patients with DLBCL
  - 30-35 years in immunocompromised patients
- More aggressive than systemic DLBCL

IMAGING

- Homogeneous enhancement (i.e., no central necrosis) in typical patient without immunocompromise
- Ring pattern in immunocompromised patients
- Can be multifocal

MICROSCOPIC

- Characteristic perivascular cuffing pattern of tumor cells
- Infiltrating component mimics infiltrating glioma, especially anaplastic astrocytoma or oligodendroglioma
- Microvascular proliferation rare
- Nonneoplastic small T cells occasionally prominent
- Corticosteroids cause extensive apoptosis and macrophage infiltrate simulating demyelination

ANCILLARY TESTS

- DLBCL
  - CD45(+), CD20(+), CD79-a(+)
- EBV(+) in immunosuppressed patients, PTLD, and in lymphomatoid granulomatosis
- High Ki-67 labeling Index
- Germinal center type
  - CD10(+) in > 30% of tumor cells
- Nongerminal center type
  - MUM1(+) and Bcl-6(+/-)
- Double-hit lymphomas: MYC(+) and Bcl-2(+)

DIAGNOSTIC CHECKLIST

- Corticosteroid treatment can melt PCNSLs
- Paucicellular areas may closely mimic infiltrating glioma
- Microvascular proliferation rare or often nonexistent

Contrast-Enhanced MR

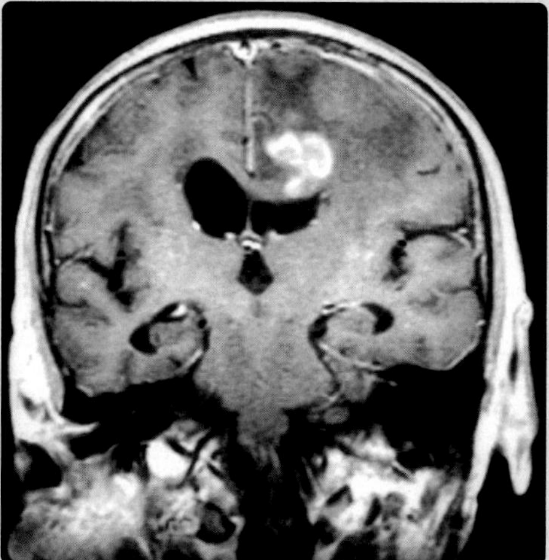

Crossing Corpus Callosum

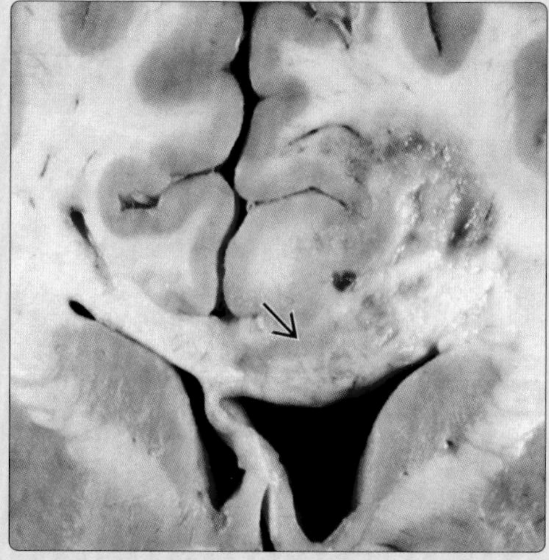

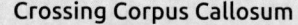

(Left) *Primary central nervous system malignant lymphomas often enhance homogeneously or in a ring pattern. Radiologically, they can mimic glioblastoma in every way, including crossing the corpus callosum.* **(Right)** *Primary central nervous system lymphoma often involves deep white matter and corpus callosum ⇒. The tumor often appears infiltrative macroscopically.*

Angiocentric Arrangement

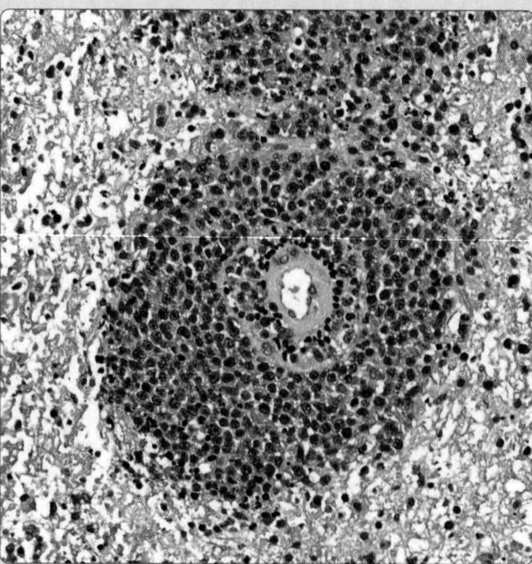

CD20 Positivity

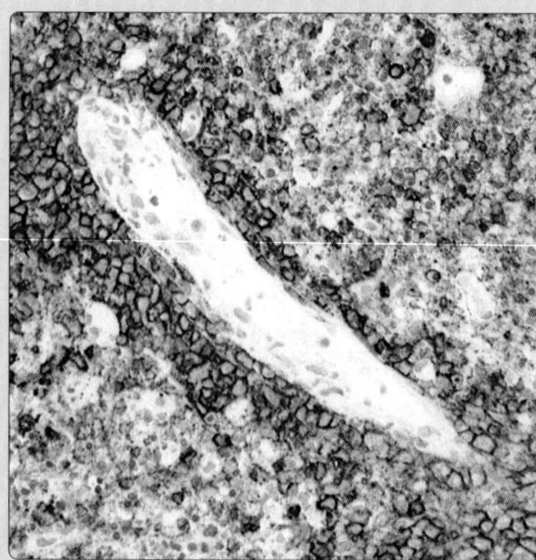

(Left) *The diagnosis is readily apparent in angiocentric and angioinvasive lesions. Metastatic carcinoma comes to mind, but the surrounding eosinophilic area is intact brain parenchyma, not necrosis.* **(Right)** *Immunohistochemical stain with antibodies against CD20 typically highlights large atypical lymphoid cells around vessels, providing support for the diagnosis of diffuse large cell B-cell lymphoma (DLBCL).*

TERMINOLOGY

Abbreviations

- Primary central nervous system lymphoma (PCNSL)

Synonyms

- Most PCNSLs are diffuse large B-cell lymphoma (DLBCL)
- Posttransplant lymphoproliferative disorder (PTLD), not considered primary CNSL

Definitions

- Rare variant of extranodal, non-Hodgkin lymphoma restricted to brain, spinal cord, eye, and meninges
- > 95% PCNSL is DLBCL

ETIOLOGY/PATHOGENESIS

Immunodeficiency States

- Increased risk for EBV-driven CNS lymphoma
  - Infections
    - HIV/AIDS
    - Epstein-Barr virus (EBV)
  - Iatrogenic immunosuppression
  - Congenital immunodeficiency syndromes
    - Wiskott-Aldrich syndrome
    - Severe combined immunodeficiency
  - Autoimmune diseases
    - Rheumatoid arthritis
    - Sjögren syndrome
    - Systemic lupus erythematosus

Unknown Etiology in Most Immunocompetent Patients

- Viruses such as EBV or HIV are absent in immunocompetent patients with PCNSL

CLINICAL ISSUES

Epidemiology

- Incidence
  - Rare, approximately 3% of all primary CNS tumors
- Age
  - Median age at presentation varies based on immune status
    - 60-70 years in immunocompetent patients
    - 30-40 years in immunocompromised patients
  - Rare in children

Presentation

- Focal neurological deficits
- Mass effects
- Neuropsychological signs
- Ocular symptoms
- Rarely seizures, fever, or night sweats
- May simulate encephalitis or leukoencephalopathy, especially in lymphomatosis cerebri type

Treatment

- Surgical approaches
  - Biopsy for diagnosis is only procedure of choice
  - Debulking to relieve mass effect, uncommon
- Drugs
  - Chemotherapy containing high-dose methotrexate
  - Rituximab (monoclonal antibody against CD20) in most combination regimens
- Radiation
  - Avoided in some centers as front line treatment
- Autologous stem cell transplantation, especially in young patients with relapse

Prognosis

- More aggressive than systemic DLBCL
- Poor survival
  - Median survival around 20-45 months for immunocompetent patients
  - Median survival around 12-18 months for immunocompromised patients
- CSF dissemination in minority of cases but can involve eye

IMAGING

MR Findings

- Majority affect cerebral hemispheres (deep brain, periventricular region, corpus callosum, cerebellum)
- ~ 1/3 multifocal
- Iso- or hypointense on T1-weighted images
- Hyperintense on T2-weighted and FLAIR images
- Variable but pronounced contrast enhancement, different between immunocompetent and immunodeficient patients
  - No dark necrotic center in sporadic cases
  - Central necrosis (rim pattern) similar to glioblastoma in immunocompromised patients
- Leakage of contrast in perfusion-weighted images
- Decreased signal in diffusion-weighted images
- Difficult to distinguish from CNS involvement by systemic lymphoma
  - Multifocal lesions and uncommon locations as well as extradural masses should prompt evaluation

MACROSCOPIC

General Features

- Solitary or multiple, large, irregular, and pale
- Soft, fish-flesh appearance, slightly darker than gray matter

MICROSCOPIC

Histologic Features

- Angiocentricity with tumor cells forming layers around vessels
- Angioinvasion, focal, sometimes with vascular necrosis
- Diffuse, single-cell invasion, without perineuronal satellitosis
- Large, round to irregular nuclei with prominent nucleoli
- Small reactive T lymphocytes, usually sparse to moderate but sometimes dominant
- Apoptosis and necrosis, especially after steroid treatment
- Necrosis, without pseudopalisading, in immunocompromised or steroid-treated patients
- No microvascular proliferation
- Corticosteroid effects
  - Increased apoptosis
  - Few, if any, viable tumor cells

- Macrophage-rich infiltrate with variable number of lymphocytes and plasma cells
- Foci of necrosis

Other Subtypes of Central Nervous System Lymphoma (< 5%)

- Posttransplant lymphoproliferative disorder (PTLD)
  - EBV(+), EBER(+)
  - Consequence of immunosuppression in allograft recipients
  - Polymorphic type does not fulfill criteria for malignant lymphoma
  - Monomorphic types may fulfill criteria for malignant lymphoma
  - Early lesions of infectious mononucleosis type may regress with reduction of immunosuppression
- Primary CNS T-cell lymphoma
  - Small, angulated cells
  - Older patients
  - T-cell associated antigens CD2, CD3, and CD5 (+)
- Anaplastic large B-cell lymphoma
  - No association with immunodeficiency
  - Extensive leptomeningeal spread
  - Large, round, pleomorphic cells with marked cytologic atypia
  - ALK(+) and t(2:5) translocation
  - Typically CD30, CD45, and EMA (+)
  - Occasionally CD3, CD43, and CD45RO (+)
  - Worst prognosis among PCNSLs
- Primary intraocular lymphoma
  - Optic nerve, retina, or vitreous
  - Usually bilateral
  - Most DLBCL
  - Vitreous cytology often helpful
- Marginal zone B-cell lymphoma and mucosa-associated tissue (MALT lymphoma)
  - Dural-based, meningioma-like mass
  - Female predominance
  - Small to medium-sized tumor cells with pale cytoplasm
  - Less cytologic atypia than DLBCL
    - Slightly irregular tumor nuclei with inconspicuous nucleoli
  - CD20, CD79-a (+)
  - Trisomy 3 most common genetic abnormality
- Lymphomatoid granulomatosis
  - EBV-driven B-cell lymphoproliferative process
  - Angiocentric, angiodestructive
  - Polymorphous background
  - Coagulation necrosis
  - Often involves the lung &/or skin in addition to CNS
- Histiocytic sarcoma
  - Histiocytic markers CD68, CD163, and lysozyme (+)
  - May be confused with glioblastoma or sarcoma
  - Aggressive, unresponsive to corticosteroids
- Primary Hodgkin lymphoma
  - Dural based, often at skull base
  - Reed-Sternberg cells, essential to diagnosis
  - Background with eosinophils & small lymphocytes
- Intravascular lymphomatosis
  - Highly aggressive form involving multiple organs without mass lesions
  - Poor prognosis, most patients diagnosed post mortem
  - Exclusively intraluminal localization of malignant B lymphocytes
- Lymphomatosis cerebri
  - MR appearance suggests leukoencephalopathy
  - No mass lesions
  - Diffuse involvement of brain parenchyma by malignant B lymphocytes

ANCILLARY TESTS

Cytology

- Dispersed individual cells
- Large, hyperchromatic nuclei with large nucleoli
- Scant amphophilic cytoplasm
- Apoptotic cells and mitotic figures
- Macrophages, some tingible body type, especially after corticosteroid treatment

Histochemistry

- Tree-ring pattern of reticulin staining in affected vessels

Immunohistochemistry

- Common markers
  - CD45(+)
  - CD20(+)
  - CD79-a(+)
  - High Ki-67 labeling index
- Germinal center phenotype
  - CD10(+) in > 30% of tumor cells
  - Bcl-6(+)
  - CD10(-)
  - MUM1(-)
- Nongerminal phenotype
  - MUM1(+) regardless of Bcl-6 or CD10 status
  - CD10(-)
  - Bcl-6(-)
  - MUM1(-)
- Double-hit lymphoma
  - Bcl-2(+) in > 50% of tumor cells
  - MYC(+) in > 40% of tumor cells

In Situ Hybridization

- EBV(+) in most CNS lymphomas in immunosuppressed patients

DIFFERENTIAL DIAGNOSIS

Systemic Malignant Lymphoma Involving CNS

- May be difficult to distinguish from PCNSL
- Prior history of systemic lymphoma or immunosuppression
- Some cases initially considered PCNSL may prove to be systemic tumors on follow-up

Glioblastoma

- Tissue fragments with fibrillar background on smears
- Variable cell size, processes
- Little angiocentricity
- Vascular endothelial proliferation and palisading necrosis
- GFAP(+), most cases

- Somewhat smaller cells in glioblastoma with PNET component; synaptophysin (+)

Anaplastic Oligodendroglioma

- Cellular monotony
- Perineuronal satellitosis
- Few lymphocytes
- CD45(-)
- S100(+)
- GFAP(+)
- IDH1(+)
- Vascular endothelial proliferation in most cases

Metastatic Carcinoma

- Tissue fragments and cells with sharply defined cytoplasm in smear preparations
- Well circumscribed, corticocentric
- Organoid patterns, cohesive architecture
- Stromal desmoplasia
- Immunostaining profile
  - Keratin (+)
  - CD45(-)
- Tissue necrosis may simulate false angiocentric pattern

Cerebral Infarction

- Slight, if any, lymphoid infiltrate, no atypia
- Ischemic, red-dead neurons in acute examples
- Abundant macrophages in subacute examples

Cerebral Abscess

- Uniform thickness; occasional multiloculate ring enhancement
- Suppuration
- Mixed lymphoplasmacytic infiltrate with neutrophils
- Capsule in well-developed, organizing lesions
- Rare CD20(+) cells

Encephalitis

- Minimal or no cytological atypia
- Principally T cells, almost no CD20(+) cells
- Microglial clusters

Demyelinating Disease

- Restricted to white matter
  - Demarcated
  - Periventricular lesions may not enhance
- Predominantly macrophages
- Perivascular small lymphocytes (T cells)
- Occasional astrocytes with multiple micronuclei (Creutzfeldt cells)

DIAGNOSTIC CHECKLIST

Clinically Relevant Pathologic Features

- Corticosteroid treatment can melt PCNSLs

Pathologic Interpretation Pearls

- Paucicellular areas may closely mimic infiltrating glioma
- Widely scattered tumor cells may be inconspicuous among small reactive lymphocytes
- Microvascular proliferation rare or often nonexistent

SELECTED REFERENCES

1. Izquierdo C et al: Lymphomatosis cerebri: a rare form of primary central nervous system lymphoma. Analysis of 7 cases and systematic review of the literature. Neuro Oncol. ePub, 2015
2. Giannini C et al: CNS lymphoma: a practical diagnostic approach. J Neuropathol Exp Neurol. 73(6):478-94, 2014
3. Scott BJ et al: A systematic approach to the diagnosis of suspected central nervous system lymphoma. JAMA Neurol. 70(3):311-9, 2013
4. Venkataraman G et al: Marginal zone lymphomas involving meningeal dura: possible link to IgG4-related diseases. Mod Pathol. 24(3):355-66, 2011
5. Gerstner ER et al: Primary central nervous system lymphoma. Arch Neurol. 67(3):291-7, 2010
6. Hattab EM et al: Most primary central nervous system diffuse large B-cell lymphomas occurring in immunocompetent individuals belong to the nongerminal center subtype: a retrospective analysis of 31 cases. Mod Pathol. 23(2):235-43, 2010
7. Raoux D et al: Primary central nervous system lymphoma: Immunohistochemical profile and prognostic significance. Neuropathology. 30(3):232-40, 2010
8. Sacho RH et al: Primary diffuse large B-cell central nervous system lymphoma presenting as an acute space-occupying subdural mass. J Neurosurg. 113(2):384-7, 2010
9. Wu D et al: "Double-Hit" mature B-cell lymphomas show a common immunophenotype by flow cytometry that includes decreased CD20 expression. Am J Clin Pathol. 134(2):258-65, 2010
10. Algazi AP et al: Biology and treatment of primary central nervous system lymphoma. Neurotherapeutics. 6(3):587-97, 2009
11. Sierra del Rio M et al: Primary CNS lymphoma in immunocompetent patients. Oncologist. 14(5):526-39, 2009
12. Fischer L et al: Meningeal dissemination in primary CNS lymphoma: prospective evaluation of 282 patients. Neurology. 71(14):1102-8, 2008
13. Rubenstein J et al: Primary lymphoma of the central nervous system: epidemiology, pathology and current approaches to diagnosis, prognosis and treatment. Leuk Lymphoma. 49 Suppl 1:43-51, 2008
14. Tu PH et al: Clinicopathologic and genetic profile of intracranial marginal zone lymphoma: a primary low-grade CNS lymphoma that mimics meningioma. J Clin Oncol. 23(24):5718-27, 2005
15. Hans CP et al: Confirmation of the molecular classification of diffuse large B-cell lymphoma by immunohistochemistry using a tissue microarray. Blood. 103(1):275-82, 2004

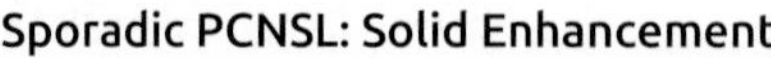

Sporadic PCNSL: Solid Enhancement | **PCNSL in HIV: Ring Enhancement**

(Left) *Sporadic diffuse large B-cell lymphomas (DLBCLs) typically enhance homogeneously without the dark necrotic center of glioblastoma or most metastases ➔. Such an image in an older patient is highly suggestive of PCNSL.* **(Right)** *Rim enhancement ➔ is common in CNS lymphomas that arise in the setting of immunosuppression. A dark zone of edema extends anteriorly from the enhancing region.*

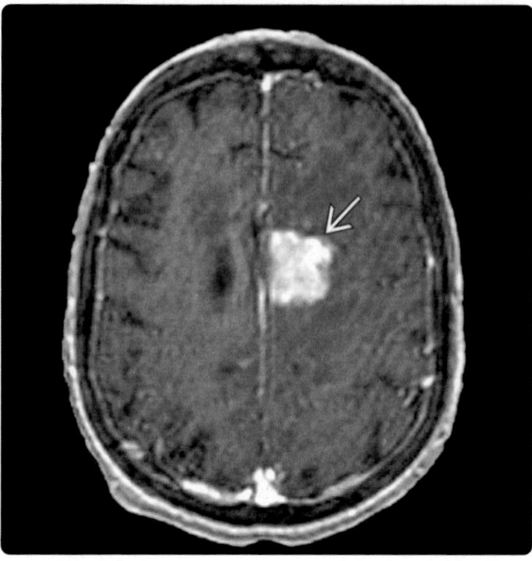

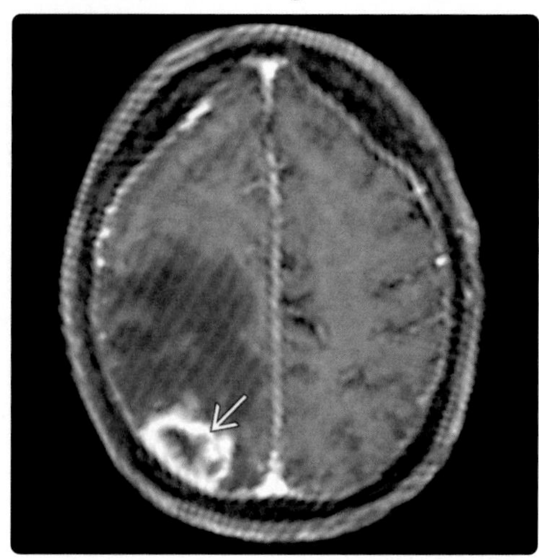

Distinctive Clustered Appearance | **Perivascular Tumor Cells and Apoptosis**

(Left) *Angiocentricity gives many primary PCNSLs a distinctive clustered unevenness. There are often scattered individual tumor cells within the parenchyma, but what strikes the eye most often is the filing of tumor cells along the Virchow-Robin spaces.* **(Right)** *Cardinal histological features of CNS DLBCLs are angiocentricity, scattered malignant cells within the neuropil, and prominent apoptosis. Microvascular proliferation is absent. Even small doses of corticosteroid treatment can induce apoptosis.*

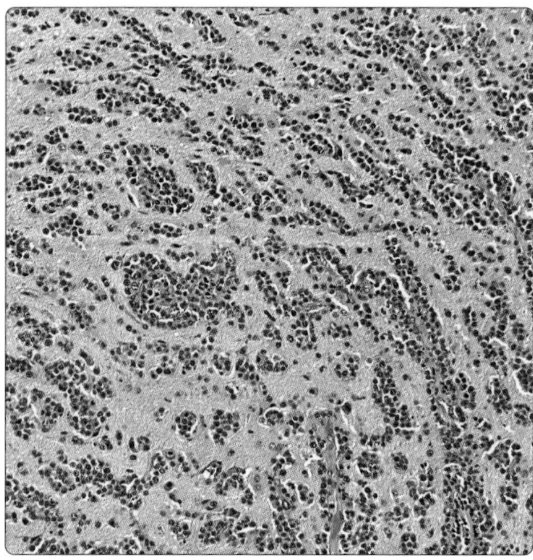

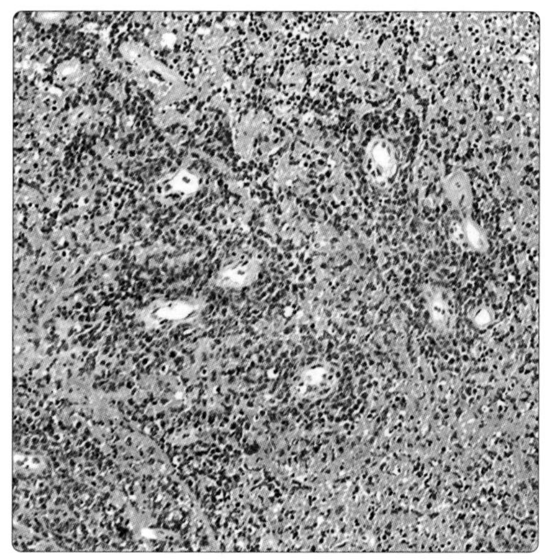

Perivascular and Parenchymal Tumor Cells | **Subtle Angiocentricity**

(Left) *While attracted to vessels, lymphoma cells also can percolate as individual cells, in glioma fashion, within the parenchyma ➔. Unlike many infiltrating gliomas, there is no perineuronal satellitosis when lymphoma infiltrates gray matter.* **(Right)** *Angiocentricity ➔ is sometimes subtle, and this diagnostic clue may be overlooked. This is especially true during frozen sections, and the infiltrative appearance of tumor cells may mislead to a diagnosis of high-grade glioma.*

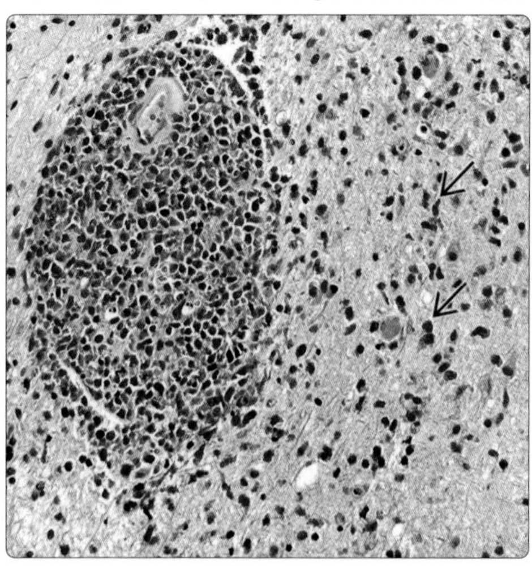

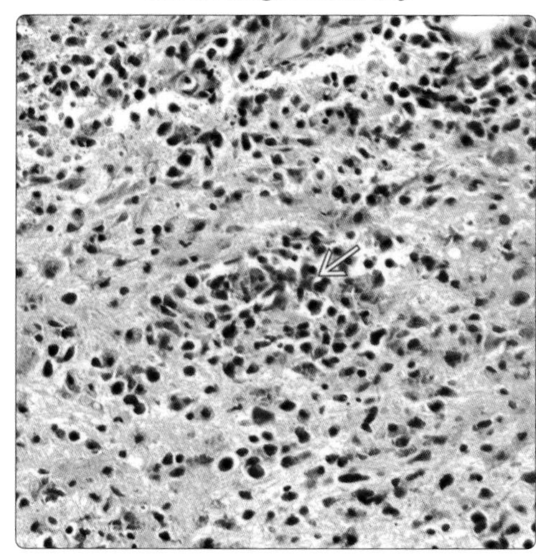

Layered Tumor Cells

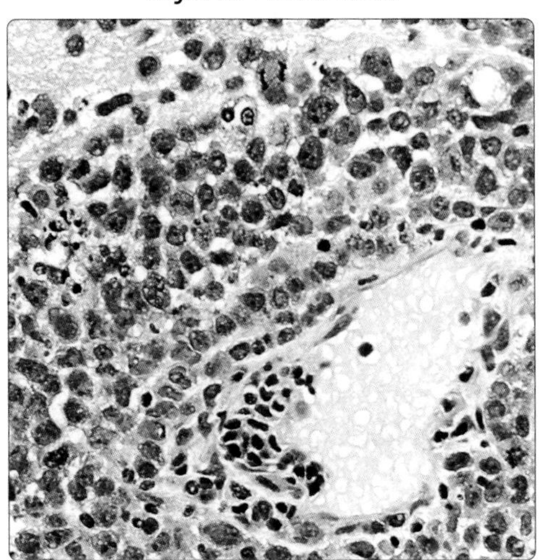

Angiocentricity on Reticulin Stains

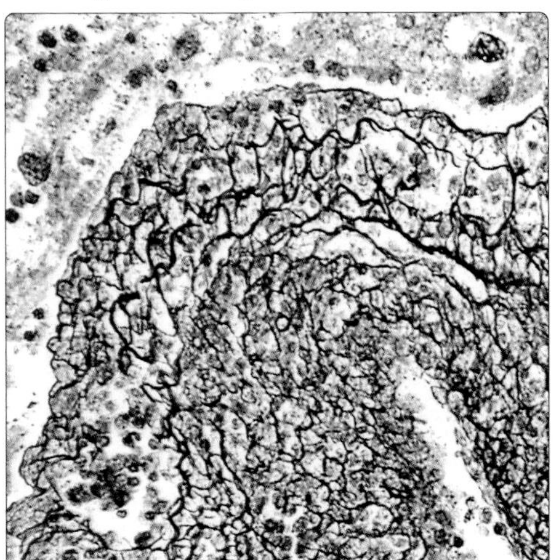

(Left) *Layering of tumor cells in and around vessels is a distinctive feature of PCNSL and extremely unusual for malignant gliomas and metastases.* **(Right)** *Rings of reticulin in and around vessel walls encompass tumor cells. This is further confirmation of the perivascular, and sometimes intramural, location of tumor cells. An old term for PCNSL was reticulum cell sarcoma because of this perivascular prominence of reticulin fibers.*

Tumor Periphery

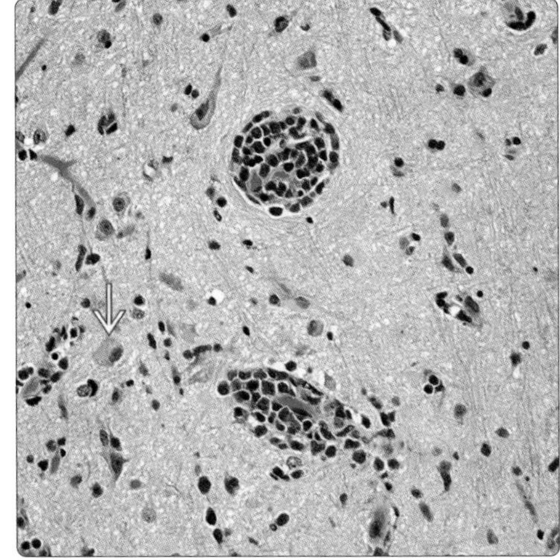

Pericapillary Distribution of Tumor Cells

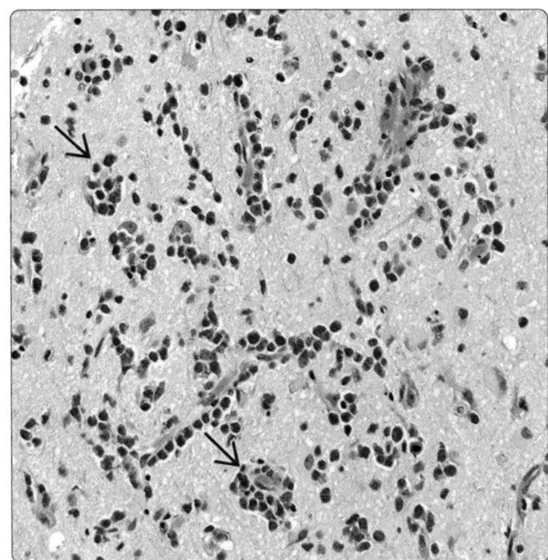

(Left) *Angiocentricity is often most obvious in paucicellular peripheral regions. Gliosis in these areas ➡ can be brisk.* **(Right)** *Capillary-tumor cell complexes ➡ can suggest perineuronal satellitosis, a phenomenon that is typically absent in PCNSL. However, unlike satellitosis, the cells do not encircle neurons.*

Oligodendroglioma-Like Features

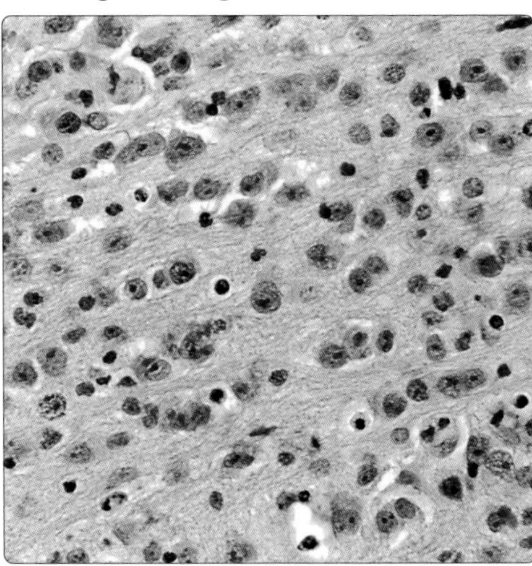

Prominent Nucleoli

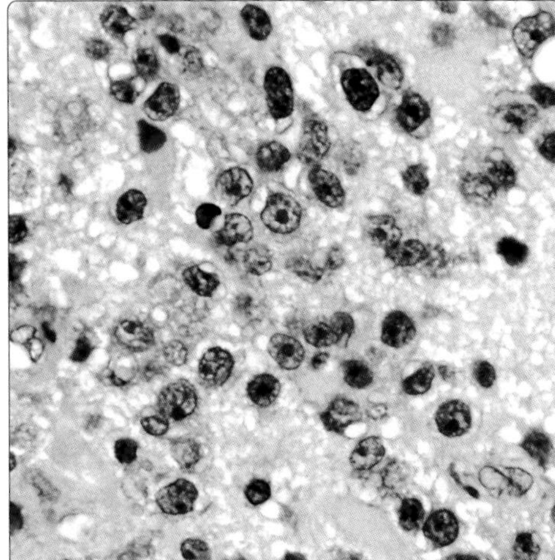

(Left) *Diffusely infiltrating cells of PCNSL resemble anaplastic oligodendroglioma, although lymphoma has somewhat more nuclear pleomorphism and larger nucleoli.* **(Right)** *Nucleoli this prominent are more typical of PCNSL than anaplastic oligodendroglioma. The dyscohesive nature of the tumor, along with the paucity of cytoplasm, are further proof of the diagnosis. Eosinophilic cytoplasm, however scant in amount, is not a feature of PCNSL.*

(Left) *PCNSL with a diffuse, sheet-like growth pattern can be mistaken for metastatic cancer or densely cellular high-grade oligodendroglioma. There is neither necrosis, as is present in most glioblastomas and metastasis, nor vascular proliferation as would be expected in a malignant glioma with this degree of cellularity.* **(Right)** *Densely cellular examples without angiocentricity may resemble cellular high-grade gliomas, especially oligodendroglioma.*

Sheets of Tumor Cells

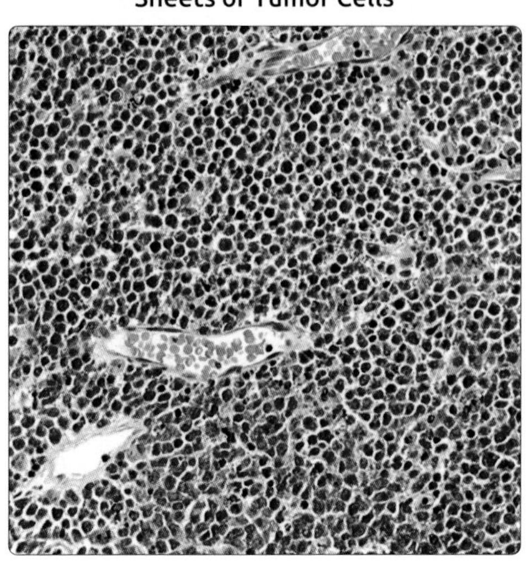

Dense Cellularity

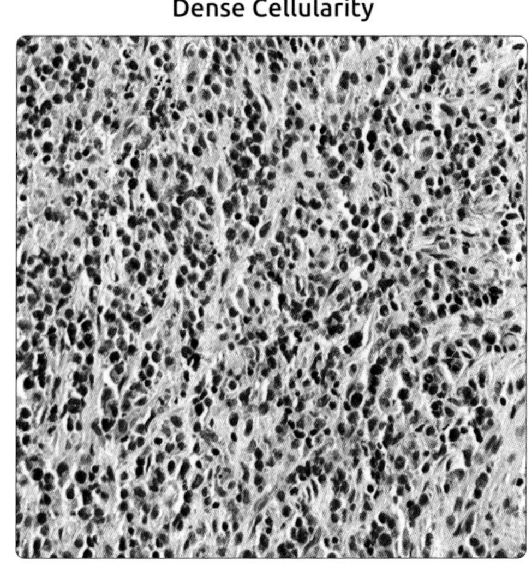

(Left) *Perivascular or angiocentric arrangement of tumor cells ⇨ may be less apparent in highly cellular areas. The hypercellular areas obscure the angiocentric pattern, which can be identified by a more careful evaluation.* **(Right)** *Irregular nuclear profiles, coarse chromatin, and prominent nucleoli are typical features. The cells often retract and create artifactual changes ➡ during tissue processing. Apoptotic cells ⇨ are usually present.*

Hypercellular Regions

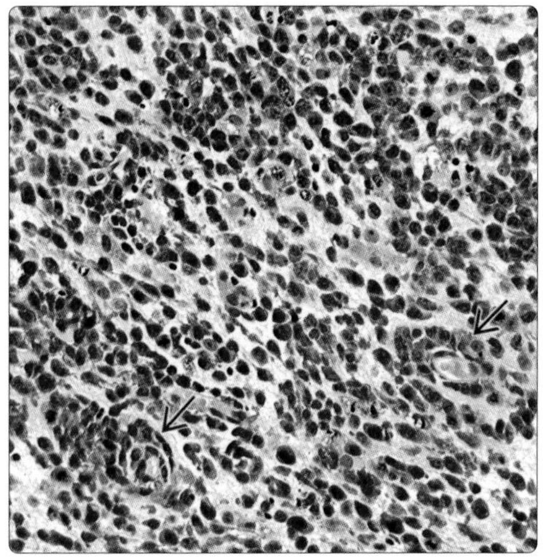

Apoptotic Cells

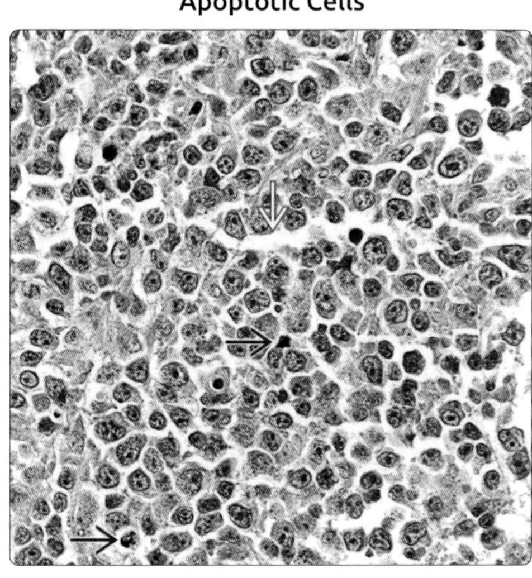

(Left) *In some DLBCLs, apoptosis and necrosis are far advanced. Tumor cells are still recognizable here despite abundant apoptosis, vascular necrosis, and nuclear debris. This picture should raise the possibility of prior treatment.* **(Right)** *Only necrosis and advanced apoptosis remain in some cases of PCNSL post steroid treatment.*

Abundant Necrosis and Apoptosis

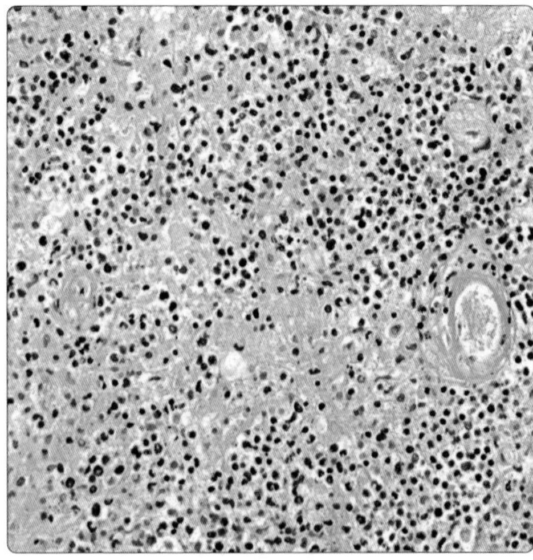

Prior Treatment: Steroids

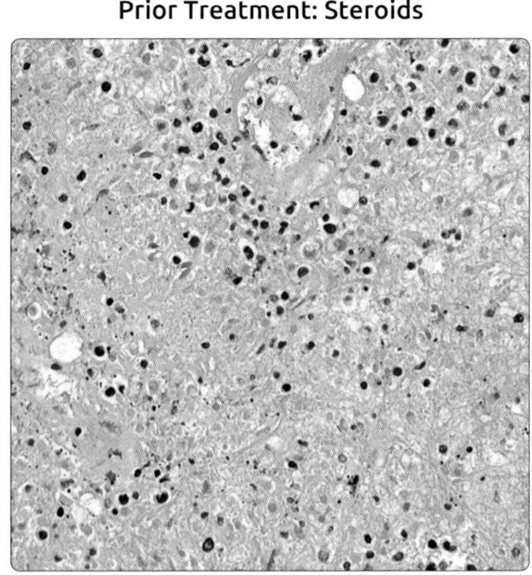

Macrophage-Rich Lesion

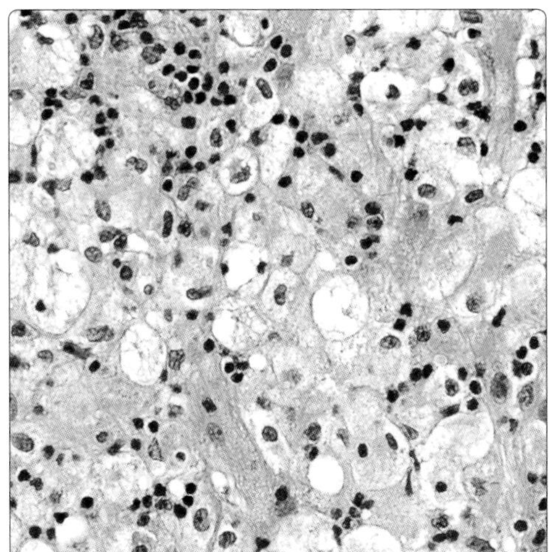

Subtle Effect of Steroid Treatment

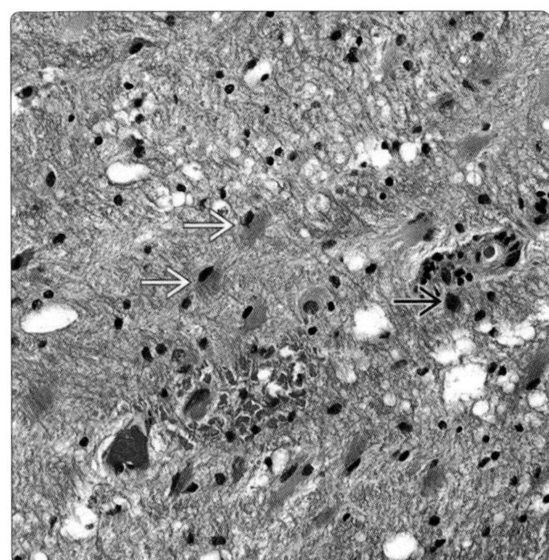

(Left) *Nothing but macrophages, reactive astrocytes, and scattered small lymphocytes remain following corticosteroid treatment in some cases.* **(Right)** *In some cases of DLBCL, the effect of corticosteroid treatment may not manifest as necrosis and apoptosis. Instead, profound gliotic reaction ➡ and only a rare perivascular atypical cell ➡ may remain.*

Anaplastic Large Cell Lymphoma

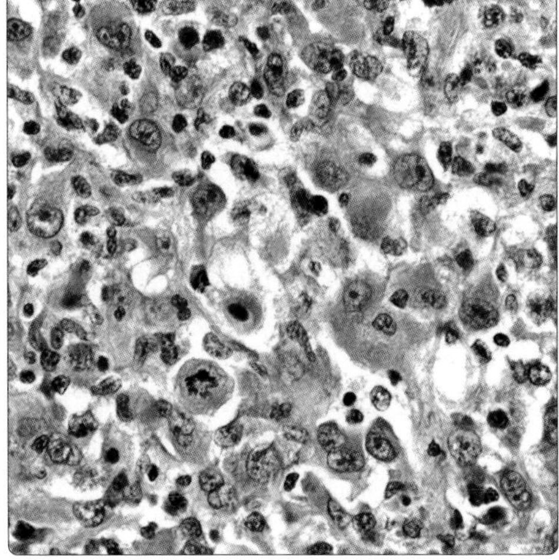

Anaplastic Large Cell Lymphoma

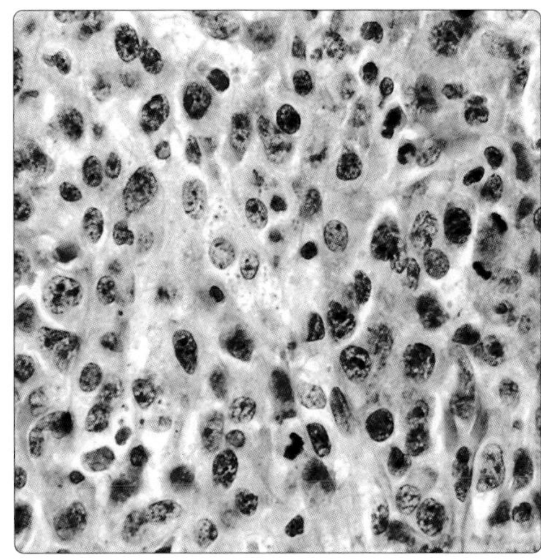

(Left) *Anaplastic large cell lymphomas show a broad morphological spectrum and are typically ALK(+) T-cell lymphomas. Morphological features can range from small cell neoplasms to large cells with abundant cytoplasm with large, irregular, and often eccentric nuclei. Most malignant cells are CD30(+).* **(Right)** *Because of their large round cells, anaplastic lymphoma may be initially misinterpreted as metastatic carcinoma or melanoma.*

MALT-Type Lymphoma

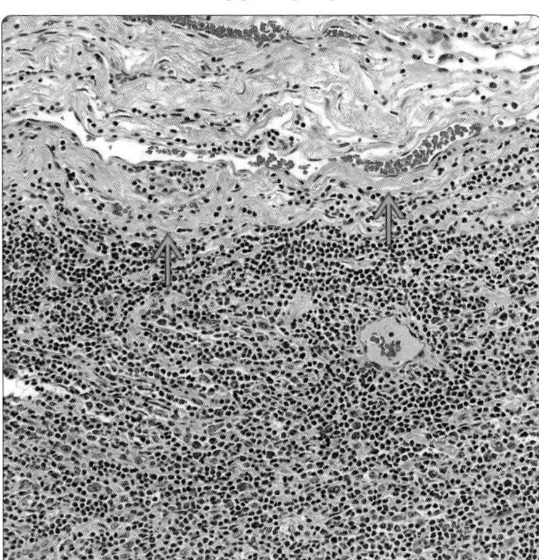

MALT-Type Lymphoma, Close-Up

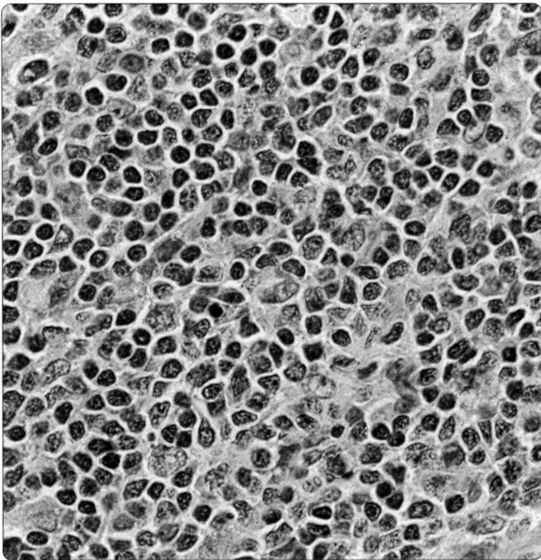

(Left) *Mucosa-associated lymphoid type (MALT) lymphomas are typically attached to the dura ➡. A homogeneous, nonnodular, sheet-like growth pattern is characteristic.* **(Right)** *Cells of MALT lymphomas are smaller, more monomorphous, and cytologically less atypical than those of the much more common, and intraparenchymal, DLBCL.*

(Left) *As in sections, smears may contain a significant number of small reactive lymphocytes ➡. The difference in size and atypia between neoplastic and nonneoplastic cells is obvious, as are large nucleoli of the malignant cells ➡.* **(Right)** *Mitotic figures ➡ are often helpful, but not necessary, in affirming the neoplastic nature of the large lymphoid cells. The dyscohesive nature of the tumor cells, along with large prominent nucleoli and little or cytoplasm, are further evidence to the diagnosis.*

Intraoperative Smear

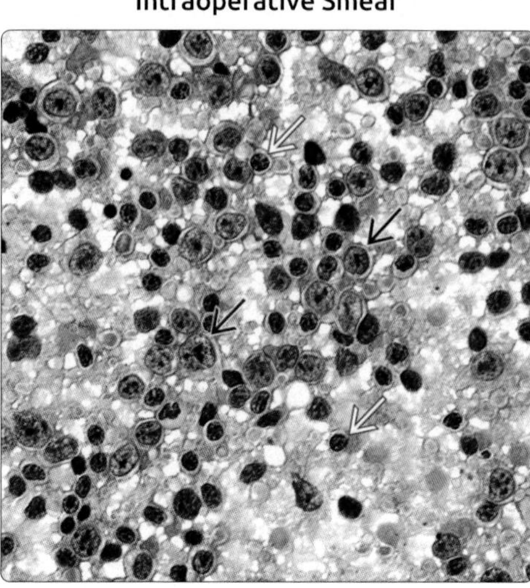

Dyscohesive Tumor Cells

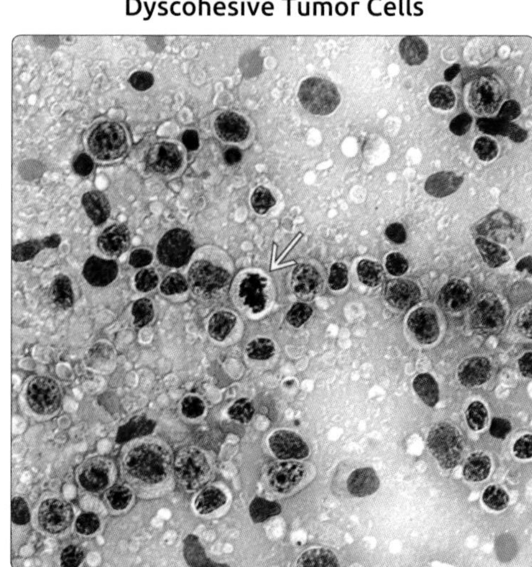

(Left) *The overwhelming majority of PCNSL cases are diffuse large cell lymphomas that are positive with the antibodies against CD20, CD79-a, as well as MUM1.* **(Right)** *Marginal zone or MALT lymphomas express strong positivity with CD20 and CD79-a antibodies, similar to DLBCL. Immunohistochemical stains also highlight the angiocentric arrangement of small neoplastic B cells.*

CD20 Positivity

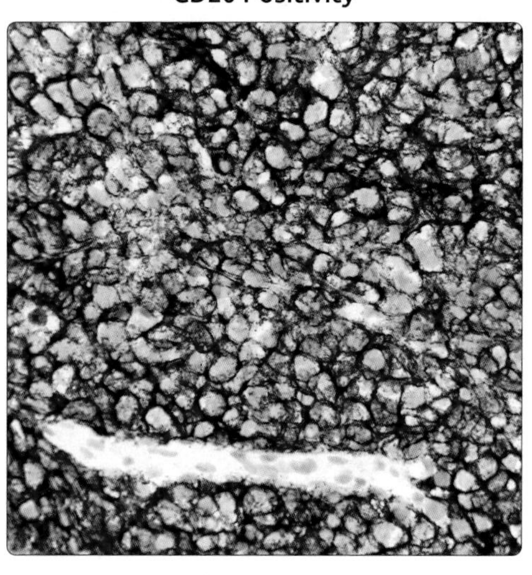

CD20 in MALT Lymphomas

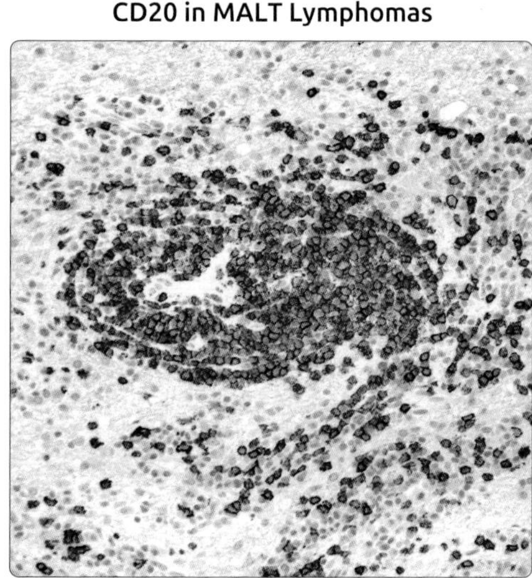

(Left) *CD20 staining helps identify lymphoma cells in a glioma-like infiltrate of individual tumor cells. Note the focal perivascular tumor cells ➡.* **(Right)** *CD79-a, the immunoglobulin-associated alpha component of the B-cell antigen, is present in the majority of B-cell lymphomas. While useful, it is a less sensitive marker than CD20.*

CD20 Staining in Parenchyma

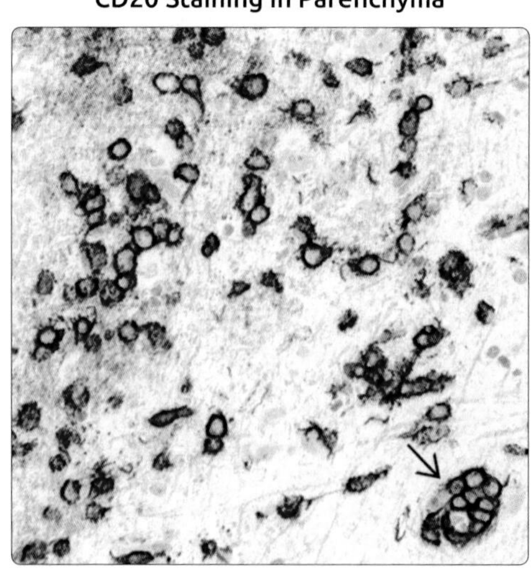

CD79-a Positivity

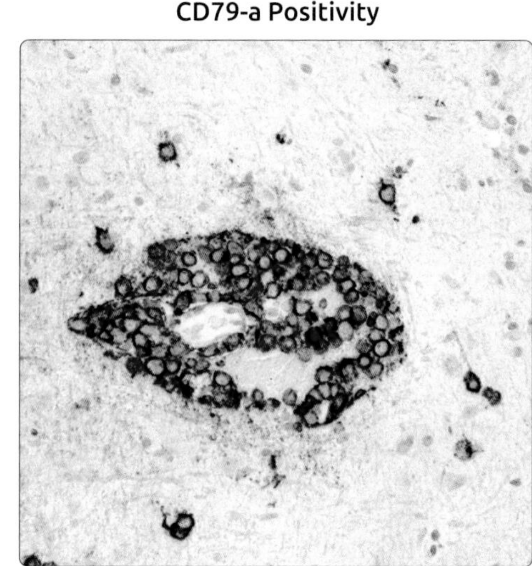

CD10 Positivity

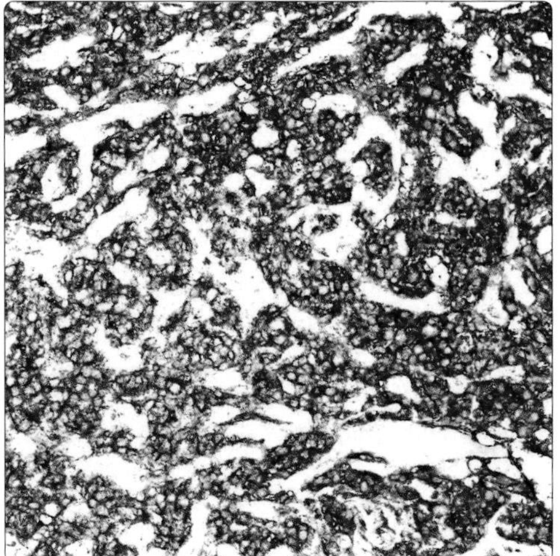

CD10 Positivity

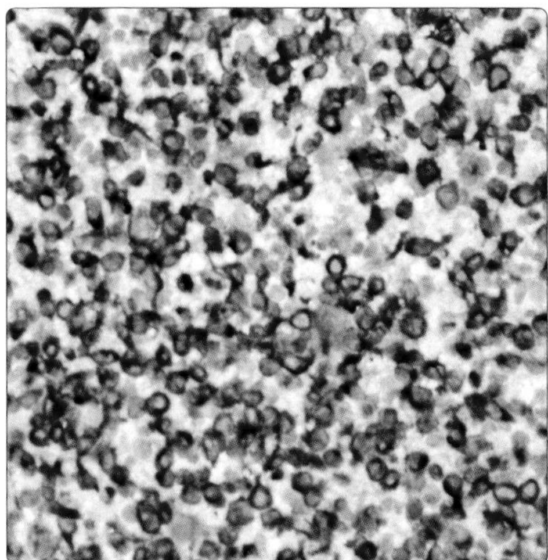

(Left) *Malignant lymphomas that demonstrate > 30% staining with CD10 are considered within the germinal center type. There is still uncertainty whether these tumors have a different prognosis compared to nongerminal center-type tumors.* **(Right)** *In most tumors, CD10 does not stain all the cells, but > 30% staining would be considered sufficient for designating the tumor in the germinal center type.*

Bcl-6 Positivity

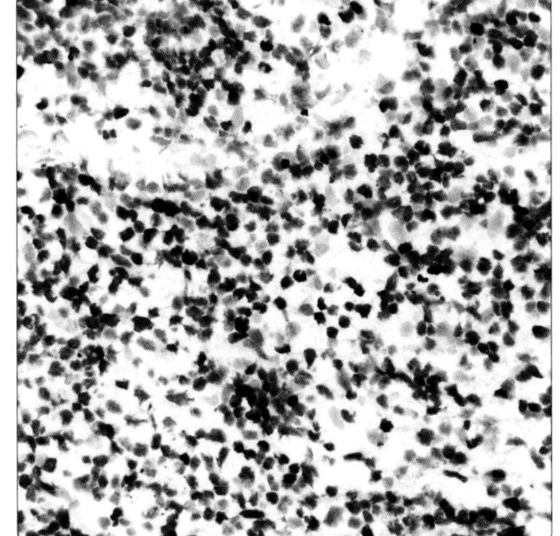

MUM1 Positivity

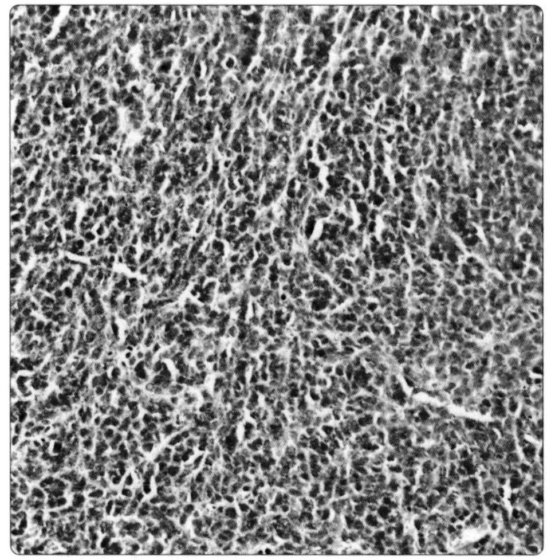

(Left) *Bcl-6 positivity would be considered as evidence for nongerminal center type DLBCL.* **(Right)** *The overwhelming majority of PCNSL cases demonstrates positivity with MUM1, which is used to classify these neoplasms as nongerminal center type, regardless of their CD10 and Bcl-6 status.*

Proliferative Index in PCNSL

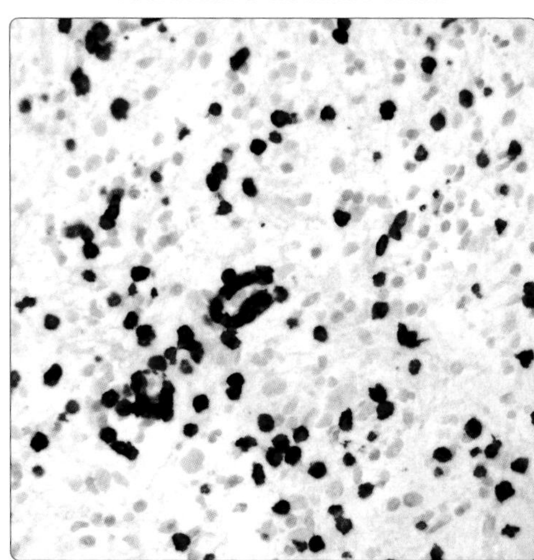

In Situ Hybridization for EBV

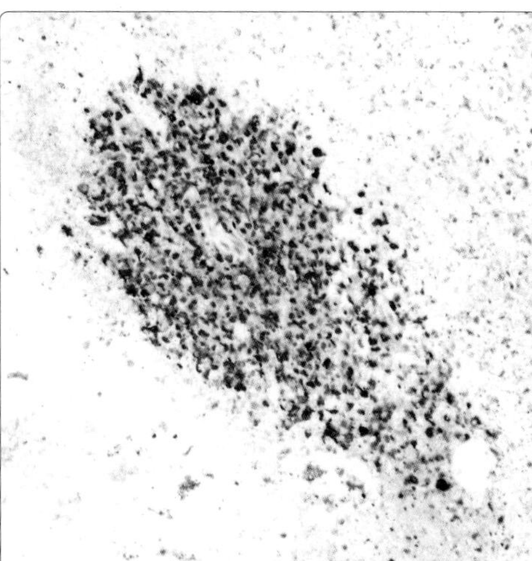

(Left) *Biopsies from PCNSL cases demonstrate very high rate of Ki-67 positivity, which often helps to distinguish them from reactive inflammatory proliferation.* **(Right)** *In situ hybridization for Epstein-Barr virus identifies EBV-encoded small RNA of the virus in this CNS lymphoma from a patient with immunodeficiency.*

KEY FACTS

CLINICAL ISSUES

- "Great imitator" with broad differential diagnosis
- Involves multiple organs (typical) or limited to CNS (uncommon)
- Prognosis poor; median survival of 5-7 months
- Many patients diagnosed at postmortem
- Western variant presents with symptoms predominantly related to single organ
- Asian variant presents with multiorgan failure

IMAGING

- Radiological studies do not reveal any mass lesion
- Multiple, bilateral FLAIR or T2W bright lesions
- Predominantly periventricular or white matter
- Patchy, sometimes punctate contrast enhancement

MICROSCOPIC

- Exclusively intraluminal location of large cytologically atypical B lymphocytes
  - CD45 and CD20 often positive in most intraluminal cells
- Involvement of small- or medium-size vessels
- Mitotic figures among clusters of intravascular tumor cells
- Involved vessels may be very focal
- There are often no associated changes in brain parenchyma, but infarct-like changes, gliosis, or even necrosis may be seen

DIAGNOSTIC CHECKLIST

- Diffuse disease with generalized, nonlocalizing symptoms
- Diagnosis often late, either at perimortem or postmortem
- No mass lesion
- Biopsies from affected sites critical in early recognition
- In some cases, obtaining additional and deeper sections from tissue is very useful
- Immunohistochemistry sometimes necessary to confirm tumor cells, and CD45 and CD20 often sufficient to establish diagnosis

Multifocal Axial FLAIR Abnormalities

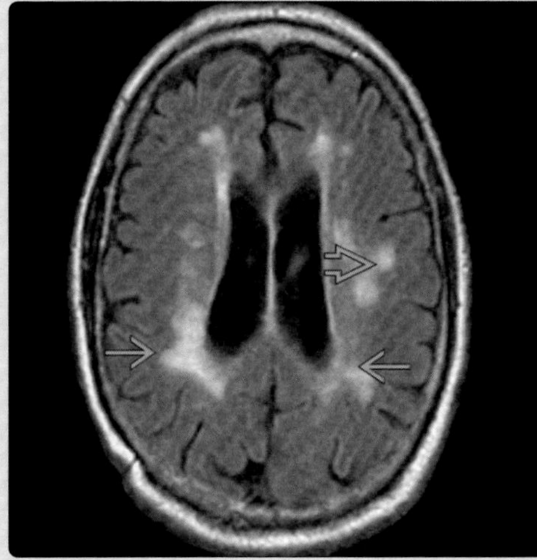

Intravascular Overtly Malignant Cells

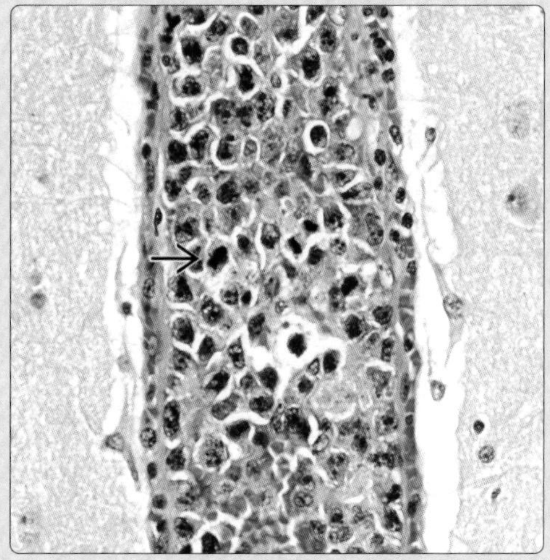

(Left) *FLAIR or T2WI demonstrate bright lesions within the deep white matter ⇒, but the lesions are especially concentrated in periventricular areas ⇒.* **(Right)** *The diagnosis is obvious when larger vessels are filled with overtly malignant cells with mitotic figures ⇒ and prominent nuclei. Involved vessels can often be found in many organs including the brain, but lymph nodes are often spared.*

Intraluminal Atypical Cells

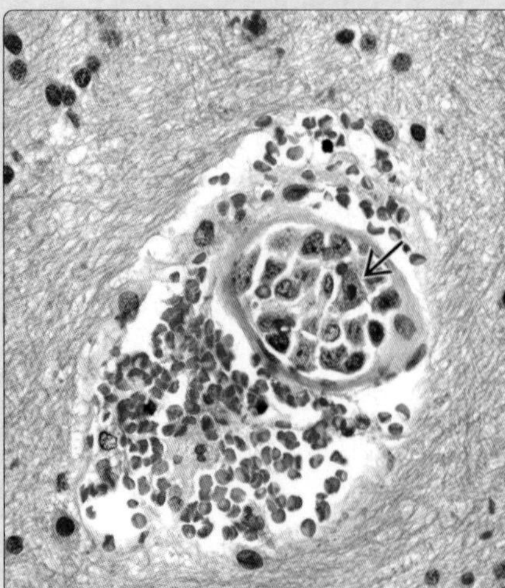

CD45(+) Intraluminal Cells

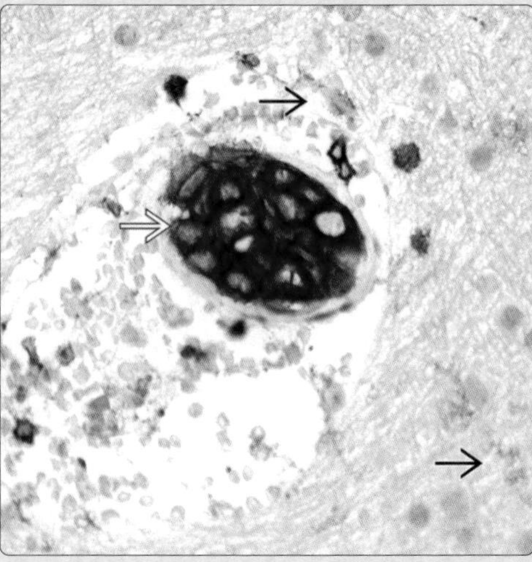

(Left) *The neoplastic lymphoid cells often fill the lumina of small or intermediary-type vessels in the CNS. Prominent nucleoli ⇒ and mitotic figures can often be observed. Note the paucity of changes in the surrounding brain parenchyma.* **(Right)** *Immunostaining with the CD45 antibody can be used to identify intraluminal tumor cells ➡ and establish the diagnosis. In addition, reactive processes and microglia can be visualized within the neurophil ⇒.*

TERMINOLOGY

Synonyms

- Angioendotheliotrophic lymphoma
- Angiotrophic large cell lymphoma
- Malignant angioendotheliomatosis
- Intravascular large B-cell lymphoma

Definitions

- Rare subtype of diffuse large B-cell lymphoma, characterized by selective proliferation of malignant B cells within lumina of small- and medium-sized vessels without parenchymal involvement

CLINICAL ISSUES

Site

- Widely disseminated at diagnosis, often involving multiple sites, but lymph nodes are often spared

Presentation

- Anemia &/or thrombocytopenia
- Hepatosplenomegaly
- Unexplained fever and confusion
- Acute cognitive decline or subacute dementia without focal neurological signs
- Spinal cord infarction or myelopathy
- Progressive myopathy
- Western variant: Symptoms related mainly to single organ involved
- Asian variant: Patients presenting with multiorgan failure

Treatment

- Adjuvant therapy
  - Historically ineffective due to rapid progression
  - Recombinant antibodies against CD20

Prognosis

- Poor; approximate median survival: 5-7 months
- Many patients succumb before diagnosis can be made

IMAGING

MR Findings

- Multiple FLAIR or T2 bright lesions
- Predominantly periventricular or white matter involvement
- Minimal, if any, enhancement
- Infarct-like lesions

MACROSCOPIC

General Features

- Dusky gray discoloration of white matter
- Some focal lesions resemble infarcts

MICROSCOPIC

Histologic Features

- Markedly atypical cells
  - Exclusively intraluminal
  - Large, round nuclei with prominent nucleoli
  - Mitoses
- Small- or medium-sized vessels affected
- Few, if any, small reactive lymphocytes
- Erythrocyte extravasation or hemosiderin focal
- Minimal, if any, perivascular change, e.g., gliosis
- Fibrin thrombi and necrosis of small vessels, occasional

ANCILLARY TESTS

Cytology

- Markedly atypical cells with scant cytoplasm
- Large nuclei with prominent nucleoli and vesicular chromatin

Immunohistochemistry

- Commonly positive for CD20, CD45, CD79-a, and MUM1
- Occasionally positive for CD5, Bcl-2, Bcl-6, and CD10

DIFFERENTIAL DIAGNOSIS

Primary Central Nervous System Lymphoma

- Tumor cells outside vessels
  - Intraparenchymal infiltrates/cohesive aggregates
  - Angioinvasive but not intraluminal

Lymphomatosis Cerebri

- Diffuse intraparenchymal, near single cell infiltration by lymphoma cells; not intravascular

Diffuse Subacute Encephalomyelitis and Nonspecific Chronic Inflammation

- Perivascular and intraparenchymal lymphocytes
- Diffuse gliosis and microglial nodules, some cases
- Largely T cells

Progressive Multifocal Leukoencephalopathy

- Macrophage infiltrate
- Intraparenchymal atypical cells with viral inclusions
- Immunoreactivity for SV40

Subacute Spinal Cord Infarction

- No brain involvement and nonprogressive

Jakob-Creutzfeldt Disease

- Predominantly cortical neuroimaging abnormality
- Spongiosis, cortex

DIAGNOSTIC CHECKLIST

Pathologic Interpretation Pearls

- Diagnosis often late, at either perimortem or postmortem
- Biopsies from affected sites critical in early recognition and intervention
- High index of suspicion and immunohistochemistry sometimes necessary to find intravascular tumor cells

SELECTED REFERENCES

1. Ponzoni M et al: Definition, diagnosis, and management of intravascular large B-cell lymphoma: proposals and perspectives from an international consensus meeting. J Clin Oncol. 25(21):3168-73, 2007
2. Gaul C et al: Intravascular lymphomatosis mimicking disseminated encephalomyelitis and encephalomyelopathy. Clin Neurol Neurosurg. 108(5):486-9, 2006
3. Ferreri AJ et al: Intravascular lymphoma: clinical presentation, natural history, management and prognostic factors in a series of 38 cases, with special emphasis on the 'cutaneous variant'. Br J Haematol. 127(2):173-83, 2004
4. Williams RL et al: Cerebral MR imaging in intravascular lymphomatosis. AJNR Am J Neuroradiol. 19(3):427-31, 1998

(Left) *Atypical lymphoid cells fill small leptomeningeal and intracortical vessels →. The cortical gliosis seen in the underlying parenchyma in this example ⇨ may not always be present.* **(Right)** *It may be difficult to distinguish intravascular tumor cells → from reactive, hypertrophic endothelial cells. Immunostaining for CD20 may be required for the diagnosis.*

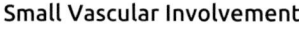

Leptomeningeal Vascular Involvement

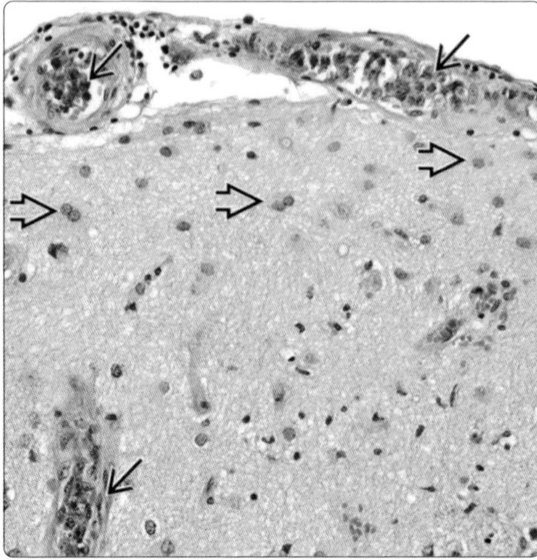

Tumor Cells or Reactive Endothelia?

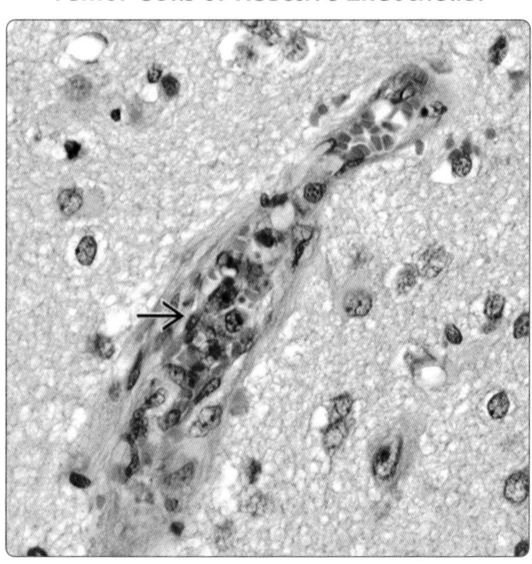

(Left) *Intravascular tumor cells may be overlooked when they are fewer, smaller, and less atypical than in the classic case. As here, the surrounding parenchyma is usually normal.* **(Right)** *Patently atypical cells fill the vessel →, while perivascular hemosiderin attests to earlier extravasation of erythrocytes. Fibrin thrombi and necrosis may also be seen around the vessels in addition to hemorrhage.*

Small Vascular Involvement

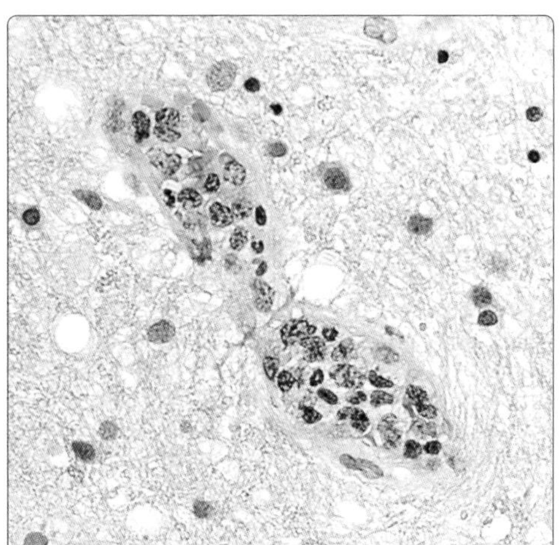

Overtly Malignant Cells

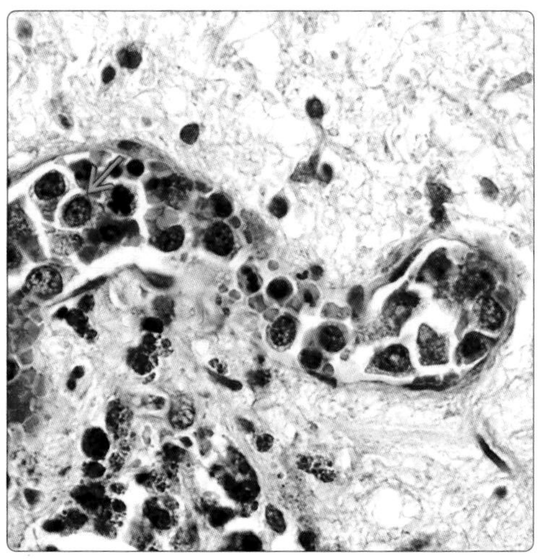

(Left) *Neoplastic cells → conform to the normal contours of the vessels rather than expanding and dilating them. Surrounding parenchyma and the neurons ⇨ often seem unaffected.* **(Right)** *Immunohistochemical staining with antibodies for CD20 makes it possible to identify 3, 2, or even 1 intravascular tumor cell →. Extravasated erythrocytes ⇨ surround the vessel. The diagnosis often requires demonstration of neoplastic tumor cells in more than 1 vessel.*

Tumor Cells Conform

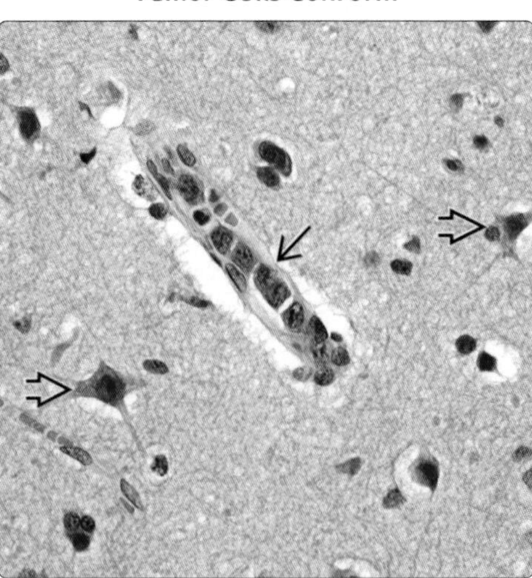

CD20 Positivity

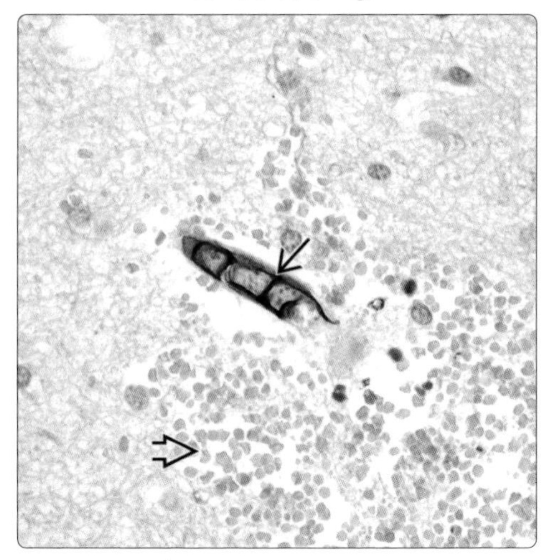

Malignant Cells in Distended Vessels

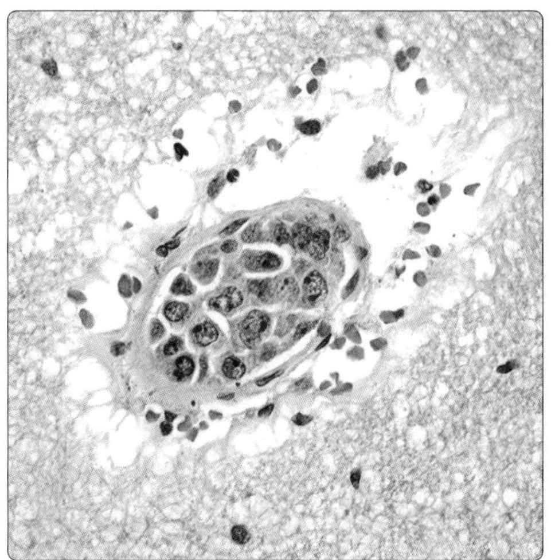

CD45 Positivity

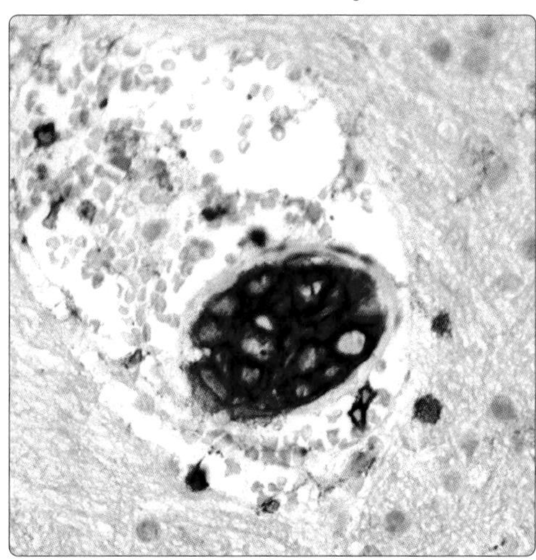

(Left) *Obviously malignant cells fill a small vessel, and, even though the tumor cells often conform to the vascular contours, some may be seen distended and give better clues for diagnosis.* **(Right)** *Immunostaining with the CD45 antibody highlights intraluminal tumor cells. This immunostain should be supplemented by CD20, which should also be positive in the tumor cells.*

CD20 Positivity

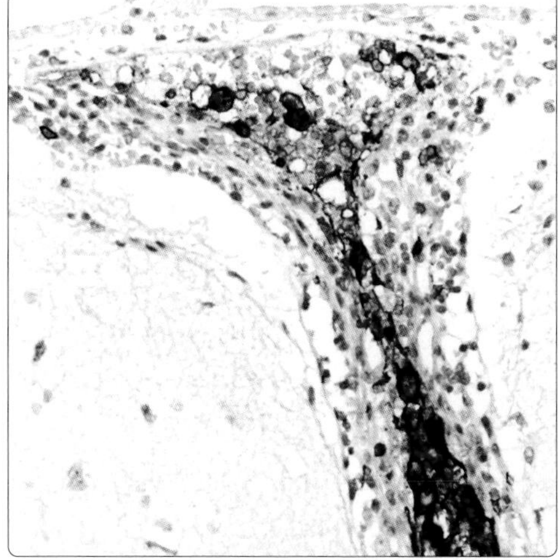

KI-67 Staining Can Be Helpful

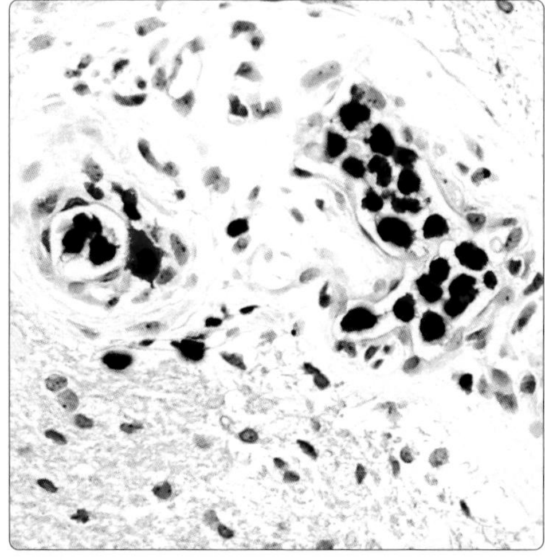

(Left) *In most patients with intravascular lymphomatosis, immunohistochemical stains highlight the CD20(+) tumor cells that obstruct a small leptomeningeal vessel.* **(Right)** *While nonspecific, the very high Ki-67 rate of intravascular lymphomatosis is comforting in the diagnosis of a malignancy, especially if based on only a few abnormal cells.*

Surrounding Ischemic/Reactive Changes

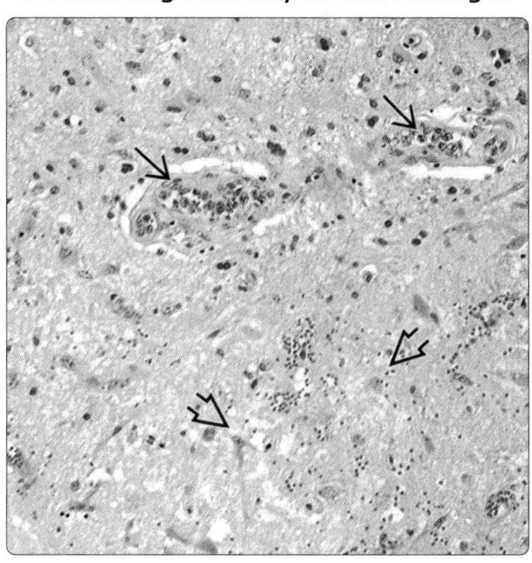

Intravascular Lymphoma in Muscle Biopsy

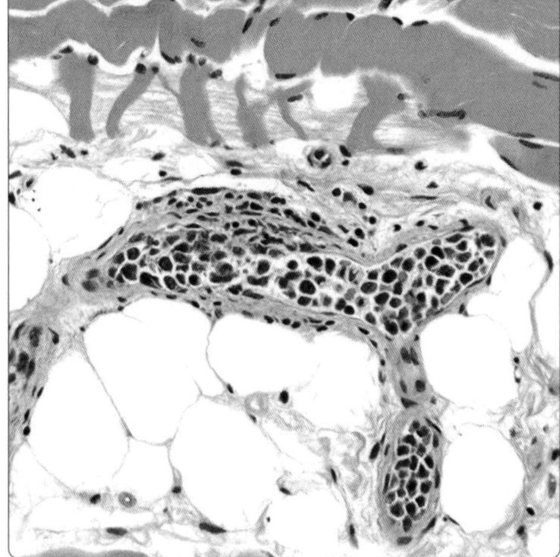

(Left) *Although surrounding parenchyma is usually unaffected, there can be ischemic damage in some cases ⇨. Tumor cells → could be overlooked easily in a section such as this.* **(Right)** *Occasionally, a fortuitous biopsy of skeletal muscle may obviate a more cumbersome brain biopsy and may reveal the diagnosis. Intravascular malignant cells stand out, even at low magnification. Skin is another site where biopsy may provide diagnosis.*

Lymphomatosis Cerebri

KEY FACTS

TERMINOLOGY

- Diffusely infiltrating primary central nervous system lymphoma without focal mass lesion

CLINICAL ISSUES

- Aggressive, often rapidly fatal

IMAGING

- Diffuse white matter hyperintensities on FLAIR and T2 images similar to leukoencephalopathy
- No discrete lesion or mass effect

MICROSCOPIC

- Diffuse infiltration by widely spaced, atypical individual neoplastic lymphocytes, usually predominantly in white matter
- Similar appearance to infiltrating glioma, especially anaplastic oligodendroglioma or gliomatosis cerebri
- No angiocentricity or angioinvasiveness

ANCILLARY TESTS

- CD20(+) and very high Ki-67 index

TOP DIFFERENTIAL DIAGNOSES

- Intravascular lymphomatosis
- Gliomatosis cerebri
- Anaplastic oligodendroglioma (paucicellular areas)
- Demyelinating disease
- Leukoencephalopathy

DIAGNOSTIC CHECKLIST

- Consider lymphomatosis cerebri when
  - Imaging features suggest leukoencephalopathy
  - There are diffusely infiltrating, round atypical cells
  - There is diffuse infiltrate with numerous Ki-67(+) cells
  - Suspected case of encephalitis shows scattered CD20 and Ki-67(+) atypical cells
  - There is progressively advancing FLAIR abnormality over time despite treatment

(Left) *FLAIR signal abnormality is typically extensive, bilateral, and largely in the white matter. Leukoencephalopathy is a common preoperative diagnosis.* **(Right)** *In contrast to classical primary central nervous system lymphoma, there is little or no contrast enhancement in lymphomatosis cerebri.*

Diffuse White Matter Abnormalities

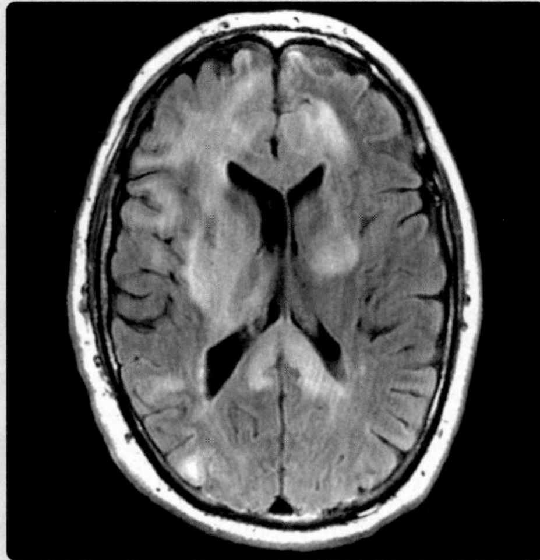

Little or No Contrast Enhancement

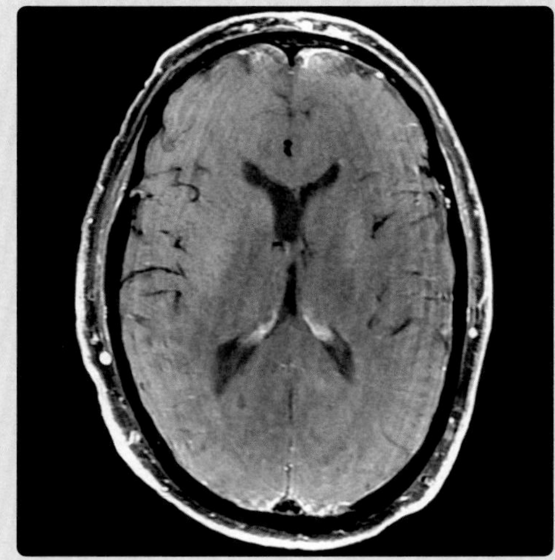

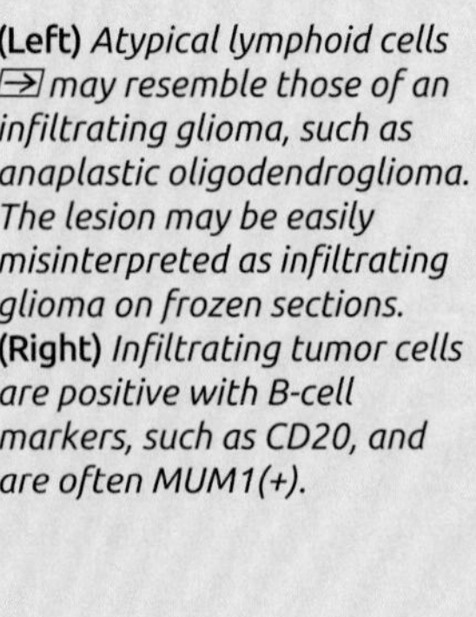

(Left) *Atypical lymphoid cells* ⇨ *may resemble those of an infiltrating glioma, such as anaplastic oligodendroglioma. The lesion may be easily misinterpreted as infiltrating glioma on frozen sections.* **(Right)** *Infiltrating tumor cells are positive with B-cell markers, such as CD20, and are often MUM1(+).*

Scattered Atypical Cells

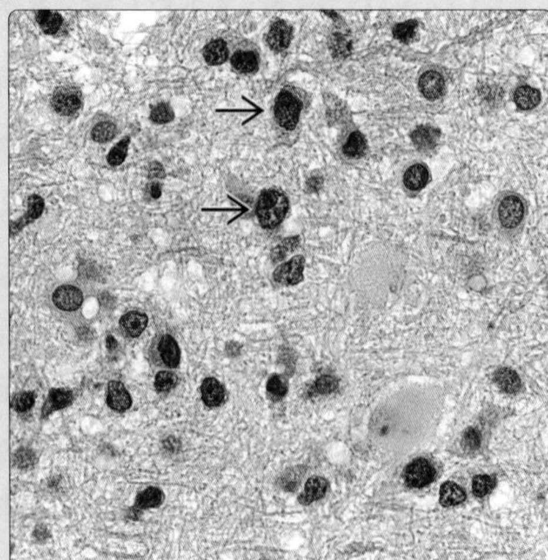

CD20 Positivity

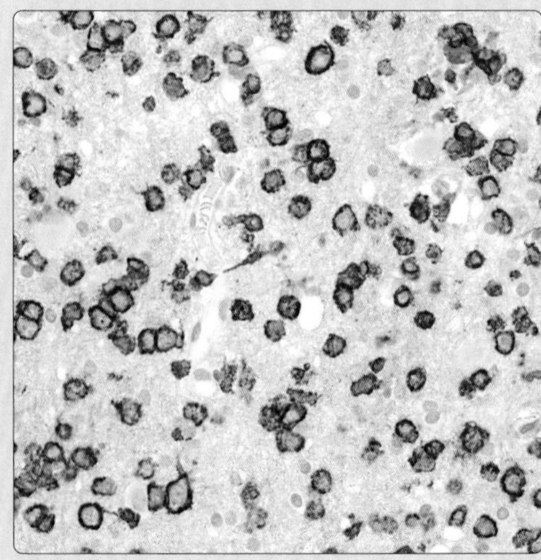

TERMINOLOGY

Definitions

- Diffusely infiltrating primary central nervous system lymphoma without focal mass lesion

CLINICAL ISSUES

Site

- Brain
- Spinal cord, rare

Presentation

- Rapidly progressive dementia
- Confusion and altered mental status
- Focal neurological deficits
- Gait disturbance
- Patients usually immunocompetent

Prognosis

- Aggressive, often rapidly fatal

IMAGING

MR Findings

- Diffuse white matter hyperintensities on FLAIR and T2 images similar to leukoencephalopathy
- No discrete lesion or mass effect
- Occasional, patchy contrast enhancement

MICROSCOPIC

Histologic Features

- Diffuse infiltration by individual, widely dispersed, cytologically atypical lymphocytes, usually predominantly in white matter
- Similar appearance to infiltrating glioma, especially anaplastic oligodendroglioma
- Variable numbers of perivascular and intraparenchymal small reactive lymphocytes
- No angiocentricity or angioinvasiveness
- No necrosis
- Reactive astrocytosis and microglial activation

ANCILLARY TESTS

Cytology

- Large, round cells with marked cytological atypia

Immunohistochemistry

- Almost always B-cell lymphoma; CD20(+)
- CD79-a(+)
- Variable numbers of CD3(+) reactive lymphocytes
- Very high Ki-67 index

DIFFERENTIAL DIAGNOSIS

Intravascular Lymphomatosis

- Tumor cells confined to vessel lumina

Gliomatosis Cerebri

- Small, usually elongated, individual infiltrating tumor cells
- Prominent gray matter involvement (usually)
- Perineuronal satellitosis common
- CD20(-), GFAP(+), Olig2(+)

Anaplastic Oligodendroglioma (Paucicellular Areas)

- Perineuronal satellitosis
- Higher cellularity overall
- Mass lesion and mass effect on MR
- Calcifications
- 1p/19q codeletion
- IDH-1(+), Olig2(+)
- CD20(-)

Demyelinating Disease

- Contrast enhancing (open ring) sign on neuroimaging, in acute and subacute phase
- More restricted to white matter
- Abundant macrophages
- Myelin loss with relative axonal sparing
- No cytologically atypical cells
- Small lymphocytes, mostly perivascular and CD3(+) T lymphocytes
- Multinucleated reactive astrocytes resembling mitotic cells (Creutzfeldt cells)

Leukoencephalopathy

- Few, if any, lymphoid cells
- No cytological atypia

Subcortical Ischemic Vascular Dementia

- Multiple distinct lesions in white matter and deep gray matter (basal ganglia and thalamus)
- Hyalinized small arteries with enlarged perivascular spaces
- Small perivascular lymphocytes only
- Lacunar infarcts
- Prominent microglial and astrocytic reaction
- Occasional small perivascular lymphocytic infiltrates
- No atypical lymphoma cells

DIAGNOSTIC CHECKLIST

Pathologic Interpretation Pearls

- Consider lymphomatosis cerebri when
  - Imaging features suggest leukoencephalopathy
  - Diffusely infiltrating, round, cytologically atypical cells
  - Diffuse, noncohesive cell infiltrates with numerous Ki-67(+) cells
  - Suspected cases of encephalitis with scattered CD20 and Ki-67(+) atypical cells
- Nondiagnostic stereotactic biopsy may necessitate additional tissue sampling

SELECTED REFERENCES

1. Izquierdo C et al: Lymphomatosis cerebri: a rare form of primary central nervous system lymphoma. Analysis of 7 cases and systematic review of the literature. Neuro Oncol. ePub, 2015
2. Pandit L et al: Lymhomatosis cerebri--a rare cause of leukoencephalopathy. J Neurol Sci. 293(1-2):122-4, 2010
3. Weaver JD et al: Lymphomatosis cerebri presenting as rapidly progressive dementia. Neurologist. 13(3):150-3, 2007
4. Rollins KE et al: Lymphomatosis cerebri as a cause of white matter dementia. Hum Pathol. 36(3):282-90, 2005
5. Bakshi R et al: Lymphomatosis cerebri presenting as a rapidly progressive dementia: clinical, neuroimaging and pathologic findings. Dement Geriatr Cogn Disord. 10(2):152-7, 1999

KEY FACTS

TERMINOLOGY

- Angiocentric and angioinvasive lymphoproliferative disorder associated with Epstein-Barr virus (EBV) infection

ETIOLOGY/PATHOGENESIS

- EBV-driven lymphoproliferative disease
- Most patients have underlying immunodeficiency

CLINICAL ISSUES

- Most common site of involvement is pulmonary followed by brain, kidney, and liver
- Lungs are often also involved in patients with CNS disease
- Aggressive disease with median survival often below 2 yr
- May progress to diffuse large B-cell lymphoma
- Regression, while exceptional, is possible

MICROSCOPIC

- Grade 1: Polymorphous lymphoid infiltrate without cytologically atypical cells
- Grade 2: Polymorphous lymphoid infiltrate with rare atypical cells
- Grade 3: Readily identifiable, numerous large, atypical EBV(+) B cells
- It is important to distinguish grade 3 lesions from grade 1 and 2 lesions

ANCILLARY TESTS

- Large cells CD20(+), EBV(+)
- Large cells variably CD30(+) and CD15(-)
- Small lymphocytes CD3(+)

TOP DIFFERENTIAL DIAGNOSES

- Dural-based mucosa-associated lymphoid tissue lymphoma
- Diffuse large B-cell lymphoma
- Extranodal NK-/T-cell lymphoma
- Infections, especially those associated with immunodeficiency

Coronal FLAIR Abnormalities

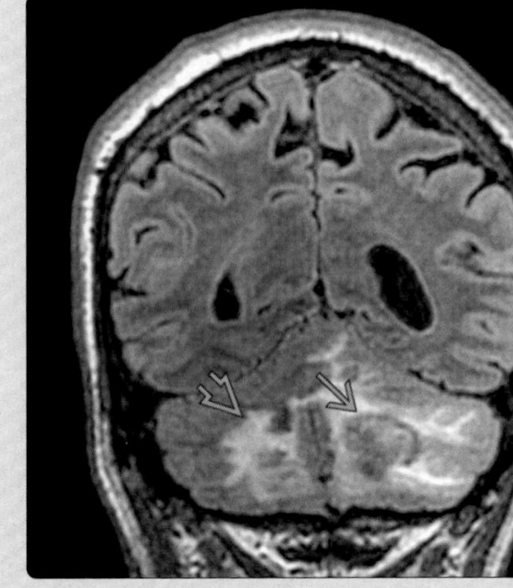

Granulomas and Mixed Lymphoid Infiltrate

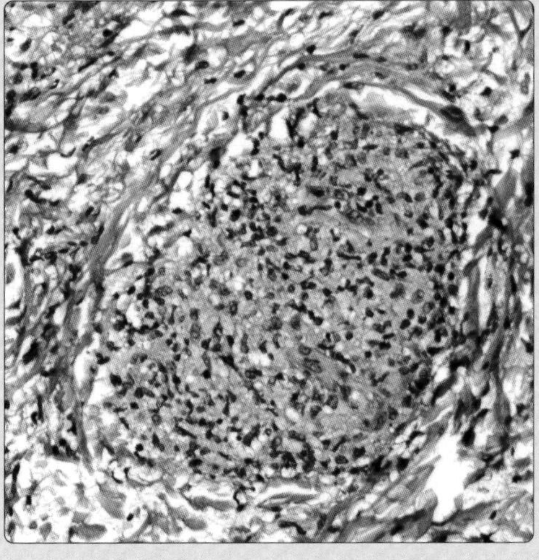

(Left) *Lymphomatoid granulomatosis can involve the cerebral or cerebellar parenchyma and is often multifocal. Coronal FLAIR image demonstrates the mass lesions ➡ and surrounding edema ➡.* **(Right)** *On initial examination, the lesions may appear indistinguishable from a granulomatous process. The number of large atypical cells is used to define the histological grade. In addition, angiocentric polymorphous destructive processes with varying amounts of lymphocytes and plasma cells are often present.*

Mixed Lymphoplasmacytic Background

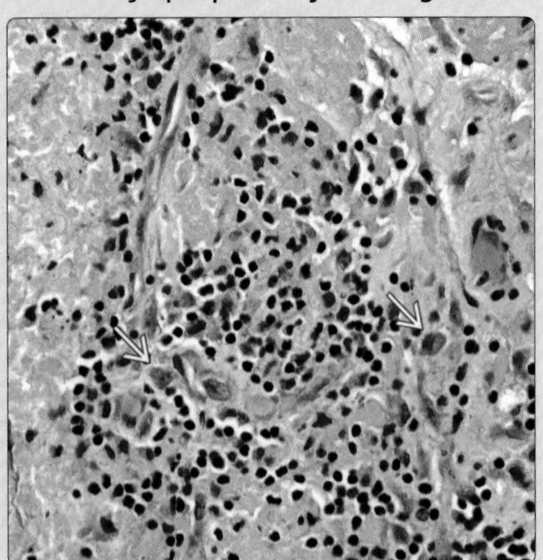

EBV Positivity on CISH

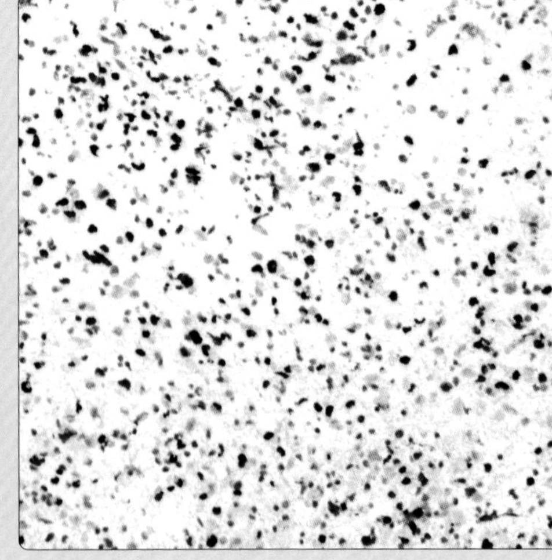

(Left) *Some lesions in the CNS may be associated with marked necrosis in addition to the mixed lymphoplasmacytic infiltrate. Atypical cells ➡ in small numbers are easy to overlook.* **(Right)** *Chromogenic in situ hybridization (CISH) for Epstein-Barr virus (EBV) often highlights viral particles within the lymphoid cell nuclei.*

TERMINOLOGY

Definitions

- Angiocentric and angioinvasive lymphoproliferative disorder associated with Epstein-Barr virus (EBV) infection

ETIOLOGY/PATHOGENESIS

Infectious Agents

- EBV-driven lymphoproliferative disease
- Most patients have underlying immunodeficiency

Predisposing Immunodeficiency Conditions

- Organ transplantation
- Wiskott-Aldrich syndrome
- HIV infection
- X-linked lymphoproliferative syndrome

CLINICAL ISSUES

Epidemiology

- Usually presents in adult life
- Male patients reportedly more commonly affected

Site

- About 1/4 of cases occur in CNS
- Lungs are most commonly involved, followed by brain, kidney, and liver
- Lungs are often also involved in patients with CNS disease
- Can involve orbit

Presentation

- Fever
- Arthralgias and myalgias
- Altered mental status
- Ataxia
- CNS involvement can be asymptomatic

Treatment

- Some cases may respond to aggressive chemotherapy with rituximab
- Low-grade lesions can respond to interferon-α

Prognosis

- Clinical aggressiveness related to proportion of large B cells
- High-grade (grade 3) lesions can behave like diffuse large B-cell lymphoma (DLBCL)
- Low-grade (grade 1 or 2) lesions can have long-term remission
- Rare cases may regress spontaneously

MICROSCOPIC

Histologic Features

- Angiocentric lymphoid infiltrate
- Predominantly lymphocytes with plasma cells and histiocytes
- Destruction of vascular walls, reminiscent of necrotizing arteritis
- Lymphocytic infiltration of vessel walls with necrosis
- Variable number of large atypical lymphocytes, some EBV(+)
- Multinucleated cells
- Uniform, large B-cell population without polymorphous background should be classified as DLBCL

Grading

- Grade 1: Polymorphous lymphoid infiltrate without cytologically atypical cells
- Grade 2: Polymorphous lymphoid infiltrate with rare atypical cells
- Grade 3: Numerous large, atypical EBV(+) B cells

ANCILLARY TESTS

Immunohistochemistry

- Large cells CD20(+), EBV(+)
- Large cells variably CD30(+) and CD15(-)
- Small lymphocytes CD3(+)

DIFFERENTIAL DIAGNOSIS

Dural-Based Mucosa-Associated Lymphoid Tissue Lymphoma

- Monomorphous, cytologically atypical B-cell neoplasm composed of small, less cytologically atypical lymphoma cells

Diffuse Large B-Cell Lymphoma

- Atypical large B cells without polymorphous background or necrosis
- EBV, mostly negative
- Some cases of lymphomatoid granulomatosis may progress to DLBCL

Extranodal NK-/T-Cell Lymphoma

- Angiodestructive and also associated with EBV

SELECTED REFERENCES

1. Gonzalez-Valcarcel J et al: Primary cerebral lymphomatoid granulomatosis as an immune reconstitution inflammatory syndrome in AIDS. J Neurol. 257(12):2106-8, 2010
2. Katzenstein AL et al: Lymphomatoid granulomatosis: insights gained over 4 decades. Am J Surg Pathol. 34(12):e35-48, 2010
3. Kobayashi Z et al: Differential diagnosis of CNS lymphomatoid granulomatosis. Neuropathology. 30(3):302; author reply 302-3, 2010
4. Araki F et al: Primary orbital lymphomatoid granulomatosis. Br J Ophthalmol. 93(4):554-6, 2009
5. Lucantoni C et al: Primary cerebral lymphomatoid granulomatosis: report of four cases and literature review. J Neurooncol. 94(2):235-42, 2009
6. Nishihara H et al: A case of central nervous system lymphomatoid granulomatosis; characteristics of PET imaging and pathological findings. J Neurooncol. 93(2):275-8, 2009
7. Takiyama A et al: CNS lymphomatoid granulomatosis with lymph node and bone marrow involvements. Erratum in: Neuropathology. 29(4):520, 2009
8. Kendi AT et al: A pediatric case of low-grade lymphomatoid granulomatosis presenting with a cerebellar mass. AJNR Am J Neuroradiol. 28(9):1803-5, 2007
9. Nishihara H et al: Immunohistochemical and gene rearrangement studies of central nervous system lymphomatoid granulomatosis. Neuropathology. 27(5):413-8, 2007
10. Sohn EH et al: Central nervous system lymphomatoid granulomatosis presenting with parkinsonism. J Clin Neurol. 3(2):108-11, 2007
11. Wyen C et al: Fatal cerebral lymphomatoid granulomatosis in an HIV-1-infected patient. J Infect. 54(3):e175-8, 2007
12. Carone DA et al: Progressive cerebral disease in lymphomatoid granulomatosis causes anterograde amnesia and neuropsychiatric disorder. J Neuroimaging. 16(2):163-6, 2006
13. Patsalides AD et al: Lymphomatoid granulomatosis: abnormalities of the brain at MR imaging. Radiology. 237(1):265-73, 2005
14. Mizuno T et al: A case of lymphomatoid granulomatosis/angiocentric immunoproliferative lesion with long clinical course and diffuse brain involvement. J Neurol Sci. 213(1-2):67-76, 2003

Primary Amyloidoma

KEY FACTS

TERMINOLOGY

- Localized mass of amyloid associated with clonal, lambda-restricted proliferation of plasma cells

ETIOLOGY/PATHOGENESIS

- Not associated with systemic disease
- Monoclonal B-cell disorder

CLINICAL ISSUES

- Adults: Brain parenchyma, deep white matter; ganglia, especially trigeminal
- Cure expected after gross total removal
- Residual mass may enlarge

IMAGING

- Marked contrast enhancement
- Hyperdense on CT
- Variable signal intensity on T1WI and T2WI
- Marked contrast enhancement
- Variable peritumoral edema
- Hyperdense

MICROSCOPIC

- Acellular, eosinophilic, homogeneous, ground-glass deposits

ANCILLARY TESTS

- AL-λ-amyloid (+)

TOP DIFFERENTIAL DIAGNOSES

- Amyloid angiopathy
- Extensively hyalinized or fibrous tumors
- Other tumefactive inflammatory lesions
- Schwannoma, ancient type
- Fibrous meningioma
- Calcifying pseudoneoplasm of neuraxis

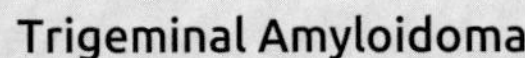

Trigeminal Amyloidoma

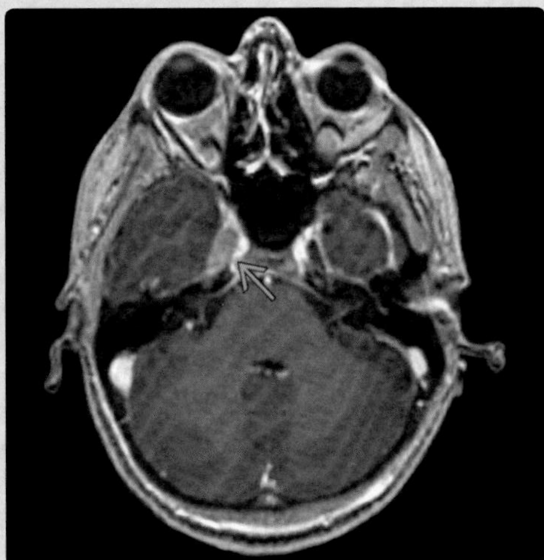

Hyalin Material With Inflammatory Cells

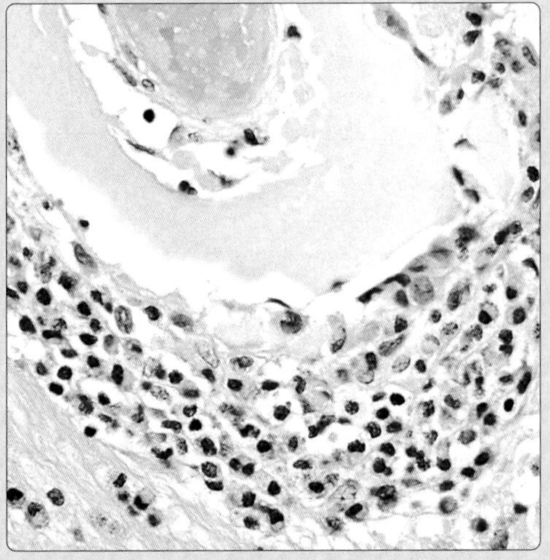

(Left) *An enhancing mass in a trigeminal ganglion that fills the cavernous sinus is one expression of this rare disease* ➡. **(Right)** *Amyloidoma is a homogeneous eosinophilic matrix surrounded by a lymphoplasmacytic infiltrate. While obvious here, the latter may be sparse.*

Ground-Glass Hyalin Substance

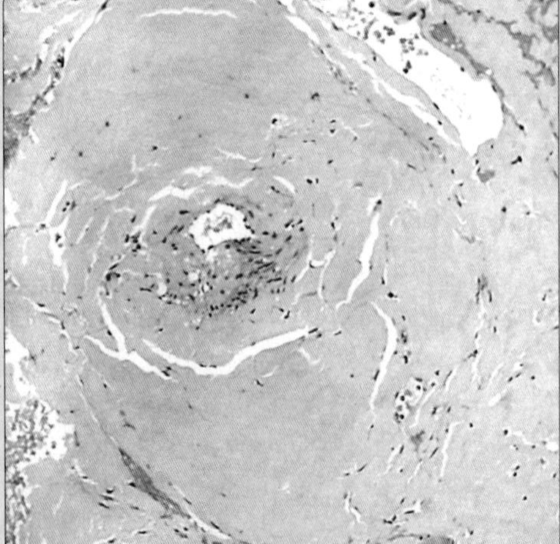

Congo Red Birefringence

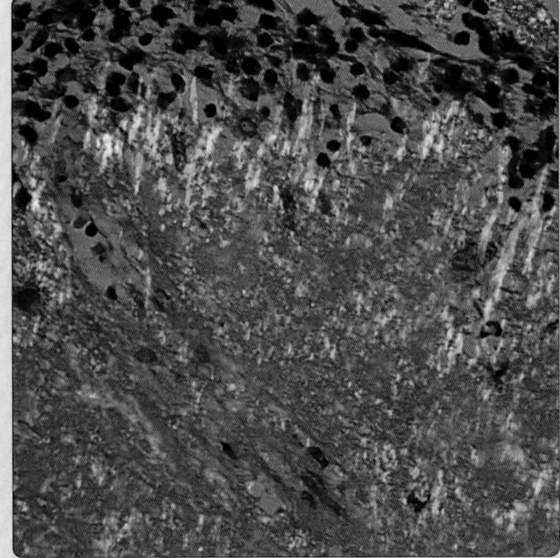

(Left) *Amyloid often appears as a homogeneous, eosinophilic substance and is often referred to as ground-glass, hyalin material.* **(Right)** *After Congo red staining, amyloid gives a characteristic apple green birefringence under polarized light.*

TERMINOLOGY

Definitions

- Localized mass of amyloid associated with clonal, lambda-restricted proliferation of plasma cells

ETIOLOGY/PATHOGENESIS

Primary

- Not associated with systemic disease
- Monoclonal B-cell disorder

CLINICAL ISSUES

Epidemiology

- Age
  - Adults

Site

- Brain parenchyma, especially deep white matter
- Ganglia, especially trigeminal, sometimes bilateral

Presentation

- Nonspecific
- Site dependent
- Spinal tumors with sensorimotor deficits or pain

Treatment

- Resection

Prognosis

- Cure expected after gross total removal
- Preexisting defects may remain
- Residual mass may enlarge

IMAGING

MR Findings

- Variable signal intensity on T1WI and T2WI
- Marked contrast enhancement
- Variable surrounding edema

CT Findings

- Hyperdense

MACROSCOPIC

General Features

- Tan or cream colored

MICROSCOPIC

Histologic Features

- Acellular, eosinophilic, homogeneous, ground-glass deposits, sometimes vascular
- Occasional surrounding lymphoplasmacytic infiltrates and macrophages
- Trapped preexisting structures, e.g., neurons, in trigeminal ganglion

ANCILLARY TESTS

Histochemistry

- Congo red (+) with apple green birefringence with polarized light
- Thioflavine-S (+)

Immunohistochemistry

- AL-λ-amyloid (+)

DIFFERENTIAL DIAGNOSIS

Amyloid Angiopathy

- Confined to vessels in subarachnoid space and cortex
- Mass lesion, hemorrhage, &/or infarct
- Aβ-amyloid

Extensively Hyalinized or Fibrous Tumors

- Schwannoma, ancient type
  - No amyloid
  - Tumor cells present
- Fibrous meningioma
  - Tumor cells present
  - No amyloid
- Calcifying pseudoneoplasm of neuraxis
  - Fibrillar rather than amorphous core
  - Superficial layer of EMA(+) cells
  - No amyloid
  - Calcifications

Demyelinating Disease

- Only rare association with amyloidoma
- Macrophage-rich lesion with loss of myelin
- Perivascular lymphocytes

Other Tumefactive Inflammatory Lesions

- More inflammation
- No amyloid

DIAGNOSTIC CHECKLIST

Pathologic Interpretation Pearls

- Consider possibility in face of acellular eosinophilic tissue

SELECTED REFERENCES

1. Foreid H et al: Intracerebral amyloidoma: case report and review of the literature. Clin Neuropathol. 29(4):217-22, 2010
2. Nossek E et al: The role of advanced MR methods in the diagnosis of cerebral amyloidoma. Amyloid. 16(2):94-8, 2009
3. Schröder R et al: Novel isolated cerebral ALlambda amyloid angiopathy with widespread subcortical distribution and leukoencephalopathy due to atypical monoclonal plasma cell proliferation, and terminal systemic gammopathy. J Neuropathol Exp Neurol. 68(3):286-99, 2009
4. Renard D et al: Primary brain amyloidoma: long-term follow-up. Arch Neurol. 65(7):979-80, 2008
5. Bookland MJ et al: Intracavernous trigeminal ganglion amyloidoma: case report. Neurosurgery. 60(3):E574; discussion E574, 2007
6. Fischer B et al: Cerebral AL lambda-amyloidoma: clinical and pathomorphological characteristics. Review of the literature and of a patient. Amyloid. 14(1):11-9, 2007
7. Laeng RH et al: Amyloidomas of the nervous system: a monoclonal B-cell disorder with monotypic amyloid light chain lambda amyloid production. Cancer. 82(2):362-74, 1998

Erdheim-Chester Disease

KEY FACTS

ETIOLOGY/PATHOGENESIS

- Inflammatory myeloid neoplasm
- More than 1/2 of cases have *BRAF V600E* mutation, indicating neoplastic origin

CLINICAL ISSUES

- 1/3 of patients present with neurological involvement
- Most frequent neurological symptoms: Ataxia, dysarthria, or hemiparesis
- Systemic findings most frequently include bone pain and diabetes insipidus
- Systemic organs need to be extensively sampled on autopsy cases
- Distinction from other non-Langerhans histiocytosis based on clinical features, location of CNS lesions, and presence of typical lesions elsewhere, especially bone

IMAGING

- Enhancing mass or infiltrative lesions, especially of posterior fossa, pituitary stalk, and meninges
- Best positive noninvasive diagnostic test is bone scintigraphy of long bones

ANCILLARY TESTS

- Cytologically normal aggregates of variably eosinophilic to foamy histiocytes
- CD68(+), CD1a(-), CD14(+), CD163(+) profile characteristic of most normal macrophages
- S100 IHC variable, may not differentiate well from other histiocytoses
- Unlike normal macrophages or many other histiocytoses, > 1/2 of all ECD cases have *BRAF V600E* mutation, BRAF VE1(+)
  - LCH and ECD share mutation

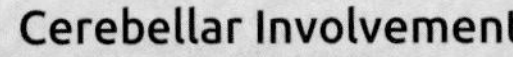

Cerebellar Involvement

Spinal Cord Involvement

(Left) *Increased FLAIR signal in the deep cerebellum around the dentate nuclei → is a classic radiological manifestation of Erdheim-Chester disease (ECD).* **(Right)** *T1-weighted MR with contrast in a patient with ECD shows several small, enhancing cervical cord lesions →. Enhancement is typical in ECD.*

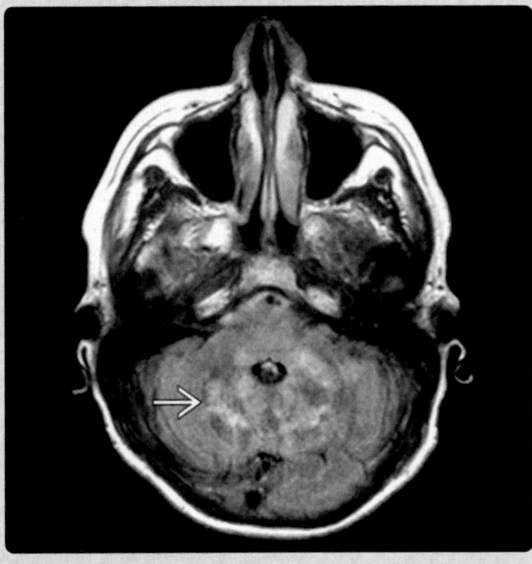

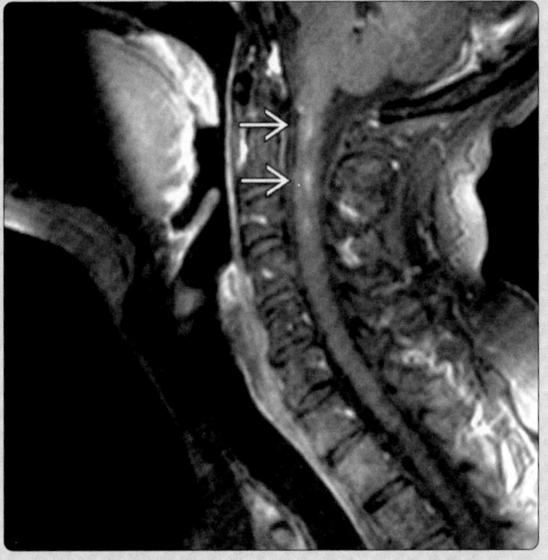

Erdheim-Chester Disease HIstiocytes

BRAF VE(+)

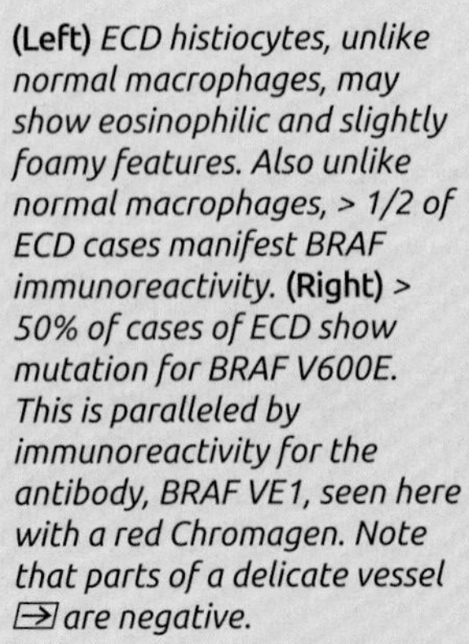

(Left) *ECD histiocytes, unlike normal macrophages, may show eosinophilic and slightly foamy features. Also unlike normal macrophages, > 1/2 of ECD cases manifest BRAF immunoreactivity.* **(Right)** *> 50% of cases of ECD show mutation for BRAF V600E. This is paralleled by immunoreactivity for the antibody, BRAF VE1, seen here with a red Chromagen. Note that parts of a delicate vessel → are negative.*

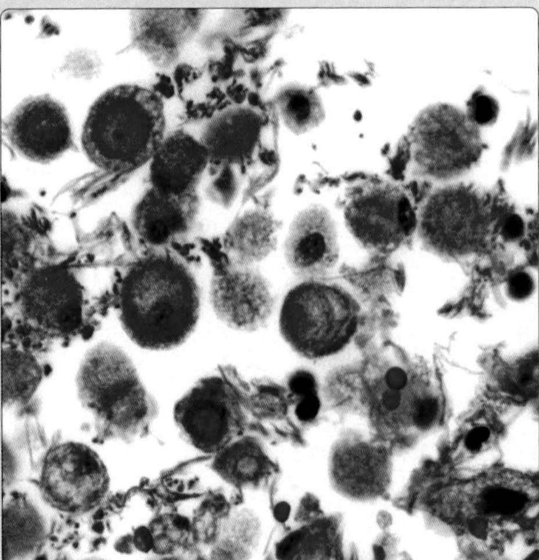

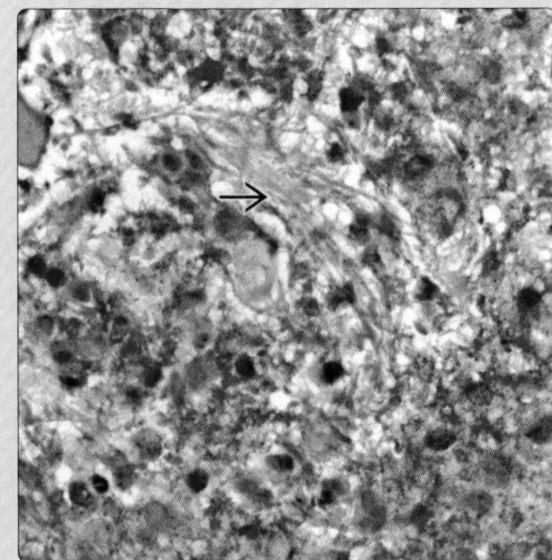

TERMINOLOGY

Abbreviations

- Erdheim-Chester disease (ECD)

Definitions

- Multiorgan, histiocytic disorder now known to be inflammatory myeloid neoplasm, with CD68(+), CD1a(-), S100(-), often BRAF VE1(+) foamy histiocytes
- Non-Langerhans histiocytosis

ETIOLOGY/PATHOGENESIS

Inflammatory Myeloid Neoplasm

- > 1/2 of all ECD patients carry the *BRAF V600E* mutation, indicating neoplastic (not reactive) disorder
- Other recurrent mutations of MAPK and PIK3 pathways (*NRAS, PIK3CA*)

CLINICAL ISSUES

Epidemiology

- Incidence
  - Uncommon
- Age
  - 30-65 years
    - Most patients with neurological symptoms

Site

- Posterior fossa, especially dentate nucleus of cerebellum, pons
- Pituitary stalk, dura, orbit, spinal cord
- Solitary CNS involvement exceedingly rare

Presentation

- Cerebellar and pyramidal syndromes most common neurological features (ataxia, gait disturbance, dysarthria, &/or hemiparesis)
- Seizures, headache, sensory disturbances
- Neuropsychiatric/cognitive difficulties
- Diabetes insipidus
- Non-CNS symptoms
  - Bone pain
  - Fever
  - Pulmonary: Septal distribution of inflammation with histiocytes
  - Cutaneous lesions, especially xanthelasma (yellowish, raised plaques near orbital areas)
  - Perinephric stranding, so-called "hairy kidney"
  - Exophthalmus
  - Periaortic infiltration
  - Pericardial thickening or effusion
  - Retroperitoneal fibrosis like infiltrate, including "coated aorta"

Treatment

- Interferon-α
- Radiotherapy generally ineffective for CNS lesions
- Chemotherapy (vinblastine, cyclophosphamide)
- Steroid efficacy inconsistent
- Targeted drug therapy now available
  - Treatment with BRAF &/or MEK inhibitors for *BRAF V600E* mutated cases can lead to dramatic response
  - Expression of PD-L1 immune checkpoint protein may suggest efficacy of immune check-point inhibitors

Prognosis

- 40-50% reported patients with neurological involvement succumb to disease
- Cardiovascular and neurological involvement worsen prognosis
- CNS involvement is strong negative prognostic factor and independent predictor of death
- Death may occur secondary to pulmonary fibrosis

Other Systemic Sites of Involvement

- Most CNS ECD patients have systemic organ involvement, including skeletal, retroperitoneal, orbital, cutaneous, cardiovascular, pulmonary systems
- Systemic involvement may only be diagnosed at autopsy and may be subtle

General Comments

- Distinction from other non-Langerhans histiocytosis based on clinical features
- Diagnosis depends on location of CNS lesions and presence of typical lesions elsewhere, especially bone
- Tissue or urine detection of *BRAF V600E* mutation can be helpful in diagnosis + treatment
- Absent Birbeck granules, negative with CD1a and langerin

IMAGING

General Features

- Infiltrative pattern with widespread parenchymal lesions or masses
- Pseudomeningioma or diffuse thickening of dura
- Combination of infiltrative and meningeal lesions

MR Findings

- Contrast enhancement
- Hyperintense lesions on T2WI

Bone Scan

- Bilateral, symmetric increased tracer uptake in metaphyses and diaphyses of long bones
- Osteosclerosis, especially of femur, tibia, usually bilateral involving metaphyses

MACROSCOPIC

General Features

- Mass lesions yellowish in proportion to number of foamy histiocytes
- Dural lesions simulate meningioma

MICROSCOPIC

Histologic Features

- Variable histological features even within same patient from site to site
  - Foamy versus eosinophilic cytoplasm to histiocytes
  - Variable Touton giant cells
  - Variable Rosenthal fibers
- Lymphoplasmacytic infiltrates

- May overshadow ECD histiocytes

ANCILLARY TESTS

Cytology

- Macrophages
  - Cytologically bland macrophages; nonreniform nuclei
  - Foamy (xanthomatous) cytoplasm but histiocytic appearance variable

Immunohistochemistry

- CD68(+), CD1a(-)
  - Variable for S100 protein, some have been IHC(+)
  - S100 immunostaining may be difficult to read in CNS histiocytes where background neuropil is strongly positive
- Also CD14(+) and CD163(+) = same immunoprofile as most macrophages
- > 1/2 of all ECD cases have *BRAF V600E* mutation, show BRAF VE1(+) IHC in histiocytes

Electron Microscopy

- No Birbeck granules

DIFFERENTIAL DIAGNOSIS

Langerhans Cell Histiocytosis

- CD1a(+)
- S100(+), but may not differentiate well from ECD
- Langerin (+)
- Birbeck granules on EM
- Most cases also have *BRAF V600E* mutation, BRAF VE(+) IHC
- Eosinophils and reniform nuclear features in histiocytes more typical of LCH than ECD
- More likely to involve craniofacial bones of skull than long bones of leg

Rosai-Dorfman Disease

- CD1a(-)
- S100(+)
- Cytoplasm less foamy
- Lack *BRAF V600E* mutation, negative BRAF VE1 IHC
- More likely to present as dural-based mass(es)

Normal Histiocytes

- Lack *BRAF V600E* mutation, negative BRAF VE1 IHC
- Share CD68(+), S100(-), CD1a(-) profile with ECD
- Usually cytoplasm more foamy than eosinophilic

DIAGNOSTIC CHECKLIST

Pathologic Interpretation Pearls

- *BRAF V600E* mutation does not distinguish between ECD and Langerhans cell histiocytosis
  - Other types of histiocytoses do not have *BRAF V600E* mutation
  - Thus, finding mutation may help distinguish ECD from other types of histiocytoses
- Absence of *BRAF V600E* mutation does not exclude diagnosis of ECD
  - Some cases have mutations in genes in MAPK and PIK3 pathways (*NRAS, PIK3CA*)
- Diagnosis can be difficult on histology alone due to variable features; finding *BRAF V600E* mutation may help
- Histiocytic appearance highly variable; may have fibrosis or polymorphous infiltrates obscuring histiocytes

SELECTED REFERENCES

1. Gatalica Z et al: Disseminated histiocytoses biomarkers beyond BRAFV600E: frequent expression of PD-L1. Oncotarget. ePub, 2015
2. Haroche J et al: The histiocytosis Erdheim-Chester disease is an inflammatory myeloid neoplasm. Expert Rev Clin Immunol. 1-10, 2015
3. Haroche J et al: Reproducible and sustained efficacy of targeted therapy with vemurafenib in patients with BRAF(V600E)-mutated Erdheim-Chester disease. J Clin Oncol. 33(5):411-8, 2015
4. Tzoulis C et al: Excellent response of intramedullary Erdheim-Chester disease to vemurafenib: a case report. BMC Res Notes. 8:171, 2015
5. Diamond EL et al: Consensus guidelines for the diagnosis and clinical management of Erdheim-Chester disease. Blood. 124(4):483-92, 2014
6. Emile JF et al: Recurrent RAS and PIK3CA mutations in Erdheim-Chester disease. Blood. 124(19):3016-9, 2014
7. Hervier B et al: Association of both Langerhans cell histiocytosis and Erdheim-Chester disease linked to the BRAFV600E mutation. Blood. 124(7):1119-26, 2014
8. Janku F et al: BRAF V600E mutations in urine and plasma cell-free DNA from patients with Erdheim-Chester disease. Oncotarget. 5(11):3607-10, 2014
9. Haroche J et al: High prevalence of BRAF V600E mutations in Erdheim-Chester disease but not in other non-Langerhans cell histiocytoses. Blood. 120(13):2700-3, 2012
10. Donaldson G et al: Erdheim-Chester disease mimicking multiple meningiomas. Br J Neurosurg. 24(3):296-7, 2010
11. Naqi R et al: Meningioma-like lesions in Erdheim Chester disease. Acta Neurochir (Wien). 152(9):1619-21, 2010
12. Suzuki HI et al: Erdheim-Chester disease: multisystem involvement and management with interferon-alpha. Leuk Res. 34(1):e21-4, 2010
13. Bianco F et al: Characteristic brain MRI appearance of Erdheim-Chester disease. Neurology. 73(24):2120-2, 2009
14. Gong L et al: Clonal status and clinicopathological feature of Erdheim-Chester disease. Pathol Res Pract. 205(9):601-7, 2009
15. Mills JA et al: Case records of the Massachusetts General Hospital. Case 25-2008. A 43-year-old man with fatigue and lesions in the pituitary and cerebellum. N Engl J Med. 359(7):736-47, 2008
16. Salsano E et al: Late-onset sporadic ataxia, pontine lesion, and retroperitoneal fibrosis: a case of Erdheim-Chester disease. Neurol Sci. 29(4):263-7, 2008
17. Shimada S et al: Intracranial lesion of Erdheim-Chester disease. Hum Pathol. 38(6):950-1, 2007
18. Vencio EF et al: Clonal cytogenetic abnormalities in Erdheim-Chester disease. Am J Surg Pathol. 31(2):319-21, 2007
19. Lachenal F et al: Neurological manifestations and neuroradiological presentation of Erdheim-Chester disease: report of 6 cases and systematic review of the literature. J Neurol. 253(10):1267-77, 2006
20. Veyssier-Belot C et al: Erdheim-Chester disease. Clinical and radiologic characteristics of 59 cases. Medicine (Baltimore). 75(3):157-69, 1996

Histiocytic Infiltrates Near Dentate Nuclei

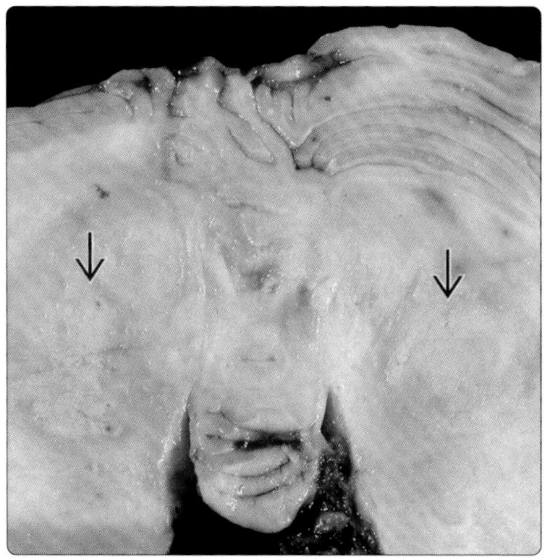

Dystrophic Mineralization

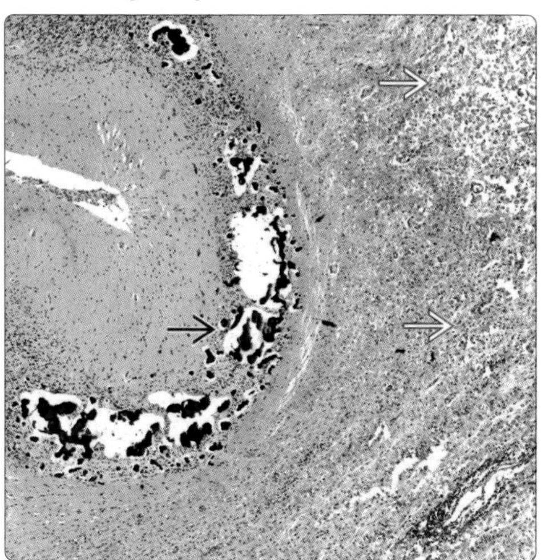

(Left) *Cerebellar dentate nuclei are classic loci for ECD ⇒. Note the bright yellow discoloration due to numerous foamy histiocytes.* **(Right)** *Low-power photomicrograph of the cerebellum in a patient with Erdheim-Chester disease shows sheets of macrophages within the white matter ➡ as well as dystrophic mineralization ⇒.*

Foamy Histiocytes

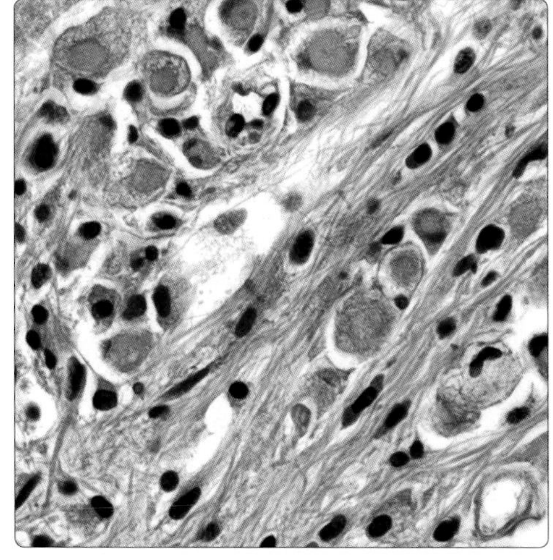

Rosenthal Fibers

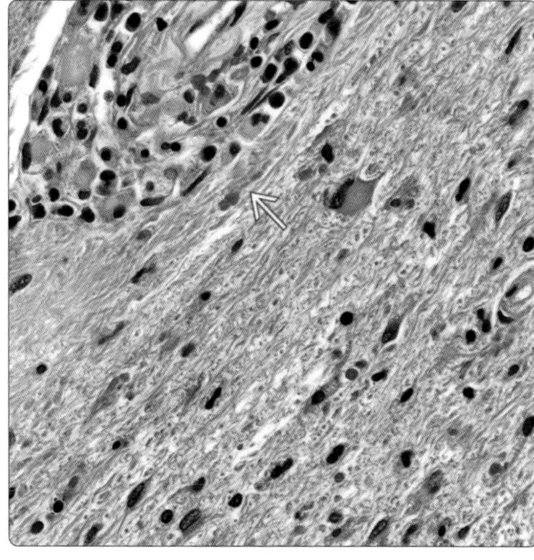

(Left) *The variably foamy histiocytes in Erdheim-Chester disease, seen here in a dentate nucleus, have cytologically normal round nuclei, unlike the grooved nuclei of Langerhans cell histiocytosis.* **(Right)** *Macrophages in ECD may be concentrated around blood vessels with Rosenthal fibers ➡ and intense gliosis in the parenchyma. Such areas are not diagnostic and cannot be distinguished from reactive processes. Intense surrounding piloid gliosis should not be misconstrued as glioma.*

Histiocytes

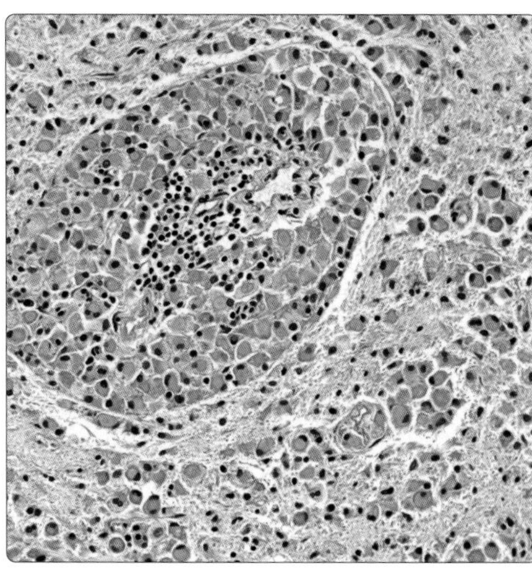

CD68(+) Histiocytes

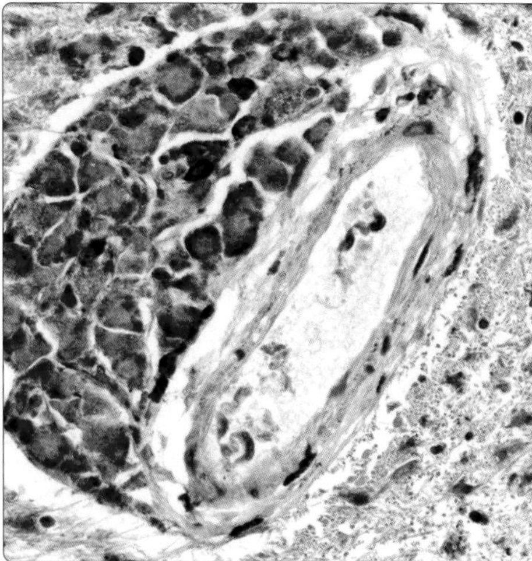

(Left) *Both perivascular and parenchymal regions may be affected. Individually, histiocytes are not unique or diagnostic of ECD. It is the distribution and systemic features that become definitive.* **(Right)** *Histiocytes in Erdheim-Chester disease are strongly immunoreactive for CD68. Since they are negative for CD1a and S100, they have the same immunoprofile as reactive macrophages in non-histiocytic disorders. Langerhans type of histiocytes are CD1a(+) and S100(+).*

Numerous Mononuclear Cells

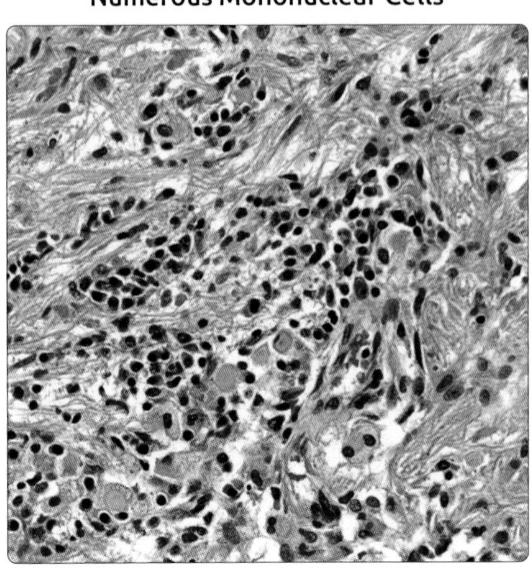

Nonspecific Collections of Histiocytes and Lymphocytes

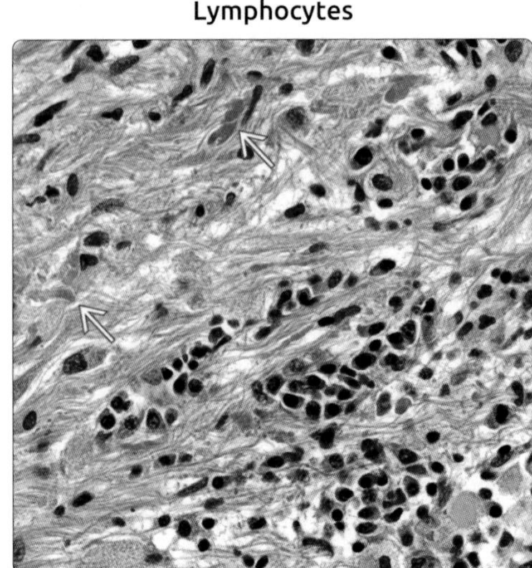

(Left) *Histiocytes and mononuclear cells intermingle in this section of hypothalamus, a frequent site of involvement in Erdheim-Chester disease.* **(Right)** *Small nests of histiocytes and lymphocytes are, in themselves, nonspecific and not diagnostic of ECD. Piloid gliosis with Rosenthal fibers ➡ surrounds this hypothalamic lesion.*

Pituitary Capsule Involvement

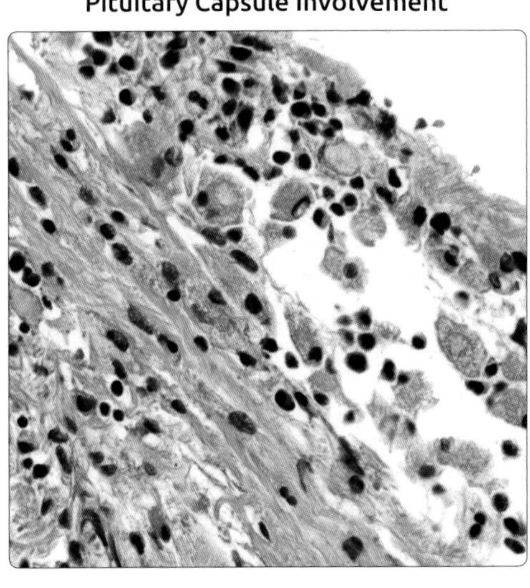

Bone Involvement

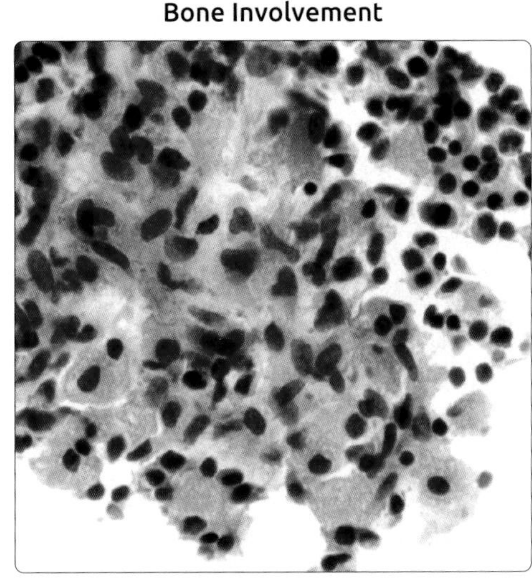

(Left) *Systemic organs are often involved in ECD, including the pituitary gland and hypothalamic stalk. Foamy histiocytes here cluster on the pituitary gland.* **(Right)** *Bone pain is the most frequent systemic symptom in ECD and bone scintigraphy is one of the best diagnostic tests. Pathological findings may be subtle, however, as illustrated by these nonspecific foamy histiocytes.*

Lung Involvement

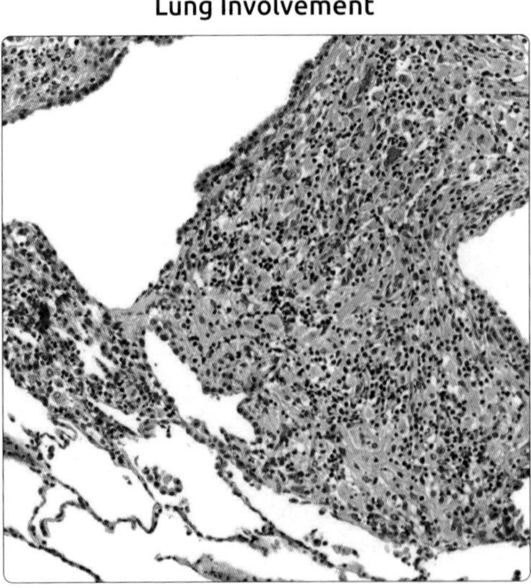

Testicular Involvement

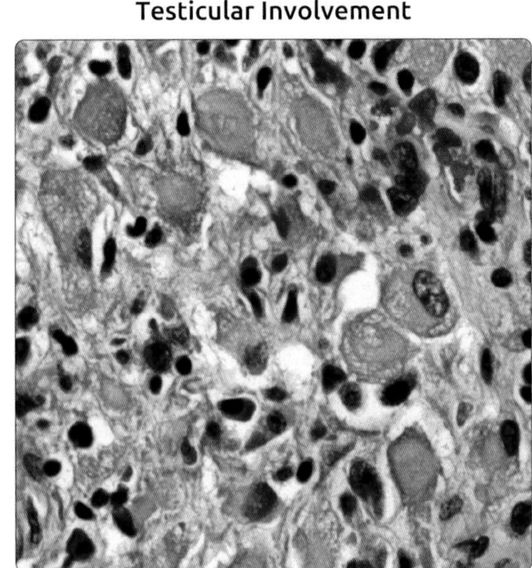

(Left) *The lung, a frequent site of systemic involvement in ECD, has a nodular interstitial infiltrate, as seen here.* **(Right)** *This cluster of histiocytes in a testicular lesion was tentatively interpreted as a sarcoid granuloma until examination of the brain revealed ECD. The foamy cells are more consistent with conventional histiocytes than epithelioid cells.*

Pontine Involvement

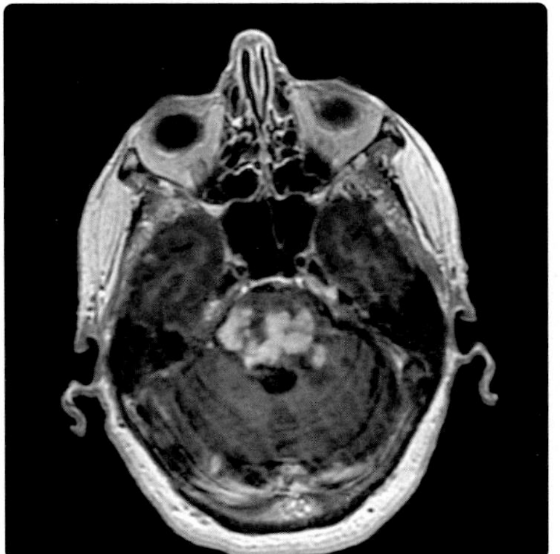

Posterior Fossa Predilection

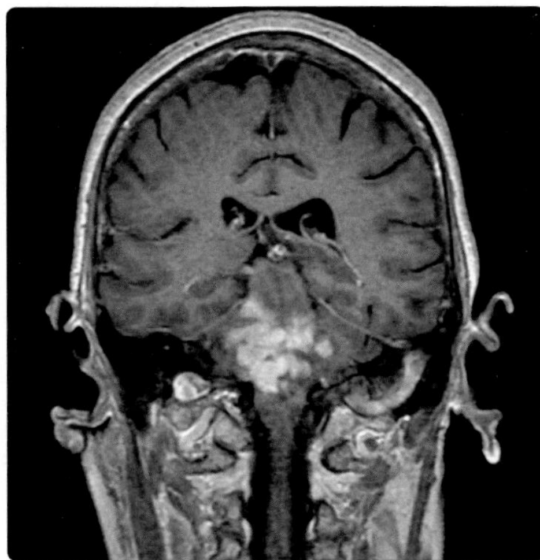

(Left) *ECD has a predilection for the posterior fossa for unexplained reasons. In this patient, the extreme nodularity of the pontine lesions simulates neoplasm.* **(Right)** *This patient was not suspected to have ECD until biopsy, underscoring the fact that ECD is a difficult diagnosis to make and biopsy may be required for confirmation.*

Polymorphous Infiltrate

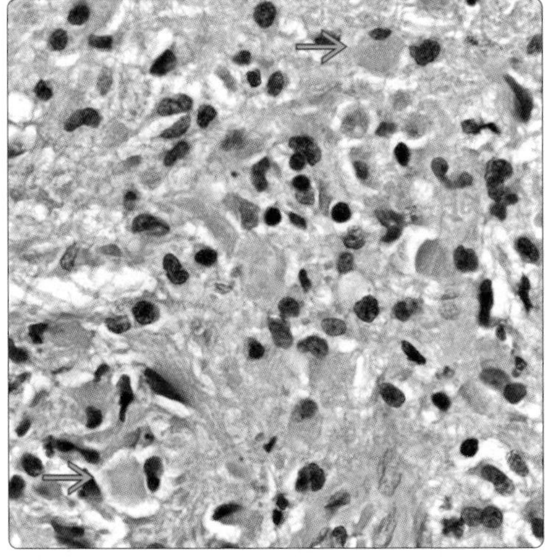

Most Erdheim-Chester BRAF VE1(+)

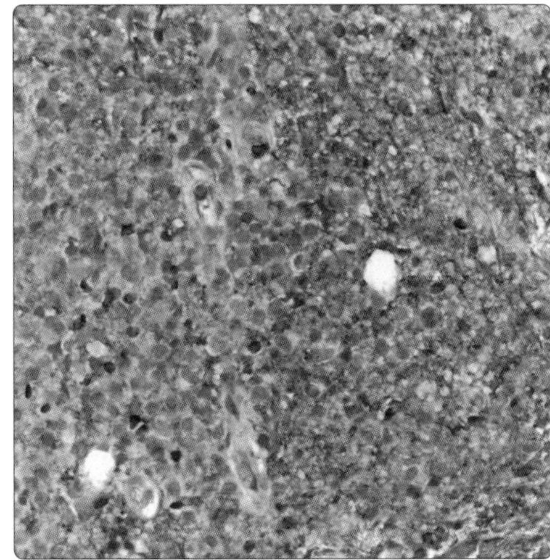

(Left) *This nonspecific polymorphous infiltrate overshadows the few histiocytes in the picture ➙.* **(Right)** *The finding of BRAF VE1 immunoreactivity as seen in this image provides diagnostic confidence in the correct clinical setting. Note that BRAF VE1 IHC(+) is shared by Langerhans cell histiocytosis but not by collections of normal macrophages.*

CD3(+) T Cells

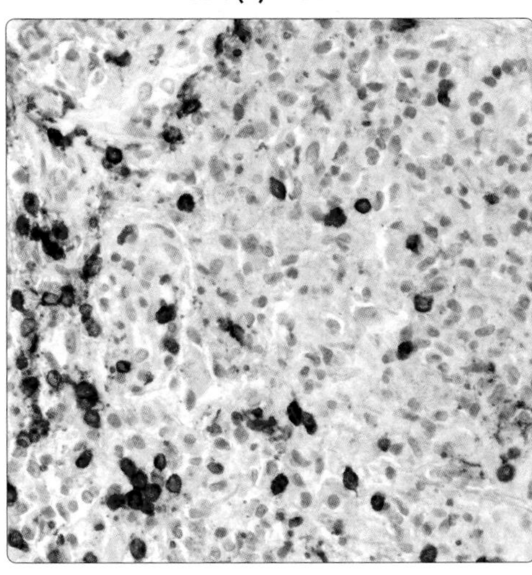

CD68(+)

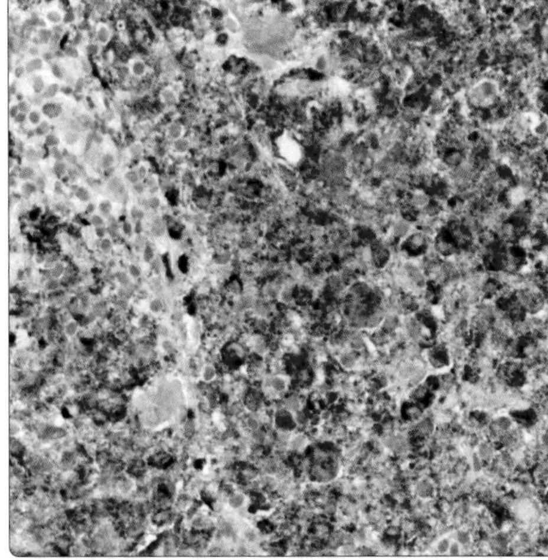

(Left) *Lymphocytes and plasma cells, as well as adjacent reactive astrocytes, can be seen in CNS collections of ECD histiocytes. These lymphocytes lack cytological atypia but can add to the misinterpretation of diffuse large cell B-cell lymphoma on H&E. ECD is of course immunonegative for CD20 or other B-cell markers.* **(Right)** *ECD histiocytes share CD68 immunoreactivity with normal macrophages, which can be seen in many CNS processes, including infarcts and demyelinating conditions.*

Langerhans Cell Histiocytosis

KEY FACTS

TERMINOLOGY

- Clonal neoplastic proliferation of Langerhans-type cells
- *BRAF V600E* mutation, BRAF VE1 IHC(+) > 50% of cases

CLINICAL ISSUES

- Solitary, lytic bone lesion, with scalp mass with lesions of vault
- Diabetes insipidus with hypothalamic involvement
- Most common in children or young adults
- Excellent prognosis for unifocal disease

IMAGING

- Discrete punched-out lytic lesion in bone that erodes cortex

MICROSCOPIC

- Langerhans cells
  - Grooved, lobulated, and clefted nuclei
  - Minimal nuclear atypia
  - Variable number of eosinophils and plasma cells, small lymphocytes, and neutrophils
- Neurodegenerative changes without Langerhans cells
  - e.g., in deep cerebellum &/or brainstem

ANCILLARY TESTS

- Langerhans cells
  - CD1a(+)
  - Langerin (+) (CD207)
  - S100 protein (+)
  - BRAF VE1(+)
- Intracytoplasmic Birbeck granules
  - 200-400 nm long
  - Racket shape with zipper-like center

(Left) *In the skull, Langerhans cell histiocytosis typically presents as a sharply defined lytic focus without sclerotic borders* ➔. **(Right)** *Nuclear grooves and clefts* ➔ *help distinguish Langerhans cells from generic histiocytes.*

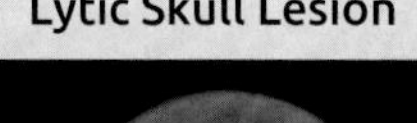

Lytic Skull Lesion

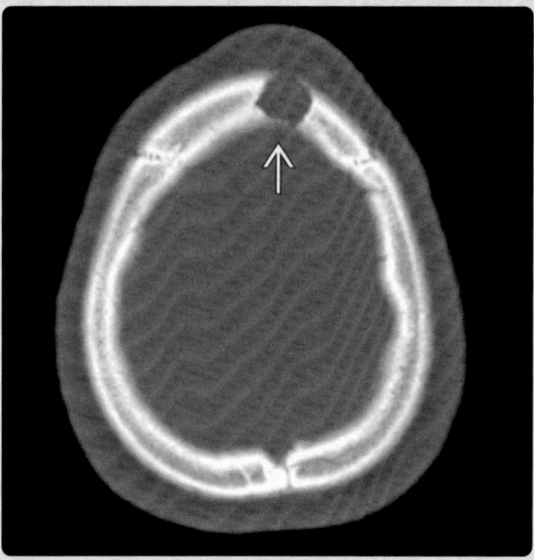

Langerhans Cells, Nuclear Grooves

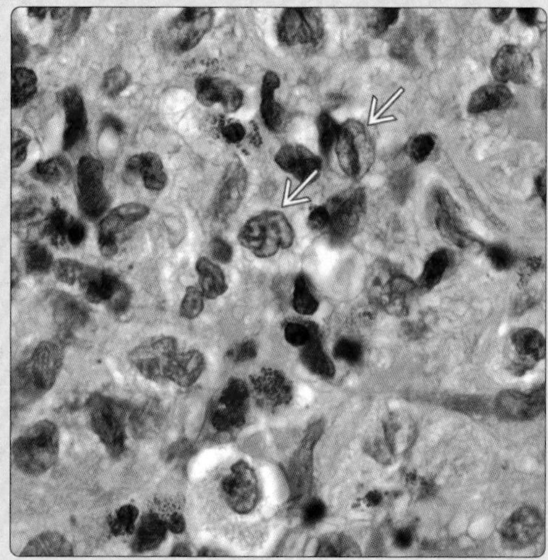

(Left) *Eosinophils admixed with macrophages suggest the possibility of Langerhans cell histiocytosis, especially with the cytological features of the histiocytes, as seen here, including nuclear grooves* ➔. **(Right)** *Most cases of Langerhans cell histiocytosis are now recognized to have BRAF V600E mutations, with BRAF VE1 immunopositivity, as seen in the histiocytes of this case (red chromogen). Presence of BRAF mutation now allows for targeted therapy with vemurafenib.*

Eosinophils

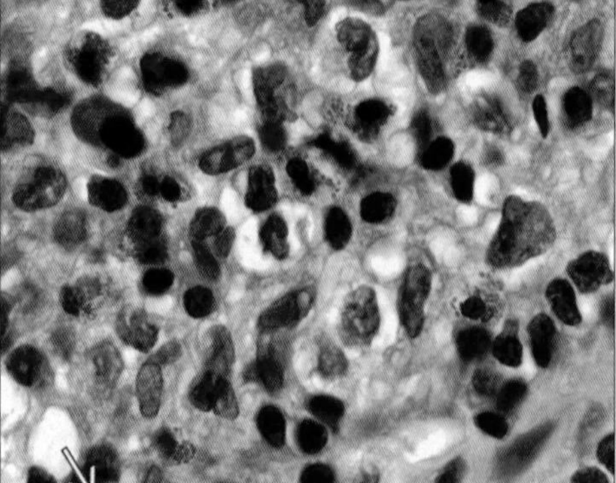

BRAF(+)

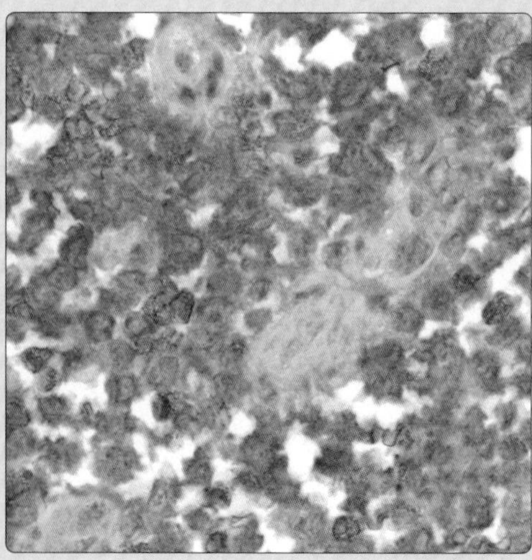

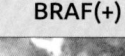

TERMINOLOGY

Abbreviations

- Langerhans cell histiocytosis (LCH)

Definitions

- Clonal neoplastic proliferation of Langerhans cells
- Most have either *BRAF V600E* or other extracellular signal-related (ERK) pathway mutations (*MAP2K1* and *MAP3K1*); mutations mutually exclusive

CLINICAL ISSUES

Epidemiology

- Age
  - Most common in children or young adults

Site

- Bone
  - LCH more likely to involve craniofacial bones, especially skull, also pelvis, proximal bones, scapula
  - Erdheim-Chester disease typically affects femur and tibia, not craniofacial bones
  - Bone lesions in Rosai-Dorfman disease are reported but uncharacteristic
- Brain
  - Hypothalamus or pituitary, especially infundibulum
  - Rarely parenchyma or other CNS sites
    - Langerhans cell proliferation
  - Cerebellar or brainstem lesions
  - Noninfiltrative neurodegeneration
- Systemic organ involvement
  - Uncommon but portends high-risk disease

Presentation

- Solitary, lytic bone lesion, scalp mass
- Diabetes insipidus with hypothalamic involvement
  - Unusual for any other sellar and parasellar lesions except germinoma
- May be subacute, several-year course before surgery
- Association with T-cell lymphoblastic leukemia (rare)
- Back pain with vertebral lesion

Treatment

- Drugs
  - Systemic chemotherapy after new onset of diabetes insipidus
  - Targeted therapy for *BRAF V600E* mutated cases (vemurafenib)

Prognosis

- Excellent prognosis for unifocal disease
- Multifocal disease and bone marrow, liver, lung involvement associated with poorer outcome
- Chronic or prolonged disease associated with increased CNS problems

IMAGING

Radiographic Findings

- Discrete punched-out lytic lesion in bone, which erodes cortex
- Enhancing suprasellar mass
  - Smaller lesions often confined to infundibulum
  - Loss of bright spot (i.e., loss of normal hyperintense signal of posterior pituitary on T1WI)
- Lytic lesion of vertebra(e)
- Hyperintense signal abnormality on FLAIR images, corresponding to nongranulomatous lesions

MACROSCOPIC

General Features

- Yellow in proportion to lipid content
- Osteolytic

MICROSCOPIC

Histologic Features

- Langerhans cells
  - Grooved, lobulated, and clefted nuclei
  - Minimal nuclear atypia
  - Variable numbers of histiocytic cells
    - Extensive in some cases but difficult to find in others
- Eosinophils and plasma cells, small lymphocytes, and neutrophils
- Multinucleated histiocytes
- Xanthoma cells
- Neurodegenerative changes, e.g., in deep cerebellum &/or brainstem
  - No Langerhans cells
  - Lymphocytes
  - Activated microglia
  - Gliosis

ANCILLARY TESTS

Immunohistochemistry

- Langerhans cells
  - CD1a, langerin (CD207), and S100 protein (+)
  - Now recognized to be *BRAF V600E* mutated tumor, with > 50% of cases showing BRAF VE1 IHC(+)

Electron Microscopy

- Intracytoplasmic Birbeck granules
  - 200-400 nm long, racket shape with zipper-like center

Cytology

- Langerhans cells with distinctive grooved or clefted nuclei
- Eosinophils

DIFFERENTIAL DIAGNOSIS

Germinoma (Suprasellar)

- Large tumor cells, CD117(+) and OCT4(+)
- Granulomatous inflammation in some cases

Lymphocytic Hypophysitis

- Usually older patients
- Often associated with pregnancy
- Epicenter on adenohypophysis in most cases
- Intraacinar lymphocytes
- No Langerhans cells

Malignant Lymphoma

- Atypia

- Appropriate immunohistochemical markers

Rosai-Dorfman Disease

- Dural-based mass(es)
- Large, pale S100(+), CD1a(-) histiocytes with emperipolesis (engulfment of lymphocytes)
- Usually BRAF VE1 IHC(-)
- Bone involvement reported but uncharacteristic

Erdheim Chester Disease

- No Langerhans cells
- Histiocytes are CD1a(-), langerin (-)
- Also often BRAF VE1 IHC(+)
- All histiocytic disorders are CD68(+), CD163(+), but Erdheim-Chester disease S100(-) or weak
- More likely to have Touton giant cells than Langerhans cell histiocytosis
- Small percentage of cases show overlap features between ECD and LCH

Nonspecific Chronic Inflammation (Inflammatory Pseudotumor)

- No Langerhans cells

Differences Amongst Histiocytoses, By Consensus Criteria

- Sites of bony involvement
  - LCH: More likely to affect craniofacial bones
  - ECD: More likely to affect femurs, tibia
  - Rosai-Dorfman: Bone involvement reported but uncharacteristic
- Skin involvement
  - LCH: Scaly erythematous patches
  - ECD: Xanthelasma
  - Rosai-Dorfman: Firm, indurated papules
- Lymph nodes
  - LCH: Uncommon but constitutes high-risk disease
  - ECD: Reported but uncharacteristic
  - Rosai-Dorfman: Cervical lymphadenopathy
- Lungs
  - LCH: Nodular and cystic changes in upper and middle lobes
  - ECD: Interlobular septal thickening, ground-glass or centrilobular opacities
  - Rosai-Dorfman: Reported but uncharacteristic
- Heart
  - LCH and Rosai-Dorfman: Reported, but uncharacteristic
  - ECD: Pericardial effusion, myocardial infiltration, periaortic sheathing (coated aorta)
- Retroperitoneum
  - LCH and Rosai-Dorfman: Reported but uncharacteristic
  - ECD: Perinephric infiltration (hairy kidney)
- CNS
  - Rosai-Dorfman: Usually dural-based masses
  - LCH and ECD: Cerebellar or brainstem lesions, dural-based lesions, brain parenchymal lesions

DIAGNOSTIC CHECKLIST

Pathologic Interpretation Pearls

- Langerhans cells may be difficult to find in small specimens from hypothalamus/infundibulum

SELECTED REFERENCES

1. Demellawy DE et al: Langerhans cell histiocytosis: a comprehensive review. Pathology. 47(4):294-301, 2015
2. Gatalica Z et al: Disseminated histiocytoses biomarkers beyond BRAFV600E: frequent expression of PD-L1. Oncotarget. ePub, 2015
3. Haroche J et al: Vemurafenib as first line therapy in BRAF-mutated Langerhans cell histiocytosis. J Am Acad Dermatol. 73(1):e29-30, 2015
4. Henderson AH et al: A case of bilateral sensorineural hearing loss from Langerhans cell histiocytosis. BMJ Case Rep. 2015, 2015
5. Hyman DM et al: Vemurafenib in Multiple Nonmelanoma Cancers with BRAF V600 Mutations. N Engl J Med. 373(8):726-36, 2015
6. Nahm JH et al: Squash smear cytology of Langerhans cell histiocytosis. Int J Clin Exp Pathol. 8(7):7998-8007, 2015
7. Nelson DS et al: MAP2K1 and MAP3K1 mutations in Langerhans cell histiocytosis. Genes Chromosomes Cancer. 54(6):361-8, 2015
8. Brown NA et al: High prevalence of somatic MAP2K1 mutations in BRAF V600E-negative Langerhans cell histiocytosis. Blood. 124(10):1655-8, 2014
9. Chakraborty R et al: Mutually exclusive recurrent somatic mutations in MAP2K1 and BRAF support a central role for ERK activation in LCH pathogenesis. Blood. 124(19):3007-15, 2014
10. Diamond EL et al: Consensus guidelines for the diagnosis and clinical management of Erdheim-Chester disease. Blood. 124(4):483-92, 2014
11. Laurencikas E et al: Incidence and pattern of radiological central nervous system Langerhans cell histiocytosis in children: a population based study. Pediatr Blood Cancer. 56(2):250-7, 2011
12. Perry VH: Central nervous system involvement in Langerhans cell histiocytosis: the importance of long term follow-up. Pediatr Blood Cancer. 56(2):175-6, 2011
13. Grois N et al: Central nervous system disease in Langerhans cell histiocytosis. J Pediatr. 156(6):873-81, 881, 2010
14. Imashuku S et al: Langerhans cell histiocytosis with multifocal bone lesions: comparative clinical features between single and multi-systems. Int J Hematol. 90(4):506-12, 2009
15. D'Ambrosio N et al: Craniofacial and intracranial manifestations of langerhans cell histiocytosis: report of findings in 100 patients. AJR Am J Roentgenol. 191(2):589-97, 2008
16. Davidson L et al: Craniospinal Langerhans cell histiocytosis in children: 30 years' experience at a single institution. J Neurosurg Pediatr. 1(3):187-95, 2008
17. Grois N et al: Neuropathology of CNS disease in Langerhans cell histiocytosis. Brain. 128(Pt 4):829-38, 2005
18. Modan-Moses D et al: Hypopituitarism in langerhans cell histiocytosis: seven cases and literature review. J Endocrinol Invest. 24(8):612-7, 2001

Infundibular Involvement

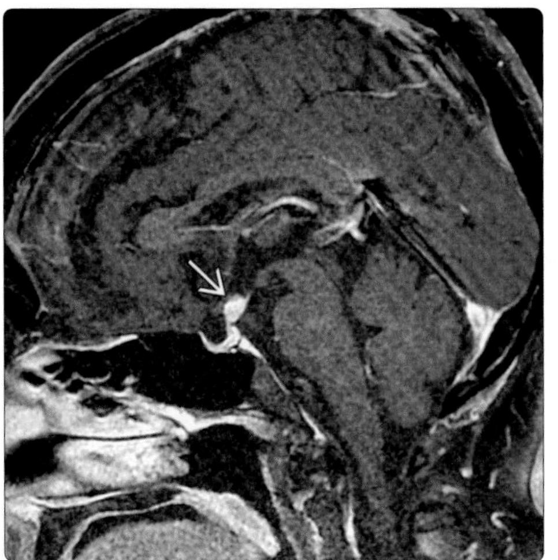

Hypercellular Mass With Eosinophils

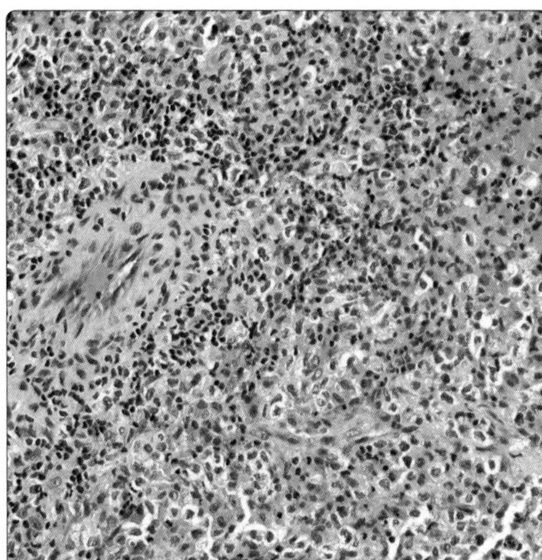

(Left) *Intracranial LCH often affects the infundibulum ➡ with early development of diabetes insipidus. Germinoma is another lymphocyte-rich lesion that frequents this same region in the young and should be considered in the differential diagnosis.* **(Right)** *A cellular mass of pale cells with scattered eosinophils is highly suspicious for LCH.*

Sheets of Monomorphous Cells

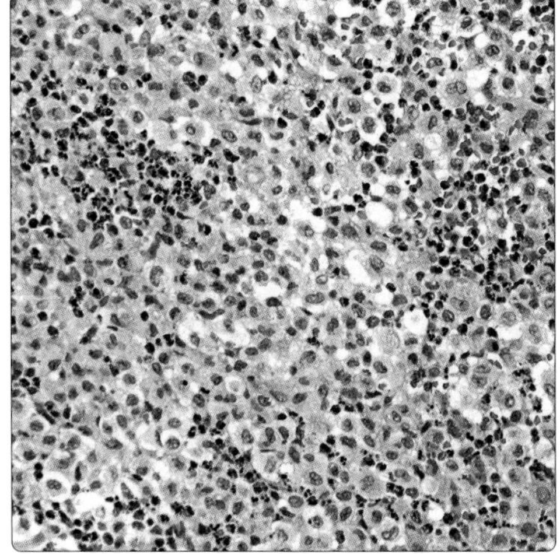

Profuse Eosinophils

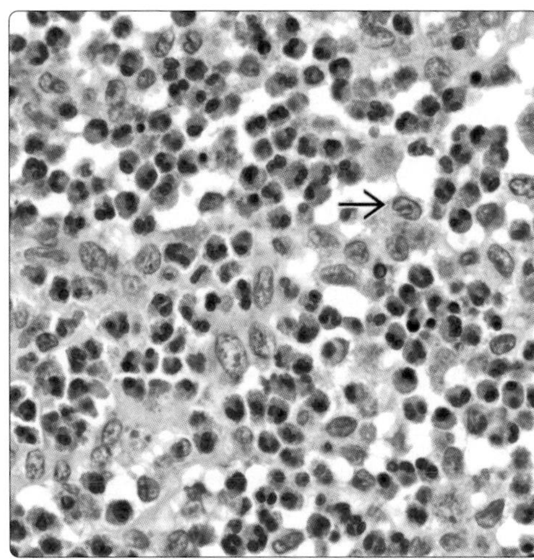

(Left) *Sheets of monomorphous cells suggest LCH but in themselves do not rule out other entities. The presence of a large number of eosinophils, however, makes LCH a prime contender at low magnification.* **(Right)** *Profuse numbers of eosinophils can be seen in some cases of Langerhans cell histiocytosis, and these may overshadow the histiocytes with grooved nuclei ➡.*

Largely Composed of Pale Histiocytes

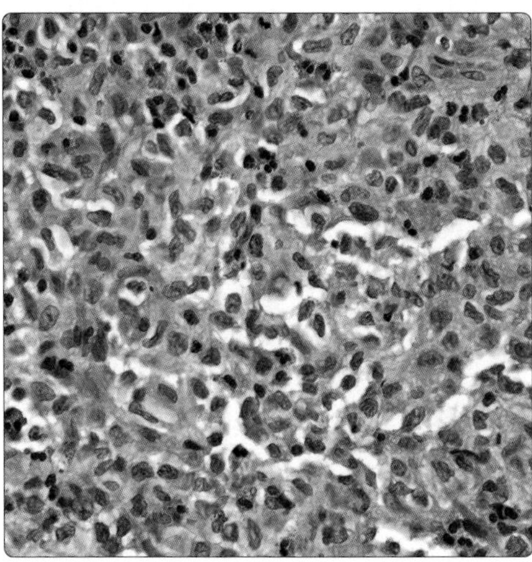

Eosinophils Obscuring Langerhans Cells

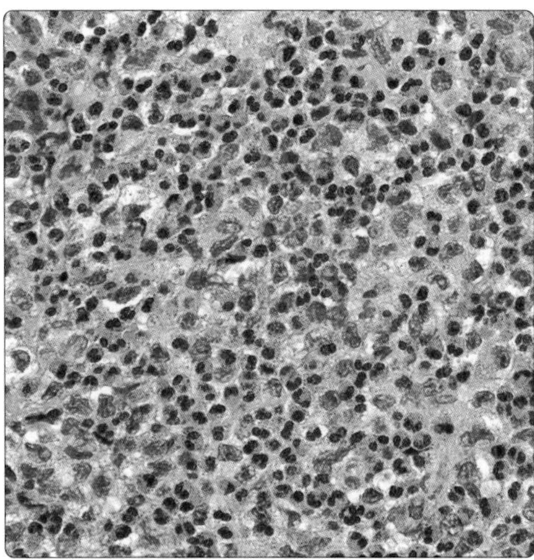

(Left) *The presence of eosinophils introduces the possibility of LCH in a lesion composed largely of pale histiocytes.* **(Right)** *Eosinophils sometimes outnumber Langerhans cells.*

(Left) *While especially prominent in certain foci of lesions within LCH ⇒, clefted and lobulated Langerhans cells may be difficult to find in some examples.* **(Right)** *Pale-staining histiocytes ⇒ and eosinophils are intermingled in LCH. Typical morphological characteristics of histiocytes in some foci may be difficult to appreciate.*

Clefted Langerhans Cells

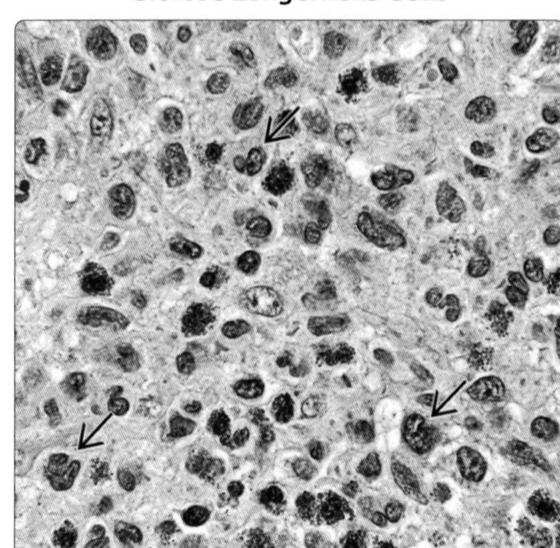

Pale Histiocytes

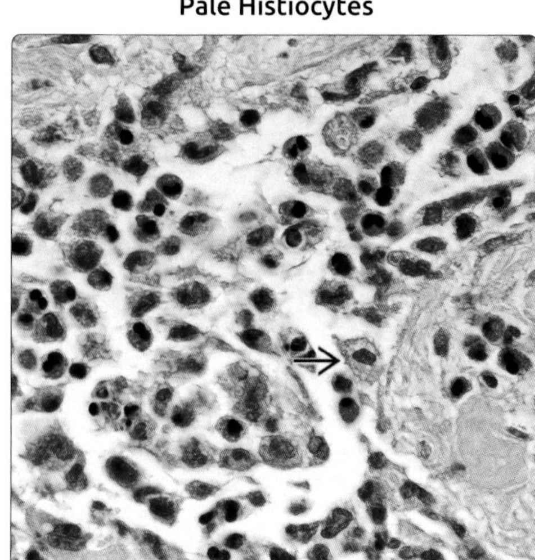

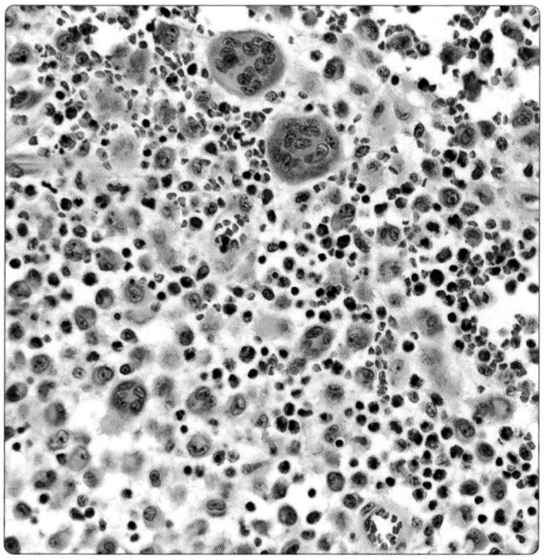

(Left) *Abundant nonspecific foamy macrophages ⇒ may obscure the nature of the lesion.* **(Right)** *A range of cells from mononuclear Langerhans cells to giant multinucleated forms can be seen in LCH.*

Nonspecific Foamy Macrophages

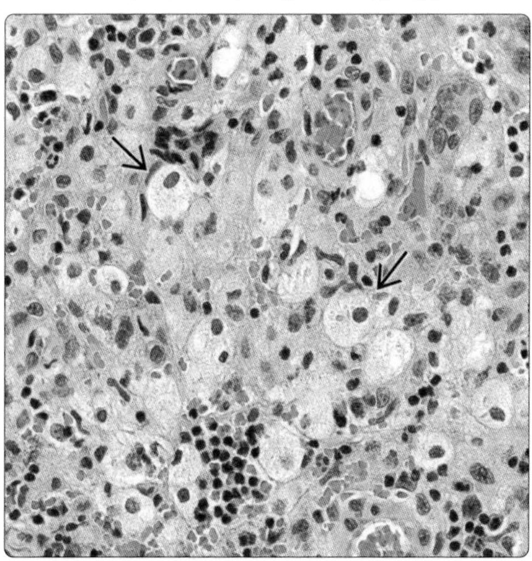

Multinucleated Langerhans Cells

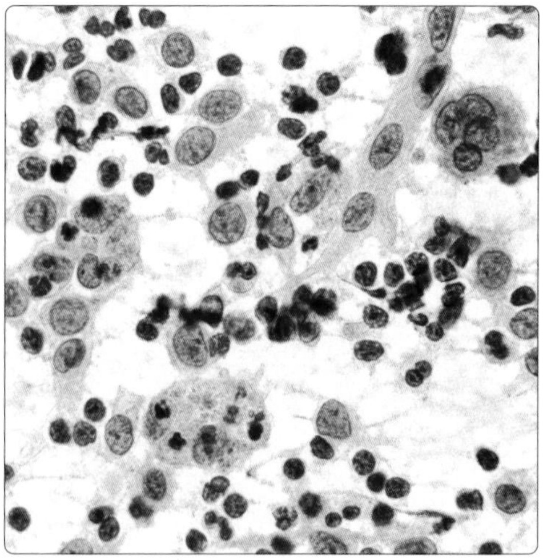

(Left) *Histiocytes with clefted or grooved nuclei are typical of LCH. Eosinophils may appear more amphophilic than eosinophilic in smears and frozen sections.* **(Right)** *Grooved and clefted nuclei are distinctive findings in a smear preparation of LCH. Multinucleated cells and lymphocytes are present in fewer numbers.*

Smear, Amphophilic-Appearing Eosinophils

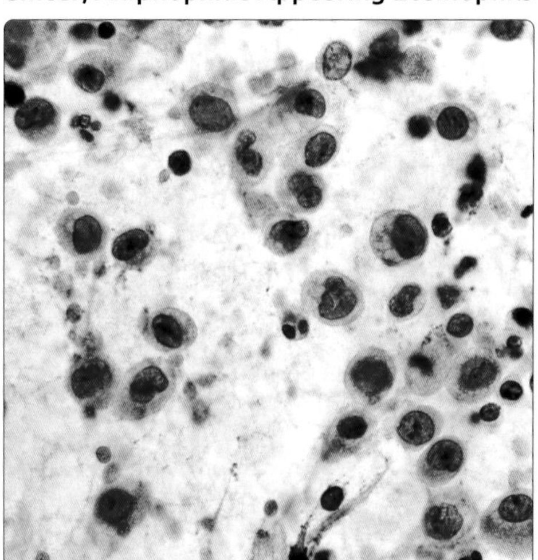

Smear, Langerhans Cells

S100(+) Histiocytes

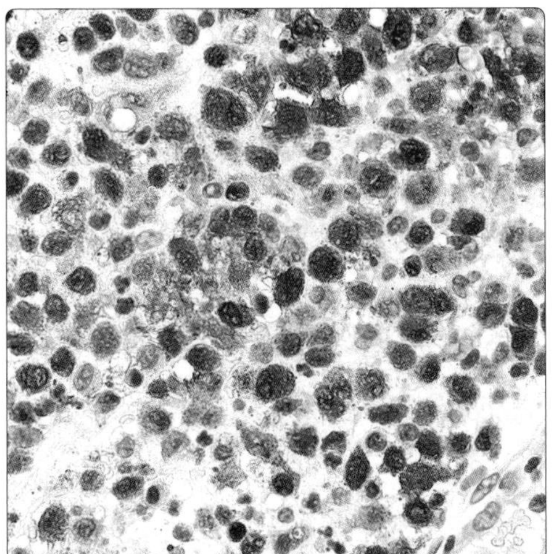

CD1a(+) Histiocytes

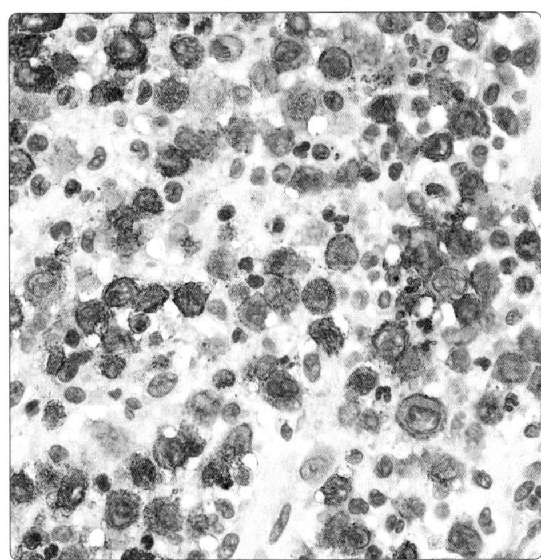

(Left) *Histiocytes in Langerhans cell histiocytosis are not only immunoreactive for CD1a but also for S100.* **(Right)** *Presence of CD1a(+) histiocytes distinguishes Langerhans cell histiocytosis from Erdheim-Chester disease or Rosai-Dorfman disease, as well as other histiocytic disorders.*

CD68(+) Histiocytes

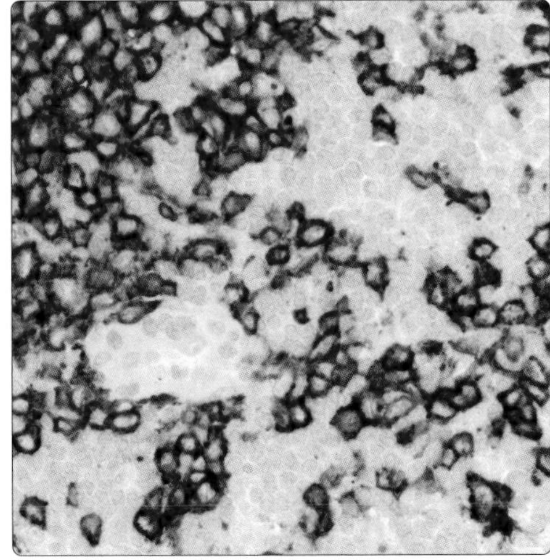

Langerin IHC(+)

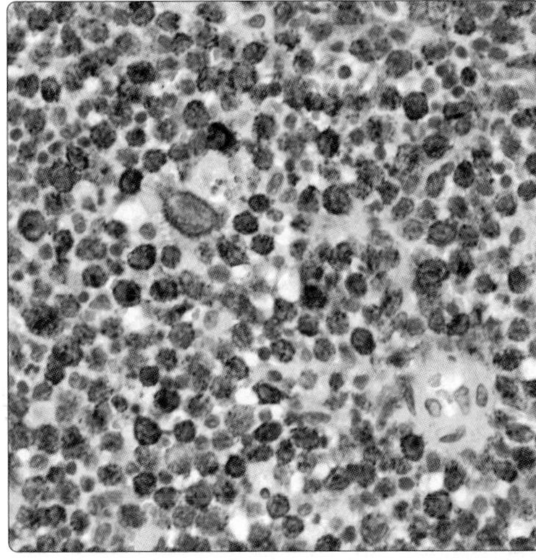

(Left) *All of the histiocytoses, Langerhans cell, Erdheim-Chester, and Rosai-Dorfman, can contain CD68(+) and CD163(+) histiocytes, as can any infectious or noninfectious granulomatous process.* **(Right)** *Langerhans cell histiocytosis is immunoreactive for langerin (CD207).*

Birbeck Granules

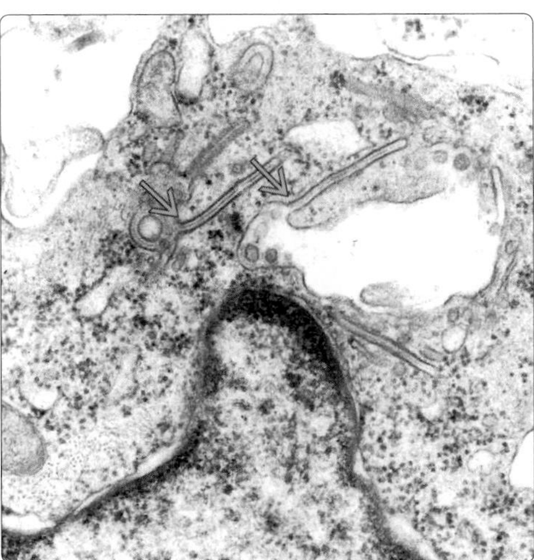

Birbeck Granules

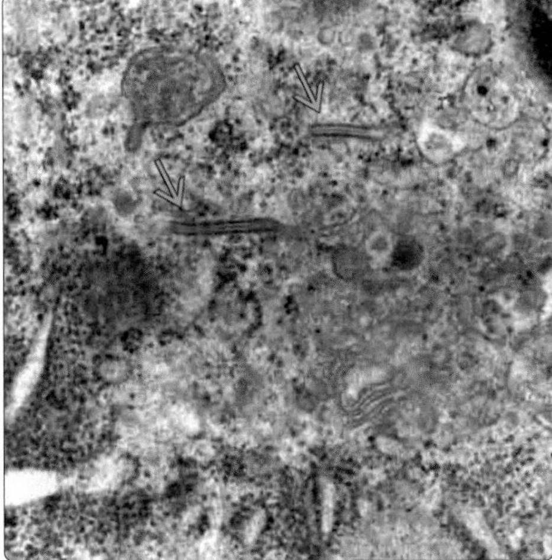

(Left) *Birbeck granules are distinctive, striated structures that arise from cell membranes ➙. They can be seen as cytoplasmic organelles with a central linear density and a striated appearance. These structures are characteristic of LCH.* **(Right)** *Although pathognomonic of LCH, Birbeck granules can be quite difficult to find, or as in this example, the Birbeck granules ➙ do not always have the tennis racket profile shown in textbooks.*

Metastatic Neoplasms, Intraparenchymal, Brain and Spinal Cord

KEY FACTS

CLINICAL ISSUES

- Throughout CNS
- Cerebral hemispheres and cerebellum most common
- Generally gray matter, especially cortex near gray-white junction
- Enhancing edema-producing mass in cerebellum in middle-aged patients is especially suspicious for metastasis
- CNS metastases usually late in disease, especially renal cell and ocular melanoma
- CNS metastasis may be initial presentation of cutaneous melanoma, lung carcinoma
- CNS metastases to unusual sites
    - Dura, often simulating meningioma
    - Infundibular stalk, resulting in diabetes insipidus
    - Pure leptomeningeal, simulating infectious meningitis
    - Intraparenchymal brainstem or spinal cord, pituitary
    - Tumor-to-tumor metastases, especially to pituitary adenoma, meningioma

IMAGING

- Almost all enhancing
- Peritumoral edema, usually prominent, steroid responsive

MICROSCOPIC

- Carcinoma (majority): Most from lung, breast, colon
- Melanoma (common, often hemorrhagic)
- Sometimes without known primary

ANCILLARY TESTS

- Cytology on intraoperative smear/touch preparation: Cohesive tissue fragments (in most cases)

TOP DIFFERENTIAL DIAGNOSES

- Glioma with epithelioid or epithelial differentiation
- Primary CNS lymphoma
- Medulloblastoma
- Hemangioblastoma (vs. renal cell carcinoma)
- Choroid plexus papilloma and carcinoma

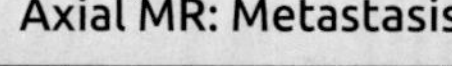

Axial MR: Metastasis

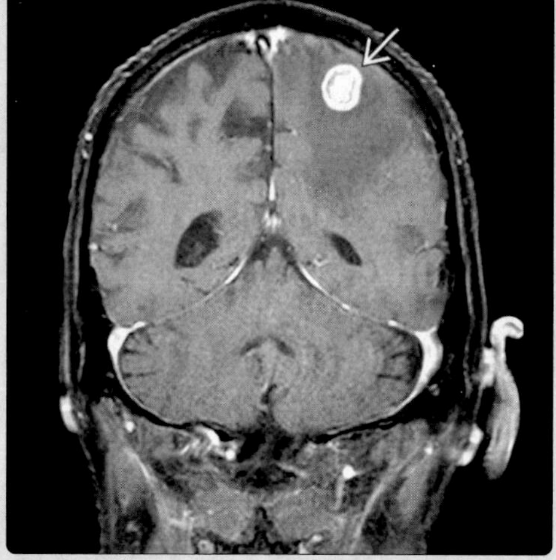

Highly Necrotic Metastasis

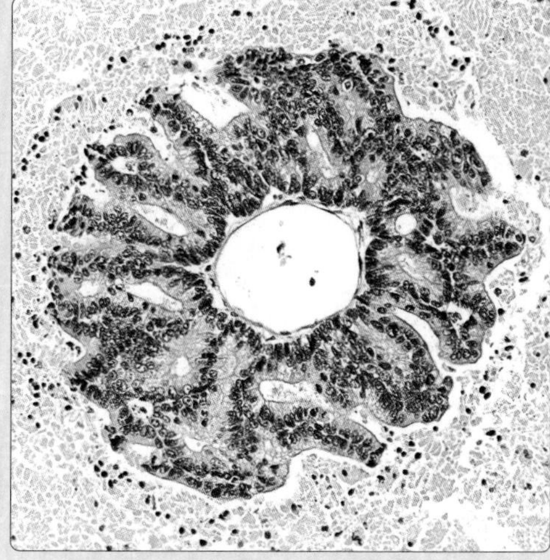

(Left) *As in this example from the colon, metastases are round, enhancing ➔, and surrounded by a considerable dark zone of cerebral edema.* **(Right)** *Necrosis in metastatic carcinomas tends to spare vessels and an isometric cuff of tumor (adenocarcinoma, in this case).*

Coronal MR: Metastasis Simulating Pituitary Adenoma

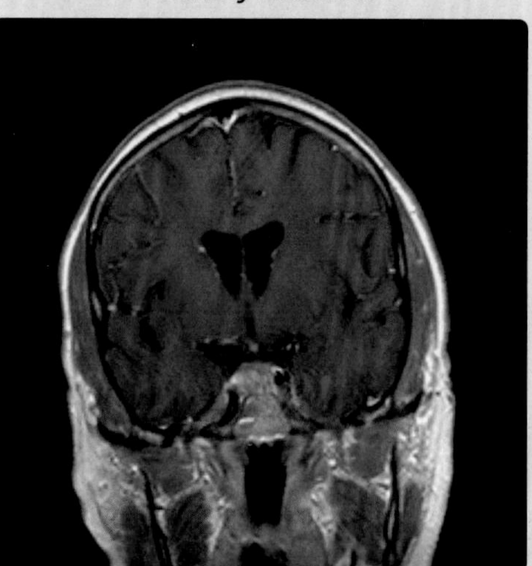

SOX10: Metastatic Melanoma

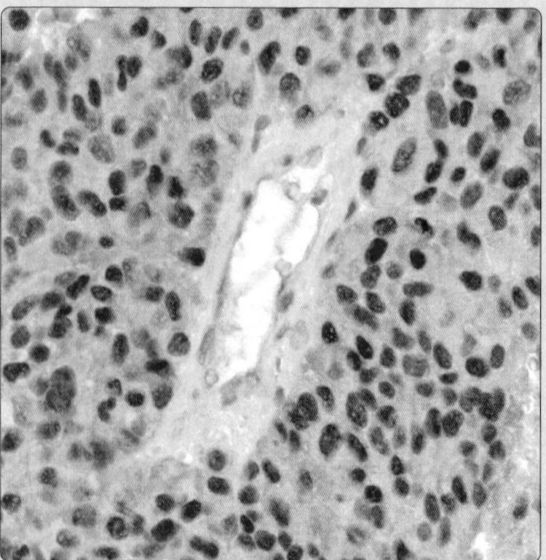

(Left) *Metastases that occur in the sella, dura, or filum terminale can mimic other tumors common to these anatomical regions, such as pituitary adenoma, meningioma, or myxopapillary ependymoma, respectively. This patient with a sellar region mass simulating pituitary adenoma proved to have metastatic thyroid carcinoma.* **(Right)** *SOX10 is an excellent IHC marker for several tumor types, including melanoma, as seen here, where all tumor nuclei are labeled. Note the negatively immunostained central vessel.*

TERMINOLOGY

Definitions

- Malignant neoplasm metastatic from distant site

CLINICAL ISSUES

Site

- Throughout CNS
  - Cerebral hemispheres and cerebellum most common
  - Rare sites
    - Pineal
    - Brainstem
    - Choroid plexus
    - Spinal cord
- Generally gray matter, especially cortex near gray-white junction
- Often multiple, occasionally miliary
- Enhancing, edema-producing mass in cerebellum in middle-aged patients is especially suspicious for metastasis

Presentation

- Usually late in disease, especially renal cell and ocular melanoma (but sometimes as initial clinical event)
- Expressions of mass effect
  - Acutely with hemorrhage (especially with melanoma)
  - From peritumoral edema typically pronounced in metastases
  - Site-dependent neurological deficits
- Seizures
- Global, nonlocalizing signs with advanced multifocal intraparenchymal disease &/or leptomeningeal dissemination

Treatment

- Surgical approaches
  - Excision
- Adjuvant therapy
  - Focal
  - Whole brain

Prognosis

- Poor

IMAGING

MR Findings

- Discrete
- Spherical
- Almost all enhancing
  - Sometimes with dark necrotic center (rim enhancement)
- Peritumoral edema, usually prominent, steroid responsive

MACROSCOPIC

General Features

- Discrete
  - Few, if any, trapped neurons or glia
- Often focally or extensively necrotic
- Firm
- Hemorrhagic (especially melanoma)
- Gray or black (some melanomas)
- Gelatinous (some mucin-producing adenocarcinomas)

MICROSCOPIC

Histologic Features

- Borders
  - Typically sharp
  - Minority infiltrative, usually along vessels
    - Especially from tumor in leptomeninges
    - Sarcomas
  - Extension along cranial nerves (especially 5th) with adenoid cystic carcinoma
- Peritumoral brain
  - Chronic inflammation
  - Gliosis
  - Edema
- Necrosis
  - Frequent, often extensive
  - Typically spares vessels and perivascular cuff of tumor
  - Usually little, if any, pseudopalisading
- Microvascular proliferation
  - Usually absent
  - Sometimes around and within renal cell carcinoma
- Tumor types
  - Carcinoma (majority)
    - Most from lung, breast, colon
  - Melanoma (common, often hemorrhagic)
    - Sometimes without known primary
  - Germ cell tumors (rare); most are primary in CNS
  - Sarcoma (rare); leiomyosarcoma, liposarcoma, rhabdosarcoma
- Fibrous septa (intratumoral)
- Lymphocytic infiltrates
  - Especially immediately surrounding brain, but also intratumoral
- Architectural patterns
  - Sheet-like
  - Lobular
  - Fascicular
  - Papillary
  - Glandular
  - Epithelioid
- Glioma-like glassy cytoplasm with processes (uncommon)
- Hemorrhage
  - In some cases, especially melanoma

ANCILLARY TESTS

Cytology

- Cohesive tissue fragments
  - In most cases
- Sharp cell borders
- Secretory product
  - Adenocarcinoma
- Prominent nucleoli
  - Especially melanoma and adenocarcinoma
- Intranuclear pseudoinclusions
  - Melanoma
- Necrotic debris

Histochemistry

- Mucicarmine
  - Staining pattern: Intracytoplasmic, globular
- Trichrome
  - Reactivity: Positive
  - Staining pattern: Intratumoral septa

Immunohistochemistry

- Carcinoma
  - Lung
    - Non-small cell: CAM5.2, CK7, BER-EP4, napsin (adenocarcinoma), TTF-1
    - Small cell: TTF-1, CD56, CAM5.2
  - Squamous cell (any site)
    - CK5/6, p63, p40 (may be superior to p63)
  - Breast
    - GCDFP, CK7, GATA3, BER-EP4, mammaglobin, ER/PR
  - Colorectal
    - CAM5.2, CK20, CDX-2, BER-EP4
  - Gastroesophageal
    - CK7, CK20, CDX-2, BER-EP4
  - Pancreatic
    - CK7, CK20, CDX-2, BER-EP4, DPC4/SMAD4 (loss)
  - Renal cell
    - pax-2, pax-8, CD10, RCCma
  - Urothelial
    - GATA3, p63
  - Thyroid
    - TTF-1, thyroglobulin, pax-8
  - Adrenal
    - Inhibin-α, Melan-A
  - Hepatocellular
    - Polyclonal CEA and CD10 (both canalicular)
  - Ovary
    - CK7, WT-1, pax-8, BER-EP4, ER/PR
  - Prostate
    - PSA, PSAP
- Melanoma
  - S100, Melan-A, HMB-45, SOX10
- Sarcoma
  - Desmin, myogenin
- Germ cell
  - CD117 (C-kit), OCT4, placental alkaline phosphatase, α-fetoprotein, β-HCG, SALL4
- Lymphoma and leukemia
  - Hematopoietic markers, especially CD20, CD79-a and CD43

Gene Expression Profiling

- May be useful in identifying tissue of origin

Mutational Testing (Often Next Generation Sequencing Panels)

- *EGFR, ALK, KRAS* testing often requested on metastatic adenocarcinoma of lung

DIFFERENTIAL DIAGNOSIS

Glioblastoma

- Conventional type
  - Infiltrating, with trapped glia and neurons
  - Small somewhat elongate cells (in most cases)
  - GFAP(+)
  - Microvascular proliferation
    - Uncommon in metastases, except for renal cell
  - Necrosis with pseudopalisading and including vessels
    - Necrosis in metastases usually spares vessels and cuff of perivascular tumor
- Epithelioid variant
  - Conventional, infiltrating tumor elsewhere in specimen (in some cases)
  - GFAP(+)
  - May be EMA(+), cytokeratins (+)
- With epithelial metaplasia
  - Conventional, infiltrating tumor elsewhere in specimen
  - GFAP(+)
  - May be EMA(+), cytokeratins (+)
  - Often with mesenchymal differentiation (gliosarcoma)
    - Reticulin rich

Anaplastic Oligodendroglioma With Epithelioid Features

- Infiltrating, with trapped glia and neurons
- Features of typical oligodendroglioma elsewhere in specimen
- Often GFAP(+)
- Epithelial markers (-)
- 1p/19q codeletion

Primary CNS Lymphoma

- Infiltrating
- Angiocentric
- Necrosis rare in sporadic lesions
- Lymphoid markers (+)
- No fibrosis

Medulloblastoma

- Nodular/desmoplastic architecture (in some cases)
- Cytokeratins, EMA, TTF-1 all (-); melanocytic markers (-)
- Nuclear and cytoplasmic staining for β-catenin (Wnt pathway)
- Staining for GAB1inclassic medulloblastomas (Shh pathway)

Hemangioblastoma

- Main differential diagnosis when considering metastatic CNS renal cell carcinoma
- Inhibin-α (+)
- pax-2, pax-8, CD10 all (-)
- EMA(-), but sometimes focally (+)
- Low Ki-67 index, but overlap

Choroid Plexus Papilloma and Carcinoma

- Intraventricular or at cerebellopontine angle
- Almost all in children
- Usually EMA(-), BER-EP4(-)
- Papillomas usually CK7(+), CK20(-)
- Synaptophysin (+)
  - In some cases

Meningioma

- Main differential diagnosis when considering dural metastasis
- Usually dural based, noninfiltrative of brain

- Atypical and anaplastic variants may show tongues of tumor extending into brain
- Vimentin (+)
- EMA variably (+), weak, focal, membranous
  - S100(+) focal in fibroblastic types
- Keratin usually (-) except high-grade examples and secretory types
- Claudin-6 (+)
- SSTR2A(+) superior to EMA
- Dual D2-40(+) + E-cadherin (+)
- Dural metastases most commonly from breast, lung, but can be prostate, other unusual sources
- Dural metastases often unassociated with parenchymal metastases

Papillary Tumor of Pineal

- Keratin positive
  - AE1/AE3, CAM5.2, CK18
- May have focal GFAP(+), dot-like EMA(+)
- Ki-67 usually low

Tumor-to-Tumor Metastasis

- Most common CNS "recipient" tumor types: Pituitary adenoma, meningioma
- Most common "donor" systemic tumor types to cause tumor-to-tumor metastasis: Breast, lung

DIAGNOSTIC CHECKLIST

Pathologic Interpretation Pearls

- Search for metastatic tumor (especially melanoma in intracranial hemorrhages)
- Use immunomarkers in panels rather than in isolation
- Antibodies often demonstrate immunostaining in tumor types outside of the originally-described specificity (example: TTF-1 in nonlung, nonthyroid cancers)
- AE1/AE3 seen in reactive astrocytes

SELECTED REFERENCES

1. Mentrikoski MJ et al: Immunohistochemical distinction of renal cell carcinoma from other carcinomas with clear-cell histomorphology: utility of CD10 and CA-125 in addition to PAX-2, PAX-8, RCCma, and adipophilin. Appl Immunohistochem Mol Morphol. 22(9):635-41, 2014
2. Ni YB et al: TTF-1 expression in breast carcinoma: an unusual but real phenomenon. Histopathology. 64(4):504-11, 2014
3. Bishop JA et al: p40 (ΔNp63) is superior to p63 for the diagnosis of pulmonary squamous cell carcinoma. Mod Pathol. 25(3):405-15, 2012
4. Karamchandani JR et al: Sox10 and S100 in the diagnosis of soft-tissue neoplasms. Appl Immunohistochem Mol Morphol. 20(5):445-50, 2012
5. Ordóñez NG: Thyroid transcription factor-1 is not expressed in squamous cell carcinomas of the lung: an immunohistochemical study with review of the literature. Appl Immunohistochem Mol Morphol. 20(6):525-30, 2012
6. Ordóñez NG: Value of thyroid transcription factor-1 immunostaining in tumor diagnosis: a review and update. Appl Immunohistochem Mol Morphol. 20(5):429-44, 2012
7. Ordóñez NG: Value of PAX 8 immunostaining in tumor diagnosis: a review and update. Adv Anat Pathol. 19(3):140-51, 2012
8. Ordóñez NG: Value of PAX2 immunostaining in tumor diagnosis: a review and update. Adv Anat Pathol. 19(6):401-9, 2012
9. Carney EM et al: PAX2(-)/PAX8(-)/inhibin A(+) immunoprofile in hemangioblastoma: A helpful combination in the differential diagnosis with metastatic clear cell renal cell carcinoma to the central nervous system. Am J Surg Pathol. 35(2):262-7, 2011
10. Sangoi AR et al: The use of immunohistochemistry in the diagnosis of metastatic clear cell renal cell carcinoma: a review of PAX-8, PAX-2, hKIM-1, RCCma, and CD10. Adv Anat Pathol. 17(6):377-93, 2010
11. Widdel L et al: Tumor-to-tumor metastasis from hematopoietic neoplasms to meningiomas: report of two patients with significant cerebral edema. World Neurosurg. 74(1):165-71, 2010
12. Wu AH et al: Gene expression profiles help identify the tissue of origin for metastatic brain cancers. Diagn Pathol. 5:26, 2010
13. Takei H et al: Tumor-to-tumor metastasis to the central nervous system. Neuropathology. 29(3):303-8, 2009
14. Ingold B et al: Renal cell carcinoma marker reliably discriminates central nervous system haemangioblastoma from brain metastases of renal cell carcinoma. Histopathology. 52(6):674-81, 2008
15. Nonaka D et al: Sox10: a pan-schwannian and melanocytic marker. Am J Surg Pathol. 32(9):1291-8, 2008
16. Siami K et al: Thyroid transcription factor-1 expression in endometrial and endocervical adenocarcinomas. Am J Surg Pathol. 31(11):1759-63, 2007
17. Becher MW et al: Immunohistochemical analysis of metastatic neoplasms of the central nervous system. J Neuropathol Exp Neurol. 65(10):935-44, 2006
18. Drlicek M et al: Immunohistochemical panel of antibodies in the diagnosis of brain metastases of the unknown primary. Pathol Res Pract. 200(10):727-34, 2004
19. Petraki C et al: Tumor to tumor metastasis: report of two cases and review of the literature. Int J Surg Pathol. 11(2):127-35, 2003
20. Espat NJ et al: Soft tissue sarcoma brain metastases. Prevalence in a cohort of 3829 patients. Cancer. 94(10):2706-11, 2002
21. Kleinschmidt-DeMasters BK: Dural metastases. A retrospective surgical and autopsy series. Arch Pathol Lab Med. 125(7):880-7, 2001
22. Gyure KA et al: Cytokeratin 7 and 20 expression in choroid plexus tumors: utility in differentiating these neoplasms from metastatic carcinomas. Mod Pathol. 13(6):638-43, 2000
23. Oh D et al: Evaluation of epithelial and keratin markers in glioblastoma multiforme: an immunohistochemical study. Arch Pathol Lab Med. 123(10):917-20, 1999
24. Gottschalk J et al: The use of immunomorphology to differentiate choroid plexus tumors from metastatic carcinomas. Cancer. 72(4):1343-9, 1993
25. Paulus W et al: Clinicopathologic correlations in epithelial choroid plexus neoplasms: a study of 52 cases. Acta Neuropathol. 80(6):635-41, 1990

(Left) *As with this melanoma, secondary CNS tumors are usually lobular, discrete masses with central necrosis. Metastatic melanomas are variably pigmented; this one is amelanotic to the naked eye.* **(Right)** *Metastases generally have sharp borders ⇨ with adjacent brain. Necrosis ➡ is common and often extensive.*

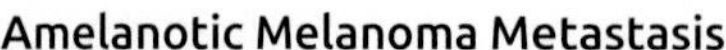

Amelanotic Melanoma Metastasis

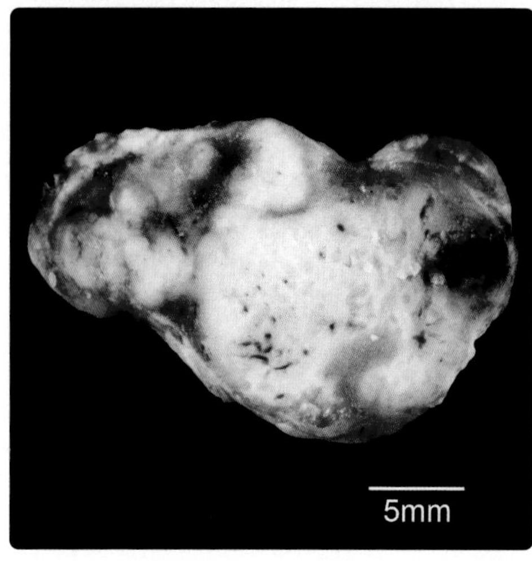

Sharply Demarcated Metastasis

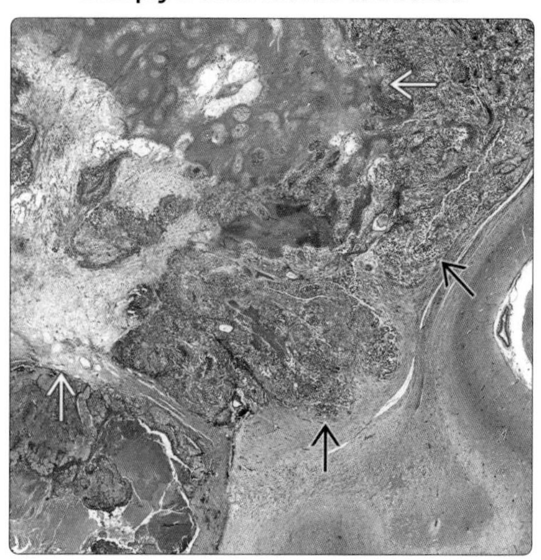

(Left) *Metastases are typically well circumscribed, with varying numbers of lymphocytes in the subjacent brain ⇨.* **(Right)** *As in this metastasis from a squamous cell carcinoma of the neck, fibrous stroma is sometimes prominent in secondary CNS tumors. Overall, it is much more prominent than in primary CNS tumors. There is sometimes a small amount in malignant gliomas, particularly gliosarcomas, but almost none in malignant lymphomas.*

Well Circumscribed

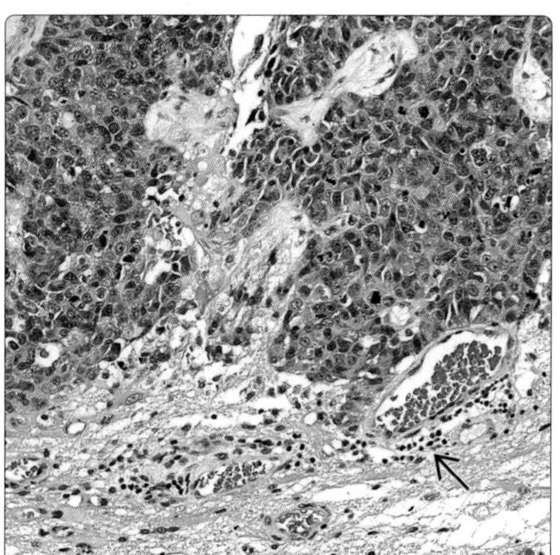

Fibrous Stroma

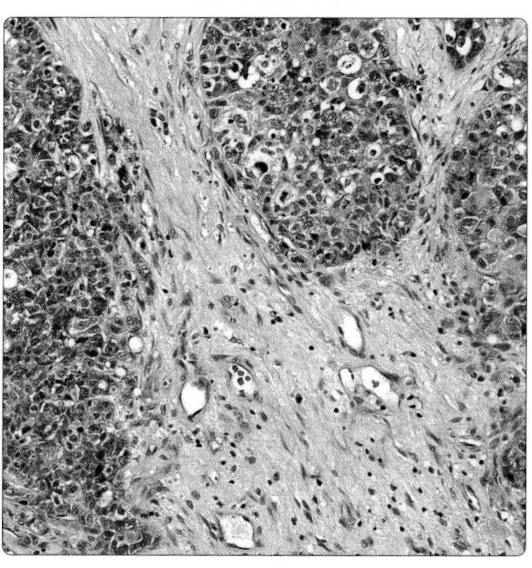

(Left) *Tumors such as this melanoma that have reached the subarachnoid space often follow Virchow-Robin spaces and vessels into the cortex.* **(Right)** *Perivascular spread gives the illusion of glioma-like diffuse infiltration, but the metastatic nature of this adenocarcinoma is not in doubt. A solid tumor mass was present elsewhere.*

Tumor Spread, Virchow-Robin Spaces

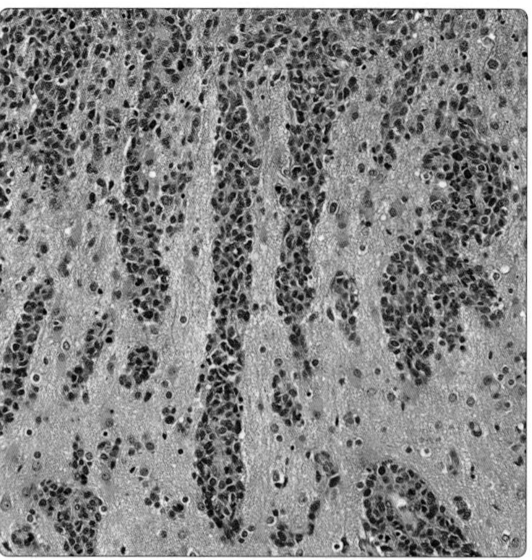

Perivascular Spread

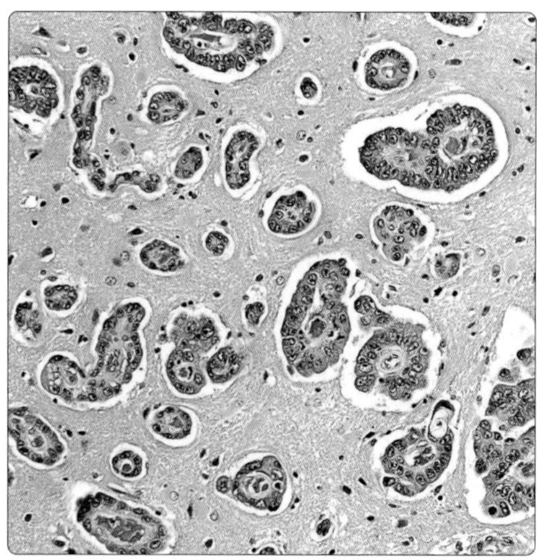

Surviving Collars of Perivascular Tumor

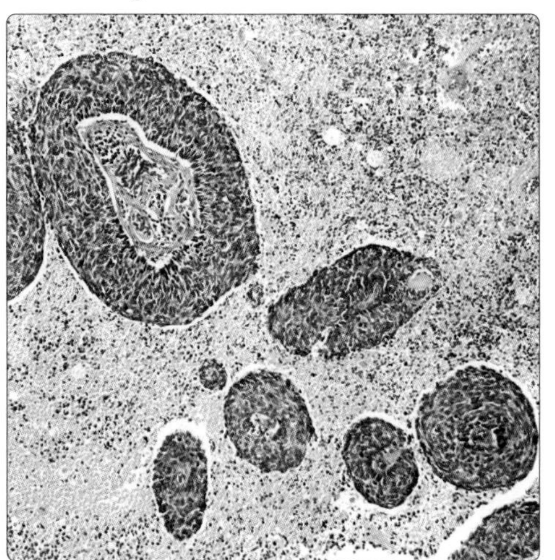

Serpiginous Necrosis Simulating Glioblastoma

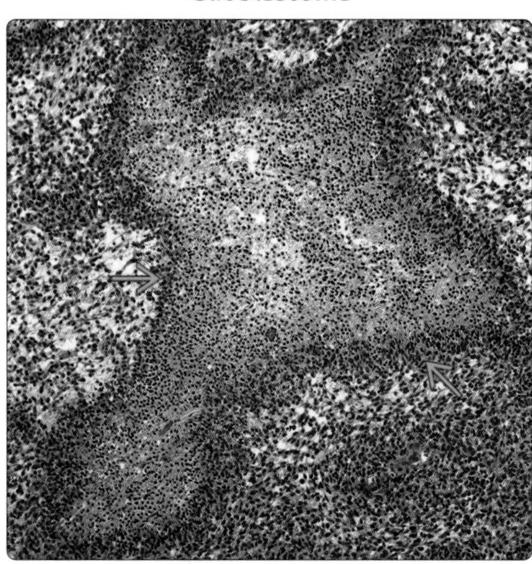

(Left) *Necrosis, prominent in most metastases, tends to spare vessels and a uniform perivascular collar of tumor.* **(Right)** *Necrosis in metastases may have a serpiginous pattern with pseudopalisading, as in this metastatic melanoma ⇒, but not usually the latter's full expression, as is iconic for glioblastoma.*

Fibrous Septa

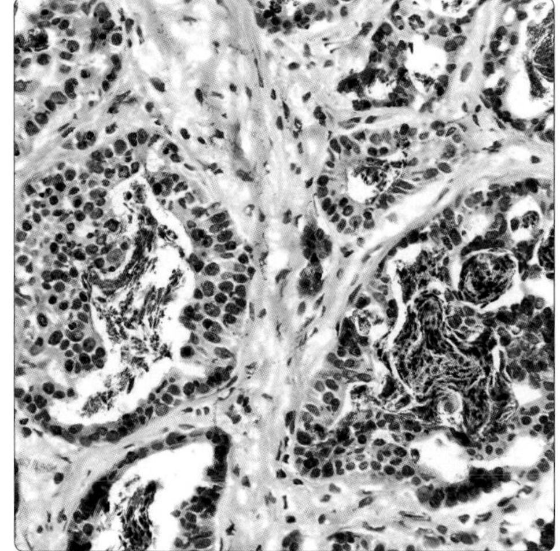

Accompanying Benign Lymphocytes

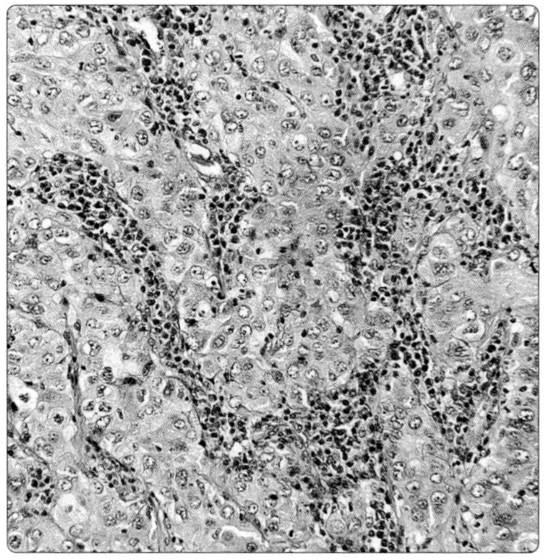

(Left) *Fibrous septa are common in metastases, as opposed to glioblastomas, except in the presence of mesenchymal differentiation (gliosarcoma). Vascular reticulin is the only connective tissue in primary CNS lymphomas.* **(Right)** *Lymphocytes are commonly identified in and around metastases (such as this squamous cancer) than in malignant gliomas (such as glioblastoma and anaplastic oligodendroglioma).*

Clear Cell Carcinoma, Kidney

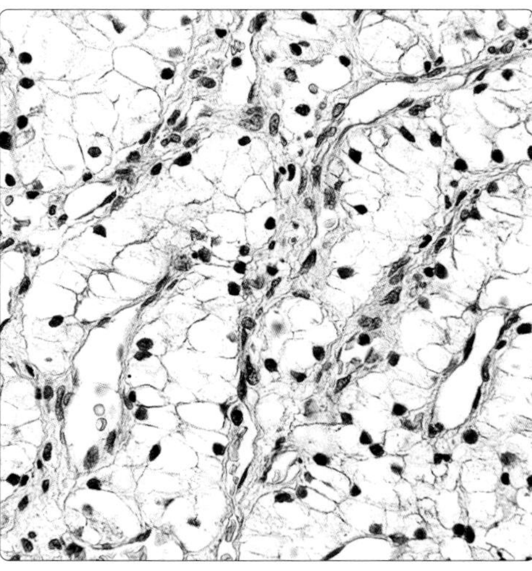

Microvascular Proliferation, Clear Cell Carcinoma, Kidney

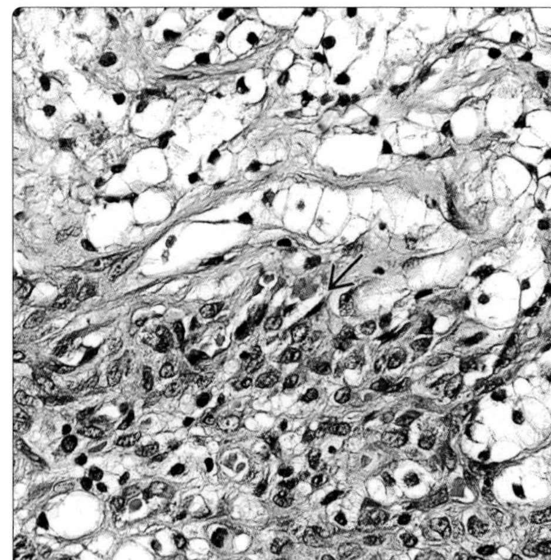

(Left) *Vacuolated, lacy cytoplasm and small uniform nuclei with little atypia or mitotic activity are typical of metastatic clear cell carcinoma from the kidney. Closely packed glands and lobules are common.* **(Right)** *Unlike high-grade gliomas, microvascular proliferation is unusual in metastases, except for renal clear cell carcinoma wherein it may be found in its glomeruloid form ⇒.*

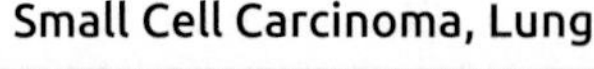

Small Cell Carcinoma, Lung

Melanophages, Melanoma

(Left) *While glioblastoma is difficult to exclude in this case from the lung, the degree of anaplasia, lobular architecture, and epithelioid features suggest small cell carcinoma.* **(Right)** *Pigment in melanomas is often more prominent in melanophages ➔ than tumor cells ⇨.*

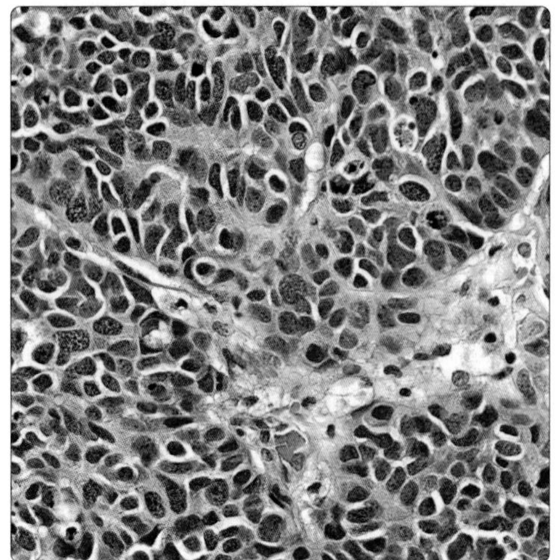

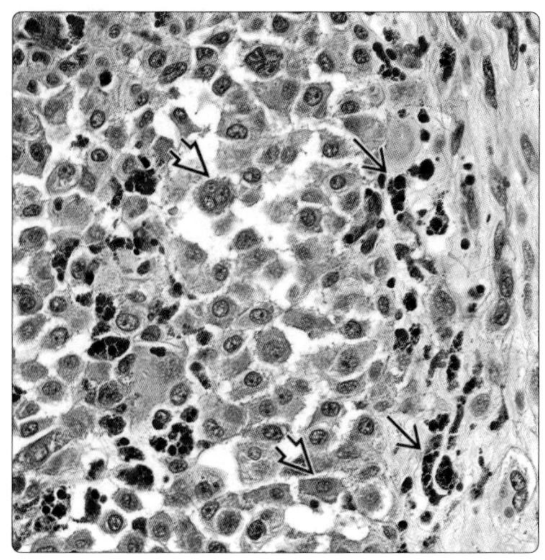

Rare Tumor Cells in Hematoma

Melan-A: Melanoma

(Left) *Intraparenchymal hematomas should be searched for malignant cells, such as those of metastatic melanoma. In this case, small and only very focal islands of malignant cells were embedded in a large intracerebellar hemorrhage.* **(Right)** *Melanoma markers, such as antibodies to Melan-A, can be used to confirm suspicions that islands of tumor cells in intracerebral hematomas could be melanoma. A prior history of melanoma is present in some, but not all, cases.*

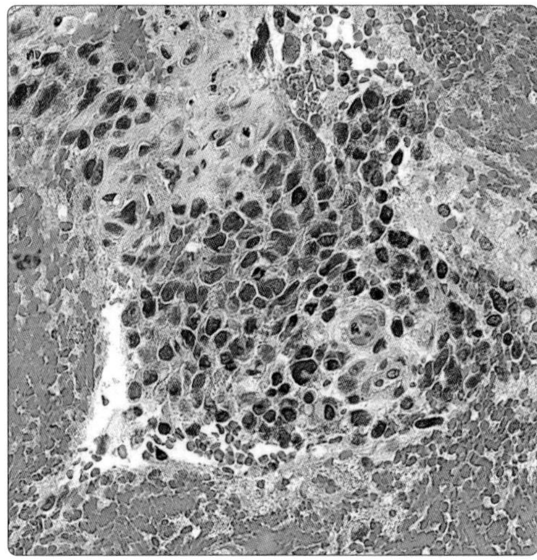

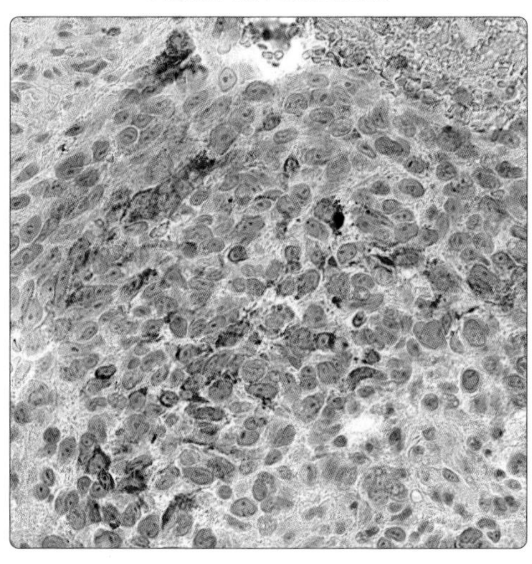

Pleomorphism in Metastasis

Metastasis With Glioma-Like Appearance

(Left) *As in this metastatic melanoma, there can be a degree of nuclear pleomorphism that might suggest glioblastoma.* **(Right)** *Glassy cytoplasm with processes creates a glioma-like appearance in some metastases. Immunostaining for GFAP, epithelial, and melanocytic markers usually resolves the problem. The issue remains in doubt in occasional cases where all antibodies are negative.*

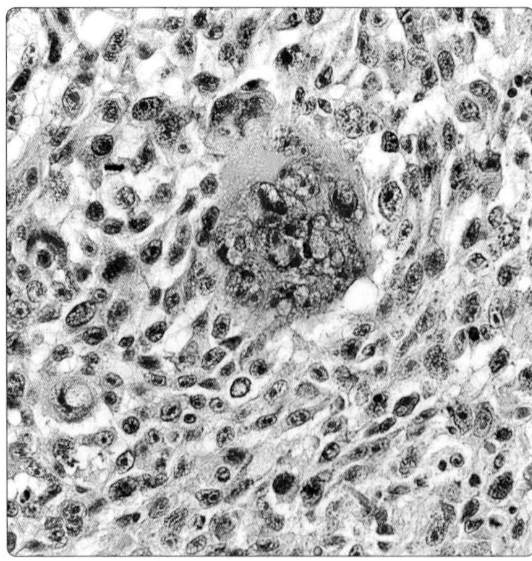

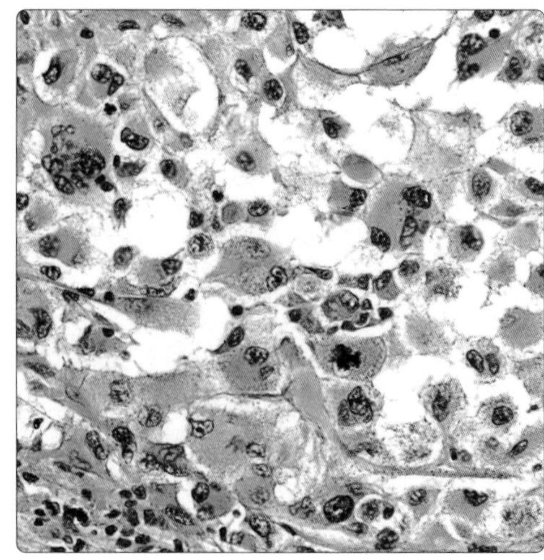

Squamous Cell Carcinoma, Neck

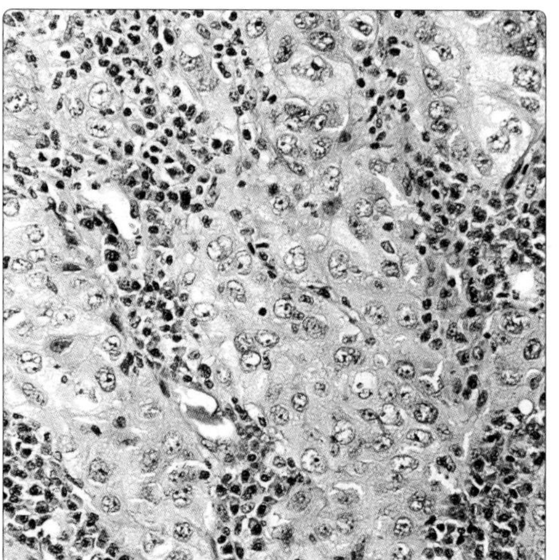

Keratins in Metastasis

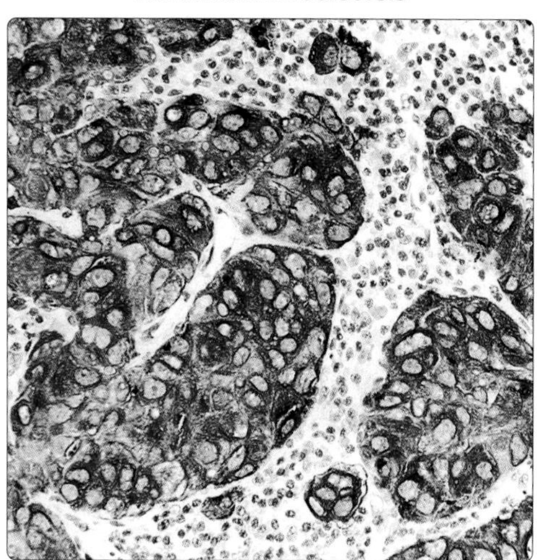

(Left) *Lobules of epithelioid cells with squamous features in a chronically inflamed stroma are very unlikely to be those of a primary CNS tumor. Squamous cell carcinoma of the neck was the primary source.* **(Right)** *Immunohistochemistry for AE1/AE3 is useful in identifying metastatic carcinomas, such as this squamous cell cancer from the neck. These antibodies must be used with caution, since they also stain reactive astrocytes (sometimes more avidly than GFAP).*

Adenocarcinoma, Lung

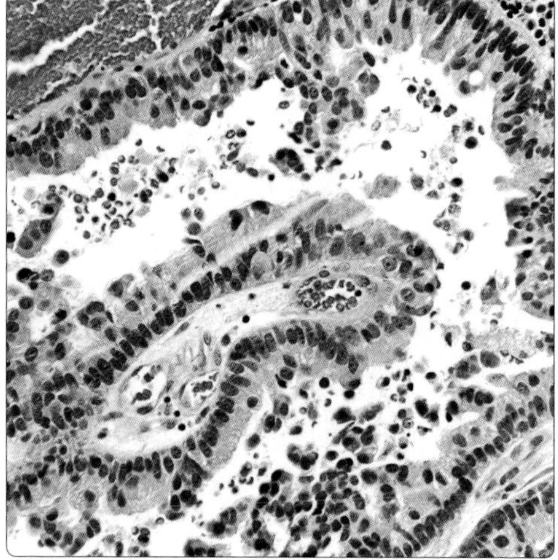

TTF-1: Metastatic Lung Carcinoma

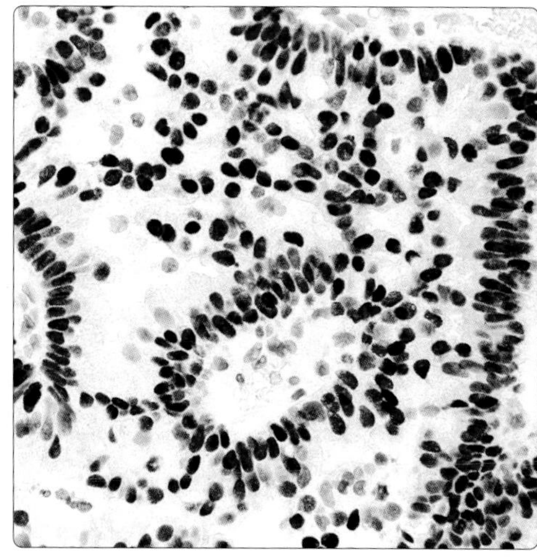

(Left) *The diagnosis of metastatic carcinoma is simple in cases with well-differentiated glandular tissue and a known primary in the lung.* **(Right)** *Antibodies to TTF-1 help identify metastases, with possible sources in the lung and thyroid. Staining is nuclear (as in this case from the lung).*

Small Cell Carcinoma, Lung

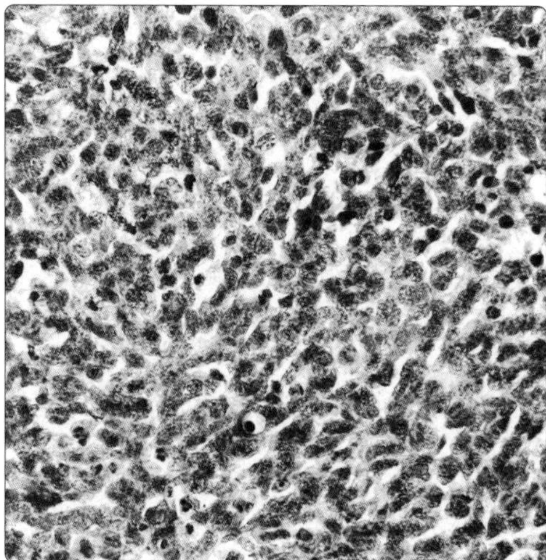

TTF-1: Small Cell Carcinoma, Lung

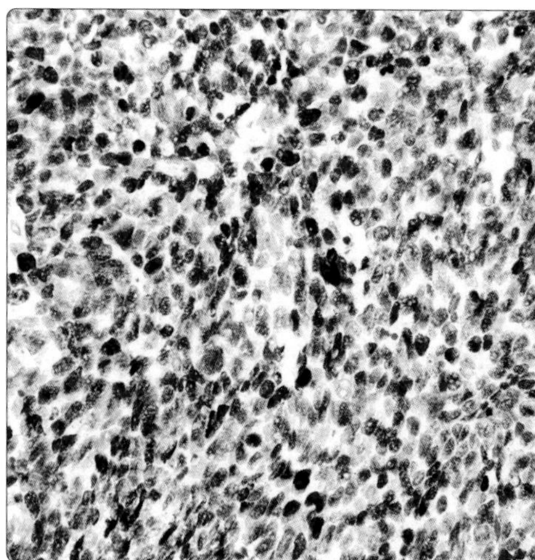

(Left) *Metastatic small cell carcinomas from the lung to the cerebellum need to be distinguished from medulloblastoma. Both can be synaptophysin positive but only the metastasis would be immunoreactive for TTF-1.* **(Right)** *Immunoreactivity of a cerebellar small cell tumor for TTF-1 supports the diagnosis of a metastasis from the lung.*

(Left) *Clear cell carcinomas have a distinctive appearance, but a confident diagnosis often requires immunohistochemistry using antibodies to pax-2 &/or pax-8.* **(Right)** *Nuclear immunostaining for pax-8 is useful in confirming that a clear cell lesion has a renal origin. Hemangioblastoma would be negative for pax-2, pax-8, and CD10.*

Clear Cell Carcinoma, Kidney

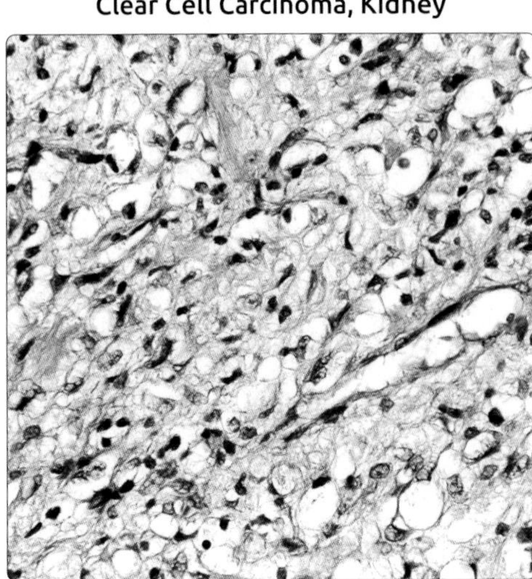

Nuclear pax-8: Clear Cell Carcinoma, Kidney

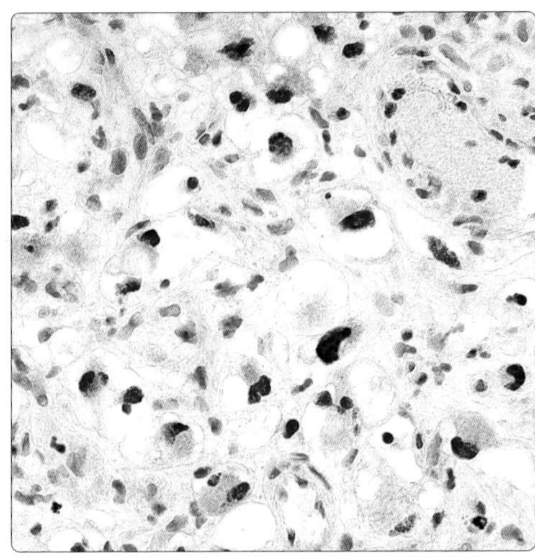

(Left) *Papillary thyroid carcinomas metastatic to the CNS are more often cranial than intraparenchymal.* **(Right)** *Antibodies to BER-EP4 stain the cytoplasm of metastases from many organs, including those of thyroid, lung, GI tract, and ovary. It is useful in identifying systemic cancer since only a rare choroid plexus tumor is positive. Lung was the primary here.*

Papillary Thyroid Carcinoma

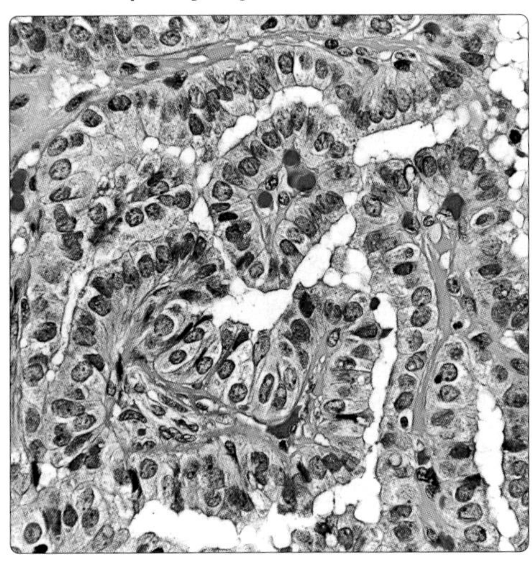

BER-EP4: Adenocarcinoma, Lung

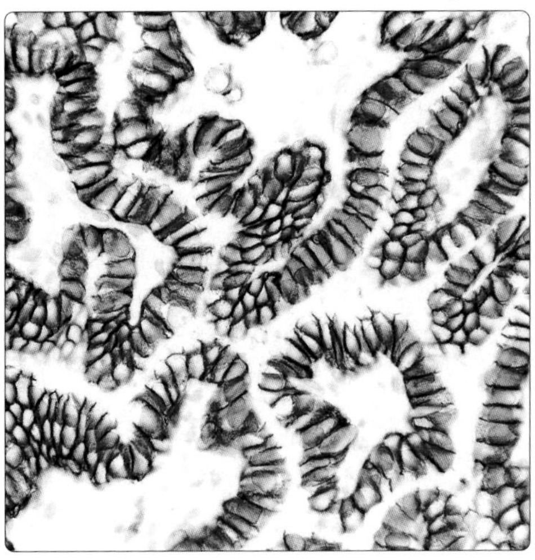

(Left) *Melanomas vary greatly in histological appearance, but are often sheets of uniform undifferentiated cells with little from which to discern the primary source (other than a general suspicion).* **(Right)** *Immunostaining for S100 protein may be the only positive melanocytic marker of poorly differentiated melanomas.*

Melanoma, Undifferentiated Cells

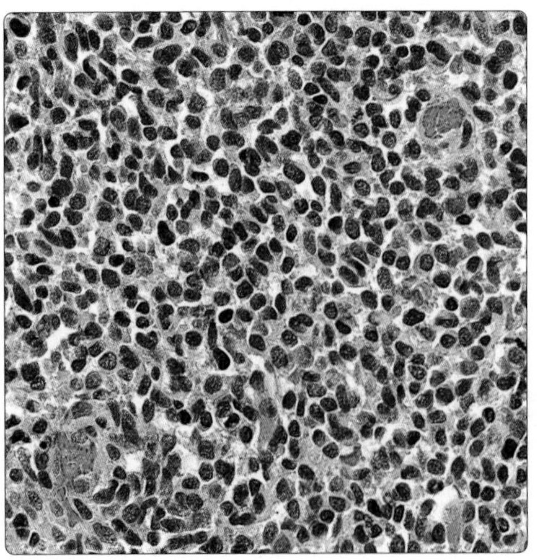

S100: Melanoma

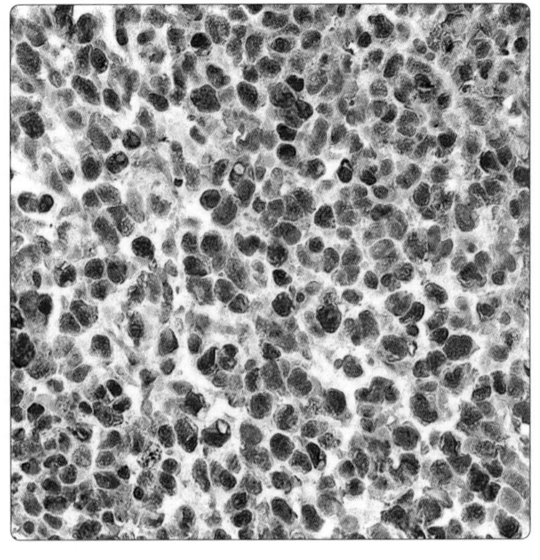

Ovarian Carcinoma

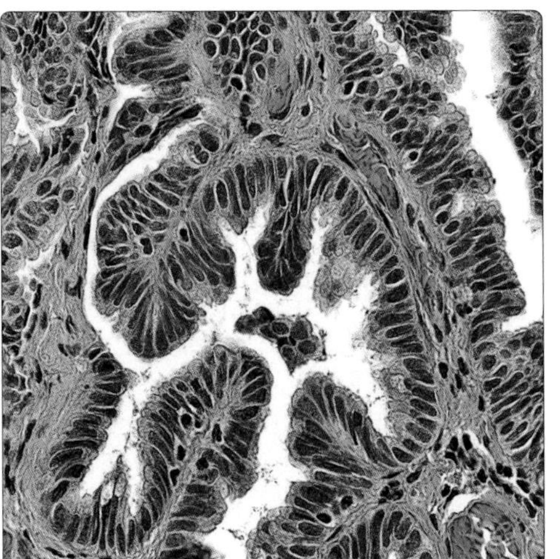

BER-EP4: Ovarian Carcinoma

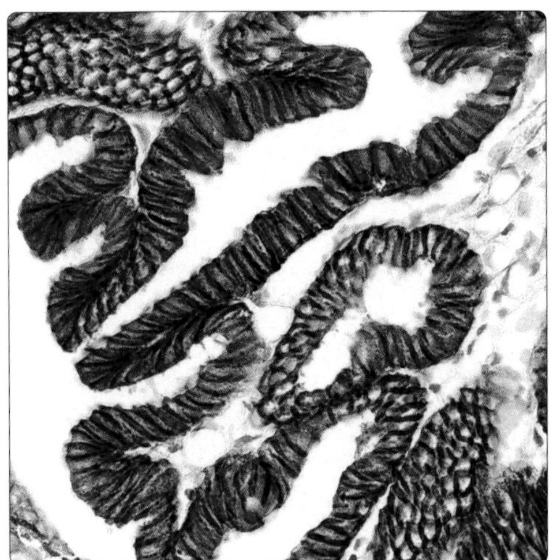

(Left) *Ovarian cancer (papillary in this example) is an unusual source of metastases to the CNS. The secondary site, spinal cord, was also uncommon.* **(Right)** *Antibodies to BER-EP4 help identify carcinomas from multiple sources, including lung, breast, colorectal, gastroesophageal, kidney, thyroid, and ovary. This was ovarian cancer metastatic to the spinal cord. Only a rare choroid plexus carcinoma is positive for BER-EP4.*

Hepatocellular Carcinoma

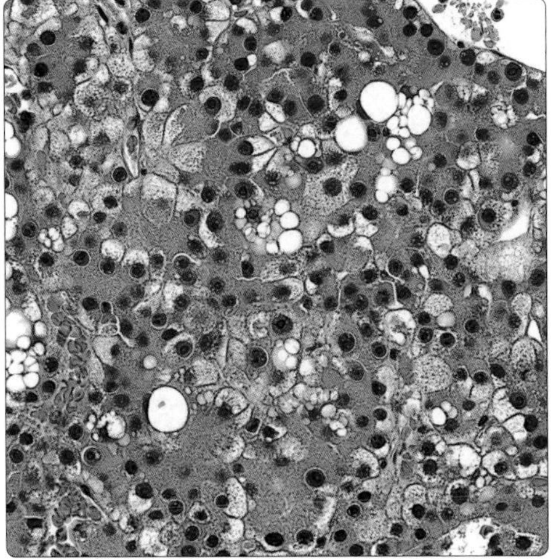

CEA: Hepatocellular Carcinoma

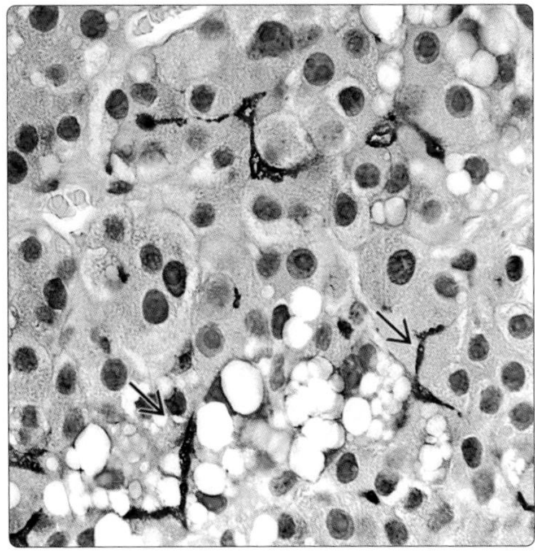

(Left) *Hepatocellular carcinoma, a most unusual form of CNS metastasis, may faithfully recreate the architecture of the parent tissue, including fatty change.* **(Right)** *Polyclonal antibodies to CEA decorate bile canaliculi ⇒ in the rare CNS metastasis of hepatocellular carcinoma.*

Adenoid Cystic Carcinoma

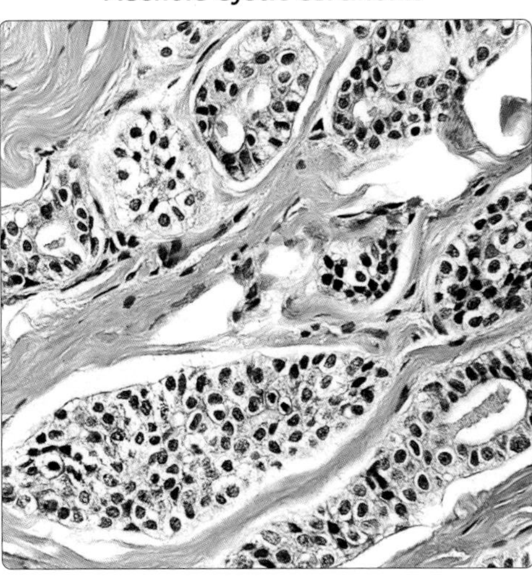

p63: Adenoid Cystic Carcinoma

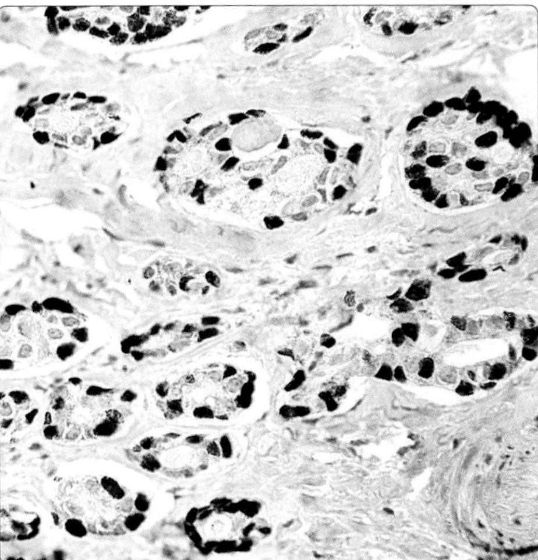

(Left) *Adenoid cystic carcinomas are often local extensions along cranial nerves than discontinuous metastases. The primary site may or may not be apparent.* **(Right)** *Immunostaining for p63 is typical of adenoid cystic carcinoma and squamous carcinomas from various sites. An outer layer of cells is stained; the inner would be positive for EMA.*

(Left) *Green-stained collagenous tissue is generally much more prominent in metastases than in primary brain tumors. Broad, dense septa, such as this, would be most unusual in glioblastoma.* **(Right)** *Histochemistry for mucin demonstrates intra- → and extracellular secretory product in a metastatic adenocarcinoma from the lung.*

Collagen More Common in Metastasis Than Primary Tumors

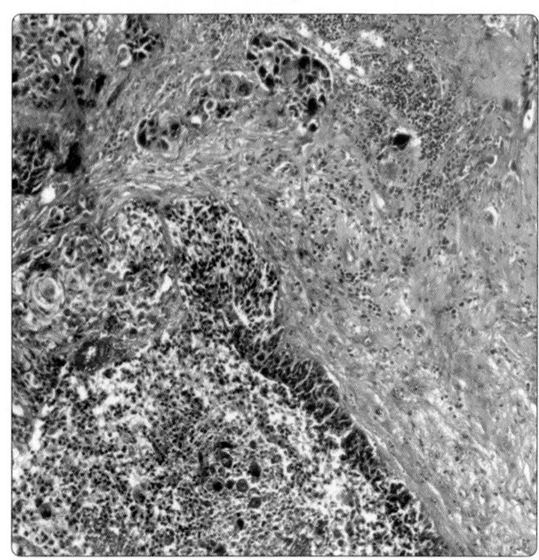

Mucicarcinoma, Adenocarcinoma, Lung

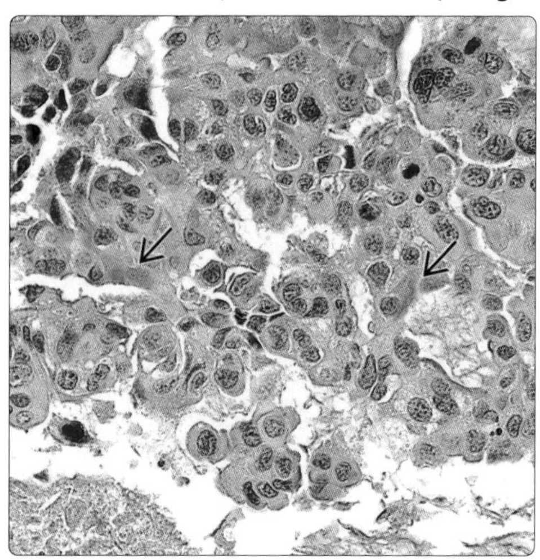

(Left) *Recent studies suggest that positive nuclear immunoreactivity to p40 may be a superior marker to p63 for identifying squamous cell carcinomas.* **(Right)** *This carcinoma of the prostate metastatic to the temporal lobe of the brain shows numerous mitotic figures; without immunostaining the primary site would be difficult to identify.*

p40: Squamous Cell Carcinoma

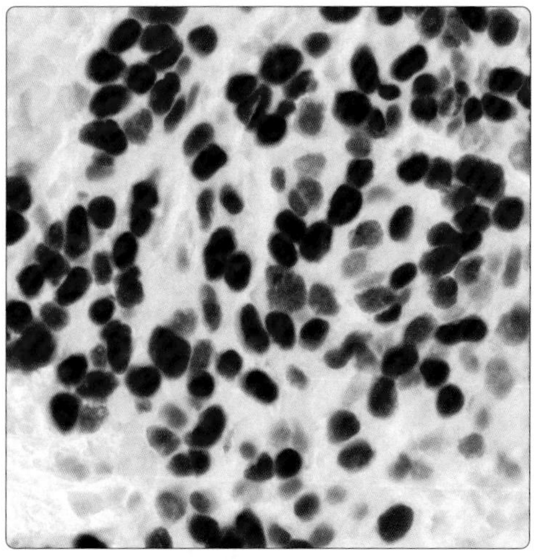

Metastatic Prostatic Carcinoma

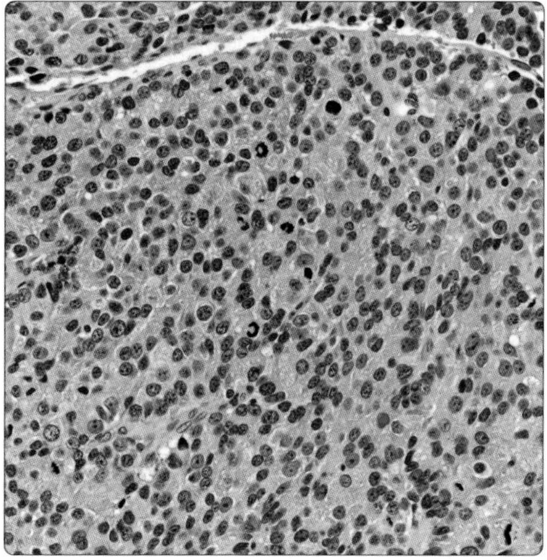

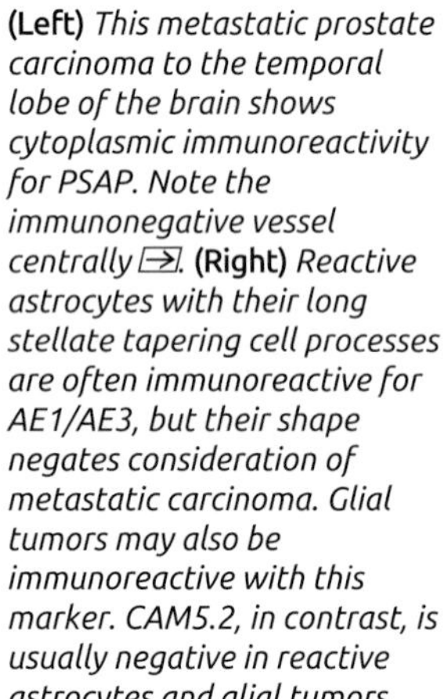

(Left) *This metastatic prostate carcinoma to the temporal lobe of the brain shows cytoplasmic immunoreactivity for PSAP. Note the immunonegative vessel centrally →.* **(Right)** *Reactive astrocytes with their long stellate tapering cell processes are often immunoreactive for AE1/AE3, but their shape negates consideration of metastatic carcinoma. Glial tumors may also be immunoreactive with this marker. CAM5.2, in contrast, is usually negative in reactive astrocytes and glial tumors.*

PSAP, Metastatic Prostate Carcinoma, Brain

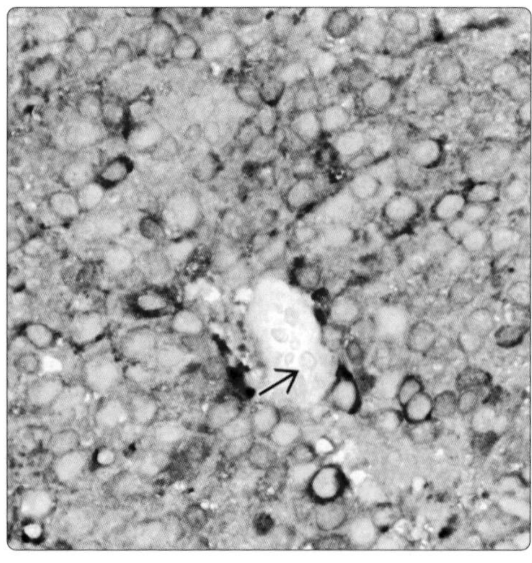

AE1/AE3

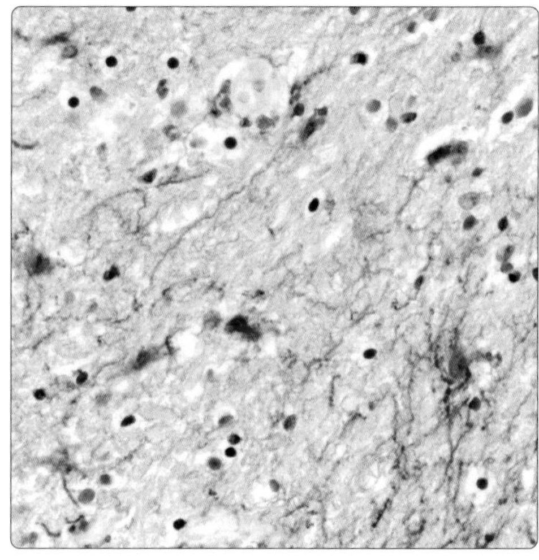

Smear: Adenocarcinoma, Lung

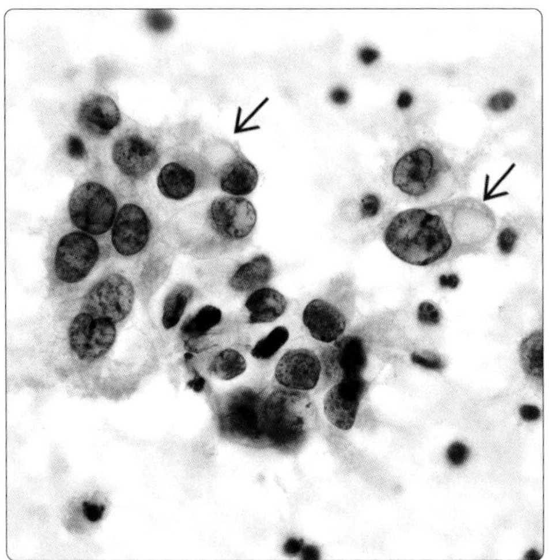

Smear: Lung With Neuroendocrine Features

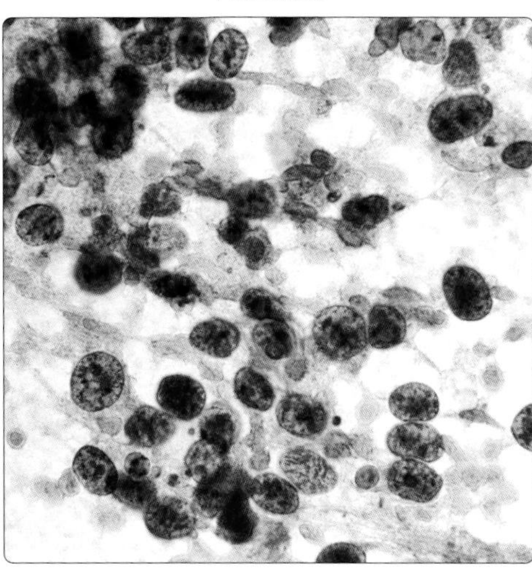

(Left) *Intracellular secretory product ⇨ helps identify the lesion as carcinoma of the adeno type. Lung was the source.* **(Right)** *This smear from lung carcinoma with neuroendocrine features shows the salt and pepper nuclear chromatin pattern and prominent nucleolus of this tumor type.*

Smear: Melanoma Without Pigment

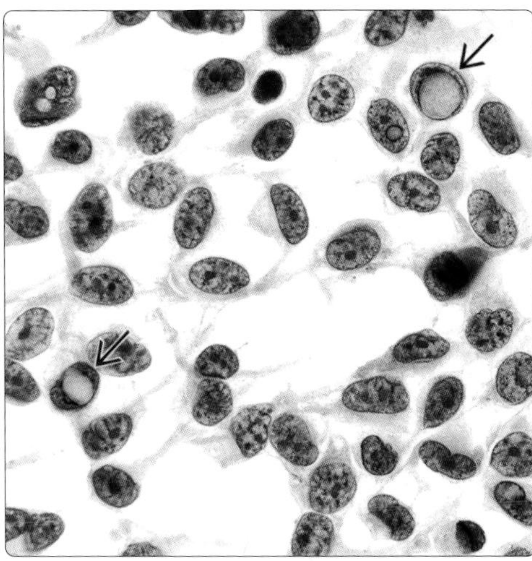

Smear: Renal Cell Carcinoma Simulating Macrophages

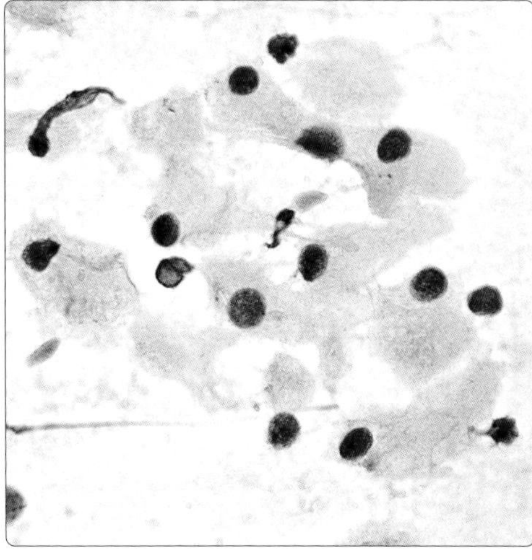

(Left) *Most melanomas in smear preparations leave monomorphous cells with short processes and oval nuclei with intranuclear inclusions ⇨. Pigmentation is variable and usually slight. There is none here.* **(Right)** *In smear preparations, deceptively bland cells of renal cell carcinoma may appear like macrophages.*

Smear: GBM

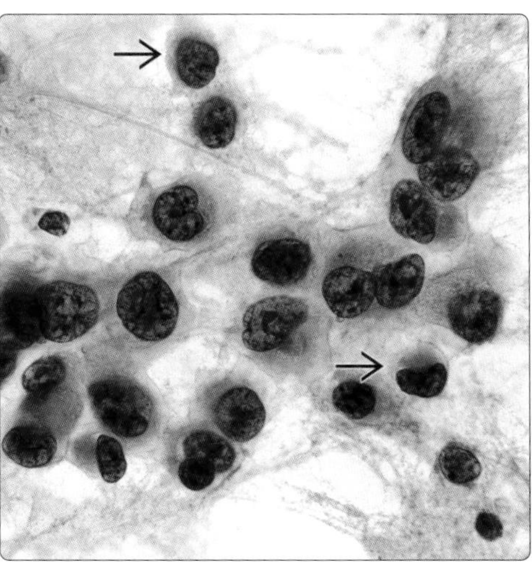

Smear: Glioblastoma With Fibrillary Cell Processes

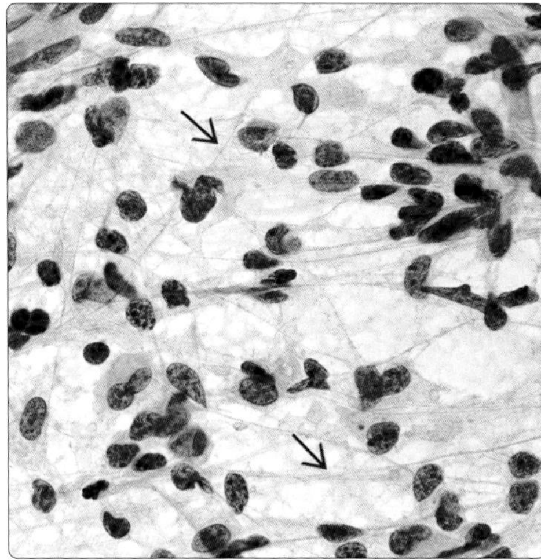

(Left) *The pleomorphic cells seen in this smear of GBM can easily simulate a metastasis, especially since some of the cells manifest rounded, cytoplasmic profiles ⇨. Some fibrillary background is present, however.* **(Right)** *In contrast to metastases, glioblastomas smear as tissue fragments with cells embedded in a fibrillar matrix created by tumor cell processes ⇨. Nuclei are smaller and more delicate than those of almost all carcinomas.*

PART I
SECTION 2
Sellar Region

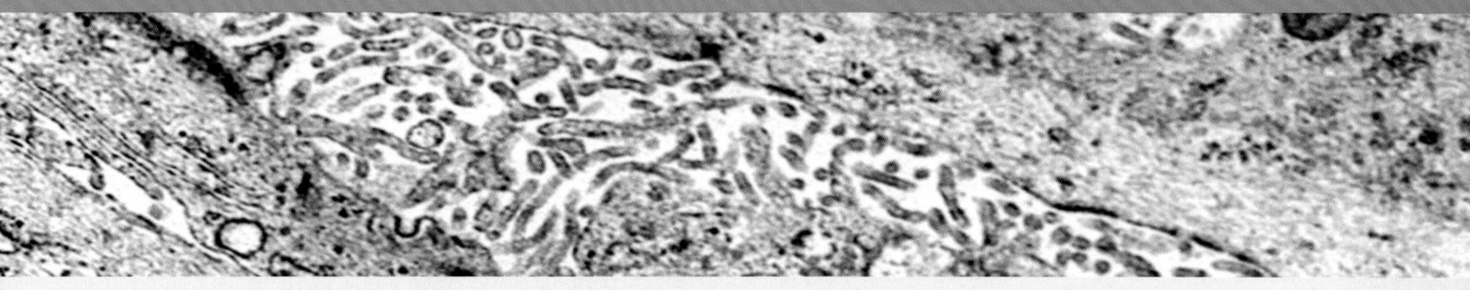

Adenohypophyseal Neoplasia and Hyperplasia

Neurohypophyseal and Hypothalamic Neoplasms

Craniopharyngiomas

Miscellaneous Neoplasms

Pituitary Adenoma

KEY FACTS

CLINICAL ISSUES

- Occur mainly in 4th-7th decade
- Often present with clinical features of hormone excess
- Larger adenomas often present with mass effects
- Typical approach via transsphenoidal route
- Drugs: Dopamine agonists, somatostatin analogs, growth hormone receptor antagonists, temozolomide
- Conventional radiotherapy for incompletely resected or recurrent tumors

IMAGING

- With rare exception (e.g., suprasellar or sphenoid sinus), arise in sella
- Extensions: Suprasellar, lateral (cavernous sinus), inferior (sphenoid sinus), posterior fossa
- Enhance, but less and delayed than normal gland

ANCILLARY TESTS

- Periodic acid-Schiff (PAS) to highlight ACTH cells and effacement of acinar architecture
- Reticulin stain reveals loss of acinar pattern
- Ultrastructural study necessary for classification in minority of cases
- Most adenomas are typical: Mitoses rare, Ki-67 < 3%
  - Atypical adenomas: Values for Ki-67 > 3%
  - Some pathologists prefer not to use atypical in diagnostic line, but rather descriptively sign out as adenoma with elevated cell cycle labeling with further comment that closer follow-up for recurrence is advised
  - Atypical adenomas should not automatically be treated with radiation therapy
- IHC has key role in clinical and biochemical correlation
  - GH, PRL, ACTH, LH, FSH, TSH, and α-subunit

Coronal MR: Sequential Images

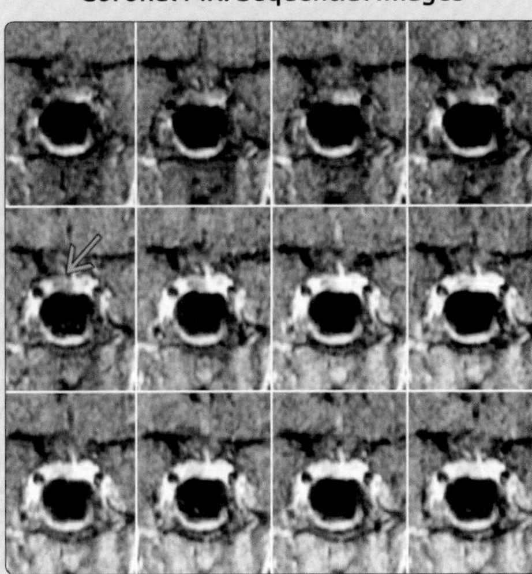

Smear: Cytological Monotony

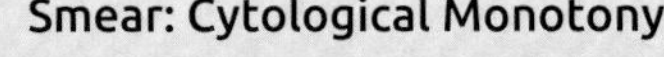

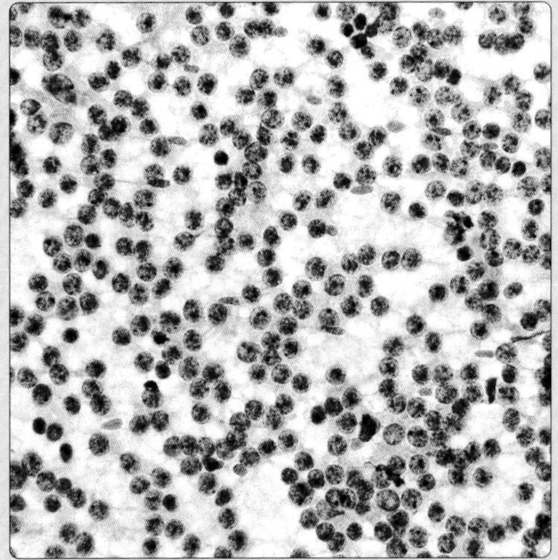

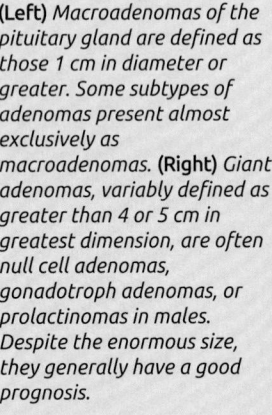

(Left) *Coronal T1 C+ MR shows multiple, rapidly sequential, dynamic images in the same plane obtained in a patient with microadenoma. The tumor* ➡ *enhances less rapidly than a normal adjacent gland.* **(Right)** *A myriad of cytologically monomorphous cells with round nuclei are characteristic of pituitary adenomas in smear preparations.*

Sagittal MR: Macroadenoma

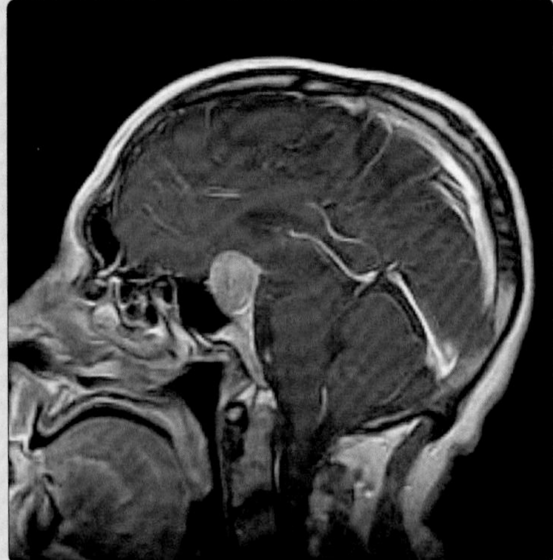

Sagittal MR: Giant Adenoma

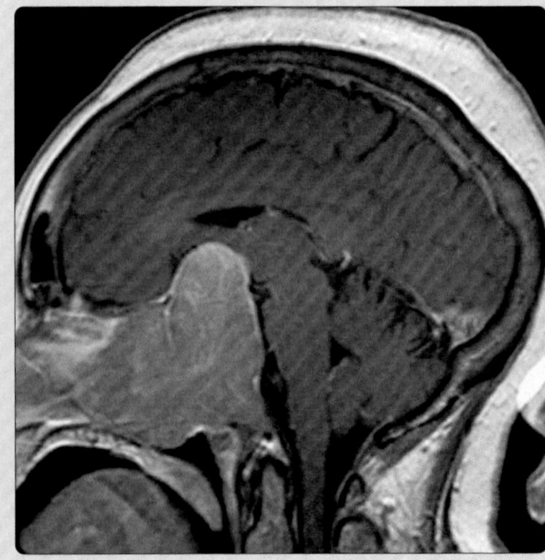

(Left) *Macroadenomas of the pituitary gland are defined as those 1 cm in diameter or greater. Some subtypes of adenomas present almost exclusively as macroadenomas.* **(Right)** *Giant adenomas, variably defined as greater than 4 or 5 cm in greatest dimension, are often null cell adenomas, gonadotroph adenomas, or prolactinomas in males. Despite the enormous size, they generally have a good prognosis.*

TERMINOLOGY

Definitions

- Adenohypophysial tumors composed of secretory cells demonstrating pituitary hormone production

ETIOLOGY/PATHOGENESIS

Pathophysiology

- Adenoma genesis is multistep, multicausal process including initiation and progression phases
- Activated oncogenes/cell cycle defects: Pituitary tumor transforming gene (PTTG) protein, Ras, p27, p18, p16, cyclins
- Loss of tumor suppressor gene function (11q13)
- Pituitary defect likely and explained by clonal nature of adenomas
  - Hormone receptor abnormality
  - Signal transduction alterations
    - Growth factors and receptors: Fibroblast growth factor receptor, nerve growth factor receptor, epidermal growth factor receptor, vascular endothelial growth factor receptor, transforming growth factor alpha and beta
- Endocrine factors (e.g., physiologic alterations at hypothalamic or systemic level) may induce cell proliferation
  - Excess production of growth hormone-releasing hormone (GHRH), corticotropin-releasing hormone (CRH), thyrotrophin-releasing hormone (TRH), or gonadotropin hormone-releasing hormone (GnRH)
  - Target organ failure with feedback disruption
- Inherited
  - MEN1 with involvement of 11q13
  - Carney complex with involvement of 2p16 and 17q
  - Familial acromegaly with involvement of 11q13 and their loci
  - McCune-Albright syndrome with involvement of 20q13.2

CLINICAL ISSUES

Epidemiology

- Incidence
  - 10-15% of intracranial and 7.5% of CNS neoplasms
  - Mainly 4th-7th decade
    - Females at somewhat greater risk
  - Adenomas uncommon in children
    - 2% of all adenomas
    - Most PRL- or ACTH-producing
  - Incidental adenomas seen in 25% of autopsies
  - Clinical classification based on biochemical, imaging, and surgical findings

Site

- Vast majority in sella turcica
  - Rare, extrasellar examples on pituitary stalk
  - Ectopic adenomas often from pharyngeal pituitary
  - Rare prolactinoma in ovarian teratoma

Presentation

- Most with clinical features of hormone excess (often microadenomas)
- Larger adenomas (macroadenomas defined as > 1 cm) with mass effects
  - Headache and visual disturbance
  - Hypopituitarism due to decreased function of LH-FSH, TSH, &/or GH cells by compression of pituitary stalk and gland
  - Causes low-level hyperprolactinemia (usually < 150 ng/mL) (stalk section effect)
- Patterns of growth and extension vary
  - Lateral extension into cavernous sinuses with resultant cranial neuropathy
  - Upward extension with resultant hypothalamic dysfunction, obstructive hydrocephalus, and brain displacement (but not invasion)
  - Downward extension into paranasal sinuses
- Hemorrhagic necrosis of large adenomas (pituitary apoplexy), may be surgical emergency
- Diabetes insipidus rarely associated with pituitary adenoma; suggests alternate diagnosis

Treatment

- Surgical approaches
  - Principal treatment
    - Via transsphenoidal route, since minimally invasive
    - Transfrontal approach for macroadenomas with large suprasellar component
  - Repeat surgery indicated in
    - Rapid progression
    - Visual loss
    - Persistent hyperfunction of ACTH adenomas (Cushing disease)
    - Failure of medical therapy
    - Massive acute hemorrhage (pituitary apoplexy)
- Drugs
  - Dopamine agonists reduce PRL level and size of PRL adenomas
  - Somatostatin analogs
    - Interact with somatostatin receptors on GH and TSH adenoma cells, reduce hormone secretion
    - Partly inhibit IGF-1 production by liver, kidney, heart, and lungs
    - Cause little reduction in tumor volume
  - Growth hormone receptor antagonists result in normalization of IGF-1 levels
  - Cyproheptadine generally fails to reduce ACTH levels in Cushing disease
    - Medical agents reducing adrenal steroid hormone production more successful
  - Clinically, nonfunctioning tumors show variable or unsatisfactory response to medical therapy
  - Chemotherapy
    - Temozolomide for aggressive tumors
    - Other conventional chemotherapies unsuccessful
- Radiation
  - Conventional radiotherapy for incompletely resected or recurrent tumors
    - In patients medically unable to undergo surgical intervention
    - In patients with hormone-secreting tumors uncontrolled by other therapies

- Complications include hypopituitarism and postirradiation glioma/sarcoma
- Stereotactic radiosurgery increasingly used
  - Optic apparatus spared

IMAGING

General Features

- Location
  - With rare exception (suprasellar location, sphenoid sinus), arise in sella
- Size
  - Tumors < 1 cm: Microadenomas
  - Larger lesions: Macroadenomas
  - Rare tumors > 5 cm: Giant adenomas (some authors use > 4 cm)
- Extensions: Suprasellar, lateral (cavernous sinus), inferior (sphenoid sinus), posterior fossa

Radiographic Findings

- Radiographic grading based on adenoma effects upon sella
  - Grade 0: Microadenomas not associated with enlargement
  - Grade 1: Intrasellar adenomas with only slight enlargement
  - Grades 2-4: Macroadenomas showing diffuse sellar enlargement without bone erosion, focal bone erosion, and extensive invasion/destruction, respectively
- Simple finding of dural invasion common when sought microscopically (up to 95%), but present in only 40% of adenomas radiographically or operatively

MR Findings

- Assessment of adenoma size best achieved by MR
- Typical MR study consists of coronal, 3 mm sections studied on T1-weighted images pre- and post-gadolinium administration
  - Adenomas enhance, but delayed and less than normal gland
  - Midline infundibulum; slight convexity of superior pituitary surface
- Sagittal imaging occasionally utilized
- CT less sensitive and specific than MR, given artifacts related to surrounding bone and, to some extent, soft tissue contrast

MICROSCOPIC

Histologic Features

- Multiple methods routinely applied
  - H&E to show tinctorial characteristics of cells (acidophilic, basophilic, chromophobic)
    - Terms not closely correlated with specific hormone production
    - Designations not intended as diagnostic terms (e.g., chromophobic adenoma)
  - Most adenomas uniform in cell makeup
    - Most have round, polygonal, or, occasionally, elongate cells with round to ovoid nuclei, delicately stippled chromatin, inconspicuous nucleoli, and moderately abundant cytoplasm
    - Atypia uncommon and mitoses rare

ANCILLARY TESTS

Histochemistry

- Periodic acid-Schiff (PAS) to highlight ACTH cells and effacement of acinar architecture
- Reticulin stain reveals loss of acinar pattern

Immunohistochemistry

- Key role in clinical and biochemical correlation
- All synaptophysin (+), but less frequently for chromogranin-A (+) (70%, mostly FSH-LH, null cell, TSH types) or low molecular weight keratin (+) (85%)
- Adenoma classification now largely based on hormonal immunotype
- Hormones routinely sought usually include
  - GH, PRL, ACTH, LH, FSH, TSH, and α-subunit
- Ki-67 elevation in atypical adenoma (defined as > 3% labeling rate)
- Pituitary adenomas show specific transcription factor expression profiles, i.e., almost all either SF1(+), PIT-1(+), or Tpit(+)

Electron Microscopy

- Specific morphologic features are original basis of classification
- Ultrastructural study still necessary for classification of several adenoma variants

Grading

- Most adenomas are typical
  - Mitoses uncommon; Ki-67 & p53 < 3%
- Atypical adenomas
  - Values for Ki-67 and p53 > above

DIFFERENTIAL DIAGNOSIS

Normal Adenohypophysis

- Normal acini by reticulin staining

Pituitary Nodular Hyperplasia

- Enlarged acini by reticulin staining

Metastatic Carcinoma

- Degree of cytological atypia incompatible with pituitary adenoma
- Cannot be diagnosed based on sellar biopsy
  - Rare carcinomas usually produce hormone (GH, ACTH)
- Clinical work-up essential

Ependymoma

- Immunoreactive for GFAP rather than synaptophysin

Pituitary Blastoma

- Early childhood
- Small blastema-like cells, true rosettes, large glandular structures
  - *DICER1* mutation

SELECTED REFERENCES

1. Gomez-Hernandez K et al: Clinical implications of accurate subtyping of pituitary adenomas: perspectives from the treating physician. Turk Patoloji Derg. 31 Suppl 1:4-17, 2015
2. Kleinschmidt-DeMasters BK et al: An algorithmic approach to sellar region masses. Arch Pathol Lab Med. 139(3):356-72, 2015

Functional Classification of Pituitary Adenomas

Adenoma Type	Frequency (%)	Male:Female	IHC Profile	Clinical Presentation
Sparsely granulated PRL-cell adenoma	27.0	1:2.5	PRL, PIT-1	Females: Amenorrhea-galactorrhea syndrome; males: Sellar mass, hypogonadism
Densely granulated PRL-cell adenoma	0.04		PRL, PIT-1	
Densely granulated GH-cell adenoma	7.1	1:0.7	GH, α-subunit (PRL, TSH, LH, FSH), PIT-1	Acromegaly (adult) or gigantism (child)
Sparsely granulated GH-cell adenoma	6.2	1:1.1	GH (PRL, α-subunit), PIT-1	Acromegaly (adult) or gigantism (child)
Mixed GH-PRL cell adenoma	3.5	1:1.1	GH, PRL (α-subunit, TSH), PIT-1	Acromegaly + hyperprolactinemia
Mammosomatotroph adenoma	1.2	1:1.1	GH, PRL (α-subunit, TSH), PIT-1	Acromegaly + hyperprolactinemia
Acidophil stem cell adenoma	1.6	1:1.5	PRL, GH, PIT-1	Hyperprolactinemia; acromegaly is uncommon
Densely granulated corticotroph adenoma	9.6	1:5.4	ACTH (LH, α-subunit), Tpit	Cushing disease, Nelson syndrome
Sparsely granulated corticotroph adenoma	Rare		ACTH, Tpit	Cushing disease, Nelson syndrome
Thyrotroph adenoma	1.1	1:1.3	TSH (GH, PRL, α-subunit), PIT-1	Hyperthyroidism
Gonadotroph adenoma	9.8	1:0.8	FSH, LH, α-subunit (ACTH), SF1	Clinically nonfunctioning sellar mass
Silent corticotroph adenoma subtype 1 apoplexy	1.5	1:1.7	ACTH, Tpit	Nonfunctioning sellar mass, pituitary
Silent corticotroph adenoma subtype 2	2.0	1:0.2	β-endorphin, ACTH, Tpit	Clinically nonfunctioning sellar mass
Silent adenoma subtype 3	1.4	1:1.1	Any combination of anterior pituitary hormones	Females: Mimics PRL-secreting adenoma; males: Nonfunctioning sellar mass
Hormone-negative adenoma (formerly null cell)	12.4	1:0.7	Usually SF1(+)	Clinically nonfunctioning sellar mass
Oncocytoma [usually SF1(+)]	13.4	1:0.5	Immunonegative (FSH, LH, TSH, α-subunit) &/or SF1	Clinically nonfunctioning sellar mass
Unclassified adenomas	1.8			Variable

3. Nishioka H et al: The complementary role of transcription factors in the accurate diagnosis of clinically nonfunctioning pituitary adenomas. Endocr Pathol. ePub, 2015
4. Kiseljak-Vassiliades K et al: Growth hormone tumor histological subtypes predict response to surgical and medical therapy. Endocrine. ePub, 2014
5. Madsen H et al: Giant pituitary adenomas: pathologic-radiographic correlations and lack of role for p53 and MIB-1 labeling. Am J Surg Pathol. 35(8):1204-13, 2011
6. Yu R et al: Pathogenesis of pituitary tumors. Prog Brain Res. 182:207-27, 2010
7. Asa SL et al: The pathogenesis of pituitary tumours. Nat Rev Cancer. 2(11):836-49, 2002
8. Meij BP et al: The long-term significance of microscopic dural invasion in 354 patients with pituitary adenomas treated with transsphenoidal surgery. J Neurosurg. 96(2):195-208, 2002
9. Woloschak M et al: Frequent inactivation of the p16 gene in human pituitary tumors by gene methylation. Mol Carcinog. 19(4):221-4, 1997
10. Young WF Jr et al: Gonadotroph adenoma of the pituitary gland: a clinicopathologic analysis of 100 cases. Mayo Clin Proc. 71(7):649-56, 1996
11. Pei L et al: Frequent loss of heterozygosity at the retinoblastoma susceptibility gene (RB) locus in aggressive pituitary tumors: evidence for a chromosome 13 tumor suppressor gene other than RB. Cancer Res. 55(8):1613-6, 1995
12. Terada T et al: Incidence, Pathology, and Recurrence of Pituitary Adenomas: Study of 647 Unselected Surgical Cases. Endocr Pathol. 6(4):301-310, 1995
13. Kane LA et al: Pituitary adenomas in childhood and adolescence. J Clin Endocrinol Metab. 79(4):1135-40, 1994
14. Pojunas KW et al: MR imaging of prolactin-secreting microadenomas. AJNR Am J Neuroradiol. 7(2):209-13, 1986
15. Scheithauer BW et al: Pathology of invasive pituitary tumors with special reference to functional classification. J Neurosurg. 65(6):733-44, 1986
16. Hardy J et al: Transsphenoidal neurosurgery of intracranial neoplasm. Adv Neurol. 15:261-73, 1976

(Left) *The midsagittal section of the sellar region shows a pituitary gland with anterior and posterior lobes. The pituitary stalk ⇨, posterior-inferior to the optic chiasm ⇨, connects the posterior lobe and hypothalamus.* **(Right)** *Horizontal cross section of a normal pituitary gland shows localizations of anterior lobe cells. LH-FSH cells are distributed diffusely. Lateral wings contain mainly GH and PRL cells. Corticotrophs and thyrotrophs are in the median mucoid wedge.*

Whole Mount, Normal Pituitary

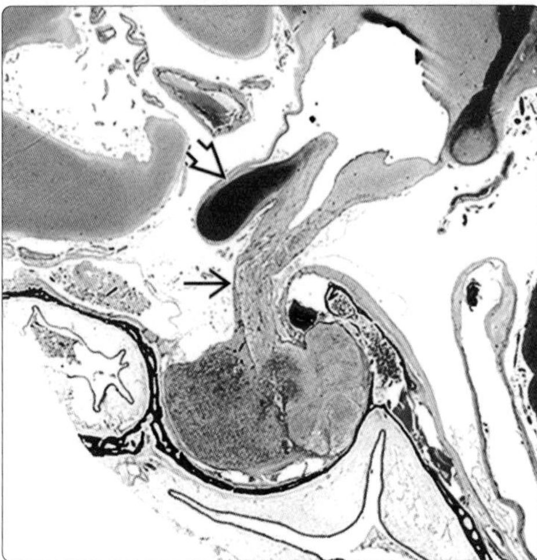

Cell Type Distribution, Normal Pituitary

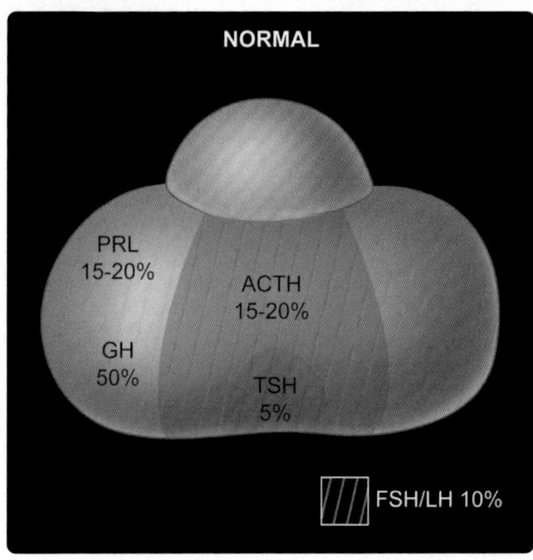

(Left) *Horizontal section of a normal pituitary gland shows a remnant of the Rathke pouch ➡, a normal developmental rest that, after formation of the anterior lobe, often persists as a cleft between the anterior ➡ and posterior lobes ⇨.* **(Right)** *Normal adenohypophysis is composed of an admixture of intraacinar eosinophilic, basophilic, and chromophobic cells.*

Normal Pituitary, Intermediate Lobe

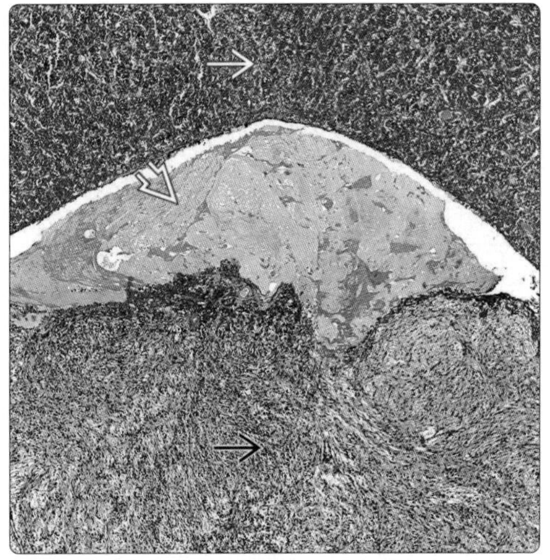

Normal Anterior Pituitary

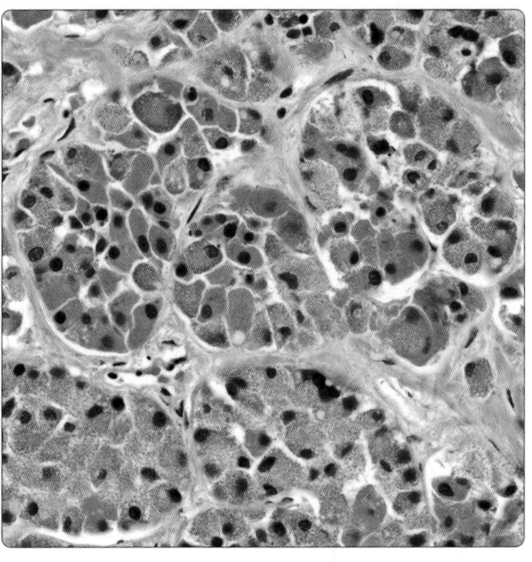

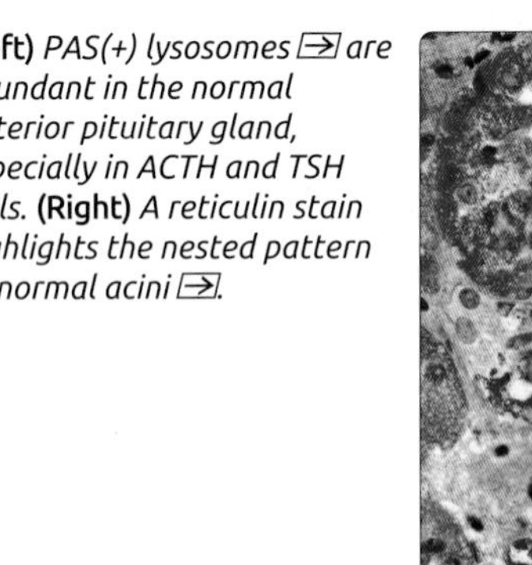

(Left) *PAS(+) lysosomes ⇨ are abundant in the normal anterior pituitary gland, especially in ACTH and TSH cells.* **(Right)** *A reticulin stain highlights the nested pattern of normal acini ⇨.*

PAS(+) Lysosomes, Normal ACTH, and TSH Cells

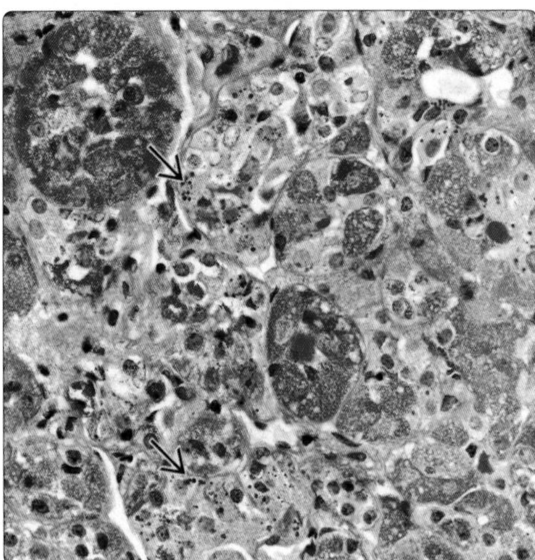

Normal Acinar Pattern, Reticulin

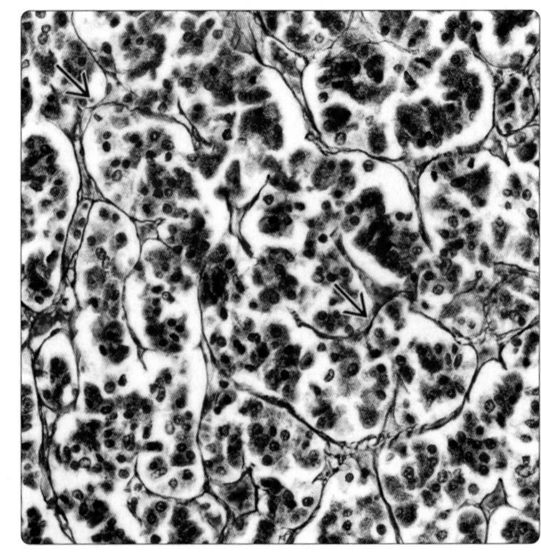

Normal Squamous Metaplasia

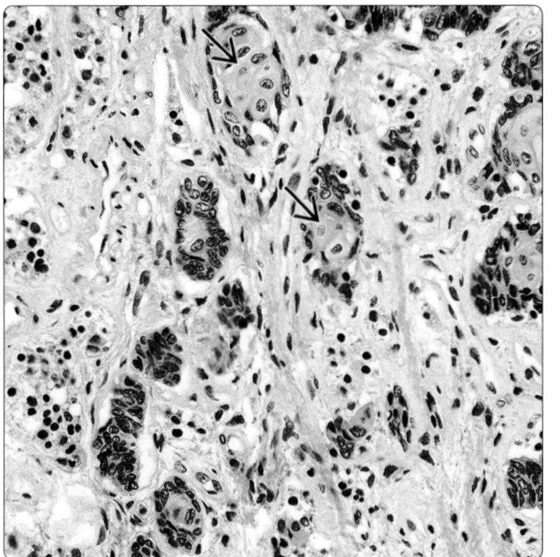

Normal Basophil Invasion

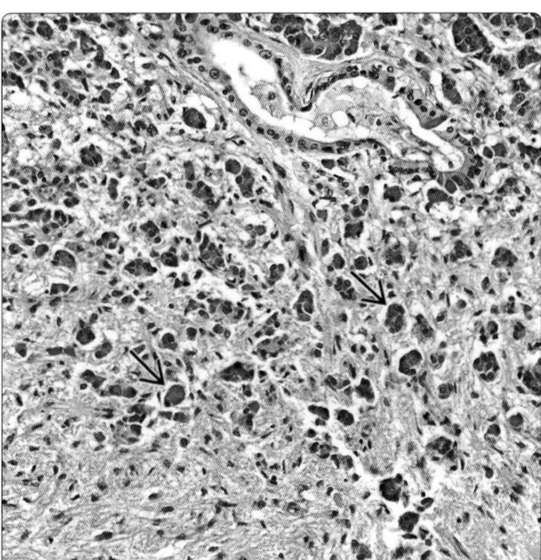

(Left) *Anterior pituitary cells along the anterior pituitary stalk may undergo squamous metaplasia ⇨. This should not be mistaken for neoplasia.* **(Right)** *Basophils ⇨ may extend into the neurohypophysis. Such cells are PAS and ACTH positive. Termed basophil invasion, this phenomenon should not be misinterpreted as infiltration of neurohypophysis by an adenoma. This phenomenon is particularly likely to be seen in older patients.*

Normal Posterior Pituitary

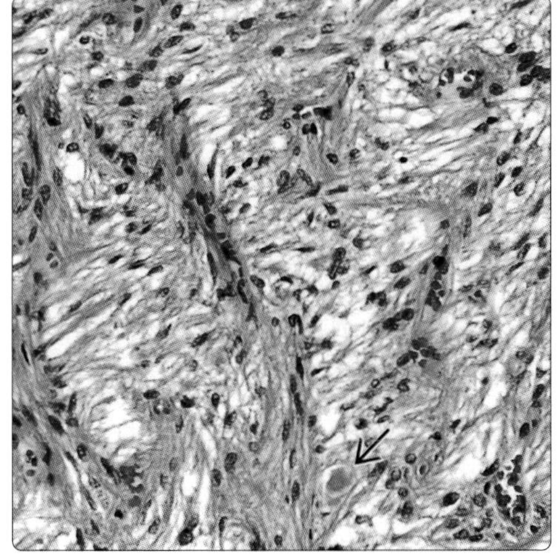

Normal Posterior Pituitary, Herring Bodies

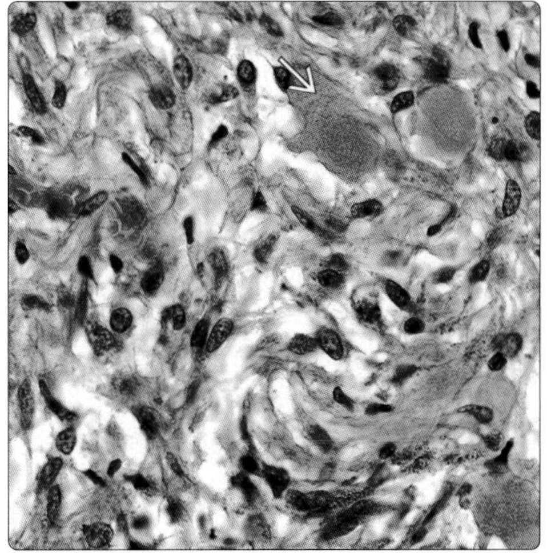

(Left) *Normal neurohypophysis is composed of unmyelinated axons of hypothalamic neurosecretory neurons, fusiform pituicytes derived from glial cells, and abundant capillaries. This part of the pituitary has a direct arterial blood supply, unlike the anterior pituitary with only its portal system. Axonal swellings (Herring bodies) ⇨ are distinctive features.* **(Right)** *Axonal swellings in neurohypophysis are known as Herring bodies ➡.*

Neurohypophysin

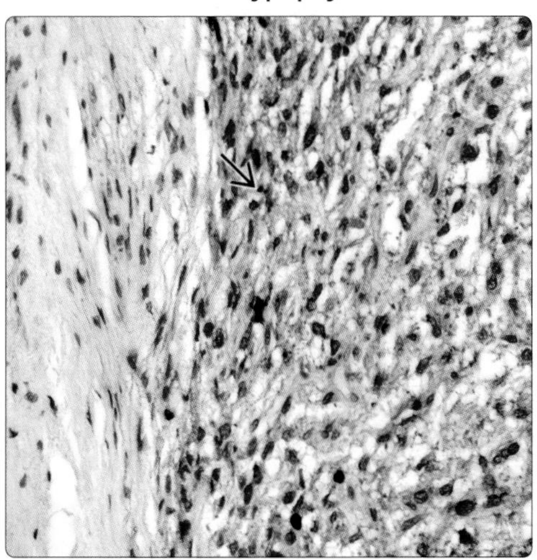

Vasopressin-Rich Axonal Processes

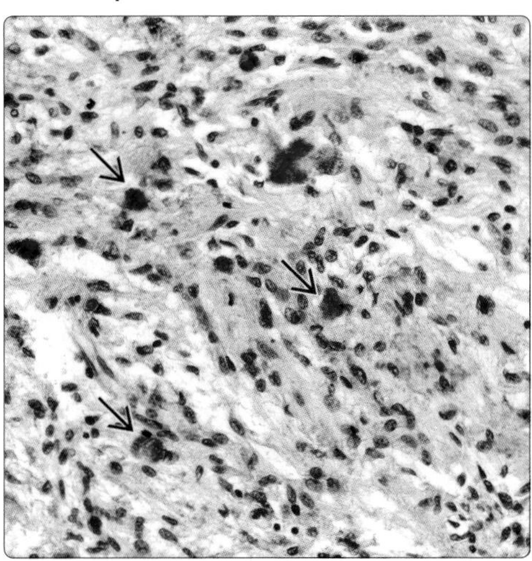

(Left) *In normal neurohypophysis, immunostaining for neurohypophysin ⇨, vasopressin, and oxytocin are noted in axons and neurosecretory vesicles.* **(Right)** *Herring bodies ⇨ and axons in neurohypophysis are rich in vasopressin, a key hormone in water metabolism.*

Adenoma

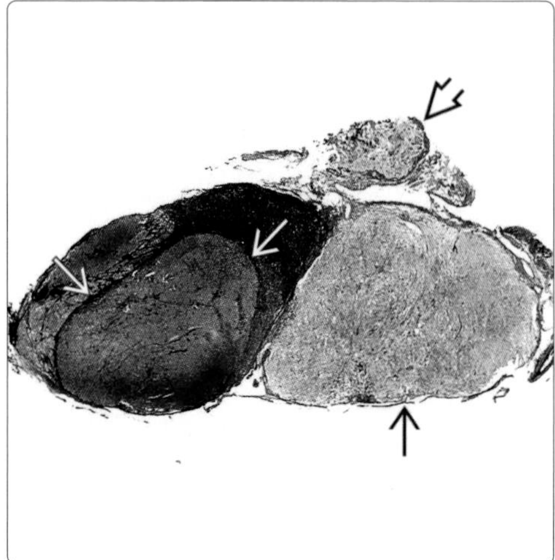

Adenoma, Reticulin

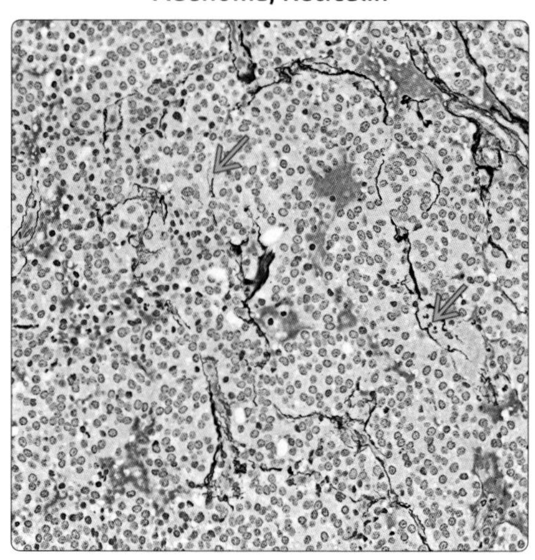

(Left) *In this sagittal section of a pituitary gland, an adenoma ➔ enlarges the anterior lobe. The posterior lobe → and stalk ⇒ are present in the same section. The discreteness of the adenoma is apparent.* **(Right)** *Reticulin staining helps to identify adenomas because of their distorted and fragmented reticulin pattern →. The gland's normal acinar architecture is missing.*

Crush Artifact, Normal Pituitary

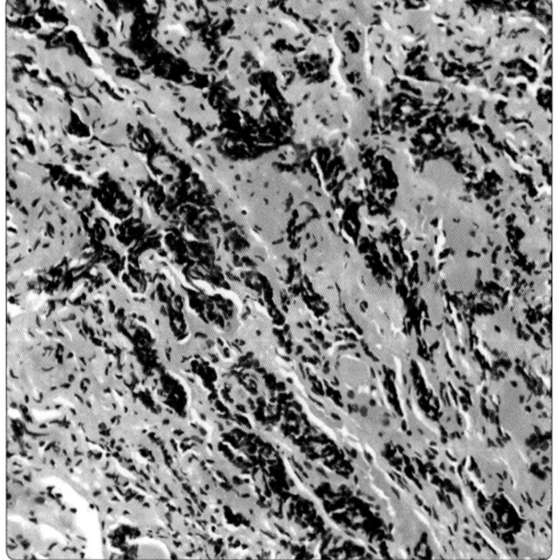

Freezing Artifact, Adenoma

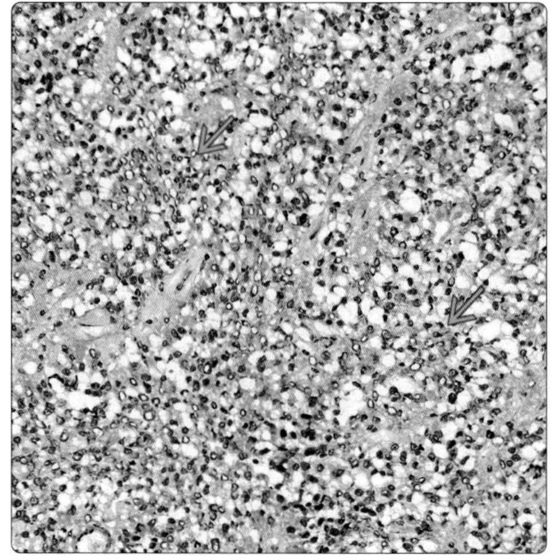

(Left) *Crush artifact of a normal anterior lobe resembles small cell carcinoma. Such artifactual compression and loss of detail is present in both frozen sections and, as seen here, in frozen tissue that had been processed for permanent sections.* **(Right)** *Freezing tissue for intraoperative diagnosis may result in interpretation challenges later, as in this case, where clustered tumor cells → simulate normal adenohypophyseal acini.*

Smear, Normal Pituitary, Admixed Cell Types

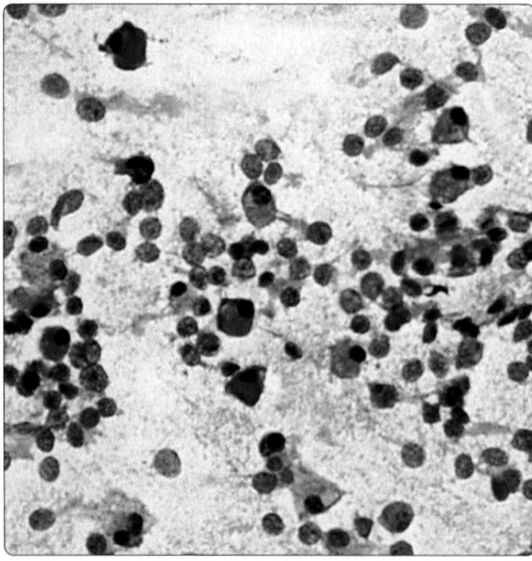

Smear, Adenoma, Mitosis

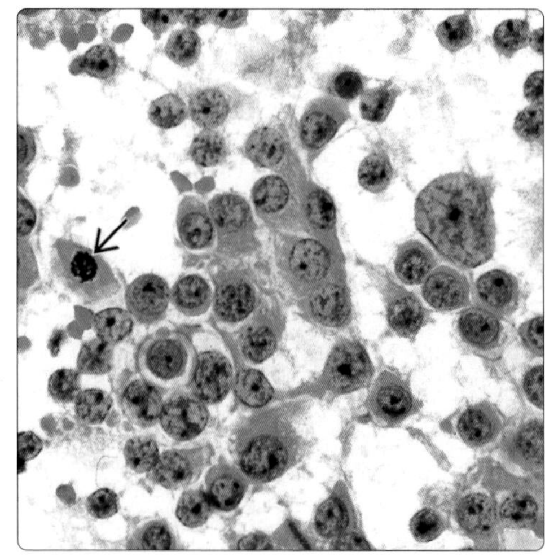

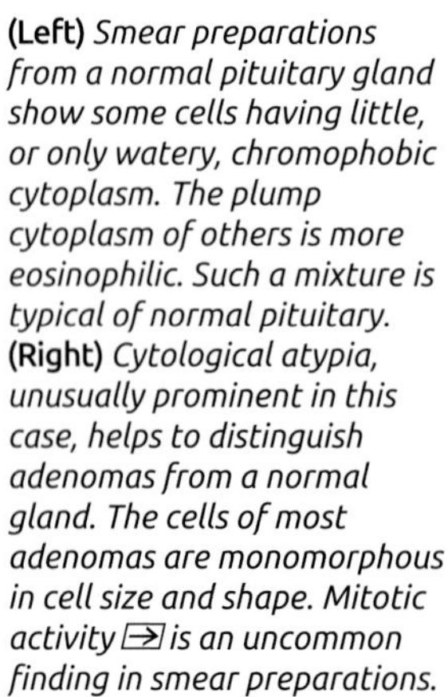

(Left) *Smear preparations from a normal pituitary gland show some cells having little, or only watery, chromophobic cytoplasm. The plump cytoplasm of others is more eosinophilic. Such a mixture is typical of normal pituitary.* **(Right)** *Cytological atypia, unusually prominent in this case, helps to distinguish adenomas from a normal gland. The cells of most adenomas are monomorphous in cell size and shape. Mitotic activity → is an uncommon finding in smear preparations.*

Adenoma, Sheet-Like Architecture

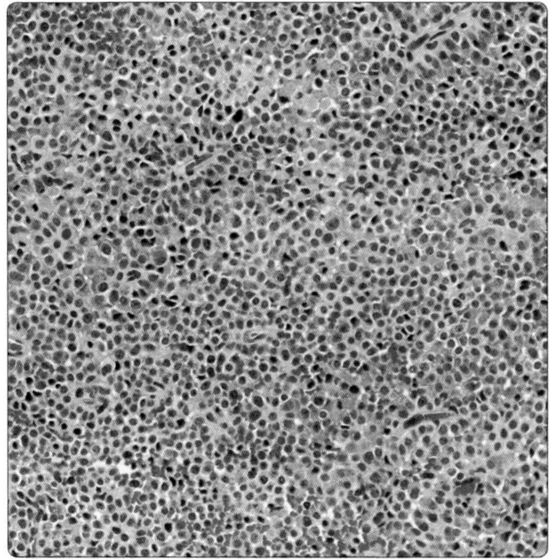

Papillary Architecture, Adenoma

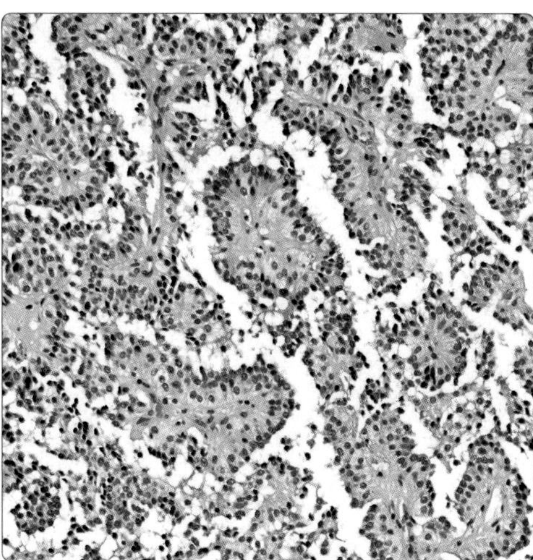

(Left) *Unlike the acinar pattern of normal adenohypophysis, a diffuse, sheet-like architecture typifies most pituitary adenomas. Synaptophysin staining can be used to remove any doubts about the nature of the lesion, since almost all adenomas are positive. There are a few alternate diagnoses in the face of a positive lesion.* **(Right)** *Papillary formation may be prominent, particularly in nonfunctioning (FSH-LH, null cell) adenomas.*

Simulating Ependymoma

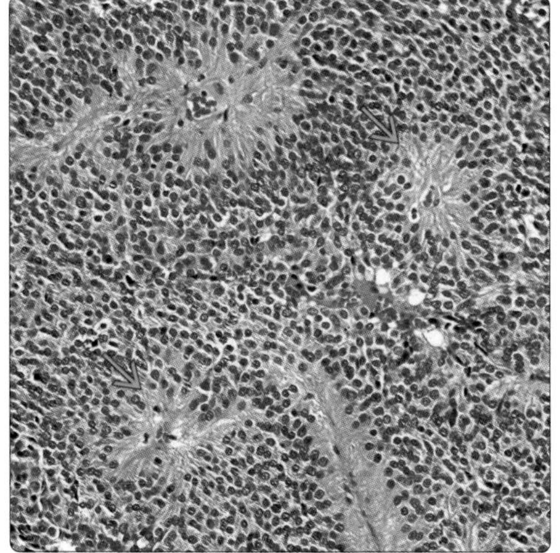

Macronodular Pattern, Adenoma

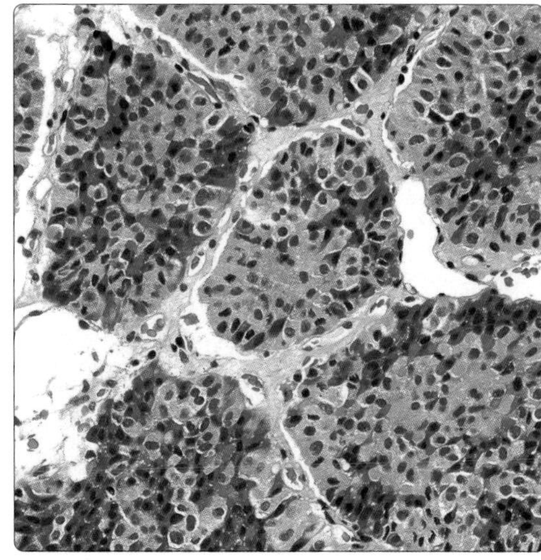

(Left) *Ependymoma-like perivascular pseudorosettes* ⇒ *are common in nonfunctioning (FSH-LH, null cell) adenomas.* **(Right)** *Adenomas may show variable patterns, including the unusual macronodular pattern in this case.*

Ribbon-Like Pattern, Adenoma

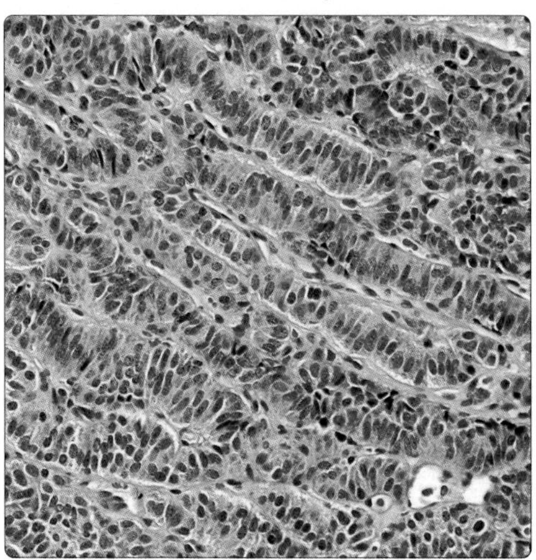

Neuronal Metaplasia, Adenoma

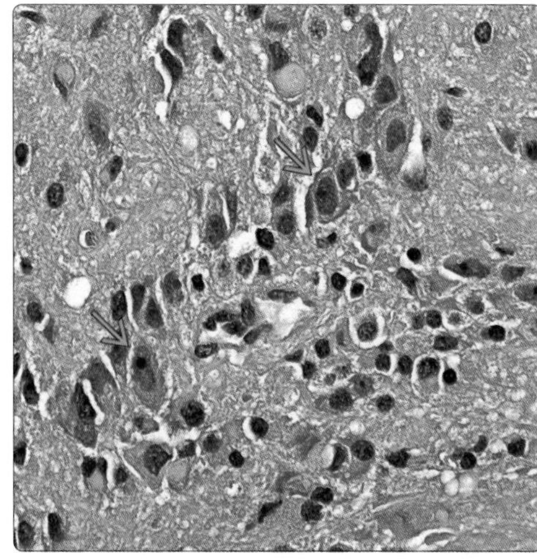

(Left) *Ribbon-like arrays are present in a minority of pituitary adenomas. These constructs are more elongate than the spherical formations of normal acini.* **(Right)** *Neuronal metaplasia of pituitary adenoma is a rare occurrence, generally appearing in growth hormone-producing types. Note ganglion cells* ⇒ *and finely fibrillar neuropil. Typical, cellular pituitary adenoma was present elsewhere.*

(Left) *Gland formation is most often seen in gonadotrophic adenomas and prolactinomas. There should be no doubt about the nature of the lesion, given sheet-like architecture and round, cytologically bland cells.* **(Right)** *Glands within pituitary adenomas may produce mucin ⇨, as is seen here with mucicarmine staining.*

Gland Formation, Adenoma

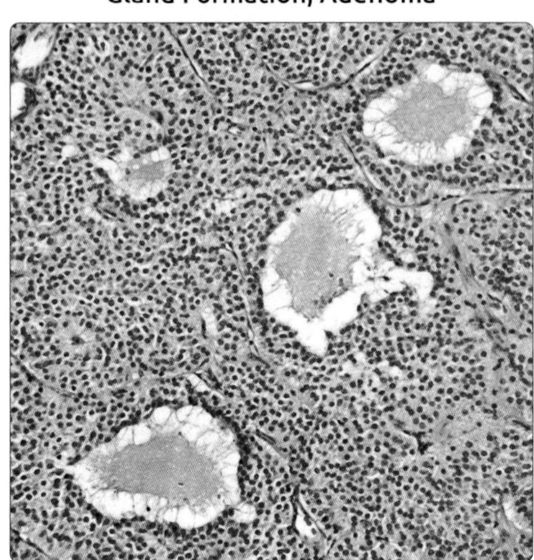

Mucin, Adenoma

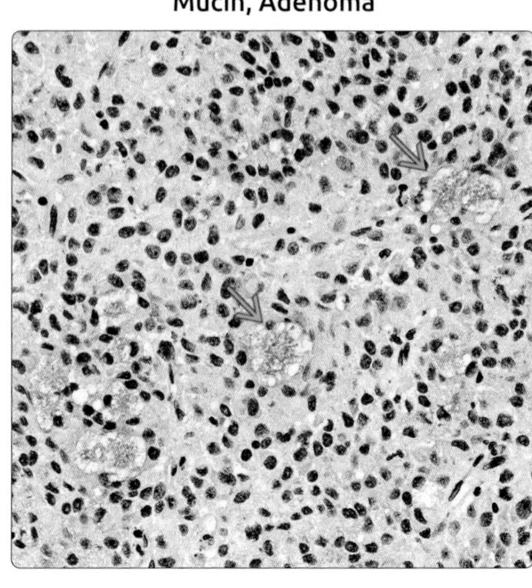

(Left) *Presenting as a surgical emergency, sudden enlargement of an adenoma associated with hemorrhagic infarction ⇨ is termed pituitary apoplexy. This small example shows peripheral organization. Surgical specimens often show only recently necrotic tumor and hemorrhage. Reticulin staining may be preserved, however, and the fragmented state typical of an adenoma may be apparent.* **(Right)** *More than an occasional mitosis ⇨ should raise the suspicion of atypical adenoma.*

Organized Hemorrhage, Adenoma

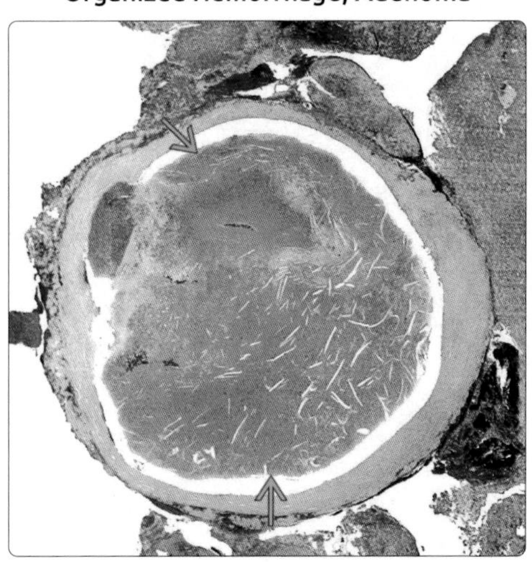

Mitosis

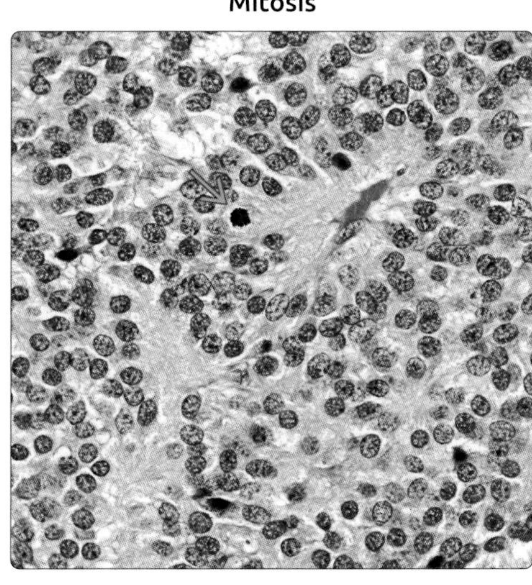

(Left) *Ki-67 labeling index is very low, except in atypical adenomas, as seen here. Nucleoli were somewhat prominent in this case. Some pathologists prefer to designate these descriptively as pituitary adenoma with elevated labeling rate rather than atypical, with the comment that closer follow-up is advised.* **(Right)** *As in this case, all pituitary adenomas are synaptophysin positive. Chromogranin immunopositivity varies in frequency and is most common in null cell, FSH/LH, and TSH cell adenomas.*

Elevated Ki-67, Atypical Adenoma

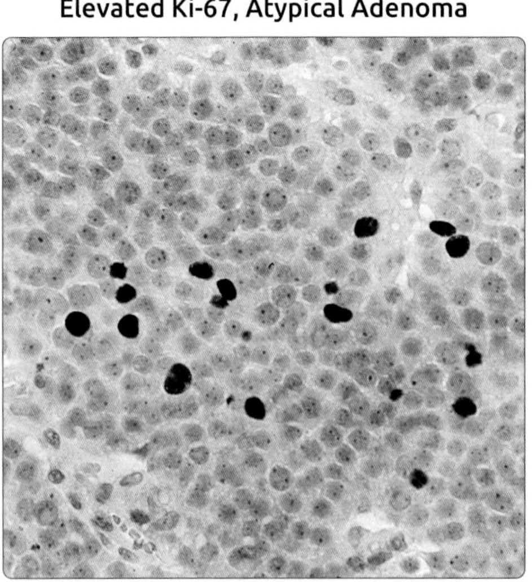

Synaptophysin, Adenoma

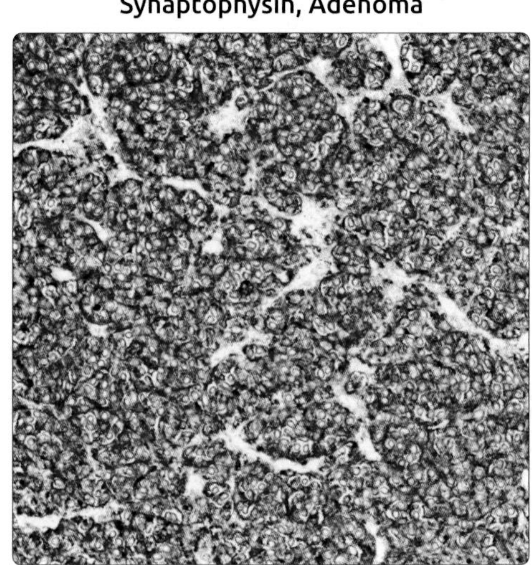

Normal Anterior Pituitary Cell Assortment

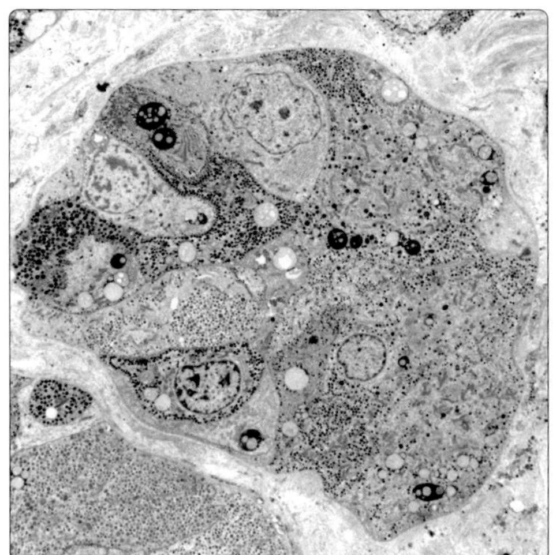

Normal Growth Hormone Cells

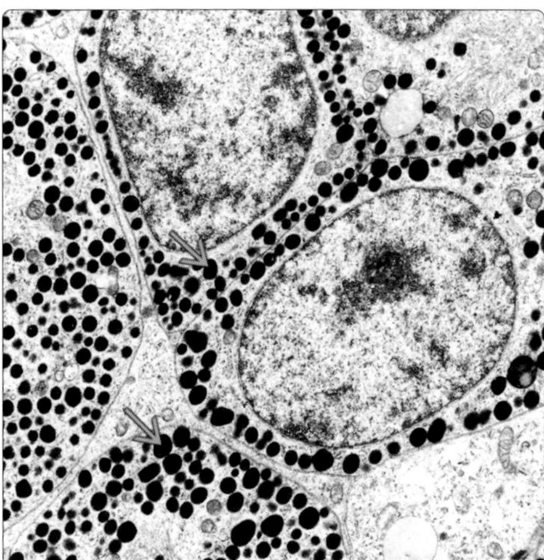

(Left) *Normal pituitary acini consists of an admixture of cells. This ultrastructural figure demonstrates the variation of each cell with different nuclear shape and diversity in the size of granules.* **(Right)** *Ultrastructurally, normal growth hormone cells are medium-sized, ovoid cells with central nuclei and numerous large secretory granules ⇒.*

Normal Prolactin Cells

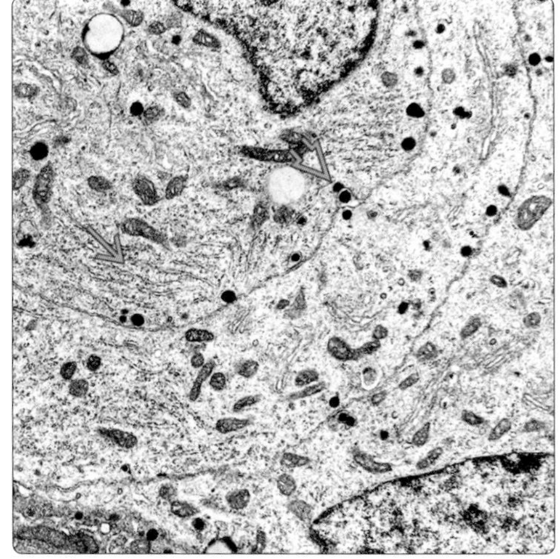

Normal Corticotroph Cells

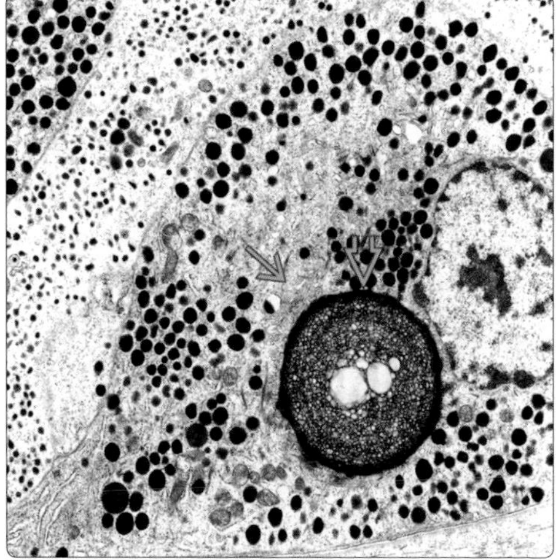

(Left) *Normal prolactin cells have abundant rough endoplasmic reticulum ⇒ and well-developed Golgi complexes. Granule extrusion (exocytosis) ⇒ is misplaced, occurring at lateral cell membranes.* **(Right)** *Normal corticotroph cells typically contain a large lysosome ⇒, secretory granules (150-450 nm) somewhat variable in morphology, and bundles of keratin filaments ⇒.*

Normal Gonadotroph Cells

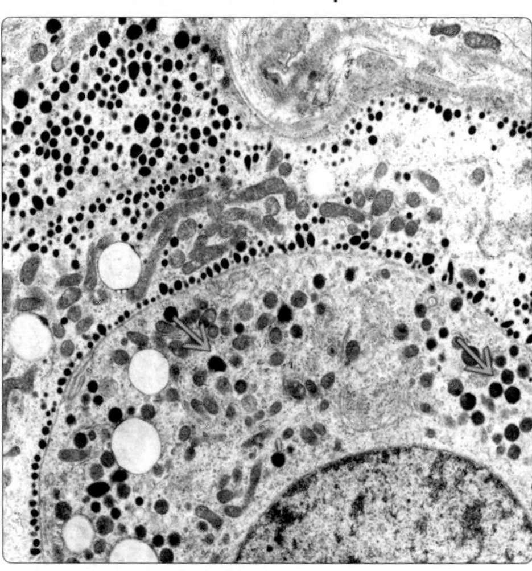

Normal TSH Cells

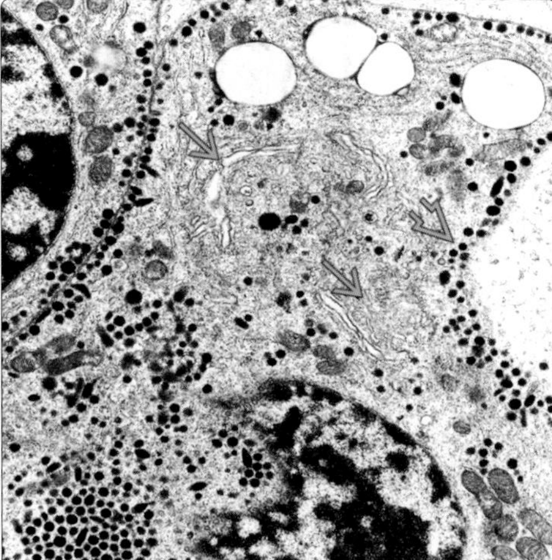

(Left) *Normal gonadotroph cells have lucent, spherical nuclei, rounded Golgi apparatus, and numerous, variably electron-dense, 200-350 nm secretory granules ⇒.* **(Right)** *Normal TSH cells are angulated and have peripherally situated secretory granules ⇒ and prominent Golgi complexes ⇒.*

KEY FACTS

CLINICAL ISSUES

- Most common pituitary adenomas
- Mostly affect young females as microadenomas
- Cause amenorrhea/galactorrhea
- Mostly affect males as invasive macroadenomas, usually lack endocrine symptoms
- Blood prolactin (PRL) levels parallel tumor size
- Dopamine agonist therapy has replaced surgery as primary treatment
  - 40% ultimately escape medical therapy

IMAGING

- MR: Hypointensity relative to pituitary
- Hemorrhage &/or cystic change (apoplexy) mainly in macroadenomas

MACROSCOPIC

- Size: 33% micro (< 1 cm), 67% macro (> 1 cm)

MICROSCOPIC

- Chromophobic adenomas (sparsely granulated) common
- Eosinophilic (densely granulated) rare
- 10% feature calcospherites
- Interstitial endocrine amyloid may form massive laminated spheres

ANCILLARY TESTS

- Sparsely granulated (chromophobic) adenomas show paranuclear PRL immunoreactivity
- Recurrence more likely if Ki-67 exceeds 3%
- Diffuse immunoreactivity for nuclear PIT-1 transcription factor

TOP DIFFERENTIAL DIAGNOSES

- Pituitary thyrotroph hyperplasia
  - Mimics PRL cell adenoma by PRL immunopositivity
  - Reticulin shows enlargement, but not destruction, of acini

(Left) *Pituitary adenomas ➔ are well-circumscribed intrasellar masses that may compress the normal gland ➔.* **(Right)** *Most prolactinomas in premenopausal females present as a microadenoma, as in this small version that erodes the sellar floor ➔ and compresses the normal gland ➔.*

Pituitary Adenoma Compressing Normal Gland

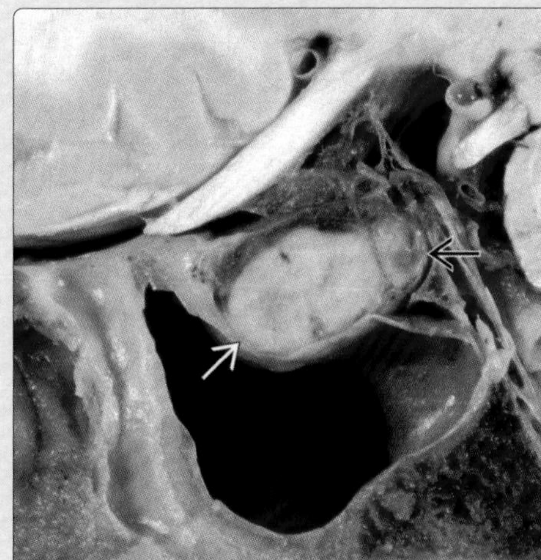

Microadenoma in Premenopausal Women

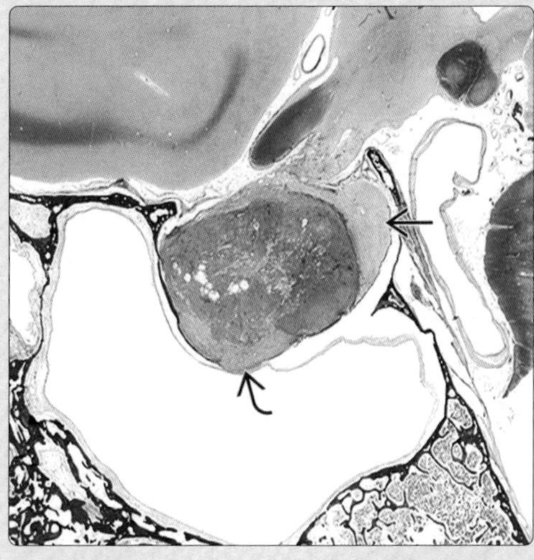

(Left) *Paranuclear Golgi pattern of prolactin (PRL) staining is characteristic of prolactinoma. Note the diffuse immunoreactivity throughout the adenoma cell population; this is typical of prolactinomas.* **(Right)** *Prolactinomas will manifest nuclear PIT-1 immunoreactivity.*

Prolactin IHC(+) Diffuse

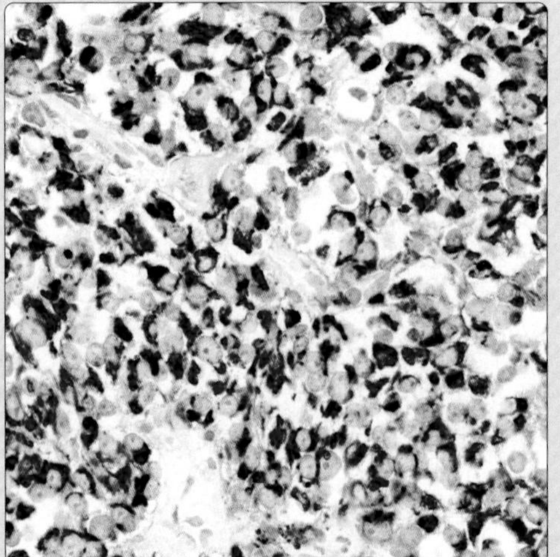

PIT-1 Nuclear Transcription Factor

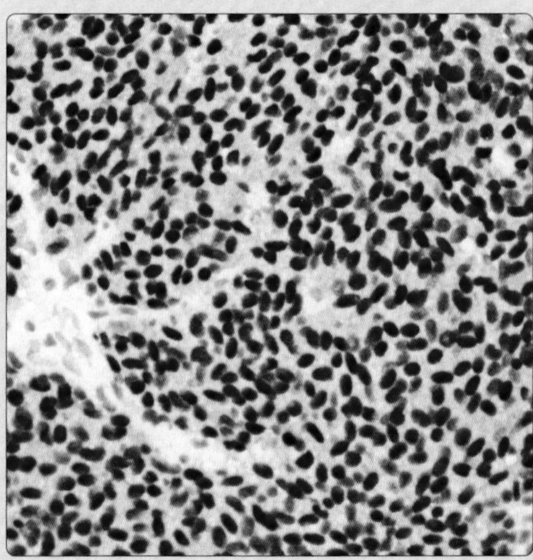

TERMINOLOGY

Synonyms

- Lactotroph adenoma

Definitions

- Benign adenohypophysial tumor composed entirely of prolactin (PRL) cells
- Positive for transcription factor PIT-1

ETIOLOGY/PATHOGENESIS

Pathophysiology

- Usually sporadic but may be MEN1 associated
- Isolated familial cases not associated with MEN1 rare
- Mechanisms of adenomagenesis unknown
  - Induced by estrogens in experimental animals but not in humans
  - Pregnancy results in marked stimulation in PRL cells but is not significant oncogenic factor
  - Rare induction after massive estrogen administration, presumably after phase of hyperplasia

Genetics

- Multiple karyotypic alterations
  - Trisomies of chromosomes 12 and less often 5, 7, 8, 9, 20
- Comparative genomic hybridization with imbalances in chromosomes, particularly in invasive and recurrent tumors
  - Imbalances in 50-80% of adenomas, more often gains of chromosomes 4q and 5q than losses of 1, 2, 11, and 13
- *RAS* oncogene mutations described in aggressive PRL cell adenomas, as well as primary PRL carcinomas and in their metastatic deposits

CLINICAL ISSUES

Epidemiology

- Incidence
  - 30% of operated pituitary adenomas
    - Frequent use of primary medical therapy (dopamine agonists) has drastically decreased number of operated adenomas
- Age
  - In females, 75% present between ages 20-40; in males, only 40% present between ages 20-40
    - Mean age in females: 25; males: 45
  - PItuitary adenomas in general are rare in children, but prolactinomas comprise significant proportion (40-50%) of pediatric adenomas
- Sex
  - Male:female = 1:5 in surgical series and 1:0.6 autopsy series

Site

- Small examples situated in posterolateral portions of anterior pituitary
- Rare ectopic sites: Suprasellar region, sphenoid sinus, or nasopharynx

Presentation

- Women present at younger ages and tend to have microadenomas, present with galactorrhea
- Males (90%) have endocrinologically inactive macroadenomas, as do postreproductive females
  - Very large PRL cell adenomas and PRL carcinomas occur almost entirely in men
- Mean serum PRL levels in men significantly higher (2,000 ng/mL) as compared to females (400 ng/mL) due to larger tumors
- Primary effect of hyperprolactinemia is secondary hypogonadism
  - In men: Decreased libido, impotence, and semen abnormalities
  - In females: Even minor PRL elevations alter function of LH/FSH cells, causing amenorrhea and infertility
- General manifestations in children include growth failure, headache, and visual disturbance
  - Pubertal females manifestations include menstrual abnormalities, galactorrhea, hypogonadism, and hypopituitarism
  - Pubertal males have visual impairment and headache since most (90%) are macroadenomas
- Present with hyperprolactinemia
  - Tumor size parallels PRL levels
    - Diagnosis requires exclusion of stalk section effect as basis of hyperprolactinemia
    - Generally < 100 ng/mL in microadenomas
    - Generally > 250 ng/mL in macroadenomas
    - Often > 1,000 ng/mL in invasive macroadenomas
    - PRL levels < 150 ng/mL can be due to compression of stalk (stalk section effect)

Treatment

- Surgery; transsphenoidal approach more effective for micro- than macroadenomas
  - Low recurrence (15%) at 10 years if postoperative normalization of PRL level
- Radiation therapy similarly effective
- Medical therapy (dopamine agonist) most effective
  - Causes dramatic shrinkage of cells and increased nuclear:cytoplasmic ratio
  - Ultrastructural correlate of cell shrinkage is marked diminution of RER and Golgi complexes, synthetic and packaging organelles of endocrine cells
  - Such treated, hyperchromatic-appearing tumors should not be mistaken for high-grade malignancy
  - PRL immunoreactivity typically decreased with treatment, only some cells remaining strongly immunopositive
  - Necrosis infrequent in medically treated examples
  - Extensive perivascular and interstitial fibrosis after protracted medical therapy (dopamine agonist)
  - Variations in D2 receptor may underlie therapeutic resistance
  - Effects of dopamine agonist treatment reversible upon discontinuance of treatment

Prognosis

- Overall recurrence rate usually under 20%
  - Macroadenomas (particularly in males and postreproductive females) show higher recurrence rates
- Significant decrease in mortality rates since introduction of dopamine agonists

- Favorable prognostic indicators include posttherapy normalization of PRL levels, be it due to surgical, medical, or radiotherapy
- Proliferation markers (mitoses and Ki-67) and p53 staining may fail to distinguish benign from aggressive or even malignant tumors
  - Recurrence more likely if Ki-67(+) and if p53 labeling index exceeds 3%

IMAGING

General Features

- Size
  - Microadenoma size often stable in reproductive females
  - In males and postreproductive females, begins as intrasellar microadenoma but comes to expand pituitary capsule and bony sella

MR Findings

- Generally hypointense relative to surrounding normal pituitary
  - Microadenomas: Less enhancement than normal anterior pituitary tissue immediately following gadolinium administration
    - After delay, differential enhancement appears, persisting in adenoma tissue
  - Macroadenomas: Generally marked contrast enhancement
- Hemorrhage and cyst formation (pituitary apoplexy) primarily in macroadenomas
- On angiography, adenomas occasionally compress carotid arteries despite their soft texture

MACROSCOPIC

General Features

- Typically soft and tan
- Macroadenomas may exhibit both fibrosis, particularly after medical therapy, and cystic change
- Extrasellar extension variable
  - Inferior extension eventually results in sphenoid sinus involvement
  - Thinning of sellar floor should not be assumed to represent invasion
  - Suprasellar growth causes elevation of sellar diaphragm and may result in chiasmal compression
  - Anterior extension may result in involvement of sphenoid sinus and nasopharynx
  - Lateral extension into cavernous sinuses may occur after invasion of dura or by growth through normally occurring dural defects

Size

- 33% micro (< 1 cm)
- 67% macro (> 1 cm)

MICROSCOPIC

Histologic Features

- Mainly chromophobic (sparsely granulated) and only rarely eosinophilic (densely granulated)
  - No clinical or biochemical differences whether sparsely or densely granulated
- Sparsely granulated tumors occasionally (10%) feature calcospherites
  - Abundance underlies formation of pituitary stone
- Acidophil stem cell adenomas may be somewhat acidophilic due to oncocytic change
  - Light microscopic cytoplasmic vacuolation occasional, corresponds to giant mitochondria
- Interstitial endocrine amyloid, occasionally disposed in massive laminated spheres (rare finding)

ANCILLARY TESTS

Immunohistochemistry

- Sparsely granulated (chromophobic) adenomas show paranuclear PRL immunoreactivity, nuclear PIT-1(+)
  - Ki-67 labeling index, although usually low, may be elevated in aggressive examples, correlates with mitotic activity
- Densely granulated (acidophilic) tumors are uncommon, show diffuse cytoplasmic PRL staining; PIT-1(+)
  - Such tumors show less mitotic activity and lower Ki-67 labeling indices than sparsely granulated adenomas
- Acidophil stem cell adenomas may also underlie hyperprolactinemia; PIT-1(+)
  - Minor staining for PRL and, to lesser extent, growth hormone

Electron Microscopy

- Release of granules, exocytosis, along lateral membranes instead of apical side of cell adjacent to perivascular space
  - Misplaced exocytosis

DIFFERENTIAL DIAGNOSIS

Pituitary Thyrotroph Hyperplasia

- Mimics PRL cell adenoma by PRL immunopositivity
- Reticulin shows enlargement, but not destruction, of acini

DIAGNOSTIC CHECKLIST

Clinically Relevant Pathologic Features

- > 250 ng/mL in macroadenomas; virtually diagnostic of PRL cell adenoma
- Macroadenomas in males and postmenopausal females are most often prolactinomas
- Microadenomas common in reproductive females and present with amenorrhea &/or galactorrhea

Pathologic Interpretation Pearls

- Paranuclear PRL staining is distinctive and typical
- Calcifications in some examples
- Massive spherical amyloid deposition in rare examples

SELECTED REFERENCES

1. Gomez-Hernandez K et al: Clinical implications of accurate subtyping of pituitary adenomas: perspectives from the treating physician. Turk Patoloji Derg. 31 Suppl 1:4-17, 2015
2. Kleinschmidt-DeMasters BK et al: An algorithmic approach to sellar region masses. Arch Pathol Lab Med. 139(3):356-72, 2015
3. Webb C et al: Pediatric pituitary adenomas. Arch Pathol Lab Med. 132(1):77-80, 2008
4. Ma W et al: Clinicopathologic study of 123 cases of prolactin-secreting pituitary adenomas with special reference to multihormone production and clonality of the adenomas. Cancer. 95(2):258-66, 2002

Incidental Pituitary Adenomas Frequent at Autopsy

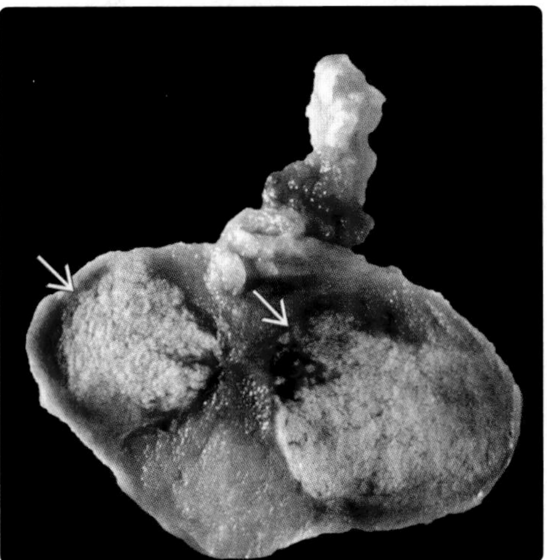

Calcospherites

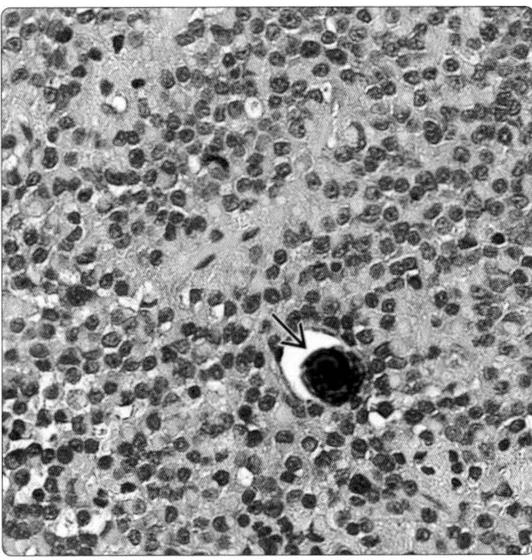

(Left) *Fully 25% of autopsies reveal incidental pituitary adenomas, nearly all subclinical. This horizontally sectioned gland shows 2 prolactinomas ➡. Most tumors found at autopsy are prolactinomas or null cell adenomas.* **(Right)** *Prolactinomas vary from chromophobic to somewhat basophilic due to abundance of rough endoplasmic reticulum. Calcospherites ➡ are present in ~ 10% of prolactinomas and are uncommon in other types.*

Amyloid Deposition

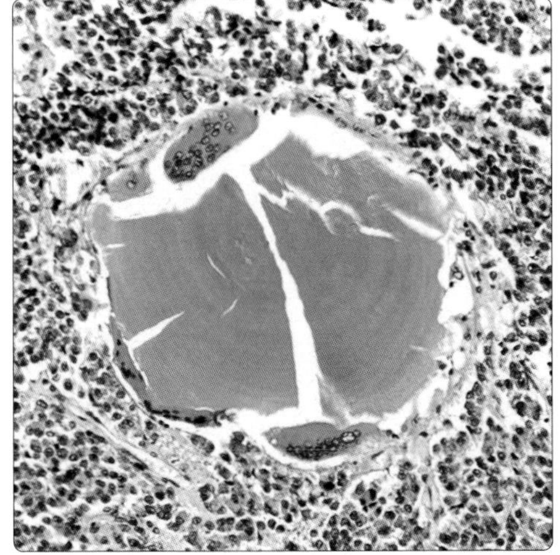

Pale Golgi Zones

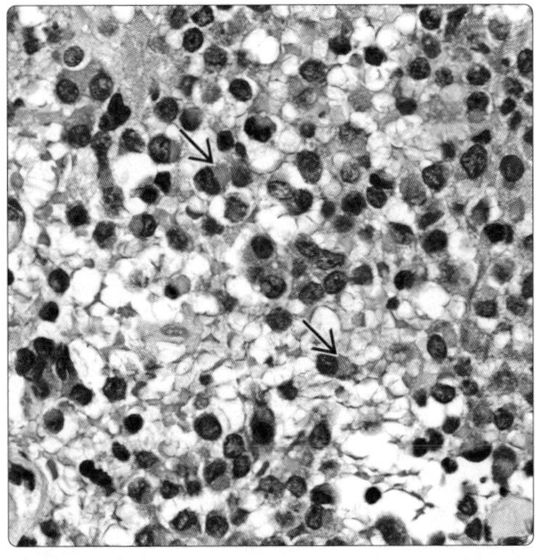

(Left) *Spherical amyloid depositions are occasionally present in prolactinomas. The concentric bodies show radial cracking. The same structures are also rarely found in corticotrophic adenomas.* **(Right)** *Prolactinoma cells have pale Golgi zones ➡ that may be apparent on light microscopy. These should not be misinterpreted as fibrous bodies, as seen in sparsely granulated growth hormone cell adenomas.*

Paranuclear Golgi Prolactin Immunoreactivity

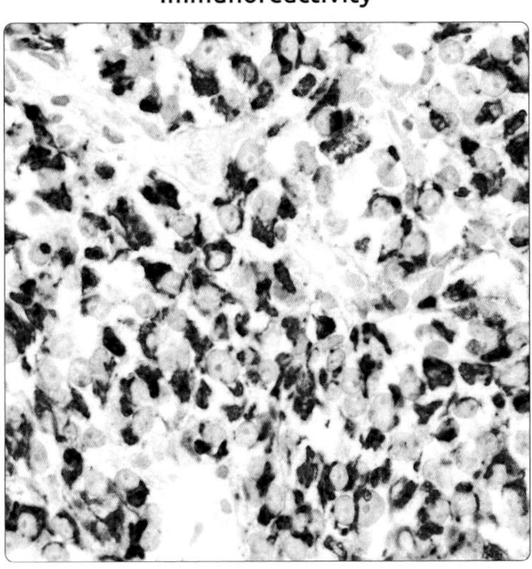

Misplaced Exocytosis

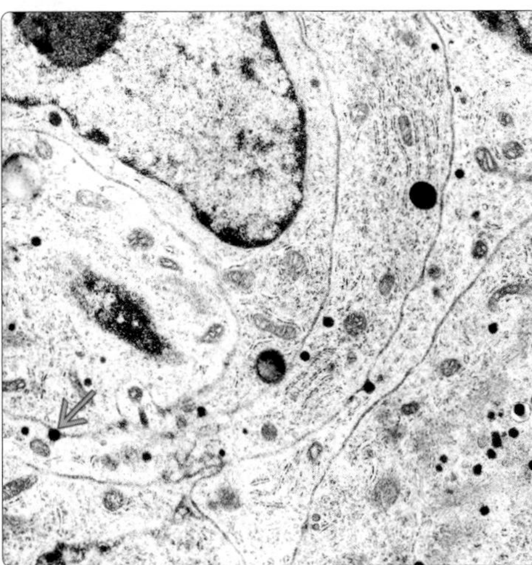

(Left) *Paranuclear Golgi pattern of PRL staining is characteristic of prolactinoma.* **(Right)** *Prolactinoma cells have ample rough endoplasmic reticulum and granules undergoing misplaced exocytosis ➡.*

Somatotroph Adenoma

KEY FACTS

ETIOLOGY/PATHOGENESIS

- Growth hormone (GH) excess causes both acromegaly and gigantism by inducing production of IGF-1 by liver, kidney, heart, and lungs

CLINICAL ISSUES

- All GH-producing tumors combined represent ≥ 20% of all adenomas
- Factors associated with outcome
  - Tumor size, invasion, basal preoperative GH level
  - Dural invasion and extrasellar growth
  - Sparsely granulated and acidophilic stem cell are acknowledged as aggressive subtypes

MICROSCOPIC

- 2 main forms: Densely and sparsely granulated
- Less common adenomas with GH(+): Mixed GH cell-PRL cell, mammosomatotroph [acidophil stem cell usually does not produce acromegaly and PRL > GH(+)]
- Rare lesions associated with GH excess
  - GH cell hyperplasia
  - Neuroendocrine neoplasms producing GH-releasing hormone

ANCILLARY TESTS

- Densely granulated: Diffusely GH(+), cytokeratin distributed throughout cytoplasm, so-called perinuclear CAM5.2; PIT-1(+)
  - Scattered fibrous bodies or intermediate forms can be identified in some cases of densely granulated GH adenomas, so-called intermediate/mixed/transitional form of GH adenoma
    - Based on keratin filament configuration in cytoplasm
    - These behave in same way as densely granulated GH adenomas
- Sparsely granulated: Weaker, patchy GH(+), with eosinophilic, rounded, cytokeratin (+) fibrous bodies in > 70% of adenoma cells; PIT-1(+)

Acromegaly

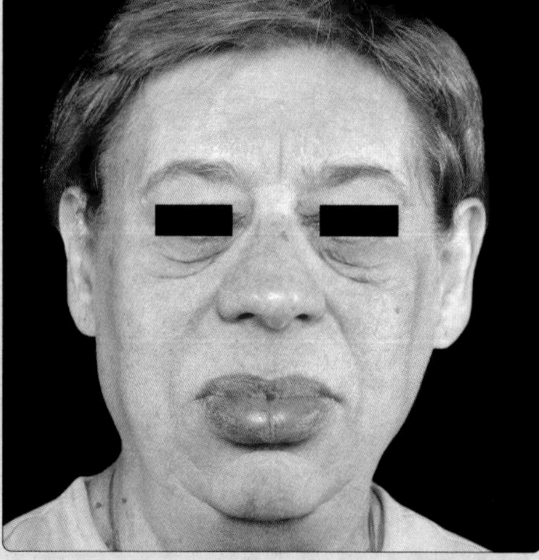

Thickened Skull, Enlarged Frontal Sinus

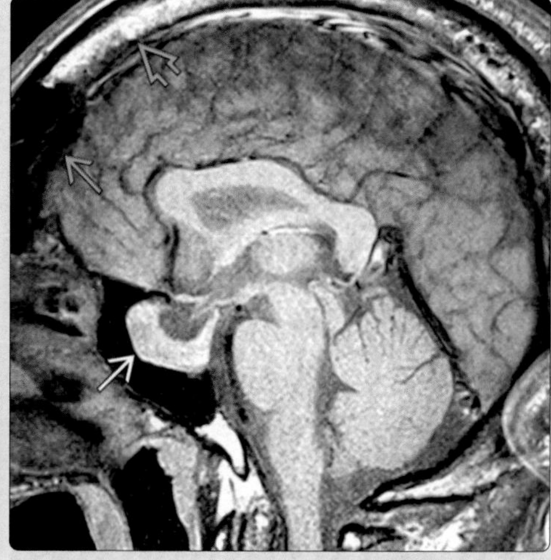

(Left) *Enlarged supraorbital ridges, wide nose, and prognathism are typical features of acromegaly.* **(Right)** *Sagittal T1WI MR in a 30-year-old man with longstanding acromegaly shows a pituitary macroadenoma invading the sphenoid sinus ➡. Note the thickened skull ⇨ and enlarged frontal sinus ⇨.*

Densely Granulated GH Adenoma, Eosinophilic, Monomorphic

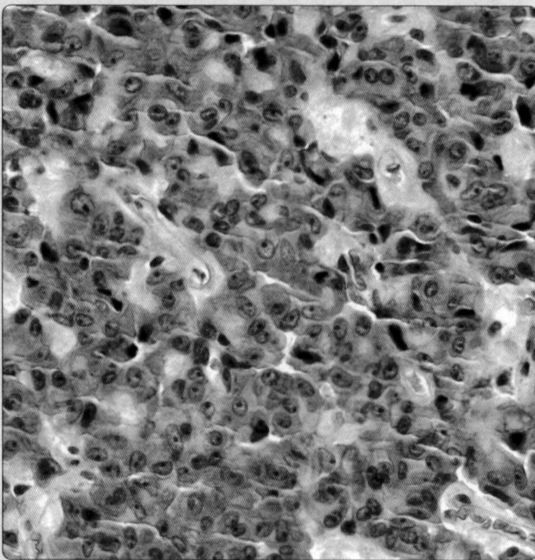

CAM5.2(+) Numerous Fibrous Bodies Seen Only in Sparsely Granulated GH Adenoma

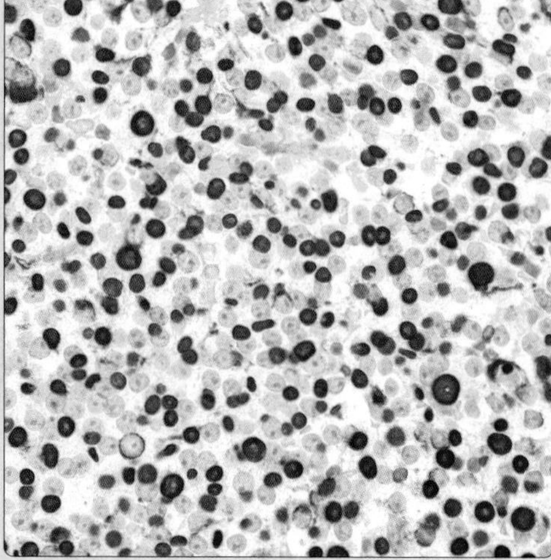

(Left) *Densely granulated growth hormone (GH) adenomas show eosinophilic cytoplasm. Note the presence of only a single-cell type, unlike normal anterior gland, which contains an assortment of eosinophils, basophils, and chromophobes.* **(Right)** *CAM5.2(+) rounded cytoplasmic collections of keratin filaments diffusely distributed throughout the adenoma in > 70% of cells are a signature hallmark of sparsely granulated GH adenoma and distinguish it from more indolent, densely granulated GH adenoma.*

TERMINOLOGY

Synonyms

- Somatotropinoma

Definitions

- Pituitary neoplasm composed of somatotrophs
  - Expressing *GH* gene and its mRNA
  - Producing, containing, and releasing growth hormone (GH)
  - Far more often endocrinologically active than silent

ETIOLOGY/PATHOGENESIS

Pathophysiology

- GH excess causes both acromegaly and gigantism by inducing production of IGF-1
  - Produced in liver, kidney, heart, and lungs
- Acromegaly
  - Postpubertal onset of GH excess results in enlargement of acral parts
  - Sometimes recognized only late in disease
- Gigantism
  - Prepubertal onset of GH excess, prior to closure of epiphyseal plates in bones, results in unrestrained somatic growth
- Coproduction of prolactin (PRL) and thyroid-stimulating hormone (TSH) may be seen due to transcription factor PIT-1
  - PIT-1 common transcription factor for all 3 hormones

CLINICAL ISSUES

Epidemiology

- Incidence
  - All GH-producing tumors combined represent 20% of all adenomas
    - All types driven by PIT-1 transcription factor
      - i.e., densely granulated, sparsely granulated, mixed GH-PRL, mammosomatotroph
      - Also driven by PIT-1: Prolactinomas, acidophil stem cell adenoma, thyrotroph adenomas
    - Densely granulated, sparsely granulated, mixed GH-PRL, mammosomatotroph adenomas present clinically with acromegaly in overwhelming majority of cases
      - Clinically silent variants are very rare
  - Densely granulated GH adenoma
    - More frequent than sparsely granulated GH adenoma
    - Generally responds better to somatostatin analogues than sparsely granulated GH adenoma
  - Sparsely granulated GH adenoma
    - More common in younger patients (< 50 years) than densely granulated GH adenoma
    - Usually larger tumors, more invasive
    - Less responsive to somatostatin analogs (SSA) than densely granulated GH adenomas
    - Aggressive behavior
      - One of few pituitary adenomas agreed upon by all experts to show more aggressive behavior
  - Mixed GH cell-PRL cell adenoma
  - Mammosomatotroph adenoma
    - 2% of overall adenomas, 8% of adenomas causing acromegaly
    - Generally indolent, although often large
  - Acidophil stem cell adenoma: 1% of adenomas; tumor usually presenting with hyperprolactinemia, not acromegaly, but also showing PRL(+) + varied GH(+)
    - Aggressive behavior
      - One of few pituitary adenomas agreed upon by all experts to show more aggressive behavior
  - Genetics
    - *MEN1* association
    - Carney complex
      - 10-20% incidence of GH-producing adenomas
    - Familial (rare)
- Age
  - 30-50 years old

Site

- Majority are sellar macroadenomas
- 15% are laterally situated microadenomas

Presentation

- Endocrine effect
  - GH/IGF-1 excess (acromegaly)
    - Hands, feet, face, jaw, tongue, sinuses, soft tissue, and bone overgrowth
    - Visceromegaly
    - Diabetes mellitus
    - Gigantism: Onset in adolescence
  - Cosecretion of PRL (30-50%) and occasionally TSH (20%) in mixed GH-PRL, mammosomatotroph adenomas, densely granulated GH adenomas, but not sparsely granulated GH adenomas
    - Acromegaly/gigantism ± amenorrhea/galactorrhea (± hyperthyroidism)
      - Mammosomatotroph adenoma usually presents with acromegaly and only mild elevation of serum PRL
      - Densely granulated and mammosomatotroph adenomas may show IHC(+) glycoprotein hormone production on paraffin (α-subunit, occasionally FSH, LH), but glycoproteins almost never clinically expressed, and are usually not detectable in serum
  - Acidophil stem cell adenoma usually nonfunctional or produces hyperprolactinemia, rarely causes mild acromegaly
    - Level of serum hyperprolactinemia is variable but differs from hyperprolactinemia in classic prolactinomas in that serum level is not as proportional to adenoma size
    - Larger acidophil stem cell adenomas produce less PRL than similar-sized PRL (i.e., sparsely granulated lactotroph) adenomas
    - With predominance of hyperprolactinemia-related symptoms, diagnosis of GH excess may be missed if GH axis is not evaluated
      - Known as fugitive acromegaly
  - Endocrinologically nonfunctional or silent GH adenomas are very rare
  - Hypopituitarism results from compression of normal anterior pituitary gland
- Mass effects

- Visual loss, obstructive hydrocephalus
- Pituitary apoplexy

Treatment

- Surgical approaches
  - Reduce hormone levels
  - Decompress optic apparatus
  - Reduce other mass effects
  - Acidophil stem cell adenomas almost always invasive, only subtotal resection is usually achieved
- Drugs
  - Somatostatin analogs (octreotide)
    - Cause decrease in GH level
    - Reduce tumor size in minority of cases
    - Mild perivascular fibrosis
    - No loss of GH immunopositivity
    - No involution of rough endoplasmic reticulum (RER) or Golgi complexes
    - Abundant, large secretory granules
    - Lysosome increase (crinophagy)
    - Sparsely granulated GH adenomas are less responsive to somatostatin analogs than densely granulated GH adenomas
  - GH receptor blocker (pegvisomant)
    - Presence of somatostatin receptors and GSP oncogene expression correlates with favorable response
  - Acidophil stem cell adenomas show no response to bromocriptine therapy
- Radiation
  - Mainly for recurrence

Prognosis

- Factors associated with outcome
  - Tumor size
  - Invasion
  - Basal preoperative GH level
  - Dural invasion and extrasellar growth univariate predictors of poor outcome
  - 8% recurrence rate at 10 years follow-up
- Overexpression of GH-releasing hormone (GHRH) mRNA transcripts is common and correlated with
  - Higher serum GH levels
  - Increased mitotic activity
  - Invasion
  - Nonremission

IMAGING

MR Findings

- Hypointense on T1 relative to normal gland
  - Enhancement initially low; increases late
  - Macroadenomas
    - Densely granulated
      - 40% are macroadenomas
    - Sparsely granulated
      - Always macroadenomas
    - Usually snowman-shaped suprasellar extension
  - Often invasive of dura, sellar bone, cavernous sinus
    - Densely granulated
      - 35% with invasion
    - Sparsely granulated
      - 65% with invasion
- Thickened skull and sellar floor as well as enlarged frontal sinuses in acromegaly

MACROSCOPIC

General Features

- Soft, tan to gray-red tumors
- Often associated with sellar bone overgrowth and large sinuses

MICROSCOPIC

Histologic Features

- 2 main forms of GH-producing adenoma (based on degree of granulation)
  - Densely granulated
    - Diffuse or solid growth pattern of eosinophilic cells, monomorphic population
  - Sparsely granulated
    - Diffuse growth pattern of chromophobic cells
    - Paranuclear eosinophilic fibrous bodies [corresponding to keratin (+)]
    - May show pleomorphism, eccentric nuclei, multinucleation, but these features are not reflective of malignant potential
- Less common GH-producing adenomas
  - Mixed GH cell-PRL cell adenoma
    - Densely granulated or sparsely granulated GH adenoma component + sparsely granulated PRL adenoma component
    - Indolent behavior usually
  - Mammosomatotroph adenoma
    - Single-cell type (producing both GH and PRL; sometimes α-subunit, TSH)
    - EM required to document single-cell type productive of all hormones, rather than mixed population as in mixed GH-PRL adenoma
    - Appears similar microscopically to densely granulated GH adenoma
  - Acidophil stem cell adenoma
    - Single-cell type (producing both PRL and GH), but cells less differentiated than single-cell population of mammosomatotroph adenoma
    - Chromophobic, some mildly eosinophilic due to oncocytic change
      - Large cytoplasmic vacuoles (giant mitochondria) can be seen on light microscopy
      - EM required to document increased/giant mitochondria
      - IHC(+) on immunostaining for mitochondria to document increased/giant mitochondria may serve as surrogate to EM
    - Occasional mild nuclear pleomorphism
    - Usually only a few scattered cells with eosinophilic fibrous bodies (keratin, i.e., CAM5.2)
    - Mitotic activity and Ki-67 index often low [mean of 8% in one study, but very broad range (1-20%)]

- Thus, cannot be diagnosed simply by elevated MIB-1 rate > 3%; not all PRL IHC(+) adenomas with elevated MIB-1 rate are acidophil stem cell adenomas
  - Immunoreactivity for PRL > for GH
    - Unlike pure prolactinomas, PRL IHC(+) usually patchy and in scattered cells, not diffuse and strong
  - Aggressive behavior: One of few pituitary adenomas agreed upon by all experts to show more aggressive behavior (along with sparsely granulated GH adenoma)
    - Usually invasive macroadenomas
- Multiple hormonal (GH/PRL/glycoprotein hormones such as FSH, LH, α-subunit)
  - Multiple hormone IHC(+) in mammosomatotroph adenomas, densely granulated GH adenomas, as well as mixed GH-PRL adenoma; almost never in sparsely granulated GH adenomas
  - Expression of multiple hormones in densely granulated/mammosomatotroph adenomas should not be considered plurihormonal
    - Unless EM shows distinctly different subsets of tumor cells in adenoma, which is rare
- Neuronal metaplasia in pituitary adenoma
  - Although uncommon, when occurs, usually found in GH adenomas, especially sparsely granulated GH adenomas
  - Clinical behavior parallels the underlying adenoma subtype
- Rare lesions associated with GH excess
  - GH cell hyperplasia
  - Neuroendocrine neoplasms producing growth hormone releasing hormone (GHRH)
    - Carcinoid, islet cell tumor, pheochromocytoma, thyroid medullary carcinoma, small cell carcinoma
    - Rare, but reason to measure GHRH in patients with GH excess

ANCILLARY TESTS

Cytology

- Widespread fibrous bodies in sparsely granulated GH adenoma involve ≥ 70% of adenoma cells

Immunohistochemistry

- Densely granulated: Diffuse and strong GH(+)
  - Perinuclear CAM5.2(+) keratin distribution throughout cytoplasm; PIT-1(+)
    - Occasionally, these tumors show a few fibrous bodies (mixed) or intermediate keratin forms
      - Tumors with intermediate/mixed/transitional keratin profiles show biologic features, including treatment response to somatostatin similar to other densely granulated GH adenomas
  - Diffuse strong E-cadherin cytoplasmic expression
  - Often show α-subunit IHC expression, may show scattered cells with PRL(+) but usually < 5%
- Sparsely granulated: May show focal, weak GH(+)
  - Fibrous bodies, i.e., dot-like CAM5.2(+) keratin expression in majority (> 70%) of adenoma cells; PIT-1(+)
  - Weak to absent E-cadherin cytoplasmic expression
  - Almost never shows α-subunit, TSH IHC(+); usually only rare scattered cells are IHC(+) for PRL, if at all
- Mixed GH-PRL adenomas
  - Patchy GH(+) in subset of adenoma cells, with usually lesser amounts of PRL(+) than GH(+), although more PRL(+) than either pure densely granulated or mammosomatotroph adenomas (% of positive cells not precisely defined); PIT-1(+)
    - 2 types: Densely granulated GH-PRL [which, like overwhelming majority (≥ 99%) of prolactinomas, are sparsely granulated prolactinoma (i.e., lactotroph adenoma)]
      - GH(+) and perinuclear CAM5.2(+) keratin distribution throughout cytoplasm in GH adenoma component
      - Express PRL and estrogen receptor (ER) in prolactin-producing component
    - Sparsely granulated GH-PRL
      - GH(+) and fibrous bodies, i.e., dot-like CAM5.2(+) keratin expression in GH adenoma component, but much less than 70% of cells, as is seen in pure sparsely granulated GH adenomas
      - Express PRL and ER in prolactin-producing component
- Mammosomatotroph adenomas
  - Appear on light microscopy identical to densely granulated GH adenoma, but often shows more admixed PRL IHC(+) than pure densely granulated GH adenomas; PIT-1(+)
  - More likely than densely granulated GH adenoma to show patchy α-subunit, TSH IHC(+)
  - Cytokeratin distribution in majority of cells is diffusely distributed throughout cytoplasm, but intermediate/transitional/mixed forms of cytoplasmic keratin distribution exist
    - Small subset of cells may contain classic fibrous bodies (<< 70%)
    - Subset of cells may contain keratin (+) cytoplasmic structures with features difficult to classify as classic fibrous bodies, yet keratin filaments fail to fill cytoplasm in perinuclear distribution, i.e., they are transitional
  - No clinical need to distinguish mammosomatotroph from densely granulated GH adenomas, have similar response to somatostatin analogs
- Acidophil stem cell adenomas
  - Appear on light microscopy chromophobic or slightly acidophilic due to increased mitochondria, PRL > GH(+), and often only PRL(+); PIT-1(+)
    - Either clinically silent or show hyperprolactinemia, although clue is that unlike ordinary pure prolactinomas, larger acidophil stem cell adenomas produce less prolactin than similar-sized PRL adenomas
    - Usually invasive macroadenomas
- PRL(+) < GH(+) in most mixed GH-PRL cell, mammosomatotroph adenomas
  - PRL exceeds GH(+) in acidophil stem cell adenomas
- Somatostatin receptor (SSTR)
  - Almost all GH tumors express SSTR2A and SSTR5 at high levels

- SSTR2A expression correlated with response to octreotide; reduced after octreotide treatment
- SSTR2A expression stronger in densely granulated than sparsely granulated GH adenomas
- IHC(+) for SSTR2A not specific for GH adenomas, since also seen in some gonadotroph (FSH/LH) adenomas, rarely other types

Electron Microscopy

- Densely granulated
  - Well-developed RER, Golgi complexes
  - Numerous large, dense, spherical granules
    - Appear similar to normal GH cells
- Sparsely granulated
  - Fibrous body consisting of intermediate filaments (keratin) and smooth endoplasmic reticulum
  - Granules and organelles often enmeshed within fibrous bodies
- Mixed GH cell-PRL cell
  - GH-secreting cells with typical EM features: Numerous large, dense, spherical granules
  - PRL-secreting cells with typical EM features: Misplaced exocytoses
- Mammosomatotroph cell
  - Large, ovoid to irregular deposits of secretory material and granules with uneven, mottled texture
  - Production of hormones by single-cell type requires verification by EM
- Acidophil stem cell
  - Cells less fully differentiated, with some features of both GH and PRL cells in each cell
    - Fibrous bodies and misplaced exocytoses
  - Oncocytic features, i.e., slight acidophilia to cytoplasm, common with giant mitochondria
    - With diminishing access to EM, IHC for mitochondria may assist in diagnosis of this mitochondrial-rich PIT-1-driven variant

DIFFERENTIAL DIAGNOSIS

Normal Adenohypophysis

- Reticulin demonstrates preserved normal acinar architecture

Pituitary Hyperplasia

- Marked expansion of acini by reticulin staining

DIAGNOSTIC CHECKLIST

Pathologic Interpretation Pearls

- Sparsely granulated GH adenoma has > 70% fibrous bodies and this is signature histological hallmark
  - Perinuclear cytoplasmic CAM5.2(+) keratin filaments fill cytoplasm in most densely granulated GH and mammosomatotroph adenomas
    - Subset with intermediate/mixed/transitional keratin profiles show biologic features including treatment response to somatostatin similar to other densely granulated GH adenomas
  - Mixed GH-PRL adenoma may be composed of dense GH-PRL or sparse GH-PRL

SELECTED REFERENCES

1. Gomez-Hernandez K et al: Clinical implications of accurate subtyping of pituitary adenomas: perspectives from the treating physician. Turk Patoloji Derg. 31 Suppl 1:4-17, 2015
2. Kiseljak-Vassiliades K et al: Differential somatostatin receptor (SSTR) 1-5 expression and downstream effectors in histologic subtypes of growth hormone pituitary tumors. Mol Cell Endocrinol. ePub, 2015
3. Kleinschmidt-DeMasters BK et al: An algorithmic approach to sellar region masses. Arch Pathol Lab Med. 139(3):356-72, 2015
4. Lee CC et al: Stereotactic radiosurgery for acromegaly: outcomes by adenoma subtype. Pituitary. 18(3):326-34, 2015
5. Nishioka H et al: The complementary role of transcription factors in the accurate diagnosis of clinically nonfunctioning pituitary adenomas. Endocr Pathol. ePub, 2015
6. Chinezu L et al: Expression of somatostatin receptors, SSTR2A and SSTR5, in 108 endocrine pituitary tumors using immunohistochemical detection with new specific monoclonal antibodies. Hum Pathol. 45(1):71-7, 2014
7. Casar-Borota O et al: Expression of SSTR2a, but not of SSTRs 1, 3, or 5 in somatotroph adenomas assessed by monoclonal antibodies was reduced by octreotide and correlated with the acute and long-term effects of octreotide. J Clin Endocrinol Metab. 98(11):E1730-9, 2013
8. Mori R et al: Clinicopathological features of growth hormone-producing pituitary adenomas in 242 acromegaly patients: classification according to hormone production and cytokeratin distribution. ISRN Endocrinol. 2013:723432, 2013
9. Zhou K et al: Expression and significance of E-cadherin and β-catenins in pituitary adenoma. Int J Surg Pathol. 21(4):363-7, 2013
10. Kiseljak-Vassiliades K et al: Clinical implications of growth hormone-secreting tumor subtypes. Endocrine. 42(1):18-28, 2012
11. Atkinson AB: From then to now: lessons from developments in our understanding of the pituitary gland. Ulster Med J. 79(2):89-94, 2010
12. Bakhtiar Y et al: Relationship between cytokeratin staining patterns and clinico-pathological features in somatotropinomae. Eur J Endocrinol. 163(4):531-9, 2010
13. Fougner SL et al: The expression of E-cadherin in somatotroph pituitary adenomas is related to tumor size, invasiveness, and somatostatin analog response. J Clin Endocrinol Metab. 95(5):2334-42, 2010
14. Lopes MB: Growth hormone-secreting adenomas: pathology and cell biology. Neurosurg Focus. 29(4):E2, 2010
15. Melmed S et al: Guidelines for acromegaly management: an update. J Clin Endocrinol Metab. 94(5):1509-17, 2009
16. Horvath A et al: Clinical and molecular genetics of acromegaly: MEN1, Carney complex, McCune-Albright syndrome, familial acromegaly and genetic defects in sporadic tumors. Rev Endocr Metab Disord. 9(1):1-11, 2008
17. Obari A et al: Clinicopathological features of growth hormone-producing pituitary adenomas: difference among various types defined by cytokeratin distribution pattern including a transitional form. Endocr Pathol. 19(2):82-91, 2008
18. Coons SW et al: Cytokeratin CK 7 and CK 20 expression in pituitary adenomas. Endocr Pathol. 16(3):201-10, 2005
19. Sano T et al: Down-regulation of E-cadherin and catenins in human pituitary growth hormone-producing adenomas. Front Horm Res. 32:127-32, 2004
20. Nishioka H et al: Fibrous bodies are associated with lower GH production and decreased expression of E-cadherin in GH-producing pituitary adenomas. Clin Endocrinol (Oxf). 59(6):768-72, 2003
21. Xu B et al: Downregulation of E-cadherin and its undercoat proteins in pituitary growth hormone cell adenomas with prominent fibrous bodies. Endocr Pathol. 13(4):341-51, 2002
22. Giustina A et al: Criteria for cure of acromegaly: a consensus statement. J Clin Endocrinol Metab. 85(2):526-9, 2000
23. Thapar K et al: Overexpression of the growth-hormone-releasing hormone gene in acromegaly-associated pituitary tumors. An event associated with neoplastic progression and aggressive behavior. Am J Pathol. 151(3):769-84, 1997
24. Yamada S et al: Growth hormone-producing pituitary adenomas: correlations between clinical characteristics and morphology. Neurosurgery. 33(1):20-7, 1993
25. Scheithauer BW et al: Pituitary adenomas of the multiple endocrine neoplasia type I syndrome. Semin Diagn Pathol. 4(3):205-11, 1987
26. Scheithauer BW et al: Plurihormonal pituitary adenomas. Semin Diagn Pathol. 3(1):69-82, 1986
27. Laws ER Jr et al: The pathogenesis of acromegaly. Clinical and immunocytochemical analysis in 75 patients. J Neurosurg. 63(1):35-8, 1985
28. Horvath E et al: Mammosomatotroph cell adenoma of the human pituitary: a morphologic entity. Virchows Arch A Pathol Anat Histopathol. 398(3):277-89, 1983

Pituitary Adenomas

Adenoma Type	Reactivity
Pituitary Adenomas Causing Acromegaly/Gigantism, With GH, CAM5.2 Pattern, IHC Pattern	
Densely granulated somatotroph adenoma	Diffuse, strong GH(+), may show α-subunit, CAM5.2 perinuclear
Intermediate/mixed/transitional growth hormone adenoma	Diffuse, strong GH(+), CAM5.2 mostly perinuclear, fibrous bodies < 70%
Sparsely granulated growth hormone adenoma	Weak, focal GH(+), CAM5.2 fibrous bodies > 70%
Mixed growth hormone-prolactinoma	GH(+) in varying degrees and distribution (small groups to scattered admixed cells); prolactin (+) stronger than in densely or sparsely granulated GH adenoma
Mammosomatotroph adenoma	Diffuse, strong GH(+), often with α-subunit, PRL, sometimes FSH, LH CAM5.2 mostly perinuclear, fibrous bodies rare if present at all
Silent subtype 3 adenoma	Some recognized as producing mild acromegaly, less commonly hyperthyroidism or mild hyperprolactinemia, CAM5.2 perinuclear in most, occasional fibrous bodies or negative CAM5.2 (rare aggressive subtype composed of monomorphic cell population and confidently diagnosed only by electron microscopy)
Pituitary Adenomas Causing Hyperprolactinemia, With PRL, CAM5.2 Pattern, IHC Pattern	
Sparsely granulated prolactin-secreting (lactotroph) adenoma	Diffuse strong PRL, Golgi pattern, CAM5.2 often moderate, no fibrous bodies
Densely granulated prolactin-secreting (lactotroph) adenoma	Diffuse, strong PRL, may be perinuclear rather than Golgi, CAM5.2, no fibrous bodies
Acidophil stem cell adenoma	Diffuse cytoplasmic PRL(+), except in rare instances where Golgi pattern present; focal GH in ~ 1/2 of cases; CAM5.2 ~ 2/3 with fibrous bodies, usually scattered rather than prominent; sometimes CAM5.2 IHC(-) or perinuclear pattern

Growth hormone = GH

Pituitary Adenoma Type by Transcription Factor Family

Adenoma Type	Comments
PIT-1 (pituitary transcription factor)	Sparsely granulated prolactin-secreting (lactotroph) adenoma, densely granulated prolactin-secreting (lactotroph) adenoma, acidophil stem cell adenoma, thyrotroph (TSH) adenoma, silent subtype 3 adenoma (variable PRL > GH or TSH), densely granulated growth hormone adenoma, intermediate/mixed/transitional growth hormone adenoma (behaves like densely granulated growth hormone adenoma), sparsely granulated growth hormone adenoma, mixed growth hormone-prolactinoma, mammosomatotroph adenoma
SF1 (steroidogenic factor)	Gonadotroph adenoma, ± IHC(+) for FSH, LH* (*presence of SF1 defines gonadotroph adenoma, even if hormone negative)
Tpit	Densely granulated ACTH (corticotroph) adenoma, sparsely granulated ACTH (corticotroph) adenoma, Crooke cell adenoma, clinically silent ACTH adenoma (either densely granulated, i.e., subtype I, or sparsely granulated, i.e., subtype II) (Tpit IHC not widely available)
Transcription factor negative for all 3 of above	Null cell adenoma (very small percentage of clinically nonfunctioning pituitary adenomas exist that are completely negative for anterior pituitary hormones **and** are further negative for all 3 transcription factors, i.e., negative for SF1, PIT-1, **and** Tpit)

Adapted from Gomez-Hernandez K et al: Clinical implications of accurate subtyping of pituitary adenomas: perspectives from the treating physician. Turk Patoloji Derg. 31 Suppl 1:4-17, 2015.

Nuclear Pleomorphism, Sparsely Granulated GH Adenoma

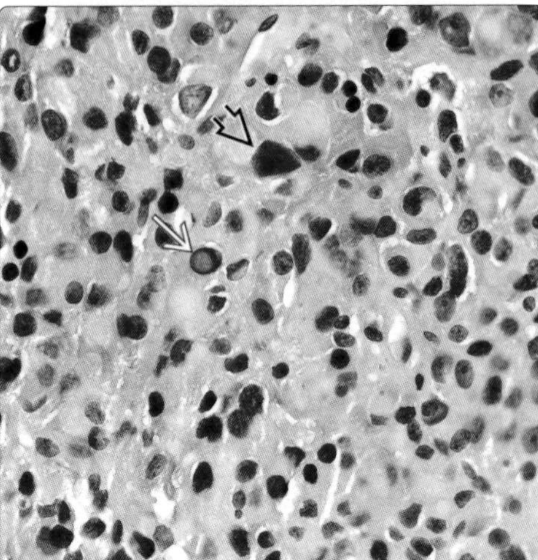

Fibrous Bodies, Paranuclear Spherical Inclusions

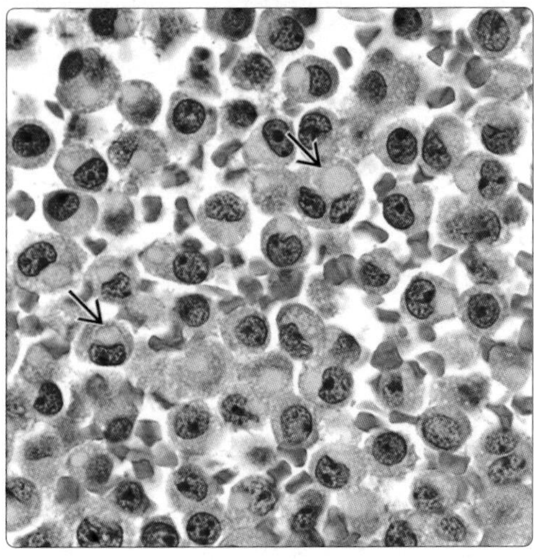

(Left) *Intranuclear pseudoinclusions ➡ & nuclear pleomorphism ⇨, while not specific, are common in GH cell adenomas, especially sparsely granulated GH adenomas. They do not impact prognosis. Pleomorphism, eccentric nuclei, and multinucleation are not reflective of malignant potential.* **(Right)** *Fibrous bodies ⇨, i.e., pale paranuclear spherical inclusions, are diagnostic features in sparsely granulated GH cell adenomas. The structures are more obvious after staining for cytokeratins, e.g., CAM5.2.*

Acidophil Stem Cell Adenoma, Chromophobic

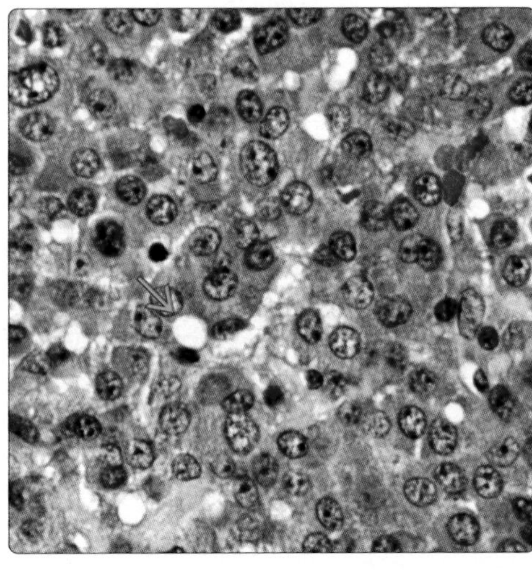

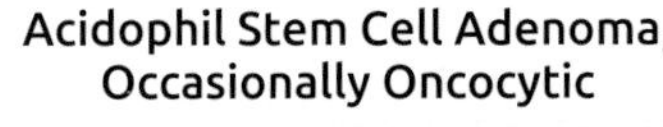

Acidophil Stem Cell Adenoma, Occasionally Oncocytic

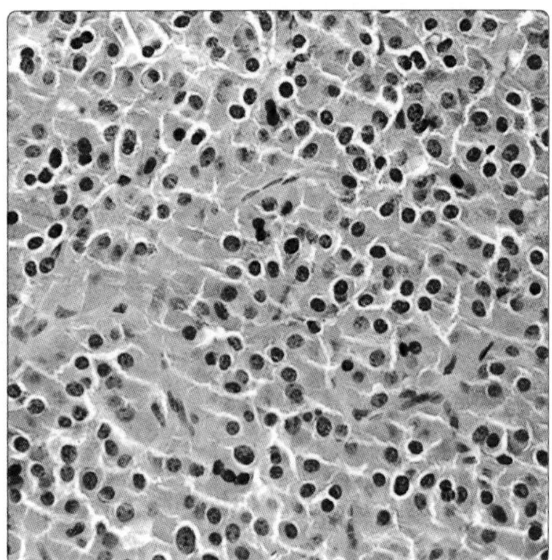

(Left) *Acidophil stem cell adenomas are mostly chromophobic. Cytoplasmic vacuoles ⇨ are due to giant mitochondria.* **(Right)** *Acidophil stem cell adenomas are occasionally oncocytic, with abundant, finely granular, slightly eosinophilic cytoplasm. The diagnosis of this rare adenoma type depends on ultrastructural identification of numerous giant mitochondria, although IHC for mitochondria may be of use in PIT-1 lineage tumors.*

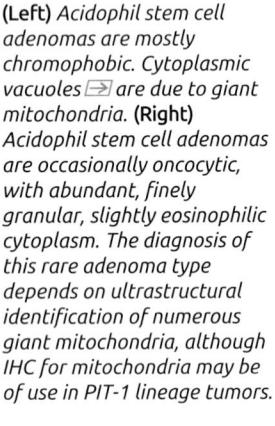

GH(+), Densely Granulated GH Adenoma

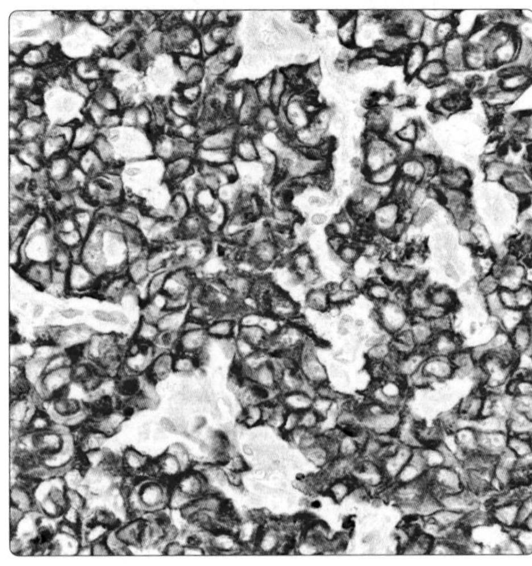

GH(+), Sparsely Granulated GH Adenoma

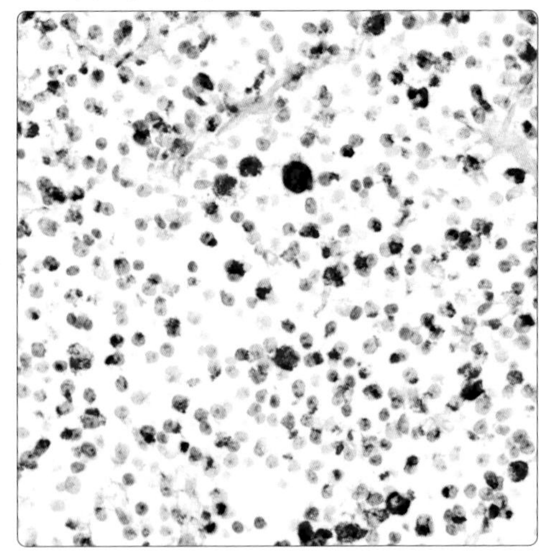

(Left) *Densely granulated somatotroph adenomas are diffusely and strongly immunopositive for growth hormone.* **(Right)** *GH staining is often scant and more focally expressed in sparsely granulated somatotroph adenomas.*

PRL(+) > GH(+), Acidophil Stem Cell Adenoma

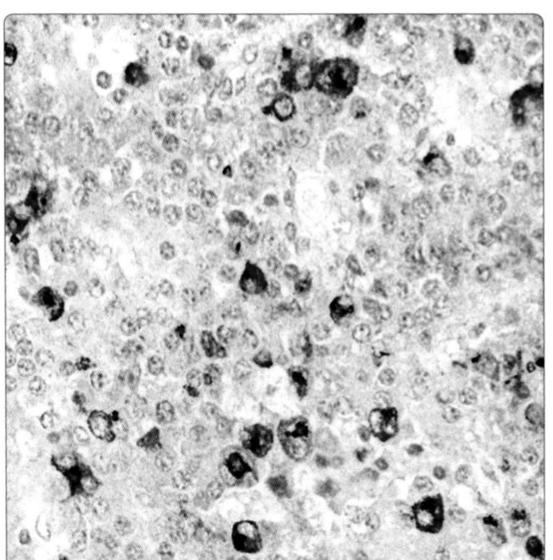

GH(+), Scant, Acidophil Stem Cell Adenoma

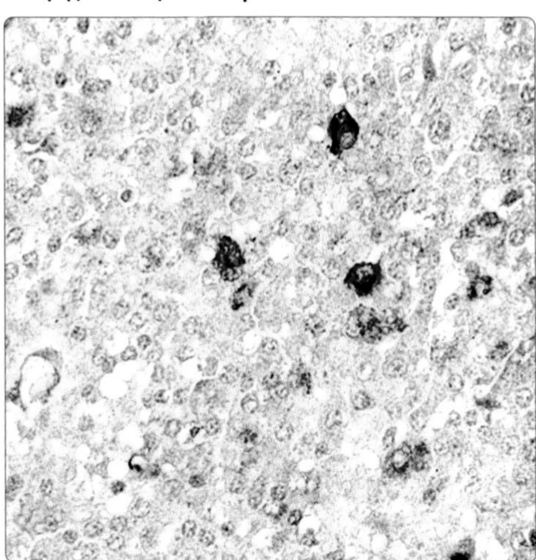

(Left) *Immunoreactivity for PRL is usually > that for GH in acidophilic stem cell adenomas; however, unlike prolactinomas, not all cells are PRL(+). Patients with acidophil stem cell adenoma usually present with hyperprolactinemia, although, unlike pure prolactinomas, the serum levels are not as proportional to tumor size, i.e., larger acidophil stem cell adenomas produce less prolactin than similar-sized pure PRL adenomas.* **(Right)** *Immunoreactivity for GH is scant in acidophil stem cell adenoma.*

CAM5.2, Densely Granulated GH Adenoma

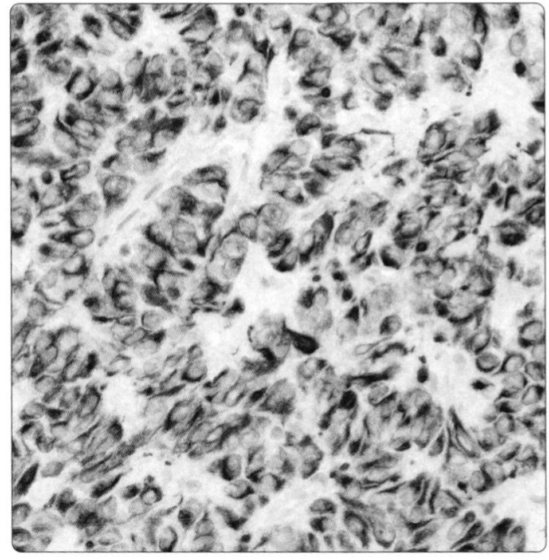

Mixed or Transitional Pattern, CAM5.2

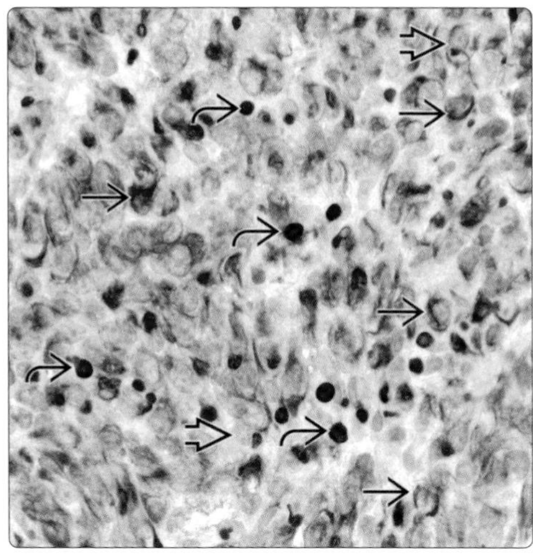

(Left) *Densely granulated GH adenomas have cytokeratin filaments throughout cytoplasm. Occasionally, these tumors show a few fibrous bodies or intermediate keratin forms, but biologic features including treatment response to somatostatin do not differ from densely granulated GH adenomas.* **(Right)** *Some GH adenomas show an admixture of fibrous bodies ↷, larger numbers of cells with perinuclear keratin →, and even a few intermediate forms ⇨. These GH adenomas behave like densely granulated GH adenomas.*

Sparsely Granulated GH Adenoma, Fibrous Bodies

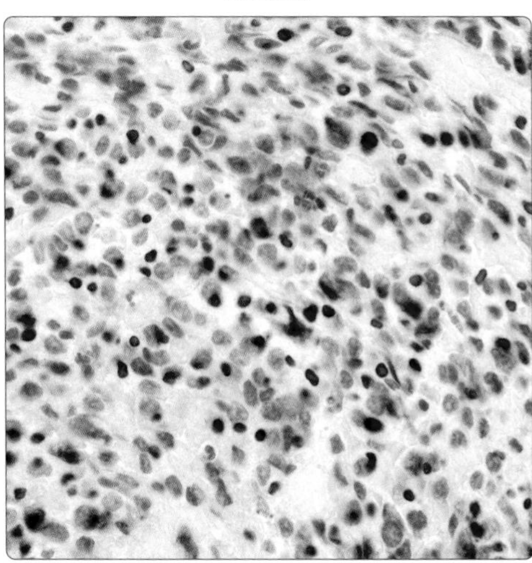

ASU(+) Can Be Seen

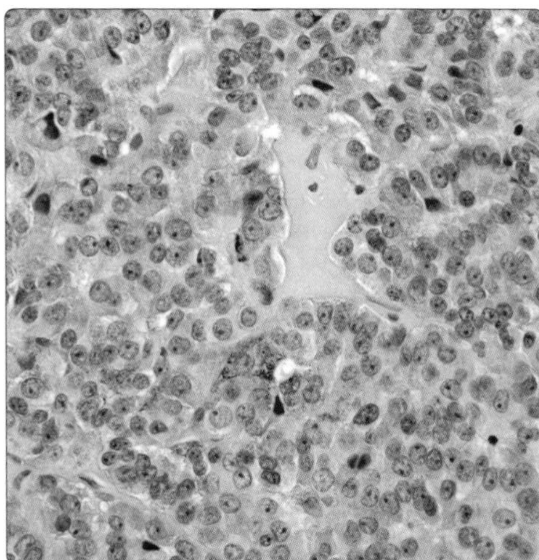

(Left) *Sparsely granulated GH adenomas have rounded keratin IHC(+) fibrous bodies in ≥ 70% adenoma cells.* **(Right)** *Densely granulated adenomas can show focal ASU(+), as can mammosomatotroph adenomas, but this is almost never found in sparsely granulated GH adenomas.*

SSTR2A Membranous IHC(+)

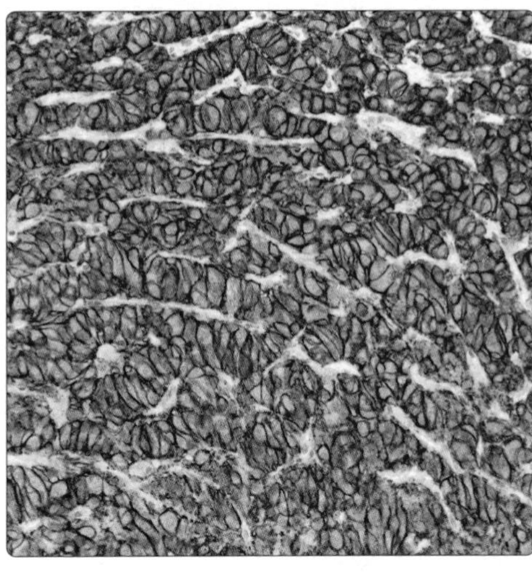

Touch Print, Sparsely Granulated GH Adenoma

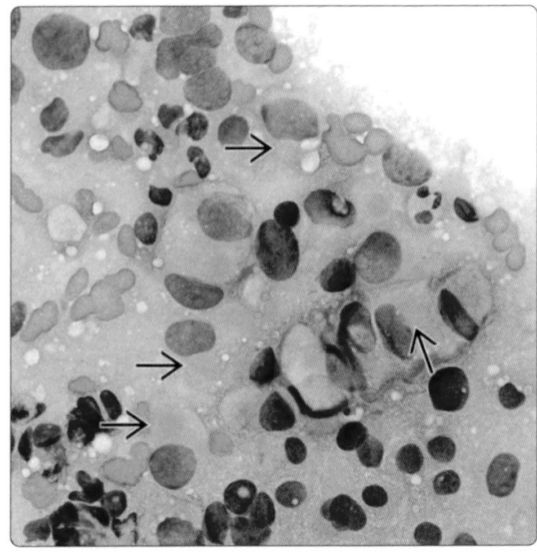

(Left) *SSTR2A expression is seen in several types of pituitary adenomas, especially GH adenomas. It is significantly higher in densely than sparsely granulated tumors.* **(Right)** *In some sparsely granulated GH adenomas, the intracytoplasmic fibrous bodies can be identified → on touch prints. Verification on permanent section with CAM5.2 IHC to identify these as fibrous bodies present in ≥ 70% of adenoma cells should be performed for diagnosis of sparsely granulated GH adenoma.*

GH(+) and PRL(+), Mammosomatotroph Adenoma, Single Adenoma Cell Type

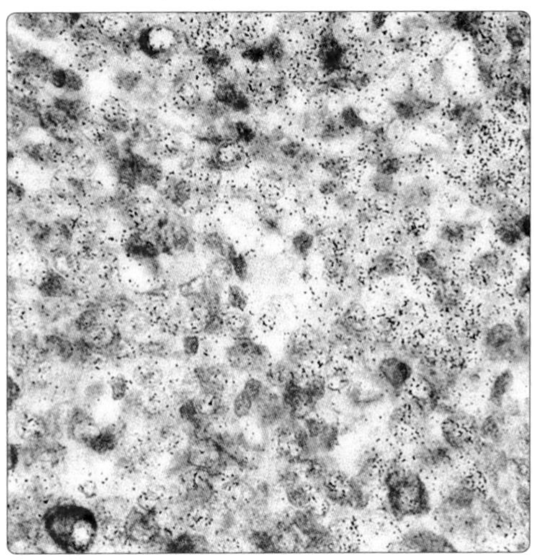

Mixed GH-PRL Adenoma, 2 Separate Adenoma Cell Populations

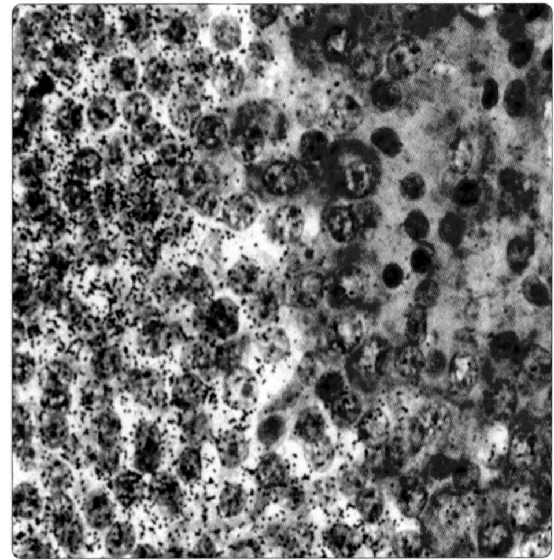

(Left) *Mammosomatotroph adenomas consist of a monomorphic cell population, secreting GH shown by immunohistochemistry (brown) and PRL by in situ hybridization (blue dot-like).* **(Right)** *In this example of mixed GH cell-PRL adenoma, GH-secreting cells are immunohistochemically brown, whereas PRL cells are overlain by blue dots by in situ hybridization.*

Interstitial Amyloid, Uncommon

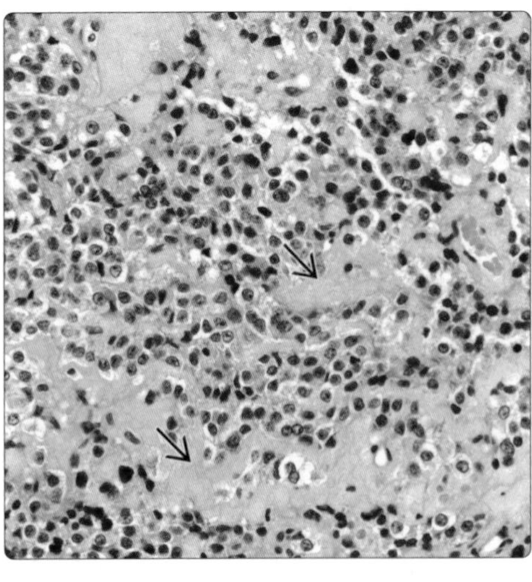

Neuronal Metaplasia

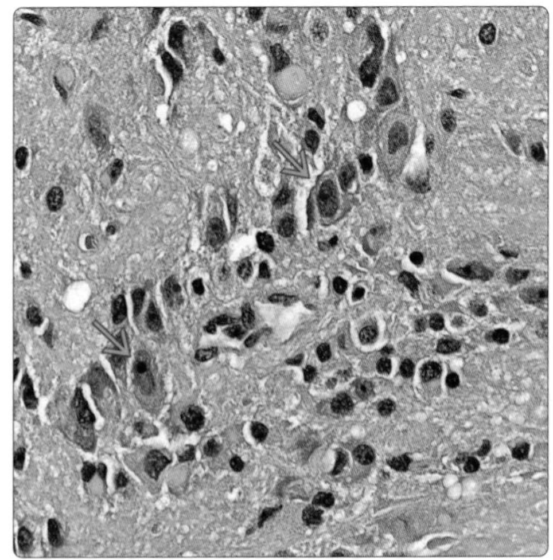

(Left) *Interstitial amyloid → is present in some GH cell adenomas.* **(Right)** *Neuronal metaplasia (hamartoma, choristoma) is the result of neuronal differentiation of GH cells →, usually in sparsely granulated growth hormone-producing adenomas. The latter, replete with innumerable fibrous bodies, was present elsewhere in this tumor.*

Densely Granulated GH Adenoma

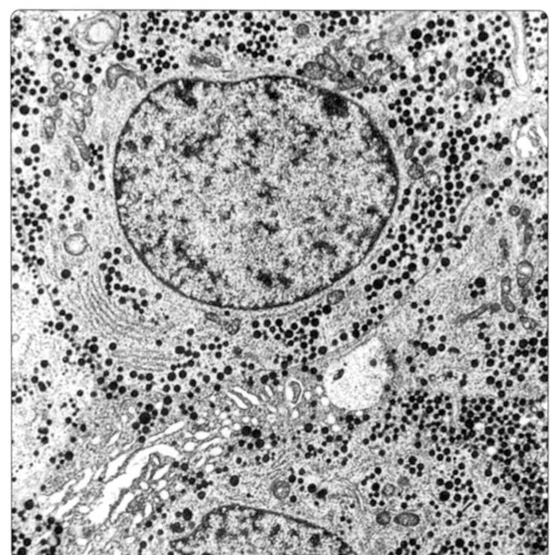

Densely Granulated, Prominent Golgi

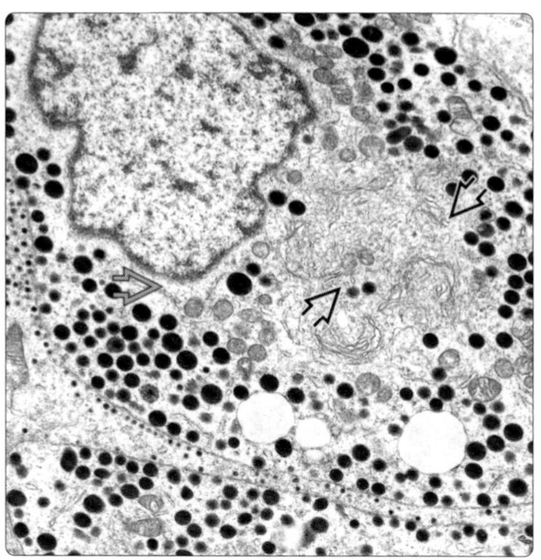

(Left) *Densely granulated GH adenomas have numerous secretory granules.* **(Right)** *Densely granulated GH cell adenomas have prominent Golgi* ➾ *and numerous large secretory granules* ➾.

Sparsely Granulated Adenoma

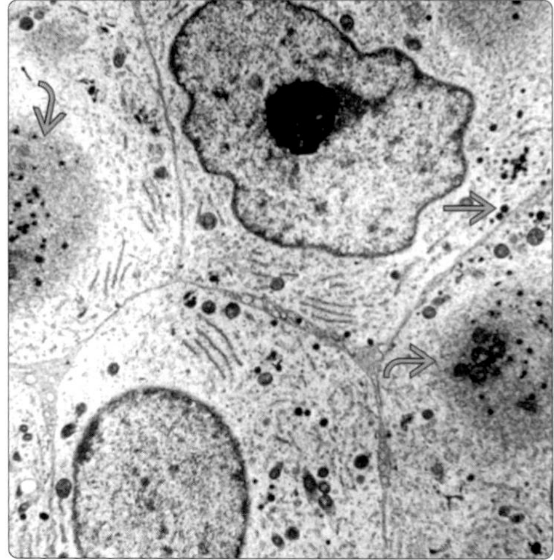

Sparsely Granulated GH Adenoma

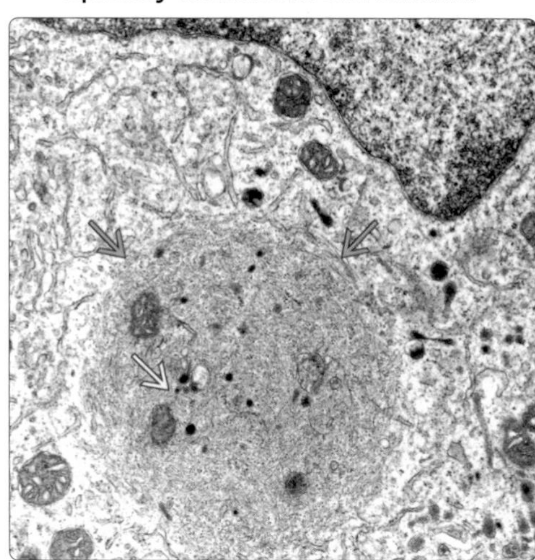

(Left) *Sparsely granulated GH adenomas have fibrous bodies* ➾ *and a paucity of small dense secretory granules* ➾. **(Right)** *Sparsely granulated GH adenomas have prominent fibrous bodies (keratin)* ➾ *that trap organelles and secretory granules* ➔.

Mammosomatotroph Adenoma

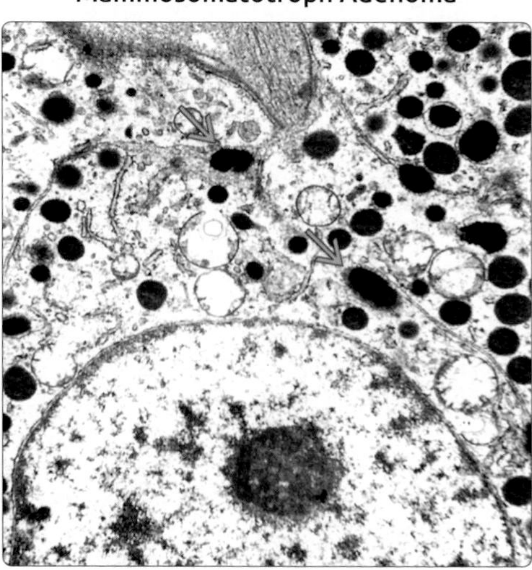

Acidophil Stem Cell Adenoma

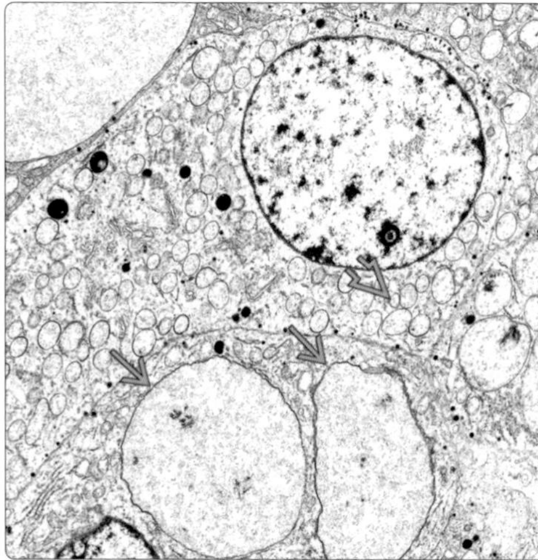

(Left) *Mammosomatotroph adenomas feature large granules* ➾ *and deposits of secretory material.* **(Right)** *Acidophil stem cell adenomas exhibit giant mitochondria* ➾ *and, occasionally, abundant conventional mitochondria (oncocytic change)* ➾.

Corticotroph Adenoma

KEY FACTS

CLINICAL ISSUES

- Most functioning ACTH adenomas are microadenomas
- Silent corticotroph adenomas tend to be macroadenomas, aggressive
- Surgery curative in 65-90%
- Clinical presentation
  - Cushing disease
  - Nelson syndrome
  - Silent corticotroph adenomas are clinically nonfunctional

MICROSCOPIC

- Basophilic to chromophobic, depending on if densely or sparsely granulated
- Accompanying normal pituitary corticotroph cells shows Crooke hyaline change in endocrinologically active ACTH adenomas
- Rare adenomas consist largely of Crooke cells
- Nelson syndrome
  - No Crooke change in normal pituitary
- Nonfunctioning or silent corticotroph adenoma
  - Apoplexy common
  - No Crooke change in accompanying normal pituitary corticotroph cells

ANCILLARY TESTS

- Ki-67 labeling index
  - Low in Cushing adenomas
  - May be increased in atypical, Nelson, Crooke cell, and silent adenomas, but not invariably
- PAS(+) in Cushing-producing, clinically active adenomas and PAS(-) in 1/2 of silent ACTH adenomas
- Keratin (+): CAM5.2 IHC(+) in all densely granulated ACTH adenomas, many sparsely granulated ACTH adenomas
- CK20 IHC(+) in nearly all densely granulated ACTH adenomas
- CAM5.2(+) extensive, positive in circumnuclear bundles of intermediate filaments in Crooke cell adenoma
- Tpit(+), but IHC not widely available

(Left) *Functional ACTH cell adenomas are typically small and noninvasive. The hypervascular nature of this example is typical. Such tumors may bleed at surgery.* **(Right)** *Densely granulated corticotroph adenomas show a monotonous population of cells with abundant basophilic cytoplasm on H&E.*

Microadenoma: Functional ACTH Adenoma

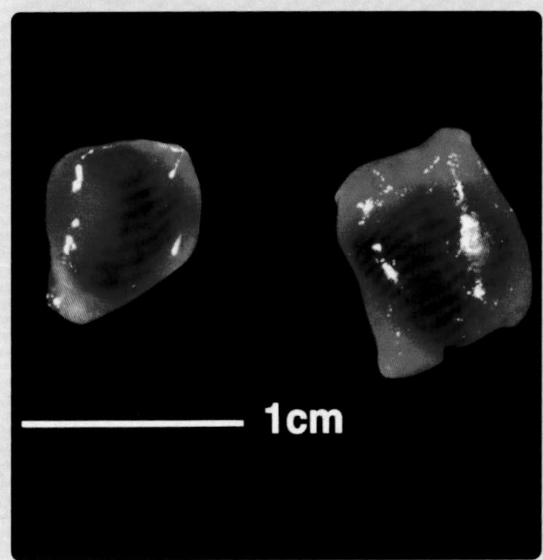

Densely Granulated, Basophilic ACTH Adenoma

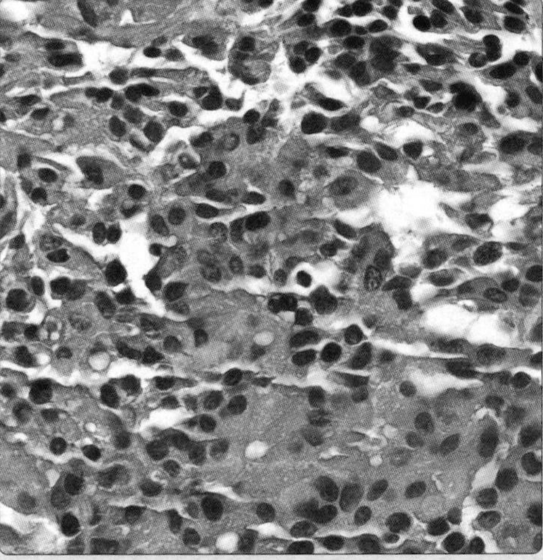

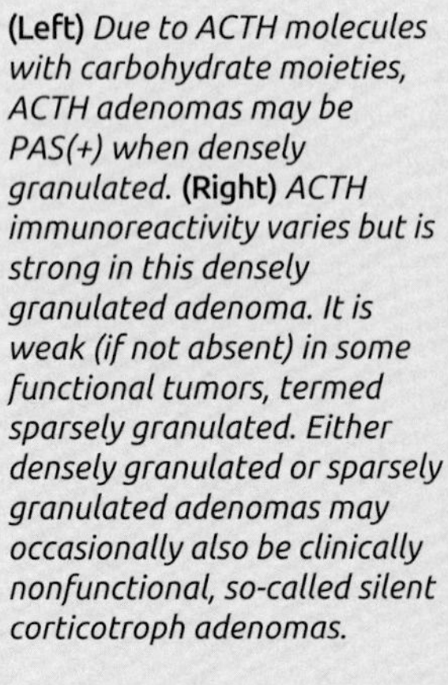
(Left) *Due to ACTH molecules with carbohydrate moieties, ACTH adenomas may be PAS(+) when densely granulated.* **(Right)** *ACTH immunoreactivity varies but is strong in this densely granulated adenoma. It is weak (if not absent) in some functional tumors, termed sparsely granulated. Either densely granulated or sparsely granulated adenomas may occasionally also be clinically nonfunctional, so-called silent corticotroph adenomas.*

PAS(+) Corticotroph Adenoma

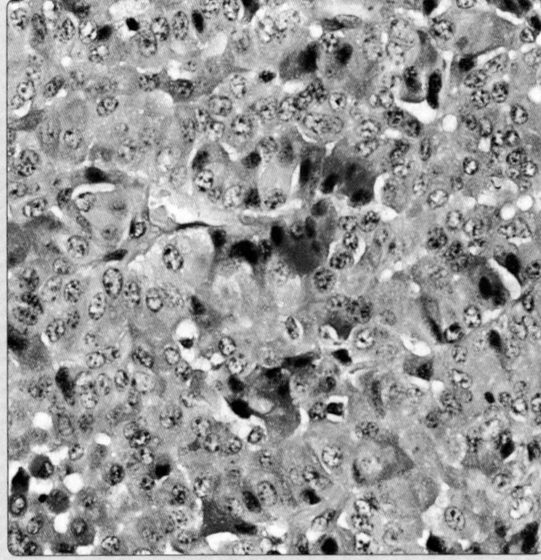

ACTH(+) Strong in Densely Granulated ACTH Adenomas

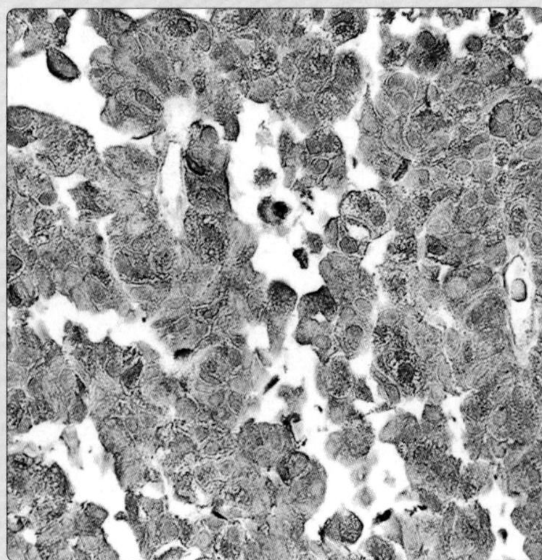

TERMINOLOGY

Synonyms

- Corticotroph cell adenoma, corticotropinoma, basophil adenoma

Definitions

- ACTH, Tpit lineage adenoma

ETIOLOGY/PATHOGENESIS

Genetics

- Sporadic in occurrence
- Minority associated with MEN1 (rare familial examples)
- Germline mutation of glucocorticoid receptor implicated in adenomagenesis
  - Somatic mutation of same receptor seen in Cushing disease and Nelson syndrome

CLINICAL ISSUES

Presentation

- Cushing disease
  - ACTH production simulates bilateral adrenal hyperplasia with cortisol overproduction
  - Should be distinguished from elevated ACTH from nonpituitary sources
  - Exhibits high level hormonal activity
  - Size of adenoma does **not** correspond to level of serum hormones
  - 80% of clinically functioning ACTH adenomas are microadenomas
- Nelson syndrome
  - Cushing disease from undetected adenoma
  - Postadrenalectomy, loss of glucocorticoid feedback, and accelerated growth of adenoma
- Silent corticotroph adenomas nonfunctional
  - Constitute ~ 20% of ACTH adenomas
  - Do not manifest clinical or biochemical evidence of hypercortisolism
  - Some have elevated serum ACTH levels with normal cortisol levels
  - Present with tumor mass effects (headache, visual disturbance, hypopituitarism)
  - Almost all silent ACTH are invasive macroadenomas

Laboratory Tests

- Endocrine testing
  - Serum ACTH, cortisol levels
    - Levels do not correlate with adenoma size, unlike prolactinomas
  - Dexamethasone suppression test
    - Adenoma-associated ACTH not suppressible
  - Petrosal sinus catheterization
    - To detect increased ACTH level in draining veins
- Other peptides derived from proopiomelanocortin (precursor of ACTH) may be produced
  - β-endorphin, β-LPH, CLIP, melanocyte stimulating hormone
- 3 histological subtypes, all driven by Tpit
  - Densely granulated corticotroph adenoma
  - Sparsely granulated corticotroph adenoma
  - Crooke cell adenoma
  - All 3 types usually endocrinologically active/functioning but can be clinically silent

Treatment

- Surgical approaches
  - Generally transsphenoidal, adrenalectomy

Prognosis

- Surgery in Cushing disease-producing adenomas: Curative in 90% of microadenomas and 65% of macroadenomas
- Crooke cell adenomas particularly aggressive; may be clinically active or silent
- Silent corticotroph adenomas
  - Often macroadenomas, prone to apoplexy
  - More aggressive than clinically active (Cushing disease-producing) ACTH adenomas
  - Cavernous sinus invasion may be more prevalent in silent corticotroph adenomas than in other types of nonfunctioning adenomas (e.g., gonadotroph or null cell adenomas)

IMAGING

MR Findings

- Enhancing lesions
- Microadenomas (85%) midline in pituitary; 10-15% locally invasive
- Macroadenoma (15%) less localized; 60% invasive

MACROSCOPIC

Size

- Microadenomas (< 1 cm) for 80% of clinically functioning ACTH adenomas; macroadenomas (> 1 cm) for most silent ACTH adenomas
- Cushing disease
  - Often microadenoma
  - Leveling of paraffin block may be necessary to detect minute adenoma fragments
  - Specimen may be lost during surgery
  - Tumor occasionally left unsampled by surgeon
- Nelson syndrome and silent corticotroph adenoma
  - Surgery yields ample specimen

MICROSCOPIC

Histologic Features

- Cushing disease; often small specimens
  - Basophilic cytoplasm in densely granulated adenomas, weakly basophilic to chromophobic in sparsely granulated ACTH adenomas
  - Accompanying normal pituitary shows ACTH cells with Crooke hyaline change (eosinophilic rings of keratin)
    - Identification of Crooke cells in adjacent nonadenomatous anterior pituitary gland verifies presence of hypercortisolism
      - However, it does not distinguish between hypercortisolism from ectopic ACTH/CRH syndrome, glucocorticoid-producing adrenocortical tumor, or prolonged treatment with glucocorticoids
  - 3 histological subtypes all driven by Tpit

- Densely granulated corticotroph adenoma: Basophilic, abundant keratin filaments
- Sparsely granulated corticotroph adenoma: Chromophobic, fewer keratin filaments
- Crooke cell adenoma (least common): Ring-like accumulation of keratin filaments
- All 3 types usually endocrinologically active, but may be silent

- Nelson syndrome
  - Histological features like Cushing adenoma
  - Variable mitotic activity
  - No Crooke change in normal pituitary
- Silent corticotroph adenoma
  - Variable amphophilia
  - Occasional cytologic atypia and variable mitotic activity
  - Apoplexy common
  - No Crooke change in adjacent normal pituitary
  - Silent corticotroph adenoma may be any of 3 histological subtypes
    - Subtype 1: Densely granulated corticotroph adenoma
    - Subtype 2: Sparsely granulated corticotroph adenoma
    - Crooke cell adenoma

ANCILLARY TESTS

Histochemistry

- PAS(+) (Cushing adenomas) or PAS(-) (1/2 of silent adenomas)
- Loss of normal anterior pituitary gland acinar pattern on reticulin staining

Immunohistochemistry

- ACTH and β-endorphin (+); Tpit(+)
  - ACTH diffuse, strong in densely granulated; focal, weak in sparsely granulated
- CAM5.2 keratin (+); extensive, present in circular bundles surrounding nucleus in Crooke cell adenoma
  - CK7 is either negative or reactive in only few scattered cells in 90% of all adenoma subtypes; not useful in adenoma identification
  - CK20 also IHC(+) in most densely granulated ACTH adenomas and nontumorous Crooke cells; do not mistake CK20 IHC(+) pituitary adenoma for metastatic tumor
- Ki-67 labeling index
  - Low in Cushing adenomas
  - May be increased in atypical, Nelson, Crooke cell, and silent adenomas but not invariably

Electron Microscopy

- Densely granulated corticotroph adenomas on EM resemble normal corticotrophs
  - Moderately developed Golgi complex and rough endoplasmic reticulum
  - Spherical to irregular 200-500 nm, variably electron-dense secretory granules
  - Perinuclear bundles of intermediate (keratin) filaments
- Crooke cell adenomas contain circumnuclear bundles of intermediate filaments
- Nonfunctioning (silent corticotrophic) adenoma
  - 150-300 nm, teardrop-shaped secretory granules
  - 2 types identified ultrastructurally
    - Silent subtype 1: Intermediate filaments identical to Cushing adenoma
    - Silent subtype 2: Lacks keratin filaments

DIFFERENTIAL DIAGNOSIS

ACTH Cell Hyperplasia

- Rare cause of Cushing disease
- Reticulin staining shows only acinar expansion

DIAGNOSTIC CHECKLIST

Pathologic Interpretation Pearls

- Crooke hyaline change in ACTH IHC(+) cells of adjacent nontumorous anterior pituitary gland documents hypercortisolemia
  - Doesn't distinguish between hypercortisolemia from corticotroph adenoma, ectopic ACTH/CRH syndrome, glucocorticoid-producing adrenocortical tumor, or prolonged treatment with glucocorticoids
- Serum levels of ACTH and cortisol do not correlate with ACTH adenoma size, unlike prolactinomas

SELECTED REFERENCES

1. Cooper O: Silent corticotroph adenomas. Pituitary. 18(2):225-31, 2015
2. Gomez-Hernandez K et al: Clinical Implications of Accurate Subtyping of Pituitary Adenomas: Perspectives from the Treating Physician. Turk Patoloji Derg. 31 Suppl 1:4-17, 2015
3. Smith TR et al: Complications after transsphenoidal surgery for patients with Cushing's disease and silent corticotroph adenomas. Neurosurg Focus. 38(2):E12, 2015
4. Zoli M et al: ACTH adenomas transforming their clinical expression: report of 5 cases. Neurosurg Focus. 38(2):E15, 2015
5. Cazabat L et al: Silent, but not unseen: multimicrocystic aspect on T2-weighted MRI in silent corticotroph adenomas. Clin Endocrinol (Oxf). 81(4):566-72, 2014
6. Dhaliwal JS et al: Orbital invasion by ACTH-secreting pituitary adenomas. Ophthal Plast Reconstr Surg. 30(2):e28-30, 2014
7. Mayson SE et al: Silent (clinically nonfunctioning) pituitary adenomas. J Neurooncol. 117(3):429-36, 2014
8. Xu Z et al: Silent corticotroph adenomas after stereotactic radiosurgery: a case-control study. Int J Radiat Oncol Biol Phys. 90(4):903-10, 2014
9. Jahangiri A et al: A comprehensive long-term retrospective analysis of silent corticotrophic adenomas vs hormone-negative adenomas. Neurosurgery. 73(1):8-17; discussion 17-8, 2013
10. Cooper O et al: Subclinical hyperfunctioning pituitary adenomas: the silent tumors. Best Pract Res Clin Endocrinol Metab. 26(4):447-60, 2012
11. Nishioka H et al: Correlation between histological subtypes and MRI findings in clinically nonfunctioning pituitary adenomas. Endocr Pathol. 23(3):151-6, 2012
12. Coons SW et al: Cytokeratin CK 7 and CK 20 expression in pituitary adenomas. Endocr Pathol. 16(3):201-10, 2005
13. Lopez JA et al: Silent corticotroph adenomas: further clinical and pathological observations. Hum Pathol. 35(9):1137-47, 2004
14. Scheithauer BW et al: Clinically silent corticotroph tumors of the pituitary gland. Neurosurgery. 47(3):723-9; discussion 729-30, 2000
15. Lloyd RV et al: The spectrum of ACTH-producing pituitary lesions. Am J Surg Pathol. 10(9):618-26, 1986
16. Robert F et al: Human corticotroph cell adenomas. Semin Diagn Pathol. 3(1):34-41, 1986

Occasional Nuclear Pseudoinclusions

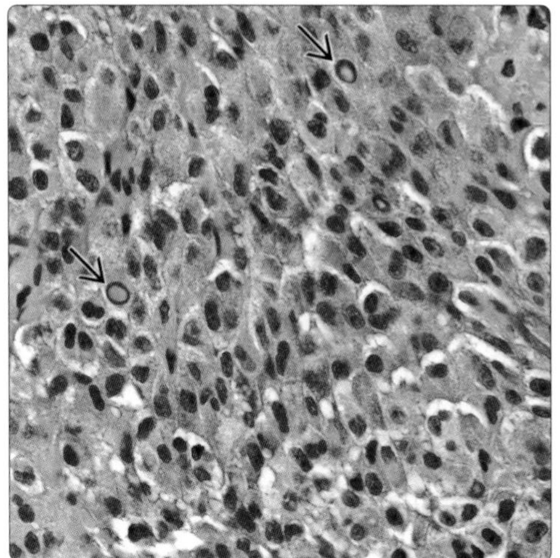

Diffuse ACTH in All Cells in Densely Granulated ACTH Adenoma

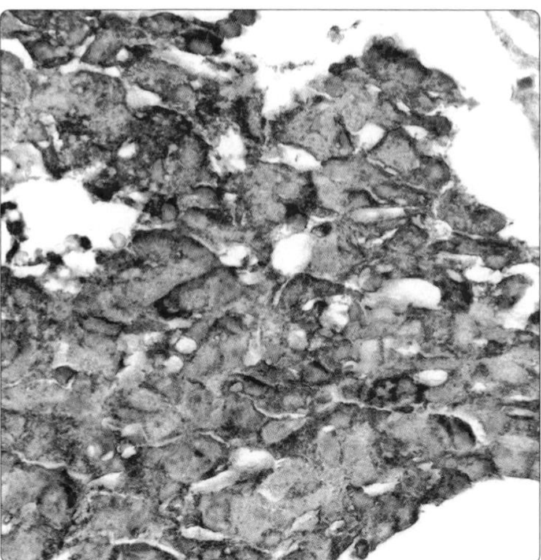

(Left) *Nuclear pseudoinclusions* ➡ *are sometimes present in, but are not specific for, ACTH adenomas. To the unwary, this may simulate meningioma, although whorls and psammoma body calcifications are absent.* **(Right)** *Strong ACTH IHC(+) is seen in all cells in a densely granulated ACTH adenoma.*

Acinar Disruption

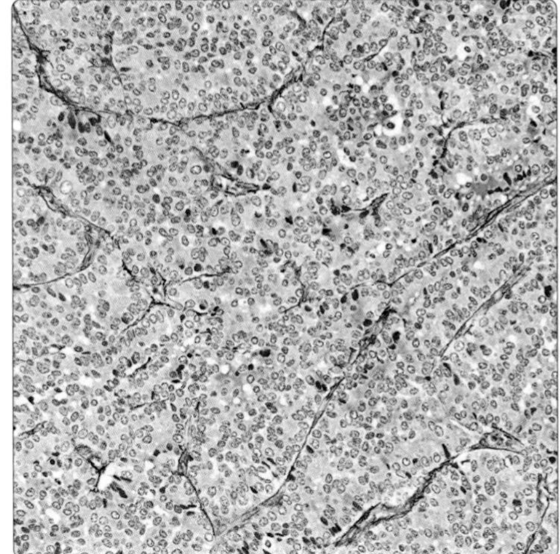

Nonneoplastic Crooke Cells

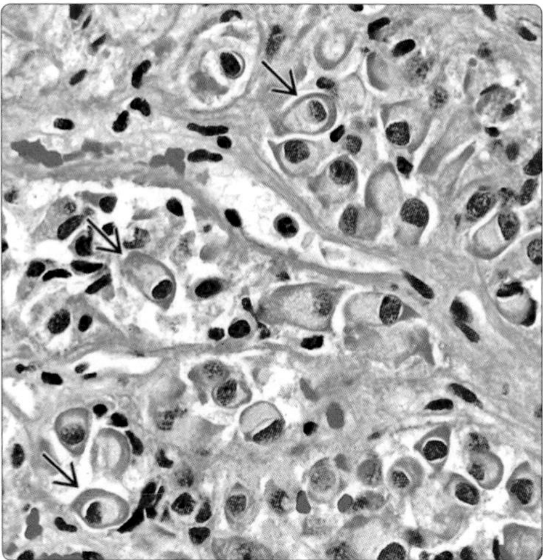

(Left) *Like all pituitary adenomas, in ACTH adenomas distortion, loss, and disruption of the pituitary gland acinar pattern are evident after staining for reticulin; this provides confirmation of adenoma diagnosis.* **(Right)** *Nonneoplastic cells with conspicuous eosinophilic rings of keratin surrounding the nucleus are termed Crooke hyaline change* ➡*. The abnormality is the result of cortisol excess from any cause. Only in the rare Crooke cell adenoma do neoplastic cells themselves have these cytokeratin-rich rings.*

ACTH in Crooke Cells in Adjacent Nontumorous Anterior Gland

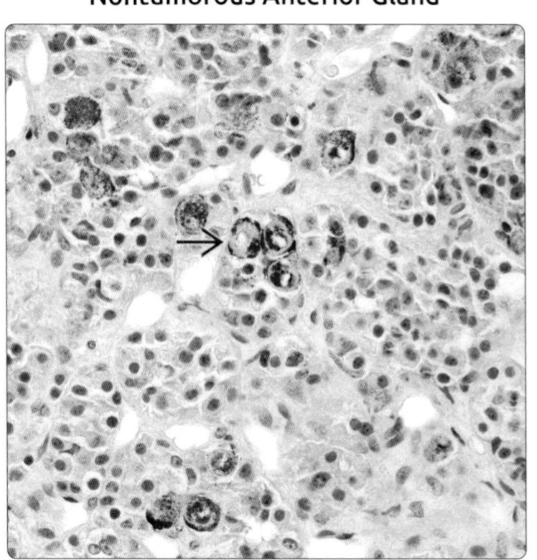

Reticulin in Normal Adjacent Nontumorous Anterior Pituitary Gland Containing Crooke Cells

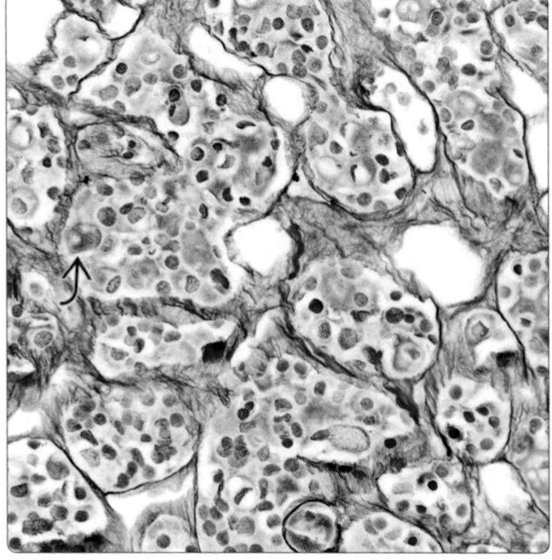

(Left) *Nonneoplastic cells with Crooke hyaline change and keratin accumulation pushes the secretory granules to the periphery of cell, as seen here on ACTH immunohistochemistry* ➡*. The abnormality is the result of cortisol excess from any cause but proves that there was indeed hypercortisolemia. They should be sought in the nontumorous anterior gland from a patient with an ACTH adenoma.* **(Right)** *Reticulin in normal adjacent gland containing Crooke cells* ➡ *shows acinar preservation.*

(Left) *Chromophobic sparsely granulated ACTH adenomas lack the cytoplasmic basophilia of densely granulated ACTH adenoma.* **(Right)** *All pituitary adenomas of all subtypes are immunoreactive for synaptophysin, even if sparsely granulated variants.*

Chromophobic Sparsely Granulated ACTH Adenoma

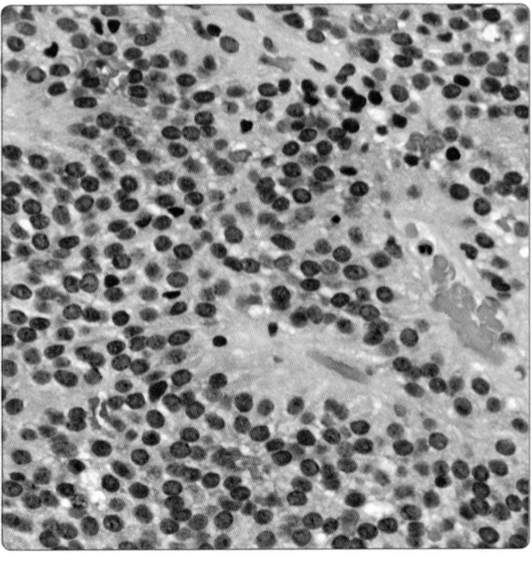

Synaptophysin IHC(+)

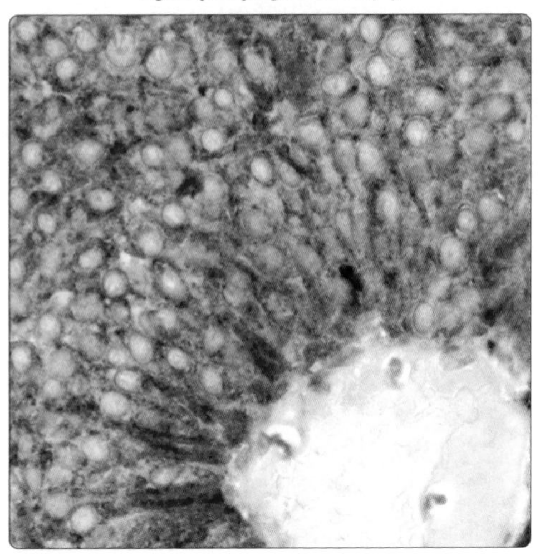

(Left) *ACTH IHC in sparsely granulated corticotroph adenomas is more focal than in densely granulated variants. This patient, however, did have Cushing disease, i.e., the adenoma was functionally active.* **(Right)** *CAM5.2(+) is identified in ~ 1/2 of sparsely granulated ACTH adenomas, as in this example. CK20(+), in contrast, is found in densely granulated ACTH adenomas, but not in sparsely granulated/focal ACTH(+) adenomas.*

ACTH, Sparsely Granulated Adenoma

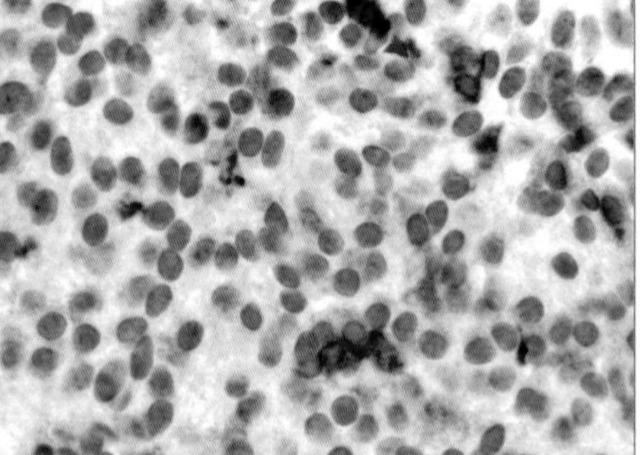

CAM5.2 in ACTH Adenoma

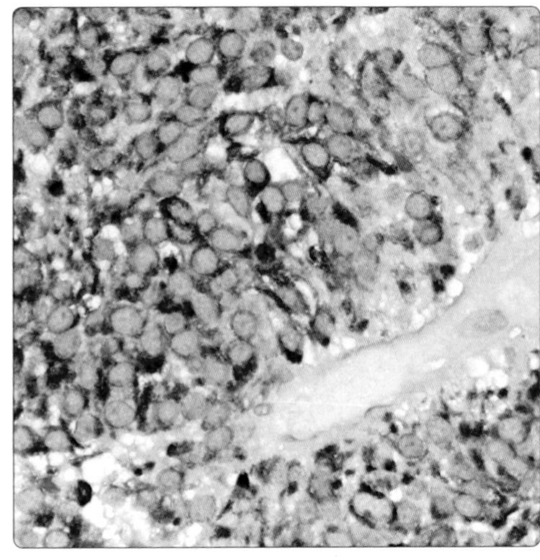

(Left) *As well as Crooke change in normal corticotrophs, rare adenomas are composed largely or entirely of Crooke cells. Such Crooke cell adenomas are often aggressive.* **(Right)** *In Crooke cell adenomas, circular bundles of keratin filaments* ➡ *are diffusely immunoreactive for low molecular weight keratins, CAM5.2 in this case.*

Rare Crooke Cell Adenoma

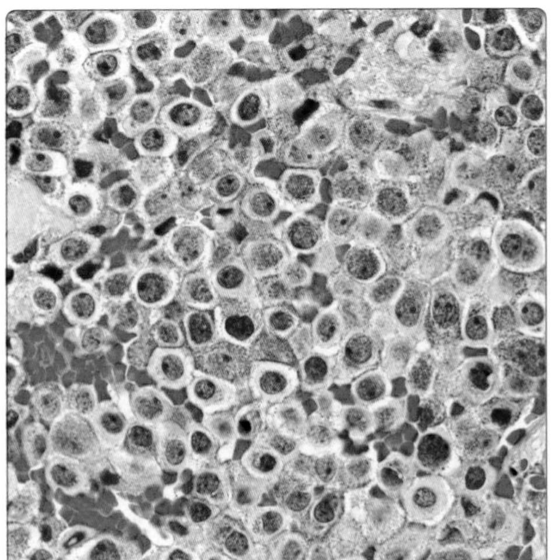

Crooke Cell Adenoma: Keratins

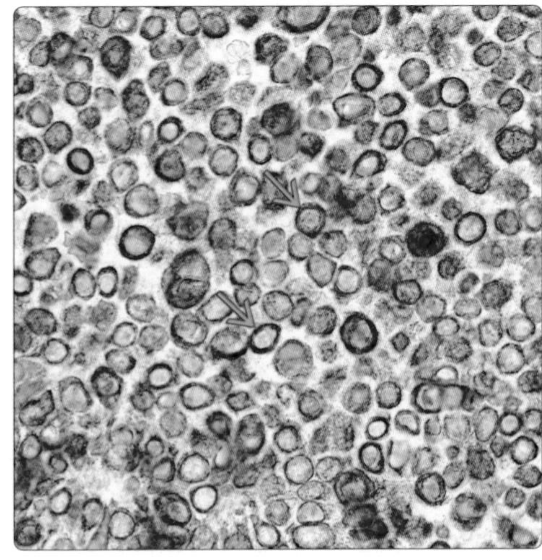

Amphophilic to Basophilic Adenoma Cells

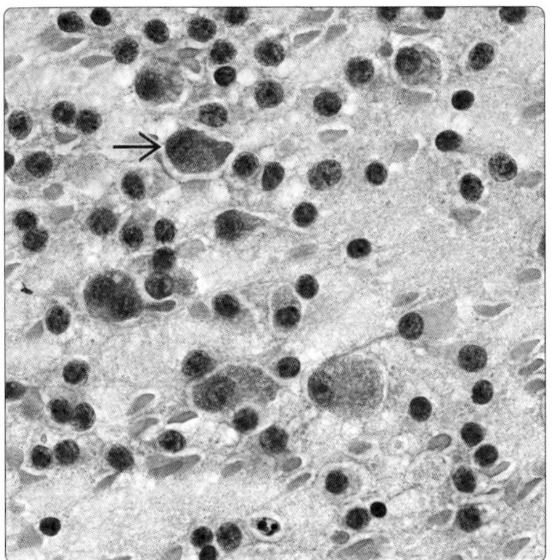

Multinucleation: Silent ACTH Adenoma

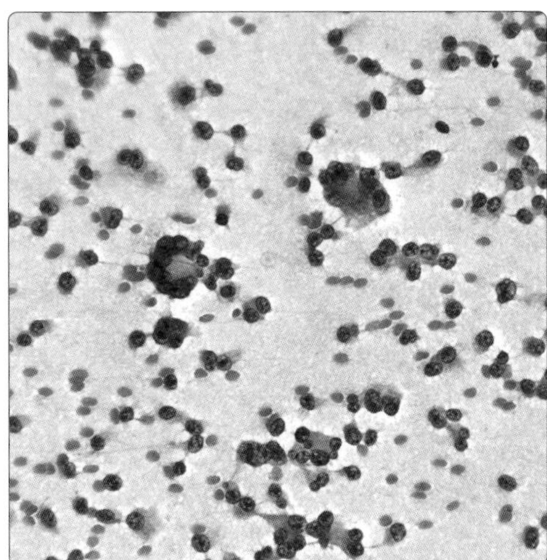

(Left) *In smear preparations, cells of corticotroph adenomas are amphophilic to basophilic* ➞. **(Right)** *Multinucleation or nuclear pleomorphism is an occasional finding in silent corticotroph adenomas. Cytological features do not affect diagnosis but silent ACTH adenomas are an acknowledged aggressive subtype of adenoma that is usually very large and invasive of structures near the sella, such as sphenoid sinus, dura, cavernous sinus, and sellar bone.*

Proopiomelanocortin (Precursor of ACTH)

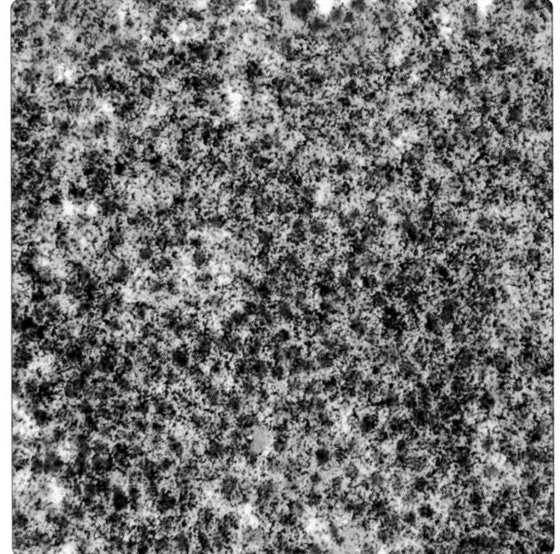

Crooke Cell Adenoma

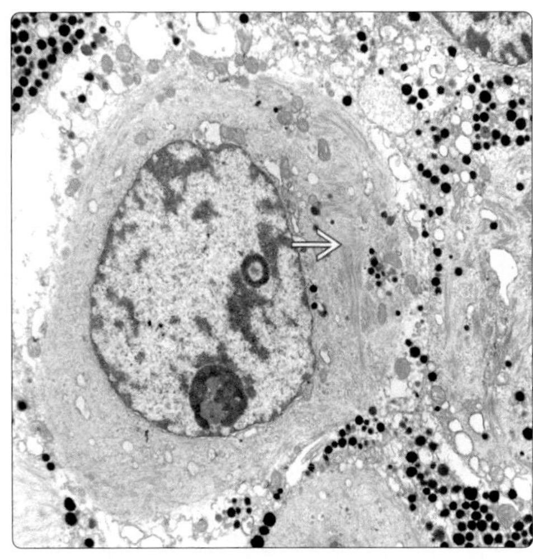

(Left) *Proopiomelanocortin (the precursor of ACTH) is shown by in situ hybridization in this ACTH cell adenoma.* **(Right)** *Crooke cell corticotroph adenoma shows keratin filaments* ➞ *that fill the cytoplasm.*

Spherical to Irregular Granules

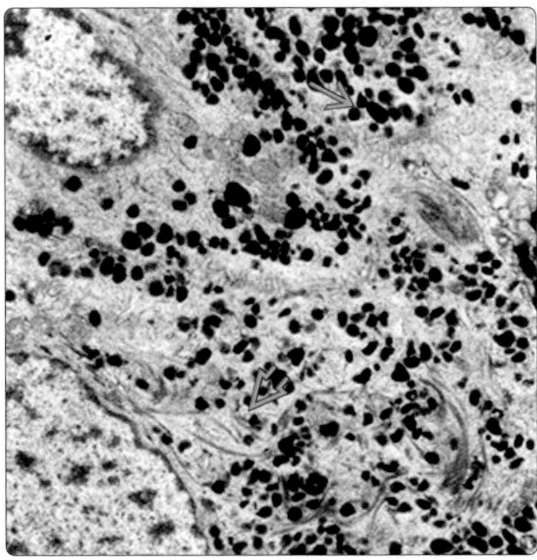

Silent ACTH Adenoma

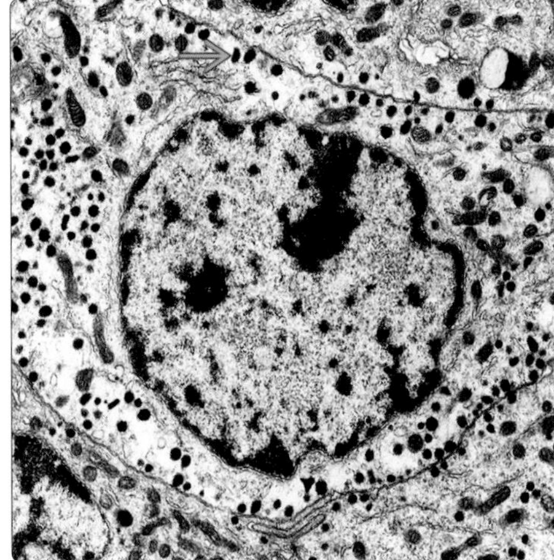

(Left) *Ultrastructurally, Cushing adenomas feature spherical to irregularly shaped secretory granules* ➞ *and numerous intermediate filaments* ➞ *in the densely granulated variant.* **(Right)** *Small secretory granules, tear or heart-shaped* ➞, *can be found in silent ACTH adenomas. No type 1 microfilaments are detected in silent ACTH adenoma, subtype II.*

Gonadotroph Adenoma

KEY FACTS

CLINICAL ISSUES

- Most common type of clinically nonfunctioning adenoma
- Many patients are elderly men
- Most common presentations due to mass effect
- Majority are clinically endocrinologically nonfunctioning
- Slow growing, more compressive than invasive
- Presentation with apoplexy common
- Biochemically, hypopituitarism
- Transsphenoidal surgery usual, but transfrontal surgery may be required
- Recurrence uncommon
- Prognosis favorable

IMAGING

- Macroadenomas demonstrating low frequency (20%) of radiographically apparent invasion
- May be associated with apoplexy on imaging studies

MICROSCOPIC

- Variable histologic patterns
  - Pseudorosetting around blood vessels, pseudopapillary-like formation, sinusoidal, diffuse patterns
- Nuclear atypia inconspicuous
- Mitotic activity absent or rare

ANCILLARY TESTS

- Staining for FSH &/or LH often patchy and highly variable in distribution within adenoma and highly variable percentage of IHC(+) cells within adenomas
- By definition, gonadotroph adenomas either IHC(+) for FSH &/or LH &/or SF1
- Chromogranin and synaptophysin reactivity strong
- Ki-67 labeling indices typically low
- α-subunit reaction frequent
  - Identification of α-subunit (+) alone requires additional confirmation of gonadotroph cell lineage with SF1(+)

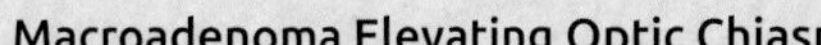

Macroadenoma Elevating Optic Chiasm

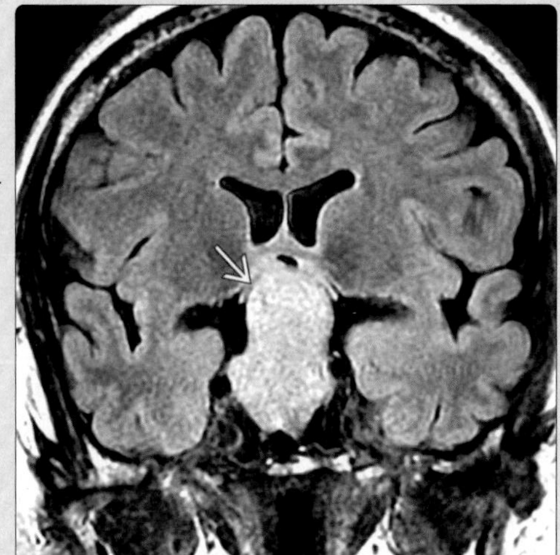

Perivascular Pseudorosette-Like Features

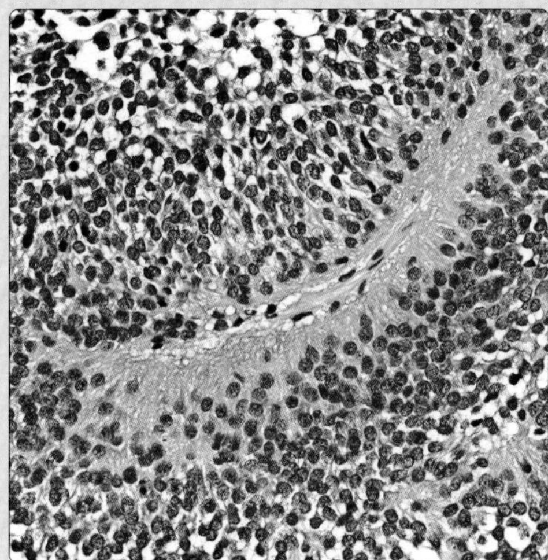

(Left) *Coronal FLAIR MR shows an example of a macroadenoma ➡ that elevates and compresses the optic chiasm. Gonadotroph adenomas are usually macroadenomas at the time of presentation.* **(Right)** *The chromophobic cells often form perivascular pseudorosette-like structures similar to those in ependymoma. These rosettes in pituitary adenomas are, however, composed of tapering cell cytoplasm rather than finely fibrillary GFAP(+) processes.*

Oncocytic Change Frequent

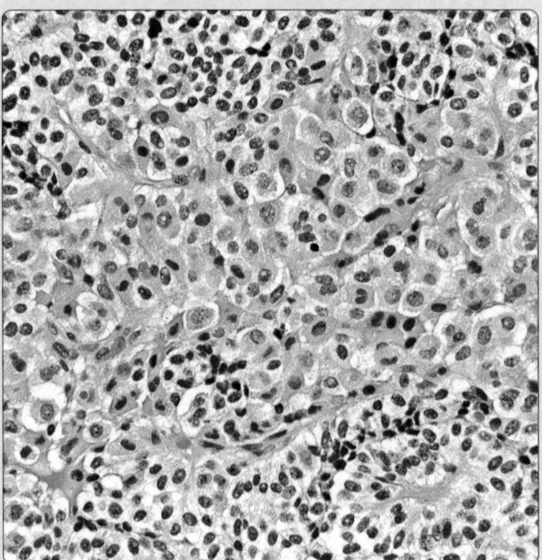

SF1(+)

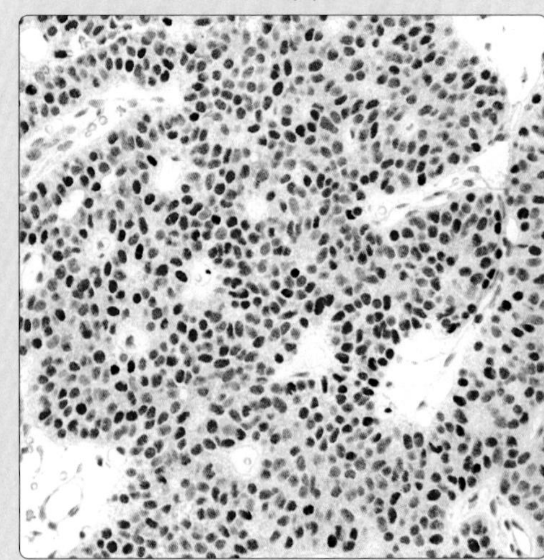

(Left) *Oncocytic change is seen in ~ 50% of gonadotroph adenomas.* **(Right)** *Gonadotroph adenomas by definition express IHC(+) for FSH &/or LH; in the absence of immunostaining for these specific anterior pituitary hormones, presence of the relevant transcription factor (SF1) also serves to define gonadotroph adenomas.*

TERMINOLOGY

Synonyms

- Gonadotropinoma

Definitions

- Adenoma producing FSH &/or LH &/or showing immunoreactivity for SF1

CLINICAL ISSUES

Epidemiology

- Incidence
  - Most common type of clinically nonfunctional adenoma
  - Increased use of more sensitive FSH/LH immunostains, coupled with SF1 IHC, shows most clinically nonfunctioning (nonsecretory) adenomas are SF1(+) gonadotroph adenomas
    - Hormone-negative adenomas with SF1 are gonadotroph adenomas; high-fidelity FSH and LH IHCs are not available in many hospitals
      - Thus, either adenoma with FSH(+) or LH(+) or both IHC(+) **or** adenoma with SF1(+) = gonadotroph adenoma
    - Hormone-negative adenomas without SF1 may have distinct clinical features; some Tpit(+)
- Age
  - Adenoma type mainly affects older adults
- Sex
  - Male patients more frequently affected

Presentation

- Most common presentations
  - Visual disturbance (70%)
  - Hypopituitarism (60%)
  - Headache (40%)
- Infrequently (20%) show clinical hormonal activities
  - Increases in serum LH/FSH infrequent (20%)
  - More readily detected in male than female patients, given postmenopausal state of most older patients
- Diagnosed on basis of immunostaining of adenoma tissues since majority are clinically nonfunctioning
- Slow growing; compressive rather than invasive lesions
- Presentation with apoplexy more commonly than many other adenoma types
- Biochemically, often associated with decreased anterior pituitary hormone levels (hypopituitarism)
- Diagnosis may be aided by TRH administration, which results in stimulation of FSH &/or LH production

Treatment

- Transsphenoidal hypophysectomy relieves mass effect
- Transfrontal surgery sometimes required to debulk large tumors with significant suprasellar component
- Only rarely, gonadotropic adenomas respond to dopamine agonist or somatostatin therapy
- Postoperative radiation therapy seldom needed or utilized
- Hormone replacement for patients with hypopituitarism

Prognosis

- Overall prognosis very favorable
- Recurrence uncommon (5% of cases)

IMAGING

General Features

- Location
  - Most large and demonstrate extrasellar extension
- Size
  - Macroadenomas demonstrating low frequency (20%) of radiographically apparent invasion

Radiographic Findings

- Suprasellar extension with chiasmal compression often seen and more common than cavernous sinus extension
- Compression or extension to cavernous sinuses, in some cases
- Given large size, compression of carotid arteries in some cases
  - Pituitary adenomas of any type almost never invade large vessel walls

MACROSCOPIC

General Features

- Gonadotropic adenomas bulky, soft, and tan
- Foci of hemorrhage, necrosis, hemosiderin, or cystic change, in some cases
  - Indicative of prior episodes of apoplexy, clinical or subclinical

MICROSCOPIC

Histologic Features

- Histologic patterns vary, sometimes within same adenoma
  - Pseudorosette-like formation around blood vessels, simulating ependymoma
  - Pseudopapillary pattern due to dyscohesion of adenoma cells
  - Sinusoidal
  - Diffuse or vaguely macronodular
  - Variable histological patterns do not correspond to immunostaining profile
- Cells medium-sized and often polygonal or polar relative to vessels (pseudorosettes)
- Limited oncocytic change due to mitochondrial accumulation (common)
- Nuclear atypia inconspicuous, and mitotic activity is absent or rare

ANCILLARY TESTS

Histochemistry

- Although normal gonadotrophs are PAS positive, gonadotroph adenomas are typically chromophobic and PAS negative

Immunohistochemistry

- Staining for FSH &/or LH often patchy and highly variable in distribution within single adenoma; widely varying percentage of immunopositive cells
  - FSH staining usually very patchy
    - FSH(+) usually not diffuse throughout entire adenoma, as in PRL(+) in prolactinomas
  - α-subunit reaction frequent in small to moderate percentage of adenoma cells

- LH immunoreactivity usually less abundant than FSH IHC(+)
- Immunophenotypic patterns do not correlate with histological pattern variations
  - i.e., pseudopapillary, macronodular, etc.
- Chromogranin and synaptophysin reactivity strong
- Ki-67 labeling indices typically low (< 2-3%)
- SF1, specific transcription factor for gonadotrophic cells, expression = in gonadotroph adenomas
  - Evaluation for SF1 necessary in adenomas without FSH or LH and only α-subunit immunoreactivity to definitively classify adenoma as gonadotroph adenoma

Genetic Testing

- Comparative genomic hybridization studies show gains and losses involving all chromosomes
- Only occasionally occur in longstanding hypogonadism
- Activin receptors expressed in gonadotropic adenomas, whereas follistatin is diminished
  - Suggesting that enhanced activin signaling may contribute to pathogenesis of gonadotrophic adenomas

Electron Microscopy

- Most tumors consist of uniform, polar cells with process formation
- Cytoplasm contains well-developed rough endoplasmic reticulum and Golgi complexes, small (50-150 nm) secretory granules often distributed along cell membranes
  - Tumors in female patients have distinctive vacuolar transformation of Golgi
  - Oncocytic change variable
- Only occasional gonadotropic adenomas resemble mature gonadotrophs in terms of morphology of secretory granules

Genetics

- Only slight increase in gonadotropic hormone-producing adenomas in *MEN1* or Carney complex

DIFFERENTIAL DIAGNOSIS

Hormone-Negative Adenoma

- Similar histologic patterns with LH/FSH adenoma
  - Pseudorosetting around blood vessels, pseudopapillary-like pattern seen, as in some gonadotroph adenomas
- May be only α-subunit immunoreactive
  - These cases require further SF1(+) to document gonadotroph adenoma lineage/diagnosis
- EM: Poorly developed organelles and few secretory granules
- Depending on sensitivity of immunostains, larger percentage of adenomas now realized to show FSH/LH immunostaining
  - i.e., gonadotroph adenomas
- SF1 immunoreactivity shared between gonadotroph adenomas and most clinically nonfunctioning (nonsecretory) adenomas
- Non-SF1 immunoreactive clinically nonfunctioning (nonsecretory) adenomas are separate entity; some Tpit(+)

SELECTED REFERENCES

1. Balogun JA et al: Null cell adenomas of the pituitary gland: an institutional review of their clinical imaging and behavioral characteristics. Endocr Pathol. 26(1):63-70, 2015
2. Gomez-Hernandez K et al: Clinical implications of accurate subtyping of pituitary adenomas: perspectives from the treating physician. Turk Patoloji Derg. 31 Suppl 1:4-17, 2015
3. Kleinschmidt-DeMasters BK et al: An algorithmic approach to sellar region masses. Arch Pathol Lab Med. 139(3):356-72, 2015
4. Nishioka H et al: The complementary role of transcription factors in the accurate diagnosis of clinically nonfunctioning pituitary adenomas. Endocr Pathol. ePub, 2015
5. Raverot G et al: Biological and radiological exploration and management of non-functioning pituitary adenoma. Ann Endocrinol (Paris). 76(3):201-9, 2015
6. Ntali G et al: Clinical review: Functioning gonadotroph adenomas. J Clin Endocrinol Metab. 99(12):4423-33, 2014
7. Newey PJ et al: Whole-exome sequencing studies of nonfunctioning pituitary adenomas. J Clin Endocrinol Metab. 98(4):E796-800, 2013
8. Baborie A et al: A clone of elusive parents: gonadotroph adenoma-female type. Ultrastruct Pathol. 36(2):85-8, 2012
9. Ersen A et al: Non-uniform response to temozolomide therapy in a pituitary gonadotroph adenoma. Can J Neurol Sci. 39(5):683-5, 2012
10. Nishioka H et al: Correlation between histological subtypes and MRI findings in clinically nonfunctioning pituitary adenomas. Endocr Pathol. 23(3):151-6, 2012
11. Xu M et al: Reprimo (RPRM) is a novel tumor suppressor in pituitary tumors and regulates survival, proliferation, and tumorigenicity. Endocrinology. 153(7):2963-73, 2012
12. Chesnokova V et al: Lineage-specific restraint of pituitary gonadotroph cell adenoma growth. PLoS One. 6(3):e17924, 2011
13. Madsen H et al: Giant pituitary adenomas: pathologic-radiographic correlations and lack of role for p53 and MIB-1 labeling. Am J Surg Pathol. 35(8):1204-13, 2011
14. Rishi A et al: A clinicopathological and immunohistochemical study of clinically non-functioning pituitary adenomas: a single institutional experience. Neurol India. 58(3):418-23, 2010
15. Lillehei KO et al: Reassessment of the role of radiation therapy in the treatment of endocrine-inactive pituitary macroadenomas. Neurosurgery. 43(3):432-8; discussion 438-9, 1998
16. Young WF Jr et al: Gonadotroph adenoma of the pituitary gland: a clinicopathologic analysis of 100 cases. Mayo Clin Proc. 71(7):649-56, 1996
17. Asa SL et al: Gonadotropin secretion in vitro by human pituitary null cell adenomas and oncocytomas. J Clin Endocrinol Metab. 62(5):1011-9, 1986

Perivascular Pseudorosette-Like Pattern, Simulating Ependymoma

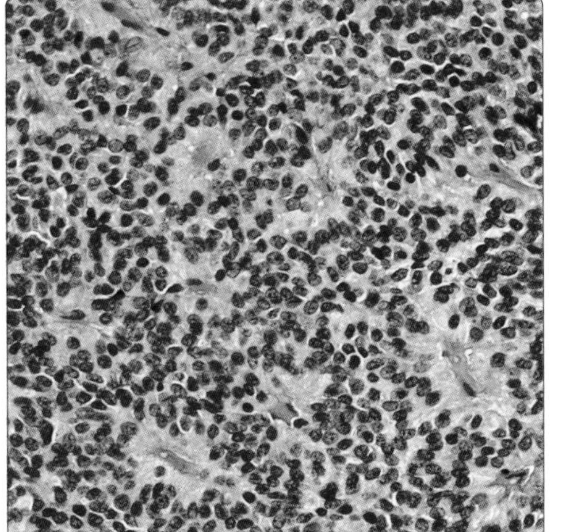

Ribbon-Like Sinusoidal Pattern

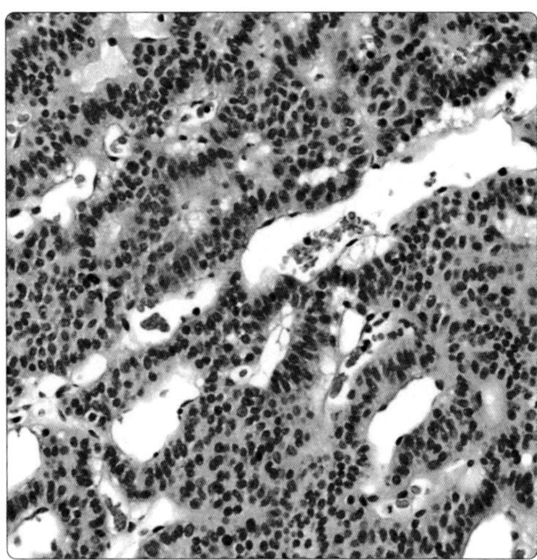

(Left) *Ependymoma-like perivascular pseudorosettes are common in gonadotroph adenomas. Pituitary adenomas are GFAP immunonegative and always synaptophysin (+), unlike ependymomas.* **(Right)** *Gonadotroph cell adenomas may assume a ribbon-like pattern. None of these histological pattern variations impact prognosis.*

Pseudopapillary-Like Structures

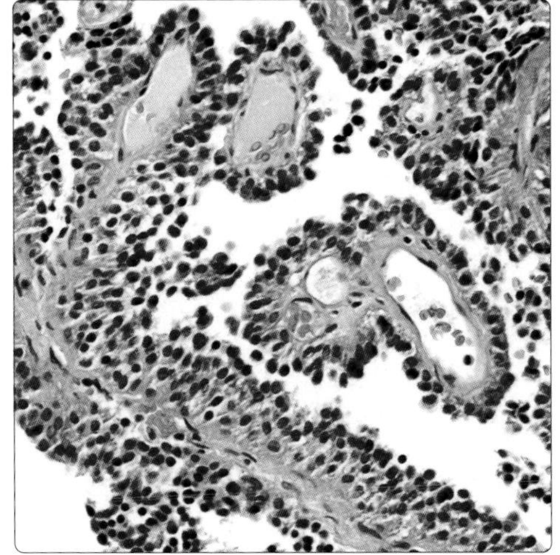

Cystic Areas

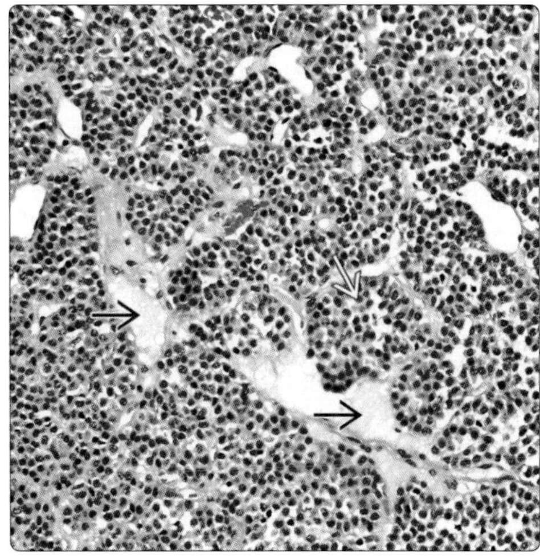

(Left) *Pseudopapillary-like structures in gonadotroph pituitary adenomas should not be misinterpreted as evidence of ependymoma. Perivascular formations in the latter neoplasm will be immunoreactive for GFAP. Those in gonadotroph cell adenomas are synaptophysin (+).* **(Right)** *Some gonadotroph adenomas have cystic areas ➙. Note how some areas of the adenoma can have a vaguely nested ➡ pattern, although most of the adenoma has sheet-like architecture.*

Oncocytic Change

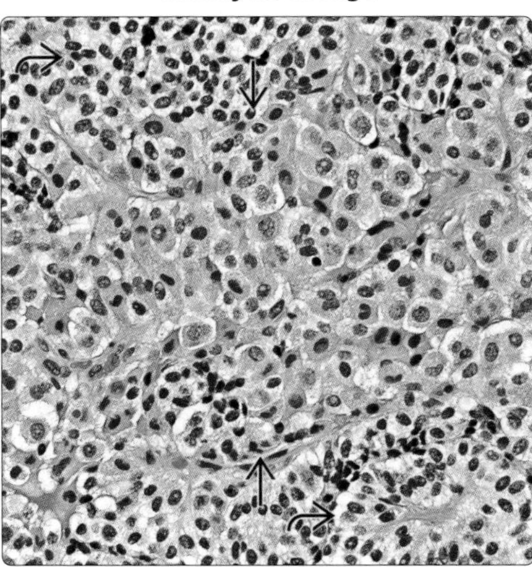

Apoplexy

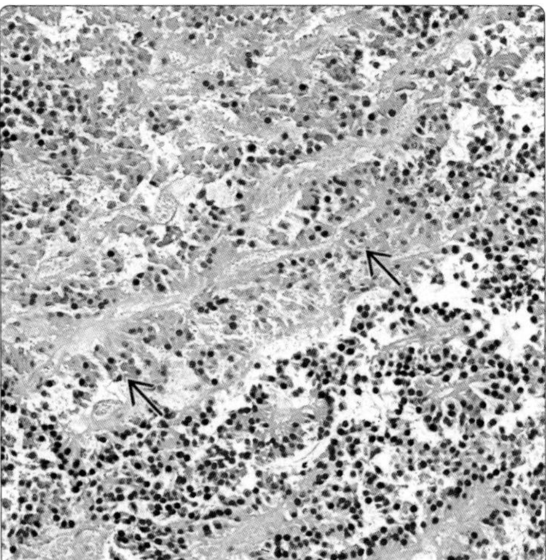

(Left) *Oncocytic change ➙ is seen in ~ 50% of gonadotroph adenomas. Note that other areas of the same adenoma show less oncocytic change ➙. These 2 different appearing areas should not be misinterpreted as "double adenoma."* **(Right)** *Gonadotroph adenomas frequently present with acute hemorrhagic infarction, resulting in clinical apoplexy. This example shows both viable and necrotic ➙ areas. Perivascular formations, visible in the viable area, are present in some gonadotroph adenomas.*

(Left) *The normal acinar pattern seen in the nonadenomatous anterior pituitary gland is usually completely lost in macroadenomas, including gonadotroph adenomas. The only remaining reticulin fibers outline blood vessels within the adenoma* ➙. **(Right)** *While the majority of gonadotroph adenomas show significant, near-total loss of reticulin, some possess a macronodular pattern. Although the reticulin appears more maintained than in some adenomas, this nevertheless is not a normal for anterior gland.*

Acinar Pattern Usually Completely Lost

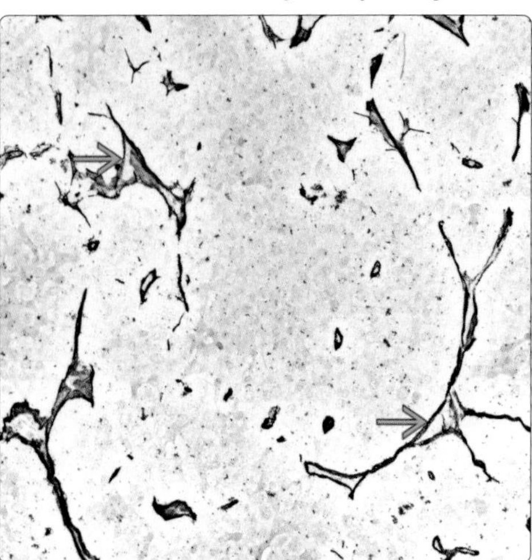

Macronodular Pattern

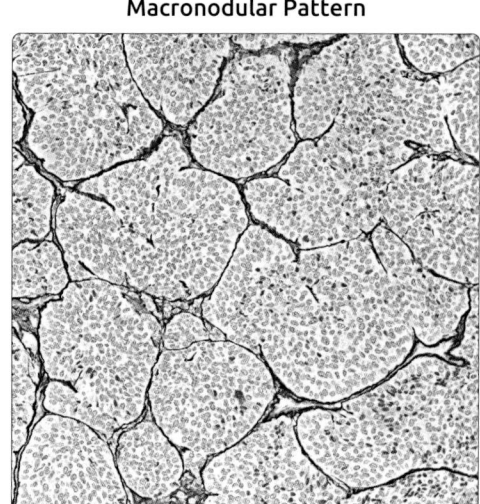

(Left) *Synaptophysin immunostaining is always positive in all types of pituitary adenomas.* **(Right)** *Most pituitary adenomas show expression of E-cadherin, seen here with a red Chromagen. The greatest exception is sparsely granulated growth hormone adenomas, in which IHC is routinely lost. Many gonadotroph adenomas also show hemosiderin pigment* ➙ *indicative of subclinical bleeding into the adenoma.*

Synaptophysin Positive in All Adenomas

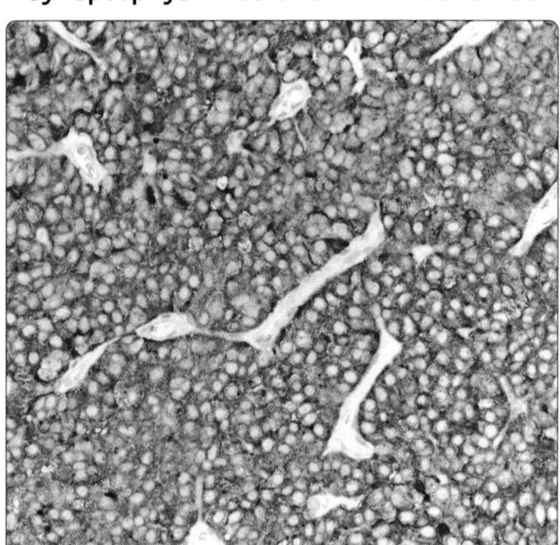

E-Cadherin (+)

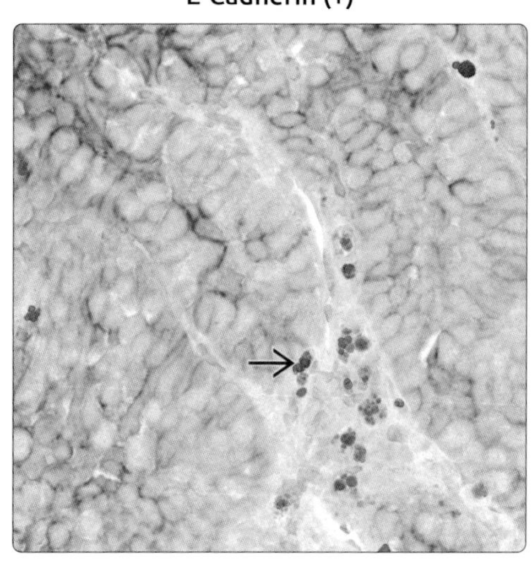

(Left) *CAM5.2 is variably immunoreactive in gonadotroph adenomas and sometimes much weaker or even negative than the case illustrated here.* **(Right)** *By definition, a gonadotroph adenoma must show either IHC(+) for SF1 or for 1 or more specific gonadotroph cell lineage hormones, i.e., FSH or LH. As in this example, in the majority of cases, FSH is stronger than LH and seen in more cells, although almost invariably patchy in distribution.*

CAM5.2 Variably Immunoreactive

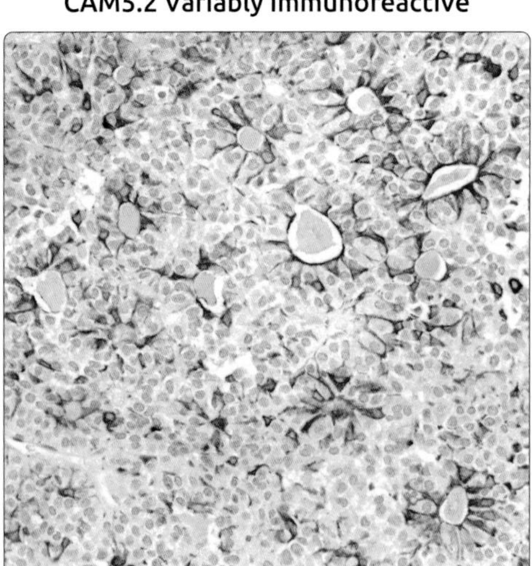

FSH Patchy

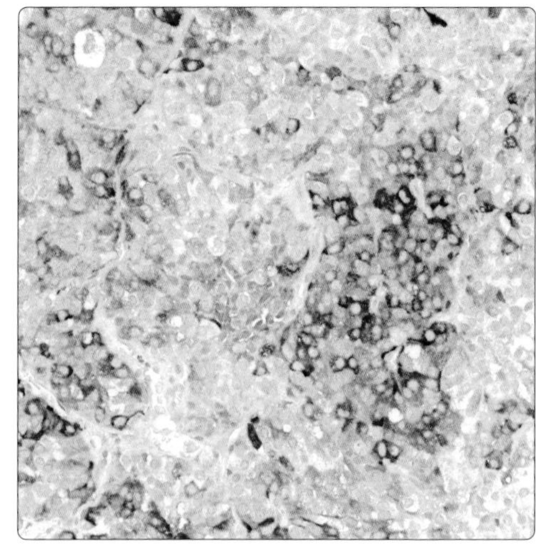

Focal LH(+)

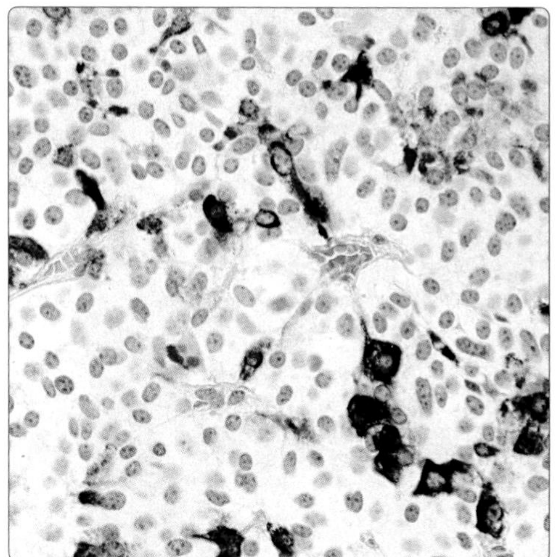

α-Subunit IHC(+)

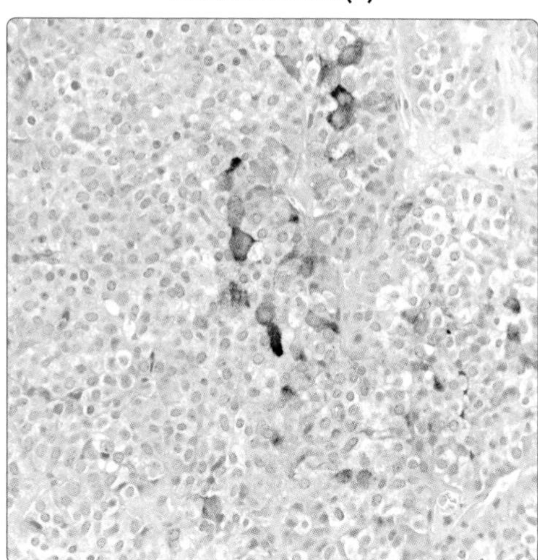

(Left) *LH reactivity is often less abundant than that for FSH and may require careful evaluation for detection. Many gonadotroph adenomas show only FSH or FSH and α-subunit immunostaining and lack LH IHC(+) altogether.* **(Right)** *Many gonadotroph adenomas will have focal patchy α-subunit immunostaining in a minority of cells, in addition to either FSH or FSH and LH IHC(+).*

Ki-67/MIB-1 Usually Low

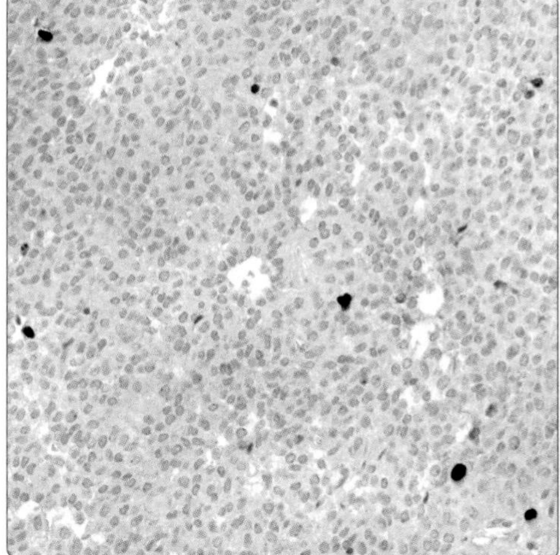

Ki-67 Elevated, Uncommon

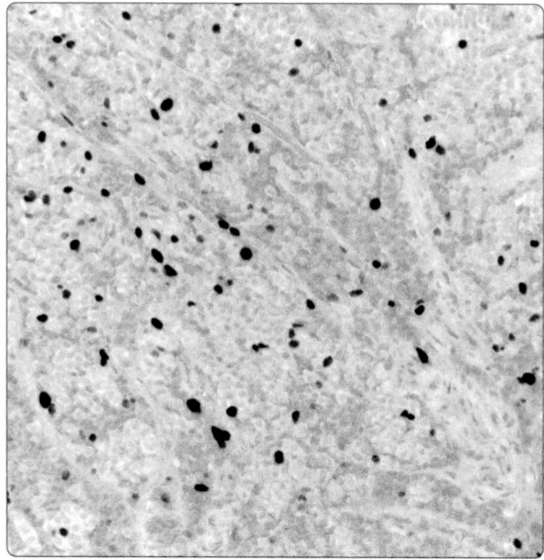

(Left) *Cell-cycle labeling rate in the majority of gonadotroph adenomas is low, paralleling their indolent growth rate.* **(Right)** *Uncommonly, gonadotroph adenomas have elevated Ki-67 rates, as shown here. Most gonadotroph adenomas are slow growing and can reach giant sizes before the patient comes to clinical presentation with mass effect, or sometimes pituitary apoplexy. Many workers eschew the term "atypical adenoma" for adenomas with Ki-67 rates > 3%, preferring instead to simply advise closer follow-up.*

Subplasmalemmal Membrane Granules

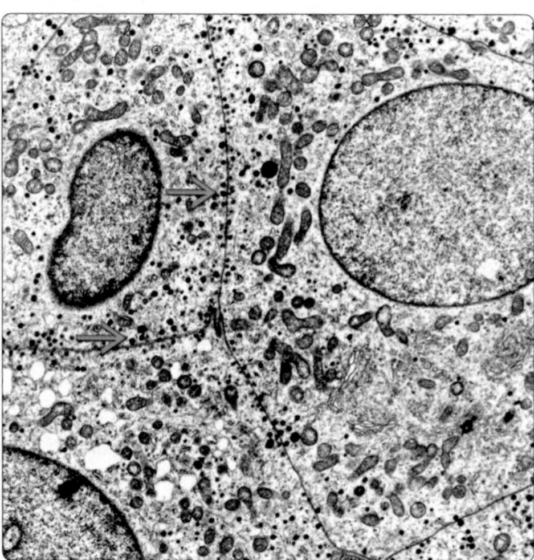

Vesicular Golgi

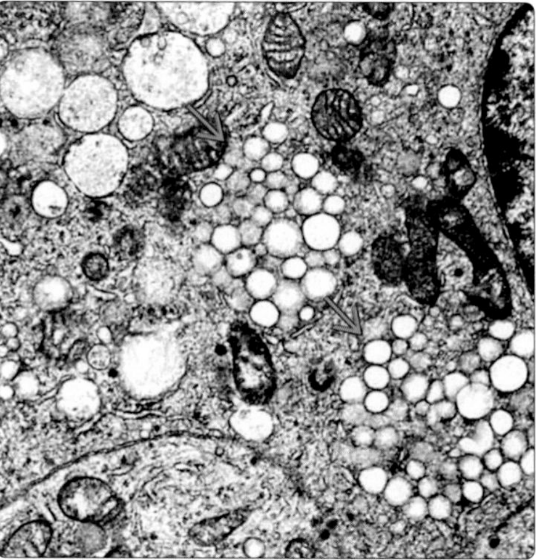

(Left) *Gonadotroph cell adenomas in male patients ultrastructurally show underdeveloped synthetic and secretory organelles, as well as increased number of mitochondria (oncocytic change). Granules are located beneath cell membranes ➡.* **(Right)** *Gonadotrophic adenomas in female patients often have vesicular Golgi ➡.*

Thyrotroph Adenoma

KEY FACTS

ETIOLOGY/PATHOGENESIS

- Patients with MEN1, as well as Carney complex, are predisposed to thyroid-stimulating hormone (TSH) adenoma

CLINICAL ISSUES

- Rarest form of adenoma (< 1% of all adenomas)
  - Most hypothyroidism is due to thyroid disease, not TSH adenoma
- Often associated with hyperthyroidism
- Often invasive and macroadenoma (75%)
- Often somatostatin-responsive
- 80% also secrete α-subunit
- Local invasion and recurrence frequent

MACROSCOPIC

- Most TSH adenomas are large and invasive adenomas by neuroimaging studies

MICROSCOPIC

- Chromophobic; often pseudorosettes
- Cells often polygonal or elongate
- Perivascular stromal fibrosis frequent
- May see small PAS(+) cytoplasmic droplets
  - Corresponds to lysosomes

ANCILLARY TESTS

- In addition to TSH, α-subunit staining frequent
- Ki-67 labeling indices often elevated above 3%
- Most ultrastructurally well differentiated and resemble normal TSH cells
- More pituitary adenomas show coexpression of GH, PRL than occur as pure TSH adenomas
  - Thyrotroph adenomas express PIT-1 transcription factor

Macroadenoma With Cavernous Sinus Invasion

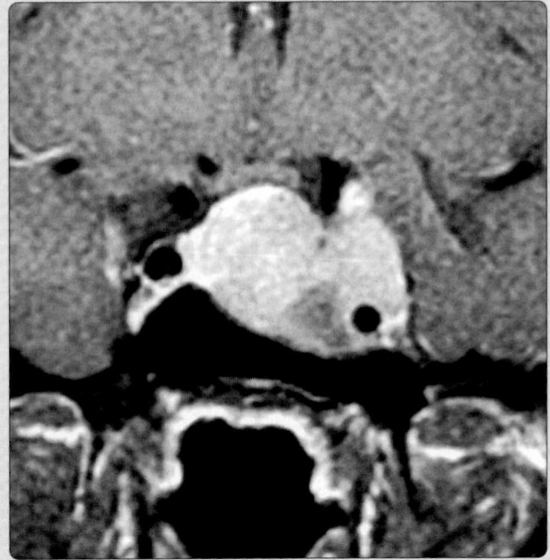

Thyroid-Stimulating Hormone Adenoma, Invasion of Bone

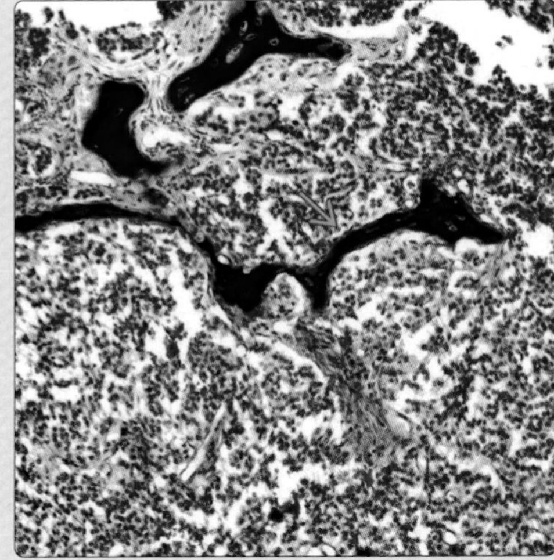

(Left) *Coronal T1 C+ MR shows a macroadenoma that enhances strongly, invades the left cavernous sinus, and erodes the sellar floor.* **(Right)** *Invasion of bone ⇨, cavernous sinus, and dura are common in thyroid-stimulating hormone (TSH) cell adenomas.*

Nuclear Pleomorphism

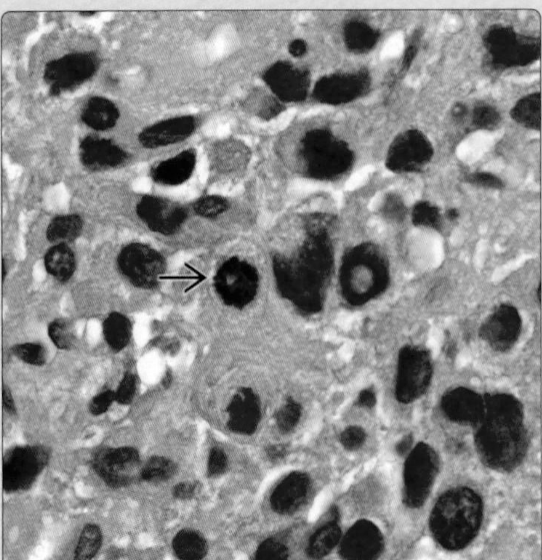

PAS(+) Cytoplasmic Globules

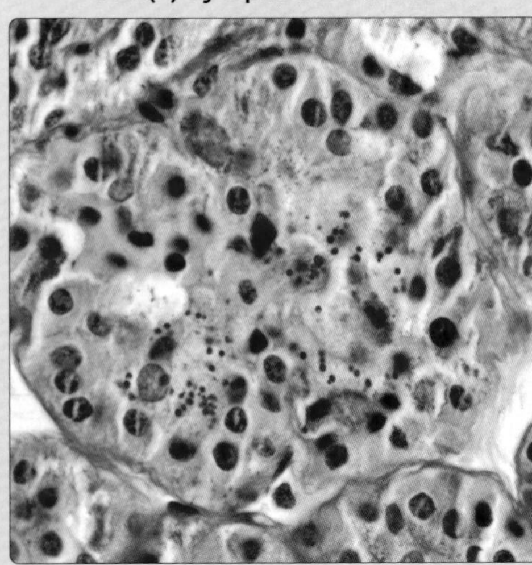

(Left) *In TSH cell adenomas, mitotic activity ⇨ is higher than other adenoma types. Nuclear irregularity is also a common feature.* **(Right)** *Cytoplasmic PAS(+) globules corresponding to large lysosomes may be seen in some examples. The cytoplasm of TSH-secreting pituitary adenomas is otherwise PAS(-).*

TERMINOLOGY

Synonyms

- Thyrotropinoma

Definitions

- Benign adenohypophysial tumor producing thyroid-stimulating hormone (TSH)

ETIOLOGY/PATHOGENESIS

Predisposing Factors

- Many arise in setting of hypothyroidism and probably preceded by TSH cell hyperplasia

Genetics

- Patients with MEN1 as well as Carney complex are predisposed

CLINICAL ISSUES

Epidemiology

- Incidence
  - TSH adenomas are rare (1% of adenomas)
- Age
  - Most occur in early adulthood to middle age
- Sex
  - Female predilection (3:1)

Site

- Microadenomas in midline
- Macroadenomas obliterate landmarks and show no favored localization

Presentation

- Rare cause of hyperthyroidism
  - Goiter and hyperthyroidism (hypermetabolism, tachycardia, tremor, proximal myopathy, and psychiatric symptoms)
- Associated with inappropriately elevated levels of TSH in presence of elevated free T4 and T3
  - 80% also secrete α-subunit
  - Ultrasensitive TSH assays now permit more ready diagnosis
- Visual field abnormalities (50%) due to mass effect
- Thyroid-directed therapy (surgical or radioiodine) may have negative effect upon TSH adenomas
  - Tumor continues to grow and become invasive (analogous to Nelson syndrome)
- Significant proportion of acromegaly associated pituitary adenomas producing GH &/or PRL cosecrete TSH as well

Treatment

- Surgery and radiotherapy induces euthyroidism in 25%
- Somatostatin analog treatment normalizes TSH levels in 75%
  - Decreases tumor volume in 40%

Prognosis

- Invasion of surrounding structures and recurrence frequent

IMAGING

General Features

- CT and MR findings
  - TSH adenomas typically invasive macroadenomas
    - ~ 60% show invasion of both cavernous sinuses

MACROSCOPIC

General Features

- Most soft and grossly invasive
  - Occasionally due to fibrosis

Size

- Most are macroadenomas (> 1 cm)

MICROSCOPIC

Histologic Features

- Chromophobic; often exhibit perivascular pseudorosettes
- Cells often polygonal or elongate
- Nuclear pleomorphism occasionally encountered, but does not impact prognosis
- Perivascular stromal fibrosis (common feature)
- Calcifications, in variable number (occasional)

ANCILLARY TESTS

Histochemistry

- PAS stains are largely negative, but focal subplasmalemmal dot-like positivity (in lysosomes) can be seen

Immunohistochemistry

- In addition to variable TSH staining, α-subunit positivity frequent
- PIT-1 transcription factor
- Ki-67 labeling indices often brisk

Electron Microscopy

- Variable features
  - Most cells well differentiated, similar to normal TSH cells
    - Medium-sized, polar cells; cytoplasmic processes
    - Sparse, small, 150-200 nm granules beneath cell membrane
    - Ample Golgi complexes and rough endoplasmic reticulum
  - Minority resemble those of null cell adenomas
    - Very few granules, with no other differential feature

SELECTED REFERENCES

1. Gomez-Hernandez K et al: Clinical implications of accurate subtyping of pituitary adenomas: perspectives from the treating physician. Turk Patoloji Derg. 31 Suppl 1:4-17, 2015
2. Rimareix F et al: Primary Medical Treatment of Thyrotropin-Secreting Pituitary Adenomas by First-Generation Somatostatin Analogs: A Case Study of Seven Patients. Thyroid. 25(8):877-82, 2015
3. Wang EL et al: Clinicopathological characterization of TSH-producing adenomas: special reference to TSH-immunoreactive but clinically non-functioning adenomas. Endocr Pathol. 20(4):209-20, 2009
4. Foppiani L et al: TSH-secreting adenomas: rare pituitary tumors with multifaceted clinical and biological features. J Endocrinol Invest. 30(7):603-9, 2007
5. Sanno N et al: Long-term surgical outcome in 16 patients with thyrotropin pituitary adenoma. J Neurosurg. 93(2):194-200, 2000

(Left) *Perivascular pseudorosettes, also frequent in gonadotroph adenomas, are common in TSH adenomas. This can superficially mimic ependymoma. However, all pituitary adenomas are immunoreactive for synaptophysin, while ependymomas are not.* **(Right)** *Neoplastic cells are often elongated as opposed to the more rounded profiles in most other adenoma types.*

Pseudorosettes Common

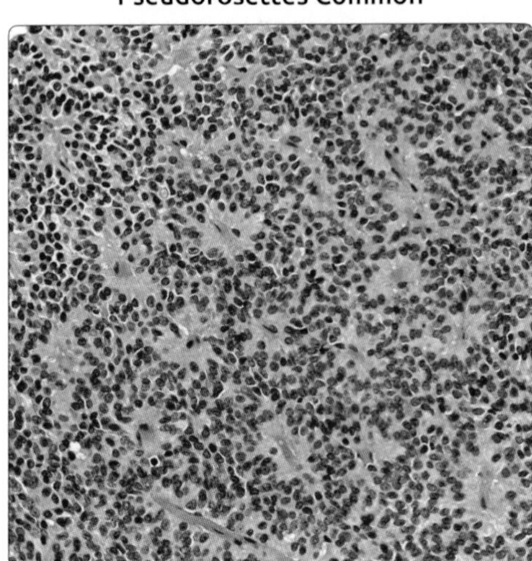

Elongated Adenoma Cells

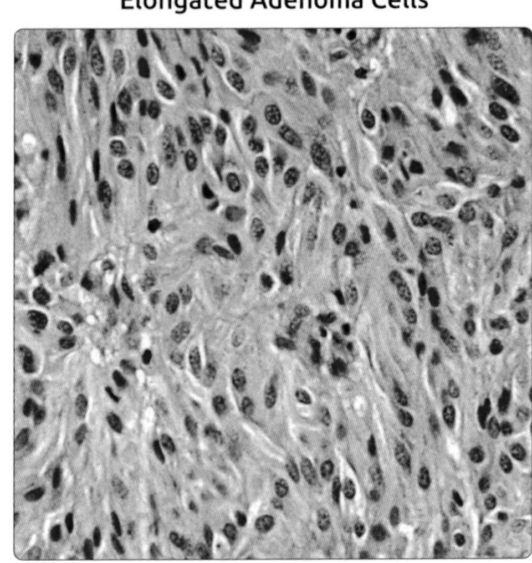

(Left) *Occasionally, TSH adenomas are sclerotic. Perivascular fibrosis ⇒ is common.* **(Right)** *TSH adenomas extending through the sellar floor reach the submucosa of the sphenoid sinus ⇒.*

Occasional Sclerosis

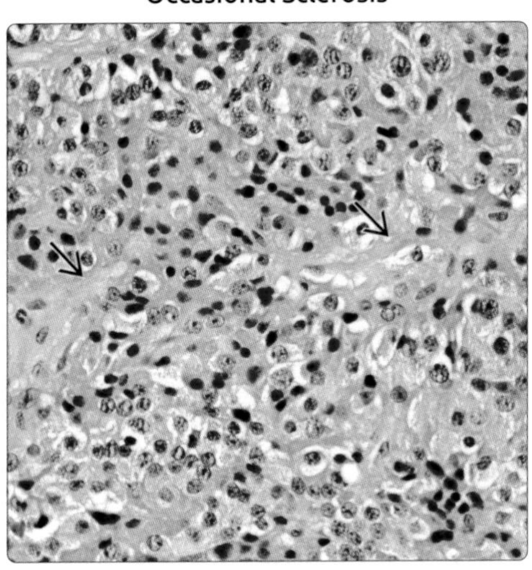

Extension Through Sellar Floor

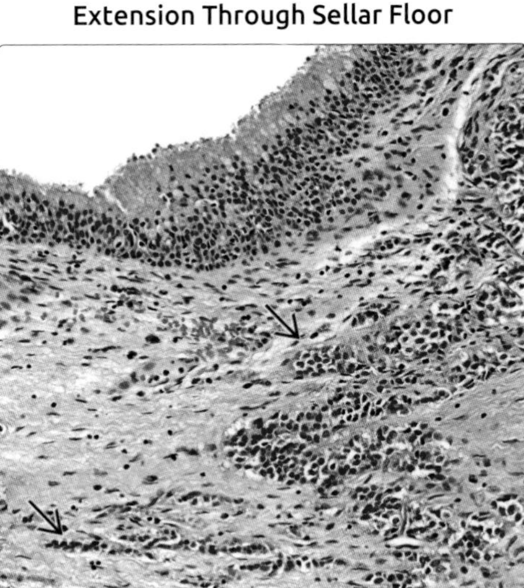

(Left) *TSH adenomas may have pseudoglandular spaces filled with mucinous material.* **(Right)** *As seen in a smear preparation, nuclear pleomorphism and prominent nucleoli mark some TSH adenomas.*

Pseudoglandular Spaces

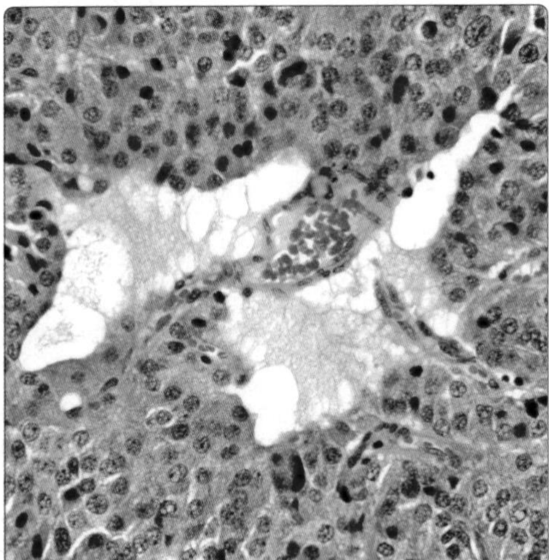

Smear, Prominent Nucleoli

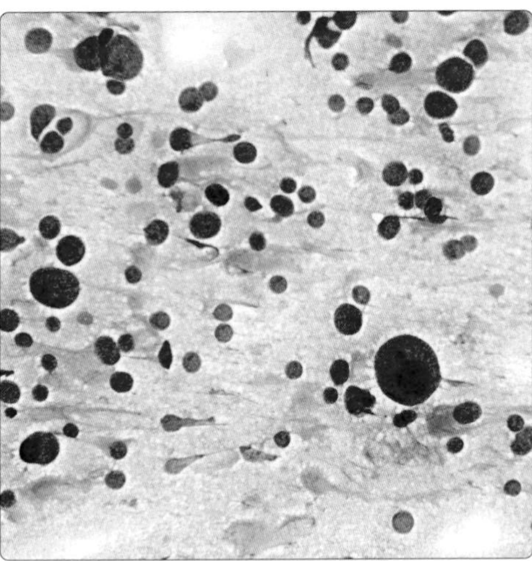

Thyroid-Stimulating Hormone Immunoreactivity: Strong

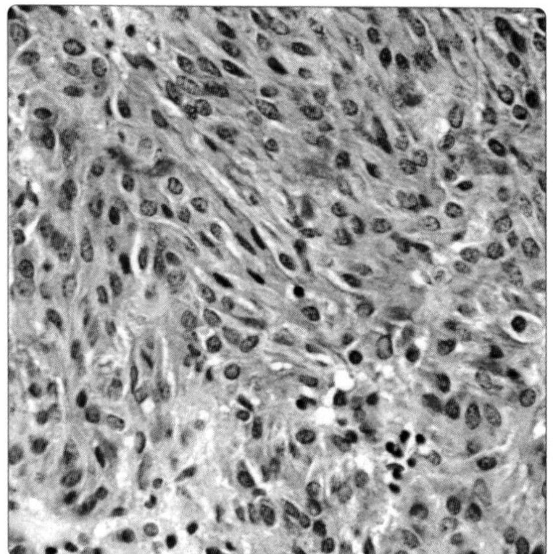

α-Subunit Immunostaining Usually Present

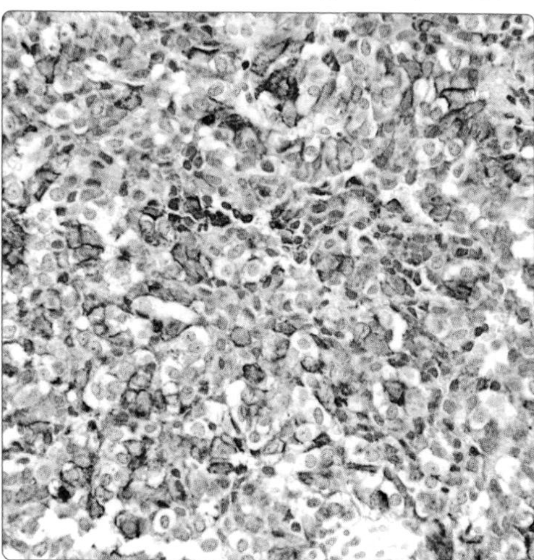

(Left) *Immunoreactivity for TSH may be strong, as illustrated here, but is usually weaker. Note the elongated cytoplasm in this TSH adenoma. Most other types of pituitary adenomas display more rounded cytoplasmic profiles.* **(Right)** *α-subunit staining is common in TSH adenomas. Blood levels of α-subunit may also be elevated.*

PAS(+) Lysosomes

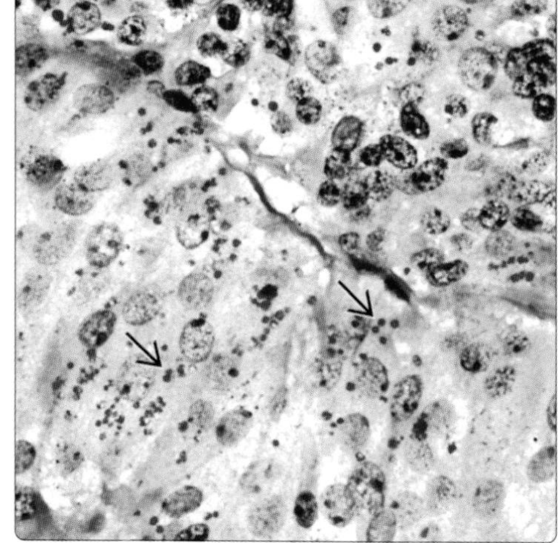

Often Brisk Ki-67 Labeling

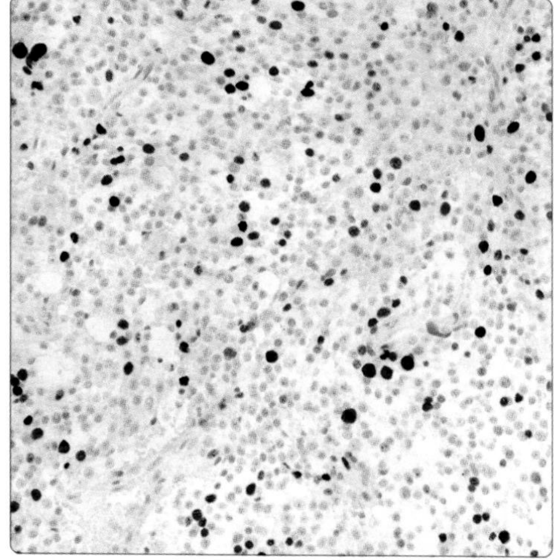

(Left) *Cytoplasmic PAS(+) globules ⇨ correspond to large lysosomes.* **(Right)** *TSH cell adenomas usually have a brisk Ki-67 rate.*

Subplasmalemmal Tiny Secretory Granules

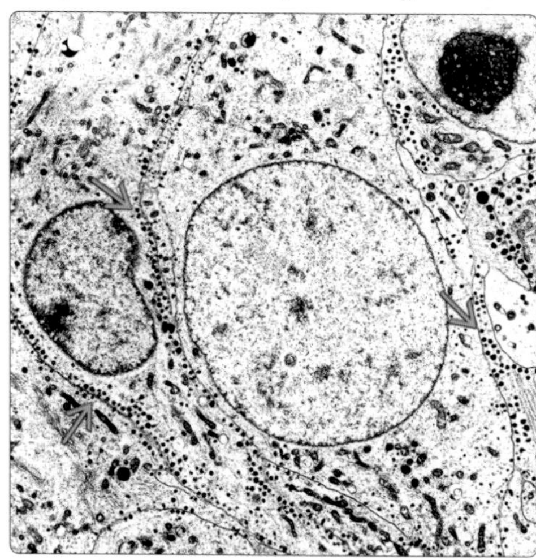

Trapped Normal Thyroid-Stimulating Hormone Cells in Null Cell Adenoma

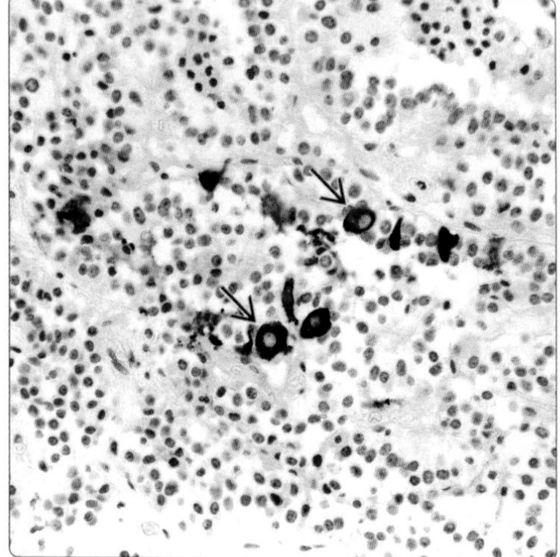

(Left) *Thyrotroph cell adenomas have euchromatic nuclei, large nucleoli, and a single subplasmalemmal layer of tiny secretory granules ⇨.* **(Right)** *Intensely stained TSH cells ⇨ within another adenoma type are trapped normal immunoreactive cells and should not be interpreted as evidence of TSH cell adenoma.*

Plurihormonal Adenoma

KEY FACTS

TERMINOLOGY

- Plurihormonal adenomas show immunoreactivities for developmentally or physiologically unrelated hormones
- Best definition of plurihormonal that of Saeger et al.
  - Type 1: Correspond on light microscopy to densely granulated GH, also expresses TSH, α-subunit, FSH, LH, PRL in various combinations; patients acromegalic; PIT-1 driven and no longer considered plurihormonal by most authors; likely mammosomatotroph lineage
  - Type 2: Structurally similar to gonadotroph adenoma but in addition to FSH/LH, additionally expresses either TSH, GH, PRL, α-subunit; ultrastructure shows plurimorphism
  - Type 3: Silent subtype 3; requires EM documentation for diagnosis; usually clinically silent, except for elevated serum prolactin levels due to pituitary stalk compression effect
    - Have unusual hormone combinations in scattered individual cells (minority of cells): GH-PRL-TSH/ACTH-GH-PRL-TSH/TSH-PRL/PRL-α-subunit

CLINICAL ISSUES

- Rare
- Nonfunctioning examples often silent subtype 3
- Aggressive, often invasive
- Frequent, but not invariable, recurrence

MICROSCOPIC

- Most chromophobic or acidophilic
- Nuclear irregularity, nucleolar prominence and mitoses especially in silent subtype 3 adenomas

ANCILLARY TESTS

- Consider silent subtype 3 when clinically nonfunctioning with scattered rare cells IHC(+) for TSH, PRL &/or GH + cytologically atypical and elevated MIB-1 rate
- EM required for diagnosis of silent subtype 3 adenoma

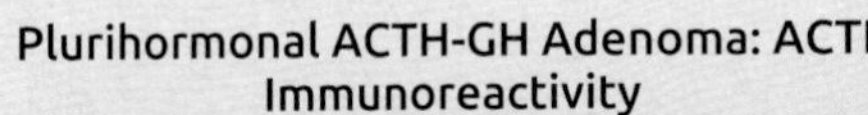

Plurihormonal ACTH-GH Adenoma: ACTH Immunoreactivity

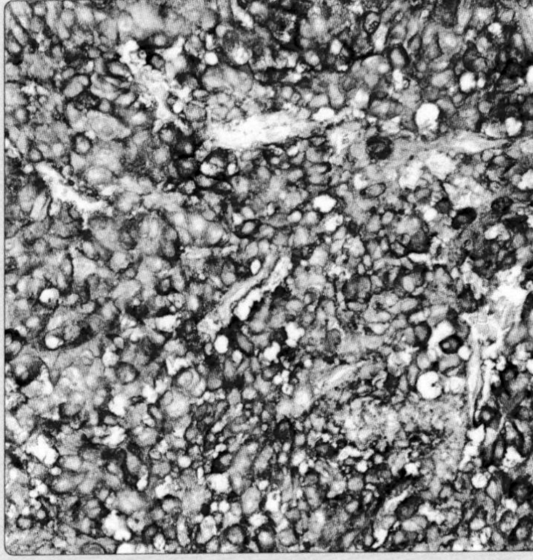

Plurihormonal ACTH-GH Adenoma: GH Immunoreactivity

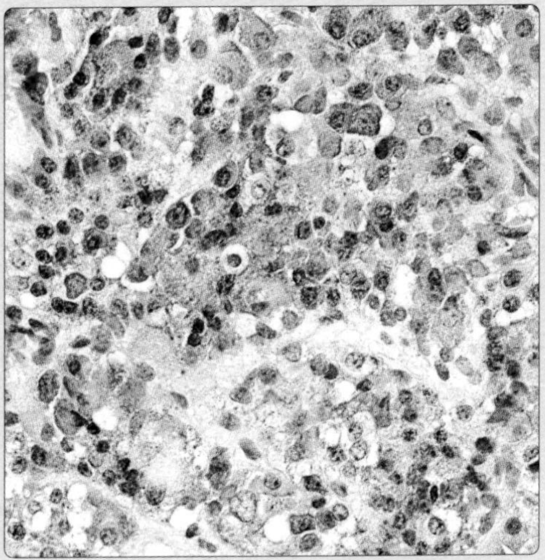

(Left) *Plurihormonal adenomas show immunoreactivities for developmentally or physiologically unrelated hormones. This example is an ACTH-GH cell adenoma, with the ACTH cell component immunostained here.* **(Right)** *GH cell component of a plurihormonal, ACTH-GH, adenoma is shown by GH immunostaining for growth hormone.*

Silent Subtype 3: Clival Destruction

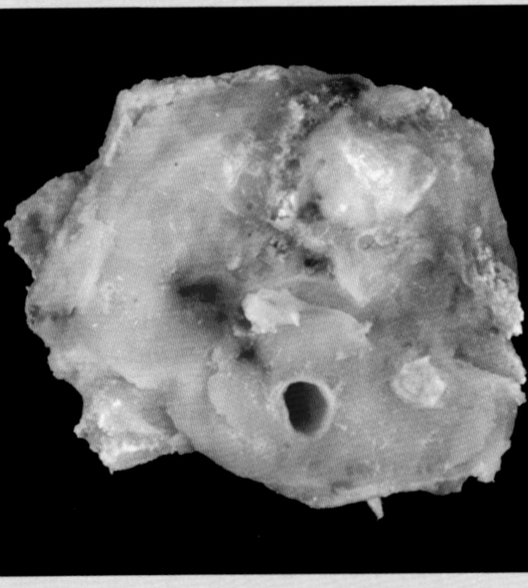

Silent Subtype 3 Adenoma

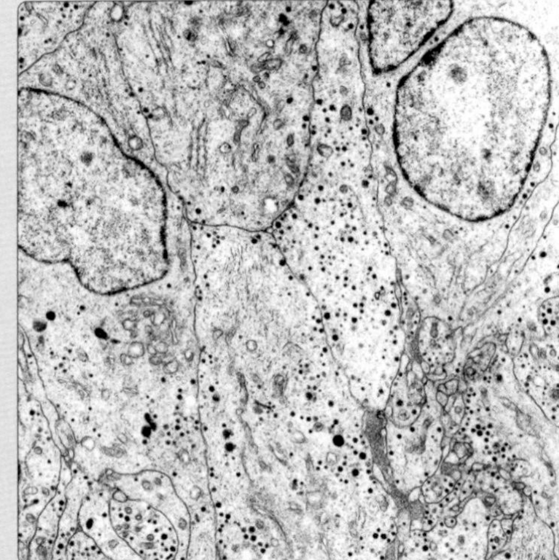

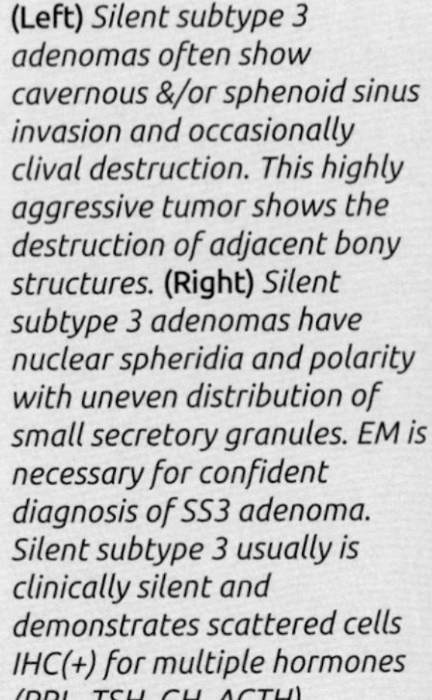

(Left) *Silent subtype 3 adenomas often show cavernous &/or sphenoid sinus invasion and occasionally clival destruction. This highly aggressive tumor shows the destruction of adjacent bony structures.* **(Right)** *Silent subtype 3 adenomas have nuclear spheridia and polarity with uneven distribution of small secretory granules. EM is necessary for confident diagnosis of SS3 adenoma. Silent subtype 3 usually is clinically silent and demonstrates scattered cells IHC(+) for multiple hormones (PRL, TSH, GH, ACTH).*

TERMINOLOGY

Synonyms

- Multihormonal adenoma

Definitions

- Variously defined by different authors as adenomas with multiple hormone production
- Best definition of plurihormonal is that of Saeger et al. who divided plurihormonal adenomas into 3 types

ETIOLOGY/PATHOGENESIS

Pathophysiology

- Transcription factor abnormalities presumed to underlie multilineage differentiation and expression of disparate hormones
- Silent subtype 3 adenomas, most common variant, associated with high levels of basic fibroblastic growth factor
  - May explain occasional occurrence of fibrosis as well as rapid growth

CLINICAL ISSUES

Epidemiology

- Incidence
  - Plurihormonal adenomas rare (< 2% of pituitary adenomas)
- Age
  - Young to middle-aged adults
  - Women with silent subtype 3 adenomas tumors present between ages 25-35; no male age predilection
- Sex
  - Both sexes equally affected

Presentation

- Most plurihormonal adenomas are macroadenomas with mass effects (visual loss, headaches)
- Combinations of hormone expression may cause spectrum of endocrine symptoms
- Nonfunctioning examples often silent subtype 3 adenomas
  - Hyperprolactinemia due to stalk effect

Treatment

- Surgical approaches
  - Transsphenoidal or transfrontal surgery
- Adjuvant therapy
  - Temozolomide
- Drugs
  - Dopamine agonists may decrease hormone overproduction by silent subtype 3 adenomas
    - Tumoral growth may be unaffected

Prognosis

- Often aggressive tumors
  - Silent subtype 3 variant aggressive with frequent invasion and recurrence (40%)
    - Rarely metastasize (6% of pituitary carcinoma)

IMAGING

Radiographic Findings

- No specific imaging features
- Most macroadenomas
- 50% invasive; sellar destruction

MACROSCOPIC

General Features

- Usually macroadenoma with extrasellar extension and frank invasion

MICROSCOPIC

Histologic Features

- **Conventional**
  - Most plurihormonal adenomas are chromophobic or acidophilic
  - Cellular pleomorphism uncommon
- **Silent subtype 3**
  - Nuclear irregularity, nucleolar prominence, and mitoses common

ANCILLARY TESTS

Immunohistochemistry

- Plurihormonality for ordinarily unrelated hormones
  - ACTH-PRL, FSH/LH-ACTH
- Silent subtype 3 requires EM for diagnosis, demonstrates scattered cells IHC(+) for various hormones in different combinations (GH, PRL, TSH, ACTH)
  - Minority entirely immunonegative
- In silent subtype 3 adenomas, transcription factor expression includes PIT-1
  - Explains underlying GH, PRL, TSH, and ACTH production
  - NeuroD1 also frequent; explains occasional ACTH production

Electron Microscopy

- Silent subtype 3 adenomas ultrastructurally distinctive
  - Large polar cells with prominent nucleoli and nuclear spheridia (inclusions of unknown function)
  - Abundance of rough and smooth endoplasmic reticulum, with rough type surrounding mitochondria
  - Massive Golgi complexes
  - Sparse small secretory granules
    - Accumulation of cell processes, hallmark of glycoprotein hormone cell differentiation
- Other plurihormonal adenomas consist of 1 or several morphologically distinct cell types, i.e., plurimorphism

DIFFERENTIAL DIAGNOSIS

Conventional Pituitary Adenomas

- Common immunophenotypic profiles

SELECTED REFERENCES

1. Erickson D et al: Silent subtype 3 pituitary adenoma: a clinicopathologic analysis of the Mayo Clinic experience. Clin Endocrinol (Oxf). 71(1):92-9, 2009
2. Saeger W et al: Pathohistological classification of pituitary tumors: 10 years of experience with the German Pituitary Tumor Registry. Eur J Endocrinol. 156(2):203-16, 2007

(Left) *A FSH/LH and GH cell plurihormonal adenoma example has both pseudopapillary structures* ⇨ *and diffuse* ⇨ *patterns.* **(Right)** *The tumor comprises somatotroph and gonadotroph cells. Note the large granules in the former* ⇨ *and small, subplasmalemmal granules* ⇨ *in the latter. This is an example of a tumor with 2 different subpopulations of cells by EM.*

Plurihormonal FSH/LH-GH Adenoma

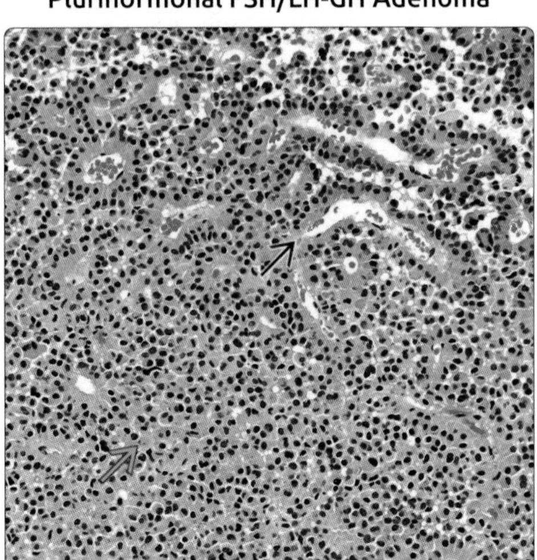

Somatotroph-Gonadotroph Adenoma

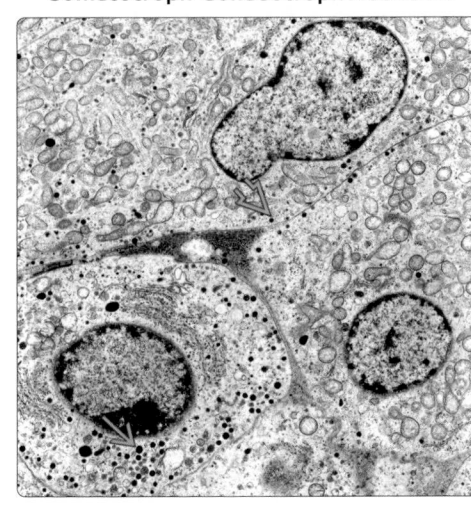

(Left) *FSH immunostaining highlights the gonadotroph cell component* ⇨ *of the FSH/LH and GH cell plurihormonal adenoma.* **(Right)** *The GH immunostain shows strong reactivity in a subset of cells of a FSH/LH and GH cell plurihormonal adenoma.*

Plurihormonal FSH/LH-GH Adenoma: FSH Immunoreactivity

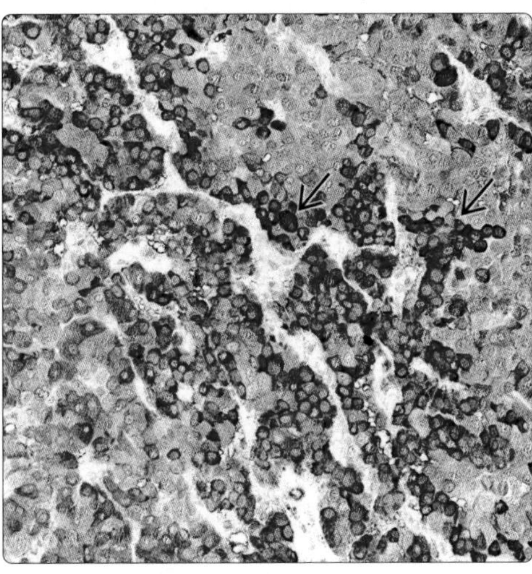

Plurihormonal FSH/LH-GH Adenoma: GH Immunoreactivity

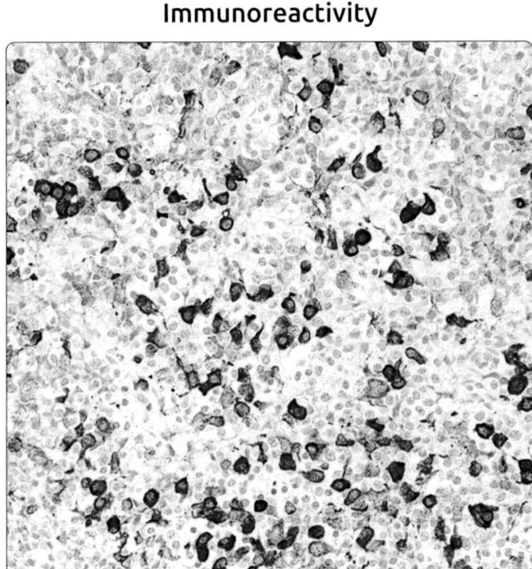

(Left) *MIB1 labeling indices are often increased in plurihormonal tumors.* **(Right)** *Nonatypical adenomas are usually immunonegative for p53, with the exception of plurihormonal types, such as this example that often may contain significant numbers of positive cells.*

MIB1 May Be Increased

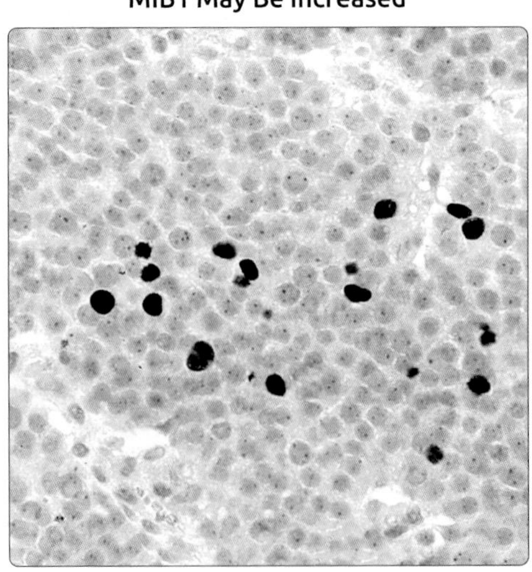

p53 May Be Increased

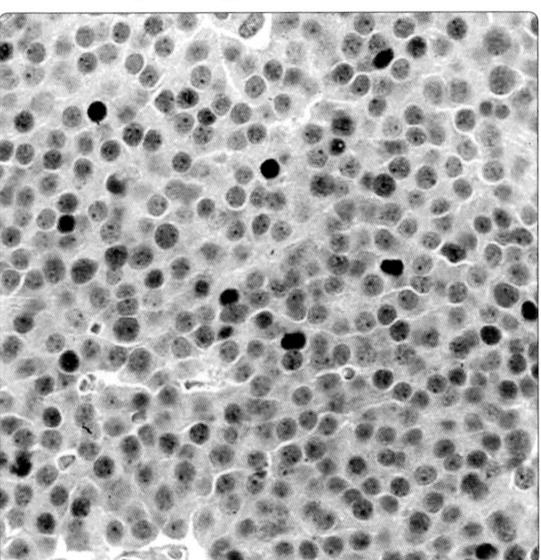

Mitoses: Silent Type 3 Adenoma

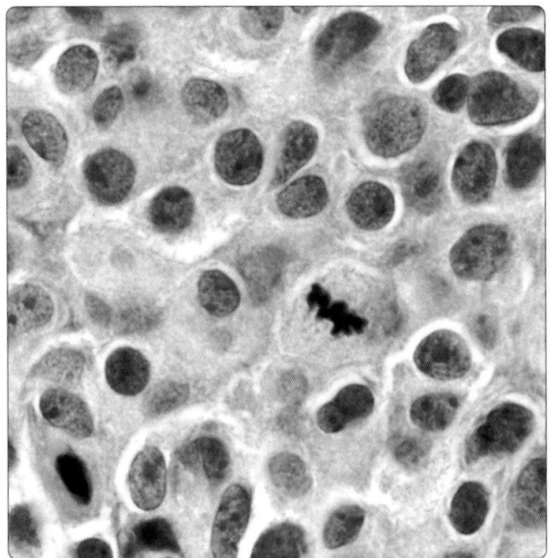

Silent Type 3 Adenoma

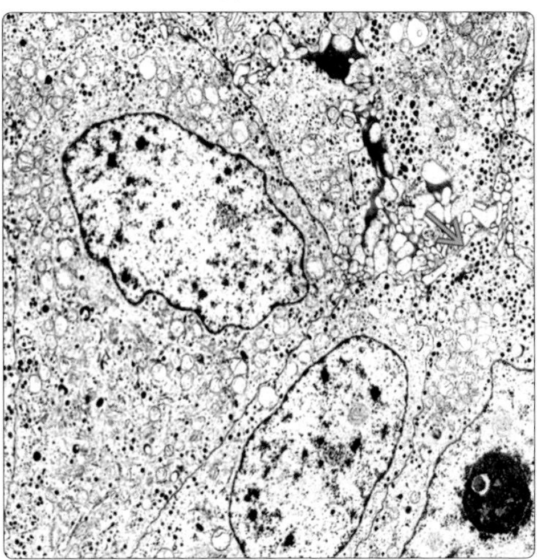

(Left) *Mitoses are common in silent subtype 3 adenomas, which are expected to behave more aggressively. Note the nuclear pleomorphism and atypia.* **(Right)** *SS3 adenomas often have elongated, large, polar-shaped cells with small secretory granules ⇒.*

Large Golgi, Silent Subtype 3 Adenoma

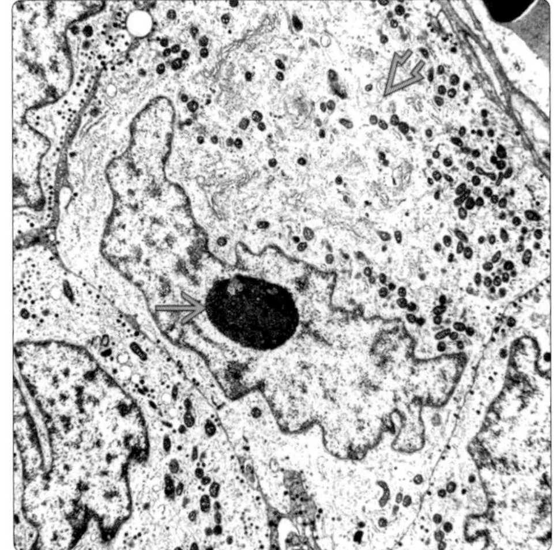

Abundant Endoplasmic Reticulum

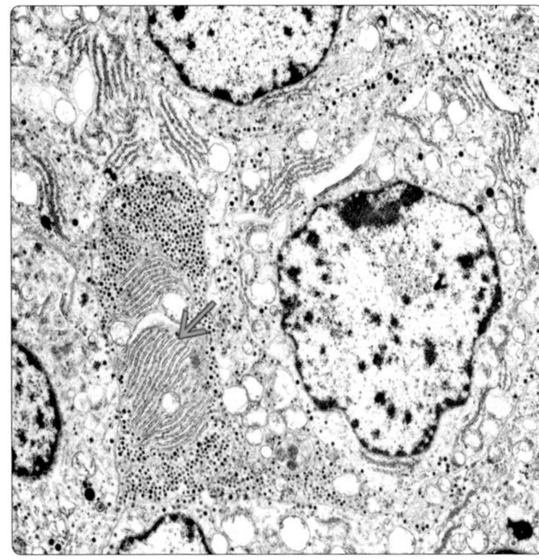

(Left) *Silent subtype 3 adenoma shows nuclear irregularity and a large Golgi zone ⇒. Note the prominent nucleoli ⇒.* **(Right)** *Silent subtype 3 adenoma features abundant, rough endoplasmic reticulum ⇒.*

Smooth Endoplasmic Reticulum

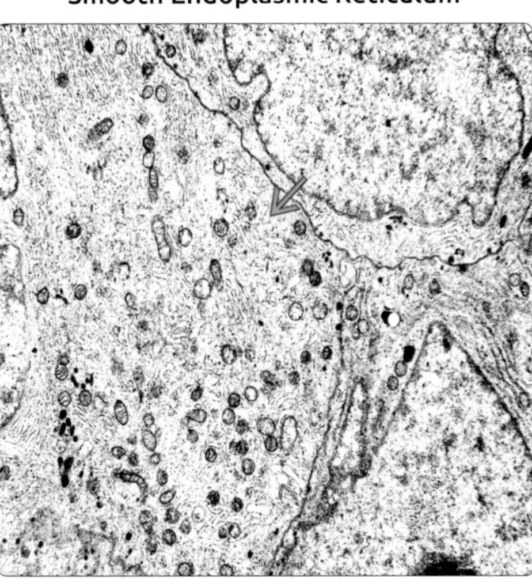

Rough Endoplasmic Reticulum

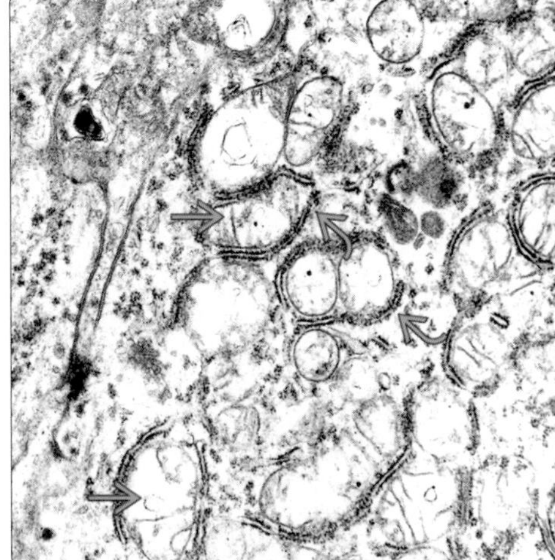

(Left) *Silent subtype 3 adenomas have abundant endoplasmic reticulum of both smooth and rough type. The former ⇒ is illustrated here.* **(Right)** *Rough endoplasmic reticulum ⇗ encircles mitochondria ⇒ in some silent subtype 3 adenomas.*

Null Cell Adenoma

KEY FACTS

CLINICAL ISSUES

- Clinically nonfunctioning (silent) adenomas are not equal to null cell adenomas
  - Term "null cell" may in future be restricted to very small minority of pituitary adenomas negative for all three transcription factors (PIT-1, SF1, Tpit)
  - ~ 3/5 of clinically nonfunctioning adenomas are gonadotroph adenomas IHC(+) for FSH, LH, 1/10 are silent ACTH IHC(+) adenomas, 1/5 are hormone-negative for **all** anterior pituitary hormones, i.e., negative for PRL, GH, ASU, FSH, LH, TSH, ACTH (Nishioka et al)
  - Of IHC hormone-negative adenomas, most (~ 2/3) are SF1 transcription factor positive, indicating gonadotroph adenoma lineage
  - 1/4 are Tpit(+) even if ACTH(-), indicating corticotroph lineage; PIT-1 lineage hormone-negative and triple-negative transcription factor negative adenomas rare (Nishioka et al)
  - More work necessary to establish prognosis of subsets
  - All types usually present with symptoms of mass effect

IMAGING

- Suprasellar extension frequent
- Marked sellar expansion/demineralization

MACROSCOPIC

- Macroadenoma
- Occasional apoplexy

MICROSCOPIC

- Most show diffuse pattern of growth
- Chromophobic or oncocytic on H&E
- PAS(-)
- Ultrastructurally poorly differentiated
  - Mitochondrial accumulation in oncocytic type

ANCILLARY TESTS

- Transcription factor IHCs not available in all laboratories, especially Tpit

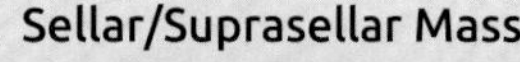

Sellar/Suprasellar Mass

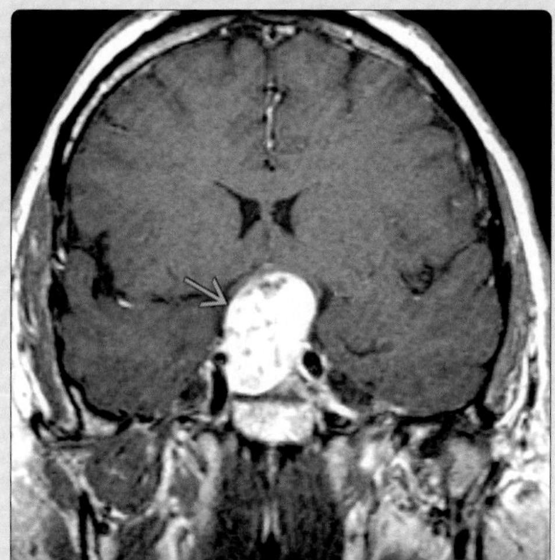

Usually Macroadenomas

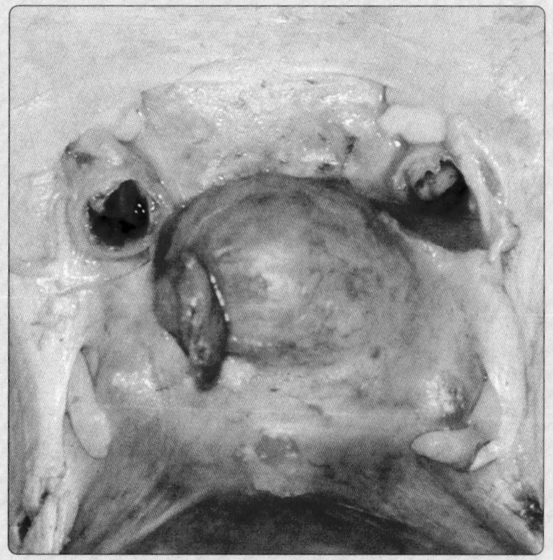

(Left) *Coronal T1 C+ MR of a macroadenoma shows an inhomogeneously enhancing intra- and suprasellar mass →. The pituitary gland cannot be found separate from the mass.* **(Right)** *Null cell adenomas, like all clinically nonfunctioning (silent) adenomas, are usually macroadenomas and their clinical presentation is due to mass effect. Hypopituitarism is also usually present.*

Diffuse Pattern

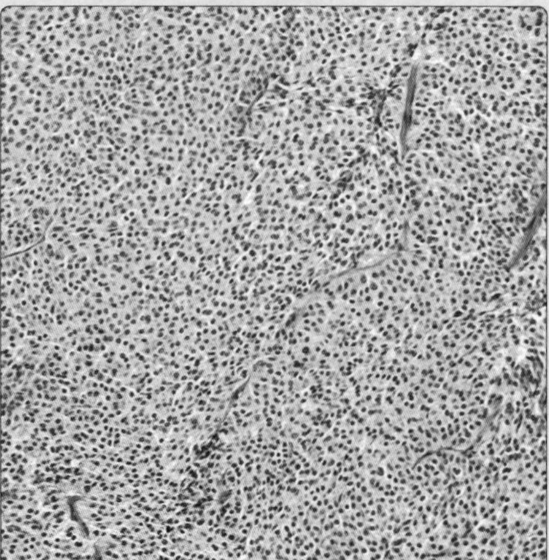

Synaptophysin Positive

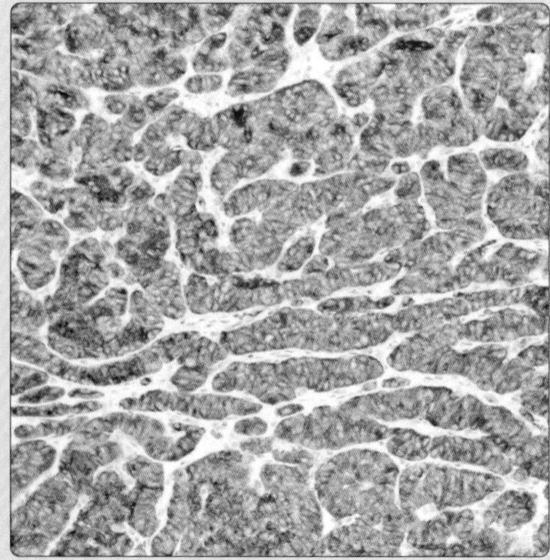

(Left) *There is no specific pattern for null cell adenomas. This chromophobic example shows a diffuse pattern.* **(Right)** *All pituitary adenomas are synaptophysin (+). This is not always true for chromogranin IHC, but many null cell adenomas are additionally chromogranin reactive.*

TERMINOLOGY

Definitions

- Null cell adenoma not synonymous with clinically nonfunctioning (silent) pituitary adenomas
  - Most (~ 3/5) of clinically nonfunctioning adenomas are gonadotroph adenomas [IHC(+) for FSH, LH], 1/10 are clinically nonfunctioning (silent) ACTH(+) adenomas, 1/5 are negative for **all** anterior pituitary hormones, i.e., negative for PRL, GH, ASU, FSH, LH, TSH, and ACTH, but most of these are still SF1 positive (~ 2/3), although 1/10 are ACTH(-) but Tpit(+)
  - Some suggest that only the very small minority IHC(-) for all anterior pituitary hormones AND all three transcription factors (PIT-1, SF1, Tpit) are true null cell adenomas

ETIOLOGY/PATHOGENESIS

Genetics

- No association of null cell adenomas with MEN1 or Carney complex

CLINICAL ISSUES

Epidemiology

- Incidence
  - Relative frequency very decreased due to increased sensitivity of immunohistochemical methods and use of SF1 (presence of SF1 indicates gonadotroph adenoma)
- Age
  - Mainly in middle-aged to older patients (mean age: 55 years)
    - Uncommon under age 40 years
- Sex
  - Slight male predilection

Site

- Virtually all arise in adenohypophysis

Presentation

- No association with endocrine hyperfunction
  - Low-level prolactin elevation due to stalk section effect
- Mass effect: Headache, visual disturbance, cranial neuropathy, hypothalamic disturbance
- Frequency of invasion relatively low (40%)
- May be incidental imaging finding

Prognosis

- Slow growing and associated with relatively favorable prognosis
- Recurrence after gross total resection in 5% at 10 years
- Resection is often subtotal given large tumor size
  - Postoperative reduction of mass effects by 75%

IMAGING

Radiographic Findings

- Nonspecific features of macroadenoma
  - Potential for downward growth into nasal cavity
- Cavernous sinus invasion in minority of cases; suprasellar extension frequent
- Marked sellar expansion and demineralization

MR Findings

- Isointense, homogeneous on T1W images
- Heterogeneous contrast enhancement but less than in normal anterior pituitary
- Cystic change or frank hemorrhage and infarction (apoplexy), occasional

CT Findings

- Contrast enhancing
  - No calcifications

MACROSCOPIC

General Features

- Generally tan and soft
- Occasional hemorrhage (apoplexy) and resultant cyst

MICROSCOPIC

Light Microscopy

- Most with diffuse pattern of growth
  - Pseudorosetting and papillation infrequent
  - Chromophobic (50%) or acidophilic due to mitochondrial accumulation (oncocytic change)
  - PAS(-)
  - Cellular pleomorphism and mitoses infrequent

ANCILLARY TESTS

Histochemistry

- PAS reactivity: Negative
- Reticulin: Disruption, or total loss, of normal anterior pituitary gland acinar pattern on reticulin

Immunohistochemistry

- Synaptophysin and chromogranin immunoreactivity strong
- Largely (-) for anterior pituitary hormones
  - Scattered cells (+) for hormones, usually β-FSH/LH or α-subunit; these adenomas can be reclassified as gonadotroph adenomas
  - Clinically nonfunctioning adenomas with immunoreactivity for steroidogenic factor 1 (SF1) are = gonadotroph adenoma
  - Those adenomas without SF1 immunoreactivity show different clinical behavior; some Tpit(+)
- Ki-67 labeling low (< 2%)

Electron Microscopy

- Polygonal cells with poorly developed organelles, including scant rough endoplasmic reticulum and Golgi
- Secretory granules small (100-250 nm) and sparse, mainly aligned beneath cell membrane

SELECTED REFERENCES

1. Balogun JA et al: Null cell adenomas of the pituitary gland: an institutional review of their clinical imaging and behavioral characteristics. Endocr Pathol. 26(1):63-70, 2015
2. Gomez-Hernandez K et al: Clinical implications of accurate subtyping of pituitary adenomas: perspectives from the treating physician. Turk Patoloji Derg. 31 Suppl 1:4-17, 2015
3. Nishioka H et al: The complementary role of transcription factors in the accurate diagnosis of clinically nonfunctioning pituitary adenomas. Endocr Pathol. ePub, 2015

(Left) *There is no specific pattern for null cell adenomas. This chromophobic example has a diffuse pattern. The sheet-like growth pattern and composition of small monomorphous cells are typical of pituitary adenomas in general.* **(Right)** *Many null cell adenomas show cellular monotony. Cellular pleomorphism and mitoses are infrequent, especially in the ones that can later be reclassified as being of gonadotroph lineage using SF1 transcription factor. Most IHC hormone-negative adenomas are SF1(+).*

Sheet-Like Growth

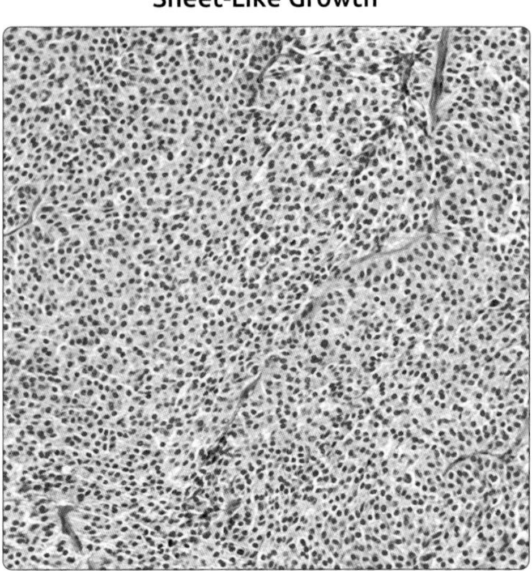

Chromophobic, Monotonous

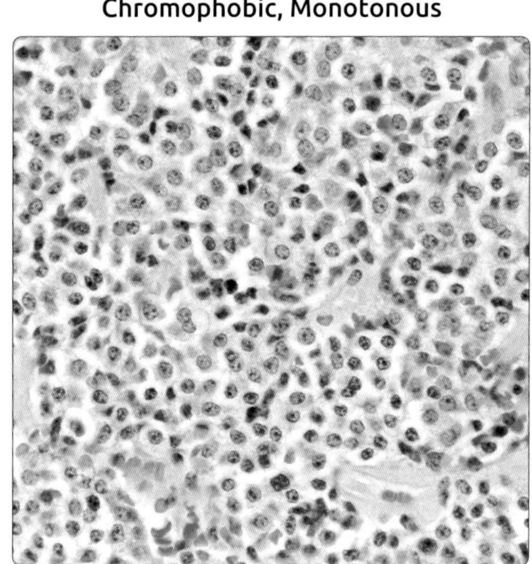

(Left) *Pink granulated cytoplasm due to mitochondrial accumulation, oncocytic change, is a frequent, but nonspecific, finding in null cell adenomas.* **(Right)** *Oncocytic change may be present focally or diffusely in null cell adenomas. This example has areas that are oncocytic → juxtaposed with those that are not (chromophobic) ⇨. This should not be misinterpreted as a true "double adenoma" which does exist in a small percentage of cases.*

Oncocytic Change Frequent

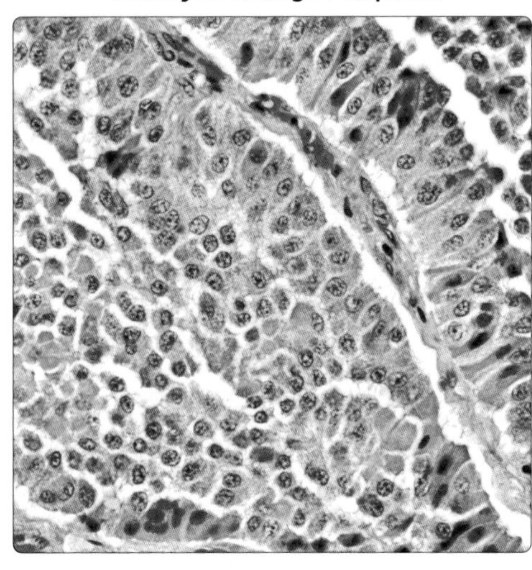

Variable Chromophobic Change

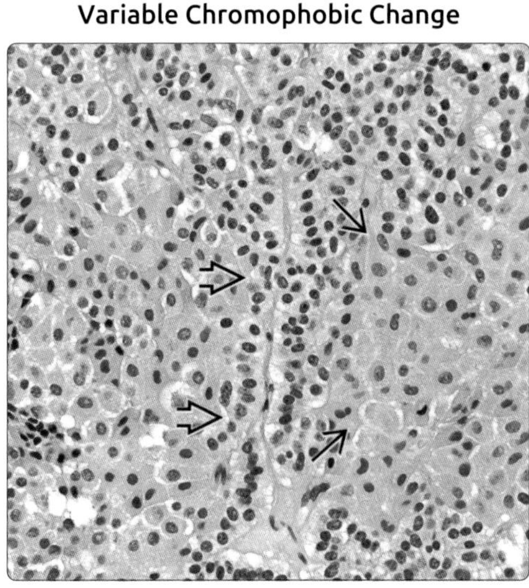

(Left) *Null cell adenomas may have a papillary pattern, but this is nonspecific since it is common in gonadotrophic adenomas (which are defined today either by the presence of FSH and/or LH IHC(+) or SF1(+).* **(Right)** *Null cell tumors behave in an indolent fashion, but apoplexy may arise due to the large size of this adenoma type. The hemorrhagic infarct → is identified by its karyolysis and, ultimately, frank loss of nuclear staining.*

Papillary Pattern

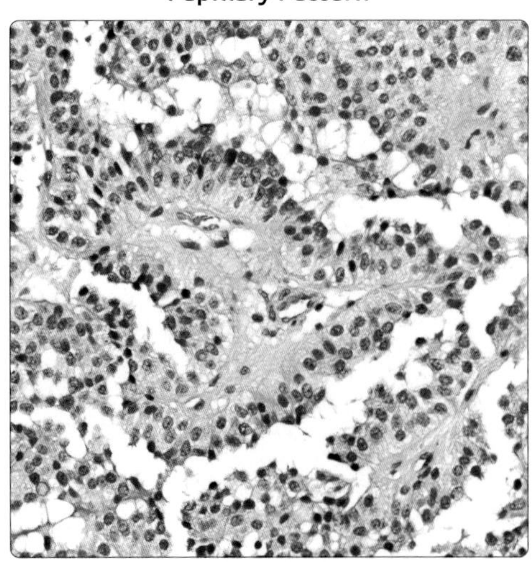

Apoplexy: Hemorrhagic Infarct

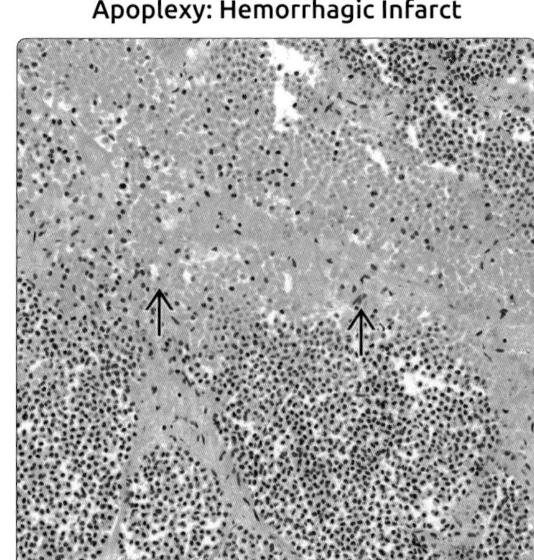

Macrolobular Pattern

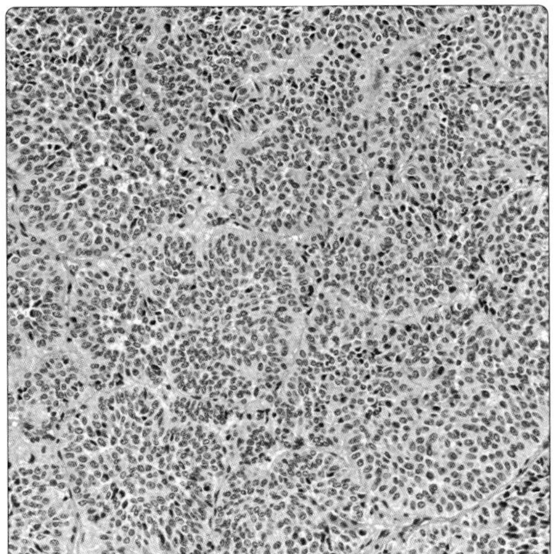

Reticulin: Macrolobular Pattern

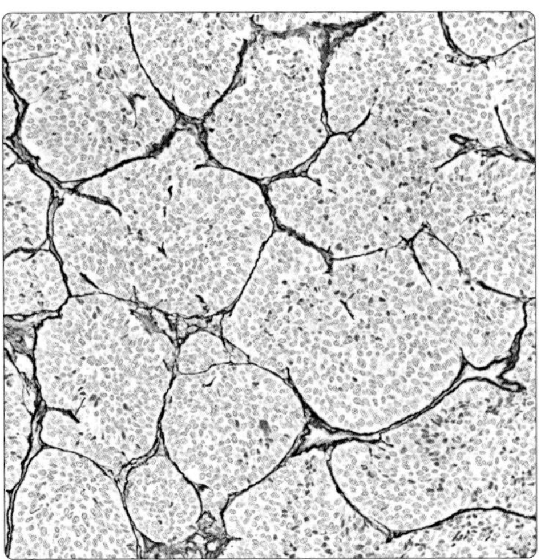

(Left) *Although nonspecific, null cell adenomas occasionally have a macrolobular pattern. This should not be misinterpreted as preservation of acinar pattern as would be seen in normal anterior gland.* **(Right)** *As expected, reticulin stain shows disruption of acinar structures in this macrolobular example. Notice that although reticulin fibers surround lobules of adenoma, there is clearly loss of normal anterior gland acinar pattern. This also should also not be misconstrued as hyperplasia.*

Chromogranin: Diffuse, Strong

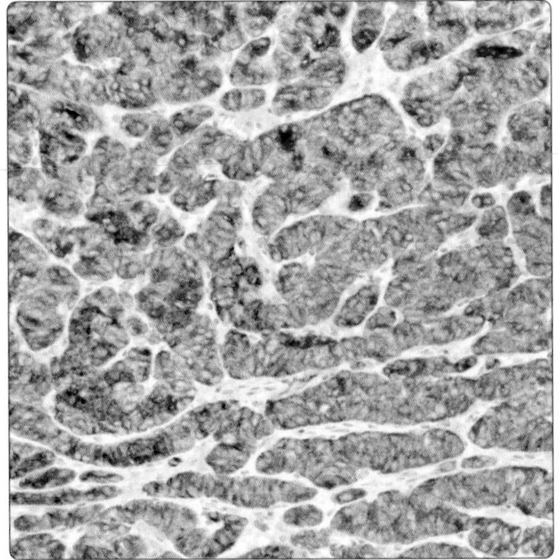

α-Subunit

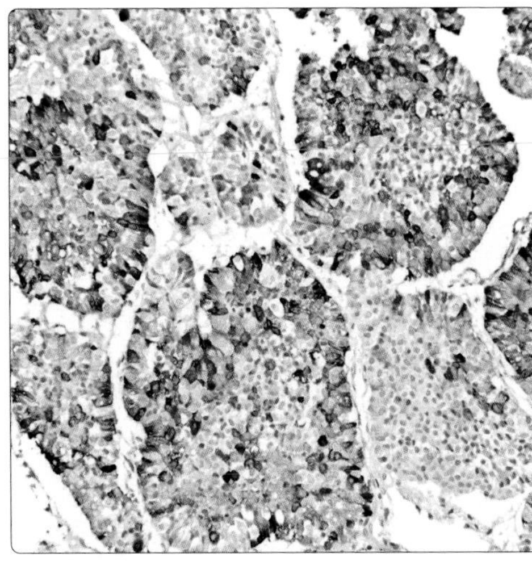

(Left) *While all pituitary adenomas are synaptophysin (+), this is not always true for chromogranin. Null cell adenomas, however, are usually chromogranin immunoreactive, particularly those of gonadotroph lineage on SF1.* **(Right)** *Null cell adenomas may show small quantities of α-subunit staining. Those with SF1 IHC(+) could be reclassified as gonadotroph adenomas. Most IHC hormone-negative adenomas are SF1(+).*

Few Secretory Granules

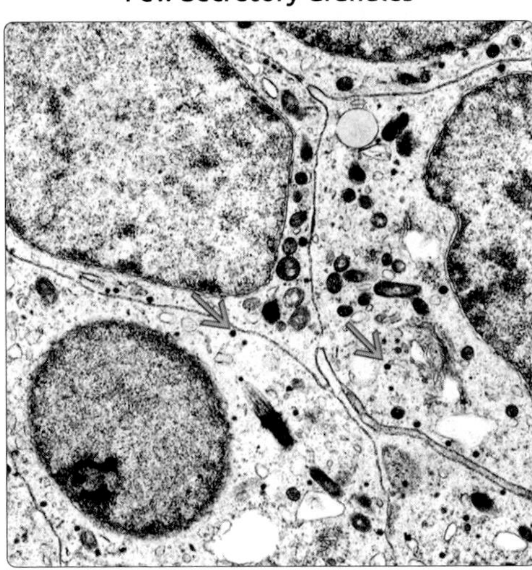

Oncocytic Change

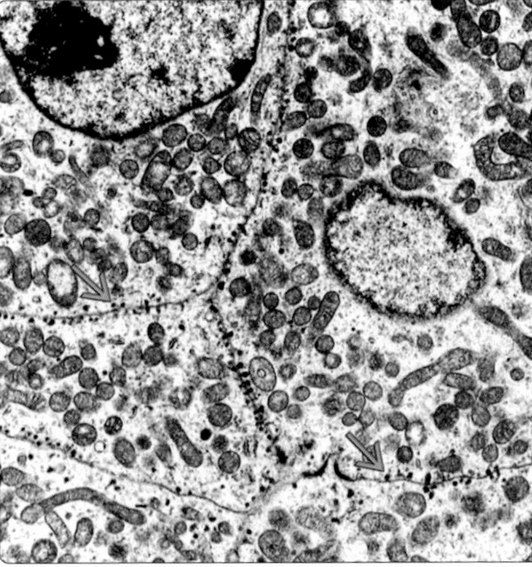

(Left) *Ultrastructurally, null cell adenomas possess few organelles, such as rough endoplasmic reticulum and Golgi complexes. There may be scant, small secretory granules ⇒ but no specific markers of functional differentiation.* **(Right)** *Oncocytic null cell adenomas may have oncocytic change expressed at the ultrastructural level as crowded mitochondria. Secretory granules ⇒ are typically located beneath the cell membrane.*

Pituitary Hyperplasia

KEY FACTS

TERMINOLOGY

- Nonneoplastic increase in adenohypophysial cell number

ETIOLOGY/PATHOGENESIS

- Most common
  - Prolactin cell hyperplasia in pregnancy
- Physiologic response to end-organ failure
- Pathologic hyperplasia associated with ectopic excess of releasing hormones
- Syndromic
- Idiopathic

CLINICAL ISSUES

- Treatment
  - Correct underlying endocrinologic cause

IMAGING

- Symmetric pituitary enlargement

MICROSCOPIC

- Diffuse hyperplasia
  - Increase in pituitary cells
  - Never truly monomorphic histology
- Nodular hyperplasia
  - Indistinct demarcation
  - Lacks compressive effects

ANCILLARY TESTS

- Reticulin
  - Highlights acinar expansion

TOP DIFFERENTIAL DIAGNOSES

- Normal adenohypophysis
  - Reticulin stains highlight normal-sized acini
- Pituitary adenoma
  - Usually larger mass, histologically
    - Greater disruption of reticulin network

Enlarged Gland, Pituitary Hyperplasia

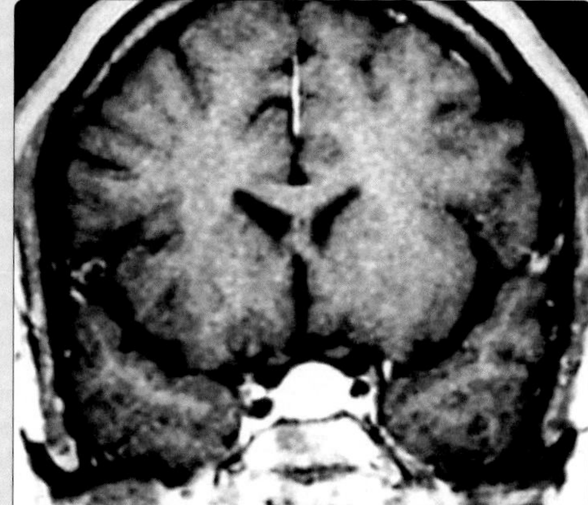

Expanded Acini

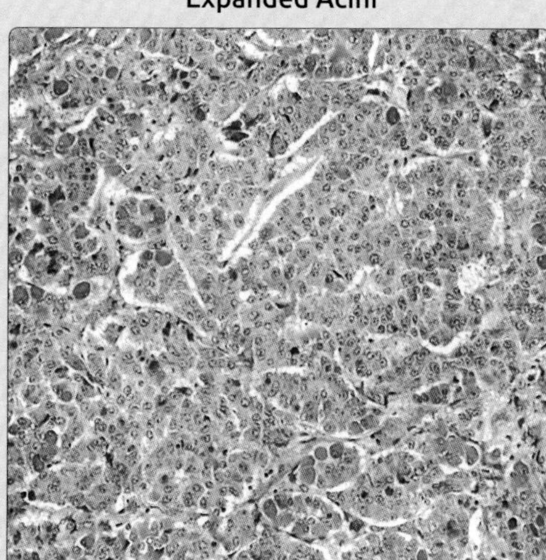

(Left) *Enlarged homogeneously enhancing pituitary gland with convex superior margin is a typical finding in pituitary hyperplasia.* **(Right)** *Pituitary hyperplasia features cytologically somewhat uniform cells in expanded acini, yet the lesion is never truly monomorphic, as is observed in this diffuse prolactin cell hyperplasia.*

Nodular Hyperplasia, Variable Acinar Size

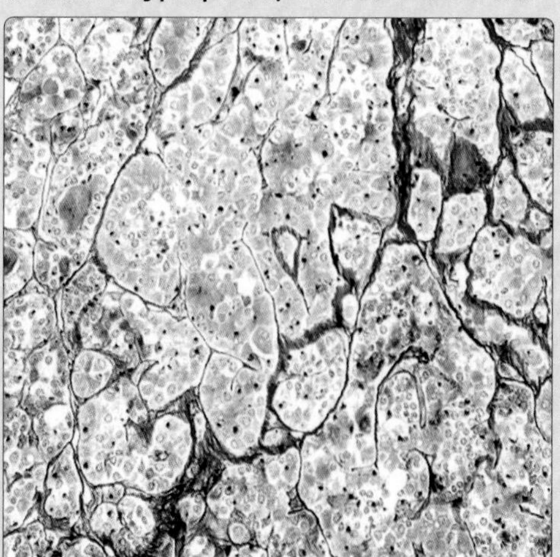

Diffuse ACTH Cell Hyperplasia

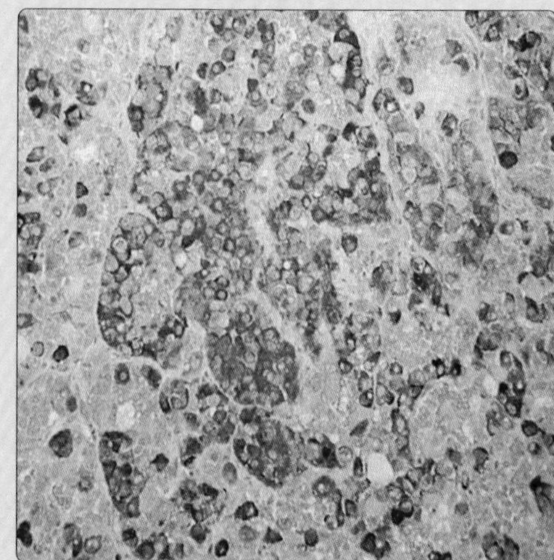

(Left) *In this nodular hyperplasia, reticulin preparation shows marked variation in the size of pituitary acini, some aggregating to form a nodule. Such nodules may be numerous.* **(Right)** *In ACTH cell hyperplasia, diffusely and strongly positive ACTH immunostain is noted.*

TERMINOLOGY

Definitions

- Nonneoplastic increase in adenohypophysial cell number

ETIOLOGY/PATHOGENESIS

Pathobiology

- Physiologic response to end-organ failure
  - Prolactin (PRL) cell hyperplasia during pregnancy, lactation, or estrogen treatment
  - ACTH cell hyperplasia due to hypocortisolism in Addison disease
  - TSH cell hyperplasia with longstanding primary hypothyroidism
  - Gonadotroph hyperplasia in primary hypogonadism due to Klinefelter or Turner syndrome
- Pathologic hyperplasia associated with ectopic excess of releasing hormones
  - Growth hormone (GH) cell hyperplasia
    - Due to increased GH-releasing hormone secreted by pancreatic islet cell tumor, pheochromocytoma, bronchial and thymic carcinoid tumor
  - ACTH cell hyperplasia
    - Secondary to corticotropin-releasing hormone secretion from hypothalamic hamartoma or neuroendocrine tumors
- Syndromic: Mammosomatotroph hyperplasia in McCune-Albright syndrome, Carney complex
- Idiopathic

CLINICAL ISSUES

Epidemiology

- Incidence
  - Rare, except for PRL cell hyperplasia in pregnancy
  - Most medically curable, no surgical specimen expected
- Age
  - Generally young adults
- Sex
  - PRL cell hyperplasia of pregnancy in women

Presentation

- Hormone-related hyperplasia
  - GH cell: Gigantism or acromegaly
  - PRL cell: Hyperprolactinemia
  - ACTH cell: Cushing disease
  - TSH cell: Hyperprolactinemia
    - In hypothyroidism, associated with PRL cell hyperplasia
  - LH-FSH: Result of early-onset hypogonadism; may cause pituitary enlargement

Treatment

- Correct underlying endocrinologic cause
- Surgical approaches
  - GH, ACTH hyperplasia: Resect hypothalamic-releasing hormone-producing tumors
- Adjuvant therapy
  - TSH hyperplasia: Medical treatment of hypothyroidism

Prognosis

- Excellent with medical treatment
- Rare association with adenoma formation

IMAGING

General Features

- Size
  - Symmetric 2-3x pituitary enlargement on CT/MR
- No sellar destruction

MICROSCOPIC

Histologic Features

- Nodular or diffuse
  - Nodularity result of acinar expansion
    - Relative cellular monomorphism in affected acini
    - Noncompressive; indistinct demarcation
    - Difficult to diagnose in fragmented specimens
  - Diffuse
    - Numerical increase in pituitary cells without alteration in architecture
- Mitoses rare
- Cytological composition
  - GH cell hyperplasia: Chromophobic to eosinophilic polygonal cells
  - PRL cell hyperplasia: Chromophobic with occasional microcalcifications
  - ACTH cell hyperplasia: Amphophilic with very large vacuole (lysosome); variable surrounding Crooke cell change
  - TSH cell hyperplasia: Chromophobic, often elongated cells with multiple large PAS+ lysosomes
  - LH-FSH hyperplasia: Hypervacuolization (castration cells)

ANCILLARY TESTS

Histochemistry

- Reticulin: Highlights acinar expansion; PAS: Stains lysosomes in TSH hyperplasia

Immunohistochemistry

- Cytoplasmic reactivity for respective hormones
- Ki-67 labeling index low level but increased over nearly immunonegative normal gland

DIFFERENTIAL DIAGNOSIS

Normal Adenohypophysis

- Heterogeneous cell populations of normal acini; reticulin stains highlight normal acini
- ACTH cells that are aggregated in normal way in lateral wings of anterior pituitary or as normal basophil invasion may mimic hyperplasia

Pituitary Adenoma

- Larger, compresses adjacent normal acini, greater disruption of reticulin network

SELECTED REFERENCES

1. De Sousa SM et al: Pituitary hyperplasia: case series and literature review of an under-recognised and heterogeneous condition. Endocrinol Diabetes Metab Case Rep. 2015:150017, 2015

(Left) *Nodular hyperplasia* ⇨ *is difficult to distinguish from adenoma. A compression effect, which is commonly seen in adenomas, is lacking.* **(Right)** *Reticulin shows enlargement of the acini, but the acinar structure is retained, unlike adenomas.*

Nodular Hyperplasia

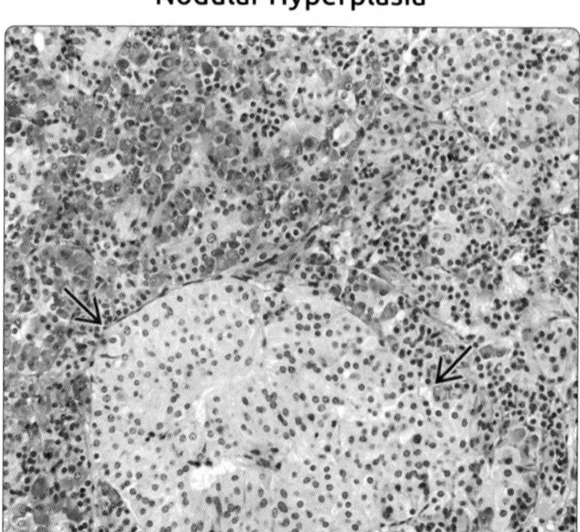

Enlargement of Acini

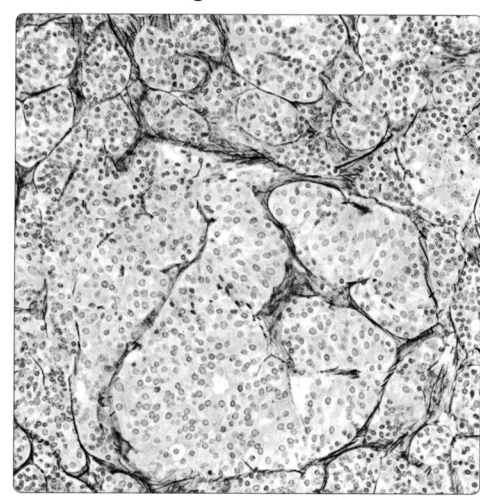

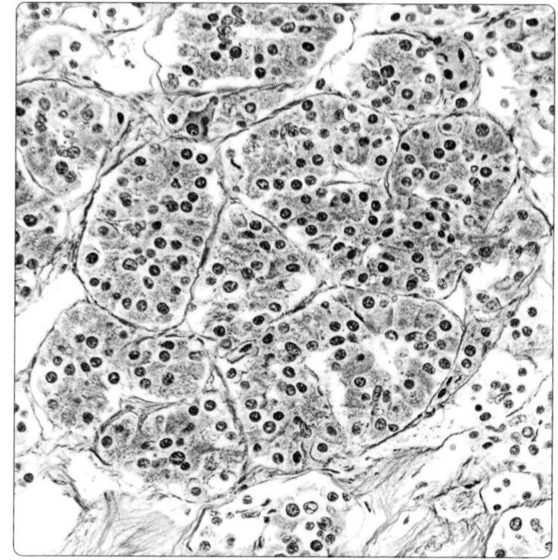

(Left) *Unlike other cell types, normal corticotroph cells tend to form sizable, hyperplasia-like aggregates.* **(Right)** *Reticulin highlights the normal acinar structures with regular size in the ACTH cell aggregations of normal pituitary.*

Normal Nodular Clusters of Corticotrophs

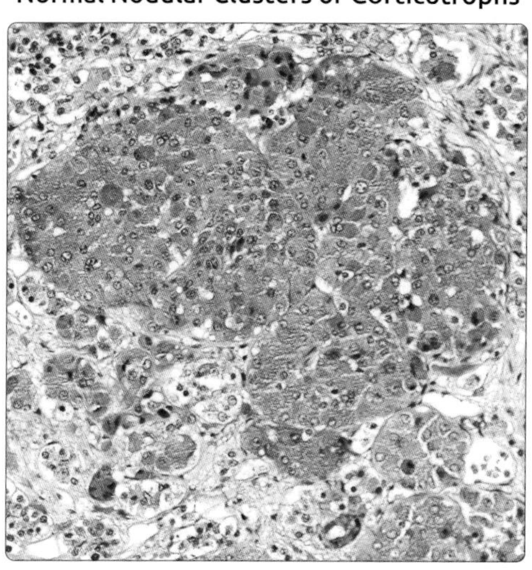

Normal Acinar Size in Corticotroph Nodules

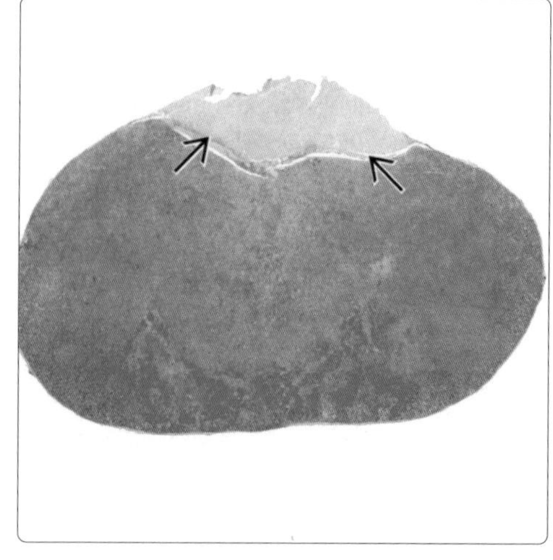

(Left) *In this example of ACTH cell hyperplasia, initial attempts to find an adenoma failed. To achieve hormone balance, the entire gland was removed.* **(Right)** *The most common physiological form of pituitary hyperplasia is the diffuse prolactin cell type in pregnancy. Here, as seen in a horizontal section, the diffusely enlarged anterior lobe dwarfs the neurohypophysis* ⇨*. The enlarged adenohypophysis is also more diffusely chromophobic than it would be in its normal state.*

ACTH Cell Hyperplasia Necessitating Hypophysectomy

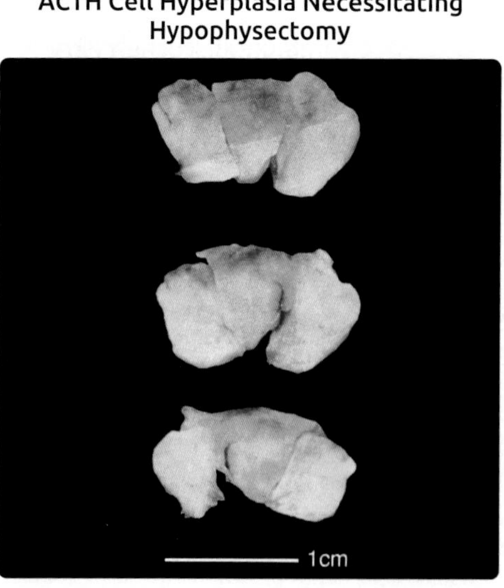

Pregnancy-Related Pituitary Hyperplasia

Gestational Prolactin Hyperplasia

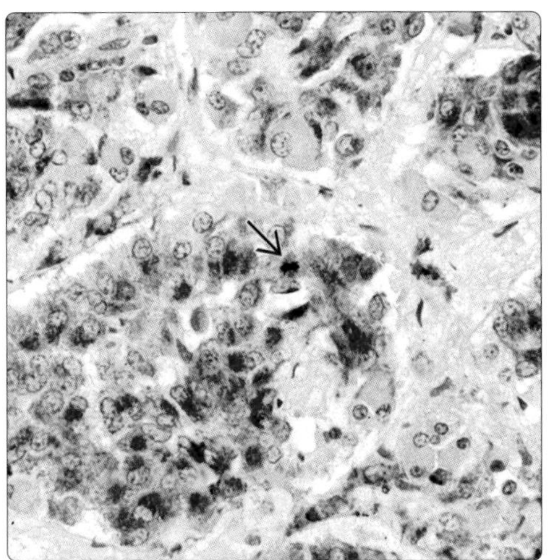

TSH Hyperplasia, Hypothyroidism

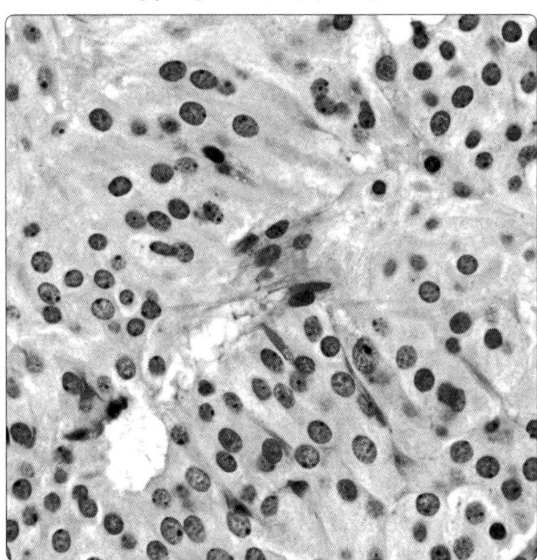

(Left) *Prolactin immunoreactivity is abundant, and occasional mitotic figures* ⇒ *may be present in gestational prolactin cell hyperplasia.* **(Right)** *TSH cell hyperplasia is seen with longstanding primary hypothyroidism. TSH cells are often angulated or spindled.*

TSH Hyperplasia

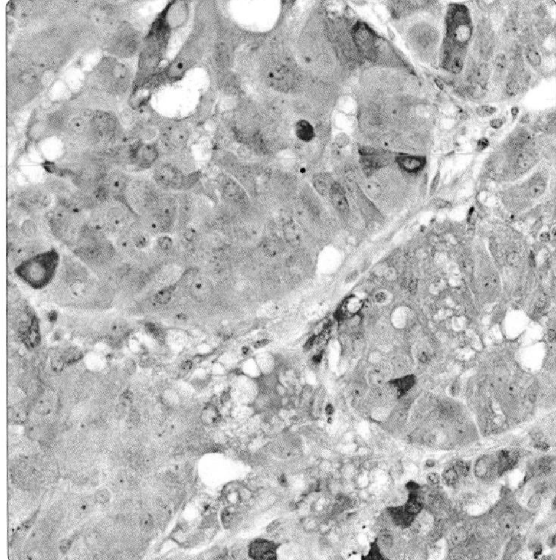

Smear, TSH Hyperplasia

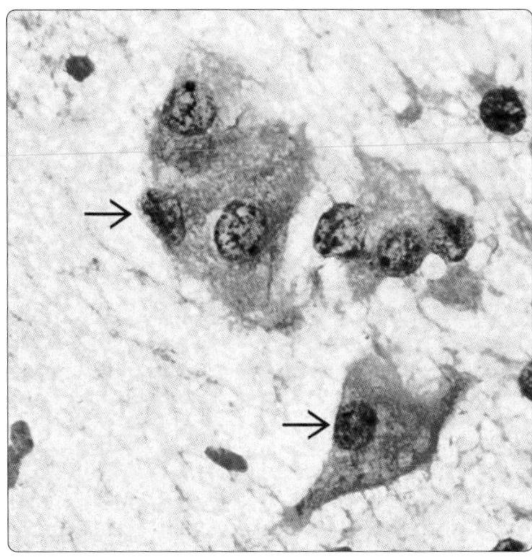

(Left) *TSH hyperplasia is not difficult to identify on immunostaining. Reactivity is widespread and varies from strong to weak among hyperplastic cells.* **(Right)** *TSH cell hyperplasia is seen with long-standing primary hypothyroidism. TSH cells* ⇒ *least frequent in the normal pituitary and often angulated or spindled are conspicuous in this smear preparation.*

Castration Cells, Hypogonadism

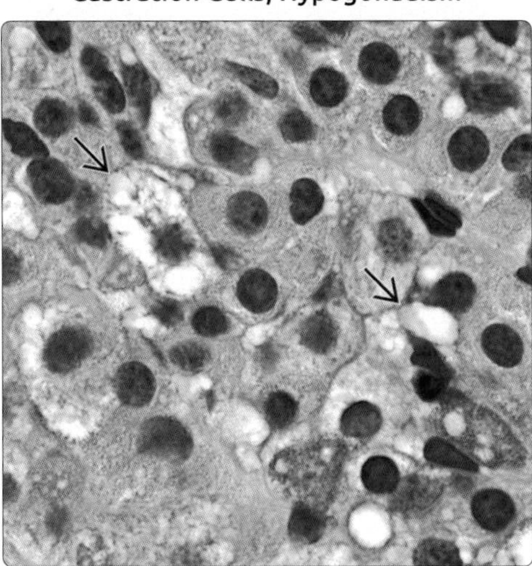

Klinefelter Syndrome, LH-FSH Hyperplasia

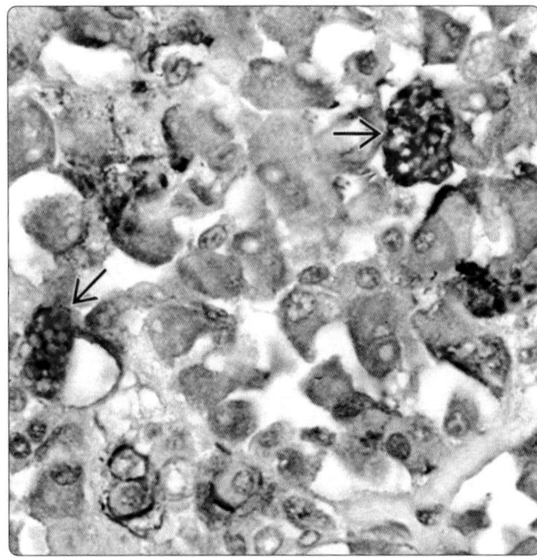

(Left) *In hypogonadism, gonadotrophic cells increase in number and acquire cytoplasmic vacuolization* ⇒ *due to dilation of the endoplasmic reticulum. These cells are known as castration cells.* **(Right)** *In Klinefelter syndrome, the pituitary gland may demonstrate LH-FSH hyperplasia, with castration cells* ⇒ *shown here by FSH immunostaining.*

Pituitary Carcinoma

KEY FACTS

TERMINOLOGY

- Adenohypophysial tumor exhibiting cerebrospinal &/or systemic metastases
    - Brain invasion also indicative of malignancy
    - Conventional morphologic malignancy criteria (nuclear atypia, pleomorphism, mitotic activity, necrosis, hemorrhage, &/or dural invasion) are insufficient for diagnosis

ETIOLOGY/PATHOGENESIS

- Arise in transition from pituitary adenoma or rarely de novo from normal adenohypophysis
- Chromosomal gains (5, 7p, 14q), losses are less frequent

CLINICAL ISSUES

- Very rare
    - Local infiltration not in itself indicator of carcinoma, but disseminating lesions, i.e., carcinomas, often arise in infiltrating adenomas
- Majority endocrinologically functional
    - Usually produce ACTH or prolactin
- Ultimate prognosis poor
    - May respond to temozolomide
- Primary sellar; rarely ectopic
- Metastatic sites
    - Craniospinal leptomeninges
    - Systemic: Mainly liver, bone, lymph node, lung

MICROSCOPIC

- Nuclear atypia absent or present
- Carcinomas may have few or many mitoses

ANCILLARY TESTS

- All synaptophysin immunopositive, chromogranin less often so
- Like adenomas, all carcinomas produce some pituitary hormones, even nonfunctional examples
- p53 and Ki-67 indices may be high

Evolving Carcinoma Identical to Invasive Adenoma

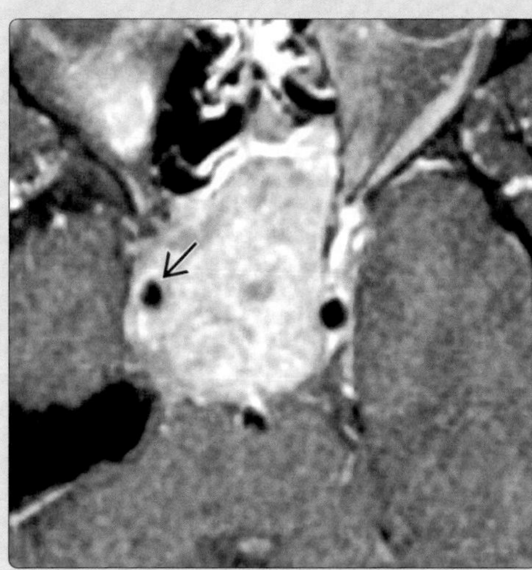

Drop Metastasis to Medulla

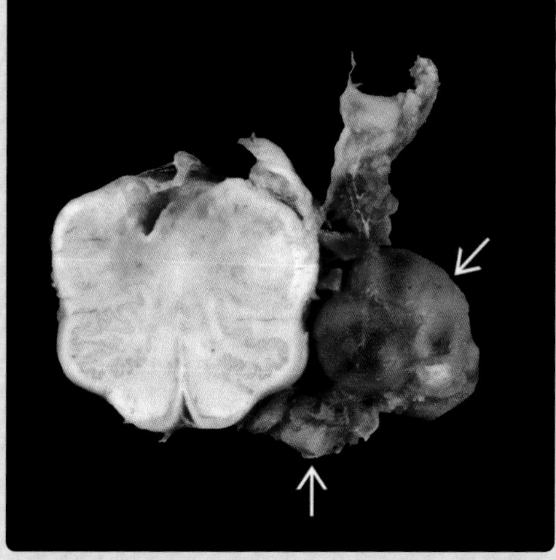

(Left) *Signs of evolving pituitary carcinoma are indistinguishable from atypical adenoma with invasion. T1WI C+ MR shows a tumor invading the clivus and encasing the right internal carotid artery* →. **(Right)** *The diagnosis of pituitary carcinoma is applied restrictively to rare lesions with drop metastasis, as here adjacent to the medulla* →, *&/or those that are disseminated to systemic sites.*

Cellular Pleomorphism in Some Carcinomas

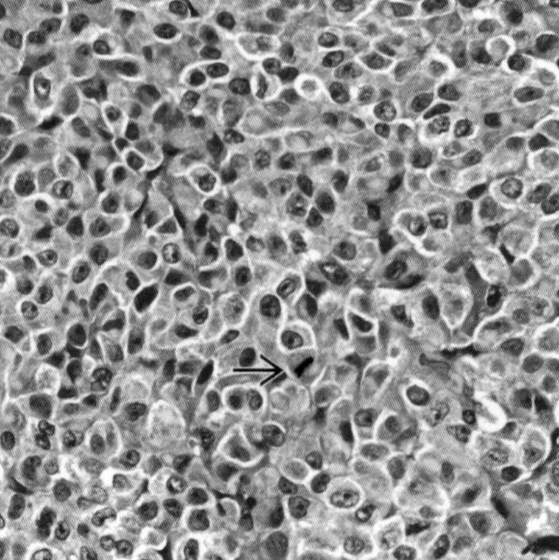

Most With High MIB-1

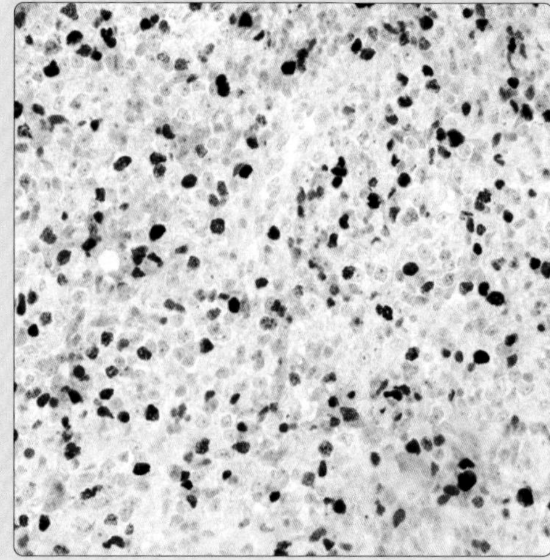

(Left) *Some pituitary carcinomas may feature cellular pleomorphism, distinct nucleoli, and mitosis* →. **(Right)** *Most pituitary carcinomas feature, not only an elevated mitotic rate, but also a high level MIB-1/Ki-67 immunolabeling.*

Pituitary Carcinoma

TERMINOLOGY

Synonyms

- Adenocarcinoma of pituitary

Definitions

- Adenohypophysial tumor exhibiting cerebrospinal &/or systemic metastases
  - Brain invasion also indicative of malignancy
- Conventional morphologic malignancy criteria (nuclear atypia, pleomorphism, mitotic activity, necrosis, hemorrhage, &/or dural invasion) are insufficient for diagnosis

ETIOLOGY/PATHOGENESIS

Pathophysiology

- Arises in transition from pituitary adenoma or de novo from previously normal adenohypophysial cells
- No evidence of pluripotent precursor cells in genesis of adenomas or carcinomas
- Invasion, e.g., dural, is common in adenomas, but malignant transformation is rare
- Latency from adenoma to carcinoma varies [ACTH > prolactin (PRL)]
- Spread to CNS is by way of cerebrospinal fluid
- Direct infiltration of brain is rare
- Systemic metastases are hematogenous, associated with cavernous sinus/jugular vein involvement
- Lymph node metastases secondary to skull base and soft tissue involvement
- Unclear whether sellar surgery facilitates metastases

Genetics

- Chromosomal gains (5, 7p, 14q), losses less frequent (comparative genomic hybridization)
- Clonality studies (X-linked gene analysis) show primary, recurrent, and metastatic carcinoma to have same allelic pattern
- Point mutations in *HRAS* in carcinomas but not their adenoma precursors
- *P53* mutations occasional
- Incidence not increased in patients with multiple endocrine neoplasia 1 syndrome or Carney complex

CLINICAL ISSUES

Epidemiology

- Incidence
  - Very rare; ~ 150 cases reported to date
  - 0.2% of operated adenohypophysial tumors
- Age
  - Adults; rare adolescents
- Sex
  - Slight female predilection

Site

- Primary sellar; rarely ectopic
- Metastatic sites
  - Craniospinal leptomeninges
  - Systemic sites: Mainly liver, bone, lymph node, lung

Presentation

- Diagnosis based on metastasis, often from multiple recurring, invasive adenomas
- De novo malignancy rare
- Interval to metastasis: 4 mo to 30 yr (mean: 10 yr)
- Malignant transformation rare in ectopic adenoma
- Majority (75%) endocrinologically functional
  - Prolactin and ACTH most frequent, followed by growth hormone (GH) and TSH
  - Presentations: Hyperprolactinemia, Nelson syndrome, Cushing disease, acromegaly, hyperthyroidism
- Pituitary hormone levels do not permit distinction of adenoma from carcinoma except for PRL (marked increase, 10-30,000 ng/mL)
- Early features of aggressive behavior: Infiltration of dura, bone, cavernous sinus, and cranial nerves
- Clinical signs specific to site of metastasis

Treatment

- Multimodality therapies (surgery, external beam radiotherapy, radiosurgery, adjuvant pharmacologic and chemotherapy)
- Temozolomide therapy efficacious
- Dopamine agonist response temporary in PRL cell carcinomas

Prognosis

- Poor prognosis; mortality 66% at 1 yr and 80% within 8 yr
- Overall mean survival: 2 yr, range: 0.25-8.00 yr
- Survival shorter in systemic vs. craniospinal metastases (1 vs. 2.6 yr)
- Long-term survival with benign histology but poor survival with anaplasia
- Loss of MGMT immunoreactivity and promoter methylation of gene associated with high response to temozolomide therapy

IMAGING

CT and MR Findings

- No features unique to pituitary carcinoma
- Bone metastases are usually osteolytic but may be osteoblastic
  - Mimic meningioma when presenting as dural-based masses
- Invasive sellar primary often extends into parasellar structures
  - Cranial nerves in cavernous sinus often affected
- Brain infrequently involved by primary tumor
- Multifocal craniospinal deposits affect leptomeninges and nerve roots, often of cauda equina

MACROSCOPIC

General Features

- Primary tumor of macroadenoma size (> 1 cm); all invasive
- Metastatic deposits may be single or multiple, nodular or diffuse
- Metastasis of pituitary carcinoma indistinguishable from metastases of carcinomas of other organs

Size

- Metastatic deposits vary from micro- to macroscopic
  - Those to spinal axis relatively small (< 2 cm)
  - Systemic metastases, particularly to liver, sometimes massive

MICROSCOPIC

Histologic Features

- May have nuclear atypia, cellular pleomorphism, mitotic activity, or necrosis
  - Also present to varying degrees in nonmetastasizing adenomas
- Most not overtly malignant histologically or cytologically

ANCILLARY TESTS

Histochemistry

- Lack of acinar architecture on reticulin staining, like adenomas

Immunohistochemistry

- All synaptophysin (+); chromogranin less often (+)
- All produce some hormones, even when clinically nonfunctional
- Ki-67 labeling index varies widely, often high in metastases
- Topoisomerase-2, an indicator of proliferation rate, often exceeds 4%
- p27, cell-cycle inhibitor, widely expressed in normal pituitary, decreased in carcinomas
- p53 expressed in most pituitary carcinomas, staining in metastatic sites highest
- VEGFR, related to angiogenesis, widely expressed
- Endoglin and CD34 (+) microvasculature increased
- Metalloproteinases increased over adenomas
- Overexpression of HER2 occasional

Electron Microscopy

- Data regarding differentiation (variable) and cytogenesis
- Does not distinguish adenoma from carcinoma

DIFFERENTIAL DIAGNOSIS

Carcinoma Metastases of Other Organs

- Anaplasia more prominent
- Negative for pituitary hormones
  - Except for rare examples that secrete ACTH or GH
- Synaptophysin (+) only in neuroendocrine carcinomas
- Organ-specific markers appropriate

DIAGNOSTIC CHECKLIST

Pathologic Interpretation Pearls

- Local infiltration not in itself indicator of carcinoma, but
- Disseminating lesions, i.e., carcinomas, often arise in infiltrating adenomas

GRADING

Grading System

- No consensus grading system established

SELECTED REFERENCES

1. Liu JK et al: The role of temozolomide in the treatment of aggressive pituitary tumors. J Clin Neurosci. 22(6):923-9, 2015
2. Sav A et al: Invasive, atypical and aggressive pituitary adenomas and carcinomas. Endocrinol Metab Clin North Am. 44(1):99-104, 2015
3. Marucci G: Treatment of pituitary neoplasms with temozolomide: A review. Cancer. 117(17):4101-2; author reply 4102, 2011
4. Syro LV et al: Treatment of pituitary neoplasms with temozolomide: a review. Cancer. 117(3):454-62, 2011
5. Roncaroli F et al: Silent corticotroph carcinoma of the adenohypophysis: a report of five cases. Am J Surg Pathol. 27(4):477-86, 2003
6. Gaffey TA et al: Corticotroph carcinoma of the pituitary: a clinicopathological study. Report of four cases. J Neurosurg. 96(2):352-60, 2002
7. Hosaka N et al: Ectopic pituitary adenoma with malignant transformation. Am J Surg Pathol. 26(8):1078-82, 2002
8. Landman RE et al: Long-term survival with ACTH-secreting carcinoma of the pituitary: a case report and review of the literature. J Clin Endocrinol Metab. 87(7):3084-9, 2002
9. Rickert CH et al: Chromosomal aberrations in pituitary carcinoma metastases. Acta Neuropathol. 102(2):117-20, 2001
10. Scheithauer BW et al: Pituitary carcinoma: an ultrastructural study of eleven cases. Ultrastruct Pathol. 25(3):227-42, 2001
11. Zahedi A et al: Distinct clonal composition of primary and metastatic adrencorticotrophic hormone-producing pituitary carcinoma. Clin Endocrinol (Oxf). 55(4):549-56, 2001
12. Nose-Alberti V et al: Adrenocorticotropin-producing pituitary carcinoma with expression of c-erbB-2 and high PCNA index: a comparative study with pituitary adenomas and normal pituitary tissues. Endocr Pathol. 9(1):53-62, 1998
13. Jin L et al: Transforming growth factor-beta, transforming growth factor-beta receptor II, and p27Kip1 expression in nontumorous and neoplastic human pituitaries. Am J Pathol. 151(2):509-19, 1997
14. Pernicone PJ et al: Pituitary carcinoma: a clinicopathologic study of 15 cases. Cancer. 79(4):804-12, 1997
15. Thapar K et al: p53 expression in pituitary adenomas and carcinomas: correlation with invasiveness and tumor growth fractions. Neurosurgery. 38(4):765-70; discussion 770-1, 1996
16. Thapar K et al: Proliferative activity and invasiveness among pituitary adenomas and carcinomas: an analysis using the MIB-1 antibody. Neurosurgery. 38(1):99-106; discussion 106-7, 1996
17. Beauchesne P et al: Gonadotropic pituitary carcinoma: case report. Neurosurgery. 37(4):810-5; discussion 815-6, 1995
18. Lubke D et al: Proliferation Markers and EGF in ACTH-Secreting Adenomas and Carcinomas of the Pituitary. Endocr Pathol. 6(1):45-55, 1995
19. Pei L et al: H-ras mutations in human pituitary carcinoma metastases. J Clin Endocrinol Metab. 78(4):842-6, 1994
20. Mixson AJ et al: Thyrotropin-secreting pituitary carcinoma. J Clin Endocrinol Metab. 76(2):529-33, 1993

Pituitary Carcinoma Drop Metastasis

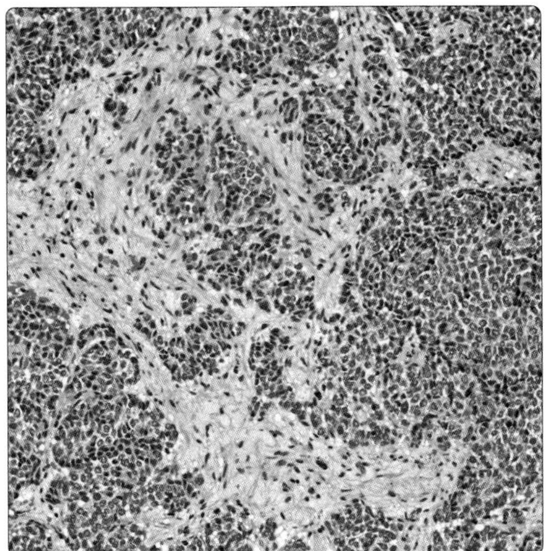

Rare Vascular Invasion

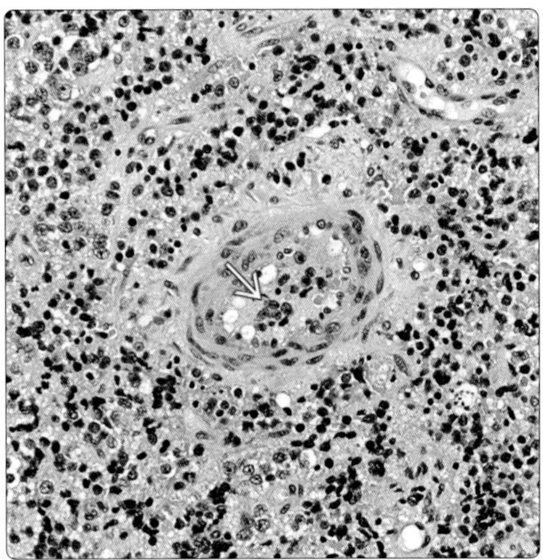

(Left) *A drop metastasis of a pituitary carcinoma to dura of lumbar spine shows solid islands of monomorphous neoplastic cells.* **(Right)** *The appearance of pituitary carcinomas varies considerably from uniform tumors to those that are more pleomorphic. Vascular invasion ➡ is rare.*

Bland Oncocytic Pituitary Carcinoma

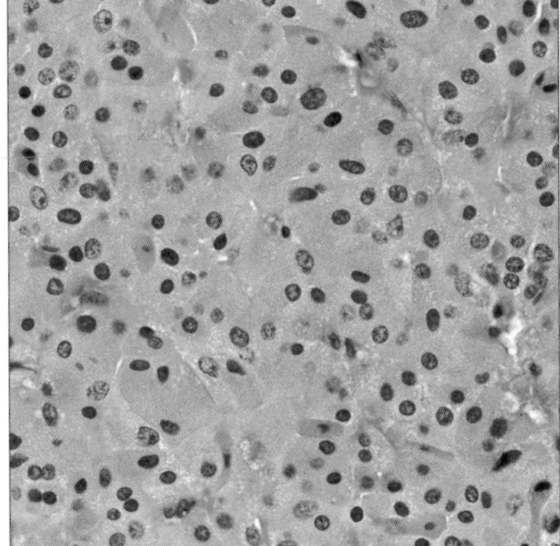

Mitotic Activity

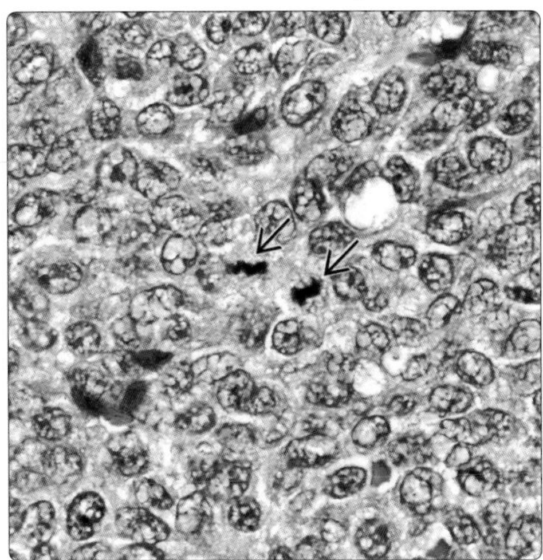

(Left) *As is the rule, this pituitary carcinoma with oncocytic features has neither significant cytological atypia nor mitotic activity.* **(Right)** *Pituitary carcinomas may have cytological atypia with cellular pleomorphism, distinct nucleoli, and mitoses ➡.*

Majority Endocrinologically Functioning

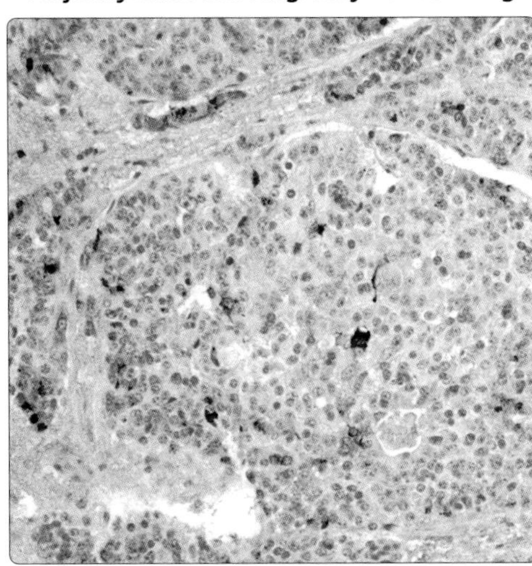

High p53 Expression, Especially in Metastatic Deposits

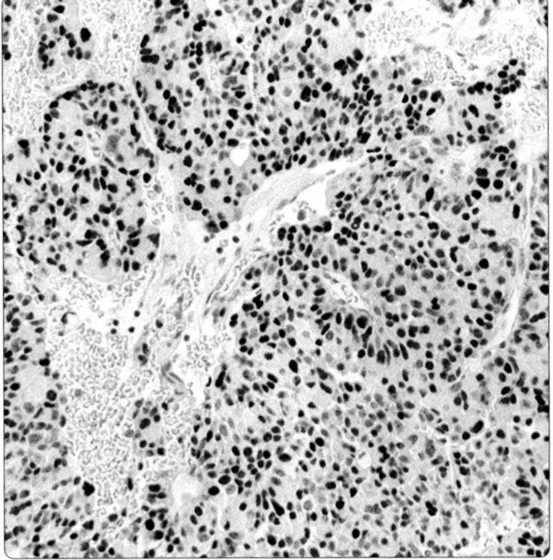

(Left) *Dural metastasis of this pituitary carcinoma is immunoreactive with prolactin. The majority of pituitary carcinomas are endocrinologically functioning.* **(Right)** *Immunoexpression of p53 is often high, especially in metastatic sites.*

Hypothalamic Hamartoma

KEY FACTS

ETIOLOGY/PATHOGENESIS

- Most sporadic
- Genetic examples uncommon: Smith-Lemli-Opitz, Pallister-Hall, Laurence Moon Biedl syndrome, holoprosencephaly

CLINICAL ISSUES

- Precocious puberty
- Uncontrollable bouts of inappropriate laughter (gelastic seizures)
- Surgery mainstay for symptomatic lesions
- Surgery/biopsy unnecessary in asymptomatic patients

IMAGING

- Floor of 3rd ventricle
- Isointense to gray matter in T1WI and T2WI sequences
- No enhancement

MACROSCOPIC

- Round, well circumscribed

MICROSCOPIC

- Mature neurons main component
  - Distributed singly (diffuse) or in clusters (nodular)

TOP DIFFERENTIAL DIAGNOSES

- Normal gray matter (correlation with imaging findings essential)
- Gangliocytoma/ganglioglioma (cytologically abnormal neurons, lymphocytes, eosinophilic granular bodies)
- Mixed pituitary adenoma-gangliocytoma (identify admixed pituitary adenoma cells)

DIAGNOSTIC CHECKLIST

- Closely resembles normal gray matter

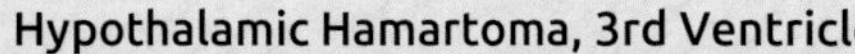

Hypothalamic Hamartoma, 3rd Ventricle

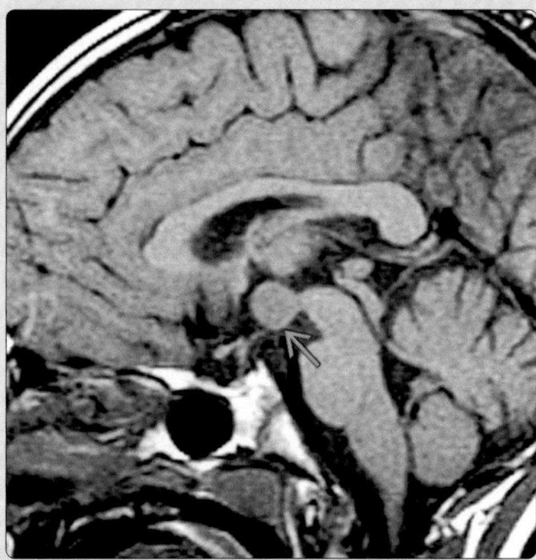

Attachment to Hypothalamus

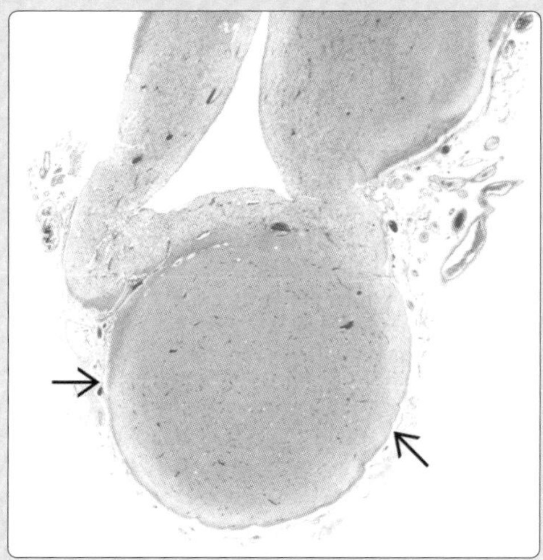

(Left) *Sagittal T1WI MR shows a hamartoma ⇨ within the 3rd ventricle. Hamartomas may extend inferiorly into the suprasellar or interpeduncular cistern or upward into the 3rd ventricle.* **(Right)** *Most hypothalamic hamartomas → are attached to the hypothalamus, either by a narrow pedicle or, as here, along a broad base. The lesion's similarity to normal gray matter is apparent even at low magnification.*

Disorganized Neurons

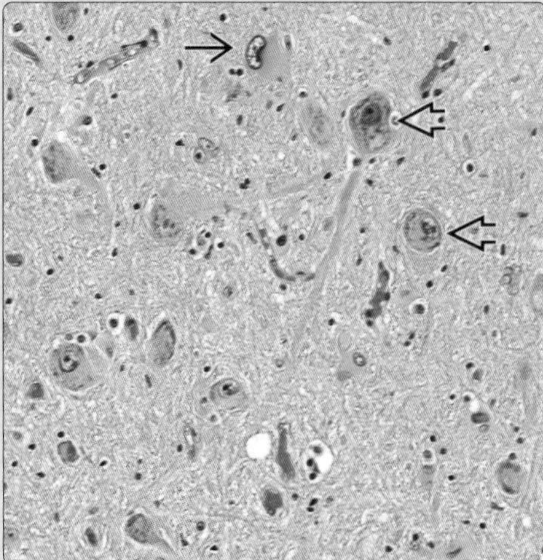

Hypertrophic Reactive Astrocytes

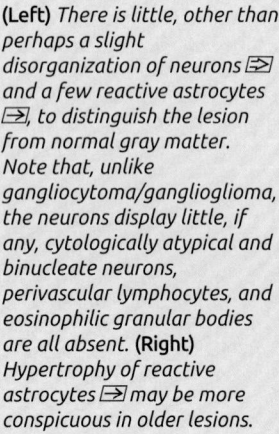

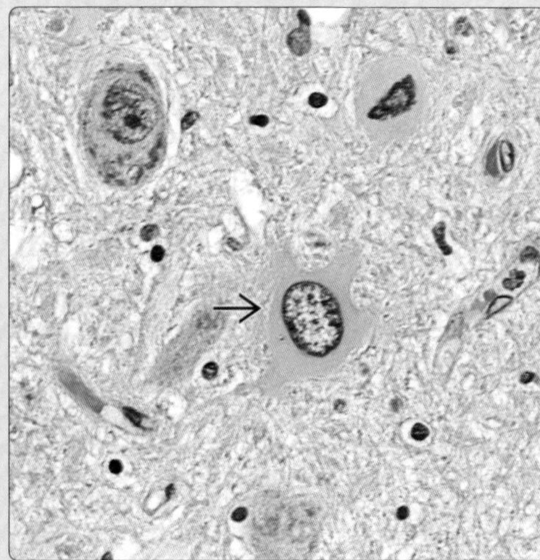

(Left) *There is little, other than perhaps a slight disorganization of neurons → and a few reactive astrocytes ⇨, to distinguish the lesion from normal gray matter. Note that, unlike gangliocytoma/ganglioglioma, the neurons display little, if any, cytologically atypical and binucleate neurons, perivascular lymphocytes, and eosinophilic granular bodies are all absent.* **(Right)** *Hypertrophy of reactive astrocytes → may be more conspicuous in older lesions.*

TERMINOLOGY

Abbreviations

- Hypothalamic hamartoma (HH)

Synonyms

- Tuber cinereum hamartoma

Definitions

- Nonneoplastic mass lesion in hypothalamus composed of gray matter (mature neurons and glia)

ETIOLOGY/PATHOGENESIS

Developmental Anomaly

- Malformative mass resulting from abnormal neuronal migration
- Those associated with genetic syndromes/malformations with germline mutations

CLINICAL ISSUES

Presentation

- Precocious puberty
- Seizures
  - Uncontrollable bouts of inappropriate laughter (gelastic seizures)
  - Other seizure types may develop with time
  - Refractory to medical treatment
- Sporadic in majority of cases
- Association with genetic syndromes and malformations
  - Pallister-Hall (5%), Smith-Lemli-Opitz, Laurence-Moon-Biedl, holoprosencephaly
  - Pallister-Hall syndrome cases tend to be less symptomatic, have minimal tumor growth

Treatment

- Surgery mainstay for symptomatic lesions; stereotactic radiosurgery, some cases
- Surgery/biopsy unnecessary in asymptomatic patients

Prognosis

- Surgery curative in symptomatic cases
- Growth over time usually not clinical concern in asymptomatic cases

IMAGING

General Features

- Location
  - Floor of 3rd ventricle
- Size
  - < 1 cm (usually); but up to 5 cm (giant)

MR Findings

- Isointense to gray matter in T1W and T2W images
- No enhancement

MACROSCOPIC

General Features

- Round, well circumscribed
- Attached to floor of 3rd ventricle; broad base (sessile) or pedunculated
- Disconnected from brain, uncommon

MICROSCOPIC

Histologic Features

- Low cellularity
- Mature neurons distributed singly (diffuse) or in clusters (nodular)
  - Cytologically normal
  - Small to intermediate size; larger neurons less frequent
  - Unmyelinated axons
- Glial component
  - Inconspicuous
  - Astrocytic hypertrophy with mild atypia, especially in older patients

ANCILLARY TESTS

Immunohistochemistry

- Neuronal markers
  - Synaptophysin, unphosphorylated neurofilament protein
  - Hypothalamic hormones and neurotransmitters
    - Growth, corticotropin, thyrotropin, and gonadotropin releasing; somatostatin and GAD-67
- Low to absent Ki-67 labeling index

DIFFERENTIAL DIAGNOSIS

Normal Brain

- Difficult distinction from normal hypothalamic tissue, especially in fragmented surgical specimen
  - No clustering of neurons and reactive gliosis
  - Correlation with imaging findings essential

Gangliocytoma/Ganglioglioma

- Architectural abnormalities more pronounced in ganglion cell tumors (clustering)
- Dysmorphic and binucleated neurons
- Perivascular lymphocytes
- Eosinophilic granular bodies

Ganglion Cell Metaplasia in Pituitary Adenoma (Mixed Pituitary Adenoma-Gangliocytoma)

- Cellular pituitary adenoma component present

DIAGNOSTIC CHECKLIST

Clinically Relevant Pathologic Features

- Mature tissue, not neoplasm

Pathologic Interpretation Pearls

- Closely resembles normal gray matter

SELECTED REFERENCES

1. Dumitrascu O et al: Teaching neuroImages: short stature, imperforate anus, and polydactyly: When is a hypothalamic mass an incidentaloma? Neurology. 84(15):e117, 2015
2. Calisto A et al: Endoscopic disconnection of hypothalamic hamartomas: safety and feasibility of robot-assisted, thulium laser-based procedures. J Neurosurg Pediatr. 14(6):563-72, 2014
3. Coons SW et al: The histopathology of hypothalamic hamartomas: study of 57 cases. J Neuropathol Exp Neurol. 66(2):131-41, 2007

Granular Cell Tumor of Infundibulum

KEY FACTS

TERMINOLOGY

- Benign (WHO grade I) intra- &/or suprasellar tumor of neurohypophysis &/or its stalk
- Granular cell tumor of infundibulum and spindle cell oncocytoma now considered variants of pituicytoma, based on shared TTF-1(+)
- Entity distinct from granular cell astrocytoma of cerebral hemispheres

CLINICAL ISSUES

- Common as incidental microscopic finding(s) in autopsies
- Mass effects; mimic pituitary adenoma
- Transsphenoidal or transfrontal resection

IMAGING

- Well-circumscribed, enhancing, supra- &/or intrasellar tumor

MICROSCOPIC

- Polygonal to elongate cells with granular, eosinophilic cytoplasm, small, eccentric nuclei

ANCILLARY TESTS

- PAS(+), diastase-resistant granularity
- CD68(+/-), S100 protein (+); pituitary hormones (-)
- Numerous electron-dense lysosomes and heterolysosomes

TOP DIFFERENTIAL DIAGNOSES

- Pituicytoma
  - TTF-1(+), but cytoplasm PAS(-), paucity of lysosomes or mitochondria
- Spindle cell oncocytoma
  - TTF-1(+) but cytoplasm granular, PAS(-), and CD68(-), mitochondrial-rich cytoplasm
- Granular cell astrocytoma of the cerebral hemispheres is different entity

Granular Cell Tumor Simulating Adenoma

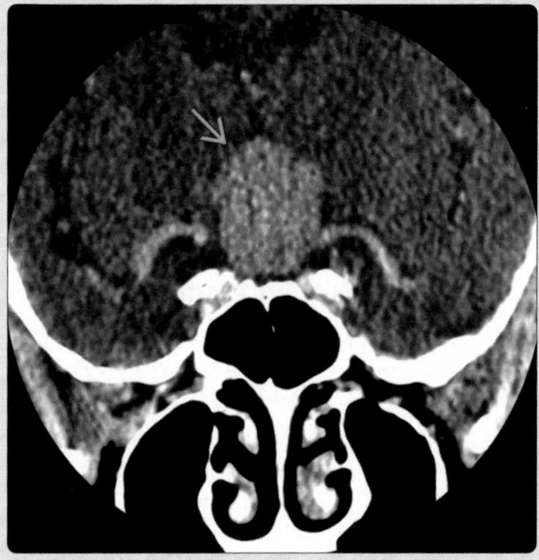

Large, Highly Granulated Cells

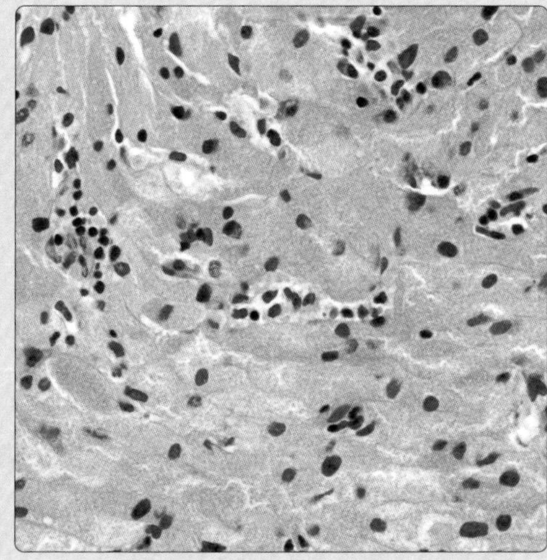

(Left) *Granular cell tumors typically present as a large sellar mass ⇒ with suprasellar extension. Radiologically, such tumors, seen here in a contrast-enhanced CT scan, resemble pituitary adenoma.* **(Right)** *Large, highly granulated cells define this rare sellar-region entity. Focal perivascular lymphocytes are common.*

Benign Inflammatory Infiltrates

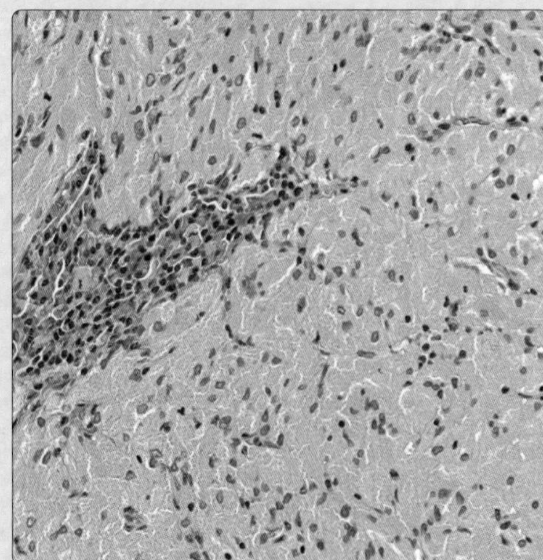

Lysosomal-Rich Tumor

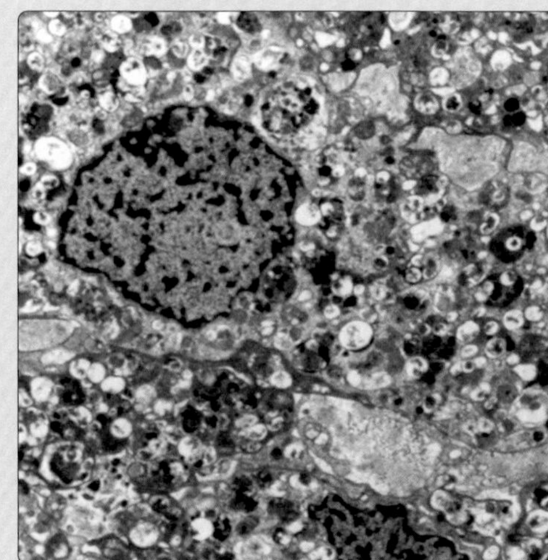

(Left) *Collections of benign plasma cells and lymphocytes are common in granular cell tumor of the infundibular stalk. Note the abundant eosinophilic cytoplasm with a granular quality.* **(Right)** *Ultrastructurally, heterolysosomes fill the cells of granular cell tumors.*

TERMINOLOGY

Definitions

- Intra- &/or suprasellar tumor of neurohypophysis &/or its stalk
- Composed of large, eosinophilic, lysosome-rich cells presumably derived from pituicytes
- WHO grade I neoplasm: Granular cell tumor of infundibulum and spindle cell oncocytoma now considered variants of pituicytoma, based on shared TTF-1(+)

CLINICAL ISSUES

Epidemiology

- Incidence
  - Uncommon as symptomatic lesion, comprises < 0.5% of sellar tumors; common as asymptomatic, incidental microscopic finding(s) in 15-20% of autopsies
- Age
  - Common in 4th-6th decades but wide age range; rare in children
- Sex
  - Female predominance (2:1) in symptomatic lesions
  - No gender predominance when asymptomatic

Presentation

- Endocrinologically nonfunctioning
  - Mass effects; mimics pituitary adenoma
  - Gradual onset of symptoms, rarely acute presentation (hemorrhage)
  - Diplopia, headache, nausea, vomiting
  - Visual field defect (chiasmal compression), panhypopituitarism, hyperprolactinemia (pituitary stalk effect) ± amenorrhea-galactorrhea syndrome
  - Diabetes insipidus (uncommon)

Treatment

- Surgical approaches
  - Transsphenoidal or transfrontal resection
- Radiation
  - Radiation therapy with subtotal removal or recurrence

Prognosis

- Resection with radiotherapy usually curative
- Outcome of symptomatic granular cell tumor poor
  - Subtotal removal followed by recurrence & unfavorable, occasionally fatal outcome
  - Survival from 2-26 months

IMAGING

Radiographic Findings

- Circumscribed intra- &/or suprasellar lesions, calcifications uncommon

MR Findings

- Nonspecific findings
  - Well circumscribed, 1-6 cm, enhancing, supra- &/or intrasellar; MR more sensitive in detecting small lesions: Isointense to gray matter on T1- and T2WI, enhancing

CT Findings

- Nonspecific findings
  - Well circumscribed, enhancing, supra- &/or intrasellar, calcification uncommon

MACROSCOPIC

General Features

- Lobulated, soft to rubbery, vascular
- Solid; gray-yellow cut surface
- Necrosis, cystic change, hemorrhage are uncommon
- Adherence to surrounding structures, infiltration of dura and cavernous sinus (uncommon)
- Intraoperative hemorrhage common

MICROSCOPIC

Histologic Features

- Classic
  - Sheets or fascicles of closely opposed polygonal to elongate cells
  - Granular, eosinophilic cytoplasm
  - Eccentric nuclei and inconspicuous nucleoli
  - Mitotic activity typically absent
  - Perivascular lymphocytes (in some cases)
- Atypical
  - Uncommon: Nuclear pleomorphism, multinucleation, prominent nucleoli, and increased mitotic activity

ANCILLARY TESTS

Cytology

- Dispersed cells with granular (lysosome-rich) cytoplasm, small eccentric nuclei, and small nucleoli

Histochemistry

- PAS(+), diastase-resistant granularity

Immunohistochemistry

- CD68(+/-), granular cytoplasm
- α-1-antitrypsin, α-1-antichymotrypsin, cathepsin-B(+), cytoplasm
- Vimentin (+) and variably S100(+)
- Rare, variable staining for galectin-3 and GFAP; TTF-1(+)
- EMA & annexin-1 (-); synaptophysin & pituitary hormones (-)

Electron Microscopy

- Numerous cytoplasmic, membrane-bound, electron-dense lysosomes and heterolysosomes
- Intermediate filaments, scant; no secretory granules

DIFFERENTIAL DIAGNOSIS

Pituicytoma

- Nongranular, variably GFAP(+) cytoplasm, TTF-1(+)

Spindle Cell Oncocytoma

- Spindle and epithelioid cells with granular, PAS(-), and CD68(-) cytoplasm due to mitochondria
- Positive for EMA, S100, vimentin, antimitochondrial antibody, annexin-1, TTF-1
- Uniformly reactive for galectin-3 but nonspecific

SELECTED REFERENCES

1. Piccirilli M et al: Granular cell tumor of the neurohypophysis: a single-institution experience. Tumori. 100(4):160e-4e, 2014

(Left) *Centered in the sellar region, this rare large granular cell tumor ⇒ extends superiorly to involve the 3rd ventricle.* **(Right)** *Granular cell tumors consist of round to polygonal cells with distinctive granular cytoplasm. The latter somewhat resembles that of another sellar region tumor, spindle cell oncocytoma. Granular cell tumors, however, attain their features from abundant lysosomes, while spindle cell oncocytomas are mitochondrial-rich.*

Granular Cell Tumor With 3rd Ventricle Extension

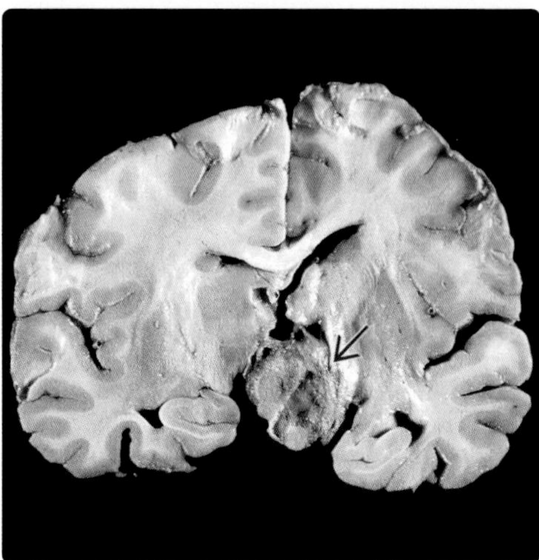

Distinctive Granular Cytoplasm

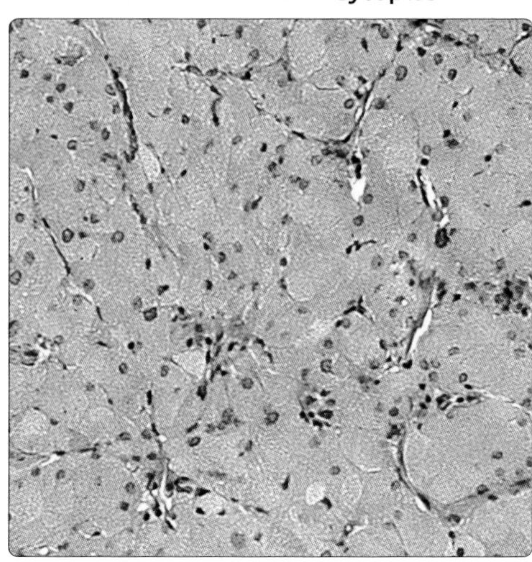

(Left) *Symptomatic granular cell tumors are large versions of granular cell tumorlets ⇒, found incidentally post mortem on the pituitary stalk.* **(Right)** *Granular cell tumorlets are well-circumscribed, compact masses of cells with ample, eosinophilic, granular cytoplasm.*

Incidental Granular Cell Tumorlets

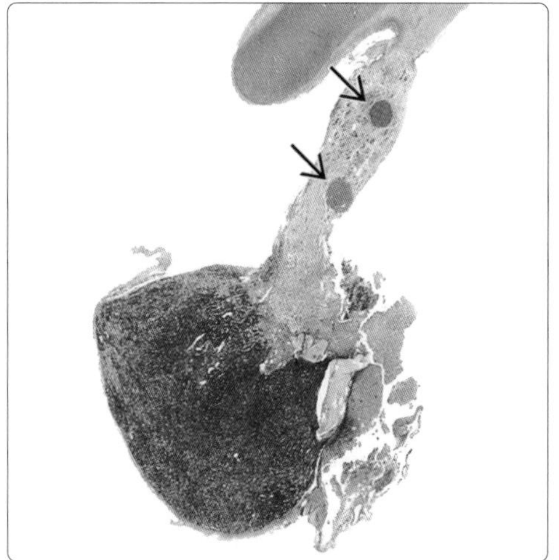

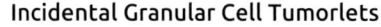

Granular Cell Tumorlet, Compact Cells

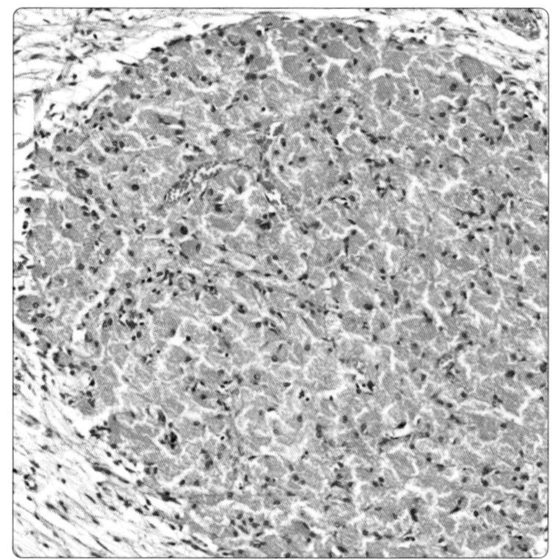

(Left) *Perivascular lymphoplasmacytic infiltrates are common in granular cell tumors of the infundibulum. Tumor cells somewhat resemble macrophages but are more elongate. The tumor cells are also coarsely granulated than are macrophages, whose cytoplasm is finely granulated or foamy.* **(Right)** *Granular cell tumor consists of polygonal to somewhat spindled cells with distinctly granular cytoplasm. A degree of nuclear pleomorphism may be present in this well-circumscribed, low-grade neoplasm.*

Granular Cells Mimicking Macrophages

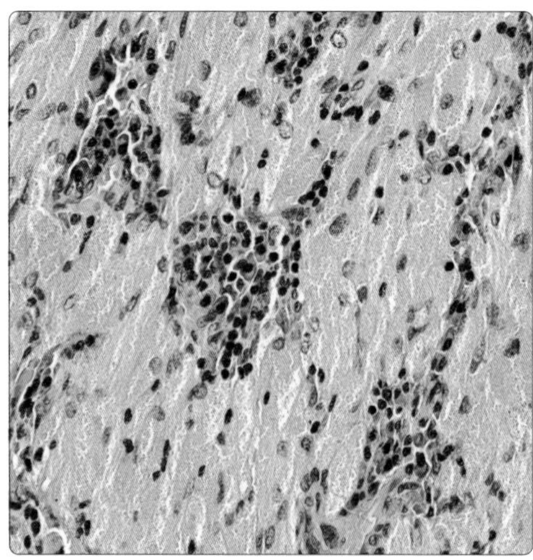

Focal Pleomorphism

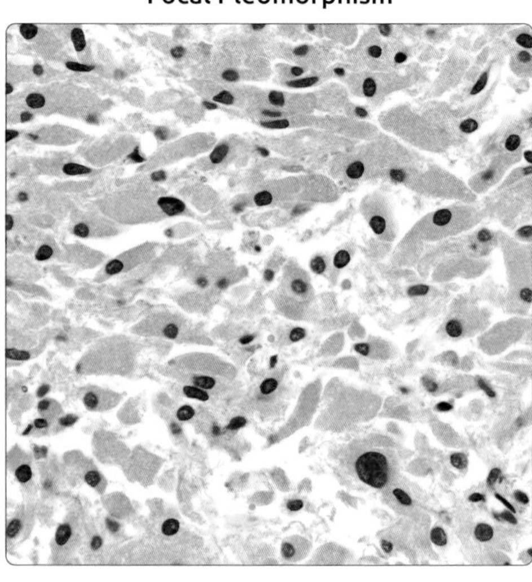

Smear, PAS(+), Diastase Resistant

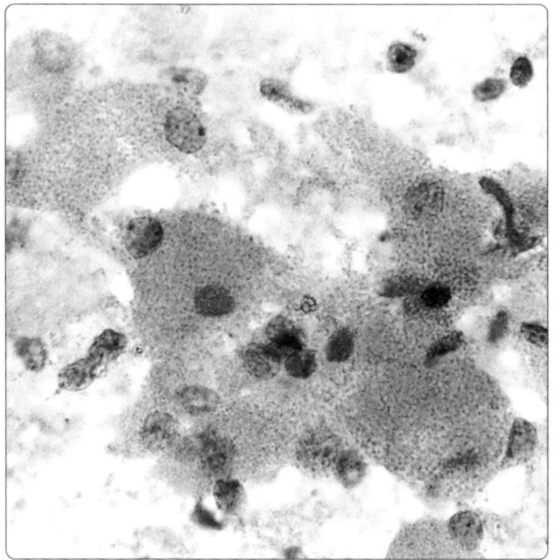

PAS(+) Due to Lysosomal-Rich Cytoplasm

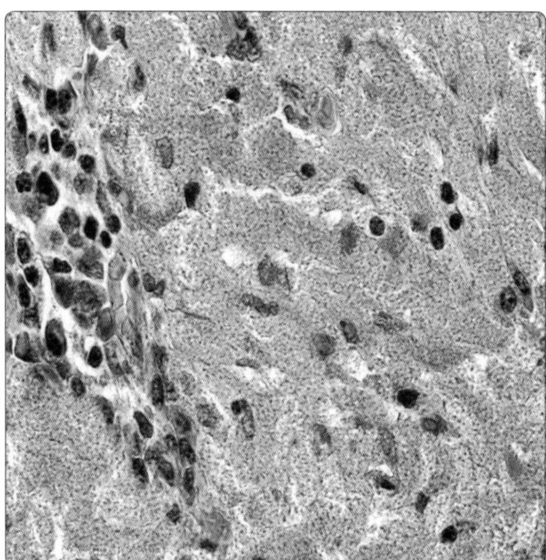

(Left) *As seen in this smear, PAS staining is resistant to diastase treatment. The sharply defined cells with bland nuclei are typical. The cytoplasm of macrophages would be more finely granular or foamy.* **(Right)** *Strong PAS positivity in the granular cell cytoplasm is due to lysosome accumulation.*

α-1-antitrypsin (+) Granular Cell Tumor

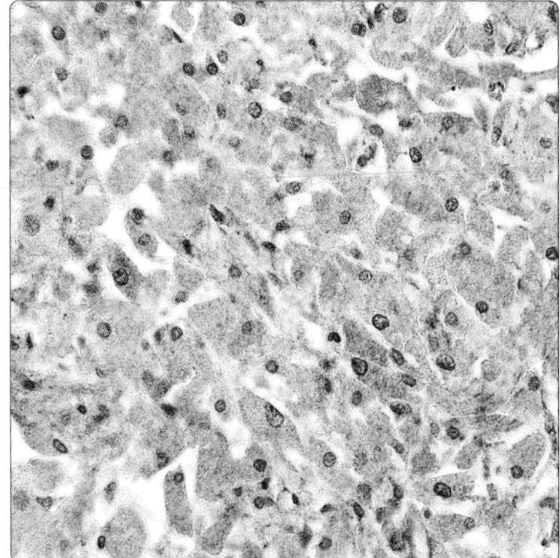

S100(+) Granular Cell Tumor

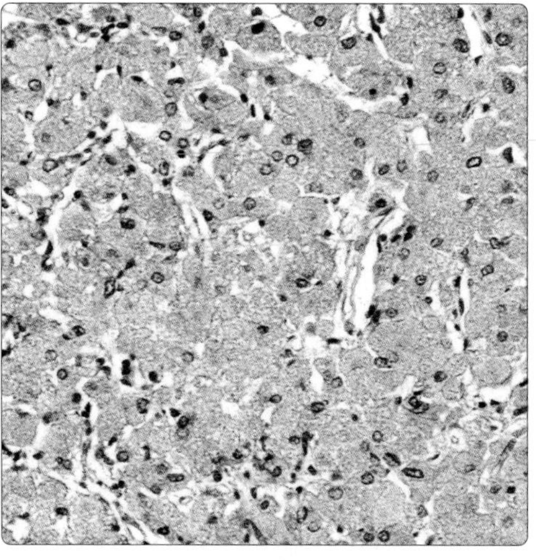

(Left) *Granular cell tumors are diffusely immunopositive for the histiocyte marker α-1-antitrypsin.* **(Right)** *Tumoral cells are immunoreactive for S100 protein, which is also the case for multiple other sellar region tumors, except for pituitary adenomas.*

Lysosomal-Rich Cytoplasm

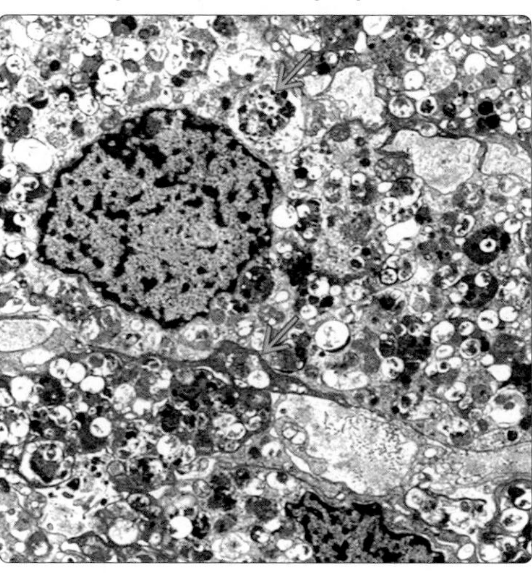

Large Lysosomes Correlate With Granularity

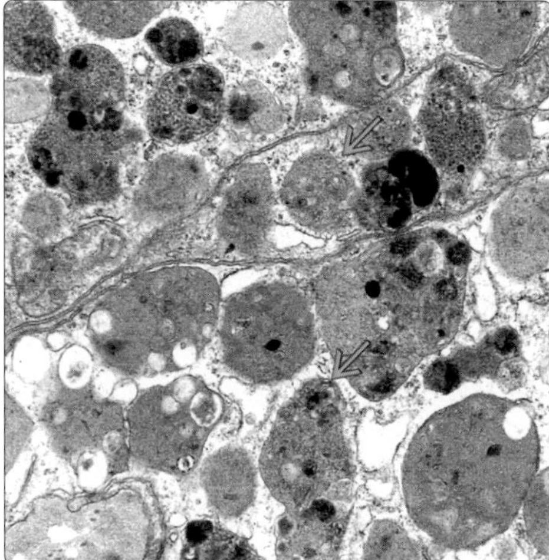

(Left) *Ultrastructurally, heterolysosomes ⇒ fill the cytoplasm of granular cell tumors.* **(Right)** *Accumulation of large lysosomes ⇒, the correlate of granular cytoplasm, is apparent in this electron micrograph at high magnification.*

Pituicytoma

KEY FACTS

TERMINOLOGY

- Rare WHO grade I, posterior pituitary &/or stalk tumor of pituicytes (modified glial cells)
- Spindle cell oncocytomas and granular cell tumors of pituitary are now considered variants of pituicytoma, based on shared nuclear TTF-1(+)

CLINICAL ISSUES

- Gross total removal curative

IMAGING

- Demarcated; solid; rarely cystic component
- Homogeneously enhancing

MICROSCOPIC

- No capsule; direct contact with surrounding structures
- Compact fascicles or storiform arrangements of bipolar, short to elongated, plump to angulated spindle cells
- Oval to elongated nuclei with little or no atypia
- Rare or no mitoses

ANCILLARY TESTS

- Vimentin, S100 protein, and TTF-1(+)
- GFAP variably (+)
- Galectin-3 variably (+)
- Ki-67 labeling: 1-2%

TOP DIFFERENTIAL DIAGNOSES

- Spindle cell oncocytoma, granular cell tumor of infundibulum [both TTF-1(+)]
  - Mitochondrial-rich (spindle cell oncocytoma) or lysosome-rich (granular cell tumor)
- Fibrous meningioma [TTF-1(-)]
- Schwannoma [TTF-1(-)]
- Pituitary adenoma [synaptophysin (+), TTF-1(-)]
  - Neurosecretory granules on electron microscopy
- Pilocytic astrocytoma [TTF-1(-)]
  - Biphasic, compact, &/or microcystic architecture, Rosenthal fibers, eosinophilic granular bodies; extensively GFAP(+)

Pituicytoma, Simulating Adenoma

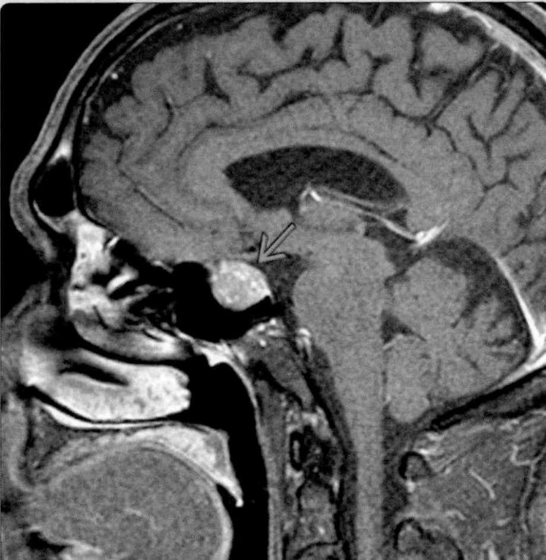

Spindled Cells, Nongranular Cytoplasm

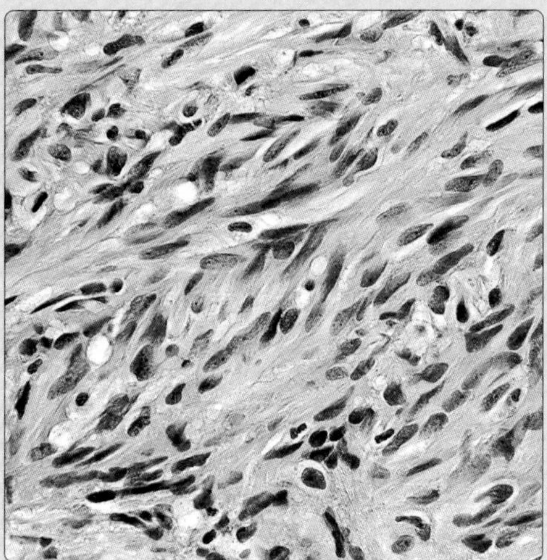

(Left) *Pituicytomas are solid, homogeneously enhancing ➡ masses that, as in this case, may occasionally be more intra- than suprasellar. Pituicytomas simulate nonfunctioning pituitary adenomas.* **(Right)** *Pituicytomas are composed of monomorphic, bipolar, spindled cells with homogeneous, nongranular, pink cytoplasm.*

S100(+) Pituicytoma

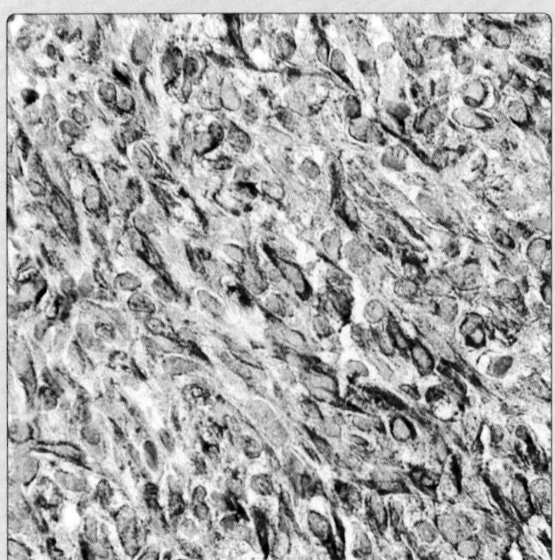

TTF-1(+) Pituicytoma

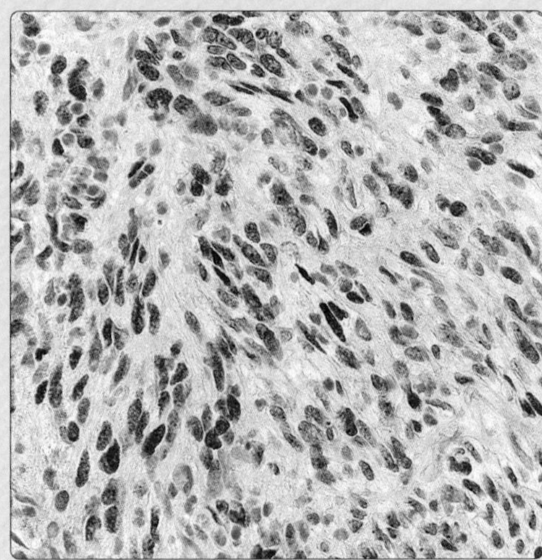

(Left) *S100 protein is often diffusely and strongly positive. This is, however, not diagnostic of pituicytoma. Fibrous meningioma, for example, an important differential for pituicytoma, may also be positive.* **(Right)** *TTF-1 immunoreactivity, which is strongly expressed in normal pituicytes, is also present in pituicytomas. Spindle cell oncocytomas and granular cell tumors are also positive and these 2 tumors are thus thought to have a shared origin with pituicytomas.*

TERMINOLOGY

Synonyms

- Infundibuloma, posterior pituitary astrocytoma

Definitions

- Rare WHO grade I, posterior pituitary &/or stalk tumor of pituicytes (modified glia)
- Spindle cell oncocytomas and granular cell tumors of pituitary are now considered variants of pituicytoma

CLINICAL ISSUES

Epidemiology

- Incidence
  - Rare
- Age
  - Adults; male predominance (M:F = 1.5:1)

Site

- Posterior lobe and pituitary stalk

Presentation

- Mimics nonfunctioning pituitary macroadenoma
  - Visual field defect (chiasmal compression), hypopituitarism, headache
- Hyperprolactinemia (pituitary stalk effect), rare presentation with hemorrhage
- Rare association with endocrine neoplasms (parathyroid adenoma, follicular thyroid carcinoma)
- Rare incidental autopsy finding

Treatment

- Resection; role of radiation unclear

Prognosis

- Subtotal removal associated with slow recurrence over years
- Gross total removal curative
- No anaplastic transformation or metastasis

IMAGING

MR and CT Findings

- Demarcated; solid; rarely cystic component, homogeneously enhancing

MACROSCOPIC

General Features

- Solid, circumscribed, rubbery mass
  - 1 to several centimeters in diameter, occasional cystic element
  - Variable adherence to adjacent suprasellar structures

MICROSCOPIC

Histologic Features

- No capsule; direct contact with surrounding structures
- Compact fascicles or storiform arrangements of bipolar, short to elongated, plump to angulated spindle cells
  - Oval to elongated nuclei with little or no atypia, rare or no mitoses
  - Herring bodies and axons at periphery represent normal surrounding posterior pituitary and stalk

ANCILLARY TESTS

Histochemistry

- PAS (Herring bodies) and Bodian or Bielschowsky (axons) limited to surrounding normal posterior pituitary gland and stalk

Immunohistochemistry

- Vimentin, S100 protein, and TTF-1(+)
- GFAP variably (+), galectin-3 variably (+)
- EMA, annexin-A1(-)
- Neurofilament protein and vasopressin positivity limited to normal axons and Herring bodies in posterior pituitary gland at periphery
- Synaptophysin and pituitary hormones (-)
- Ki-67 labeling 1-2%

DIFFERENTIAL DIAGNOSIS

Spindle Cell Oncocytoma

- Epithelioid and spindle cells; occasional multinucleated giant cells
- Frequent, patchy chronic inflammation
- Granular cytoplasm, PAS(-) and PTAH(+)
- EMA, antimitochondrial antibody, annexin-A1, and TTF-1 all (+), GFAP(-)
- Ultrastructure: Mitochondrion-rich, no neurosecretory granules (unlike pituitary adenoma), occasional desmosomes or primitive junctions

Granular Cell Tumor of Infundibulum

- PAS(+) and CD68(+) granular cytoplasm
- α-1-antitrypsin, α-1-antichymotrypsin, cathepsin-B (+), TTF-1(+)
- Rare, variable staining for galectin-3, GFAP
- Ultrastructure: Phagolysosome-rich cytoplasm, no neurosecretory granules (unlike pituitary adenoma)

Fibrous Meningioma

- Variable whorls, psammoma bodies, but may be rare or absent in fibrous subtype
- Nuclear cytoplasmic pseudoinclusions, but may be rare or absent in fibrous subtype
- Thick vessels and stromal calcifications
- EMA(+) but may be weak; progesterone receptors usually, but not always (+); SSTR2A(+), GFAP(-), TTF-1(-)

Schwannoma

- Antoni A and B patterns, intercellular reticulin and pericellular collagen IV(+); caution: Occasionally GFAP(+)

Pituitary Adenoma

- More epithelial cytology, infrequently spindle celled
- Synaptophysin IHC(+) in 100%; variably IHC(+) for pituitary hormones, chromogranin; low molecular weight keratin
  - TTF-1, S100 protein, GFAP all (-)

SELECTED REFERENCES

1. Kleinschmidt-DeMasters BK et al: Update on hypophysitis and TTF-1 expressing sellar region masses. Brain Pathol. 23(5):495-514, 2013

(Left) *While pituicytomas are unencapsulated, they are also noninvasive. There is, thus, a discrete border* → *with adjacent tissue.* **(Right)** *Pituicytomas are composed of interlacing fascicles of elongated, eosinophilic spindle cells.*

Pituicytoma Noninvasive

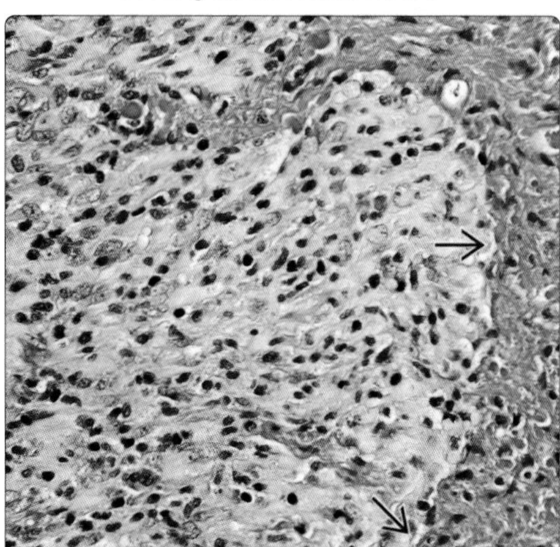

Interlacing Fascicles

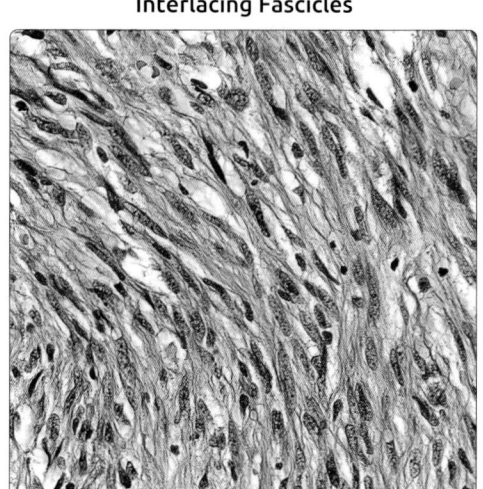

(Left) *Nuclei are oval to elongated and have slightly irregular borders. Vasculature* → *is delicate, without the hyalinization of fibrous meningiomas. The illustrated tissue is too cellular to be normal infundibulum or neurohypophysis.* **(Right)** *Elongated, bipolar spindle cells may form only crude fascicles. A degree of nuclear pleomorphism* → *&/or mitoses are occasionally present, but the lesions are histologically low grade.*

Vasculature Nonhyalinized

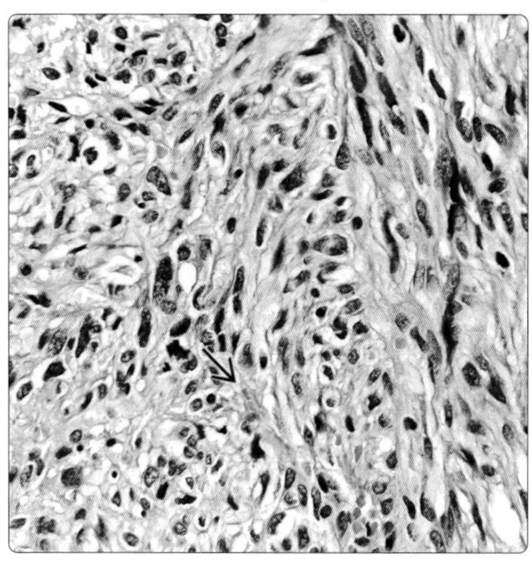

Nuclear Pleomorphism

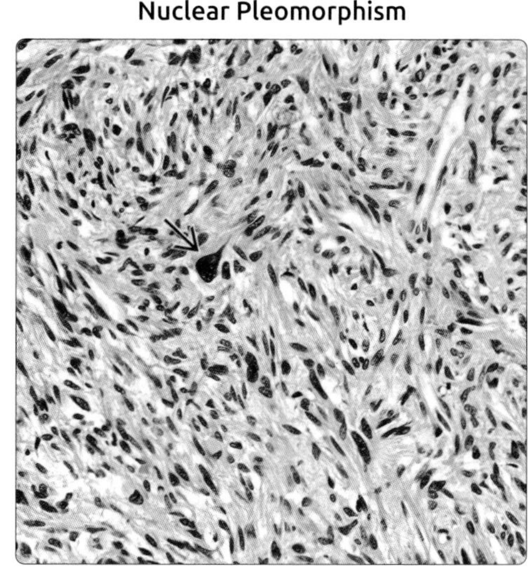

(Left) *S100 is often diffusely and strongly positive.* **(Right)** *GFAP staining varies from moderate and diffuse to focal and weak. It is strong in this area of this case.*

S100 Diffuse, Positive

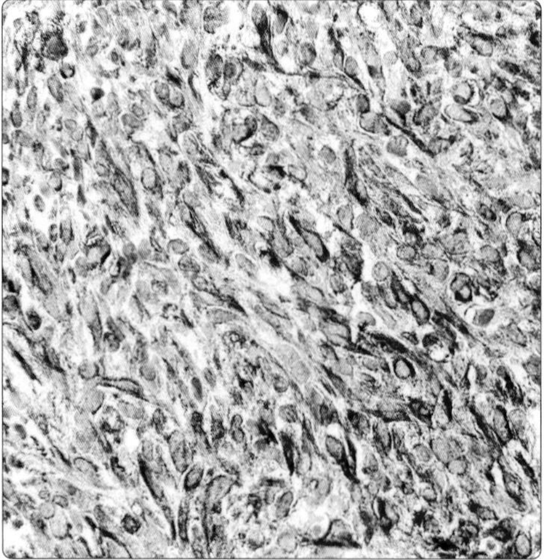

Pituicytoma GFAP(+), Strong

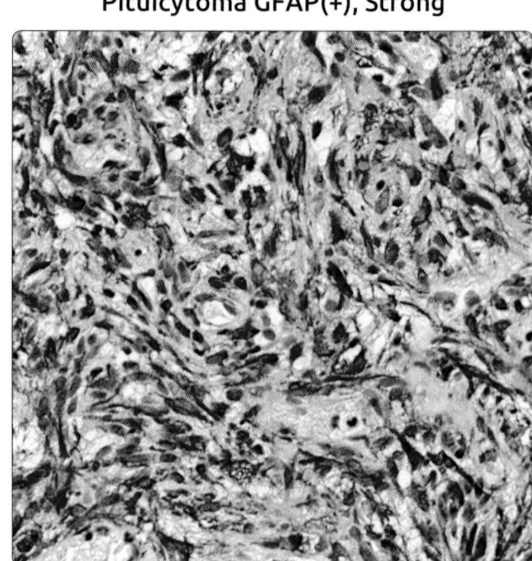

Secretory Granules

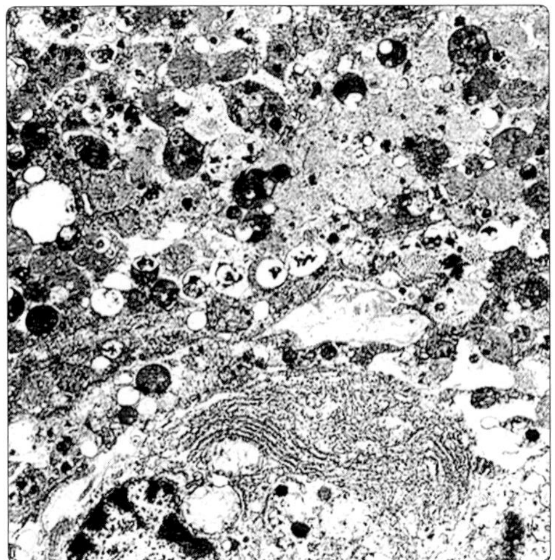

Smear, Pituicytoma Spindle Cells

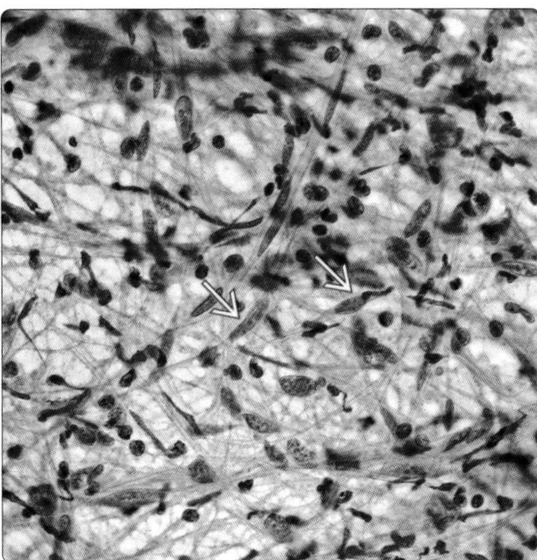

(Left) *Ultrastructurally, pituicytoma cells have no secretory granules, as would be expected in pituitary adenoma. Instead, there are varying numbers of intermediate (glial) filaments and abundant lysosomes.* **(Right)** *Tumor spindle cells ➔ are most apparent in smear preparations.*

Smear, Bipolar Spindle Cells

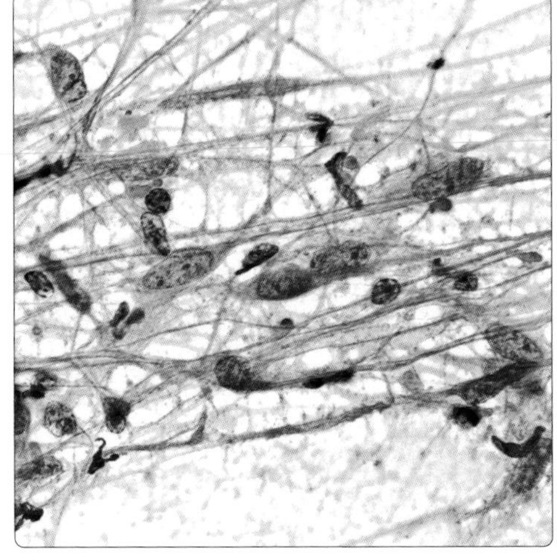

Normal Neurohypophysis

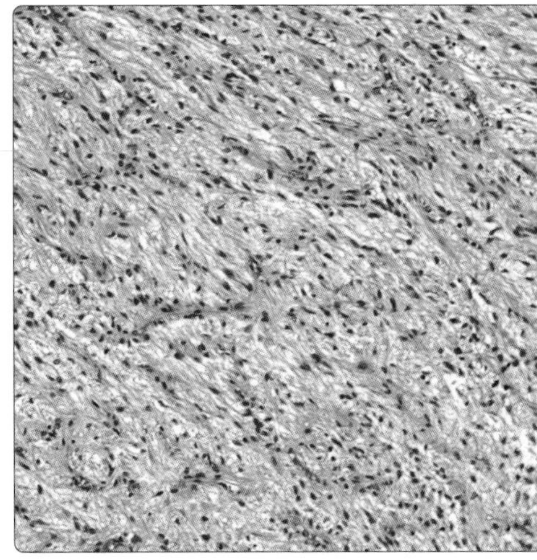

(Left) *Tumoral cells have oval to elongated nuclei with small nucleoli and long bipolar processes.* **(Right)** *Normal neurohypophysis can simulate a pituicytoma due to its fibrillary features. Normal neurohypophysis is also TTF-1(+), but, unlike pituicytoma, it contains axons.*

Normal Posterior Lobe

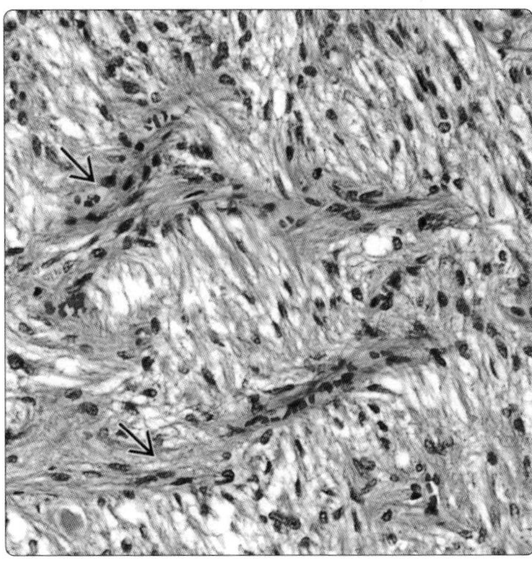

GFAP, Normal Posterior Lobe

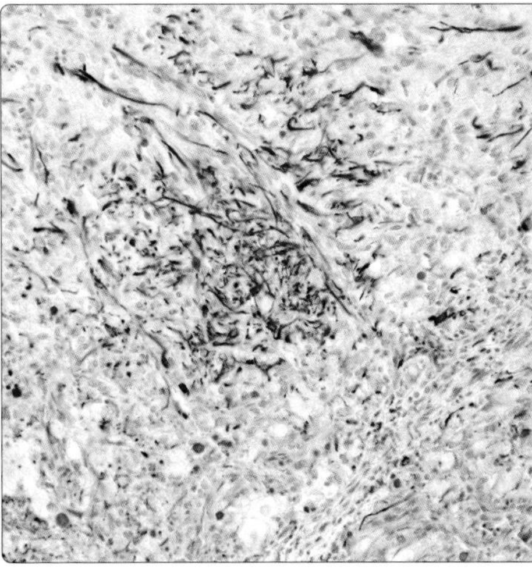

(Left) *Normal neurohypophysis consists of axons and pituicytes, the latter ➔ mainly concentrating around vessels.* **(Right)** *The pituicyte is a specialized glial cell of the stalk and posterior lobe of the pituitary gland. The glial feature is demonstrated by GFAP stain in this normal postlobe section.*

KEY FACTS

TERMINOLOGY

- (Supra)sellar epithelial neoplasm resembling ameloblastoma or keratinizing and calcifying odontogenic cyst

CLINICAL ISSUES

- Bimodal with peaks at 5-10 years and 50-60 years
- More common, even in adults, than papillary craniopharyngioma
- Recur after incomplete excision

IMAGING

- CT: Partially Ca++, partially cystic and solid, cystic suprasellar mass

MICROSCOPIC

- Distinctive palisading epithelium, loose stellate reticulum and "wet" keratin in most cases
- Peritumoral piloid gliosis, Rosenthal fibers common
- "Wet" keratin diagnostic even in absence of viable epithelium
- Xanthomatous cells only suggest diagnosis

ANCILLARY TESTS

- Immunopositive for β-catenin but IHC+ focal and maximal in whorls; β-catenin intranuclear (nuclear translocation) and cytoplasmic
- Immunonegative for mutant BRAF (BRAF V600E)

DIAGNOSTIC CHECKLIST

- Adamantinomatous or papillary type?
    - Nuclear palisades and "wet" keratin favor adamantinomatous
    - β-catenin nuclear immunoreactivity in adamantinomatous
    - Papillary type lacks xanthogranulomatous reaction

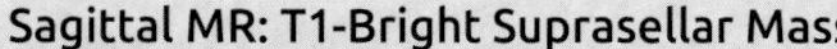

Sagittal MR: T1-Bright Suprasellar Mass

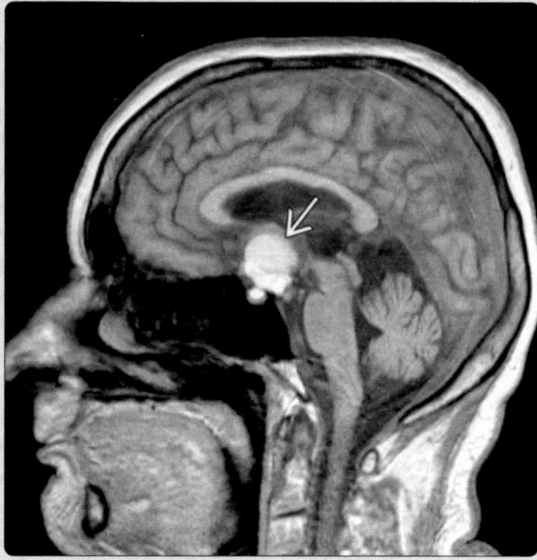

Peripheral Palisading of Epithelium

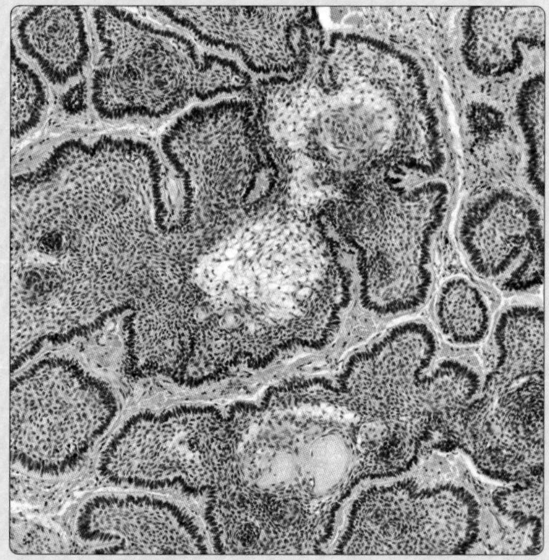

(Left) *The high protein content of encysted fluid makes many adamantinomatous craniopharyngiomas bright → on precontrast T1-weighted MR images.* **(Right)** *Lobular architecture, peripheral palisading, loose stellate reticulum, and nodules of "wet" keratin characterize this instantly recognizable lesion.*

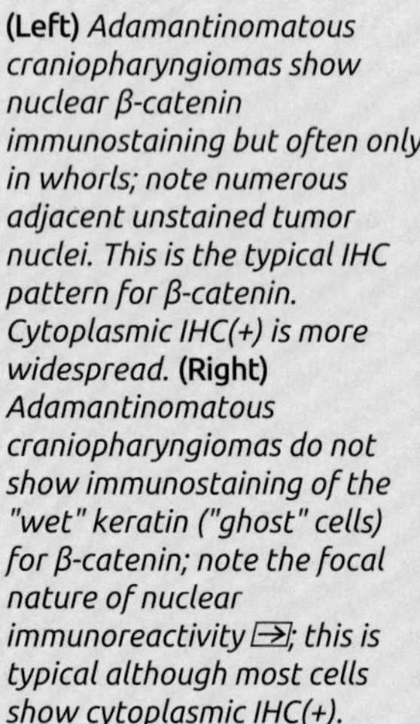

Nuclear β-Catenin

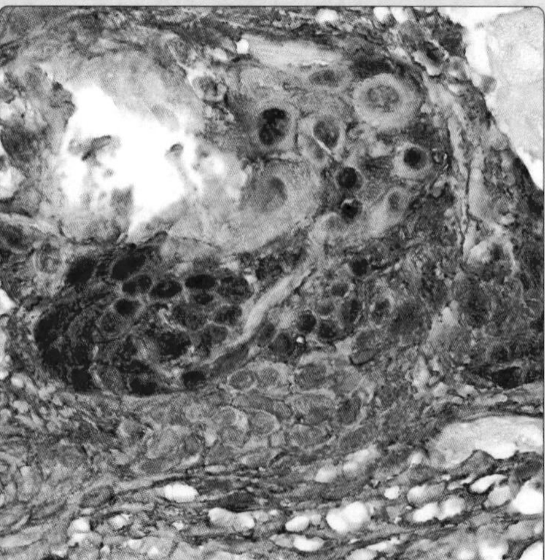

"Wet" Keratin Negative for β-Catenin

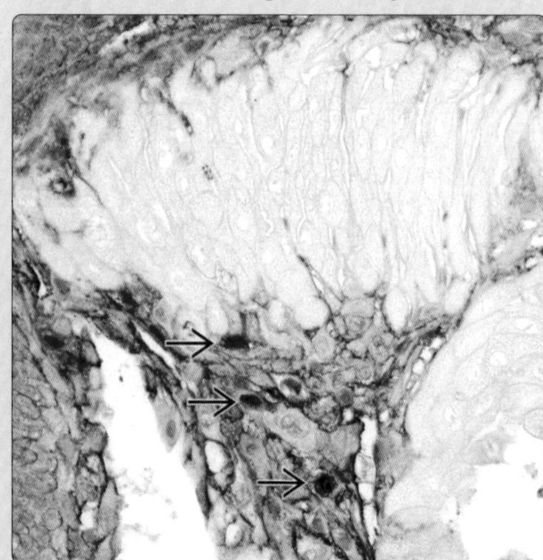

(Left) *Adamantinomatous craniopharyngiomas show nuclear β-catenin immunostaining but often only in whorls; note numerous adjacent unstained tumor nuclei. This is the typical IHC pattern for β-catenin. Cytoplasmic IHC(+) is more widespread.* **(Right)** *Adamantinomatous craniopharyngiomas do not show immunostaining of the "wet" keratin ("ghost" cells) for β-catenin; note the focal nature of nuclear immunoreactivity →; this is typical although most cells show cytoplasmic IHC(+).*

TERMINOLOGY

Definitions

- (Supra)sellar epithelial neoplasm resembling ameloblastoma as well as keratinizing and calcifying odontogenic cyst
- WHO grade I

ETIOLOGY/PATHOGENESIS

Developmental Anomaly

- Possible origin in remnants of Rathke pouch epithelium or misplaced odontogenic rests along pituitary stalk

CLINICAL ISSUES

Epidemiology

- Incidence
  - Low
- Age
  - Bimodal with peaks at 5-10 years and 50-60 years
  - Rarely, congenital or in senescence
  - More common, even in adults, than papillary craniopharyngioma
- Ethnicity
  - Higher frequency in Africa and Far East

Site

- Suprasellar
  - Infrequent intrasellar component
  - Extension into neighboring structures
  - Posterior extension to prepontine and interpeduncular cisterns, cerebellopontine angle, even foramen magnum
- Intranasal, sphenoid sinus, cerebellopontine angle, and pineal region are rare primary sites

Presentation

- Visual disturbances
- Endocrine deficiencies
  - Growth failure and delayed puberty in children
  - Deficiencies of GH > LH/FSH > ACTH > TSH
  - Diabetes insipidus (adults > children)
- Headache
- Cognitive impairment and personality changes
- Rare chemical meningitis with cyst spillage

Treatment

- Options, risks, complications
  - Treatment controversial
- Surgical approaches
  - Complete resection, but technically challenging, and with risk of operative damage to hypothalamus and neighboring structures with need for lifelong pituitary hormone replacement
  - Subtotal resection with observation
  - Cyst aspiration, repeated, for recurrent lesions
- Adjuvant therapy
  - Intracystic bleomycin to control recurrence
- Radiation
  - Radiation (conventional or stereotactic) for subtotally resected tumors
  - Intralesional, to control cysts in some cases

Prognosis

- Cystic recurrences common after incomplete excision
  - Debatable relationship between Ki-67 index and likelihood of recurrence
- 5-year survival excellent
  - Variable incidence of endocrinologic deficiencies
- Rarely undergo malignant transformation
  - Multiple recurrences and radiation increase risk
    - Prior radiotherapy in almost all cases

IMAGING

General Features

- Best diagnostic clue
  - CT: Partially calcified, cystic/solid, suprasellar mass
  - MR: High signal intensity on pre-T1
- Location
  - Extraaxial, suprasellar at interface with pituitary stalk and pituitary gland
    - Supra- and infra-, rarely intrasellar
- Size
  - Variable, often > 5 cm
  - May be massive in recurrence
- Morphology
  - Multilobulated and multicystic

MR Findings

- T1-weighted images: Hyperintense with fluid levels consistent with cystic nature
  - Heterogeneous with 3 components: Large hyperintense cyst superiorly, isointense sold mass inferiorly, and calcified nodule with solid area
  - Occasionally, hypointense
- Most hyperintense on T2W imaging
- Heterogeneous enhancement

CT Findings

- Mixed low-density and isointense signals
  - Solid portion enhances or forms peripheral ring enhancement surrounding cyst
- CT superior to MR for detection of calcification

MACROSCOPIC

General Features

- Irregular interface with surrounding brain
  - Densely adherent to adjacent structures
- Lobular, partly cystic, often calcified
  - Cysts with dark "motor oil" fluid, rich in glistening cholesterol crystals
    - Potential for chemical meningitis with spillage

MICROSCOPIC

Histologic Features

- Borders
  - Generally circumscribed but often microscopic brain invasion
    - Small tongues of tissue extend into hypothalamic parenchyma
- Patterns of spread
  - Usually expansion and local infiltration

  - Dissemination in CSF or surgical tract, rare
- Compact sheets, nodules, anastomosing trabeculae, and "clover leafs" of squamous epithelium
- Peripheral layer of palisaded epithelium surrounds loose stellate reticulum
- Nodules of plump anucleate squames "ghost" cells, "wet" keratin
- Intralobular whorl-like formations
- Degenerative changes, often in recurrences
  - Cysts with flat epithelium, squamous debris
  - Fibrosis, chronic inflammation, cholesterol clefts
  - Extensive calcification, or rarely, ossification
  - Often scant epithelium postirradiation
- Piloid gliosis in surrounding brain
- Rarely, melanin pigment
- Rarely, collision tumor with pituitary adenoma
- Malignant features transformation
  - Postirradiation > spontaneous

ANCILLARY TESTS

Cytology

- Cohesive clumps or sheets of epithelium
- Nodules of "wet" keratin
- Macrophages, amorphous debris, calcifications, reactive pilocytes

Immunohistochemistry

- CK7, CK8, CK14 (+)
- β-catenin (+) in whorls; intranuclear (nuclear translocation) and cytoplasmic
- Ki-67 low
- Rarely immunopositive for mutant BRAF (BRAF V600E)

Genetic Testing

- β-catenin mutations
- Rarely mutated for BRAF V600E

DIFFERENTIAL DIAGNOSIS

Papillary Craniopharyngioma

- Lacks prominent palisading, "wet" keratin, stellate reticulum, calcifications, fibrosis
- No "machinery oil"-like fluid
  - No cholesterol in cyst fluid
- No xanthogranulomatous reaction
- Nuclear β-catenin (-), CK8(-) and CK20(-)
- Immunopositive for cytoplasmic mutant BRAF (BRAF V600E)

Rathke Cleft Cyst With Squamous Metaplasia

- More intra- than suprasellar
- Squamous tissue often focally overlain by ciliated &/or mucus-containing cells
- No "wet" keratin or calcification
- β-catenin (-) nuclei
- CK8(+) and CK20(+)

Epidermoid Cyst

- Uniloculate, thin layer of keratinizing squamous epithelium
- Flaky or "dry" keratin principal component
- Keratohyaline granules
- No nuclear palisades
- No "wet" keratin
- Almost no fibrous tissue

Pilocytic Astrocytoma

- Greater cellularity than piloid gliosis
- Often biphasic or with loose, spongy, microcystic tissue
- Eosinophilic granular bodies in some cases

Xanthogranuloma of Sellar Region

- Cholesterol clefts, macrophages, giant cells, inflammation, hemosiderin, necrosis, and cysts
- No epithelium
- Reactive process; not an entity

DIAGNOSTIC CHECKLIST

Clinically Relevant Pathologic Features

- Adherence to local structures minimizes chance of total excision without postoperative neurological/neuroendocrine deficits

Pathologic Interpretation Pearls

- Complex epithelial tumor with ribbons of palisaded cells, calcification
- "Wet" keratin alone diagnostic
- Piloid gliosis with Rosenthal fibers may surround craniopharyngioma and mimic glioma

SELECTED REFERENCES

1. Brastianos PK et al: Exome sequencing identifies BRAF mutations in papillary craniopharyngiomas. Nat Genet. 46(2):161-5, 2014
2. Larkin SJ et al: BRAF V600E mutations are characteristic for papillary craniopharyngioma and may coexist with CTNNB1-mutated adamantinomatous craniopharyngioma. Acta Neuropathol. 127(6):927-9, 2014
3. Ishida M et al: Malignant transformation in craniopharyngioma after radiation therapy: a case report and review of the literature. Clin Neuropathol. 29(1):2-8, 2010
4. Rodriguez FJ et al: The spectrum of malignancy in craniopharyngioma. Am J Surg Pathol. 31(7):1020-8, 2007
5. Haupt R et al: Epidemiological aspects of craniopharyngioma. J Pediatr Endocrinol Metab. 19 Suppl 1:289-93, 2006
6. Hofmann BM et al: Nuclear beta-catenin accumulation as reliable marker for the differentiation between cystic craniopharyngiomas and rathke cleft cysts: a clinico-pathologic approach. Am J Surg Pathol. 30(12):1595-603, 2006
7. Kato K et al: Possible linkage between specific histological structures and aberrant reactivation of the Wnt pathway in adamantinomatous craniopharyngioma. J Pathol. 203(3):814-21, 2004
8. Losa M et al: Correlation between clinical characteristics and proliferative activity in patients with craniopharyngioma. J Neurol Neurosurg Psychiatry. 75(6):889-92, 2004
9. Sekine S et al: Craniopharyngiomas of adamantinomatous type harbor beta-catenin gene mutations. Am J Pathol. 161(6):1997-2001, 2002
10. Xin W et al: Differential expression of cytokeratins 8 and 20 distinguishes craniopharyngioma from rathke cleft cyst. Arch Pathol Lab Med. 126(10):1174-8, 2002
11. Kurosaki M et al: Immunohistochemical localisation of cytokeratins in craniopharyngioma. Acta Neurochir (Wien). 143(2):147-51, 2001
12. Tateyama H et al: Different keratin profiles in craniopharyngioma subtypes and ameloblastomas. Pathol Res Pract. 197(11):735-42, 2001
13. Paulus W et al: Odontogenic classification of craniopharyngiomas: a clinicopathological study of 54 cases. Histopathology. 30(2):172-6, 1997

Axial CT: Calcification

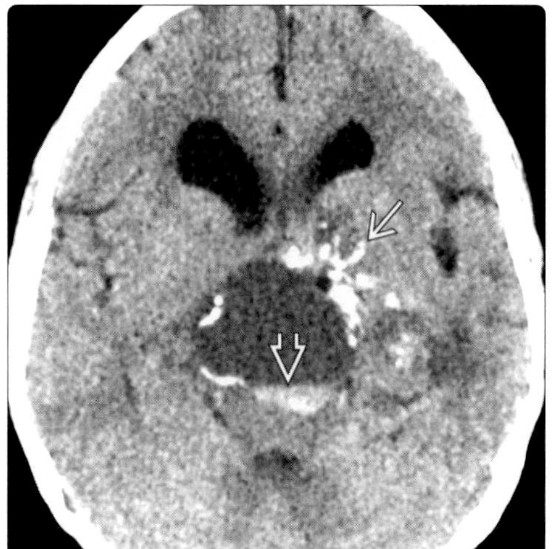

Prominent Calcification

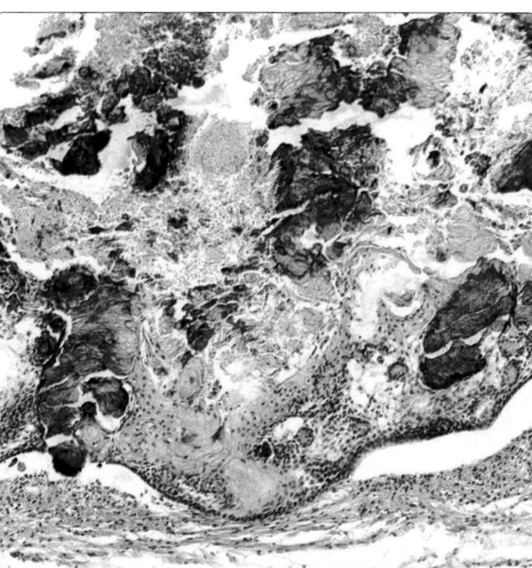

(Left) *The preoperative diagnosis is made on the basis of a cystic sellar region lesion with peripheral calcifications ➡ and a fluid-fluid ➡ level.* **(Right)** *Calcification is present in almost all examples and is often deposited on "wet" keratin.*

Multicystic

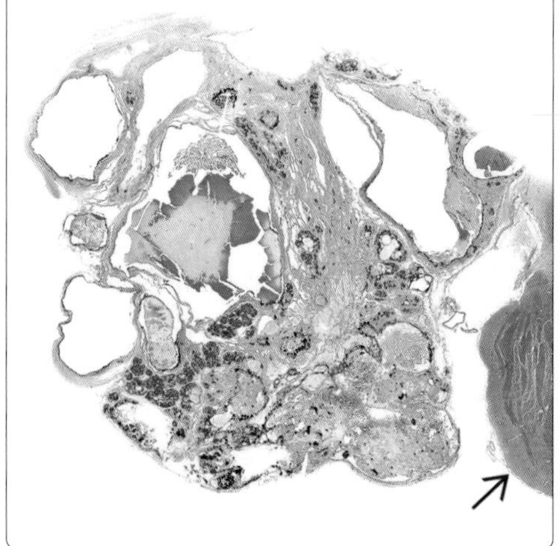

Focal "Wet" Keratin

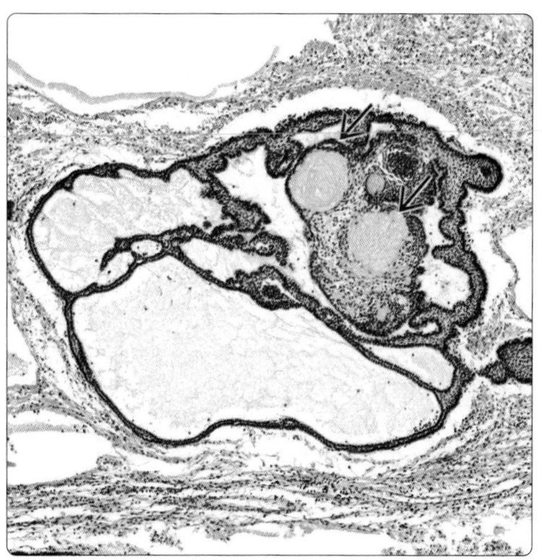

(Left) *A complex, multicystic suprasellar mass with cellular nodules may be a craniopharyngioma or a teratoma. Generally circumscribed, the lesion adheres to the brain, so total excision without hypothalamic damage is often difficult. The pons is on the right ➡.* **(Right)** *Instantly recognizable is a cystic craniopharyngioma with palisading epithelium and "wet" keratin ➡.*

Stellate Reticulum

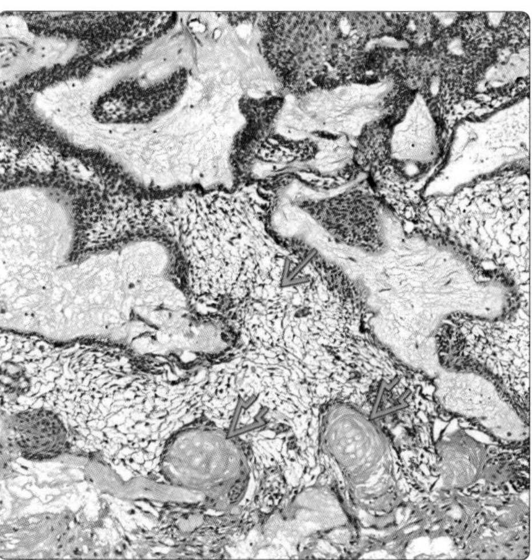

Subtle Pseudopalisading

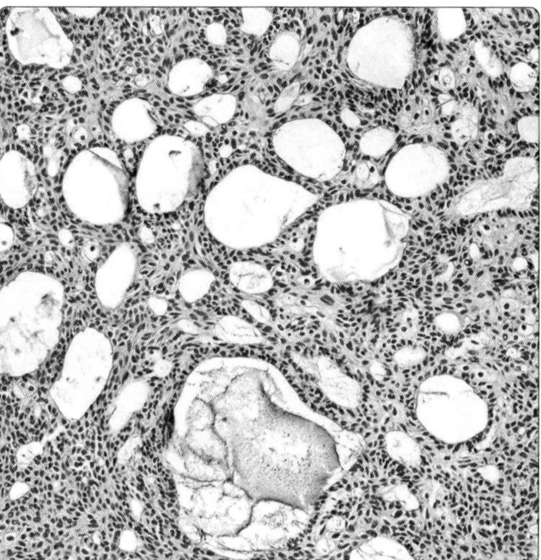

(Left) *Stellate reticulum ➡ is present in tumor lobules. Diagnostic acellular nodules of "wet" keratin ➡ are also present. Palisading cells at the tumor-stroma interface may be inconspicuous.* **(Right)** *Multicystic architecture and a hint of palisading, but no "wet" keratin or stellate reticulum, create a less diagnostic picture of adamantinomatous craniopharyngioma.*

(Left) *Palisading ⇨, "wet" keratin ⇨, and stellate reticulum ➡ are key features of adamantinomatous craniopharyngioma. Palisading is present in papillary craniopharyngioma, but is not as developed as in the adamantinomatous lesion.* **(Right)** *A nodule of anuclear "ghost" cells termed "wet" keratin ⇨ lies in the stellate reticulum. The combination is diagnostic. Note the reactive astrocytosis and Rosenthal fibers in adjacent brain tissue at right.*

Prominent Pseudopalisading

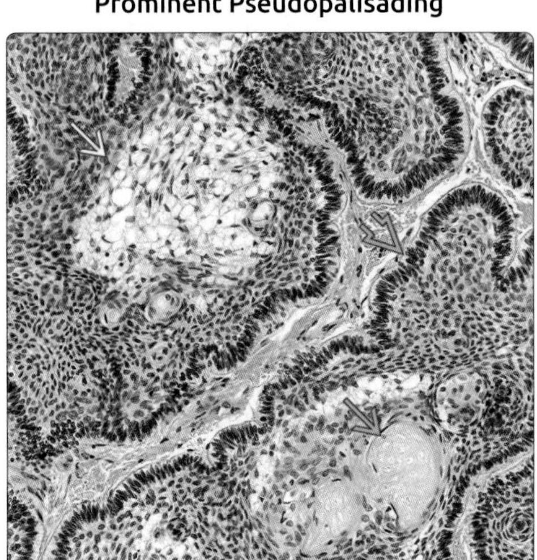

"Ghost" Cells

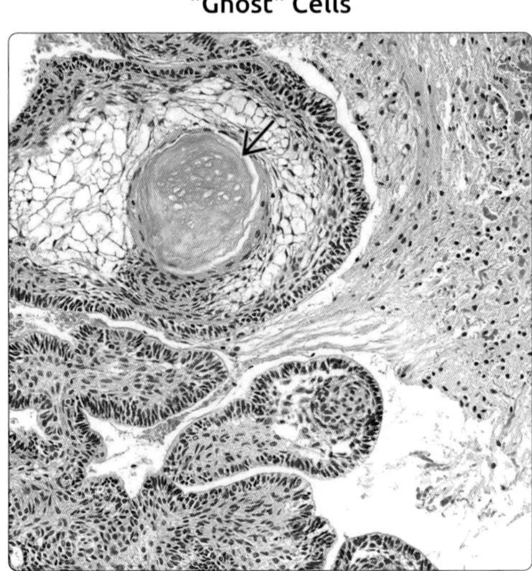

(Left) *Complex epithelial ribbons surround the interstitial basophilic myxoid matrix.* **(Right)** *Convoluted ribbons of cells with peripheral palisading are one of many tissue patterns of adamantinomatous craniopharyngioma.*

Interstitial Myxoid Matrix

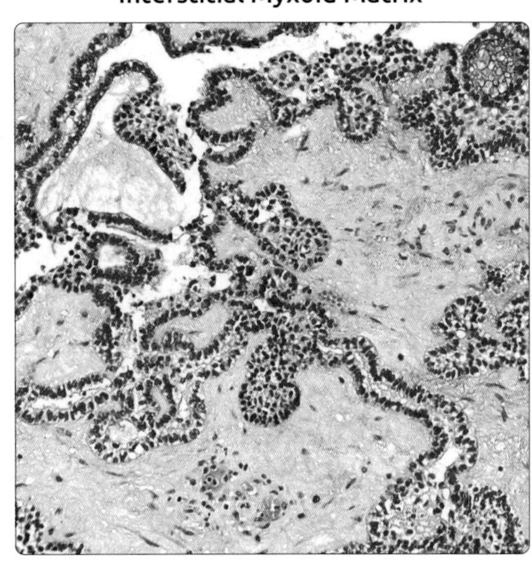

Ribbons of Tumor Cells

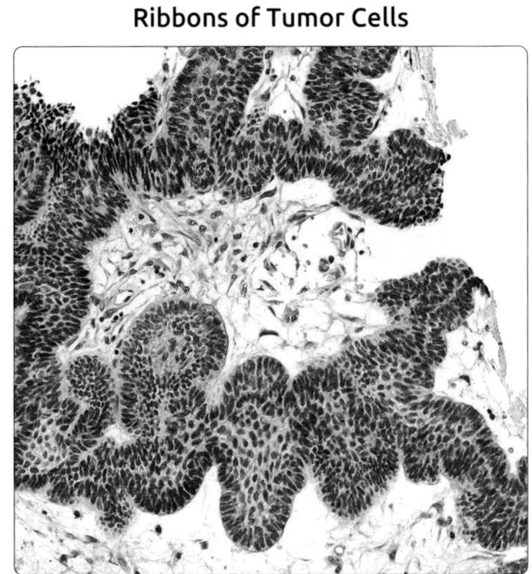

(Left) *Peripheral palisading ⇨ gives the lesion its distinctive adamantinomatous quality. A centrally placed epithelial whorl is also present ⇨.* **(Right)** *Loose stellate reticulum and palisading are 2 features excluding papillary craniopharyngioma and a Rathke cleft cyst with squamous metaplasia.*

Epithelial Whorl

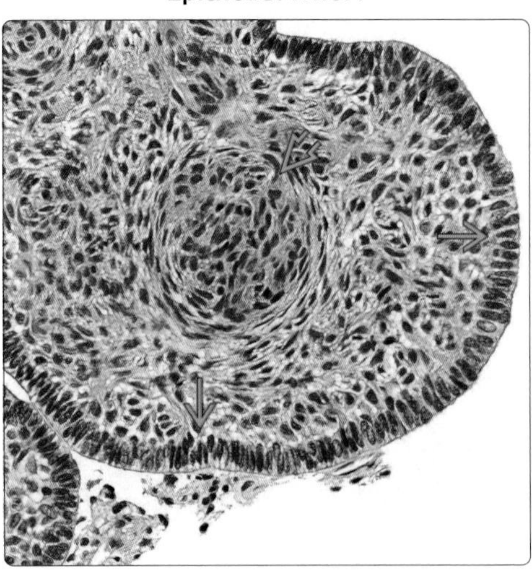

Loose Stellate Reticulum

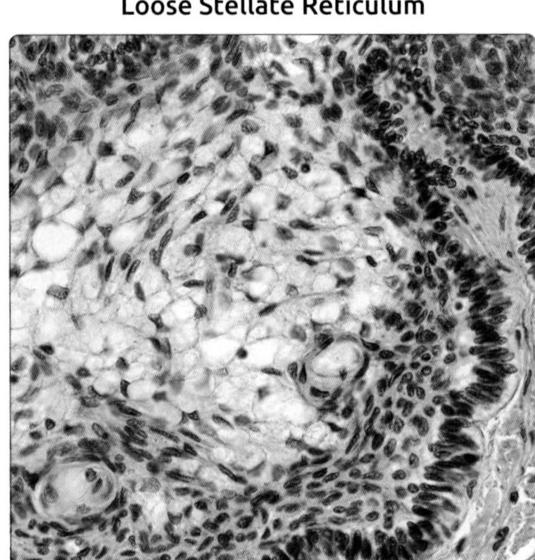

"Ghost" Cells

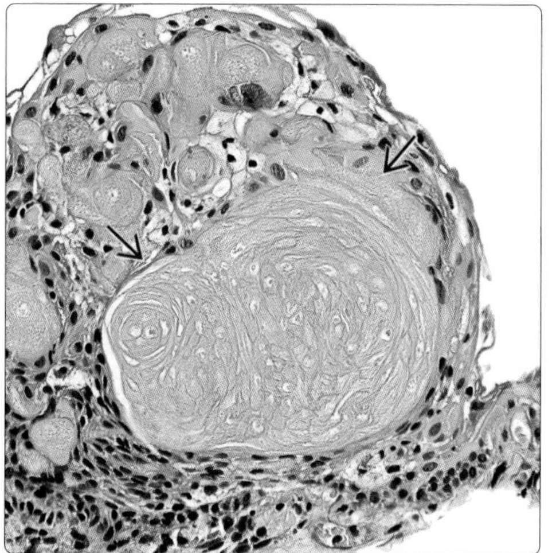

Calcifying "Wet" Keratin

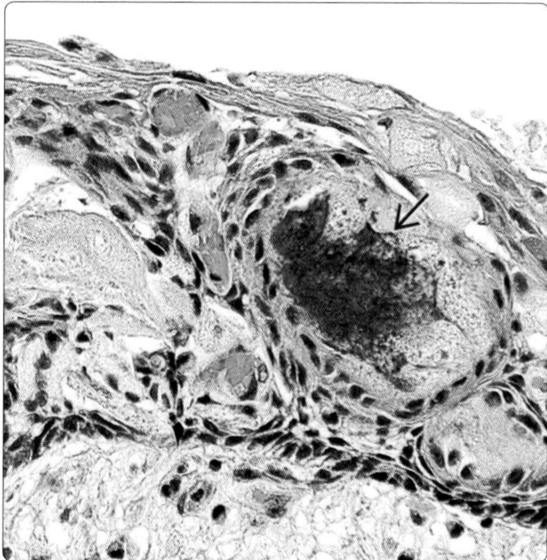

(Left) *Excrescences in the cyst wall may be formed largely of anuclear "ghost" cells ("wet" keratin) ⇨. The latter is distinct from the "dry," flaky keratin composed of flat squames in epidermoid cysts. "Wet" keratin is absent also in papillary craniopharyngiomas.* **(Right)** *Calcium ⇨ is usually deposited on keratin nodules.*

Attenuated Epithelium

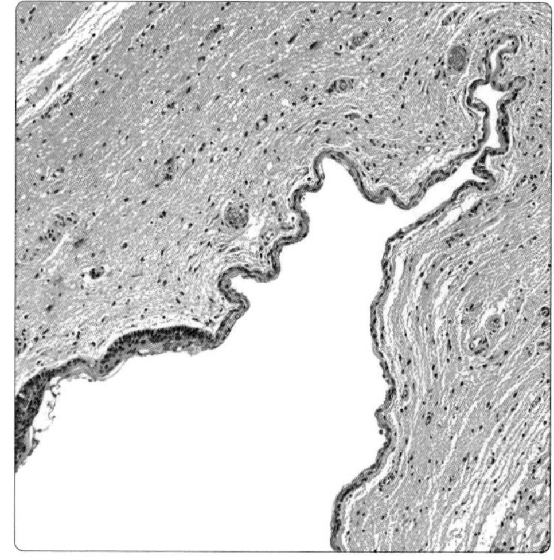

Flattened Single-Layer Epithelium

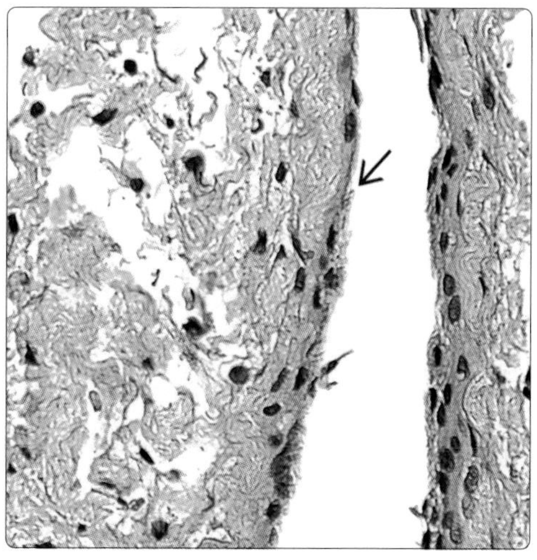

(Left) *Particularly in the chronic, recurrent lesions, epithelium is intimately related to surrounding brain without a surgically exploitable cleavage plane. Note the thinning of the epithelium.* **(Right)** *Only a single-cell layered epithelium ⇨ may persist in the wall of large cystic craniopharyngiomas. The diagnosis of an adamantinomatous craniopharyngioma depends on the presence of classic epithelial patterns elsewhere or of "wet" keratin.*

Piloid Gliosis

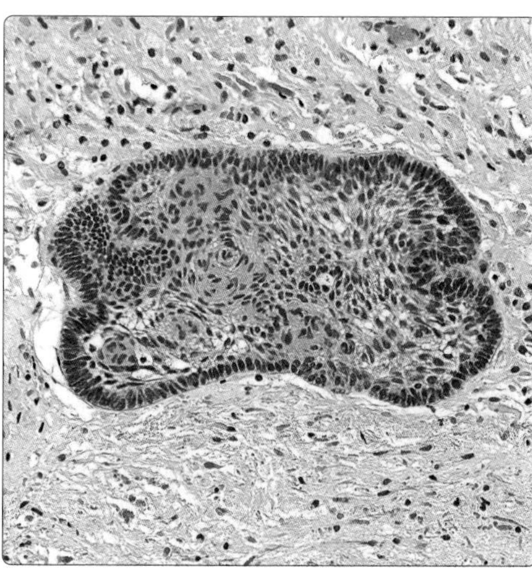

"Wet" Keratin Devoid of Surrounding Inflammation

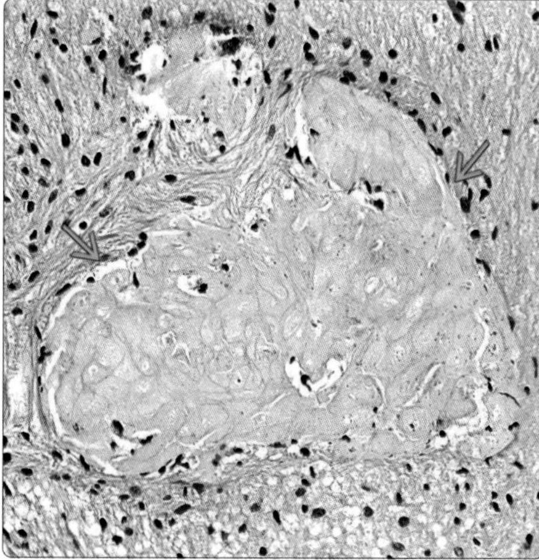

(Left) *Nodules of adamantinomatous epithelium with peripheral palisading often extend into adjacent brain. Piloid gliosis typically surrounds these nests.* **(Right)** *Nodules of anuclear squames ⇨ may excite little inflammatory reaction (as in this case), or produce a granulomatous response.*

(Left) *Multiple nodules of "wet" keratin may be compacted into solid, faintly calcified sheets of anuclear squames.* **(Right)** *Dead, anuclear "ghost" cells are diagnostic of adamantinomatous craniopharyngioma. Squames occurring in epidermoid cysts are much thinner.*

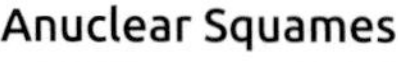

Anuclear Squames

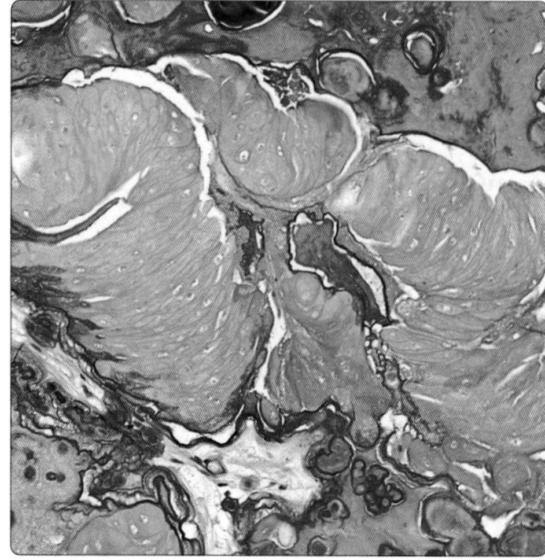

Dead "Ghost" Cells

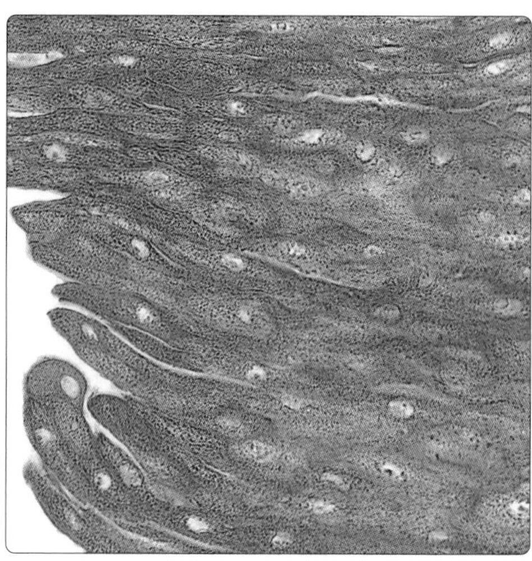

(Left) *Only attenuated epithelium → may be present in surgical specimens of chronic lesions. A lymphocytic and granulomatous reaction with multinucleated foreign body-type giant cells → to cyst contents is common. Cysts in recurrent craniopharyngiomas may be massive and multiloculate.* **(Right)** *A lymphoplasmacytic infiltrate may partially obscure the attenuated epithelium, which in longstanding tumors has lost its diagnostic features.*

Multinucleated Foreign Body Giant Cells

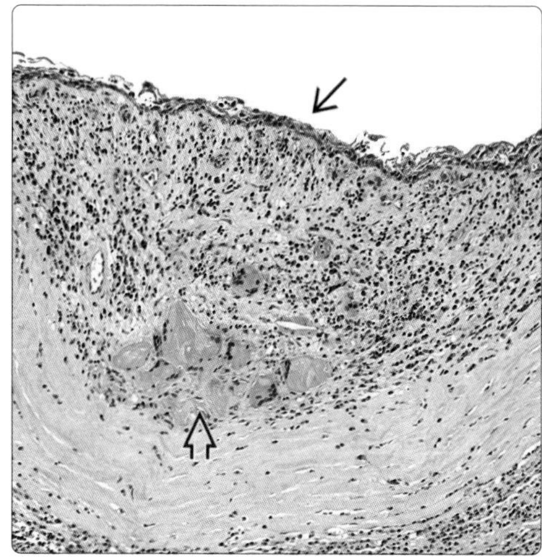

Lymphoplasmacytic Reaction

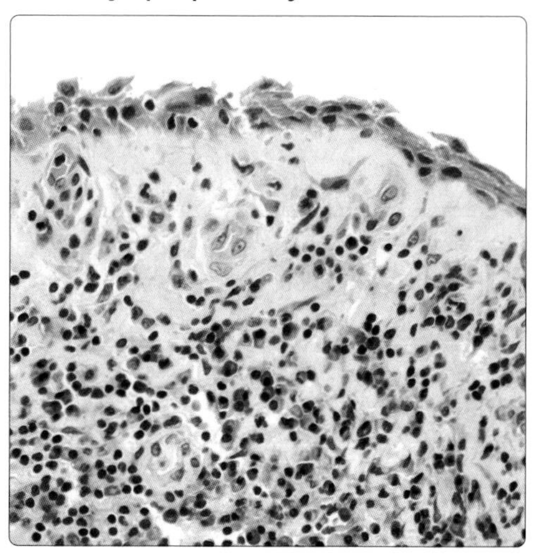

(Left) *A xanthogranulomatous reaction to ruptured cyst contents, with cholesterol clefts → and multinucleated giant cells, is not uncommon and also occurs in other sella-region lesions such as Rathke cleft cyst.* **(Right)** *Dense piloid gliosis with Rosenthal fibers → adjacent to a craniopharyngioma may simulate pilocytic astrocytoma. The absence of loose, microcystic tissue common in astrocytoma helps distinguish the two.*

Xanthogranulomatous Reaction

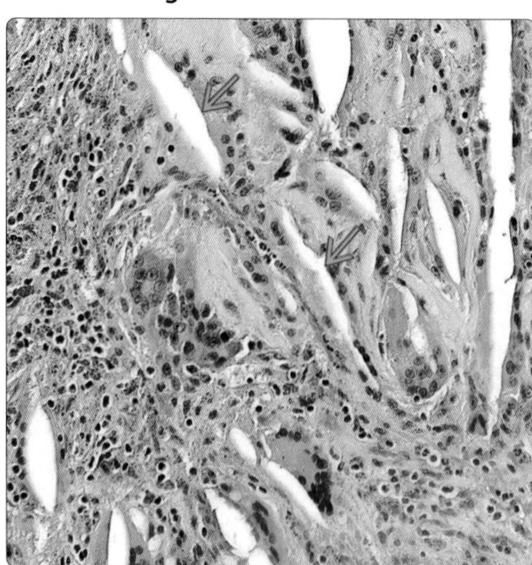

Rosenthal Fibers

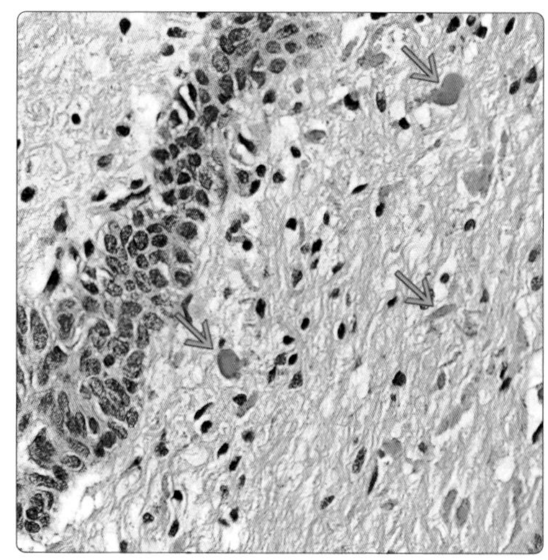

Clumps of Cells on Smear Preparation

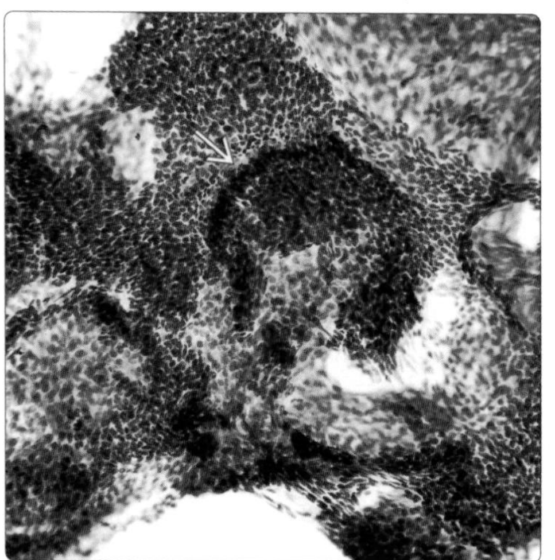

"Wet" Keratin on Smear Preparation

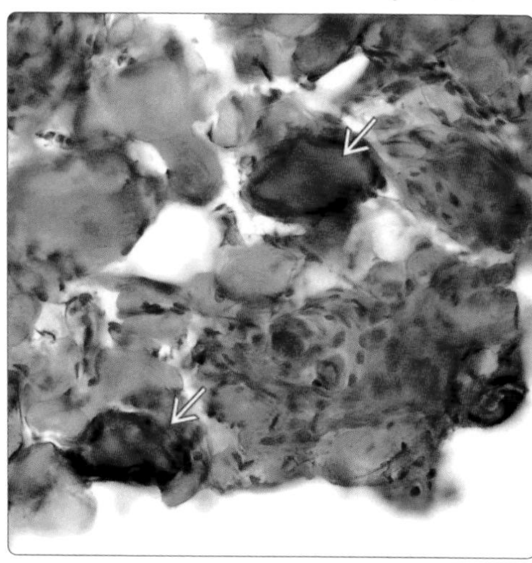

(Left) *Craniopharyngiomas smear out reluctantly, remaining in cohesive clumps of uniform epithelial cells with peripheral palisading* ➡*.* **(Right)** *In smear preparations from lesions in the sellar region, clumps of anucleate squames, "wet" keratin* ➡*, alone are diagnostic of craniopharyngioma of the adamantinomatous type. They are absent in papillary craniopharyngiomas.*

Cholesterol Flakes, Intraoperative View

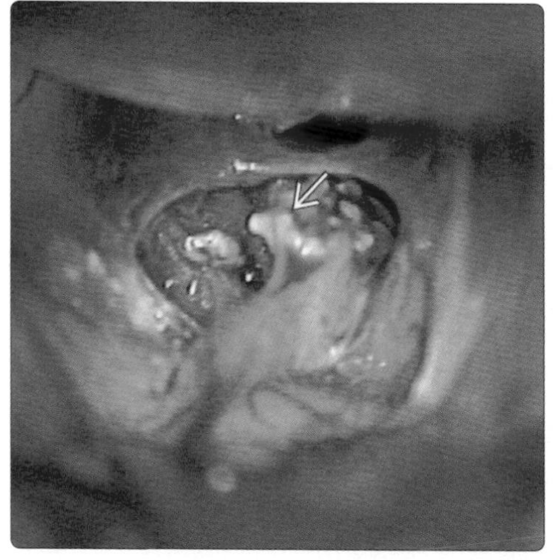

Cholesterol Crystals, Polarized Light

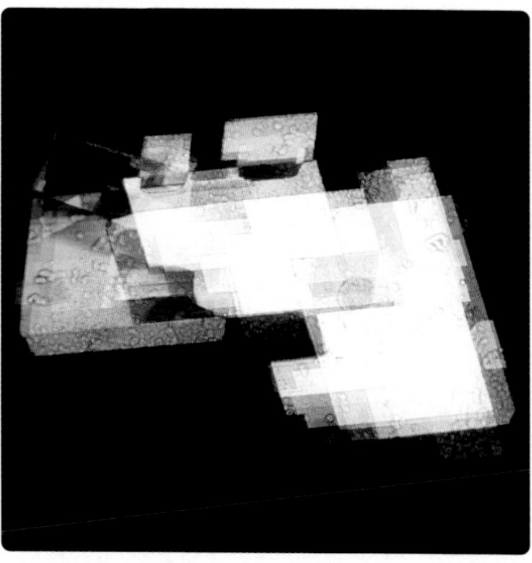

(Left) *Yellow cholesterol flakes* ➡ *are typical intraoperative findings in craniopharyngiomas of the adamantinomatous (but not papillary) type. (Courtesy G. Jallo, MD.)* **(Right)** *As visualized with polarized light, cholesterol crystals from the "motor oil" fluid have a distinctive gray, multilaminar structure and notched, "state of Utah" configuration.*

CAM5.2-Positive Whorls

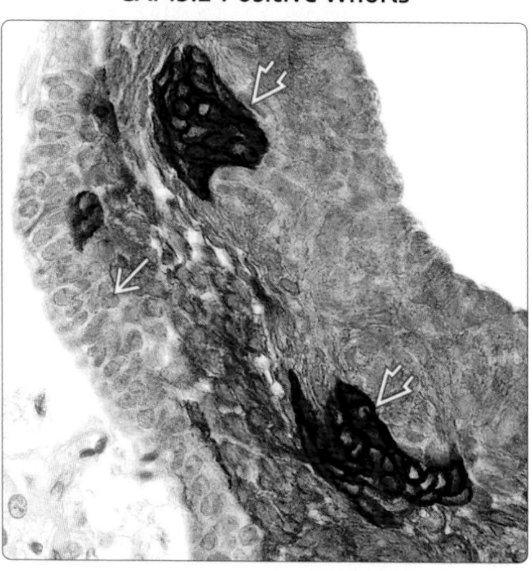

β-Catenin-Positive Whorls

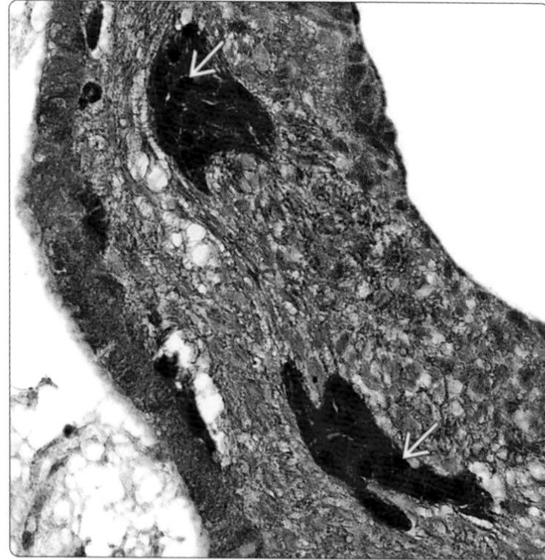

(Left) *Whorl-like islands of epithelial cells are immunoreactive for CK8/18 (CAM5.2)* ➡*, but the palisading epithelium* ➡ *is not.* **(Right)** *Presumed to reflect mutations in the β-catenin gene in adamantinomatous craniopharyngiomas, nuclei* ➡*, not just cytoplasm, are immunoreactive for β-catenin. Positivity is especially prominent in whorl-like structures. Rathke cleft cysts and papillary craniopharyngiomas are negative.*

Papillary Craniopharyngioma

KEY FACTS

ETIOLOGY/PATHOGENESIS

- 10% of craniopharyngiomas
- Now known to have *BRAF* V600E mutation in almost all cases, distinguishing it from *CTNNB1*-mutated adamantinomatous craniopharyngioma

CLINICAL ISSUES

- Affects adults
- Frequent suprasellar/3rd ventricular involvement
- Prognosis may be more favorable than that of adamantinomatous variant

IMAGING

- Contrast-enhancing solid or cystic mass
- No calcification (unlike adamantinomatous variant)

MACROSCOPIC

- Encapsulated
- Lack adhesions with brain

MICROSCOPIC

- Well-differentiated nonkeratinizing squamous epithelium
- Papillary fibrovascular stroma

ANCILLARY TESTS

- BRAF VE1: Cytoplasm (+)
- β-catenin: Membranous (+), nuclei (-) [unlike adamantinomatous craniopharyngioma where focal nuclear IHC(+) found]

TOP DIFFERENTIAL DIAGNOSES

- Rathke cleft cyst with squamous metaplasia

DIAGNOSTIC CHECKLIST

- Well-circumscribed, mostly solid lesion, supratentorial or intraventricular
- Do not misinterpret collagenous whorls as keratin whorls
- Beware of possible scant goblet cells, unlike extensive mucin-producing epithelium in Rathke cleft cyst

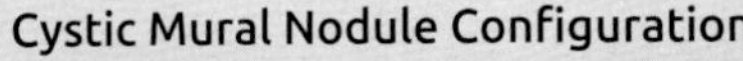

Cystic Mural Nodule Configuration

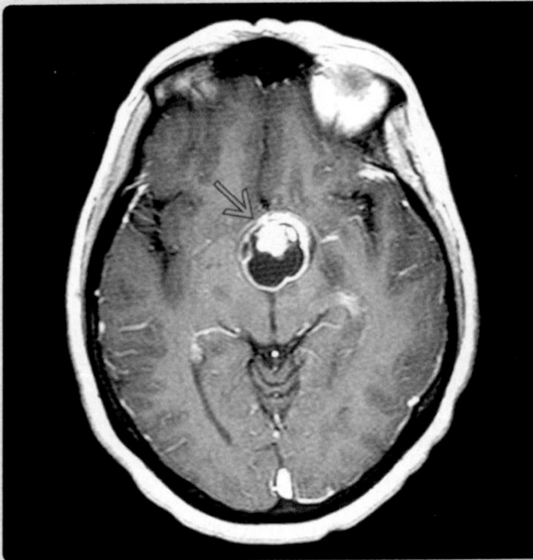

Nodules in Cyst Wall

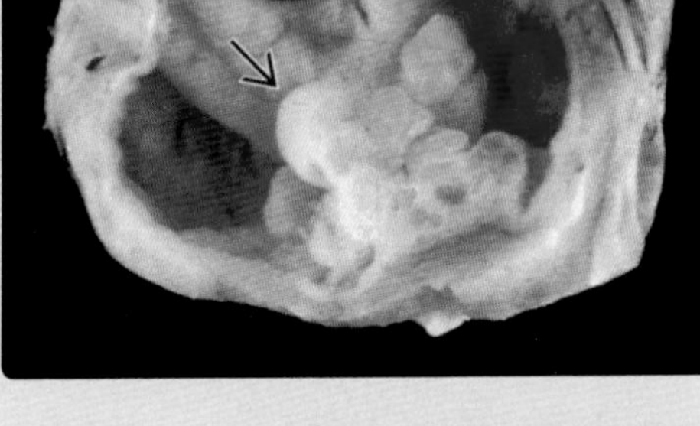

(Left) *Papillary craniopharyngiomas are enhancing, usually cystic suprasellar masses, sometimes with a mural nodule →.* **(Right)** *Grossly, this example nicely shows the cystic nature of the lesion and intrusive epithelial nodules → in the cyst wall.*

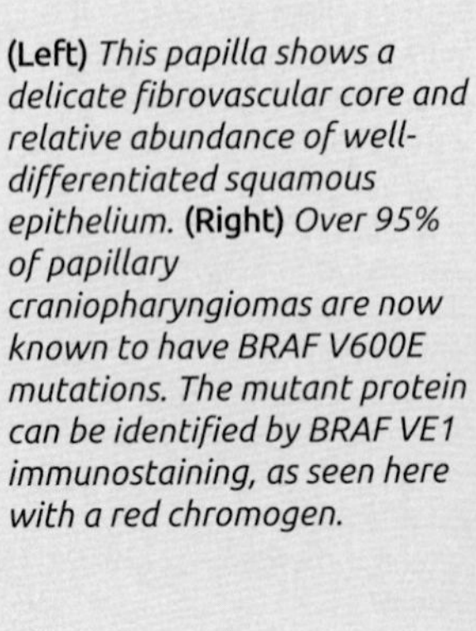

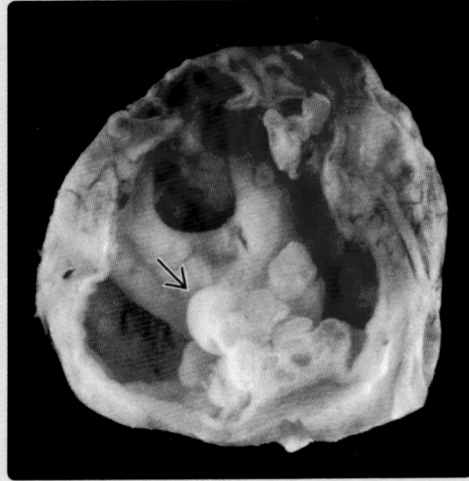

Well-Differentiated Squamous Epithelium

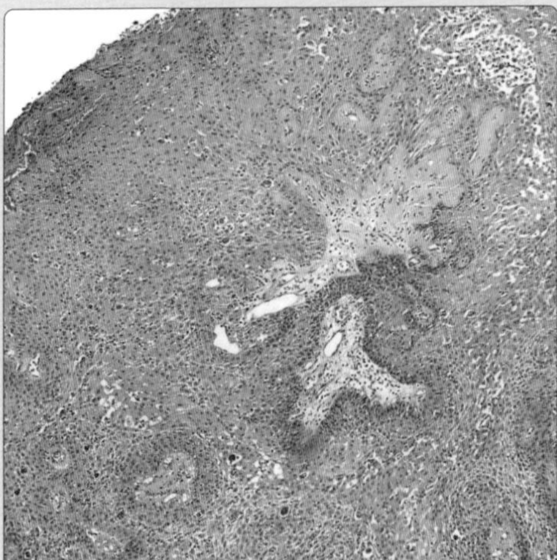

Papillary Craniopharyngioma: BRAF VE1 IHC(+)

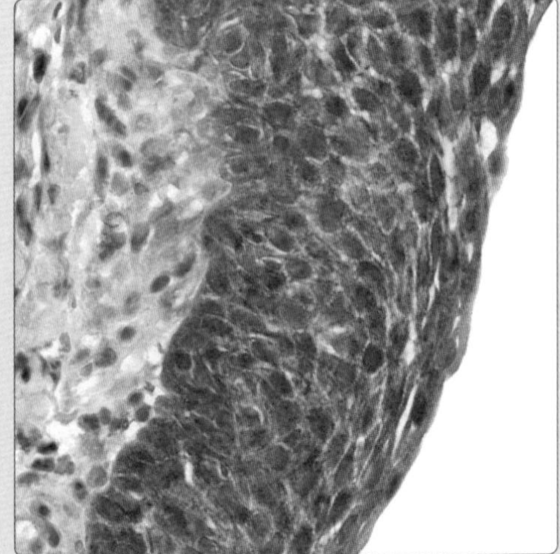

(Left) *This papilla shows a delicate fibrovascular core and relative abundance of well-differentiated squamous epithelium.* **(Right)** *Over 95% of papillary craniopharyngiomas are now known to have BRAF V600E mutations. The mutant protein can be identified by BRAF VE1 immunostaining, as seen here with a red chromogen.*

TERMINOLOGY

Synonyms

- Suprasellar papillary squamous epithelioma
- Ciliated craniopharyngioma
- Ciliated and goblet cell craniopharyngioma

Definitions

- Well-differentiated, pseudopapillary, squamous epithelial tumor of sella &/or suprasellar region
- WHO grade I

ETIOLOGY/PATHOGENESIS

Pathogenesis

- Possible transition from Rathke cleft cyst
- *BRAF V600E* mutation
  - Distinguishes papillary craniopharyngioma origin from that of *CTNNB1*-mutated adamantinomatous craniopharyngioma

CLINICAL ISSUES

Epidemiology

- Incidence
  - 10% of all craniopharyngiomas
- Age
  - Almost always in adults
- Sex
  - No predilection

Site

- Suprasellar or intraventricular (3rd ventricle)

Presentation

- Visual disturbance
- Obstructive hydrocephalus
- Mental/personality changes
- Hyperprolactinemia
  - Pituitary stalk effect
- Diencephalic syndrome, uncommon

Treatment

- Options, risks, complications
  - Optimal therapy
    - Gross total resection
      - Facilitated by smooth surface
  - May respond to targeted therapies due to *BRAF V600E* mutation (vemurafenib)

Prognosis

- Gross total resection often safely achieved
  - Decreases complications and recurrence rate
- Somewhat better than for adamantinomatous variant
- Meningeal seeding along prior resection tract or to remote leptomeningeal site (exceptional)
- Increased Ki-67 labeling indices associated with greater likelihood of recurrence

IMAGING

Radiographic Findings

- More often supra- than intrasellar
- Infrequently entirely within 3rd ventricle
- Lesions variably solid
  - When cystic, may have mural nodule
- More often circumscribed and solid
- No calcification (unlike adamantinomatous variant)

MR Findings

- Contrast-enhancing solid or cystic mass

CT Findings

- Contrast enhancing
- No calcification

MACROSCOPIC

General Features

- Discrete, encapsulated, often solid
- Not densely adherent to brain-like adamantinomatous variant
- No cholesterol-rich, machinery oil-like content
- Clear fluid contents when cystic

MICROSCOPIC

Histologic Features

- Solid sheets of well-differentiated epithelium
- Crude papillae result from dehiscence of epithelium around fibrovascular stromal cores
- Scant goblet/ciliated cells in cyst lining, in some cases
- Small whorls, in some cases

ANCILLARY TESTS

Cytology

- Sheets of epithelial cells
- Individual nucleated squames
- Whorls, focal

Histochemistry

- PAS(+) goblet cells, focal, in some cases

Immunohistochemistry

- Cytokeratins and epithelial membrane antigen (+)
- CK7(+) in all but basal layer
  - Unlike Rathke cleft cysts, CK8(-), and CK20(-)
- Ki-67 labeling indices low, with rare exception
- BRAF VE1
  - Cytoplasm (+)
    - Parallels presence of *BRAF V600E* mutation in 95% of cases
- β-catenin
  - Membranous (+), nuclei (-)
    - Differs from adamantinomatous craniopharyngioma where nuclei focally (+)

DIFFERENTIAL DIAGNOSIS

Rathke Cleft Cyst With Squamous Metaplasia

- Cystic
  - No solid component
- Ciliated or mucin-producing epithelium usually extensive but may be focal

Adamantinomatous Craniopharyngioma

- Irregular, infiltrative interface
- Complex architecture
- Wet keratin
- Calcification
- Conspicuous columnar basal layer
- Loose-textured stellate reticulum
- β-catenin
  - Nuclei (+)
    - Especially near wet keratin whorls

Epidermoid and Dermoid Cyst

- Nonpapillary
- Keratohyaline granules and anucleate squames

DIAGNOSTIC CHECKLIST

Clinically Relevant Pathologic Features

- Circumscribed nature permits complete excision in some cases
- Almost all patients are adults
- May have cyst and mural nodule configuration on neuroimaging
  - Can lead to preoperative diagnostic confusion

Pathologic Interpretation Pearls

- Difficult distinction in some cases from Rathke cleft cyst with prominent squamous metaplasia
- BRAF VE1
  - Cytoplasm (+)
    - Parallels presence of *BRAF V600E* mutation in 95% of cases
    - May respond to targeted therapies due to *BRAF V600E* mutation (vemurafenib)
- *BRAF V600E* mutation may be useful marker for differentiating Rathke cleft cysts with squamous metaplasia from papillary craniopharyngioma
- β-catenin
  - Membranous (+), nuclei (-)
    - Differs from adamantinomatous craniopharyngioma where focal nuclei are (+)
- Do not misinterpret collagenous whorls as keratin whorls
- Beware of possible scant goblet cells
  - Contrasts with extensive mucin-producing epithelium in Rathke cleft cyst
- No calcification, unlike adamantinomatous craniopharyngioma

SELECTED REFERENCES

1. Aylwin SJ et al: Pronounced response of papillary craniopharyngioma to treatment with vemurafenib, a BRAF inhibitor. Pituitary. ePub, 2015
2. Chaohu W et al: Calretinin is expressed in the stroma of adamantinomatous craniopharyngioma and may induce calcification. Clin Neurol Neurosurg. 138:124-128, 2015
3. Daubenbüchel AM et al: Neuroendocrine Disorders in Pediatric Craniopharyngioma Patients. J Clin Med. 4(3):389-413, 2015
4. Esheba GE et al: Comparative immunohistochemical expression of β-catenin, EGFR, ErbB2, and p63 in adamantinomatous and papillary craniopharyngiomas. J Egypt Natl Canc Inst. 27(3):139-45, 2015
5. Kim JH et al: BRAF V600E mutation is a useful marker for differentiating Rathke's cleft cyst with squamous metaplasia from papillary craniopharyngioma. J Neurooncol. ePub, 2015
6. Scagliotti V et al: Histopathology and molecular characterisation of intrauterine-diagnosed congenital craniopharyngioma. Pituitary. ePub, 2015
7. Özyurt J et al: A systematic review of cognitive performance in patients with childhood craniopharyngioma. J Neurooncol. ePub, 2015
8. Brastianos PK et al: Exome sequencing identifies BRAF mutations in papillary craniopharyngiomas. Nat Genet. 46(2):161-5, 2014
9. Schweizer L et al: BRAF V600E analysis for the differentiation of papillary craniopharyngiomas and Rathke's cleft cysts. Neuropathol Appl Neurobiol. ePub, 2014
10. Pekmezci M et al: Clinicopathological characteristics of adamantinomatous and papillary craniopharyngiomas: University of California, San Francisco experience 1985-2005. Neurosurgery. 67(5):1341-9; discussion 1349, 2010
11. Zada G et al: Craniopharyngioma and other cystic epithelial lesions of the sellar region: a review of clinical, imaging, and histopathological relationships. Neurosurg Focus. 28(4):E4, 2010
12. Prabhu VC et al: The pathogenesis of craniopharyngiomas. Childs Nerv Syst. 21(8-9):622-7, 2005
13. Elmaci L et al: Metastatic papillary craniopharyngioma: case study and study of tumor angiogenesis. Neuro Oncol. 4(2):123-8, 2002
14. Xin W et al: Differential expression of cytokeratins 8 and 20 distinguishes craniopharyngioma from rathke cleft cyst. Arch Pathol Lab Med. 126(10):1174-8, 2002
15. Lee DK et al: Postoperative spinal seeding of craniopharyngioma. Case report. J Neurosurg. 94(4):617-20, 2001
16. Crotty TB et al: Papillary craniopharyngioma: a clinicopathological study of 48 cases. J Neurosurg. 83(2):206-14, 1995
17. Yasargil MG et al: Total removal of craniopharyngiomas. Approaches and long-term results in 144 patients. J Neurosurg. 73(1):3-11, 1990
18. Giangaspero F et al: Suprasellar papillary squamous epithelioma ("papillary craniopharyngioma"). Am J Surg Pathol. 8(1):57-64, 1984

Mixed Solid and Cystic Mass Above Pituitary

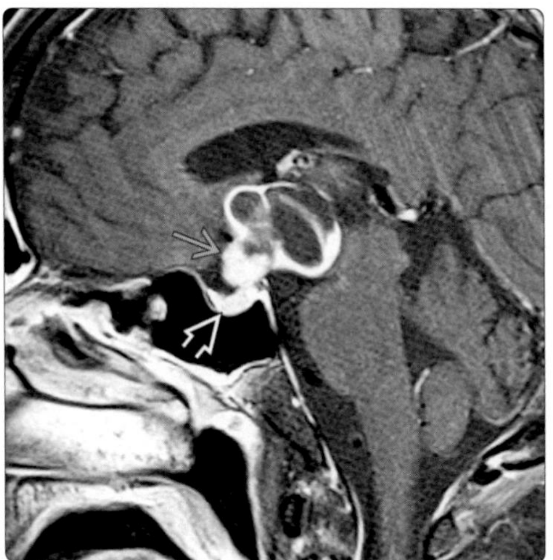

Obstructive Hydrocephalus

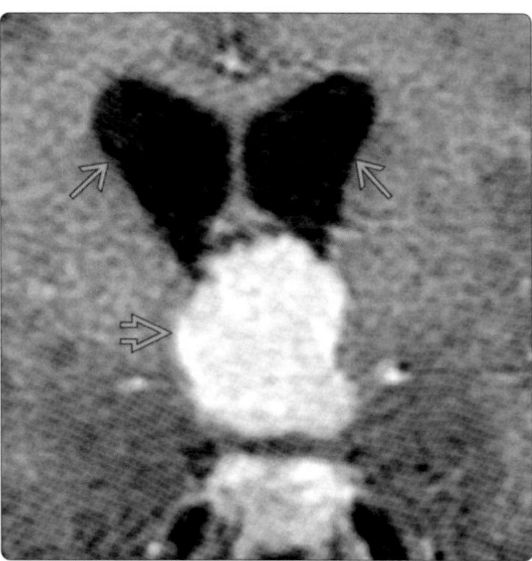

(Left) *Sagittal T1 C+ MR shows a mixed solid and cystic suprasellar mass with a mural nodule ➙. The lesion is separate from the pituitary ➙, as is typical of both craniopharyngioma types.* **(Right)** *Papillary craniopharyngiomas are usually solid and contrast enhancing with a frequent suprasellar or ventricular ⇨ location. Note the symmetric hydrocephalus ➙.*

Largely Within 3rd Ventricle

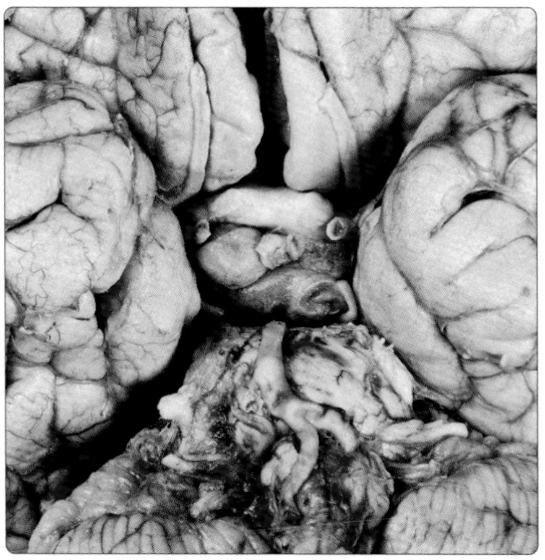

Absence of Machine Oil Content

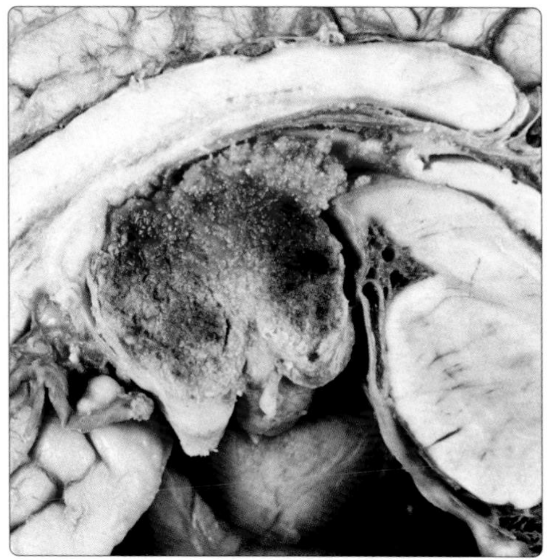

(Left) *As viewed from the base of the brain, papillary craniopharyngiomas may appear largely internal, within the 3rd ventricle.* **(Right)** *Papillary craniopharyngiomas are solid or cystic masses that may lie largely within the 3rd ventricle. Such a location, and the absence of machinery oil fluid, help distinguish the rare papillary lesion from the more common adamantinomatous type.*

Papillary Configuration

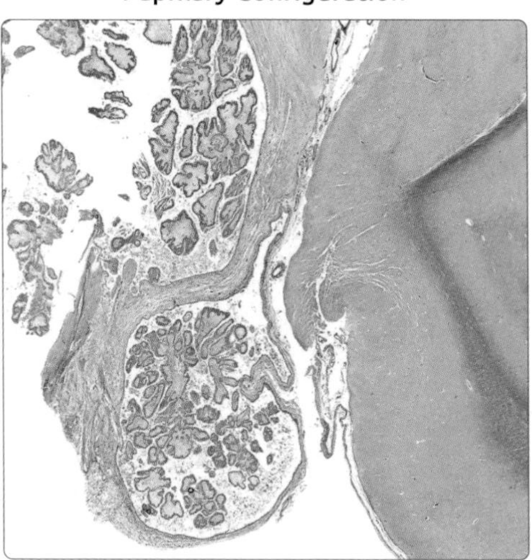

Cauliflower-Like Configuration

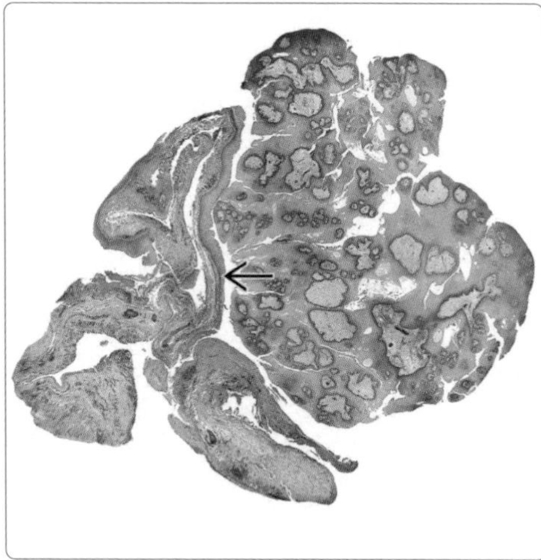

(Left) *Whole-mount section of the tumor highlights its papillary nature. The squamous epithelial covering distinguishes papillary craniopharyngioma from choroid plexus papilloma.* **(Right)** *Classic histopathology features include a papillary, cauliflower-like configuration, often surrounded by a squamous epithelium-lined cyst wall ➙.*

(**Left**) *The epithelial lining ⇨ should prompt a search for pseudopapillae ⇨. In this case, the epithelial lining is far too thick to be that of an epidermoid cyst. It is also nonkeratinized.* (**Right**) *Dehiscence of the epithelium is the basis of pseudopapillae formation. Mature cells retain their nuclei unlike anuclear squames in an epidermoid cyst.*

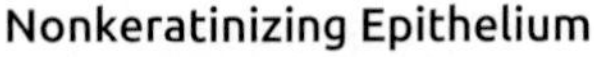

Nonkeratinizing Epithelium

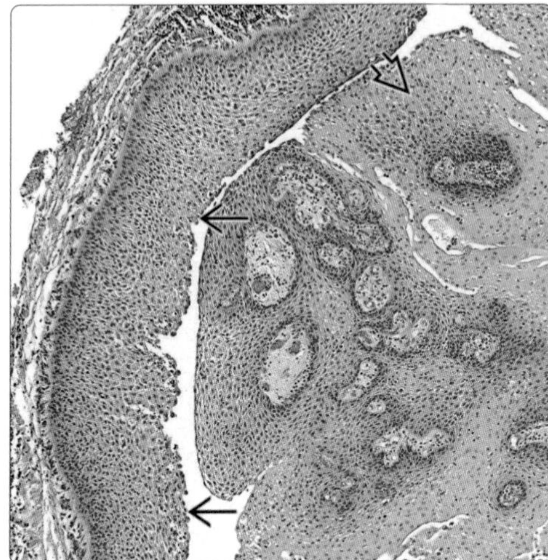

Nuclear Retention in Epithelial Cells

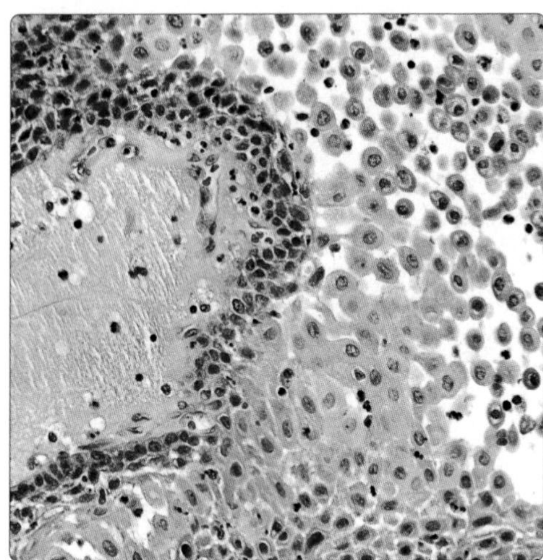

(**Left**) *This well-differentiated squamous epithelium is nonkeratinizing unlike that of epidermoid cysts, which generate innumerable anuclear squames.* (**Right**) *Palisading, if any, in the basal layer of papillary craniopharyngiomas is not as pronounced as in the adamantinomatous counterpart.*

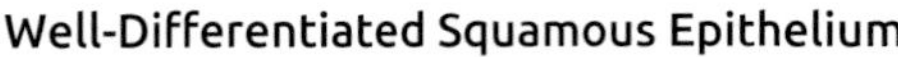

Well-Differentiated Squamous Epithelium

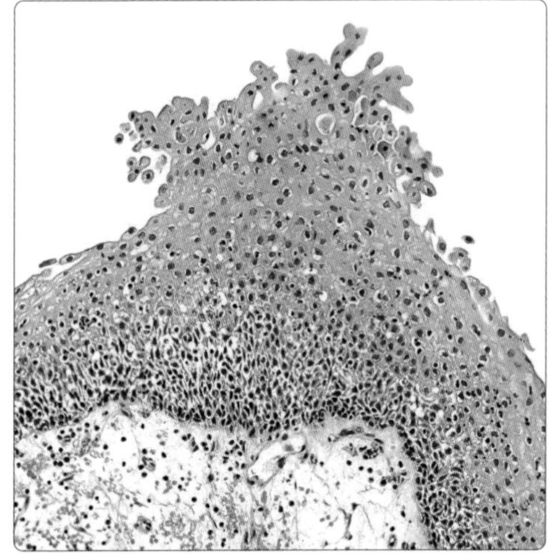

Minimal Basal Layer Palisading

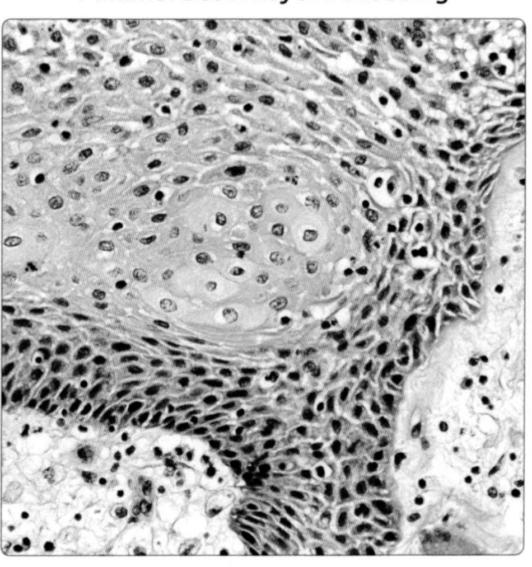

(**Left**) *Well-formed epithelial whorls ➡ are not uncommon in papillary craniopharyngiomas.* (**Right**) *Collagenous whorl-like structures that project from the stroma into the epithelium should not be mistaken for keratin whorls.*

Epithelial Whorls

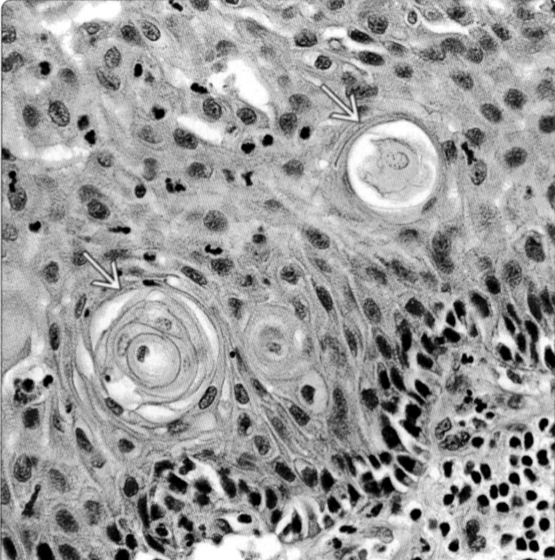

Collagenous Whorls Simulating Keratin

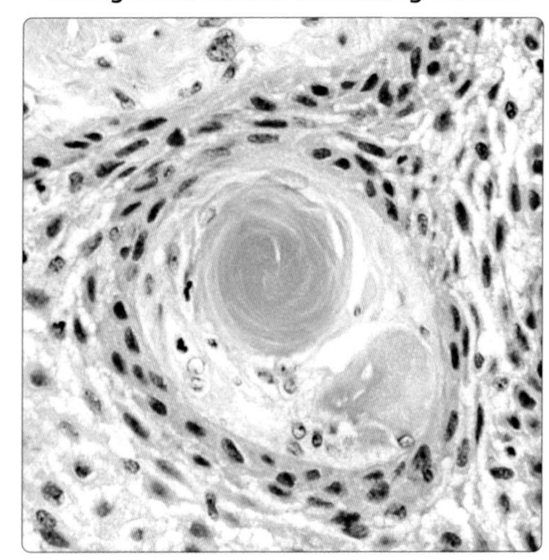

Focal Goblet Cells

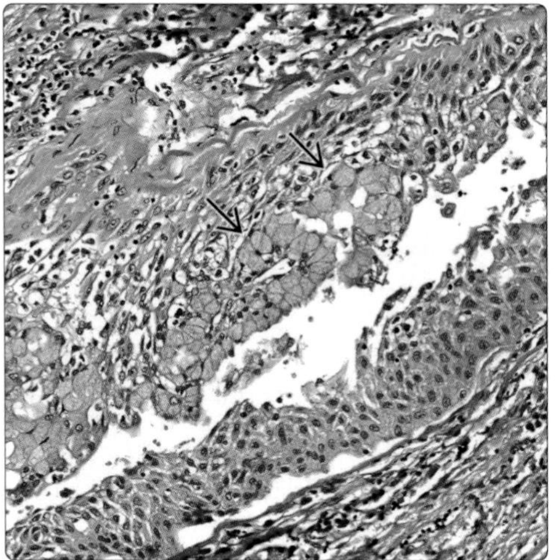

PAS, Focal Goblet Cells

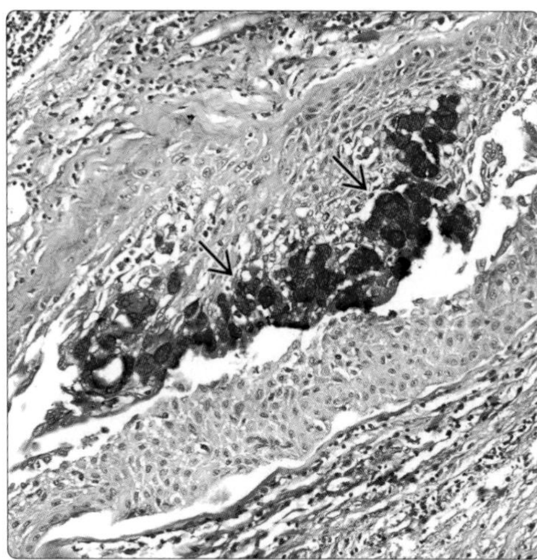

(Left) *The presence of goblet cells* ⇨ *overlying the squamous epithelium creates a diagnostic dilemma as to whether such lesions are papillary craniopharyngioma or Rathke cleft cyst with prominent squamous metaplasia. Tissue suggesting papillary craniopharyngioma dominated this lesion elsewhere.* **(Right)** *PAS stain highlights the goblet cells* ⇨ *with underlying squamous epithelium.*

Edematous Stroma, Epithelial Dehiscence

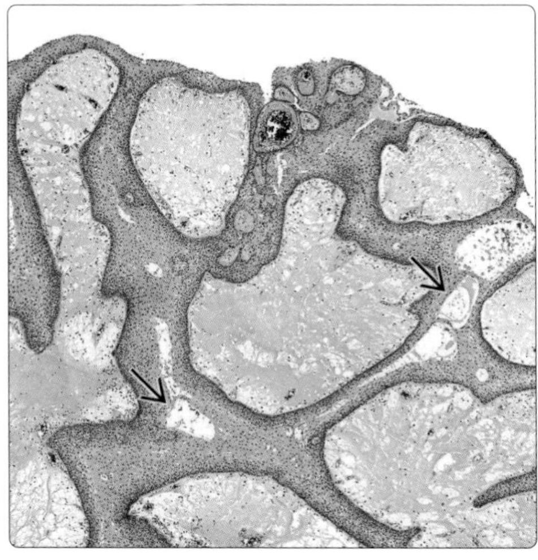

Fibrotic Stroma, Established Lesion

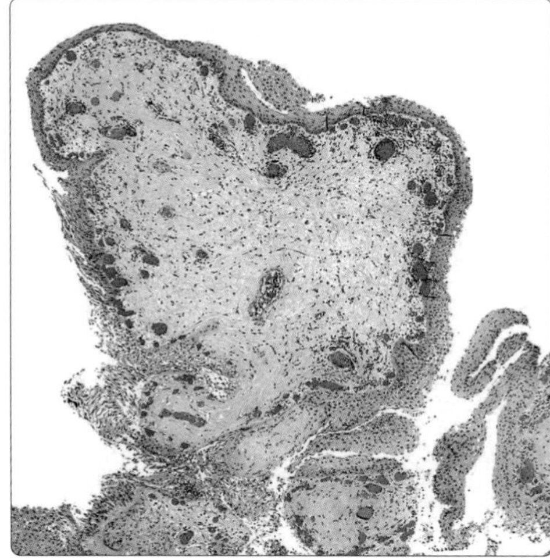

(Left) *The stroma of what will be papillary structures are edematous in early-phase lesions. Dehiscence of epithelium* ⇨ *is another early finding.* **(Right)** *Pseudopapillae in established lesions have variably fibrotic and vascular cores.*

Smear, Well-Differentiated Squamous Cells

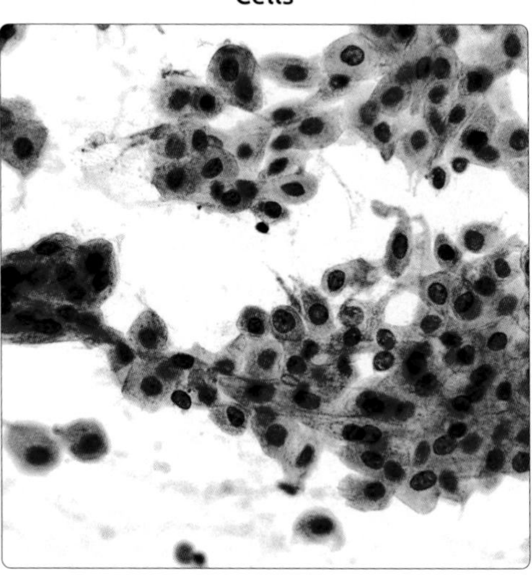

Smear, Occasional Whorls

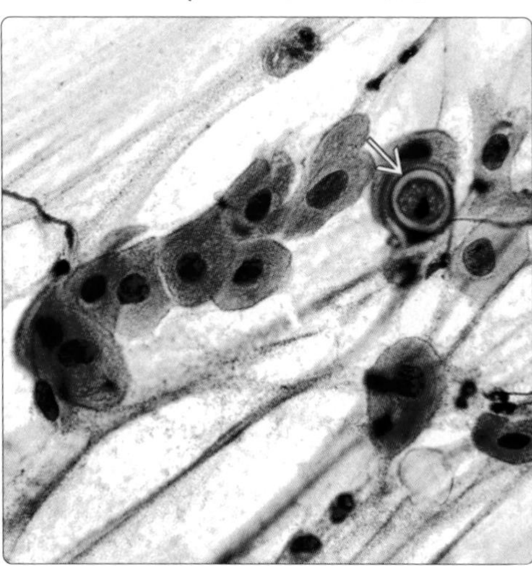

(Left) *Cytologically, the somewhat cohesive well-differentiated squamous cells have discrete cell borders, typical of an epithelial lesion.* **(Right)** *Obviously, squamous cells form occasional whorls* ➡ *as are typically absent in adamantinomatous craniopharyngiomas and epidermoid cysts.*

(Left) *The lesions sometimes show moderate chronic inflammatory cells and loss of epithelium associated with stromal iron deposition →.* **(Right)** *Iron deposition associated with chronic inflammation is highlighted by Prussian blue staining →.*

Hemosiderin Deposits

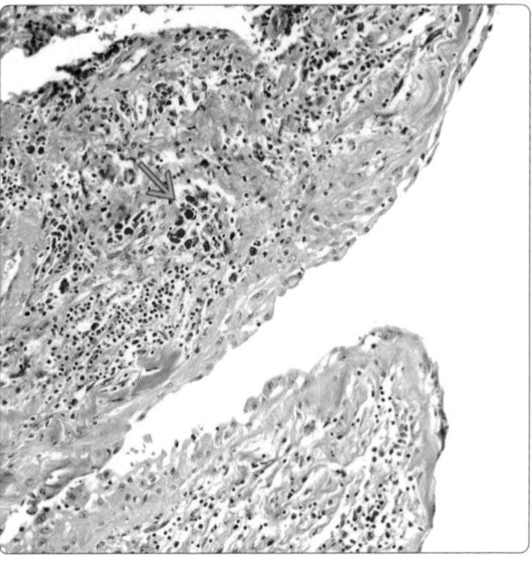

Prussian Blue, Hemosiderin Deposits

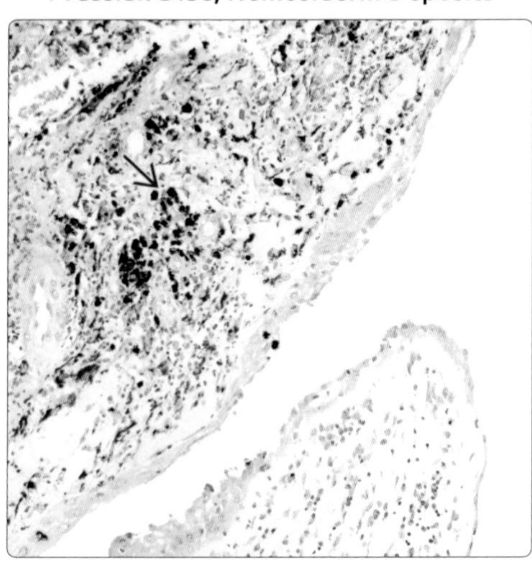

(Left) *Pancytokeratin is diffusely positive in all layers of the papillary epithelium.* **(Right)** *Immunostaining for Ki-67 is restricted to the basal layer →, as is consistent with the very well-differentiated nature of papillary craniopharyngioma.*

Pankeratin, Diffuse

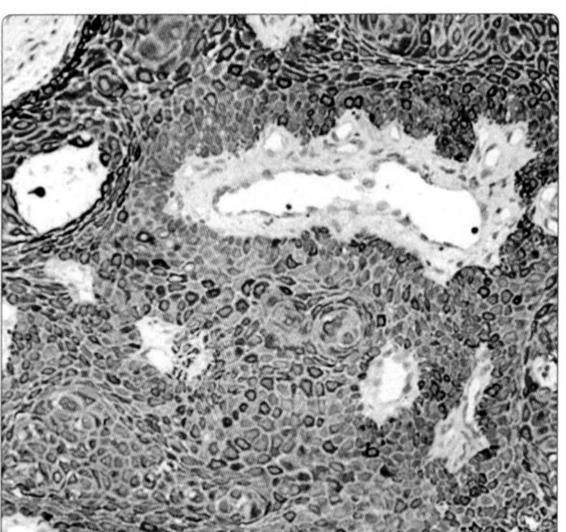

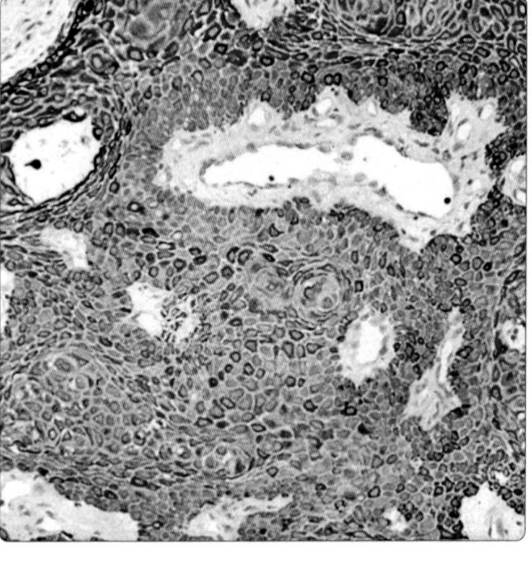

Ki-67 Restricted to Basal Layer

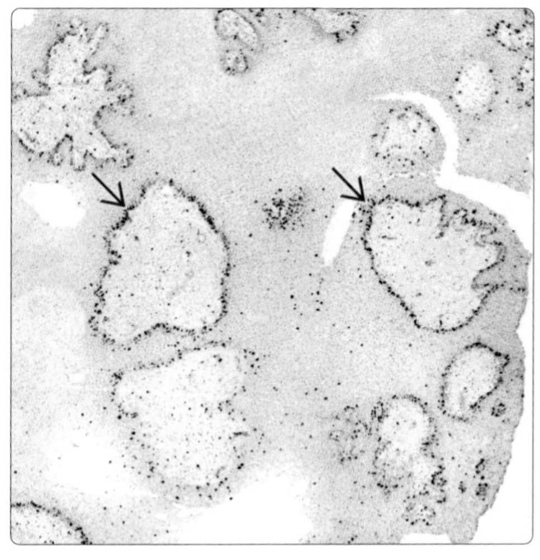

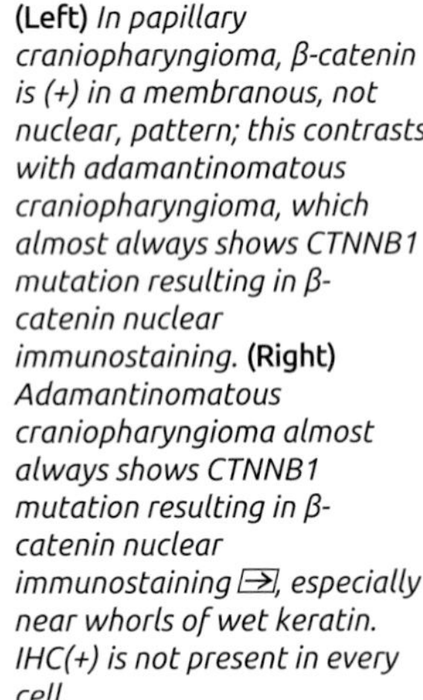

(Left) *In papillary craniopharyngioma, β-catenin is (+) in a membranous, not nuclear, pattern; this contrasts with adamantinomatous craniopharyngioma, which almost always shows CTNNB1 mutation resulting in β-catenin nuclear immunostaining.* **(Right)** *Adamantinomatous craniopharyngioma almost always shows CTNNB1 mutation resulting in β-catenin nuclear immunostaining →, especially near whorls of wet keratin. IHC(+) is not present in every cell.*

Papillary Craniopharyngioma, β-Catenin Membranous IHC

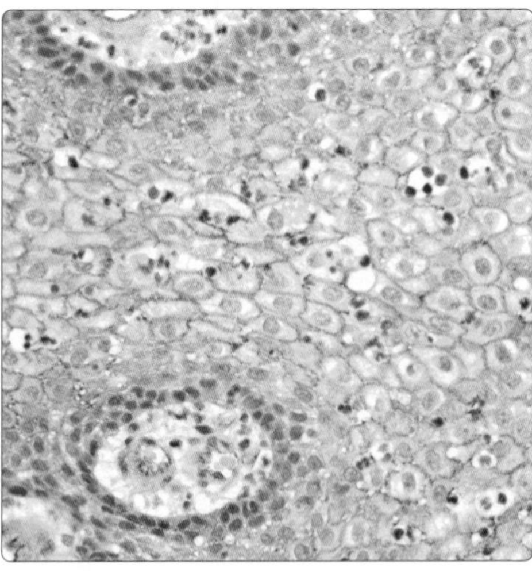

Adamantinomatous Craniopharyngioma, β-Catenin Focal Nuclear IHC

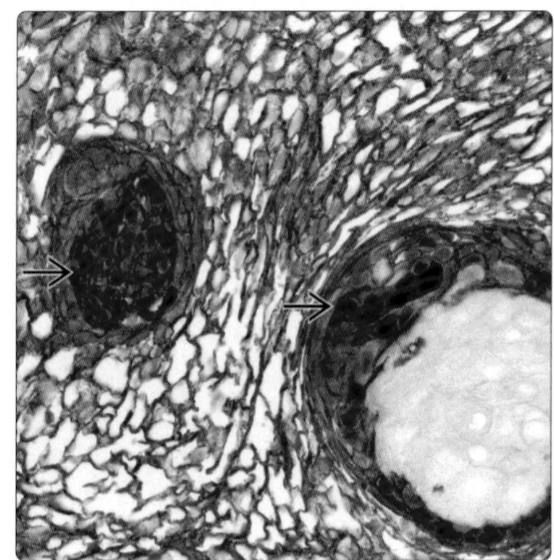

Cystic, No Solid Component

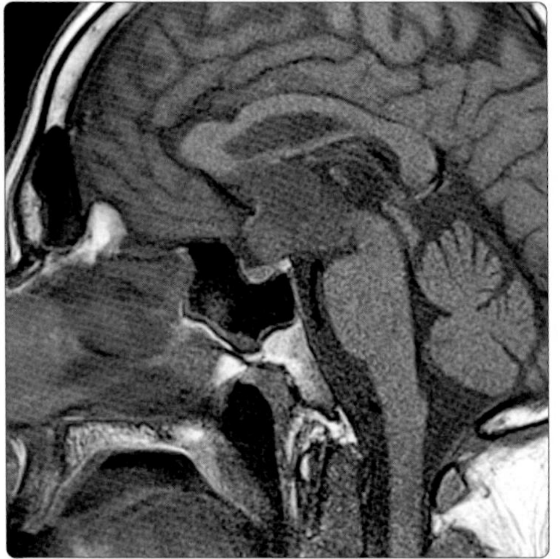

Solid, No Cystic Component

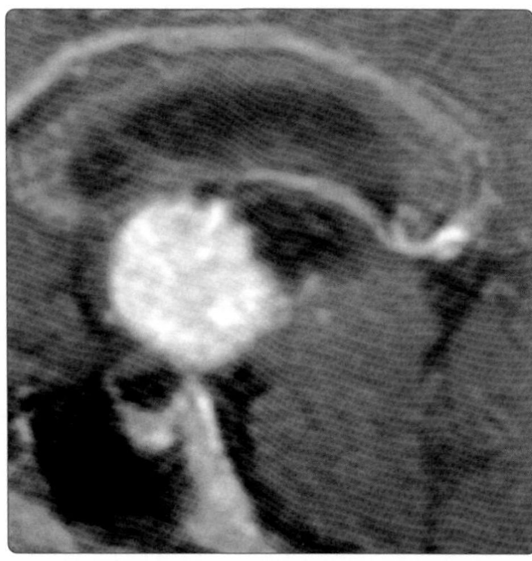

(Left) *Some tumors are cystic with only a minimal solid component.* **(Right)** *MR scan showing solid, contrast enhancing tumor in the 3rd ventricle is a frequent imaging finding of papillary craniopharyngiomas.*

Rare Seeded Deposit

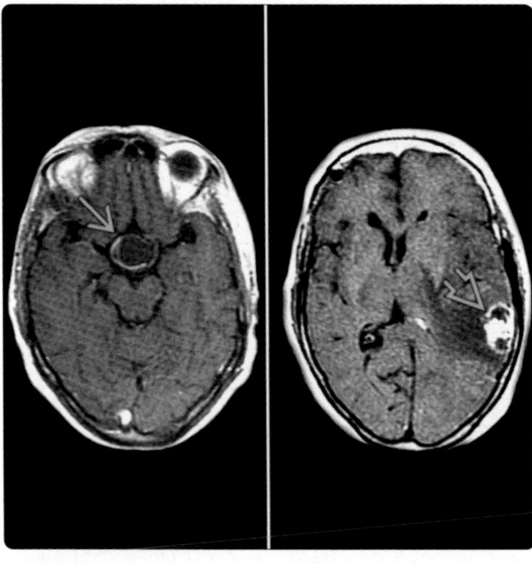

Solid 3rd Ventricular Example

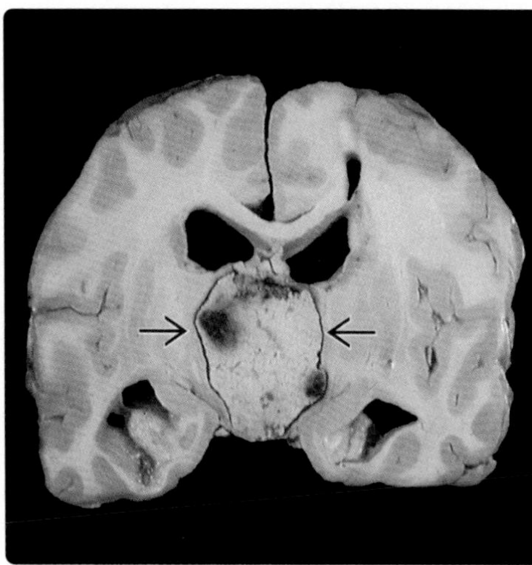

(Left) *Imaging shows a rare complication of papillary craniopharyngioma: Seeded deposit. The original lesion ⇨ was a cystic hypothalamic region mass. After an interval, a seeded deposit established itself on the cortical surface ⇨. A biopsy of the latter lesion showed classic papillary craniopharyngioma.* **(Right)** *A superficial biopsy of this solid 3rd ventricular example ➔ of a papillary craniopharyngioma yielded only arachnoidal tissue that had been mistaken for meningioma.*

Well-Formed Desmosomes

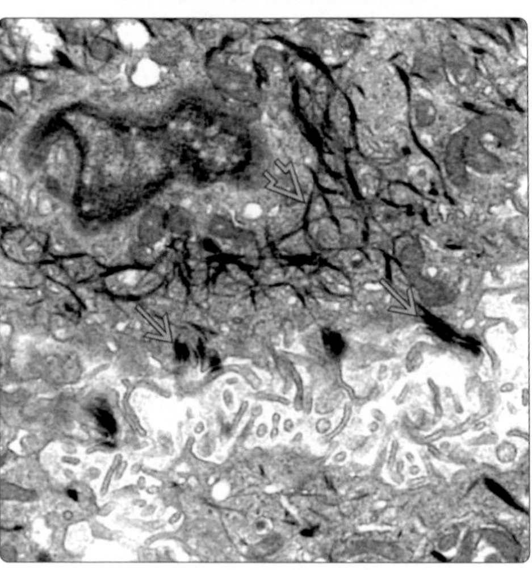

Cell Surface Features

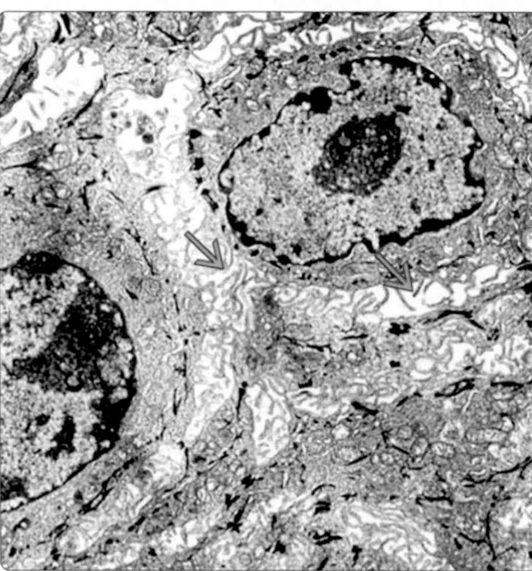

(Left) *Intracytoplasmic tonofilament bundles ⇨ and well-formed desmosomes ⇨ are well seen at high magnification in these cells with features of overt squamous differentiation.* **(Right)** *Ultrastructurally, apposed tumor cells have delicate surface specializations ⇨.*

Spindle Cell Oncocytoma

KEY FACTS

ETIOLOGY/PATHOGENESIS

- Spindle cell oncocytomas (SCOs) and granular cell tumors of pituitary now considered variants of pituicytoma based on shared TTF-1(+)

CLINICAL ISSUES

- Indistinguishable from nonfunctioning pituitary macroadenomas

IMAGING

- Demarcated, solid, contrast enhancing
- Intra- and suprasellar mass, occasionally hemorrhagic
- Only occasional skull base destruction

MICROSCOPIC

- Fascicles of eosinophilic spindle cells admixed with epithelioid cells
- Mild to marked nuclear pleomorphism, occasional nucleolar prominence
- < 2/10 HPF mitosis in primary tumors
- Patchy lymphocytic inflammation in most tumors
- May have focal hemosiderin

ANCILLARY TESTS

- Negative for pituitary hormones
- Positive for TTF-1, vimentin, EMA, S100 protein, antimitochondrial antibody, galactin-3, and annexin-A1
- Ki-67: 1-10% (mean: ~ 3%)
- Negative for synaptophysin, chromogranin, cytokeratin, CD34, Bcl-2, smooth muscle actin, and desmin

TOP DIFFERENTIAL DIAGNOSES

- Pituitary adenoma: Synaptophysin (+), TTF-1(-)
- Meningioma: Progesterone receptors (+), TTF-1(-)
- Pituicytoma: Also TTF-1(+) but usually EMA(-), variably GFAP(+), less mitochondrial-rich

Spindle Cell Oncocytoma Simulating Macroadenoma

Fascicled Architecture Simulating Meningioma

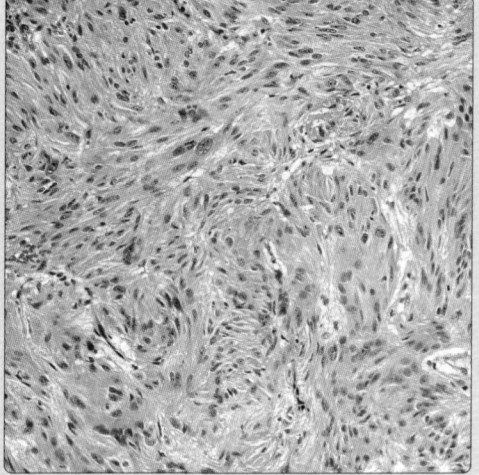

(Left) *T1WI MR shows a contrast-enhancing spindle cell oncocytoma (SCO) with suprasellar extension ⇒.* **(Right)** *Spindle cells with eosinophilic cytoplasm due to oncocytic change tend to form fascicles. This appearance in SCO may prompt strong consideration of meningioma in the differential diagnosis but TTF-1(+) IHC in SCO and negative in meningioma.*

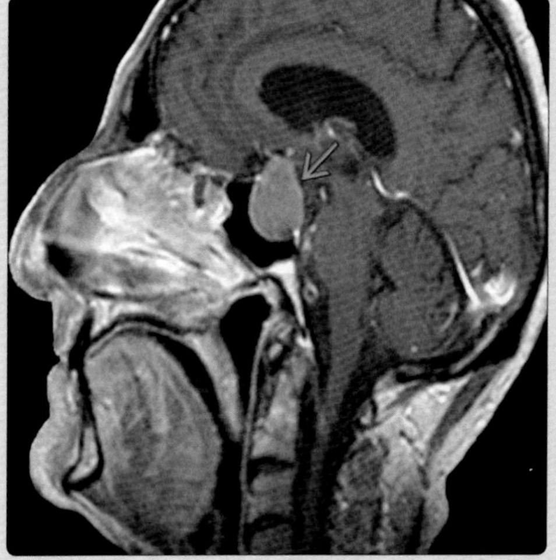

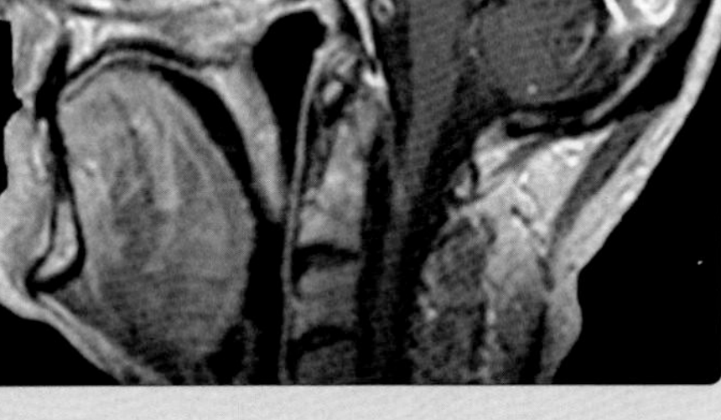

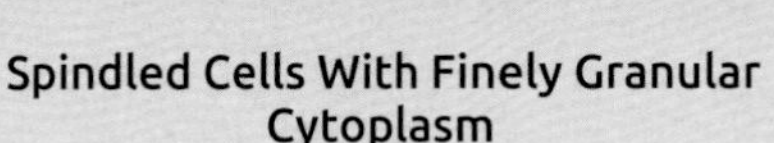

Spindled Cells With Finely Granular Cytoplasm

TTF-1(+), Shared With Pituicytoma

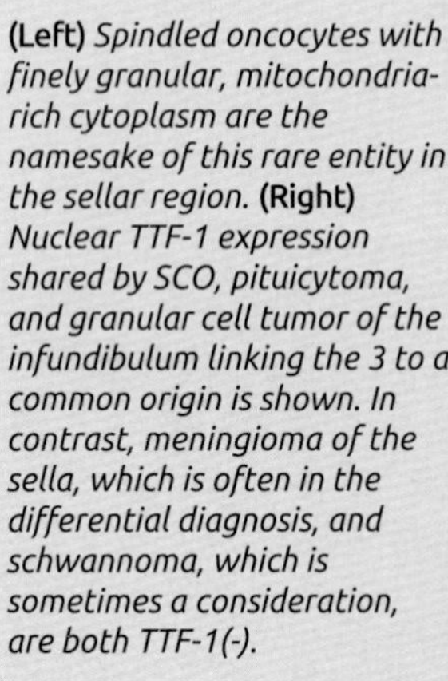

(Left) *Spindled oncocytes with finely granular, mitochondria-rich cytoplasm are the namesake of this rare entity in the sellar region.* **(Right)** *Nuclear TTF-1 expression shared by SCO, pituicytoma, and granular cell tumor of the infundibulum linking the 3 to a common origin is shown. In contrast, meningioma of the sella, which is often in the differential diagnosis, and schwannoma, which is sometimes a consideration, are both TTF-1(-).*

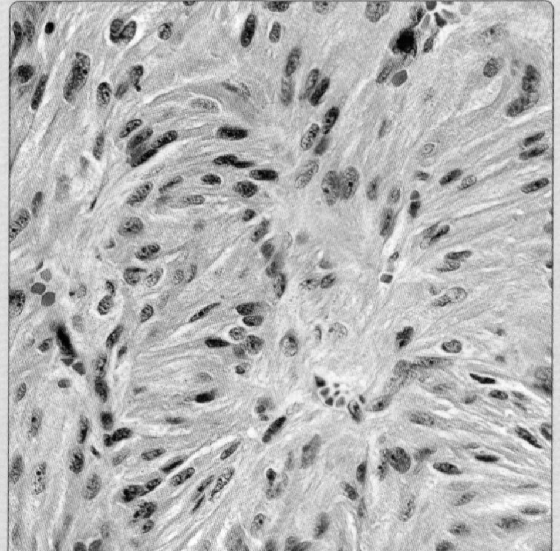

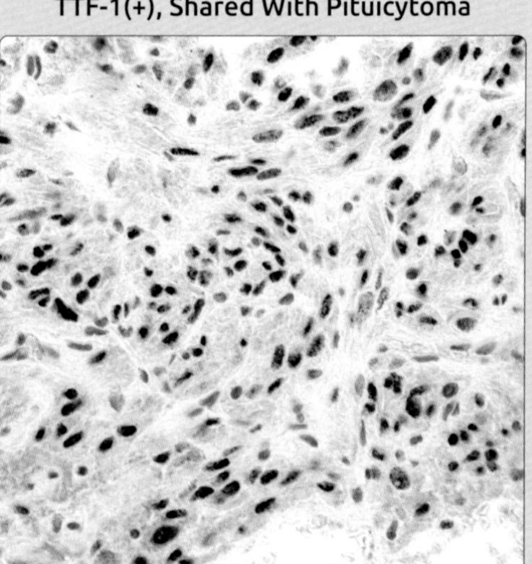

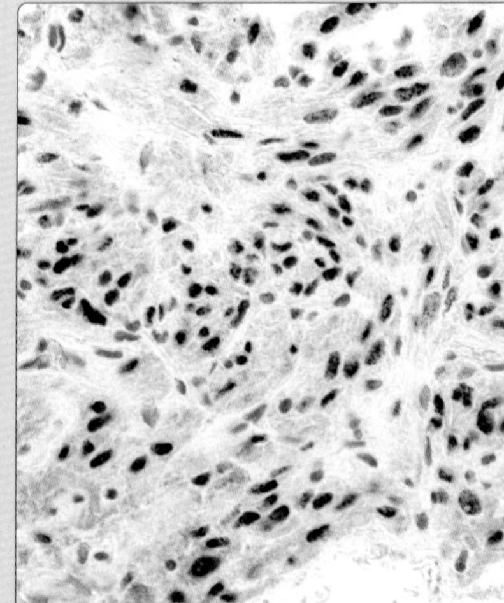

Spindle Cell Oncocytoma

TERMINOLOGY

Abbreviations

- Spindle cell oncocytoma (SCO)

Definitions

- Benign sellar tumor of adenohypophysis consisting of granular, mitochondria-rich, spindle to epithelioid cells
- SCOs and granular cell tumors of pituitary now considered variants of pituicytoma based on shared TTF-1(+)

CLINICAL ISSUES

Epidemiology

- Incidence
  - Rare (< 1% of sellar tumors)
- Age
  - Adults 25-70 years
- Sex
  - No predilection

Presentation

- Mass effect
  - Pituitary hypofunction, visual symptoms, headache
- Features indistinguishable from nonfunctioning pituitary macroadenomas except for possible increased bleeding

Treatment

- Surgical approaches
  - Gross total resection
- Radiation
  - Role not firmly established

Prognosis

- May show recurrence(s)
- Locally aggressive behavior, occasionally

IMAGING

MR Findings

- Demarcated, solid, contrast enhancing
- Intra- and suprasellar mass
- ± sellar &/or skull base destruction

MACROSCOPIC

General Features

- 1- to 6.5-cm lesion consisting of soft, creamy tissue resembling pituitary adenoma
- Firm-textured areas of dural involvement or sellar floor invasion
- No sharp demarcation from pituitary parenchyma

MICROSCOPIC

Histologic Features

- Fascicles of spindle cells admixed with epithelioid cells, both featuring eosinophilic, granular cytoplasm due to mitochondrial accumulation
- Mild to marked nuclear pleomorphism, open or dense chromatin, occasional nucleolar prominence
  - Osteoclast-like giant cells
- No or scant mitoses (< 2/10 HPF) in primary tumors
  - More mitotic activity in recurrences
- Patchy lymphocytic inflammation in most tumors

ANCILLARY TESTS

Cytology

- Spindle to polygonal, densely opposed cells containing abundant mitochondria

Histochemistry

- PTAH
  - Reactivity: Positive
  - Staining pattern: Cytoplasmic
- Alcian blue/periodic acid-Schiff
  - Reactivity: Negative

Immunohistochemistry

- Positive for EMA, S100 protein, vimentin, antimitochondrial antibody, galectin-3, and annexin-A1
- TTF-1(+) expression, shared with pituicytoma, granular cell tumor of infundibulum, linking the 3
- Negative for GFAP, cytokeratin, CD34, Bcl-2, smooth muscle actin, and desmin
- Negative for pituitary hormones, synaptophysin, chromogranin
- Ki-67: 1-10% (mean: 2.8%)
  - Rarely 20%, in recurrence

Electron Microscopy

- Abundant mitochondria
- Well-formed desmosomes without tonofilaments and intermediate junctions
- No secretory granules

DIFFERENTIAL DIAGNOSIS

Pituicytoma

- Also TTF-1(+); variable GFAP, galectin-3 immunoreactivity
- EMA(-), annexin-A1 (-); less mitochondrial-rich than SCO

Granular Cell Tumor of Infundibulum

- Cytoplasm coarsely granular and PAS(+), not oncocytic
- Perivascular lymphocytes, in some case, more lysosomal-rich than SCO
- EMA(-), annexin-A1 (-), galectin-3: Rare positivity

Pituitary Adenoma

- Epithelial features, cellular uniformity
- Synaptophysin and pituitary hormone (+), TTF1(-)
- Endocrine organelles (well-formed rough endoplasmic reticulum, Golgi, and secretory granules) on ultrastructure
- Rarely oncocytic

Meningioma

- Cellular whorls, psammoma bodies, collagenous stroma, and vessels
- S100 protein (+) (20%, patchy), progesterone receptors (+), TTF-1(-)
- Annexin-A1 (+)

SELECTED REFERENCES

1. Kleinschmidt-DeMasters BK et al: Update on hypophysitis and TTF-1 expressing sellar region masses. Brain Pathol. 23(5):495-514, 2013

(Left) *Spindle cells with prominent eosinophilic cytoplasm due to oncocytic change are assembled in vaguely formed fascicles.* **(Right)** *Not all cases are formed of closely packed cells in fascicles. Open chromatin and distinct nucleoli are present in some cases.*

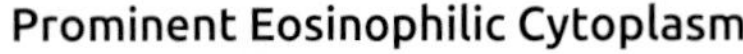

Prominent Eosinophilic Cytoplasm

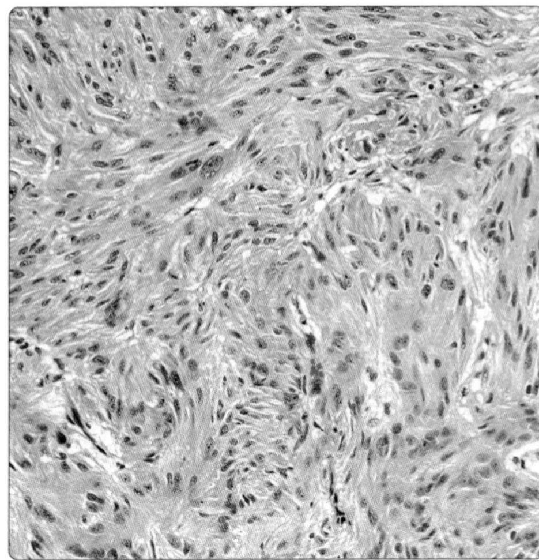

Distinct Nucleoli in Some Cases

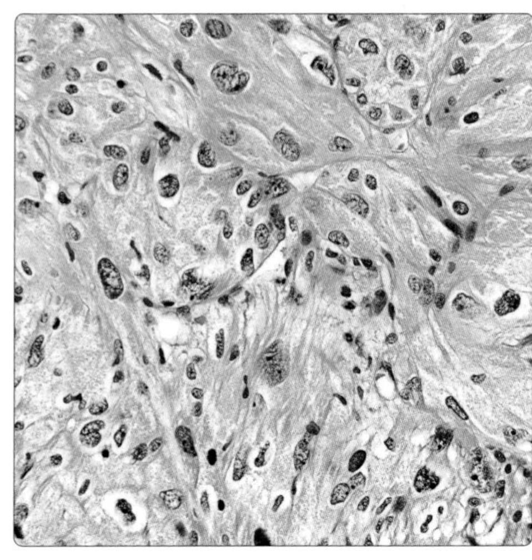

(Left) *There may be considerable nuclear pleomorphism, including giant cells ⇒ with prominent nucleoli. More objective measures of anaplasia, i.e., multiple mitoses and a high Ki-67 rate, will be absent.* **(Right)** *Smudgy, dark, pleomorphic nuclei express a prognostically insignificant degenerative form of atypia.*

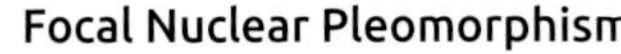

Focal Nuclear Pleomorphism

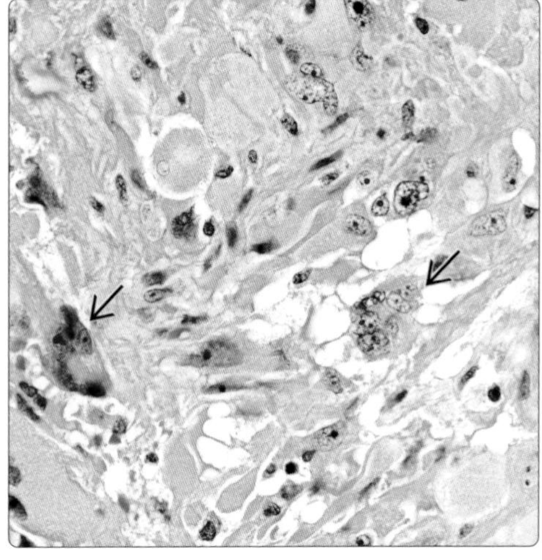

Prognostically Insignificant Pleomorphism

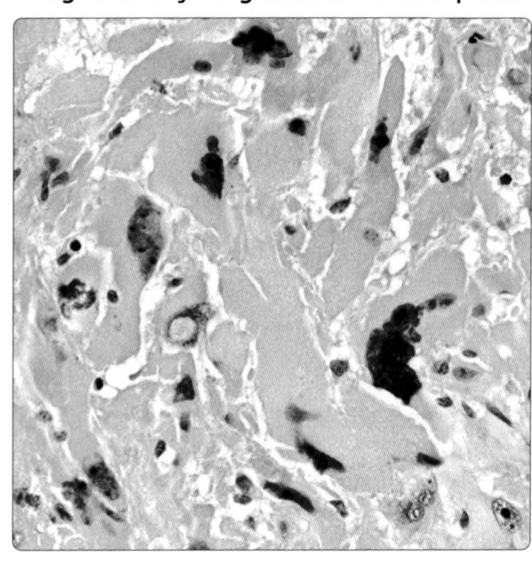

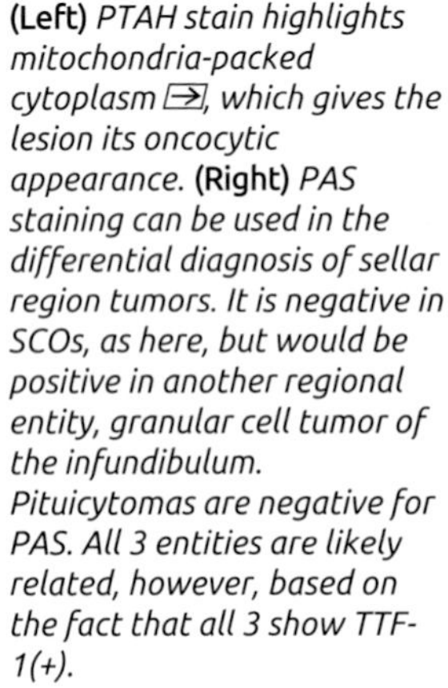

(Left) *PTAH stain highlights mitochondria-packed cytoplasm ⇒, which gives the lesion its oncocytic appearance.* **(Right)** *PAS staining can be used in the differential diagnosis of sellar region tumors. It is negative in SCOs, as here, but would be positive in another regional entity, granular cell tumor of the infundibulum. Pituicytomas are negative for PAS. All 3 entities are likely related, however, based on the fact that all 3 show TTF-1(+).*

PTAH Highlights Mitochondrial-Rich Cytoplasm

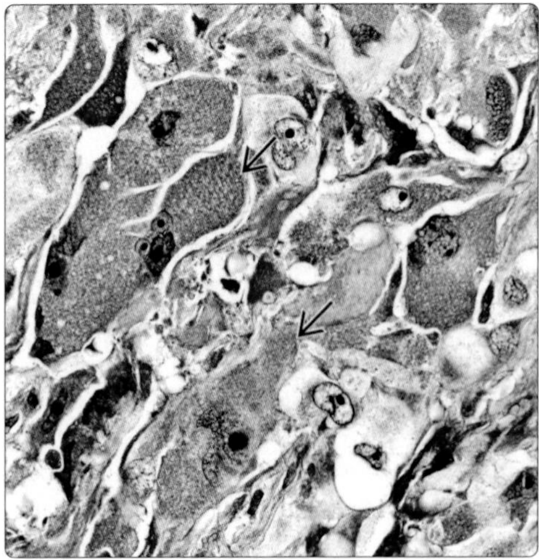

PAS(-) Unlike Granular Cell Tumor

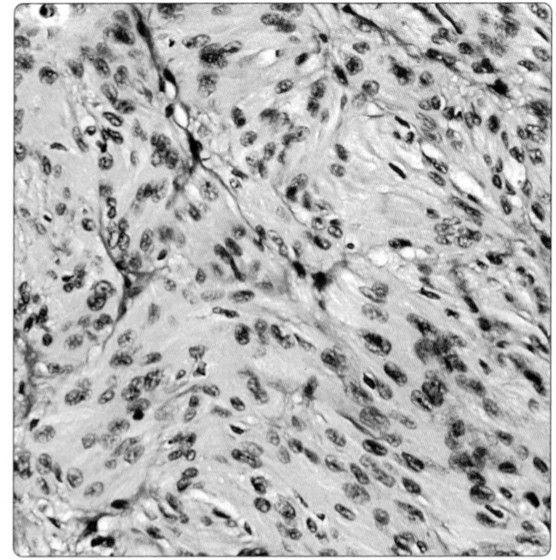

S100(+)

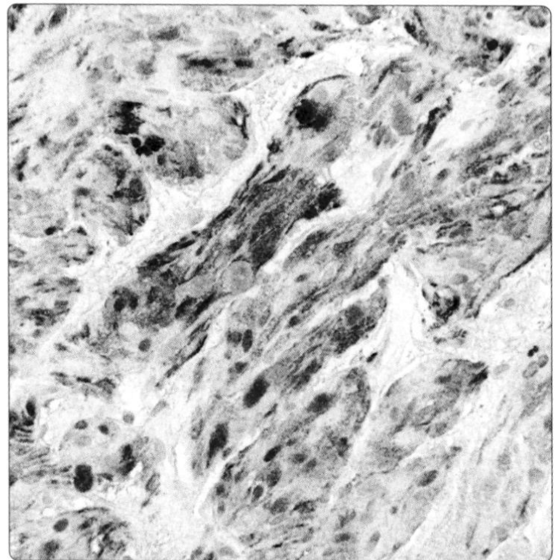

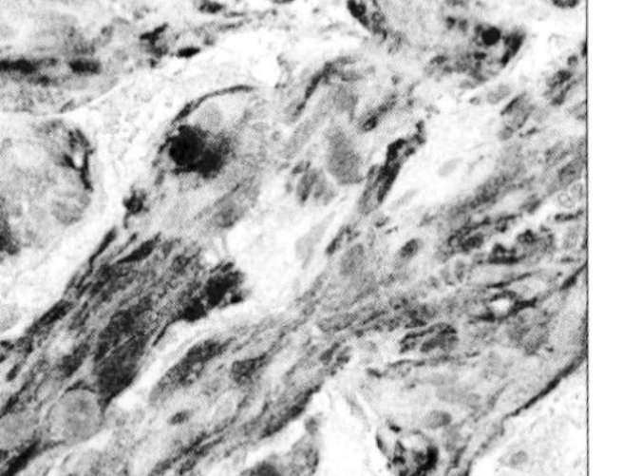

EMA(+) Distinguishes Spindle Cell Oncocytoma From Pituicytoma

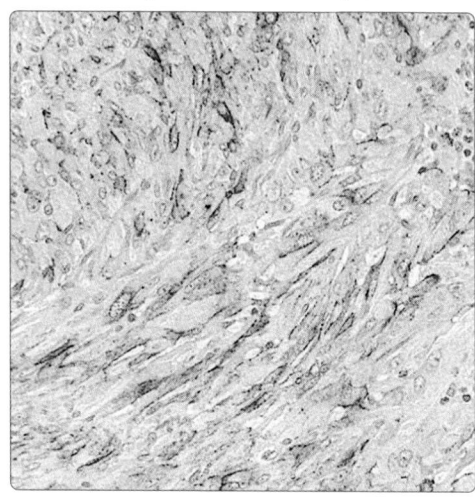

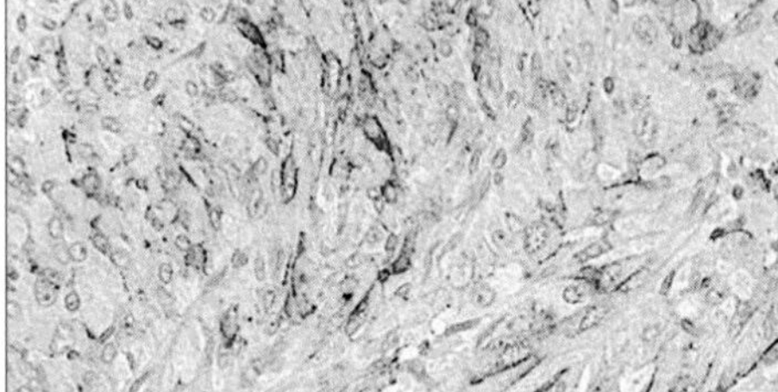

(Left) *Neoplastic cells are immunoreactive for the S100 protein. The 2 differential diagnostic entities, granular cell tumor of infundibulum and pituicytoma, are also usually positive. A 3rd, fibrous meningioma, is usually negative but can be positive. However, a fibrous meningioma would be TTF-1(-), unlike the other 3.* **(Right)** *The positivity on an EMA immunostain may be a helpful feature for distinguishing SCO from pituicytoma and granular cell tumor, which are generally negative for EMA protein.*

Galectin-3 (+), Characteristic but Nonspecific

Annexin-A1 (+) Distinguishes Spindle Cell Oncocytoma From Pituicytoma

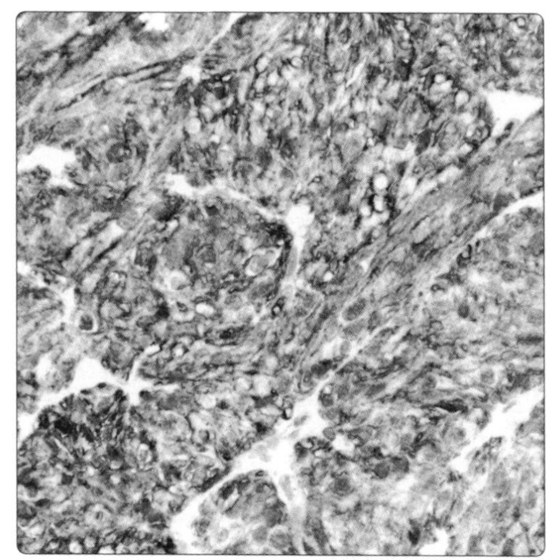

(Left) *Galectin-3 immunostaining is characteristic but nonspecific. It is found to be positive in a variety of tumors in the central nervous system and sella. In a normal pituitary gland, galectin-3 is expressed in folliculostellate cells and ACTH cells.* **(Right)** *Immunoreactivity for annexin-A1, also expressed in normal folliculostellate cells, is characteristic of SPC. Other sellar region tumors, such as pituicytoma and granular cell tumor of the infundibulum, are negative.*

TTF-1(+) Nuclear Expression

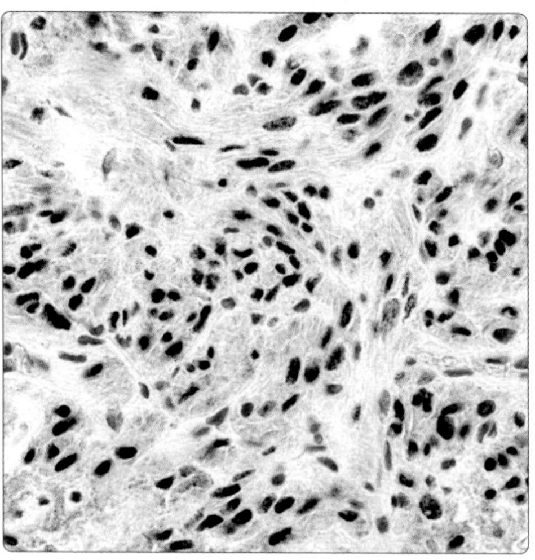

Abundant Mitochondria

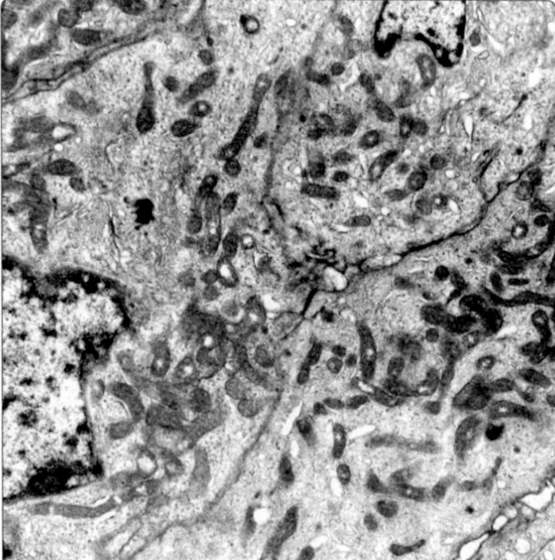

(Left) *Nuclear expression of TTF-1 should not cause a misdiagnosis of pituicytoma, a spindle cell lesion of the sellar region that is also immunoreactive. Local granular cell tumors may be positive as well.* **(Right)** *By definition, mitochondria are abundant at the ultrastructural level in an oncocytic neoplasm.*

Pituitary Blastoma

KEY FACTS

TERMINOLOGY
- Neonatal pituitary tumor exhibiting differentiation to Rathke epithelium, adenohypophysial, secretory cells

ETIOLOGY/PATHOGENESIS
- Part of the *DICER1*-pleuropulmonary blastoma familial tumor predisposition syndrome

CLINICAL ISSUES
- Infantile presentation
- ACTH secretion common
- Transsphenoidal surgery, reexcisions
- Temozolomide, polychemotherapy
- Aggressive behavior, but limited experience

IMAGING
- Large enhancing, invasive mass with suprasellar extension

MICROSCOPIC
- Moderate to highly cellular tumor
- Small and large glandular structures
- Secretory cells
- Small blastema-like cells
- Folliculostellate
- Mitotic activity from 0-16/10 HPF

ANCILLARY TESTS
- Synaptophysin, chromogranin (+)
- Hormonal immunoreactivity variable-majority ACTH(+)
- Annexin-1, CAM5.2, galectin-3, p27, and p53 (+)

TOP DIFFERENTIAL DIAGNOSES
- Pituitary adenoma
- Immature teratomas

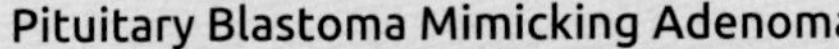

Pituitary Blastoma Mimicking Adenoma

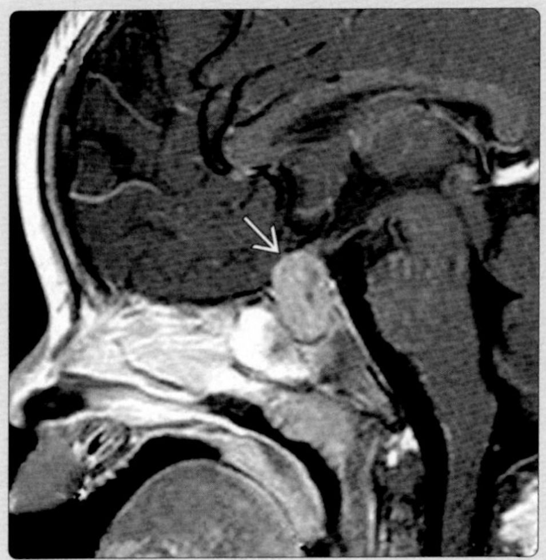

Glandular Structures With Secretory Cells

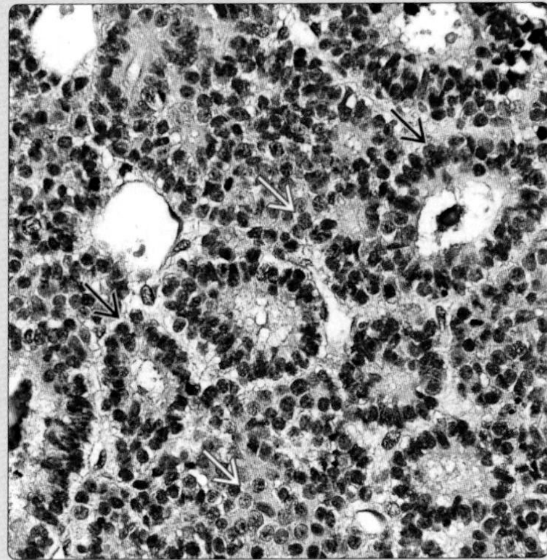

(Left) *As a contrast-enhancing mass with suprasellar extension* ➡, *a pituitary blastoma mimics pituitary macroadenoma, except for the very young age of the patient.* **(Right)** *Glandular structures resembling Rathke epithelium* ⇨ *among diffuse, larger secretory cells* ➡ *are typical components of this rare entity.*

Pale Secretory Cells, Small Blastema Cells

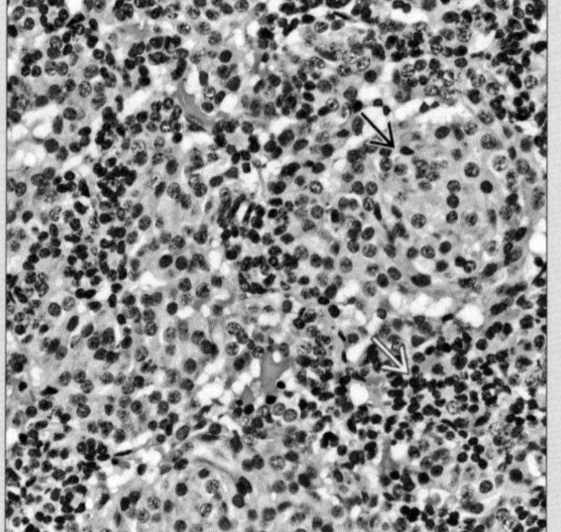

ACTH(+) Secretory With Neuroendocrine Cells

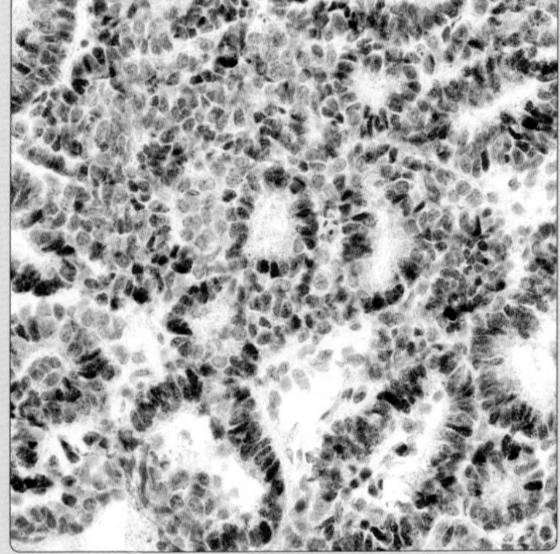

(Left) *Zones of large pale secretory cells* ⇨ *are surrounded by streams of small blastema-like cells* ➡. **(Right)** *The secretory and neuroendocrine cells are weakly immunoreactive for ACTH.*

TERMINOLOGY

Definitions

- Neonatal pituitary tumor with differentiation to Rathke, adenohypophysial cells of secretory type, and folliculostellate cells

ETIOLOGY/PATHOGENESIS

Associating Syndromes

- Familial *DICER1* cancer syndrome: Associated with other blastomas (pleuropulmonary blastoma), cystic nephroma
  - Pituitary blastoma is pathognomonic feature of germ-line *DICER1* mutation and tumor harbors 2nd somatic mutation in *DICER1*
- Appears to be embryonal tumor originating in utero

Cellular Origin

- Embryonal tumor of pituitary anlage cells

Pathobiology

- Order of hormonal appearance as in embryogenesis
- Correlates with early stage (8-12 week) pituitary
- Hormone expression linked to specific transcription factors and respective hormones

CLINICAL ISSUES

Epidemiology

- Incidence
  - Rare (~ 12 cases reported to date)
- Age
  - Early childhood (< 2 years) presentation

Presentation

- Ophthalmoplegia, visual disturbances
- Most hormonally functioning
  - ACTH secretion (Cushing disease) common
  - No clinical GH excess

Treatment

- Surgical approaches
  - Transsphenoidal approach
- Adjuvant therapy
  - Temozolomide
  - Polychemotherapy

Prognosis

- Aggressive behavior in most but limited experience

IMAGING

General Features

- Large enhancing sellar mass
  - Suprasellar extension
  - Cavernous sinus invasion

MICROSCOPIC

Histologic Features

- Moderate to highly cellular lesion
- Large and small glandular structures resembling Rathke epithelium
- Clusters of large pituitary secretory cells
  - Round to oval nuclei, inconspicuous nucleoli, moderate cytoplasm
- Small blastema-like cells
  - Undifferentiated chromophobic cells
- Variable mitotic activity (0-16/10 HPF)
- Necrosis rare
- Rare microcalcification in glands
- No normal acinar pituitary architecture
- No Crooke cells

ANCILLARY TESTS

Histochemistry

- Weak PAS(+) secretory cells
- PAS(+) basal lamina surrounds glandular structures
- One tumor showed PAS(+) mucin-secreting cells

Immunohistochemistry

- Small cells and glandular structures
  - Vimentin, keratin, EMA, S100 (+)
  - CAM5.2(+)
  - Galectin-3 (+)
  - Annexin-1 (+)
  - Synaptophysin (-)
  - p53: Abundantly (+) in glands
  - MGMT: Frequently (+), variable degree
  - Collagen IV (+) basal lamina around glands
- Secretory cells
  - Synaptophysin, chromogranin (+)
  - Keratins (+)
  - ACTH, β-endorphin; CRH(+) to lesser extent
  - GH: Rare (+)
  - p27: Frequently (+)
- Ki-67 positivity ranges from < 1-60%
- Germ cell markers negative

Electron Microscopy

- Undifferentiated small polyhedral cells containing only polyribosomes
- Secretory cells: Granules and filaments (keratin)
- Typical pituitary follicles formed by folliculostellate cells

DIFFERENTIAL DIAGNOSIS

Pituitary Adenoma

- Late childhood to adulthood
  - Only rare ACTH cell adenomas in infancy
- Monomorphous
- Lack Rathke epithelium and primitive elements

Immature Teratoma

- All 3 germ cell layers represented

SELECTED REFERENCES

1. de Kock L et al: Pituitary blastoma: a pathognomonic feature of germ-line DICER1 mutations. Acta Neuropathol. 128(1):111-22, 2014
2. Sahakitrungruang T et al: Germline and somatic DICER1 mutations in a pituitary blastoma causing infantile-onset Cushing's disease. J Clin Endocrinol Metab. 99(8):E1487-92, 2014
3. Schultz KA et al: *DICER1*-pleuropulmonary blastoma familial tumor predisposition syndrome: a unique constellation of neoplastic conditions. Pathol Case Rev. 19(2):90-100, 2014
4. Scheithauer BW et al: Pituitary blastoma: a unique embryonal tumor. Pituitary. 15(3):365-73, 2012

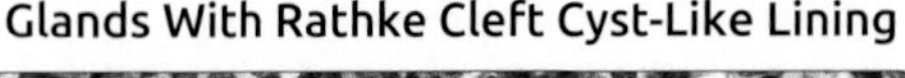

Glands With Rathke Cleft Cyst-Like Lining

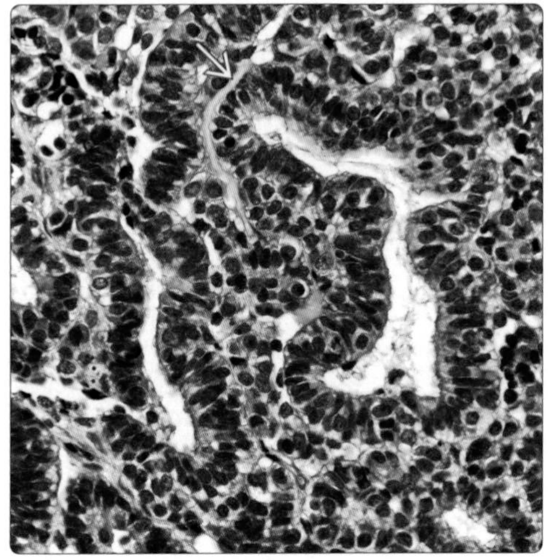

Brisk Mitotic Activity

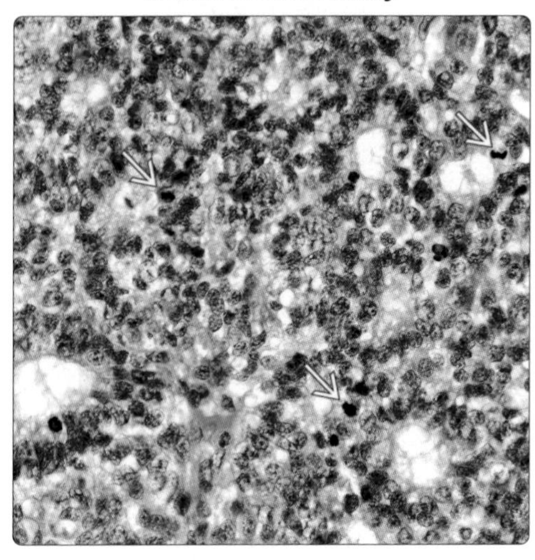

(Left) *Larger glandular structures → are separated by a compact, nonglandular component. The epithelium resembles that of Rathke cleft cyst but is more cytologically atypical and more mitotically active. The Ki-67 rate is high as well.* **(Right)** *An occasional tumor shows brisk mitotic activity →. The latter has ranged from 0-16/10 HPF among reported examples.*

Necrosis Possible

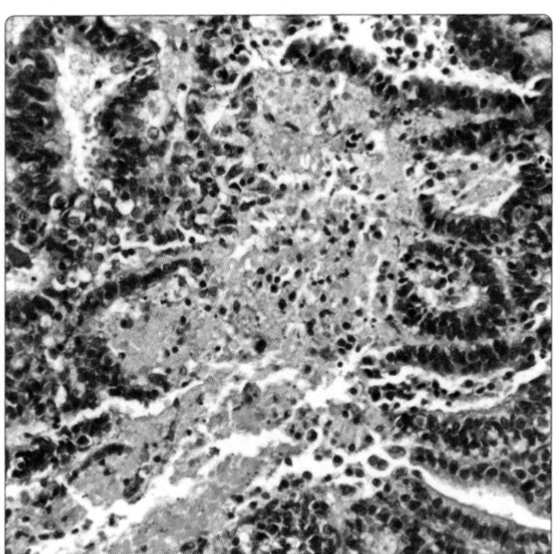

Rare Goblet Cell Transformation

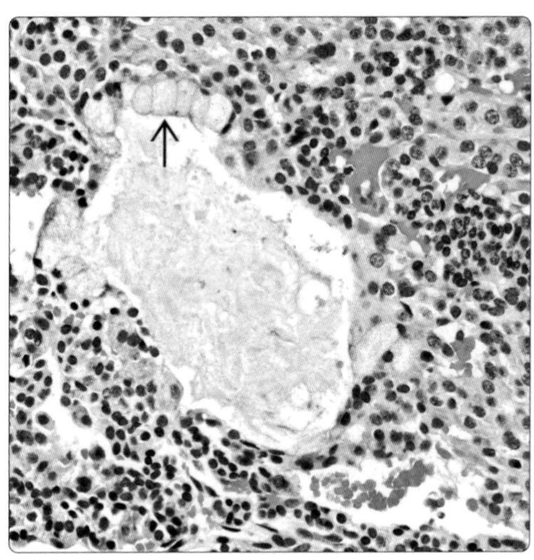

(Left) *Necrosis may be present in accord with mitotic activity of some lesions. The possibility of a malignant germ cell tumor could be entertained and appropriate immunostains applied.* **(Right)** *A rare feature of pituitary blastomas is focal goblet cell transformation → within larger glands that resembles Rathke cleft cyst epithelium.*

Reticulin Outlines Clusters of Epithelial Cells

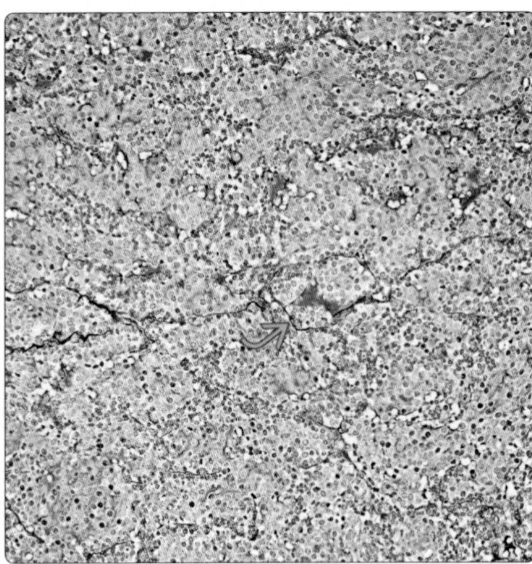

Synaptophysin (+) Secretory Cells

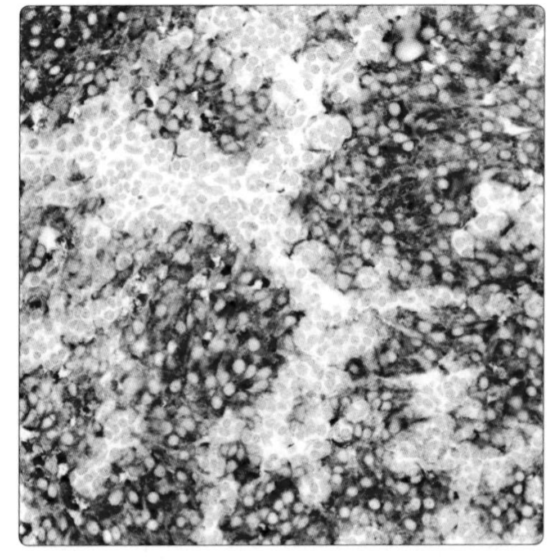

(Left) *Reticulin shows a positivity mainly around clusters of epithelial cells →.* **(Right)** *Zones of secretory cells are immunoreactive for synaptophysin. The Rathke-like epithelium (not shown) would be negative.*

Pancytokeratin (+) Glandular Epithelium

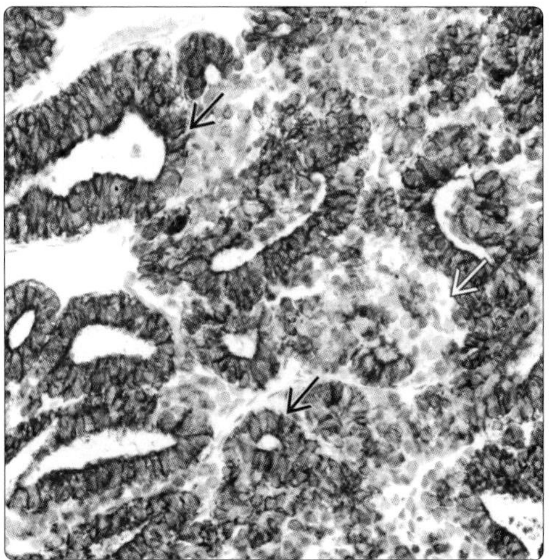

Annexin (+) Suggesting Folliculostellate Cell Differentiation

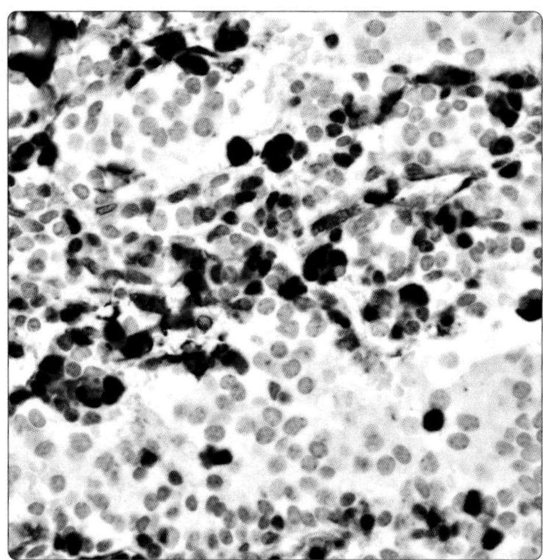

(Left) *Glandular epithelial cells resembling Rathke epithelium are immunoreactive for pankeratins* ⇒. *Intervening secretory cells* ➡ *are negative.* **(Right)** *Annexin-1 positivity, mainly in small glands and in blastema-like cells, suggests folliculostellate cell differentiation in the nonepithelial component of this very rare entity.*

ACTH(+), Secretory With Neuroendocrine Cells

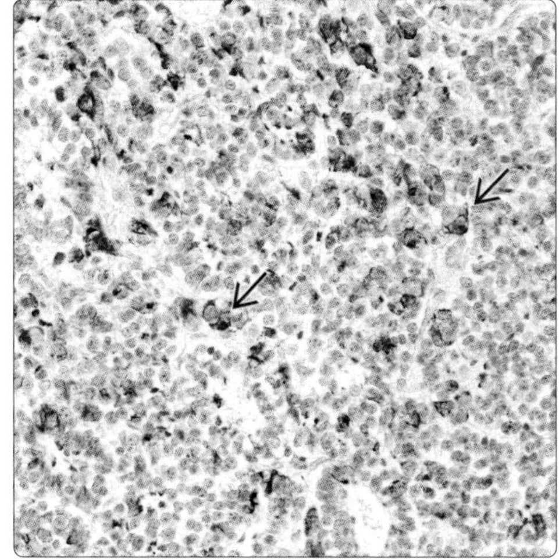

Ki-67, Highest in Glandular Epithelium

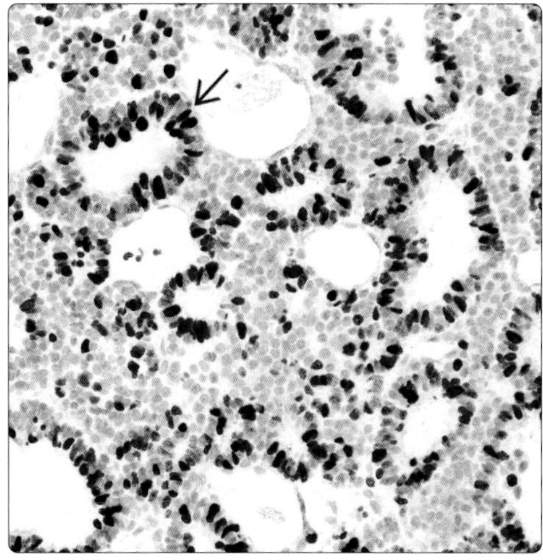

(Left) *Secretory and neuroendocrine cells are weakly immunoreactive for ACTH* ⇒. **(Right)** *Ki-67 labeling index varies considerably, ranging from low to as high as 60%. Labeling indices are highest in glandular cells* ⇒.

Folliculostellate Cells

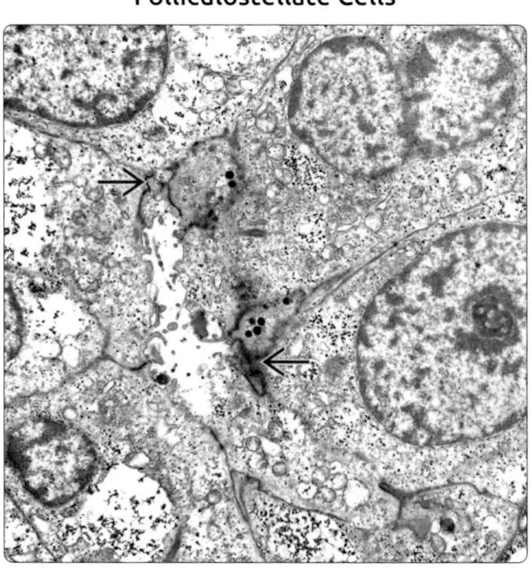

Corticotroph Cell

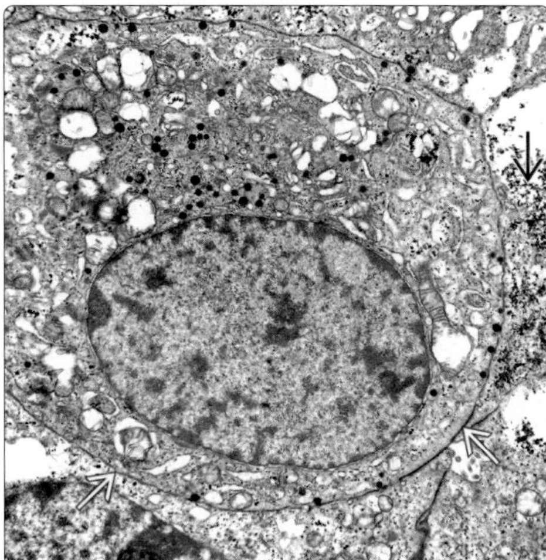

(Left) *A follicle composed of folliculostellate cells is shown. Note the intercellular junctions* ⇒ *between these relatively undifferentiated cells.* **(Right)** *Electron micrograph depicts small, glycogen-rich undifferentiated cells* ⇒, *as well as a large, granulated corticotroph cell* ➡.

Secondary Neoplasms of the Pituitary and Sellar Region

KEY FACTS

TERMINOLOGY

- Tumors with nonpituitary origin involving pituitary gland via hematogenous spread or direct sellar extension

CLINICAL ISSUES

- Affects older adults
- Carcinoma of breast and lung are the most frequent primary tumors
- Mostly starts from sellar bony structures
  - Extends to posterior lobe
- Obvious evidence of systemic malignancy
- Visual field disturbance (ophthalmoplegia, ptosis)
- Diabetes insipidus
- Hyperprolactinemia due to stalk compression effect
- Prognosis poor
  - Survival < 1 year

IMAGING

- Metastasis suggested by irregular destruction of bone

MACROSCOPIC

- Grossly inapparent in general

MICROSCOPIC

- Microscopic features typically those of primary tumor
- 2 patterns of anterior lobe involvement
  - Filling of sinusoids
  - Replacement of secretory cells in somewhat expanded acini
- Vascular invasion

TOP DIFFERENTIAL DIAGNOSES

- Pituitary carcinoma
- Meningioma

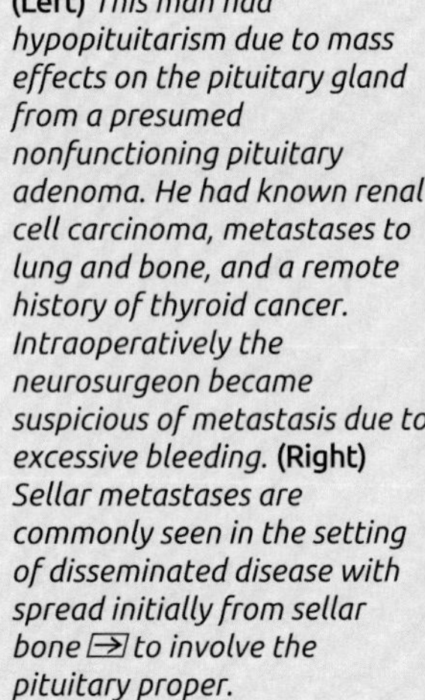

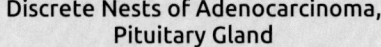

(Left) *This man had hypopituitarism due to mass effects on the pituitary gland from a presumed nonfunctioning pituitary adenoma. He had known renal cell carcinoma, metastases to lung and bone, and a remote history of thyroid cancer. Intraoperatively the neurosurgeon became suspicious of metastasis due to excessive bleeding.* **(Right)** *Sellar metastases are commonly seen in the setting of disseminated disease with spread initially from sellar bone* → *to involve the pituitary proper.*

Metastatic Thyroid Carcinoma Simulating Adenoma

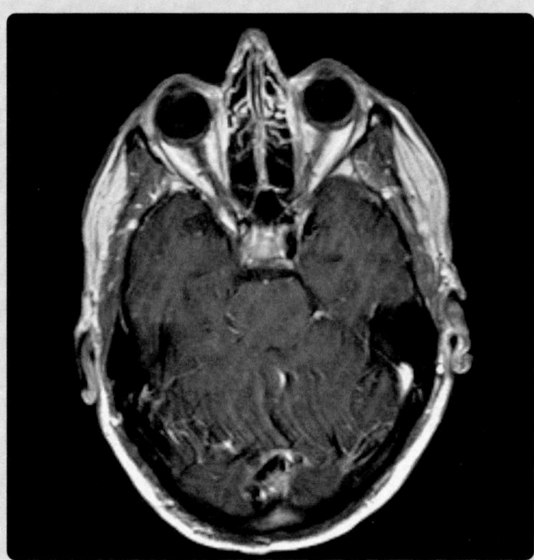

Metastatic Disease, Sellar Bone

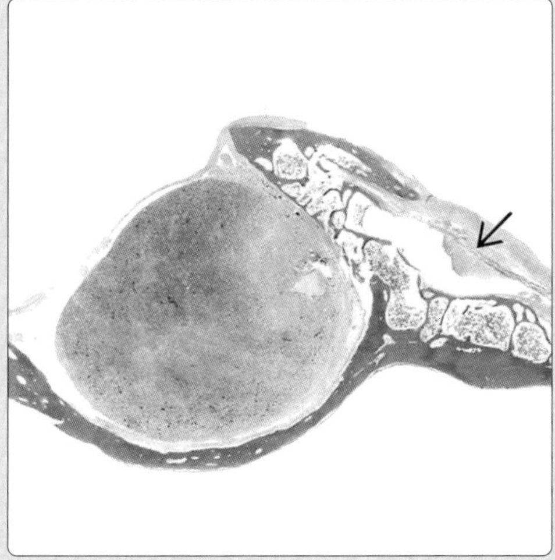

(Left) *This patient had invasive adenocarcinoma of the lung involving left lower lobe and left upper lobe and at autopsy was found to have widespread metastatic leptomeningeal carcinoma (meningeal carcinomatosis) with microfoci of tumor in numerous sites, including pituitary gland* →*. Note the assortment of cell types in the normal anterior gland.* **(Right)** *Metastatic tumor cells fill adenohypophyseal sinusoids* → *in this case, intimately admixed with normal cells. Normal pituitary cells are bright pink.*

Discrete Nests of Adenocarcinoma, Pituitary Gland

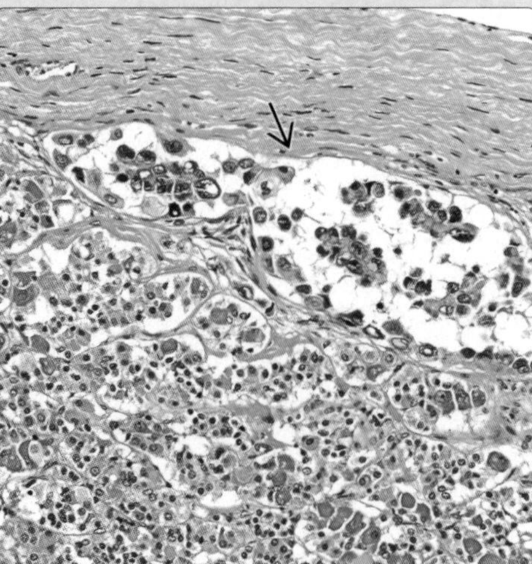

Metastatic Cells Filling Pituitary Acinus

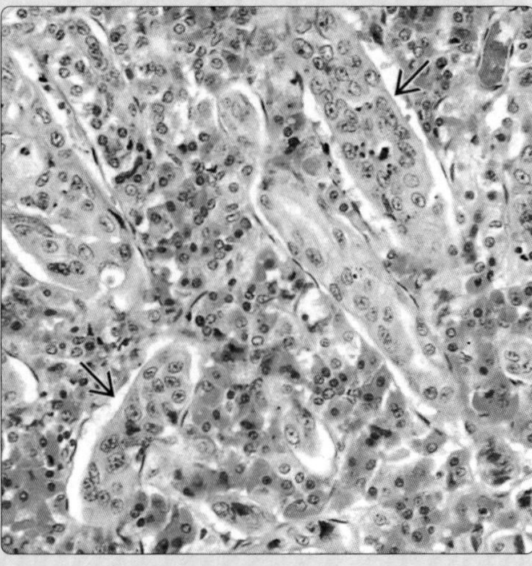

TERMINOLOGY

Synonyms

- Metastatic tumor

Definitions

- Tumors with nonpituitary origin involving pituitary and sellar organs via hematogenous spread or direct sellar extension

ETIOLOGY/PATHOGENESIS

Involvement of Sellar Organs by Malignant Tumor

- Most pituitary involvement is secondary spread from adjacent bony or dural deposit
- From sellar bony structures, tumor extends to posterior lobe
- Extension from posterior to anterior lobe by direct spread via short portal vessels
  - Or via long portal vessels originating in hypothalamus
- Diffuse spread in hematogenous malignancies
  - Lymphoma, leukemia
- Most common tumor types to metastasize to pituitary
  - Breast, lung

CLINICAL ISSUES

Epidemiology

- Incidence
  - Secondary involvement of sellar region
    - In ~ 25% of cancer patients
  - Hematopoietic tumors far more often secondary than primary in sella
  - Overall rare condition
    - 1 study showed incidence of pituitary metastases among all intracranial metastases was < 1%
    - Pituitary metastases among all autopsied cancer cases is 11-12%
- Age
  - Middle-aged or elderly
- Sex
  - F > M

Site

- Primary tumor
  - Female patients
    - Breast (65%)
    - Lung (15%)
    - Stomach (10%)
  - Male patients
    - Lung (65%)
    - Prostate (10%)
    - Bladder (5%)
- Metastasis
  - Most extensions from sellar bony structures, extends to posterior lobe
  - Hematologic spread
    - More often to posterior lobe (45%) (direct arterial supply) than anterior lobe (20%) (indirect portal blood supply)
      - Both lobes involved in 30% of cases
      - Pituitary stalk capsule involved in 10% of cases
  - Hypothalamic involvement more often due to extension from sellar bone than direct metastasis

Presentation

- Obvious evidence of systemic malignancy
  - Metastases in terminal phase
  - Occasionally occur with no prior history of malignancy
  - Pituitary symptoms usually overshadowed by manifestations of generalized disease
- Visual field disturbance
  - Ophthalmoplegia, ptosis
  - Results of cavernous sinus involvement
  - Rapid development of cranial neuropathies more suggestive of secondary disease than of pituitary adenoma
- Diabetes insipidus most frequent endocrinopathy
- Hyperprolactinemia due to stalk compression
- Hypopituitarism rare
- Pituitary adenomas rarely recipients of metastases
  - Result in rapid worsening of mass effects

Treatment

- Surgical decompression ± radiotherapy possibly beneficial

Prognosis

- Metastatic tumor involvement of sella occurs late
  - Prognosis poor
    - Survival < 1 year

IMAGING

MR Findings

- Enhancing sellar mass
- Involvement in pituitary stalk by invasion rather than by displacement as seen in pituitary adenoma

CT Findings

- Metastasis suggested by irregular destruction of bone
  - In comparison, large pituitary adenomas tend to symmetrically expand and remodel bone

MACROSCOPIC

General Features

- Direct invasion from adjacent structures
- Tumor usually emanates from sellar bone/dura
- Most metastases to pituitary gland grossly inapparent
  - Metastases often firm in texture due to accompanying fibrosis
- Carcinomas may form expanding masses

MICROSCOPIC

Histologic Features

- Microscopic features typically those of primary tumor
- 2 patterns of anterior lobe involvement
  - Sinusoidal filling
  - Replacement of secretory cells in somewhat expanded acini

Lymphatic/Vascular Invasion

- Vascular invasion may be prominent

ANCILLARY TESTS

Immunohistochemistry

- Many tumors with distinctive profiles
  - In carcinomas of a variety of sites
    - Keratin, EMA, and CEA (+)
  - In mammary carcinoma
    - Estrogen, progesterone, and HER-2 NEU expression
  - Thyroid and lung
    - TTF-1(+)
  - Prostate
    - Prostate-specific antigen and prostatic acid phosphatase (+)
  - Enteric carcinoma, particularly colon
    - CD1a(+)
  - Neuroendocrine carcinomas
    - Chromogranin and synaptophysin (+)
  - Common hematopoietic tumors
    - LCA, CD20, CD3, and monotypic immunoglobulin light chain (+)

DIFFERENTIAL DIAGNOSIS

Pituitary Carcinoma

- Histologic anaplasia not severe
- Synaptophysin (+)
  - Pituitary hormones may be (+)

Meningioma

- Presentation with hypopituitarism or diabetes insipidus
- Basal cranial or sellar diaphragm is tumor source
  - Pituitary stalk compression
  - Intrasellar extension

DIAGNOSTIC CHECKLIST

Clinically Relevant Pathologic Features

- Most patients with sellar region metastasis have known systemic malignancy
- Rare patients reported with 1st clinical presentation as sellar region metastasis
- Hyperprolactinemia can occur secondary to stalk compression effect
- Prognosis is generally poor with sellar region metastasis

SELECTED REFERENCES

1. Fortunati N et al: Pituitary lesions in breast cancer patients: A report of three cases. Oncol Lett. 9(6):2762-2766, 2015
2. Habu M et al: Pituitary metastases: current practice in Japan. J Neurosurg. 1-10, 2015
3. He W et al: Metastatic involvement of the pituitary gland: a systematic review with pooled individual patient data analysis. Pituitary. 18(1):159-68, 2015
4. Shah N et al: An unusual initial presentation of hepatocellular carcinoma as a sellar mass. J Nat Sci Biol Med. 6(2):471-4, 2015
5. Al-Aridi R et al: Clinical and biochemical characteristic features of metastatic cancer to the sella turcica: an analytical review. Pituitary. 17(6):575-87, 2014
6. Dropcho EJ: Neurologic complications of lung cancer. Handb Clin Neurol. 119:335-61, 2014
7. Gormally JF et al: Pituitary metastasis from breast cancer presenting as diabetes insipidus. BMJ Case Rep. 2014, 2014
8. Magnoli F et al: Renal cell carcinoma metastatic to a pituitary FSH/LH adenoma: case report and review of the literature. Ultrastruct Pathol. 38(6):430-7, 2014
9. Sogani J et al: Sellar collision tumor involving metastatic lung cancer and pituitary adenoma: radiologic-pathologic correlation and review of the literature. Clin Imaging. 38(3):318-21, 2014
10. Thewjitcharoen Y et al: Colorectal cancer manifesting with metastasis to prolactinoma: report of a case involving symptoms mimicking pituitary apoplexy. Intern Med. 53(17):1965-9, 2014
11. Ariel D et al: Clinical characteristics and pituitary dysfunction in patients with metastatic cancer to the sella. Endocr Pract. 19(6):914-9, 2013
12. Besic N et al: Sites of metastases of anaplastic thyroid carcinoma: autopsy findings in 45 cases from a single institution. Thyroid. 23(6):709-13, 2013
13. Chikani V et al: Pituitary metastases from papillary carcinoma of thyroid: a case report and literature review. Endocrinol Diabetes Metab Case Rep. 2013:130024, 2013
14. Ithimakin S et al: Pituitary metastasis from renal cell carcinoma: a case report with literature review. J Med Assoc Thai. 96 Suppl 2:S257-61, 2013
15. Masui K et al: Pituitary apoplexy caused by hemorrhage from pituitary metastatic melanoma: case report. Neurol Med Chir (Tokyo). 53(10):695-8, 2013
16. Ratti M et al: Pituitary gland metastasis from rectal cancer: report of a case and literature review. Springerplus. 2:467, 2013
17. Senetta R et al: Pituitary metastasis of an unknown neuroendocrine breast carcinoma mimicking a pituitary adenoma. Pathology. 45(4):422-4, 2013
18. McCutcheon IE et al: Metastatic melanoma to the pituitary gland. Can J Neurol Sci. 34(3):322-7, 2007
19. Branch CL Jr et al: Metastatic tumors of the sella turcica masquerading as primary pituitary tumors. J Clin Endocrinol Metab. 65(3):469-74, 1987
20. Juan D et al: Case report of vasopressin-responsive diabetes insipidus associated with chronic myelogenous leukemia. Cancer. 56(6):1468-9, 1985
21. Scheithauer BW: Pathology of the pituitary and sellar region: exclusive of pituitary adenoma. Pathol Annu. 20 Pt 1:67-155, 1985
22. Kimmel DW et al: Systemic cancer presenting as diabetes insipidus. Clinical and radiographic features of 11 patients with a review of metastatic-induced diabetes insipidus. Cancer. 52(12):2355-8, 1983

Metastatic Breast Carcinoma

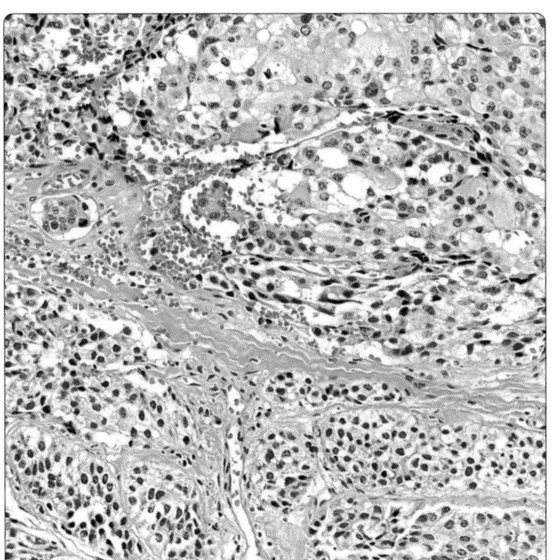

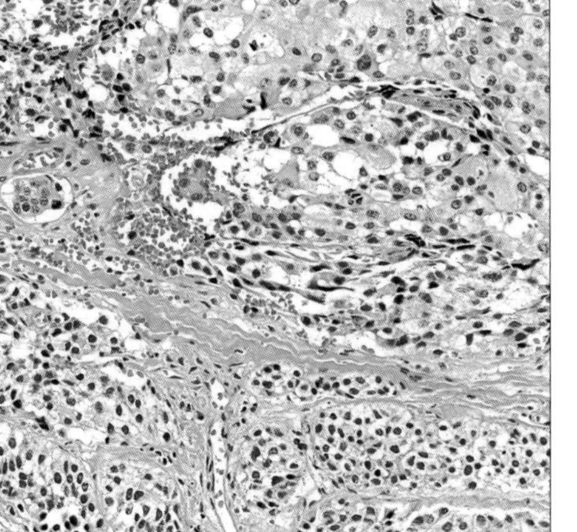

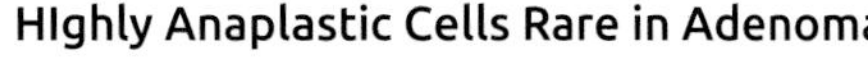

HIghly Anaplastic Cells Rare in Adenoma

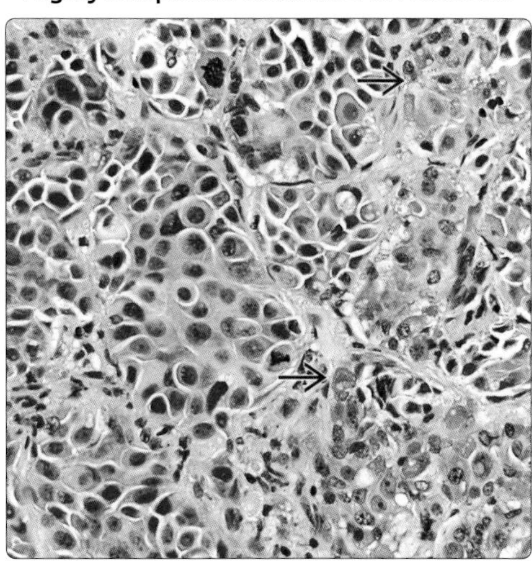

(Left) *Metastases to the pituitary gland, mammary carcinoma in this example, initially involve sellar bone and secondarily extend into the gland.* **(Right)** *Primary pituitary tumors, either benign or malignant, are almost never highly anaplastic. Anaplastic cells along with normal adenohypophyseal cells ➔ suggest secondary malignancy, as in this metastatic breast carcinoma.*

Mammaglobin (+) Metastatic Breast Carcinoma

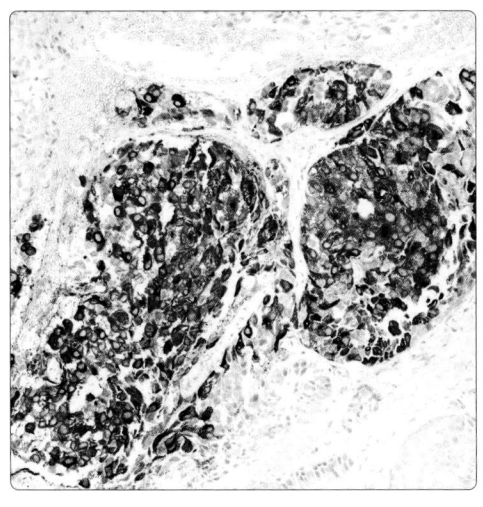

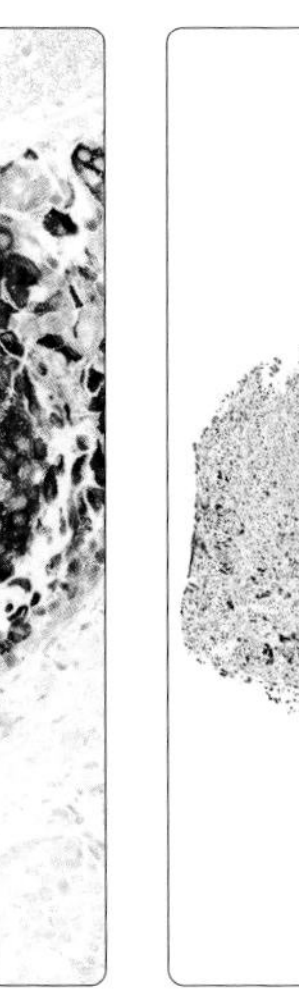

ACTH(+) Residual Normal Pituitary Cells

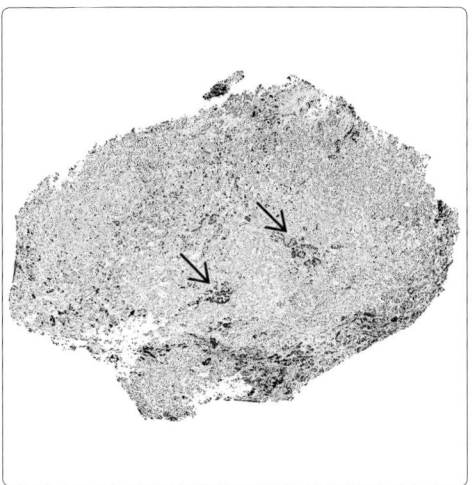

(Left) *Malignant tumor cells in metastatic breast carcinoma are immunoreactive for mammaglobin protein.* **(Right)** *Remaining normal ACTH immunoreactive corticotrophs ➔ are overrun by metastatic cells of breast carcinoma.*

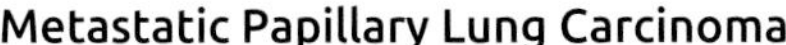

Metastatic Papillary Lung Carcinoma

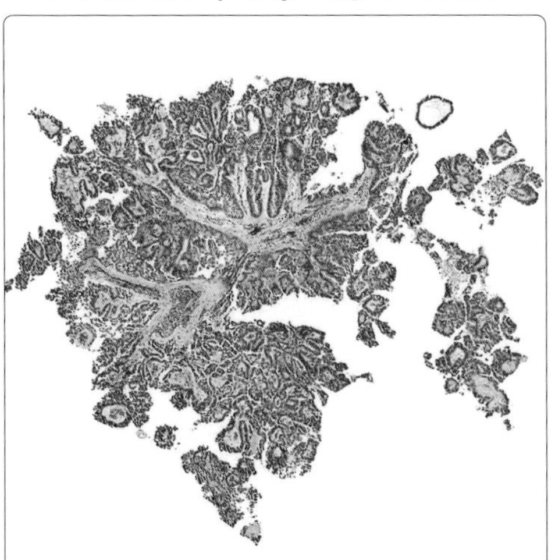

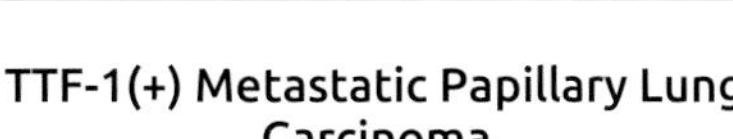

TTF-1(+) Metastatic Papillary Lung Carcinoma

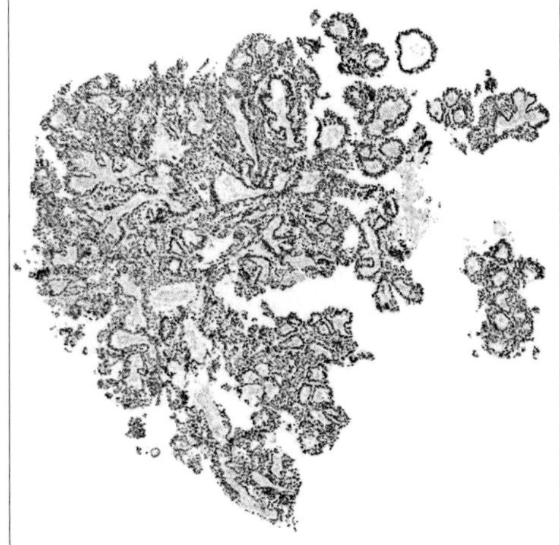

(Left) *A papillary lung carcinoma metastasized to the pituitary. In most cases, patients are known to have an extracranial primary. It is rare for a pituitary metastasis to be the initial presentation of systemic cancer, as it was in this case.* **(Right)** *Immunoreactivity for TTF-1 supports the diagnosis of metastatic lung cancer in this papillary intrasellar mass.*

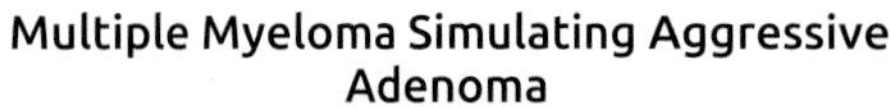

Multiple Myeloma Simulating Aggressive Adenoma

Myeloma Plasmacytoid Cells

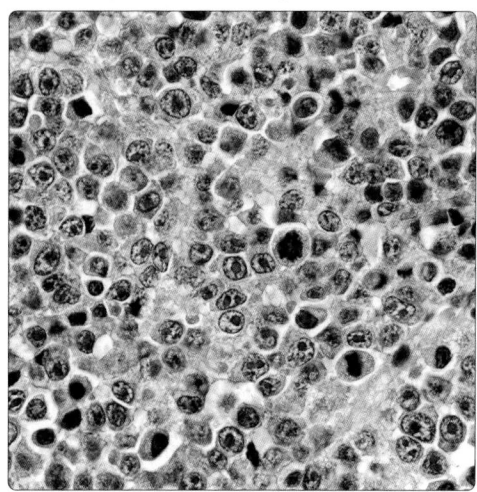

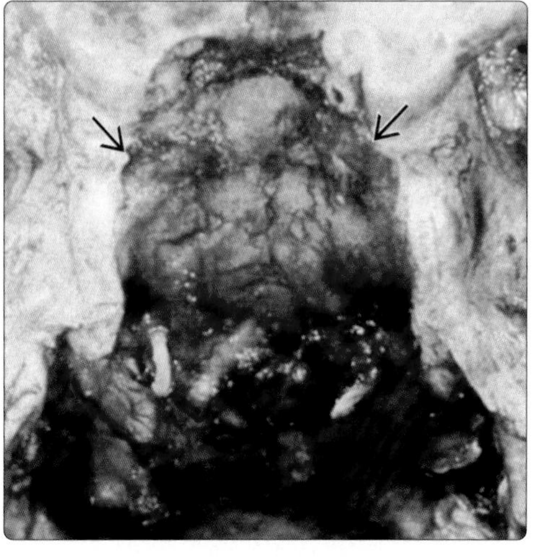

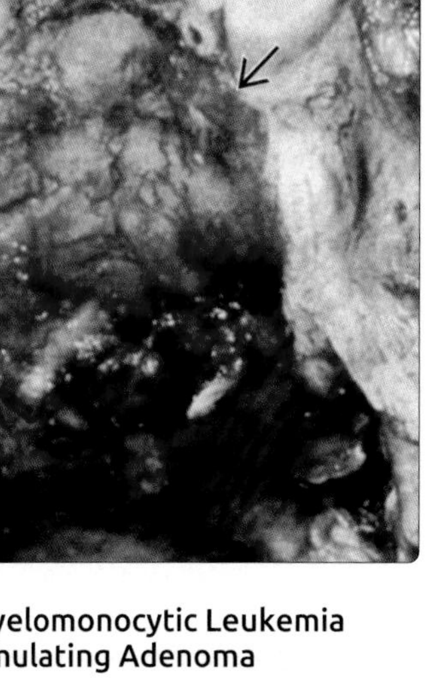

(Left) *Multiple myeloma presented as a pituitary mass* → *that was thought clinically to be an aggressive pituitary adenoma.* **(Right)** *Dyscohesive, mitotically active, and obviously plasmacytoid cells comprise myeloma of the pituitary region. In plasmacytoma the differential should include prolactinoma, which can have distinctively plasmacytoid features, including prominent nucleoli.*

Acute Myelomonocytic Leukemia Simulating Adenoma

Metastatic Small Cell Carcinoma

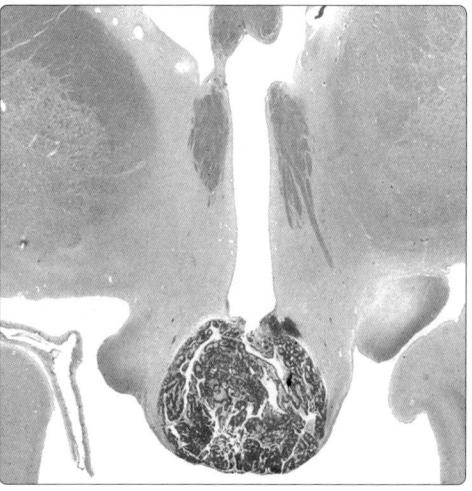

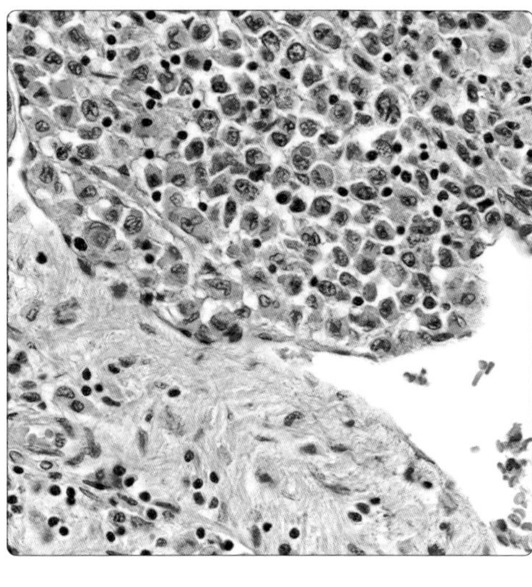

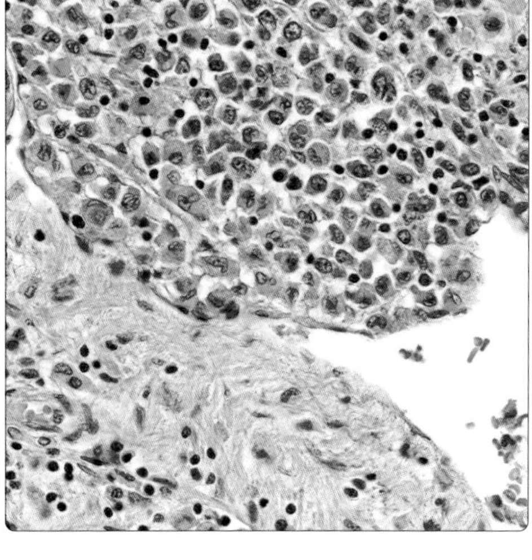

(Left) *Acute myelomonocytic leukemia has dyscohesive tumor cells that could be mistaken for those of an adenoma.* **(Right)** *In this coronal whole-mount section, metastatic small cell carcinoma involves the hypothalamus posterior to the chiasm. Although infrequent, this is a classic pattern of metastatic spread. The patient's pituitary showed remarkable corticotroph cell hyperplasia as a result of the lesion's release of corticotrophin-releasing hormones.*

Anaplastic Astrocytoma Extending Into Sella

Anaplastic Astrocytoma Extending Into Pituitary Gland

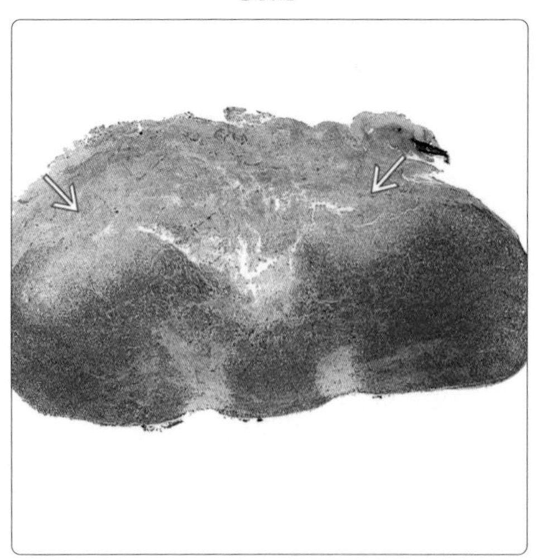

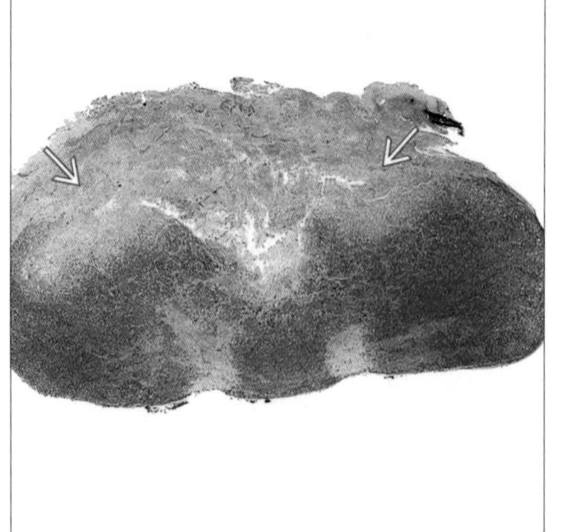

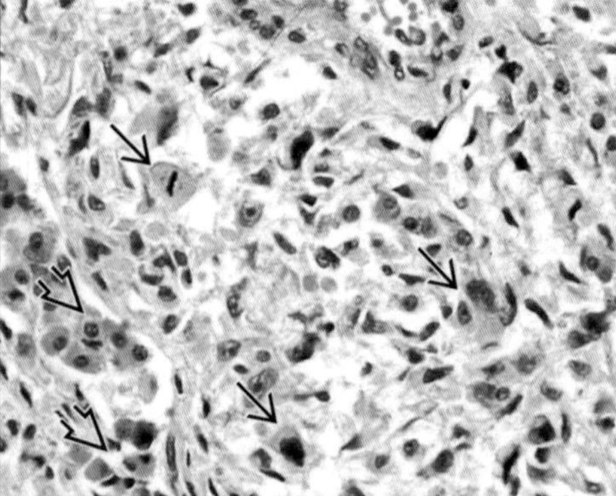

(Left) *Anaplastic astrocytoma of hypothalamus may undergo sellar extension to involve pituitary gland. In this case, the lighter staining tumor* ➔ *extends from posterior lobe into the darker staining adenohypophysis.* **(Right)** *Astrocytic cells* → *from a hypothalamic anaplastic astrocytoma intermingle with more eosinophilic, better circumscribed cells of the normal gland* ⇒*.*

Autopsy, Metastasis to Pituitary

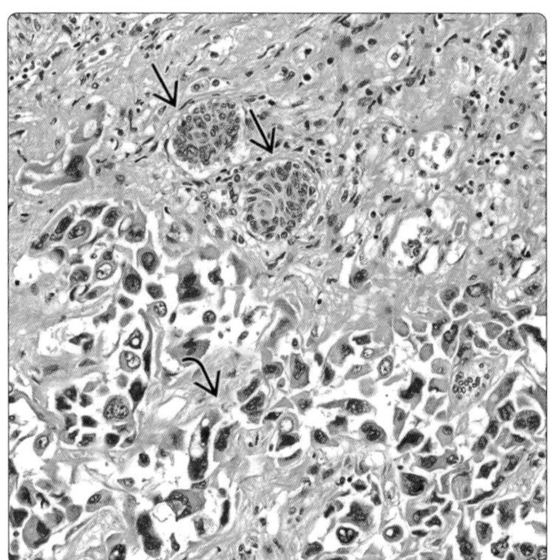

Pars Tuberalis, Normal

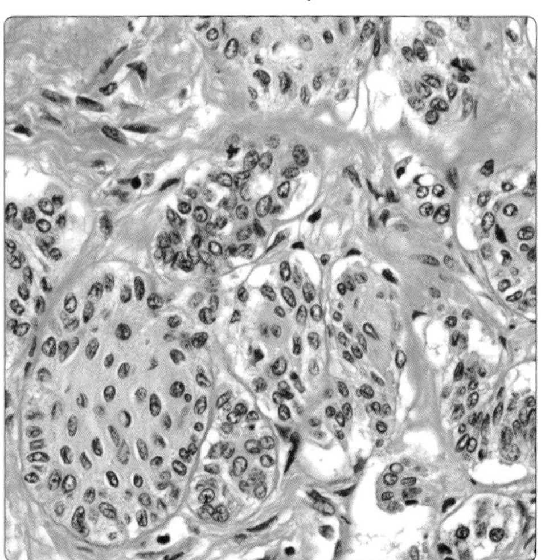

(Left) *Normal pituitary gland pars tuberalis contains nests of cells with squamous metaplasia ➙, and these should not be mistaken for metastatic tumor. Contrast the benign appearance of these cells with the invasive lung adenocarcinoma cells nearby ➙.* **(Right)** *Normal pituitary gland pars tuberalis contains nests of pituitary cells that can undergo squamous metaplasia. These should not be mistaken for a metastasis at time of autopsy or biopsy.*

Metastasis, Severe Cytological Atypia

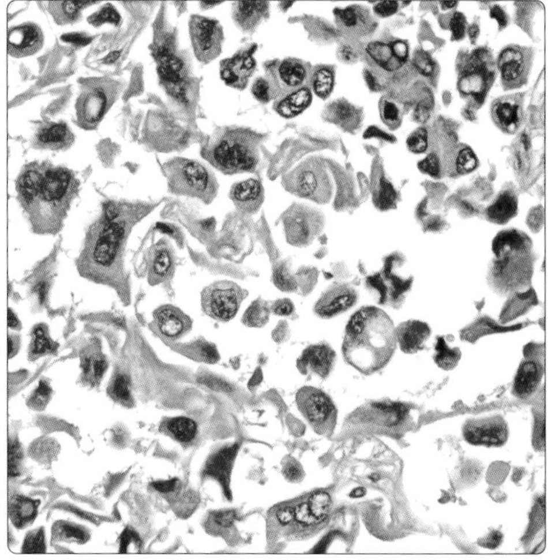

Smear, Metastatic Thyroid Carcinoma

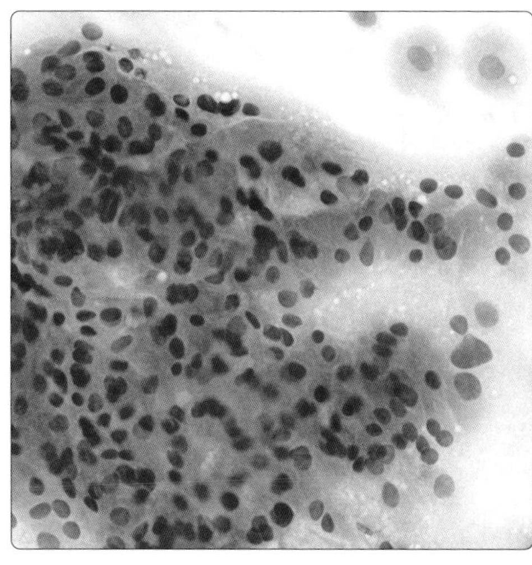

(Left) *Invasive adenocarcinoma of the lung in this case not only caused leptomeningeal carcinomatosis at autopsy, but also produced metastatic deposits in the pituitary gland. This degree of cytologically atypia is almost never seen in pituitary adenomas.* **(Right)** *This intraoperative smear preparation from a patient with metastatic follicular thyroid carcinoma to the pituitary gland simulating adenoma shows significant cohesiveness of cells.*

Metastatic Thyroid Carcinoma, Pituitary Gland

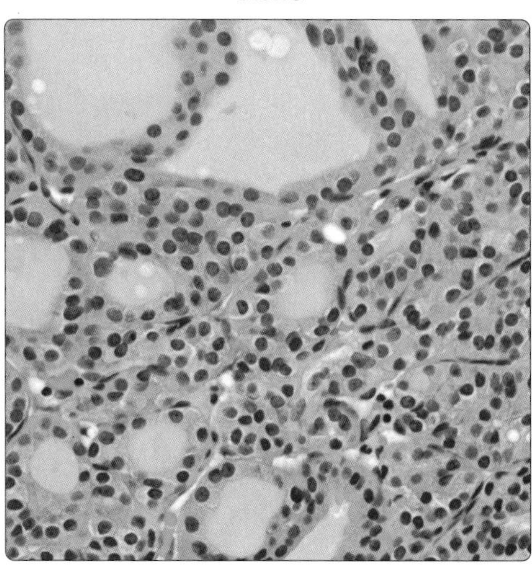

TTF-1(+) Metastatic Thyroid Carcinoma

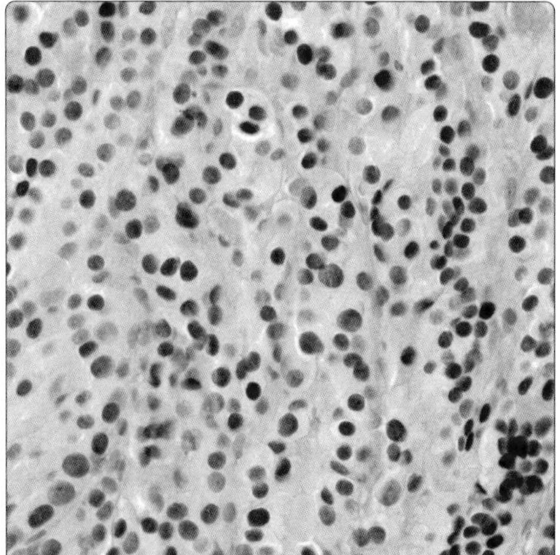

(Left) *This metastasis to the pituitary gland was from thyroid carcinoma. Endocrine metastases to the pituitary gland, like pituitary adenomas, may show relative nuclear monotony, minimal pleomorphism, absence of necrosis, and lack of brisk mitotic activity.* **(Right)** *Although several sellar region masses manifest TTF-1 IHC(+), including pituicytoma, spindle cell oncocytoma, granular cell tumor of infundibulum, and even normal posterior pituitary gland, TTF-1(+) is also seen in some metastatic cancers.*

PART I
SECTION 3

Meninges

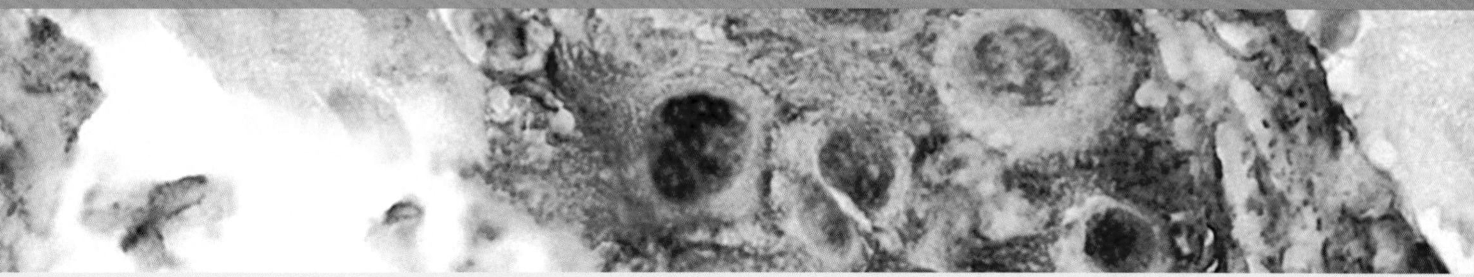

Meningioma

KEY FACTS

ETIOLOGY/PATHOGENESIS

- Most sporadic, few after irradiation, rare tumors associated with neurofibromatosis 2 (NF2), schwannomatosis
- Clear cell meningiomas seen in germline mutations of *SMARCE1*

CLINICAL ISSUES

- Peak: 65-75 years
- Located throughout CNS
- Recurrence risk increases with grade and incomplete resection

IMAGING

- Intensely enhancing with extension along dura (dural tail)
- Peritumoral edema may be seen with grade II or III, secretory, or adherent microcystic subtype

MICROSCOPIC

- Grading based on histological subtype, brain invasion, mitotic rate, or algorithm using 5 histological features

ANCILLARY TESTS

- EMA(+) (may be weak or focal), SSTR2A(+), dual E-cadherin/D2-40(+), vimentin (+), cytokeratin (±), S100(±)
  - SSTR2A (somatostatin receptor 2a) is more sensitive diagnostic marker than EMA
  - Dual IHC(+) for D2-40, E-cadherin in most meningiomas, even atypical, anaplastic
- Monosomy 22 or Ch22q deletions most frequent genetic abnormality, usually involving deletion *NF2* gene
  - More common in fibroblastic, transitional, and psammomatous types (80%) than in meningothelial (25%); mutations in genes *TRAF7*, *KLF4*, *AKT1*, *SMO* in other subtypes
- Unlike SFT/hemangiopericytoma, negative for STAT6 nuclear IHC(+)

DIAGNOSTIC CHECKLIST

- Anaplastic meningiomas often cytokeratin (+), can be confused with metastatic carcinoma

Dural Tail

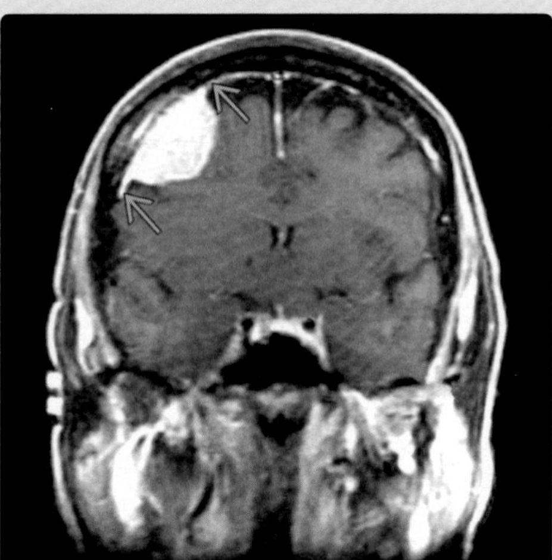

Smear, Whorls

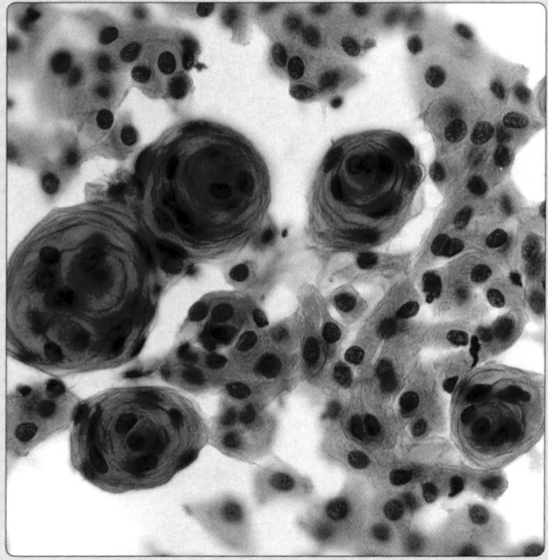

(Left) *Most meningiomas are homogeneously enhancing, discrete masses, with lateral extensions along the inner surface of the dura known as dural tails ⇨.* **(Right)** *Well-formed whorls in a cytologically bland tumor are unmistakable evidence of meningioma in smear preparations.*

D2-40 (Podoplanin) (+) Meningioma; E-Cadherin IHC(+) Meningioma

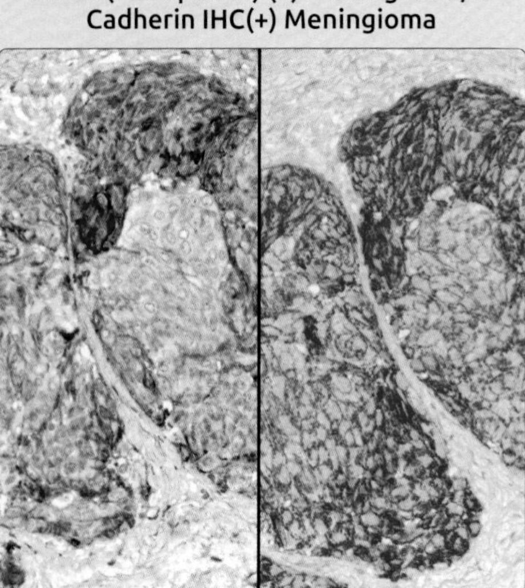

SSTR2A(+), Diffuse Membranous, Cytoplasmic

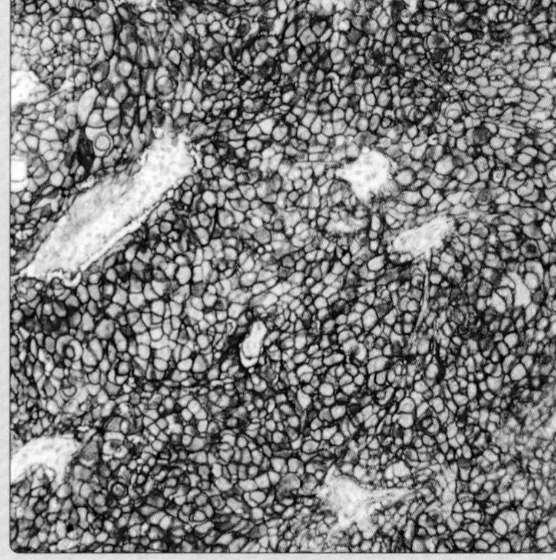

(Left) *D2-40 (podoplanin) (+) meningiomas have dual mesenchymal and epithelial features, and, thus, it is not surprising that they have dual immunoreactivity for D2-40 and E-cadherin. Many tumor types are immunoreactive for one or the other but not both. This paired IHC(+) can be helpful in cases with weak or negligible EMA IHC.* **(Right)** *Diffuse membranous and cytoplasmic immunoreactivity for somatostatin receptor 2a has been shown to be a more sensitive diagnostic marker of meningioma than EMA.*

TERMINOLOGY

Definitions

- Neoplasm arising from meningothelial (arachnoid) cells, usually dural based
- WHO grade I, II (atypical), or III (anaplastic)

ETIOLOGY/PATHOGENESIS

Environmental Exposure

- Radiation
  - Survivors of childhood leukemia and brain tumors, often interval of decade or more

Other Risk Factors/Syndromes

- Neurofibromatosis 2 (NF2)
  - Multiple, potentially innumerable
  - Early onset, childhood
- Schwannomatosis
  - 5% of patients
  - *SMARCB1* germline mutation

CLINICAL ISSUES

Epidemiology

- Incidence
  - Common, ~ 30% of primary intracranial tumors
- Age
  - Peak: 65-75 years
    - Uncommon in children, often associated with NF2
- Sex
  - F:M = 2:1
    - Spinal, F:M ~ 10:1
  - In childhood, males preferentially affected
  - Equal gender in hereditary syndromes
  - In atypical and anaplastic tumors, M > F

Site

- Parasagittal, convexities, sphenoid ridge
  - Falcine tumors sometimes bilateral
- Posterior fossa (10%)
- Optic nerve sheath (uncommon)
- Intraventricular (uncommon)
- Spinal (10%)
  - Rare below thoracic level, then often clear cell type
- Ectopic: Intraosseous, scalp, sinuses, parotid, parapharyngeal space, mediastinum, lung, adrenal

Presentation

- Location dependent
  - Parasagittal: Headache, seizures, monoparesis of contralateral leg
  - Anterior falx: Headache, optic atrophy, personality changes
  - Frontal skull base: Impaired vision, headache, anosmia, mental changes
  - Lateral sphenoid wing: Painless unilateral exophthalmos, unilateral loss of vision and hearing
  - Optic nerve: Exophthalmos, monocular loss of vision
  - Spinal cord: Pain, Brown-Séquard syndrome

Natural History

- Grade I: Grows slowly and compresses adjacent structures
- Grade II: Variable, some recur or invade brain
- Grade III: Sarcoma-like; recur, invade, and may metastasize to lung, liver, bone, lymph nodes, etc.

Treatment

- Surgical approaches
  - Observation, when stable, especially if densely calcified
  - Gross total resection is treatment of choice
- Drugs
  - Limited efficacy in recurrent tumors
- Radiation
  - Most incompletely excised grade II tumors, all grade III tumors
  - Stereotactic radiosurgery (gamma knife) for critically located and skull base tumors

Prognosis

- Excellent for completely excised WHO grade I and II tumors
- Poor for grade III, anaplastic tumors
- Recurrence risk increases with grade and presence of residual tumor
- Skull base meningiomas often recur

IMAGING

MR Findings

- Isointense to gray matter on T1WI
- Isointense to cortex on T2WI (most cases)
  - Most CNS tumors hyperintense (i.e., bright)
- Hypointense, dark, fibrous type, due to collagen and calcium
- Intensely enhancing
  - Extension along dura (dural tail)
    - Most meningiomas but not specific
- Peritumoral edema
  - Common in
    - Grades II and III
    - Microcystic or other types attached to brain
    - Secretory type
- Macrocyst, in some cases, especially microcystic type

CT Findings

- Calcifications, highest incidence in spinal tumors
- Hyperostosis of adjacent skull but not spine

MACROSCOPIC

General Features

- Broad based, with dural attachment in most cases
  - Gritty, especially psammomatous spinal tumors
  - Sometimes gelatinous or cystic
- Solid, globular, circumscribed
  - Flat, plate-like (en plaque) variant
- Bilobed, dumbbell-shaped (falcine or tentorial)
- Atypical and anaplastic types often attached to brain, infrequent in grade I except for microcystic subtype
- Fibrous types especially smooth surfaced
- Microcystic types
  - Macrocystic in minority of cases

- Often attached to edematous brain
- Sometimes embedded in brain
- Adjacent skull often thickened
  - ± tumor invasion
- Invasion of superior sagittal sinus with parasagittal tumors

MICROSCOPIC

Histologic Features

- Borders
  - With brain
    - Generally sharp, pushing
    - Perivascular extension difficult to distinguish from true invasion in random sections
    - Cortical invasion, grade II (and III)
  - With bone, soft tissues
    - Even grade I meningiomas often infiltrate skull but rarely spine
    - Associated hyperostosis, not osteolysis
- Meningothelial subtype
  - Lobules of cells with ample cytoplasm and indistinct borders (syncytia)
  - Nuclear pseudoinclusions (cytoplasmic invaginations)
  - Homogeneous light-gray nuclei
- Fibrous (fibroblastic)
  - Spindle-shaped cells in fascicles
  - Variable collagen and reticulin content
  - Linear stromal calcifications
- Transitional
  - Mixed meningothelial and fibrous features
  - Whorls and psammoma bodies common
- Psammomatous
  - Abundant psammoma bodies
    - Few meningothelial cells in some cases
- Angiomatous
  - Innumerable blood vessels
    - Large, thick blood vessels mimic vascular malformation; small vessels mimic hemangioblastoma
- Microcystic
  - Broad attachment to brain (common)
  - Loose texture, intercellular spaces
  - Foci of classical meningioma patterns present or not
  - Foamy cells
  - Nuclear pleomorphism, scattered cells, mimic hemangioblastoma
  - Thickened, hyalinized vessels
- Secretory
  - Pseudopsammoma bodies in meningothelial cells
    - Small, eosinophilic spheres
    - Sometimes multiple per cell
- Lymphoplasmacyte rich
  - Classic meningioma with abundant chronic inflammation
  - Plasma cells with Russell bodies
- Metaplastic
  - Not single histologic type
  - Lipomatous, xanthomatous, cartilaginous, myxoid, osseous
    - Lipomatous closely resembles normal adipose tissue
- Chordoid, grade II
  - Epithelial, chordoma-like formations
  - Percentage of chordoid component required unclear but more than just focal
    - May increase in percentage with multiple recurrences
  - Rarely pure, usually associated with conventional meningioma
- Clear cell, grade II
  - Monomorphous
  - Clear, glycogen-rich, PAS(+) cytoplasm
  - Often exists in pure form
  - Collagen blocks obliterate pattern with time
  - Few if any whorls, no psammoma bodies or nuclear inclusions
- Rhabdoid, grade III
  - Rhabdoid cells
    - Eccentric nuclei, prominent nucleoli
  - Eosinophilic cytoplasmic paranuclear whorl
  - Increased mitoses and Ki-67 index
  - Rarely pure, usually associated with conventional meningioma
  - Significance of rhabdoid features in absence of concomitant atypia and mitoses unclear
    - May not be prognostically adverse
  - Percent rhabdoid component required unclear but more than focal
  - Sometimes associated with papillary features
- Papillary, grade III
  - Perivascular pseudorosettes
  - Rarely pure, usually associated with atypical meningioma element
  - Sometimes associated with rhabdoid features
- Rare tissue patterns
  - Oncocytic (mitochondrion rich)
    - Granular cytoplasm
  - Meningioma with meningioangiomatosis
    - Usually children or young adults
    - Perivascular proliferation of elongated, fibroblast-like cells and meningothelial cells
    - May mimic brain invasion and thus meningioma grade II
    - Trapped islands of cortex with preserved ganglion cells; neurofibrillary tangles in some; psammoma bodies
  - Epithelioid
    - Cords or small lobules resembling glandular differentiation (rare)
    - Secretory subtype
  - Metastasis to meningioma
    - Breast carcinoma most common
- Miscellaneous features
  - Vascular invasion of no prognostic significance
    - Dural venous sinuses, especially superior sagittal, are common
  - Systemic metastases
    - Usually grade III, but "benign metastasizing meningioma" reported
    - Lung most common site
    - Other sites: Liver, lymph nodes, bone
  - Postembolization, intravascular embolic material
    - Increased perinecrotic, mitoses, and Ki-67
  - Dural tail on imaging

- Clustered vessels or tumor
- Petaloid, tyrosine-rich crystals
- Mitoses
  - ≤ 3 mitoses per 10 HPF: Grade I
  - ≥ 4 mitoses per 10 HPF: Grade II
  - ≥ 20 mitoses per 10 HPF: Grade III
  - Mitoses increased around foci of embolic necrosis

ANCILLARY TESTS

Cytology

- Often more specific than frozen sections
  - Smears well: Tissue fragments and some individual cells
  - Whorls, psammoma bodies
  - Nuclear pseudoinclusions
  - Clear (washed out) chromatin
  - Linear cytoplasmic streaking
  - Degenerative atypia (in some cases)
  - Nucleoli
    - Small: Grade I
    - Larger: Some grades II and III
- Cellular elongation, fibrous type
- Nuclear pleomorphism and vacuolated tumor cells, microcystic variant
- Small cell change, some grade II types
- Pseudopsammoma bodies, secretory variant
- Short cords of cells in myxoid matrix, chordoid subtype
- Perivascular pseudorosettes, papillary subtype
- Rhabdoid phenotype, rhabdoid variant
- Mitoses in grades II and III

Immunohistochemistry

- EMA(+)
  - Almost all, but may be focal/weak (e.g., in fibrous type)
  - Membrane pattern
- Cytokeratins
  - CK18(+), in ~ 2/3 of cases
  - CK20(-)
  - Other CKs variably and focally (+)
  - Secretory type, routinely (+) in pseudopsammoma bodies, CK7, CK8, CK18, CK19, and AE1/AE3
- CEA
  - Secretory subtype (+) in and around pseudopsammoma bodies
- Steroid receptors
  - Progesterone receptors
    - Variable percentage of (+) cells, from none to almost all
    - (-) staining does not rule out meningioma
    - Less likely (+) in anaplastic types
  - Estrogen receptors
    - Usually (-)
- S100 variably (+)
  - Usually not strongly and diffusely, including nuclei, like schwannoma
- Vimentin (+) in almost all cases, little diagnostic value
- Ki-67
  - Considerable intra- and intertumoral variation
  - Grade I lesions usually ≤ 5%
  - No defined threshold for grade I vs. II or II vs. III
  - High in grade III
- Meningiomas have dual immunoreactivity for D2-40 (podoplanin) and E-cadherin
  - Many tumor types are immunoreactive for one or the other, but not both
  - Paired IHC(+) can be superior to EMA IHC, even in unusual meningioma subtypes
- Somatostatin receptor type IIA (SSTR2A)
  - Diffuse strong membranous, cytoplasmic immunoreactivity
  - May be superior to EMA IHC, even in unusual meningioma subtypes
- Unlike SFT/hemangiopericytoma, (-) for STAT6 nuclear IHC(+)

Genetic Testing

- LOH 22q12.2 (monosomy 22) most frequent abnormality
  - *NF2* gene near universal target of deletion
  - Occurs in 60-80% of cases
  - More common in fibroblastic, transitional, and psammomatous types (80%) than in meningothelial (25%)
  - Mutations in *TRAF7*, *KLF4*, *AKT1*, *SMO* identified in meningiomas lacking *NF2* alterations
  - Combined *TRAF7* and *KLF4* mutations characterize secretory type
  - Angiomatous meningiomas have distinct genetic profile, have multiple chromosomal polysomes, especially chromosomes 5, 13, 20
- Losses of 1p, 6q, 10, 14q, and 18q: Atypical or anaplastic types
  - Losses of 6q and 14q (e.g., *MEG3*, *NDRG2*) especially important
- Gains or amplifications of 1q, 9q, 12q, 15q, 17q, and 20q: Atypical or anaplastic types
- *TERT* promoter mutations associated with malignant progression
- Loss of 1p and 7p in radiation-induced tumors
- Germline mutations in *SMARCE1* identified as cause of multiple clear cell meningiomas
- 5% of individuals with schwannomatosis develop meningiomas through mutation of SWI/SNF chromatin remodeling complex subunit, *SMARCB1*

Electron Microscopy

- Interdigitating cell membranes
- Cytoplasmic intermediate filaments, vimentin
- Desmosomes
- Microlumina with microvilli (secretory subtype)
- Intracytoplasmic mass of intermediate filaments (rhabdoid subtype)

DIFFERENTIAL DIAGNOSIS

Meningothelial Hyperplasia

- Adjacent lesion prompting proliferation
  - Adjacent hemorrhage
  - Inflammation
    - Difficult distinction from lymphoplasmacytic meningioma (in some cases)
- Small, not large compact mass of meningothelial cells

Schwannoma

- Smears poorly
  - Tissue fragments only
    - Fascicular architecture
    - Club-shaped nuclei
- S100(+), EMA(-), SSTR2A(-)
- Collagen type IV (+), pericellular
- Reticulin (+), pericellular

Chordoma

- Midline
- Bone destruction
- Physaliphorous cells
- Brachyury (+), keratin (+), EMA(+)
- S100(±)

Hemangioblastoma

- Rare supratentorially
- No whorls or psammoma bodies
- Extensive reticulin in reticular variant
- Inhibin-α (+) stromal cells
- Few if any EMA(+) cells

Melanocytoma

- Nested architecture
- Melanin variable
- HMB-45(+), Melan-A(+), S100(+), SOX10(+)
- EMA(-)

Meningioangiomatosis

- Intracortical, plaque-like
- Abundant trapped brain with ganglion cells
- Perivascular meningothelial and spindle cells
- Associated with meningioma in some cases

Solitary Fibrous Tumor/Hemangiopericytoma

- Reticulin-rich, hemangiopericytoma (HPC)
- Collagen strips between spindle cells, solitary fibrous tumor (SFT)
- No calcifications or psammoma bodies
- CD34(+)
  - SFT: Diffuse
  - HPC: Variable, may be (-)
- EMA(-), except focally in loose textured areas, HPCs
- STAT 6 nuclear IHC(+) due to *STAT6-NAB2* fusion and STAT6 nuclear translocation (not seen in meningiomas)

Metastatic Carcinoma

- Strong cytokeratin (+) vs. mostly (-) meningiomas

Primary Hematopoietic Diseases

- Rosai-Dorfman disease
  - Large, S100(+) histiocytes
  - Emperipolesis

Meningeal Fibrosarcoma

- Monomorphous, often spindle cells
- Herringbone pattern (some)
- Abundant pericellular reticulin, EMA(-)

Gemistocytic Astrocytoma

- More differential issue in frozen sections
- Intraparenchymal, infiltrating
- Fibrillar background
- Perivascular chronic inflammation
- GFAP(+)

Astroblastoma

- Intraparenchymal
- Often cystic
- Vessel hyalinization
- GFAP usually (+), but not always
- Some focally EMA(+), surface staining, microlumina

Vascular Malformation (Angiomatous and Microcystic Meningiomas)

- No neoplastic meningothelial cells

Superficial Glioblastoma/Gliosarcoma

- GFAP(+) component
- Abundant pericellular reticulin in sarcoma component
- EMA(-), except for rare example with epithelial differentiation

DIAGNOSTIC CHECKLIST

Pathologic Interpretation Pearls

- Highly variable histologic patterns
- Cytology (smears) often more specific than frozen sections
- Anaplastic meningiomas often cytokeratin (+), can be confused with metastatic carcinoma

GRADING

WHO Grade I

- Meningothelial, fibrous, transitional, angiomatous, microcystic, secretory, metaplastic, lymphoplasmacyte rich, psammomatous
  - ≤ 3 mitoses per 10 HPFs
  - No brain invasion

WHO Grade II

- ≥ 4 mitoses/10 HPFs **or**
- 3 of the following
  - High cellularity
  - Small cells with high N:C ratio, clustered
  - Prominent nucleoli
  - Uninterrupted growth pattern (sheeting)
  - Spontaneous necrosis ± palisading
- Brain invasion or chordoid or clear cell subtype

WHO Grade III

- ≥ 20 mitoses per 10 HPF or
- Overt malignant features resembling carcinoma, melanoma, sarcoma, or
- Rhabdoid or papillary subtype
- Spontaneous necrosis frequent but not required

SELECTED REFERENCES

1. Menke JR et al: Somatostatin receptor 2a is a more sensitive diagnostic marker of meningioma than epithelial membrane antigen. Acta Neuropathol. 130(3):441-3, 2015
2. Clark VE et al: Genomic analysis of non-NF2 meningiomas reveals mutations in TRAF7, KLF4, AKT1, and SMO. Science. 339(6123):1077-80, 2013
3. Nagaishi M et al: Slug, twist, and E-cadherin as immunohistochemical biomarkers in meningeal tumors. PLoS One. 7(9):e46053, 2012

Occasionally Completely Intraosseous

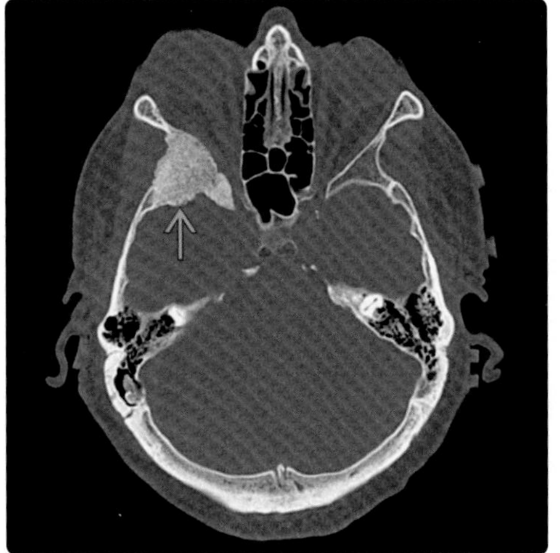

Bone Invasion Does Not Impact Grading

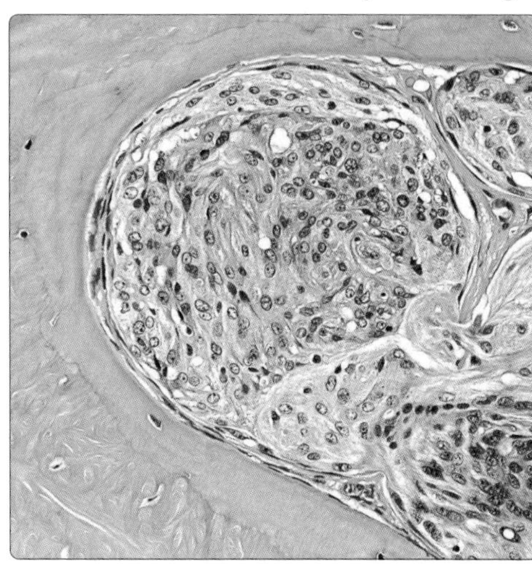

(Left) *Meningiomas are sometimes principally or exclusively intraosseous ⇒, as seen here in the sphenoid bone.* **(Right)** *Bone invasion is not a factor in tumor grading, but it may complicate resection and increase the likelihood of recurrence. Most osseoinvasive meningiomas are grade I.*

Falcine Meningioma

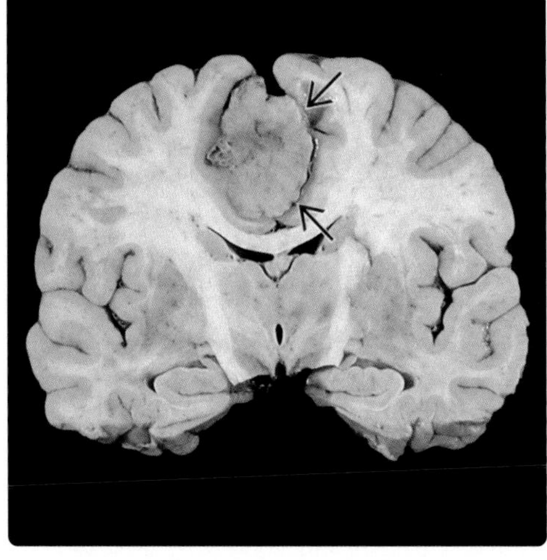

Intraspinal, Extramedullary Mass

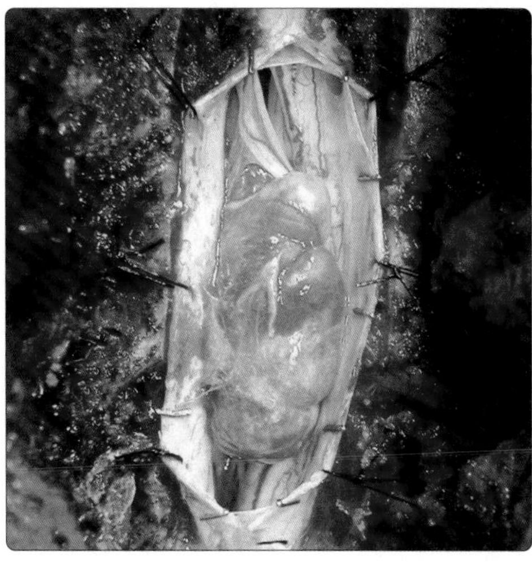

(Left) *This falcine tumor ⇒ extends both right and left to displace brain. (Courtesy K. Ligon, MD.)* **(Right)** *Intraspinal meningiomas are dural-based, well-circumscribed masses that lend themselves to total excision. Schwannoma is the principal differential diagnostic concern. Myxopapillary ependymoma and the rare paraganglioma would be added for a tumor in the cauda equina. (Courtesy Z. Gokaslan, MD.)*

Dural Tail May Be Extension of Meningioma

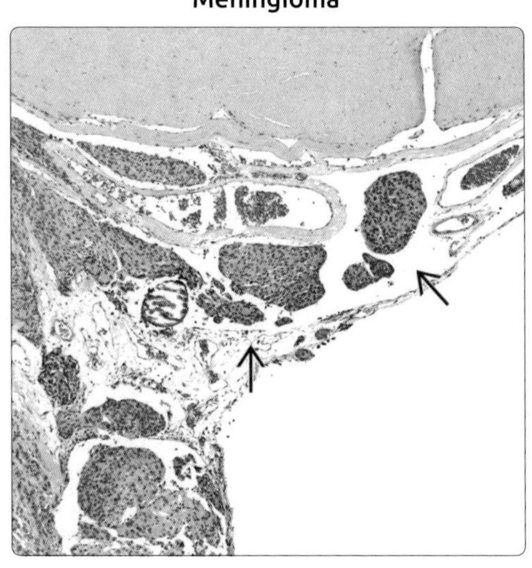

Dural Tail, (-) for Meningioma

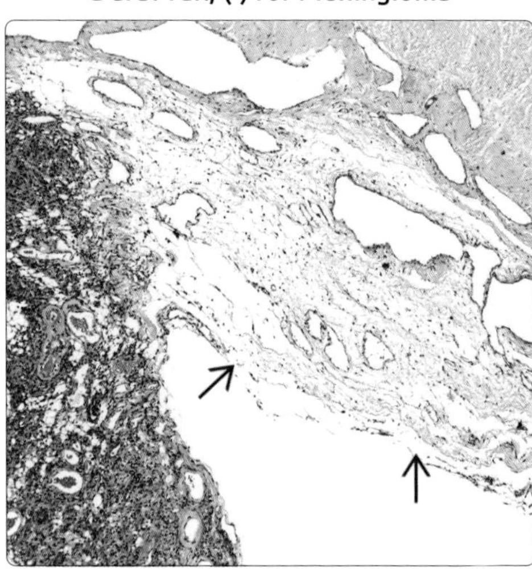

(Left) *The dural tail is, in many cases, an extension of the tumor ⇒ along the inner aspect of the dura. In other tumors, it is only loose vessels and stroma but still contrast enhancing.* **(Right)** *The dural tail is, in some instances, nothing but a peripheral triangle of vessels and loose stroma ⇒ at the lateral margin of the tumor-dura interface.*

(Left) *Washed-out nuclei* → *and pseudoinclusions are common in meningothelial meningiomas.* **(Right)** *Meningothelial meningiomas have oval nuclei, often with nuclear grooves* →*.*

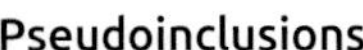

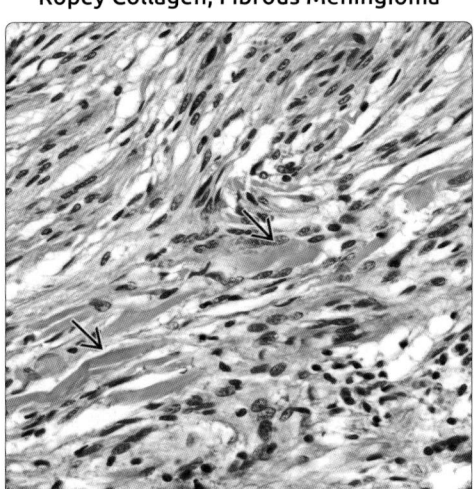

Pseudoinclusions

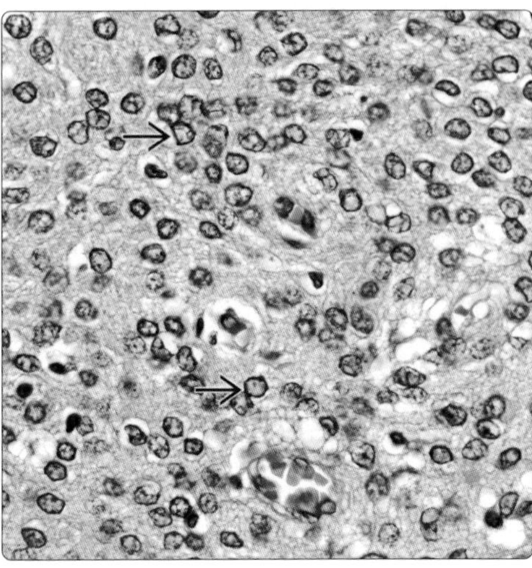

Meningothelial Meningioma, Nuclear Grooves

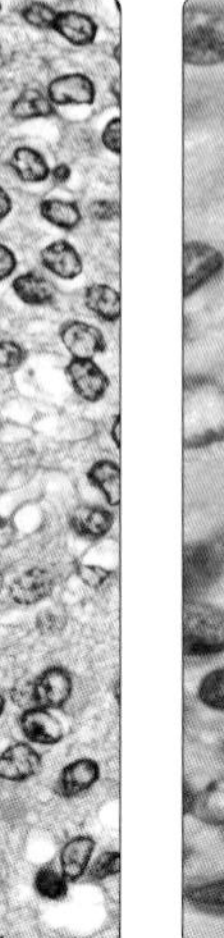

(Left) *Linear stromal calcifications* → *are common in meningiomas of the fibrous subtype. Whorls and psammoma bodies are often scant or absent.* **(Right)** *Some fibrous meningiomas contain ropey collagen* → *of the type seen in solitary fibrous tumor (SFT). SFT should show nuclear STAT6 and immunoreactivity for CD34. CD34 is confined to vessels in meningiomas, which would additionally have immunopositivity for EMA, dual D2-40/E-cadherin, and SSTR2A.*

Linear Stromal Calcifications, Fibrous Subtype

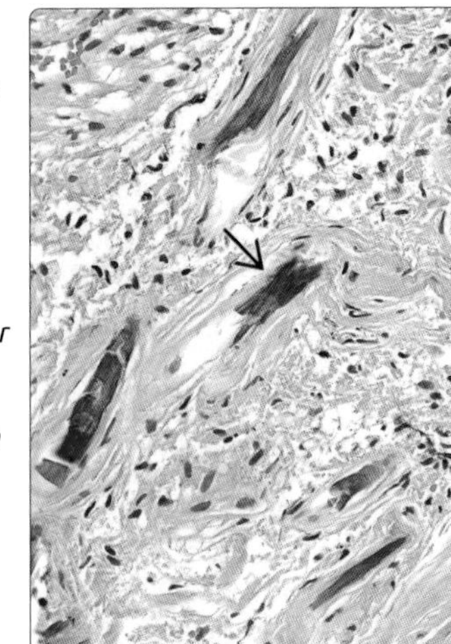

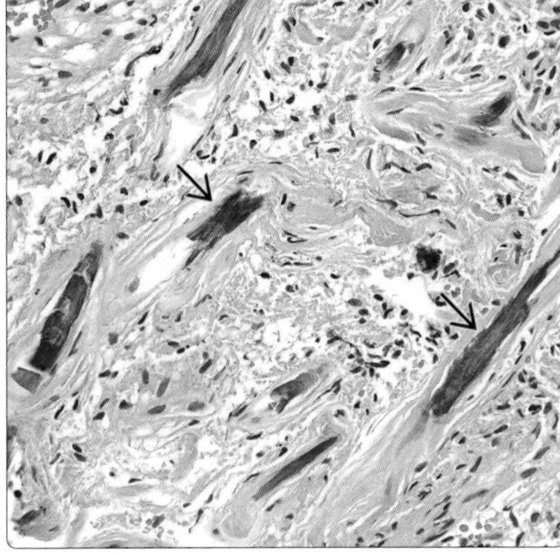

Ropey Collagen, Fibrous Meningioma

(Left) *Meningothelial whorls and lobules are conspicuous in transitional meningiomas, which, by definition, have features of both fibrous and meningothelial variants.* **(Right)** *Compact multilayered whorls are definitive evidence of meningioma, as seen here in a transitional subtype with its requisite features of both meningothelial and fibrous subtypes.*

Whorls and Lobules, Transitional Subtype

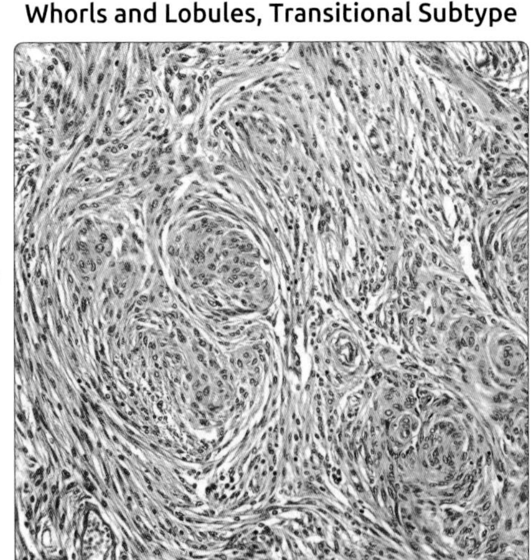

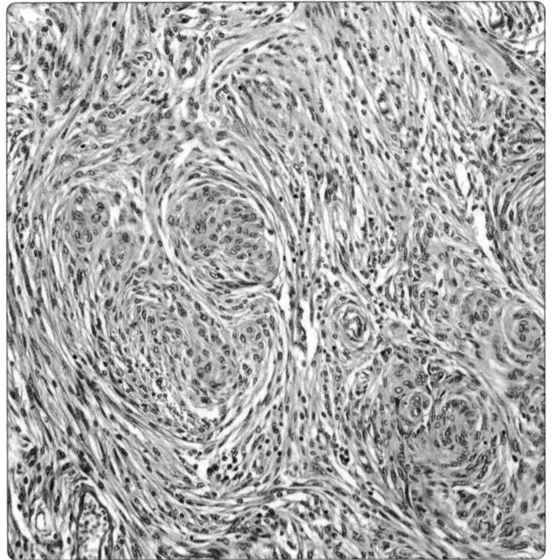

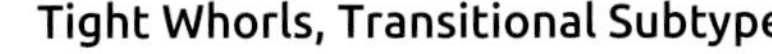

Tight Whorls, Transitional Subtype

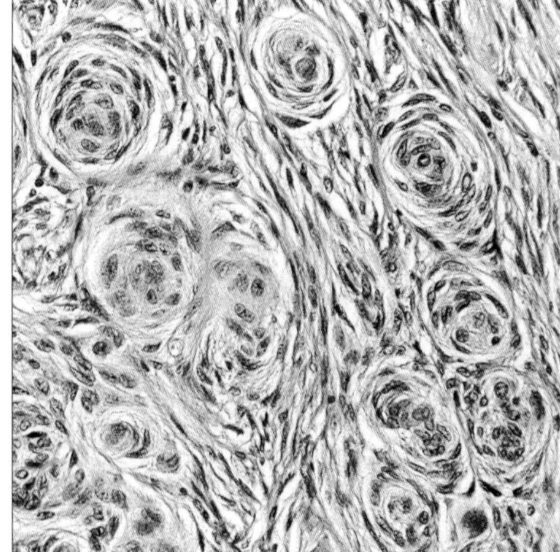

Psammomatous Meningioma, Common Intraspinally in Women

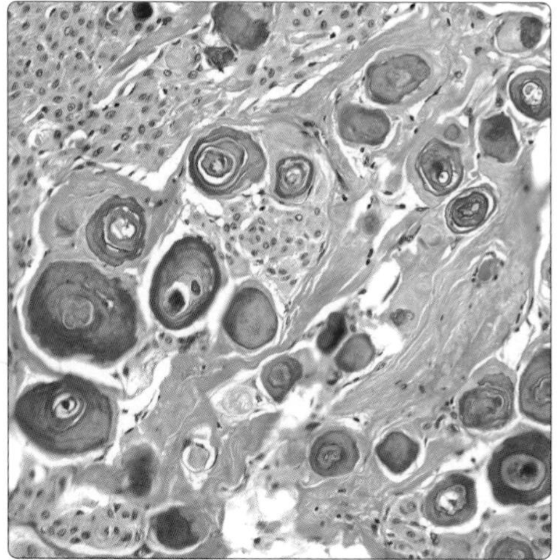

Laminated Psammoma Bodies

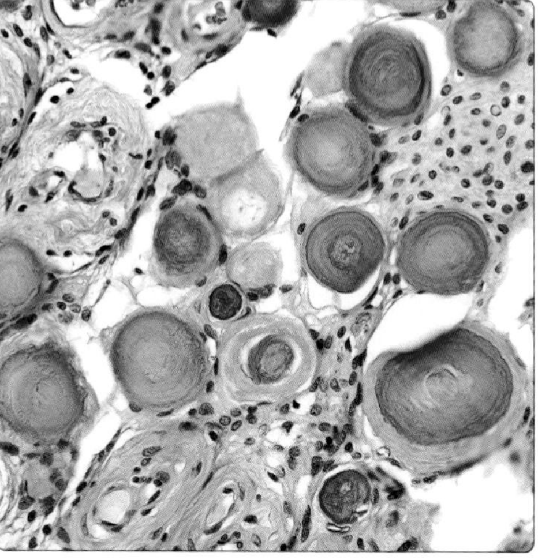

(Left) *Psammomatous meningiomas are laden with iconic laminated eosinophilic or slightly basophilic bodies that often begin in a whorl. This subtype is common intraspinally, wherein almost all meningiomas arise in women.* **(Right)** *Distinctively laminated, round psammoma bodies should be distinguished from the more irregular, whorl-free calcospherites that populate intraparenchymal lesions, such as astrocytomas and oligodendrogliomas.*

Microcystic Meningioma

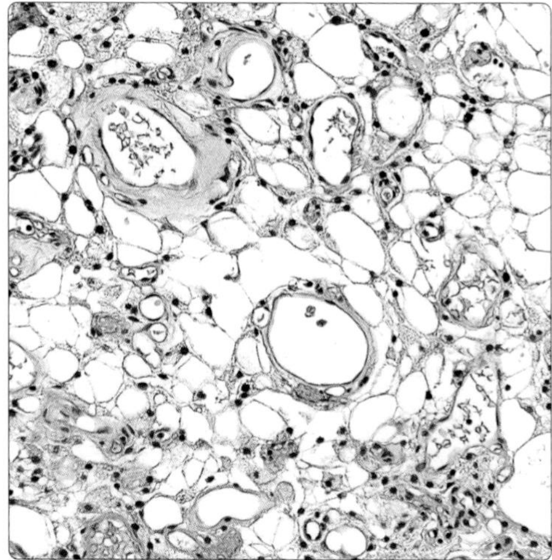

Microcystic Meningioma Simulating Hemangioblastoma

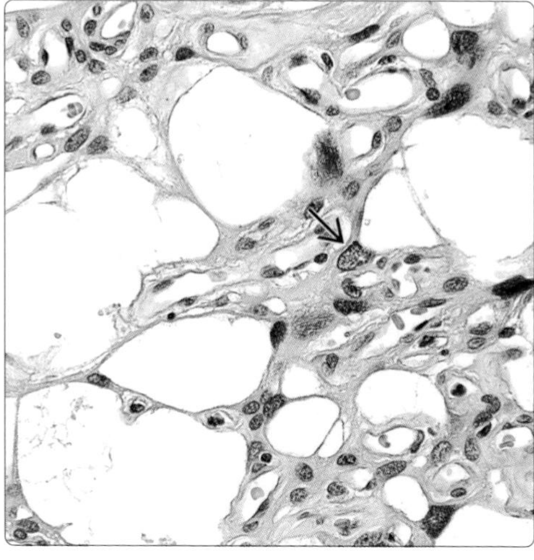

(Left) *A cobweb architecture with xanthoma and xanthoma-like cells is one of the many phenotypes of microcystic meningioma.* **(Right)** *Microcystic spaces and scattered large hyperchromatic nuclei ⇨ in microcystic meningiomas create a resemblance to hemangioblastoma. Immunostaining would be (+) for EMA and SSTR2A in the meningioma and (-) in hemangioblastoma. The latter tumor would be (+) for inhibin-a, a meningioma would not. A newer marker for HBL is cytoplasmic brachyury.*

Numerous Hyalinized Vessels Simulating Vascular Malformation

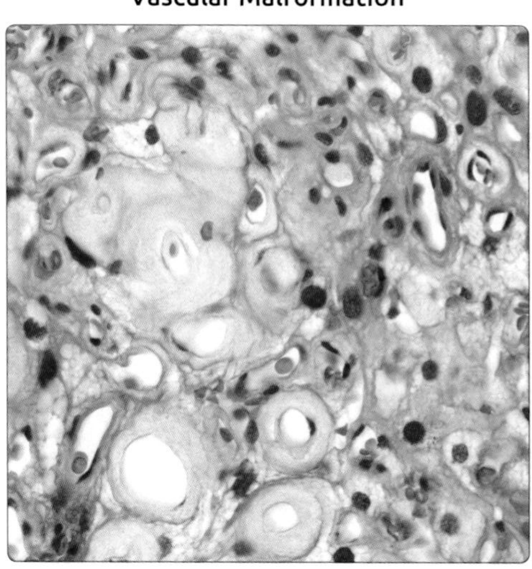

Subtle Meningioma Cells

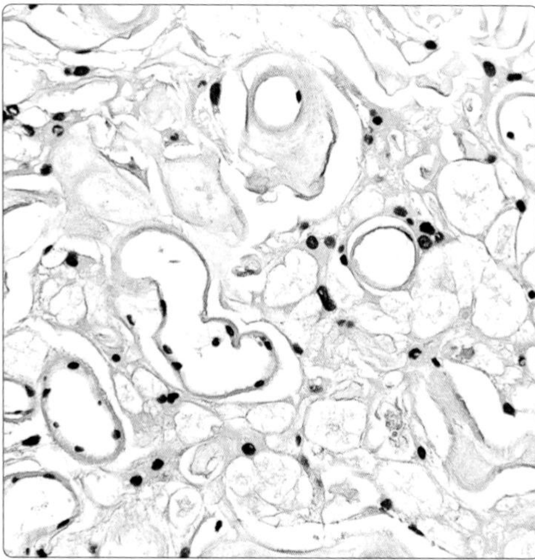

(Left) *Numerous hyalinized blood vessels dominate some meningiomas, microcystic in this case, which then also could be considered angiomatous. The possibility of a vascular malformation sometimes arises in such lesions, although tumor cells are obvious here.* **(Right)** *Thickened vessels and pale tumor cells create a distinctive pattern that superficially does not appear meningothelial. Immunostaining for EMA and SSTR2A would be appropriate.*

Pseudopsammoma Bodies, Secretory Meningioma

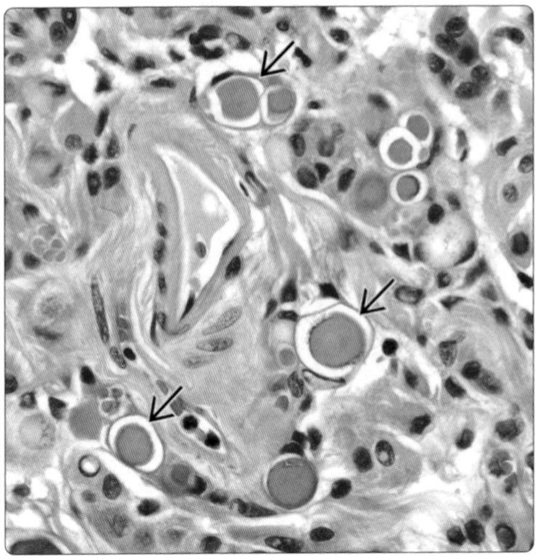

PAS(+), Pseudopsammoma Bodies

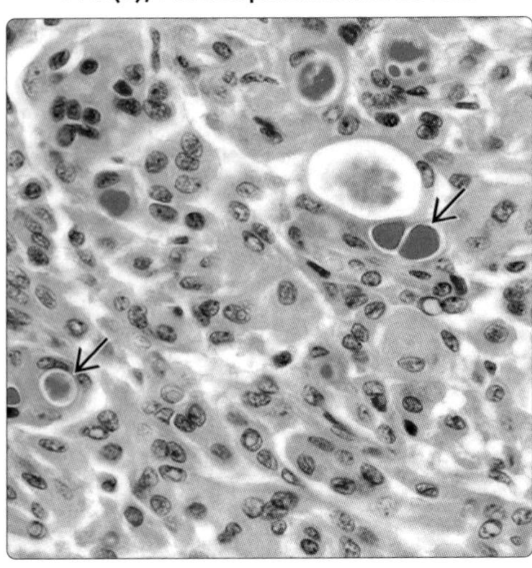

(Left) *Eosinophilic globules, known as pseudopsammoma bodies →, are defining features of secretory meningioma. Ultrastructural examination would be notable for lumina replete with epithelial features, such as tight junctions and microvilli.* **(Right)** *Not surprisingly given their glycogen content, pseudopsammoma bodies → are PAS(+). Unlike psammoma bodies, they are not laminated or mineralized.*

CEA(+), Secretory Meningioma

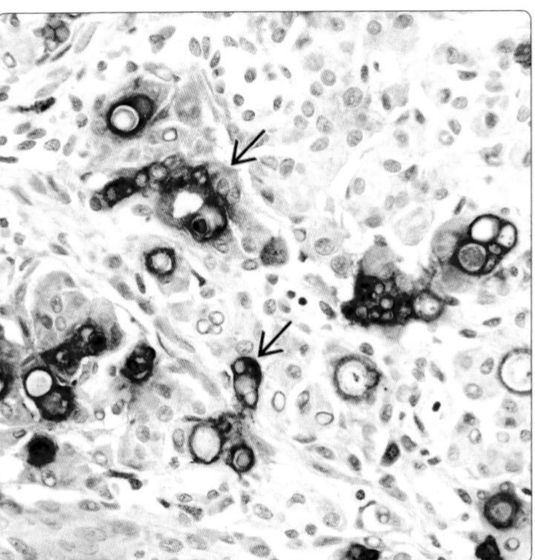

Keratin, Secretory Meningioma

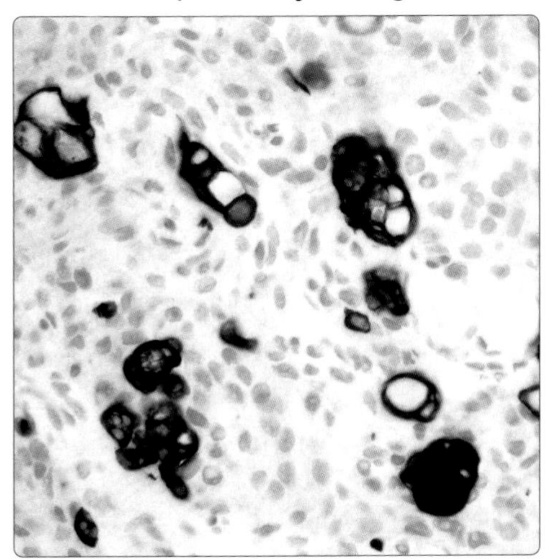

(Left) *Carcinoembryonic antigen is present in and around pseudopsammoma bodies →. It may even find its way into the bloodstream in detectable amounts.* **(Right)** *Tumor cells associated with the gland-like spaces of pseudopsammoma bodies are cytokeratin (+) in a secretory meningioma.*

Lymphoplasmacytic Meningioma

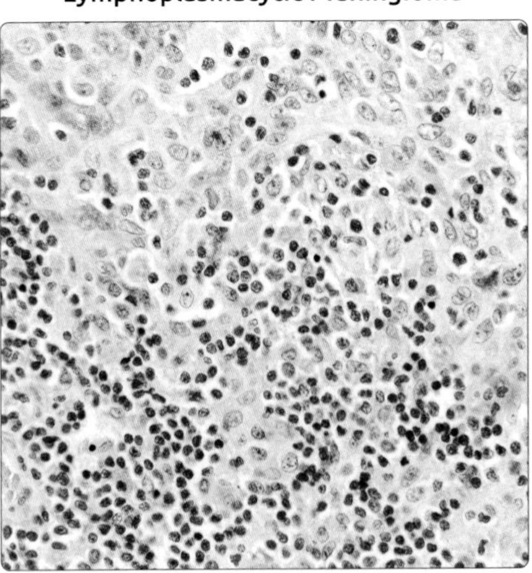

Meningothelial Whorl

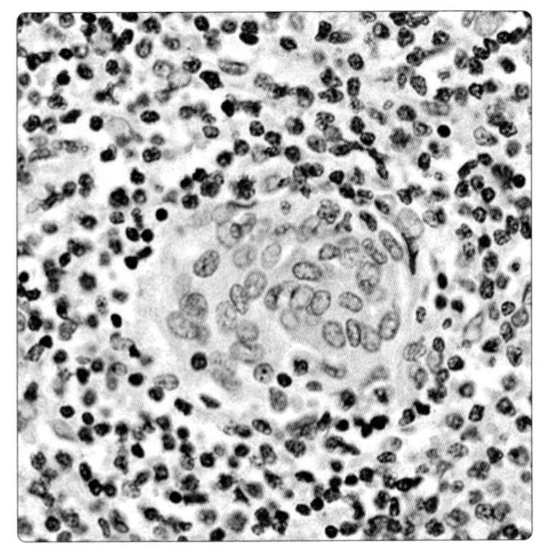

(Left) *Mixed meningothelial cells and chronic inflammatory cells can sometimes create a confusing combination. In this case, there are enough of the former to be sure that the meningothelial cells are neoplastic.* **(Right)** *EMA or SSTR2A positivity within a meningothelial whorl would help confirm the presence of meningothelial cells but not necessarily meningioma. Small nodules, such as this, may be normal or hyperplastic meningothelium caught up in a meningeal inflammatory process.*

Osseous Metaplasia

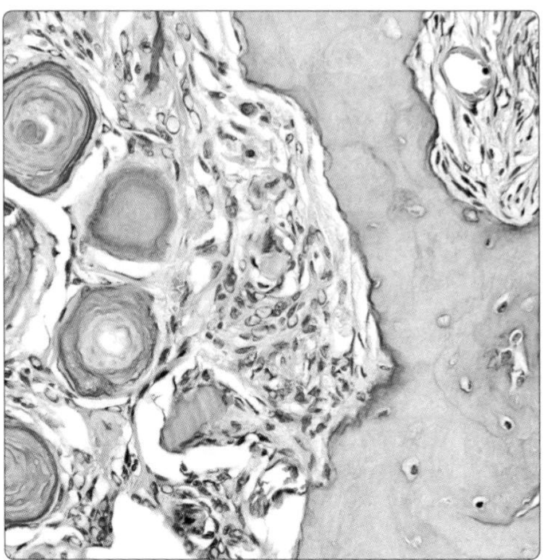

Rare Cartilaginous Differentiation

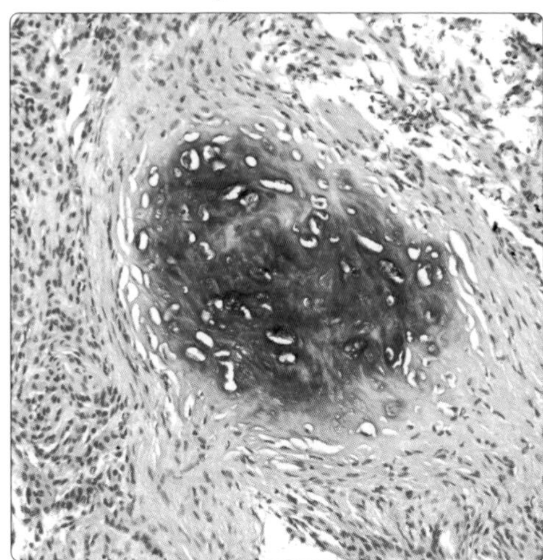

(Left) *Psammoma body-rich meningiomas are prone to osseous metaplasia.* **(Right)** *Meningioma with cartilaginous differentiation, an uncommon variant, should not cause confusion with mesenchymal chondrosarcoma. The absence of the latter's small cell, reticulin-rich anaplastic element resolves the issue in this case.*

Metaplastic Lipomatous Meningioma

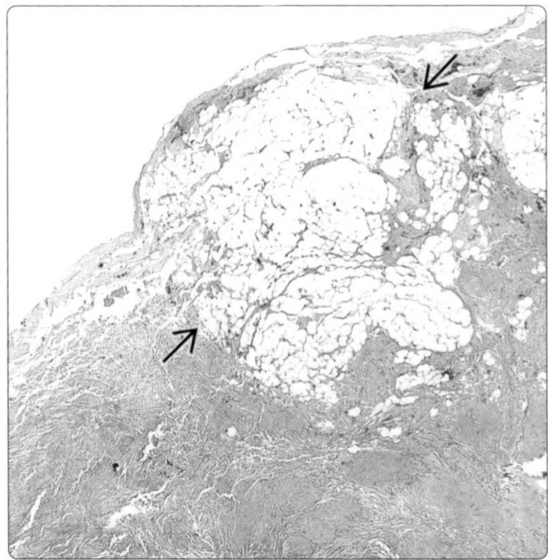

Clear Cells Resembling Adipocytes

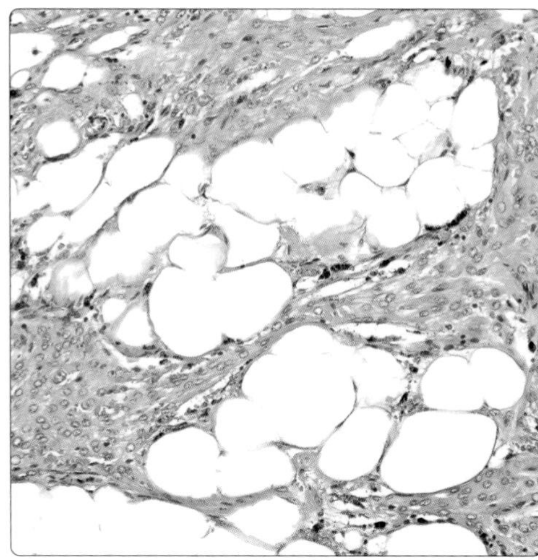

(Left) *Lobulated cells closely resembling those of adipose tissue* ➙ *are not uncommon in meningiomas. The clear cell component was entirely intradural and, therefore, was not adipose tissue invaded by tumor.* **(Right)** *Clear cells closely resemble adipocytes but can be distinguished in some cases by their surface immunopositivity for EMA. Thus, they often appear to represent intracytoplasmic fat.*

Chordoid Meningioma

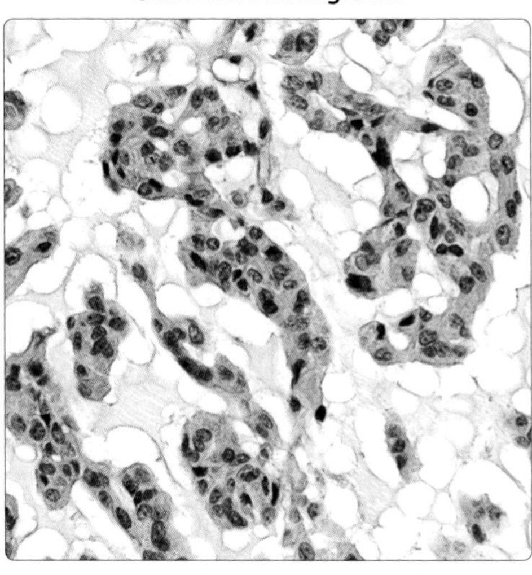

Chordoid Areas

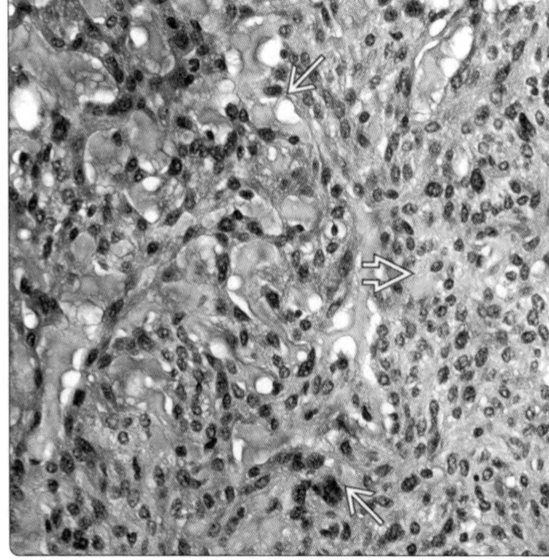

(Left) *Cords of epithelioid cells in a myxoid background create the chordoid subtype that is, by definition, grade II. Histologically similar formations occur intracranially in chordoid gliomas of the 3rd ventricle and chordomas of the clivus. Chordoid gliomas have recently been recognized to show nuclear TTF-1 IHC(+), and additionally are GFAP(+), while chordoid meningiomas are not.* **(Right)** *Chordoid tissue* ➙ *is commonly associated with conventional meningioma* ➙ *that is often grade II in its own right.*

(Left) *Cytological blandness and low-level mitotic activity belie the grade II nature of clear cell meningioma, a recurrence-prone subtype. Whorls, and especially psammoma bodies, are uncommon.* (Right) *Small, circular collagenous knots* → *are a distinctive feature of clear cell meningiomas. Tumor cells are monomorphous, round, and cytologically bland in this lesion that at first, and even at second glance, may not appear meningothelial.*

Clear Cell Meningioma

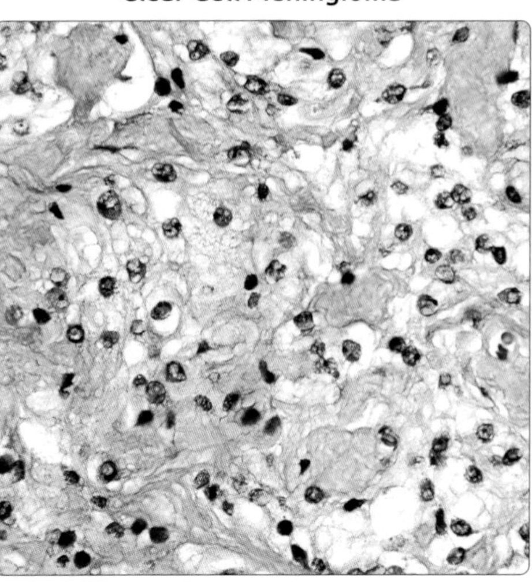

Knots of Collagen, Clear Cell Meningioma

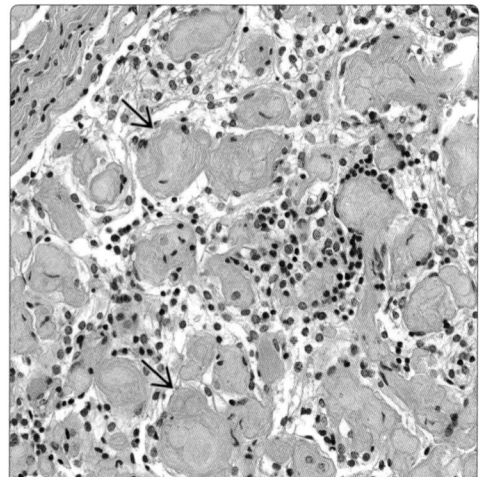

(Left) *Densely hyalinized tissue encroaches on neoplastic cells in many clear cell meningiomas. Astroblastomas often contain similar hyalinized components.* (Right) *The clear cell appearance is due largely to PAS(+) cytoplasmic glycogen that would be removed by diastase digestion.*

Clear Cell Meningioma Dominated by Hyalinization

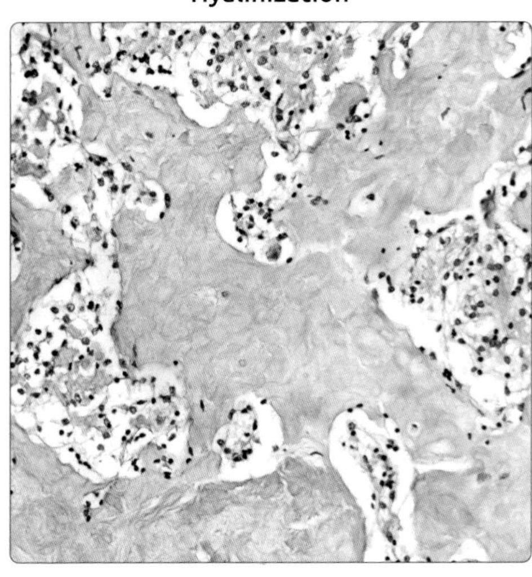

Clear Cell Meningioma, PAS(+) Glycogen

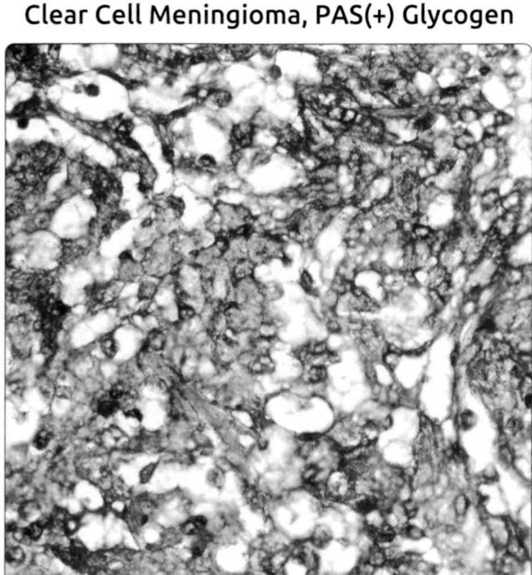

(Left) *Rhabdoid/epithelioid cells have well-circumscribed eosinophilic inclusions* → *and nuclei with prominent nucleoli. Mitoses* ⇨ *are often present. The significance of rhabdoid tumors without dividing cells is unclear, but such tumors may not be considered grade III.* (Right) *Round nuclei with prominent nucleoli in combination with eosinophilic intracytoplasmic inclusions* → *create the rhabdoid phenotype. Mitoses* ⇨ *are common. These tumors do not show SMARCB1 mutation (i.e., no INI1 IHC nuclear loss).*

Rhabdoid Meningioma

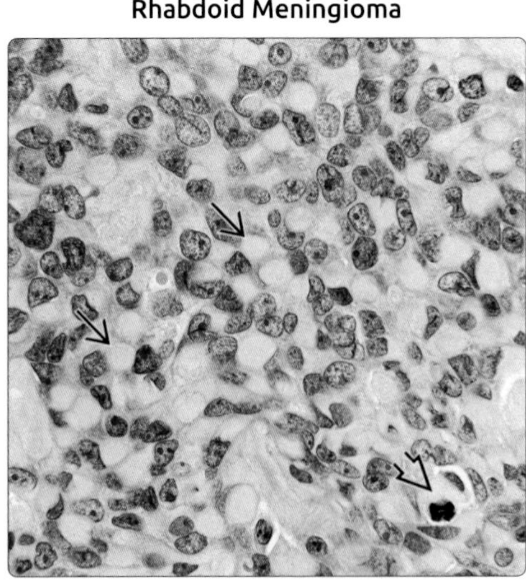

Rhabdoid Cells

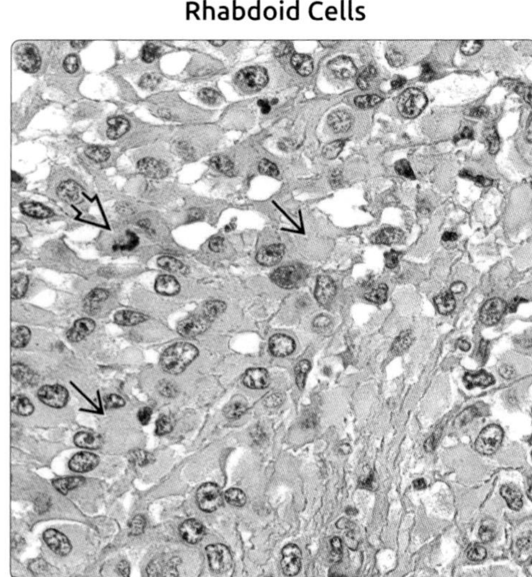

Papillary Meningioma

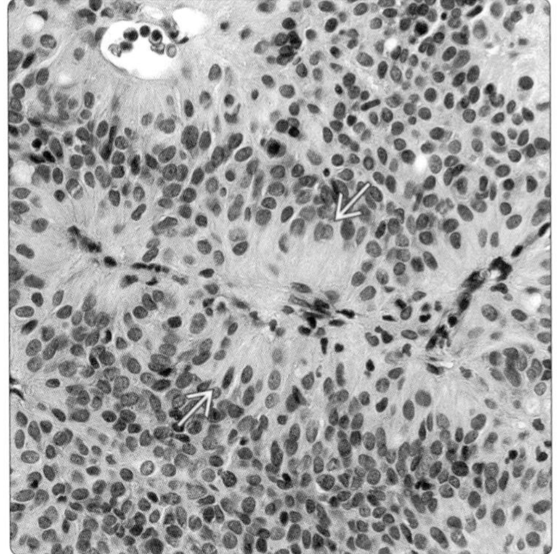

Papillary Meningioma Simulating Ependymoma

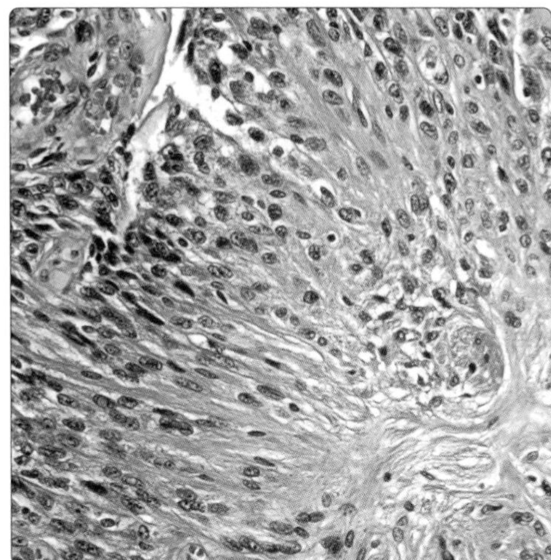

(Left) *Ependymoma-like perivascular pseudorosettes ➡ define papillary meningioma. Pseudopapillae that result from artifactual tissue dehiscence may occur in ordinary meningiomas and should not be considered papillary meningioma.* **(Right)** *In aggregate, fibrillary processes forming perivascular pseudorosettes in papillary meningiomas may suggest ependymoma. The issue is resolved by GFAP staining, which is (-) in meningiomas.*

Meningioangiomatosis

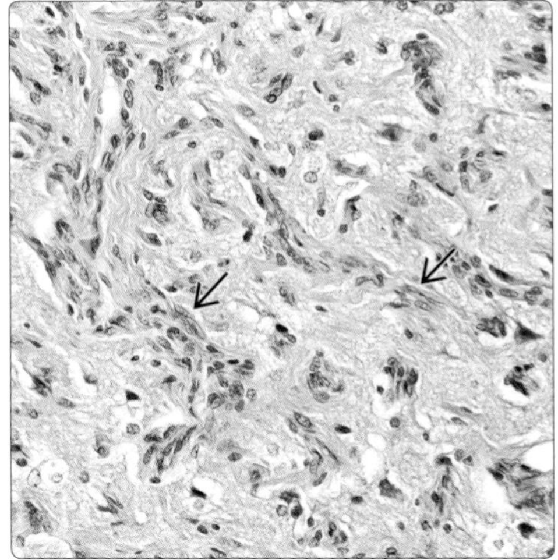

Smear, Elongate Cells

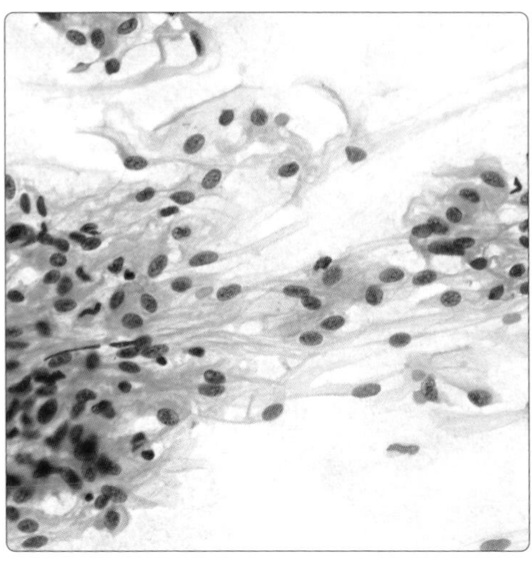

(Left) *In the condition known as meningioma with meningioangiomatosis, meningothelial or fibroblast-like cells ➡ extend from a superficial meningioma along intracortical vessels into the cortex. Intracortical extension along Virchow-Robin spaces does not define the tumor as grade II.* **(Right)** *Meningioma on smear preparation often shows the low N:C ratio and tapering eosinophilic cell processes. Schwannomas in contrast do not smear well and usually show more elongate nuclei with tapering ends.*

Simulating Glandular Tissue

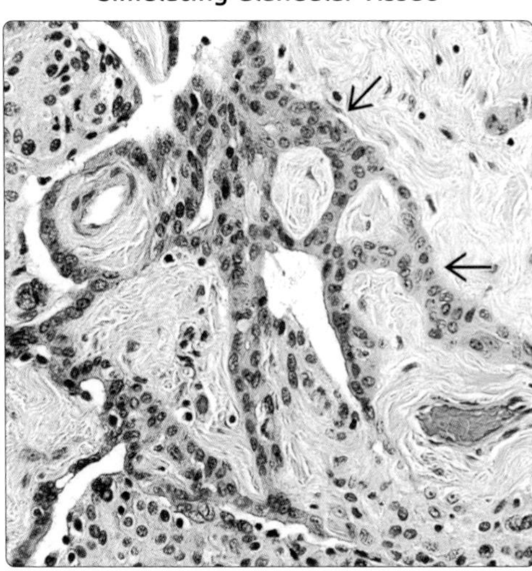

Tumor-to-Tumor Metastasis

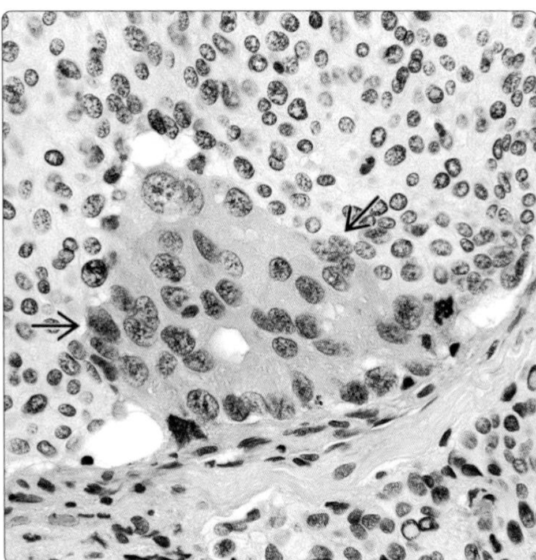

(Left) *Rare meningiomas, both low and high grade, have a focal epithelial differentiation resembling glandular tissue ➡. The possibility of a metastasis to a meningioma must be considered.* **(Right)** *Occasional meningiomas host metastatic cancer ➡, breast cancer being the most common source. Immunohistochemistry and clinical history become important in distinguishing such foci from innocent epithelioid change.*

(Left) *Petal-like, tyrosine-rich crystals* → *are a rare feature in meningiomas, usually found in the uncommon clear cell subtype.* **(Right)** *Invasive meningiomas may incorporate large, heavily pigmented, nonneoplastic melanocytes* →*. Staining for EMA and melanocytic markers can be used to exclude a melanocytic tumor.*

Rare Tyrosine-Rich Crystals, Clear Cell Type

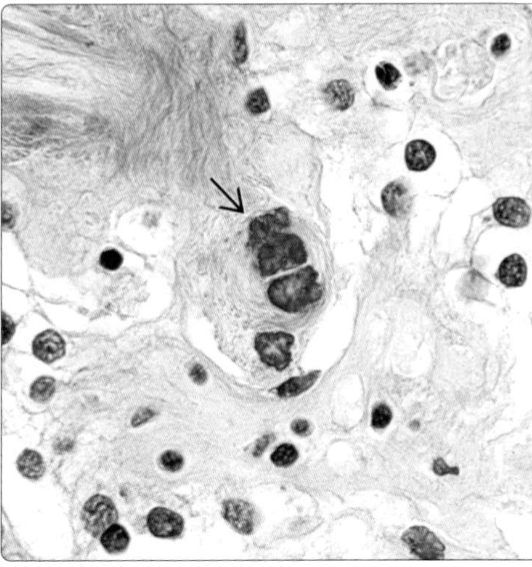

Invasive Meningioma Incorporating Melanocytes

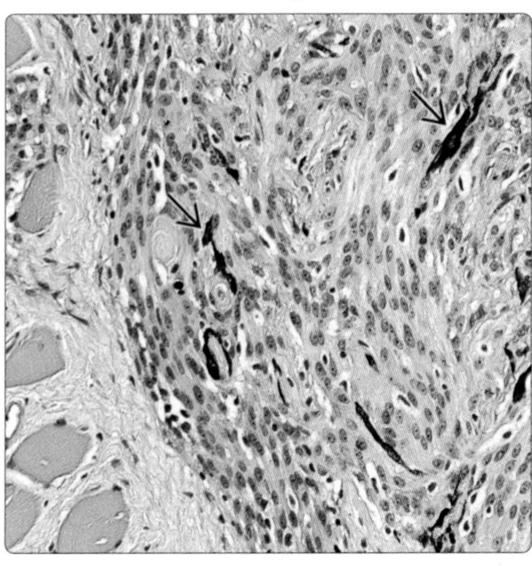

(Left) *Copious, streaked cytoplasm is characteristic of meningiomas in smear preparations. Nuclei, typically ovoid and bland, contain Barr bodies* → *in meningiomas in women. Cells in meningioma are more likely to be dispersed individually than in schwannoma, a common differential lesion.* **(Right)** *Intranuclear cytoplasmic intrusions* ➡ *are a helpful, and common, diagnostic feature. Smears often provide more definitive evidence of meningiomas than frozen sections.*

Smear, Cells Dispersed

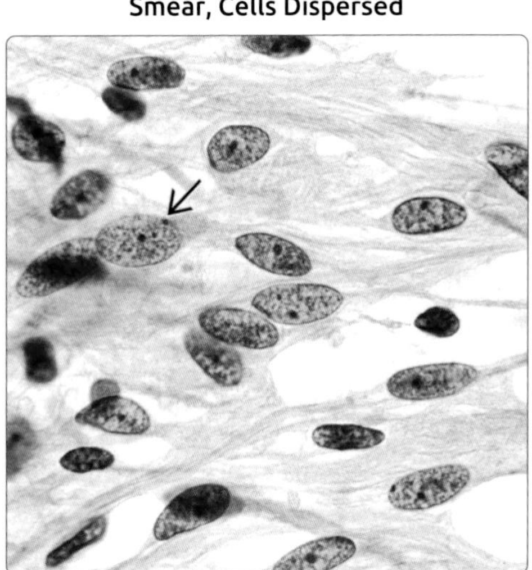

Smear, Intranuclear Cytoplasmic Inclusions

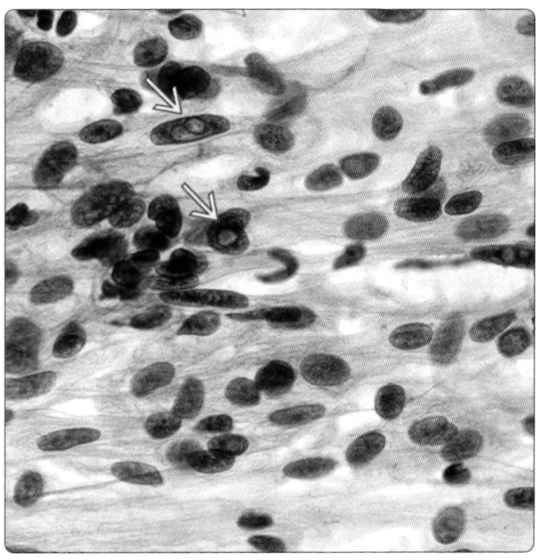

(Left) *Ependymoma-like perivascular pseudorosettes in papillary meningiomas are well seen in smear preparations.* **(Right)** *Marked atypia and mitoses* → *raise suspicion for a grade III meningioma. Cytoplasm is typically scant in the round epithelioid cells of anaplastic meningioma, which comprises only a small percentage of all meningiomas.*

Smear, Papillary Meningioma

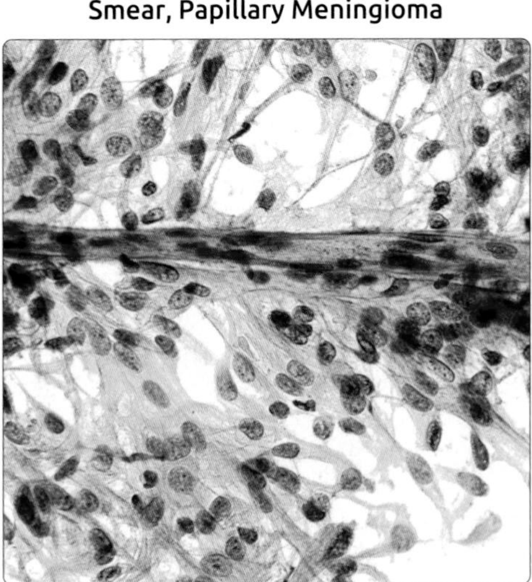

Smear, Marked Atypia, Mitoses

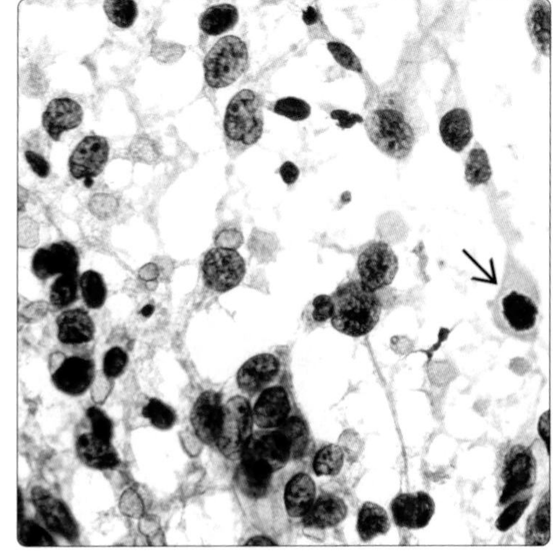

Focal EMA(+), Fibrous Meningioma

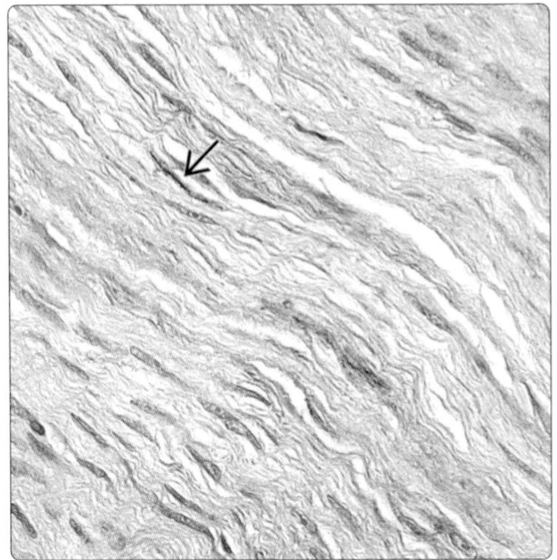

EMA(+), Clear Cell Meningioma

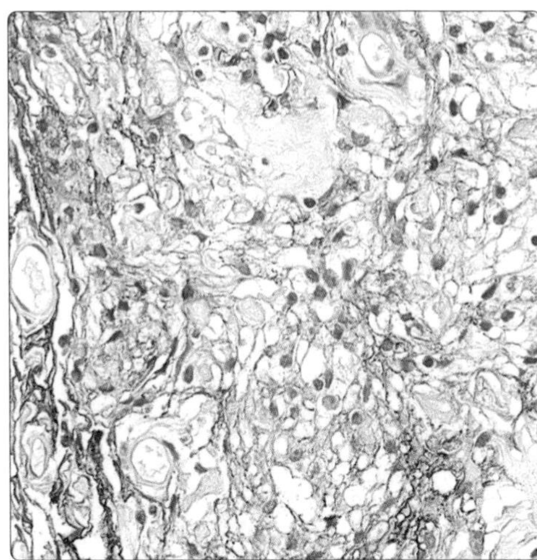

(Left) *Fibrous meningiomas are often only faintly and focally, if at all, EMA(+). Focal accentuations ➡ are reassuring evidence that the immunostaining is real.* **(Right)** *Reaction product traces cell surfaces in meningioma as in this clear cell variant. Immunopositivity is most pronounced in meningothelial and transitional subtypes, less so in fibroblastic and clear cell types. Overall, EMA immunopositivity in meningiomas is less robust than in metastatic carcinoma. SSTR2A IHC is superior to EMA for meningioma.*

Nuclear Progesterone Receptor Variable

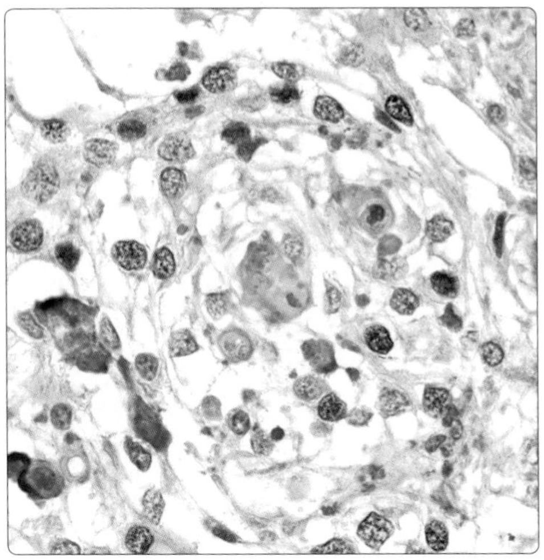

CAM5.2(+) Anaplastic Meningioma Simulating Metastatic Carcinoma

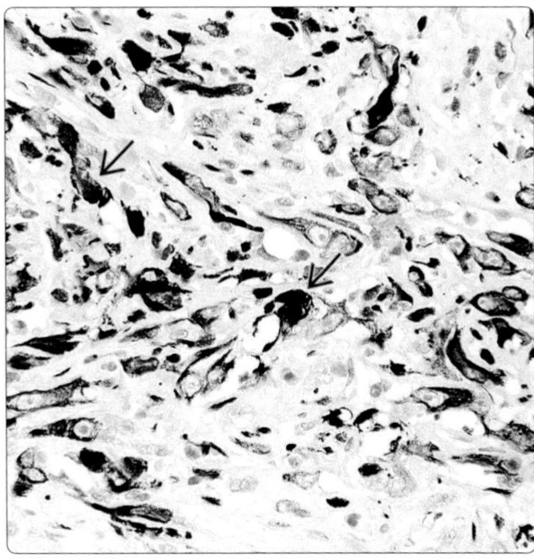

(Left) *There is considerable inter- and intratumoral variation in staining for progesterone receptors. For example, in this clear cell meningioma some nuclei are (+) and others are not. Some otherwise classical meningiomas are (-) throughout.* **(Right)** *Complicating the distinction of anaplastic meningioma from metastatic carcinoma is the former's common immunoreactivity for cytokeratins ➡, CAM5.2 in this case.*

Sheeting Architecture, Atypical Meningioma

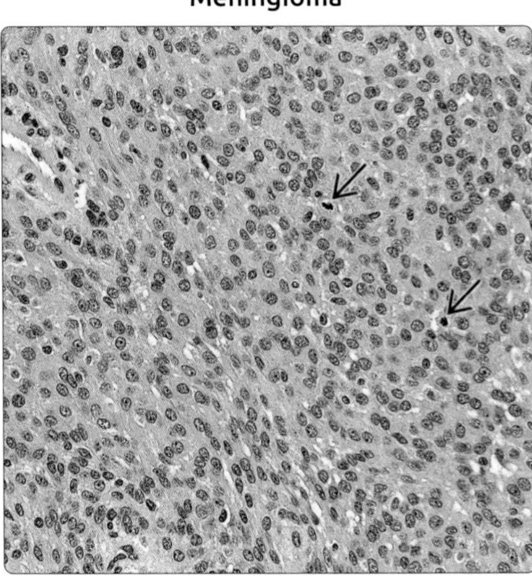

Mitoses, Prominent Nucleoli, Atypical Meningioma

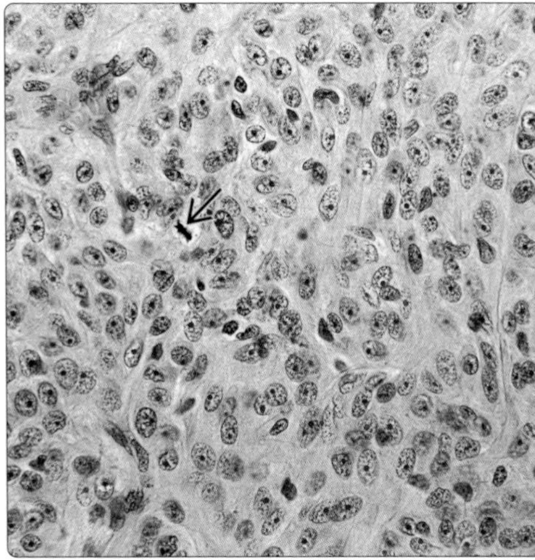

(Left) *Loss of lobularity (sheeting) is a common feature of grade II meningiomas. Mitoses ➡ are often increased above the grade I level in such cases.* **(Right)** *Mitoses ➡ and cells with prominent nucleoli are typical of most grade II meningiomas.*

(Left) *The presence of aggregates of small cells with high nuclear:cytoplasmic ratios (small cell change)* → *is 1 of 5 grading parameters used in an algorithm to distinguish grade II from grade I meningiomas. Mitoses* ⇨ *are present in this grade II lesion.* (Right) *Small foci of spontaneous necrosis, such as this, should be distinguished from large, geographic areas due to preoperative embolization.*

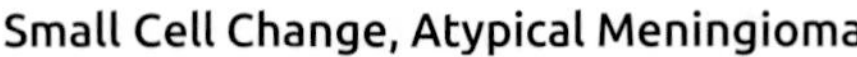

Small Cell Change, Atypical Meningioma

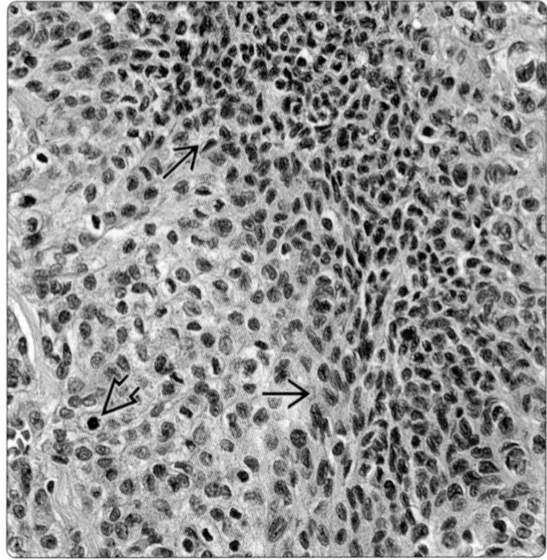

Spontaneous Necrosis, Atypical Meningioma

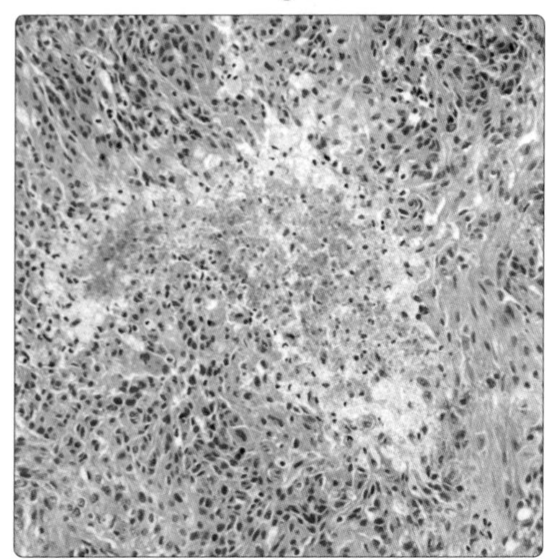

(Left) *Embolization, with polyvinyl alcohol* → *in this case, often leads to extensive necrosis, especially in perivascular zones* ⇨*.* (Right) *The distinction between true brain invasion and mere pushing is sometimes challenging. In the former, tumor cells extend beyond the pial surface into the brain parenchyma, as seen in this example.*

Embolization With Necrosis

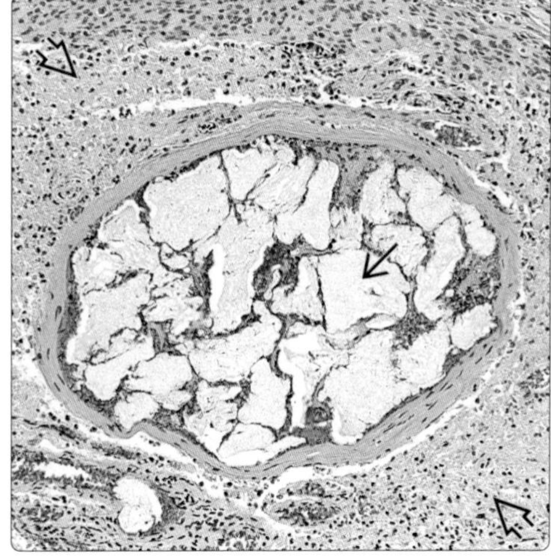

True Invasion With Breaching of Pial Surface

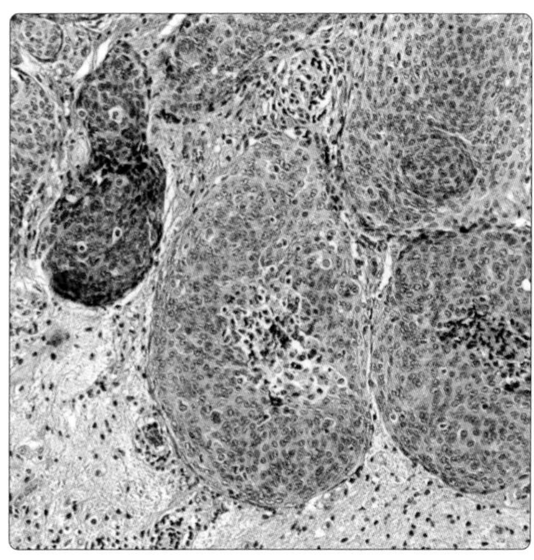

(Left) *Small foci of necrosis* ➡ *are often present in the center of invading papillae of grade II or III meningiomas.* (Right) *Immunostaining for GFAP helps identify trapped CNS parenchyma* → *and establishes brain invasion, making this meningioma at least grade II.*

Necrosis in Brain-Invasive Nodules of Atypical Meningioma

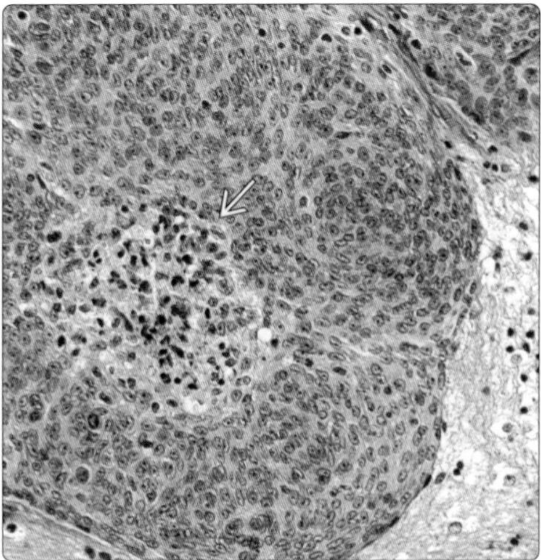

Brain Invasion Highlighted by GFAP

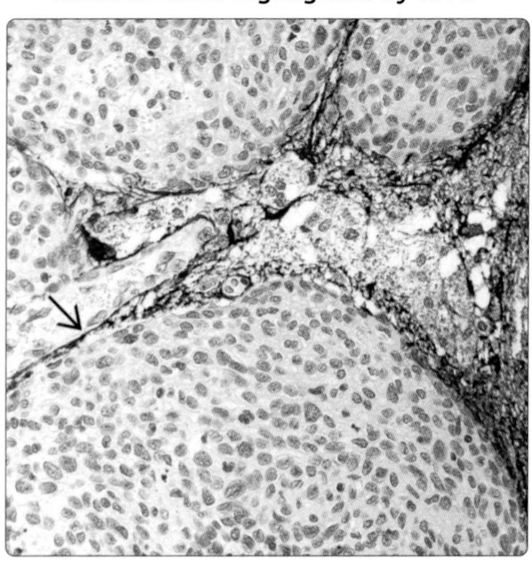

Brain Invasion by Small Groups of Cells Rare

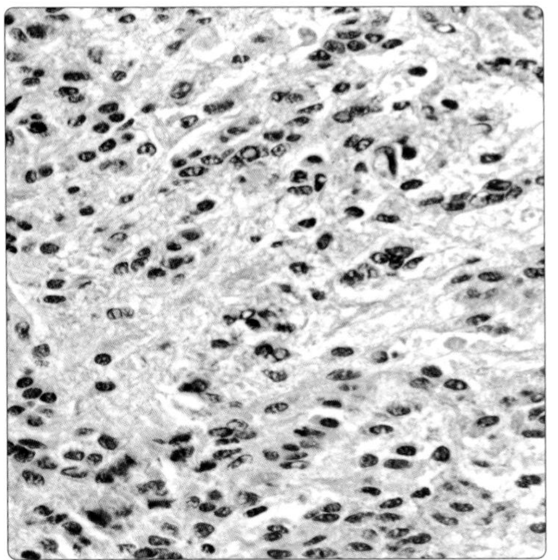

Perivascular Extension Along Virchow-Robin Spaces Not True Brain Invasion

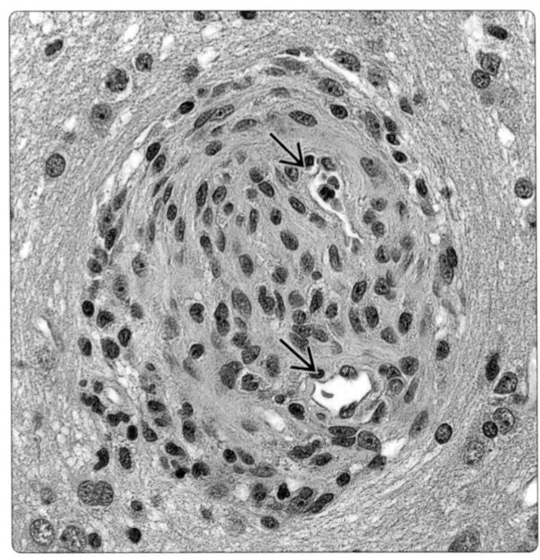

(Left) *Infiltration by small groups or even individual cells is unusual in meningiomas, wherein the invading tumor-brain interface is usually better defined.* **(Right)** *While perhaps prognostically unfavorable, extension along cortical vessels ⮕ is not considered true brain invasion.*

Sagittal Sinus Occlusion

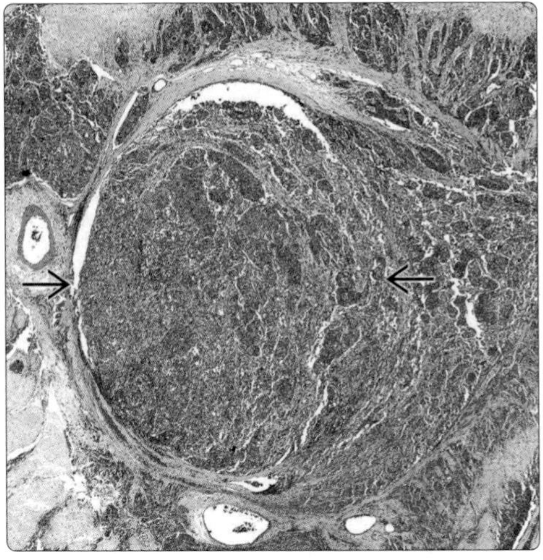

Benign Meningioma in Dural Venous Sinuses

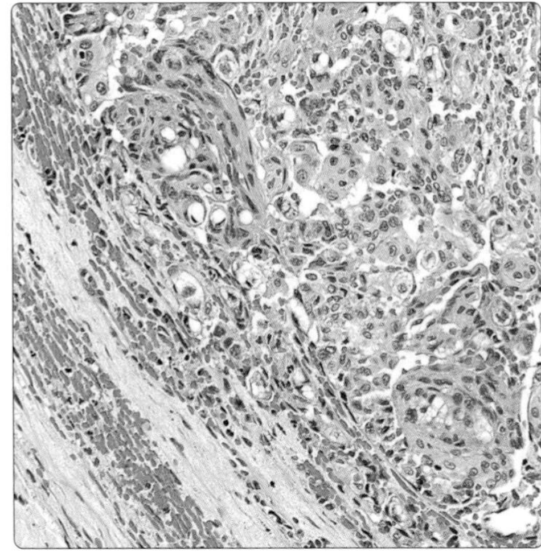

(Left) *Parasagittal meningiomas of any grade are prone to invade and eventually occlude the superior sagittal sinus ⮕. Since this happens slowly, collaterals can be recruited and infarction avoided. On the other hand, abrupt surgical removal of a patent or only partially occluded sinus may produce parasagittal venous infarction.* **(Right)** *As in this whorl-forming case, meningiomas involving dural venous sinuses are often well differentiated, grade I.*

Dural Invasion Benign Meningioma

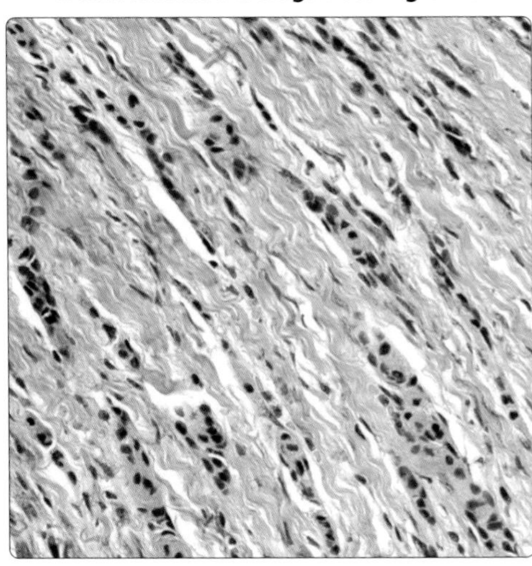

Soft Tissue/Muscle Invasion Not Grading Criterion

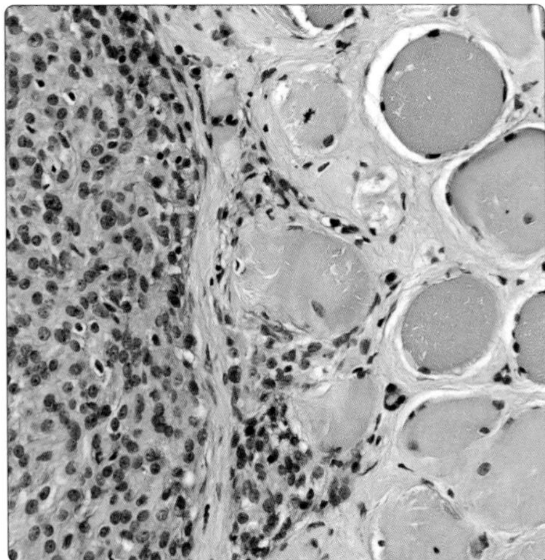

(Left) *Invasion of the dura may preclude total resection, but it is not a grading determinant, in contrast to invasion of the brain. Most dura-invasive meningiomas are grade I.* **(Right)** *Having penetrated the skull, meningiomas readily infiltrate cranial skeletal muscle. While this may affect ability to achieve gross total resection, such invasion is not a grading criterion.*

(Left) *Tumor nodules within the dura usually lie within tissue clefts but occasionally invade vessels, such as this venule* →*. The presence of endothelial cells certifies that the hollow structure is indeed a vessel.* **(Right)** *Immunostaining for CD34 can be used to confirm vascular invasion by establishing the presence of endothelial cells* →*. This intrusion is largely of academic interest; however, impressive as it is, it has no known prognostic significance.*

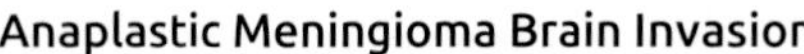

Anaplastic Meningioma Brain Invasion

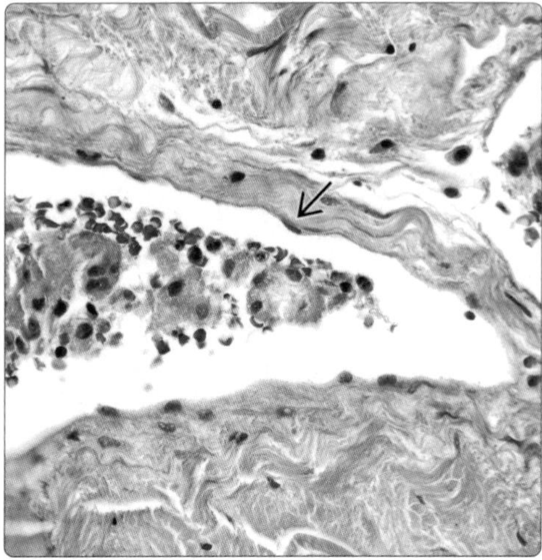

Meningioma Within Dural Venule, CD34

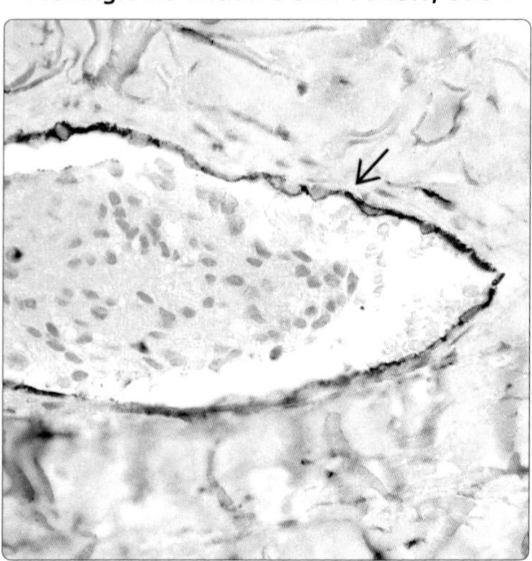

(Left) *Epithelioid cytological features and multiple mitoses* → *are common in anaplastic, grade III meningiomas. Twenty or more mitoses per 10 high-power fields is the threshold. Necrosis (not shown) is often prominent.* **(Right)** *Mitotically active, markedly atypical epithelioid cells and necrosis point to the diagnosis of grade III meningioma.*

Anaplastic Meningioma

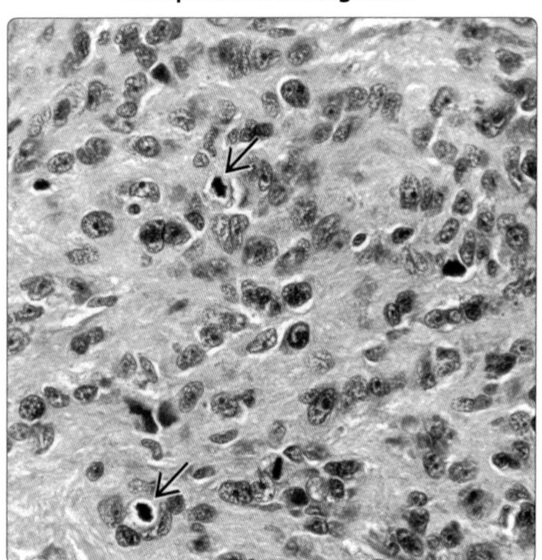

Anaplastic Meningioma

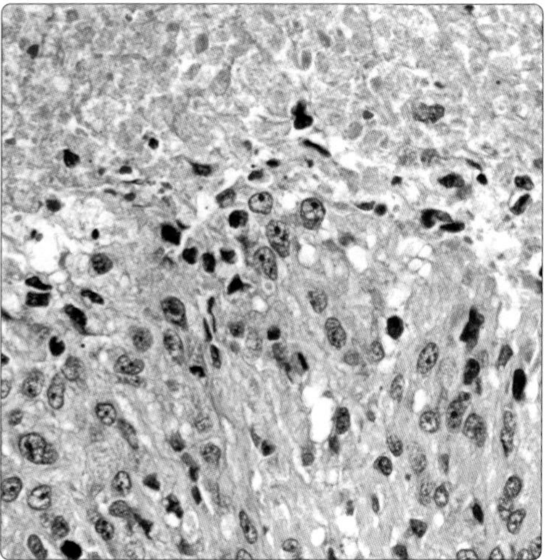

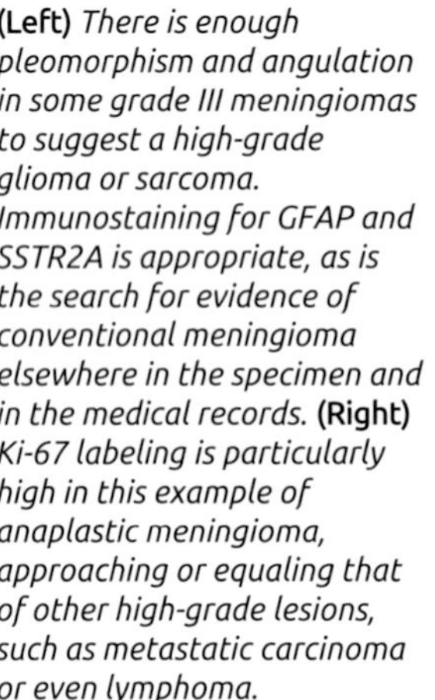

(Left) *There is enough pleomorphism and angulation in some grade III meningiomas to suggest a high-grade glioma or sarcoma. Immunostaining for GFAP and SSTR2A is appropriate, as is the search for evidence of conventional meningioma elsewhere in the specimen and in the medical records.* **(Right)** *Ki-67 labeling is particularly high in this example of anaplastic meningioma, approaching or equaling that of other high-grade lesions, such as metastatic carcinoma or even lymphoma.*

Anaplastic Meningioma Simulating Glioblastoma

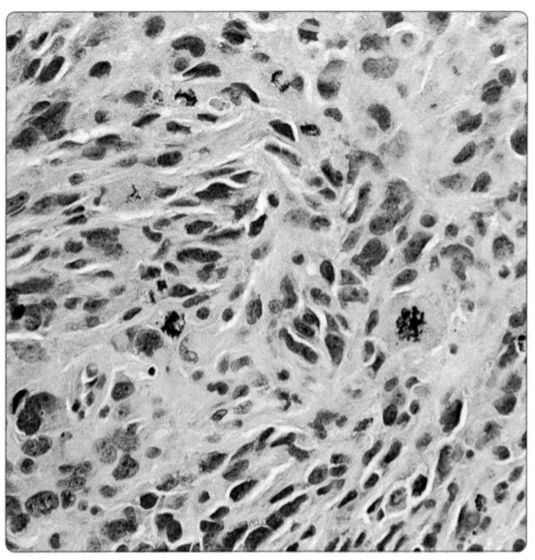

Anaplastic Meningioma, Ki-67 Elevated

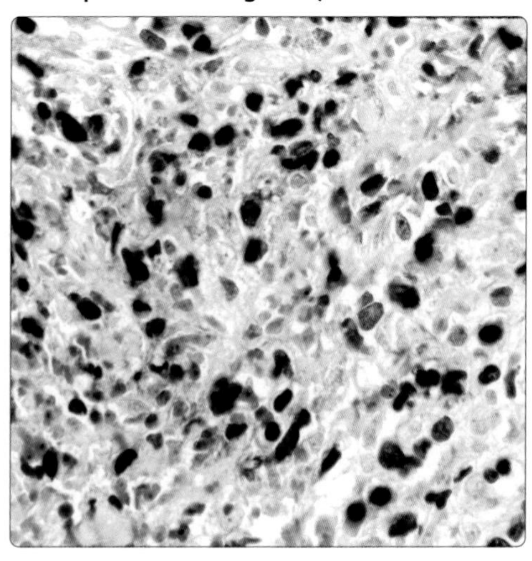

Meningioma Within Dural Venule

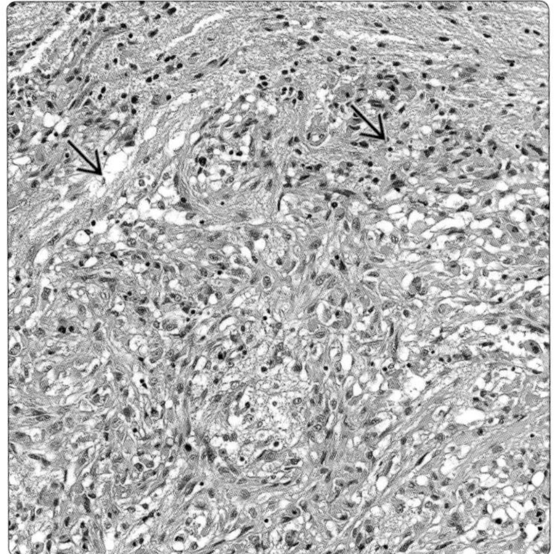

Brain Invasion, Anaplastic Meningioma, GFAP

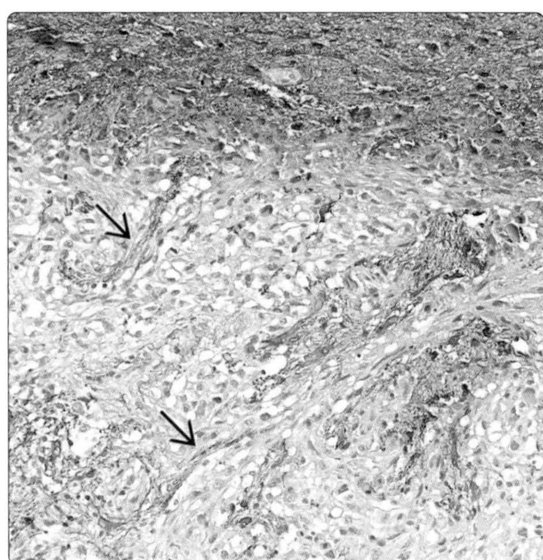

(Left) *Grade III anaplastic meningiomas freely invade underlying brain ➡, often producing a more intricate, less discrete tumor-brain interface than the grade II type with its sometimes more pushing margin. The extent and depth of infiltration would be better seen after immunostaining for GFAP.* **(Right)** *Anaplastic, grade III meningiomas are often especially invasive of the brain, trapping GFAP(+) parenchyma ➡ deep within the lesion.*

Low-Grade Area in Anaplastic Meningioma

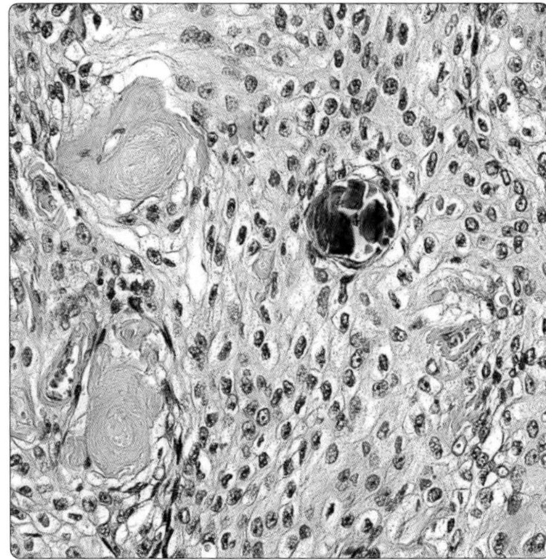

Anaplastic Meningioma

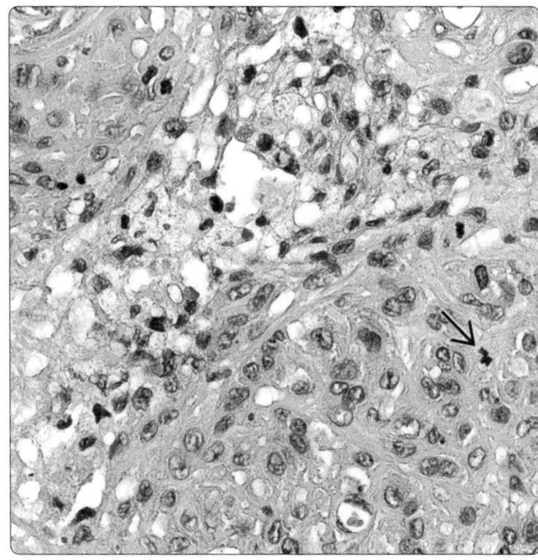

(Left) *Meningiomas often show evidence of tumor progression by association of both well-differentiated and anaplastic tissue within the same lesion. The latter was found elsewhere in this grade I tumor.* **(Right)** *Epithelioid features, mitoses ➡, and necrosis form a common triad in grade III meningiomas. Grade I tumor was present elsewhere in the specimen.*

Metastatic Dural Implant

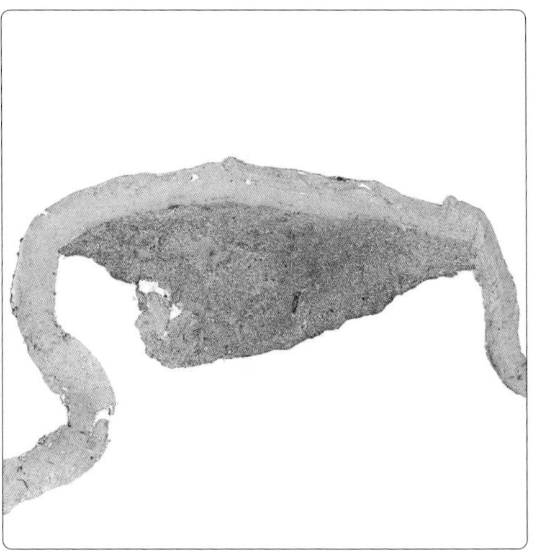

Lung Metastasis

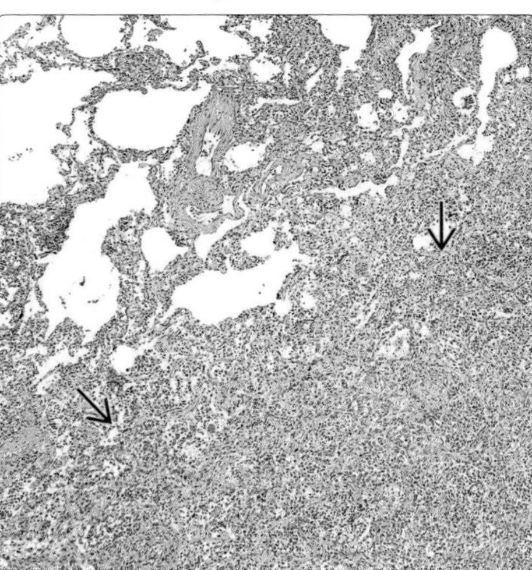

(Left) *Metastatic dural implants are 1 complication of grade III meningiomas. Others include local invasion and, uncommonly, distant metastases.* **(Right)** *Only infrequently do meningiomas metastasize to systemic sites, such as the lung ➡, as seen in this grade III example. Other but considerably less common secondary sites include liver, lymph nodes, and bone. (Courtesy W. M. Klein, MD.)*

Solitary Fibrous Tumor

KEY FACTS

TERMINOLOGY

- In CNS, solitary fibrous tumor (SFT)/hemangiopericytoma (HPC) terminology still utilized; considered to exist in spectrum; most SFT/HPCs harbor *NAB2/STAT6* fusion
  - Grade I (most are classic SFT type), grade II (mixture of both types), grade III (most are classic HPC type)

CLINICAL ISSUES

- Dural based, rarely parenchymal or intraventricular
- Favorable prognosis with gross total resection, but tend to recur if incompletely excised
- Tumors previously considered as SFT represent lower end of spectrum, with more indolent behavior
- Tumors previously considered as HPC in CNS represent higher end of spectrum, with less favorable prognosis

IMAGING

- Circumscribed, usually dural based with dural tail

MICROSCOPIC

- Compact, noninfiltrating unless anaplastic
- Biphasic with alternating paucicellular and hypercellular areas
- Bands of brightly eosinophilic wire-like collagen

ANCILLARY TESTS

- Diffusely CD34(+), but may be reduced or negative in malignant type
- Bcl-2(+), CD99(+), SSTR2A(-)
- STAT6(+), nuclear

TOP DIFFERENTIAL DIAGNOSES

- Fibrous meningioma
- Schwannoma
- Melanocytic neoplasm

DIAGNOSTIC CHECKLIST

- High mitotic rate and necrosis, poor prognostic factors

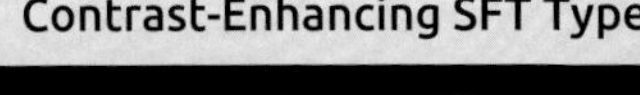
Contrast-Enhancing SFT Type

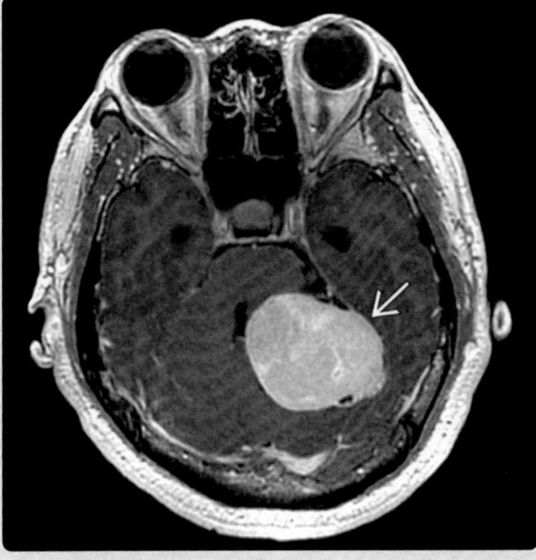

SFT Type

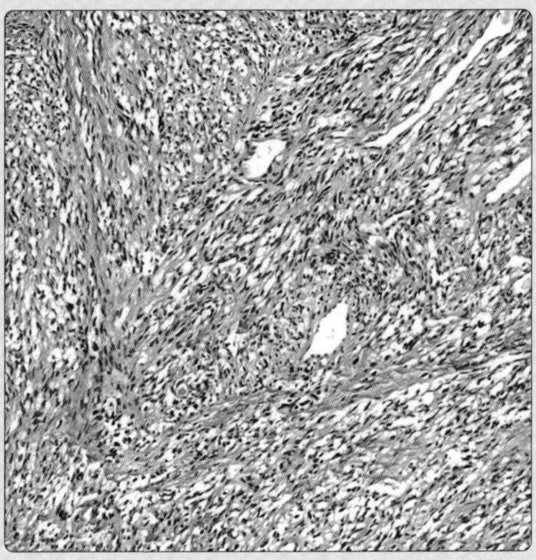

(Left) *In this axial contrast-enhanced T1-weighted MR, solitary fibrous tumor (SFT) appears as a diffusely enhancing tumor with a broad attachment to dura mater ➡. There is associated mass effect with compression of the 4th ventricle.* **(Right)** *Many CNS tumors in this category demonstrate a spindle cell appearance with abundant collagen fibers invested in between tumor cells, creating a vaguely fascicular and often a patternless architecture. The vessels typically demonstrate the so-called staghorn structure.*

Contrast-Enhancing HPC Type

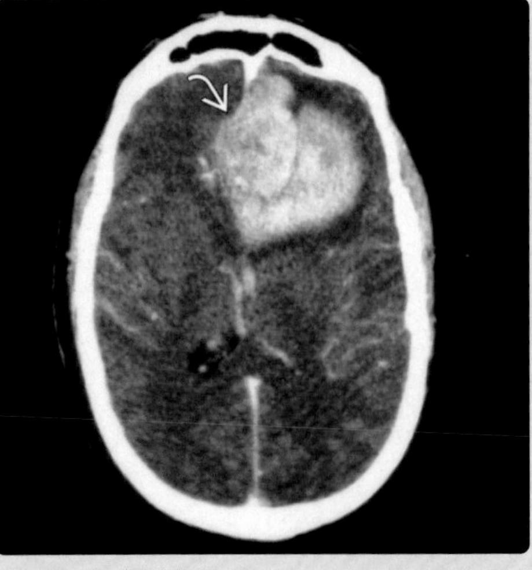

Hemangiopericytoma Type

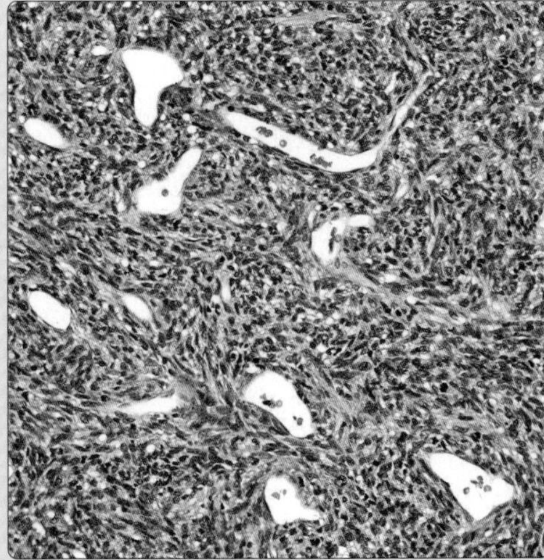

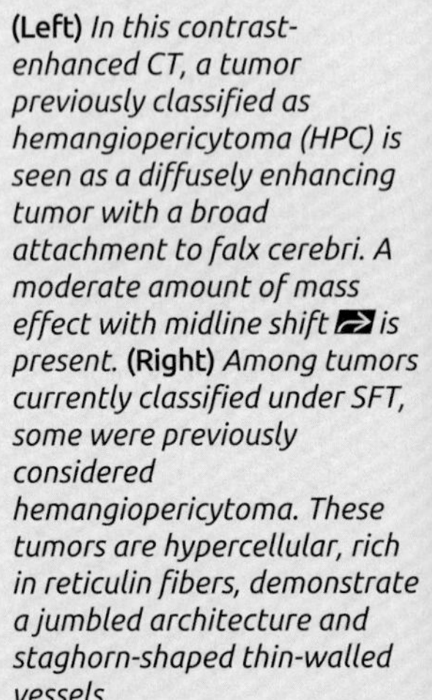
(Left) *In this contrast-enhanced CT, a tumor previously classified as hemangiopericytoma (HPC) is seen as a diffusely enhancing tumor with a broad attachment to falx cerebri. A moderate amount of mass effect with midline shift ➡ is present.* **(Right)** *Among tumors currently classified under SFT, some were previously considered hemangiopericytoma. These tumors are hypercellular, rich in reticulin fibers, demonstrate a jumbled architecture and staghorn-shaped thin-walled vessels.*

TERMINOLOGY

Abbreviations

- Solitary fibrous tumor (SFT)
- Hemangiopericytoma (HPC) or solitary fibrous tumor, hemangiopericytoma-type (SFT/HPC)

Definitions

- Ubiquitous mesenchymal neoplasm of fibroblastic nature with prominent hemangiopericytoma (HPC)-like vessels
  - Tumors previously considered under HPC are currently classified as SFT according to current WHO soft tissue classification, but two entities; SFT and HPC are recognized in WHO CNS 2007
  - Most SFT/HPCs harbor *NAB2/STAT6* fusion

CLINICAL ISSUES

Epidemiology

- Incidence
  - Uncommon; most common is HPC type, followed by SFT type
- Age
  - Mean: ~ 50 years
- Now considered spectrum of neoplasms from low grade to frankly anaplastic
  - Tumors previously considered as SFT represent lower end of spectrum, with more indolent behavior
  - Tumors previously considered as HPC in CNS have less favorable prognosis

Site

- Dural based in most cases
  - Usually falx cerebri or tentorium cerebelli
- Extraaxial
  - Cerebrum
  - Cerebellum and cerebellopontine angle
  - Spinal cord
- Intraventricular

Presentation

- Depending on tumor location
  - Headaches
  - Seizures
  - Focal deficits

Treatment

- Gross total resection

Prognosis

- Low-grade tumors with classic SFT pattern have favorable prognosis after gross total resection
- Intermediate prognosis for more mitotically active lesions
- Unfavorable for malignant or high-grade examples or those with HPC pattern
- Potential for progression from low-grade tumors to anaplastic
- Systemic metastases
  - Lung, liver, and bone metastases
- Cerebrospinal/leptomeningeal spread, rare

IMAGING

MR Findings

- Circumscribed, usually dural based
  - Dural tail (some)
- Isointense to gray matter on T1WI
- Variable and mixed areas of high and low signal intensity on T2WI
  - Low signal in collagen-rich areas
- Avid, heterogeneous contrast enhancement
- Variable peritumoral edema &/or mass effect

MACROSCOPIC

General Features

- White-tan, firm, and rubbery
- Smooth or bosselated, unencapsulated surface
- Vascular spaces and hemorrhage on cut section
- Cysts, in some cases, are rare
- Traps regional vessels and nerves
- Compresses surrounding CNS parenchyma without gross invasion
- Potential for parenchymal invasion in anaplastic examples, rare

MICROSCOPIC

Histologic Features

- 2 major histological patterns
  - SFT type
    - Low to moderate cellularity
    - Noninfiltrative, discrete borders
    - Patternless pattern
    - Rich amount of brightly eosinophilic collagen invested in strips in between tumor cells
      - Rarely keloid-like or amianthoid fibers
    - Biphasic, paucicellular hyalinized areas and cellular regions
    - Occasionally fascicular or storiform architecture
    - Loose spongy tissue with occasional myxoid change
    - Often delicate and thin-walled vessels
      - Focally thick-walled, hyalinized vessels, especially in low-cellularity areas
      - HPC-like vessels, focal
      - Slit-like vessels with bland endothelial cells
    - Strong collagen staining on trichrome
    - Patchy irregular reticulin staining
    - Low mitotic rate, except in rare anaplastic tumors
  - Anaplasia [uncommon in SFT (SFT with anaplastic features)]
    - Necrosis
    - Mitoses > 5/10 HPF
    - High cellularity and marked nuclear pleomorphism
    - Fascicular, sometimes herringbone architecture
    - Variable loss of CD34 immunoreactivity
  - HPC type
    - Highly cellular tumor, jumbled pattern
    - Round oval nuclei
    - Delicate and prominent HPC-like staghorn vessels
    - Prominent reticulin staining surrounding individual or small clusters of cells

  - Collagen bundles focally present
- Tumors with hybrid features reported
  - Some SFT types may recur as HPC type or vice versa

ANCILLARY TESTS

Cytology

- Bland, oval cells with dark nuclei and homogeneous chromatin
  - More hyperchromatic than meningioma
- Sparse cytoplasm
  - Less than meningioma
- Nucleoli usually inconspicuous
- No intranuclear pseudoinclusions

Immunohistochemistry

- STAT6(+), nuclear
- CD34
  - Diffusely positive in common SFT type
  - Often limited to vessels in HPC type
- Bcl-2 variably positive
- CD99(+)
- Collagen IV, pericellular
  - More prominent in SFT type
  - Focal or limited tumor cells positive in HPC type
- S100(-), desmin (-), EMA(-), most keratins (-), claudin (-)
- FXIIIA, variable, may be negative
- Mostly low Ki-67 rate (1-4%) but higher (> 10%) in malignant/anaplastic types

Genetic Testing

- *NAB2/STAT6* fusion recognized as molecular signature of these tumors
  - Recent studies in soft tissues suggest that SFT-type and HPC-type tumors may have different fusion types

Electron Microscopy

- Fibroblastic features
- Abundant, rough endoplasmic reticulum
- No junctions or basal lamina

DIFFERENTIAL DIAGNOSIS

Fibrous Meningioma

- Whorls and psammoma bodies, but may be scant or absent in this subtype
- Nuclear pseudoinclusions, but often scant or absent
- Stromal calcifications, common
- EMA(+), SSTR2A(+), nuclear STAT6(-)
- Progesterone receptors (+), E cadherin (+) in some cases
- CD34(+) in vessels only

Schwannoma

- Relation to peripheral nerve
- Antoni A and Antoni B tissues
- S100, CD57, collagen IV, nuclear SOX10 all diffusely positive

Melanocytic Neoplasms

- Uniformly hypercellular, nested pattern
- Cells more epithelioid
- Prominent nucleoli and intranuclear inclusions
- Melanin but may be scarce or absent
- Less collagen
- MITF, HMB-45, Melan-A, S100 all positive

Gliosarcoma

- Glial component without reticulin
- More anaplasia and often parenchymal infiltration in glial component
- Microvascular proliferation
- Necrosis common
- Often p53(+) and always nuclear STAT6(-)
- GFAP(+) at least focally, S100(+)

Fibrosarcoma

- Herringbone pattern
- Cytological monomorphism
- Little vessel hyalinization
- Only vessels CD34(+), nuclear STAT6(-)

DIAGNOSTIC CHECKLIST

Pathologic Interpretation Pearls

- Cases borderline between SFT and HPC not uncommon
- Use STAT6, EMA, and CD34 to distinguish from fibrous meningioma
- High mitotic rate and necrosis are poor prognostic factors

GRADING

SFT to Cellular SFT (HPC) Spectrum (Suggested Marseille System)

- Grade I (most are classic SFT type)
  - Low cellularity, no necrosis, and ≤ 5 mitoses/10 HPF
- Grade II (mixture of both types)
  - IIa: High cellularity, no necrosis, and ≤ 5 mitoses/10 HPF
  - IIb: High cellularity, no necrosis, and > 5 mitoses/10 HPF
- Grade III (most are classic HPC type)
  - High cellularity, necrosis, > 5 mitoses/10 HPF

SELECTED REFERENCES

1. Barthelmeß S et al: Solitary fibrous tumors/hemangiopericytomas with different variants of the NAB2-STAT6 gene fusion are characterized by specific histomorphology and distinct clinicopathological features. Am J Pathol. 184(4):1209-18, 2014
2. Chmielecki J et al: Whole-exome sequencing identifies a recurrent NAB2-STAT6 fusion in solitary fibrous tumors. Nat Genet. 45(2):131-2, 2013
3. Fargen KM et al: The central nervous system solitary fibrous tumor: a review of clinical, imaging and pathologic findings among all reported cases from 1996 to 2010. Clin Neurol Neurosurg. 113(9):703-10, 2011
4. Bouvier C et al: Solitary fibrous tumors and haemangiopericytomas of the meninges: overlapping pathological features and common prognostic factors suggest the same spectrum of tumors. Brain Pathol. 22(4):511-21, 2011
5. Hayashi Y et al: A reevaluation of the primary diagnosis of hemangiopericytoma and the clinical importance of differential diagnosis from solitary fibrous tumor of the central nervous system. Clin Neurol Neurosurg. 111(1):34-8, 2009
6. Tihan T et al: Solitary fibrous tumors in the central nervous system. A clinicopathologic review of 18 cases and comparison to meningeal hemangiopericytomas. Arch Pathol Lab Med. 127(4):432-9, 2003
7. Carneiro SS et al: Solitary fibrous tumor of the meninges: a lesion distinct from fibrous meningioma. A clinicopathologic and immunohistochemical study. Am J Clin Pathol. 106(2):217-24, 1996
8. Mena H et al: Hemangiopericytoma of the central nervous system: a review of 94 cases. Hum Pathol. 22(1):84-91, 1991
9. Fletcher CDM, World Health Organization., International Agency for Research on Cancer. Who classification of tumours of soft tissue and bone. Lyon: IARC Press; 2013

Intraventricular Tumor

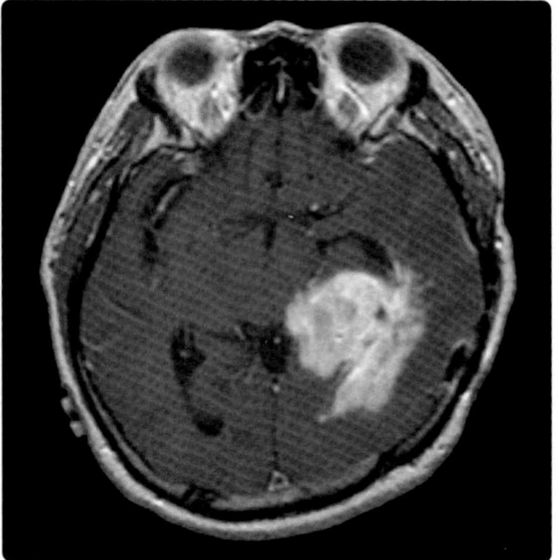

Liver Metastasis, HPC Type

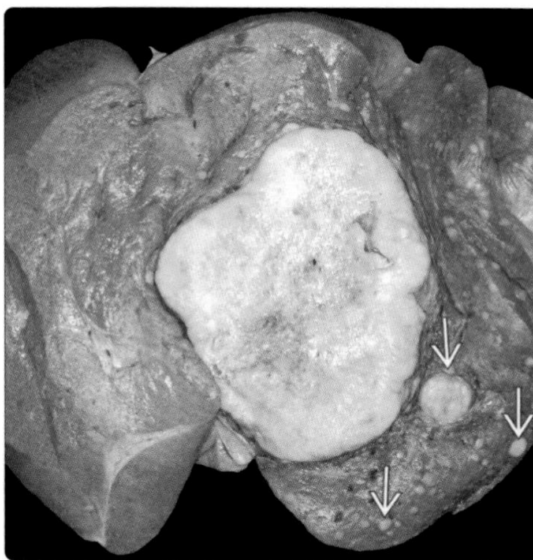

(Left) *This axial contrast-enhanced T1-weighted MR demonstrates a large left frontoparietal tumor with ventricular extension. Intraoperatively, the tumor was well demarcated from the surrounding parenchyma.* **(Right)** *This large metastatic liver tumor was discovered almost a decade after the initial resection of a brain tumor. The original tumor had been diagnosed as angiomatous meningioma and was later recognized to be hemangiopericytoma. Note the numerous smaller metastatic foci* ➡*.*

Macroscopic Appearance, SFT Type

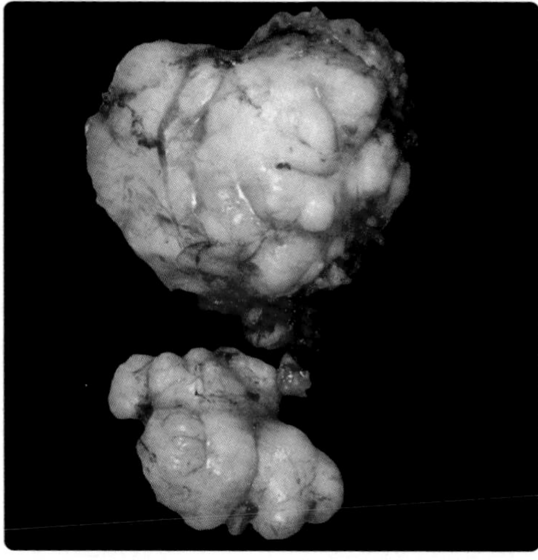

Macroscopic Appearance, SFT Type

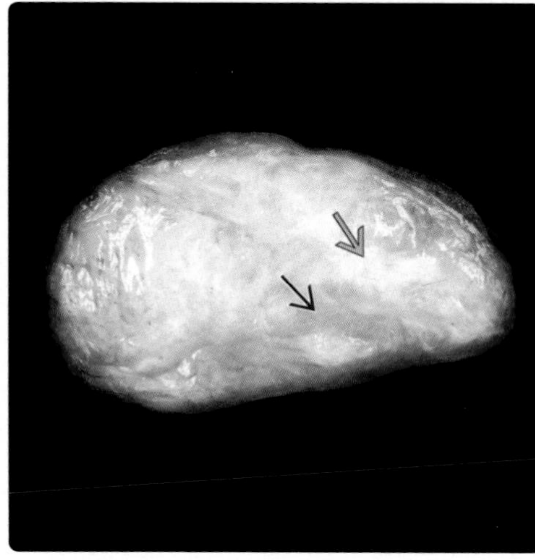

(Left) *Solitary fibrous tumors are firm, well-circumscribed masses that may be macroscopically confused with meningioma.* **(Right)** *This cross section of a well-defined tumor demonstrates the prominent tan-white fibrous bands* ➡ *within the mass and areas that appear more fleshy* ➡*. Despite its clear demarcation, there was no recognizable fibrous capsule.*

Dural-Based Tumor, HPC Type

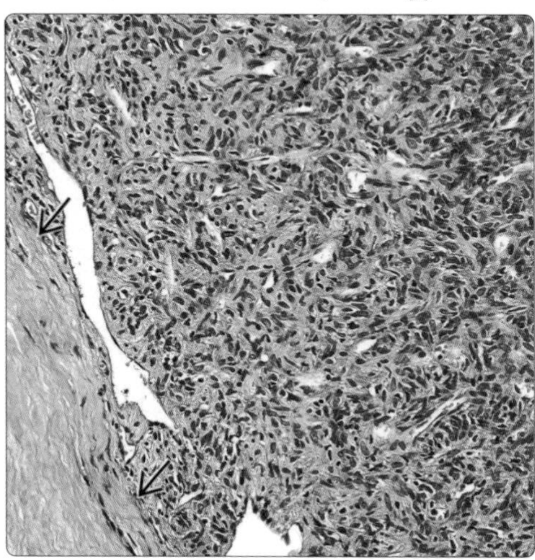

Intraoperative Smear

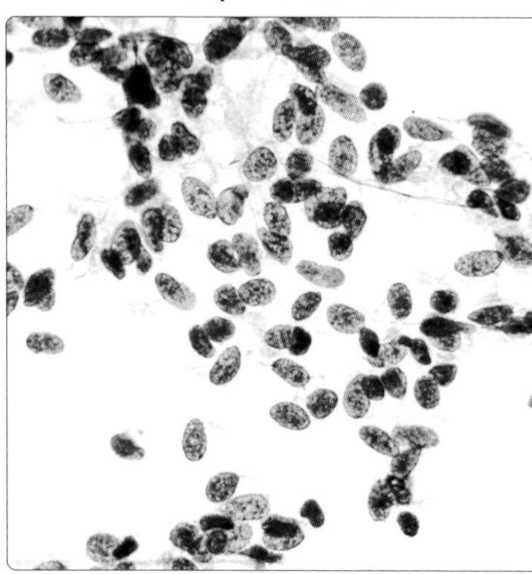

(Left) *Like meningiomas, HPC-type lesions are usually firmly adherent to dura* ➡*. The densely cellular tissue interrupted by slit-like vessels is typical of HPC. The paucity of perivascular collagen helps exclude meningioma.* **(Right)** *Uniform cells with inconspicuous cytoplasm and small, dark, oval nuclei distinguish SFT/HPC from meningioma in smear preparations. Nuclear pseudoinclusions and psammoma bodies are not features of the former.*

(Left) *Fusiform cells in fascicles separated by dense bands of collagen are typical of SFT.* **(Right)** *Elongated, cytologically bland, somewhat wavy cells separated by collagen bundles are classic features of solitary fibrous tumors. Fibrous meningioma would be in the differential but can be excluded in part by lack of reaction for CD34 and positive staining with SSTR2A and EMA.*

Rich Collagen Bands, SFT Type

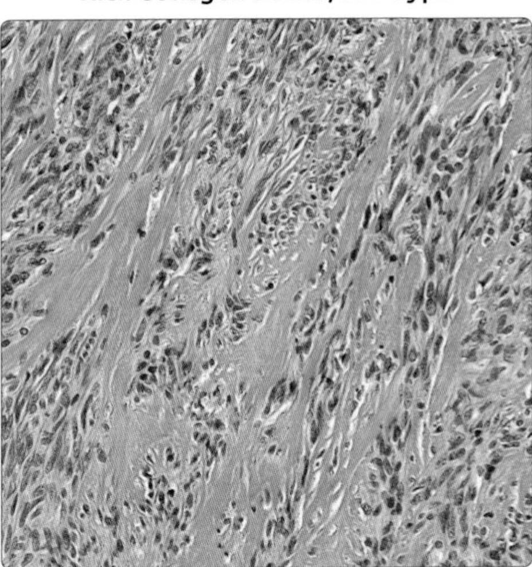

Spindle Cells, SFT Type

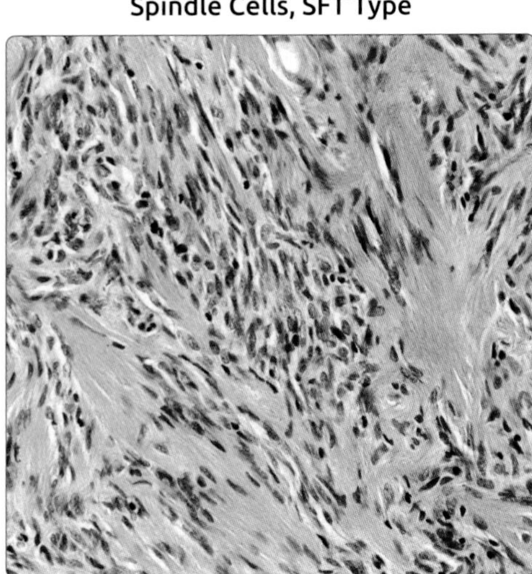

(Left) *Bands of trichrome-positive collagen can be seen in SFT-type tumors.* **(Right)** *Staghorn vessels ⇨ and dense, patternless cellularity help distinguish HPC type from meningioma. While the borders are often discrete, there may be a slight suggestion of parenchymal involvement in some tumors ➡.*

Trichome, SFT Type

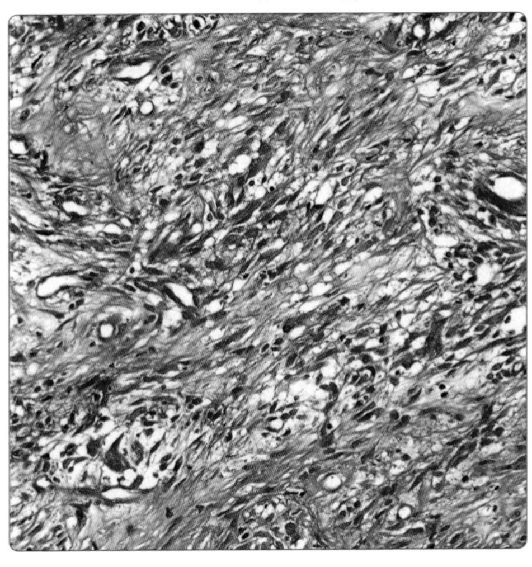

Low Magnification, HPC Type

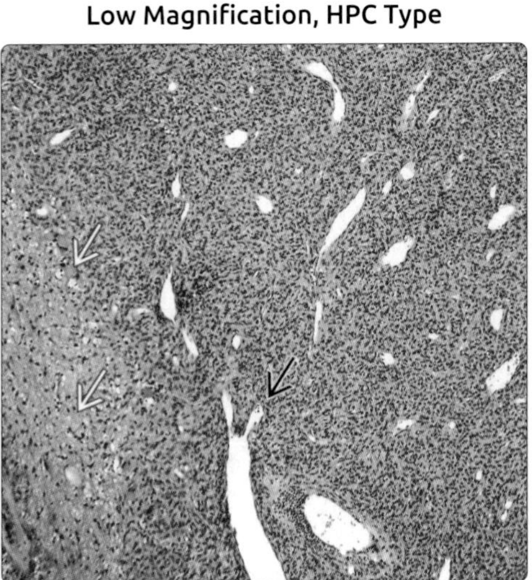

(Left) *The HPC type of tumors shows brisk cellularity, less conspicuous collagen, and prominent vasculature with the staghorn vessels ⇨. There is usually only a moderate amount of cellular pleomorphism except in anaplastic tumors.* **(Right)** *Coarse, pale-staining collagen bundles ⇨, rather than fine, black reticulin fibers, fill the interstitium in most SFTs. Delicate, pervasive, intensely staining reticulin fibers are more typical of the HPC type.*

Jumbled Pattern, HPC Type

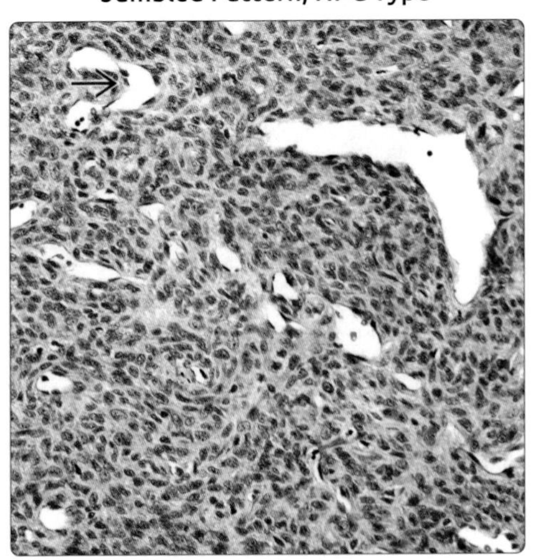

Elaborate Reticulin, HPC Type

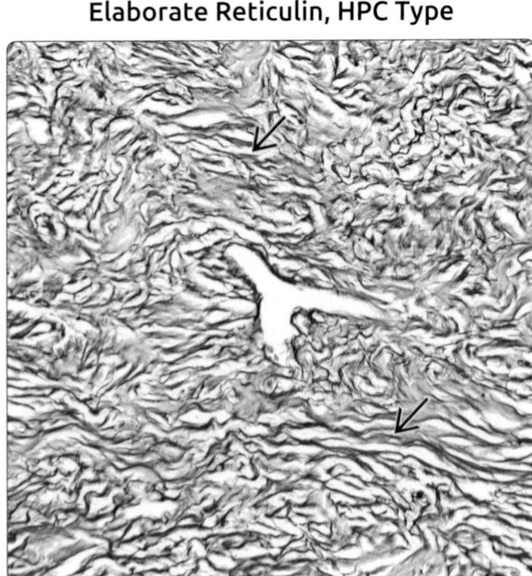

Dense Sclerotic Areas, SFT Type

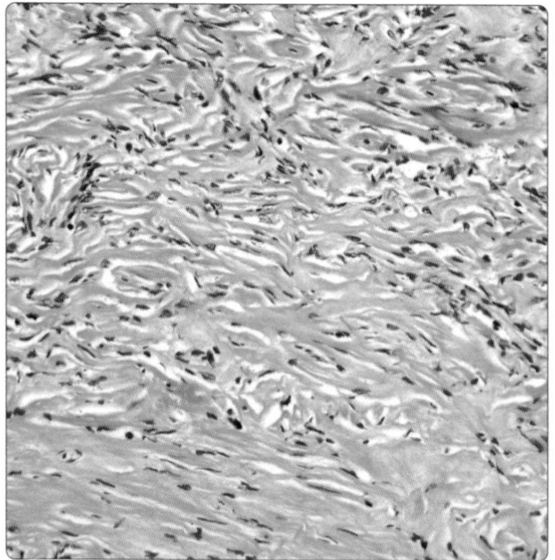

SFT, Hybrid Patterns

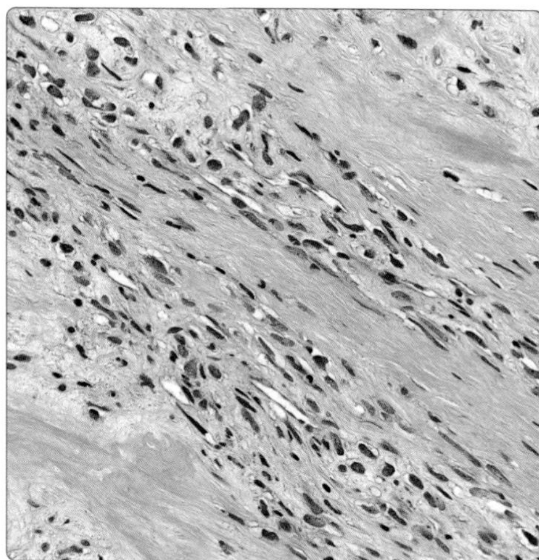

(Left) *In this paucicellular, diagnostically ambiguous sclerotic area, differential diagnosis ranges from SFT to fibrous meningioma to collagenous scar. Classic features of SFT were present elsewhere in this meningeal tumor.* **(Right)** *A nexus between the SFT and HPC types is found in some tumors. Elsewhere, the tumor was typical of HPC type with jumbled pattern. These hybrid examples reinforce the concept of SFT as a single entity with 2 prominent histological patterns.*

Pale Hypocellular Zones

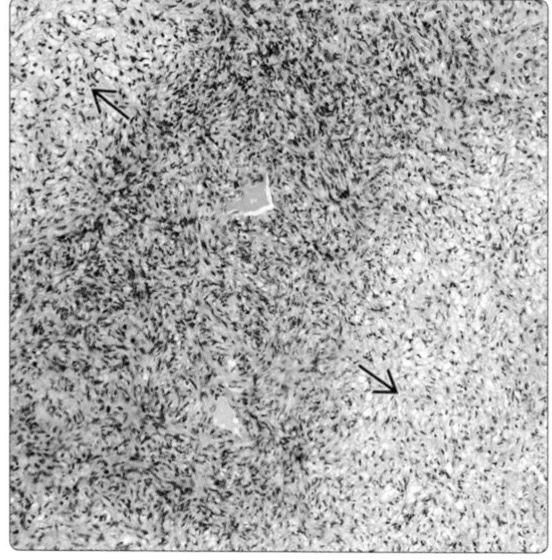

Vague Whorl-Like Structures, HPC Type

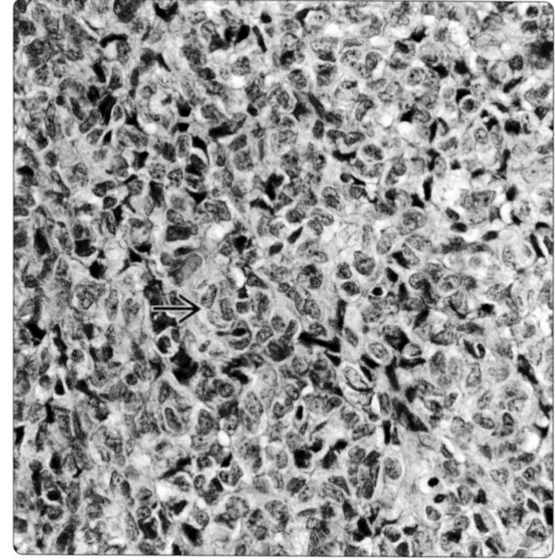

(Left) *Pale, hypocellular zones ⊡ are common in both SFT and HPC types. The absence of thick hyalinized vessels or of a particular pattern, especially of whorls, is not consistent with meningioma. Nevertheless, immunostaining in such cases is useful.* **(Right)** *Vague, whorl-like structures in HPCs ⊡ might suggest meningioma, but the plump, disorganized cells are not typical features of the latter tumor. The nested architecture in this case also somewhat resembles that of a primary meningeal melanocytic tumor.*

Uncommon Patterns, Virchow-Robin Spaces

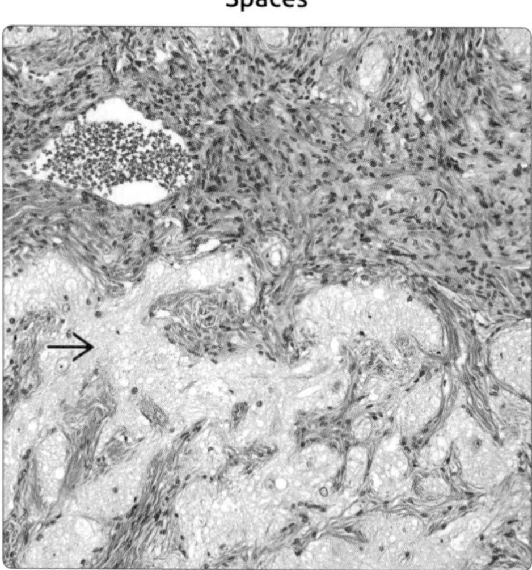

Discrete Borders, HPC Type

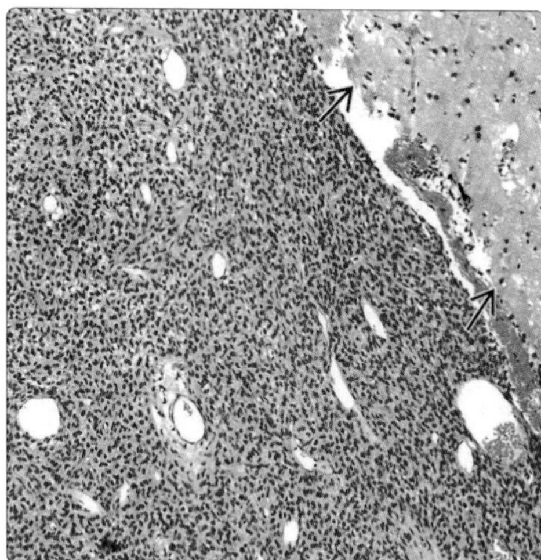

(Left) *SFTs can involve the Virchow-Robin spaces in the adjacent brain ⊡, simulating a meningioangiomatosis-like pattern. While this may be difficult to distinguish from brain parenchymal invasion, perivascular spread of tumor cells creates a distinctive appearance.* **(Right)** *The pia, shown juxtaposed ⊡ with the brain-tumor interface, has not been breached in this case. Despite their deceptively circumscribed appearance in some cases, tumors of the HPC type often recur locally and are prone to late distant metastasis.*

(Left) *Features of anaplastic SFT, such as increased cellularity and mitotic activity ⇨, are apparent even at low magnification. The bright collagen in between tumor cells is still recognizable in this tumor, which showed NAB2/STAT6 fusion.* **(Right)** *Aggressiveness in SFTs is defined largely by mitotic activity ➡, specifically > 5 mitoses/10 HPF. High cellularity and increased atypia are also present. Necrosis is also a poor prognostic factor in association with increased mitoses and high cellularity.*

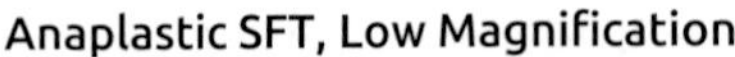

Anaplastic SFT, Low Magnification

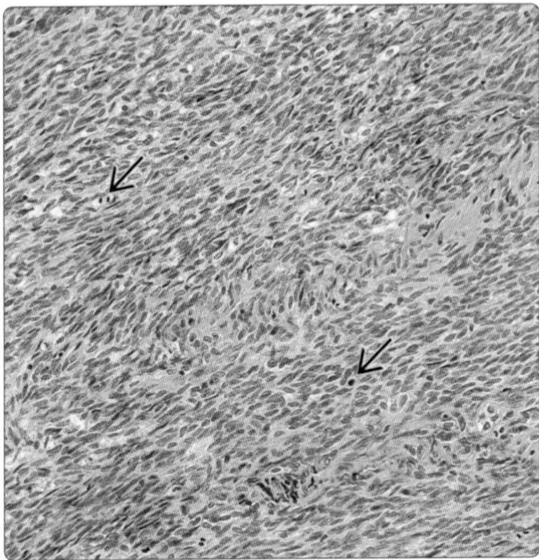

Anaplastic SFT, Pleomorphism and Mitoses

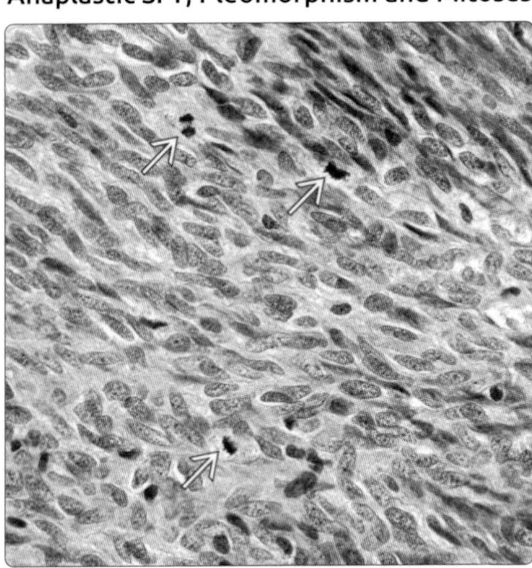

(Left) *Necrosis is present in some solitary fibrous tumors, generally those that are mitotically active ⇨. Necrosis ➡ is a poor prognostic factor in SFTs.* **(Right)** *While atypia is generally greater in anaplastic SFTs, mitotic activity ⇨ is the key feature. Multiple mitoses are present here. Presence of > 5 mitoses/10 HPF has been suggested to predict more aggressive behavior in tumors along the SFT-HPC spectrum. Necrosis is also an important grading parameter.*

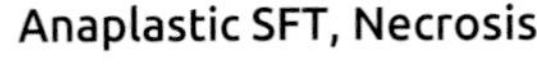

Anaplastic SFT, Necrosis

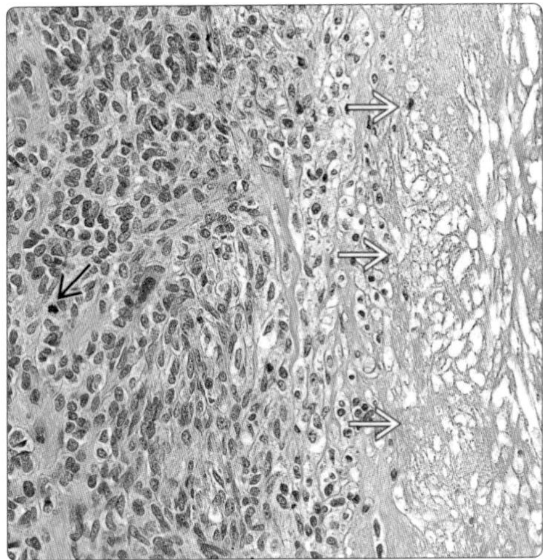

Anaplastic SFT, Mitoses

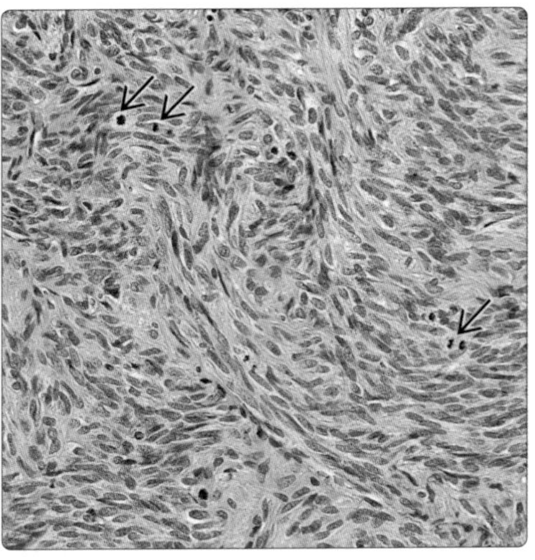

(Left) *Cytologic atypia is generally not marked in SFTs but may be considerable, especially in the presence of other features, such as high cellularity, increased mitotic activity, and necrosis. The illustrated turbulent architecture is common in the HPC type.* **(Right)** *While quite inconspicuous in typical SFT, the nucleoli can be quite prominent ➡ in anaplastic examples. This anaplastic example is of the HPC type, with large vesicular nuclei and abundant mitoses ⇨.*

Anaplastic SFT, Turbulent Architecture

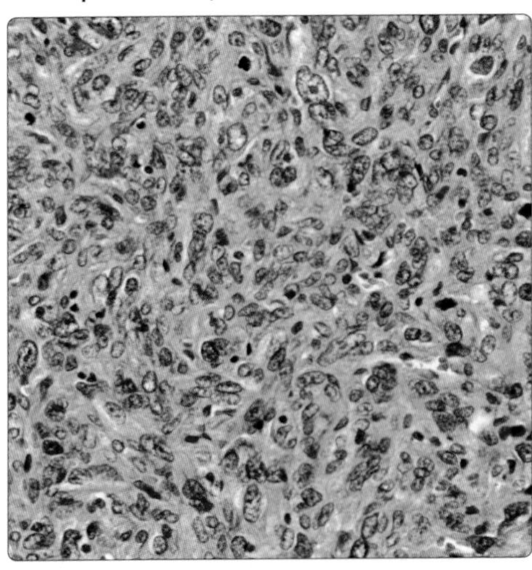

Anaplastic SFT, Macronucleoli

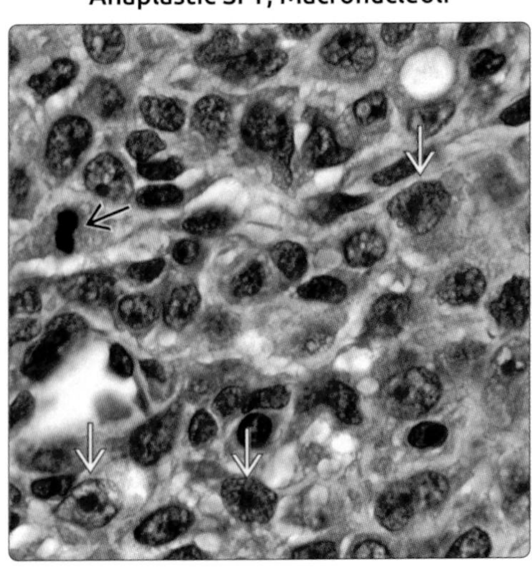

SFT, Diffuse Strong CD34 Staining

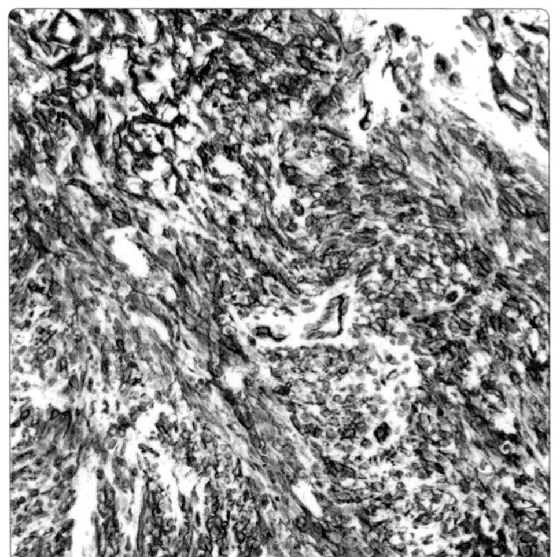

HPC, CD34 Staining Highlights Vasculature

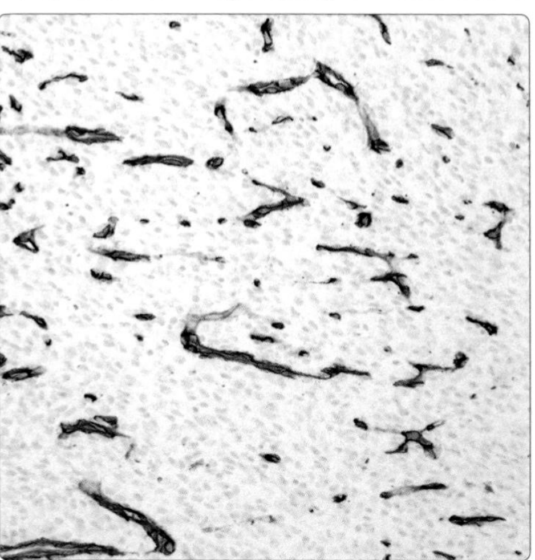

(Left) *The typical SFT demonstrates diffuse strong staining with CD34. This operational definition of SFT has excluded tumors with the typical HPC type from the diagnosis in the past.* **(Right)** *While the CD34 staining is diffuse and strong in the tumors with the classical SFT-type morphology, this staining highlights only the vasculature in cases with the typical HPC-type morphology. The type of NAB2/STAT6 fusion in these tumors may be distinct.*

Bcl-2 Positivity

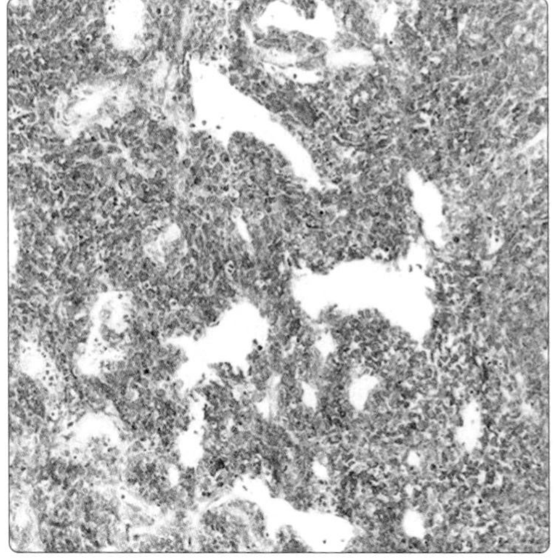

CD99 Staining

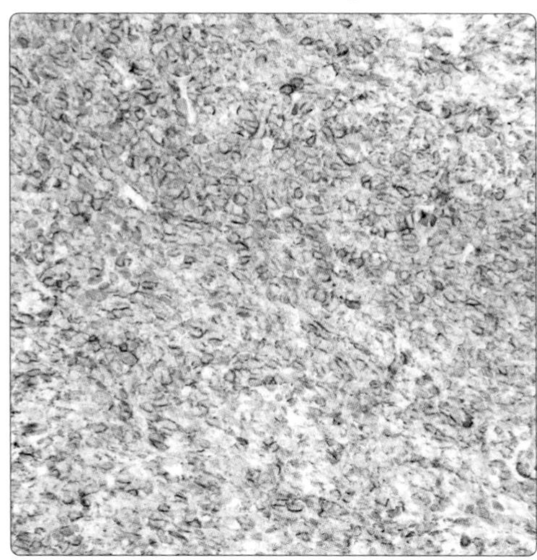

(Left) *Both the SFT and the HPC types of this tumor entity show strong positivity with the Bcl-2 antibodies. This staining is also positive in many other entities but provides a helpful distinction from meningiomas and schwannomas, which are often Bcl-2 negative.* **(Right)** *Like many other tumors that can be in the differential diagnosis of SFT, the tumors in this category also show positivity with CD99 antibodies.*

Nuclear STAT6 Positivity, SFT Type

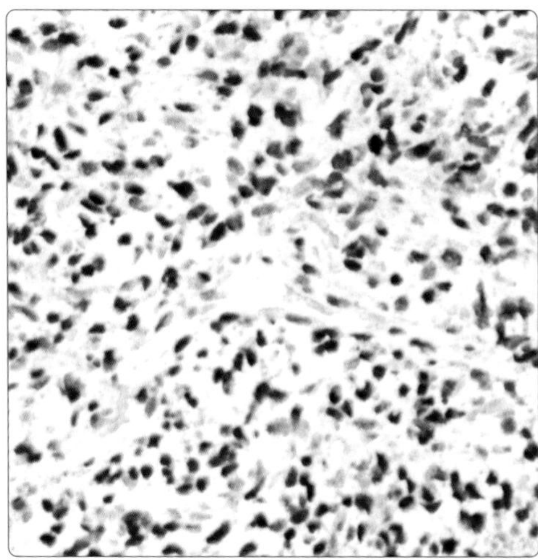

HPC Type, STAT6 Nuclear Positivity

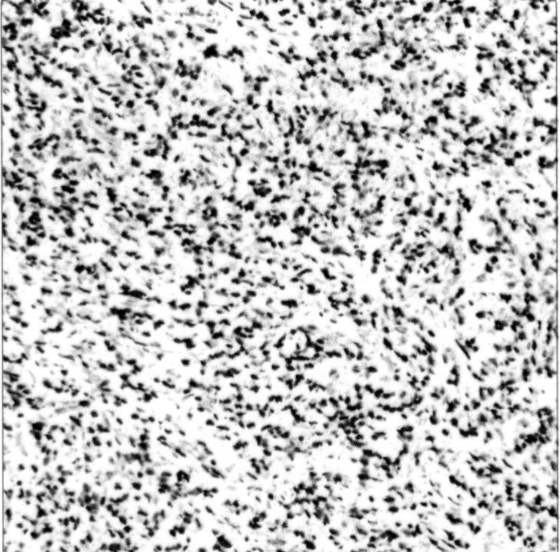

(Left) *Almost all SFTs, regardless of their histological pattern of subtype, demonstrate strong diffuse nuclear positivity with the STAT6 antibodies. This staining underscores the fusion that is often the NAB2/STAT6 fusion that translocates the STAT6 to the nucleus of the cell.* **(Right)** *HPCs of the CNS show translocation of STAT6 from the cytoplasm to the nucleus and therefore nuclear expression of STAT6 protein. In contrast, a meningioma would have only cytoplasmic STAT6 immunoreactivity.*

Primary Melanocytic Neoplasms

KEY FACTS

TERMINOLOGY

- Spectrum from low-grade melanocytoma to malignant melanoma
  - No consensus grading system

CLINICAL ISSUES

- Sites
  - Posterior fossa, spinal cord, supratentorial
- Prognosis
  - Good for melanocytoma
  - Guarded for intermediate lesions
  - Poor for melanoma, but better than for metastatic melanoma to CNS

IMAGING

- Heavily pigmented cases are dark on T2WI and bright on precontrast T1WI

MICROSCOPIC

- Mitotic activity minimal or absent in melanocytoma
- Nested architecture, in some cases, especially lower grade
- Meningioma-like, sheet-like, or lobular architecture in some cases
- Spindled or epithelioid cells more likely in melanoma
- Nucleoli small in most melanocytomas; large, eosinophilic in melanomas but also in some melanocytomas and intermediate lesions
- Necrosis and invasion in melanoma
- Ill-defined intermediate category

TOP DIFFERENTIAL DIAGNOSES

- Melanotic schwannoma
- Meningioma
- Solitary fibrous tumor/hemangiopericytoma
- Metastatic melanoma
- Metastatic carcinoma

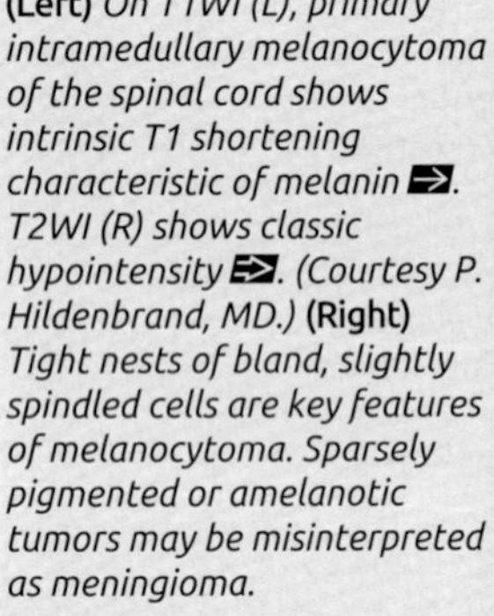

(Left) *On T1WI (L), primary intramedullary melanocytoma of the spinal cord shows intrinsic T1 shortening characteristic of melanin ➔. T2WI (R) shows classic hypointensity ➔. (Courtesy P. Hildenbrand, MD.)* **(Right)** *Tight nests of bland, slightly spindled cells are key features of melanocytoma. Sparsely pigmented or amelanotic tumors may be misinterpreted as meningioma.*

Intramedullary Melanocytoma

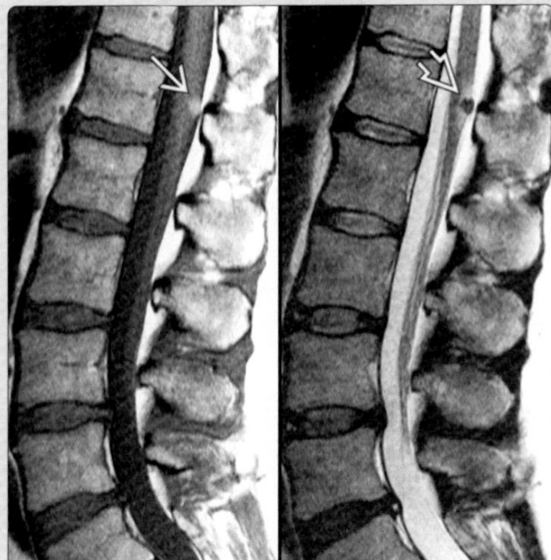

Nests of Spindled Cells

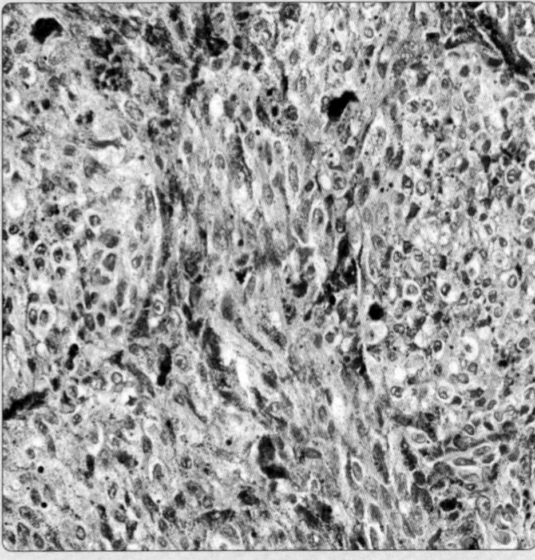

(Left) *Some melanomas are focally necrotic ➔. Mitoses ➔ were present in this lesion with a degree of pleomorphism that would be atypical for a lower grade melanocytic tumor.* **(Right)** *Most primary CNS melanocytomas and melanomas show strong immunolabeling for a variety of melanocytic markers. A red chromogen is helpful in heavily pigmented tumors.*

Focal Necrosis

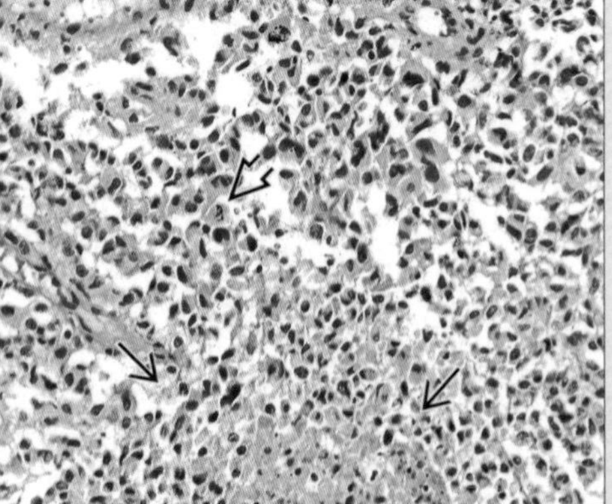

MART-1 Immunoreactivity

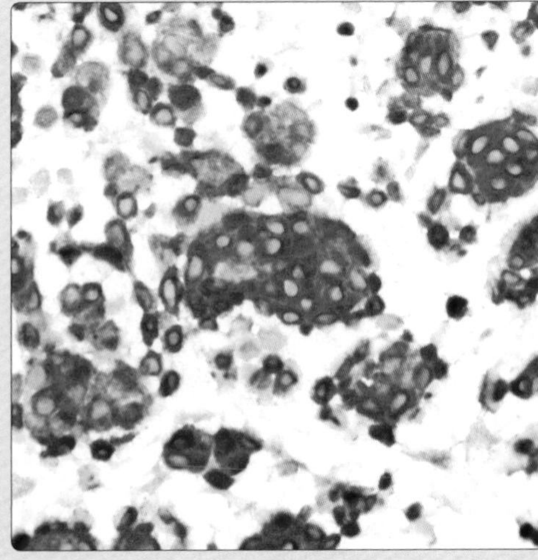

TERMINOLOGY

Definitions

- Uncommon neoplasms derived from normal leptomeningeal melanocytes
  - Nodular mass
    - Morphologic spectrum from low-grade melanocytoma to melanocytic tumor of intermediate differentiation to malignant melanoma
    - No consensus on precise criteria distinguishing these subdivisions
  - Diffuse leptomeningeal infiltrate
    - Meningeal melanocytosis/melanomatosis (neurocutaneous melanosis) (rare)

ETIOLOGY/PATHOGENESIS

Developmental Anomaly

- Neurocutaneous melanosis
  - Aberrant expression of hepatocyte growth factor/scatter factor (*HGF*) implicated

CLINICAL ISSUES

Epidemiology

- Incidence
  - Rare
- Age
  - Mostly adults
    - 5th decade for focal malignant melanoma
    - 4th decade for diffuse melanomatosis
  - Children with neurocutaneous melanosis syndrome
    - Symptomatic by 2 years of age
- Sex
  - Primary CNS nodular melanoma more common in male patients
  - No preference for neurocutaneous melanosis
- Ethnicity
  - Caucasians > other races

Site

- Posterior fossa
  - Base of skull
  - Cerebellopontine angle
  - Meckel cave
    - Melanocytoma in this site associated with nevus of Ota
- Spinal cord
  - Intradural extramedullary
    - Most melanocytomas arise at cervical and thoracic levels
  - Largely intramedullary (rare)
- Supratentorial
  - Leptomeninges
  - Intraventricular (rare)

Presentation

- Nodular mass
  - Site-dependent deficits
- Diffuse leptomeningeal infiltrate
  - Seizures
  - Signs/symptoms of increased intracranial pressure
  - Myelopathy with spinal cord involvement

Treatment

- Complete surgical resection for melanocytoma
- No effective therapy for others

Prognosis

- Good for melanocytoma
  - Rarely undergo malignant transformation
- Guarded for melanocytic tumors of intermediate differentiation
- Poor for melanoma, but
  - Better prognosis for primary CNS than metastatic melanoma
- Poor for neurocutaneous melanosis
  - Majority undergo malignant transformation with death by 4 years of age

IMAGING

MR Findings

- Nodular mass
  - Extraaxial and well circumscribed
  - Iso-, hypointense on T2WI and hyperintense on precontrast T1WI
  - Homogeneous enhancement
  - T1 and T2 signal characteristics dependent on melanin content
    - Highly pigmented lesions bright on precontrast T1WI and dark on T2WI
    - Most lesions not sufficiently pigmented to generate these signal characteristics
- Diffuse leptomeningeal infiltrate
  - T1 shortening within brain parenchyma & meninges
  - Leptomeningeal or intraparenchymal enhancement heralds malignant transformation

MACROSCOPIC

General Features

- Nodular mass
  - Solitary mass lesions, pigmented or nonpigmented
  - Hemorrhage or necrosis in some cases
- Diffuse leptomeningeal infiltrate
  - Dense, black subarachnoid staining

MICROSCOPIC

Histologic Features

- Nodular mass
  - Compact, circumscribed
    - Can extend along Virchow-Robin spaces (melanocytic tumor with intermediate differentiation and melanoma)
  - Nested architecture in some cases, especially ↓ grade
  - Meningioma-like sheet-like or lobular architecture in some cases
  - Vasocentric fascicles
  - Spindled or epithelioid cells (more likely in melanoma)
  - Uniform, bean-shaped nuclei
    - With longitudinal grooves, focal
  - Nucleoli

- Small in most melanocytomas
- Large, eosinophilic in melanomas but also in some melanocytomas and intermediate lesions
- Variable pigment (dense to absent)
  - Often heaviest along periphery
  - Sometimes largely in melanophages
  - Histochemical stains (e.g., Fontana-Masson) may be applied to confirm melanin on cases of questionable pigment
- Mitotic activity variable by grade
- Necrosis uncommon
- Diffuse leptomeningeal infiltrate
  - Benign or malignant melanocytes in leptomeninges and Virchow-Robin spaces

ANCILLARY TESTS

Cytology

- Melanocytoma and melanocytic tumor of intermediate differentiation
  - Uniform epithelioid or bipolar spindled cells
  - Bean-shaped or grooved nucleoli
  - Small, but sometimes large, eosinophilic nucleoli
  - Variable pigmentation, intra- and extracellular
- Melanoma
  - Dyscohesive
  - Greater cellular pleomorphism and nuclear atypia
  - Large nucleoli, coarse chromatin
  - Variable pigmentation, intra- and extracellular
  - Melanophages

Immunohistochemistry

- S100(+), HMB-45(+), MART-1/Melan-A(+)
  - S100 most sensitive but least specific
- SOX9, SOX10 (+)
- Tyrosinase (+) and MITF(+)
- Cytokeratin and EMA(-)

Genetic Testing

- *GNAQ/11* mutations frequent in primary leptomeningeal melanocytic lesions, particularly melanocytoma

DIFFERENTIAL DIAGNOSIS

Melanotic Schwannoma

- Obvious relation to nerve in some cases
- Pericellular reticulin and collagen IV (+)
- Psammoma bodies in psammomatous variant
- Not always clear distinction

Meningioma

- Whorls and psammoma bodies
- May contain trapped meningeal melanocytes
- EMA(+)
- No such entity as melanotic meningioma; most formerly reported as such likely represent melanocytoma

Solitary Fibrous Tumor/Hemangiopericytoma

- Wire-like collagen
- Dense cellularity; staghorn vessels
- CD34(+) (variable in hemangiopericytoma)/nuclear STAT6 reactivity

Metastatic Melanoma

- More likely intraparenchymal and multiple
- History of primary in most cases
- Often more pleomorphic and necrotic

Metastatic Carcinoma

- Usually not discrete leptomeningeal
- Positive for keratin and negative for melanocytic markers

DIAGNOSTIC CHECKLIST

Clinically Relevant Pathologic Features

- Tumors with invasive pattern more likely to recur

Pathologic Interpretation Pearls

- May closely resemble meningioma
- May be amelanotic

GRADING

General Considerations

- No established cut-offs, much overlap

Melanocytoma

- Nested architecture in many but not all cases
- Minimal atypia
- Small, single nucleoli
- Few mitoses (≤ 1/10 HPF), but no established cut-off point from melanoma; overlap with intermediate lesions in some cases
- Low Ki-67 labeling index (< 2%)

Intermediate Grade

- Ill-defined category
  - Sometimes employed for lesions with focal mitoses > 2/10 HPF, but not other features of melanoma
    - e.g., lesions with little cytological atypia, no necrosis
- Invasion is significant, but perivascular extension is more frequent and should not be mistaken for invasion
  - Invasion sometimes present in tumor with rare, if any, mitoses
- Ki-67 index ↑ over melanocytoma

Malignant Melanoma

- Less nested, more sheet-like than melanocytoma
- Nuclear enlargement, macronucleoli and atypia usually increased over melanocytoma
- Necrosis &/or invasion in some cases
- Mitoses (> 2/10 HPF) but not precisely defined
- Ki-67 indices, mean ~ 8%

SELECTED REFERENCES

1. Koelsche C et al: Melanotic tumors of the nervous system are characterized by distinct mutational, chromosomal and epigenomic profiles. Brain Pathol. 25(2):202-8, 2015
2. Küsters-Vandevelde HV et al: Activating mutations of the GNAQ gene: a frequent event in primary melanocytic neoplasms of the central nervous system. Acta Neuropathol. 119(3):317-23, 2010
3. Smith AB et al: Pigmented lesions of the central nervous system: radiologic-pathologic correlation. Radiographics. 29(5):1503-24, 2009
4. Brat DJ et al: Primary melanocytic neoplasms of the central nervous systems. Am J Surg Pathol. 23(7):745-54, 1999

Minimal Nuclear Variation

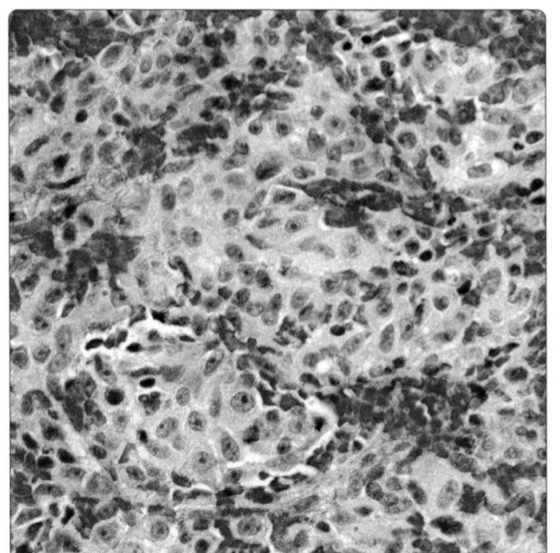

Nuclear Grooves

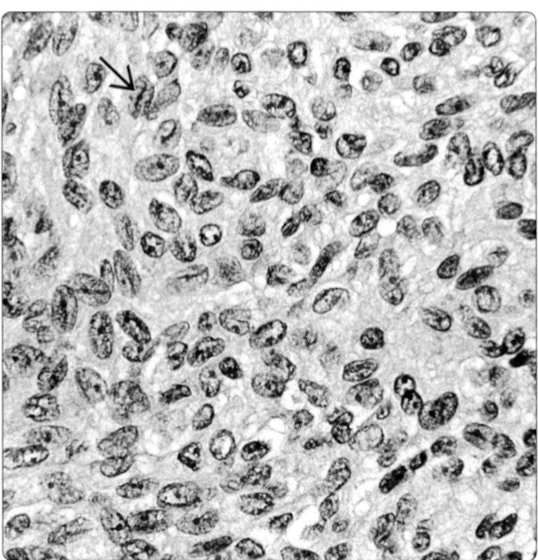

(Left) *Melanocytomas exhibit minimal variation in nuclear size and shape; they often contain small, but not inconspicuous, nucleoli. A nested pattern is common. Mitotic figures are exceptional.* **(Right)** *While usually only focal, if present at all, longitudinal nuclear grooves ➲ are useful in suggesting the melanocytic nature of a leptomeningeal tumor that, in the absence of pigment, could possibly be confused with meningioma.*

Cytologically Bland Neoplasm

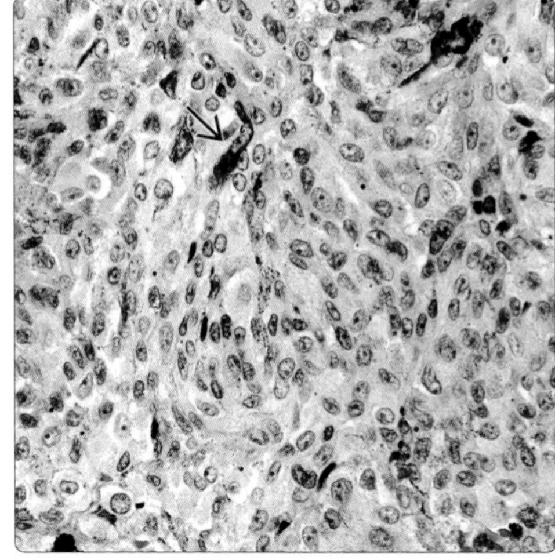

Dense Pigmentation

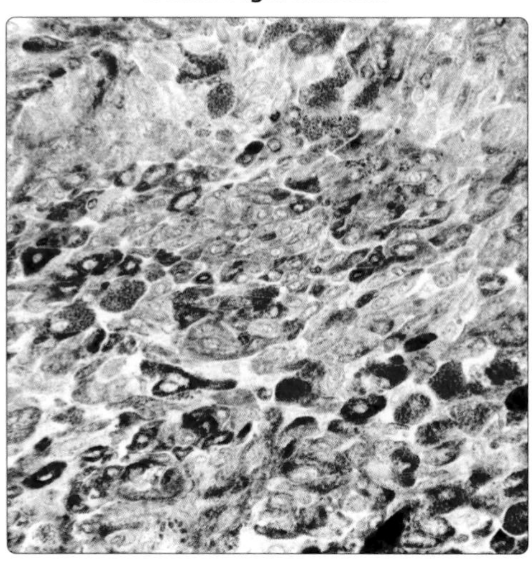

(Left) *But for the pigment ➲, cytologically bland melanocytic neoplasms such as this can be mistaken easily for meningioma. No mitoses were identified in this lesion with small nucleoli.* **(Right)** *Dense pigmentation obscuring cytological details may require bleaching to assess cytological atypia and mitotic activity. This mitosis-free melanocytoma had a low Ki-67 index. Nucleoli may be small as in this case, yet prominent in melanocytic tumors with few if any mitoses.*

Nested Architecture

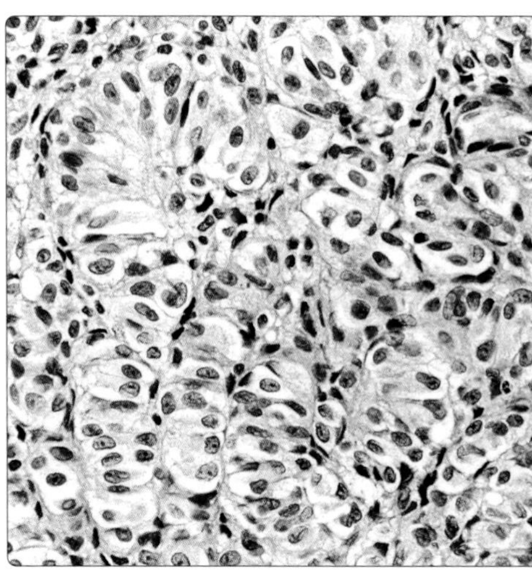

Nested Architecture

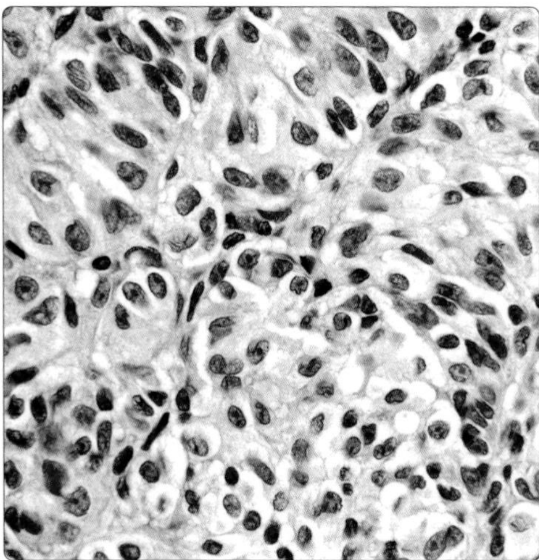

(Left) *Nested architecture is highly suspicious for melanocytic neoplasm, lack of pigment notwithstanding. On the basis of low-level mitotic activity, this difficult-to-grade melanocytic tumor was placed in the ill-defined intermediate category.* **(Right)** *A nested architecture is common in primary CNS melanocytic tumors, especially those of lower grade but in some melanomas as well. This lesion was intermediate, an attractive category in some cases but one that lacks a precise definition.*

(Left) *Sheet-like, rather nested architecture is present in some cases. Areas such as this without mitoses would qualify as melanocytoma. Mitoses elsewhere in this tumor warranted the designation of intermediate grade in this invasive lesion.* **(Right)** *Primary melanocytic tumors are often difficult to grade, as in this example with prominent nucleoli but rare mitoses. Cytologically, the lesions are prime melanoma suspects, but they have low proliferative potential. The pigment might be dismissed as hemosiderin.*

Sheet-Like Architecture

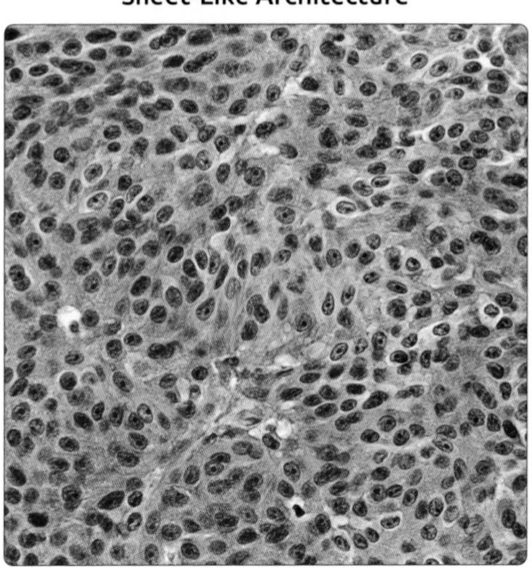

Prominent Nucleoli

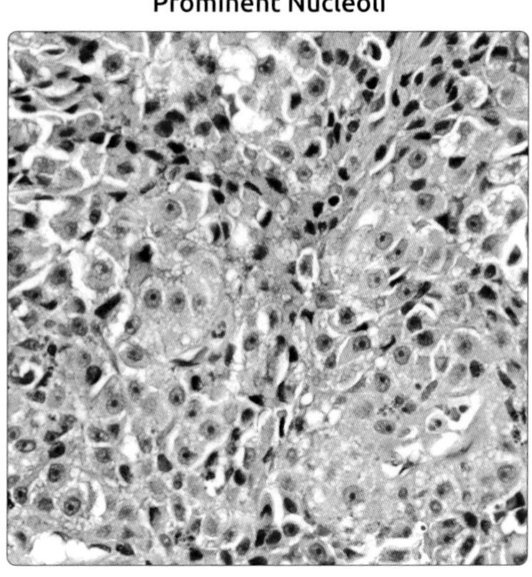

(Left) *Cellular but cytologically bland melanocytic tumors can resemble meningiomas. Scattered mitoses* ⇒ *were present in this tumor that was too mitotically active to be melanocytoma but fell short of melanoma.* **(Right)** *The distinction between melanocytoma of intermediate differentiation and melanoma is not always clear. Generally, any more than a rare mitosis* ⇒ *is grounds for diagnosis as the intermediate lesion, and more than a few is evidence for melanoma.*

Bland Melanocytic Tumor

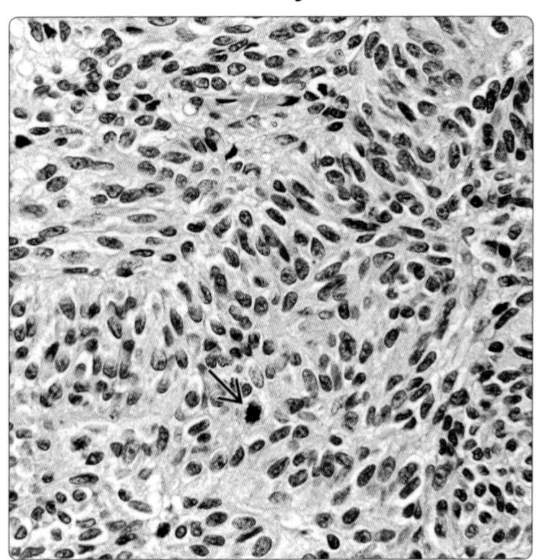

Rare Mitosis

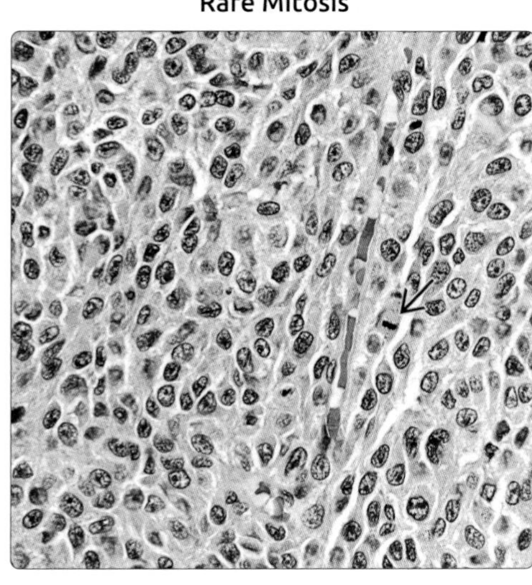

(Left) *Although a cytologically bland melanocytoma, this lesion invaded the brain, earning the designation intermediate. Similar grading issues are encountered in invasive meningiomas that are otherwise grade I tumors.* **(Right)** *Cytological features and multiple mitoses* ⇒ *leave no doubt that this tumor is melanoma, not melanocytic tumor of lower grade. Immunostains such as S100 and HMB-45 would help establish its melanocytic nature.*

Brain Invasion

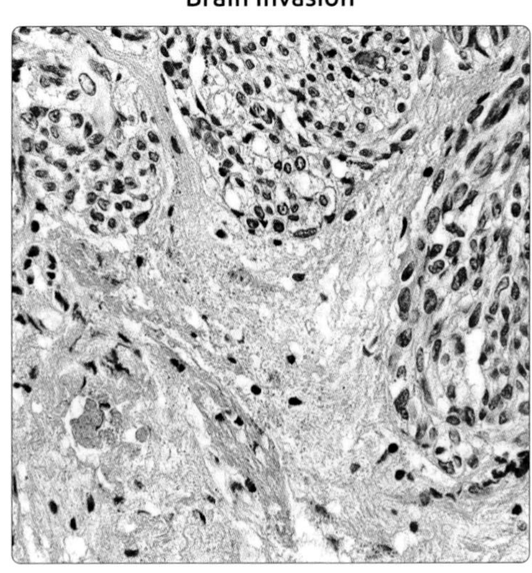

Multiple Mitoses

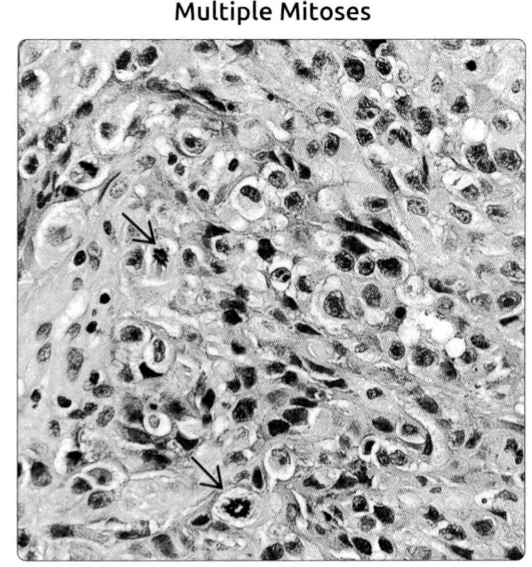

Nuclear Pleomorphism

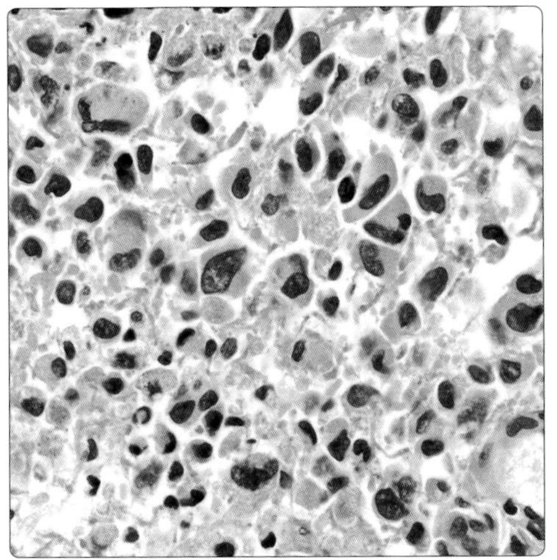

Heavy Pigmentation

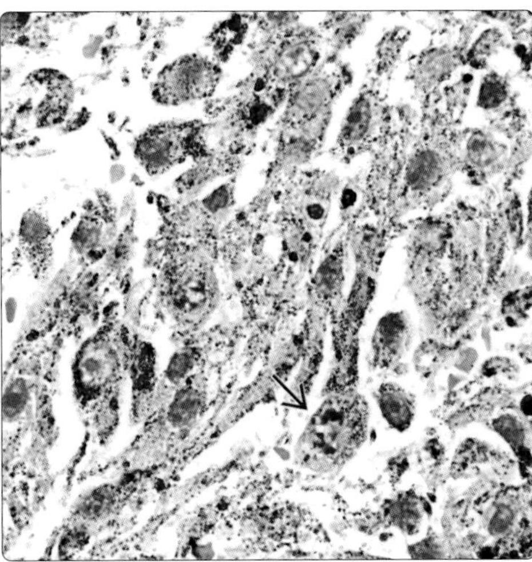

(Left) *Some melanomas feature considerable nuclear pleomorphism, which prompts instant consideration of a high-grade lesion. The melanocytic nature may be more subtle. Multiple mitoses were present.* **(Right)** *Without bleaching, mitoses ➔ may be difficult to identify in heavily pigmented melanomas such as this. Prominent nucleoli are typical of melanoma, but they are present in some mitosis-poor lower grade primary CNS melanocytic tumors as well.*

Delicate, Uniform Nuclei

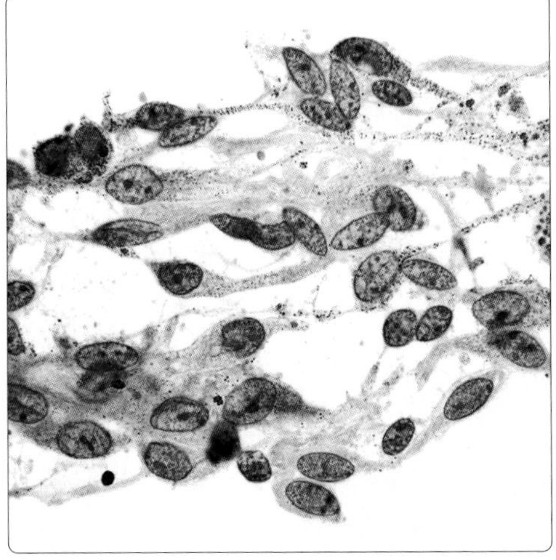

Monotonous Epithelioid Appearance

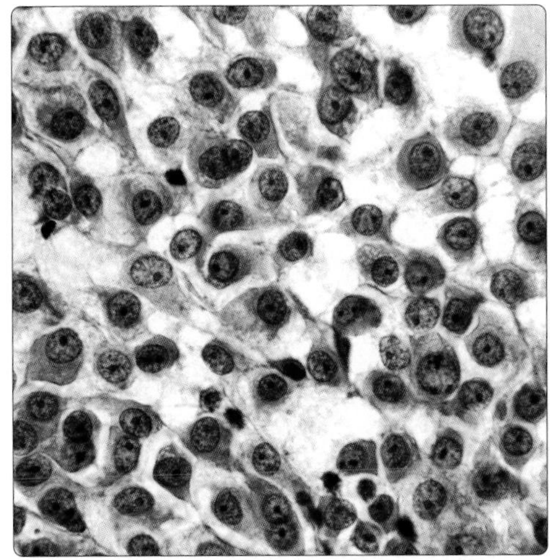

(Left) *Delicate, uniform nuclei and pigment-laden bipolar processes are common findings in melanocytoma. Nuclei are somewhat more hyperchromatic, and nucleoli are larger than those seen in meningiomas. Occasional meningiomas contain hemosiderin, which can be confused with melanin.* **(Right)** *In smear preparations, primary CNS melanocytic tumors often have a monotonous epithelioid appearance with round nuclei and prominent nucleoli.*

Neurocutaneous Melanosis

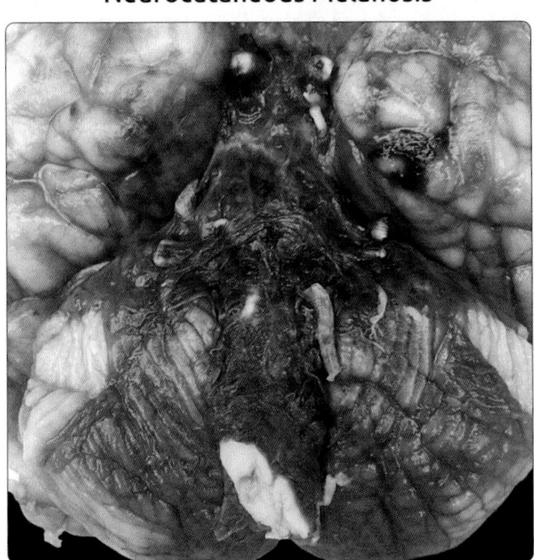

Leptomeningeal Involvement

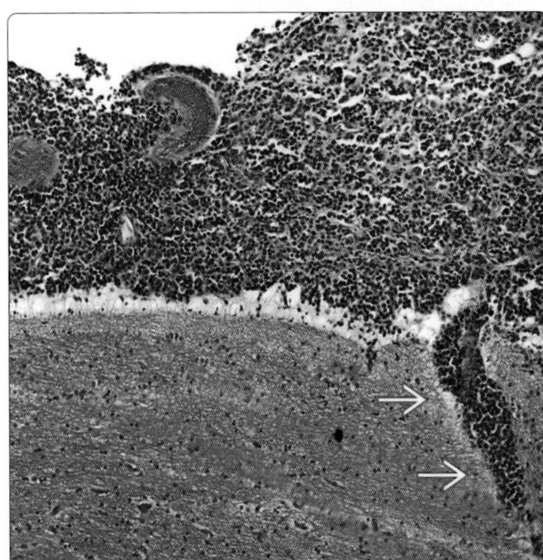

(Left) *Diffuse involvement of the basal leptomeninges is shown in a patient with neurocutaneous melanosis.* **(Right)** *Diffuse leptomeningeal involvement is 1 of the features of neurocutaneous melanosis. Spread into Virchow-Robin spaces may be present ➔.*

KEY FACTS

TERMINOLOGY

- Primary neoplasms of skull and spine that contain bone, cartilage, or notochordal tissue
  - Exhibit varying degrees of aggressiveness

ETIOLOGY/PATHOGENESIS

- Ewing sarcoma (EWS) translocation (*EWS/FLI1*) on 22q12; other less common translocations reported

CLINICAL ISSUES

- Postradiation osteosarcoma arises in younger population and Paget disease-associated in older population
- Chordoma arises along axial skeleton and midline skull base (sacrum > clivus)
- Mortality higher for mesenchymal chondrosarcoma and tumors of higher grade
- Osteosarcoma: Prognosis generally poor for axial skeletal and skull
- EWS: Overall survival 60-75%
- Chordoma: High incidence of local recurrence
- Clinical presentation (fever, leucocytosis) of EWS may mimic osteomyelitis

IMAGING

- Parafalcine chondrosarcoma may masquerade as meningioma

ANCILLARY TESTS

- EWS CD99(+), but nonspecific; interpret with caution
- Chondrosarcoma: Positive for S100, D2-40 (podoplanin); negative for nuclear brachyury, keratins, EMA
  - Subset shows mutation for *IDH1/IDH2*, but not always R132H and thus not always IDH1 IHC(+)
- Chordoma: Positive for S100, cytokeratins (CK8, CK18, CK19), EMA nuclear brachyury; negative for D2-40 (podoplanin)
- Chordoid meningioma: Positive for S100, D2-40 (podoplanin), SSTR2A; negative for keratins, nuclear brachyury

(Left) *Sagittal T1WI C+ FS MR shows a large, heterogeneously enhancing midline mass that has destroyed most of the clivus and extends posteriorly ⇨ to indent the pons.* **(Right)** *Sagittal graphic shows an expansile, destructive mass originating from the clivus, displacing the pons ⇨ and elevating the pituitary gland. Note the intratumoral free-floating bone fragments.*

Erosive Clival Mass

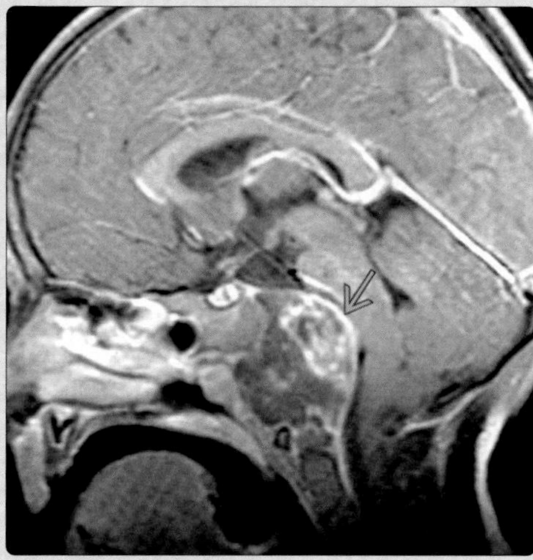

Erosive Clival Mass

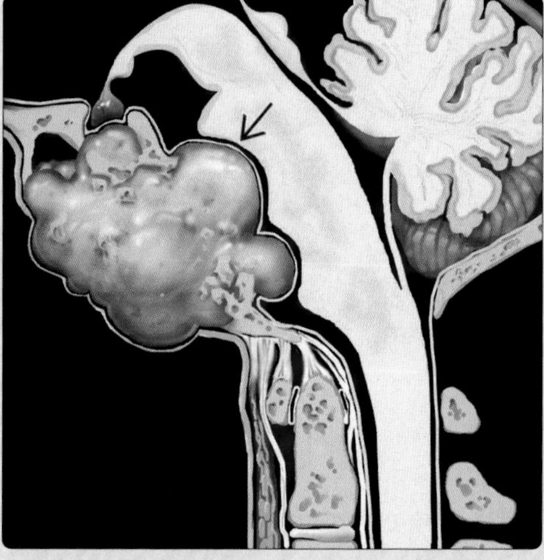

(Left) *D2-40 functions as an effective chondroid marker distinguishing true chondroid tumors from chordoma. In 1 study, 94% of grades I and II chondrosarcomas, but not chordomas, showed this cytoplasmic IHC profile.* **(Right)** *Chordoma, but not chondrosarcomas or chordoid meningiomas, show nuclear immunoreactivity for brachyury.*

Podoplanin (D2-40) (+) in Myxoid Chondrosarcoma

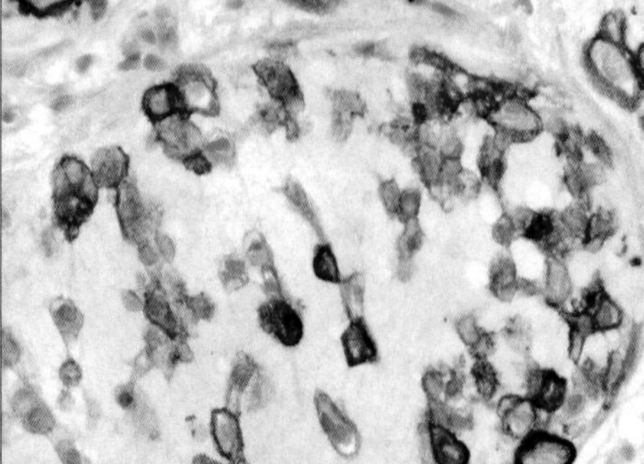

Chordoma, Brachyury Nuclear IHC(+)

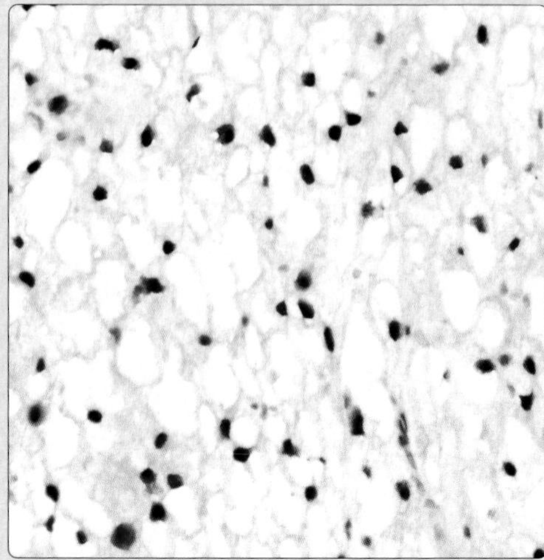

TERMINOLOGY

Synonyms

- Osteosarcoma: Osteogenic sarcoma

Definitions

- Primary neoplasms of skull and spine that contain bone, cartilage, or notochordal tissue
  - Osteosarcoma
    - Malignant, bone-forming tumor
  - Ewing sarcoma (EWS)
  - Chondrosarcoma
    - Malignant neoplasm producing hyaline cartilage
  - Chordoma
    - Low-grade, malignant neoplasm of notochordal origin

ETIOLOGY/PATHOGENESIS

Genetics

- Osteosarcoma
  - Hereditary retinoblastoma *RB1* gene on 13q14
  - Li-Fraumeni syndrome (germline mutation of *TP53*)
- EWS: (*EWSR1/FLI1*) on 22q12; other less common translocations reported
- Myxoid chondrosarcoma: Chromosome 13 and 21 [(der(13;21)(q10;q10)] translocation
- T (brachyury) gene duplication on 6q27 in familial chordoma
- *IDH1*/*IDH2* mutations in chondrosarcomas, but not chordomas
  - Most, but not all, *IDH1 R132H*
  - Only those with *IDH1 R132H* mutation recognized by immunostain

Pathogenesis

- Osteosarcomas
  - Most arise de novo
  - Occur in patients with Paget disease and fibrous dysplasia
  - Follow radiation therapy

CLINICAL ISSUES

Epidemiology

- Incidence
  - All uncommon to rare
- Age
  - Osteosarcoma: Mostly during first 2 decades
    - Except those arising in Paget disease
  - EWS: Peaks in 20s but wide range
  - Chondrosarcoma: Adults and children
  - Chordoma: Peaks in 50s and 60s
- Sex
  - Osteosarcoma: More common in males
  - EWS: Slightly more common in males
  - Chondrosarcoma: More common in males
  - Chordoma: 2x more frequent in males

Site

- Osteosarcoma: Spine and skull
- EWS: Spinal canal and skull, occasionally intradural
- Chondrosarcoma: Mostly skull based
  - Mesenchymal variant often dural based, rarely intraparenchymal
  - Parafalcine tumors occur in younger patients
- Chordoma: Along axial skeleton and midline skull base (sacrum > clivus)
  - Chondroid variant exclusively skull base
  - Skull base involvement more midline than chondrosarcoma

Presentation

- Osteosarcoma
  - Pathologic fractures
  - Pain
- EWS
  - Fever, leucocytosis, elevated sedimentation rate (mimicking osteomyelitis)
- Chondrosarcoma
  - Site-dependent mass effects
- Chordoma
  - Headaches, visual disturbances for clivus tumors
  - Pain, pathologic fractures for spinal tumors

Treatment

- Surgery for osteosarcoma, chondrosarcoma, chordoma
  - Adjuvant radiotherapy &/or chemotherapy often necessary
- Surgery and chemotherapy mainstays for Ewing sarcoma

Prognosis

- Osteosarcoma: Generally poor for axial skeletal and skull
  - Chemotherapy-induced necrosis correlates with improved prognosis
  - Poor prognosis for patients with metastases
- EWS: Overall survival 60-75%
  - Worse for spinal location because of difficulty of resection
  - Systemic symptoms associated with poor prognosis
- Chondrosarcoma
  - Mortality higher for mesenchymal type and tumors of higher grade
- Chordoma: High incidence of local recurrence
  - Up to 30% metastasize, most to lungs

IMAGING

Osteosarcoma

- Poorly defined, mixed lytic and blastic
- Involves vertebral body or neural arch
- Heterogeneous on CT and MR

Ewing Sarcoma

- Centered on vertebral body or sacrum
- Permeative, moth-eaten destruction
- MR best tool to assess extent of involvement

Chondrosarcoma

- Intracranial: Dura or skull based
- Skull-based lesions more lateralized than chordoma
- Destructive
- Parafalcine tumors mimic meningiomas

Chordoma

- CT shows lytic, destructive lesion

- More midline than chondrosarcoma
- Iso- or hypointense to brain on T1WI and hyperintense on T2WI
- Avid enhancement
- Clivus tumors may extend into sella
- Sacral tumors extend into soft tissue anteriorly

MACROSCOPIC

General Features

- Osteosarcoma and chondrosarcoma
  - Multilobulated, circumscribed
  - Fleshy, gray-white with flecks of cartilage or bone
  - Hemorrhage and necrosis in some cases
- EWS
  - Poorly demarcated
  - Sometimes associated soft tissue mass
  - Grayish-yellow, soft, and necrotic; may resemble pus
- Chordoma
  - Firm, solid, multinodular mass
  - Sections show shiny, blue-gray, translucent areas
  - Hemorrhagic

MICROSCOPIC

Histologic Features

- Osteosarcoma
  - Malignant cells depositing coarse, lace-like bone (osteoid)
  - May contain malignant-appearing cartilage or fibroblasts
  - Variants include osteoblastic, chondroblastic, fibroblastic, and mixed
  - Osteoclast-like giant cells in some tumors
  - Pleomorphism variable
  - Atypical mitoses common
  - Necrosis
- EWS
  - Uniform dark blue cells with inconspicuous cytoplasmic borders
  - Large, round nuclei with evenly dispersed chromatin
    - Small, hyperchromatic, but not overtly anaplastic
  - Mitotically active but not always highly
  - Necrosis
  - Rosette-like structures, sometimes Homer Wright
  - Delicate fibrous septa but lack extracellular matrix
- Chondrosarcoma
  - Mesenchymal
    - Hemangiopericytoma-like tissue with small, round, oval, or spindle-shaped cells with high nuclear:cytoplasmic ratios
    - Staghorn vessels
    - Islands of hyaline cartilage with linear progression of chondrocytes: Resting → proliferative → hypertrophic
    - Central calcification or ossification of cartilaginous islands
  - Conventional
    - Lobular pattern
    - Hyaline cartilage with large chondrocytes
    - Other examples show evenly spaced, uniform cells in basophilic matrix
    - Spindling of chondrocytes
    - Nuclear pleomorphism
    - Binucleation
    - Mitoses rare
- Chordoma
  - Lobules separated by fibrovascular bands
  - Tumor cells grow in cords and nests
  - Blue myxoid stroma
  - Small, round nuclei with abundant bubbly cytoplasm (physaliferous)
  - Rarely, mitoses, pleomorphic nuclei (malignant transformation)
  - Chondroid variant with chondroid tissue
    - Stains with epithelial markers
  - Pleomorphism variable, sometimes prominent
  - Necrosis seen in 35% of sacral tumors

ANCILLARY TESTS

Cytology

- Osteosarcoma
  - Cytology difficult due to bone matrix
- EWS
  - Uniform small round blue cells
  - Inconspicuous nucleoli
  - Dirty background due to necrosis
- Chondrosarcoma
  - Mesenchymal
    - Densely cellular, hemangiopericytoma-like round cells
    - Hyaline cartilage
  - Conventional
    - Fragments of basophilic cartilage with evenly distributed chondrocytes
    - Round or spindled cells with sharp borders
    - Binucleation and small distinct nucleoli
    - Lacks cytoplasmic vacuolation
- Chordoma
  - Myxoid matrix imparts blue background
  - Bland, round to ovoid epithelial cells with distinct borders
  - Pale, eosinophilic cytoplasm growing in cords, strands, or clusters
  - Physaliphorous cells with intracytoplasmic vacuoles

Histochemistry

- PAS-diastase sensitive cytoplasm in EWS
  - Reactivity: Positive
  - Staining pattern: Cytoplasmic

Immunohistochemistry

- Osteosarcoma
  - IHC not helpful in identifying osteoid
- EWS
  - CD99(+) [*CD99* (*MIC2*) gene product] membranous staining, vimentin, focal keratin (+)
    - Nonspecific, interpret with caution
- Chondrosarcoma
  - S100(+)
  - D2-40 (podoplanin) (+)
  - EMA(-)
  - Nuclear brachyury (-)
  - Cytokeratins (-)

- Chordoma
  - Nuclear brachyury (+)
  - Cytokeratins (CK8, CK18, CK19), EMA, S100 all (+)
  - Podoplanin (D2-40) (-)
  - Poorly differentiated variants may show loss of nuclear SMARCB1/INI1 protein expression
- Mesenchymal chondrosarcoma
  - EMA and desmin were expressed focally in 35% and 50% of cases, respectively
  - INI1 retained
  - Round cells (-) for MYOD1, myogenin, SMA, GFAP, keratins, estrogen receptor

DIFFERENTIAL DIAGNOSIS

DDx of Osteosarcoma

- Fibrous dysplasia
- Osteoblastoma
- Stress fracture
  - Osteoid and woven bone trabeculae have parallel arrangement with osteoblastic rimming
    - Disorganized in osteosarcoma
  - Lacks nuclear atypia and atypical mitoses
- EWS
  - Small cell osteosarcoma more pleomorphic

DDx of Ewing Sarcoma

- Lymphomas/leukemias
  - Precursor B-cell lymphoma may contain rosettes and be PAS(+), CD99(+), and rarely, vimentin and keratin (+)
    - CD79-α(+), CD43(+), TdT(+), CD10(+), CD34(+)
    - *IGH* gene rearrangement in 90%
- Small cell osteosarcoma produces osteoid or bone, though distinction controversial
- Embryonal rhabdomyosarcoma
  - Larger cells with distinct eosinophilic cytoplasm
  - Mostly CD99(-) and muscle antigens (+)
- Mesenchymal chondrosarcoma contains cartilage, but may not be seen in small biopsy specimens
- Metastatic neuroblastoma
  - (+) for neuronal markers
- Desmoplastic small round cell tumor
  - Specific reciprocal translocation t(11;22) (p13;q12)
  - *EWSR1-WT1* fusion transcript
  - Polyphenotypia with coexpression of epithelial, mesenchymal, myogenic, and neural markers
  - Desmoplastic stroma

DDx of Chondrosarcoma

- Chordoma
  - Shows more cytoplasmic vacuolation, tissue fragments with polygonal cells
- Mucin-producing metastatic adenocarcinoma
  - Shows more epithelial features

DDx of Chordoma

- Chondrosarcoma
  - More cartilaginous, less epithelial
  - Nuclear brachyury, EMA, keratins all (-)
  - D2-40 reliably IHC(+) in low-grade chondroid neoplasms (100% of enchondromas and 94% of grades I and II chondrosarcomas), but not chordomas
- Mucin-producing metastatic adenocarcinoma
  - Lacks lobular growth
  - Greater atypia, mitoses, necrosis
  - Brachyury (-)
- Giant notochordal rest (variant of ecchordosis physalifora)
  - On imaging, not destructive
  - Lacks lobular growth
  - Lacks cytologic atypia
- Chordoid meningioma
  - Whorls and nuclear pseudoinclusions
  - Positive for D2-40 (podoplanin) as is chondrosarcoma, but unlike chordoma, negative for nuclear brachyury
  - SSTR2A(+) (membranous)

DIAGNOSTIC CHECKLIST

Pathologic Interpretation Pearls

- CD99 staining nonspecific; interpret with caution
- S100(+) does not distinguish between chordoma and chondrosarcoma

SELECTED REFERENCES

1. Tinoco G et al: The biology and management of cartilaginous tumors: a role for targeting isocitrate dehydrogenase. Am Soc Clin Oncol Educ Book. 35:e648-55, 2015
2. Chavez JA et al: Anaplastic chordoma with loss of INI1 and brachyury expression in a 2-year-old girl. Clin Neuropathol. 33(6):418-420, 2014
3. Arai M et al: Frequent IDH1/2 mutations in intracranial chondrosarcoma: a possible diagnostic clue for its differentiation from chordoma. Brain Tumor Pathol. 29(4):201-6, 2012
4. Patel AJ et al: Radiation-induced osteosarcomas of the calvarium and skull base. Cancer. 117(10):2120-6, 2011
5. Presneau N et al: Role of the transcription factor T (brachyury) in the pathogenesis of sporadic chordoma: a genetic and functional-based study. J Pathol. 223(3):327-35, 2011
6. Sadeghi SM et al: Spontaneous conversion of fibrous dysplasia into osteosarcoma. J Craniofac Surg. 22(3):959-61, 2011
7. Fanburg-Smith JC et al: Immunoprofile of mesenchymal chondrosarcoma: aberrant desmin and EMA expression, retention of INI1, and negative estrogen receptor in 22 female-predominant central nervous system and musculoskeletal cases. Ann Diagn Pathol. 14(1):8-14, 2010
8. Fanburg-Smith JC et al: Reappraisal of mesenchymal chondrosarcoma: novel morphologic observations of the hyaline cartilage and endochondral ossification and beta-catenin, Sox9, and osteocalcin immunostaining of 22 cases. Hum Pathol. 41(5):653-62, 2010
9. Indelicato DJ et al: Spinal and paraspinal Ewing tumors. Int J Radiat Oncol Biol Phys. 76(5):1463-71, 2010
10. Mobley BC et al: Loss of SMARCB1/INI1 expression in poorly differentiated chordomas. Acta Neuropathol. 120(6):745-53, 2010
11. Schoenfeld AJ et al: Osteosarcoma of the spine: experience in 26 patients treated at the Massachusetts General Hospital. Spine J. 10(8):708-14, 2010
12. Whaley JT et al: Ewing tumors of the head and neck. Am J Clin Oncol. 33(4):321-6, 2010
13. Bloch OG et al: A systematic review of intracranial chondrosarcoma and survival. J Clin Neurosci. 16(12):1547-51, 2009
14. Boccardo M et al: Parafalcine chondrosarcoma: report of a case and review of the literature. J Neurosurg Sci. 53(3):137-40, 2009
15. Oakley GJ et al: Brachyury, SOX-9, and podoplanin, new markers in the skull base chordoma vs chondrosarcoma differential: a tissue microarray-based comparative analysis. Mod Pathol. 21(12):1461-9, 2008
16. Tirabosco R et al: Brachyury expression in extra-axial skeletal and soft tissue chordomas: a marker that distinguishes chordoma from mixed tumor/myoepithelioma/parachordoma in soft tissue. Am J Surg Pathol. 32(4):572-80, 2008
17. Huse JT et al: D2-40 functions as an effective chondroid marker distinguishing true chondroid tumors from chordoma. Acta Neuropathol. 113(1):87-94, 2007

(Left) *The 2 basic components of osteosarcoma are sarcomatous tumor cells and tumor bone matrix (osteoid). Tumor cells within the loose, myxoid matrix elaborate the trabeculae of immature osteoid.* **(Right)** *Virtually all osteosarcomas affecting the CNS are high grade. This classic example contains pleomorphic tumor cells and numerous mitoses.*

Osteosarcoma

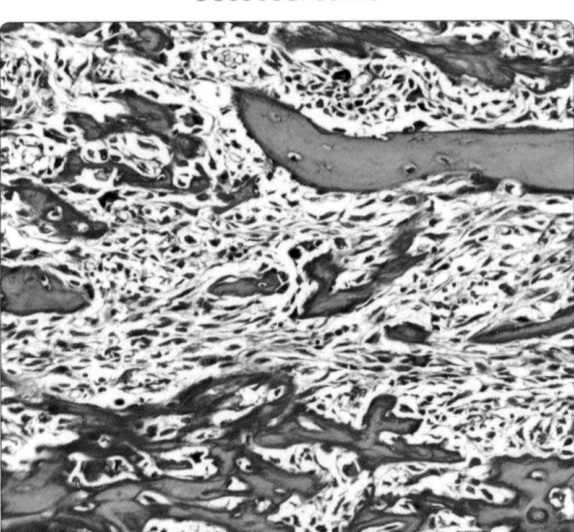

Osteosarcoma, Pleomorphism

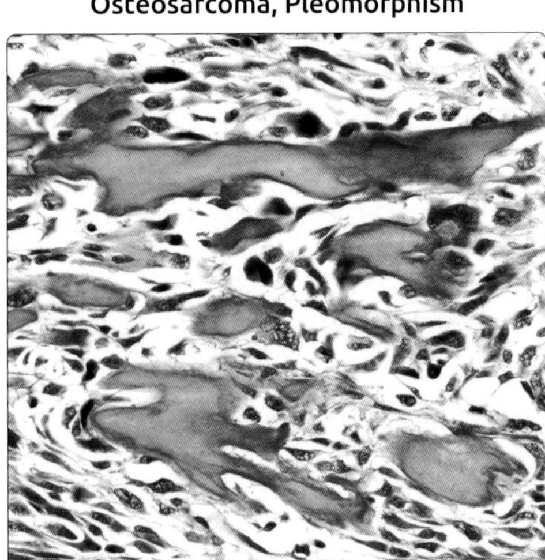

(Left) *Identifying the bone-forming component in an osteosarcoma may require extensive sampling if spindle cells dominate. Osteoclast-like giant cells ⇨ may be widely distributed throughout the tumor.* **(Right)** *Microscopic features of osteosarcoma can vary among different lesions and even in different areas of the same tumor. Tumor cells can appear epithelioid, spindled, or even simulate a small blue cell neoplasm. Osteoid ⇨ is present.*

Osteosarcoma, Paucity of Osteoid

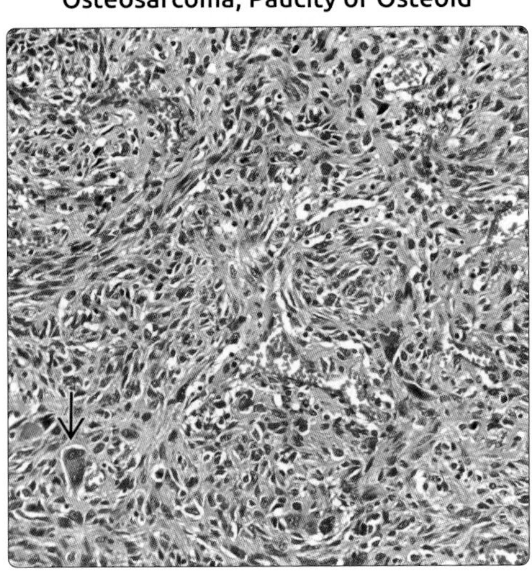

Osteoid

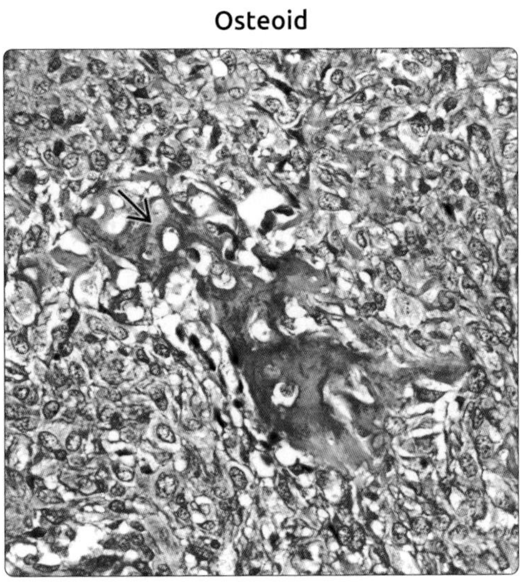

(Left) *Ewing sarcoma (EWS) often features a solidly packed, lobular growth pattern. The histopathological findings are reminiscent of other embryonal tumors. Cells are uniform.* **(Right)** *The cytoplasm in EWS may be pale staining or vacuolated as a result of intracellular glycogen. Glycogen is present in variable amounts in a majority of tumors.*

Ewing Sarcoma

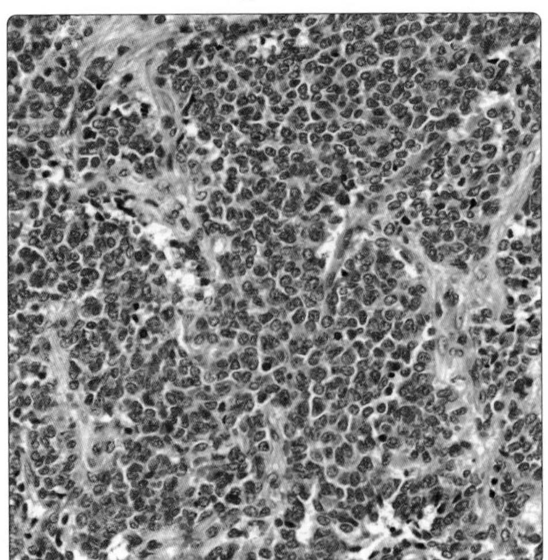

Ewing Sarcoma, Glycogen-Rich Cytoplasm

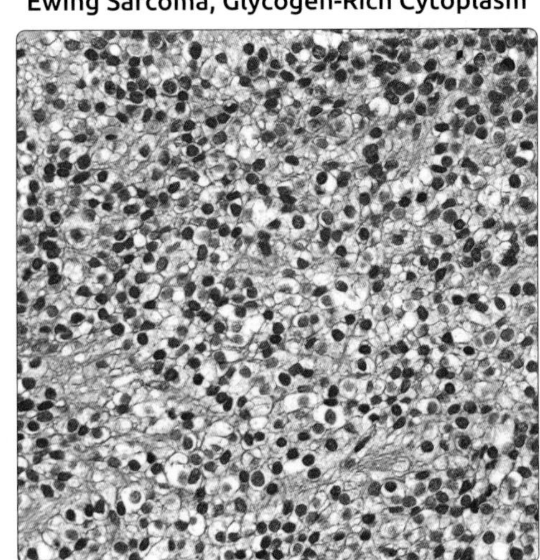

Ewing Sarcoma, Paucity of Mitotic Figures

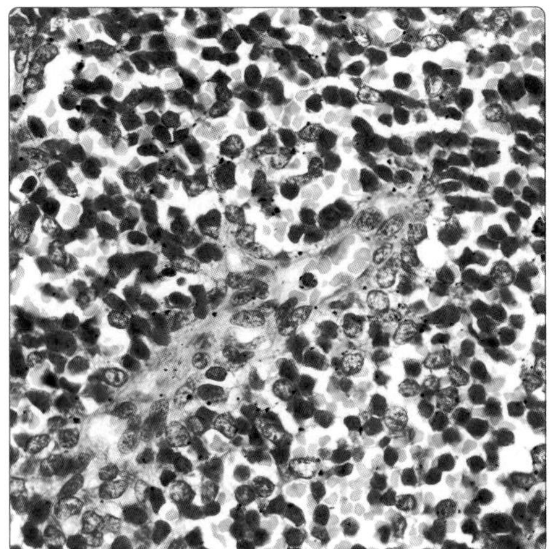

Ewing Sarcoma, CD99(+)

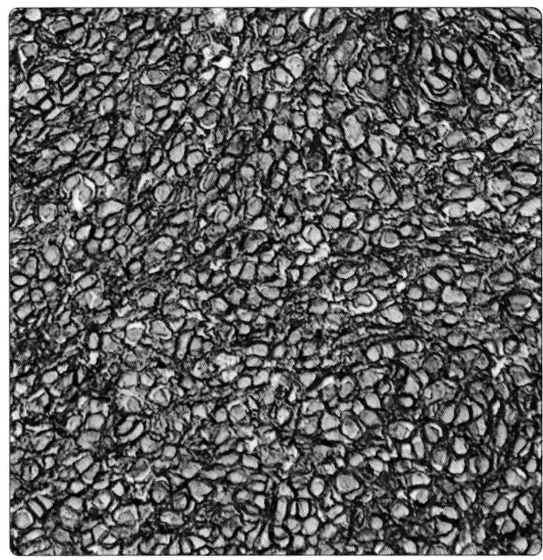

(Left) *The number of mitotic figures varies in EWS. In many cases, the paucity of mitoses contrasts sharply with the tumors' high cellularity and overall primitive appearance.* **(Right)** *Although not diagnostic, tumor cells diffusely express CD99 in EWS. Tumors may also stain positively for synaptophysin.*

Chondrosarcoma

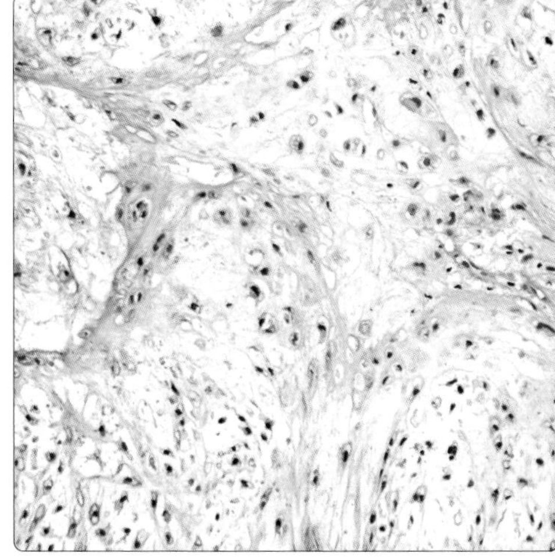

Chondrosarcoma, Hyaline Cartilage

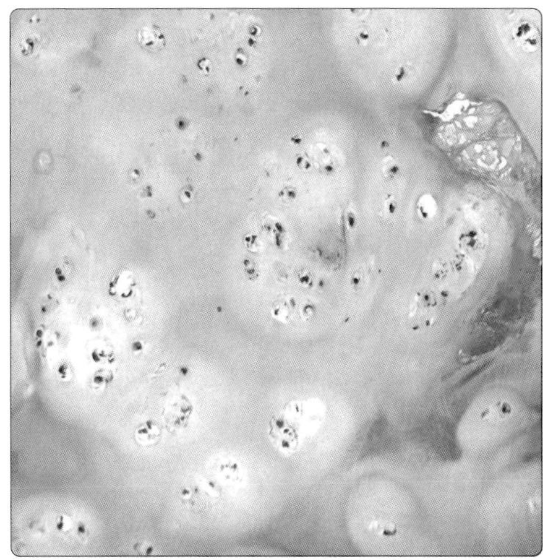

(Left) *Conventional chondrosarcoma demonstrates lobules separated by delicate fibrovascular bands. Parafalcine tumors favor younger patients and can be confused radiologically with meningioma, a neoplasm that only rarely has metaplastic cartilage.* **(Right)** *This chondrosarcoma shows hyaline cartilage matrix disposed in irregular lobules. Ossification may be seen at the periphery of the lobules.*

Chondrosarcoma Simulating Chordoma

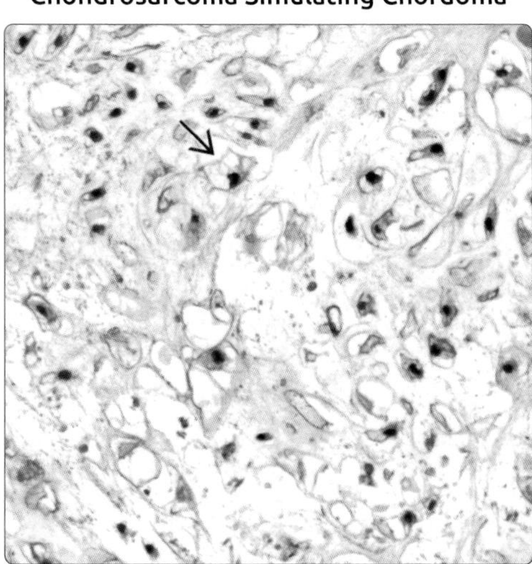

Chondrosarcoma Immunonegative for IDH1 (R132H) but IDH1 Mutated (R132S)

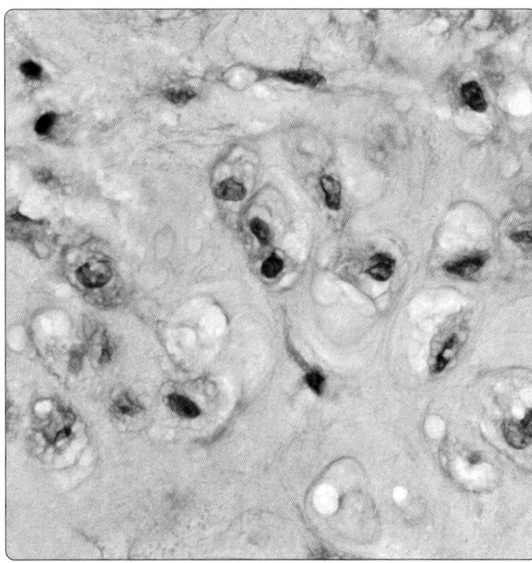

(Left) *Neoplastic chondrocytes ➔ with vacuolated cytoplasm in conventional chondrosarcoma can resemble physaliphorous cells of chordoma.* **(Right)** *Mildly increased cellularity and atypia are signature features of low-grade conventional chondrosarcoma. Note the hyperchromatic nuclei that vary in size and shape. This chondrosarcoma was immunonegative for IDH1 (R132H) but was found by mutational analysis to have a noncanonical mutation at R132S that is unrecognized by the IDH1 antibody.*

(Left) *Chondrosarcomas that qualify as grade II are more cellular and more cytologically atypical than grade I tumors.* **(Right)** *Dedifferentiated chondrosarcoma, rarely primary to the CNS, is distinguished by the presence of a low-grade cartilaginous precursor lesion that transitions abruptly to a high-grade sarcomatous component with mitoses →.*

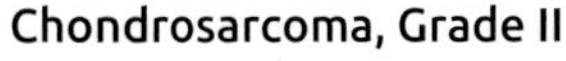

Chondrosarcoma, Grade II

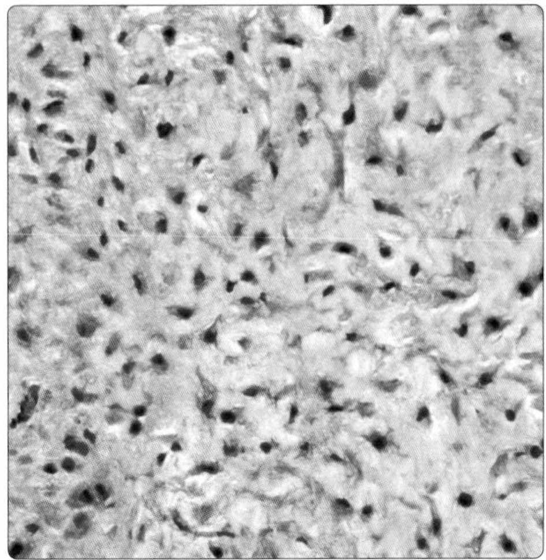

Chondrosarcoma, Dedifferentiated

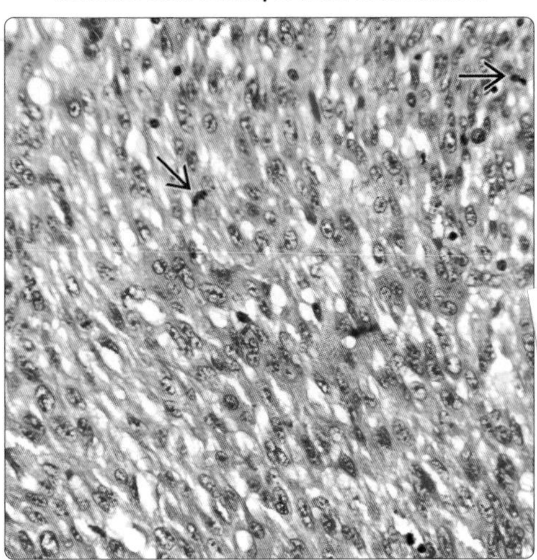

(Left) *Mesenchymal chondrosarcomas contain confluent islands of chondroid matrix admixed with hemangiopericytoma-like tissue →.* **(Right)** *Sheaths of closely packed oval or spindle-shaped → cells interdigitate with benign-appearing cartilaginous tissue.*

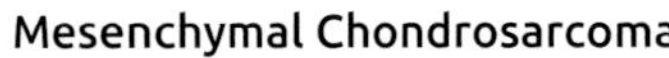

Mesenchymal Chondrosarcoma

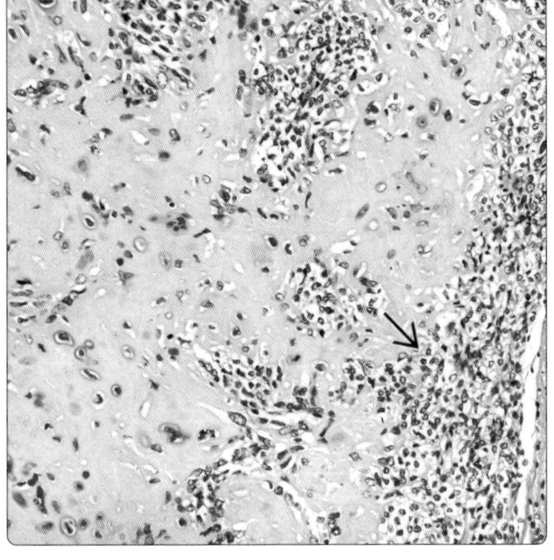

Mesenchymal Chondrosarcoma

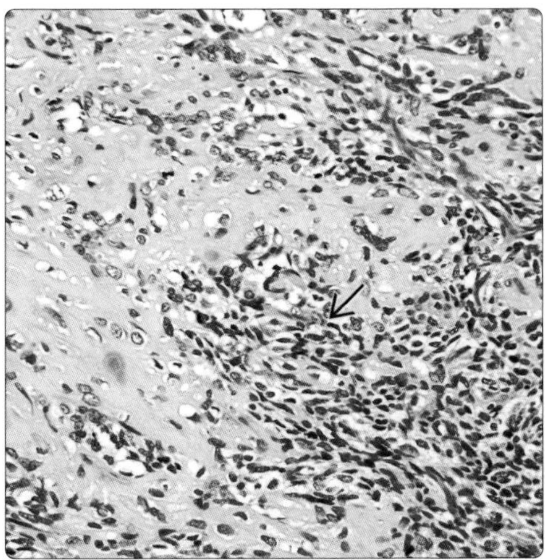

(Left) *Although usually well defined, cartilaginous foci → in mesenchymal chondrosarcoma sometimes blend with surrounding undifferentiated cells.* **(Right)** *Immunohistochemical preparations are helpful in the diagnosis of chordoma. Most tumors are immunoreactive for nuclear brachyury, vimentin, S100, cytokeratin and EMA. They are negative for D2-40, unlike almost all low-grade chondroid tumors. Strong, diffuse keratin IHC(+) is seen here.*

Mesenchymal Chondrosarcoma, Inconspicuous Cartilage

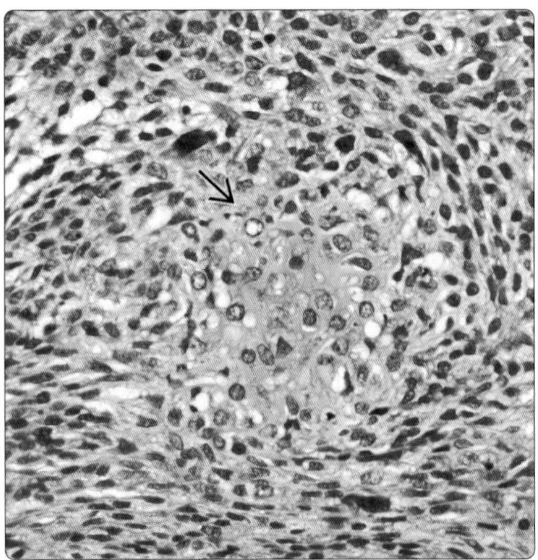

CK18(+) Distinguishes Chordoma From Chondrosarcoma

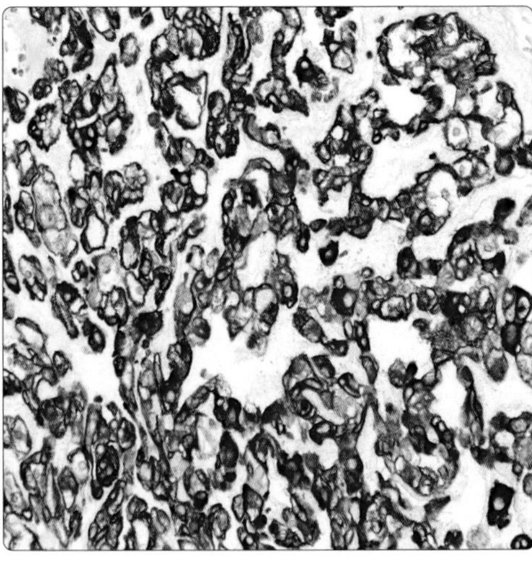

Chordoma, Lobular Architecture

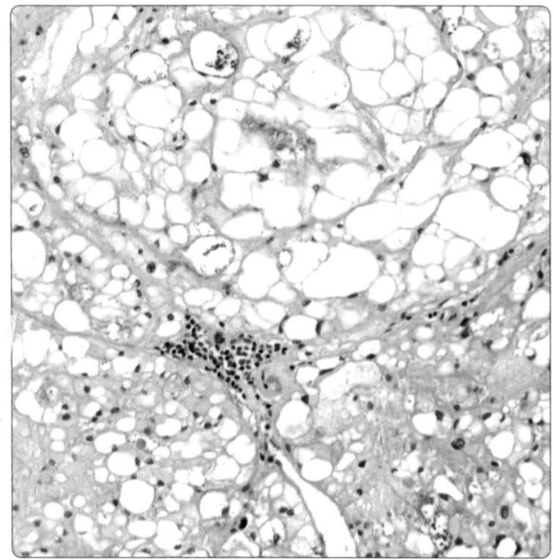

Chordoma, Anastomosing Cords of Cells

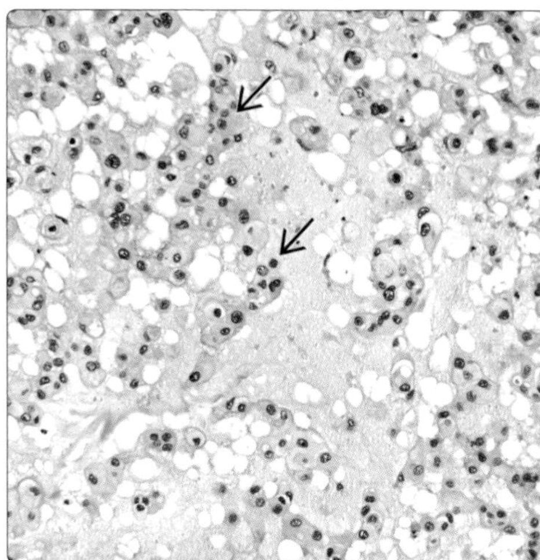

(Left) *Similar to chondrosarcoma, tumor cells in chordoma are disposed in irregular lobules. Variable amounts of intracellular and extracellular mucin are present. Foci of cartilaginous differentiation may be seen in chordoma, which may obscure the distinction from chondrosarcoma.* **(Right)** *The epithelioid tumor cells in chordomas are arranged in distinctive anastomosing cords ⇒. Extracellular mucin can be extensive.*

Chordoma Simulating Adenocarcinoma

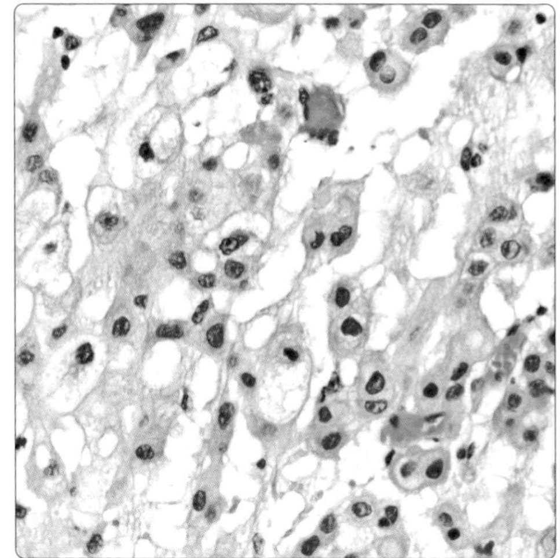

Chordoma, Cytoplasmic Vacuolization

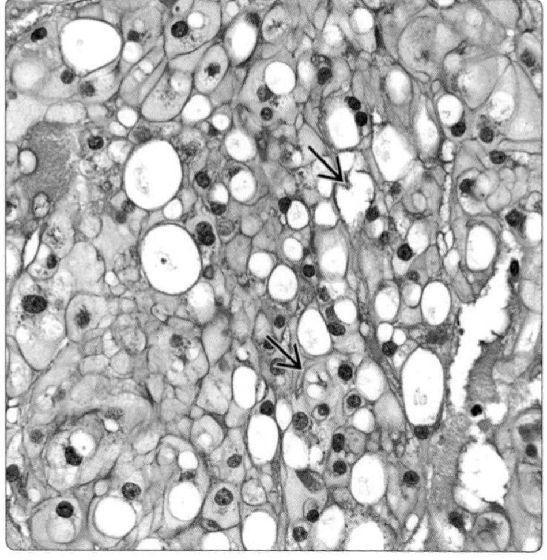

(Left) *The overtly epithelial appearance of the tumor cells in chordoma may sometimes lead to confusion with mucin-producing adenocarcinoma.* **(Right)** *Individual cells in chordoma are often larger and more polygonal than the small round cells with discrete borders that are common in chondrosarcoma. Although not a classic example, tell-tale cytoplasmic vacuolation ⇒ assists in the correct diagnosis of chordoma in this case.*

Physaliphorous Cells, Vacuolated

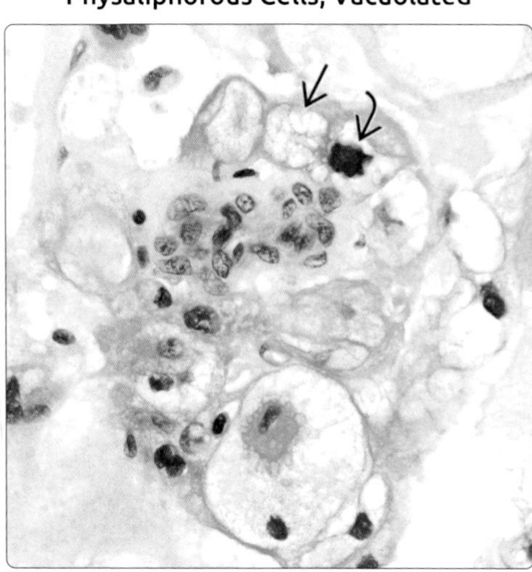

Chordoma, Nuclear Pleomorphism

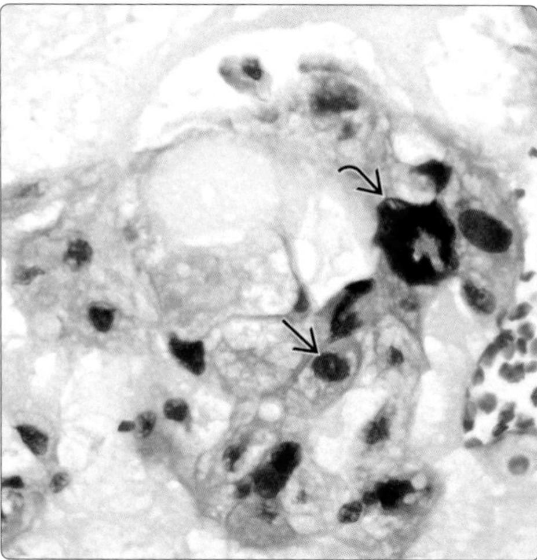

(Left) *Physaliphorous cells are filled with vacuoles ⇒. Nuclei are typically bland, but mild pleomorphism ⇗ may be present in otherwise low-grade chordomas. Rarely, increasing atypia and mitoses signify malignant transformation.* **(Right)** *Physaliphorous cells have bubbly cytoplasm and the nuclei are typically bland ⇒, but pleomorphism ⇗ may be present in otherwise low-grade chordomas. This does not impact prognosis.*

Fibrosarcoma

KEY FACTS

TERMINOLOGY

- Collagen-forming, malignant spindle cell tumor that cannot be assigned to another sarcoma category
- Largely diagnosis of exclusion

ETIOLOGY/PATHOGENESIS

- Spontaneous/sporadic
- Radiation induced
- Metastatic from soft tissues, may not be dural based

CLINICAL ISSUES

- Recur and metastasize outside CNS

MICROSCOPIC

- Monomorphic spindle cells with high N:C ratios
  - Isolated pleomorphic nuclei, uncommon
- Typical herringbone architecture
- Storiform pattern, less common
- Abundant reticulin
- Variable stromal collagen, keloid-like or hyalinized areas

ANCILLARY TESTS

- Mitotically active spindle cells with tapered hyperchromatic nuclei
- Typically, only positive immunostain is vimentin
  - Occasionally focal and weak positivity with smooth muscle antibodies
  - Focal CD34 positivity, rare
- Multiple numerical and structural, but nonspecific, chromosomal aberrations

TOP DIFFERENTIAL DIAGNOSES

- Anaplastic meningioma
- Hemangiopericytoma/solitary fibrous tumor
- Gliosarcoma
- Inflammatory myofibroblastic tumor
- Other high-grade sarcomas, primary or metastatic

Uniform Spindle Cells: Herringbone Pattern

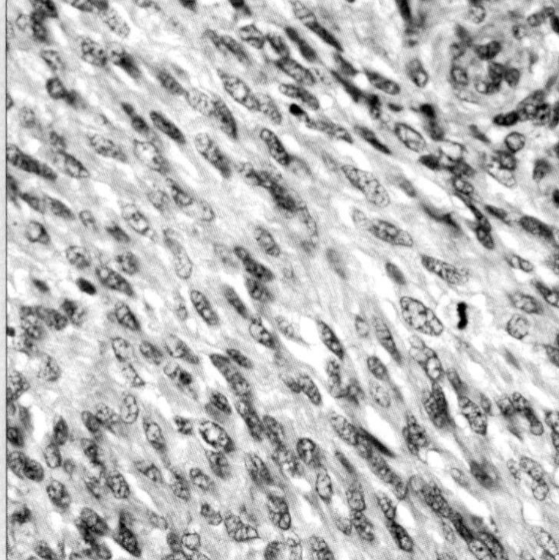

Abundant Reticulin

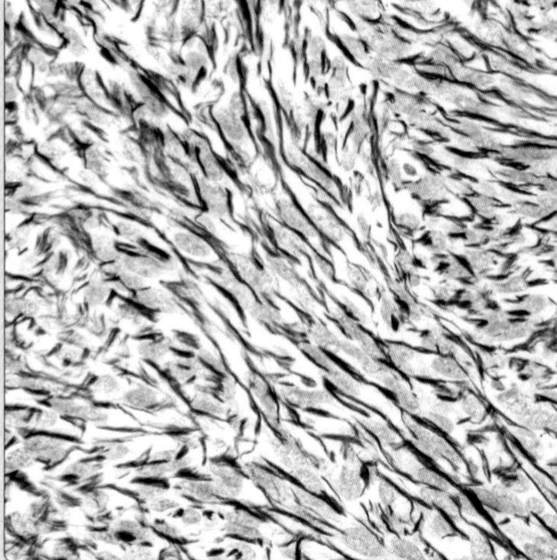

(Left) *Fibrosarcomas have uniform spindle cells arranged in intersecting fascicles. Negative immunostaining for S100 protein and nuclear SOX10 helps separate this entity from malignant melanoma and schwannoma.* **(Right)** *Reticulin fibers surround individual neoplastic cells.*

Fibrosarcoma: Radiation Induced

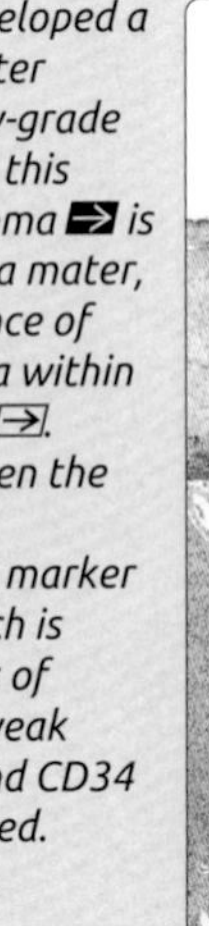

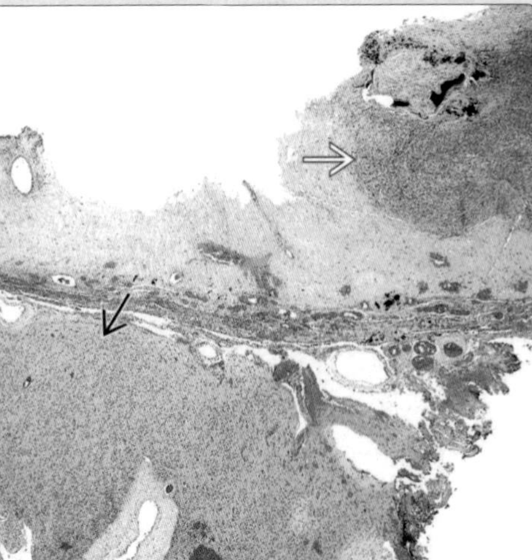

Vimentin Positivity in Fibrosarcoma

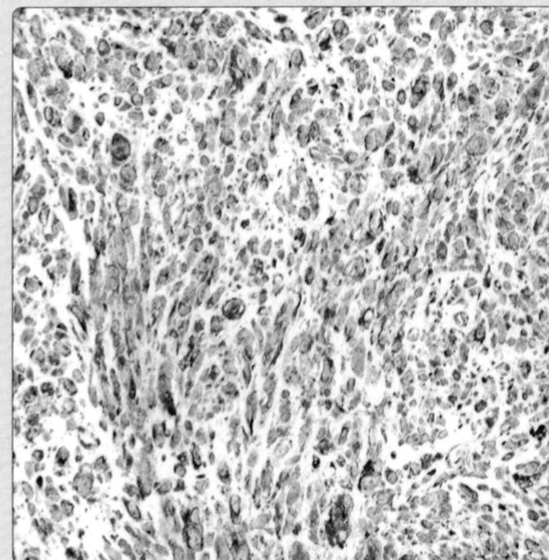

(Left) *This patient developed a fibrosarcoma years after radiotherapy for a low-grade oligodendroglioma. In this section, the fibrosarcoma ➡ is seen involving the dura mater, while there is recurrence of the oligodendroglioma within the underlying cortex ⇒.* **(Right)** *Vimentin is often the only positive immunohistochemical marker in fibrosarcomas, which is essentially a diagnosis of exclusion. Focal and weak positivity with SMA and CD34 can also be encountered.*

TERMINOLOGY

Definitions

- Collagen-forming, malignant spindle cell tumor that cannot be assigned to another sarcoma category
- Largely diagnosis of exclusion

ETIOLOGY/PATHOGENESIS

Etiology

- Spontaneous
- Post irradiation
  - Following treatment of primary intraaxial tumors
- Metastatic
  - Always consider local extension or metastatic disease

CLINICAL ISSUES

Epidemiology

- Incidence
  - < 1% intracranial neoplasms
- Age
  - All ages
- Sex
  - Male = female

Site

- Dural based, some spontaneous cases
- Skull base (e.g., after irradiation of pituitary adenoma)

Presentation

- Location dependent

Natural History

- Recur and metastasize outside CNS

Treatment

- Adjuvant therapy
  - Radiation offers limited benefit
- Surgical resection

Prognosis

- Poor

MACROSCOPIC

General Features

- Discrete mass
- Fleshy cut surface with hemorrhage, cysts, and necrosis

MICROSCOPIC

Histologic Features

- Typical herringbone architecture
- Storiform pattern, less common
- Collagen-rich stroma
- Monomorphic fusiform cells with high N:C ratios
- Pleomorphic, multinuclear cells (uncommon)
- Necrosis in some cases

ANCILLARY TESTS

Histochemistry

- Reticulin
  - Often demonstrates rich network around individual cells

Immunohistochemistry

- Vimentin (+)
- S100(-), Leu-7(-), EMA(-), ALK1(-), cytokeratin (-)

Electron Microscopy

- Fibroblasts with abundant rough endoplasmic reticulum
- Lacks myofilaments, external lamina, intercellular junctions

Cytology

- Mitotically active spindle cells
- Tapered, darkly staining nuclei

DIFFERENTIAL DIAGNOSIS

Anaplastic Meningioma, WHO Grade III

- Usually retains some meningothelial features
- Lacks herringbone pattern
- SSTR2A(+); EMA(+), may be focal or absent
- Cytokeratins (+) in some cases

Hemangiopericytoma/Solitary Fibrous Tumor

- Turbulent rather than herringbone architecture
- Biphasic with areas of reduced cellular density
- Thin-walled, staghorn vessels
- CD34(+), nuclear STAT6(+)

Gliosarcoma

- GFAP(+) glial component

Malignant Peripheral Nerve Sheath Tumor

- Relation to peripheral nerve
- Marked histologic variation
- Many are S100(+)

Cellular Schwannoma

- Relation to peripheral nerve
- Schwannian cytology
- Lacks herringbone pattern
- Extensively S100(+), nuclear SOX10(+)

Desmoplastic Infantile Ganglioglioma

- Prominent desmoplasia
- Small ganglion cells and glassy astrocytes
- Lacks herringbone pattern
- GFAP(+), synaptophysin (+), chromogranin (+)

Melanocytic Neoplasm

- Less cellular elongation
- Less cellular without herringbone pattern
- S100(+), HMB-45(+), Melan-A(+)

Inflammatory Myofibroblastic Tumor

- Abundant lymphoplasmacytic cells
- ALK-1(+)

SELECTED REFERENCES

1. Oliveira AM et al: Primary sarcomas of the brain and spinal cord: a study of 18 cases. Am J Surg Pathol. 26(8):1056-63, 2002
2. Paulus W et al: Primary intracranial sarcomas: histopathological features of 19 cases. Histopathology. 18(5):395-402, 1991
3. Mena H et al: Primary brain sarcomas: light and electron microscopic features. Cancer. 42(3):1298-307, 1978

Smooth Muscle Neoplasms

KEY FACTS

TERMINOLOGY

- Rare, mostly malignant smooth muscle tumors that resemble their soft tissue counterparts
- Some lesions borderline between leiomyoma and leiomyosarcoma

ETIOLOGY/PATHOGENESIS

- Association with EBV infection in immunosuppressed patients
  - AIDS patients
  - Organ transplant recipients
  - Children with primary immunodeficiency syndromes

CLINICAL ISSUES

- May occur as single or multiple lesions
- Treated with surgical excision, but no single standard of care
- AIDS patients with smooth muscle tumors and virological and immunological responses to combined antiretroviral therapy (cART) survive, even with partial resection

MICROSCOPIC

- Fascicular architecture
- Criss-crossing or whorling bundles of smooth muscle cells in leiomyoma
- Necrosis and mitoses in leiomyosarcoma

ANCILLARY TESTS

- Diffuse vimentin, smooth muscle actin, desmin, H-caldesmon (+)
- In situ hybridization (+) for Epstein-Barr virus (Epstein-Barr virus-encoded small RNAs [EBER]) in smooth muscle tumors from immunocompromised patients

TOP DIFFERENTIAL DIAGNOSES

- Schwannoma
- Meningioma

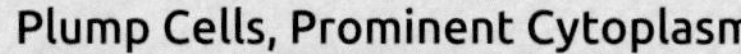

Plump Cells, Prominent Cytoplasm

Muscle-Specific Actin

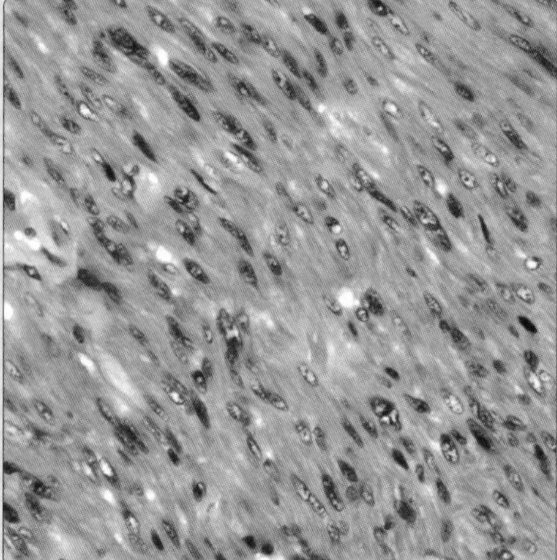

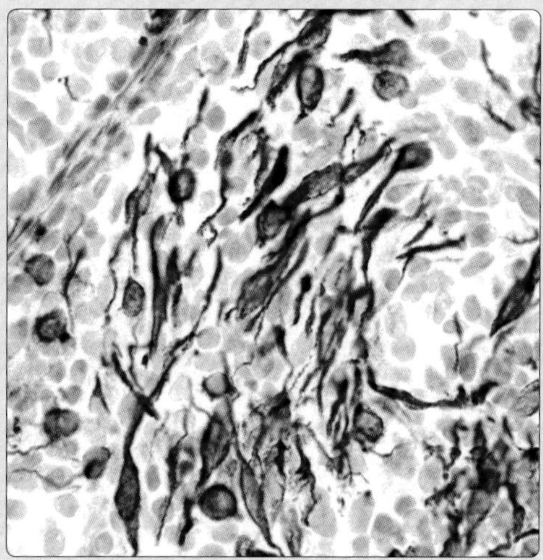

(Left) *A spindle cell neoplasm with plump cells with prominent cytoplasm is suspicious for smooth muscle tumor, especially in the setting of immunodeficiency. Most examples are dural based and mimic the imaging and gross appearance of meningioma.* **(Right)** *Immunohistochemistry, here for muscle-specific actin, can be used to establish the myoid nature of the lesion.*

Leiomyosarcoma, Mitoses

EBER In Situ Hybridization, Immunosuppressed Patient

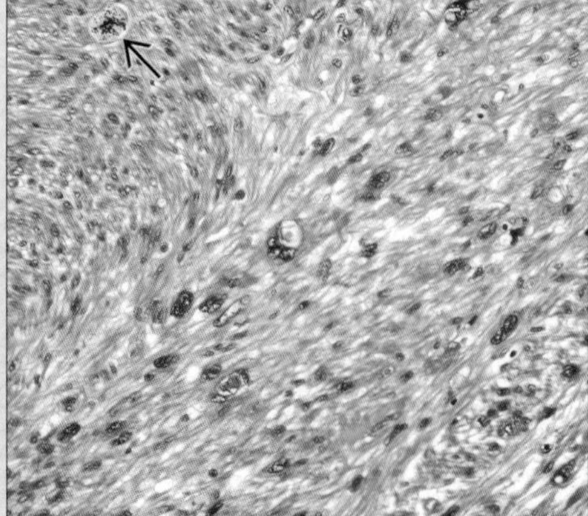

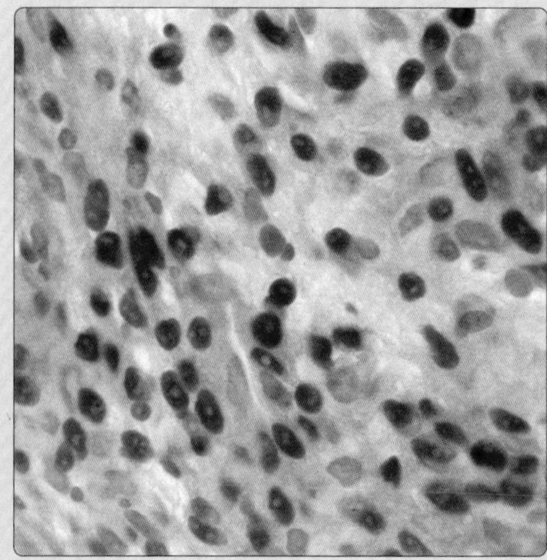

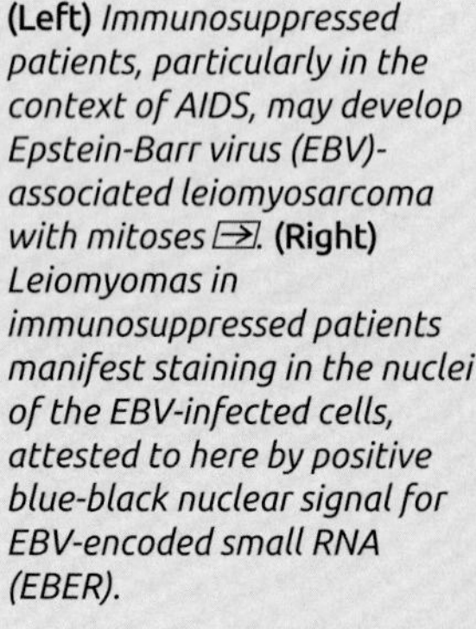

(Left) *Immunosuppressed patients, particularly in the context of AIDS, may develop Epstein-Barr virus (EBV)-associated leiomyosarcoma with mitoses* ➙. **(Right)** *Leiomyomas in immunosuppressed patients manifest staining in the nuclei of the EBV-infected cells, attested to here by positive blue-black nuclear signal for EBV-encoded small RNA (EBER).*

TERMINOLOGY

Definitions

- Rare, usually malignant smooth muscle tumors that resemble their soft tissue counterparts

ETIOLOGY/PATHOGENESIS

Infectious Agents

- Association with Epstein-Barr virus (EBV) infection in immunosuppressed patients

CLINICAL ISSUES

Epidemiology

- Incidence
  - Rare

Presentation

- Headaches and signs of increased intracranial pressure

Treatment

- Excision sufficient for benign tumors

Prognosis

- Often low grade, with corresponding good prognosis
- Malignant tumors recur or metastasize
  - Depends on location, size, histologic features

IMAGING

General Features

- Extraaxial
- Resemble meningioma
- Location of EBV-driven smooth muscle tumors appears related to type of immunodeficiency
  - In AIDS they are frequently located intracranially or intraspinally
  - In posttransplant patients, often involve liver, lung
  - In children, may also occur in setting of primary immune disorders, i.e., severe combined and common variable immunodeficiency syndromes

MACROSCOPIC

General Features

- May occur as single or multiple well-circumscribed lesions
- Hemorrhage and necrosis in some malignant examples

MICROSCOPIC

Histologic Features

- Leiomyoma
  - Criss-crossing or whorling bundles of smooth muscle cells
  - Variable cellularity and vascularity
  - Generally little atypia or mitotic activity
- Leiomyosarcoma
  - Compact fascicular architecture
  - Focal pleomorphism common
  - Necrosis and mitoses
- Some lesions borderline between leiomyoma and leiomyosarcoma

ANCILLARY TESTS

Cytology

- Leiomyoma
  - Cohesive clusters
  - Fine to moderately granular chromatin, multiple nucleoli and chromocenters
  - Granular, ill-defined cytoplasm with tapering ends
- Leiomyosarcoma
  - Loose clusters and individual cells
  - Large, hyperchromatic, club-like nuclei with coarse chromatin and bipolar cytoplasm
  - Multinucleation, cellular pleomorphism, and tumor necrosis, mitoses

Immunohistochemistry

- Diffuse vimentin, smooth muscle actin, desmin, H-caldesmon all (+)
- Focally cytokeratin, EMA, CD34 (+)

In Situ Hybridization

- EBV(+) examples in immunosuppressed hosts

DIFFERENTIAL DIAGNOSIS

Meningioma

- Whorls, psammoma bodies
- Stromal calcifications (fibrous subtype)
- EMA(+), SSTR2A(+)
- Muscle markers (-)

Schwannoma

- Antoni A and B tissues
- Diffusely S100(+), nuclear SOX10(+)
- Muscle markers (-)

Primary Melanocytic Tumor

- Less spindled
- Prominent nucleoli
- Melanocytic markers (+)
- Muscle markers (-)

DIAGNOSTIC CHECKLIST

Pathologic Interpretation Pearls

- Spindle cells with blunt or cigar-shaped nuclei typical of this rare, often immunosuppression-associated CNS tumor
- Mitoses, pleomorphism, and necrosis in malignant examples

SELECTED REFERENCES

1. Arva NC et al: Rare presentations of Epstein-Barr virus-associated smooth muscle tumor in children. Pediatr Dev Pathol. ePub, 2015
2. Jossen J et al: Epstein-Barr virus-associated smooth muscle tumors in children following solid organ transplantation: A review. Pediatr Transplant. 19(2):235-43, 2015
3. Issarachaikul R et al: Epstein-Barr virus-associated smooth muscle tumors in AIDS patients: a largest case (series). Intern Med. 53(20):2391-6, 2014
4. Sivendran S et al: Primary intracranial leiomyosarcoma in an HIV-infected patient. Int J Clin Oncol. 16(1):63-6, 2011
5. Gupta S et al: Epstein-Barr virus-associated intracranial leiomyosarcoma in an HIV-positive adolescent. J Pediatr Hematol Oncol. 32(4):e144-7, 2010
6. Hua W et al: Primary intracranial leiomyomas: Report of two cases and review of the literature. Clin Neurol Neurosurg. 111(10):907-12, 2009

Adipocytic Neoplasms

KEY FACTS

ETIOLOGY/PATHOGENESIS

- Lipomas thought to represent congenital malformations derived from meninx primitiva, but recent genetic data favor neoplastic origin for some
- In one study of peripheral and CNS lipomatous lesions, *HMGA2* rearrangements were almost never identified; thus PNS/CNS lesions may be different from conventional lipomas

CLINICAL ISSUES

- Intracranial (majority supratentorial and midline)
- Spinal (mostly lumbosacral)
- Symptoms
  - Lipomas rarely symptomatic, usually incidental neuroradiological or autopsy finding
  - Occasional mass effect and compression of adjacent structures
- Treatment of lipoma
  - Usually none
  - Simple excision if symptomatic

MACROSCOPIC

- Yellow, soft, lobulated mass attached to meninges, sometimes adherent to brain

MICROSCOPIC

- Classic lipoma
- Variants: Angiolipoma, lipoma with heterologous elements, hibernoma, spindle cell/pleomorphic lipoma, lipoblastoma, atypical lipoma, liposarcoma
  - Many of these variants are extremely rare (or even never encountered) in nervous system

DIAGNOSTIC CHECKLIST

- Lipoma of 8th cranial nerve
  - Mimics schwannoma clinically, but distinguished radiologically
- Rule out meningioma with areas of adiposytic metaplasia

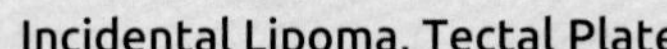

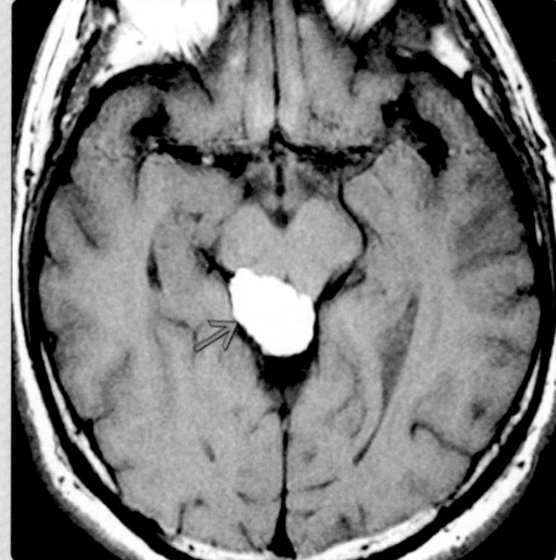

Incidental Lipoma, Tectal Plate

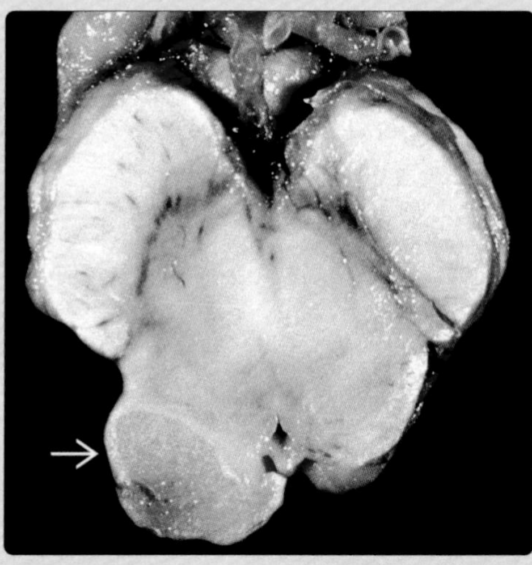

(Left) *Axial T1WI MR scan found an incidental large, lobulated hyperintense mass ⇨ dorsal to the midbrain. The signal intensity is identical to that of fat in the scalp and orbit.* **(Right)** *Autopsied brain sectioned in the axial plane shows a subpial lipoma ➡ of the dorsal midbrain, with a characteristic gross, bright yellow appearance typical of benign adipose tissue. (Courtesy E. Hedley-Whyte, MD.)*

Lipoma

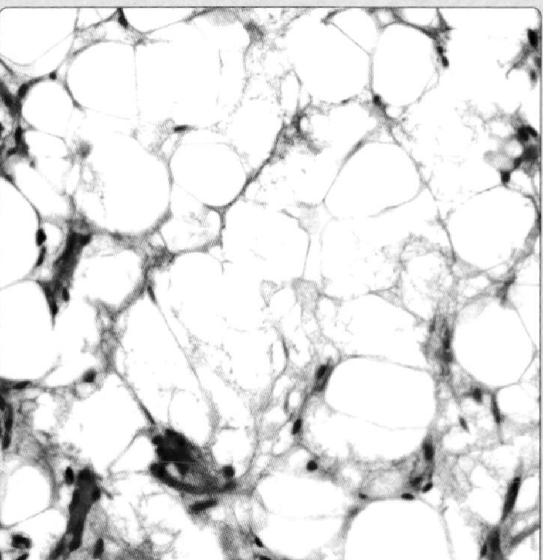

Hibernoma

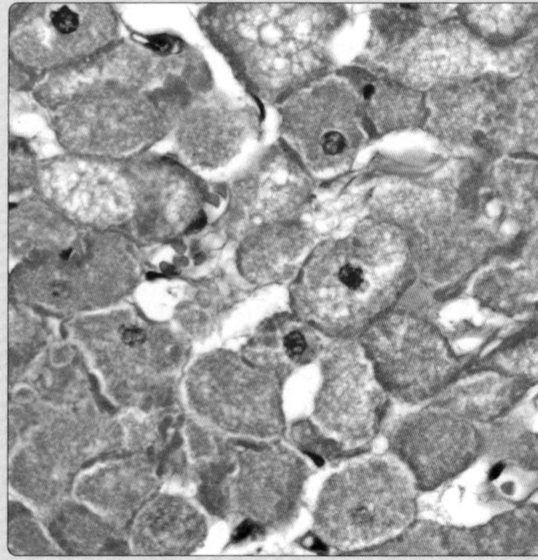

(Left) *Lipomas are composed of mature fat and most commonly are found in the supratentorial pericallosal region but also near the quadrigeminal plate, interpeduncular cistern, suprasellar area, and cerebellopontine angle.* **(Right)** *Hibernoma is a distinctive benign tumor of childhood that resembles brown fat. It contains small, centrally placed nuclei and cytoplasm that varies from pale multivacuolated to granular eosinophilic. Mature white fat is often admixed.*

TERMINOLOGY

Synonyms

- Lipomatous hamartoma

Definitions

- Lipoma
  - Tumors that resemble mature adipose tissue
- Liposarcoma
  - Rare malignant mesenchymal tumor of adipose tissue

ETIOLOGY/PATHOGENESIS

Developmental Anomaly

- Lipomas thought to represent congenital malformations derived from meninx primitiva
  - Recent genetic data favor neoplastic origin for some

Other Common Risk Factors/Syndromes

- Agenesis/hypoplasia of corpus callosum most common, malformative
- Epidermal nevus syndrome
- Goldenhar syndrome
- Spinal dysraphism and encephaloceles
- Fishman syndrome (encephalocraniocutaneous lipomatosis)
- Pai syndrome
  - Facial clefts, skin, and, rarely, interhemispheric lipomas

Genetics

- 12q13-15 rearrangements in conventional lipoma
  - Gene on 12q that is in involved in lipomas is *HMGA2* (through rearrangments)
  - In 1 study of limited numbers of CNS cases of lipomatous lesions of CNS, *HMGA2* rearrangements not identified; thus, CNS lesions may be different from conventional lipomas
- 16q in spindle cell/pleomorphic lipoma
- 11q13 in hibernoma
- 8q in lipoblastoma

CLINICAL ISSUES

Epidemiology

- Incidence
  - Rare
- Age
  - All
- Sex
  - Slightly ↑ in females

Site

- Intracranial (majority supratentorial and midline)
  - Interhemispheric (pericallosal) 40-50%
  - Quadrigeminal plate/superior cerebellar area
  - Suprasellar/interpeduncular
  - Cerebellopontine angle
  - Sylvian cistern
  - 8th cranial nerve: Mimics schwannoma clinically, but distinguished radiologically
- Spinal (mostly lumbosacral)
  - Intradural, epidural, or intramedullary
    - Cervical or thoracic cord, when not associated with dysraphism
    - Lumbar cord (filum terminale), common, with tethered cord, malformative

Presentation

- Lipomas rarely symptomatic, usually incidental neuroradiological or autopsy finding
- Mass effect and compression of adjacent structures
  - Intracranial
    - Headaches
    - Seizures
    - Hypothalamic disturbances
    - Cranial nerve deficits
  - Spinal
    - Pain
    - Sphincter, motor, and sensory deficits

Treatment

- Lipoma
  - Usually none
  - Simple excision if symptomatic
- Liposarcoma
  - Multimodality

Prognosis

- Excellent for lipoma and variants
- Less favorable for liposarcoma, though data limited

IMAGING

General Features

- Best diagnostic clue
  - Well-demarcated extraaxial mass with fat attenuation/intensity

MR Findings

- Homogeneous, hyperintense T1WI
- Hypointense on T2WI
- Fat-suppression sequences confirm

CT Findings

- Circumscribed, nonenhancing hypodensity
- ± calcification, prominent in corpus callosum examples

MACROSCOPIC

General Features

- Yellow, soft, lobulated mass attached to meninges, sometimes adherent to brain
- Greasy
- Circumscribed or diffuse
- Thin membranous capsule
- May encase blood vessels and nerves

Size

- Varies from tiny to large, most < 5 cm

MICROSCOPIC

Histologic Features

- Mature adipocytes
- Mild to moderate variation in size

- Variable hyalinization, vascularity
- ± skeletal/smooth muscle, cartilage, bone
- Myxoid matrix: Myxoid lipoma
- Prominent fibrous septa: Fibrolipoma

Cytologic Features

- Balloon-like cells with clear cytoplasm, eccentric nuclei

Variants of Lipoma

- Many of these are extremely rare (or even never encountered) in CNS
  - Angiolipoma
    - Variable capillary caliber
      - Hyalinization common; fibrin microthrombi
  - Lipoma with heterologous elements
    - Myolipoma: Especially in internal auditory canal
    - Chondrolipoma, osteolipoma
  - Hibernoma
    - Composed of brown fat
  - Spindle cell/pleomorphic lipoma
    - Variable numbers of spindle or giant cells
    - Coarse collagen bands between spindle cells
    - ± mast cells, lymphocytes, plasma cells
    - Pseudoangiomatoid spaces
  - Lipoblastoma
    - Lobulated, myxoid immature fat
  - Atypical lipoma
    - Well-differentiated lipoma with significant nuclear atypia
    - Essentially identical to well-differentiated liposarcoma
    - Tendency to undergo malignant transformation
  - Liposarcoma
    - Widened fibrous septa, hypercellularity, nuclear pleomorphism
    - ± lymphocytic infiltrates, single cell necrosis
    - Myxoid, round cell, or pleomorphic elements may be present
      - Sheets of round cells may resemble lymphoma in small biopsy
      - Pleomorphic variant sometimes composed of epithelioid cells

ANCILLARY TESTS

Cytology

- Adipocytes with small, peripherally located nuclei

Immunohistochemistry

- Lipogenic tumors variably S100(+)
- Spindle/pleomorphic liposarcoma may be CD34(+), CK7, 8, 18(+)

DIFFERENTIAL DIAGNOSIS

Lipidized CNS Neoplasms

- Meningioma
  - Most common lipidized tumor
  - Classic meningioma features present and usually predominant
  - EMA(+), SSTR2A(+)
  - Meningothelial-like whorls rare in dedifferentiated liposarcoma
- Neurocytomas
  - Central and extraventricular
    - Intraventricular and intraparenchymal, not leptomeningeal; synaptophysin (+)
    - Classic neurocytoma features, usually predominant
  - Cerebellar
    - Intraparenchymal, not leptomeningeal
    - Classic neurocytoma features, usually predominant
- Gliomas
  - Glioblastoma
    - Intraparenchymal, not leptomeningeal
    - Lipidization rare, focal
  - Gliosarcoma
    - Lipidized cells only focal
    - Cellular, GFAP(+) glioma
    - Reticulin-rich tissue with mesenchymal differentiation
  - Ependymoma
    - Lipidized cells only focal
  - Astrocytoma
    - Lipidized cells focal in tumor with classic ependymoma features
  - Pleomorphic xanthoastrocytoma
    - Only focal xanthomatous change, not adipocyte-like lipidization
    - Eosinophilic granular bodies
    - GFAP(+)
- Hemangioblastoma
  - Highly vascular
  - Small lipid droplets in stromal, interstitial cells, not adipose-like tissue

Teratoma

- Tissue elements from all 3 germinal layers

Other Sarcomas

- Liposarcoma, especially dedifferentiated, may mimic other sarcomas
- Immunohistochemistry &/or ultrastructural study sometimes helpful

Metastatic Carcinoma

- Immunoprofile distinguishes from pleomorphic liposarcoma

DIAGNOSTIC CHECKLIST

Pathologic Interpretation Pearls

- Myxoid, round cell, or pleomorphic components indicate higher grade liposarcoma (rare)

GRADING

Liposarcoma

- Graded same as soft tissue counterpart
- Adequate sampling important, may harbor areas identical to lipoma

SELECTED REFERENCES

1. Zhang H et al: Molecular testing for lipomatous tumors: critical analysis and test recommendations based on the analysis of 405 extremity-based tumors. Am J Surg Pathol. 34(9):1304-11, 2010
2. Rodriguez FJ et al: HMGA2 rearrangements are rare in benign lipomatous lesions of the nervous system. Acta Neuropathol. 116(3):337-8, 2008

Dural-Based Lipoma

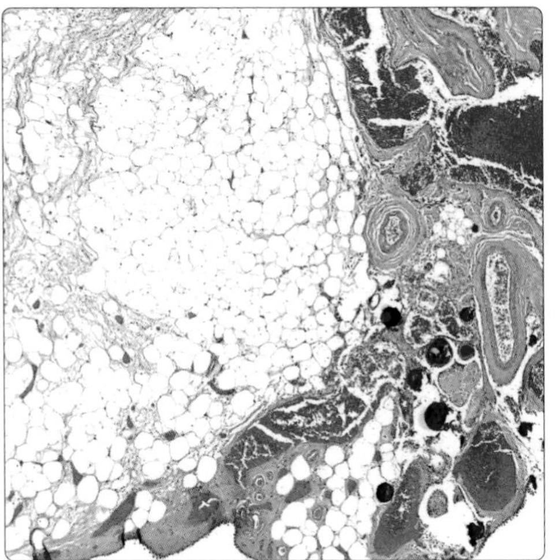

Angiolipoma

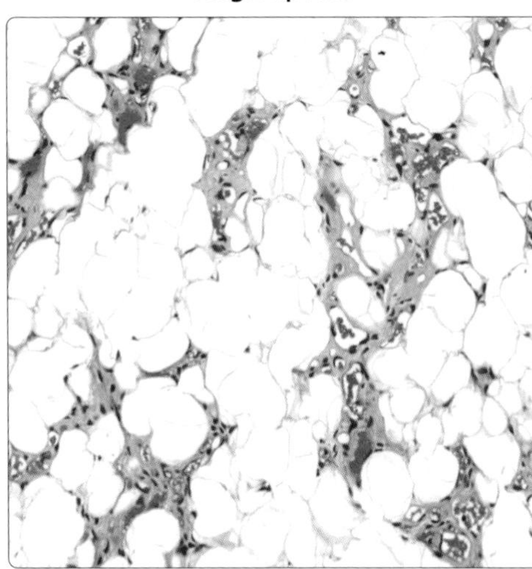

(Left) *This dural-based lipoma was situated deep in the interhemispheric fissure. Partial or complete agenesis of the corpus callosum may accompany such a midline lipoma.* **(Right)** *Angiolipomas have thick-walled capillaries with slender endothelial cells, often as clusters along the periphery of the tumor. Fibrin microthrombi and erythrocytes typically fill the lumina.*

Spindle Cell Lipoma

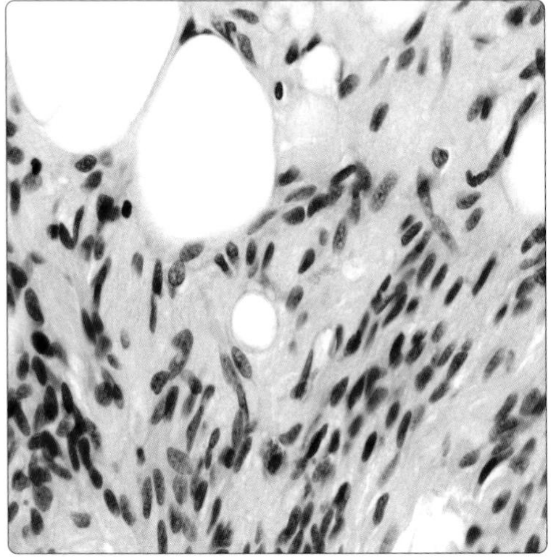

Pleomorphic Lipoma

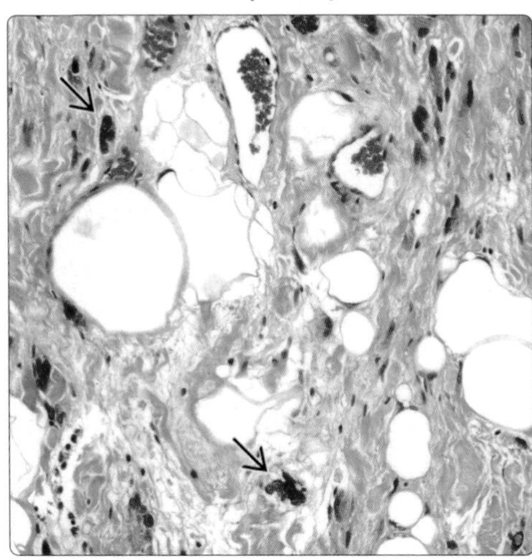

(Left) *An admixture of mature fat, uniform bland spindle cells, and coarse, rope-like collagen supports the diagnosis of spindle cell lipoma. Despite the increased cellularity, these tumors have a benign behavior.* **(Right)** *Pleomorphic lipomas contain floret-like giant cells ⇒ that consist of radially arranged nuclei resembling petals of a flower. Like spindle cell lipoma, these tumors are strongly CD34(+).*

CNS Liposarcoma, Well Differentiated

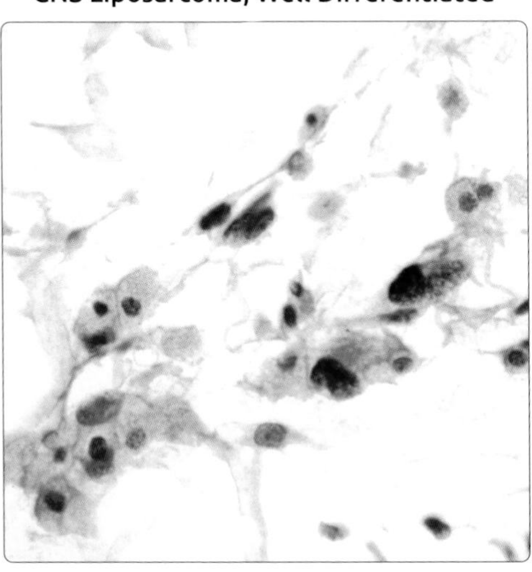

Pleomorphic Liposarcoma

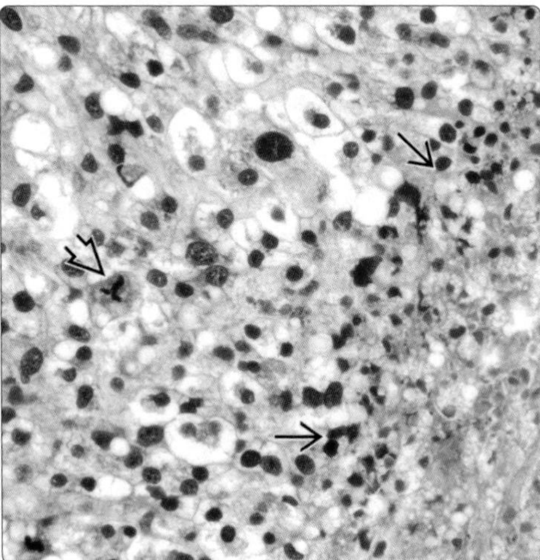

(Left) *Rare CNS liposarcomas are well-differentiated. They are distinguished from their benign counterparts by the presence of occasional cells with enlarged, hyperchromatic nuclei.* **(Right)** *Pleomorphic liposarcoma is a high-grade sarcoma with bizarre, pleomorphic lipoblasts. Note the necrosis → and atypical mitoses ⇨. Such tumors can mimic epithelial neoplasms or even a high-grade pleomorphic xanthoastrocytoma.*

Meningeal Glioma and Gliomatosis

KEY FACTS

TERMINOLOGY

- Diffuse or localized glioma within leptomeninges
- Often difficult, if not impossible in many cases, to exclude origin from small intraparenchymal primary

CLINICAL ISSUES

- Poor prognosis
  - Median survival: 38 months
- Present with meningeal signs/symptoms
- Chronic meningitis, especially tuberculous, a common clinical diagnosis

IMAGING

- Gadolinium enhancement of leptomeninges on T1WI
- No evidence of parenchymal involvement

MACROSCOPIC

- Solitary, multinodular, or diffuse leptomeningeal thickening

MICROSCOPIC

- Astrocytic phenotype most common
- Rare reports of meningeal gliomatosis with anaplastic oligodendroglioma, ependymoma, gliosarcoma

ANCILLARY TESTS

- GFAP, Olig2(+) immunohistochemistry

TOP DIFFERENTIAL DIAGNOSES

- Leptomeningeal carcinomatosis
- Meningioma
- Meningeal sarcoma

DIAGNOSTIC CHECKLIST

- Recognize fibrillar background to help identify glial nature

(Left) *The diffuse disease encases both spinal cord and nerve roots ⊟. Multiple neoplastic and inflammatory diseases are possibilities at the macroscopic level.* **(Right)** *The lesion, which fills the subarachnoid space, often has a somewhat fascicular architecture that can resemble that of many other neoplasms.*

Meningeal Gliomatosis Encasing Spinal Cord, Nerve Roots

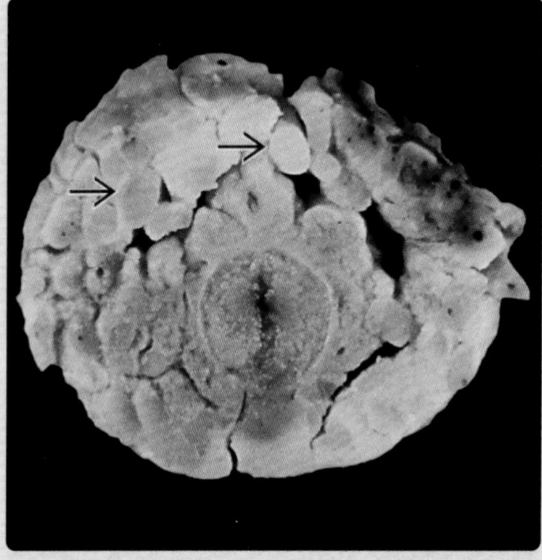

Fascicled Architecture Mimicking Meningioma or Sarcoma

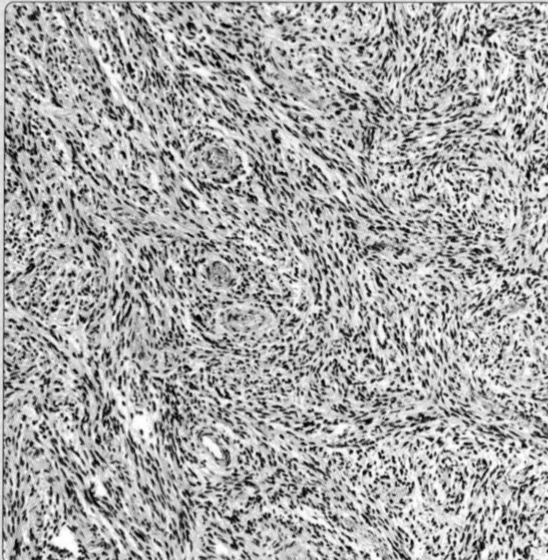

(Left) *The possibility of an astrocytoma should be entertained when the specimen contains jumbled pleomorphic nuclei embedded in an eosinophilic fibrillar background.* **(Right)** *Immunoreactivity for glial fibrillary acidic protein ⊟ helps define the glial nature of this rare neoplasm.*

Meningeal Gliomatosis, Fibrillar Background

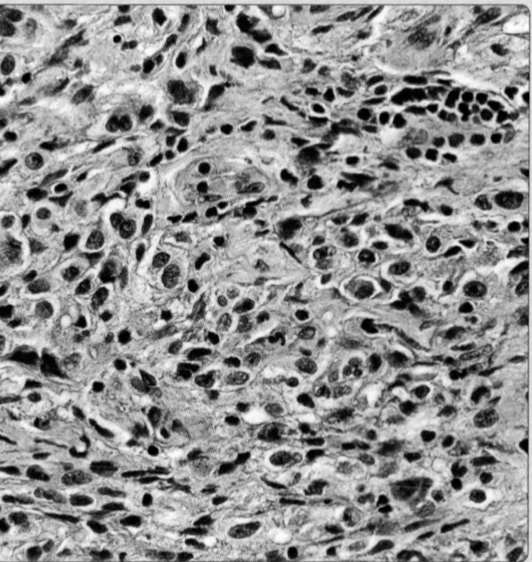

Meningeal Gliomatosis, GFAP(+)

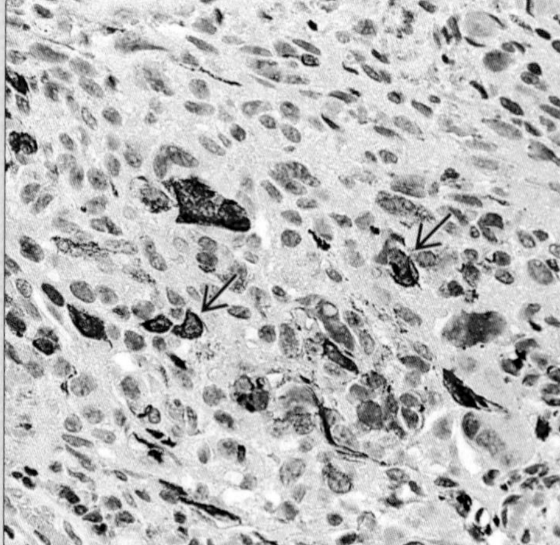

Meningeal Glioma and Gliomatosis

TERMINOLOGY

Definitions

- Diffuse or localized glioma within leptomeninges
- Often difficult, if not impossible in many cases, to exclude origin from small intraparenchymal primary

ETIOLOGY/PATHOGENESIS

Etiology

- Thought to arise from heterotopic neuroglial rests within leptomeninges
- Majority found along anterior medulla or lumbosacral spinal cord

CLINICAL ISSUES

Epidemiology

- Incidence
  - Exceedingly rare
- Age
  - Mean: 35 years; range: 9-71 years
- Sex
  - No predilection

Presentation

- Meningeal signs/symptoms
  - Headache, stiff neck
- Multiple cranial nerve palsies
- Seizures
- Intracranial hypertension

Treatment

- Surgical approaches
  - Meningeal biopsy
  - Shunting to reduce intracranial pressure
- Adjuvant therapy
  - Chemotherapy
- Radiation
  - Temporary remission reported after craniospinal radiation

Prognosis

- Poor (median survival: 38 months)

IMAGING

MR Findings

- Gadolinium enhancement of leptomeninges on T1WI MR
- Hydrocephalus
- No evidence of parenchymal involvement

MACROSCOPIC

General Features

- Solitary, multinodular, or diffuse leptomeningeal thickening

MICROSCOPIC

Histologic Features

- Astrocytic
  - Pleomorphism
  - Glassy cytoplasm, fibrillar background
- Oligodendroglioma
  - Back-to-back uniform round, cytologically bland cells with perinuclear halos
  - Poorly characterized disease
- Ependymoma
  - Perivascular pseudorosettes and true rosettes

Cytologic Features

- Depends on glial phenotype

ANCILLARY TESTS

Immunohistochemistry

- GFAP(+), in astrocytic and ependymal types

CSF

- Pleocytosis, increased protein
- Positive cytology rare

DIFFERENTIAL DIAGNOSIS

Chronic Meningitis

- Infectious organism present in some cases, but may be difficult to identify/isolate
- Inflammation, e.g., granulomatous (sarcoidosis, tuberculosis)

Meningeal Carcinomatosis/Lymphomatosis

- Discrete, GFAP(-) tumor cells
- No fibrillar background
- Appropriate epithelial, melanocytic, or lymphoid markers positive

Secondary Invasion of Meninges by Primary Intraparenchymal Glioma

- Difficult to exclude ante- or even postmortem
- Intraparenchymal primary focus may be small

Meningioma

- Whorls, nuclear pseudoinclusions
- EMA(+), SSTR2A(+)

DIAGNOSTIC CHECKLIST

Pathologic Interpretation Pearls

- Recognize fibrillar background to help identify glial nature

SELECTED REFERENCES

1. Moon JH et al: Primary diffuse leptomeningeal gliosarcomatosis. Brain Tumor Res Treat. 3(1):34-8, 2015
2. Iunes EA et al: Multifocal intradural extramedullary ependymoma. Case report. J Neurosurg Spine. 14(1):65-70, 2011
3. Keith T et al: A report of the natural history of leptomeningeal gliomatosis. J Clin Neurosci. 18(4):582-5, 2011
4. Dörner L et al: Primary diffuse leptomeningeal gliomatosis in a 2-year-old girl. Surg Neurol. 71(6):713-9, discussion 719, 2009
5. Michotte A et al: Primary leptomeningeal anaplastic oligodendroglioma with a 1p36-19q13 deletion: report of a unique case successfully treated with Temozolomide. J Neurol Sci. 287(1-2):267-70, 2009
6. Ozkul A et al: Primary diffuse leptomeningeal oligodendrogliomatosis causing sudden death. J Neurooncol. 81(1):75-9, 2007
7. Debono B et al: Primary diffuse multinodular leptomeningeal gliomatosis: case report and review of the literature. Surg Neurol. 65(3):273-82; discussion 282, 2006
8. Bohner G et al: Pilocytic astrocytoma presenting as primary diffuse leptomeningeal gliomatosis: report of a unique case and review of the literature. Acta Neuropathol. 110(3):306-11, 2005

Metastatic Neoplasms, Intracranial and Intraspinal Meninges

KEY FACTS

TERMINOLOGY

- Leptomeningeal carcinomatosis, carcinomatous meningitis, lymphomatous meningitis, leukemic meningitis, etc.
- Diffuse infiltration of subarachnoid space or focal mass from
  - Systemic cancer (at any cancer stage but usually late)
  - Primary CNS tumor
- Dural metastasis
  - Often from breast, lung, prostate, sarcoma
  - Usually not coassociated with leptomeningeal carcinomatosis
  - Not able to be detected by cerebrospinal fluid cytology
  - Mimics meningioma

IMAGING

- Diffuse leptomeningeal enhancement or focal nodular leptomeningeal spinal deposits on MR
- Thickening of cranial nerves, especially VII and VIII
- Focal, nodular, leptomeningeal spinal deposits

MICROSCOPIC

- Diffuse leptomeningeal from systemic primary
  - Free-floating, usually round, individual cells
  - Epithelial structures, e.g., glands, uncommon
- Dural metastases: Globoid or en plaque subdural metastasis from systemic primary
  - Undifferentiated, glandular, squamous differentiation, etc. depending on site and degree of anaplasia
- Diffuse leptomeningeal from CNS primary, e.g., medulloblastoma, pilocytic astrocytoma, glioblastoma

DIAGNOSTIC CHECKLIST

- Disseminated leptomeningeal adenocarcinoma cells may closely resemble macrophages

(Left) *Axial T1-weighted MR with gadolinium shows enhancing metastatic tumor filling the subarachnoid space ➡. (Right) Axial graphic depicts metastatic tumor involving the subarachnoid spaces, including the insular regions bilaterally ➡.*

Leptomeningeal Carcinomatosis

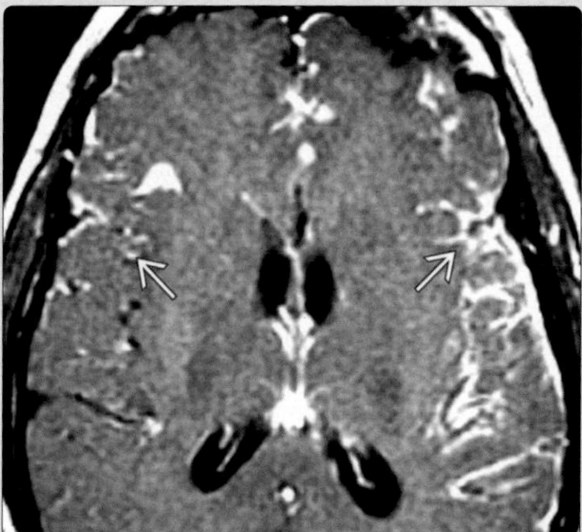

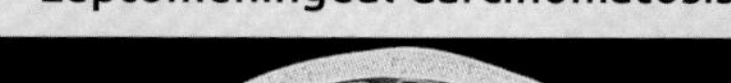

Leptomeningeal Carcinomatosis

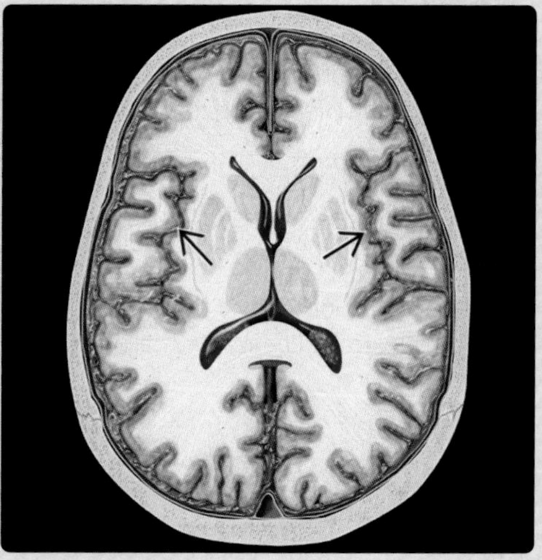

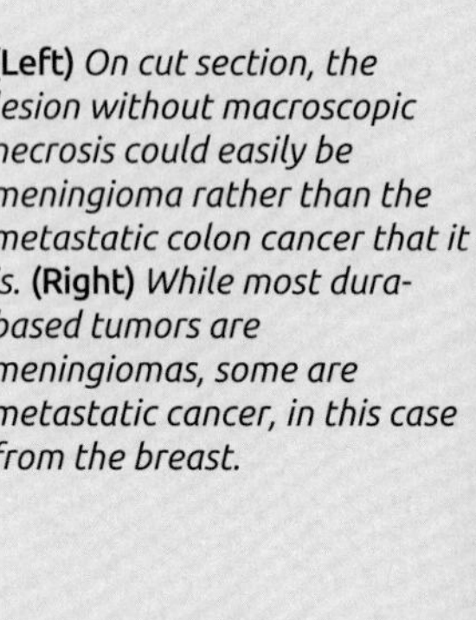

(Left) *On cut section, the lesion without macroscopic necrosis could easily be meningioma rather than the metastatic colon cancer that it is.* **(Right)** *While most dura-based tumors are meningiomas, some are metastatic cancer, in this case from the breast.*

Dural Metastasis Simulating Meningioma

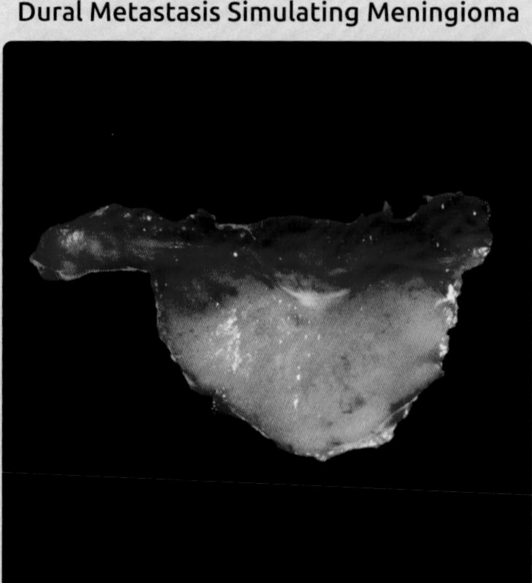

Dural Metastasis, Breast Cancer

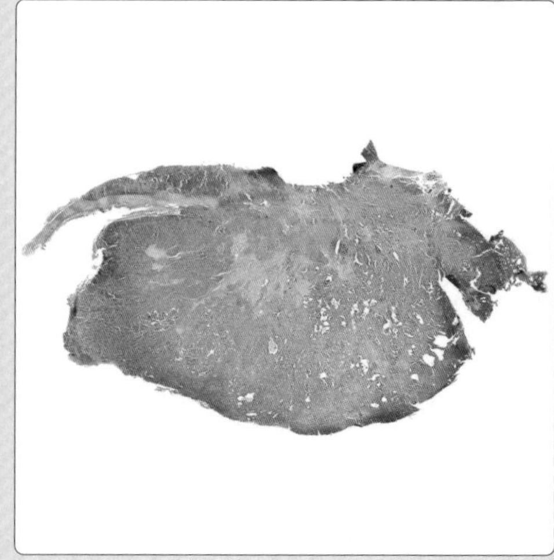

TERMINOLOGY

Synonyms

- Leptomeningeal carcinomatosis
- Carcinomatous meningitis
- Neoplastic meningitis
- Lymphomatous meningitis
- Leukemic meningitis
- Drop metastases

Definitions

- Diffuse infiltration of subarachnoid space of brain &/or spinal cord from
  - Systemic cancer (at any stage but usually late)
  - Primary CNS tumor
- Globoid or en plaque dural-based mass, single or multiple, from systemic primary
  - ± involvement of adjacent skull

ETIOLOGY/PATHOGENESIS

Mode of Access

- Hematogenous
- Direct extension of metastasis to skull or brain
- Cerebrospinal fluid (CSF) dissemination of primary CNS tumor

Neurocutaneous Melanosis (Rare)

- Large, "bathing trunk" nevus
- Leptomeningeal melanoma/melanosis

CLINICAL ISSUES

Epidemiology

- Incidence
  - Uncommon, 5% of patients with cancer
- Age
  - Adults more common
  - Children, especially those with leukemia, medulloblastoma, pilocytic astrocytoma

Presentation

- Headache
- Mental status changes
- Cranial nerve dysfunction
  - CNS dysfunction sometimes isolated
- Seizures
- Radiculopathy
- Myelopathy

Treatment

- Surgical approaches
  - Ventriculoperitoneal shunting to relieve obstructive hydrocephalus
- Adjuvant therapy
  - Intrathecal/systemic chemotherapy
    - EGFR(+) tyrosine kinase inhibitors for non-small cell lung cancer
- Radiation
  - Involved-field radiotherapy

Prognosis

- Overall poor (< 6 months)
- Better prognosis for lung cancer with *EGFR* mutations

IMAGING

MR Findings

- Hydrocephalus
- Diffuse leptomeningeal enhancement
- Thickening of cranial nerves, especially VII and VIII
- Focal nodular, "lumpy bumpy," leptomeningeal spinal deposits

CT Findings

- Hydrocephalus
- Enhancement of tentorium, sylvian fissures, basal cisterns, cortical subarachnoid space, and ventricular walls

MACROSCOPIC

General Features

- Diffuse leptomeningeal disease
  - Meningeal studding or thickening with opacification
  - Thickened cranial &/or spinal nerves
  - Melanosis
  - Sometimes with discrete, solid intraparenchymal metastasis
- Globular, meningioma-like mass
  - Sometimes focally necrotic
  - May be solitary
- En plaque subdural mass

MICROSCOPIC

Histologic Features

- Diffuse leptomeningeal from systemic primary
  - Common features
    - Infiltrate and enlarge cranial and spinal nerves
    - Superficial parenchymal invasion (in some cases)
    - May follow Virchow-Robin spaces for short distances
  - Free-floating, usually round, individual cells
    - With secretory product, signet ring cells (in some cases)
    - Cytologically bland and resemble macrophages in some cases
    - Melanoma: Intranuclear pseudoinclusions, prominent nucleoli, pigmentation variable and may be absent
    - Lymphoma or leukemia
  - Epithelial structures, e.g., glands (uncommon)
- Globoid or en plaque subdural metastasis from systemic primary
  - Undifferentiated, glandular, squamous differentiation, etc., depending on site and degree of anaplasia
  - Necrosis (variable)
- Common sources
  - Breast
  - Lung
  - Stomach (classic but now uncommon)
  - Prostate
- Diffuse leptomeningeal from CNS primary
  - Undifferentiated or nodular/desmoplastic tissue: Medulloblastoma
  - Piloid tissue: Pilocytic or pilomyxoid astrocytoma

- Perivascular pseudorosettes, myxoid substance: Myxopapillary ependymoma, rostral spread
- Perivascular pseudorosettes: Ependymoma, cellular type
- Melanocytic, variably pigmented
- Germ cell tumor
  - Germinoma
  - Nongerminomatous

Cytologic Features

- Variable atypia and nuclear pleomorphism
  - Atypia sometimes slight in renal cell, breast, prostate, stomach carcinomas
  - May resemble macrophages
- Discrete cell borders
- Prominent nucleoli
  - Adenocarcinoma
  - Melanoma
- Secretory product, signet ring cells
- Chronic inflammatory reaction
  - Exaggerated mononuclear reaction: "Encephalitic variant"
- Negative cytology not uncommon
  - Multiple examinations may be required
  - Subsequent taps also sometimes negative in spite of later, autopsy-proven disease
  - Possibly higher yield with cisternal sampling, though not routine
- Leukemia, lymphoma

ANCILLARY TESTS

Immunohistochemistry

- Carcinoma
  - Lung
    - Non-small cell: CAM5.2, CK7, BER-EP4, napsin (adenocarcinoma), TTF-1
    - Small cell: TTF-1, CD56, CAM5.2
  - Squamous cell, any site: CK5/6, p63
  - Breast: GCDFP, CK7, GATA3, BER-EP4, mammaglobin, ER/PR
  - Colorectal: CAM5.2, CK20, CDX-2, BER-EP4
  - Gastroesophageal: CK7, CK20, CDX-2, BER-EP4
  - Pancreatic: CK7, CK20, CDX-2, BER-EP4, DPC4/SMAD4 (loss)
  - Renal cell: pax-2, pax-8, CD10, RCCma
  - Urothelial: GATA3, p63
  - Thyroid: TTF-1, thyroglobulin, pax-8
  - Adrenal: Inhibin-α, Melan-A
  - Hepatocellular: Polyclonal CEA and CD10 (both canalicular)
  - Ovary: CK7, WT1, pax-8, BER-EP4, ER/PR
- Melanoma: S100, Melan-A, HMB-45, SOX10
- Lymphoma and leukemia: Hematopoietic markers, especially CD20, CD79-a, and CD43
- Sarcoma: Desmin, myogenin
- Germ cell: CD117 (c-kit), OCT4, placental alkaline phosphatase, α-fetoprotein, HCG-β, SALL4
- Medulloblastoma, pineoblastoma, supratentorial primitive neuroectodermal tumors (PNETs)
  - Synaptophysin
- Glioma
  - GFAP

DIFFERENTIAL DIAGNOSIS

Diffuse Leptomeningeal Tumor

- Inflammatory, macrophage-rich disease
  - Little if any cytological atypia
  - Immunopositivity for lymphocyte and macrophage markers
- Intracranial hypotension with diffuse dural enhancement
  - Dural, not leptomeningeal, enhancement as in meningeal carcinomatosis
  - Biopsy findings: Delicate vessels on inner surface of dura

Globoid or En Plaque Dural Mass

- Anaplastic meningioma
  - Can be difficult when cytokeratin (+); SSTR2A(+)
  - Lower grade meningioma elsewhere in specimen
  - Generally less epithelial than well- or moderately well-differentiated carcinomas
  - Body scan (-)
- Inflammatory pseudotumor
  - No neoplastic cells
  - Granulomatous inflammation (in some cases)
- Cellular solitary fibrous tumor/hemangiopericytoma
  - Fascicular architecture
  - Variably CD34(+), nuclear STAT6(+)
  - EMA and cytokeratin (-)
  - Abundant reticulin

DIAGNOSTIC CHECKLIST

Pathologic Interpretation Pearls

- Disseminated leptomeningeal adenocarcinoma cells may closely resemble macrophages

SELECTED REFERENCES

1. Chen H et al: Expression and significance of transforming growth factor-β receptor type II and DPC4/Smad4 in non-small cell lung cancer. Exp Ther Med. 9(1):227-231, 2015
2. Demagny H et al: The tumor suppressor Smad4/DPC4 is regulated by phosphorylations that integrate FGF, Wnt, and TGF-β signaling. Cell Rep. 9(2):688-700, 2014
3. Chamberlain MC: Lymphomatous meningitis as a presentation of non-Hodgkin lymphoma. Clin Adv Hematol Oncol. 9(5):419-20, 2011
4. de Azevedo CR et al: Meningeal carcinomatosis in breast cancer: prognostic factors and outcome. J Neurooncol. 104(2):565-72, 2011
5. Meriggi F et al: Newer avenues for the treatment of leptomeningeal carcinomatosis. Cent Nerv Syst Agents Med Chem. 11(1):38-44, 2011
6. Quadri SA et al: Primary central nervous system lymphoma causing multiple spinal cord compression and carcinomatous meningitis in a 6-year-old: a case report. J Pediatr Hematol Oncol. 33(4):312-5, 2011
7. Chamberlain MC: Leptomeningeal metastasis. Curr Opin Neurol. 22(6):665-74, 2009
8. Yi HG et al: Epidermal growth factor receptor (EGFR) tyrosine kinase inhibitors (TKIs) are effective for leptomeningeal metastasis from non-small cell lung cancer patients with sensitive EGFR mutation or other predictive factors of good response for EGFR TKI. Lung Cancer. 65(1):80-4, 2009
9. Edgar MA et al: The differential diagnosis of central nervous system tumors: a critical examination of some recent immunohistochemical applications. Arch Pathol Lab Med. 132(3):500-9, 2008
10. Becher MW et al: Immunohistochemical analysis of metastatic neoplasms of the central nervous system. J Neuropathol Exp Neurol. 65(10):935-44, 2006
11. Jaeckle KA: Neoplastic meningitis from systemic malignancies: diagnosis, prognosis and treatment. Semin Oncol. 33(3):312-23, 2006
12. DeAngelis LM et al: Leptomeningeal metastasis. Cancer Invest. 23(2):145-54, 2005
13. Mehta M et al: Radiation therapy for leptomeningeal cancer. Cancer Treat Res. 125:147-58, 2005

Severe Leptomeningeal Opacification

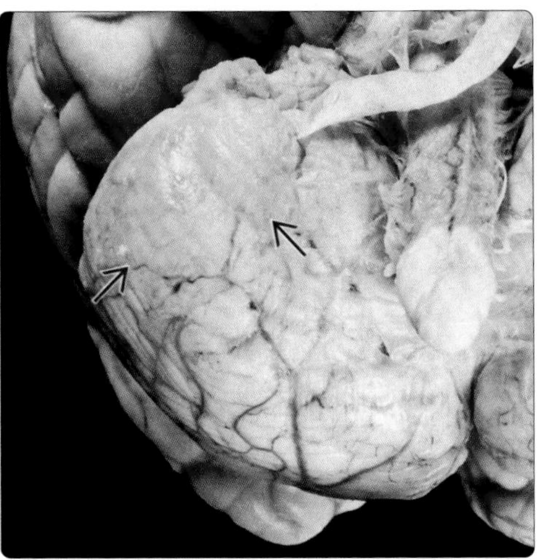

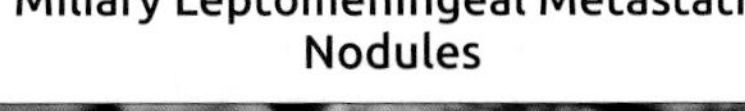

Miliary Leptomeningeal Metastatic Nodules

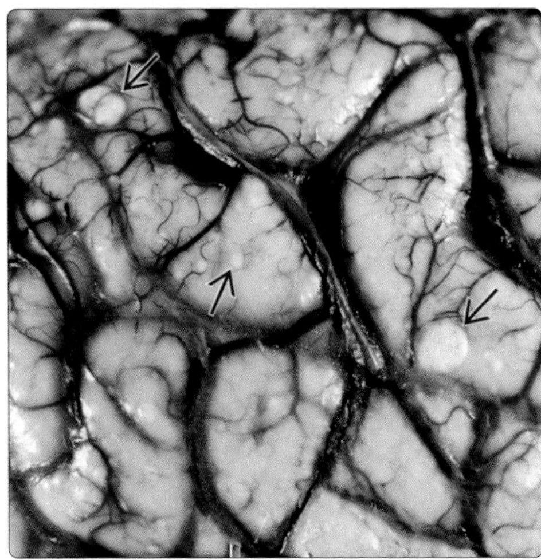

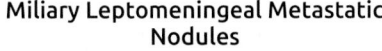

(Left) *Metastatic cancer, from the stomach in this case, may focally or diffusely thicken the leptomeninges →. Although obvious here, opacification may be subtle.* **(Right)** *Miliary leptomeningeal nodules → are 1 form of diffuse meningeal metastatic cancer, mammary in this case.*

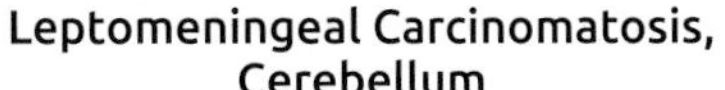

Leptomeningeal Carcinomatosis, Cerebellum

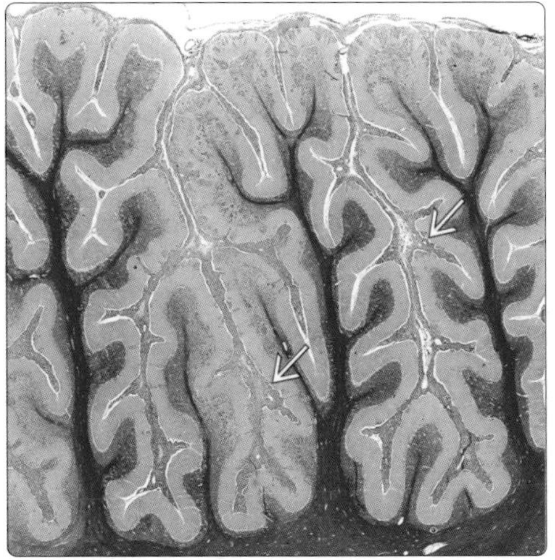

Extension Into Underlying Brain

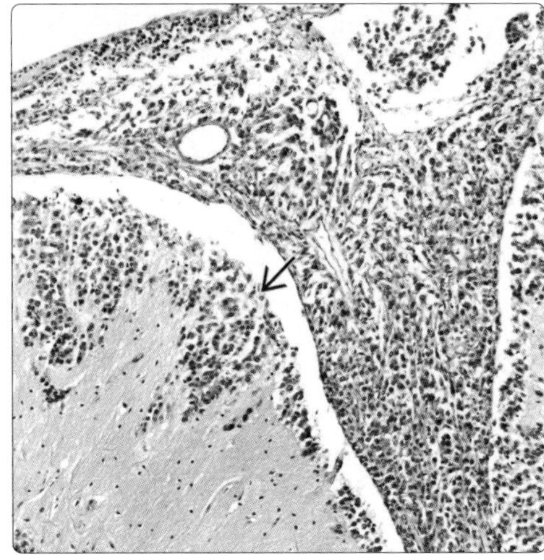

(Left) *Metastatic carcinoma from the stomach fills the subarachnoid space → overlying the cerebellum in this diffuse form of metastatic cancer, which is usually adenocarcinoma. Melanoma is another tumor type prone to such dissemination. Note how tumor involves deep sulcal spaces.* **(Right)** *Leptomeningeal metastatic carcinoma can extend secondarily into the underlying brain &/or extend along perivascular spaces →.*

Signet Ring Adenocarcinoma Simulating Macrophages

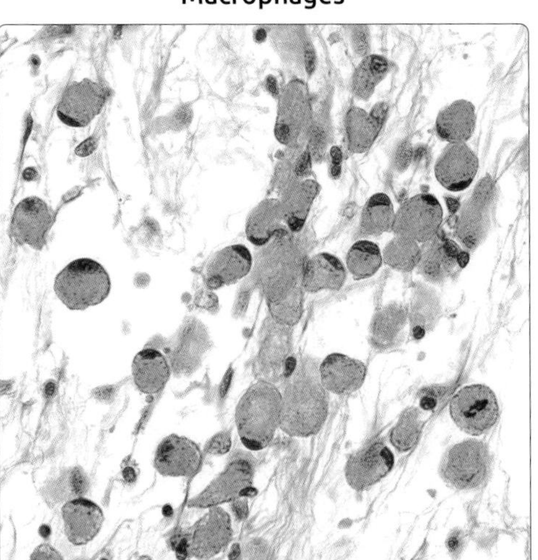

CSF Cytology, Adenocarcinoma

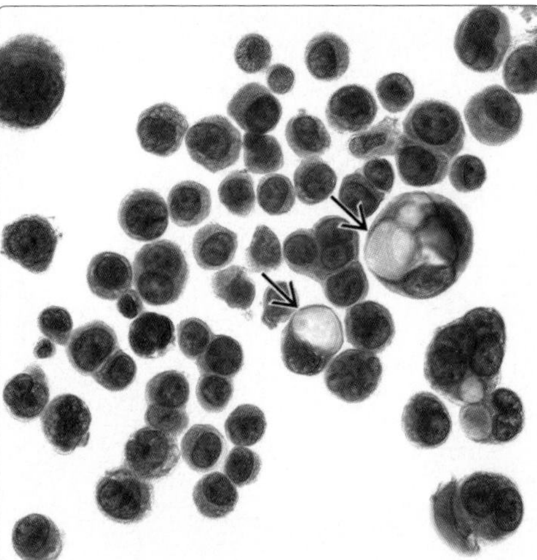

(Left) *Cytologically bland carcinoma cells should not be interpreted as macrophages. Although the cells here have classic signet ring configurations, their cytoplasm is deceptively granular rather than clear or mucoid.* **(Right)** *Coarse chromatin, prominent nucleoli, and nuclear pleomorphism establish the neoplastic nature of these cells, obtained by a lumbar puncture from a woman with a history of breast cancer. Intracytoplasmic vacuoles → help identify the lesion as adenocarcinoma.*

(Left) *Cerebrospinal fluid (CSF) cytology in fluid from an HIV-positive patient shows the pleomorphic cells with scant cytoplasm and clefted or notched nuclei that are typical of large cell malignant lymphoma.* **(Right)** *Leptomeningeal involvement in a patient with acute myelogenous leukemia was documented by CSF cytology.*

CSF Cytology, Large Cell Lymphoma

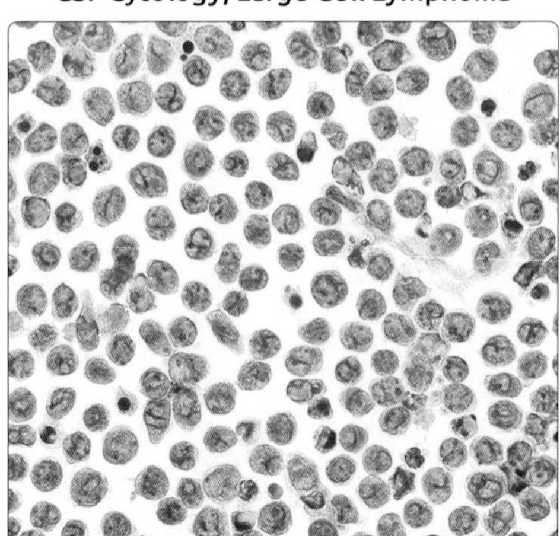

CSF Cytology, Acute Myelogenous Leukemia

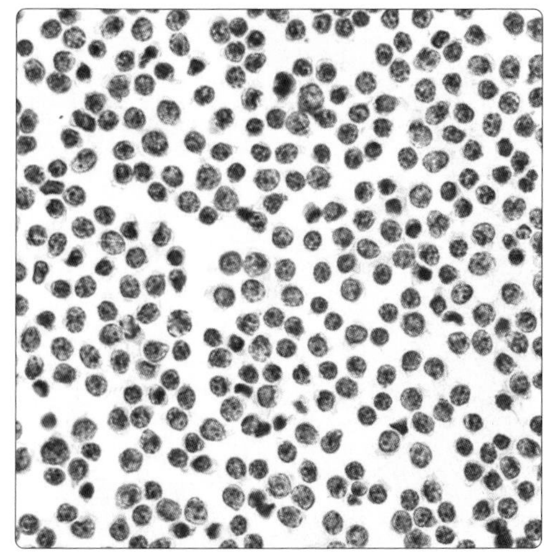

(Left) *Penetrating the dura and narrowing the superior sagittal sinus, this metastatic squamous cell carcinoma shares some properties with meningioma, a lesion well known for its propensity to invade and occlude the sinus. The overlying skull was also involved.* **(Right)** *Squamous differentiation is evident at high magnification ⇒ in this dural metastasis in a chronic smoker.*

Dural Metastasis Simulating Meningioma

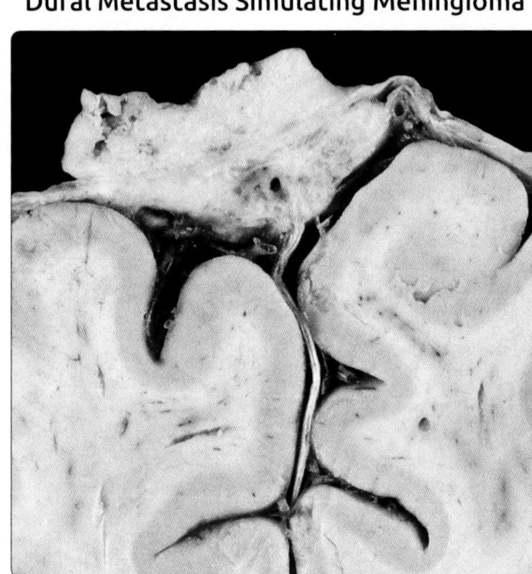

Dural Metastasis, Metastatic Squamous Cell Carcinoma

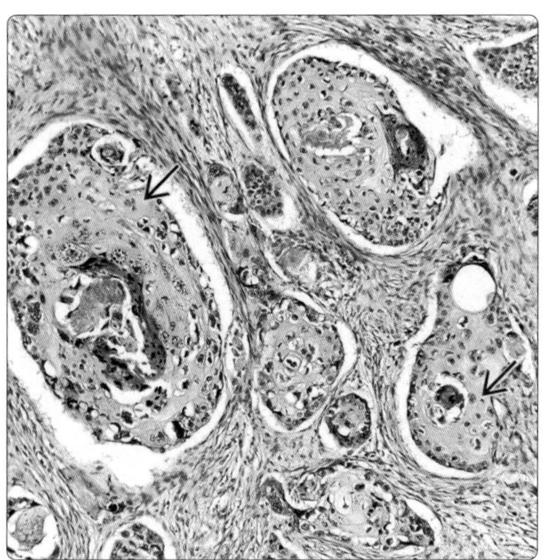

(Left) *Dural metastases, in this case from a primary in the colon, may macroscopically resemble meningioma. Such lesions from the colon, as with many other primaries, usually occur late in the disease.* **(Right)** *Small nests and a cribriform pattern in larger lobules make the breast a prime suspect for the primary of this globular metastasis to the dura.*

Dural Metastasis, Colon Cancer

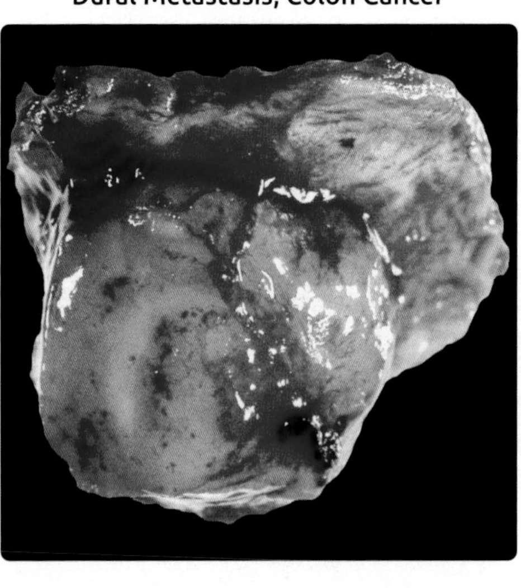

Dural Metastasis, Breast Cancer

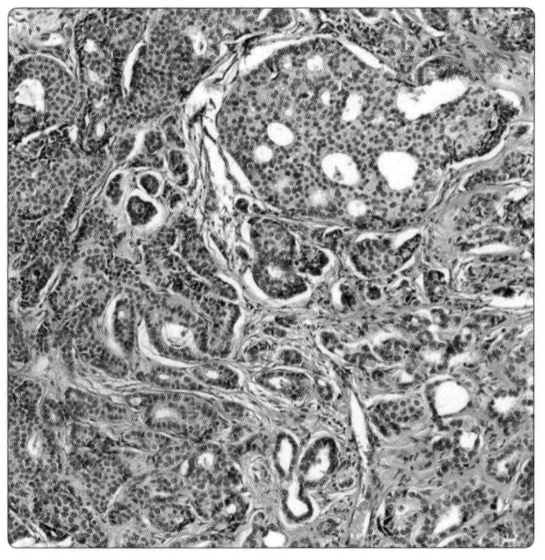

Dural Metastasis, Prostate Cancer

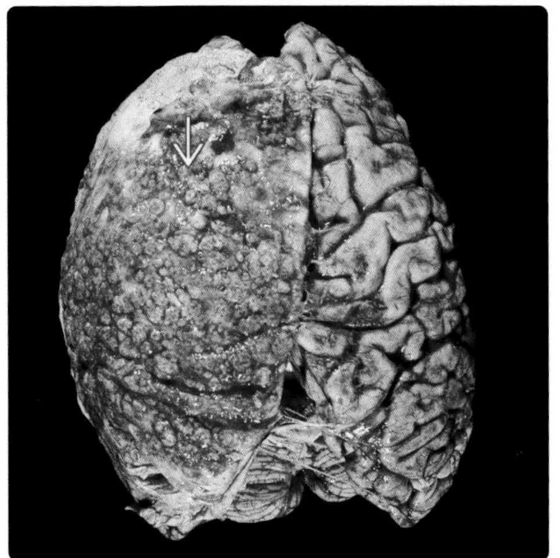

Dural Metastasis With Extension Into Subarachnoid Space

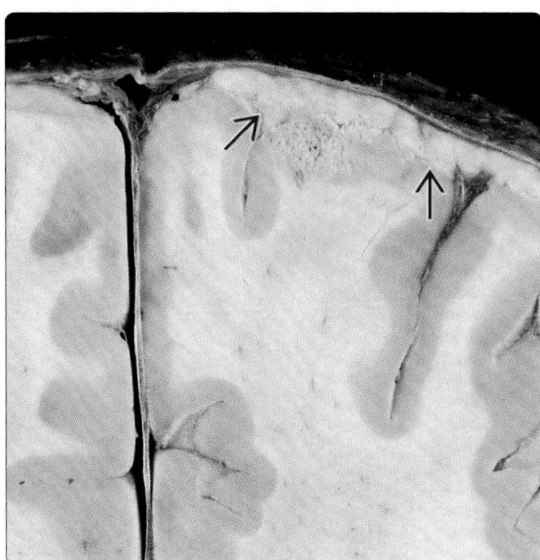

(Left) *Some metastases carpet the dura ➡ rather than form a large exophytic mass. Prostate was the source in this case.* **(Right)** *A dural-based tumor from the prostate ⇨ binds dura and pial surface, in the process obliterating the intervening subarachnoid space.*

CSF Dissemination, Medulloblastoma

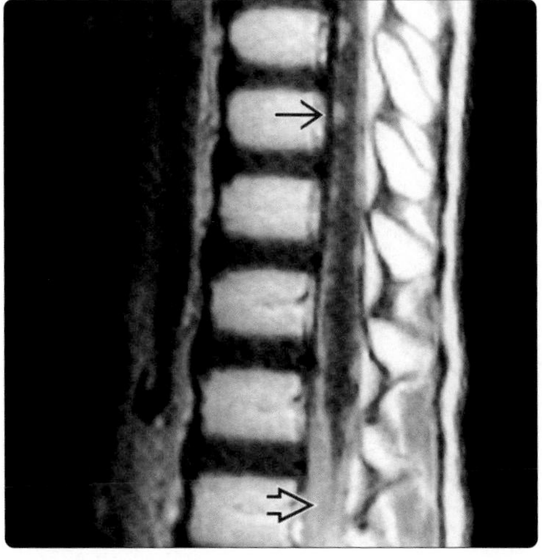

CSF Dissemination, Medulloblastoma

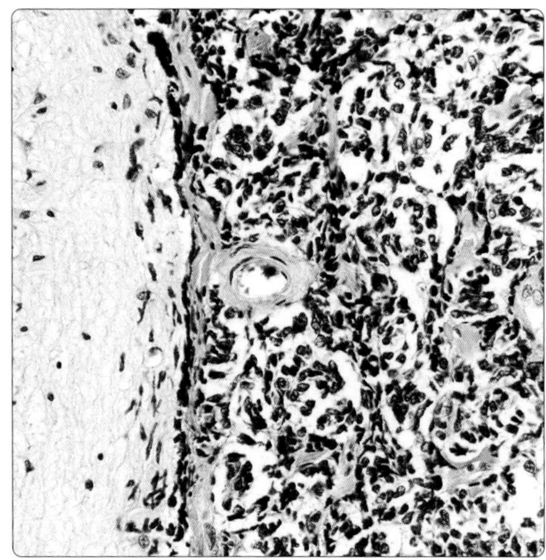

(Left) *Medulloblastomas are especially prone to CSF dissemination. This lesion has nodular leptomeningeal foci ⇨ and confluent tumor in the caudal thecal sac ⇨. CSF cytology and spine imaging are part of the staging work-up for medulloblastoma.* **(Right)** *Although occasional disseminated medulloblastoma will be from nodular/desmoplastic types, CSF dissemination is more frequent with large cell/anaplastic medulloblastomas.*

CSF Drop Metastases, Pediatric Pontine Glioblastoma

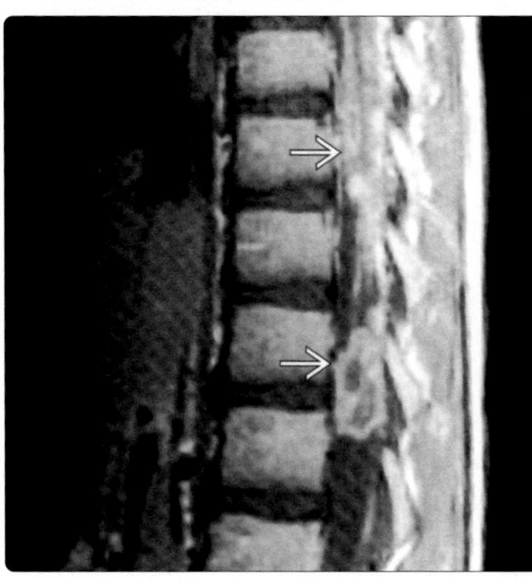

Drop Metastases, Nerve Root Involvement

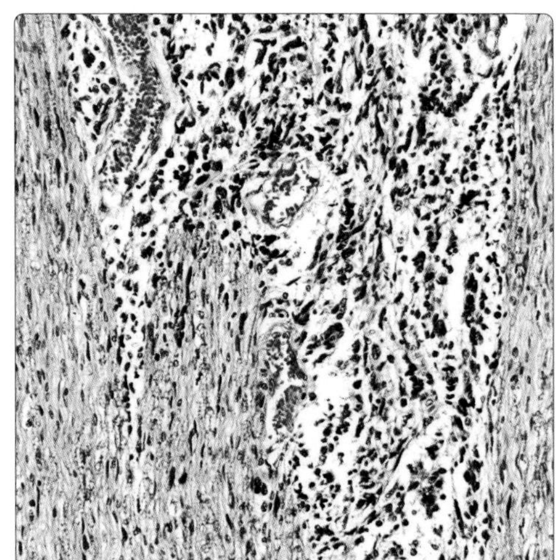

(Left) *Glioblastomas, especially from the pons as in this pediatric case, occasionally spread throughout CSF pathways as contrast-enhancing deposits, if not bulky masses ➡.* **(Right)** *Undifferentiated cells of a drop metastasis separate and infiltrate blue myelin-stained spinal nerve roots. A glioblastoma in the pons of a young child was the source. Glioblastomas are less prone to such dissemination than medulloblastomas.*

PART I
SECTION 4
Cranial, Spinal, and Peripheral Nerves

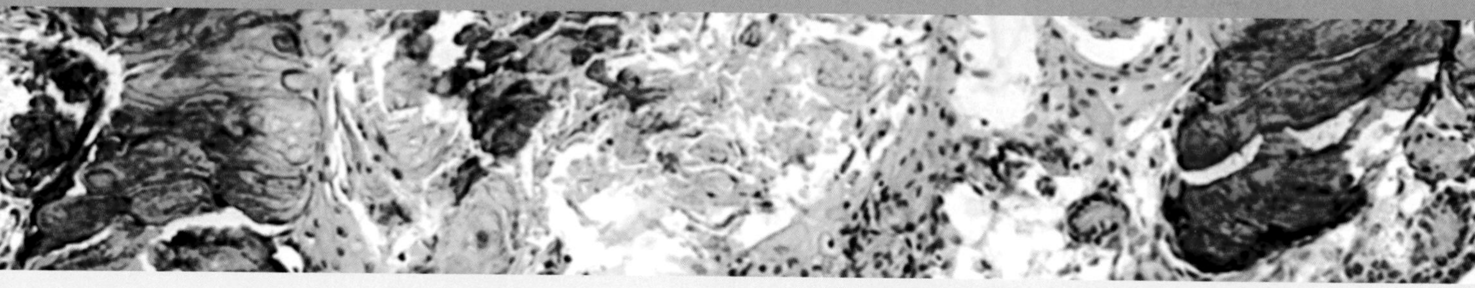

Schwannoma Variants

Neurofibroma

Primary Malignant Neoplasms of Nerve

Perineurioma

Lipoma of 8th Cranial Nerve

Conventional Schwannoma

KEY FACTS

TERMINOLOGY
- Benign nerve sheath tumor of Schwann cells

CLINICAL ISSUES
- NF2, schwannomatosis association (when multiple)
- Head, neck, flexor extremities common locations
- Gross total removal curative
- Malignant transformation extremely rare

IMAGING
- MR: Circumscribed, heterogeneous enhancement

MACROSCOPIC
- Often solitary; nodular, encapsulated
- Cystic change, yellow discoloration

MICROSCOPIC
- Capsule of perineurium and epineurial collagen
- Compact spindle cells ± Verocay bodies (Antoni A)
- Loose-textured cell processes (Antoni B)
- Hyalinized vessels, mucin deposition
- Degenerative nuclear atypia (ancient schwannoma)

ANCILLARY TESTS
- S100 protein
  - Tumoral Schwann cells
- EMA
  - Capsular perineurial cells
- Collagen IV
  - Pericellular basal lamina
- EM
  - Continuous pericellular basal lamina, long-spacing collagen

TOP DIFFERENTIAL DIAGNOSES
- Neurofibroma
- Nerve sheath myxoma
- Leiomyoma
- Malignant peripheral nerve sheath tumor

Eccentric Growth Pattern

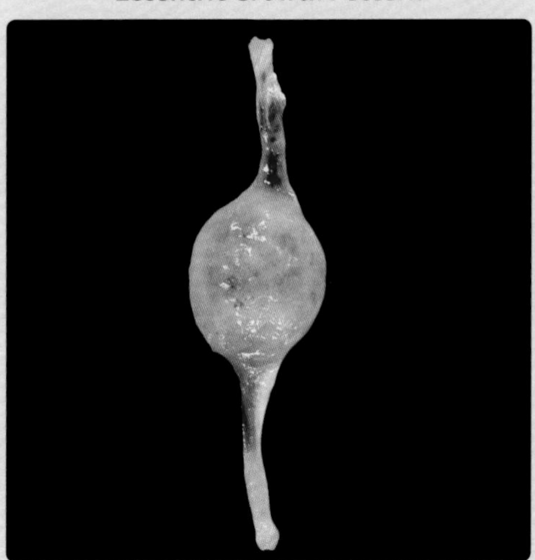

Verocay Bodies

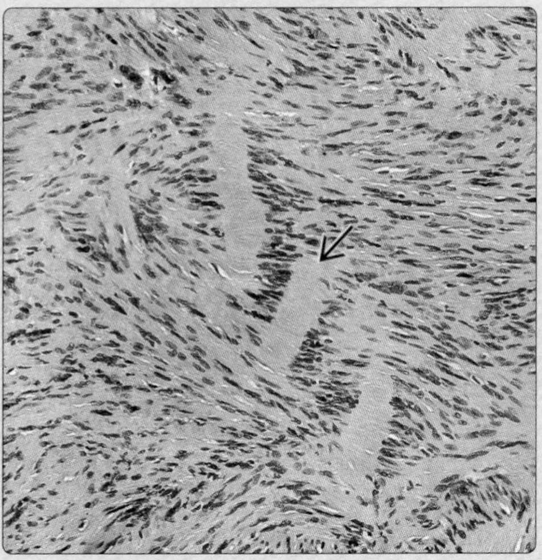

(Left) *Schwannomas are globoid masses eccentric to the nerve of origin.* **(Right)** *Verocay bodies, a distinctive feature of schwannomas, result from the regimentation of Schwann cells and their processes* ➙*.*

Eccentric Growth Pattern

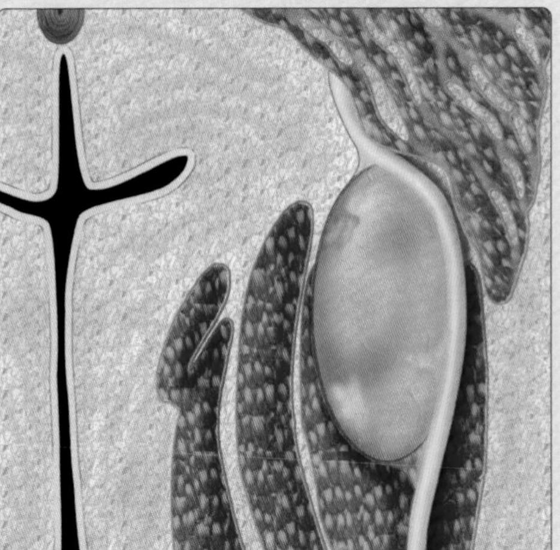

SOX10 Expression

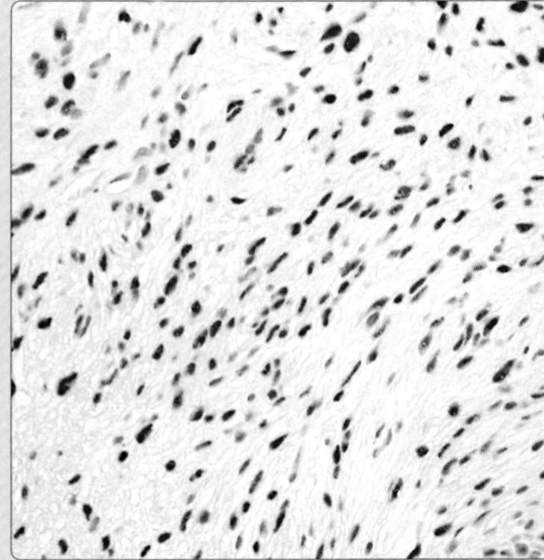

(Left) *An eccentric growth pattern to the parent nerve is an architectural gross feature of schwannoma, as illustrated in this example arising in the thigh.* **(Right)** *SOX10 immunoexpression is frequent in schwannomas, a diagnostically useful marker that recognizes neural crest-derived neoplasms.*

TERMINOLOGY

Synonyms

- Neurilemmoma, neurinoma

Definitions

- Benign, typically encapsulated, nonmelanotic nerve sheath tumor composed of Schwann cells alone

ETIOLOGY/PATHOGENESIS

Environmental Exposure

- Irradiation predisposing factor

Chromosomal Alterations

- Majority show aberrations of neurofibromatosis 2 (*NF2*) gene located in chromosome region 22q12.2

CLINICAL ISSUES

Epidemiology

- Incidence
  - NF2 association
    - Bilateral vestibular schwannomas
    - Multiple schwannomas
  - Schwannomatosis association
    - Sporadic (85%), hereditary (15%)
    - No vestibular nerve tumors
  - Neurofibromatosis type 1 (NF1) association very rare
    - Solitary
  - Most schwannomas are sporadic (asyndromic)
- Age
  - All ages affected; peak incidence 3rd-6th decade

Site

- Head and neck
- Flexor surface of extremities
- Cranial and spinal nerve roots
  - Sensory (vestibular root affected)
- Mediastinal, retroperitoneal tumors often massive
- Autonomic nerves uncommonly involved
- Intraparenchymal
  - Spinal cord > brain examples (rare)
- Intraosseous schwannomas (rare)

Presentation

- Asymptomatic mass in most cases
- Slow-growing
- Size varies from microscopic (intrafascicular) to large, compressive, bone-erosive tumors
- Paraspinous: Sensory symptoms
- Intraspinal: Cord compression with motor signs
- Pain in schwannomatosis-associated tumors
- Rare examples act as host for metastases of various malignant tumors (breast, lung, etc.)

Treatment

- Excision of tumor with parent nerve preserved when possible
- Gamma knife radiosurgery option for vestibular schwannomas

Prognosis

- Site-related
  - Gross total removal curative
  - Subtotal removal, slow recurrence
    - Cranial, spinal, and giant sacral schwannoma
  - NF2 tumors larger and more prone to recur
  - Malignant transformation extremely rare

IMAGING

Radiographic Findings

- Conventional x-ray: Sharply circumscribed, focal calcification occasional

MR Findings

- Circumscribed, heterogeneous enhancement, high T2 signal; cystic change
- Remodeling of bone
  - Vestibular: Auditory canal
  - Spinal: Foraminal, "dumbbell" configuration
  - Giant sacral schwannoma: Compressive bone destruction
- Brain displacement in intracranial examples
- Imaging characteristics related to proportions of Antoni A & B areas and degenerative changes

CT Findings

- Circumscribed, low attenuation, enhancement, cystic change/focal calcification

MACROSCOPIC

General Features

- Solitary: Multifocality in nerve is rare (NF2 and schwannomatosis association)
- Nodular, smooth contoured
- Encapsulation: Lacking in mucosal, visceral, and intraparenchymal tumors, scant in some intradural examples
- Eccentric growth relative to parent nerve
- Cystic change common
- Yellow discoloration due to lipidization
- Hemorrhage ± extensive infarct-like necrosis
- Calcification focal but rarely extensive

MICROSCOPIC

Histologic Features

- Capsule of perineurium and epineurial collagen
  - May contain parent nerve or nearby ganglion
- Schwann cells (exclusive component)
  - Antoni A arrangement
    - Compact spindle cells ± Verocay bodies of alternating, aligned nuclei and processes
    - Verocay bodies uncommon in 8th nerve examples
    - Whorl formation or tight cell clusters (occasional)
    - Rosetted cells with centrally directed processes (neuroblastoma-like schwannoma)
    - Predominates in spinal canal tumors
  - Antoni B arrangement
    - Multipolar, loose-textured, haphazardly arranged cell processes, pseudogland formation
    - Degenerative nuclear atypia (ancient schwannoma)

- Plump cells in rare epithelioid schwannoma
- Granular cell change uncommon and patchy
- Miscellaneous
  - Nonpalisading infarct-like necrosis in large examples
    - No prognostic significance
  - Lipid-rich, histiocyte infiltrates, perivascular or patchy
  - Chondroosseous or adipose metaplasia
  - Rare mitotic figures
  - Hyalinized vessels with associated hemosiderin deposition
  - Vascular ectasia ± thrombosis, recanalization
  - Necrotic debris ± cholesterol crystals
  - Diffuse hyalinization
  - Mucin deposition rarely widespread
  - Scant intratumoral axons
  - Cutaneous adnexal entrapment
  - Associated arachnoidal cell reaction rare and NF2 associated (mixed schwannoma-meningioma)
  - Lipofuscin commonly seen
  - Gastrointestinal schwannomas show peripheral cuff-like lymphoid aggregates
- Some tumors may show hybrid features of schwannoma and other peripheral nerve sheath tumors, particularly perineurioma

Cytologic Features

- Elongate to plump nuclei
- Inconspicuous nucleoli
- Intranuclear cytoplasmic pseudoinclusions

ANCILLARY TESTS

Histochemistry

- Periodic acid-Schiff: Pericellular basal lamina, debris-containing histiocytes
- Reticulin: Pericellular basal lamina
- Trichrome: Capsular, perivascular, and patchy stromal collagen deposits
- Oil red O: Lipid-laden histiocytes
- Alcian blue: Mucin accumulation (Antoni B > Antoni A), rarely diffuse and abundant
- Bodian and Bielschowsky: Intratumoral axons and in peritumoral nerve fascicles

Immunohistochemistry

- CD57, S100, and SOX10 protein: Tumoral Schwann cells
- Neurofilament protein: Scattered axons often peripherally located, also in peritumoral fascicles
- Epithelial membrane antigen: Capsular perineurial cells
- Collagen IV: Pericellular basal lamina of Schwann cells
- GFAP: Variably positive in some schwannomas
  - More common in retroperitoneal schwannomas
- CD68: Histiocytes and granular cells
- CD34: Scant in perivascular region of Antoni B tissue
- Keratin: May be positive in some examples
  - Cross reaction of antibody with GFAP
- Mosaic pattern of SMARCB1/INI1 immunostaining more frequent in syndrome-associated (NF2, schwannomatosis) schwannomas

Genetic Testing

- Somatic inactivation of *NF2* tumor suppressor gene common genetic alteration
- Germline *NF2* gene mutation in NF2
- Germline alteration in schwannomatosis associated cases unknown in most cases
  - *SMARCB1* or *LZTR1* germline mutations in subset

Electron Microscopy

- Scant organelles: Golgi, rough endoplasmic reticulum, mitochondria, lysosomes, lipid droplets
- Rudimentary junctions
- Pericellular continuous basal lamina
- Long-spacing collagen in stroma

DIFFERENTIAL DIAGNOSIS

Neurofibroma

- May resemble Antoni B tissue of schwannoma
- Lacks thick capsule
- S100, SOX10: Partial staining
- NF immunoreactive axons often grouped/aligned

Nerve Sheath Myxoma

- Unencapsulated, superficially located
- Also composed of Schwann cells
- No Antoni A/B areas
- No Verocay bodies

Malignant Peripheral Nerve Sheath Tumors

- Malignant cytologic features
  - Unlike degenerative atypia (bizarre hyperchromatic cells, intranuclear cytoplasmic inclusions) of schwannomas
- Necrosis often with palisading cells

Leiomyoma

- Lacks thick hyaline capsule
- Blunted nuclei rather than tapered
- More dense eosinophilic cytoplasm, distinct cell borders
- Nuclear palisading may be seen
- S100(-)
- Reactive for myogenic markers (SMA, desmin)

Ganglioneuroma

- Should be differentiated from schwannoma affecting dorsal root ganglia
- Haphazardly arranged, cytologically dysmorphic ganglion cells
- Spindle cell component less cellular; axon-containing throughout

Palisaded Myofibroblastoma

- Typically involves lymph nodes
- S100(-)

SELECTED REFERENCES

1. Karamchandani JR et al: Sox10 and S100 in the diagnosis of soft-tissue neoplasms. Appl Immunohistochem Mol Morphol. 20(5):445-50, 2012
2. Hornick JL et al: Hybrid schwannoma/perineurioma: clinicopathologic analysis of 42 distinctive benign nerve sheath tumors. Am J Surg Pathol. 33(10):1554-61, 2009

Yellow Appearance

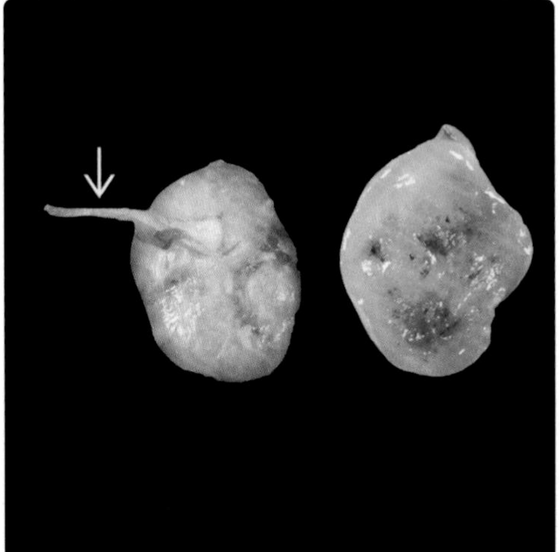

Attachment to Parent Nerve

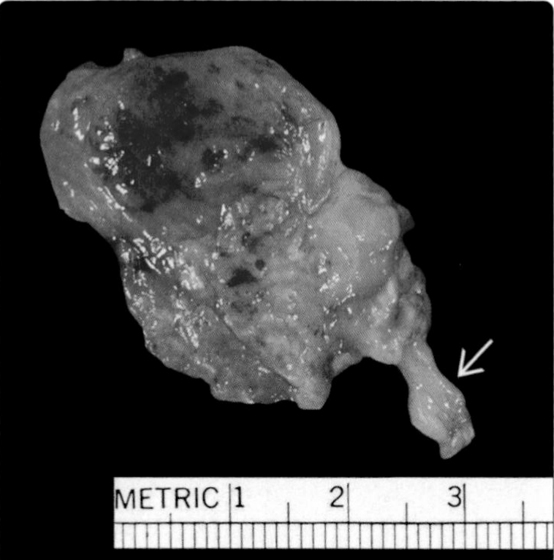

(Left) *Schwannomas may be yellow due to their lipid content. Note the nerve of origin ➡.* **(Right)** *The parent nerve ➡ is often attached to the tumor.*

Hemorrhage

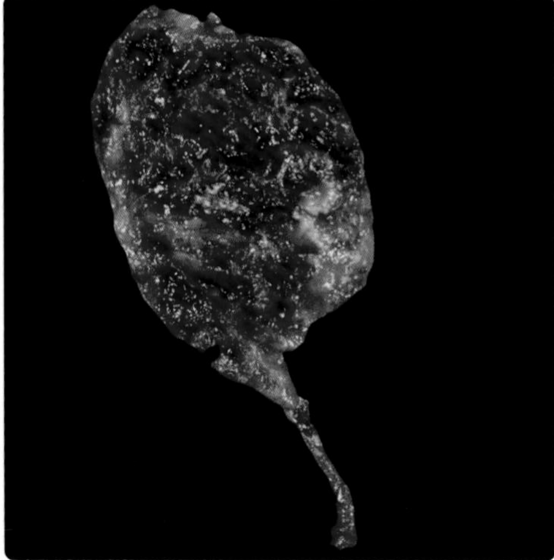

Translucency

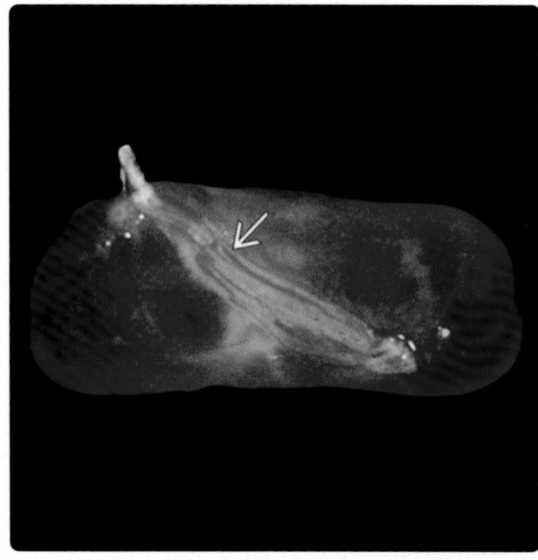

(Left) *Hemorrhage as a degenerative change is sometimes prominent.* **(Right)** *Extensive cystic degeneration produces a translucency in this lumbar root schwannoma. Note the superficial, displaced nerve ➡.*

Spinal Cord Compression

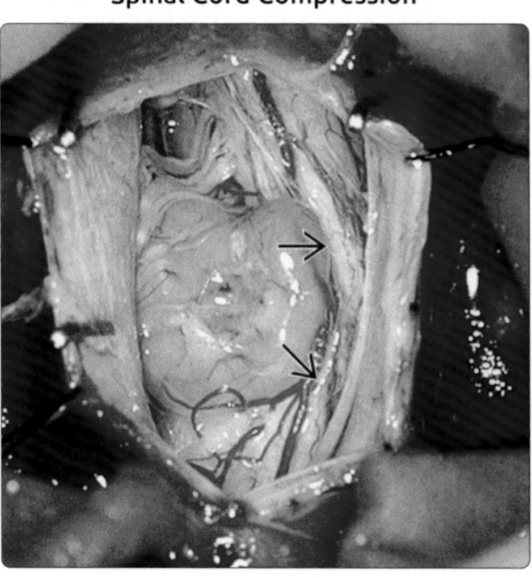

Visceral Schwannoma

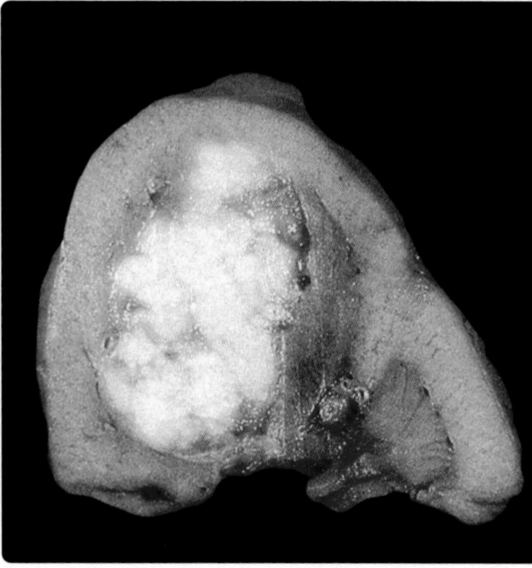

(Left) *This discrete, nodular lumbar intradural schwannoma compresses the spinal cord ➡. Surgical excision was curative.* **(Right)** *Infrequent visceral examples are mainly seen in the gastrointestinal system. This much less common example arose in the kidney. Visceral schwannomas are typically unencapsulated.*

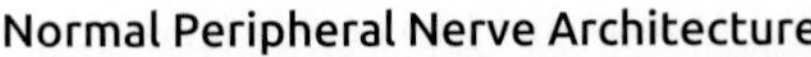

Normal Peripheral Nerve Architecture

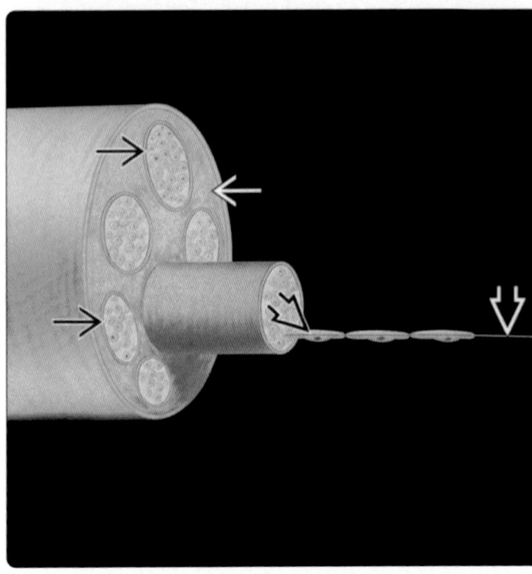

Schwannoma, Eccentric Growth Pattern

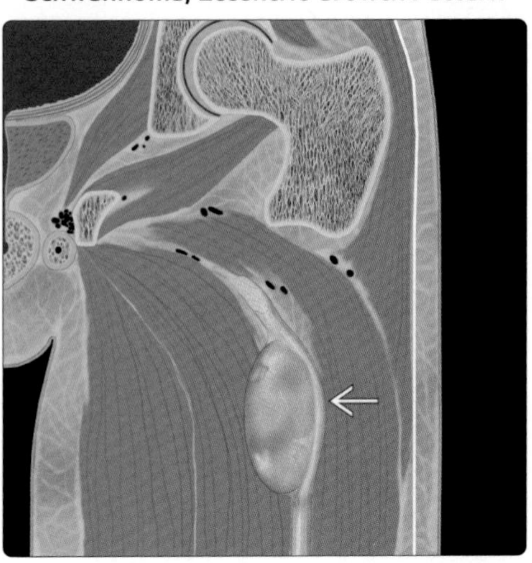

(Left) *A nerve trunk is composed of multiple fascicles, each surrounded by perineurium and the surrounding epineurium. Fascicles are composed of nerve fibers (axons) surrounded by Schwann cells. The intrafascicular endoneurium contains nerve fibers and blood vessels.* **(Right)** *This illustration of a typical schwannoma in the thigh shows the typical eccentricity of a schwannoma to the parent nerve.*

Unifascicular Nerve Schwannoma

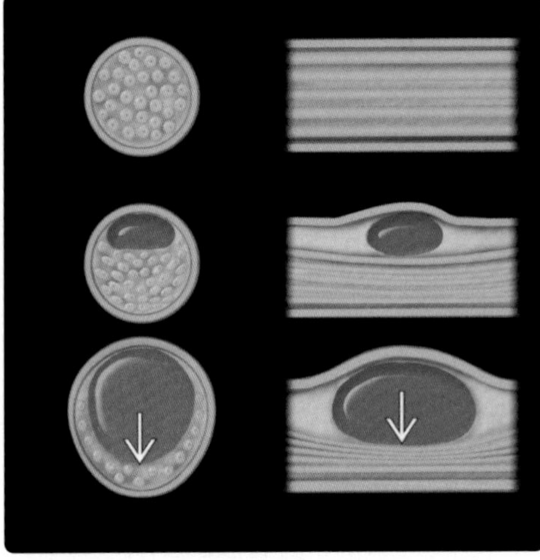

Nerve Fascicle Displacement

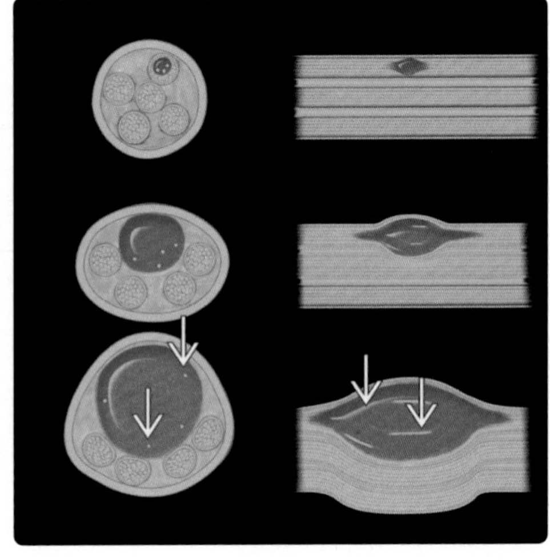

(Left) *This illustration shows a schwannoma arising within a unifascicular nerve. The tumor displaces other nerve fibers peripherally.* **(Right)** *Schwannomas often entrap axons in the affected fascicle of a multifascicular nerve. Adjacent nerve fascicles are displaced peripherally. The tumor evolves into an eccentric globoid mass.*

Antoni A and Antoni B Patterns

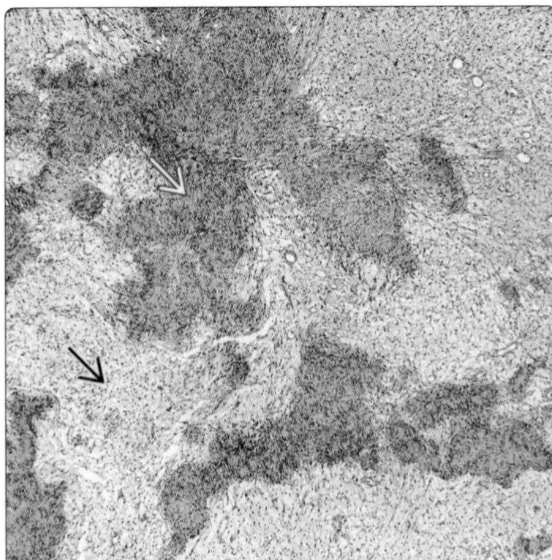

Antoni A and Antoni B Juxtaposition

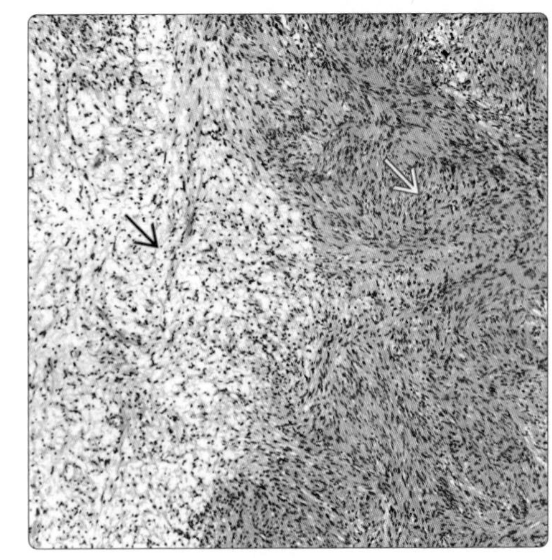

(Left) *Schwannomas contain Antoni A tissue composed of compact spindle cells and loose-textured Antoni B areas. The relative percentage of these 2 components varies from case to case. The B tissue is prominent here.* **(Right)** *The juxtaposition of cellular Antoni A and loose Antoni B patterns is classic for conventional schwannoma.*

Verocay Body-Rich Schwannoma

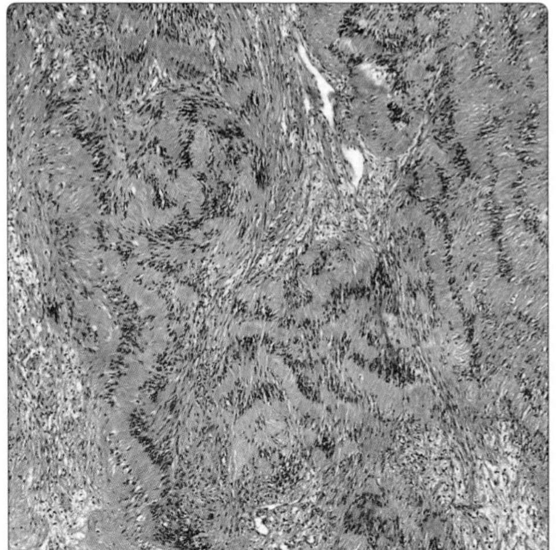

Whorls

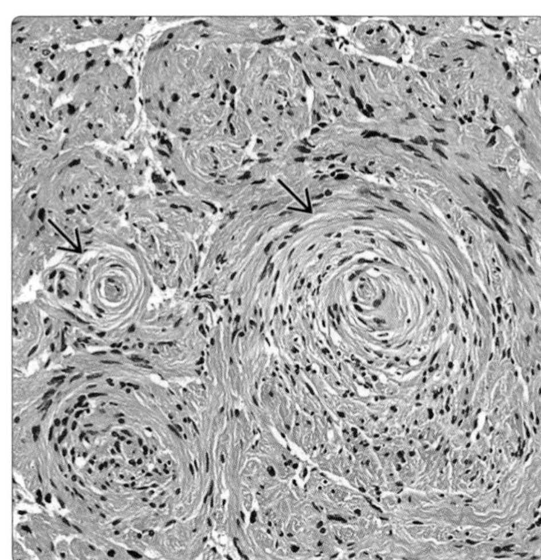

(Left) *Although uncommon overall, Verocay body-rich schwannomas are frequent in the spinal intradural compartment.* **(Right)** *Whorls ➡ are more common in NF2-associated schwannomas.*

PAS(+) Basement Membranes

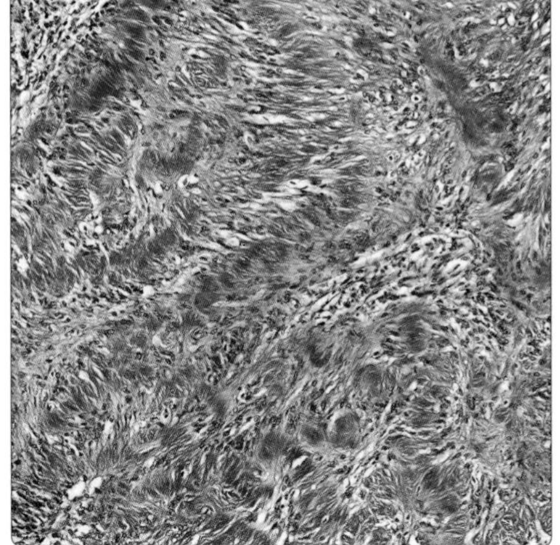

Collagen in Verocay Bodies

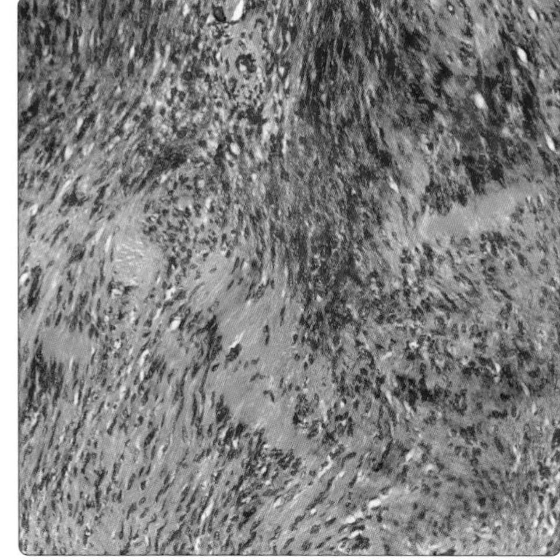

(Left) *The fibrillar component of Verocay bodies show aggregates of PAS(+) basement membranes.* **(Right)** *The collagen component of Verocay bodies is demonstrated by Masson trichrome staining.*

Collagenous Capsule

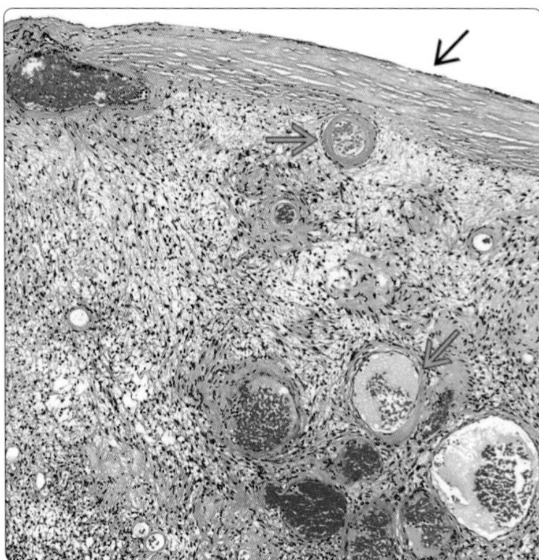

Collagen Bands

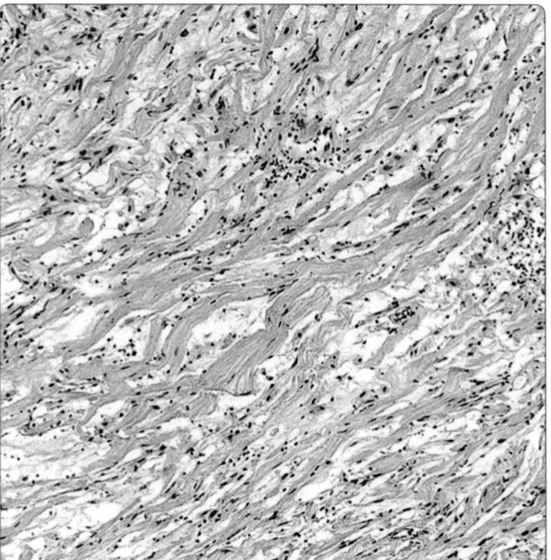

(Left) *Schwannomas often possess a thick collagenous capsule ➡ and hyalinized vessels ➡ in which thrombosis and recanalization are common.* **(Right)** *Schwannomas, particularly of the cauda equina, often show collagen bands resembling the "shredded carrots" of neurofibroma. Adequate sampling is important for the findings to support diagnosis of schwannoma.*

(Left) *Foamy phagocytic Schwann cells* → *and, rarely, adipocyte-like cells* ➡*, are present in some schwannomas.* **(Right)** *Some schwannomas may be extensively infiltrated by histiocytes, seen here after immunostaining for CD68.*

Foamy Schwann Cells

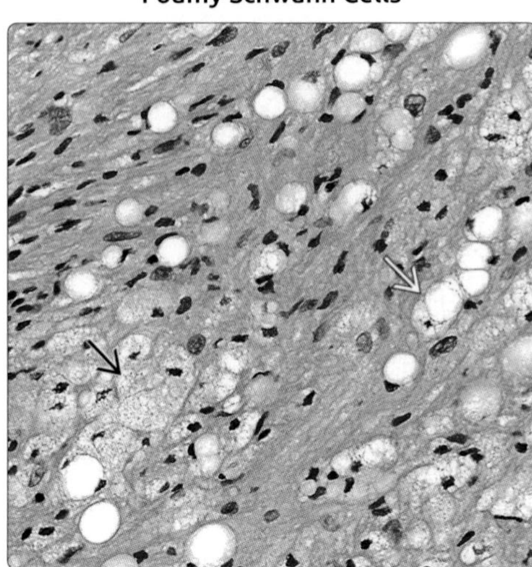

Histiocytic Infiltration

(Left) *Longstanding schwannomas may be extensively calcified* →*.* **(Right)** *Schwannomas may contain large hemorrhagic zones so as to mimic metastatic tumor.*

Calcification

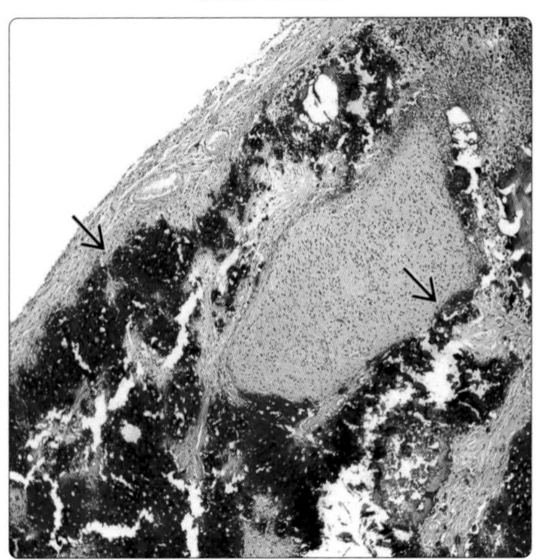

Hemorrhagic Zone

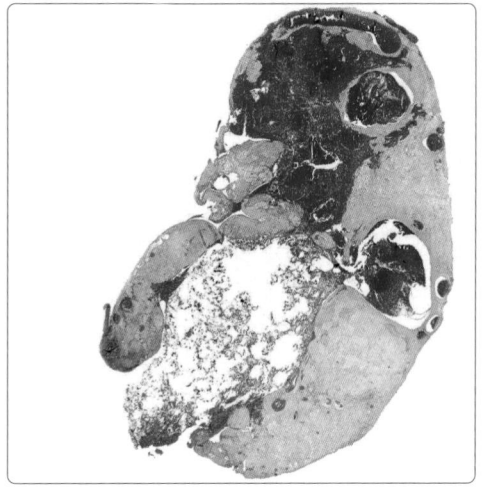

(Left) *Schwannomas may have cystic degeneration that, when extensive, produces a multilocular appearance.* **(Right)** *Cysts within schwannomas may have a pseudoepithelial lining* →*.*

Cystic Degeneration

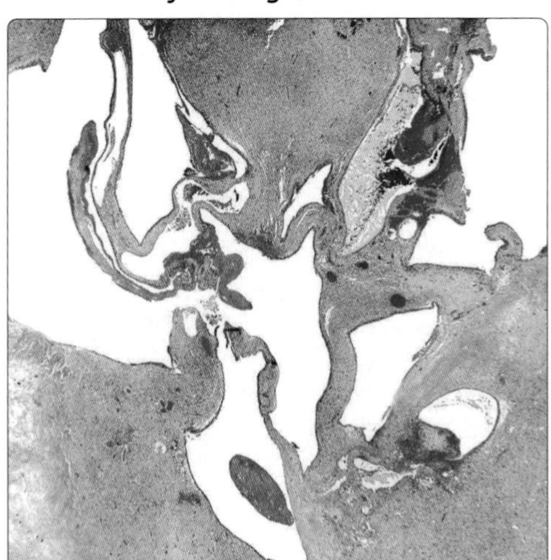

Pseudoepithelial Lining

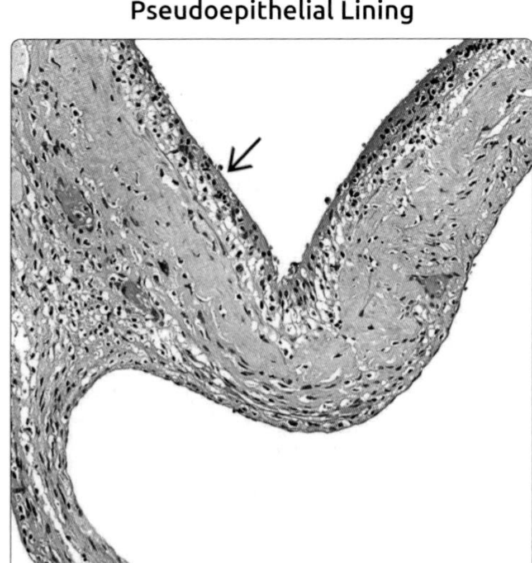

Ancient Change, Lipofusion

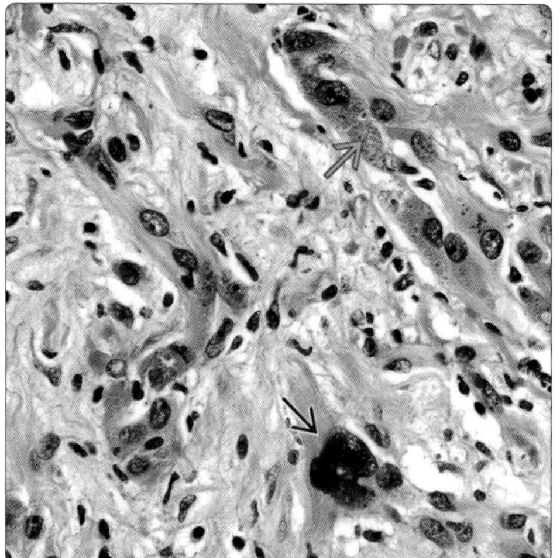

Lipofuscin Pigment, PAS(+)

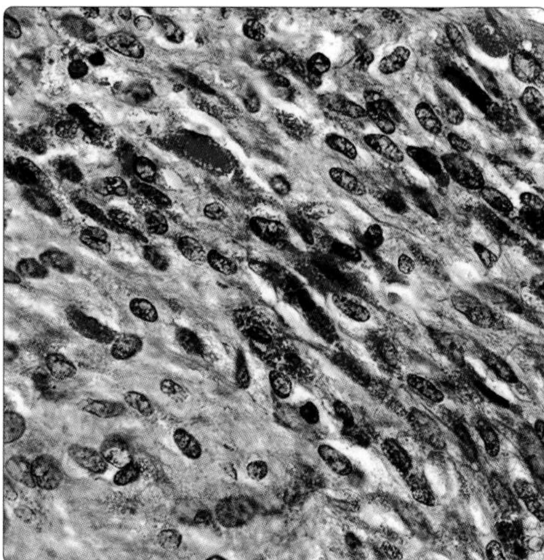

(Left) *Degenerative nuclear atypia (ancient change) is characterized by marked pleomorphism and smudgy hyperchromasia ⇒. Lipofuscin pigment ⇒ is common in schwannomas.* **(Right)** *Lipofuscin pigment's PAS-positivity helps in its differential from melanin, as in melanotic schwannomas.*

Neurofibromatosis Type 2

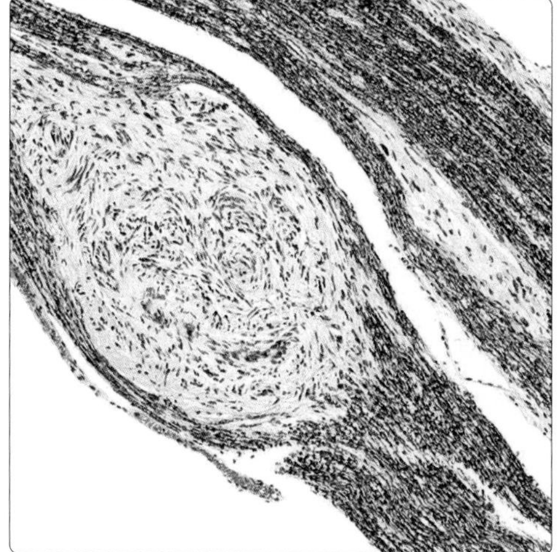

Epithelioid Schwann Cells

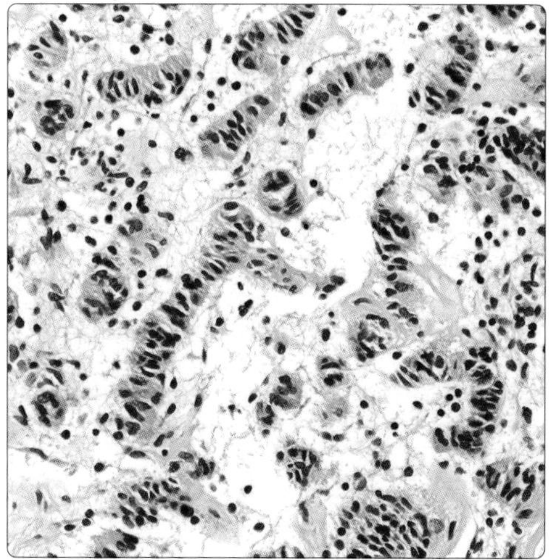

(Left) *Multiple spinal intradural nerve root schwannomas are common in neurofibromatosis type 2. This example is stained with Luxol fast blue for myelin and Bodian for peritumoral nerve fibers.* **(Right)** *Tight clusters of epithelioid Schwann cells, an infrequent finding, cause diagnostic confusion in small specimens. Epithelial tumors may be in the differential; however, the tumor would be S100 and SOX10 positive. Epithelioid MPNSTs, another possibility, would be anaplastic and mitotically active.*

Pseudorosettes

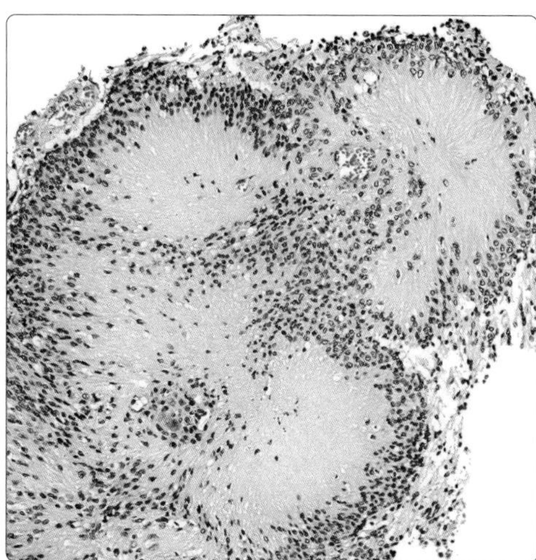

Amianthoid Collagen Fibers

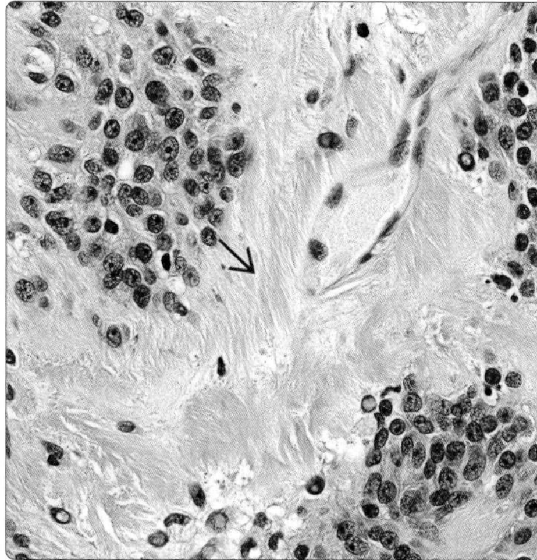

(Left) *Processes of small Schwann cells radiate toward a center, resulting in pseudorosette formation in neuroblastoma-like schwannoma.* **(Right)** *Amianthoid collagen fibers ⇒ are often present in neuroblastoma-like schwannomas.*

(Left) *Schwannomas such as this with extensive myxoid change must be differentiated from myxoma. The latter is superficially located, unencapsulated, and multinodular.* **(Right)** *Myxoid change in schwannoma is highlighted on this Alcian blue stain.*

Myxoid Change

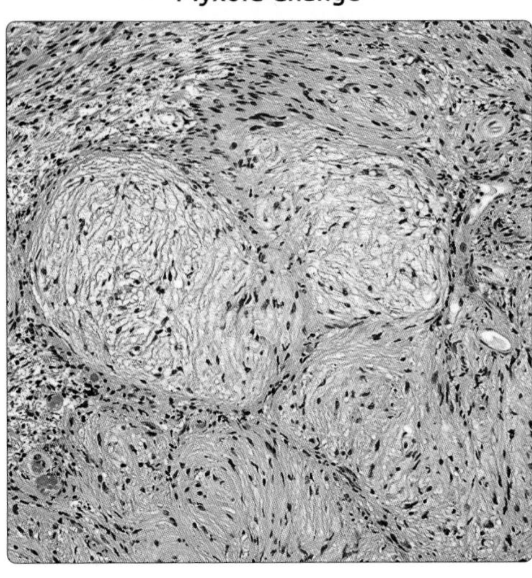

Myxoid Change

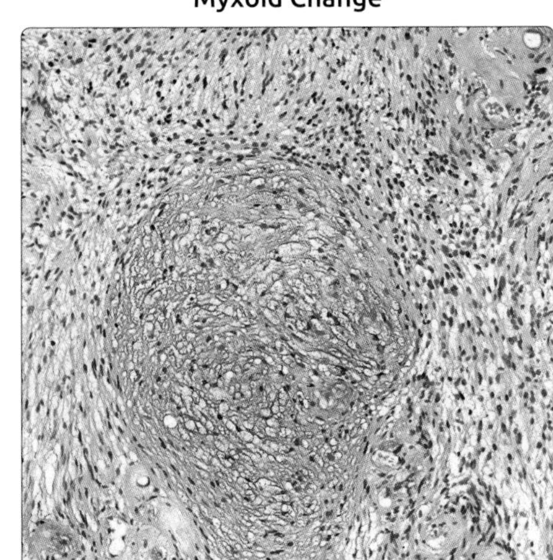

(Left) *Gastrointestinal schwannomas commonly feature a peripheral cuff of lymphocytes ⇒. Note the lack of a capsule.* **(Right)** *The reticular/microcystic schwannoma is a rare variant of schwannoma with a predilection for viscera, especially the gastrointestinal tract. Its tumoral cells, with clear cytoplasm mimicking signet ring cells, are immunoreactive for S100 protein.*

Lymphocyte Cuff

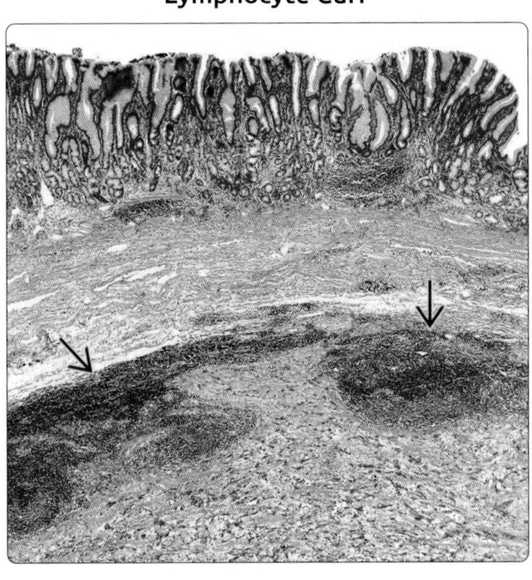

Reticular/Microcystic Variant

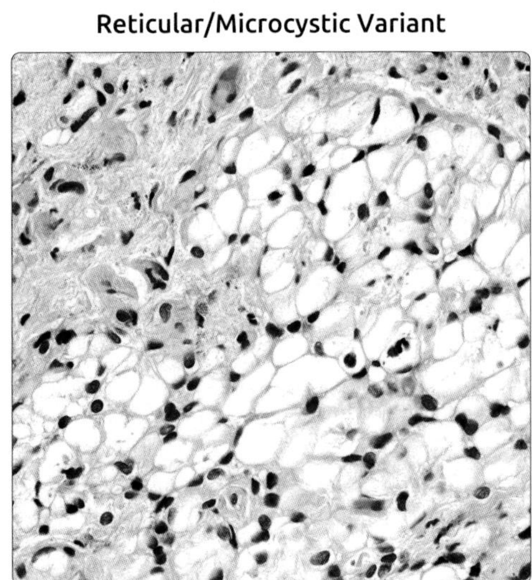

(Left) *A smear preparation from schwannoma shows neoplastic cells with elongate, tapered, club-shaped nuclei, inconspicuous nucleoli, and delicate cell processes. Schwannomas typically do not smear out as individual cells, but only as small tissue fragments.* **(Right)** *On frozen sections, hyalinized vessels may be an important clue. The cells with blunt nuclei have a tendency toward parallel arrangement.*

Club-Shaped Nuclei

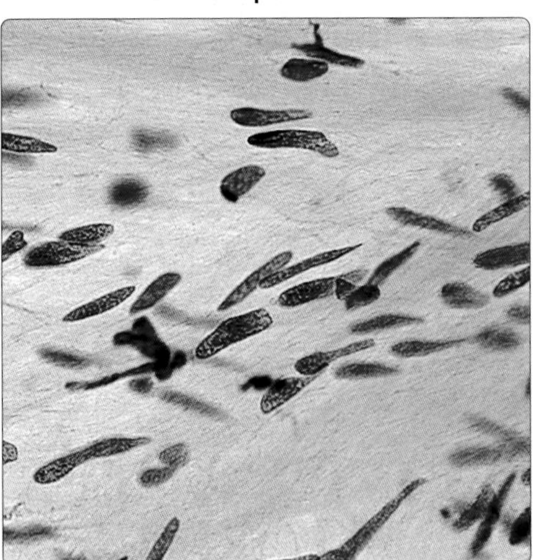

Hyalinized Vessels

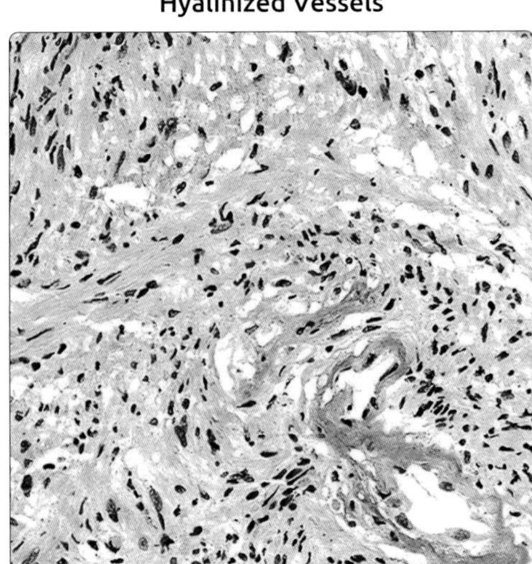

S100 Expression

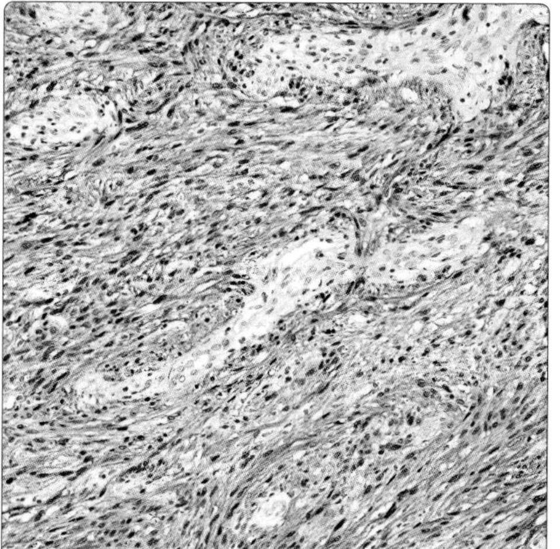

GFAP Expression

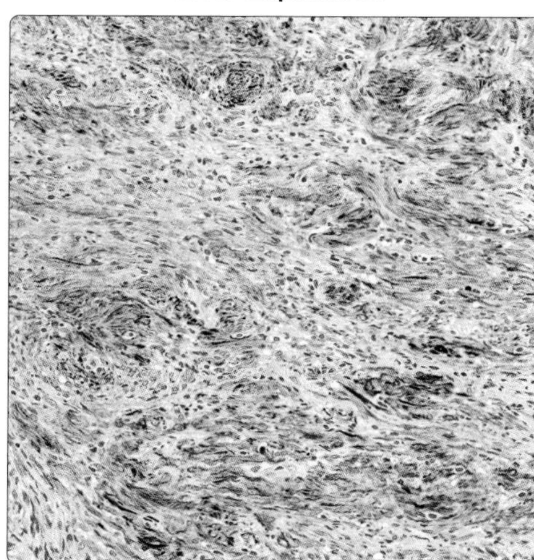

(Left) *Neoplastic Schwann cells in schwannomas are diffusely and strongly immunoreactive with S100 protein. Both cytoplasm and nuclei are stained.* **(Right)** *GFAP may be variably positive in schwannomas, especially retroperitoneal examples. Such immunoreactivity can be misinterpreted as conclusive evidence of glioma in the case of a tumor in the cauda equina, where myxopapillary ependymoma is an important differential diagnosis entity.*

Collagen IV Immunostaining

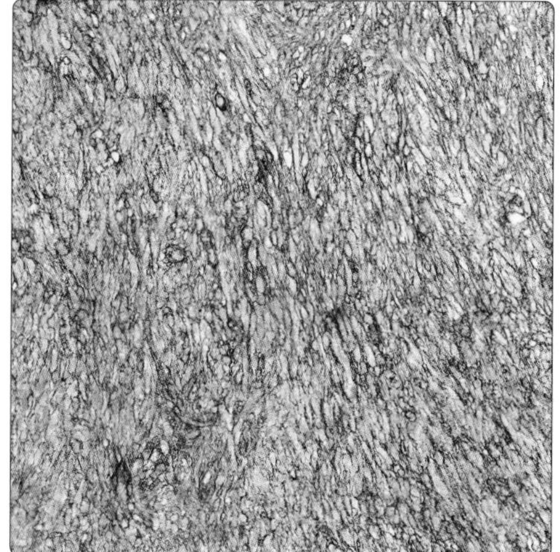

Pericellular Reticulin

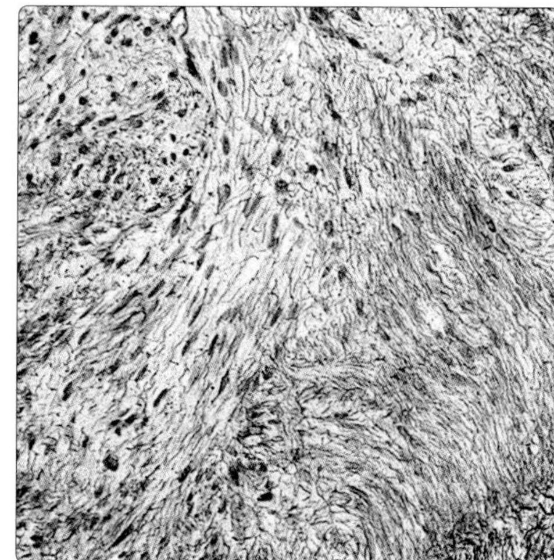

(Left) *Collagen IV immunostaining in schwannomas may be variable, i.e., delicate or strong, focal or diffuse.* **(Right)** *Abundant delicate, pericellular reticulin staining is typical of schwannomas.*

EMA Immunostaining

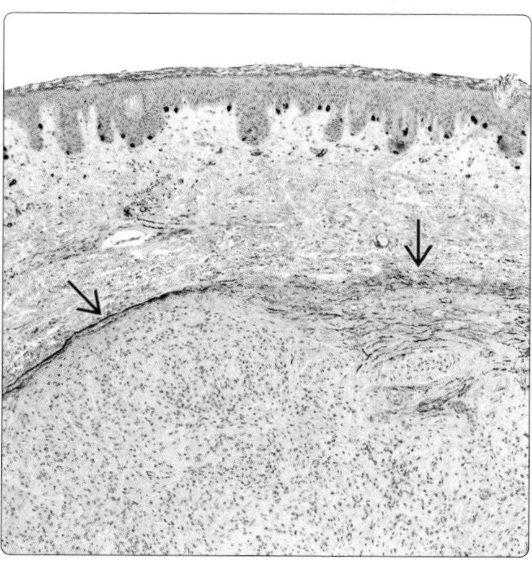

Basal Lamina Enshrouded Processes

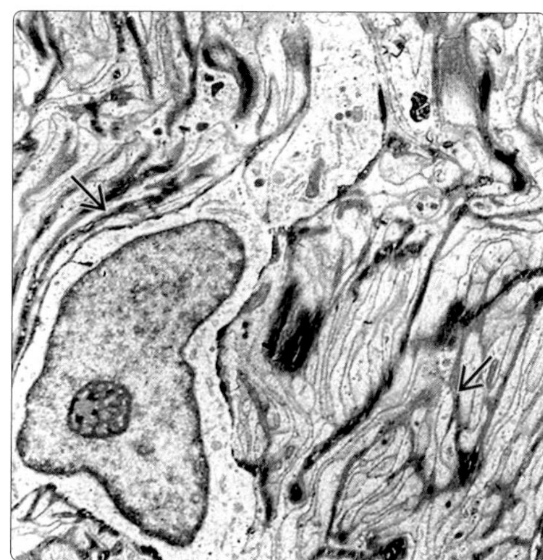

(Left) *EMA immunostaining highlights peripherally perineurial cells ⇨. Tumoral cells are negative.* **(Right)** *Long, thin, entwined, basal lamina-enshrouded ⇨ processes are typical ultrastructural features of schwannoma.*

Cellular Schwannoma

KEY FACTS

CLINICAL ISSUES

- 5% of benign peripheral nerve sheath tumors
- Female predominance (F:M = 2:1)
- Slow growing
- Asymptomatic > pain, sensorimotor symptoms
- Paravertebral (mediastinum, pelvis, retroperitoneum), intraspinous, peripheral nerves
- Gross total resection curative
- Not metastatic

MACROSCOPIC

- Well circumscribed, encapsulated

MICROSCOPIC

- Hyalinized vasculature
- Antoni A pattern without Verocay bodies
- Subcapsular chronic inflammation
- Minor nuclear atypia
- Mitotic figures frequent (1-10/10 HPF); may be higher in tumors in young children

ANCILLARY TESTS

- S100, SOX10: Strong and diffusely (+)
- Collagen IV: (+), but may not be uniform
- Reticulin: Surrounds individual cells

TOP DIFFERENTIAL DIAGNOSES

- Malignant peripheral nerve sheath tumor
  - Mitotic counts > 10/10 HPF
  - S100 and CD57 (+) in scattered cells in 50% of tumors
  - Complete loss of SOX10 neurofibromin or p16 seen in MPNST, not cellular schwannoma
- Leiomyosarcoma
  - S100(-) or scant
  - SMA(+), desmin(+)

Eccentric Pattern of Growth

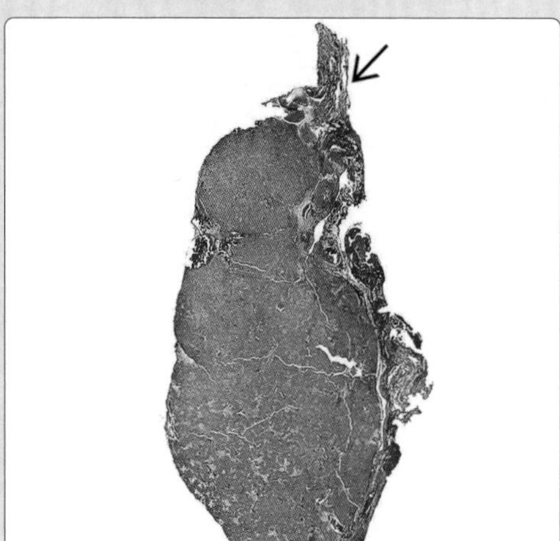

Mitotic Activity

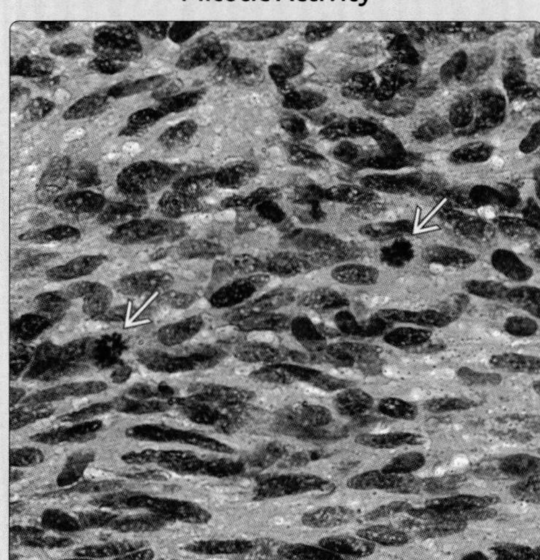

(Left) *Cellular schwannomas of the nonmucosal types are, like conventional schwannomas, discrete masses largely eccentric to the nerve of origin ➡.* **(Right)** *Antoni A pattern, hypercellularity, mitoses ➡, and spindling of hyperchromatic tumor cells typify the tumor.*

Histiocytes

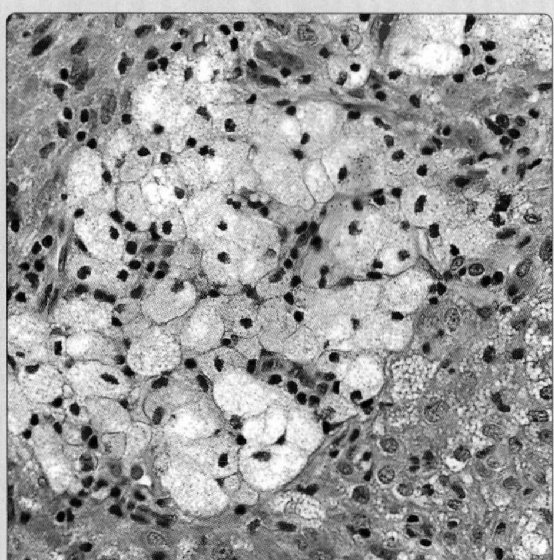

S100 Expression

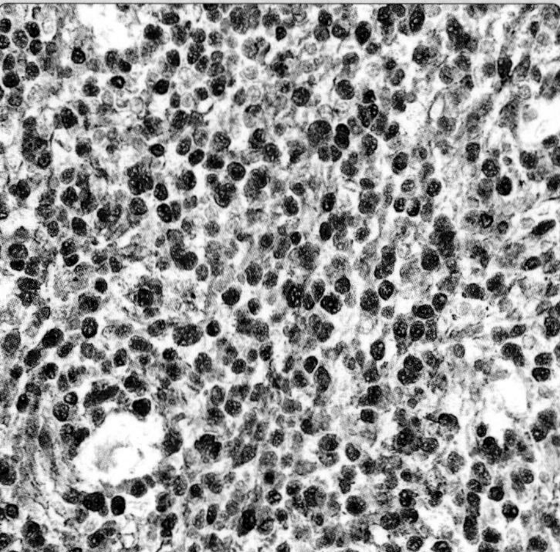

(Left) *Infiltrates or aggregates of foamy histiocytes populate a subset of cellular schwannomas and may be a subtle clue to the diagnosis.* **(Right)** *Strong, uniform S100 expression is a universal feature of cellular schwannoma and useful to distinguish it from malignant peripheral nerve sheath tumors and other neoplasms in the differential diagnosis.*

TERMINOLOGY

Definitions

- Benign schwannoma characterized by high cellularity and increased proliferative activity

ETIOLOGY/PATHOGENESIS

Associated Syndromes

- Rare association with neurofibromatosis type 1 or 2

CLINICAL ISSUES

Epidemiology

- Incidence
  - 5% of benign peripheral nerve sheath tumors
- Age
  - Peak incidence in 4th decade
  - 5% pediatric
- Sex
  - Female predominance (F:M = 2:1)

Presentation

- Slow growing
- Asymptomatic > painful, sensorimotor symptoms
  - Occasional incidental radiographic finding
- Sensory nerve roots
  - Paravertebral
  - Mediastinum, pelvis, retroperitoneum
  - Intraspinous
    - 30% dumbbell configuration
    - 30% bone erosion
  - 10% intracranial (cranial nerves 5, 8, etc.)

Treatment

- Surgical approaches
  - Gross total resection optimal
- Radiation
  - Infrequently needed for recurrence

Prognosis

- Gross total resection curative
- Subtotal resection: Recurrence (30-40% in intracranial, intraspinal, sacral)
- No malignant transformation; not metastatic

MACROSCOPIC

General Features

- Most resemble conventional schwannomas
  - Well circumscribed, encapsulated
  - Usually solid, no yellow lipidization
  - Minority multinodular/plexiform
- 1-20 cm (mean: 5 cm)
- Gross necrosis lacking
- Destructive bone erosion in spinal/sacral examples
- Focal soft tissue infiltration when capsule partly incomplete

MICROSCOPIC

Histologic Features

- Essential features of conventional schwannoma
  - Well-formed capsule
  - Hyalinized vasculature
  - Patchy lipid-laden histiocytes
- Hypercellularity
- Antoni A pattern without Verocay bodies
  - Antoni B pattern scant (10%) or absent
- Minor nuclear atypia
- Mitotic figures frequent (1-10/10 HPF); perhaps higher in tumors in young children
  - Occasionally may have greater proliferative indices in this age group
- Microcysts uncommon
- Micronecrosis uncommon
  - Lacks pseudopalisading
- Subcapsular chronic inflammation
- Scant intratumoral axons

Cytologic Features

- Spindle cells with tapered nuclei and eosinophilic, afibrillar cytoplasm
- Mild pleomorphism and nuclear hyperchromasia

ANCILLARY TESTS

Histochemistry

- Reticulin
  - Surrounds individual cells

Immunohistochemistry

- S100, SOX10: Strongly, diffusely (+)
- Collagen IV (+)
- GFAP: Variably (+) in up to 1/2 of cases
- Neurofilament protein (+) in scant axons
- EMA(+) in capsular perineurial cells
- Ki-67 as high as 25% (median index: 5%); higher in rare examples in infants

Electron Microscopy

- Full spectrum of Schwann cell features, continuous basement membrane

DIFFERENTIAL DIAGNOSIS

Malignant Peripheral Nerve Sheath Tumors

- Infiltrative or pseudoencapsulated
- Geographic necrosis common
- Mitotic counts > 10/10 HPF
- S100 and CD57 (+) often in scattered or no cells
- GFAP very rarely (+)
- Collagen IV generally (-)
- Complete loss of SOX10, neurofibromin, or p16 seen in MPNST, not cellular schwannoma
- Ultrastructural Schwann cell features usually lacking

Leiomyosarcoma

- Lacks fibrous capsule
- Cut surface whorled
- Blunt-ended nuclei
- S100 usually (-); muscle markers (+)

SELECTED REFERENCES

1. Pekmezci M et al: Morphologic and immunohistochemical features of malignant peripheral nerve sheath tumors and cellular schwannomas. Mod Pathol. 28 (2):187-200, 2015

(Left) *Tumoral cells are arranged in fascicles or whorls in this highly cellular tumor composed largely of Antoni A tissue. Verocay bodies are typically absent in this schwannoma variant.* **(Right)** *While often only a focal feature, hyalinized vessels ➡ help establish a schwannian nature.*

Antoni A, Verocay Bodies Absent

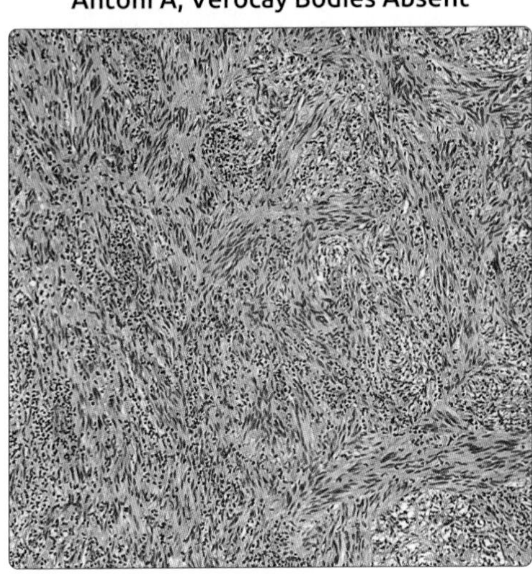

Hyalinized Vessels

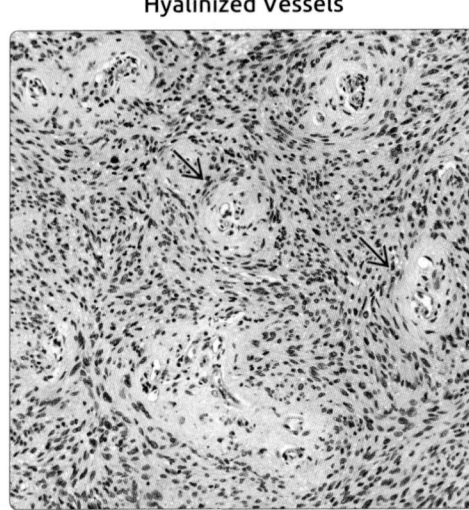

(Left) *Subcapsular ➡ and perivascular chronic inflammation is common and more characteristic of cellular schwannomas as opposed to conventional types.* **(Right)** *The diagnosis of schwannoma may not immediately come to mind in cellular schwannomas with unusual patterns such as cell clustering.*

Chronic Inflammation

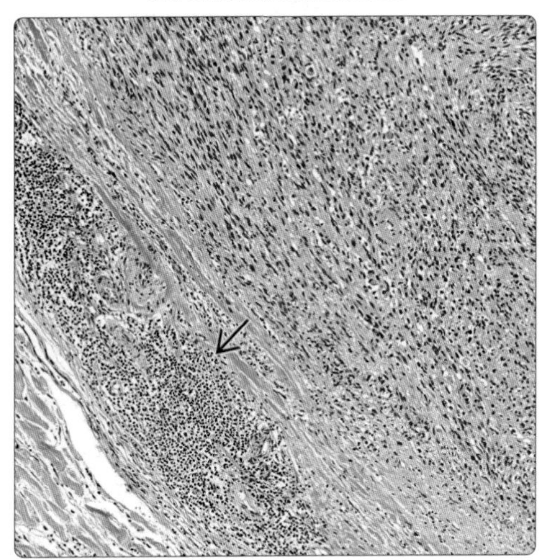

Cell Clustering

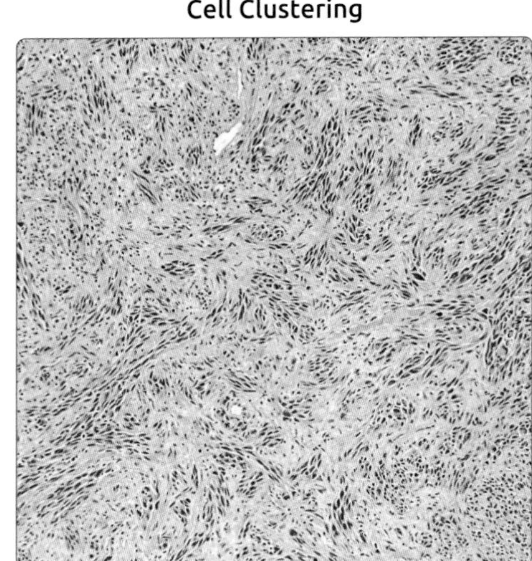

(Left) *Cellular schwannomas are, by definition, mitotically active. Mitoses ➡ up to 4/10 HPFs are common; occasionally, even more may be found.* **(Right)** *Focal nonpalisading necrosis is not a sign of malignancy in cellular schwannomas. Conversely, pseudopalisading necrosis is not a feature of cellular schwannoma and should raise the possibility of malignant peripheral nerve sheath tumor.*

Mitotic Activity

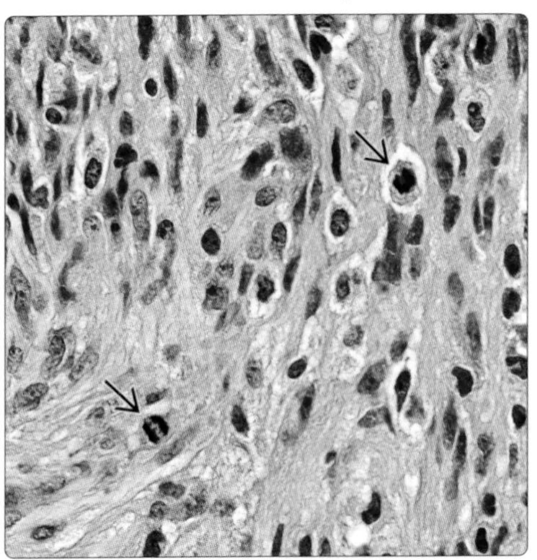

Nonpalisading Necrosis

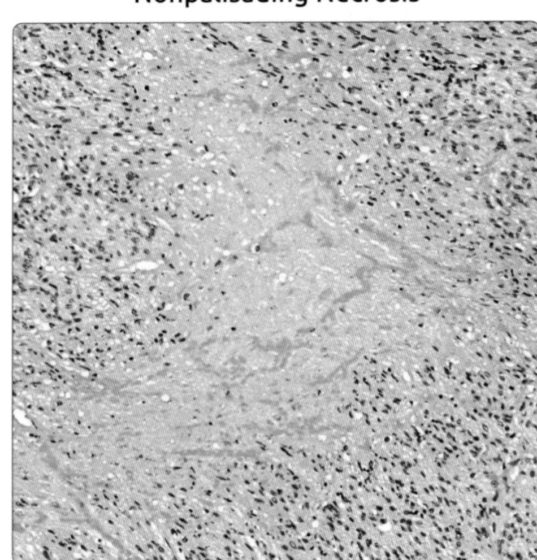

Cell Crowding

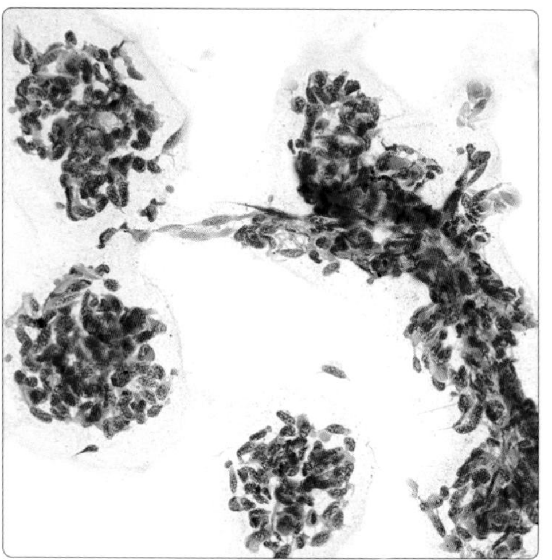

S100 Immunopositivity

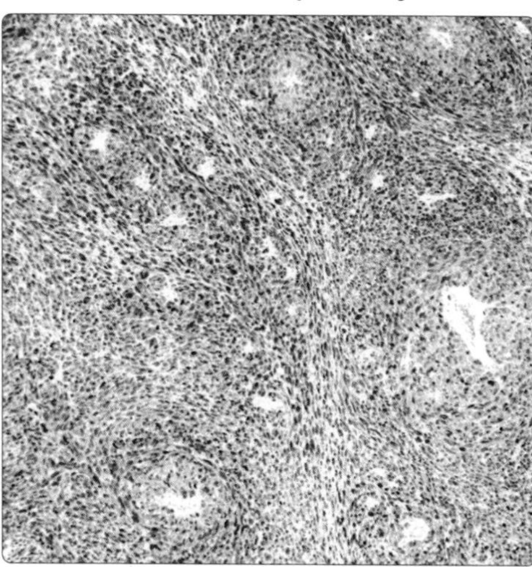

(Left) *In smear preparations, cells are more crowded as opposed to those in conventional schwannomas. Despite the hypercellularity, nuclear uniformity is typical.* **(Right)** *Diffuse and robust immunopositivity for S100 protein helps to differentiate cellular schwannoma from malignant peripheral nerve sheath tumor.*

Intercellular Collagen IV Positivity

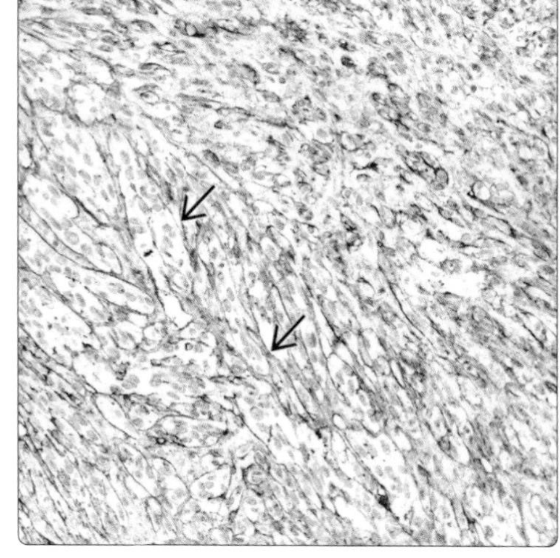

Intercellular Reticulin

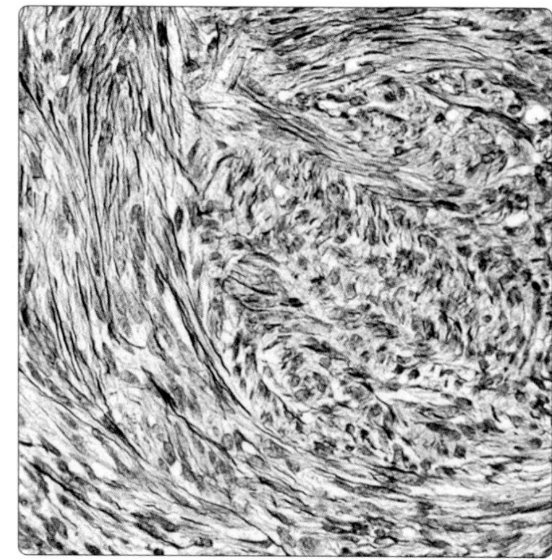

(Left) *Linear intercellular collagen IV positivity ➙, although often patchy, is typical of cellular schwannoma as it is for conventional types.* **(Right)** *As with conventional schwannomas, cells are individually surrounded by reticulin, a reflection of both the presence of basement membrane and deposition of intercellular collagen.*

Ki-67 Stain

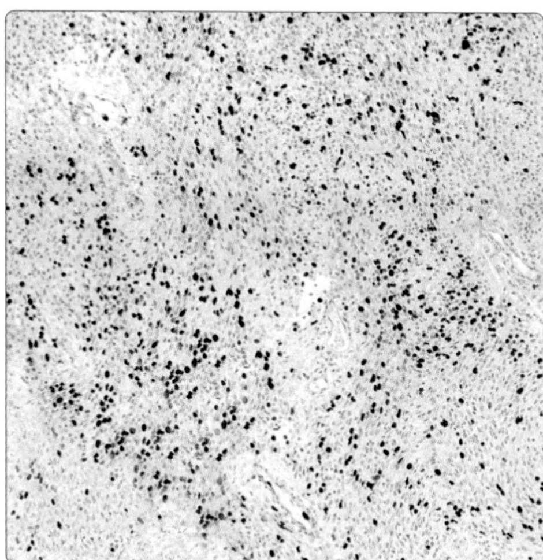

Basement Membrane

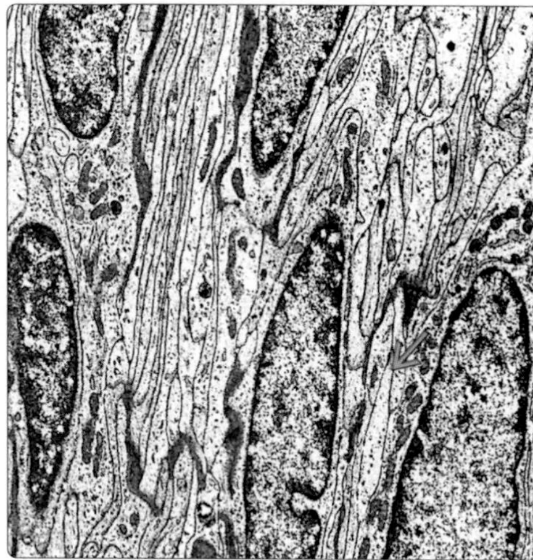

(Left) *Ki-67 staining may be moderate to focally high.* **(Right)** *Ultrastructurally, basement membrane ➙ continuously surrounds tumor cells.*

Melanotic Schwannoma

KEY FACTS

CLINICAL ISSUES

- Sporadic or syndromic (Carney complex)
- Syndromic (Carney complex)
  - Frequent mutation of tumor suppressor gene *PRKAR1A*
- Distant metastases not infrequent (15-44%)

MACROSCOPIC

- No encapsulation; occasionally interrupted, thin collagen layer with soft tissue invasion

MICROSCOPIC

- Delicate chromatin/small nucleoli/rare mitoses (benign)
- Vesicular nuclei/coarse chromatin/violaceous macronucleoli, frequent mitoses (malignant)
- Pigmentation variable or patchy
- Psammomatous calcifications in psammomatous variant

ANCILLARY TESTS

- Reticulin outlines lobules
- S100, HMB-45, SOX10, Melan-A, tyrosinase positive
- Collagen IV and laminin outline basal lamina around lobules
- Frequent 22q loss
- Frequent whole chromosome gains (Ch4-9)
- Global methylation and gene expression profiles different from schwannoma, melanocytoma, and melanoma
- Lack of *GNAQ* or *GNA11* mutations in most instances

TOP DIFFERENTIAL DIAGNOSES

- Conventional schwannoma
  - Contain lipofuscin [PAS(+)] but lack melanin
- Pigmented neurofibroma
  - Typically diffusely infiltrative
- Melanocytoma
  - Lack long-spacing collagen
- Primary or metastatic melanoma
  - Cytologically malignant
- Clear cell sarcoma (soft tissue melanoma)
  - No immunohistochemical or ultrastructural basal lamina

Pigmentation

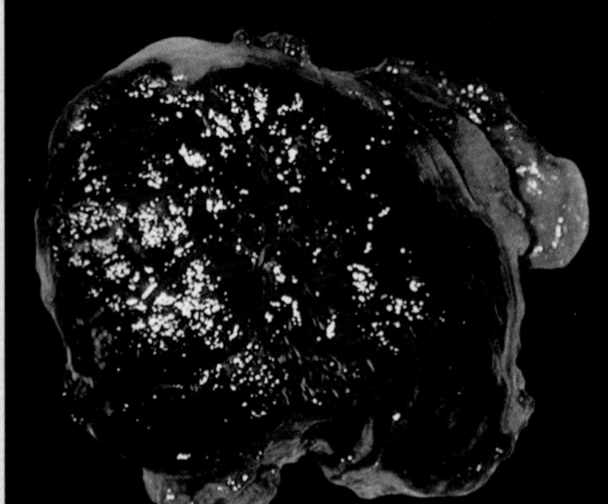

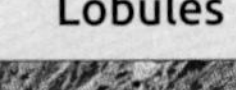

Lobules

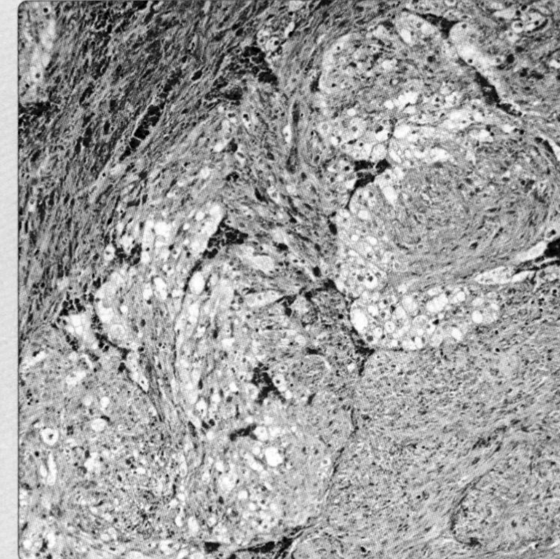

(Left) *Circumscribed and ovoid like other schwannomas, melanocytic variants are variably pigmented, extremely so in this case.* **(Right)** *Pigmented spindle-shaped or epithelioid cells often form lobules.*

Variable Pigmentation

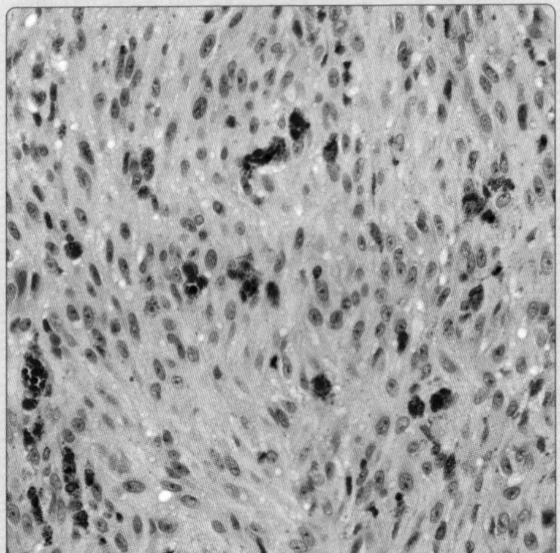

Small Lobules

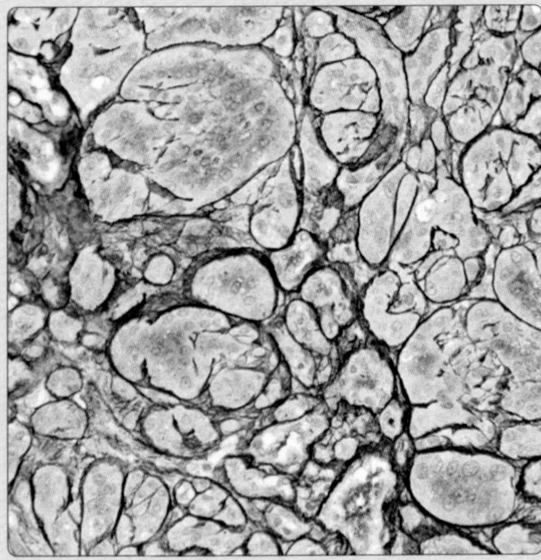

(Left) *Spindle cells with round nuclei and a small distinct nucleolus are usual features. Pigmentation degree may show variation in different tumors.* **(Right)** *Reticulin circumscribes small lobules, whereas it would be more pericellular in conventional schwannomas.*

TERMINOLOGY

Synonyms

- Pigmented schwannoma
- Melanogenic schwannoma
- Melanogenic nerve sheath tumor

Definitions

- Often circumscribed tumor of melanin-producing Schwann cells

CLINICAL ISSUES

Epidemiology

- Incidence
  - Sporadic
  - Syndromic (Carney complex)
    - Frequent mutation of tumor suppressor gene *PRKAR1A*
- Age
  - Childhood to senescence (mean: 35 years)
    - Decade younger in patients with Carney complex
- Sex
  - Slight female predominance (1.5:1) in both sporadic and syndromic types

Site

- Sporadic
  - Spinal nerves and ganglia (cervicothoracic)
  - Rarely multiple
- Syndromic (Carney complex)
  - Alimentary tract
  - Viscera (heart, liver, lung)
  - Bone
  - 15% multiple

Presentation

- Sporadic
  - Nerve root associated tumors: Pain or sensory disturbance
- Syndromic (Carney complex; autosomal dominant)
  - Psammomatous melanotic schwannoma: Mass effects
  - Lentigines (65%) of face, lips, caruncle, & female genitalia
  - Myxomas of heart (65%), skin (25%), breast (20%)
  - Blue nevi of extremities and trunk
  - Endocrine overactivity
    - Cushing syndrome (25%): Pigmented nodular adrenocortical disease
    - Acromegaly: Pituitary adenoma, mammosomatotroph type
    - Precocious puberty (30%): Large cell Sertoli tumor of testis

Treatment

- Surgical approaches
  - Resection with tumor-free margins for all lesions

Prognosis

- Recurrence with subtotal resection
- Malignant
  - Metastasis
    - Not infrequent (15-44%)
    - Distinguish metastases from 2nd primary
    - Prognosis same in conventional and psammomatous variants
    - 15% die of tumor

IMAGING

MR Findings

- Features depend on paramagnetic free radicals in melanin
  - Hyperintense on T1-weighted MR
  - Hypointense in T2-weighted MR
- Contrast enhancing
- Solid > cystic
- Demarcated, ± nerve association
- Benign tumors may erode bone (spinal foramina)
- Malignant tumors less demarcated; invasive destruction of bone

CT Findings

- Calcification/ossification on CT in some psammomatous tumors

MACROSCOPIC

General Features

- 0.5-26.0 cm (median: 5 cm)
- Circumscribed
- Round to sausage shaped
  - Spinal nerve root tumors: Dumbbell shaped
- Occasionally lobulated or cystic
- No encapsulation
  - Occasionally thin collagen layer with soft tissue invasion
- Effects of bone
  - Erosion (benign tumors)
  - Invasive destruction (malignant tumors)
- Cut surface gray to tar black
  - Infrequently cystic
  - Occasional hemorrhage or necrosis
  - Occasional subcapsular grittiness (psammomatous variant)
- Soft to rubbery; occasionally hard
- Maybe multifocal, usually when malignant

MICROSCOPIC

Histologic Features

- Melanotic schwannoma
  - High cellularity, lobules and fascicles
  - Spindle to epithelioid cells
    - Eosinophilic to amphophilic cytoplasm
    - Clear cells occasional
    - Occasional multinucleation
    - Variable pigmentation
  - Nuclear/cytoplasmic pseudoinclusions
  - Pigmentation variable or patchy
  - Thin-walled vessels
  - Scan often incomplete collagenous capsule
  - Palisading, Verocay bodies, microcysts (very uncommon)
  - Melanophages frequent and most pigmented of cells
- Features associated with more aggressive behavior
  - Vesicular nuclei and coarse chromatin

- Violaceous macronucleoli
- Frequent mitoses
  - Mitotic activity > 1 mitosis per 10 HPF correlated with metastases in large study
- Geographic necrosis
- No single feature diagnostic
- Metastases may have more epithelioid features and increased mitotic rate compared to primary tumor
- Psammomatous melanotic schwannoma
  - Conventional features with psammomatous calcifications
  - Cytoplasmic vacuolation (60%)
  - Infrequent peripheral osseous metaplasia

ANCILLARY TESTS

Histochemistry

- Fontana-Masson
  - Staining pattern: Granular
  - Stains for melanin
- Potassium permanganate bleach removes melanin
  - Permits appreciation of cytologic detail
  - May interfere with immunoreactivities
- Reticulin outlines lobules
- Periodic acid-Schiff (PAS) stains psammoma bodies

Immunohistochemistry

- S100(+) (with rare exceptions)
- HMB-45, Melan-A, tyrosinase all (+)
- Collagen IV and laminin (+)
  - Outline perilobular basal lamina
  - Not pericellular as in other schwannoma variants
- Vimentin (+)
- GFAP usually (-)
- EMA(-)
- SMARCB1 retained
- PRKAR1A lost in ~ 1/3 of cases

Genetic Testing

- Complex karyotype in one study
  - Frequent 22q loss
  - Recurrent losses in Ch1, Ch17p arm, and Ch21
  - Frequent whole chromosome gains (Ch4-9)
- Global methylation and gene expression profiles different from schwannoma, melanocytoma, and melanoma
- Lack of *GNAQ* or *GNA11* mutations in most instances

Electron Microscopy

- Clusters of spindle-shaped or plump cells; some dendritic cells
- Cell processes
- Melanosomes in variable stages (II-IV) of maturation
- Occasional intermediate filaments
- Variable surface basal lamina
- Rudimentary junctions
- Extracellular long-spacing collagen (Luse bodies)

DIFFERENTIAL DIAGNOSIS

Conventional Schwannoma

- Thick, continuous
- Antoni A and B patterns
- Verocay bodies
- Contain lipofuscin [PAS(+)] but lack melanin
- Has distinct capsule
- Lack psammoma bodies
- Lack adipose-like cells
- Rarely involve alimentary tract

Pigmented Neurofibroma

- Typically diffusely infiltrative
- Pigmentation largely microscopic
- Small nuclei, scant cytoplasm
- Lack distinct nucleolus
- S100 protein not uniformly (+)
- Ultrastructure heterogeneous; includes perineurial-like cells and fibroblasts

Melanocytoma

- Tumors of cranial or spinal leptomeninges
- Compressive of surroundings
- Elongated to polygonal cells
- Small to relatively prominent nucleoli
- Few mitoses
- Lack psammoma bodies and adipose-like cells
- Lack long-spacing collagen

Primary or Metastatic Melanoma

- Cytologically malignant
- Lack of psammoma bodies and adipose-like cells
- Lack collagen IV (+) basal lamina
- Rare basal lamina on electron microscopy

Clear Cell Sarcoma (Soft Tissue Melanoma)

- Grossly and microscopically invasive
- Cytologically malignant
- Scant or no melanin pigment
- Clear cells, no psammoma bodies
- No immunohistochemical or ultrastructural basal lamina
- *EWSR1-ATF1* fusion (90% of soft tissue cases)

DIAGNOSTIC CHECKLIST

Clinically Relevant Pathologic Features

- Distant metastases in 15-44%
- May be associated with Carney complex

Pathologic Interpretation Pearls

- Differential diagnosis from malignant melanoma may be challenging
  - Psammomatous calcification and basal lamina around lobules favor melanotic schwannoma
- Lack distinct capsule, Antoni A and Antoni B areas, Verocay bodies

SELECTED REFERENCES

1. Koelsche C et al: Melanotic tumors of the nervous system are characterized by distinct mutational, chromosomal and epigenomic profiles. Brain Pathol. 25(2):202-8, 2015
2. Torres-Mora J et al: Malignant melanotic schwannian tumor: a clinicopathologic, immunohistochemical, and gene expression profiling study of 40 cases, with a proposal for the reclassification of "melanotic schwannoma". Am J Surg Pathol. 38(1):94-105, 2014

Fascicular Pattern

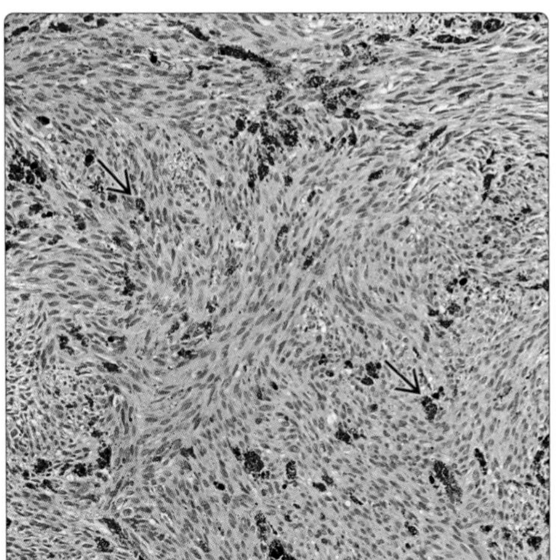

Abundant Pigment in Macrophages

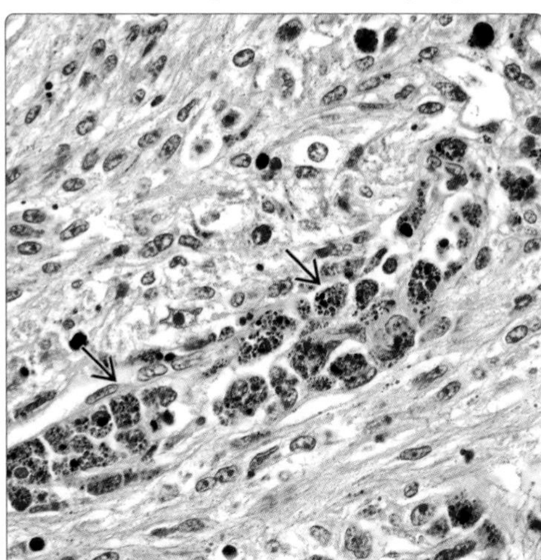

(Left) *Melanotic schwannomas often have a fascicular pattern similar to that of differential diagnostic entities such as melanocytic tumors and fibrous meningioma. Melanin* ⇒ *is variable in extent.* **(Right)** *Spindle cells with round nuclei and small distinct nucleoli are common features. As here, pigment is often more abundant in melanophages* ⇒ *than in tumoral cells.*

Melanin Pigment

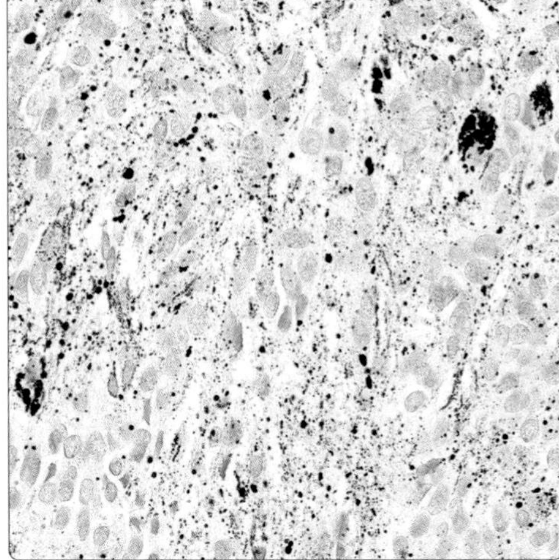

Degenerative Nuclear Atypia

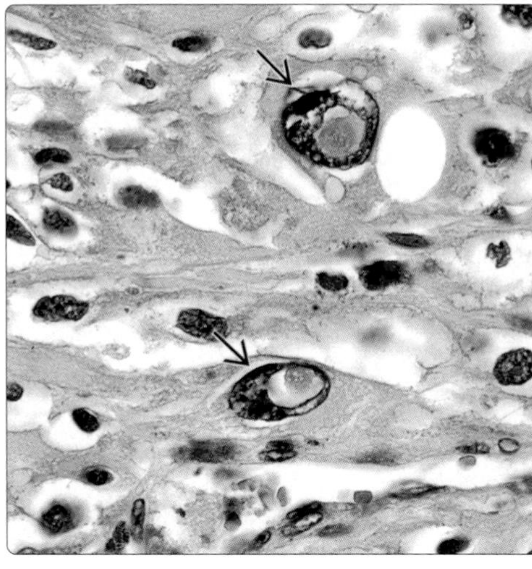

(Left) *Granular melanin pigment is present in both tumoral cells and melanophages. Free melanin, best seen on Fontana staining, helps in differentiation from hemosiderin.* **(Right)** *Degenerative nuclear atypia with nuclear-cytoplasmic pseudoinclusions* ⇒ *is common in melanocytic schwannomas. Abundant mitotic activity, an objective index of anaplasia, is lacking.*

Abundant Melanin

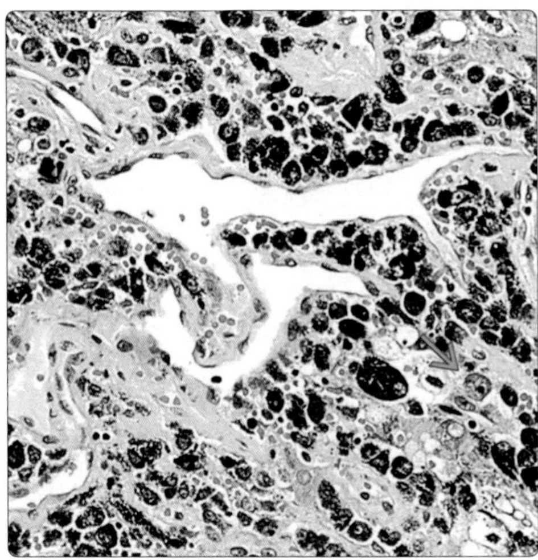

Thin-Walled Vessels

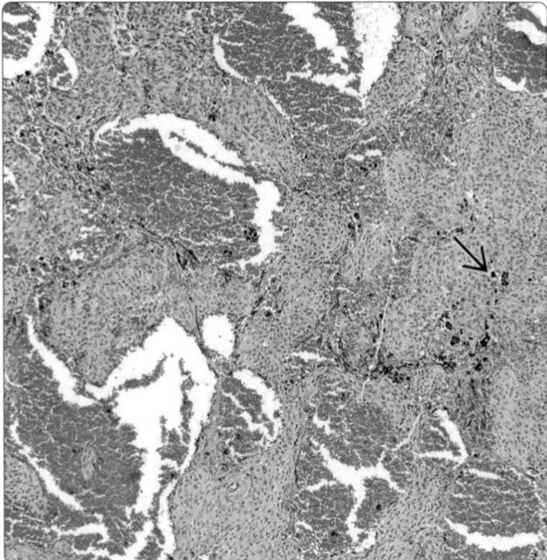

(Left) *When abundant, melanin can obscure cytologic details, leaving only a few unpigmented cells* ⇒ *with which to assess the nature and grade of the lesion. Unlike conventional schwannomas, vessels are thin walled.* **(Right)** *Congested thin-walled vessels may produce a hemangiopericytoma-like appearance. The presence of pigment* ⇒ *helps one entertain the possibility of melanocytic schwannoma and melanocytoma.*

(Left) *Typically unencapsulated, melanotic schwannomas can infiltrate surrounding soft tissue* →. *This tumor is extensively calcified* →. **(Right)** *Malignant melanotic schwannomas have prominent cytologic atypia, with vesicular nuclei and distinct eosinophilic nucleoli. Mitotic activity* → *is brisk.*

Soft Tissue Infiltration

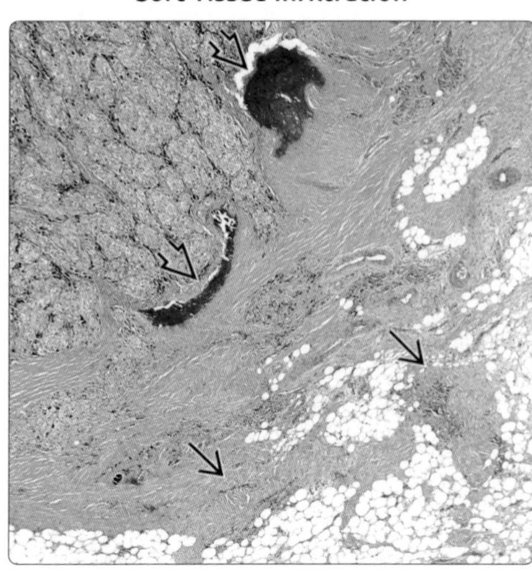

Cytologic Atypia

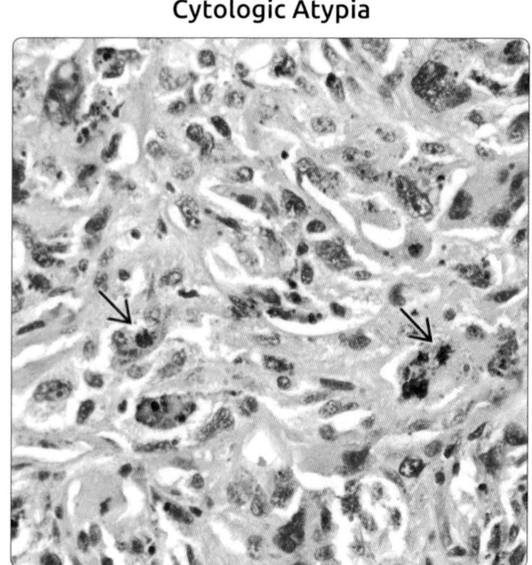

(Left) *Lentiginous pigmentation of the face and lips is typical of Carney complex, which also includes myxomas of heart, skin, and breast.* **(Right)** *Myxomas of the breast are one component of Carney complex. Note the intralobular deposition of myxoid substance* →. *Fibroadenomas may show similar changes.*

Lentiginous Pigmentation

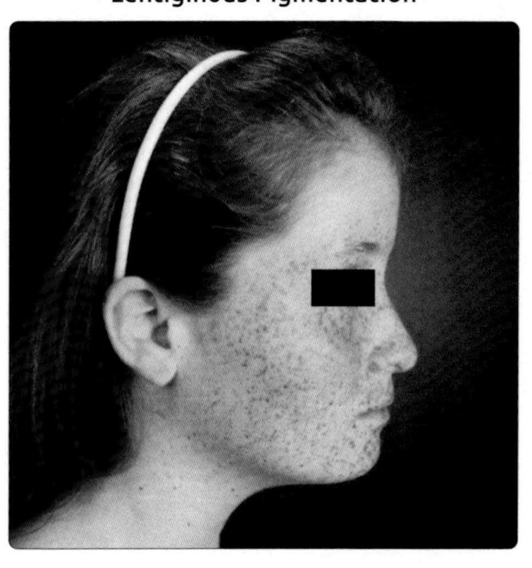

Breast Myxoma

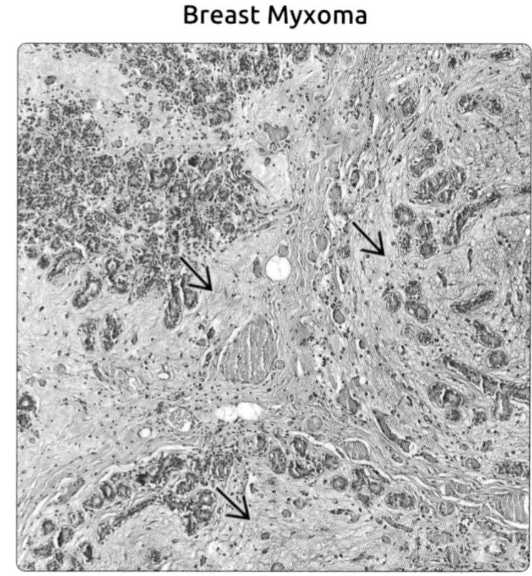

(Left) *Psammomatous melanotic schwannomas typically have clear adipocyte-like cells* →. *Note the nucleolar enlargement* ➡, *which should prompt a search for mitoses since such a lesion may be a malignant variant of melanocytic schwannoma.* **(Right)** *Psammomatous melanotic schwannomas have psammomatous calcifications* ➡ *in varying numbers.*

Adipocyte-Like Cells

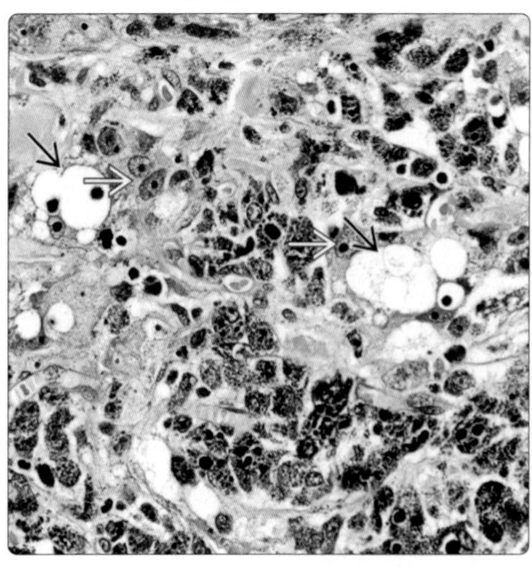

Psammomatous Calcifications

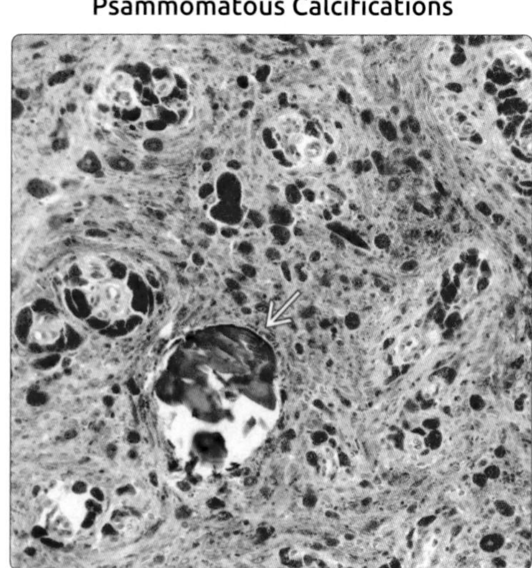

Melanophages

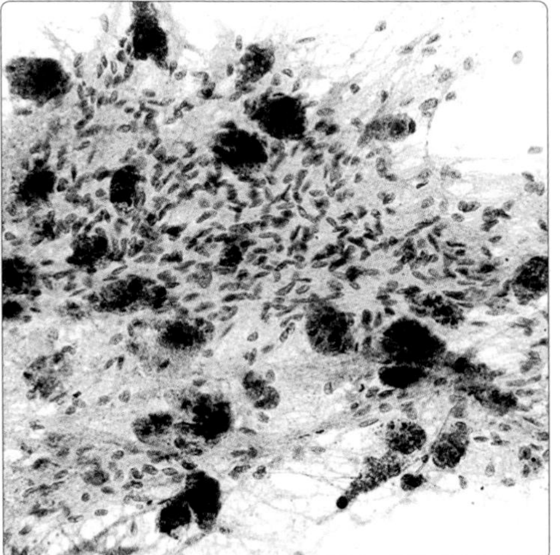

Low Ki-67 Indices

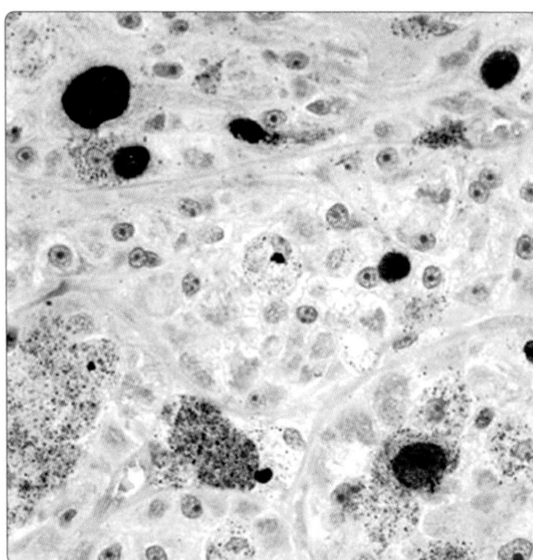

(Left) *A cytologic preparation of melanotic schwannoma shows abundant melanophages among less pigmented spindle-shaped tumor cells.* **(Right)** *Ki-67 indices are low in melanotic schwannomas other than the rare anaplastic variants. An increase, as in this example, may raise the question of malignant transformation.*

S100 Positivity

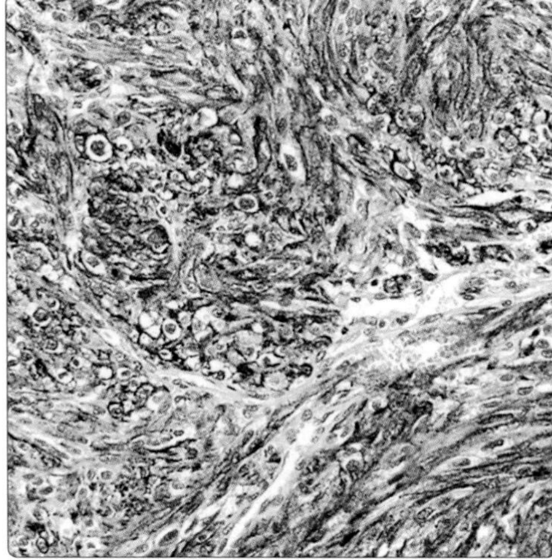

Perilobular Collagen IV Staining

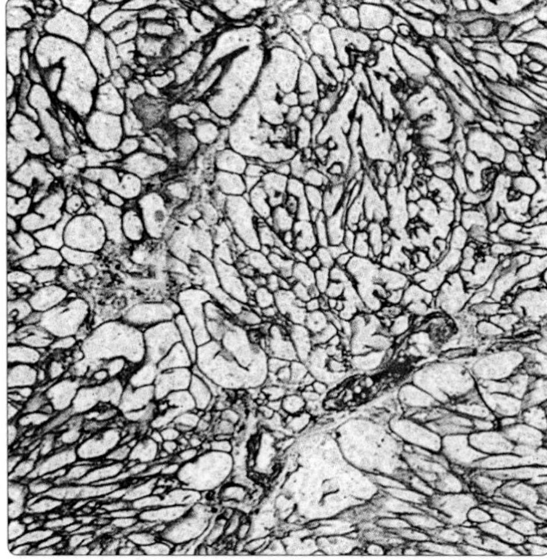

(Left) *As with other variants of schwannoma, melanotic types are diffusely positive for S100 protein.* **(Right)** *Collagen IV staining in melanocytic schwannomas is more perilobular than pericellular as would be the case in a conventional schwannoma.*

Basal Lamina

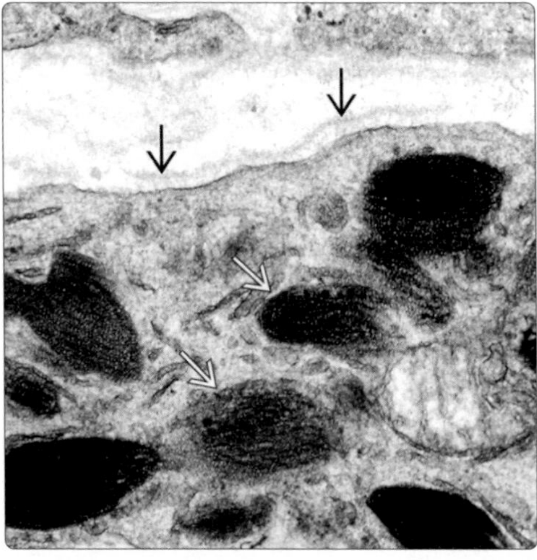

Melanocytoma

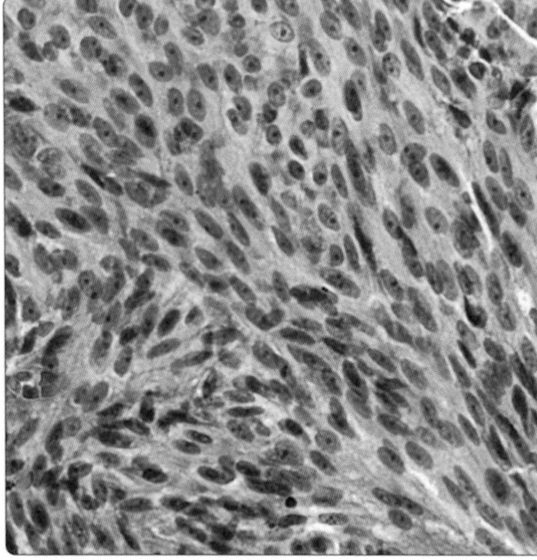

(Left) *Basal lamina ⇨ around single or grouped cells is a typical ultrastructural feature of melanocytic schwannoma. Melanosomes ➡ are also prominent in this case.* **(Right)** *Melanocytic neoplasms, melanocytoma seen here, represent main differential diagnosis of melanotic schwannoma. Anatomic location and ancillary studies (e.g., collagen IV immunohistochemistry) may help in this distinction. Melanocytoma has less abundant collagen IV immunostaining, mostly perivascular.*

Plexiform Schwannoma

KEY FACTS

CLINICAL ISSUES

- Dermal-subcutaneous (90%)
- Prognosis excellent with simple excision
- Sporadic (90%)
- NF2 associated (5%)
- Schwannomatosis associated (5%)

MACROSCOPIC

- Circumscribed lesion(s) but may be extensive
- Plexiform to multinodular expanded fascicle(s)

MICROSCOPIC

- Antoni A > B tissue
- Scant mitoses (except in cellular tumors)
- Peripheral perineurial ensheathment
- Multiple (2-50) nodules

ANCILLARY TESTS

- Reticulin (+) around individual cells
- S100 diffusely (+), SOX10(+)

TOP DIFFERENTIAL DIAGNOSES

- Plexiform neurofibroma
  - Smaller cells
  - Frequent interfascicular diffuse neurofibroma element
  - Abundant stromal mucin
  - S100 partially (+)
- Palisaded encapsulated neuroma (PEN)
  - Abundant axons
- Traumatic neuroma
  - Lacks circumscription
  - Numerous microfascicles
- Cutaneous leiomyoma
  - S100(-), SOX10(-)
  - SMA and desmin (+)

Multinodularity

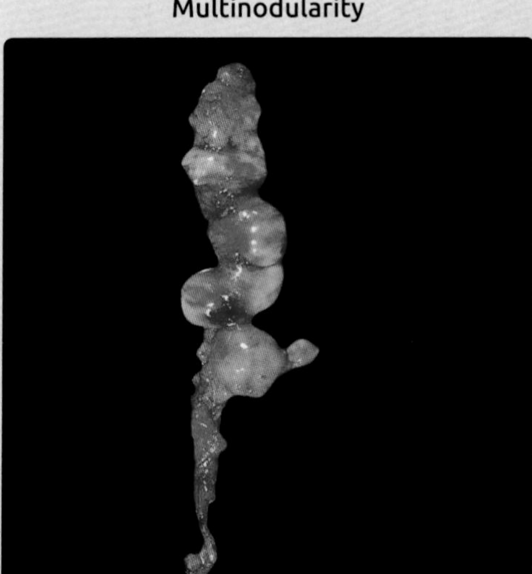

Plexiform Nature

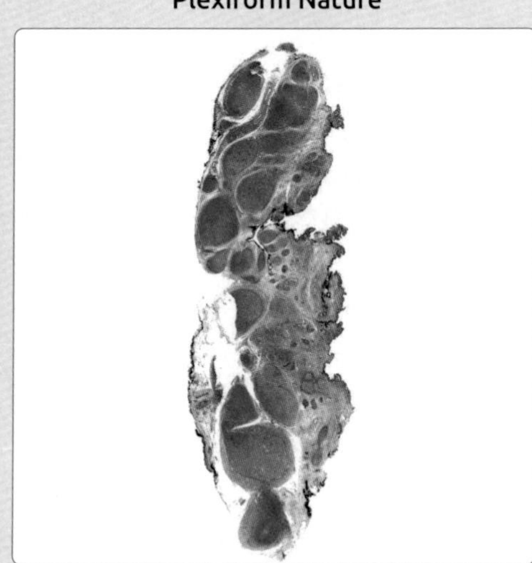

(Left) *A plexiform multinodularity is typical of plexiform schwannoma.* **(Right)** *Microsections demonstrate the plexiform nature of the tumor at low magnification.*

Multiple Nodules

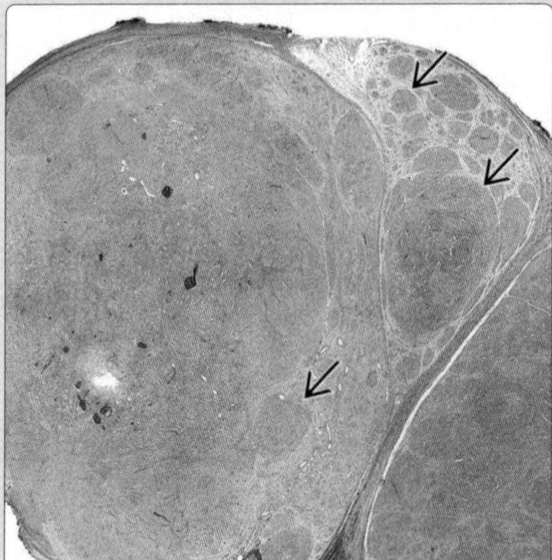

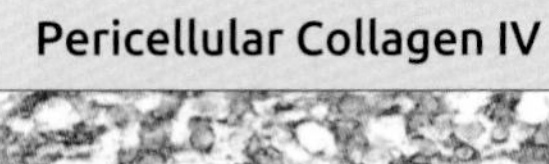

Pericellular Collagen IV

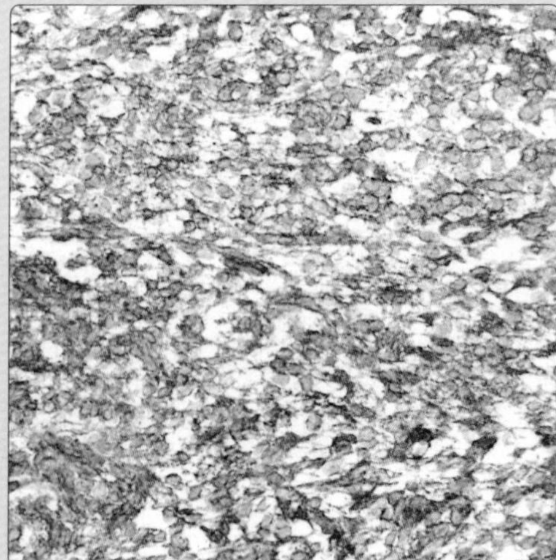

(Left) *The number of nodules → in a plexiform schwannoma varies from few to many. There are many of varying sizes in this case.* **(Right)** *Plexiform schwannomas share immunohistochemical features with other well differentiated Schwann cell neoplasms, including pericellular immunoreactivity for collagen IV.*

TERMINOLOGY

Synonyms

- Multinodular schwannoma

Definitions

- Tumor of Schwann cells with plexiform or multinodular growth

CLINICAL ISSUES

Epidemiology

- Incidence
  - Sporadic (90%)
  - NF2 associated (5%)
  - Schwannomatosis associated (5%)
  - Solitary; occasionally multiple in NF2 and schwannomatosis
    - Asymptomatic > painful or tender (schwannomatosis)
  - Location varies
    - Dermal/subcutaneous (90%)
    - Extremity, trunk, head and neck
    - Mucosal sites
    - Visceral rare
  - Rare examples of conventional schwannoma contiguous with deep plexiform component
- Age
  - Childhood to old age (mean: 35 years)
    - Rarely congenital
- Sex
  - No predilection

Prognosis

- Adults
  - Excellent with simple excision
  - Infrequent recurrence of large, cellular &/or mitotically active examples
- Children
  - Recurrence (50%) if infiltrative or poorly circumscribed
  - No deaths of disease or metastases

MACROSCOPIC

General Features

- Few grossly obvious; rarely > 10 cm
  - Bone erosion infrequent
  - Soft tissue infiltration uncommon (childhood)
- Circumscribed
- Plexiform to multinodular expanded fascicle(s)
- No necrosis or hemorrhage
- Cut surface may be yellow due to lipid accumulation

MICROSCOPIC

Histologic Features

- Round to oval contours of schwannoma-affected nerve fascicle(s)
- Multiple (2-50) nodules or foci of fascicular expansion
- Occasional cellular-type schwannoma
  - Hypercellularity
  - Mitotically active
  - Tendency for local recurrence
- Antoni A > B tissue
  - Some nodules entirely Antoni A
  - Arrays of palisaded nuclei more common than well-formed Verocay body
- Minor degenerative atypia
- Scant mitoses (except in cellular tumors)
- Peripheral perineurial ensheathment
- Occasional scattered or displaced intratumoral axons
- Large nodules show thickened capsule
- Necrosis absent

Cytologic Features

- Typical schwannoma features
  - Spindle cells with tapered nuclei

ANCILLARY TESTS

Histochemistry

- Reticulin (+) around individual cells
- Occasional Bodian or Bielschowsky (+) axons, with LFB/PAS(+) Schwann cell sheaths

Immunohistochemistry

- S100 diffusely (+), SOX10(+)
- GFAP(+) in most cases
- Neurofilament protein (+) residual axons

Electron Microscopy

- Features of typical Schwann cells
  - Cytoplasmic intermediate filaments
  - Processes covered by basement membrane
  - Scant junctions
- Long-spacing collagen (Luse bodies)

DIFFERENTIAL DIAGNOSIS

Plexiform Neurofibroma

- Spindled smaller nuclei
- Thick collagen bundles
- Abundant mucinous matrix
- S100 subtotally (+)
- Frequent interfascicular diffuse element

Palisaded Encapsulated Neuroma (PEN)

- Uni- and occasionally multinodularity
- Relatively abundant axons
- Apical irregular loss of perineurial capsule
- Deep nerve entry zone

Traumatic Neuroma

- Lacks circumscription
- Parent nerve obvious
- Abundant microfascicles

Cutaneous Leiomyoma

- Blunt-ended nuclei
- S100 minor staining at best; SOX10(-)
- Smooth muscle actin and desmin (+)

SELECTED REFERENCES

1. Hébert-Blouin MN et al: Multinodular/plexiform (multifascicular) schwannomas of major peripheral nerves: an underrecognized part of the spectrum of schwannomas. J Neurosurg. 112(2):372-82, 2010

(Left) *Long-axis MR of the thigh shows a hyperintense plexiform schwannoma* ➔ *superior and posterior to the knee.* **(Right)** *Plexiform schwannomas are frequent in the head and neck. This orbital tumor* ➔ *was misdiagnosed as malignant peripheral nerve sheath tumor.*

Long-Axis MR

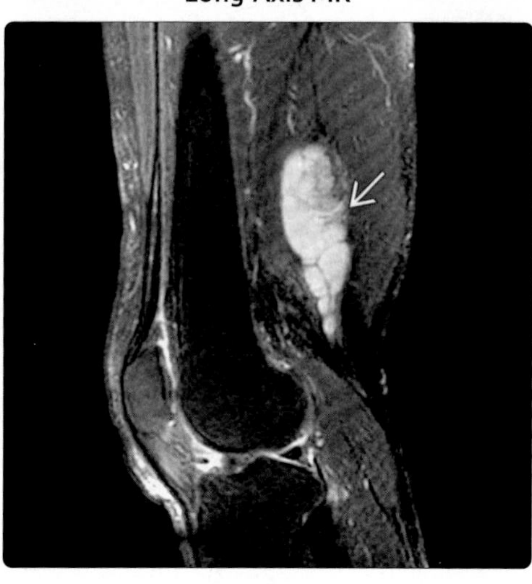

Orbital Location

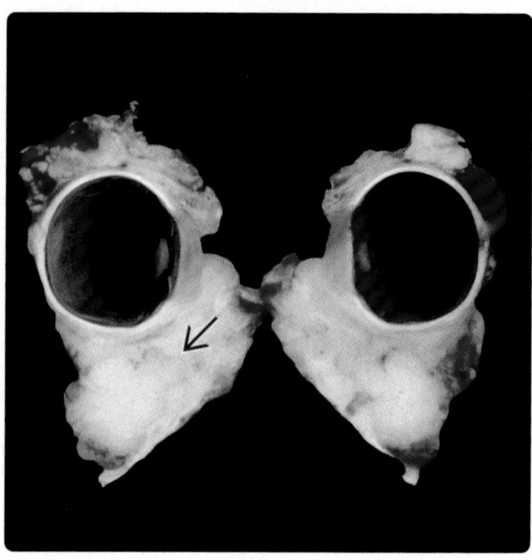

(Left) *Nodules in plexiform schwannoma vary in number and size, as demonstrated in this example.* **(Right)** *Small nodules often have thin capsules of expanded perineurium, while larger nodules have relatively thicker capsules* ➔*.*

Nodules

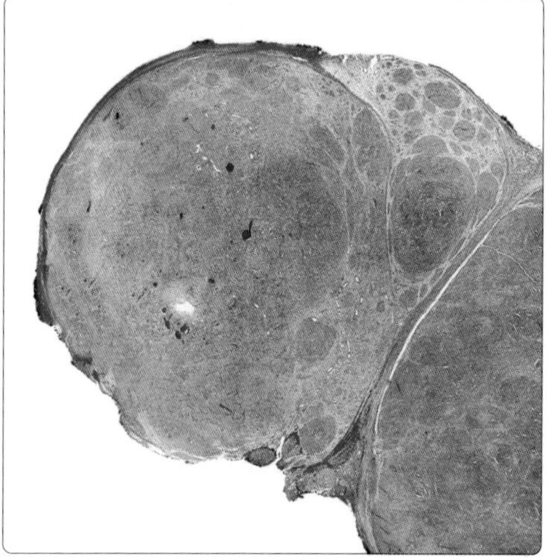

Capsule

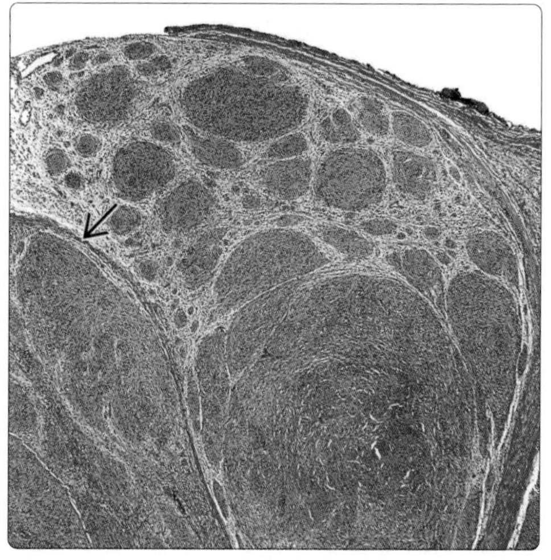

(Left) *Many plexiform schwannomas are subcutaneous masses with nodules interrelating like pieces of a jig-saw puzzle.* **(Right)** *Although classically spindle-shaped, tumoral cells can rarely have epithelioid cytologic features.*

Subcutaneous Mass

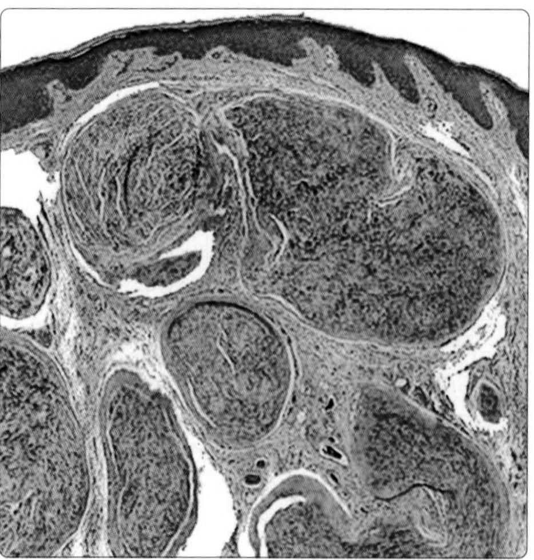

Rare Epithelioid Features

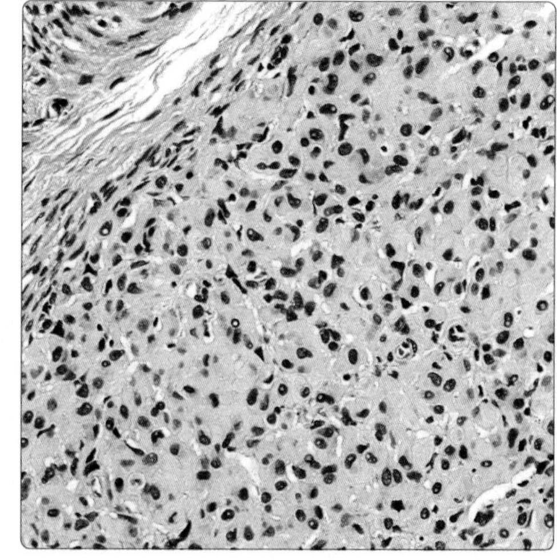

Internodular Tissue

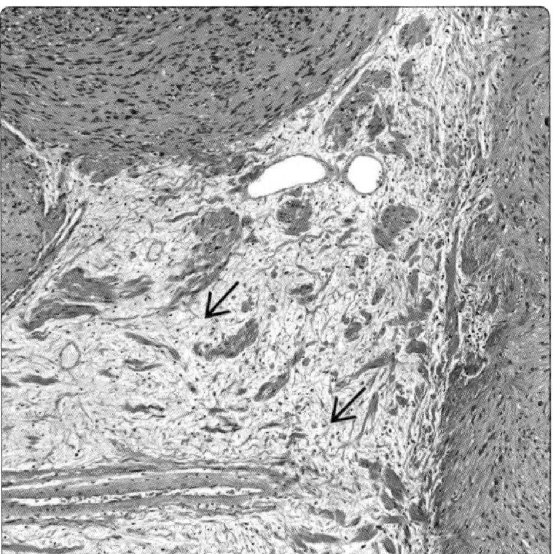

Small Nodules

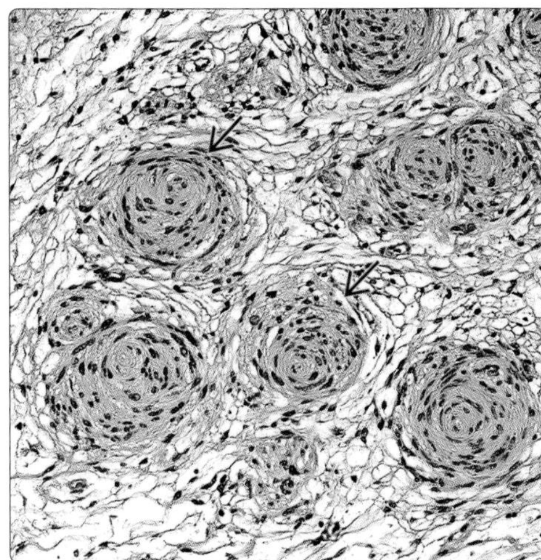

(Left) *Loose-textured internodular tissue ⇒ may resemble neurofibroma.* **(Right)** *Small nodules ⇒ may mimic onion bulbs in conventional schwannomas, or pseudo-onion bulbs as in intraneural perineurioma.*

Antoni A Tissue

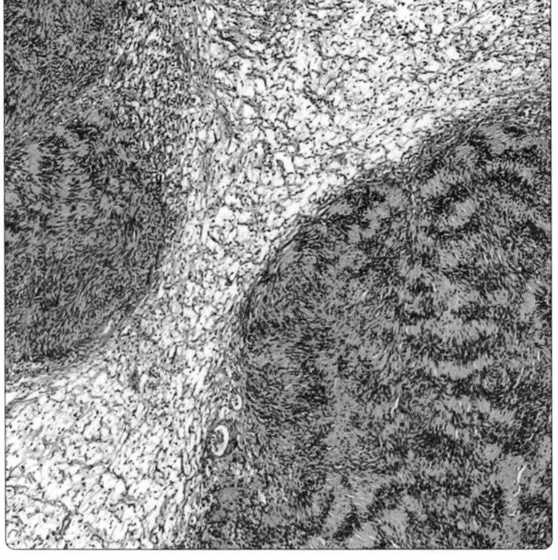

S100 Positivity

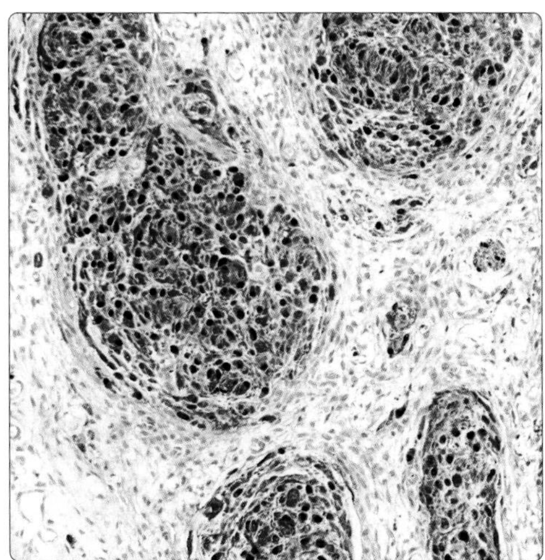

(Left) *Nodules are mostly composed of Antoni A tissue, sometimes with palisaded nuclei (Verocay bodies).* **(Right)** *Tumoral cells are diffusely positive for S100 protein, whereas intranodular cells are not.*

EMA(+) Perineurium

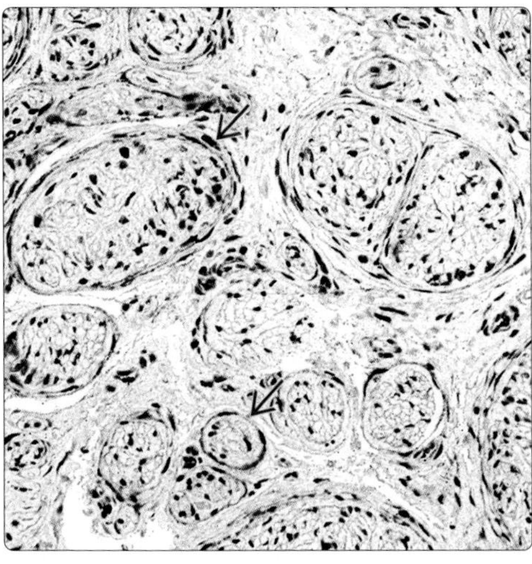

Long-Spacing Collagen (Luse Bodies)

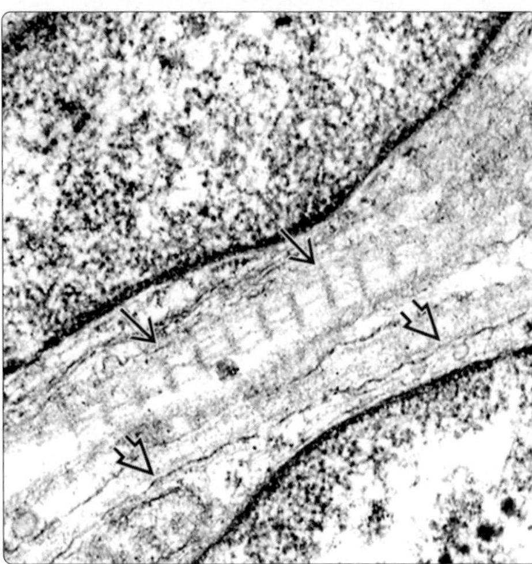

(Left) *EMA-positive perineurial cells ⇒ circumscribe nodules in plexiform schwannoma.* **(Right)** *The intercellular compartment may contain long-spacing collagen (Luse bodies) ⇒. As is typical of Schwann cell tumors, basal lamina ⇒ covers tumor cells.*

Plexiform Neurofibroma

KEY FACTS

CLINICAL ISSUES

- Epidemiology
  - Frequent NF1 association
  - Congenital onset
- Site
  - Head and neck, chest, abdomen common sites
- Presentation
  - Often asymptomatic
  - Overlying café au lait pigmentation
- Treatment
  - Debulking of tumor optimal therapy
- Prognosis
  - Recurrence in 50% of cases
  - 5% undergo malignant change

MACROSCOPIC

- Multifascicle involvement of nerve

MICROSCOPIC

- Nondestructive involvement of interfascicular and perineural soft tissue common
- Pseudomeissnerian corpuscles or melanin-producing Schwann cells in interfascicular tissue common
- Variation of histology from conventional to atypical or cellular neurofibroma

ANCILLARY TESTS

- Variably S100(+), SOX10(+)
- Leu-7(+)
- Rare cells membrane labeled for EMA; also highlights perineurium
- CD34(+) in cells other than those expressing S100
- Collagen IV surrounds individual cells and highlights perineurium
- EM: Cellular heterogeneity

(Left) *The majority of neurofibromas affecting the mesentery are of plexiform type, as this example found adjacent to the small intestine. The multinodular appearance is typical.* **(Right)** *Plexiform neurofibromas, as here adjacent to the small bowel, show multiple, enlarged, pale fascicles.*

Multinodular Appearance in Mesentery

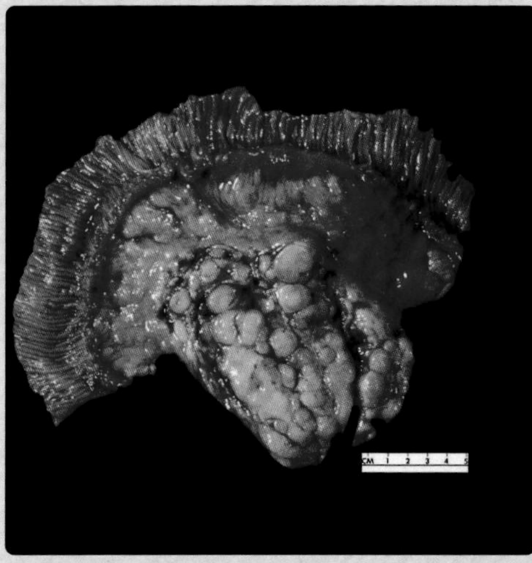

Multiple Enlarged Nerve Fascicles

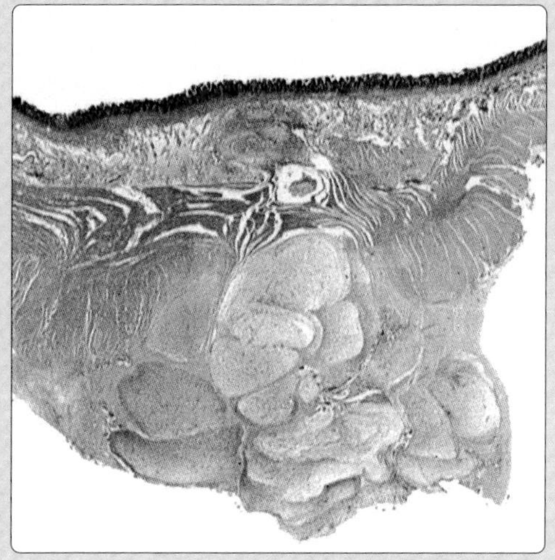

(Left) *Fascicles involved by plexiform neurofibroma may show the nerve fiber bundles* ⇒ *in their center.* **(Right)** *S100 immunostain is positive in neurofibromas, but not in all cells.*

Nerve Fiber Bundles

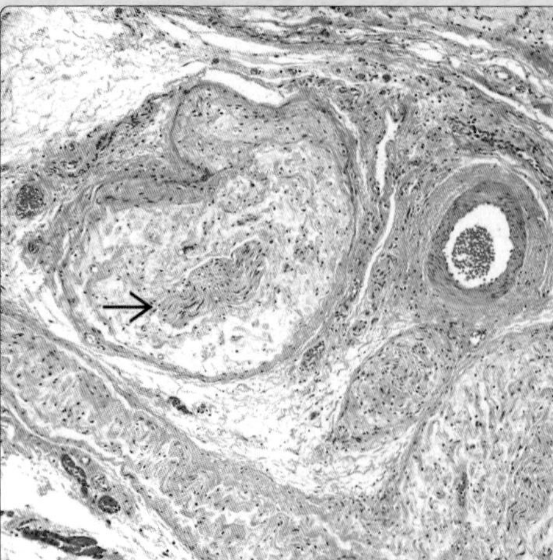

S100 Immunostaining

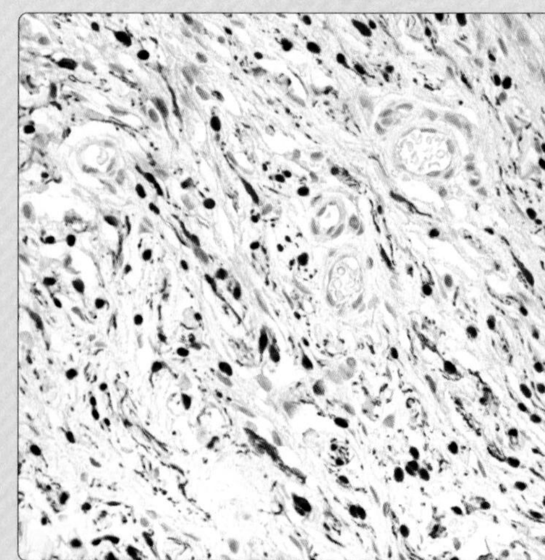

TERMINOLOGY

Definitions

- Architecturally complex neurofibroma involving multiple nerve fascicles
  - Often (but not invariably) those of branched nerve

CLINICAL ISSUES

Epidemiology

- Incidence
  - NF1 association (chromosome 17q11.2)
    - 33% of all patients
  - Asyndromic examples may occur as segmental neurofibromatosis (local somatic mutation)
- Age
  - Congenital onset
- Sex
  - No predilection

Site

- Regions: 35% head and neck, 20% chest, 45% abdominal
- Nerves: Spinal, cranial (mainly 5, 9, 10), autonomic

Presentation

- Apparent in neonates or young children
- Growth in childhood, subsequent stabilization
- Often asymptomatic but may cause disfigurement or mass effect
- Little neurologic loss or dysfunction
- May be overlain by café au lait pigmentation or hair
  - May cause hypertrophy of skin, surrounding soft tissue, or bone
- Occasional growth in pregnancy
- Painful enlargement suggests malignant transformation

Treatment

- Surgical approaches
  - Debulking of large, disfiguring, and particularly painful tumors
    - Total removal often not impossible
- Drugs
  - MEK inhibition has shown efficacy in targeting NF1-associated nerve sheath neoplasms in preclinical studies

Prognosis

- Most plexiform tumors benign
- Resection of brachial or pelvic plexus and spinal tumors fraught with neurologic complications
- Postoperative regrowth at 5 years seen in 50% of cases
- Improvement in 20% with partial resection
- 5% undergo malignant change

IMAGING

Radiographic Findings

- Irregularly demarcated mass

MR Findings

- Poorly delineated, worm-like, soft tissue mass
- T1WI: Isointense; T2WI: Hyperintense

MACROSCOPIC

General Features

- Multifascicle involvement of nerve
  - Worm-like enlargement of branching nerves
  - Rope-like enlargement of aligned fascicles in nonbranching nerves (e.g., sciatic)
  - Diffuse infiltration of extraneural tissue as well (some cases)

MICROSCOPIC

Histologic Features

- Multiple fascicle involvement
  - Permeation by neurofibroma
  - Occasional involvement of spinal, cranial, or autonomic ganglia
- Frequent nondestructive neurofibromatous involvement of interfascicular and perineural soft tissue
  - Pseudomeissnerian corpuscles or melanin-producing Schwann cells often seen
- Variation of histology from conventional to atypical or cellular neurofibroma
- Malignant transformation in 5% of plexiform neurofibroma
  - Crowded cellularity
  - Nuclear enlargement
  - Hyperchromasia
  - Mitotic activity variable (not an essential diagnostic feature)

ANCILLARY TESTS

Immunohistochemistry

- Pseudomeissnerian corpuscles
  - S100(+)
  - Peripheral cells EMA(+); not seen in normal Wagner-Meissner corpuscles
- Variably S100(+), SOX10(+), Leu-7(+) throughout
- p53 low level (+), weak to moderate
  - Reactivity increases in cellular neurofibroma
- NFP shows grouped axons at center of involved fascicles; (-) in diffuse extraneural component
- Ki-67 labeling index: Range 1-15% (cellular neurofibroma); mean 5%

DIFFERENTIAL DIAGNOSIS

Plexiform Schwannoma

- Pure Schwann cell process
- Diffusely S100(+), SOX10(+)
- Scant peripherally displaced axons
- Ultrastructurally uniform Schwann cell features

Plexiform Fibrohistiocytic Tumor

- Biphasic histology with myofibroblasts and osteoclast-like giant cells
- No nerve association
- S100(-)

SELECTED REFERENCES

1. Jessen WJ et al: MEK inhibition exhibits efficacy in human and mouse neurofibromatosis tumors. J Clin Invest. 123(1):340-7, 2013

(Left) *Neurofibromatous change in multiple nerve fascicles creates a plexiform configuration that has been likened to a bag of worms.* **(Right)** *The plexiform architecture created by enlarged nerve fascicles* ⇨ *is readily seen at low magnification. This example also has a dermal and subcutaneous component* ➡.

Bag of Worms

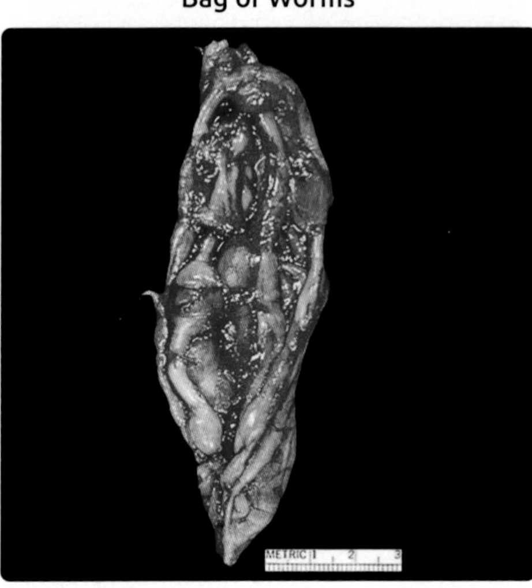

Enlarged Nerve Fascicles

(Left) *Collagen bundles forming shredded carrots* ⇨ *are common features of many neurofibromas, including the plexiform variant.* **(Right)** *Plexiform neurofibromas often extend into extrafascicular soft tissue* ⇨.

Shredded Carrots

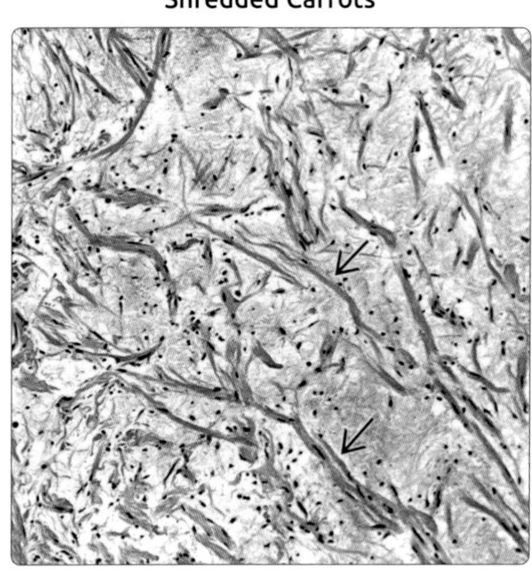

Extrafascicular Soft Tissue Extension

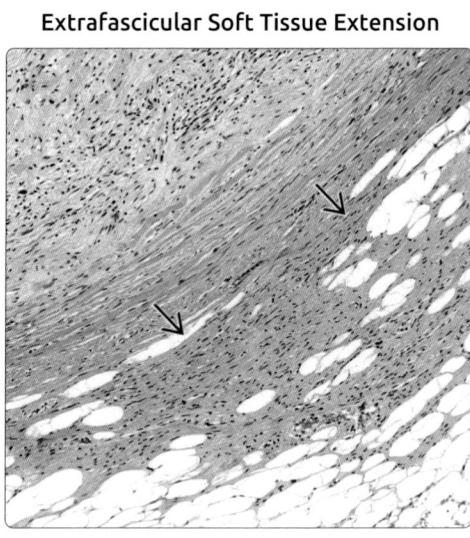

(Left) *Mucopolysaccharide-rich enlarged fascicles of neurofibroma are pale in H&E-stained sections.* **(Right)** *The mucoid matrix within the enlarged fascicles filled with tumor reacts strongly with Alcian blue* ⇨. *The subcutaneous component* ➡ *is less strongly positive.*

Enlarged Fascicles

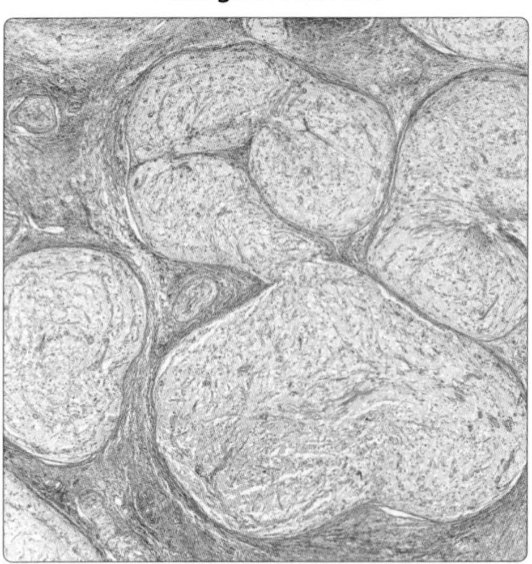

Mucoid Matrix

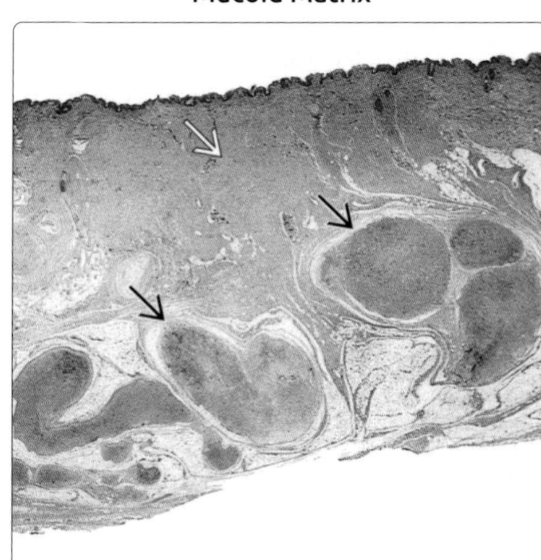

Unaffected Nerve Fibers

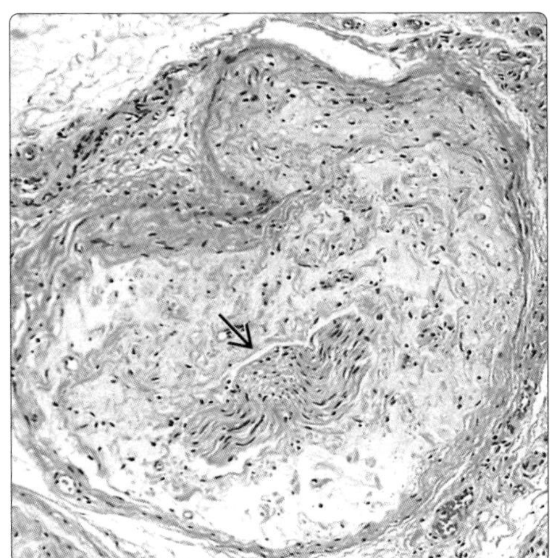

Nerve Fiber Bundles

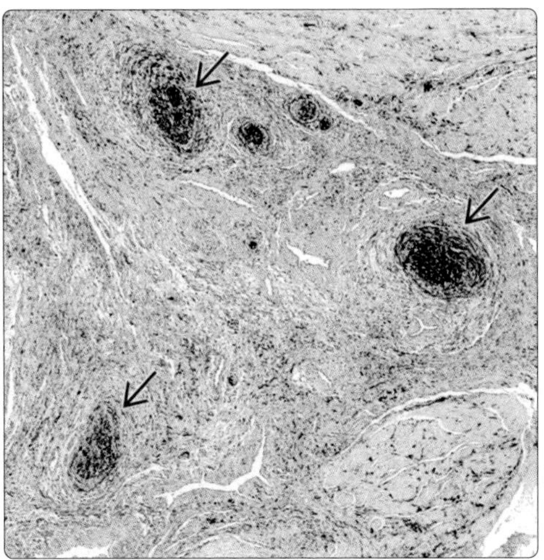

(Left) *Unaffected nerve fibers ⇒ often sit centrally within enlarged fascicles overrun by the myxoid substance-rich tumor.* **(Right)** *Nerve fiber bundles ⇒ trapped within the neoplasm are highlighted by S100 staining.*

Pseudomeissnerian Corpuscles

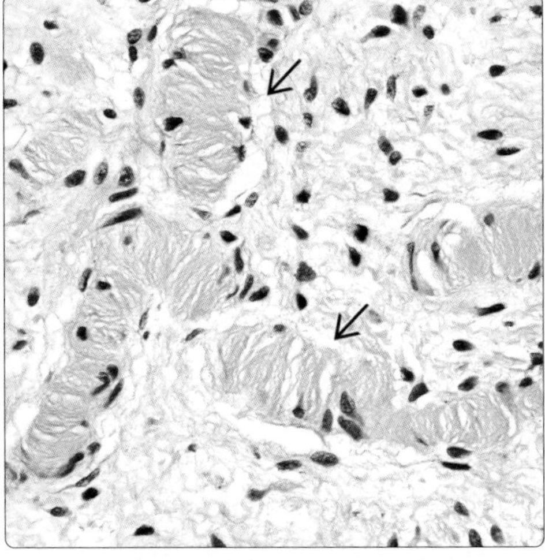

Onion Bulbs

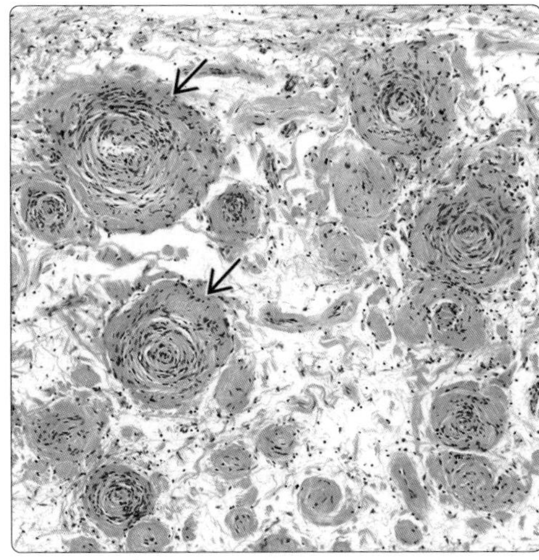

(Left) *Pseudomeissnerian corpuscles ⇒ are important features of neurofibromas. These distinctive structures abound in some plexiform neurofibromas.* **(Right)** *Schwann cell onion bulbs ⇒ are occasionally present in plexiform neurofibromas.*

Entrapped Ganglion Cells

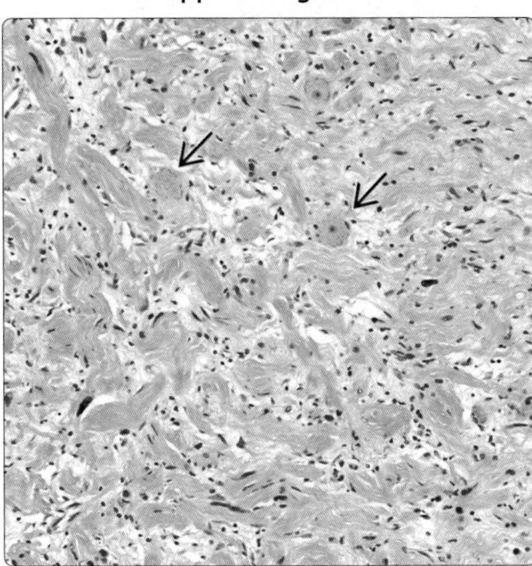

S100 Immunostaining

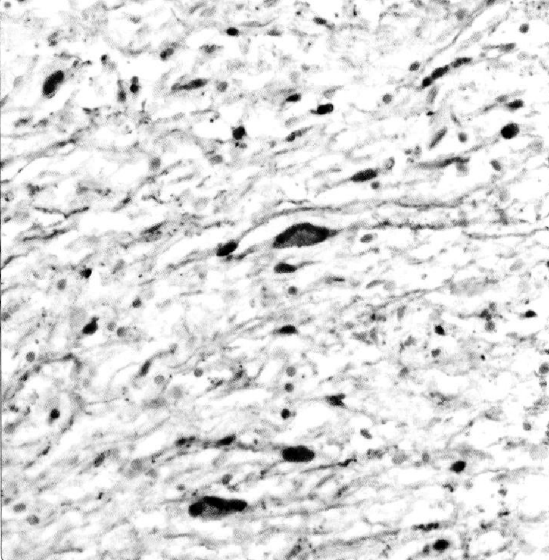

(Left) *Trapping ganglion cells ⇒ in the process, paraspinal plexiform neurofibromas often overrun dorsal root ganglia. Ganglion cells are focal in this context, not dispersed throughout the lesion as is usually the case in ganglioneuroma.* **(Right)** *S100 immunostaining is variably positive in neurofibromas, often with a mixture of positive and negative cells.*

Localized Intraneural Neurofibroma

KEY FACTS

TERMINOLOGY

- Intraneural, affecting grossly apparent nerves

CLINICAL ISSUES

- 2nd most frequent form of neurofibroma
- Multiple lesions usually neurofibromatosis type 1 associated
- Spinal, cranial, and autonomic nerves affected
- Resection of parent nerve with tumor-free margins
- Malignant transformation rare

MACROSCOPIC

- Usually fusiform with thin capsule
- Translucent cut surface
- 1 to several cm

MICROSCOPIC

- Small Schwann cells with elongate nuclei
- Occasional degenerative nuclear atypia
- No or low-level mitotic activity
- Stromal mucin &/or collagen bundles
- Delicate vasculature
- Mast cells

ANCILLARY TESTS

- S100(+), SOX10(+), EMA(-) or rare, NFP(+) axons variable
- Electron microscopy: Schwann cells, perineurial-like cells, fibroblasts

TOP DIFFERENTIAL DIAGNOSES

- Low-grade malignant peripheral nerve sheath tumor: Nuclear atypia, higher mitotic activity
- Nerve sheath myxoma: Multinodular
- Schwannoma: Diffusely S100 and SOX10(+)

Intraspinal Component

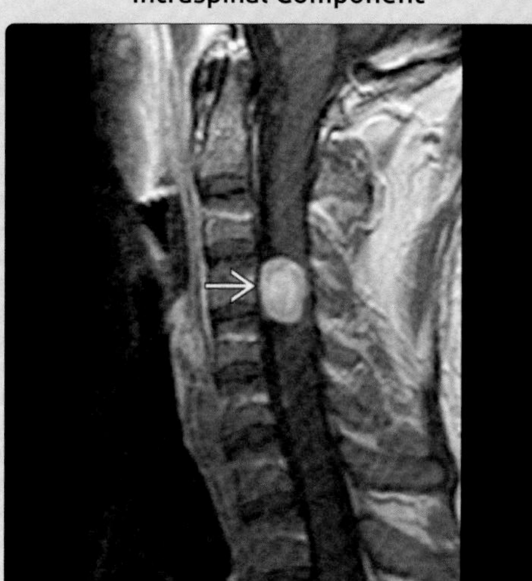

Fusiform Neurofibroma

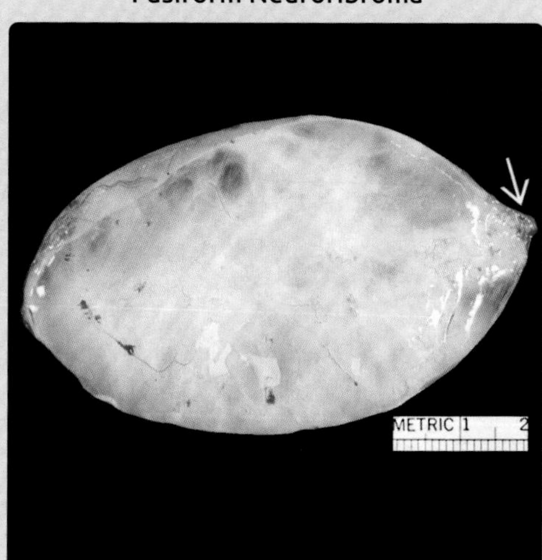

(Left) *Sagittal T1WI C+ MR shows the intraspinal component of a neurofibroma ➡. The enhancement pattern is notable for a concentric or target appearance, analogous to the classic target sign seen with neurofibromas on T2WI.* **(Right)** *A thin capsule delineates a typically fusiform neurofibroma with an almost translucent cut surface. The parent nerve ➡ is present at one end.*

Thin Fibrous Capsule

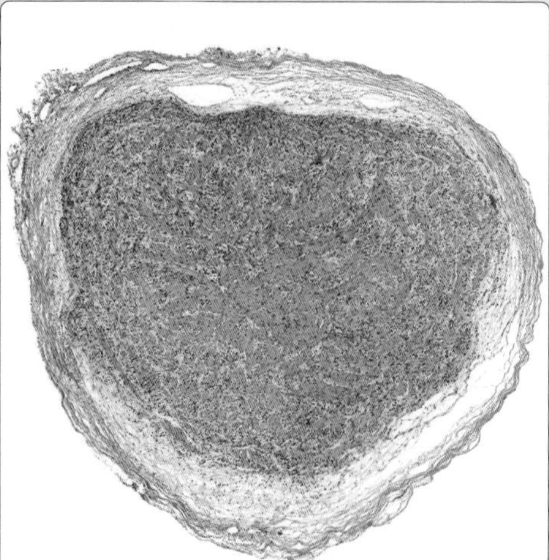

Entrapped Ganglion Cells

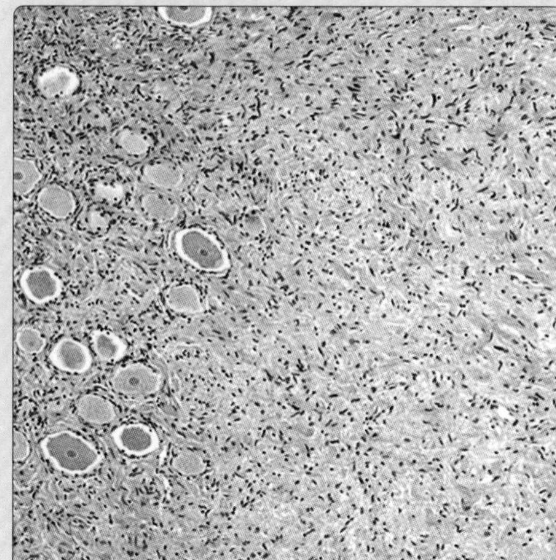

(Left) *The thin fibrous capsule around the tumor is best observed microscopically. This relatively old lesion is centrally more collagenous, rather than myxoid.* **(Right)** *Intraneural neurofibromas in the spine may infiltrate sensory ganglia. Entrapped ganglion cells should not be mistaken for a ganglioneuroma.*

TERMINOLOGY

Definitions

- Entirely intraneural neurofibroma affecting grossly apparent nerves, small to large
  - Intradermal nerves excluded

CLINICAL ISSUES

Epidemiology

- Incidence
  - 2nd most frequent form of neurofibroma after cutaneous neurofibroma
  - Multifocality suggests neurofibromatosis type 1 (NF1) association
- Age
  - Young adults
- Sex
  - No predilection

Site

- Spinal, cranial, and autonomic nerves affected
- Spinal root tumors usually cervical in NF1
  - Often dumbbell-shaped (intra- and extraspinal)

Presentation

- Superficial tumors often palpable, laterally mobile lesion
- Deep tumors of larger nerves produce sensory disturbance &/or pain
- Intraspinal tumors may compress spinal cord with weakness, loss of sensation, and pain

Treatment

- Surgical approaches
  - Resection of parent nerve with tumor-free margins
    - Neurologically functioning nerves often spared

Prognosis

- Resection of benign tumors curative
- Malignant transformation
  - Relatively rare; incidence considerably lower than that for plexiform neurofibroma
  - Heralded by tumor enlargement and pain

IMAGING

Radiographic Findings

- Discrete, fusiform/ovoid or lobulated mass
- Enlargement of vertebral foramen in "dumbbell" tumors

MR Findings

- Bright signal on T2 image
  - Target sign in most deep tumors and in minority of superficial tumors

MACROSCOPIC

General Features

- Solid, segmental fusiform to ovoid or lobulated intraneural tumor
- Tumor involves single fascicle; other fascicles displaced
- Translucent, gray-white, mucin-rich stroma (early lesions)
- Gray-tan, collagen-rich stroma (older tumors)
- Thin collagenous capsule

Size

- Variable (ranging from < 1 cm to several cm

MICROSCOPIC

Histologic Features

- Low to medium cellularity
  - Cellular forms seen less frequently
- Small Schwann cells with often elongated, curved, or ovoid nuclei; no discernible nucleoli
- Some tumors show degenerative nuclear atypia (atypical neurofibroma subgroup)
  - Large, hyperchromatic nuclei with smudgy chromatin
  - Inconspicuous nucleoli
  - No or low-level mitotic activity
- Stromal mucin (diffuse) &/or collagen bundles ("shredded carrots")
- Occasional hyalinized stroma
- Delicate vasculature; no hyalinized, hemosiderin-associated vessels
- Residual axons dispersed &/or centrally situated in affected fascicle
- Mast cells frequent

ANCILLARY TESTS

Histochemistry

- Alcian blue
  - Variable mucopolysaccharide content
- Trichrome
  - Variable collagen content
- Bielschowsky or Bodian stains label axons
- Luxol fast blue labels residual Schwann sheaths

Immunohistochemistry

- S100 and SOX10: Schwann cells (+)
  - Not all tumoral cells are (+)
- EMA: Perineurial cells in tumor capsule and rare perineurial-like tumor cells (+)
- CD34: Occasional (+) fibroblasts
- NFP: Scant or aligned axons
- Collagen IV: Variable delicate cell surface staining

DIFFERENTIAL DIAGNOSIS

Low-Grade Malignant Peripheral Nerve Sheath Tumor

- Hypercellularity, nuclear enlargement, and hyperchromasia
- Mitoses variable

Schwannoma

- S100, SOX10 diffusely (+)

Nerve Sheath Myxoma

- Multinodularity, abundant mucin

SELECTED REFERENCES

1. Woodruff JM: Pathology of tumors of the peripheral nerve sheath in type 1 neurofibromatosis. Am J Med Genet. 89(1):23-30, 1999
2. Woodruff JM: Pathology of the major peripheral nerve sheath neoplasms. Monogr Pathol. 38:129-61, 1996

(Left) *Intraneural neurofibromas arise from a nerve fascicle and develop into a fusiform lesion. Attempts at total resection may produce neurological deficits if neurologically functioning fascicles are included in the specimen.* **(Right)** *At surgery, uninvolved fascicles should be spared if possible. The tumor can often be resected with negative proximal and distal margins.*

Fusiform Lesion

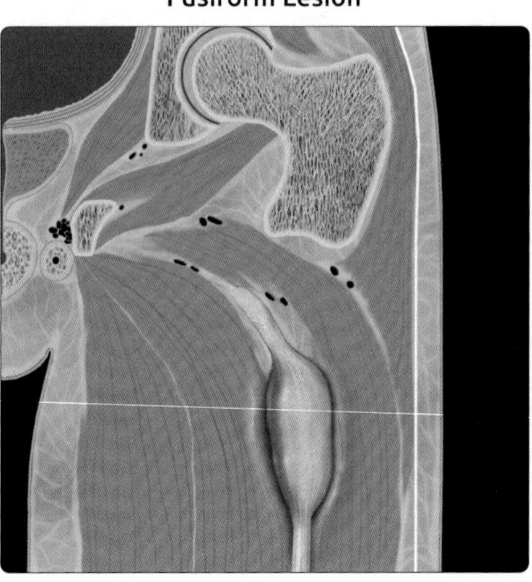

Tumor and Parent Nerve

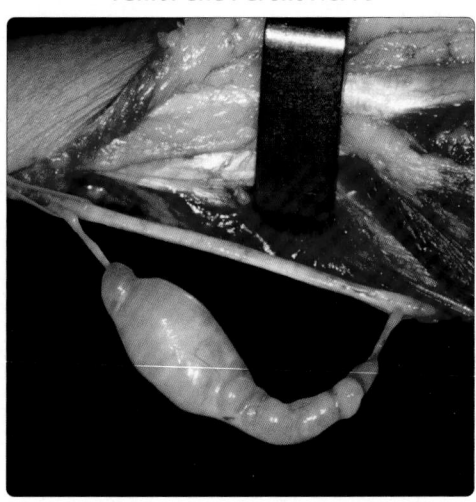

(Left) *Target sign, a mass with low signal intensity centrally and surrounded by high signal intensity ➡, is a characteristic imaging finding of intraneural neurofibromas on T2WI MR.* **(Right)** *When neurofibromas involve large nerves, aligned residual nerve fibers may be observed. Note bundles of residual myelinated axons ⇨ in this tumor stained with Luxol fast blue.*

Target Sign

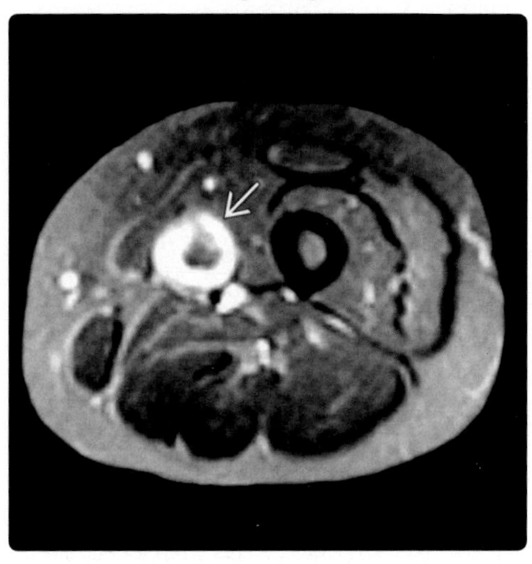

Residual Myelinated Axons

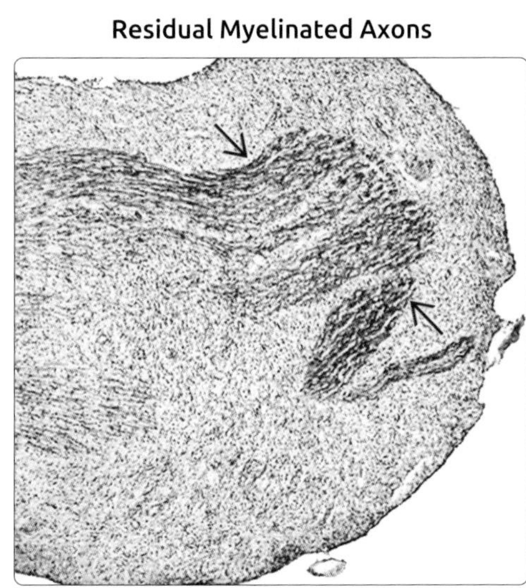

(Left) *Heavy collagen bundles in neurofibromas have been likened to "shredded carrots."* **(Right)** *In early collagen deposition, residual nerve fiber sheaths are more abundant, demonstrated by S100 immunostain.*

"Shredded Carrots"

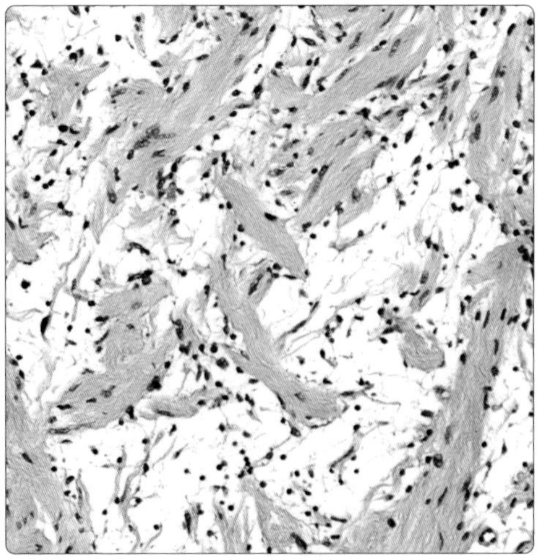

Residual Nerve Fiber Sheaths

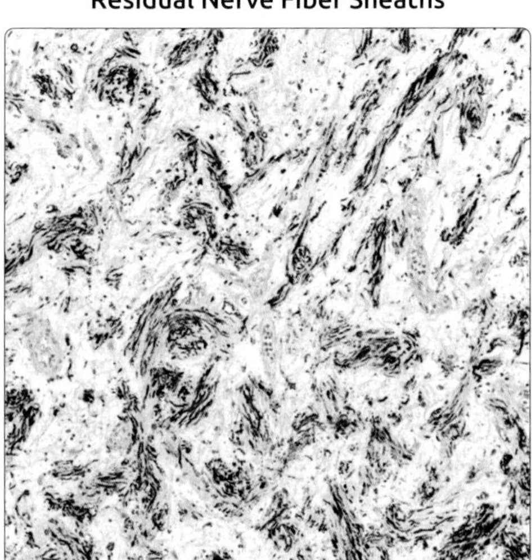

Loose Textured Matrix

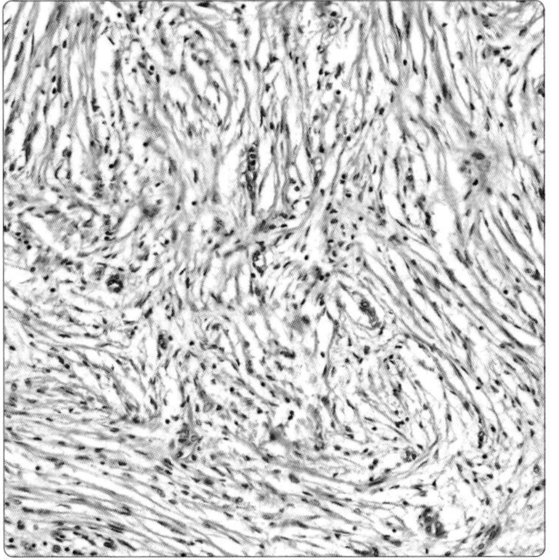

Nerve Sheath Myxoma

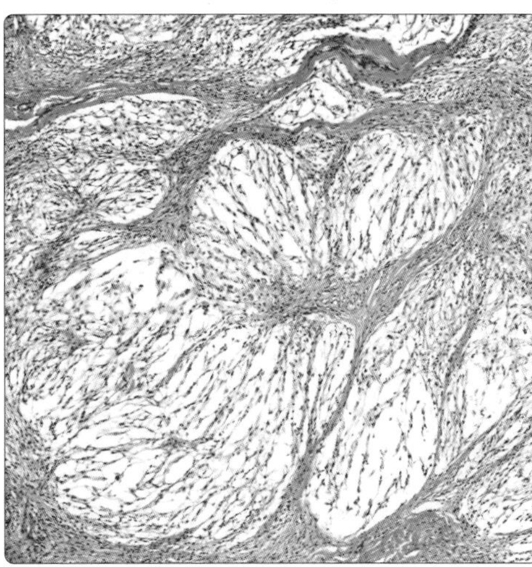

(Left) *The stroma of neurofibroma can be a loose-textured matrix that surrounds the spindle cells.* **(Right)** *Nerve sheath myxomas such as this are differentiated from intraneural neurofibromas by their multinodular architecture and uniform composition of Schwann cells. Unlike neurofibromas, all cells would be S100 positive.*

Small and Curved Cells

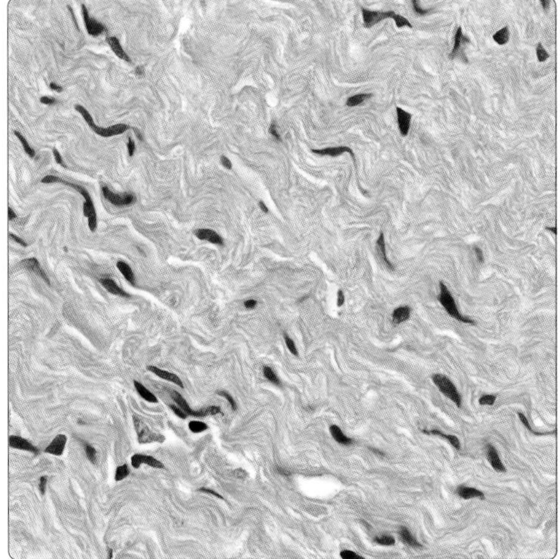

Degenerative Atypia

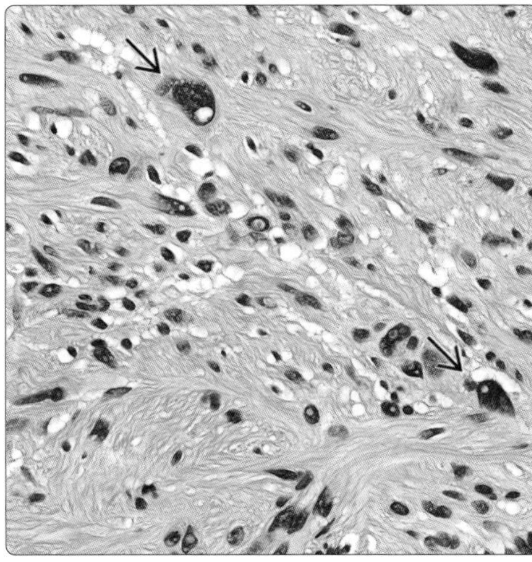

(Left) *Typical neurofibroma cells are small and curved. In older lesions such as this, stroma may be extensively collagenous.* **(Right)** *Nuclei in neurofibromas with degenerative atypia (atypical neurofibroma) are often pleomorphic and have smudgy chromatin. Nuclear pseudoinclusions ⇒ are common.*

Subtotal S100 Protein Staining

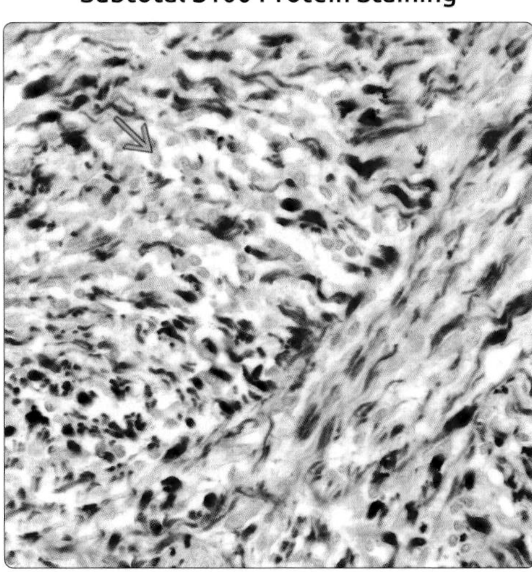

EMA-Positive Perineurial Cells

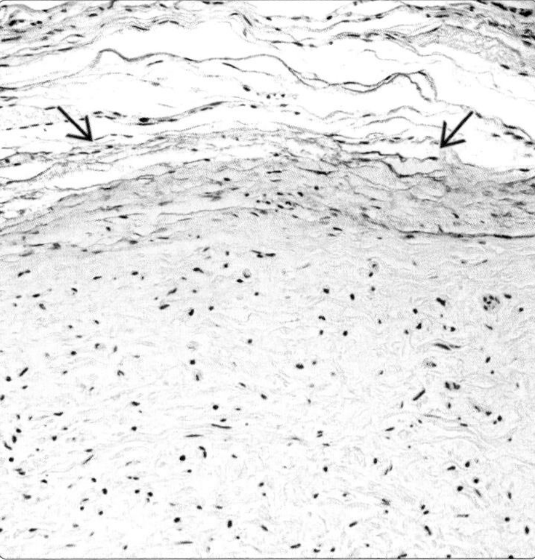

(Left) *Subtotal S100 protein staining characterizes neurofibromas. Unlike schwannomas, not all the tumor cells are S100 immunoreactive ⇒.* **(Right)** *EMA typically stains the perineurial cells ⇒ in the delicate capsule. This tumor is negative.*

TERMINOLOGY

Definitions

- Benign nerve sheath tumor composed of mixture of Schwann, perineurial-like, and fibroblastic cells outside confines of nerve

EPIDEMIOLOGY

Age Range

- Broad (children to adults)

ETIOLOGY/PATHOGENESIS

Associated Syndromes

- Most sporadic, nonsyndrome associated
- Neurofibromatosis type 1 (NF1) association frequent in visceral, multiple cutaneous, and massive soft tissue neurofibromas
- Neurofibromatosis type 2 (NF2) association rare, cutaneous

CLINICAL IMPLICATIONS

Clinical Presentation

- Cutaneous
  - Solitary or multiple nodular to polypoid lesions
  - Diffuse infiltrate, subcutaneous extension
- Massive soft tissue
  - Often limb girdle involvement
- Visceral neurofibromas
  - Most upper gastrointestinal

Imaging Findings

- General Features
  - Circumscribed or infiltrative in soft tissue lesions
  - MR isointense on T1WI, hyperintense on T2WI

MACROSCOPIC

Localized Cutaneous

- Nodular or polypoid, dermal
- Gray-tan cut surface

Diffuse Cutaneous

- Ill-defined, plaque-like thickening of dermis and subcutaneous tissue

Massive Soft Tissue

- Large diffuse tumor
- Often with muscle involvement

Pigmented

- Often, diffuse cutaneous lesion with pigmented, hypertrichosis overlying skin

Dendritic Cell

- Questionably true neurofibroma
- Intradermal
- Oval masses lying perpendicular to epidermis

MICROSCOPIC

General Features

- Schwann cells with elongate, curved, or ovoid nuclei
- Melanin production in Schwann cells (pigmented neurofibroma)
- Pseudomeissnerian &/or Pacinian-like corpuscles
- Mast cells frequent
- Stroma myxoid or collagenous
- Collagen bundles forming "shredded carrots"
- Focal schwannoma-like nodules with nuclear palisading
- Mitosis scant or absent
- No necrosis
- Malignant transformation rare

Atypical Neurofibroma

- Cells with large, pleomorphic nuclei, smudgy chromatin, nuclear-cytoplasmic pseudoinclusions, inconspicuous nucleoli
  - Degenerative changes with no correlation of biological behavior
  - Mitotic activity absent or low

Cellular Neurofibroma

- Focally or diffuse hypercellularity

Multiple Polypoid Lesions

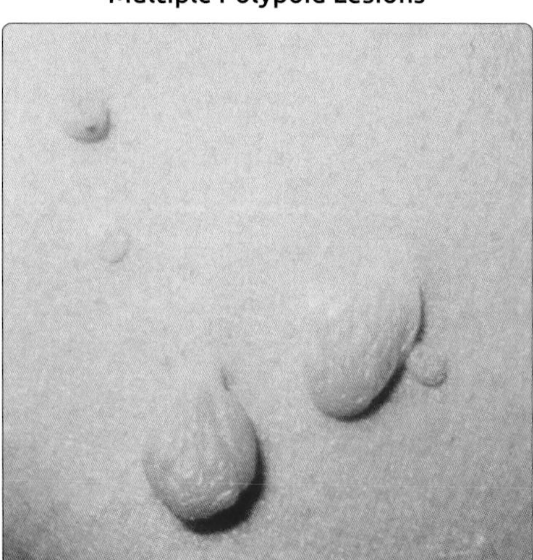

Polypoid Shape

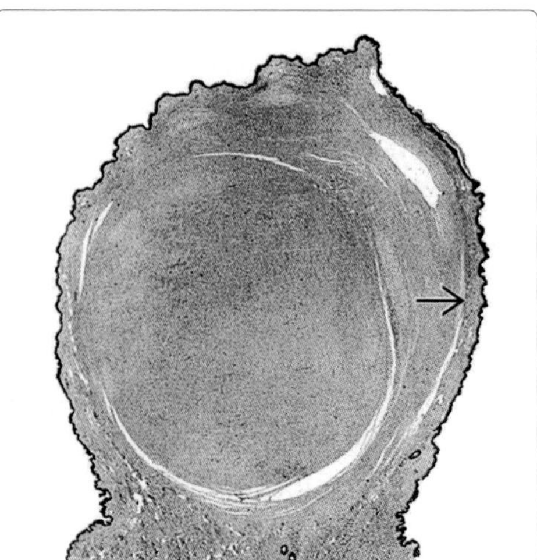

(Left) *Pedunculated cutaneous neurofibromas are multiple polypoid lesions mostly affecting the trunk in neurofibromatosis type 1 (NF1).* **(Right)** *Localized cutaneous neurofibromas are polypoid in shape. There is usually a grenz zone ➙ between the tumor and epidermis.*

- Mitotic activity absent or low

VARIANTS

Localized Cutaneous

- Often separated from epidermis by grenz zone
- Involves dermis and superficial subcutaneous tissue

Diffuse Cutaneous

- Nondestructive
- Permeate dermis and subcutaneous fat
- Cutaneous adnexa entrapped
- Pseudomeissnerian corpuscles frequent
- Minor deep plexiform element (some)

Massive Soft Tissue

- Large, infiltrative of soft tissue and muscle

Pigmented

- Patchy pigmentation
- Pigmented cells dendritic, spindle, or epithelioid

Dendritic Cell

- Multinodular arrangement with 2 cell types
  - Type I
    - Circumferential small, dark, lymphocyte-like
  - Type II
    - Central, larger vesicular nuclei; intranuclear inclusions; eosinophilic cytoplasm; stellate configuration

ANCILLARY TESTS

Immunohistochemistry

- S100 protein (+)
  - Subtotal staining of cells
  - Type I and II cells in dendritic cell variant
- SOX10(+), collagen IV(+)
- Schwann cells EMA(-), some perineurial-like (+)
- CD34(-) variable positivity in nonneoplastic fibroblast component
- Melan-A and HMB-45 both (+) in Schwann cells of pigmented variant
- Ki-67 labeling index very low or (-), p53(-), or rare cells (+)

Electron Microscopy

- Schwann cells with continuous basal lamina
- Perineurial-like cells with pinocytic vesicles, discontinuous basal lamina
- Fibroblasts with abundant rough endoplasmic reticulum, no basal lamina

DIFFERENTIAL DIAGNOSIS

Malignant Peripheral Nerve Sheath Tumor (MPNST)

- Often intraneural
- High cellularity
- Nuclei 3x size of neurofibroma cells
- Nuclear hyperchromasia
- High mitotic index (often), but mitotic activity not required for low-grade MPNST diagnosis
- Necrosis common
- p53(+)

Schwannoma

- Uniformly S100(+), SOX10(+)
- Thick perineurial capsule EMA(+)
- Collagenous vessels
- Occasional axons

Spindle Cell Lipoma

- Spindle cells CD34(+)
- S100(-)

Congenital or Neurotized Nevi

- Diffuse S100(+), SOX10(+)
- Nevoid architecture

Nerve Sheath Myxoma

- Lobular architecture
- Diffusely S100(+), SOX10(+)
- High mucin content

Dermatofibrosarcoma Protuberans and Bednar Tumor

- Storiform pattern
- CD34(+) uniform
- S100(-)

Desmoplastic Melanoma

- In situ element
- Large hyperchromatic cells
- Usually CD34(-)

SELECTED REFERENCES

1. Schaefer IM et al: Malignant peripheral nerve sheath tumor (MPNST) arising in diffuse-type neurofibroma: clinicopathologic characterization in a series of 9 cases. Am J Surg Pathol. ePub, 2015
2. Yeh I et al: Distinguishing neurofibroma from desmoplastic melanoma: the value of the CD34 fingerprint. J Cutan Pathol. 38(8):625-30, 2011
3. Michal M et al: Dendritic cell neurofibroma with pseudorosettes: a report of 18 cases of a distinct and hitherto unrecognized neurofibroma variant. Am J Surg Pathol. 25(5):587-94, 2001
4. Fetsch JF et al: Pigmented (melanotic) neurofibroma: a clinicopathologic and immunohistochemical analysis of 19 lesions from 17 patients. Am J Surg Pathol. 24(3):331-43, 2000
5. Khalifa MA et al: What are the CD34+ cells in benign peripheral nerve sheath tumors? Double immunostaining study of CD34 and S-100 protein. Am J Clin Pathol. 114(1):123-6, 2000
6. Lin BT et al: Neurofibroma and cellular neurofibroma with atypia: a report of 14 tumors. Am J Surg Pathol. 21(12):1443-9, 1997
7. Skuse GR et al: The neurofibroma in von Recklinghausen neurofibromatosis has a unicellular origin. Am J Hum Genet. 49(3):600-7, 1991
8. Theaker JM et al: Epithelial membrane antigen expression by the perineurial cell: further studies of peripheral nerve lesions. Histopathology. 14(6):581-92, 1989
9. Erlandson RA et al: Peripheral nerve sheath tumors: an electron microscopic study of 43 cases. Cancer. 49(2):273-87, 1982
10. Smith TW et al: Tactile-like structures in neurofibromas. An ultrastructural study. Acta Neuropathol. 50(3):233-6, 1980

(Left) *Cutaneous neurofibromas may be diffuse and occupy all of a localized lesion.* **(Right)** *A dermal neurofibroma is composed of bland spindle cells with curved or elongate nuclei.*

Diffuse Pattern

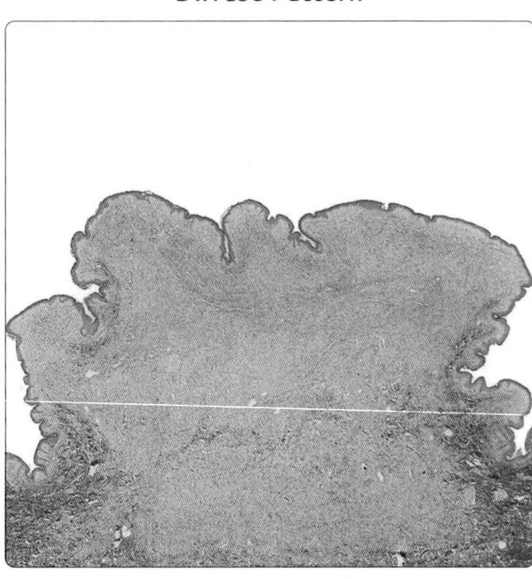

Bland Spindle Cells

(Left) *Diffuse cutaneous neurofibromas are seen as thickened brawny lesions.* **(Right)** *Diffuse cutaneous neurofibromas on a cut section show involvement of subcutaneous tissue.*

Thickened Brawny Lesion

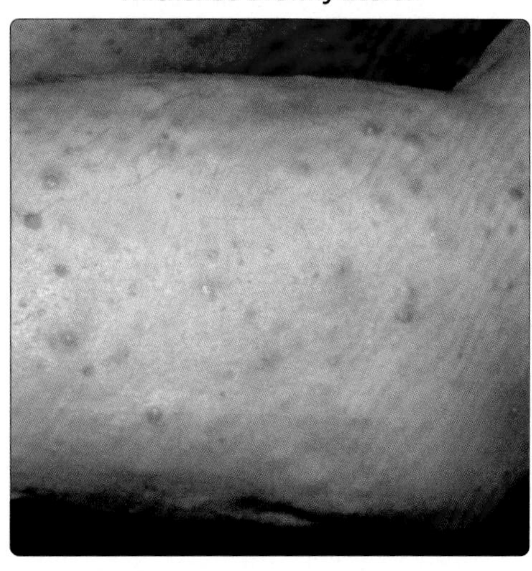

Subcutaneous Tissue Involvement

(Left) *Neurofibromas of a cutaneous type leave a grenz zone* → *between the epidermis and the involved dermis.* **(Right)** *Dermal neurofibromas overrun the skin adnexa. Note the entrapped adnexa* →.

Grenz Zone

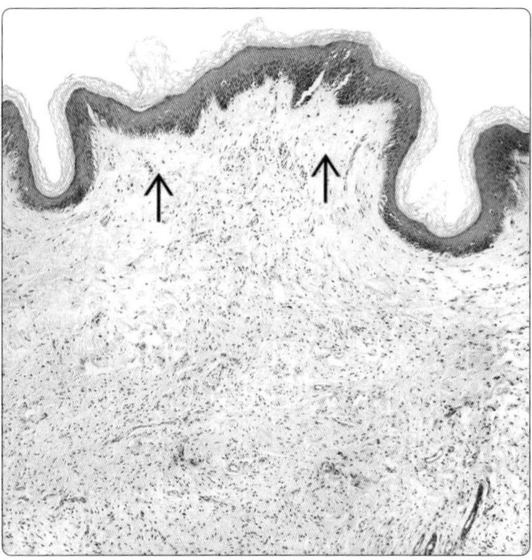

Entrapped Adnexa

Dermal and Subcutaneous Involvement

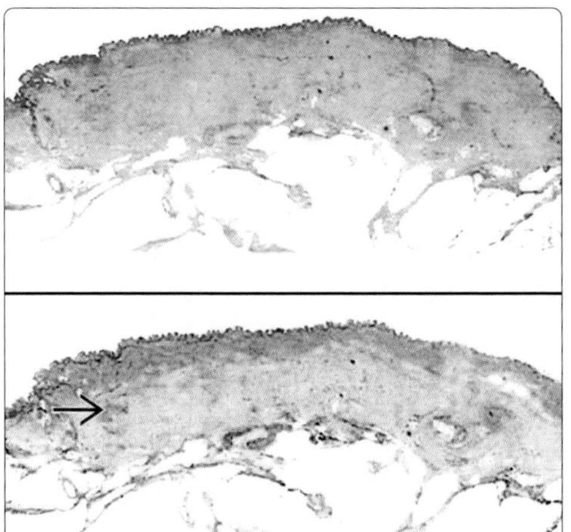

Infiltration of Subcutaneous Fat

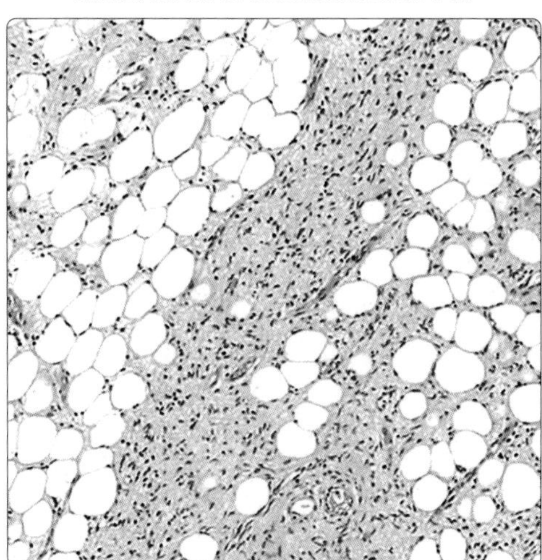

(Left) *Diffuse cutaneous neurofibromas involve the dermis and subcutaneous tissues. The thickness seen in this example is more apparent on a trichrome stain* ⇨. **(Right)** *Infiltration of subcutaneous fat is a conspicuous feature of diffuse cutaneous neurofibromas. This lesion extends through septa and also intercellular spaces.*

Café Au Lait Pigmentation

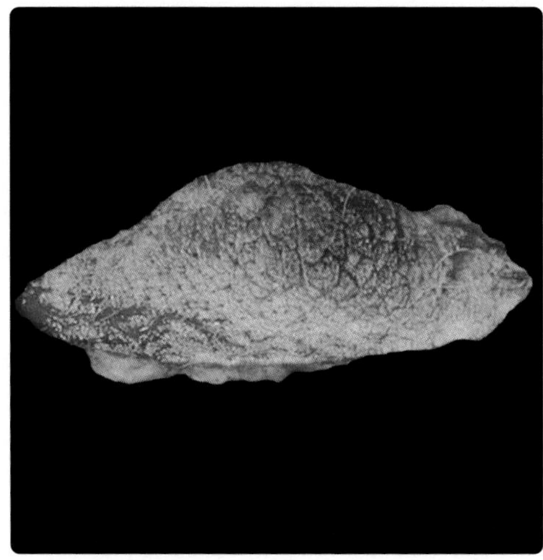

Pigmented Schwann Cells

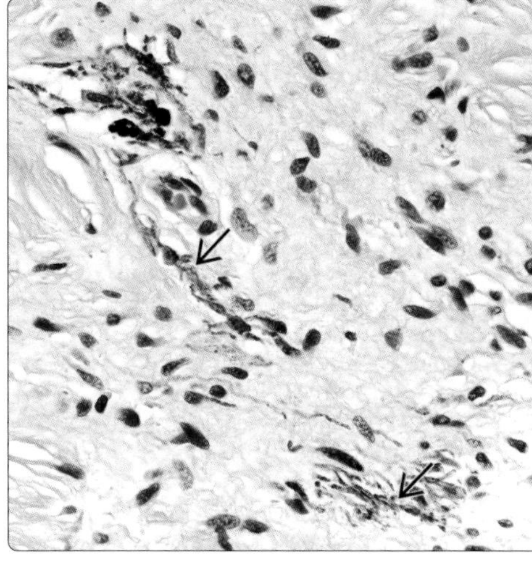

(Left) *Skin overlying pigmented neurofibromas may show café au lait type pigmentation and hypertrichosis.* **(Right)** *Schwann cells in a pigmented neurofibroma* ⇨ *are spindle-shaped. They may also be epithelioid. Pigmentation is found focally throughout the lesion.*

Pseudorosettes

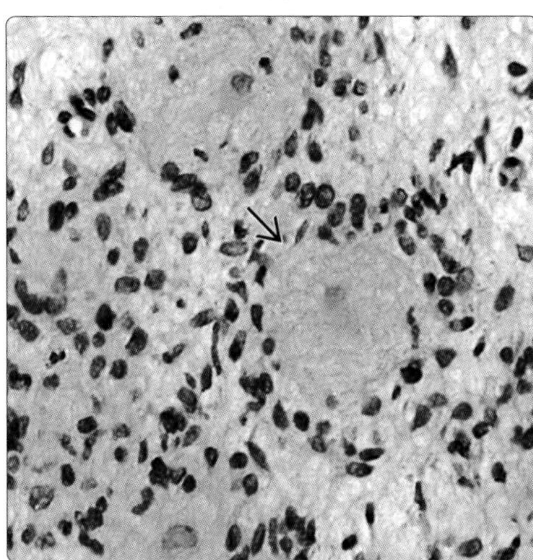

S100(+) Type II Cells

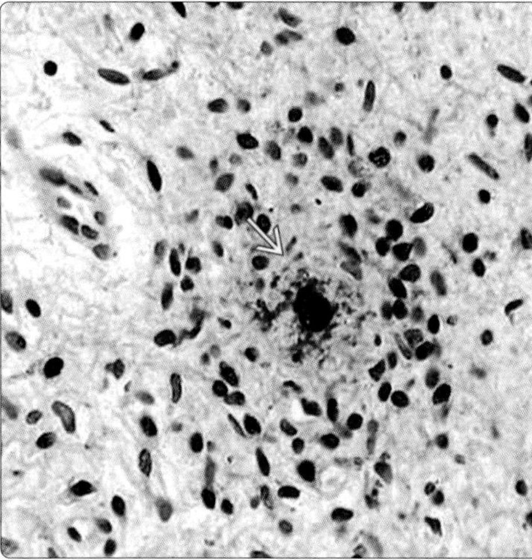

(Left) *So-called "dendritic cell neurofibromas" have pseudorosettes formed of small, dark, lymphocyte-like (type I) cells arranged concentrically around larger type II cells, with pale-staining, vesicular nuclei and eosinophilic cytoplasm* ⇨. **(Right)** *Type II cells in dendritic cell neurofibroma show strong immunoreactivity for S100 protein* ➡. *Note the positivity of type I cells as well.*

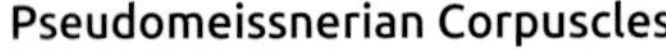

Pseudomeissnerian Corpuscles

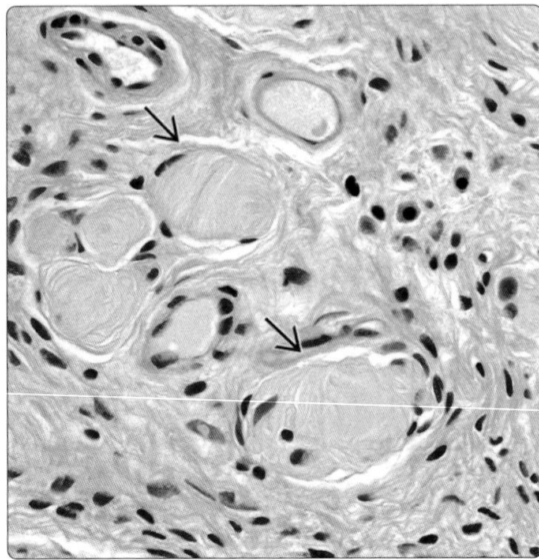

Pseudomeissnerian Corpuscles

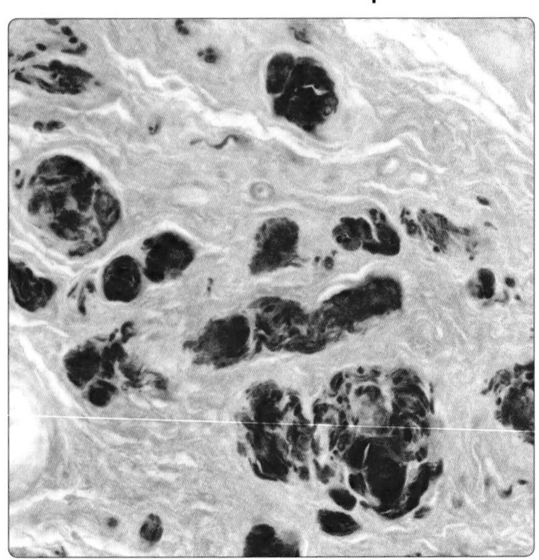

(Left) *Neurofibromas may have pseudomeissnerian corpuscles ⇨. Such corpuscles, as well as whorls resembling Pacinian corpuscles, are considered examples of tactile differentiation.* **(Right)** *Pseudomeissnerian corpuscles are S100 immunoreactive.*

Whorls

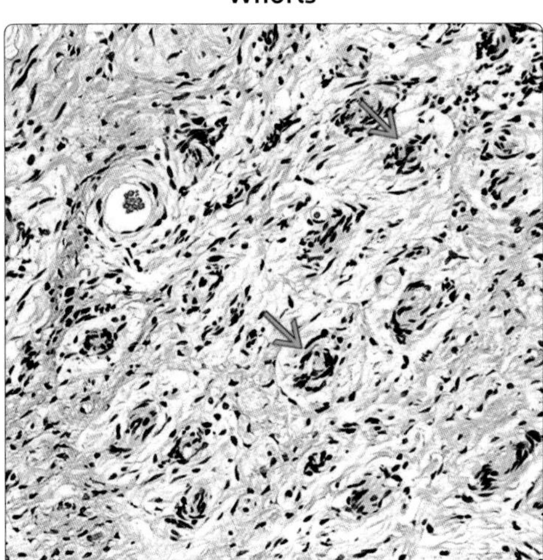

S100 Immunoreactivity

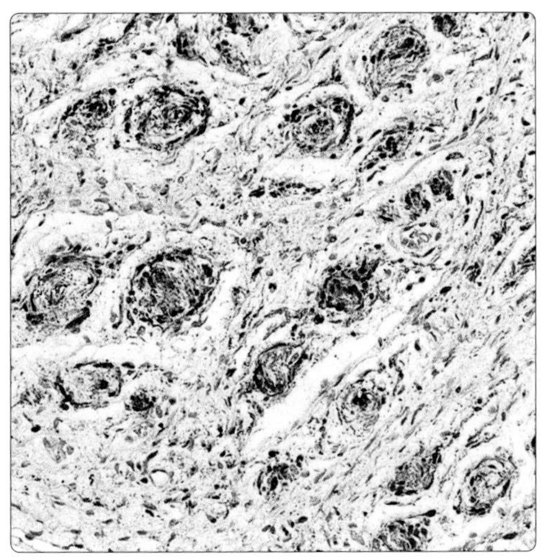

(Left) *Whorls ⇨ reminiscent of true onion bulbs of localized hypertrophic neuropathy are uncommon features of neurofibroma.* **(Right)** *S100 protein immunoreactivity shows the schwannian nature of the cells forming whorls in a neurofibroma. Neurofilament protein stains may show a central axon.*

Soft Tissue and Muscle Infiltration

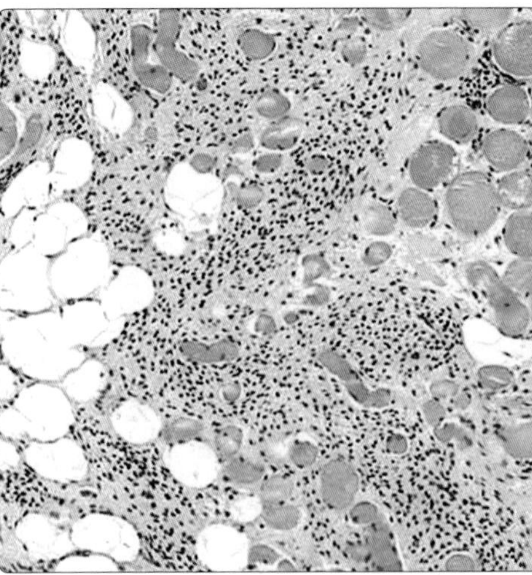

Hypercellularity

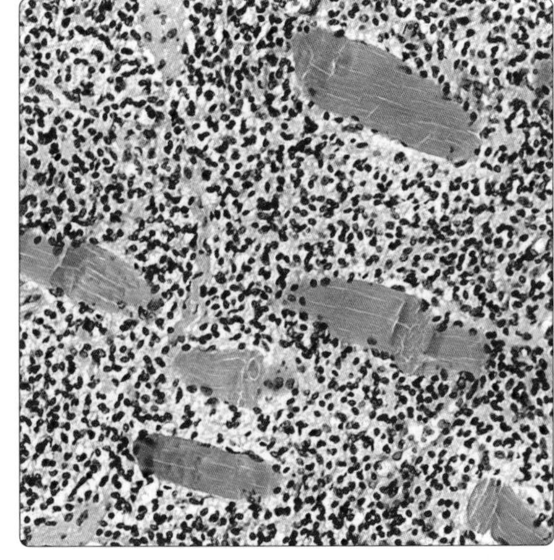

(Left) *Massive soft tissue neurofibromas infiltrate surrounding adipose tissue and muscle.* **(Right)** *Hypercellularity and infiltration in massive soft tissue neurofibromas should not be misinterpreted as evidence of malignancy.*

Thin-Walled Blood Vessels

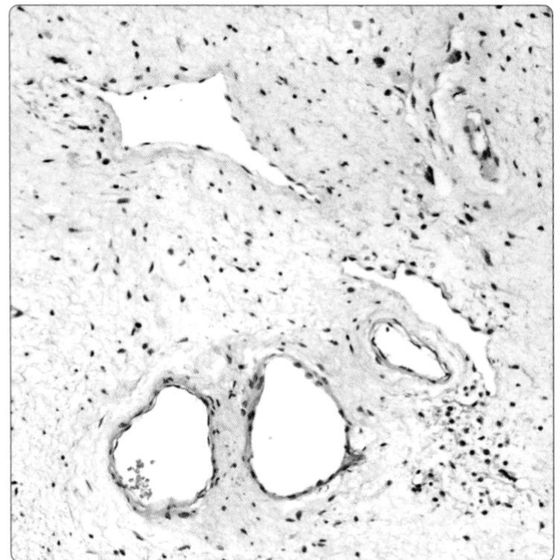

Mast Cells

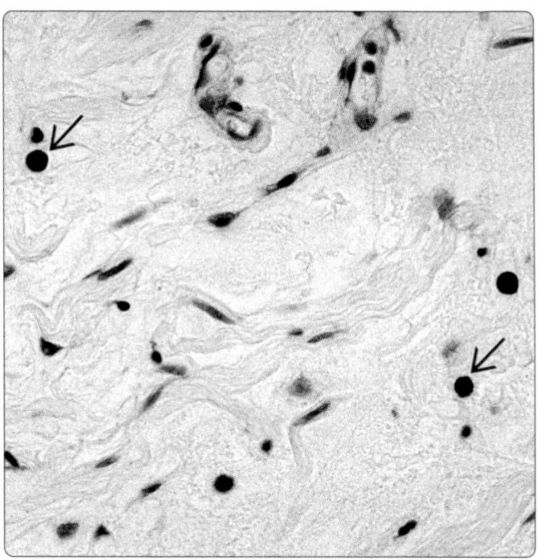

(Left) *Neurofibromas feature thin-walled blood vessels that should be contrasted with the hyalinized vasculature that is typical of schwannoma.* **(Right)** *A toluidine blue stain highlights frequent mast cells ➙ in neurofibromas of all types.*

Cellular Crowding

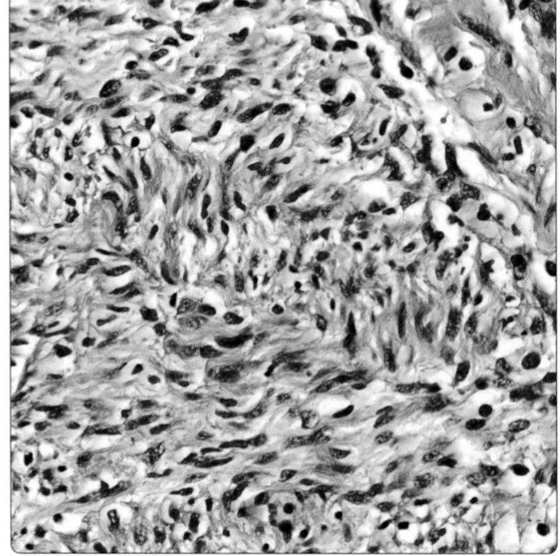

Pleomorphic Nuclei

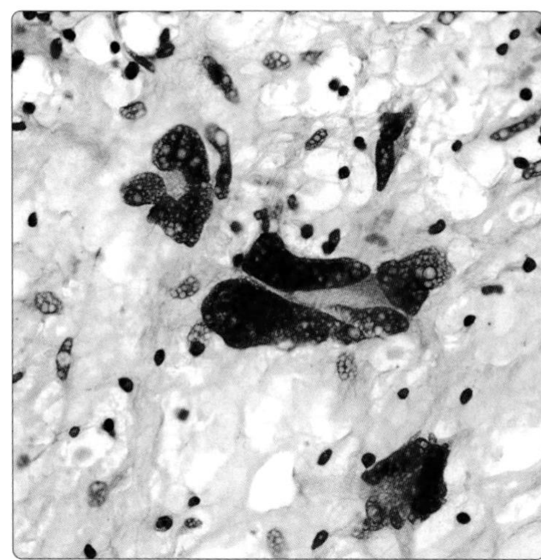

(Left) *Cellular neurofibromas show cellular crowding but no significant cellular enlargement and only minor hyperchromasia. Note the lack of mitotic activity.* **(Right)** *Atypical neurofibromas have pleomorphic, large nuclei and smudgy chromatin. Nucleoli are inconspicuous. Such cells lack proliferative activity.*

Subtotal S100 Immunostaining

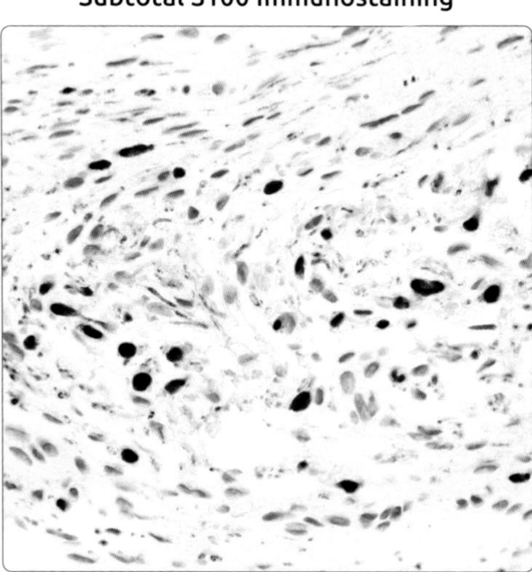

Perineurial-Like Cells

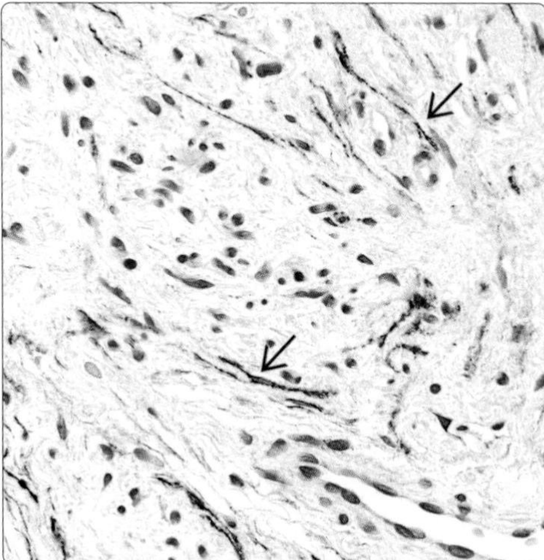

(Left) *Subtotal S100 immunostaining is an important diagnostic feature of neurofibromas. Not all cells are positive.* **(Right)** *EMA immunopositivity, which is not a frequent finding in neurofibromas, reflects the presence of tumoral perineurial-like cells ➙.*

Malignant Peripheral Nerve Sheath Tumor

KEY FACTS

TERMINOLOGY

- Malignant neoplasm originating from, or demonstrating differentiation toward, nerve sheath elements

ETIOLOGY/PATHOGENESIS

- Ionizing radiation
- 2-3% of patients with NF1 have MPNST
- 50% of MPNST occur in NF1

CLINICAL ISSUES

- Young adults; rarely pediatric
- Buttock, thigh, brachial plexus, upper arm, paraspinal

IMAGING

- Infiltrative, heterogeneously enhancing mass

MACROSCOPIC

- Surrounded by pseudocapsule
- Majority > 5 cm

MICROSCOPIC

- Pattern and cytologic variation
- Mitoses high (usually > 4/10 HPF)
- Geographic necrosis ± pseudopalisading
- Heterologous elements (10% of cases)
  - Epithelial glandular, squamous, neuroendocrine, rhabdomyoblastic, cartilage, bone

ANCILLARY TESTS

- S100, CD57(+); EMA(+) with perineurial differentiation
- SOX10(+) frequent but not uniform

TOP DIFFERENTIAL DIAGNOSES

- Neurofibroma
- Cellular schwannoma
- Fibrosarcoma
- Synovial sarcoma

MPNST Nerve Association

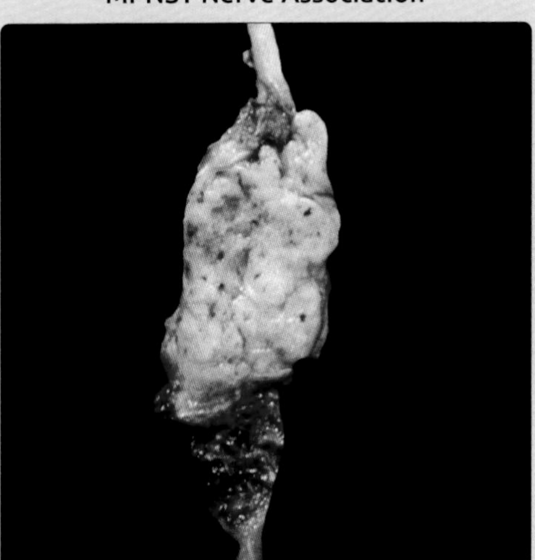

Herringbone Pattern

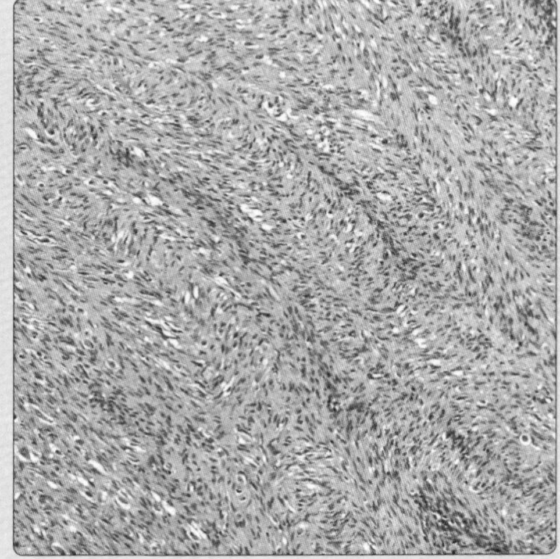

(Left) *Malignant peripheral nerve sheath tumor (MPNSTs) usually arise within large nerves, most commonly the sciatic. The tumor typically has irregular borders with surrounding tissue.* **(Right)** *A herringbone pattern is not uncommon in MPNST, which provides a close resemblance to fibrosarcoma.*

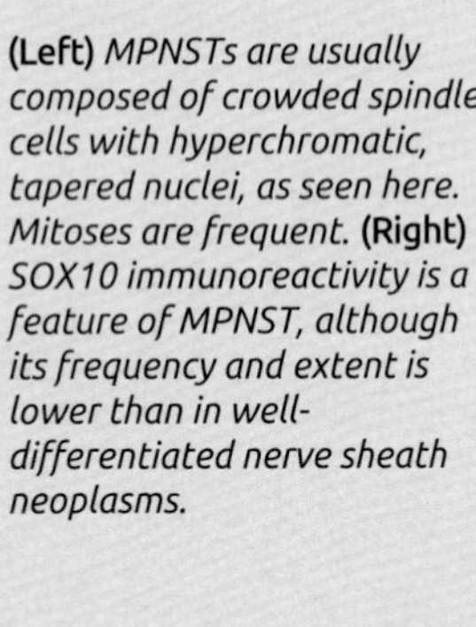

(Left) *MPNSTs are usually composed of crowded spindle cells with hyperchromatic, tapered nuclei, as seen here. Mitoses are frequent.* **(Right)** *SOX10 immunoreactivity is a feature of MPNST, although its frequency and extent is lower than in well-differentiated nerve sheath neoplasms.*

Spindle Cells in MPNST

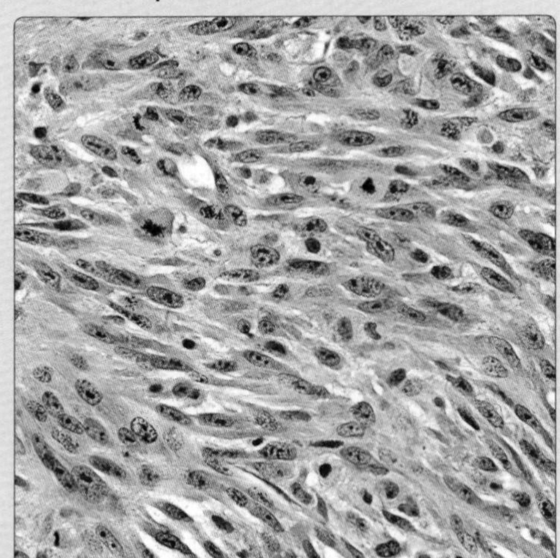

SOX10 Immunoreactivity in MPNST

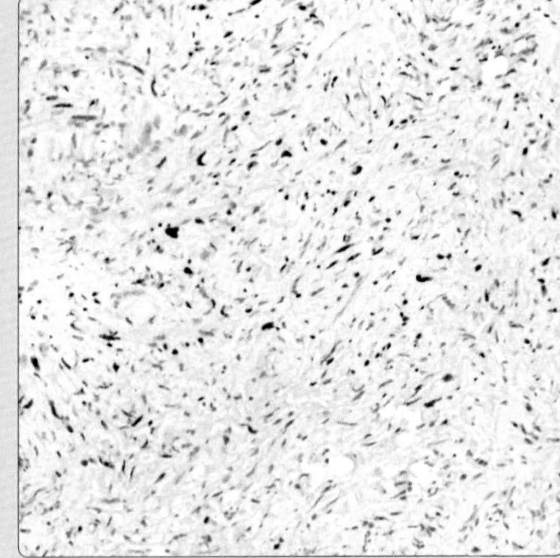

TERMINOLOGY

Abbreviations

- Malignant peripheral nerve sheath tumor (MPNST)

Synonyms

- Antiquated terms
  - Neurogenic sarcoma
  - Neurofibrosarcoma
  - Malignant schwannoma

Definitions

- Malignant tumor of nerve sheath elements (Schwann or perineurial cell differentiation)
  - Originating in nerve
  - Arising in transition from benign peripheral nerve sheath tumor (neurofibroma much more common than schwannoma) or de novo
  - Arising in transition from other neuroectodermal tumors (ganglioneuroma/ganglioneuroblastoma or pheochromocytoma)
  - Developing in setting of neurofibromatosis type 1 (NF1) (von Recklinghausen disease)
  - Developing sporadically, unassociated with nerve or precursor but with histologic, immunohistochemical, &/or ultrastructural features of MPNST

ETIOLOGY/PATHOGENESIS

Radiation

- Ionizing radiation underlies ~ 10% of MPNST
  - Reported mean latency: 15-18 years

Chemical Carcinogens

- No apparent association

Associated Syndromes

- ~ 50% of MPNST occur in NF1
- 2-3% of patients with NF1 develop MPNST
- All reported multiple MPNSTs occur in NF1

CLINICAL ISSUES

Epidemiology

- Incidence
  - 0.0001% of general population
  - ~ 5% of all soft tissue tumors
- Age
  - Adulthood (20-50 years)
    - Mean age
      - Sporadic tumors 40-44 years
    - Mean age
      - NF1-associated tumors 20-35 years
  - Pediatric tumors (rare)
    - NF1 associated in 50-60%
- Sex
  - Slight female predominance

Site

- Large and medium-sized nerves
  - Sciatic most frequently affected
- Common sites include
  - Buttock
  - Thigh
  - Brachial plexus
  - Upper arm
  - Paraspinal
- Cranial nerves and visceral examples rare

Presentation

- Rapidly growing mass
- Pain, motor weakness, sensory loss
- Sudden enlargement of preexisting neurofibroma

Treatment

- Surgical approaches
  - Wide en bloc resection
- Adjuvant therapy
  - No effective chemotherapeutic regimen
- Radiation
  - Retards and reduces incidence of local recurrence

Prognosis

- Recurrence frequent (40-70%)
- Overall rate of metastasis: 30-45%
  - Higher at particular sites
    - Buttock
    - Lower extremity
    - Paraspinal
  - Higher in NF1 patients
- Common metastatic sites include
  - Lung
  - Bone
  - Pleura
  - Soft tissue
  - Liver
  - Brain
- ~ 70% die of tumor
- 5-year survival rate
  - 53-50%
- 10-year survival rate
  - ~ 30%

IMAGING

General Features

- Large, infiltrative, heterogeneous (viable/necrotic) mass

MR Findings

- Architecture best seen in longitudinal axis
- T1 with contrast
  - Marked enhancement
- T1WI
  - Isointense compared to muscle
- T2WI
  - Hyperintense compared to fat

CT Findings

- Soft tissue mass hypodense to muscle
- Heterogeneous areas corresponding to hemorrhage and necrosis

MACROSCOPIC

General Features

- Tumors involving a nerve
  - Fusiform
- Tumors unassociated with nerve
  - Globoid
- Arising from neurofibroma
  - Intraneural, plexiform neurofibroma or diffuse (rare)
    - MPNST often focal; multiple sections recommended
- Cut surface firm, gray-tan
- Pseudocapsule
- Necrosis and hemorrhage common

Size

- Majority > 5 cm

MICROSCOPIC

Histologic Features

- Associated nerve or neurofibroma (50%)
- Hypercellular, mainly spindle cells
- Herringbone, storiform, tissue culture-like patterns
- Fibrous or myxoid stroma
- Nuclear palisading (rare)
- Hyperchromatic, crowded nuclei; mitoses (usually > 4/10 HPF)
- Geographic necrosis ± pseudopalisading
- Perivascular aggregation of viable tumor cells
- Multinucleated, large, pleomorphic cells (occasional)
- Malignant heterologous elements in 10% of cases
  - Skeletal muscle, smooth muscle, cartilage, bone
  - Epithelial glandular, squamous, neuroendocrine
- Histologic variants
  - MPNST with epithelial differentiation
  - MPNST with rhabdomyoblastic (Triton tumor) or osteocartilaginous differentiation
  - MPNST with angiosarcoma
  - Epithelioid MPNST
    - Distinctive variant of MPNST usually arising in superficial sites
    - Usually not NF1 associated
    - Round or polygonal cells with voluminous cytoplasm, well-defined borders, vesicular nuclei, and macronucleoli
    - Multilobular growth pattern
    - 1 of morphologic forms of MPNST developing in schwannoma
    - Strong expression of schwannian markers (unlike conventional MPNST), including S100, SOX10, collagen IV
    - INI1 loss in subset
  - MPNST with perineurial differentiation
    - Whorl formation characteristic
    - EMA expression
- Low-grade tumors: Less cellular, lower mitotic activity, no necrosis
  - Cell crowding, nuclear enlargement, hyperchromasia are essential diagnostic features
- MPNST ex-schwannoma rare
  - Usually in form of epithelioid change, primitive round blue cell tumor, or angiosarcoma

ANCILLARY TESTS

Cytology

- Highly varied, none diagnostic

Immunohistochemistry

- S100 and CD57 (+) both about 1/2, may be focal
- SOX10 (+) frequent but not positive in all tumors and usually positive in subset of tumor cells
- Collagen IV variably (+); negative in high-grade examples
- EMA(+) with perineurial differentiation
- NFP identifies associated axons, if any
- TLE1 weak and focal positivity
- Desmin (+) with rhabdomyoblastic differentiation
- Cytokeratin, CEA (+) with glandular differentiation
- Chromogranin (+) with neuroendocrine differentiation
- Ki-67 labeling index: Moderate to high
- p53(+), p27 often (-)
- Loss of neurofibromin reactivity using specific antibody helps differentiate from similar spindle cell neoplasms
- EGFR immunoreactivity and p16 loss frequent

Flow Cytometry

- Aneuploidy common

In Situ Hybridization

- CDKN2A deletion may be helpful in identifying early transition to MPNST in neurofibromas
- EGFR amplification in subset

Genetic Testing

- Frequent inactivating mutations in components of polycomb repressive complex (PRC2), *EED*, or *SUZ12*, in majority of cases
  - Mutations results in loss of histone H3 lysine 27 trimethylation (H3K27me3)
- Frequent alterations in *CDKN2A* and NF1 tumor suppressors
- *BRAF* (V600E) mutation present in subset of sporadic MPNST (up to 20%), but very rare in NF1-associated MPNST

Electron Microscopy

- Variable differentiation (basal lamina) or undifferentiated cells

DIFFERENTIAL DIAGNOSIS

Cellular Neurofibroma

- Small cells, 1/3 size of MPNST
- Mitotic indices usually not higher than 4/10 HPF
- No necrosis

Atypical Neurofibroma

- Degenerative atypia (bizarre giant cells) with nuclear pseudoinclusions; smudgy chromatin
- Mitotic activity usually not higher than 4/10 HPF
- No necrosis

Cellular Schwannoma

- Collagenous capsule and vessels
- Antoni A tissue dominant

- Collagen IV and S100 diffusely (+)
- Neurofibromin usually preserved
- No gross necrosis

Perineurioma

- Bland nuclear features
- Few or scant mitoses
- Elongate narrow processes
- EMA(+), collagen IV (+); S100(-)

Fibrosarcoma

- S100(-)
- Lack of nerve association

Leiomyosarcoma

- SMA(+), desmin (+)
- S100 only minor positivity

Synovial Sarcoma

- *SS18-SSX1* or *SS18-SSX2* gene fusions usually resulting from t(X;18) translocation
- TLE1 diffuse, strong nuclear positivity; minor S100 positivity (20%)
- Keratin and EMA (+) in 20%

Epithelioid Sarcoma

- EMA(+), keratin (+), S100(-)
- INI1 loss of nuclear staining

Gastrointestinal Stromal Tumor

- KIT(+)

Ossifying Fibromyxoid Tumor of Soft Parts

- Shares S100 expression with Schwann cell neoplasms
- Usually develop in superficial locations
- Peripheral bony shell in most cases
- Desmin expression in subset
- Mosaic pattern of INI1 loss

Irradiation-Induced Atypia in Normal Nerve

- No proliferative activity

DIAGNOSTIC CHECKLIST

Clinically Relevant Pathologic Features

- Always think of MPNST when encountering cellular spindle cell neoplasms in patients with NF1
- Sudden enlargement or pain in large NF1-associated neurofibroma is always alarming clinical sign

Pathologic Interpretation Pearls

- Important to sample large/plexiform neurofibromas since malignant change may be focal and difficult to recognize
- Partial S100 expression in cellular Schwann cell neoplasm is characteristic

SELECTED REFERENCES

1. Jo VY et al: Epithelioid Malignant Peripheral Nerve Sheath Tumor: Clinicopathologic Analysis of 63 Cases. Am J Surg Pathol. ePub, 2015
2. Schaefer IM et al: Malignant Peripheral Nerve Sheath Tumor (MPNST) Arising in Diffuse-type Neurofibroma: Clinicopathologic Characterization in a Series of 9 Cases. Am J Surg Pathol. ePub, 2015
3. Hirbe AC et al: BRAFV600E mutation in sporadic and neurofibromatosis type 1-related malignant peripheral nerve sheath tumors. Neuro Oncol. 16(3):466-7, 2014
4. Lee W et al: PRC2 is recurrently inactivated through EED or SUZ12 loss in malignant peripheral nerve sheath tumors. Nat Genet. 46(11):1227-32, 2014
5. Pekmezci M et al: Morphologic and immunohistochemical features of malignant peripheral nerve sheath tumors and cellular schwannomas. Mod Pathol. ePub, 2014
6. Reuss DE et al: Neurofibromin specific antibody differentiates malignant peripheral nerve sheath tumors (MPNST) from other spindle cell neoplasms. Acta Neuropathol. 127(4):565-72, 2014
7. Zhang M et al: Somatic mutations of SUZ12 in malignant peripheral nerve sheath tumors. Nat Genet. 46(11):1170-2, 2014
8. Beert E et al: Atypical neurofibromas in neurofibromatosis type 1 are premalignant tumors. Genes Chromosomes Cancer. 50(12):1021-32, 2011
9. Kosemehmetoglu K et al: TLE1 expression is not specific for synovial sarcoma: a whole section study of 163 soft tissue and bone neoplasms. Mod Pathol. 22(7):872-8, 2009
10. Scheithauer BW et al: Malignant peripheral nerve sheath tumors of cranial nerves and intracranial contents: a clinicopathologic study of 17 cases. Am J Surg Pathol. 33(3):325-38, 2009
11. Woodruff JM et al: Congenital and childhood plexiform (multinodular) cellular schwannoma: a troublesome mimic of malignant peripheral nerve sheath tumor. Am J Surg Pathol. 27(10):1321-9, 2003
12. Rosenberg AS et al: Malignant peripheral nerve sheath tumor with perineurial differentiation: "malignant perineurioma". J Cutan Pathol. 29(6):362-7, 2002
13. Hirose T et al: Perineurial malignant peripheral nerve sheath tumor (MPNST): a clinicopathologic, immunohistochemical, and ultrastructural study of seven cases. Am J Surg Pathol. 22(11):1368-78, 1998
14. Wong WW et al: Malignant peripheral nerve sheath tumor: analysis of treatment outcome. Int J Radiat Oncol Biol Phys. 42(2):351-60, 1998
15. Woodruff JM: Pathology of the major peripheral nerve sheath neoplasms. Monogr Pathol. 38:129-61, 1996
16. Vauthey JN et al: Extremity malignant peripheral nerve sheath tumors (neurogenic sarcomas): a 10-year experience. Ann Surg Oncol. 2(2):126-31, 1995
17. Woodruff JM et al: Nerve sheath tumors. Am J Surg Pathol. 19(5):608-11, 1995
18. Woodruff JM et al: Glandular peripheral nerve sheath tumors. Cancer. 72(12):3618-28, 1993
19. Hruban RH et al: Malignant peripheral nerve sheath tumors of the buttock and lower extremity. A study of 43 cases. Cancer. 66(6):1253-65, 1990
20. Christensen WN et al: Neuroendocrine differentiation in the glandular peripheral nerve sheath tumor. Pathologic distinction from the biphasic synovial sarcoma with glands. Am J Surg Pathol. 12(6):417-26, 1988
21. Wick MR et al: Malignant peripheral nerve sheath tumor. An immunohistochemical study of 62 cases. Am J Clin Pathol. 87(4):425-33, 1987
22. DiCarlo EF et al: The purely epithelioid malignant peripheral nerve sheath tumor. Am J Surg Pathol. 10(7):478-90, 1986
23. Ducatman BS et al: Malignant peripheral nerve sheath tumors. A clinicopathologic study of 120 cases. Cancer. 57(10):2006-21, 1986
24. Debruyne FM et al: Results of a Dutch Phase II trial with the LHRH agonist buserelin in patients with metastatic prostatic cancer. Prog Clin Biol Res. 185A:251-70, 1985
25. Ducatman BS et al: Malignant peripheral nerve sheath tumors with divergent differentiation. Cancer. 54(6):1049-57, 1984
26. Ricci A Jr et al: Malignant peripheral nerve sheath tumors arising from ganglioneuromas. Am J Surg Pathol. 8(1):19-29, 1984
27. Ducatman BS et al: Postirradiation neurofibrosarcoma. Cancer. 51(6):1028-33, 1983
28. Foley KM et al: Radiation-induced malignant and atypical peripheral nerve sheath tumors. Ann Neurol. 7(4):311-8, 1980

(Left) *Coronal T1 C+ MR shows an enhancing mass ➔ in the right medial thigh. Central nonenhancing areas are consistent with necrosis in this rapidly growing lesion.* **(Right)** *NF1 patients are prone to MPNST, as seen in this mass ➔ originating in the flank region. Note generalized hyperpigmentation and café au lait spots ➔.*

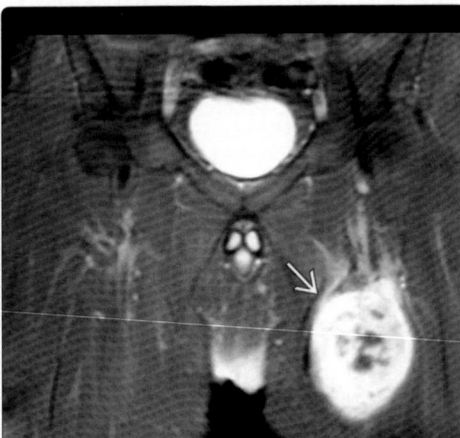

MR Image Findings

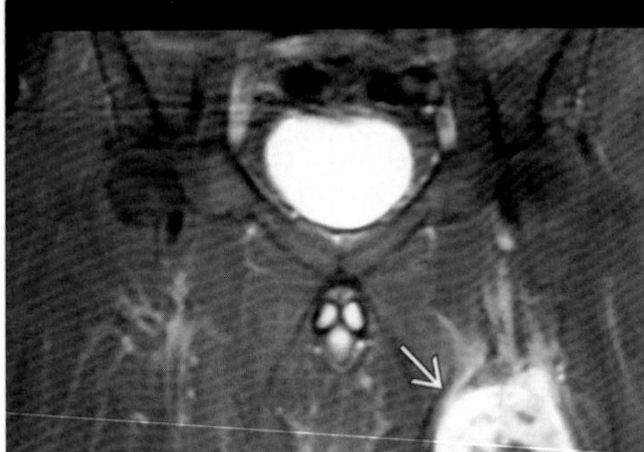

NF1 Association

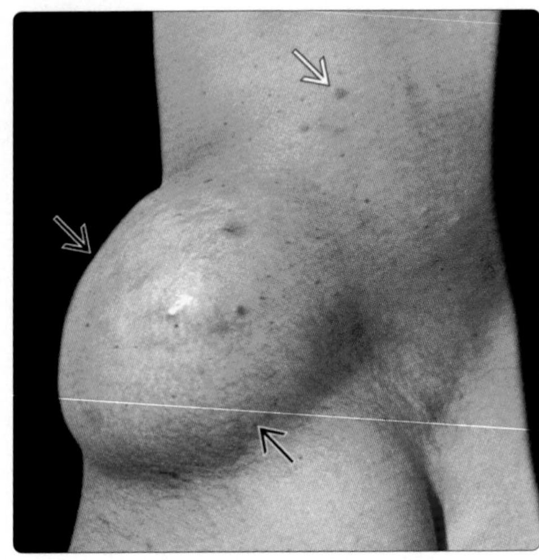

(Left) *As shown here, MPNST may have a pseudocapsule ➔ formed by reactive fibrosis that is admixed with tumor.* **(Right)** *Cut surfaces of MPNSTs are heterogeneous in appearance due to hemorrhage and necrosis, as seen in this highly cellular fleshy mass.*

Pseudocapsule

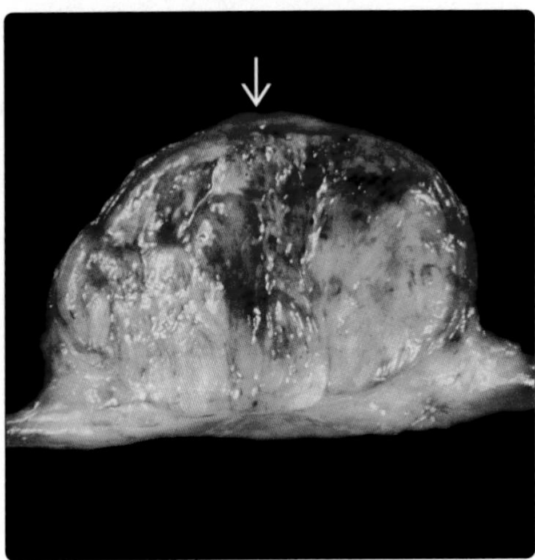

Heterogeneous Cut Surface

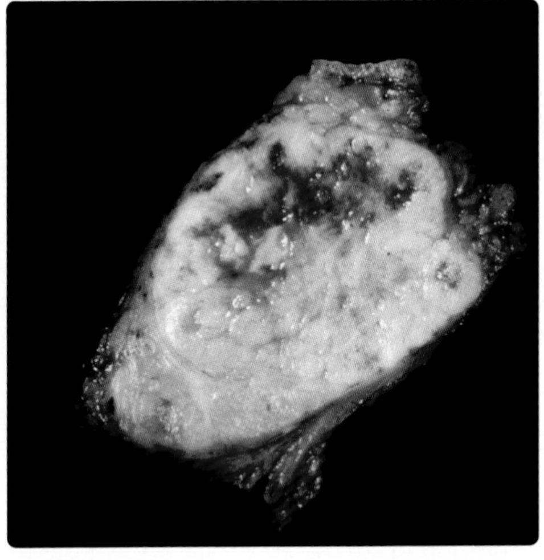

(Left) *MPNSTs are locally aggressive, as exemplified by this chest wall example of MPNSTs invading the ribs ➔.* **(Right)** *In this example, MPNST arises in a ganglioneuroma. Note the necrosis of the MPNST element ➔, the latter being relatively well demarcated from the parent lesion.*

Chest Wall Involvement

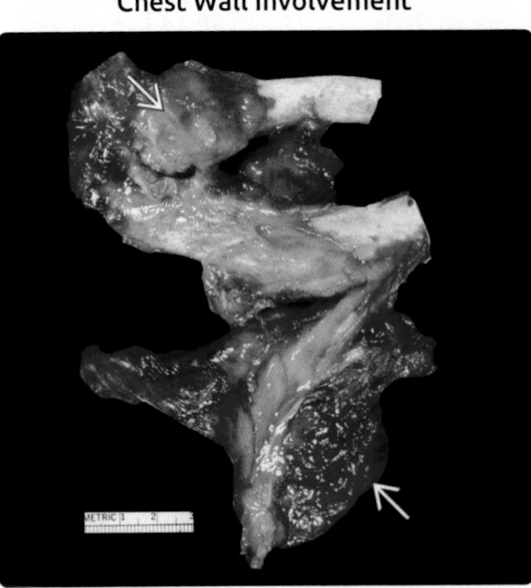

MPNST Developing From Ganglioneuroma

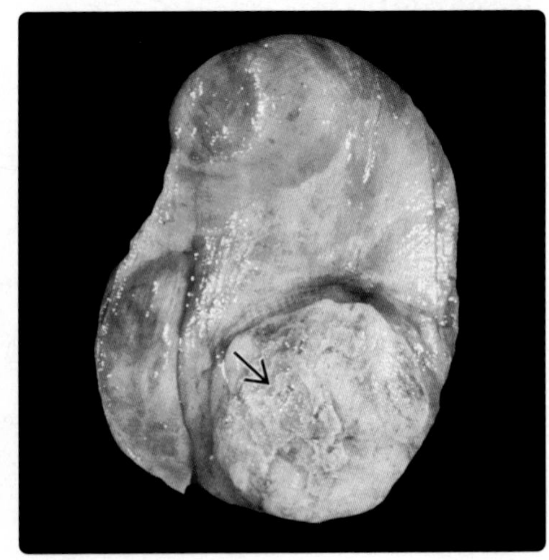

Fascicular Architecture

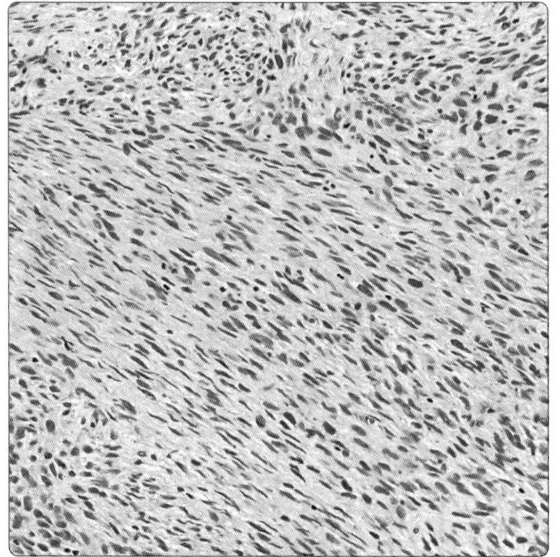

Staghorn-Like Vasculature

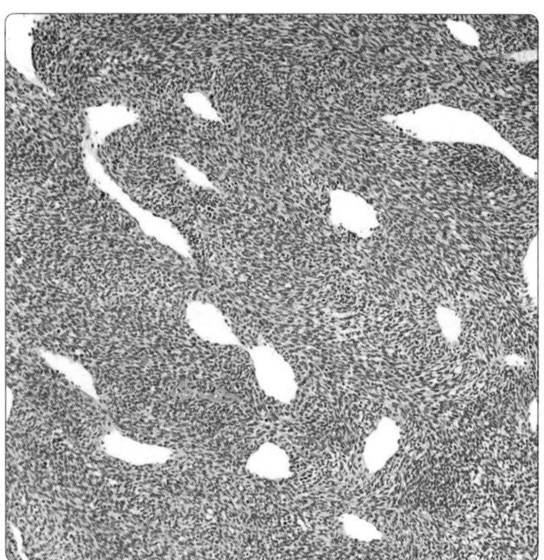

(Left) *Most MPNSTs demonstrate a fascicular architecture, and therefore morphologically overlap with fibrosarcoma.* **(Right)** *Because of their high cellularity and staghorn-like vasculature, some MPNSTs mimic hemangiopericytoma. Both are rich in reticulin. Distinction in such cases is made, in part, by S100 immunoreactivity in at least the focal areas of MPNSTs.*

Lobular Architecture

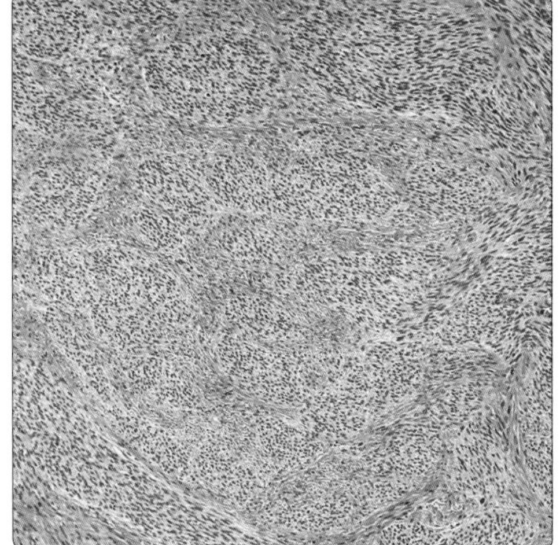

Tissue Culture-Like Pattern

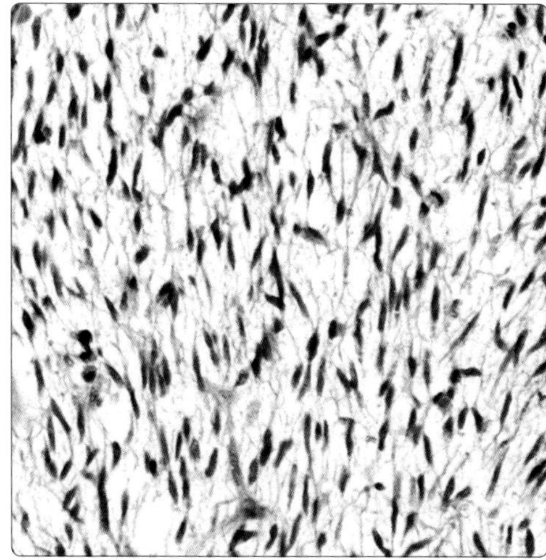

(Left) *MPNSTs have many patterns, including a lobulated, somewhat fascicular cellular mass.* **(Right)** *Rare tumors have a tissue culture-like pattern produced by independent spindle cells that one can imagine migrating over the surface of a Petri dish.*

Pseudopapillary Architecture

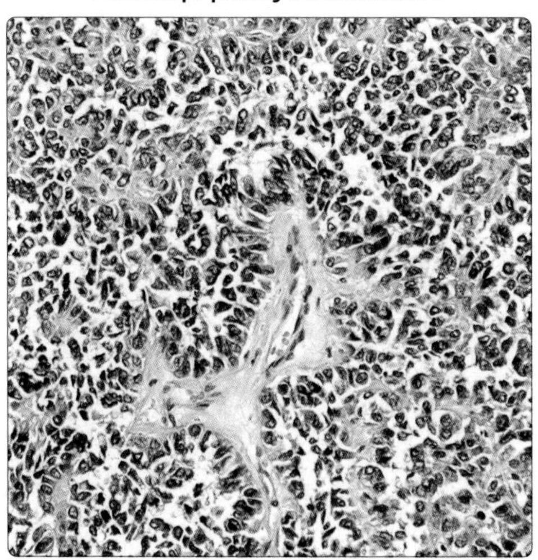

Chordoma-Like Architecture

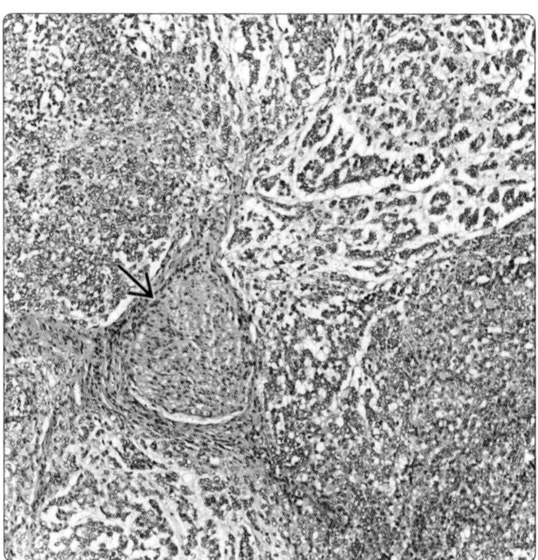

(Left) *Perivascular, somewhat epithelioid cells create pseudopapillary architecture in some cases, as seen here.* **(Right)** *MPNSTs may have prominent myxoid stroma and a somewhat chordoma-like architecture. An overrun nerve ⇨ is present in the center of the field.*

(Left) *MPNSTs are aggressive lesions with the capacity to invade bone* → *and soft tissues. Distant metastases are common.* **(Right)** *MPNSTs often infiltrate surrounding soft tissue* →*. By contrast, schwannomas are encapsulated tumors and do not infiltrate surrounding soft tissue, unless they arise in a mucosa.*

Bone Invasion

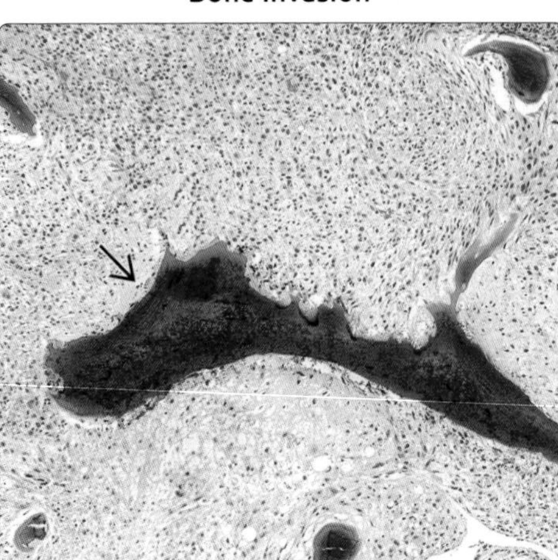

Soft Tissue Infiltration

(Left) *Necrosis, frequent in MPNST, may be either infarct-like or with pseudopalisading* →*, as in this case.* **(Right)** *Large areas of geographic necrosis are characteristic of high-grade MPNST.*

Pseudopalisading Necrosis

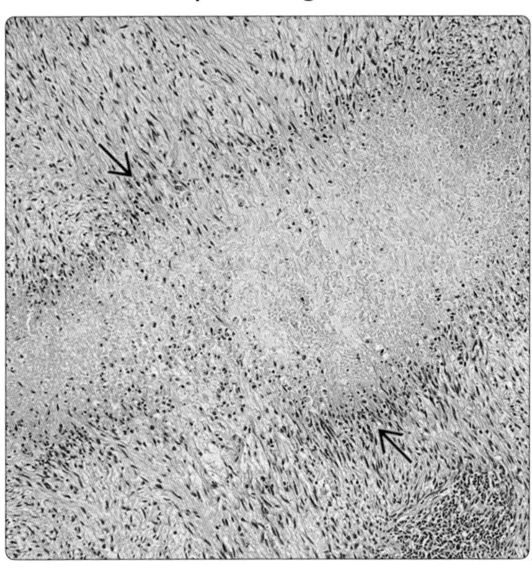

Geographic Necrosis

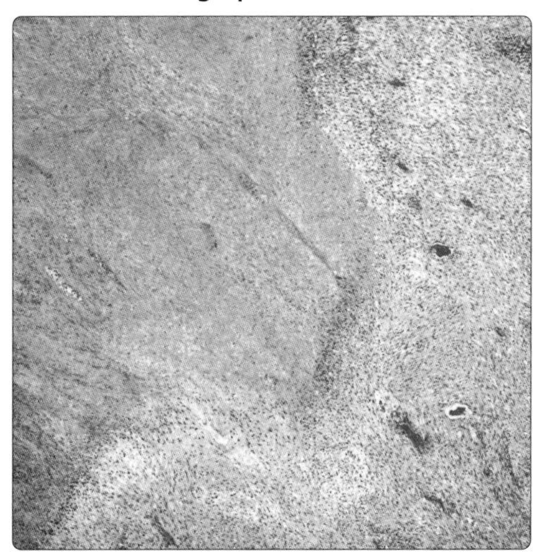

(Left) *Necrosis tends to spare perivascular tumor cells.* **(Right)** *Microvascular proliferation* → *is common in MPNSTs, as seen in this case.*

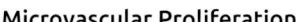

Viable Perivascular Tumor Cells

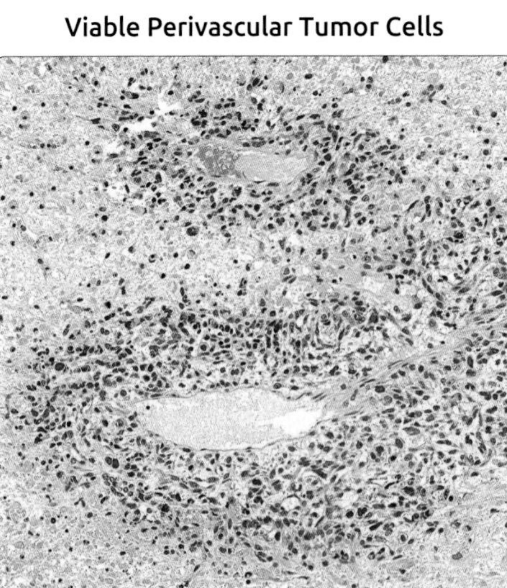

Microvascular Proliferation

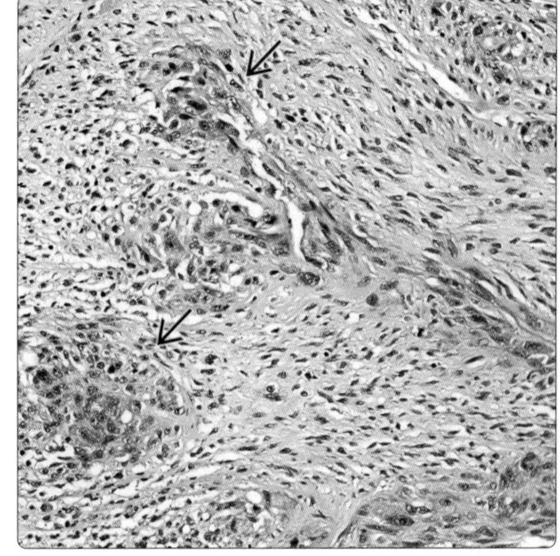

Microvascular Infiltration

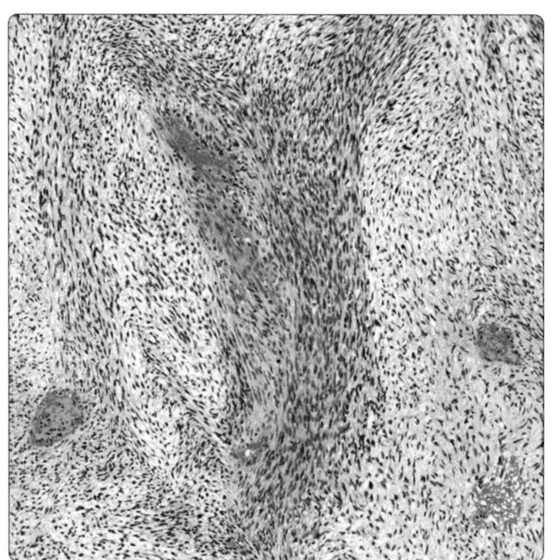

Vascular Invasion

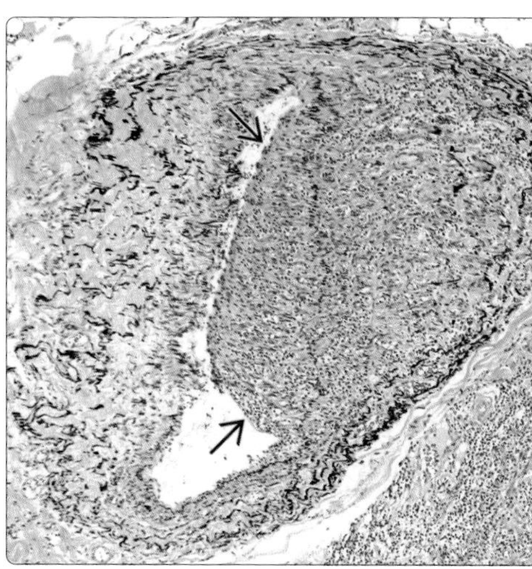

(Left) *Perivascular hypercellularity and frank invasion of microvascular walls may be present in MPNST, and is more typical of MPNST when compared to morphologically similar mimics.* **(Right)** *Vascular invasion ⇨ occurs in a subset of MPNST.*

MPNST Arising in Schwannoma

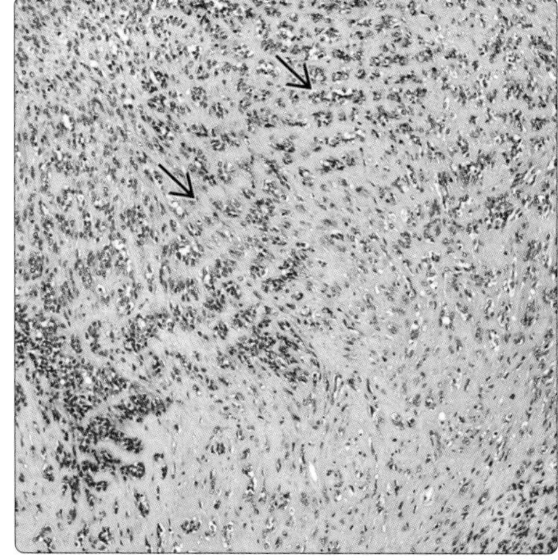

Nodular, Myxoid-Rich Areas

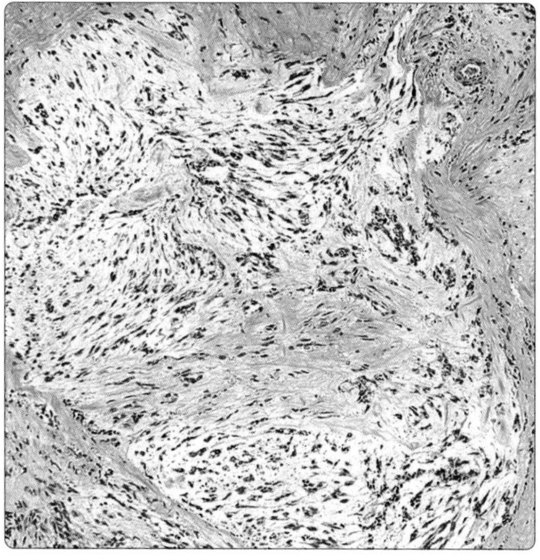

(Left) *The presence of Verocay bodies ⇨ helps establish the origin of a rare MPNST arising in a schwannoma.* **(Right)** *Some MPNSTs arising from schwannomas have nodular, myxoid tissue-rich areas, as seen here.*

Collagenous Stroma

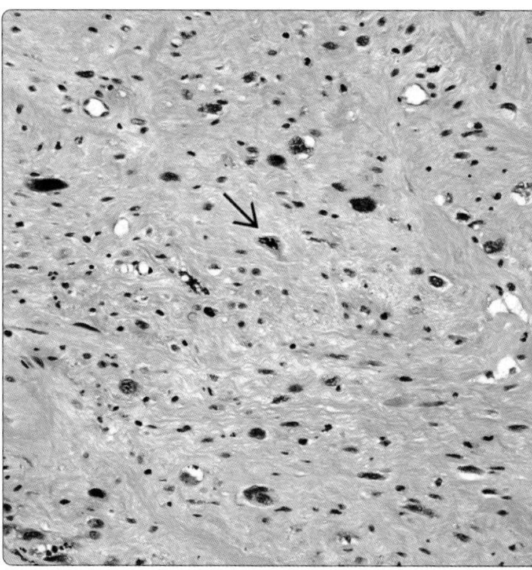

Schwann Cell Atypia in Irradiated Nerve

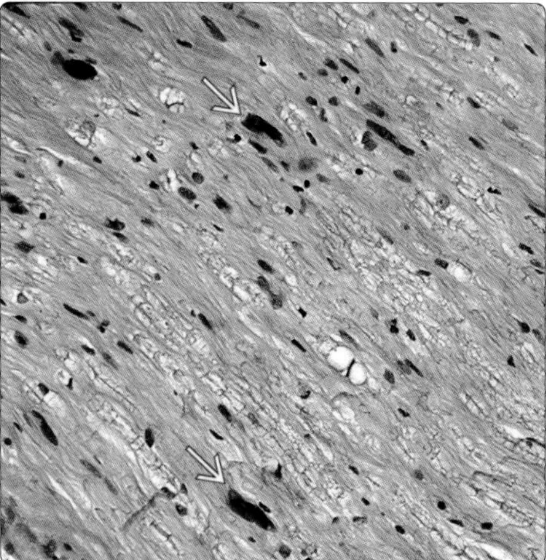

(Left) *Stroma of MPNSTs may be largely collagenous. Prominent hyperchromasia and mitotic figures ⇨ are helpful in the diagnosis.* **(Right)** *Previously irradiated normal nerves may have pleomorphic Schwann cells and nuclear atypia ➡ that might suggest MPNST. As a rule, such radiation-affected cells do not show proliferative activity.*

(Left) *Rhabdomyoblasts ➡ are classic examples of mesenchymal differentiation in MPNSTs in which such cells may form fascicle-like clusters. Such tumors are known as Triton tumors.* **(Right)** *Residual normal muscle fibers ➡ may be incorporated in an invasive MPNST. Linear shape, bland peripheral nuclei, and abundant striations help distinguish these normal cells from rare rhabdomyoblastic differentiation.*

Rhabdomyoblasts in Triton Tumor

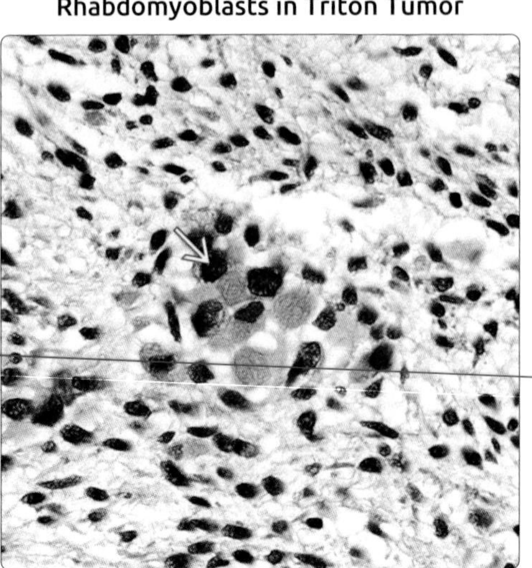

Entrapped Skeletal Muscle

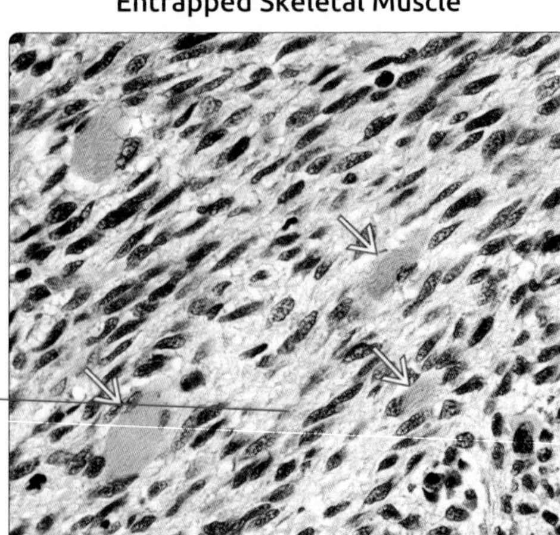

(Left) *Neoplastic cells with rhabdomyoblastic differentiation are immunoreactive for desmin.* **(Right)** *Chondrosarcoma ➡ is one form of mesenchymal differentiation in MPNST. Rhabdo-, osteo-, lipo-, or angiosarcomatous differentiation may also be present. Rhabdomyosarcomatous is the most common.*

Desmin Expression in Triton Tumor

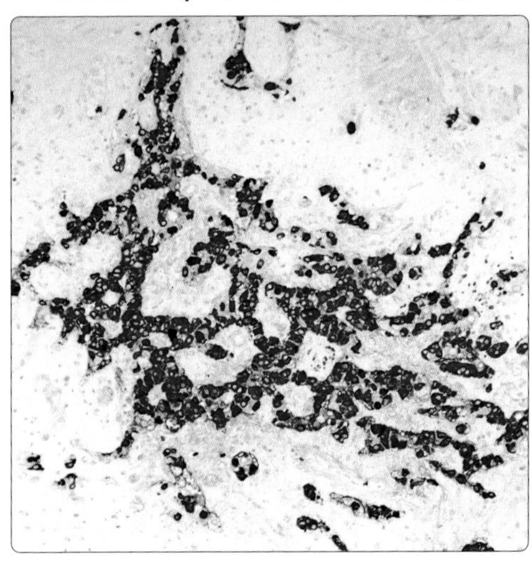

Cartilaginous Differentiation

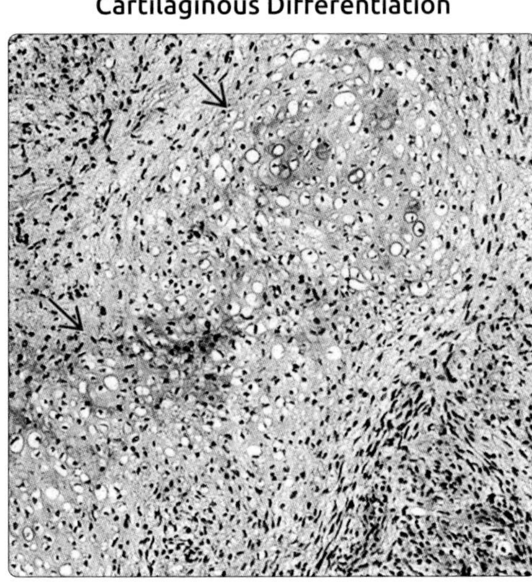

(Left) *Although most MPNSTs demonstrate evidence of schwannian origin or differentiation, a rare subset show evidence of perineurial differentiation. Residual axons are present within this example of an infiltrating nerve ➡.* **(Right)** *EMA is a useful marker to identify perineurial differentiation in this rare MPNST subtype.*

MPNST With Perineurial Differentiation

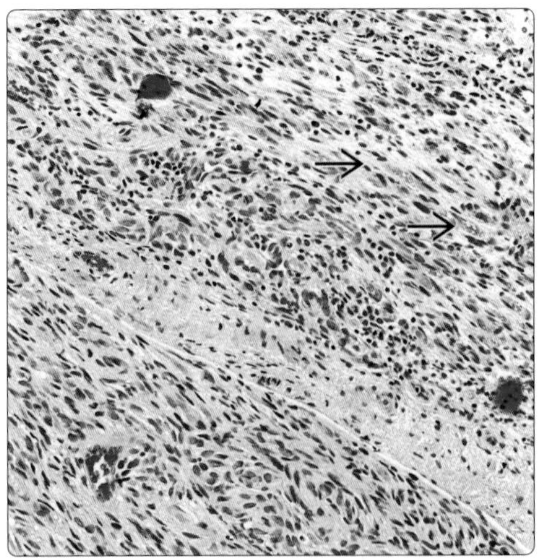

EMA Expression in MPNST

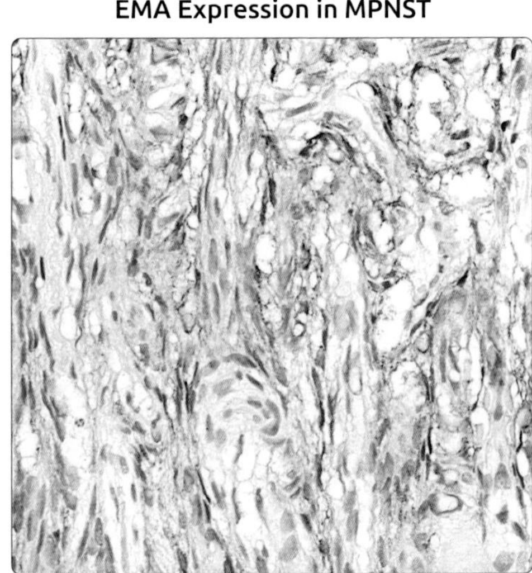

Whorl-Like Structures

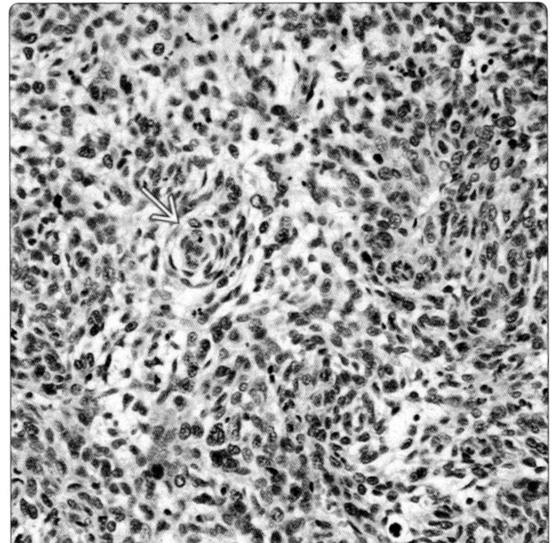

Whorls

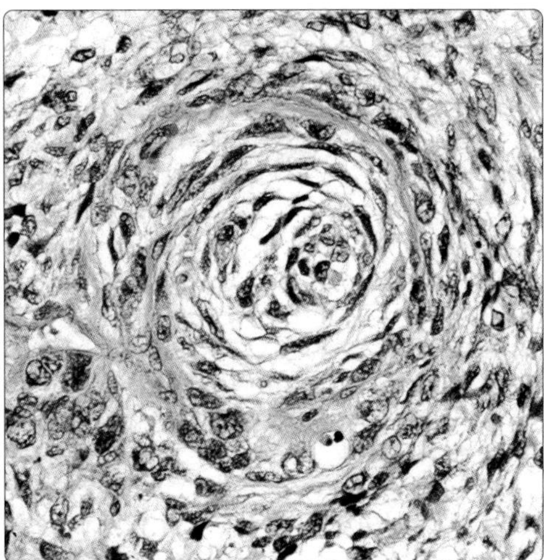

(Left) *MPNSTs with perineurial differentiation may have whorl-like structures* ➡. **(Right)** *Whorls, a suggestive feature of perineurial differentiation, should not be misinterpreted as tactile bodies.*

Glandular Differentiation

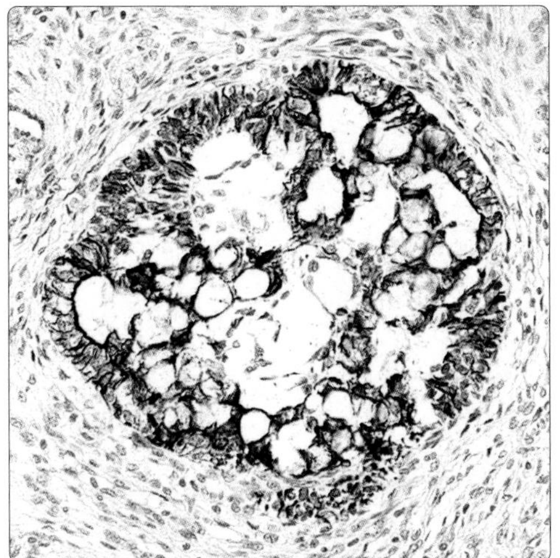

Glands With Neuroendocrine Differentiation

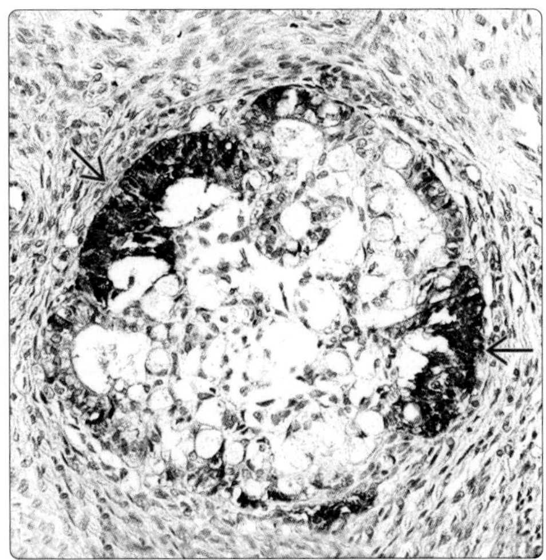

(Left) *Glandular differentiation in MPNSTs may be immunoreactive for CAM5.2.* **(Right)** *Glands in MPNST may have neuroendocrine differentiation, reflected in their immunoreactivity for chromogranin* ➡.

Periglandular S100 Expression

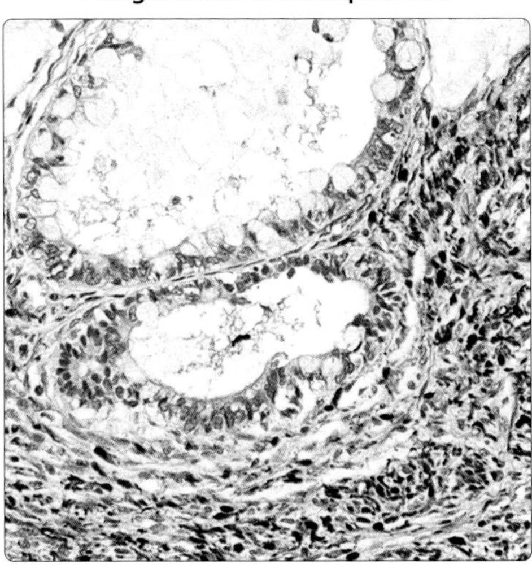

Glands Within Mucin Pools

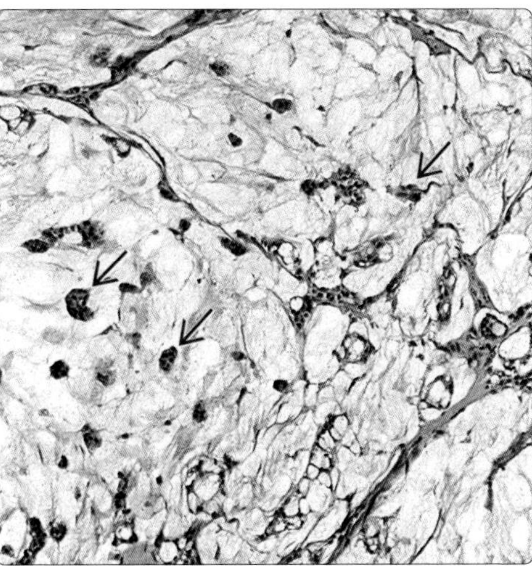

(Left) *Spindle cells surrounding glandular structures in some MPNSTs are immunoreactive for S100.* **(Right)** *Small glands* ➡ *may be suspended in large pools of extracellular mucin.*

(Left) *Although usually arising in peripheral nerves, MPNSTs may also begin in neuroectodermal tumors such as pheochromocytoma →.* **(Right)** *Low- to intermediate-grade MPNSTs may be extensively immunoreactive for S100 protein. Others are only focally positive, if at all.*

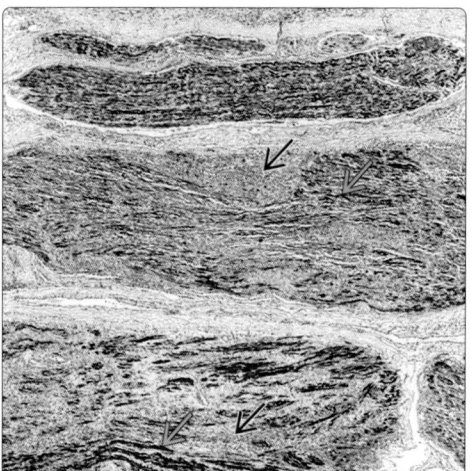

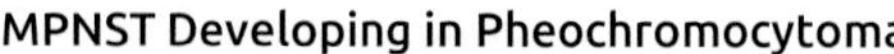

MPNST Developing in Pheochromocytoma

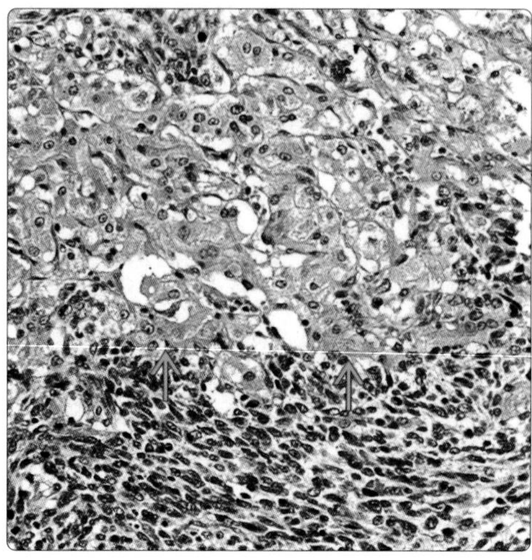

S100 Expression in Low-Grade MPNST

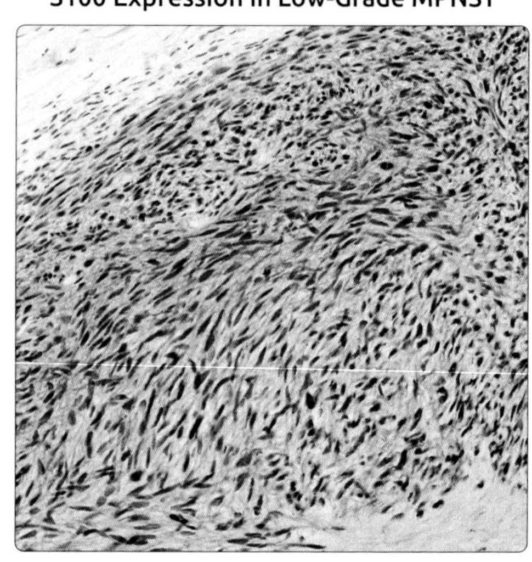

(Left) *MPNSTs → may spread along nerves, as is apparent here in tumor cells that extend between axons immunostained for neurofilament protein →.* **(Right)** *Some MPNSTs are immunoreactive for CD57. The marker should be applied in conjunction with S100. Expression of either protein is evidence in favor of peripheral nerve sheath tumor.*

Nerve Spread

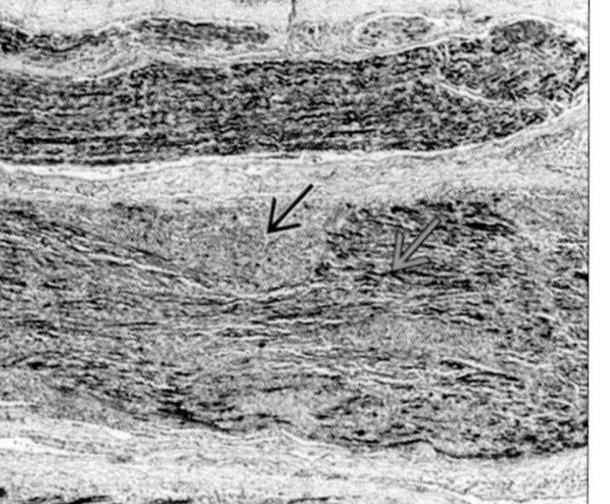

CD57 Expression

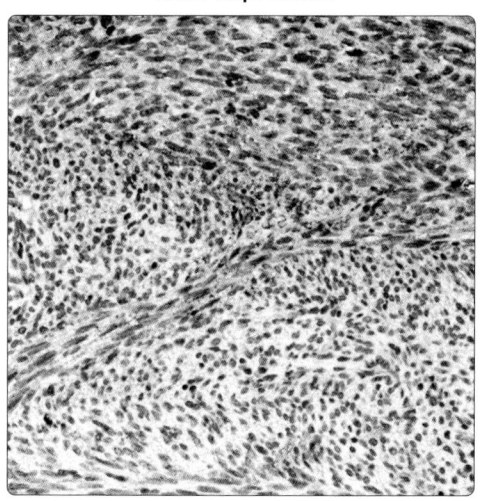

(Left) *Pericellular collagen IV staining → may be focal or diffuse. Vessels are darkly stained.* **(Right)** *SOX10 is a useful marker in the recognition of tumors derived from the neural crest, including Schwann cell and melanocytic neoplasms. Expression in MPNST is variable.*

Pericellular Collagen IV

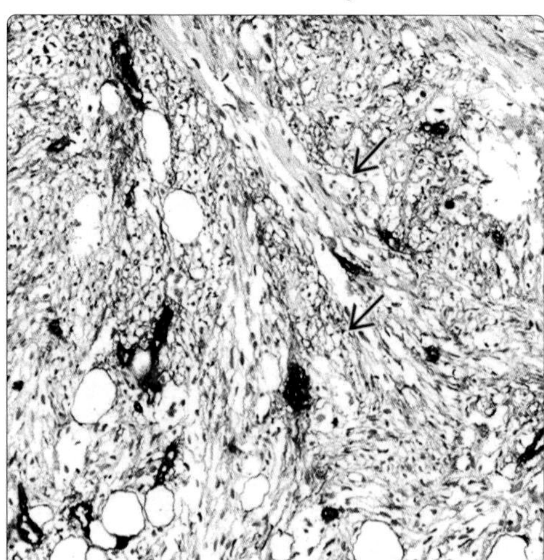

SOX10 Expression

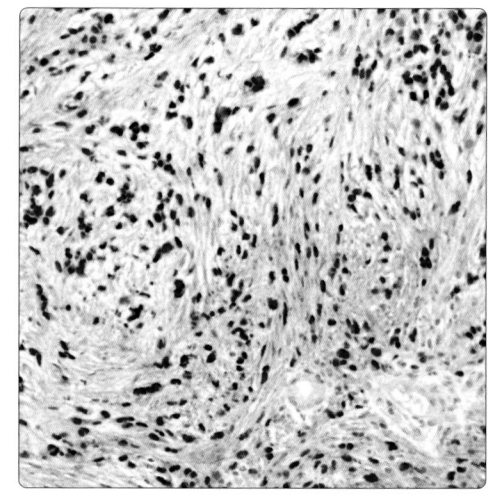

Hypercellularity in Neurofibroma

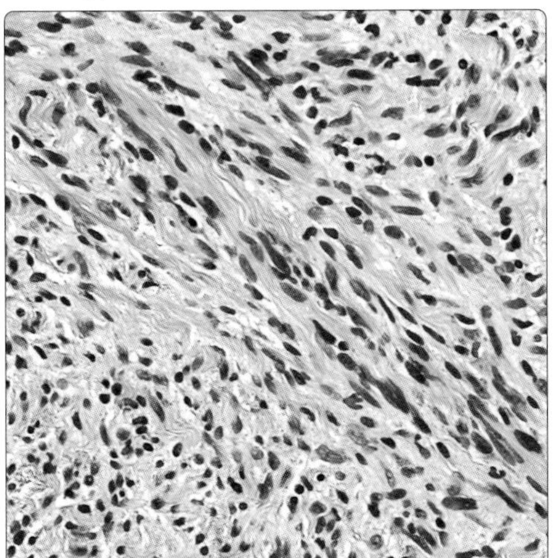

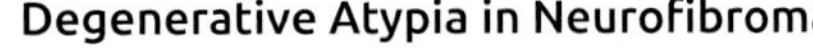

Degenerative Atypia in Neurofibroma

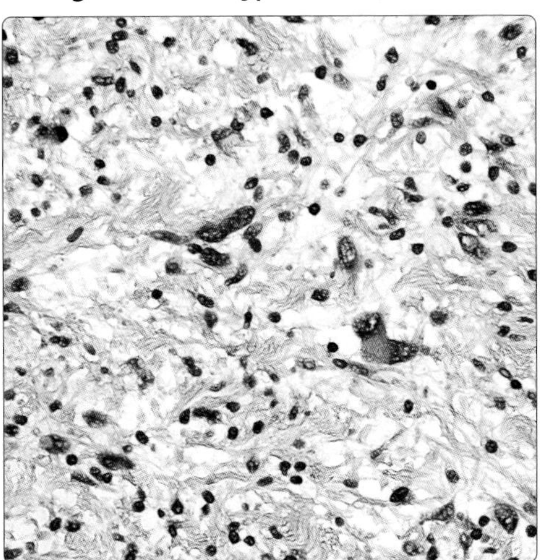

(Left) *Areas of increased cellularity in neurofibroma are worrisome, particularly when developing in the setting of NF1. This neurofibroma demonstrates increased nuclear crowding but does not yet satisfy criteria for MPNST.* **(Right)** *Isolated degenerative atypia in neurofibroma should not be interpreted as malignant change. However, systematic examination is recommended in these cases, given that transition into MPNST may be focal.*

Atypical Neurofibroma With Transition to MPNST

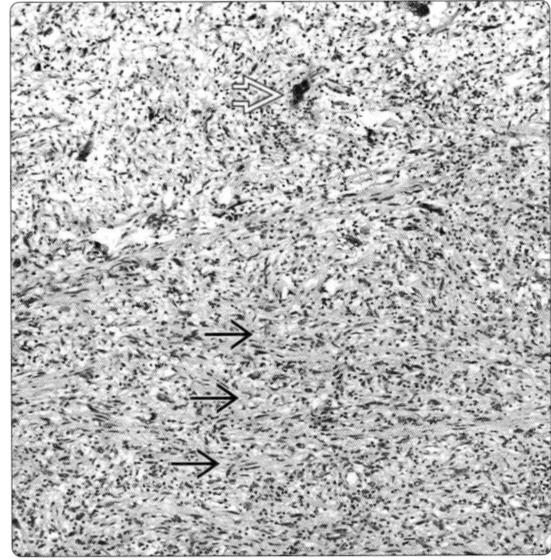

MPNST Developing in Neurofibroma

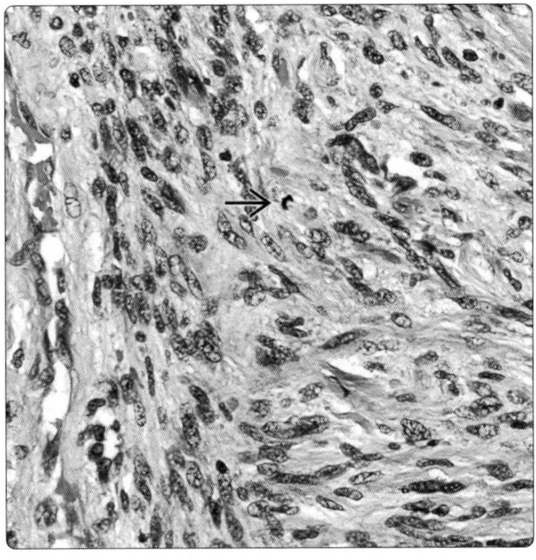

(Left) *The transition to MPNST in neurofibroma may be gradual and difficult to recognize. In this example, areas of atypical neurofibroma with degenerative atypia* ⇨ *transition into areas of uniform nuclear enlargement, nuclear hyperchromasia and crowding* →*, satisfying criteria for MPNST.* **(Right)** *In this case, overt diagnostic features of MPNST developing within neurofibroma, including severe nuclear atypia, hypercellularity, and mitotic activity* → *are seen. However, the latter is not required for diagnosis of MPNST.*

p53 Positivity in MPNST

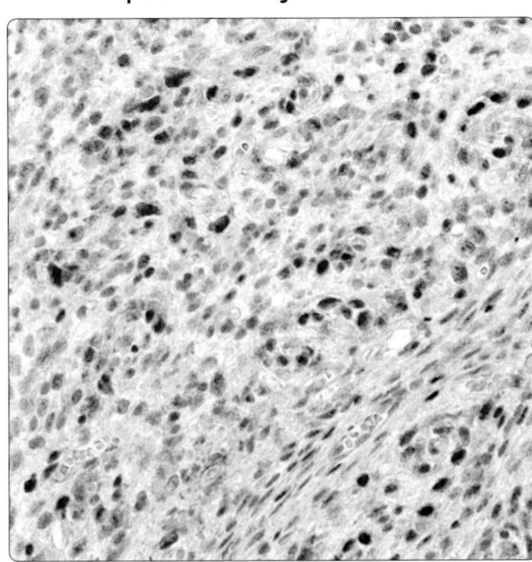

p16 Loss in MPNST

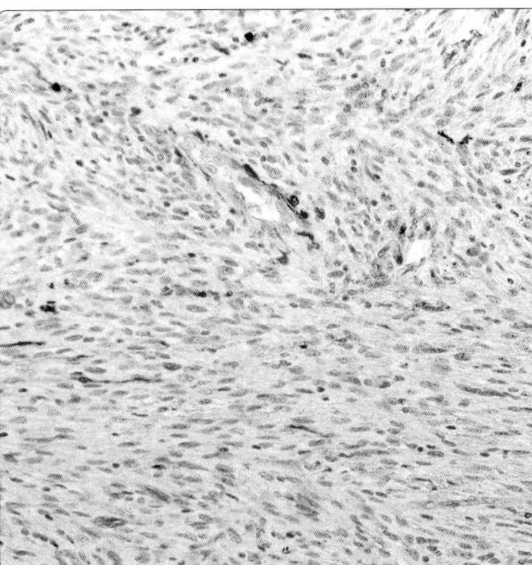

(Left) *The presence of strong p53 immunostaining is helpful as an adjunct to recognize the transformation of neurofibromas into MPNST.* **(Right)** *p16 is usually inactivated by genetic mechanisms in MPNST evolution, and protein loss may be recognized by immunohistochemistry in some cases. In contrast, p16 is usually expressed in neurofibromas, where it represents a marker of senescence.*

(Left) *MPNSTs more commonly arise in transition from a neurofibroma* ➔*, as shown in this example, than from any other benign peripheral nerve sheath tumor. An origin in a schwannoma is rare.* **(Right)** *Ki-67 labeling index is apparently increased in the MPNST foci compared to the foci of neurofibroma.*

Transition From Neurofibroma

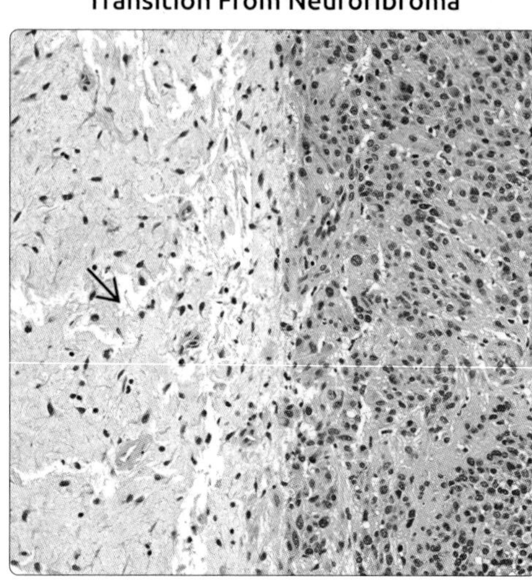

Transition From Neurofibroma: Ki-67

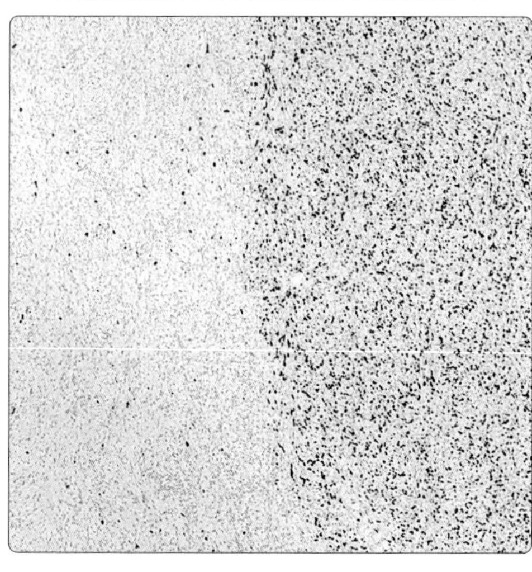

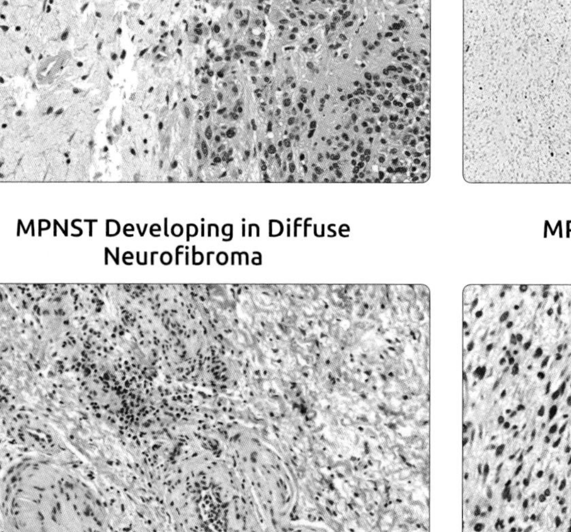

(Left) *MPNST usually develops from plexiform neurofibromas, but as this example shows, it may develop from diffuse neurofibromas in the context of NF1 on rare occasions.* **(Right)** *A focus of nuclear crowding, enlargement, and hyperchromasia in an MPNST developing within a diffuse neurofibroma is seen in this NF1 patient.*

MPNST Developing in Diffuse Neurofibroma

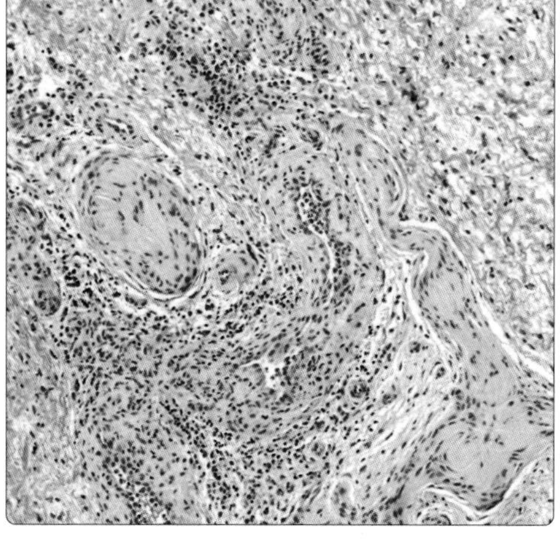

MPNST Developing in Diffuse Neurofibroma

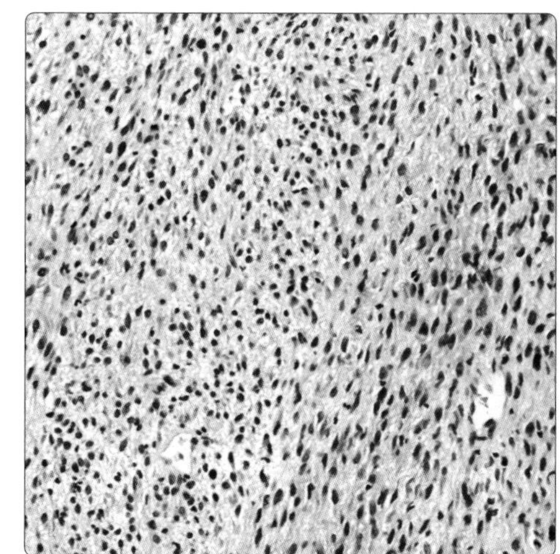

(Left) *Cannibalism of cells, nuclear hyperchromasia, nucleolar prominence, and pleomorphism are present in some epithelioid MPNSTs.* **(Right)** *In this case, MPNST cells with epithelial differentiation may be immunoreactive for cytokeratins.*

Cannibalism

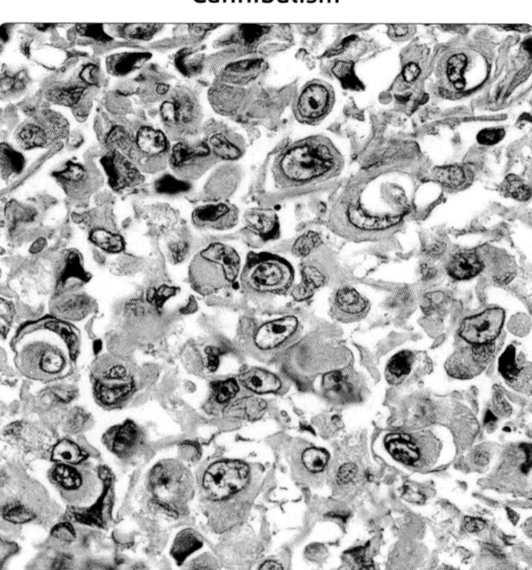

Cytokeratin Expression

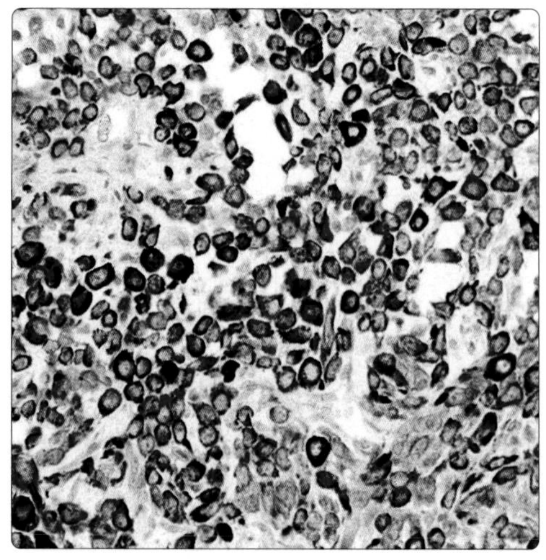

Lobular Architecture

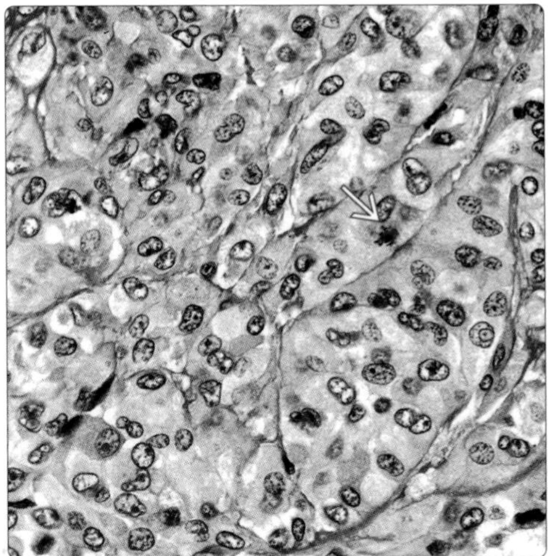

Myxoid Stroma

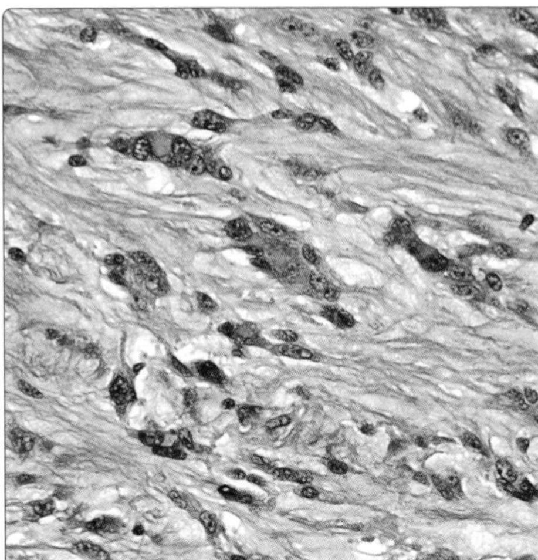

(Left) *Epithelioid MPNSTs may have a lobular architecture. Cytologic atypia and mitotic activity* ➔ *are consistent features.* **(Right)** *Epithelioid MPNST is often composed by cells arranged in cords and small nests that are embedded in a myxoid stroma.*

Epithelioid MPNST Ex-Schwannoma

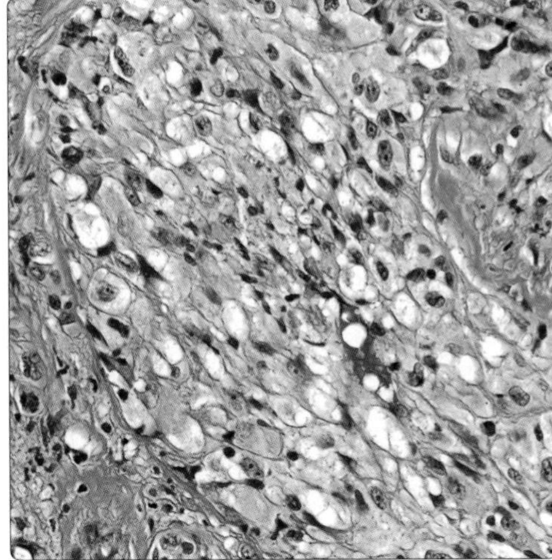

Epithelioid MPNST in Schwannomatosis

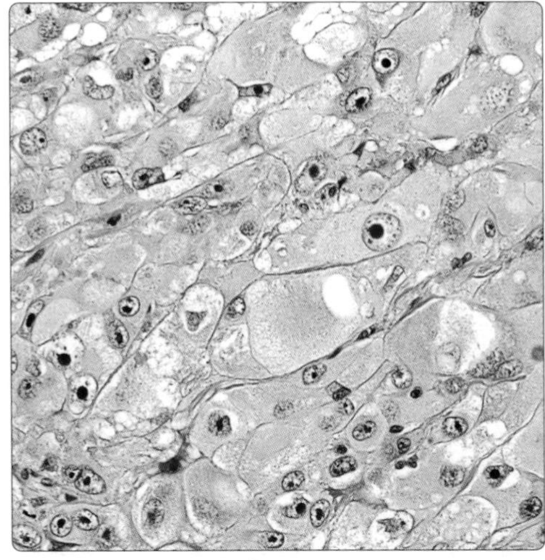

(Left) *Epithelioid MPNST is one of the morphologic variations encountered in the rare schwannomas that develop malignant degeneration.* **(Right)** *Pronounced cytologic atypia, including macronucleoli, characterizes this epithelioid MPNST that arose within a schwannoma in a patient satisfying clinical criteria for schwannomatosis.*

Strong S100 Expression

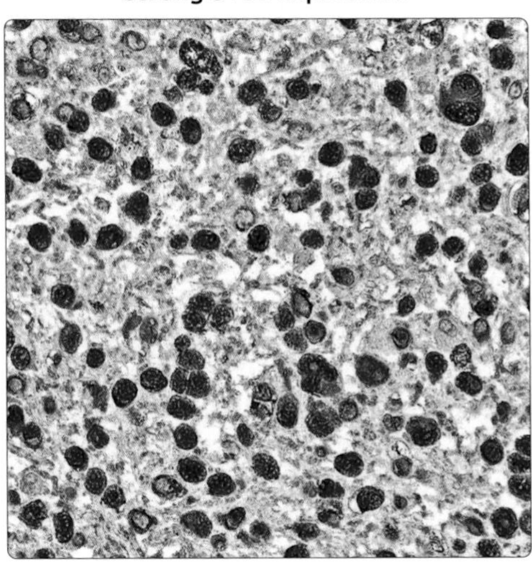

Pericellular Collagen IV

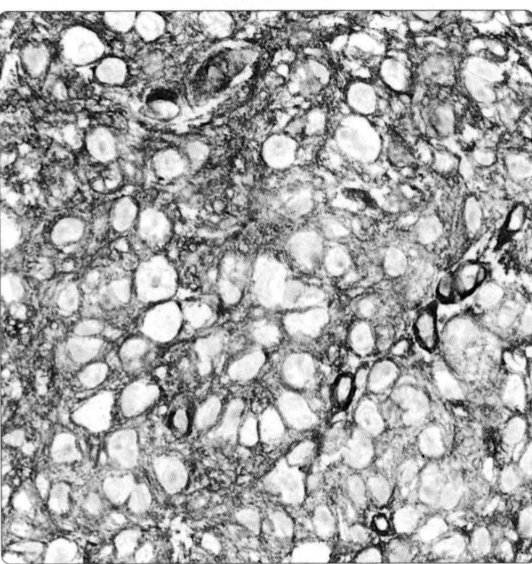

(Left) *Unlike conventional MPNST, the epithelioid variant demonstrates consistently strong, uniform S100 expression. Strong cytoplasmic and nuclear expression, as illustrated here, is characteristic. The lack of specific melanocytic markers (e.g., Melan-A, HMB-45) is required to exclude melanoma in many instances.* **(Right)** *Strong pericellular collagen IV is another immunohistochemical feature of epithelioid MPNST.*

Intraneural Perineurioma

KEY FACTS

TERMINOLOGY

- Benign intraneural neoplasms composed of perineurial cells forming pseudoonion bulbs

ETIOLOGY/PATHOGENESIS

- Deletion of chromosome region 22q11

CLINICAL ISSUES

- No syndrome association
- Progressive muscle weakness
- No recurrence or malignant transformation

MACROSCOPIC

- Segmental, uniform expansion of nerve

MICROSCOPIC

- Pseudoonion bulbs surround nerve fibers
- Rare mitoses
- Rope-like bundles of perineurial cells seen in longitudinal sections

ANCILLARY TESTS

- S100: Labels nonneoplastic Schwann sheaths
- Neurofilament protein: Labels axons
- EMA(+)/S100(-) perineurial cell processes
- Claudin-1(+), GLUT1(+)

TOP DIFFERENTIAL DIAGNOSES

- Localized hypertrophic neuropathy
  - True onion bulbs composed of S100(+) Schwann cell processes
- Neurofibroma
- Malignant peripheral nerve sheath tumor
- Inherited polyneuropathies
- Chronic inflammatory demyelinating polyneuropathy
  - S100(+), EMA(-) onion bulbs

Nerve Enlargement

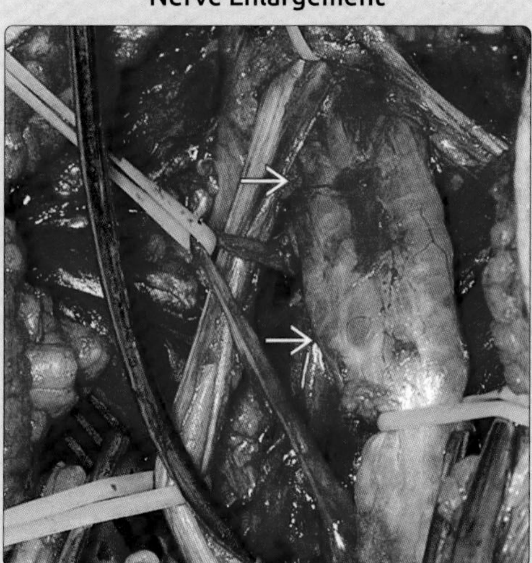

Fascicular Involvement

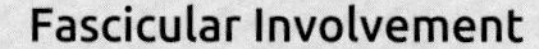

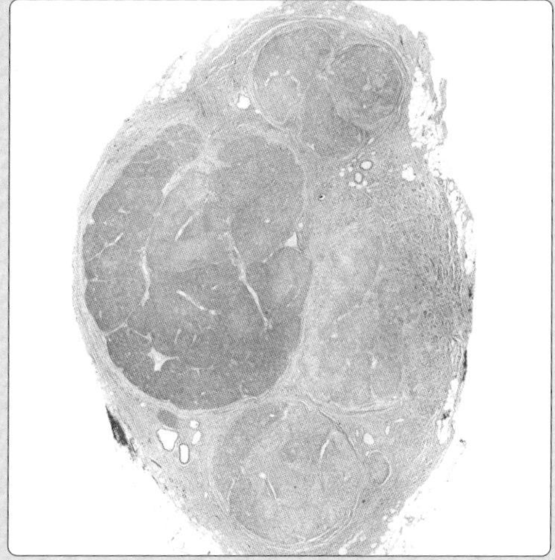

(Left) *Intraoperatively, the enlarged nerve ➔ has an irregular, almost nodular appearance.* **(Right)** *Intraneural perineurioma is characterized by enlargement of individual nerve fascicles by a predominant endoneurial neoplastic perineurial cell proliferation.*

Pseudoonion Bulbs

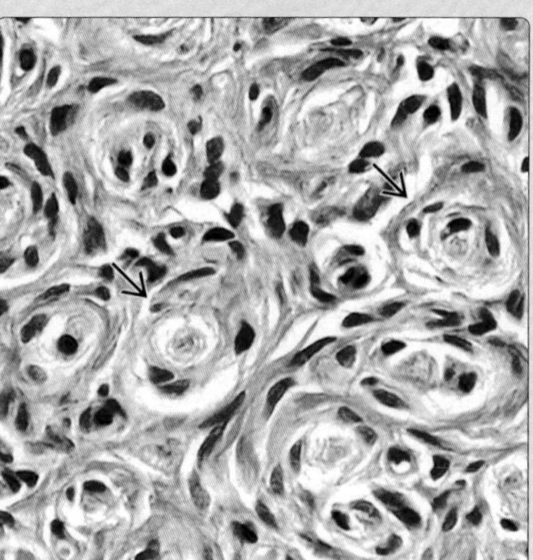

Residual Axons

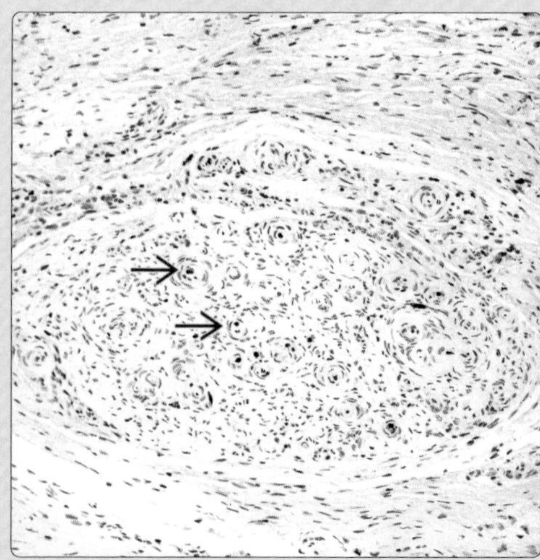

(Left) *Nerve fibers surrounded by multilayered perineurial cells are known as pseudoonion bulbs ➔. Some perineurial cells connect ("bridge") one bulb to another.* **(Right)** *Residual axons identified within pseudoonion bulbs ➔ with neurofilament protein immunostain represent a constant feature of intraneural perineurioma.*

TERMINOLOGY

Definitions

- Benign intraneural neoplasm composed of perineurial cells forming pseudoonion bulbs

ETIOLOGY/PATHOGENESIS

Chromosomal Abnormalities

- Deletion of chromosome region 22q11/monosomy 22
  - Supports lesion being neoplastic rather than reactive

CLINICAL ISSUES

Epidemiology

- Incidence
  - Rare (< 100 reported cases)
  - No syndrome association
- Age
  - Adolescence to early adulthood
- Sex
  - No predilection

Site

- Spinal nerve roots, trunks, or branches
  - Median, tibial, peroneal, sciatic often affected
- Solitary; rarely multiple adjacent nerves
- Cranial nerves rarely involved

Presentation

- Progressive muscle weakness
  - Localized muscle atrophy
- Sensory disturbance less frequent
- Nonpalpable mass

Treatment

- Options, risks, complications
  - Biopsy of electromyographically confirmed, nonfunctional fascicle

Prognosis

- Very slow growth
- Eventual loss of sensorimotor function
- No recurrence
- No malignant transformation

IMAGING

MR Findings

- Segmental, tubular enlargement of nerve

MACROSCOPIC

General Features

- Segmental, uniform expansion of nerve
- Thickened, coarse, pale, firm fascicles
- 2-10 cm long (rarely as long as 30 cm)
- Multifascicle (plexiform) involvement may occur

MICROSCOPIC

Histologic Features

- Multiple fascicles involved on cross section of nerve
- Variably hypercellular fascicles
- Pseudoonion bulbs
  - Perineurial cells ensheathing nerve fibers (axons and Schwann sheaths)
    - 3-6 layers
    - Nerve fibers: Myelinated or unmyelinated
  - Interconnection of pseudoonion bulbs (bridging)
  - Hypercellular perineurial septa contain perineurial cells
  - Occasional perineurial whorls surround endoneurial vessels
  - No significant cytologic atypia
- Rare mitoses
- Rope-like bundles of perineurial cells in longitudinal sections
- No epineurial involvement
- Chronic lesions show endoneurial collagen deposition

ANCILLARY TESTS

Immunohistochemistry

- S100(+), SOX10(+) nonneoplastic Schwann cell sheaths
- Neurofilament protein (+) axons
  - Axonal density lower in intraneural perineurioma compared with true neuropathies, but variable
- Neoplastic perineurial cells
  - EMA(+)/S100(-) perineurial cell processes; claudin-1(+) ~ 42%; GLUT1(+) ~ 90%
- Ki-67: Usually low labeling index but up to 15% in individual cases
- p53 protein: Frequent low-level staining

Genetic Testing

- Deletion of chromosome region 22q11/monosomy 22

Electron Microscopy

- Perineurial cells
  - Thin cell processes, numerous pinocytotic vesicles, incomplete surface basal lamina, intercellular collagen fibers

DIFFERENTIAL DIAGNOSIS

Localized Hypertrophic Neuropathy

- True onion bulbs composed of S100(+), EMA(-) Schwann cell processes

Neurofibroma

- May have onion bulb-like structures (Schwann cells)
- S100 positivity strong, EMA(-) or scant

Malignant Peripheral Nerve Sheath Tumor

- No pseudoonion bulbs
- Longitudinal sections of intraneural perineurioma may be challenging due to apparent high cellularity

Inherited Polyneuropathies of Charcot-Marie-Tooth/Dejerine Sottas

- S100(+), EMA(-) onion bulbs

SELECTED REFERENCES

1. Mauermann ML et al: Longitudinal study of intraneural perineurioma–a benign, focal hypertrophic neuropathy of youth. Brain. 132(8):2265-76, 2009

(Left) *Cross section of a nerve fascicle shows the numerous pseudoonion bulbs* ⇒ *that, in aggregate, give the lesion its distinctive appearance.* **(Right)** *The number of perineurial cell layers in pseudoonion bulbs varies from one structure to another. The cytologically bland component cells have little or no mitotic activity.*

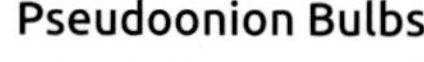

Pseudoonion Bulbs

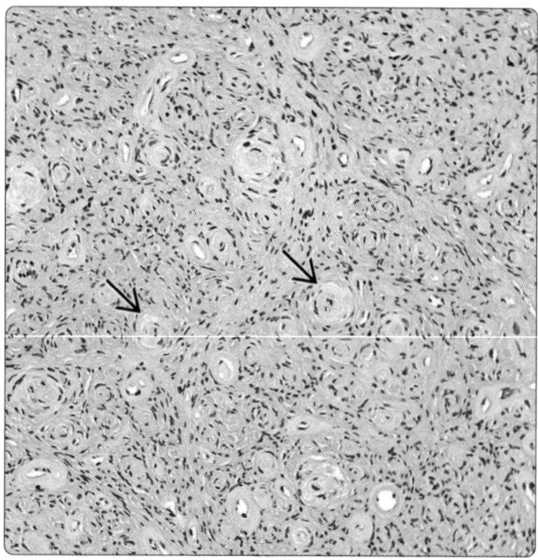

Pseudoonion Bulbs, Cross Section

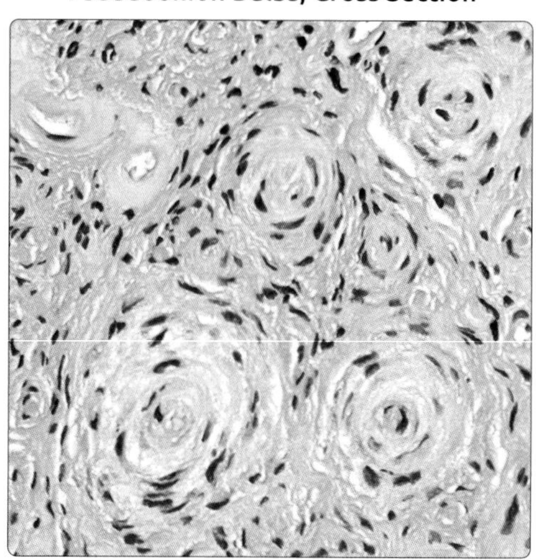

(Left) *It is more difficult to identify pseudoonion bulbs in longitudinal sections (such as this) than in cross sections. Rope-like bundles of perineurial cells are readily seen, however. The hypercellularity might raise concern for a malignant peripheral nerve sheath tumor. Mitoses are sparse though.* **(Right)** *Chronic lesions show collagenization on Masson trichrome staining.*

Hypercellularity, Longitudinal Section

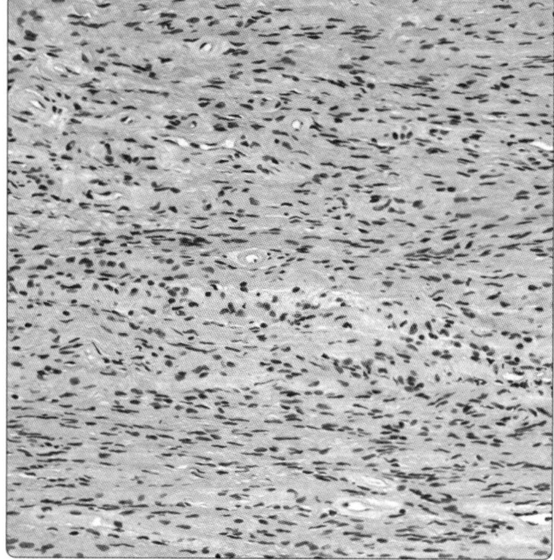

Collagenization

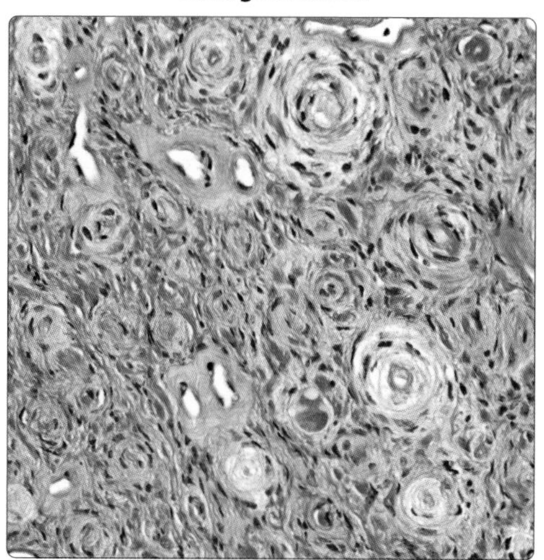

(Left) *Axons are often depleted and abnormally clustered* ⇒ *within pseudoonion bulbs.* **(Right)** *Normal nerve fascicles are composed of myelinated or unmyelinated nerve fibers surrounded by Schwann cells as seen here in a cross section stained with Luxol fast blue for myelin and Bielschowsky for axons.*

Axon Depletion

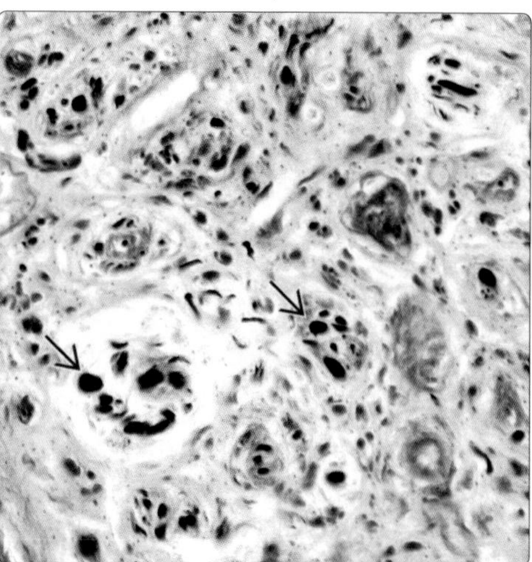

Nerve Fascicles

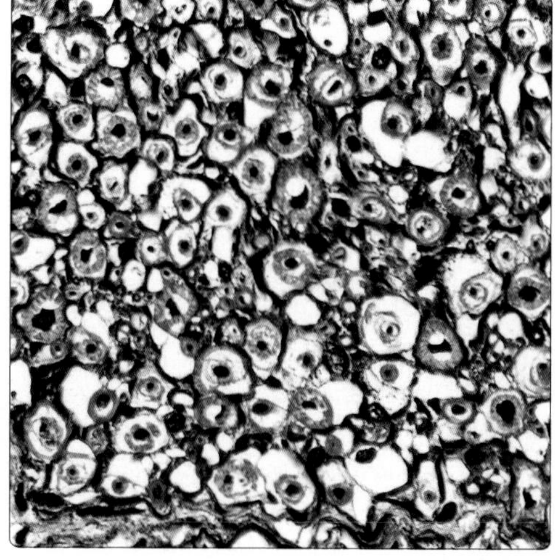

Sparing of Epineurium

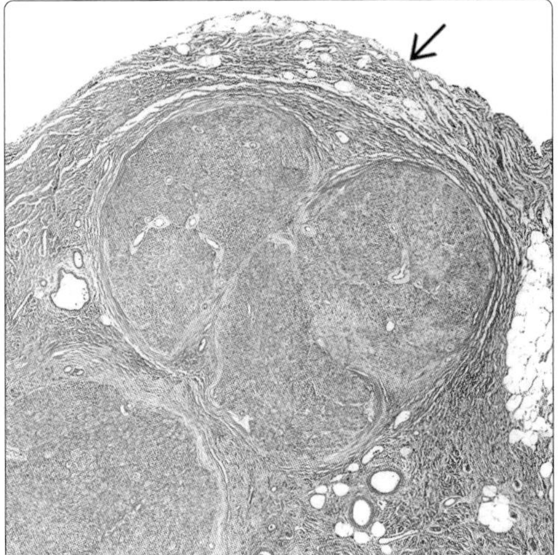

Whorls

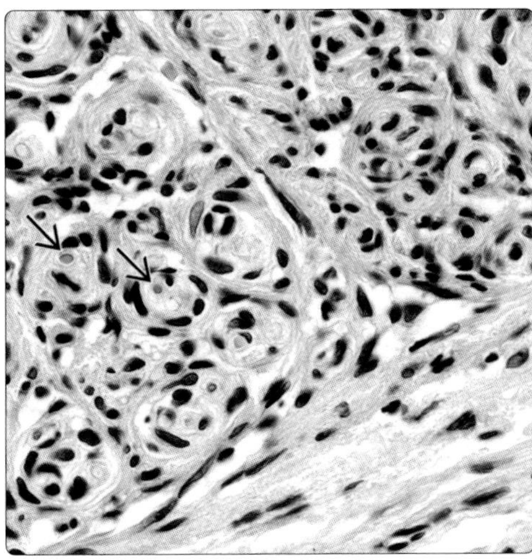

(Left) *Despite the involvement of endoneurium, and possibly perineurium, the epineurium ➔ is not affected.* **(Right)** *Whorls may also enwrap endoneurial capillaries ➔.*

EMA Expression

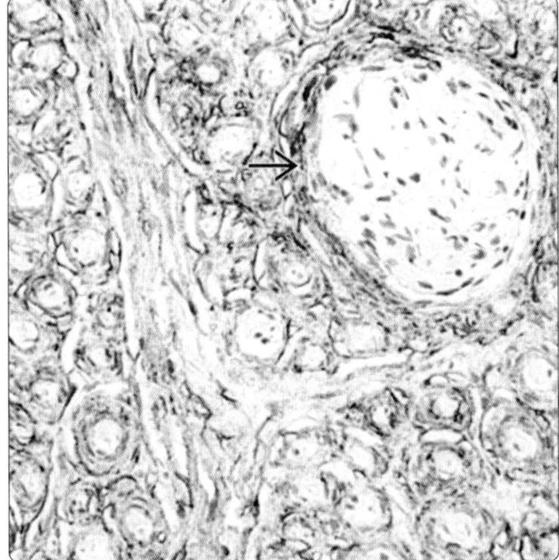

Axons

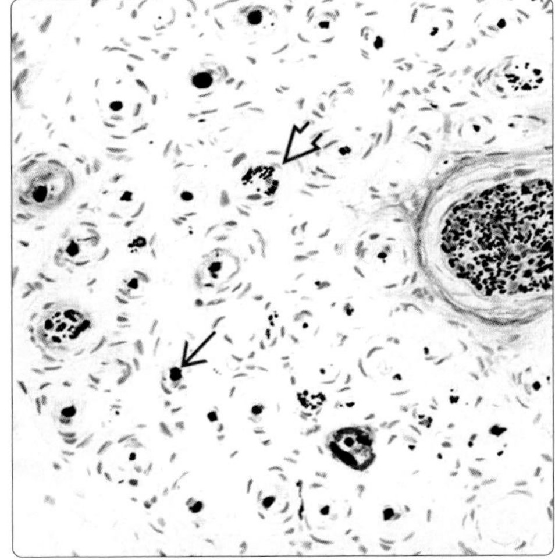

(Left) *EMA typically stains pseudoonion bulbs. An unaffected nerve fascicle ➔ is present.* **(Right)** *Staining for neurofilament protein shows axons to be single in some pseudoonion bulbs ➔ and multiple ➔ in others.*

S100(+) Schwann Cells

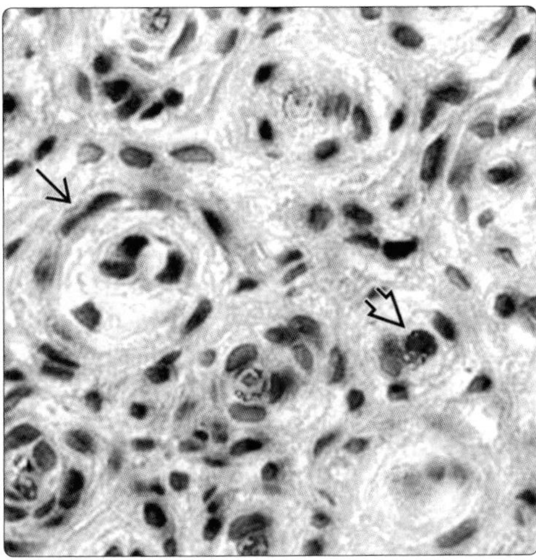

Layered Perineurial Cells

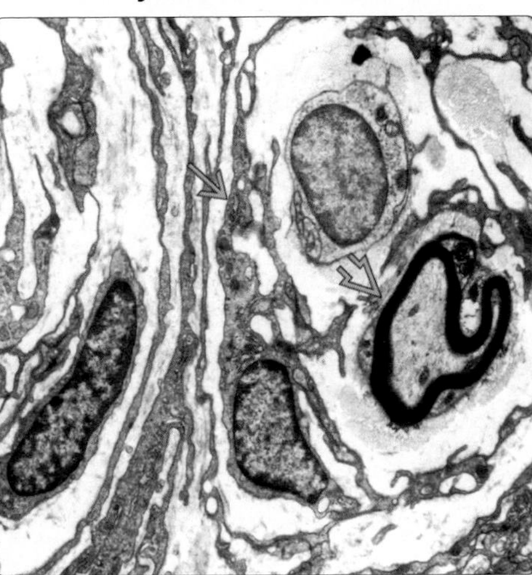

(Left) *Concentric layers of pseudoonion bulbs ➔ formed from S100 protein (-) cells are shown surrounding residual (+) Schwann cells ➔. These centrally placed axon-Schwann cell complexes help in the identification of perineurioma-associated pseudoonion bulbs.* **(Right)** *Layered perineurial cells ➔ surrounding a myelinated nerve fiber ➔ create pseudoonion bulbs at the ultrastructural level.*

Soft Tissue Perineurioma

KEY FACTS

TERMINOLOGY

- Benign soft tissue neoplasm of perineurial cells

ETIOLOGY/PATHOGENESIS

- Partial deletion of chromosome 22 in some cases

CLINICAL ISSUES

- No definite syndrome association
- Subcutaneous more common than soft tissue
- Less commonly deep soft tissues of extremities, trunk
- Complete excision curative

MACROSCOPIC

- Unencapsulated but well circumscribed
- No nerve association

MICROSCOPIC

- Long, narrow processes
- Fascicles, whorls, or storiform pattern
- Collagen or mucin-rich stroma
- Mitosis scant or absent

ANCILLARY TESTS

- EMA, GLUT1, and claudin (+)
- S100 and neurofilament protein (-)
- Collagen IV: Abundant basement membrane

TOP DIFFERENTIAL DIAGNOSES

- Neurofibroma
- Extracranial fibrous meningioma
- Solitary fibrous tumor
- Dermatofibrosarcoma protuberans
- Low-grade fibromyxoid sarcoma

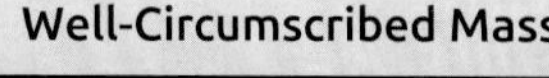

Well-Circumscribed Mass

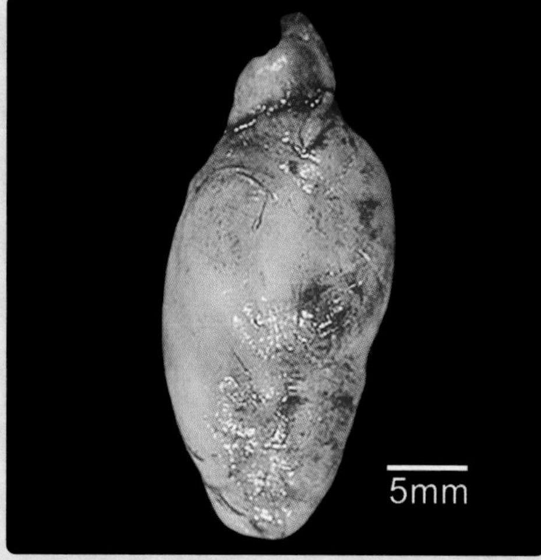

Vague Fasciculation

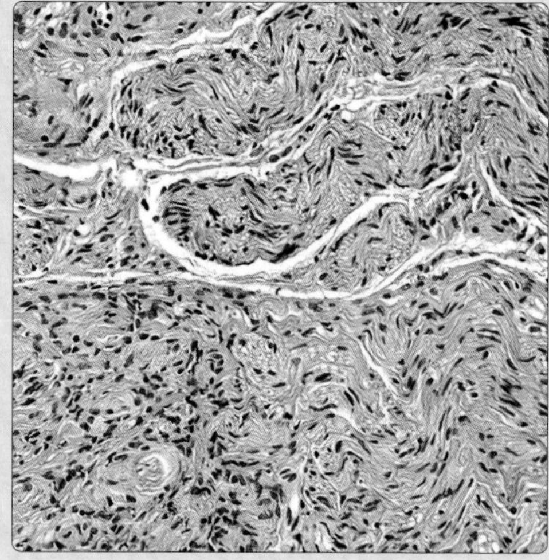

(Left) *Soft tissue perineuriomas are well-circumscribed, ovoid masses.* **(Right)** *Vague fasciculation of spindle cells in a dense stroma is frequently observed in soft tissue perineuriomas.*

Collagenous Stroma

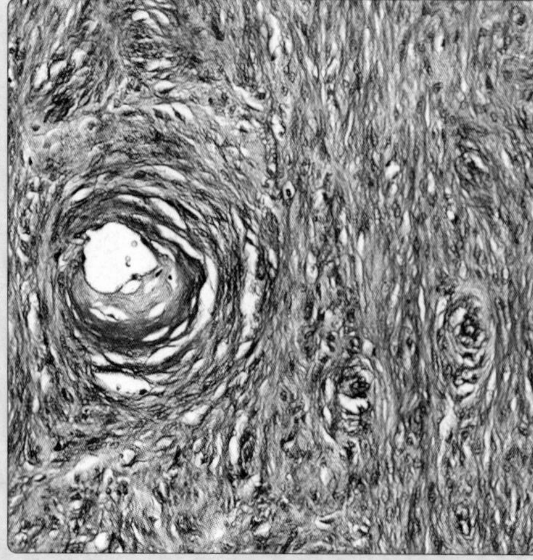

Elongated Cells With Narrow Processes

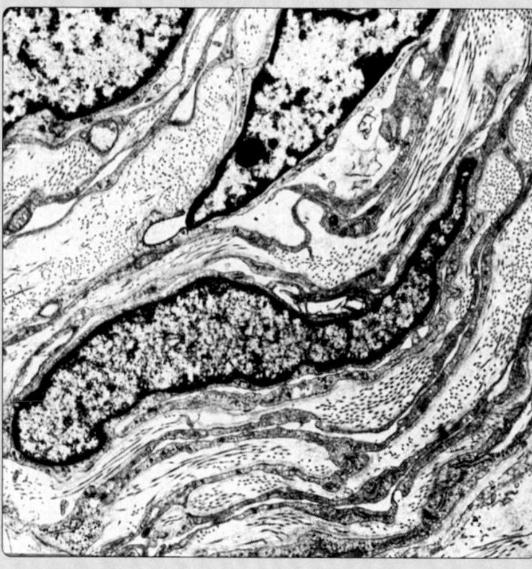

(Left) *Collagenous stroma varies from subtle to frank sclerosis in soft tissue perineurioma. Here, a Masson trichrome stain highlights collagen in a chronic lesion.* **(Right)** *Ultrastructurally, neoplastic cells in perineurioma feature elongated, narrow processes in a collagenous stroma, nucleus with clumped chromatin, and inconspicuous nucleoli.*

TERMINOLOGY

Definitions

- Benign soft tissue neoplasm composed of perineurial cells

ETIOLOGY/PATHOGENESIS

Chromosomal Abnormalities

- At least partial deletion of chromosome 22

CLINICAL ISSUES

Epidemiology

- Incidence
  - No syndrome association
    - Rarely reported in neurofibromatosis type 1 or neurofibromatosis type 2 patients, but biologic association unclear
- Age
  - Middle-aged adults
- Sex
  - Female predominance (F:M = 4:1)

Site

- Subcutaneous common
- Less common in deep soft tissues of extremities, trunk
- Rare in viscera

Presentation

- Painless mass
- Neurologically asymptomatic

Treatment

- Complete excision

Prognosis

- No recurrence/metastases after total resection

IMAGING

General Features

- Well delineated

MR Findings

- T2: Homogeneous high signal intensity
- T1: Homogeneous low signal intensity

MACROSCOPIC

General Features

- Unencapsulated but well circumscribed
- Nodular or ovoid, rubbery to firm
- Cut surface white-tan
- No nerve association

MICROSCOPIC

Histologic Features

- No associated nerve
- Neither distinct capsule nor significant infiltration
- Elongated bundles, interweaving fascicles, loose whorls, or vague storiform arrangements
- Myxoid change in subset
- Cells with curved, wavy, or disc-shaped nuclei
- Nuclear pleomorphism and hyperchromasia, occasional
- Narrow, long processes
- Mitosis scant or absent
- No necrosis
- Collagen-rich stroma
  - Dissection of collagen by tumor cells
- Longstanding lesions potentially sclerotic
- Sclerosing perineurioma variant
  - Most frequent in hands of young men
  - Extensive collagen deposition, epithelioid morphology
- Reticular/retiform perineurioma variant
  - Lace-like pattern of growth, collagenous to myxoid stroma
- Rare hybrid tumors with features of both perineurioma and schwannoma

ANCILLARY TESTS

Immunohistochemistry

- EMA, GLUT1, and claudin (+)
- S100(-)
- Collagen IV: Abundant basement membrane
- Neurofilament protein (-)
- Actin and desmin (-)

In Situ Hybridization

- Chromosome 22q11 loss

Electron Microscopy

- Normal-appearing perineurial cells: Long, narrow processes, pinocytotic vesicles, incomplete surface basal lamina, tight junctions
- Dissection and encirclement of collagen bundles

DIFFERENTIAL DIAGNOSIS

Neurofibroma

- S100 protein (+), SOX10(+), only rare EMA(+) cells

Solitary Fibrous Tumor

- CD34 and Bcl-2 (+), EMA(-)
- Nuclear STAT6 immunoreactivity

Dermatofibrosarcoma Protuberans

- CD34(+), EMA(-)

Myoepithelioma

- Actin (+), CK(+)

Fibrous Meningioma

- Similar immunophenotype
- Dural attachment

Low-Grade Fibromyxoid Sarcoma

- Prominent stromal collagen, transition into myxoid nodules abrupt
- EMA expression in up to 40%, but MUC4 expression in all cases (while negative in perineurioma)
- FUS rearrangements

SELECTED REFERENCES

1. Hornick JL et al: Soft tissue perineurioma: clinicopathologic analysis of 81 cases including those with atypical histologic features. Am J Surg Pathol. 29(7):845-58, 2005

(Left) *Perineuriomas may have parallel spindle cells in a myxoid stroma.* **(Right)** *Storiform pattern and whorls are common in soft tissue perineuriomas. Blood vessels are usually inconspicuous but may be hyalinized in longstanding examples.*

Parallel Spindle Cells in Myxoid Stroma

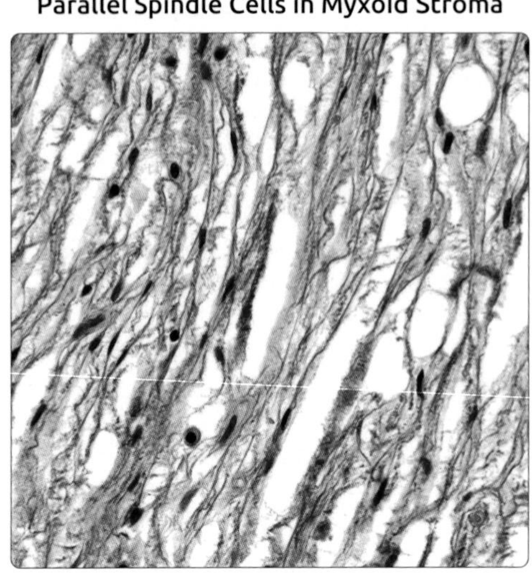

Storiform Pattern

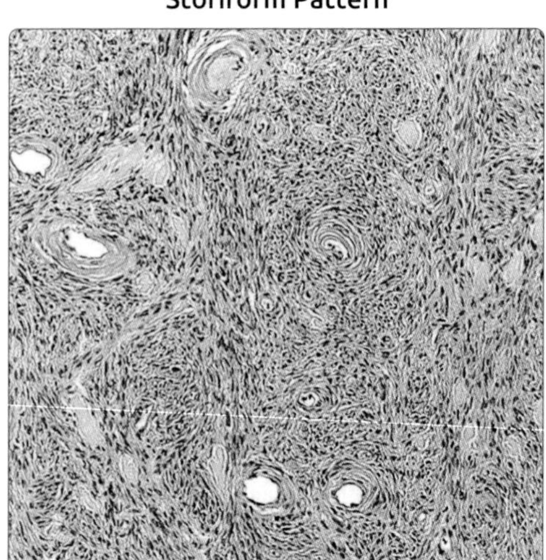

(Left) *Note lack of a capsule in this subcutaneous perineurioma. The overlying epidermis may show pseudoepitheliomatous hyperplasia.* **(Right)** *Rare perineuriomas appear in the head and neck. This example is just beneath the mucosal epithelium of a maxillary sinus. As is typical, there is no capsule.*

Absent Capsule

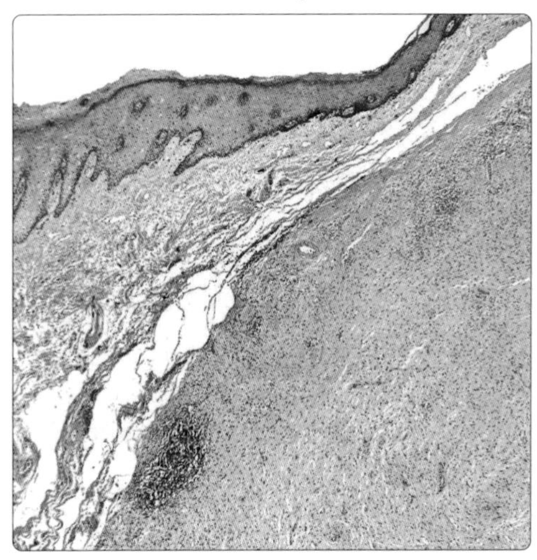

Sinonasal Location

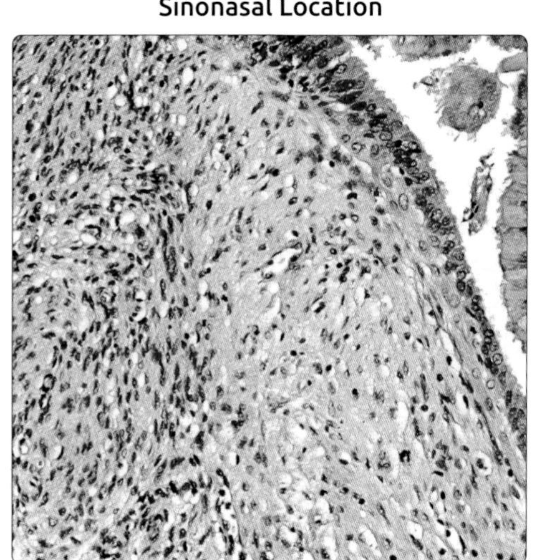

(Left) *Neoplastic perineural cells may form whorls ➔. Cells have bland, wavy, or disc-shaped nuclei.* **(Right)** *Longstanding lesions, particularly in the hands of male patients, show extensive sclerosis. Note dissection into collagen bundles by neoplastic cells ⇨.*

Whorls

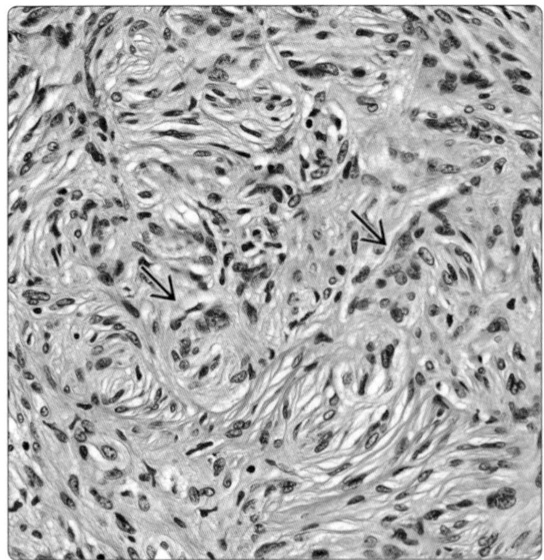

Sclerosing Perineurioma

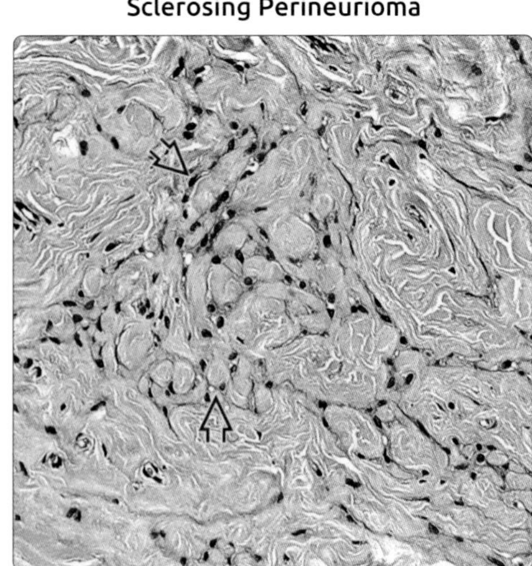

EMA Positivity

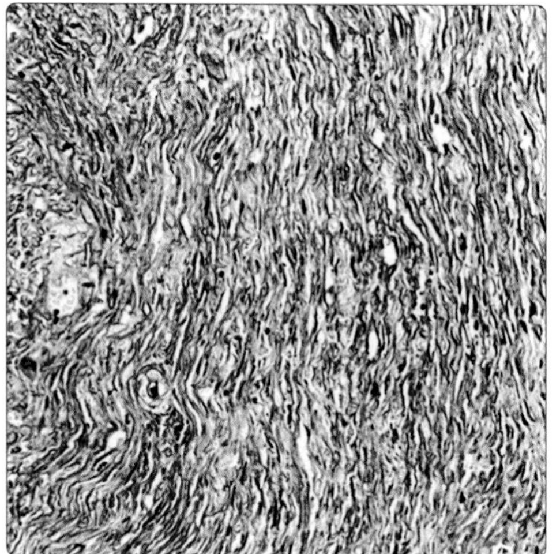

GLUT1 Positivity

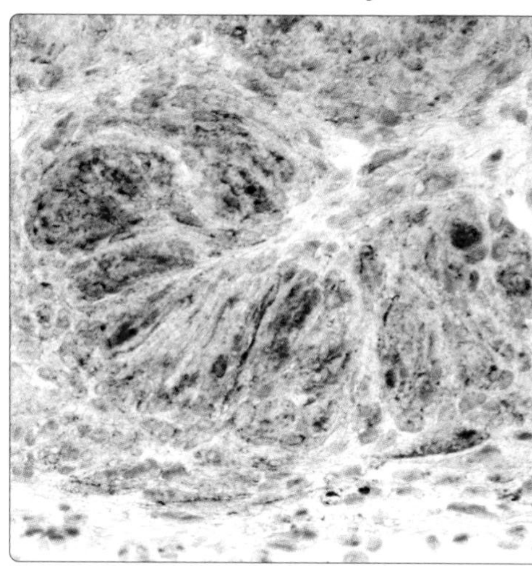

(Left) *Diffuse EMA positivity is a diagnostically helpful feature of soft tissue perineuriomas.* **(Right)** *GLUT1 labels neoplastic perineurial cells. It is not a specific marker for perineurial differentiation, yet it is a helpful tool for the differential diagnosis of low-grade fibromyxoid sarcoma, dermatofibrosarcoma protuberans, and myxofibrosarcoma, which are all negative.*

Claudin-1 Immunopositivity

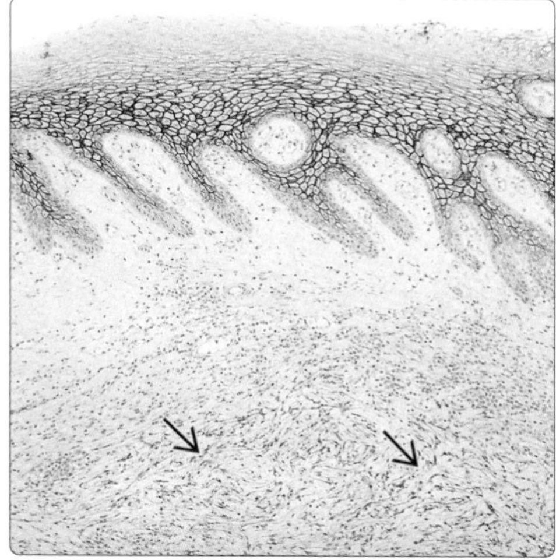

Collagen IV Immunostaining

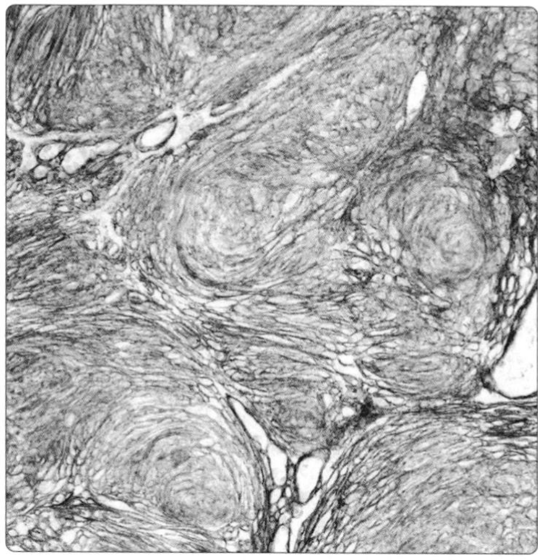

(Left) *Variable claudin-1 immunopositivity ➔ is seen in soft tissue perineuriomas.* **(Right)** *Collagen IV immunostaining highlights abundant pericellular basement membranes.*

Ch22 Loss

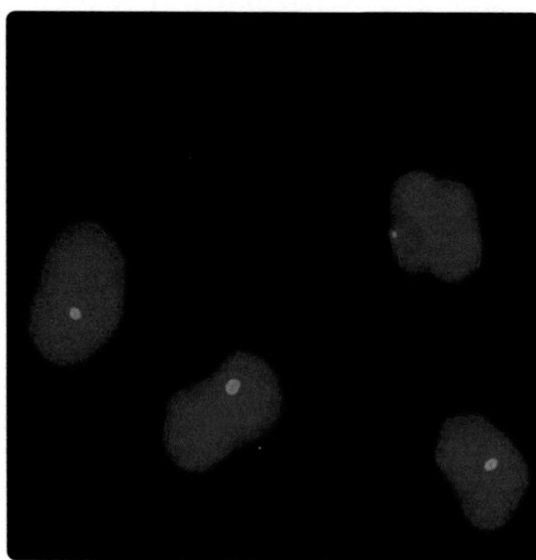

Micropinocytic Vesicles

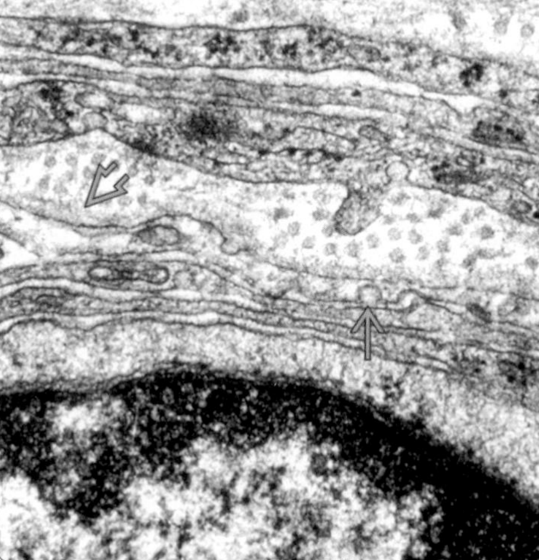

(Left) *Fluorescence in situ hybridization with a probe specific for the M-bcr locus, which maps to the chromosome band 22q11, shows Ch22/22q loss in perineurioma cells.* **(Right)** *Narrow cell processes with micropinocytic vesicles ➔ are covered by interrupted basal lamina ⇨.*

Lipoma of 8th Cranial Nerve

KEY FACTS

TERMINOLOGY

- Lipoma of internal auditory canal, lipochoristoma, lipomatous choristoma, 8th nerve choristoma, myolipoma, rhabdomyoma
- Benign adiposytic lesion usually involving 8th cranial nerve, occasionally containing mature muscle (myolipoma or rhabdomyoma)

ETIOLOGY/PATHOGENESIS

- Intimate admixture with cranial nerve, stability over time, and presence of other mesenchymal elements suggest malformation

CLINICAL ISSUES

- Almost always confined to internal auditory canal
- Excellent prognosis
- Hearing loss, dizziness, tinnitus, cranial nerve neuropathy
- Favorable; indolent behavior

IMAGING

- Variable imaging characteristics depending on presence of additional nonadipositic components

MICROSCOPIC

- Predominant component of mature adipose tissue
- May dissect along cranial nerve fascicles
- Myogenic component may predominate (rare)

ANCILLARY TESTS

- Lack *HMGA2* rearrangements by FISH (in contrast to conventional lipomas)

TOP DIFFERENTIAL DIAGNOSES

- Schwannoma
- Teratoma
- Meningioma
- Traumatic neuroma

(Left) *Unlike vestibular schwannoma, the lipomas of the 8th cranial nerve ➔ have the bright signal of adipose tissue on this precontrast T1WI MR.* **(Right)** *Adipose tissue, ganglion cells, and H&E/Luxol fast blue stained myelinated nerve fibers ⇨ are classic components.*

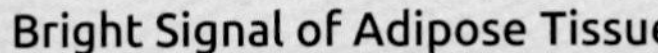
Bright Signal of Adipose Tissue

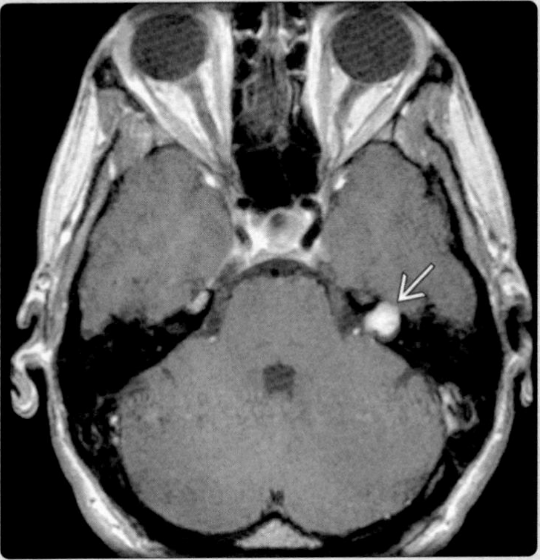

Myelinated Nerve Fibers

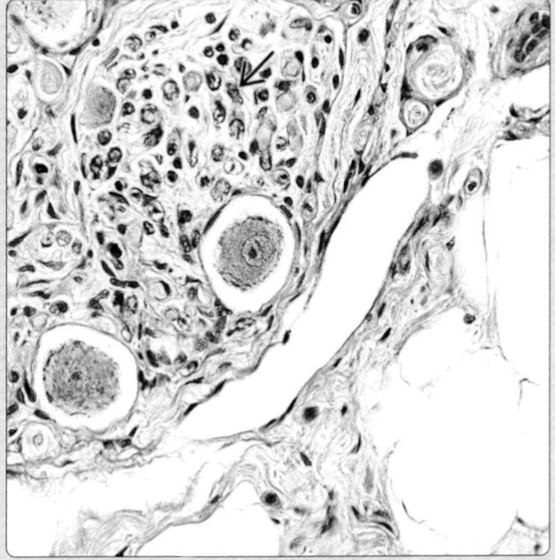

(Left) *Bundles composed of peripheral nerve axons ⇨ are surrounded by mature adipose tissue.* **(Right)** *Striated muscle cells ⇨ add interest to more complex mesenchymal lesions. When striated muscle predominates, the term rhabdomyoma may be appropriate.*

Peripheral Nerve Axons

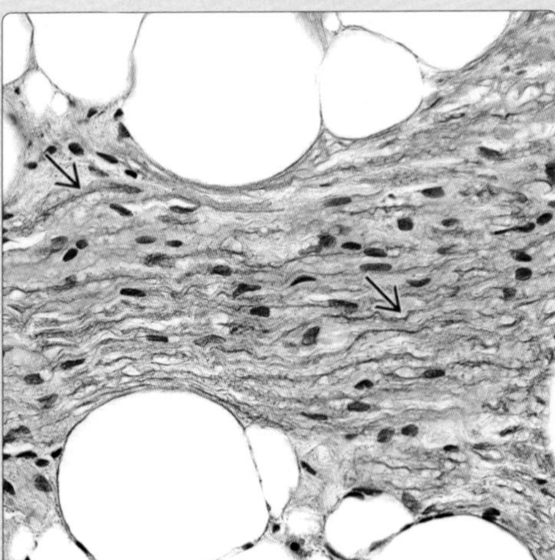

Striated Muscle

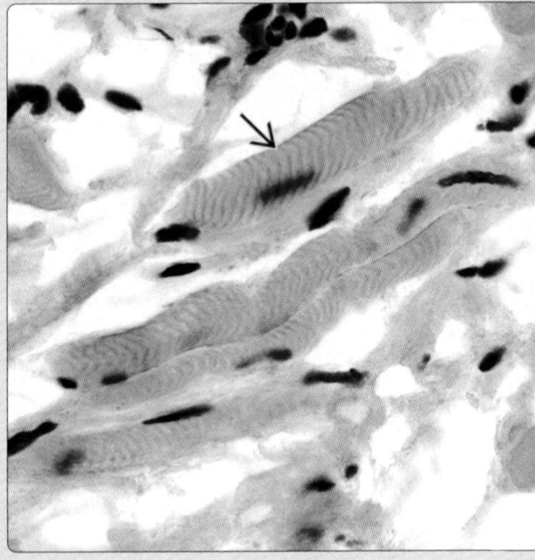

Lipoma of 8th Cranial Nerve

TERMINOLOGY

Synonyms

- Lipoma of internal auditory canal, lipochoristoma, lipomatous choristoma, 8th nerve choristoma, myolipoma, rhabdomyoma

Definitions

- Benign adiposytic lesion usually involving 8th cranial nerve, occasionally containing mature muscle (myolipoma or rhabdomyoma)

ETIOLOGY/PATHOGENESIS

Malformative vs. Neoplastic

- Intimate admixture with cranial nerve, stability over time, and presence of other mesenchymal elements suggest malformation

CLINICAL ISSUES

Site

- Almost always confined to internal auditory canal
- Larger lesions may extend to cerebellopontine angle to involve multiple cranial nerves

Presentation

- Hearing loss, dizziness, tinnitus, cranial nerve neuropathy
- Bilateral in minority of cases
- Multiple additional body lipomas reported in 1 case

Treatment

- Observation sufficient in most cases given diagnostic accuracy of current imaging modalities
- Sometimes approached surgically in expectation of vestibular schwannoma

Prognosis

- Favorable; indolent behavior
- Frequent stabilization after subtotal resection or even without intervention

IMAGING

MR Findings

- Variable imaging characteristics depending on presence of additional nonadipositic components
  - Predominantly fatty: T1 hyperintense, lack of contrast enhancement
  - Nonfatty components: T1 iso- to hypointense to brain, variable enhancement
  - Fat suppression MR sequences increase precision of preoperative diagnosis

MICROSCOPIC

Histologic Features

- Predominant component of mature adipose tissue
- May dissect along cranial nerve fascicles
- Myelinated peripheral nerve fibers
- Tortuous vessels
- Variable mesenchymal components, including fibrous tissue, cartilage, and smooth and skeletal muscle
  - Myogenic component may predominate (rare)
  - Cartilage (rare)
- Disruption of adjacent ganglia in some cases

ANCILLARY TESTS

Genetic Testing

- 3 lipomas of 8th cranial nerve lacked *HMGA2* rearrangements by FISH
  - Suggests biological distinction from conventional soft tissue lipomas, which usually have *HMGA2* rearrangements

DIFFERENTIAL DIAGNOSIS

Schwannoma

- Most common neoplasm of 8th cranial nerve
- Not intrinsically bright on precontrast T1WI MR
- Presence of mature fat uncommon

Teratoma

- Additional elements of all 3 germ cell layers

Meningioma

- May contain adipose tissue as metaplastic phenomenon but meningothelial tissue predominant

Traumatic Neuroma

- Disorganized nerve twigs, but no adiposytic component

DIAGNOSTIC CHECKLIST

Clinically Relevant Pathologic Features

- Can be identified radiologically because of adipose tissue

Pathologic Interpretation Pearls

- Exclude teratoma by searching for additional somatic components

SELECTED REFERENCES

1. Rodriguez FJ et al: HMGA2 rearrangements are rare in benign lipomatous lesions of the nervous system. Acta Neuropathol. 116(3):337-8, 2008
2. Brodsky JR et al: Lipoma of the cerebellopontine angle. Am J Otolaryngol. 27(4):271-4, 2006
3. Dazert S et al: Rare tumors of the internal auditory canal. Eur Arch Otorhinolaryngol. 262(7):550-4, 2005
4. Wu SS et al: Lipochoristomas (lipomatous tumors) of the acoustic nerve. Arch Pathol Lab Med. 127(11):1475-9, 2003
5. Hilton MP et al: Facial nerve paralysis and meningioma of the internal auditory canal. J Laryngol Otol. 116(2):132-4, 2002
6. Krainik A et al: MRI of unusual lesions in the internal auditory canal. Neuroradiology. 43(1):52-7, 2001
7. Wang CC et al: Diagnosis and treatment of lipomas of the internal auditory canal. Ear Nose Throat J. 80(5):340-2, 345, 2001
8. Bigelow DC et al: Lipomas of the internal auditory canal and cerebellopontine angle. Laryngoscope. 108(10):1459-69, 1998
9. Greinwald JH Jr et al: Lipomas of the internal auditory canal. Laryngoscope. 107(3):364-8, 1997

PART I
SECTION 5
Familial Tumor Syndromes

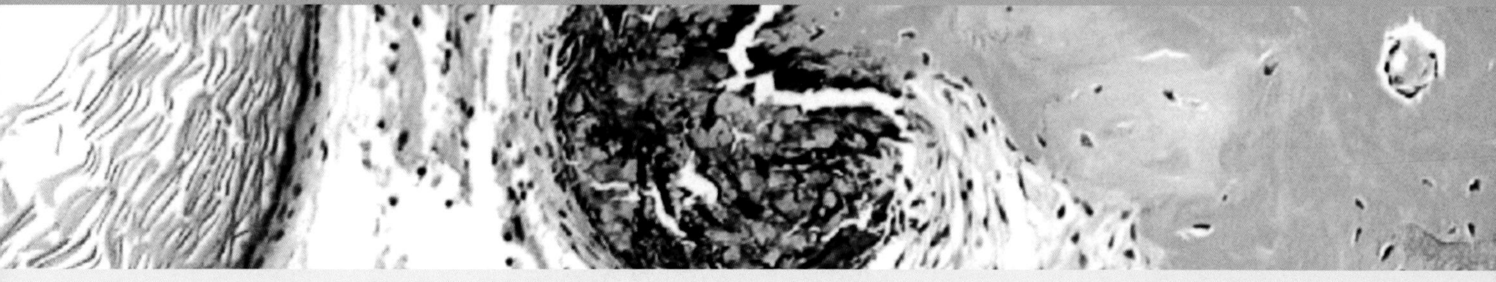

Neurofibromatosis

Other

Neurofibromatosis 1

KEY FACTS

ETIOLOGY/PATHOGENESIS

- ~ 1/3,000
- Autosomal dominant
- 50% sporadic occurrence
- Mutations in *NF1* gene (at 17q11.2)
- Functions as tumor suppressor, plays role in cell proliferation and differentiation

CLINICAL ISSUES

- Manifestations usually evident in childhood
- ≥ 2 of criteria
  - ≥ 6 café au lait spots
  - ≥ 2 neurofibromas
  - ≥ 1 plexiform neurofibroma
  - Freckling in axilla and groin
  - Optic nerve glioma (pilocytic astrocytoma)
  - ≥ 2 Lisch nodules
  - Distinctive bony lesion(s)
  - 1st-degree relative with neurofibromatosis type 1
- Neurogenic-associated neoplasms
  - Neurofibromas
  - Malignant peripheral nerve sheath tumor
  - Optic glioma (pilocytic astrocytoma)
  - Diffusely infiltrating astrocytomas of all grades
- Nonneurogenic-associated neoplasms
  - Rhabdomyosarcoma
  - Juvenile myelomonocytic leukemia
  - Pheochromocytoma
- CNS nontumoral manifestations
  - Occasionally neuroglial hamartomas (e.g., gliofibrillary nodules)
  - Aqueductal stenosis, hydrocephalus
  - Macrocephaly
  - Intellectual impairment common
  - Unknown bright objects: Asymptomatic focal areas of ↑ T2 signal on MR

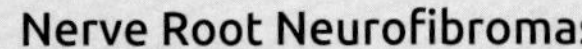

Nerve Root Neurofibromas

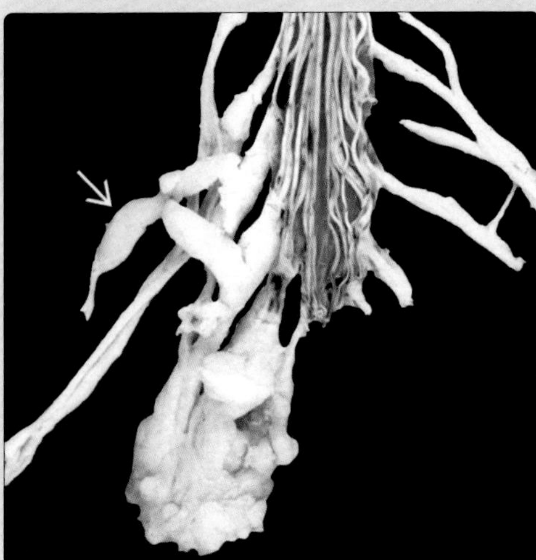

Pilocytic Astrocytoma of Optic Nerve

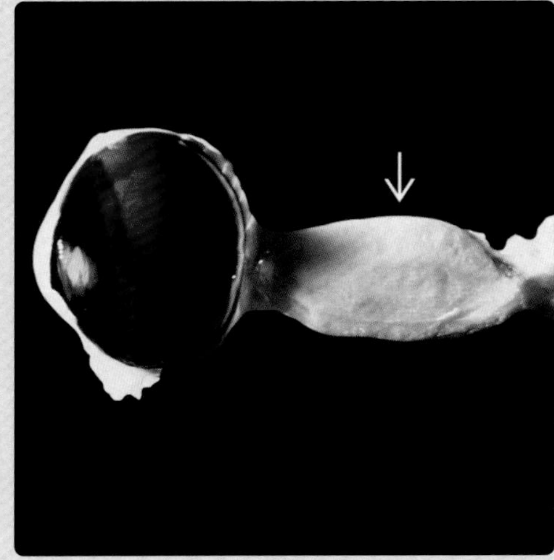

(Left) *Neurofibromas developing in multiple spinal nerve roots ➔ are limited to patients with neurofibromatosis type 1 (NF1).* **(Right)** *The most common glioma in NF1 is pilocytic astrocytoma, classically of the optic nerve ➔ and its leptomeninges. Such bilateral tumors are restricted to patients with NF1.*

Lisch Nodules

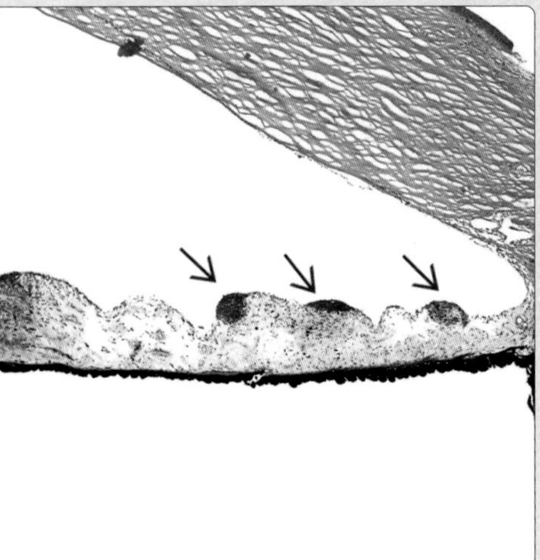

Plexiform Neurofibroma

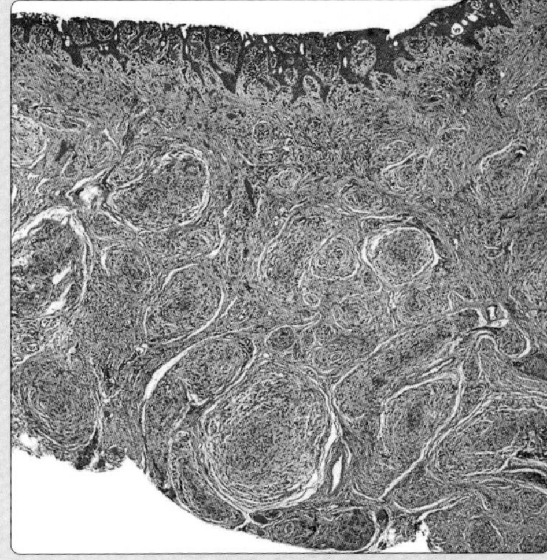

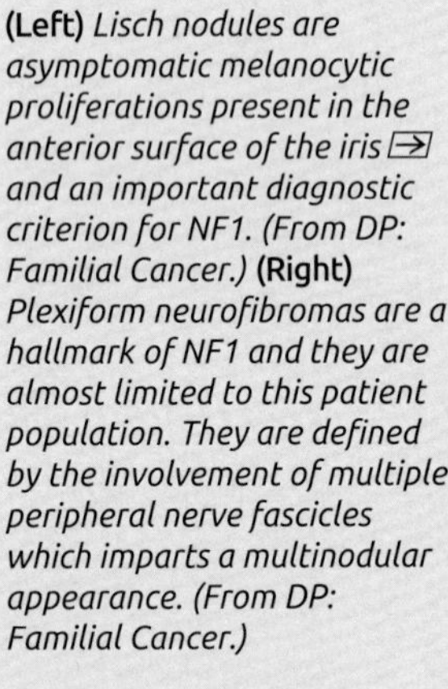

(Left) *Lisch nodules are asymptomatic melanocytic proliferations present in the anterior surface of the iris ➔ and an important diagnostic criterion for NF1. (From DP: Familial Cancer.)* **(Right)** *Plexiform neurofibromas are a hallmark of NF1 and they are almost limited to this patient population. They are defined by the involvement of multiple peripheral nerve fascicles which imparts a multinodular appearance. (From DP: Familial Cancer.)*

Neurofibromatosis 1

TERMINOLOGY

Abbreviations

- Neurofibromatosis 1 (NF1)

Synonyms

- Peripheral neurofibromatosis
- von Recklinghausen disease

Definitions

- Cancer predisposition syndrome due to genetic alterations of *NF1*

ETIOLOGY/PATHOGENESIS

Inheritance

- Autosomal dominant

Nonhereditary Incidence

- 50% sporadic occurrence

Chromosomal Alterations

- Mutations at 17q11.2
  - Encoded protein: Neurofibromin
    - Functions as tumor suppressor, plays role in cell proliferation and differentiation

CLINICAL ISSUES

Epidemiology

- Incidence
  - ~ 1/3,000
- Age
  - Manifestations usually evident in childhood
- Sex
  - M = F

Presentation

- ≥ 2 criteria
  - ≥ 6 café au lait spots; earliest manifestation
    - Postpubertal: ≥ 1.5 cm; prepubertal: ≥ 0.5 cm
  - ≥ 2 neurofibromas
  - ≥ 1 plexiform neurofibroma
  - Freckling in axilla and groin
    - Pigmentation of intertriginous skin
  - Optic nerve glioma (pilocytic astrocytoma)
  - ≥ 2 Lisch nodules
    - Pigmented iris hamartomas
  - Distinctive bony lesion(s)
    - Dysplasia of sphenoid bone
    - Dysplasia or thinning of long bone cortex
  - 1st-degree relative with NF1
- Localized NF1
  - 1 limb or single dermatome
  - Local somatic mutation
  - No genetic transmission
- Neurogenic-associated neoplasms
  - Neurofibromas
    - Localized cutaneous
    - Diffuse cutaneous
    - Localized intraneural
    - Plexiform
    - Massive soft tissue
    - Visceral, mainly gastrointestinal
  - Malignant peripheral nerve sheath tumor (MPNST)
  - Ganglioneuromatosis: gastrointestinal
    - Not specific, also a feature of other syndromes (multiple endocrine neoplasia type 2B, Cowden)
  - Optic glioma
    - Bilateral examples only in NF1
    - 80% diagnosed by age 11
  - Diffusely infiltrating astrocytomas of any grade
- Nonneurogenic-associated neoplasms
  - Rhabdomyosarcoma
  - Juvenile myelomonocytic leukemia
  - Juvenile xanthogranuloma
  - Gastrointestinal stromal tumor
  - Glomus tumor
  - Pheochromocytoma
- CNS nontumoral manifestations
  - Unknown bright objects: Asymptomatic focal areas of ↑ T2 signal on MR
  - Occasionally neuroglial hamartomas (e.g., gliofibrillary nodules)
  - Aqueductal stenosis, hydrocephalus
  - Macrocephaly
  - Intellectual impairment common
- Miscellaneous associated lesions
  - Skeletal dysplasias
    - Scalloping of vertebral bodies, kyphoscoliosis
    - Overgrowth of long bones
    - Pseudoarthroses
    - Bone cysts
    - Lower thoracic acute angular scoliosis, exclusively in NF1
    - Facial asymmetry and proptosis
  - Mesodermal dysplasias
    - Arterial intimal fibrosis, vascular stenosis
    - Aneurysms
    - Hypertrophic cardiomyopathy

Prognosis

- Risk of malignant neoplasm 10x > normal population
- Loss or mutation of tumor suppressor genes in addition to *NF1* gene with transformation of neurofibroma to MPNST
  - 5% of NF1 patients
- Hyperpigmentation in café au lait spot extending across the midline associated with increased risk of MPNST development

IMAGING

MR Findings

- T2WI MR: Unidentified bright objects

CT Findings

- PET/CT: Helpful to detect malignant transition of plexiform neurofibroma

SELECTED REFERENCES

1. Riccardi VM: Neurofibromatosis type 1 is a disorder of dysplasia: the importance of distinguishing features, consequences, and complications. Birth Defects Res A Clin Mol Teratol. 88(1):9-14, 2010

Neurofibromatosis 2

KEY FACTS

ETIOLOGY/PATHOGENESIS

- Autosomal dominant or sporadic
- Mutations at 22q12, *NF2* gene
- Sporadic occurrence (50%)

CLINICAL ISSUES

- Incidence: 1/50,000
- 2nd or 3rd decade
- Schwannoma
  - Bilateral vestibular schwannomas, hallmark
  - Similar histologic features as sporadic tumors
  - Features occurring more frequently in neurofibromatosis 2 (NF2)-associated schwannomas include whorl formation, multiple tumors involving single nerve, and juxtaposition to meningioma
- Meningioma, often multiple; ependymoma, intraspinal; juvenile posterior subcapsular lenticular opacities/juvenile cortical cataract
- Meningiomas not higher grade than sporadic lesions, less often brain invasive
- Ependymoma
  - Cervical cord and cervicomedullary junction are favored sites in NF2
  - Majority of NF2-associated ependymomas are low grade and asymptomatic
- Mortality due to CNS complications
  - Increased risk of mortality with early-onset disease
- Associated nonneoplastic CNS lesions
  - Meningioangiomatosis
  - Glial microhamartomas, S100(+)
  - Intramedullary schwannosis
- Associated nonneoplastic peripheral manifestations
  - Posterior subcapsular lens opacity
  - Mononeuropathy/polyneuropathy

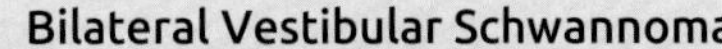

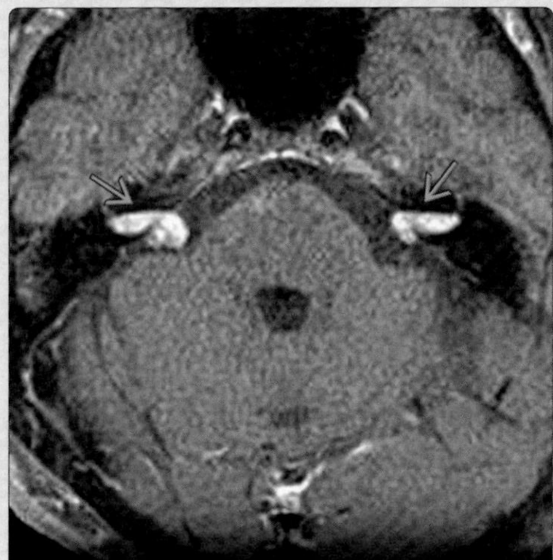

Multiple Meningiomas

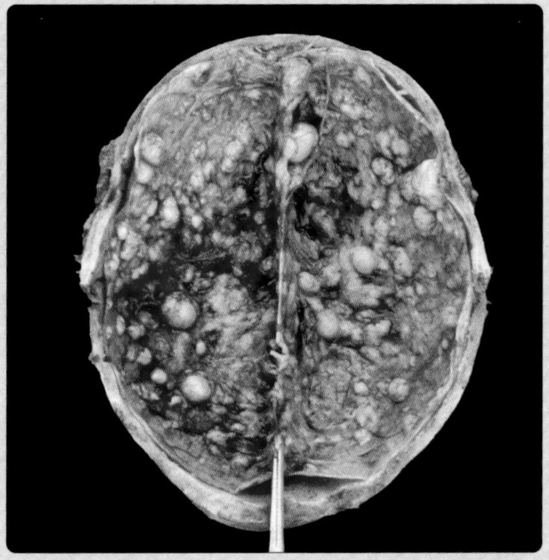

(Left) *Bilateral vestibular schwannomas are pathognomonic of neurofibromatosis 2 (NF2), presenting as enhancing masses in the cerebellopontine angle →. (From: DP: Familial Cancer.)* **(Right)** *Meningiomas of this multitude are consistent with NF2 but may rarely be a component of other familial genetic syndromes.*

Multiple Schwannomas

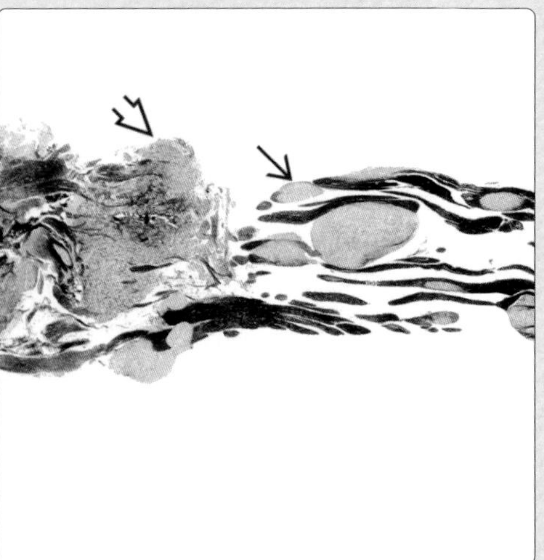

Whorls in Schwannoma

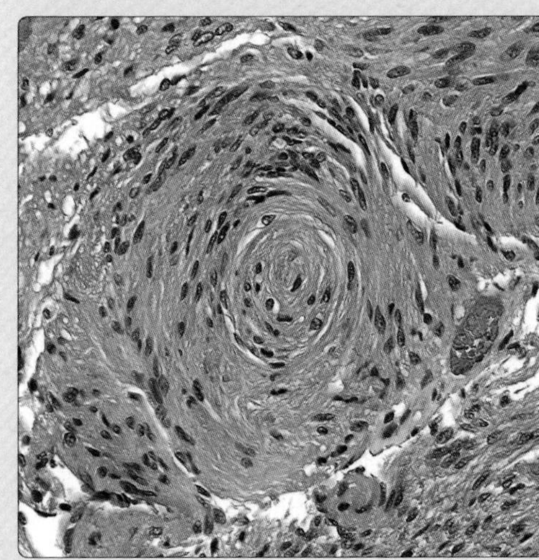

(Left) *Multiple schwannomas are seen arising from trigeminal ganglion ⇨ and nerve →. Schwannoma is the principal peripheral nervous system tumor in NF2, whereas neurofibroma is the principal PNS tumor in NF1.* **(Right)** *Whorls resembling those encountered in meningiomas may be more frequent in NF2-associated schwannomas than in sporadic tumors. IHC may help in their distinction, particularly in small biopsies. (From: DP: Familial Cancer.)*

TERMINOLOGY

Abbreviations

- Neurofibromatosis 2 (NF2)

Synonyms

- Central neurofibromatosis
- Bilateral acoustic neurofibromatosis

Definitions

- Cancer predisposition syndrome due to genetic alterations in *NF2* gene

ETIOLOGY/PATHOGENESIS

Inheritance

- Autosomal dominant

Nonhereditary Incidence

- 50% sporadic occurrence

Chromosomal Alterations

- Mutations in *NF2* gene at 22q12
  - Encoded protein: Merlin (schwannomin)
  - Functions as tumor suppressor, mediates communication between extracellular milieu and cytoskeleton
- 30% of de novo NF2 patients have mosaic genetic alterations

CLINICAL ISSUES

Epidemiology

- Incidence
  - 1/50,000
- Age
  - 2nd or 3rd decade

Presentation

- Diagnostic criteria for NF2 (Manchester criteria, 1992)
  - Bilateral vestibular schwannomas
  - Or
    - 1st-degree relative with NF2 and unilateral vestibular schwannoma, or any 2 of following: Meningioma, glioma, schwannoma, juvenile posterior subcapsular lenticular opacities/juvenile cortical cataract
  - Or
    - Unilateral vestibular schwannoma and any 2 of following: Neurofibroma, meningioma, glioma, schwannoma, posterior subcapsular lens opacity
  - Or
    - 2 or more meningiomas + unilateral vestibular schwannoma or any 2 of: Neurofibroma, glioma, schwannoma, or cataract
- Baser criteria (2011) incorporate genetic information to clinical information
- NF2 with rapid disease course
  - Early onset
  - Multiple tumors in addition to bilateral vestibular schwannomas
- Features of associated neoplasms
  - Schwannoma
    - Bilateral vestibular schwannomas; hallmark
    - Cutaneous and spinal schwannomas common
    - Plexiform schwannomas (but not specific to syndrome)
    - Multifocal within nerve with prominent myxoid change
    - Similar histologic features as sporadic tumors
    - Features occurring more frequently in NF2-associated schwannomas include whorl formation, multiple tumors involving single nerve, and juxtaposition to meningioma
  - Meningioma
    - Multiple
    - Meningiomatosis, when multifocal involves both cranial and spinal meninges
    - Intraventricular, uncommon
  - Ependymoma
    - Cervical cord and cervicomedullary junction are favored sites in NF2
    - Majority of NF2-associated ependymomas are low grade and asymptomatic
  - Admixture of schwannoma and meningioma
- Associated nonneoplastic CNS lesions
  - Meningioangiomatosis
  - Glial microhamartomas, S100(+)
  - Cellular ependymal ectopias
  - Intramedullary schwannosis
  - Syringomyelia
  - Cerebral, cerebellar, periventricular, choroid plexus calcifications
- Associated nonneoplastic peripheral manifestations
  - Posterior subcapsular lens opacity
  - Mononeuropathy/polyneuropathy

Prognosis

- All vestibular schwannomas, benign
- Meningiomas not higher grade than sporadic lesions, less often brain invasive
- Increased risk of mortality with early-onset disease
- Mortality due to CNS complications

IMAGING

MR Findings

- Demonstration of vestibular schwannomas may require thin slices

DIAGNOSTIC CHECKLIST

Pathologic Interpretation Pearls

- NF2 frequently undiagnosed in children; therefore, further assessment for NF2 features may be recommended in children presenting with meningiomas

SELECTED REFERENCES

1. Baser ME et al: Empirical development of improved diagnostic criteria for neurofibromatosis 2. Genet Med. 13(6):576-81, 2011
2. Smith MJ et al: Cranial meningiomas in 411 neurofibromatosis type 2 (NF2) patients with proven gene mutations: clear positional effect of mutations, but absence of female severity effect on age at onset. J Med Genet. 48(4):261-5, 2011
3. Perry A et al: Aggressive phenotypic and genotypic features in pediatric and NF2-associated meningiomas: a clinicopathologic study of 53 cases. J Neuropathol Exp Neurol. 60(10):994-1003, 2001

Schwannomatosis

KEY FACTS

TERMINOLOGY

- Neurofibromatosis with multiple nonvestibular schwannomas

ETIOLOGY/PATHOGENESIS

- 75-85% sporadic, 15-25% inherited
- Alterations in chromosome 22q
  - Biallelic somatic inactivation of *NF2* gene
  - Germline mutations of *SMARCB1*/INI1 gene
  - Germline mutations in *LZTR1* in subset

CLINICAL ISSUES

- 1:40,000
- 2nd and 3rd decades
- Pain (may be disabling)
- Less frequently associated with meningiomas
- Rare examples with malignant rhabdoid tumor
- Diagnostic criteria
  - Several clinical criteria proposed to distinguish schwannomatosis from neurofibromatosis 2 (NF2)
  - Lack of bilateral vestibular schwannoma; lack of NF2 in 1st-degree relative; lack of germline *NF2* mutation
  - Recent proposals incorporate molecular testing

MICROSCOPIC

- Schwannoma
  - Schwannomas with classic features
  - Prominent myxoid change
  - Peritumoral edema
- Tumors with hybrid neurofibroma/schwannoma features overrepresented in syndrome-associated peripheral nerve tumors, particularly in schwannomatosis

ANCILLARY TESTS

- Mosaicism for INI1 IHC in 93% of tumors from familial schwannomatosis, only 55% of sporadic schwannomatosis
  - Variable in practice, does not distinguish NF2 from schwannomatosis-associated schwannomas

(Left) *Multiple schwannomas are the hallmark of schwannomatosis ➡. The spinal nerves are frequently involved in these patients. (From: DP: Familial Cancer.)* **(Right)** *Surgical specimen from a patient with schwannomatosis demonstrates multiple schwannoma nodules ➡. Multiple foci of expansion may occur along the same or nearby fascicles.*

Multiple Schwannomas

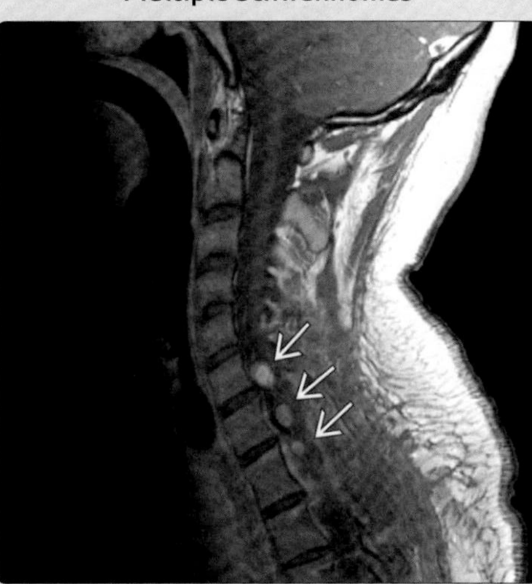

Multiple Schwannomas

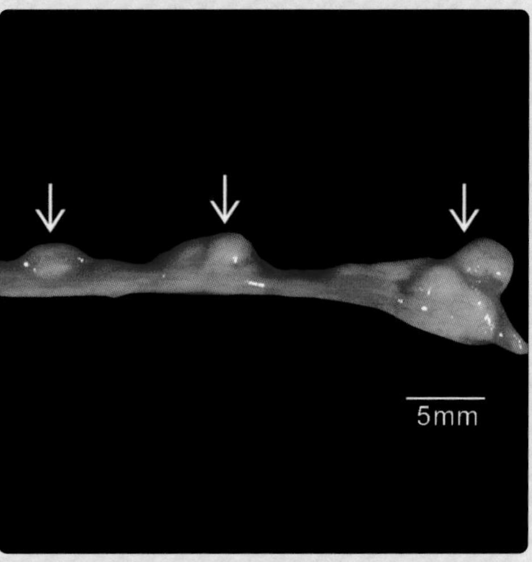

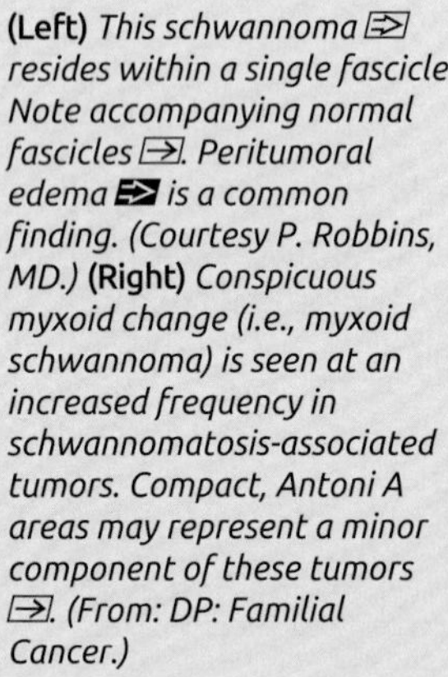

(Left) *This schwannoma ➡ resides within a single fascicle. Note accompanying normal fascicles ➡. Peritumoral edema ➡ is a common finding. (Courtesy P. Robbins, MD.)* **(Right)** *Conspicuous myxoid change (i.e., myxoid schwannoma) is seen at an increased frequency in schwannomatosis-associated tumors. Compact, Antoni A areas may represent a minor component of these tumors ➡. (From: DP: Familial Cancer.)*

Schwannoma Within Single Fascicle

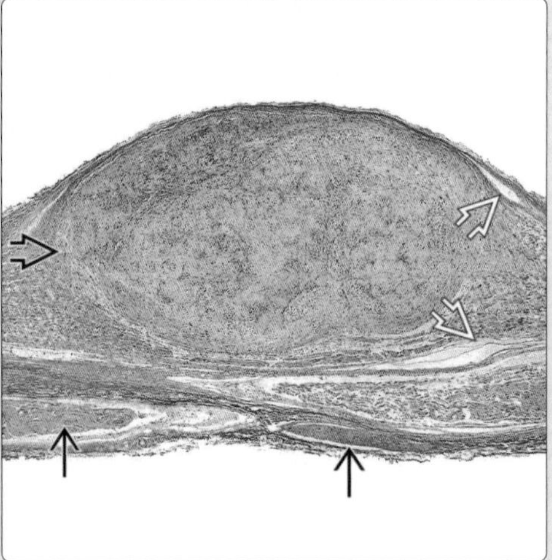

Myxoid Change

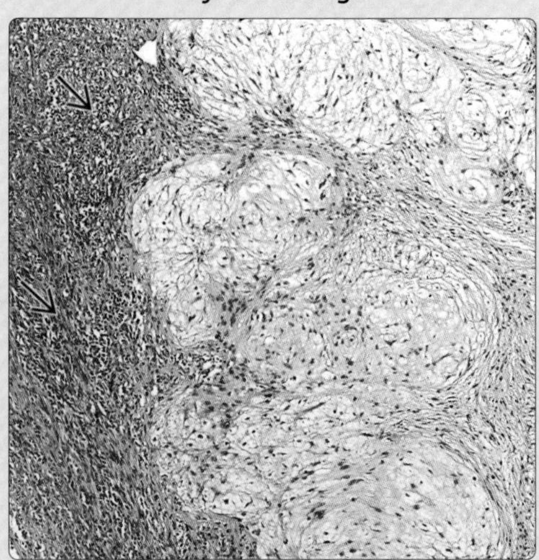

TERMINOLOGY

Definitions

- Non-neurofibromatosis 1 (NF1)/NF2 syndrome with multiple, nonvestibular schwannomas

ETIOLOGY/PATHOGENESIS

Chromosomal Alterations

- Germline mutations of *SMARCB1*/INI1 gene (in subset of cases)
  - 40-50% of familial cases, 8-10% of sporadic cases
  - 4-hit hypothesis: (1) germline *SMARCB1* mutation → loss of Chr 22 with remaining (2) *SMARCB1* allele and (3) *NF2* gene → loss of remaining (4) *NF2* allele
- Germline mutations in *LZTR1* in subset

Inheritance

- 75-85% sporadic, 15-25% inherited

CLINICAL ISSUES

Epidemiology

- Incidence
  - 1:40,000
- Age
  - 2nd and 3rd decade

Site

- Multiple schwannomas of spinal (75%), subcutaneous (15%), and cranial nerves (10%)
- Segmental in 30% cases

Presentation

- Pain (may be disabling)
- Rarely associated with meningiomas
- Infrequently with superficial neurofibromas
- Rare examples with malignant rhabdoid tumor
- No nonneoplastic manifestations
- Diagnostic criteria
  - Several clinical criteria proposed to distinguish schwannomatosis from NF2
  - Lack of bilateral vestibular schwannoma; lack of NF2 in 1st-degree relative; lack of germline *NF2* mutation
  - Recent proposals incorporate molecular testing

Treatment

- Surgery and pain management

Prognosis

- Good
- Anaplastic transformation rare

IMAGING

General Features

- Plexiform/multinodular lesions common

MACROSCOPIC

General Features

- Schwannomas vary from globular, multiple in fascicles, to plexiform

MICROSCOPIC

Histologic Features

- Schwannoma
  - Schwannomas with classic features
  - Prominent myxoid change
  - Peritumoral edema
- Tumors with hybrid neurofibroma/schwannoma features overrepresented in syndrome-associated peripheral nerve tumors, particularly in schwannomatosis

ANCILLARY TESTS

Immunohistochemistry

- Schwannomas positive for S100, collagen IV, SOX10; negative for EMA
- Schwannomas with mosaic pattern of INI1 staining
  - 93% of familial, 55% of sporadic schwannomatosis
  - Also in rare, solitary schwannomas not associated with schwannomatosis
  - Variable in practice, does not distinguish NF2 from schwannomatosis-associated schwannomas

DIFFERENTIAL DIAGNOSIS

Neurofibromatosis 2

- Multiple schwannomas with bilateral vestibular schwannomas
- May also have mosaic pattern of INI1 staining (83%)

Neurofibromatosis 1

- Multiple neurofibromas
  - Prominent myxoid change
  - Tumors painless
  - Subtotal S100 positivity

SELECTED REFERENCES

1. Piotrowski A et al: Germline loss-of-function mutations in LZTR1 predispose to an inherited disorder of multiple schwannomas. Nat Genet. 46(2):182-7, 2014
2. Plotkin SR et al: Update from the 2011 International Schwannomatosis Workshop: From genetics to diagnostic criteria. Am J Med Genet A. 161(3):405-16, 2013
3. Harder A et al: Hybrid neurofibroma/schwannoma is overrepresented among schwannomatosis and neurofibromatosis patients. Am J Surg Pathol. 36(5):702-9, 2012
4. Baser ME et al: Empirical development of improved diagnostic criteria for neurofibromatosis 2. Genet Med. 13(6):576-81, 2011
5. Rodriguez FJ et al: Superficial neurofibromas in the setting of schwannomatosis: nosologic implications. Acta Neuropathol. 121(5):663-8, 2011
6. Rousseau G et al: SMARCB1/INI1 germline mutations contribute to 10% of sporadic schwannomatosis. BMC Neurol. 11:9, 2011
7. Bacci C et al: Schwannomatosis associated with multiple meningiomas due to a familial SMARCB1 mutation. Neurogenetics. 11(1):73-80, 2010
8. Hulsebos TJ et al: SMARCB1/INI1 maternal germ line mosaicism in schwannomatosis. Clin Genet. 77(1):86-91, 2010
9. Swensen JJ et al: Familial occurrence of schwannomas and malignant rhabdoid tumour associated with a duplication in SMARCB1. J Med Genet. 46(1):68-72, 2009
10. Patil S et al: Immunohistochemical analysis supports a role for INI1/SMARCB1 in hereditary forms of schwannomas, but not in solitary, sporadic schwannomas. Brain Pathol. 18(4):517-9, 2008
11. Baser ME et al: Increasing the specificity of diagnostic criteria for schwannomatosis. Neurology. 66(5):730-2, 2006
12. MacCollin M et al: Diagnostic criteria for schwannomatosis. Neurology. 64(11):1838-45, 2005

von Hippel-Lindau Syndrome

KEY FACTS

TERMINOLOGY

- Autosomal dominant, germline mutation of *VHL* gene located on chromosome 3p25-p26
- Incidence ~ 1:40.000 population; > 90% penetrance by 65 yr

CLINICAL ISSUES

- 80% of individuals with von Hippel-Lindau (VHL) syndrome have affected parent
- Molecular genetic testing indicated in all suspected individuals
- Poorer prognosis with renal cell carcinoma
- Clinical criteria for diagnosis
  - Known family history: Diagnosis made on presence of single retinal or cerebellar hemangioblastoma (HBL), RCC, or pheochromocytoma
  - Clear cell carcinoma of kidney, endolymphatic sac tumor, pheochromocytoma, epididymal cystadenoma, renal cysts, pancreatic cysts, pancreatic neuroendocrine tumor, or adenoma
  - No family history: Diagnosis requires ≥ 2 retinal or cerebellar HBLs or single HBL and additional characteristic lesion

MICROSCOPIC

- Hemangioblastomas
- Endolymphatic sac tumor
  - Bone destructive, papillary, and well-differentiated adenocarcinoma with low mitotic rate
  - Bland, often single-layered atypical epithelium with sclerotic and cystic components
  - Typically cytokeratin (+), EMA(+), GFAP(+), S100(+)

ANCILLARY TESTS

- 4 molecular subtypes are recognized
- Type 1: Without pheochromocytoma
- Type 2: With pheochromocytoma but without RCC
- Type 3: With pheochromocytoma and RCC
- Type 4: With pheochromocytoma only

Multiple Hemangioblastomas

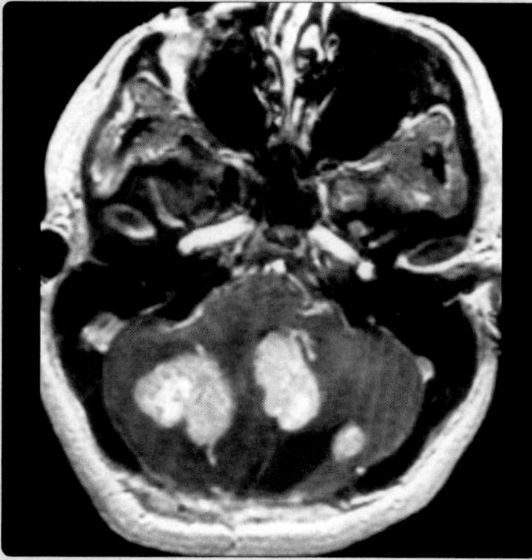

Endolymphatic Sac Tumor

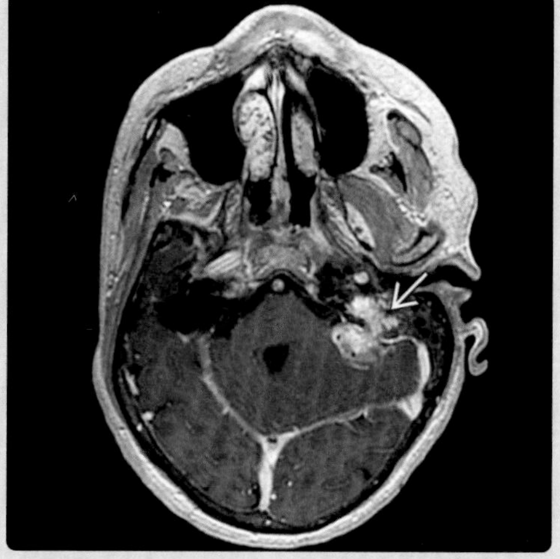

(Left) *Patients with von Hippel-Lindau (VHL) syndrome can have multiple hemangioblastomas that are either solid or solid-cystic. Axial contrast-enhanced T1WI MR demonstrates predominantly solid posterior fossa tumors.* **(Right)** *Axial contrast-enhanced T1WI MR shows a papillary endolymphatic sac tumor ➔ in a patient with VHL syndrome. In most instances, the tumor enhances avidly but variably, and mass effect can be seen.*

Typical Hemangioblastomas

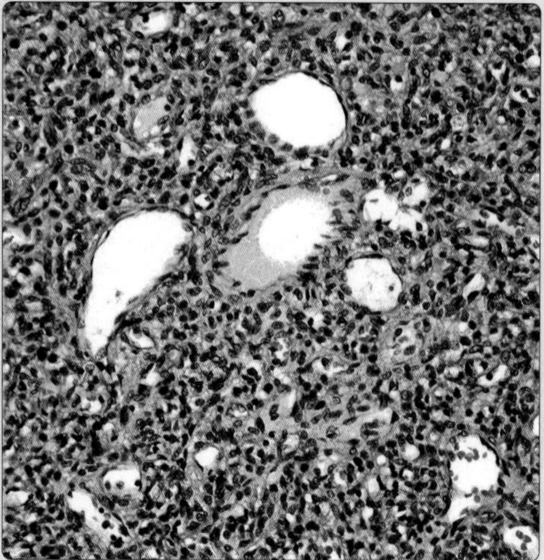

Endolymphatic Sac Tumor

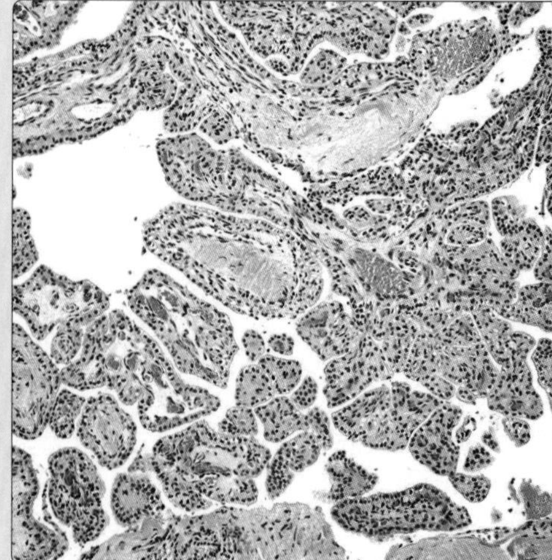

(Left) *Retinal hemangioblastomas are histologically identical to cerebellar examples, and some may appear cellular and compact. VHL patients can have metachronous cerebellar, cerebral, and spinal hemangioblastomas.* **(Right)** *Endolymphatic sac tumors are histologically well-differentiated papillary carcinomas with minimal anaplasia. The immunohistochemical staining pattern is only suggestive of a low-grade adenocarcinoma without special features.*

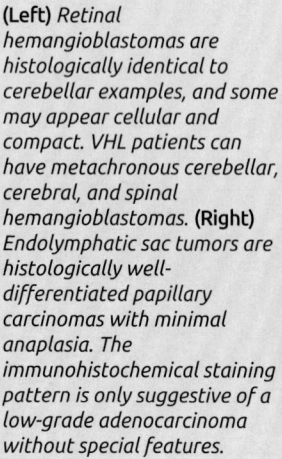

TERMINOLOGY

Abbreviations

- von Hippel-Lindau (VHL) disease

Definitions

- Germline mutation of *VHL* gene on chromosome 3p25-p26
- Autosomal dominant
- Diagnosis based on CNS hemangioblastoma and 1 other VHL-associated tumor or previous family history

CLINICAL ISSUES

Epidemiology

- Incidence
  - ~ 1:40,000 population
  - > 90% penetrance by age 65
  - 80% of individuals with VHL syndrome have affected parent
- Age
  - Young adults
    - Mean age: ~ 30 years

Presentation

- Visual loss due to retinal hemangioblastoma
- Nausea, vomiting, and ataxia due to cerebellar hemangioblastoma
- Deafness, vertigo, or tinnitus due to endolymphatic sac tumors
- Myelopathy with spinal cord tumor
- Presentation with kidney tumor or paraganglioma rare

Laboratory Tests

- Molecular genetic testing is indicated in all suspected individuals
- Sequence analysis of all 3 exons of *VHL* gene
- Measurement of urinary catecholamine metabolites

Treatment

- Surgical approaches
  - CNS neoplasms: Gross total resection is goal
  - Early detection and removal of renal, adrenal tumors as well as endolymphatic sac tumors, regardless of symptoms
- Drugs
  - Rare, unresectable pheochromocytomas may be treated with tyrosine kinase inhibitors
- Radiation
  - Local radiation for inoperable or subtotally resected tumors
  - Laser photocoagulation for retinal tumors

Prognosis

- Poorer with renal cell carcinoma
- Multiple recurrent and new tumors
- Endolymphatic sac tumors can recur
- Potential for CSF spread, uncommon
- Paraplegia may complicate management of spinal tumors

Diagnostic Criteria

- Hemangioblastomas in CNS or retina and
- Family history of VHL syndrome or
- Other associated tumor
  - Clear cell carcinoma of kidney
  - Endolymphatic sac tumor
  - Pheochromocytoma
  - Epididymal cystadenoma
  - Pancreatic neuroendocrine tumor or adenoma

IMAGING

Radiographic Findings

- Hemangioblastoma
  - Sites
    - Retina
    - Cerebellum
    - Medulla
    - Supratentorial brain (rare)
    - Spinal cord
    - Spinal nerve roots
    - Extraspinal peripheral nerve
  - Discrete, sometimes cystic mass
  - Highly vascular, flow voids
- Endolymphatic sac tumor
  - Site
    - Temporal bone
    - Sometimes bilateral
  - Often erosive
  - Hypervascular, contrast enhancing
  - May be hyperintense on noncontrast T1WI

ANCILLARY TESTS

Genetic Testing

- 4 molecular subtypes
  - Type 1: Without pheochromocytoma
  - Type 2: With pheochromocytoma but without renal cell carcinoma
  - Type 3: With pheochromocytoma and renal cell carcinoma
  - Type 4: With pheochromocytoma only
- Biallelic mutational inactivation of *VHL* gene is typical of all tumors in all types
- Missense mutation most common in all subtypes, but type of missense mutations correlates with disease subtype
- Close correlation between type of germline mutations and spectrum of clinical manifestations
- Deletion of *VHL* is associated with lower risk of renal cell carcinoma and is typical in type 2 patients
- Anticipation (tendency for individuals in successive generations to present at earlier age) is not observed

SELECTED REFERENCES

1. Maher ER et al: von Hippel-Lindau disease: a clinical and scientific review. Eur J Hum Genet. 19(6):617-23, 2011
2. Calzada MJ: Von Hippel-Lindau syndrome: molecular mechanisms of the disease. Clin Transl Oncol. 12(3):160-5, 2010
3. Leung RS et al: Imaging features of von Hippel-Lindau disease. Radiographics. 28(1):65-79; quiz 323, 2008
4. Shehata BM et al: Von Hippel-Lindau (VHL) disease: an update on the clinico-pathologic and genetic aspects. Adv Anat Pathol. 15(3):165-71, 2008
5. Wong WT et al: Ocular von Hippel-Lindau disease: clinical update and emerging treatments. Curr Opin Ophthalmol. 19(3):213-7, 2008
6. Mukherji SK et al: Papillary endolymphatic sac tumors: CT, MR imaging, and angiographic findings in 20 patients. Radiology. 202(3):801-8, 1997

Tuberous Sclerosis Complex

KEY FACTS

TERMINOLOGY

- Autosomal dominant; mutations in *TSC1* or *TSC2*
  - 2/3 of patients with spontaneous mutations
- Principally affects CNS, kidney, and heart

CLINICAL ISSUES

- Major features
  - Cortical tuber
  - Subependymal nodule
  - Subependymal giant cell astrocytoma
  - Retinal astrocytic proliferations (hamartomas)
  - Non-CNS: Facial angiofibroma, hypomelanotic nodules (> 3), cardiac rhabdomyoma, renal angiomyolipoma, Shagreen patch
- Recent use of mTOR inhibitors has been promising in patients with subependymal giant cell astrocytomas and other tumors such as renal angiomyolipoma
  - Not all lesions of tuberous sclerosis complex regress under mTOR inhibitors

IMAGING

- Cortical tubers: Low signal on T1-weighted and contrast-enhanced images, with underlying hyperintense white matter lesions on FLAIR
- Subependymal giant cell astrocytoma
- Subependymal nodules/hamartomas

ANCILLARY TESTS

- *TSC1* (hamartin), located on chromosome 9q34
  - Most are truncation mutations
  - More common in familial cases
- *TSC2* (tuberin), located on chromosome 16p13
  - Deletions, missense, nonsense, and frameshift insertions
  - More common in sporadic cases
- TSC1and TSC2 proteins form functional complex to suppress mTOR activity

Tuberous Sclerosis Brain

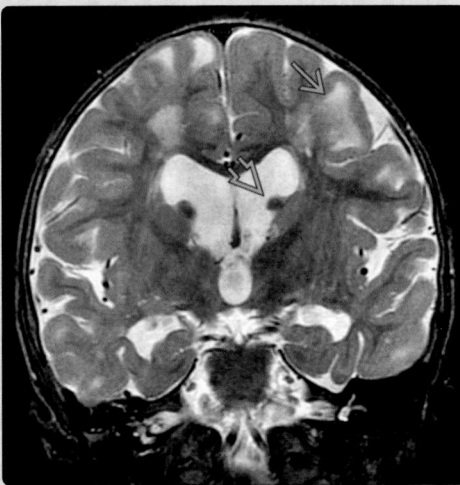

Autopsy Image of Subependymal Nodule

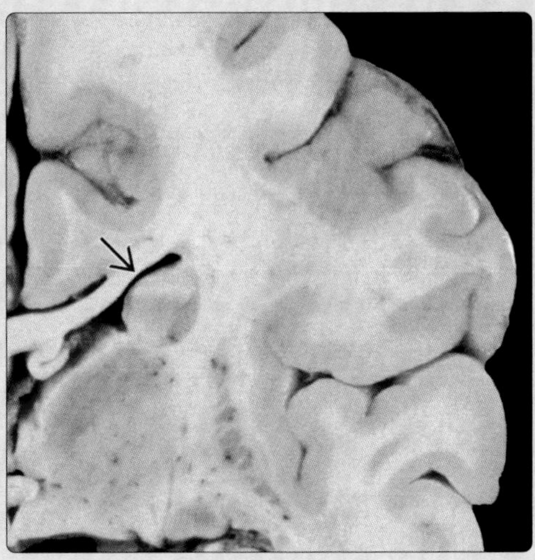

(Left) *Cerebral lesions present in tuberous sclerosis complex (TSC) include tubers with underlying white matter hyperintensity and calcified subependymal nodules that are often hypointense on T2-weighted images.* **(Right)** *Gross autopsy section from a patient with TSC illustrates a subependymal nodule near the body of the caudate nucleus. (Courtesy A. T. Yachnis, MD.)*

Retinal Astrocytoma in Tuberous Sclerosis

Balloon Cells of Cortical Tubers

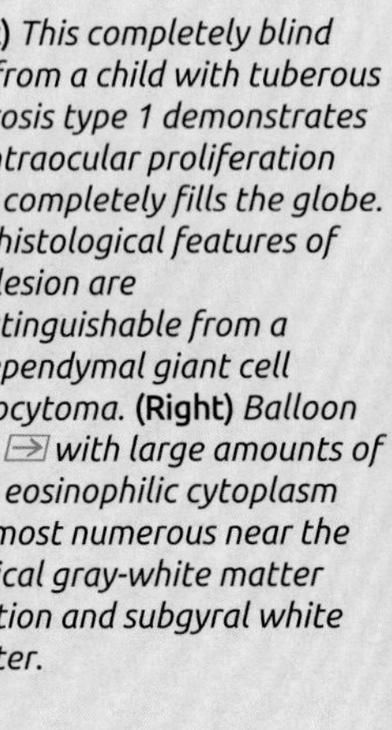

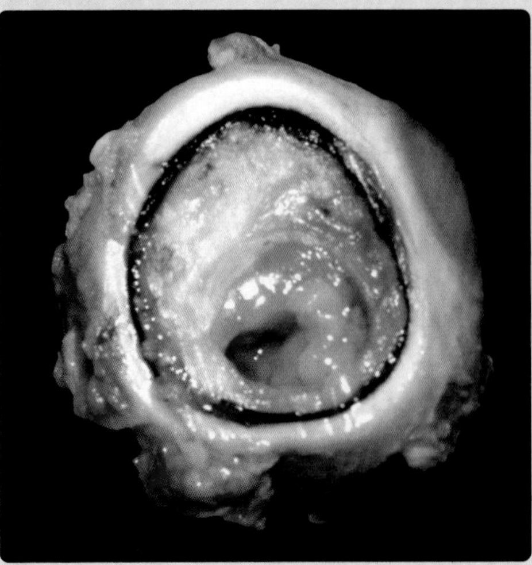

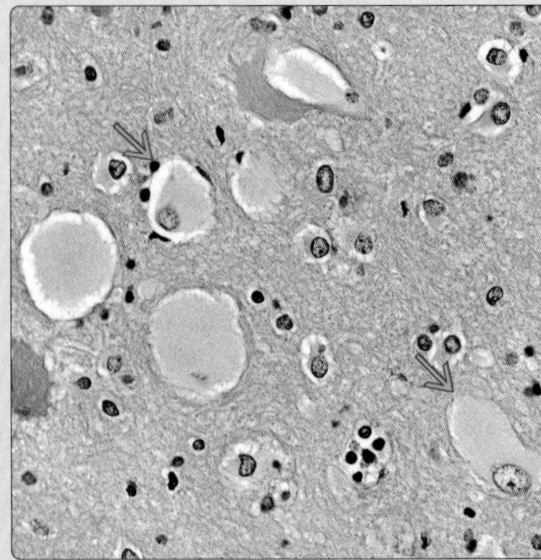

(Left) *This completely blind eye from a child with tuberous sclerosis type 1 demonstrates an intraocular proliferation that completely fills the globe. The histological features of this lesion are indistinguishable from a subependymal giant cell astrocytoma.* **(Right)** *Balloon cells with large amounts of pale eosinophilic cytoplasm are most numerous near the cortical gray-white matter junction and subgyral white matter.*

TERMINOLOGY

Abbreviations

- Tuberous sclerosis complex (TSC)

Definitions

- Autosomal dominant; mutations in *TSC1* or *TSC2*
  - 2/3 of patients with spontaneous mutations
- Principally affects CNS, kidney, and heart

CLINICAL ISSUES

Epidemiology

- Incidence
  - 2nd most common neurocutaneous disorder: 1:8,000 in general population

Presentation

- Most common within 1st decade of life
- Neurological symptoms most common presentation
- Seizures or autistic behavior in majority of patients
- Subependymal giant cell astrocytoma (SEGA) usually 1st recognized feature

Diagnostic Criteria

- Definitive: 2 major or 1 major and 2 minor features
- Probable: 1 major and 1 minor feature
- Possible: 1 major or ≥ 2 minor features
  - Major features
    - Cortical tuber
    - Subependymal nodule
    - Subependymal giant cell astrocytoma
    - Facial angiofibroma
    - Ungual/periungual fibroma
    - > 3 hypomelanotic macules
    - Connective tissue nevi (Shagreen patch)
    - Retinal astrocytic proliferations (hamartomas)
    - Cardiac rhabdomyoma
    - Renal angiomyolipoma
    - Lymphangiomatosis
  - Minor features
    - White matter linear migration lines (cyst-like lesions)
    - Transmantle cortical dysplasia
    - Retinal patch
    - Non-CNS lesions: Hamartomatous rectal polyps; gingival fibroma, hypomelanotic clustered skin lesions, bone cysts, renal cysts, nonrenal hamartomas

Miscellaneous Associated Lesions

- Corpus callosum agenesis, hemimegalencephaly, schizencephaly, cerebrovascular anomalies, e.g., aneurysms, vermian agenesis or hypoplasia, linear gyriform cerebellar calcifications, cerebellar hemispheric hyperplasia

IMAGING

Radiographic Findings

- Calcified subependymal nodules: Classic appearance
- Early stage cortical tubers are T2 hypointense and later become hyperintense
- Cortical tubers: Low signal on T1-weighted and contrast-enhanced images
- Streaky hyperintense white matter lesions on FLAIR
- SEGA and subependymal nodules enhance

MACROSCOPIC

Cortical Tubers

- Firm, nodular gray matter lesions, few millimeters to a centimeter
- More common in cerebral cortex, typically multiple; can occur in cerebellar cortex

Subependymal Nodules

- Nodular protrusions of ventricular walls
- Most common near foramen of Monro

SEGA

- Well-circumscribed mass near foramen of Monro

MICROSCOPIC

Histologic Features

- Cortical tubers
  - Proliferation of glial cells imparting haphazard appearance to cortex
  - Giant cells (balloon cells) as well as dysmorphic neurons
  - Irregular lamination pattern
  - Calcifications
- Subependymal nodules
  - Calcifications
  - Haphazard arrangement of glial cells and giant cells
  - Giant cells with both astrocytic and neuronal differentiation
  - Elongated cells with streaming eosinophilic cytoplasm, arranged in fascicles
- Retinal astrocytic proliferations (hamartomas)
  - Identical to subependymal nodules or SEGA

ANCILLARY TESTS

Immunohistochemistry

- Tuber
  - Balloon cells
    - Variably immunoreactive to vimentin, S100 protein, glial fibrillary acidic protein
    - Variably immunoreactive to class III β-tubulin, nestin, neurofilament, synaptophysin
- Subependymal hamartoma: Similar to SEGA

Genetic Testing

- *TSC1* (hamartin), located on chromosome 9q34
  - Most mutations truncations
  - More common in familial cases
- *TSC2* (tuberin), located on chromosome 16p13
  - Deletions, missense, nonsense, and frameshift insertions
  - Majority of cases
- TSC1and TSC2 proteins form functional complex to suppress mTOR activity

SELECTED REFERENCES

1. Han CW et al: Immunohistochemical analysis of developmental neural antigen expression in the balloon cells of focal cortical dysplasia. J Clin Neurosci. 18(1):114-8, 2011

Turcot Syndrome

KEY FACTS

TERMINOLOGY

- Germline mutations characterized by gastrointestinal and central nervous system neoplasms
- Recent findings of patients with *MUTYH* gene mutation may suggest yet a 3rd type in this group of familial tumor disposition syndromes

CLINICAL ISSUES

- Type 1
  - Glioblastoma (presentation earlier than peak incidence in general population)
  - Small and large intestinal polyps and colorectal cancer
  - Often autosomal recessive
  - Distinction from constitutional mismatch repair deficiency syndrome may not be possible
- Type 2
  - Medulloblastoma (presentation later than peak incidence in general population)
  - Numerous intestinal polyps with family history of polyposis
  - Often autosomal dominant

ANCILLARY TESTS

- Type 1: Germline mutations of mismatch repair genes
  - *MLH1* (chr 3p21.3)
  - *MSH2* (chr 2p16)
  - *PMS2* (chr 7p22
- Less commonly, *MSH3* (chr 5q11), *PMS1* (2q32)
- Type 2: Germline mutations in *APC* gene
  - *APC* gene (chr 5q21)

TOP DIFFERENTIAL DIAGNOSES

- Li-Fraumeni syndrome
- Constitutional mismatch repair deficiency syndrome
  - May not be easily distinguishable from type 1

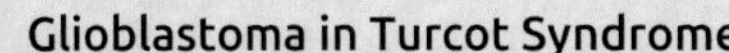

Glioblastoma in Turcot Syndrome | **Medulloblastoma in Turcot Syndrome**

(Left) *Astrocytic tumors in Turcot syndrome type 1 are clinically indistinguishable from sporadic tumors. These neoplasms are typically high grade, mostly glioblastoma, with significant mass effect as seen in this FLAIR image.* **(Right)** *Turcot syndrome type 2 associated with germline APC mutations typically harbors medulloblastomas. As in most medulloblastomas with Wnt pathway alterations, the tumors are usually located centrally.*

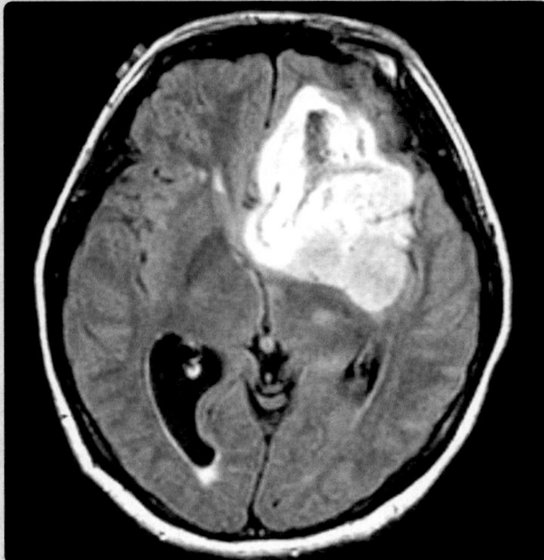

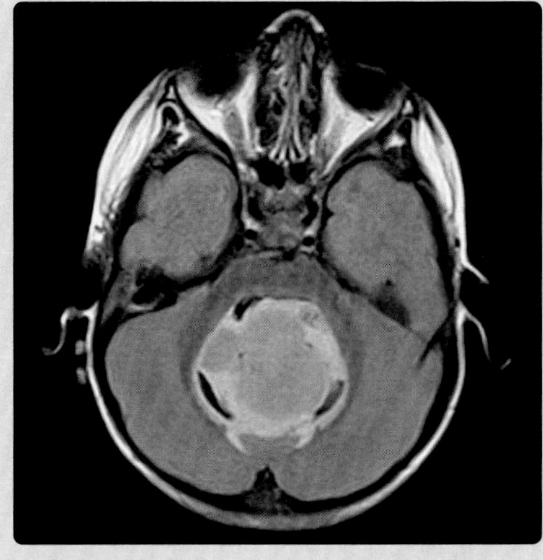

Glioblastoma in Turcot Syndrome | **Medulloblastoma in Turcot Syndrome**

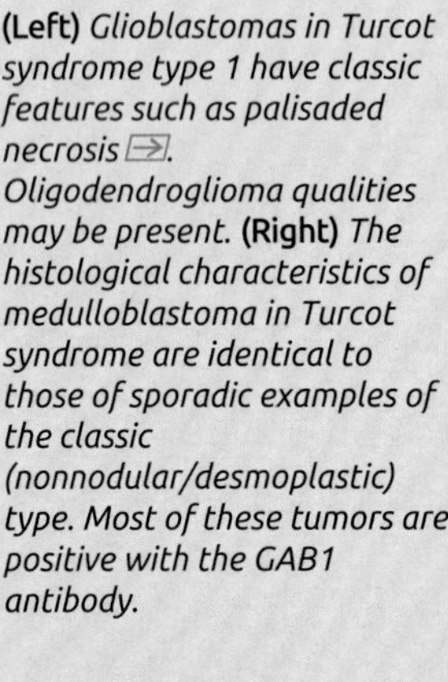

(Left) *Glioblastomas in Turcot syndrome type 1 have classic features such as palisaded necrosis ⇒. Oligodendroglioma qualities may be present.* **(Right)** *The histological characteristics of medulloblastoma in Turcot syndrome are identical to those of sporadic examples of the classic (nonnodular/desmoplastic) type. Most of these tumors are positive with the GAB1 antibody.*

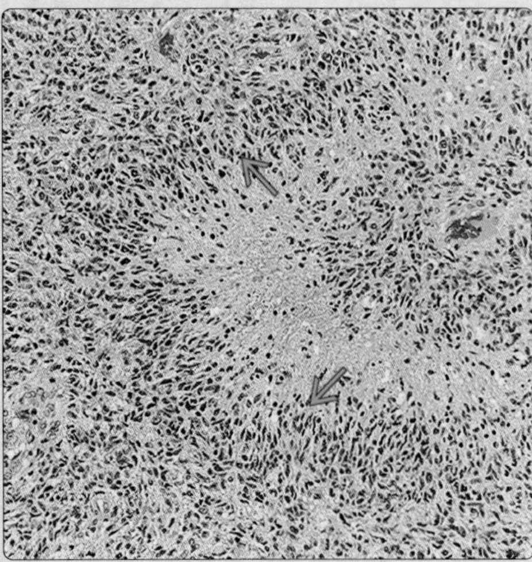

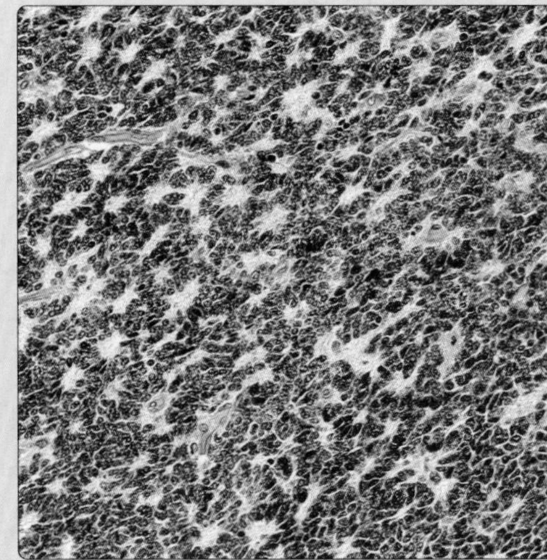

TERMINOLOGY

Definitions

- Autosomal dominant disorders characterized by gastrointestinal and CNS neoplasms
  - Type 1 hereditary nonpolyposis colorectal cancer (Lynch syndrome) and glioblastoma
  - Type 2 familial adenomatous polyposis and medulloblastoma
    - In addition: Skin lesions such as epidermoid cysts, craniofacial exostosis

ETIOLOGY/PATHOGENESIS

Germline Mutation in Tumor Suppressor or DNA Mismatch Repair Genes

- Type 1: DNA mismatch repair genes *(MLH1, MSH2, PMS2)*
- Type 2: Adenomatous polyposis coli (*APC*) gene

CLINICAL ISSUES

Presentation

- Glioblastoma (in type 1): Presentation earlier than peak incidence in general population
  - Median age: 18 years
- Medulloblastoma (in type 2): Presentation later than peak incidence in general population
  - Median age: 15 years
- No family history of polyposis in type 1, frequent family history of polyposis in type 2

Prognosis

- Presentation of CNS tumors at younger age = poor prognostic sign

Diagnostic Criteria

- Type 1
  - Glioblastoma
  - Small and large intestinal polyps and colorectal cancer
  - Often autosomal recessive
- Type 2
  - Medulloblastoma
  - Numerous intestinal polyps with family history of polyposis
  - Often autosomal dominant

MACROSCOPIC

Colorectal Lesions

- Type 1: Small number of polyps with occasional large (> 3 cm) polyps
- Type 2: Innumerable small polyps

MICROSCOPIC

Histologic Features

- Type 1
  - Anaplastic astrocytoma or glioblastoma, sometimes with oligodendroglioma qualities
  - Other types such as oligodendroglioma, ependymoma, glioneuronal tumors (all rare)
- Type 2
  - Medulloblastoma
    - Classic (nonnodular) type GAB1 positive

ANCILLARY TESTS

Genetic Testing

- Type 1
  - Germline mutations of mismatch repair genes
    - Most commonly, *PMS2* (chr 7p22), *MLH1* (chr 3p21.3), or *MSH2* (chr 2p16)
    - Less commonly, *MSH3* (chr 5q11), *PMS*1 (2q32)
    - None of the genes commonly implicated in sporadic glioblastomas
- Type 2
  - *APC* gene (chr 5q21)
  - *APC* also mutated in some sporadic medulloblastomas of classic (nonnodular/desmoplastic) type
- Some patients have neither *APC* nor mismatch repair gene mutations

DIFFERENTIAL DIAGNOSIS

Li-Fraumeni Syndrome

- Colorectal and CNS tumors can also occur
- Choroid plexus tumors, especially carcinomas, common
- Germline *TP53* gene mutations
- No *APC* or mismatch repair gene mutations
- Colorectal tumors typically carcinomas, not polyps

Constitutional Mismatch Repair Deficiency Syndrome

- Distinct childhood cancer predisposition syndrome due to biallelic germline mutations in mismatch repair genes
  - *MLH1, MSH2, MSH6, PMS2*
- Associated with consanguinity
- Most patients have high-grade gliomas, and some have colonic carcinomas
- May not be easily distinguishable from type 1

SELECTED REFERENCES

1. Wimmer K et al: Diagnostic criteria for constitutional mismatch repair deficiency syndrome: suggestions of the European consortium 'care for CMMRD' (C4CMMRD). J Med Genet. 51(6):355-65, 2014
2. Lusis EA et al: Glioblastomas with giant cell and sarcomatous features in patients with Turcot syndrome type 1: a clinicopathological study of 3 cases. Neurosurgery. 67(3):811-7; discussion 817, 2010
3. Baehring J et al: Anaplastic oligoastrocytoma in Turcot syndrome. J Neurooncol. 95(2):293-8, 2009
4. Giunti L et al: Type A microsatellite instability in pediatric gliomas as an indicator of Turcot syndrome. Eur J Hum Genet. 17(7):919-27, 2009
5. Hottinger AF et al: Neurooncology of familial cancer syndromes. J Child Neurol. 24(12):1526-35, 2009
6. Sjursen W et al: A homozygote splice site PMS2 mutation as cause of Turcot syndrome gives rise to two different abnormal transcripts. Fam Cancer. 8(3):179-86, 2009
7. Agostini M et al: Two PMS2 mutations in a Turcot syndrome family with small bowel cancers. Am J Gastroenterol. 100(8):1886-91, 2005
8. Hegde MR et al: A homozygous mutation in MSH6 causes Turcot syndrome. Clin Cancer Res. 11(13):4689-93, 2005
9. Qualman SJ et al: Molecular basis of the brain tumor-polyposis (Turcot) syndrome. Pediatr Dev Pathol. 6(6):574-6, 2003
10. Hamilton SR et al: The molecular basis of Turcot's syndrome. N Engl J Med. 332(13):839-47, 1995
11. Mori T et al: Germ-line and somatic mutations of the APC gene in patients with Turcot syndrome and analysis of APC mutations in brain tumors. Genes Chromosomes Cancer. 9(3):168-72, 1994
12. Munden PM et al: Ocular findings in Turcot syndrome (glioma-polyposis). Ophthalmology. 98(1):111-4, 1991

PART II
SECTION 1
Benign Cysts

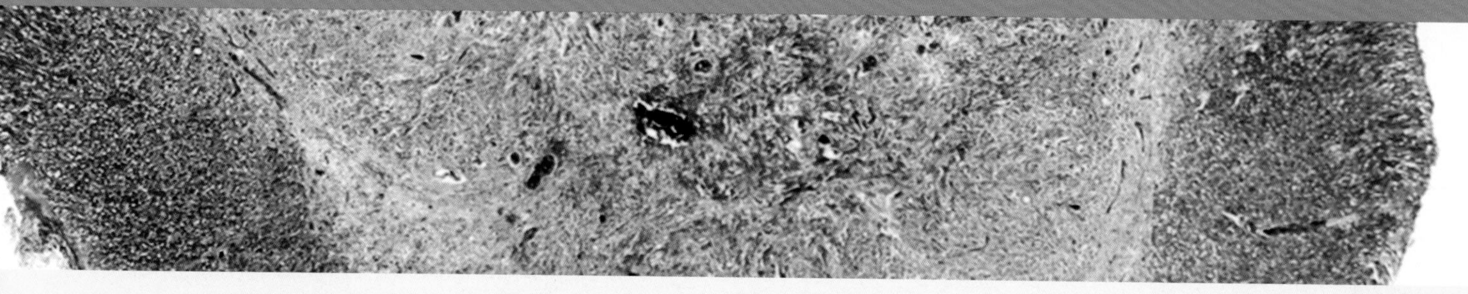

Arachnoid Cyst

KEY FACTS

ETIOLOGY/PATHOGENESIS

- Majority congenital

CLINICAL ISSUES

- More common in children and young adults
- Most supratentorial, often in sylvian fissure
- Majority asymptomatic
- Asymptomatic cysts do not require treatment
- Surgery when symptomatic

IMAGING

- Contents of arachnoid cyst isointense to CSF
- Hyperintense on T2 and FLAIR (as CSF)
- No enhancement
- No restricted diffusion (in contrast to epidermoid cyst)

MICROSCOPIC

- Lined by single layer of mature arachnoid cells, although cells not always apparent

ANCILLARY TESTS

- Cyst lining cells EMA(+)

TOP DIFFERENTIAL DIAGNOSES

- Epidermoid cyst
  - Squamous epithelium, keratinous content
- Neurenteric (endodermal, enterogenous) cyst
  - Columnar epithelium, variably ciliated
  - Occasionally with goblet cells, surface glycocalyx
  - Recapitulate bronchogenic/respiratory or gastrointestinal epithelium, even with muscularis mucosa
  - EMA(+), cytokeratins (+), CEA(+), sometimes S100(+)
- Porencephalic cyst without arachnoidal lining
  - Porencephalic cyst intraparenchymal, not meningeal
  - May have surrounding gliosis
- Ependymal cyst
  - Lacks cilia, S100(+), occasionally focal GFAP(+) cells
  - Cells rest on neuropil/glial tissue, without basal lamina

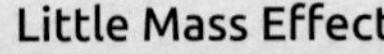

Little Mass Effect

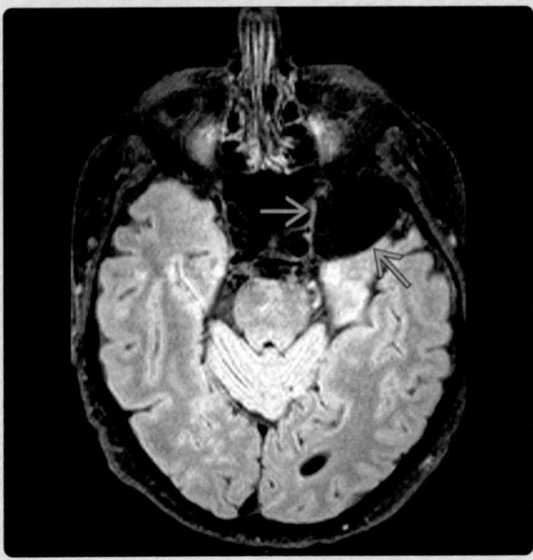

Cyst Wall

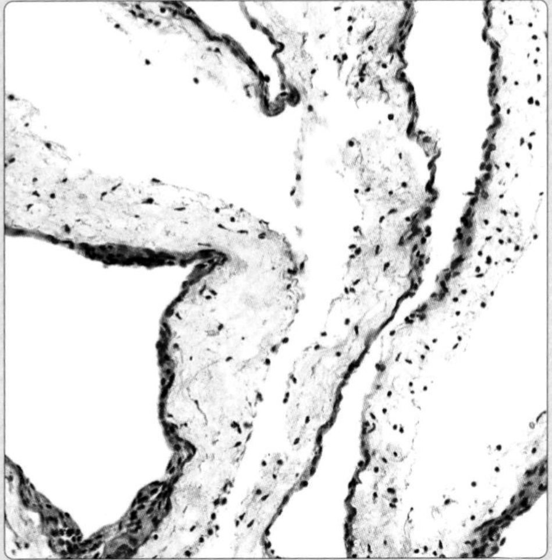

(Left) *Arachnoid cysts (AC) → have the same signal intensity as cerebrospinal fluid (CSF) and typically exert little, if any, mass effect.* **(Right)** *ACs may so closely resemble the normal arachnoid membrane that they may not be recognized as lesional. Correlation with neuroimaging is helpful in this context.*

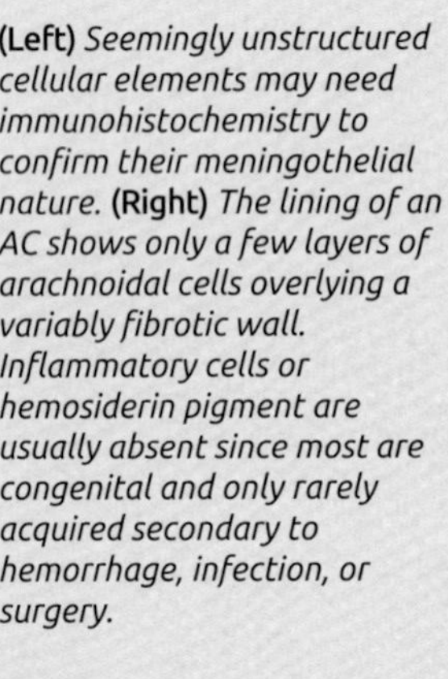

(Left) *Seemingly unstructured cellular elements may need immunohistochemistry to confirm their meningothelial nature.* **(Right)** *The lining of an AC shows only a few layers of arachnoidal cells overlying a variably fibrotic wall. Inflammatory cells or hemosiderin pigment are usually absent since most are congenital and only rarely acquired secondary to hemorrhage, infection, or surgery.*

Cells Not Obviously Meningothelial

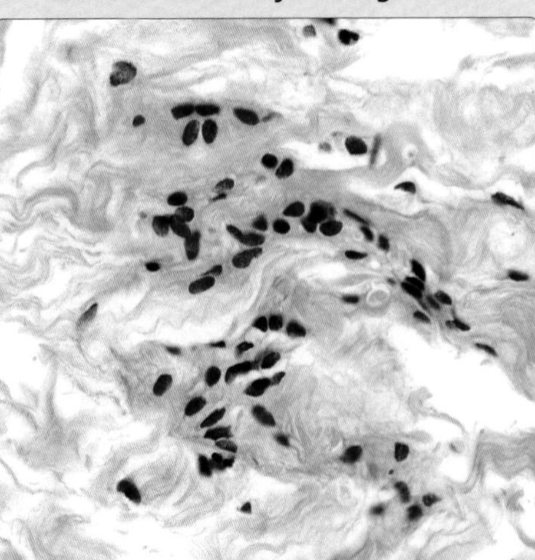

Cyst Wall With Collagen

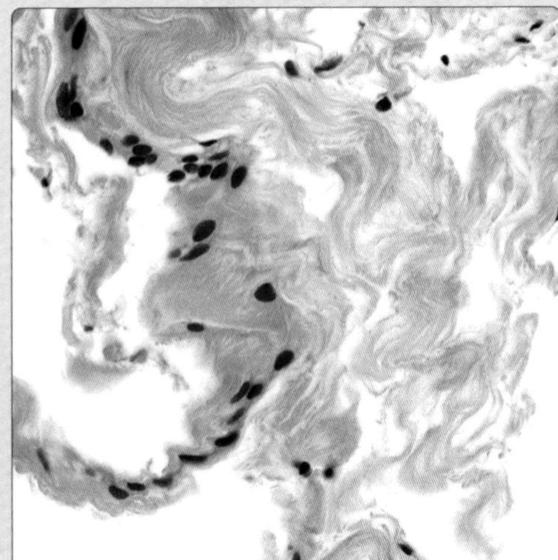

TERMINOLOGY

Abbreviations

- Arachnoid cyst (AC)

Synonyms

- Meningeal cyst

Definitions

- Collection of cerebrospinal fluid (CSF) lined by layer of arachnoid cells

ETIOLOGY/PATHOGENESIS

Developmental Anomaly

- Majority congenital
- Benign, nonneoplastic
- Rarely coexist with other lesions, such as meningiomas

Other Etiologies

- Rarely acquired subsequent to hemorrhage, infection, or surgery

CLINICAL ISSUES

Epidemiology

- Incidence
  - Any age
  - More common in children and young adults
  - ~ 2% of young adults
  - Rarely familial
- Sex
  - Male predominance reported in some studies

Site

- Mostly supratentorial, often involves sylvian fissure
- Occasionally intraspinal or posterior fossa

Presentation

- Majority asymptomatic
- Craniomegaly in young children
- Headache (most common)
- Weakness
- Hydrocephalus
- Reversible cognitive dysfunction
- Hemiparesis, seizures, visual loss, or cranial nerve dysfunction (rare)
- May coexist with subdural hematoma (rare)

Treatment

- Options, risks, complications
  - Children with macrocephaly more likely to require shunts
  - Subdural hematoma or hygromas rare complications
- Surgical approaches
  - Asymptomatic cysts do not require treatment
  - Surgery when symptomatic
  - Surgical options
    - Surgical fenestration
    - Resection of cyst, partial or total
    - Cystoperitoneal or ventriculoperitoneal shunting in minority

Prognosis

- Most remain asymptomatic without complications
- Occasionally regress spontaneously
- Rarely enlarge
- Resection and fenestration often curative

IMAGING

MR Findings

- Contents isointense to cerebrospinal fluid (CSF)
- Hyperintense on T2 and FLAIR (as CSF)
- No restricted diffusion (in contrast to epidermoid cyst)
- No enhancement
- Displace surrounding structures (occasionally)
- Remodeling of inner table of skull (occasionally)

MACROSCOPIC

General Features

- Clear to translucent

MICROSCOPIC

Histologic Features

- Lined by single layer of mature arachnoid cells, although arachnoid cells not always apparent
- Rare foci of meningothelial hyperplasia
- Delicate fibrous membrane
- Rare small inflammatory infiltrates

ANCILLARY TESTS

Immunohistochemistry

- Lining cells EMA(+)

DIFFERENTIAL DIAGNOSIS

Epidermoid Cyst

- Squamous epithelium
- Keratinous content

Neurenteric Cyst

- Columnar epithelium

Porencephaly or Schizencephaly

- Intraparenchymal
- No arachnoidal lining

SELECTED REFERENCES

1. Wang Y et al: Clinical and radiological outcomes of surgical treatment for symptomatic arachnoid cysts in adults. J Clin Neurosci. ePub, 2015
2. Petridis AK et al: Spinal cord compression caused by idiopathic intradural arachnoid cysts of the spine: review of the literature and illustrated case. Eur Spine J. 19 Suppl 2:S124-9, 2010
3. Martínez-Lage JF et al: CSF overdrainage in shunted intracranial arachnoid cysts: a series and review. Childs Nerv Syst. 25(9):1061-9, 2009
4. Russo N et al: Spontaneous reduction of intracranial arachnoid cysts: a complete review. Br J Neurosurg. 22(5):626-9, 2008
5. Pradilla G et al: Arachnoid cysts: case series and review of the literature. Neurosurg Focus. 22(2):E7, 2007
6. Alehan FK et al: Familial arachnoid cysts in association with autosomal dominant polycystic kidney disease. Pediatrics. 110(1 Pt 1):e13, 2002
7. Jallo GI et al: Arachnoid cysts of the cerebellopontine angle: diagnosis and surgery. Neurosurgery. 40(1):31-7; discussion 37-8, 1997
8. Parsch CS et al: Arachnoid cysts associated with subdural hematomas and hygromas: analysis of 16 cases, long-term follow-up, and review of the literature. Neurosurgery. 40(3):483-90, 1997

Epidermoid and Dermoid Cysts

KEY FACTS

TERMINOLOGY

- Epidermoid cyst (EC)
- Dermoid cyst (DC)
- Cholesteatoma: Ruptured cystic mass composed primarily of keratinous debris and xanthogranulomatous reaction

CLINICAL ISSUES

- EC more common than DC
- Cerebellopontine angle most common site
- Gross total resection curative but may be difficult because of cranial nerve and vascular involvement

IMAGING

- Bright on diffusion-weighted images
- Typically do not enhance

MACROSCOPIC

- EC: Distinctive mother of pearl sheen; keratinous, flaky contents
- DC: Matted hair and "cheesy" keratinous contents

MICROSCOPIC

- EC: Simple stratified squamous epithelium with no adnexal structures
- Mature epidermis, dermis, and adnexa in DC
- Foreign-body giant cell reaction to ruptured cyst contents
- Progression to squamous cell carcinoma (rare)

TOP DIFFERENTIAL DIAGNOSES

- Teratoma
- Rathke cleft cyst with squamous metaplasia
- Papillary craniopharyngioma

DIAGNOSTIC CHECKLIST

- Some surgical specimens from EC contain only anuclear squames
  - These should not be given an insufficient diagnosis

Epidermoid Cyst, Cerebellopontine Angle

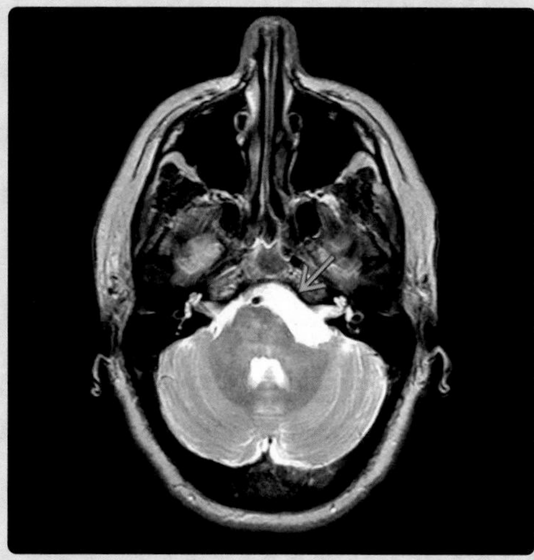

Epidermoid/Dermoid Cysts Distinguishable From Arachnoid Cysts

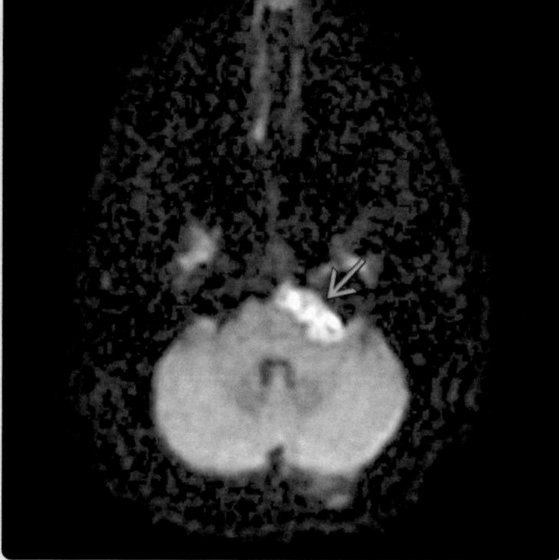

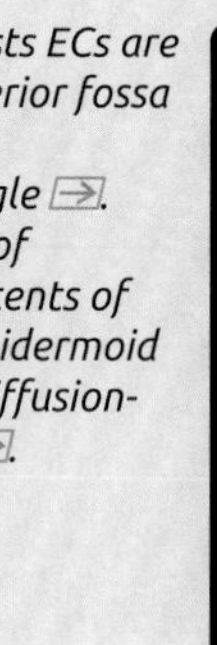

(Left) *Epidermoid cysts ECs are common in the posterior fossa in and around the cerebellopontine angle.* **(Right)** *Unlike those of arachnoid cysts, contents of both dermoid and epidermoid cysts are bright on diffusion-weighted imaging.*

Epidermoid Cyst, Anuclear Laminate Keratin

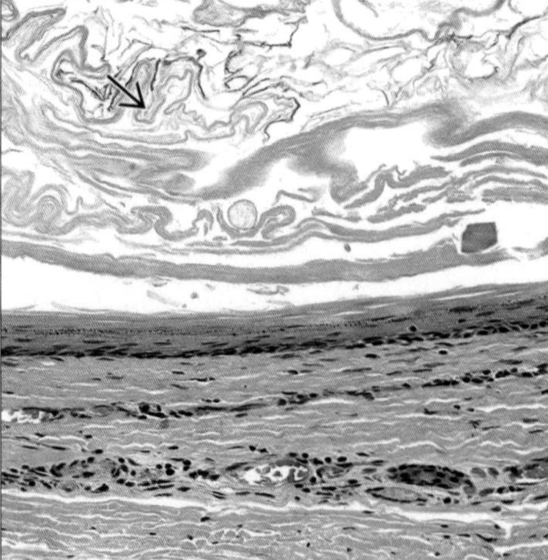

Dermoid Cyst, Adnexal Glands

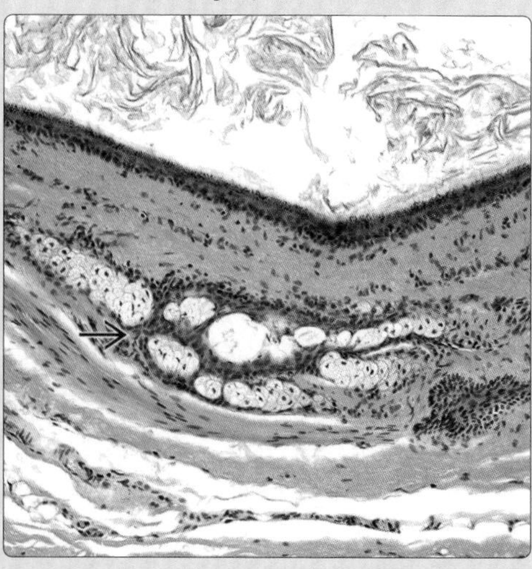

(Left) *Like ECs elsewhere in the body, those in the CNS contain anuclear laminate keratin and are lined by cytologically benign squamous epithelium.* **(Right)** *Adnexal glands are found in the wall of dermoid, but not CNS epidermoid, cysts. Note the prominent sebaceous glands seen here.*

TERMINOLOGY

Abbreviations

- Epidermoid cyst (EC); dermoid cyst (DC)

Definitions

- EC: Histologically benign cystic mass with mature epidermis and keratinous material without adnexal structures
- DC: Histologically benign cystic mass with mature skin, keratinous material, and adnexal structures

CLINICAL ISSUES

Epidemiology

- Incidence
  - EC more common than DC
- Age
  - ECs usually in adults
  - DCs usually in children

Site

- Throughout CNS
- Almost all extraaxial, leptomeningeal
- DC more often midline, posterior fossa
- EC most common in cerebellopontine angle
- Other sites: Supra/parasellar region, calvaria, spinal cord; all usually EC
- Rare examples intraosseous (intradiploic), especially EC

Presentation

- Slowly progressive symptoms
- Headache (most common)
- Cranial nerve dysfunction with cerebellopontine angle cysts (usually EC)
- Intracalvarial (intraosseous) examples asymptomatic or present as scalp mass
- Infection via sinus tract (DC) (uncommon)

Treatment

- Gross total resection curative but may be difficult with cranial nerve and vascular involvement

Prognosis

- Excellent long-term survival
- Frequent recurrence after subtotal resection, especially EC
- Rare dissemination of cyst contents in subarachnoid space after surgery
- Chemical meningitis or cyst rupture (rare)
- Malignant degeneration (rare)

IMAGING

MR Findings

- Variable intensity on T1-weighted images
- Often hyperintense on FLAIR and T2-weighted images
- ↓ diffusion (bright) on diffusion-weighted images
- Nonenhancing
- DC with contents with signal equivalent to that of fat
- Calcifications, some cases, especially DC
- Intradiploic examples bone-erosive with sclerotic rim

MACROSCOPIC

General Features

- ECs frequently incorporate adjacent nerves and vessels
- Smooth, partly translucent cyst wall
- EC: Distinctive mother of pearl sheen; keratinous, flaky contents
- DC: "Cheesy" keratinous contents; matted hair; sinus tract (some DCs)

MICROSCOPIC

Histologic Features

- Mature keratinizing squamous epithelium with keratohyaline granules
- No adnexal structures in EC
- Mature epidermis, dermis, and adnexa, DC
- Osseous metaplasia, occasional DC
- Foreign-body giant cell reaction to ruptured cyst contents
- Mitoses absent or rare
- Progression to squamous cell carcinoma, rare

ANCILLARY TESTS

Cytology

- Anuclear squames

Immunohistochemistry

- Cyst lining epithelial membrane antigen and keratin (+)

DIFFERENTIAL DIAGNOSIS

Arachnoid Cyst

- Very low, simple, nonstratified, nonkeratinizing epithelium

Teratoma

- Mature ectodermal elements and adnexa
- Usually also immature elements
- Includes endodermal & mesenchymal elements (cartilage)

Rathke Cleft Cyst With Squamous Metaplasia

- Partly columnar, ciliated epithelial lining
- Squamous metaplasia continuous with ciliated epithelium
- No anuclear squames
- Proteinaceous and colloidal cyst contents

Papillary Craniopharyngioma

- Solid, with pseudopapillae
- No anuclear squames
- No adnexa

DIAGNOSTIC CHECKLIST

Clinically Relevant Pathologic Features

- Total excision of EC often difficult due to incorporation of regional nerves and vessels

Pathologic Interpretation Pearls

- As surgical specimens, ECs usually consist of little but anuclear squames

SELECTED REFERENCES

1. Osborn AG et al: Intracranial cysts: radiologic-pathologic correlation and imaging approach. Radiology. 239(3):650-64, 2006

(Left) *Unable to fully exfoliate, pale-staining anuclear squames create a mass that stretches the thin, germinative epithelium.* (Right) *The keratinous contents of epidermoid cysts are identical to those of cutaneous epidermal inclusion cysts.*

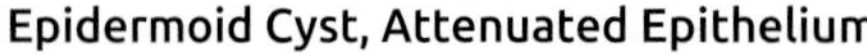

Epidermoid Cyst, Attenuated Epithelium

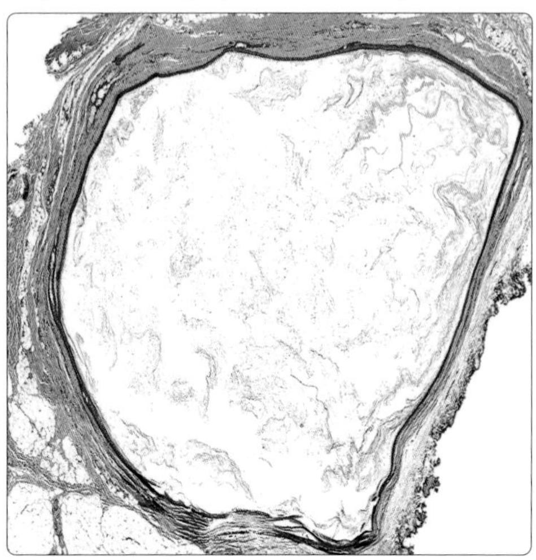

Keratinous Contents

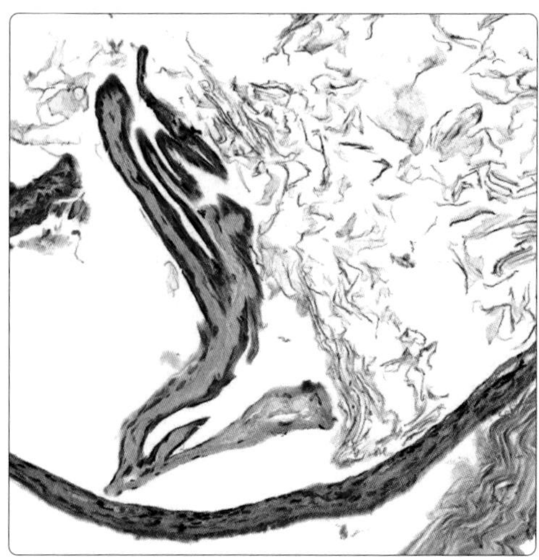

(Left) *The epidermoid cyst squamous epithelium resembles that of the skin. Unlike the latter, however, there is no equivalent of the dermis and its adnexa.* (Right) *Epidermoid cysts are commonly found at the cerebellopontine angle, where they may be intimately attached to the surface of the cerebellum →. Note the granule cell layer of cerebellum ↪. Purkinje cell neurons have disappeared in this area adjacent to the cyst.*

Epidermoid Cyst, No Dermis, No Adnexa

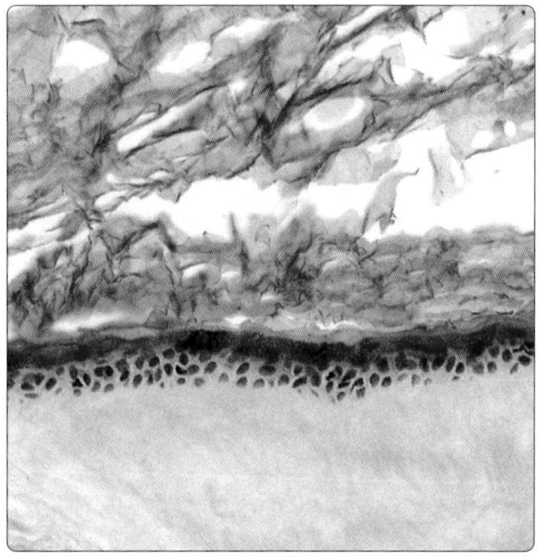

Intimate Attachment to Cerebellum

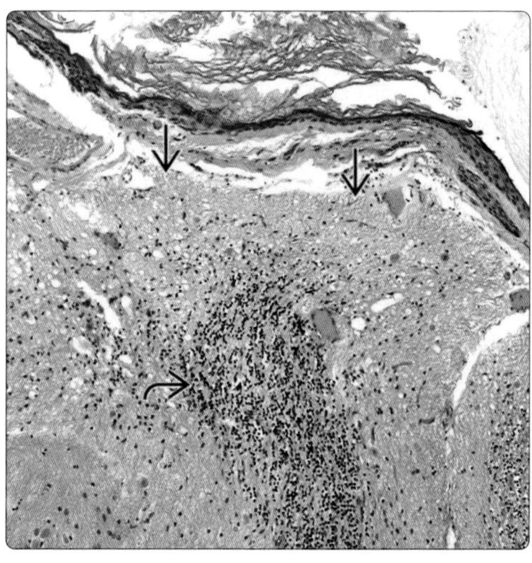

(Left) *Dermoid and epidermoid cysts contain anuclear ghosts of squamous cells, in contrast to homogeneous proteinaceous contents of colloid and Rathke cleft cysts.* (Right) *Detached anuclear squames or "cell ghosts" are typical of both epidermoid and dermoid cysts.*

Anuclear Contents

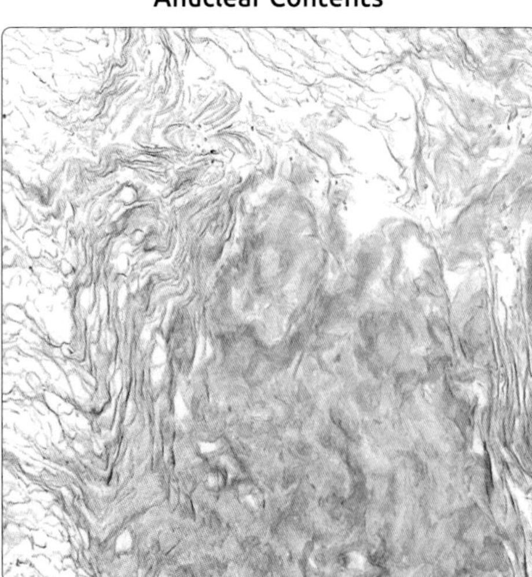

Smear, Anuclear Squames

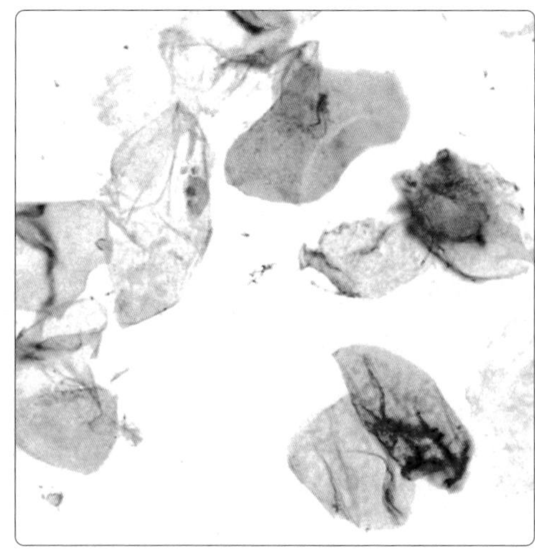

Dermoid Cyst, Adnexal Structures

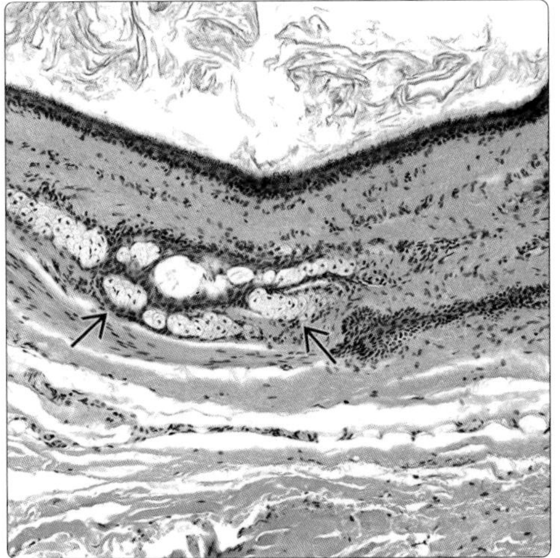

Dermoid Cyst, Complex Cyst Wall

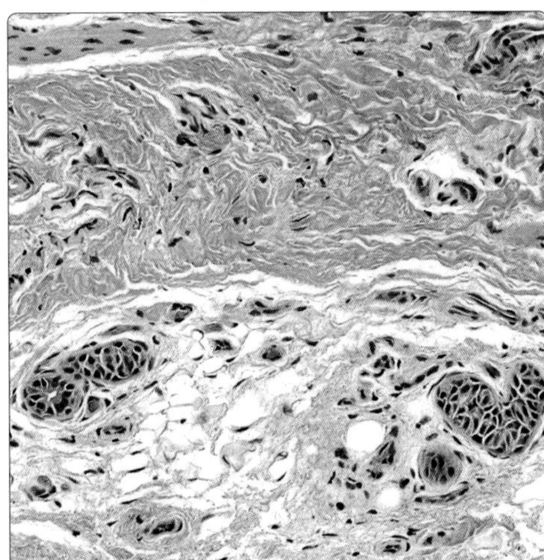

(Left) *Dermoid cysts (DCs) have surface epithelium and keratinous contents but also adnexal elements, such as sebaceous glands ⇒ and an amount of dermal collagen not expected in an epidermoid. A thicker wall is the result.* **(Right)** *The complex wall of the DC has glands of eccrine, apocrine, or sebaceous types. The cyst wall can also contain adipose tissue and considerable collagen.*

Dermoid Cyst, Hair Shafts

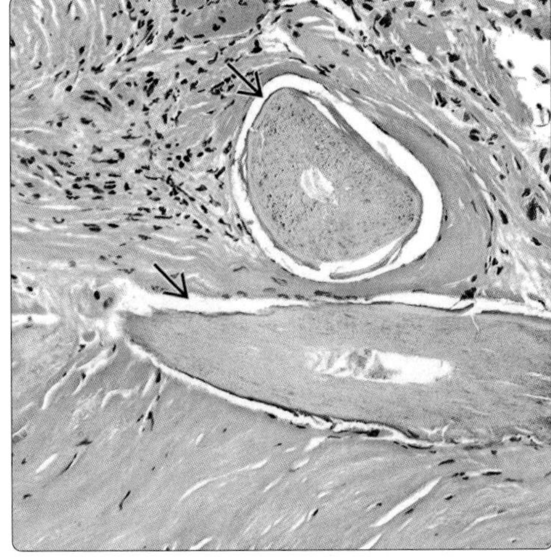

Uncommon Calcification, Bone

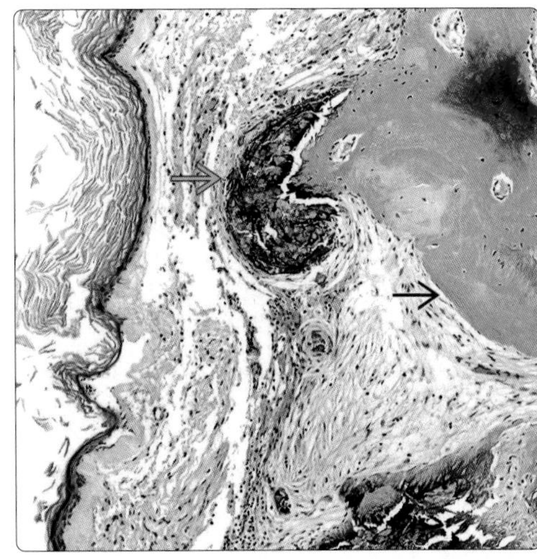

(Left) *The cyst wall in DCs often contains well-formed follicular bulbs and hair shafts ⇒ similar to those in teratomas. Hair follicles may be associated with inflammation and fibrosis.* **(Right)** *Dystrophic calcifications ⇒ and bone ⇒ are uncommon in ECs and DCs. No teratomatous immature elements are present, however.*

Granulomatous Response to Rupture

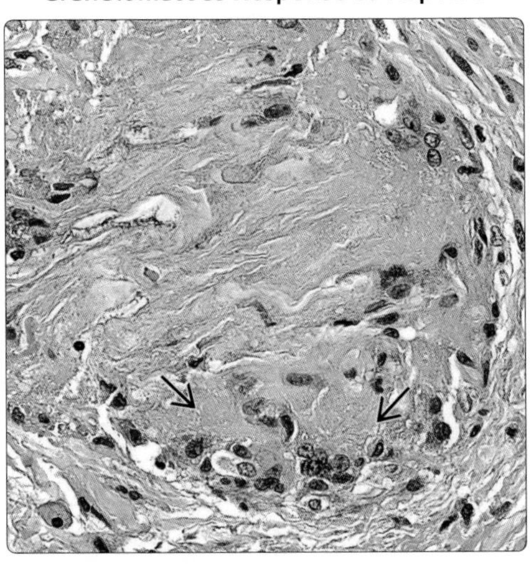

Cholesterol Clefts After Rupture

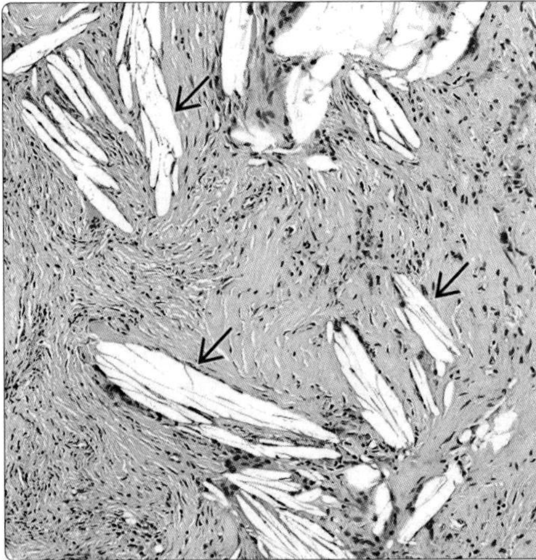

(Left) *Ruptured contents of ECs or DCs may elicit a granulomatous reaction with giant cells ⇒ that simulates a primary inflammatory process.* **(Right)** *Ruptured cysts can release content that evokes a xanthogranulomatous response with cholesterol clefts ⇒.*

Colloid Cyst

KEY FACTS

TERMINOLOGY

- Benign cyst lined by columnar epithelium residing near the foramen of Monro, usually in 3rd ventricle

CLINICAL ISSUES

- Treated by excision or cyst drainage
- Prognosis excellent
- Rare examples associated with sudden death

MACROSCOPIC

- Smooth surfaced
- Clear to turbid contents
- Liquid to gelatinous or firm depending upon hydration

MICROSCOPIC

- Pseudostratified epithelium with both ciliated and goblet cells
- Cuboidal or flattened with pressure atrophy
- Amorphous proteinaceous material
- Xanthogranulomatous reaction

ANCILLARY TESTS

- EMA, uniformly positive
- Cytokeratins, low- and high-molecular weight often positive
- GFAP and S-100(-)

TOP DIFFERENTIAL DIAGNOSES

- Normal choroid plexus
- Choroid plexus papilloma
- Rathke cleft cyst
- Craniopharyngioma
- Xanthogranuloma

DIAGNOSTIC CHECKLIST

- Step sections may be necessary to find epithelium
- Normal choroid plexus sometimes dominant part of specimen

Colloid Cyst With Hydrocephalus

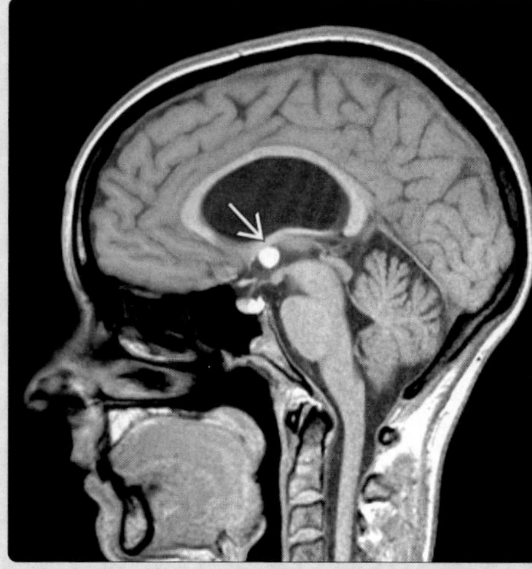

Lateral Ventricle Colloid Cyst

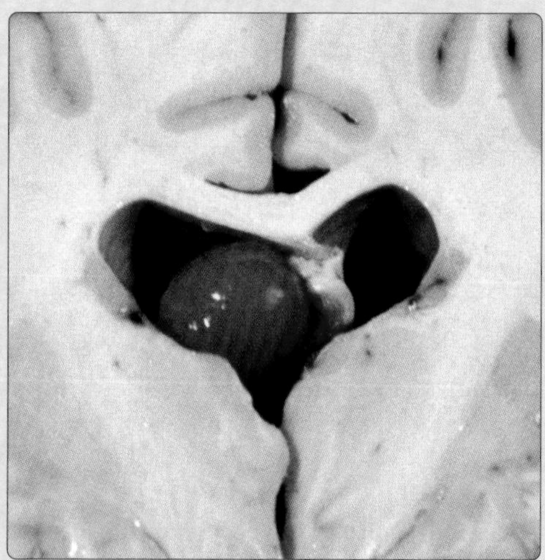

(Left) *Colloid cysts are benign cysts lined by columnar epithelium residing near foramen of Monro, usually in 3rd ventricle. As is apparent in this T1W precontrast image, colloid cysts ➡ are critically positioned to obstruct cerebrospinal fluid flow and produce hydrocephalus, even when small.* **(Right)** *Colloid cysts are smooth-surfaced benign cysts lined by columnar epithelium residing near the foramen of Monro, usually in the 3rd ventricle. This example, however, is positioned within the lateral ventricle.*

Incidental in Septum Pellucidum

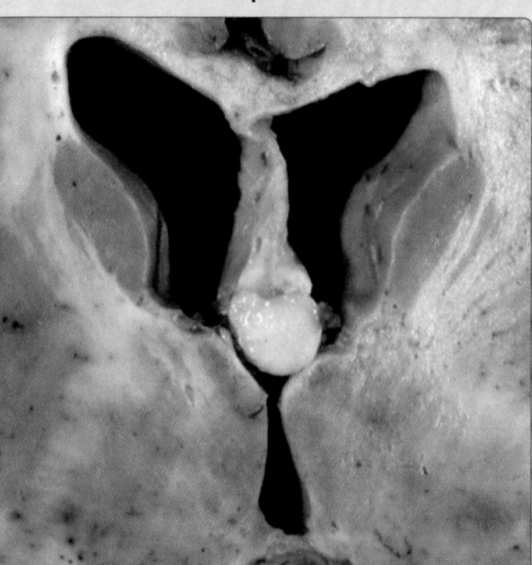

Ciliated Epithelium of Colloid Cyst

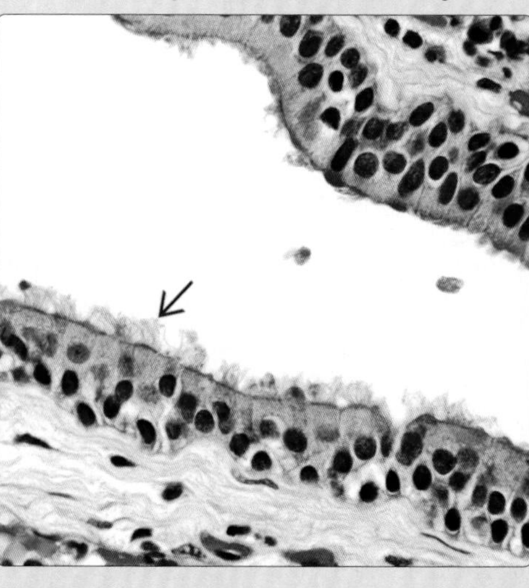

(Left) *Colloid cysts are benign cysts lined by columnar epithelium residing near foramen of Monro, usually in the 3rd ventricle and may be incidentally identified at autopsy.* **(Right)** *Without pressure atrophy, the lining of the colloid cyst is ciliated ➡ and pseudostratified. Normal choroid plexus, often included in the specimen, is neither. Normal ependyma is simple low columnar and nonciliated.*

TERMINOLOGY

Definitions

- Benign cyst lined by columnar epithelium residing near foramen of Monro, usually in 3rd ventricle

CLINICAL ISSUES

Presentation

- Signs/symptoms of obstructive hydrocephalus
  - Headaches &/or drop attacks
- Some associated with sudden death

Natural History

- Most are stable and some may enlarge slowly over time

Treatment

- Surgical approaches
  - Excision, preferred
  - Drainage only (uncommon, potential for cyst recurrence)
  - Observation and serial imaging
    - Reasonable when stable, asymptomatic, and without associated hydrocephalus

Prognosis

- Excellent

IMAGING

MR Findings

- Well-circumscribed midline "cyst" may involve septum pellucidum
- Variable, usually hyperintense on T1- and iso- or hyperintense on T2-weighted images
- Nonenhancing and does not suppress on FLAIR

MACROSCOPIC

General Features

- Smooth surfaced
- Clear to turbid contents
  - Liquid to gelatinous or firm depending upon hydration

MICROSCOPIC

Histologic Features

- Epithelium
  - Pseudostratified and ciliated
  - Simple cuboidal or flattened with pressure atrophy
  - No squamous metaplasia, unlike Rathke cleft cyst
  - Variable number of goblet cells
- Delicate capsule
- Contents
  - Amorphous proteinaceous material
  - Scattered exfoliated cells
  - Scattered filamentous, *Actinomyces*-like arrays of nucleoprotein (uncommon)
- Attached normal choroid plexus is common
- Xanthogranulomatous reaction (uncommon)
  - Cholesterol clefts, multinucleated giant cells, macrophages, and hemosiderin

ANCILLARY TESTS

Cytology

- Cohesive sheets of epithelial cells
- Individual ciliated and goblet cells
- Amorphous proteinaceous material with *Actinomyces*-like nucleoprotein arrays

Immunohistochemistry

- EMA, uniformly positive
- Cytokeratins, low- and high-molecular weight often positive
- GFAP(-), S100(-)

DIFFERENTIAL DIAGNOSIS

Normal Choroid Plexus

- Sometimes dominant, or only, epithelial tissue
- "Cobblestone" epithelium and papillary appearance
- No ciliated or goblet cells
- EMA generally negative; cytokeratins only sparsely positive

Choroid Plexus Papilloma

- Redundant pseudostratified epithelium, papillations

Rathke Cleft Cyst

- Sellar or suprasellar
- Prone to squamous metaplasia

Craniopharyngiomas: Papillary and Adamantinomatous

- Adamantinomatous: Wet keratin, solid component, palisading cells, nuclear β-catenin (+)
- Papillary: Solid squamous component, BRAF V600E(+)

Xanthogranuloma

- No epithelium, this is reactive change, not entity
- Mostly sellar location

DIAGNOSTIC CHECKLIST

Pathologic Interpretation Pearls

- Deeper sections of tissue may be necessary to find ciliated epithelium
- Knowing exact location is helpful in diagnosis

SELECTED REFERENCES

1. Boogaarts HD et al: Long-term results of the neuroendoscopic management of colloid cysts of the third ventricle: a series of 90 cases. Neurosurgery. 68(1):179-87, 2011
2. Hellwig D et al: Neuroendoscopic treatment for colloid cysts of the third ventricle: the experience of a decade. Neurosurgery. 62(6 Suppl 3):1101-9, 2008
3. Pollock BE et al: Natural history of asymptomatic colloid cysts of the third ventricle. J Neurosurg. 91(3):364-9, 1999
4. Lach B et al: Colloid cyst of the third ventricle. A comparative immunohistochemical study of neuraxis cysts and choroid plexus epithelium. J Neurosurg. 78(1):101-11, 1993

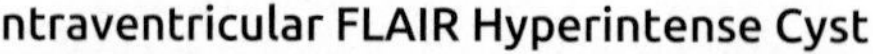

Intraventricular FLAIR Hyperintense Cyst

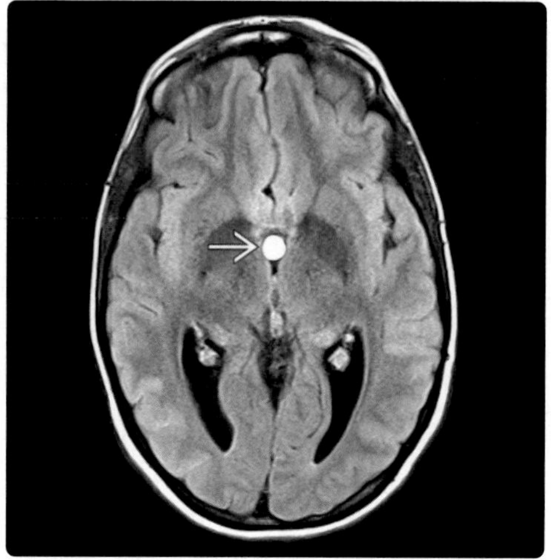

Acellular Cyst Contents

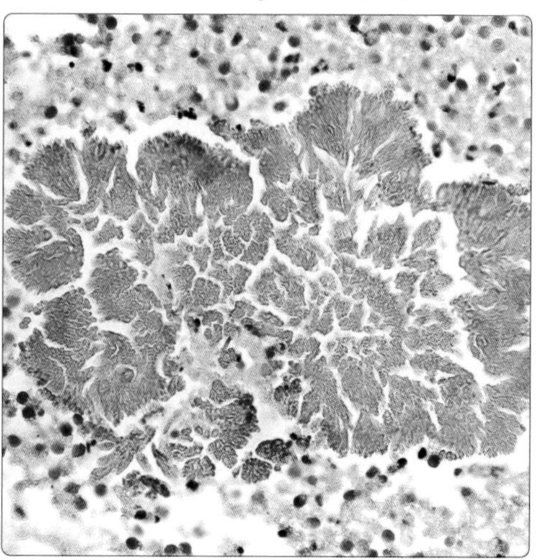

(Left) *The solid intraventricular colloid cyst ➡ does not show suppression of the signal on FLAIR images and appears as a solid intraventricular lesion. Colloid cysts have characteristic anatomical locations, namely residing near the foramen of Monro, usually in the 3rd ventricle.* **(Right)** *Intracystic, eosinophilic, branching arrays of nucleoprotein may mislead the observer that some colloid cysts harbor infectious organisms, such as Actinomyces.*

Adjacent Choroid Plexus

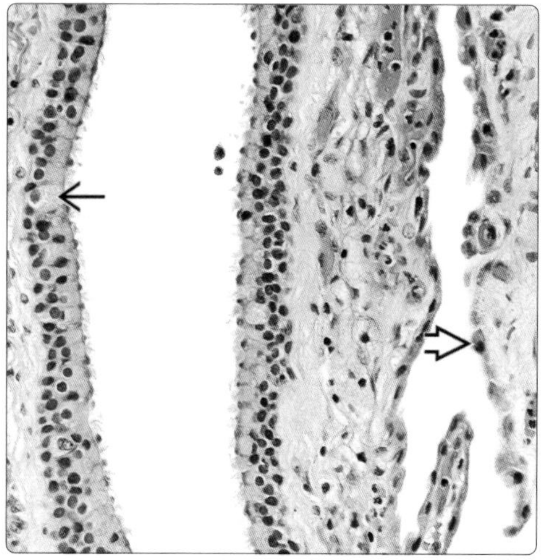

Attenuated Epithelium in Colloid Cyst

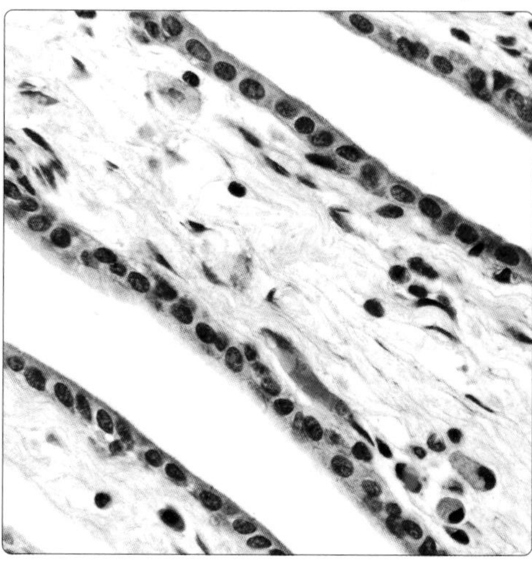

(Left) *Normal choroid plexus is often included in surgical specimens of colloid cysts. The lining of the latter is pseudostratified columnar with scattered goblet cells ⇨. A simple, low cobblestoned layer ⇨ covers the choroid plexus.* **(Right)** *Showing "pressure atrophy," the epithelium of colloid cysts may be low columnar or even flattened. Cilia are sparse and often absent in such cases.*

Papillary-Like Fronds

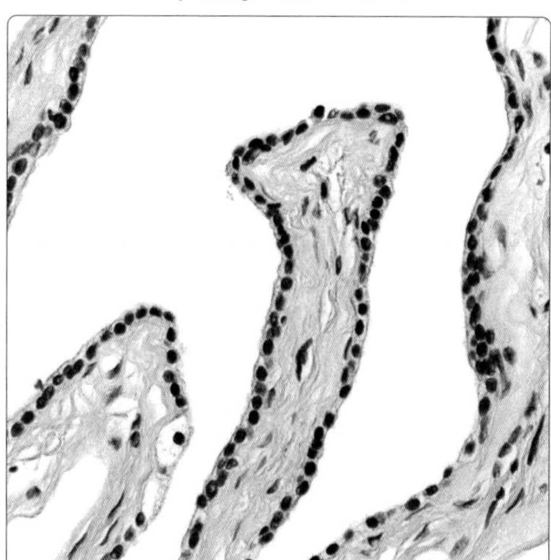

Attenuated Epithelium and Cyst Wall

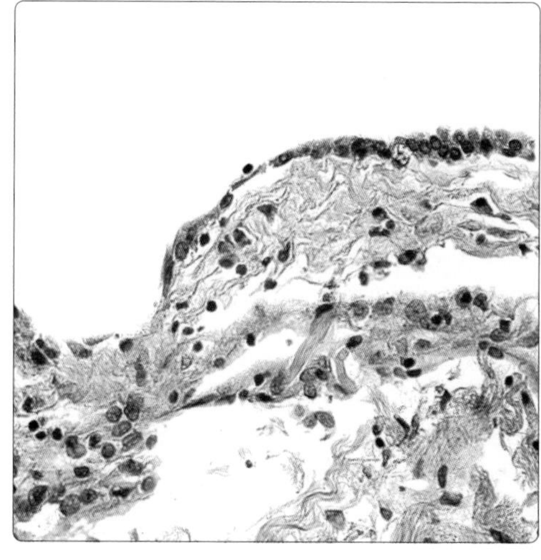

(Left) *Infoldings in collapsed colloid cysts may suggest normal or neoplastic choroid plexus epithelium. The cyst lining here is too simple for either and lacks the cobblestone profile of normal plexus.* **(Right)** *The cyst wall often contains a number of reactive cells and fibrous tissue. In this section, the epithelium is also attenuated with little or no evidence of cilia.*

Colloid Cyst: Intraoperative Smear

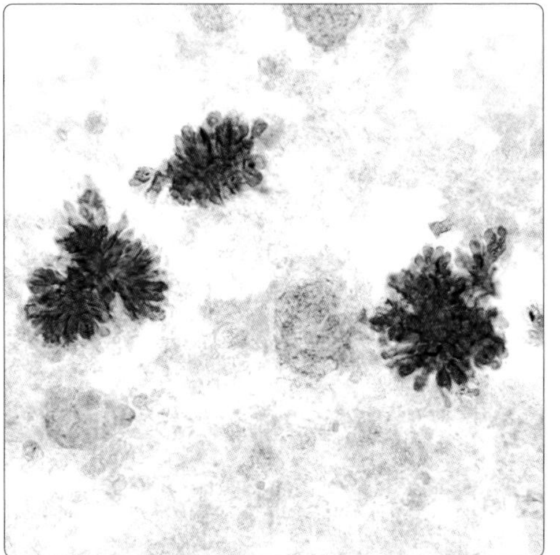

Colloid Cyst: Tissue Fragments

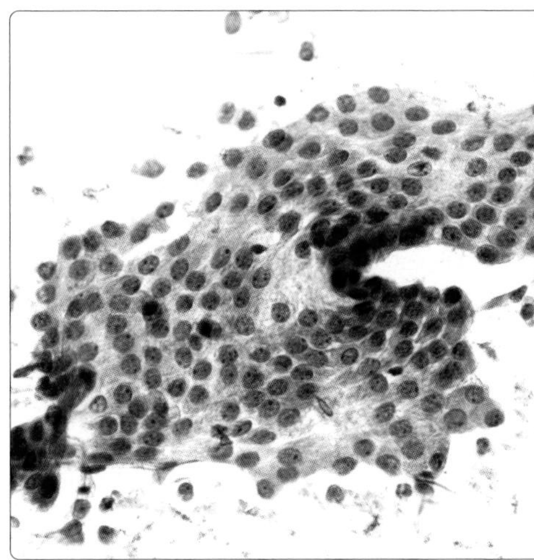

(Left) *As here, in a smear preparation, the contents of a colloid cyst may contain branching basophilic aggregates of nucleoprotein that closely resemble colonies of Actinomyces.* **(Right)** *Tissue fragments of benign epithelium are typical findings in smear preparations of colloid cysts.*

Colloid Cyst Cells vs. Choroid Plexus

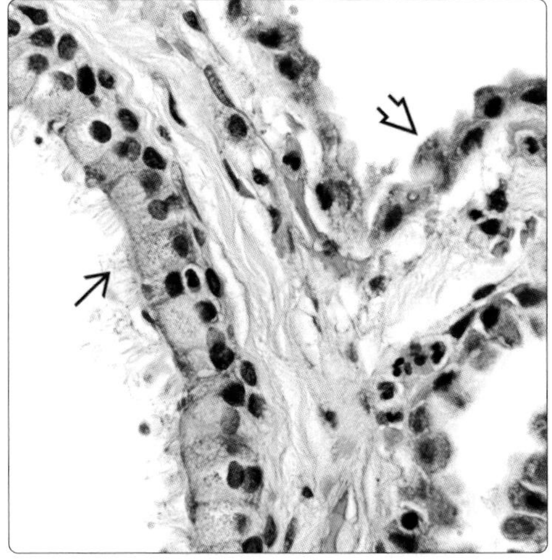

Ciliated Epithelium and Macrophages

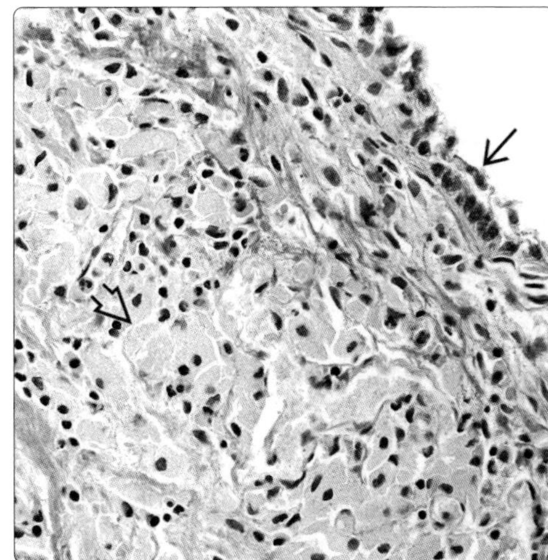

(Left) *The distinction between the tall, ciliated epithelium → of a colloid cyst and that of attached normal choroid plexus with its cuboidal, "cobblestone" profile ⇒ is generally easy.* **(Right)** *A surrounding macrophage-rich response ⇒ can partially, or totally, obscure the cyst's columnar epithelium →.*

Xanthogranulomatous Reaction

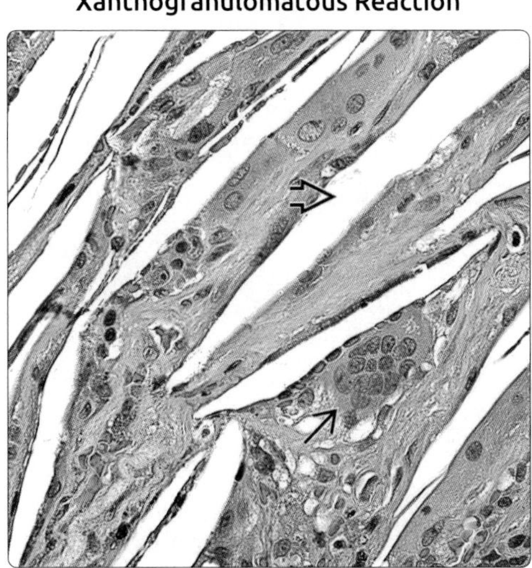

Colloid Cyst: Cytokeratin (+)

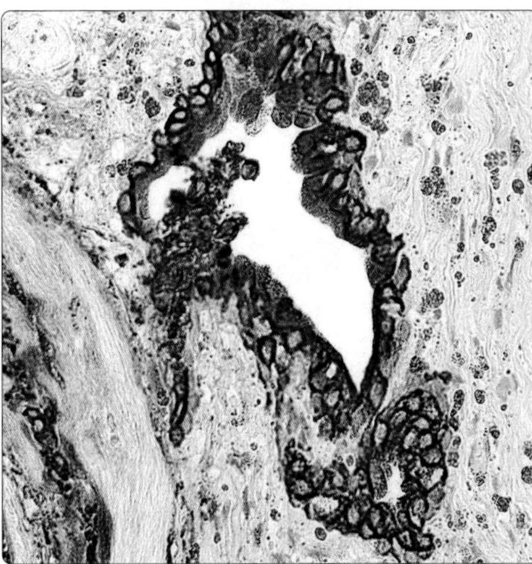

(Left) *Some colloid cysts may contain a mural xanthogranulomatous reaction with multinucleated giant cells → and cholesterol clefts ⇒.* **(Right)** *Colloid cysts are immunoreactive for CK7, as in this case. Immunoreactivity of normal choroid plexus is patchy at best.*

Rathke Cleft Cyst

KEY FACTS

TERMINOLOGY

- Benign sellar region cyst lined by ciliated, mucus-producing epithelium

CLINICAL ISSUES

- Common cause for negative biopsy of suspected pituitary adenoma
- Rare evolution to papillary craniopharyngioma
- Excellent prognosis, even with partial resection or drainage
- Recurrence possible with partial resection

IMAGING

- Supra/intrasellar
- Discrete
- Variable signal characteristics of cyst contents
    - Variable enhancement of rim, usually none (sometimes compressed pituitary)
    - Compressed pituitary around cyst may create image of rim enhancement (claw sign)
- Many have central white nodule
    - More than 2/3 of cysts have small T2 hypointense intracystic nodule

MICROSCOPIC

- Well-differentiated epithelium, usually ciliated, often with goblet cells, but sometimes cuboidal or simple squamous
- Myxoid/mucoid material may be prominent, if not exclusive, component
- High magnification and step sections sometimes necessary to find epithelium
- Extensive squamous metaplasia in some cases
- Overlap with papillary craniopharyngioma in some cases
- Xanthogranulomatous change (uncommon)

DIAGNOSTIC CHECKLIST

- Consider Rathke cleft cyst in face of myxoid material, but no neoplasm, in sellar region mass
- Remember to consider other cystic lesions if not intra or suprasellar

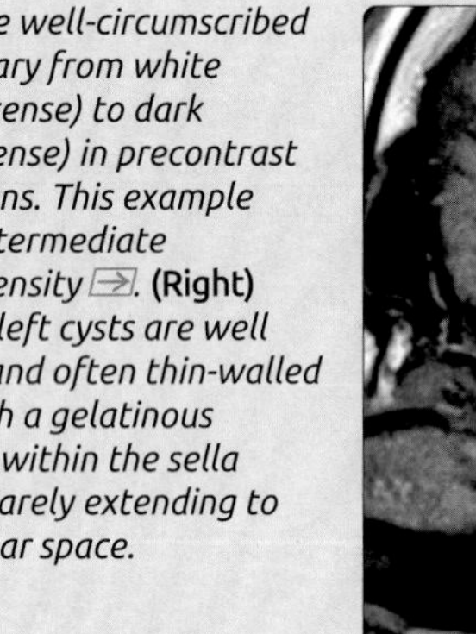

(Left) *The well-circumscribed lesions vary from white (hyperintense) to dark (hypointense) in precontrast T1WI scans. This example shows intermediate hyperintensity →.* **(Right)** *Rathke cleft cysts are well defined and often thin-walled cysts with a gelatinous material within the sella turcica, rarely extending to suprasellar space.*

Intrasellar Cyst on Sagittal Image

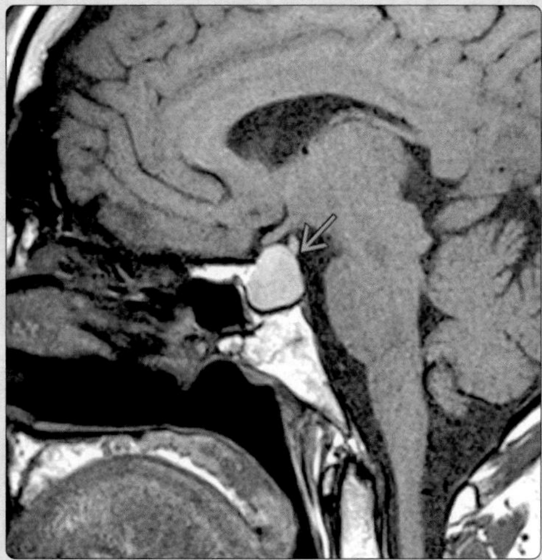

Macroscopic Appearance

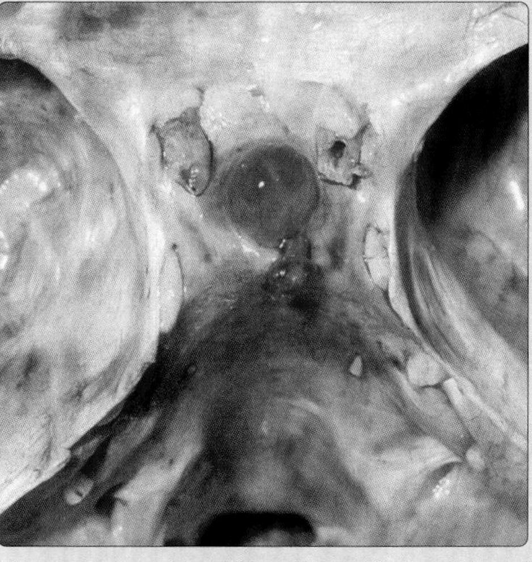

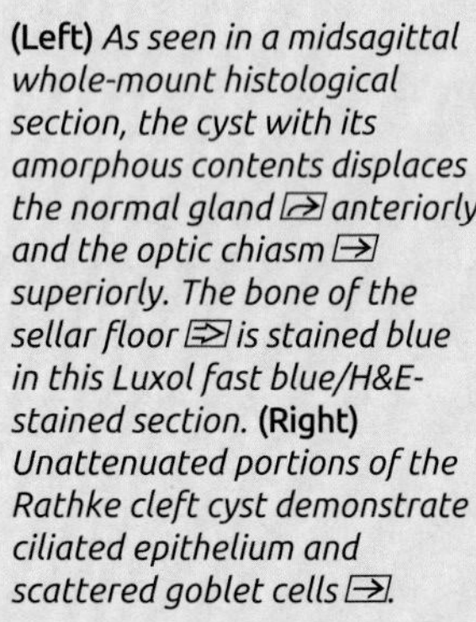

(Left) *As seen in a midsagittal whole-mount histological section, the cyst with its amorphous contents displaces the normal gland → anteriorly and the optic chiasm → superiorly. The bone of the sellar floor → is stained blue in this Luxol fast blue/H&E-stained section.* **(Right)** *Unattenuated portions of the Rathke cleft cyst demonstrate ciliated epithelium and scattered goblet cells →.*

Well-Defined Intrasellar Cyst

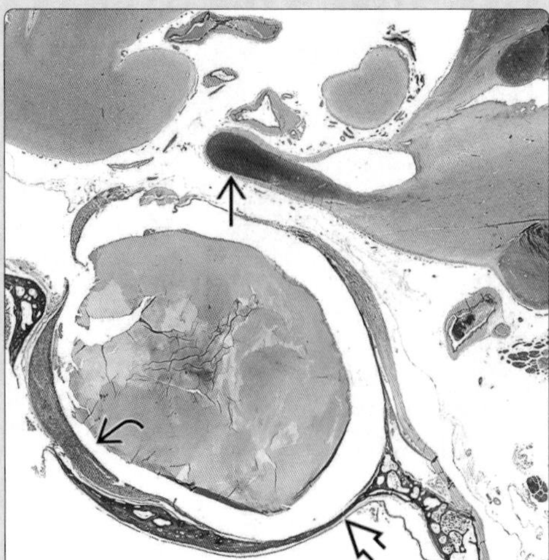

Ciliated Epithelium With Goblet Cells

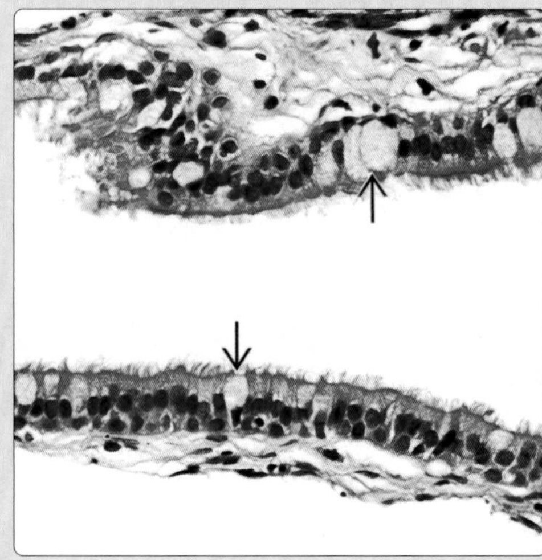

TERMINOLOGY

Abbreviations

- Rathke cleft cyst (RCC)

Definitions

- Benign sellar region cyst lined by ciliated, mucus-producing epithelium

CLINICAL ISSUES

Presentation

- Headache
- Galactorrhea
- Hypopituitarism
- Visual field loss

Treatment

- Surgical approaches
  - Excision, partial resection, or cyst drainage

Prognosis

- Excellent, even with partial resection or drainage
- Recurrence possible with partial resection

IMAGING

MR Findings

- Supra/intrasellar
- Discrete
- Variable signal characteristics of cyst contents
  - T1WI: ~ 1/2 bright/white in precontrast images, ~ 1/2 black or gray
  - T2WI: Some hyperintense (white), others dark
    - Many have central white nodule
- Variable enhancement of rim, usually none (sometimes compressed pituitary)

MACROSCOPIC

- Well-circumscribed cyst with delicate capsule
- Clear cerebrospinal fluid (CSF)-like, mucoid, or gelatinous contents

MICROSCOPIC

Histologic Features

- Mucoid cyst contents prominent, may be only component in surgical specimen
- Simple or pseudostratified, ciliated columnar epithelium, may be scanty &/or often distorted (if present)
- Goblet cells (some cases)
- Simple squamous epithelium (pressure atrophy) similar to craniopharyngiomas
- Squamous metaplasia (some cases) may be prominent or even dominant
- Collagenous layer external to epithelium; variable but thicker than in normal intermediate lobe cysts
- Chronic inflammation (some cases)
- Xanthogranulomatous change (uncommon)
  - Cholesterol clefts, multinucleated giant cells, hemosiderin, and fibrosis
- Overlap with papillary craniopharyngioma (rare)

ANCILLARY TESTS

Cytology

- Ciliated columnar cells (most cases)
- Goblet cells (some cases)
- Myxoid/mucoid background

Immunohistochemistry

- Cytokeratin (+)
- Epithelial membrane antigen (+)

DIFFERENTIAL DIAGNOSIS

Normal Intermediate Lobe Cysts

- Small and may be multiple
- Less collagen and fewer (if any) goblet cells

Craniopharyngioma

- Adamantinomatous
  - Palisading cells, stellate reticulin, wet keratin, calcifications
  - "Motor oil fluid" with floating, notched, laminated cholesterol crystals
  - Attenuated cyst wall, similar to RCC (in some cases)
- Papillary
  - Large, solid mass of squamous epithelium
  - Few (if any) goblet cells in most cases
  - Attenuated cyst wall similar to RCC (in some cases)
  - Craniopharyngioma with goblet cell and ciliated cell and RCC with squamous metaplasia may overlap

Epidermoid Cyst

- Surface maturation with anuclear squames
- No ciliated or goblet cells
- Cyst contents: Anuclear squames rather than amorphous material

Xanthogranuloma of Sellar Region

- With adamantinomatous craniopharyngioma
  - Focal craniopharyngioma epithelium
- Pure xanthogranuloma
  - No epithelium

DIAGNOSTIC CHECKLIST

Pathologic Interpretation Pearls

- Consider RCC in sellar region mass, with
  - Mucin-rich or xanthomatous lesion
  - Mucoid/myxoid material but no neoplasm

SELECTED REFERENCES

1. Kim JH et al: BRAF V600E mutation is a useful marker for differentiating Rathke's cleft cyst with squamous metaplasia from papillary craniopharyngioma. J Neurooncol. 123(1):189-91, 2015
2. Wen L et al: Rathke's cleft cyst: clinicopathological and MRI findings in 22 patients. Clin Radiol. 65(1):47-55, 2010
3. Hama S et al: Changes in the epithelium of Rathke cleft cyst associated with inflammation. J Neurosurg. 96(2):209-16, 2002
4. Paulus W et al: Xanthogranuloma of the sellar region: a clinicopathological entity different from adamantinomatous craniopharyngioma. Acta Neuropathol. 97(4):377-82, 1999
5. Kleinschmidt-DeMasters BK et al: The pathologic, surgical, and MR spectrum of Rathke cleft cysts. Surg Neurol. 44(1):19-26; discussion 26-7, 1995

(Left) *In the absence of pressure atrophy or advanced squamous metaplasia, the pseudostratified epithelium bristles with cilia ➩.* **(Right)** *The epithelium may be simple rather than pseudostratified. While ciliated cells are present here ➩, they may be scanty or absent. In most instances, pressure atrophy may prevent visualization of cilia on sections.*

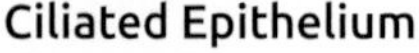

Ciliated Epithelium

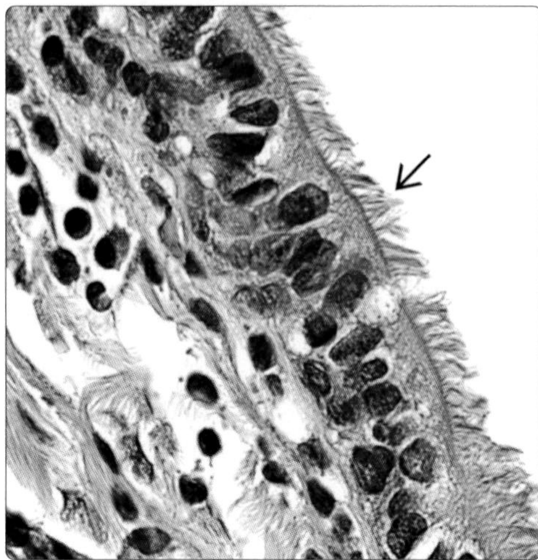

Stunted Cilia, Simple Epithelium

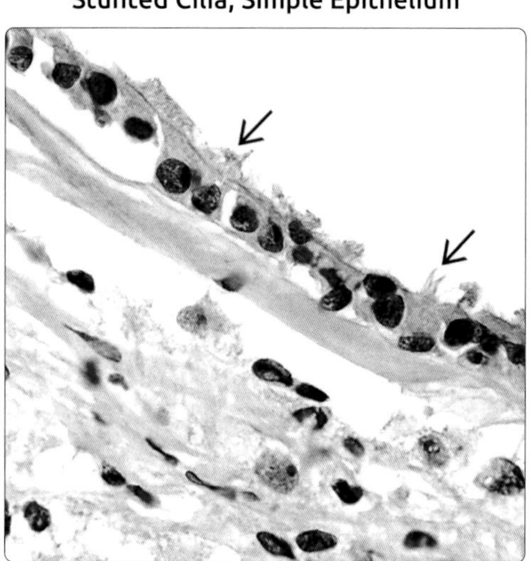

(Left) *Ciliated cells ➩ and goblet cells ➡ are diagnostic features of Rathke cleft cysts in this tissue fragment in a smear preparation.* **(Right)** *A cell bristling with cilia ➩ sits among distended goblet cells ➡ on a smear preparation. Goblet cells can be scant in a smear or frozen section of a Rathke cleft cyst.*

Smear Preparation

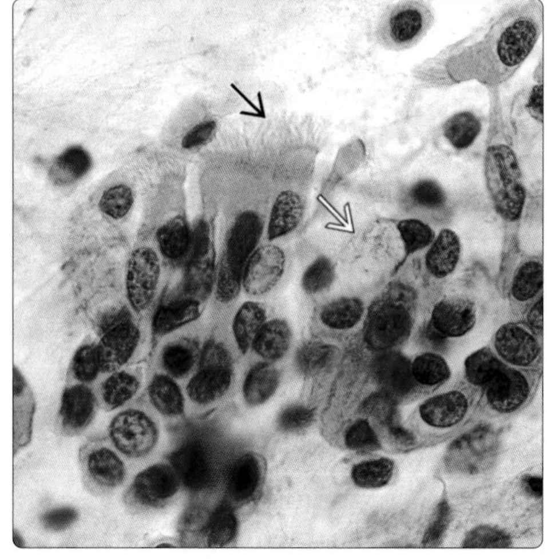

Goblet Cell on Smear

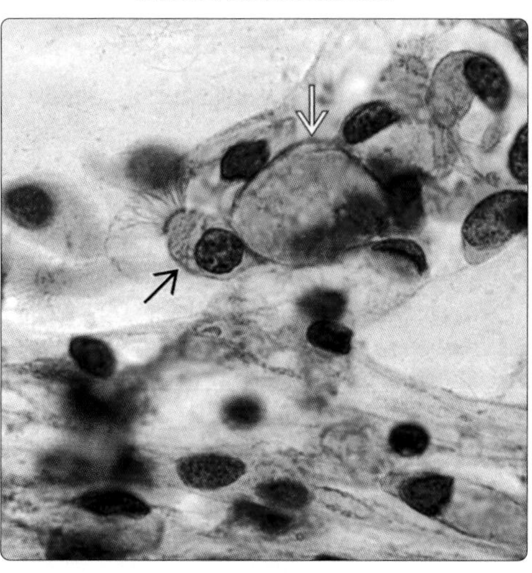

(Left) *Only small fragments of a low columnar or cuboidal epithelium may be found, with step sections/levels necessary for detection in some cases. The amount of underlying collagen helps distinguish Rathke cleft cysts from normal intermediate lobe cysts. The latter have only the most delicate layer.* **(Right)** *The ciliated epithelium of Rathke cleft cysts can appear flat, and cilia or the goblet cells may not be readily discernible.*

Low Columnar Epithelium

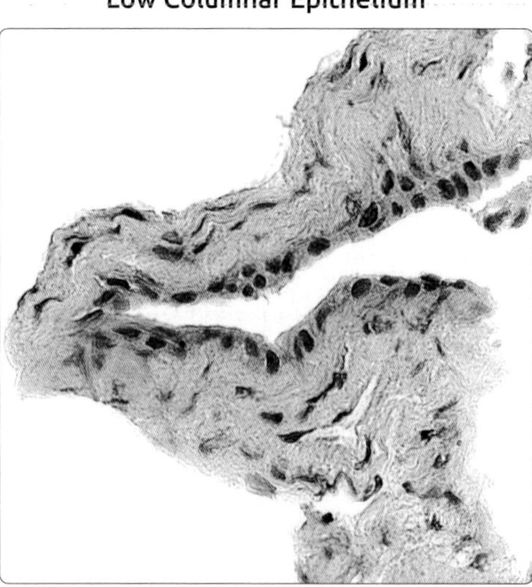

Attenuated Epithelium

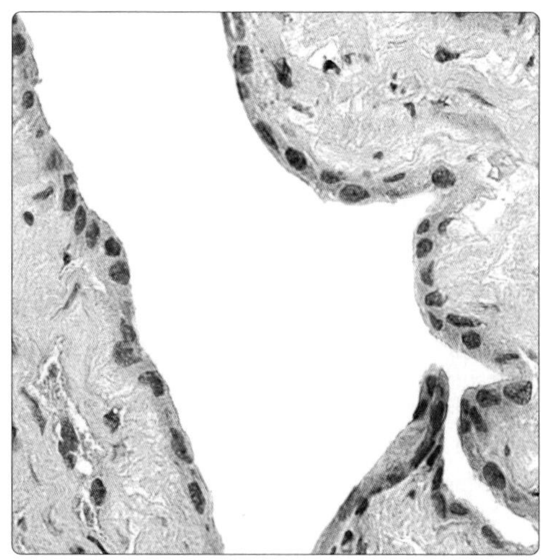

Squamous Metaplasia

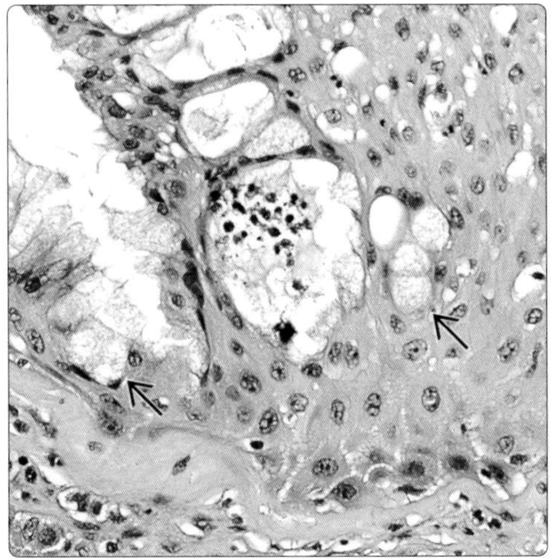

Squamous Metaplasia and Goblet Cells

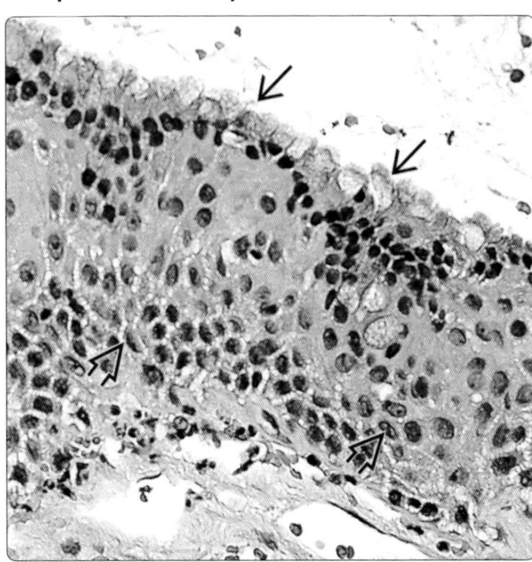

(Left) *Prominent squamous metaplasia may simulate papillary craniopharyngioma. Goblet cells ➡, prominent here, help identify the lesion as a Rathke cleft cyst.* **(Right)** *Proliferating squamous cells ⇒ lift off the native epithelium ➡, the latter with its ciliated and goblet cells. This diagnostic surface layer is very focal in some cases.*

Florid Squamous Metaplasia

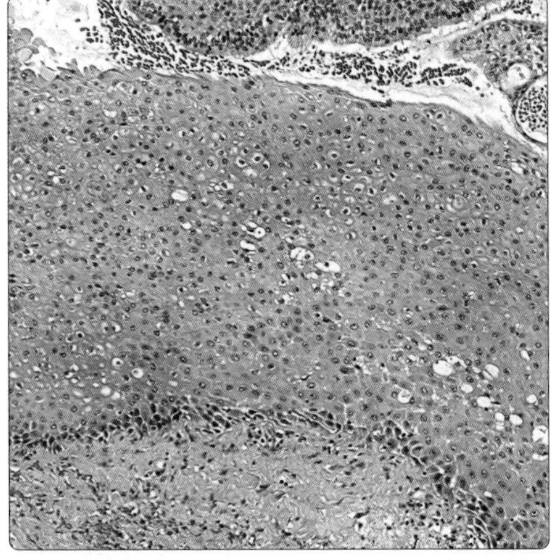

Xanthogranulomatous Change

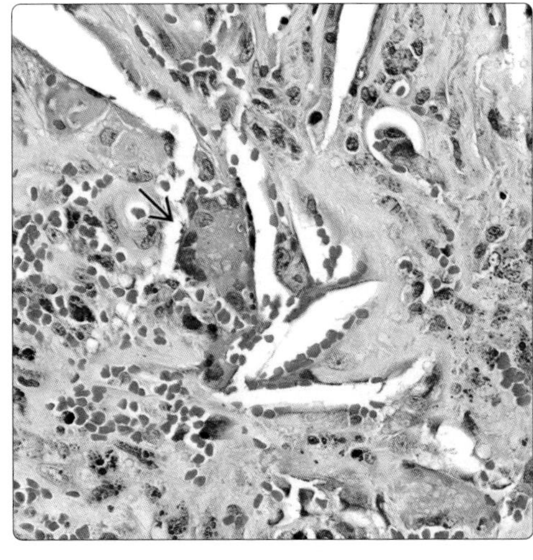

(Left) *In some cysts, the extent of squamous metaplasia makes the lesion difficult to distinguish from a papillary craniopharyngioma.* **(Right)** *Xanthogranulomatous reactions with giant cells ➡ and cholesterol clefts dominate some cases in which the epithelium may be only focal, if detectable at all.*

Inflammatory Cells and Ciliated Epithelium

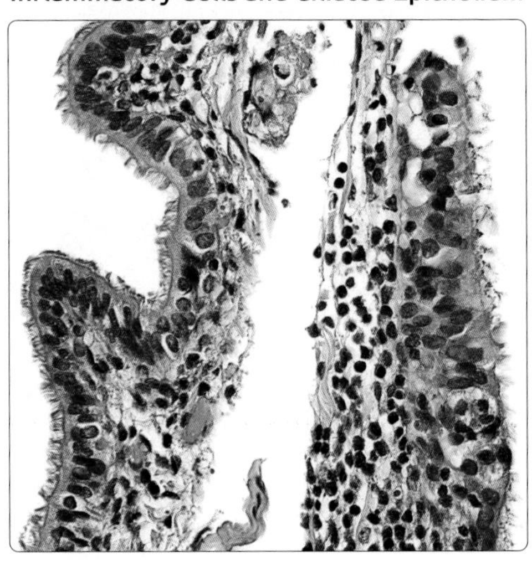

Acellular Cyst Content

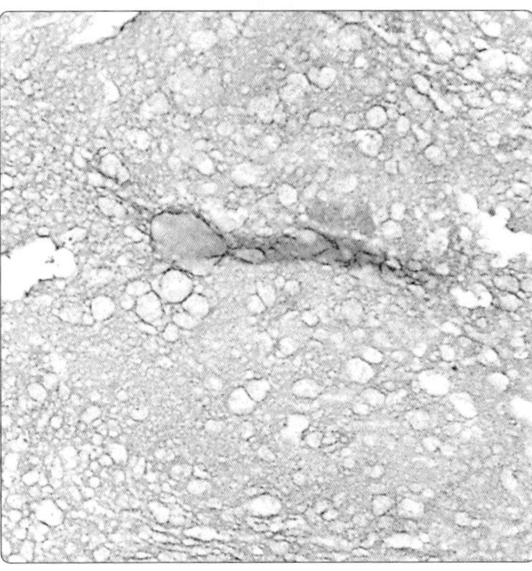

(Left) *Chronic inflammatory cells, sometimes in large numbers, may populate the underlying tissue and invade the epithelium.* **(Right)** *There may be nothing but amorphous content without an epithelial lining in some cases, in which only a descriptive diagnosis is possible.*

Endodermal Cyst

KEY FACTS

TERMINOLOGY

- Nonneoplastic cyst with well-differentiated epithelium, presumably derived from misplaced endoderm
- Synonyms
    - Enterogenous, neurenteric, bronchiogenic, foregut, epithelial

CLINICAL ISSUES

- Intraspinal (intradural extramedullary) most common location
- Posterior fossa, most common intracranial site, usually anterior to brainstem
- Prognosis
    - Excellent in most cases; less favorable if malignant change &/or cerebrospinal fluid dissemination

MICROSCOPIC

- Pseudostratified columnar epithelium with ciliated cells usually predominating, goblet cells variable in number
- Malignant change (rare)

TOP DIFFERENTIAL DIAGNOSES

- Ependymal cyst
- Rathke cleft cyst
- Epidermoid and dermoid cysts
- Arachnoid cyst
- Cystic dilatation of ventriculus terminalis
- Papillary endolymphatic sac tumor (cerebellopontine angle)
- Papillary craniopharyngioma
- True cystic teratoma
    - Admixture of 2-3 ectodermal/mesodermal/endodermal lineage tissues, as well as possible germ cell components

DIAGNOSTIC CHECKLIST

- Epithelium may be low cuboidal or even simple squamous

(Left) *This slightly hyperintense, well-delineated mass ➙ sits anterior to the brainstem, a common site.* **(Right)** *Endodermal cysts may rarely occur in supratentorial locations. Despite the massive size, note the smooth contour of the homogeneous cyst and absence of mass effect or herniation.*

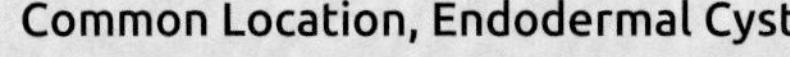

Common Location, Endodermal Cyst

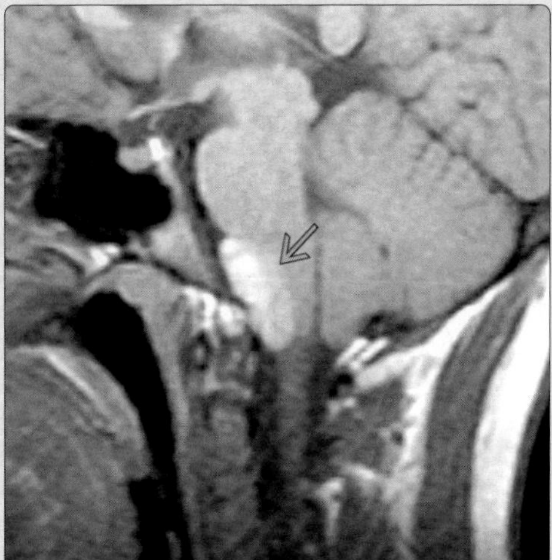

Rare Frontal Lobe Cyst

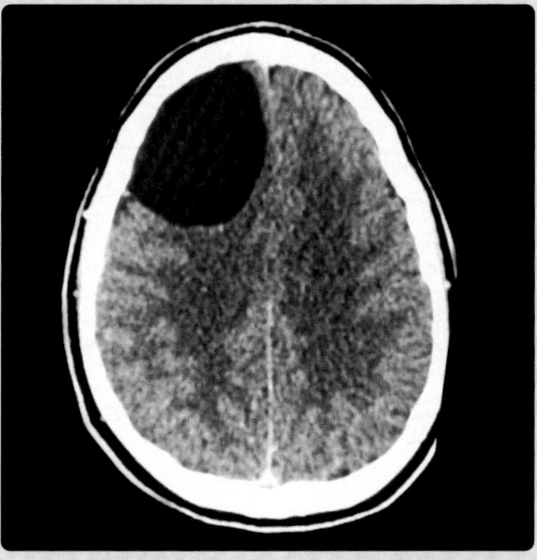

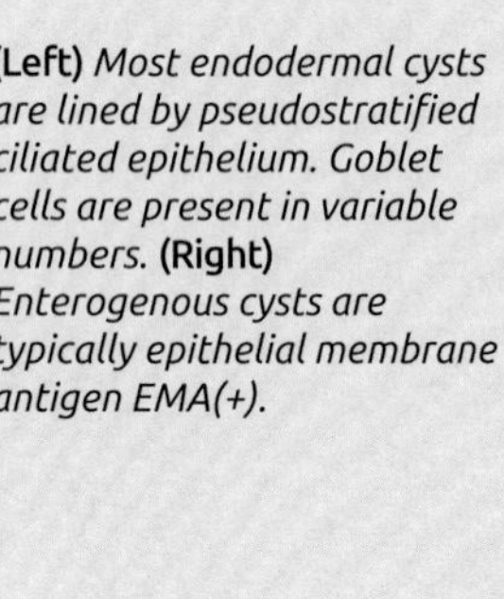

(Left) *Most endodermal cysts are lined by pseudostratified ciliated epithelium. Goblet cells are present in variable numbers.* **(Right)** *Enterogenous cysts are typically epithelial membrane antigen EMA(+).*

Pseudostratified Ciliated Epithelium

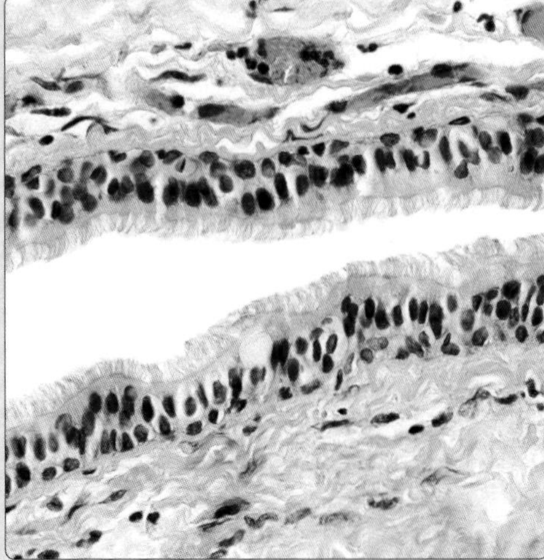

Epithelial Membrane Antigen, Endodermal Cyst

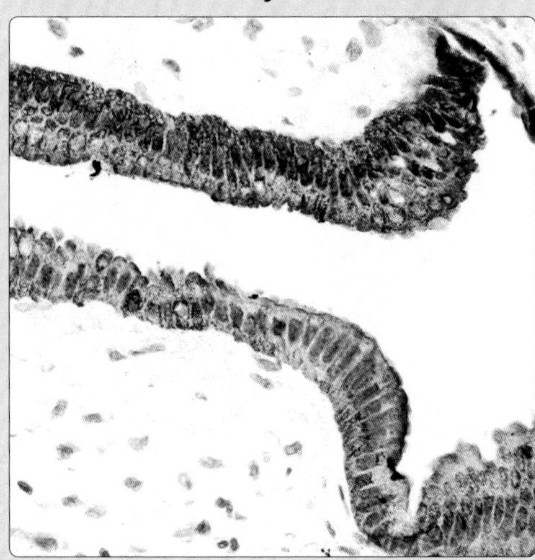

TERMINOLOGY

Synonyms

- Enterogenous, neurenteric, enteric, bronchogenic, foregut, epithelial

Definitions

- Nonneoplastic cyst with well-differentiated epithelium, presumably derived from misplaced endoderm

CLINICAL ISSUES

Site

- Intraspinal (intradural extramedullary) (most)
- Intracranial
  - Posterior fossa, most common intracranial site, usually anterior to brainstem
  - Supratentorial (rare)

Presentation

- Spinal: Pain, sensorimotor deficits
- Intracranial: Headache, cranial nerve deficits, cerebellar signs

Treatment

- Gross total excision curative; cyst drainage

Prognosis

- Excellent, most cases
- Less favorable with rare malignant change &/or cerebrospinal fluid (CSF) dissemination

IMAGING

MR Findings

- Contents
  - Hyperintense, bright to CSF on FLAIR and T2WI
  - Isointense to slightly hyperintense to CSF on T1WI
- Nonenhancing

CT Findings

- Abnormal vertebral bodies slightly caudal to level of mass in some cases

MACROSCOPIC

General Features

- Discrete, smooth surfaced
- Gray-white liquid to turbid viscous contents

MICROSCOPIC

Histologic Features

- Endodermal cyst
  - Pseudostratified columnar epithelium with
    - Ciliated cells, usually predominant
    - Goblet cells, periodic acid-Schiff, and mucicarmine (+)
  - Cuboidal epithelium, "pressure atrophy"
  - Subepithelial basement membrane
  - Xanthogranulomatous change (rare)
  - Squamous metaplasia (rare)
- With features of lung (bronchogenic cyst)
  - Pseudostratified columnar epithelium with ciliated cells &/or goblet cells
  - Cartilage &/or smooth muscle
  - Mucous and serous glands
- With features of intestinal/gastric differentiation
  - Glands &/or muscularis mucosa
- Malignant change (rare)
  - Benign epithelium
  - Transitional intraepithelial neoplasia
  - Carcinoma: Papillary, few if any cilia, invasion, atypia, high mitotic activity, necrosis in some cases, high Ki-67
  - CSF dissemination

ANCILLARY TESTS

Cytology

- Ciliated cells and goblet cells in varying proportions

Immunohistochemistry

- Epithelial membrane antigen (EMA)(+)
- Cytokeratin (+)
- CEA(+) in some cases

DIFFERENTIAL DIAGNOSIS

Ependymal Cyst

- S100(+); some focal glial fibrillary acidic protein (+); EMA and cytokeratin (-), but (+) cases overlap with some reported endodermal cysts
- Cyst rests on neuropil/glial base without basement membrane

Rathke Cleft Cyst

- Sella region, midline; can be histologically identical to endodermal cyst
- Squamous metaplasia and xanthogranulomatous reaction more likely

Epidermoid and Dermoid Cysts

- Keratinizing squamous epithelium

Arachnoid Cyst

- Leptomeningeal; flat, often inconspicuous, epithelium

Cystic Dilatation of Ventriculus Terminalis

- In conus medullaris, no goblet cells, no cilia in adults (light microscopy)

Papillary Endolymphatic Sac Tumor (Cerebellopontine Angle)

- von Hippel-Lindau syndrome, papillary, bone erosion all characteristic

Papillary Craniopharyngioma

- Usually prominent solid component, nonkeratinizing epithelium, focal goblet cells in some cases

True Cystic Teratoma

- Admixture of 2-3 ectodermal/mesodermal/endodermal lineage tissues, as well as possible germ cell components

SELECTED REFERENCES

1. Mittal S et al: Supratentorial neurenteric cysts. A fascinating entity of uncertain embryopathogenesis. Clin Neurol Neurosurg. 112(2):89-97, 2010
2. Dunham CP et al: Malignant transformation of an intraaxial-supratentorial neurenteric cyst--case report and review of the literature. Clin Neuropathol. 28(6):460-6, 2009

(Left) *Cilia ⇒ are inescapable at high magnification in a lesion that can be histologically identical to a Rathke cleft cyst.* **(Right)** *In a close facsimile of bronchial epithelium, the lining of this benign cyst has both ciliated ⇒ and goblet cells ⇒.*

Cilia

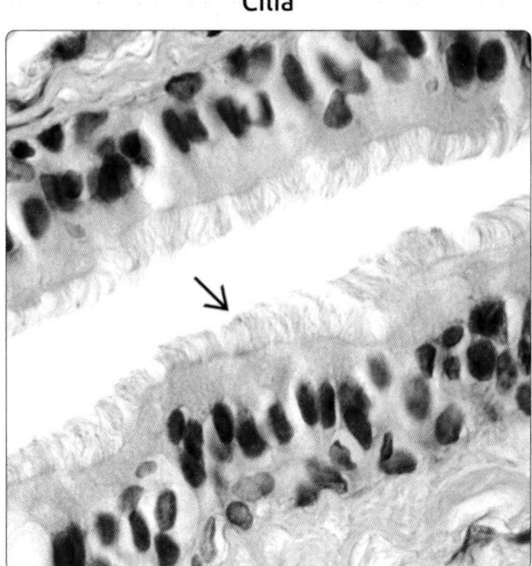

Predominance of Ciliated Cells

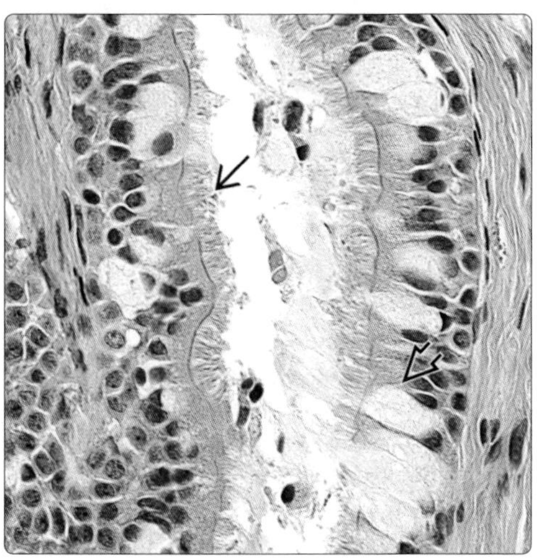

(Left) *Goblet cells abound in some cases, such as this, but it is the ciliated cell that usually predominates.* **(Right)** *The lining of some endodermal cysts is more complicated than the simple epithelium of the classic lesion. Submucosal glands are present in this case. The presence of goblet cells clearly distinguishes this lesion from ependymal cyst.*

Predominance of Goblet Cells

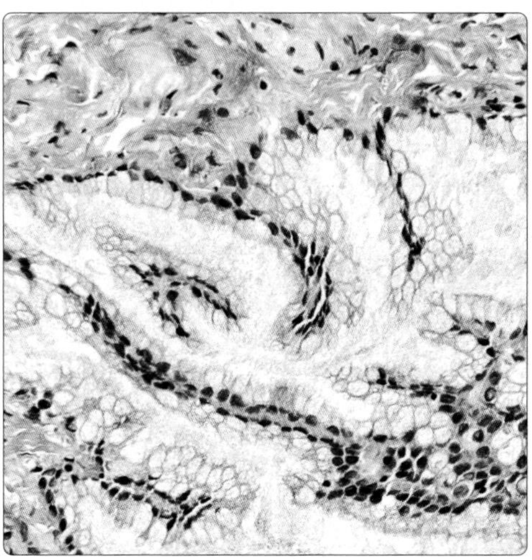

Submucosal-Type Glands

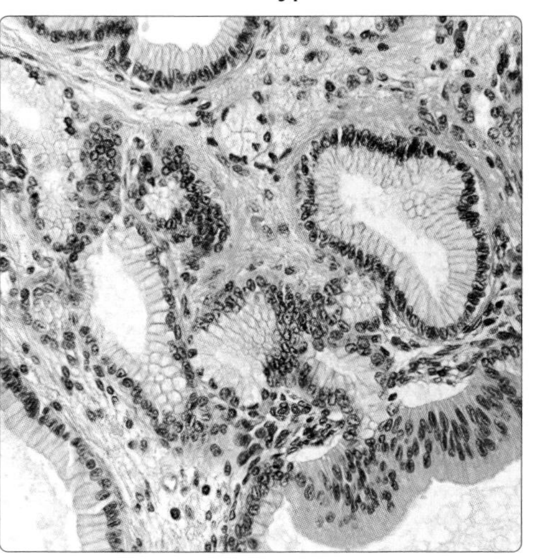

(Left) *Glands in a submucosa-like layer help create a more complex form of endodermal cysts. Goblet cells ⇒ are a principal component of some glands. Such complex endodermal cysts should be distinguished from true cystic teratomas that contain an admixture of 2-3 ectodermal/mesodermal/endodermal lineage tissues, as well as possible germ cell components.* **(Right)** *The epithelium ranges from tall, almost pseudostratified ⇒, to low and cuboidal ⇒. Cilia are absent in this case.*

Complex Endodermal Cyst

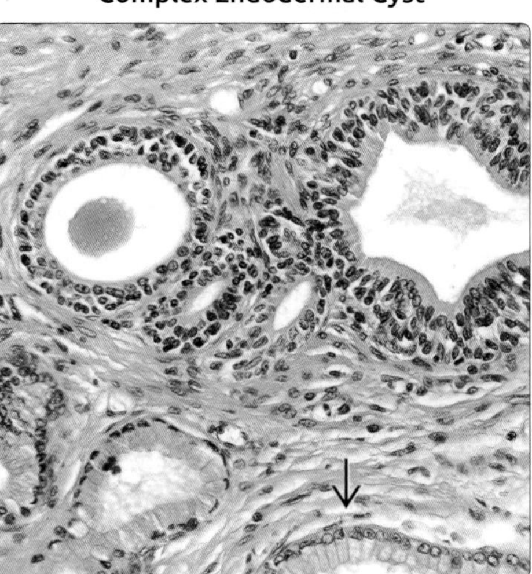

Low Cuboidal Epithelium

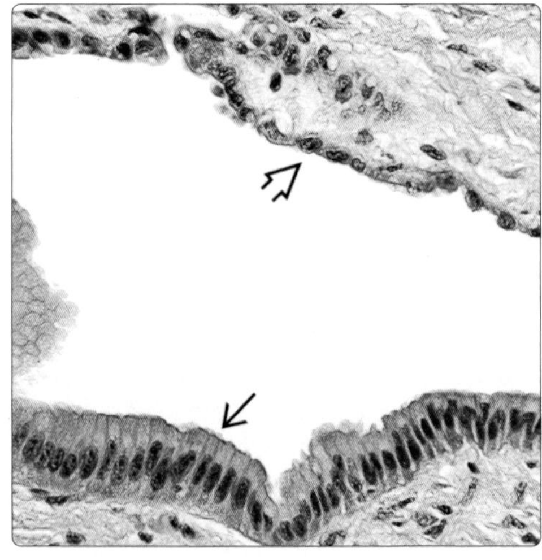

Benign Ciliated Epithelium

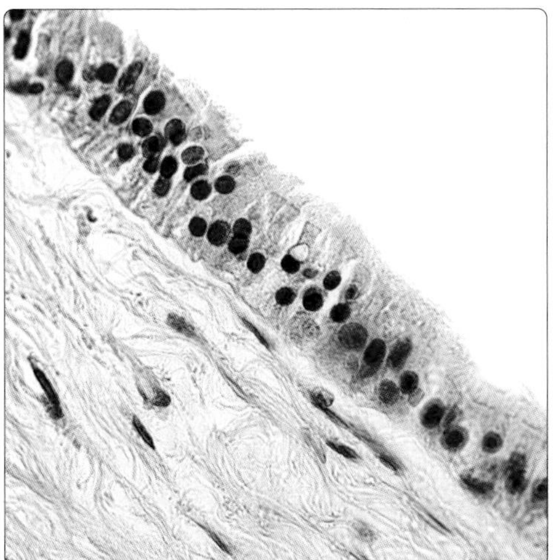

Malignant Transformation

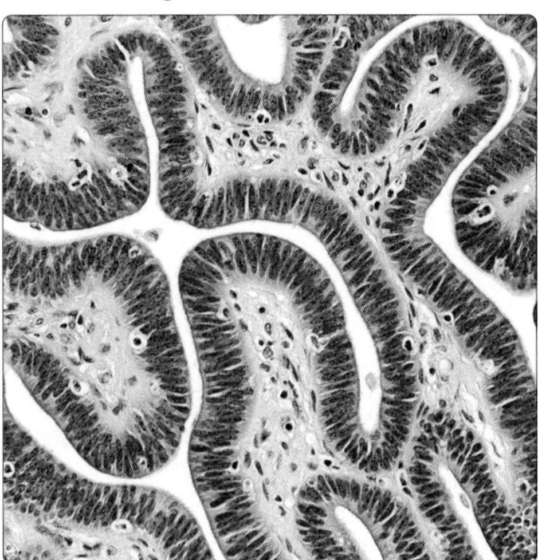

(Left) *Malignant transformation is rare in endodermal cysts. This benign ciliated epithelium was associated elsewhere with well-differentiated papillary carcinoma.* **(Right)** *This well-differentiated papillary adenocarcinoma arose in a typical highly differentiated endodermal cyst. The malignant epithelium is crowded, atypical, and nonciliated.*

CAM5.2 Endodermal Cyst

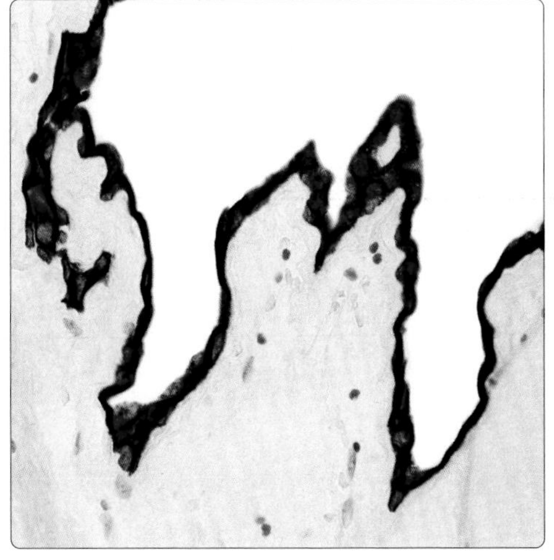

Ber-EP4 Endodermal Cyst

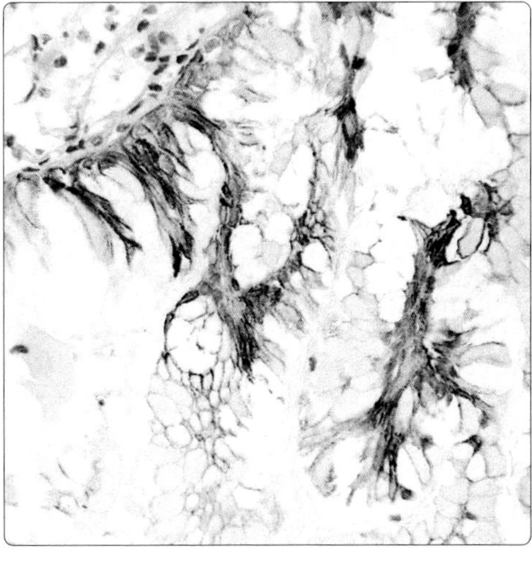

(Left) *Strong reactivity for CAM5.2 is common in enterogenous cysts.* **(Right)** *Immunoreactivity for Ber-EP4 in this goblet cell-rich lesion accords with its endodermal derivation.*

Smear, Abundant Shedding

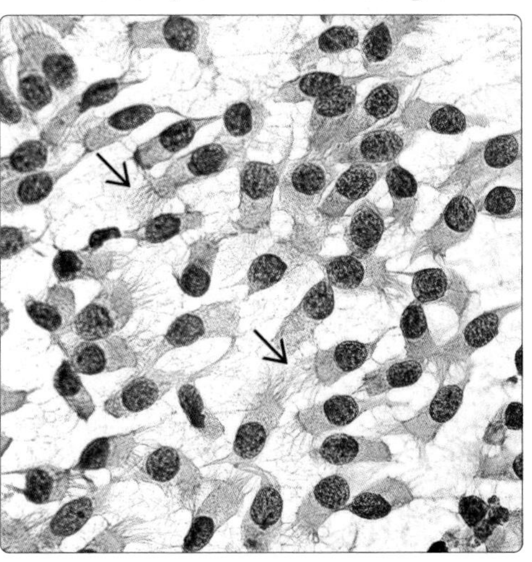

Electron Micrograph, Cilia

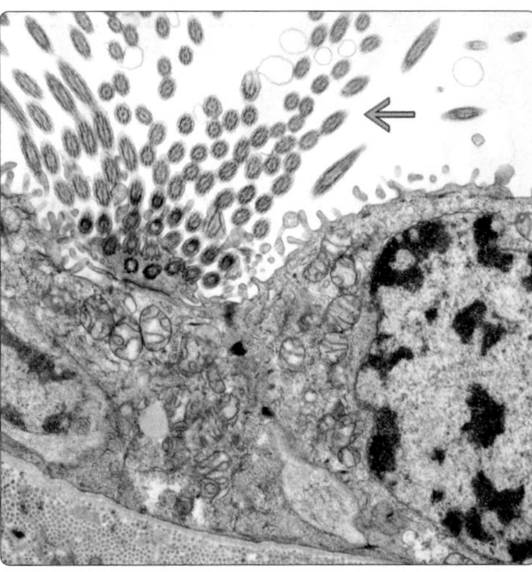

(Left) *Luxuriantly ciliated columnar epithelial cells ⇨ shed freely in smears. Goblet cells are typically less common.* **(Right)** *Ultrastructurally, cilia ⇨ fan out into the cyst lumen. A nonciliated cell with microvilli abuts at the right.*

Ependymal Cyst

KEY FACTS

TERMINOLOGY

- Benign ependymal-lined cyst
- Overlap in histological and immunohistochemical features with some reported cases of endodermal (neurenteric) cysts
- Entity best defined when restricted to intraparenchymal lesions, especially supratentorial and paraventricular, and EMA(-) and cytokeratin (-)

CLINICAL ISSUES

- Usually supratentorial
- Paraventricular, rarely intraventricular
- Prognosis good with excision

MACROSCOPIC

- Discrete, smooth walled

MICROSCOPIC

- Simple epithelial lining

TOP DIFFERENTIAL DIAGNOSES

- Endodermal (neurenteric) cyst
  - Ciliated epithelium but may be cuboidal with pressure atrophy
  - Variable goblet cells
- Epidermoid cyst
  - Stratified squamous epithelium, anucleate keratin contents
- Dermoid cyst
  - Stratified squamous epithelium, adnexal component
- Cystic ependymoma
  - Solid tumor component

DIAGNOSTIC CHECKLIST

- Not always clear distinction from endodermal (neurenteric) cysts in published cases

Ependymal Cyst, Well Circumscribed

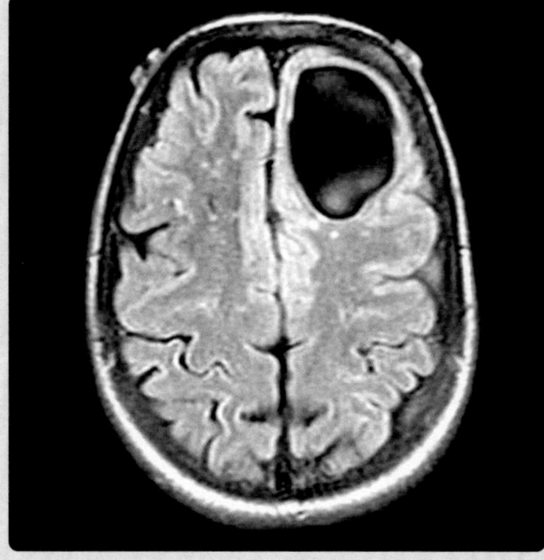

Ependymal Cyst, Low Cuboidal Lining

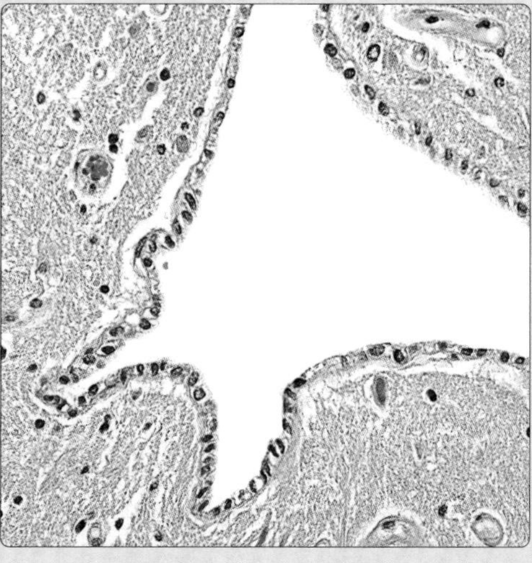

(Left) *As seen in this FLAIR image, ependymal cysts are well-circumscribed, fluid-filled masses, often supratentorial and paraventricular.* **(Right)** *A simple, nonstratified low-columnar/cuboidal epithelium is typical. Cilia are not usually as prominent as they are in endodermal (neurenteric) cysts if they are present at all.*

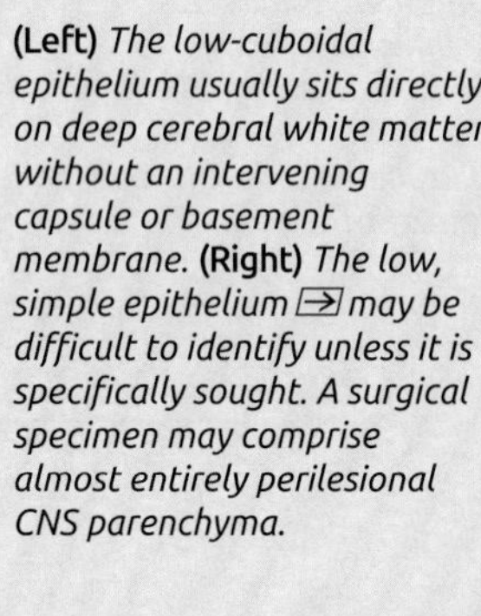

(Left) *The low-cuboidal epithelium usually sits directly on deep cerebral white matter without an intervening capsule or basement membrane.* **(Right)** *The low, simple epithelium ➡ may be difficult to identify unless it is specifically sought. A surgical specimen may comprise almost entirely perilesional CNS parenchyma.*

Epithelium Lying on Glial Tissue

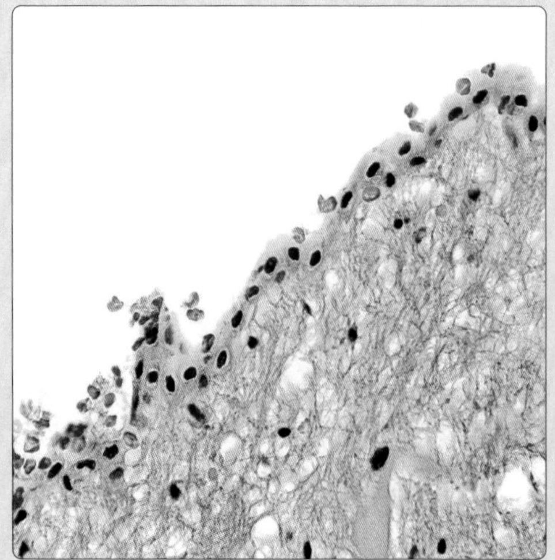

Inconspicuous Low, Simple Epithelium

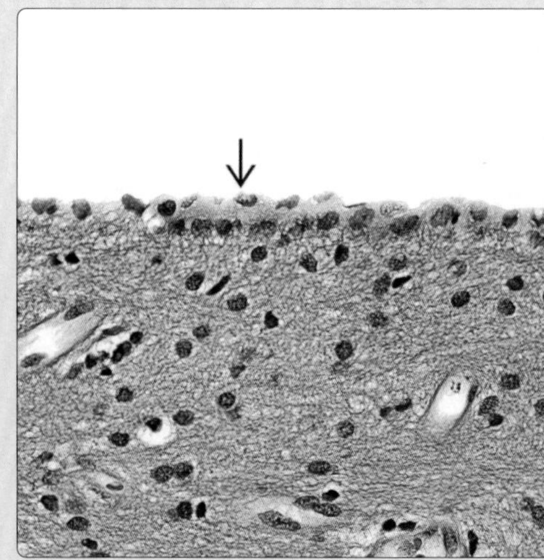

TERMINOLOGY

Synonyms

- Glioependymal, neuroepithelial, epithelial cyst

Definitions

- Benign, usually intraparenchymal cyst lined by ependyma
- Overlaps in pathological features with endodermal (neurenteric) cyst in some reported cases
- Entity best defined when restricted to EMA(-) and cytokeratin (-) intraparenchymal lesions, especially when supratentorial and paraventricular

CLINICAL ISSUES

Site

- Throughout CNS
- Usually supratentorial
  - Paraventricular
  - Rarely intraventricular

Presentation

- Variable depending on location
- Headaches
- Seizures

Treatment

- Surgical approaches
  - Excision
  - Drainage, fenestration
  - Spinal intramedullary ependymal cysts may require cyst-subarachnoid shunt placement

Prognosis

- Good

IMAGING

MR Findings

- Fluid filled
- No enhancement

MACROSCOPIC

General Features

- Discrete
- Smooth walled
- Clear or opalescent contents

MICROSCOPIC

Histologic Features

- Epithelial lining
  - Ciliated or nonciliated
  - Columnar to cuboidal to simple squamous (nonkeratinizing)
- Usually little if any surrounding gliosis
- Generally no basement membrane

ANCILLARY TESTS

Immunohistochemistry

- GFAP(+)
- S100(+)
- EMA(±); positive cases overlap with endodermal (neurenteric) cyst
- Cytokeratins (±); positive cases overlap with endodermal (neurenteric) cyst

Electron Microscopy

- Cilia
- Microvilli
- Glycocalyx
- Zonulae adherentes

DIFFERENTIAL DIAGNOSIS

Normal Ependyma

- May be difficult distinction
  - Location of sampled tissue important

Ependymoma

- Solid component

Cystic Dilatation of Ventriculus Terminalis

- In conus medullaris

Endodermal (Neurenteric) Cyst

- Ciliated epithelium but may be cuboidal with pressure atrophy
- Goblet cells
- EMA and cytokeratins (+) but overlap in features with ependymal cyst in some reported cases

Rathke Cleft Cyst

- Midline, sella region
- Goblet cells
- Frequent squamous metaplasia
- Xanthogranulomatous reaction, in some cases
- EMA and cytokeratins (+)

Epidermoid and Dermoid Cysts

- Stratified squamous epithelium, anucleate keratin contents
- Adnexa (dermoid cyst)

DIAGNOSTIC CHECKLIST

Pathologic Interpretation Pearls

- Not always clear distinction from endodermal (neurenteric) cysts in published cases

SELECTED REFERENCES

1. Jones RT et al: Cross-reactivity of the BRAF VE1 antibody with epitopes in axonemal dyneins leads to staining of cilia. Mod Pathol. 28(4):596-606, 2015
2. Yang T et al: Clinical characteristics and surgical outcomes of spinal intramedullary ependymal cysts. Acta Neurochir (Wien). 156(2):269-75, 2014
3. Prieto R et al: Ependymal cyst of the midbrain. Clin Neuropathol. 32(3):183-8, 2013
4. Conrad J et al: Mesencephalic ependymal cysts: treatment under pure endoscopic or endoscope-assisted keyhole conditions. J Neurosurg. 109(4):723-8, 2008
5. de Moura Batista L et al: Cystic lesion of the ventriculus terminalis: proposal for a new clinical classification. J Neurosurg Spine. 8(2):163-8, 2008
6. Balasubramaniam C et al: Intramedullary glioependymal cyst and tethered cord in an infant. Childs Nerv Syst. 20(7):496-8, 2004
7. Sidhu M et al: Histological analysis of cystic tumour like lesions of central nervous system. Indian J Pathol Microbiol. 45(1):7-14, 2002
8. Boockvar JA et al: Symptomatic lateral ventricular ependymal cysts: criteria for distinguishing these rare cysts from other symptomatic cysts of the ventricles: case report. Neurosurgery. 46(5):1229-32; discussion 1232-3, 2000

Pineal Cyst

KEY FACTS

CLINICAL ISSUES

- Incidence
  - ~ 2-4%
    - Higher in young women
- Usually incidental finding during work-up for other conditions
  - e.g., head trauma, unrelated headache

IMAGING

- Cystic pineal region mass
- Fluid-fluid level in some cases

MACROSCOPIC

- Often hemosiderin stained
- Cyst contents variably clear, murky, brown

MICROSCOPIC

- Lobular architecture
  - Pineal gland component
- Frequent calcifications
  - Normal "brain sand"
- Sharp interface
  - Glial component often with Rosenthal fibers
- No mitoses
- No epithelial or ependymal lining to cyst wall

DIAGNOSTIC CHECKLIST

- Lobular architecture in compressed adjacent normal pineal gland
- Calcifications more common in normal compressed adjacent pineal gland than in pineocytoma
- Pineal gland component easily misinterpreted histologically as pineocytoma
- Rosenthal fiber-rich gliotic component easily misinterpreted histologically as pilocytic astrocytoma if pineal gland not recognized
- Ki-67(+) cells confined largely to vessels

(Left) *FLAIR MR shows a fluid-fluid level ➡, which is not uncommon, as the result of intralesional hemorrhage.* **(Right)** *Pineal cysts seldom come to biopsy, but when they do, the presence of numerous Rosenthal fibers ➡ may lead to mistaken diagnosis of pilocytic astrocytoma. Note the absence of a cyst wall lining.*

Fluid-Fluid Level, Pineal Cyst

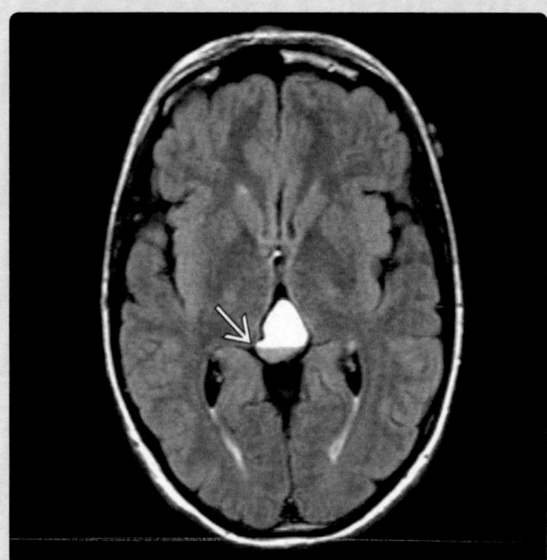

Pineal Cyst, Biopsy

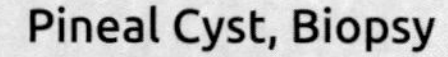

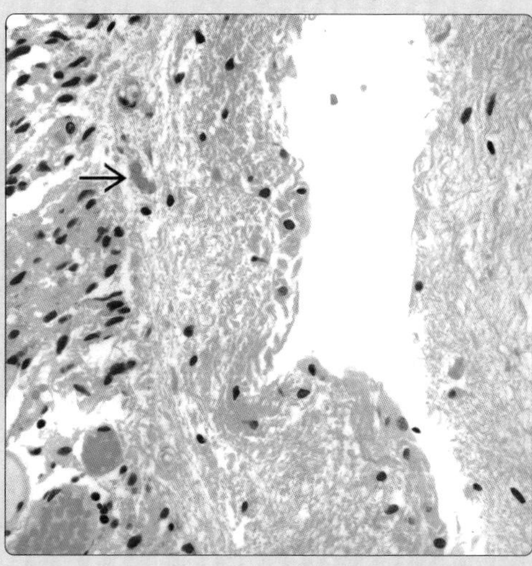

(Left) *Iron-laden cells are usually most abundant near the cavity.* **(Right)** *Most autopsies will contain pineal glands with cysts, which, by the time the patient reaches later adult life, are unilocular. These cysts are not lined by epithelium and are surrounded by normal pineal gland ➡.*

Pineal Cyst, Perl Iron

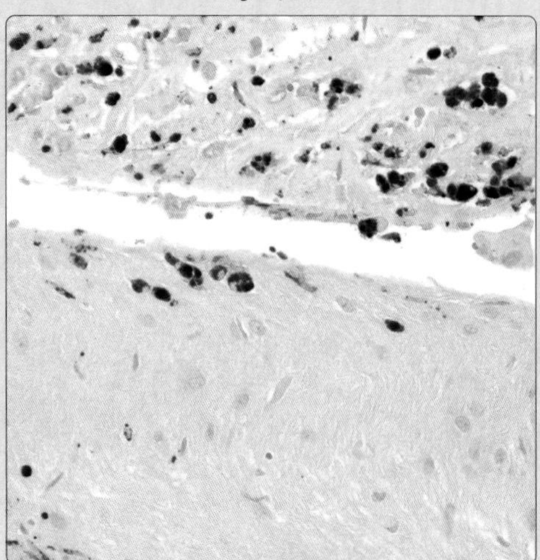

Pineal Cyst, Autopsy

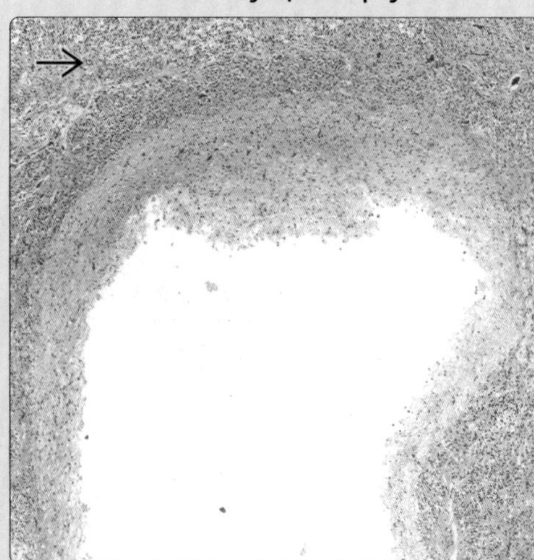

TERMINOLOGY

Definitions

- Nonneoplastic cyst of pineal gland

ETIOLOGY/PATHOGENESIS

Developmental Anomaly

- Likely represents one end of spectrum of normally occurring cyst(s) within pineal gland
- Not strongly associated with underlying genetic condition

CLINICAL ISSUES

Epidemiology

- Incidence
  - ~ 2-4%
    - Higher incidence in young women
  - Uncommon late in life as symptomatic lesions but small pineal cyst found frequently at autopsy
  - May occur in normal children but asymptomatic
    - Cysts often septated
    - In one study using 3 Tesla (3T) imaging, incidental pineal cysts were identified in 57% of children
- Sex
  - Female predilection

Presentation

- Usually incidental finding during work-up of other conditions
  - e.g., head trauma, headache
- Symptomatic due to CSF flow obstruction
  - Headaches
  - Nausea and vomiting
  - Unsteadiness of gait
  - Cranial nerve dysfunction
- Symptoms potentially precipitated by intracystic hemorrhage
  - Pineal apoplexy

Treatment

- Surgical approaches
  - Excision, complete or partial

Prognosis

- Excellent

IMAGING

MR Findings

- Midline, pineal region
- Smooth-surfaced, round or ovoid mass
- Obstructive hydrocephalus (some cases)
- Evidence of acute or subacute hemorrhage (some cases)
- Fluid-fluid level (some cases)
- Enlargement over time seen in minority, usually younger children
  - In one study
    - Mean age of patients with cysts that changed or grew was 5.5 years
    - Mean age of patients with stable pineal cysts was 12.2 years
- Cysts often septated when found incidentally in children

MACROSCOPIC

General Features

- Smooth surface
- Hemosiderin-stained inner surface
- Contents variably clear, murky, brown

Size

- Majority of patients harboring pineal cyst require no treatment
  - Incidental pineal cysts identified in 57% of children
    - Mean maximum linear dimension of 4.2 mm (range: 1.5-16 mm)
  - Surgery is option for subset of adult or pediatric patients with secondary hydrocephalus or Parinaud syndrome
- Some studies suggest pineal cyst resection in absence of ventriculomegaly or Parinaud syndrome may still be warranted
  - Pineal cyst may cause intermittent occlusion of cerebrospinal fluid pathways, causing some small pineal cysts to become intermittently symptomatic
  - In one study, mean preoperative cyst diameter of those undergoing surgical resection was 1.5 cm (range: 0.9-2.2 cm)

MICROSCOPIC

Histologic Features

- Attenuated pineal parenchyma, outer layer
  - Lobular architecture
  - Rosette-like structures
    - Lobules of parenchymal cells
  - Calcifications
    - Corpora arenacea, "brain sand"
  - Uniform, cytologically bland nuclei
  - No mitoses
- Sharply defined zone of finely fibrillar, glial tissue with
  - Rosenthal fibers
  - Hemosiderin staining, siderophages
  - No microcysts or biphasic pattern
  - Degenerative atypia (±)
- No ependymal or epithelial lining in cyst wall

ANCILLARY TESTS

Cytology

- Clumps of cohesive cells
- Oval, cytologically bland nuclei of pineal gland
- Moderate cytoplasm with bipolar processes
- No mitoses

Immunohistochemistry

- Synaptophysin (+)
  - Strong, diffuse, in pineal parenchyma
- GFAP(+) scattered inter- and intralobular astrocytes in pineal gland
  - Also cyst wall
- Ki-67 labeling index low
  - More in endothelial cells than in pinealocytes

DIFFERENTIAL DIAGNOSIS

Pineocytoma

- More cellular
- Sheet-like rather than lobular architecture
- Pineocytomatous rosettes (some cases)
- Higher Ki-67 index
- Large pleomorphic cells (some cases)
- GFAP(-)

Papillary Tumor of the Pineal Region

- Epithelial features
- Higher cellularity
- Mitoses
- Higher Ki-67 index
- Necrosis (some cases)
- Immunohistochemistry
  - Cytokeratin (+)
  - Synaptophysin (-)

Ependymoma

- Sheet-like rather than lobular architecture
- Perivascular pseudorosettes
- GFAP(+)
- Largely synaptophysin (-)
- EMA(+)
  - Especially dot-like or circular profiles of microlumina

Pilocytic Astrocytoma

- Spongy/microcystic and compact tissues
- Hyalinized vessels
- Eosinophilic granular bodies
- Greater degenerative atypia in chronic examples
- Higher Ki-67 index
- No epithelial-like or lobular component

Ganglion Cell Tumor

- More complex architecture, ganglioglioma
- Dysmorphic cells
- Microcystic tissue with eosinophilic granular bodies
- Perivascular lymphocytes

Cystic Teratoma

- Need to recognize endodermal, ectodermal, mesenchymal elements in noncystic portion of mass
- Cysts lined by tall columnar, ciliated, cuboidal, goblet cell epithelium
- No gliotic cyst wall with Rosenthal fibers, hemosiderin as in pineal cyst

DIAGNOSTIC CHECKLIST

Clinically Relevant Pathologic Features

- Normal compressed pineal gland adjacent to pineal cyst easily misinterpreted histologically as pineocytoma
  - Normal gland has lobular architecture
    - Uniform size to lobules
    - Synaptophysin (+)
- Rosenthal fiber-rich gliotic component easily misinterpreted histologically as pilocytic astrocytoma if compressed normal pineal gland not recognized

Pathologic Interpretation Pearls

- Cyst wall composed of glial layer with hemosiderin deposition
- Ki-67(+) cells confined largely to vessels
- Calcifications often seen in normal pineal gland compressed at edge of cyst more common than in pineocytoma
  - Calcifications far more common in normal pineal gland than in pineocytoma
- No epithelial or ependymal lining to pineal cyst wall

SELECTED REFERENCES

1. Kalani MY et al: Pineal cyst resection in the absence of ventriculomegaly or Parinaud's syndrome: clinical outcomes and implications for patient selection. J Neurosurg. 1-5, 2015
2. Berhouma M et al: Update on the management of pineal cysts: Case series and a review of the literature. Neurochirurgie. ePub, 2014
3. Whitehead MT et al: Incidental pineal cysts in children who undergo 3-T MRI. Pediatr Radiol. 43(12):1577-83, 2013
4. Lacroix-Boudhrioua V et al: Pineal cysts in children. Insights Imaging. 2(6):671-678, 2011
5. Al-Holou WN et al: The natural history of pineal cysts in children and young adults. J Neurosurg Pediatr. 5(2):162-6, 2010
6. Al-Holou WN et al: Prevalence of pineal cysts in children and young adults. Clinical article. J Neurosurg Pediatr. 4(3):230-6, 2009
7. Sarikaya-Seiwert S et al: Symptomatic intracystic hemorrhage in pineal cysts. Report of 3 cases. J Neurosurg Pediatr. 4(2):130-6, 2009
8. Scheithauer BW: Pathobiology of the pineal gland with emphasis on parenchymal tumors. Brain Tumor Pathol. 16(1):1-9, 1999
9. Sawamura Y et al: Magnetic resonance images reveal a high incidence of asymptomatic pineal cysts in young women. Neurosurgery. 37(1):11-5; discussion 15-6, 1995

Pineal Cyst, Siderophages

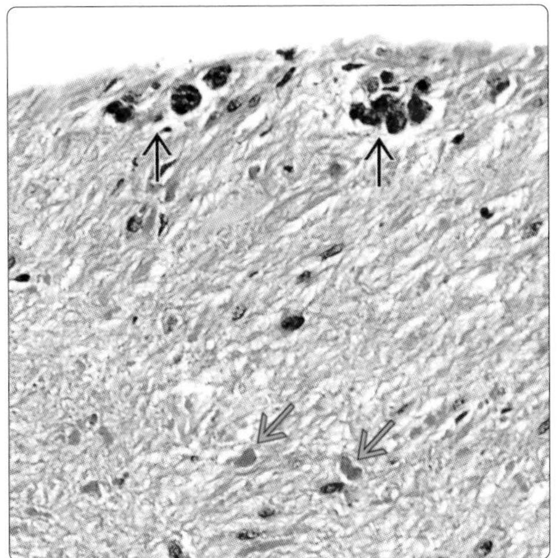

Pineal Cyst, Ferrugination Secondary to Hemorrhage

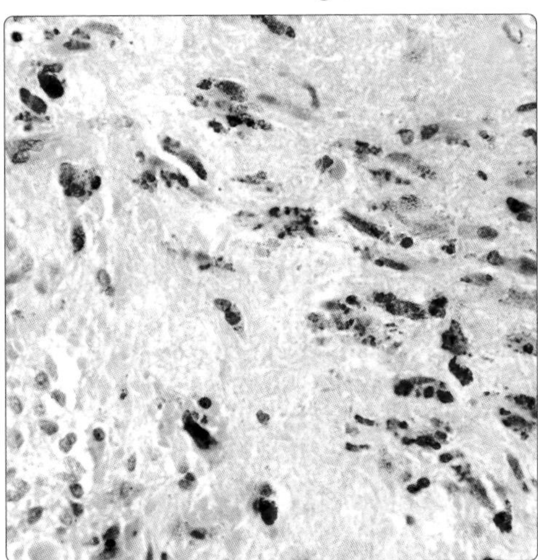

(Left) *The glial component lacks the usual spongy quality of pilocytic astrocytoma. Siderophages ➡ abut the cavity. Rosenthal fibers ➡ are not specific for pilocytic astrocytoma.* **(Right)** *Gliotic tissue in the pineal region with this degree of ferrugination is highly suspicious for pineal cyst. As a consequence of hemorrhage, sometimes large and acute enough to precipitate symptomatic enlargement, pineal cysts are often macroscopically brown.*

Pineal Cyst, Incidental Autopsy Finding

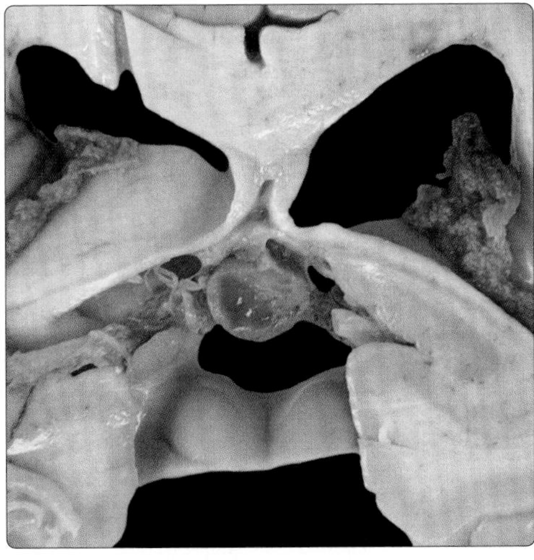

Severe Liver Disease, Elevated Bilirubin

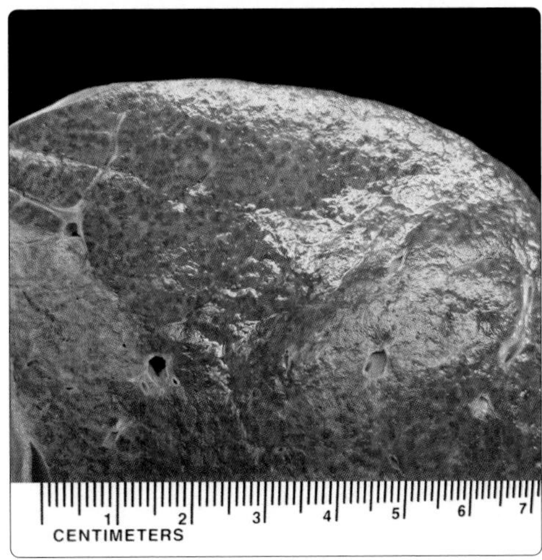

(Left) *This adult patient with an incidental pineal cyst at autopsy also suffered from terminal liver failure and elevated bilirubin. Note that the pineal gland does not possess a blood-brain barrier and thus becomes bilirubin-stained when blood levels are elevated.* **(Right)** *Patients with elevated bilirubin can show greenish staining not only in the liver, as seen here, but in brain sites devoid of a blood brain barrier, such as the pineal gland or choroid plexi.*

Autopsy Pineal Cyst, Child

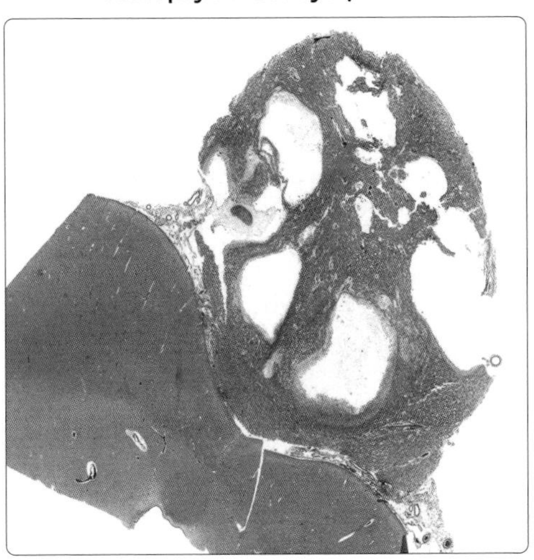

Autopsy Pineal Cyst, Older Adult

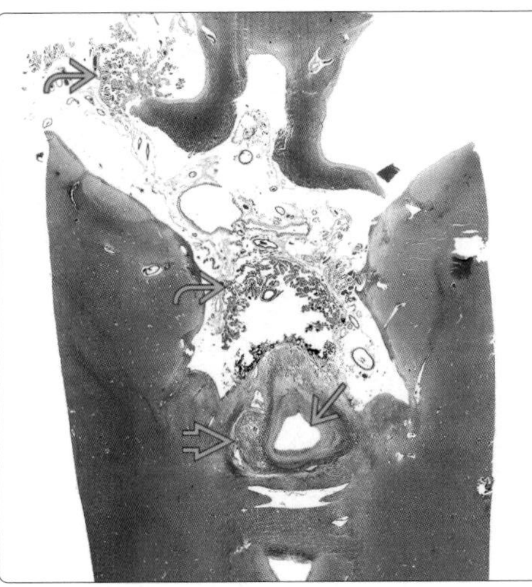

(Left) *Pineal cysts can be found incidentally at autopsy in children as well as adults, but may have a septated/multiloculated appearance as seen here in a 12-year-old patient who succumbed to cancer.* **(Right)** *This whole mount section of a pineal cyst found incidentally at autopsy shows the single cystic configuration typical for an older adult ➡. Note the compressed, distorted pineal gland at the perimeter ➡, as well as choroid plexus ➡.*

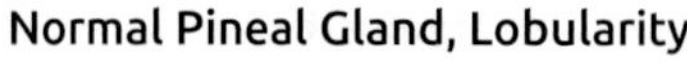

(Left) *The tissue's lobularity is a distinctive feature, although superficial fibrillar intralobular tissue lends an ependymomatous quality. The latter areas would be synaptophysin (+) rather than GFAP(+), however.* **(Right)** *The pineal gland's neuronal qualities may be interpreted as evidence of a ganglion cell tumor. Such an impression would be seemingly confirmed by the tissue's immunoreactivity for synaptophysin, except for the tissue's distinctive, uniform lobularity.*

Normal Pineal Gland, Lobularity

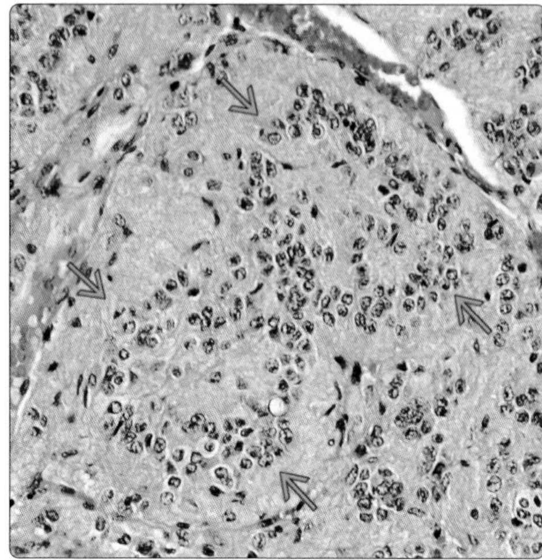

Normal Pineal Gland, Neuronal Features

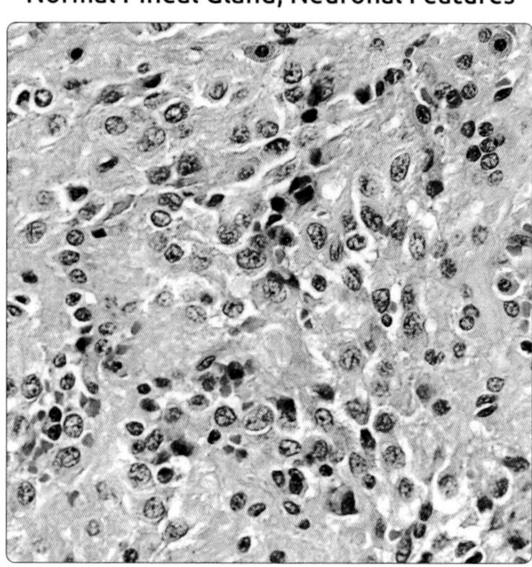

(Left) *At high magnification, it is easy to focus on the normal pineal gland's mildly pleomorphic nuclei and assume a neoplasm. Note the Rosenthal fiber in the glial component.* **(Right)** *The sharp divide between pineal parenchyma and glial tissue is best appreciated at low magnification.*

Normal Pineal Gland Mimicking Tumor

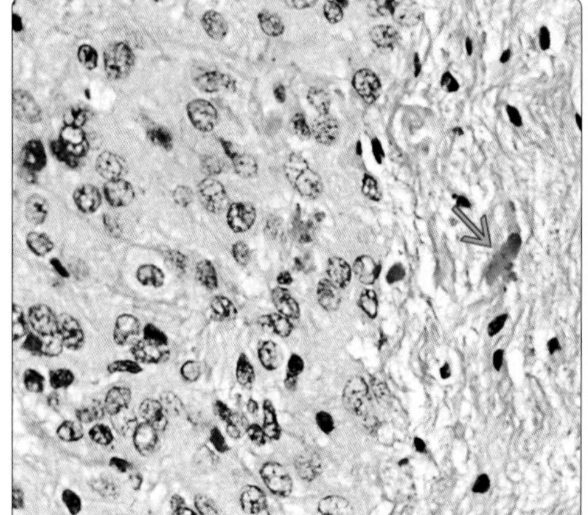

Normal Pineal Gland

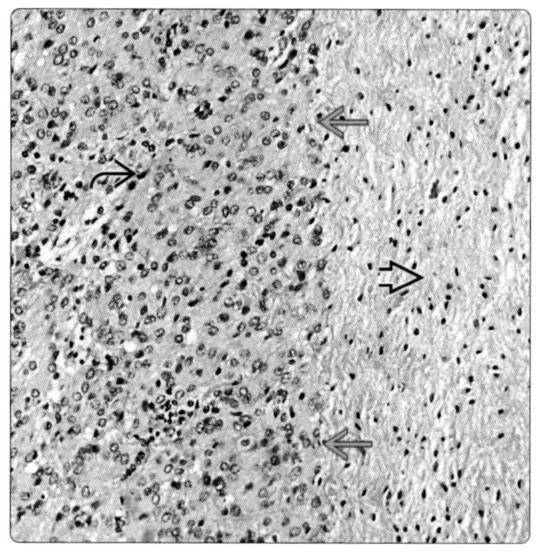

(Left) *Normal pineal gland is sharply divided from adjacent glial tissue.* **(Right)** *Calcified bodies, corpora arenacea or "brain sand," are more likely in a normal pineal gland than pineocytomas. They may be present, however, in the normal gland that is often attached to other pineal region tumors.*

Normal Pineal Gland, Sharp Divide

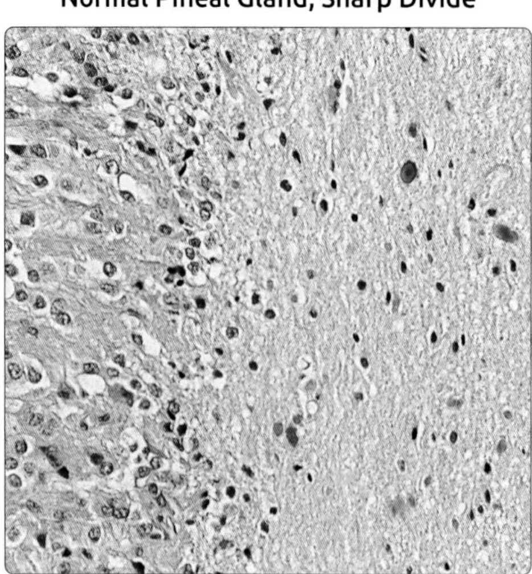

Corpora Arenacea

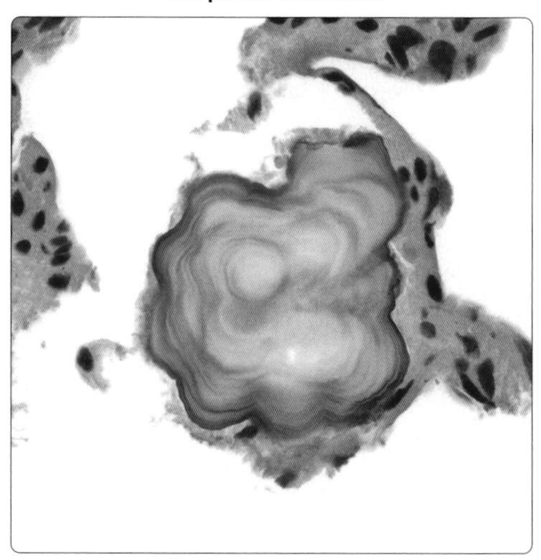

Pineal Cyst, Rosenthal Fibers

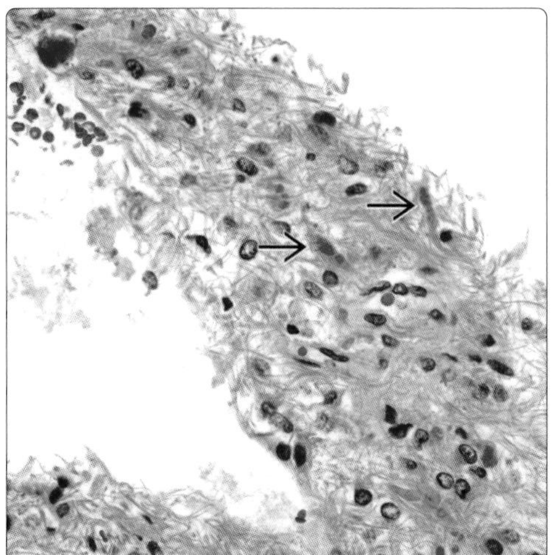

Smear, Normal Pinealocytes, Normal Gland

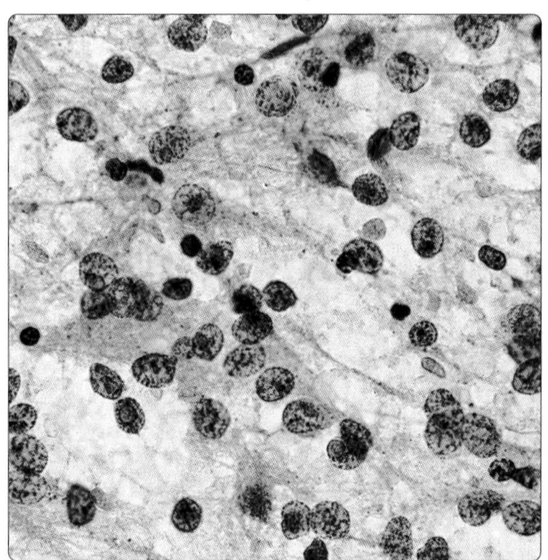

(Left) *Pineal cysts often show numerous Rosenthal fibers* → *in the gliotic cyst wall and this may lead to mistaken diagnosis of pilocytic astrocytoma.* **(Right)** *The character of the nuclei and fibrillar background misrepresent the lesion as a neoplasm, such as astrocytoma or neuronal tumor. The uniform, round-to-oval nuclei with nucleoli are, however, typical of normal pinealocytes. Familiarity with clinical history and radiological findings are important in entertaining the possibility of pineal cyst.*

Synaptophysin, Normal Pineal Gland

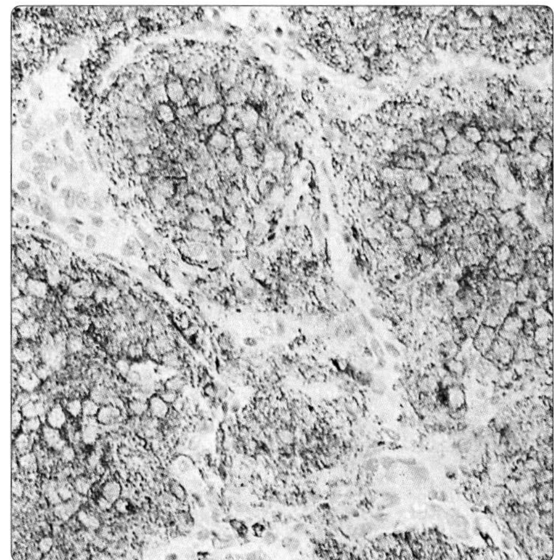

Normal Pineal Gland, Synaptophysin, Lobularity

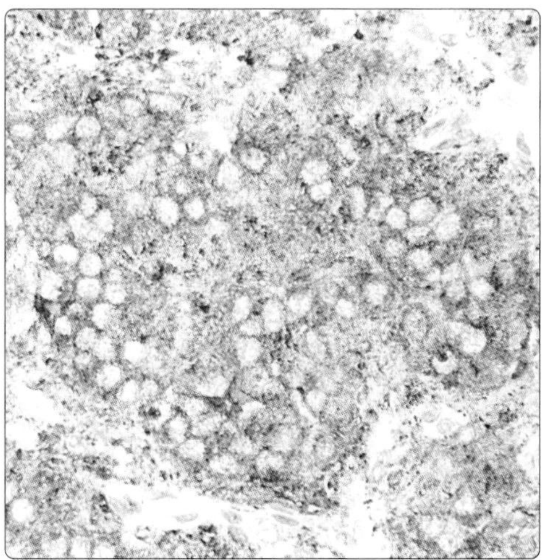

(Left) *Synaptophysin staining emphasizes the lobular architecture of the normal gland. Pineocytomas are more sheet-like.* **(Right)** *Intense, finely granular staining is typical for the normal pineal gland and is not in itself evidence of a neuronal neoplasm. Note the lobular architecture of the normal gland highlighted by the immunostaining.*

Normal Gland, Rare Cell Cycling

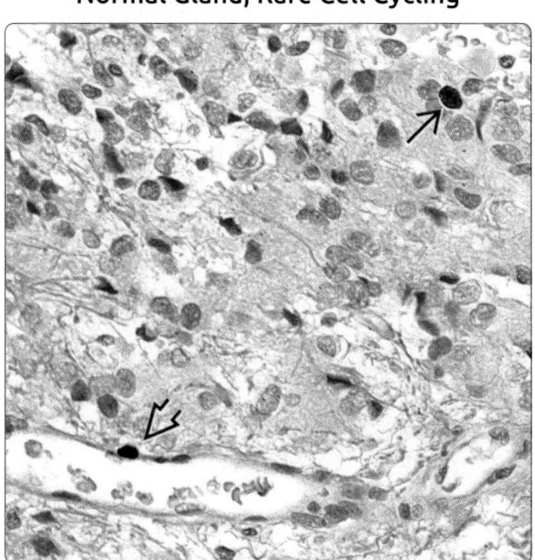

Normal Pineal Gland, GFAP(+) Cells Within Lobules

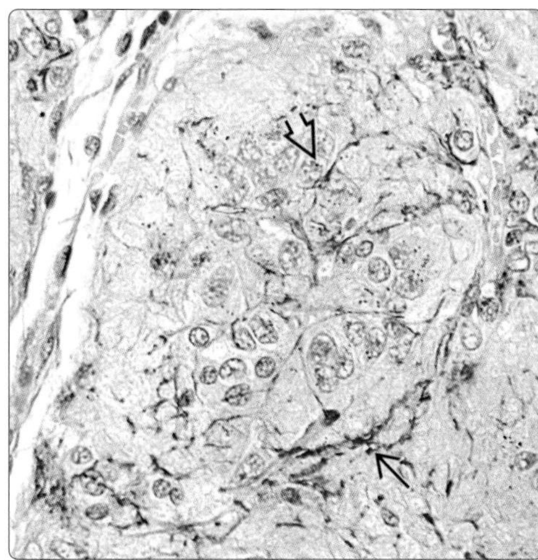

(Left) *Only a rare parenchymal cell* → *is immunoreactive for Ki-67. More often, only endothelial cells* ⇨ *are positive.* **(Right)** *GFAP(+) cells between* → *and within* ⇨ *the lobules help identify normality. Lobules of neurons with such fine intercalated glial processes would be unusual in a glioneuronal tumor.*

Facet Joint Synovial Cyst

KEY FACTS

TERMINOLOGY

- Synonyms: Synovial cyst, synovial excrescence

ETIOLOGY/PATHOGENESIS

- Degeneration of facet joint leads to fluid escape from joint capsule, which remains within synovium, creating sac-like protrusion

CLINICAL ISSUES

- Older adults
- Lower spine, L4-S5 in almost all cases
- In communication with facet joint
- Leg pain
- Myelopathy in some cases
- Excision is curative

IMAGING

- Discrete, 1-2 cm smooth walled

MACROSCOPIC

- Intraspinal, extradural
- In continuity with facet joint

MICROSCOPIC

- Lumen lined by synovial epithelium but inconstant and not always present in small fragments of tissue

TOP DIFFERENTIAL DIAGNOSES

- Extruded intervertebral disc
- Schwannoma, cystic
- Perineural (Tarlov) cyst

DIAGNOSTIC CHECKLIST

- Epithelium may be inconspicuous or absent
- Calcium pyrophosphate in some cases
  - Does not imply systemic calcium disorder

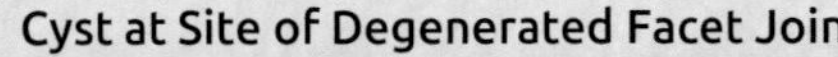

Cyst at Site of Degenerated Facet Joint

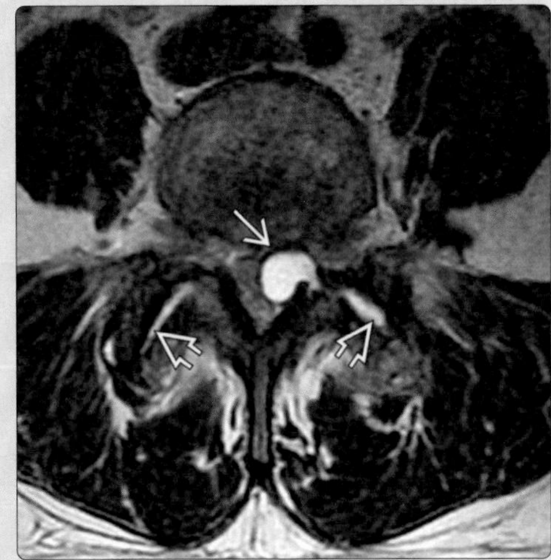

Fluid Escape From Joint Capsule

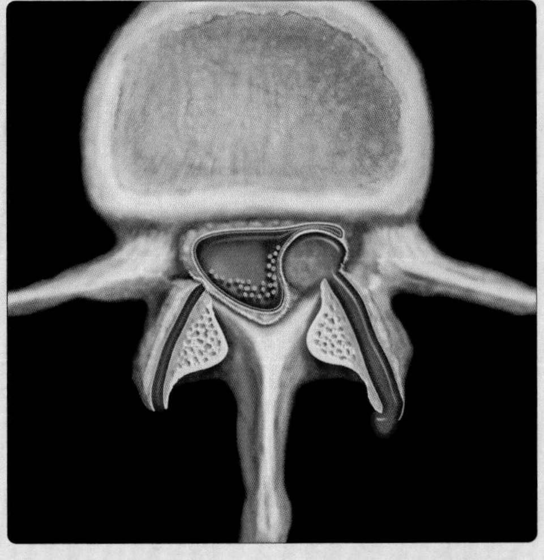

(Left) *Axial T2WI demonstrates a classic synovial cyst ➡ extending anteromedially from the degenerated left facet joint. Note the fluid in both facet joints ⇨.* **(Right)** *Degeneration of the facet joint leads to fluid escape from the joint capsule, which remains within the synovium, creating a sac-like protrusion.*

Granulation Tissue

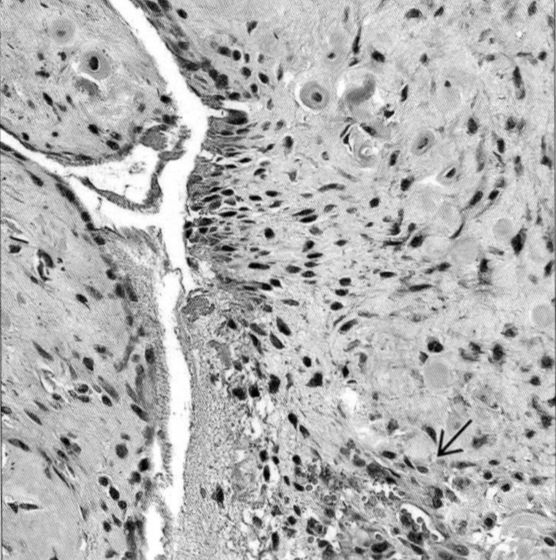

Only Focal Epithelium

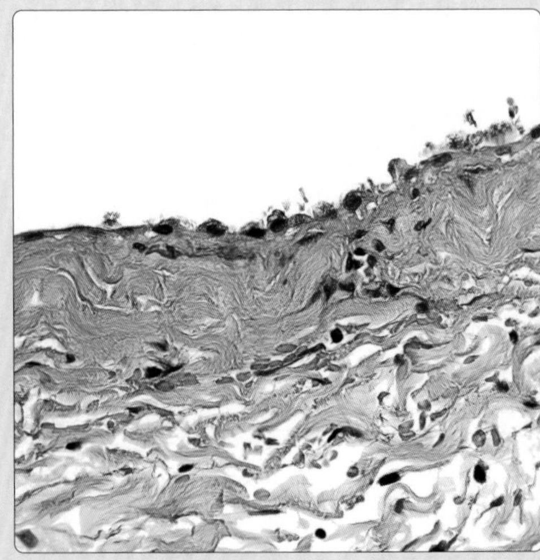

(Left) *Reactive changes, such as granulation tissue →, may be present around the cyst. The cyst lining is relatively prominent in this area.* **(Right)** *A careful search is sometimes necessary to find the epithelium.*

TERMINOLOGY

Definitions

- Synovial cyst formed from degenerative facet joint

CLINICAL ISSUES

Epidemiology

- Age
  - Older adults, 60 years or more

Site

- Spine
  - Lower spine, especially L4-S5 (almost all cases)
  - Cervical (occasional)
  - In communication with facet joint
  - Dorsolateral to thecal sac

Presentation

- Pain
  - Leg &/or back
  - Often radiating
- Myelopathy in some cases

Treatment

- Surgical approaches
  - Excision, curative

Prognosis

- Excellent

Associated Local Conditions

- Spondylolisthesis
- Hypermobility
- Tumoral calcinosis (calcium pyrophosphate) in some cases

IMAGING

MR Findings

- Discrete, 1-2 cm, smooth walled
- T1WI
  - Hypointense similar to cerebrospinal fluid
  - Hyperintense with hemorrhagic or proteinaceous contents
- T2WI
  - Hyperintense if in communication with facet joint
- T1WI C+
  - Enhancing wall

CT Findings

- Degenerative disc disease
- Arthritic changes with hypertrophy of facet joints
- Spondylolisthesis

MACROSCOPIC

General Features

- Intraspinal, extradural
- In continuity with facet joint
- Fibrous wall
- Smooth lining
- Fluid contents
  - Viscid or mucoid
  - Clear or yellow
  - Sometimes evidence of hemorrhage

MICROSCOPIC

Histologic Features

- Lumen lined by synovial epithelium but inconstant and not always present
- Surrounding reactive changes
- Associated calcium pyrophosphate deposition in some cases

DIFFERENTIAL DIAGNOSIS

Extruded Intervertebral Disc

- Fragments of fibrocartilage only
- No synovial epithelium
- No contact with facet joint

Tumoral Calcinosis

- Calcific debris
- Vague granulomatous response

Perineural (Tarlov) Cyst

- Associated with nerve root
- Thin wall
- No synovial epithelium

Schwannoma

- Associated with sensory nerve root
- Antoni A and B tissue
- SOX10 nuclear (+)
- S100(+)

DIAGNOSTIC CHECKLIST

Pathologic Interpretation Pearls

- Epithelium may be inconspicuous or absent

SELECTED REFERENCES

1. Scholz C et al: Incomplete resection of lumbar synovial cysts - Evaluating the risk of recurrence. Clin Neurol Neurosurg. 136:29-32, 2015
2. Lyons MK et al: Subaxial cervical synovial cysts: report of 35 histologically confirmed surgically treated cases and review of the literature. Spine (Phila Pa 1976). 36(20):E1285-9, 2011
3. Harries A et al: Synovial cyst presenting as a C1/2 tumour. Br J Neurosurg. 24(5):595-6, 2010
4. Arantes M et al: Spontaneous hemorrhage in a lumbar ganglion cyst. Spine (Phila Pa 1976). 33(15):E521-4, 2008
5. Sandhu FA et al: Minimally invasive surgical treatment of lumbar synovial cysts. Neurosurgery. 54(1):107-11; discussion 111-2, 2004
6. Sze CI et al: Synovial excrescences and cysts of the spine: clinicopathological features and contributions to spinal stenosis. Clin Neuropathol. 23(2):80-90, 2004
7. Gadgil AA et al: Bilateral symptomatic synovial cysts of the lumbar spine caused by calcium pyrophosphate deposition disease: a case report. Spine (Phila Pa 1976). 27(19):E428-31, 2002
8. Durant DM et al: Tumoral calcinosis of the spine: a study of 21 cases. Spine (Phila Pa 1976). 26(15):1673-9, 2001
9. Radatz M et al: Synovial cysts of the lumbar spine: a review. Br J Neurosurg. 11(6):520-4, 1997
10. Yarde WL et al: Synovial cysts of the lumbar spine: diagnosis, surgical management, and pathogenesis. Report of eight cases. Surg Neurol. 43(5):459-64; discussion 465, 1995
11. Gorey MT et al: Lumbar synovial cysts eroding bone. AJNR Am J Neuroradiol. 13(1):161-3, 1992
12. Sachdev VP et al: Synovial cysts of the lumbar facet joint. Mt Sinai J Med. 58(2):125-8, 1991

PART II
SECTION 2

Infectious, Inflammatory, and Reactive Lesions

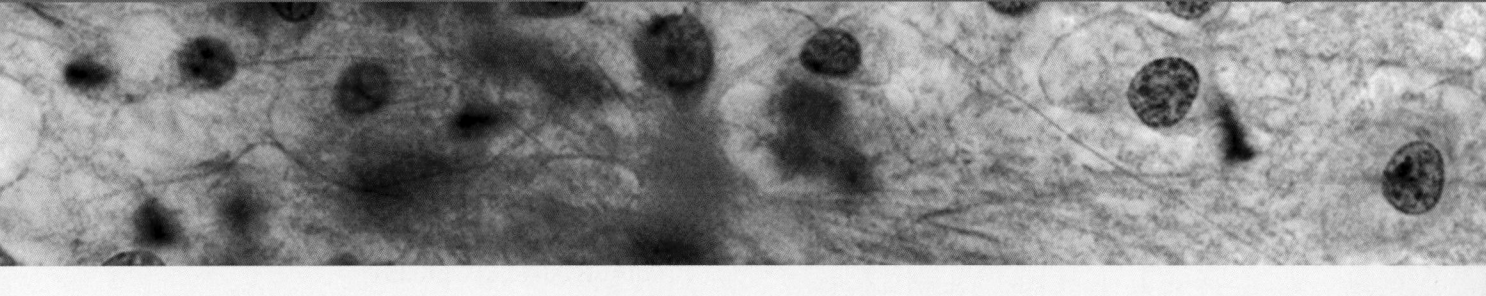

Demyelinating Diseases

Bacterial Infections

Viral Infections

Fungal Infections

Protozoal and Parasitic Infections

Other Inflammatory Diseases

Reactive Conditions and Noninflammatory Pseudoneoplasms

Demyelinating Disease (Multiple Sclerosis-Tumefactive Demyelination)

KEY FACTS

TERMINOLOGY

- Acute demyelinating disease prompting biopsy due to enhancement, prominent surrounding edema, and tumor or abscess-like appearance
- Most patients with demyelinating disease prompting biopsy eventually develop relapsing-remitting multiple sclerosis (MS)
- Disease course in most patients, once MS diagnosis is made by clinical/neuroimaging criteria, similar to that of "ordinary" MS

IMAGING

- Open ring sign is characteristic MR enhancement feature
- Inconsistent with pathological diagnosis of grade II infiltrating gliomas

MICROSCOPIC

- Sharp border
- Numerous foamy macrophages
- Admixed reactive astrocytes with long processes
- Loss of myelin on special stains
- Relatively greater preservation of axons than myelin
- Variable perivascular lymphocytic cuffing

TOP DIFFERENTIAL DIAGNOSES

- Astrocytoma, oligodendroglioma
- Glioblastoma
- Lymphocytic vasculitis
- Infarct
- Acute disseminated encephalomyelitis
- Steroid-treated CNS lymphoma

DIAGNOSTIC CHECKLIST

- May closely resemble astrocytoma or oligodendroglioma in H&E sections
- Recognition of macrophages on touch and smear preparations during intraoperative consultation aids in diagnosis

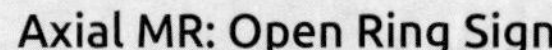

Axial MR: Open Ring Sign

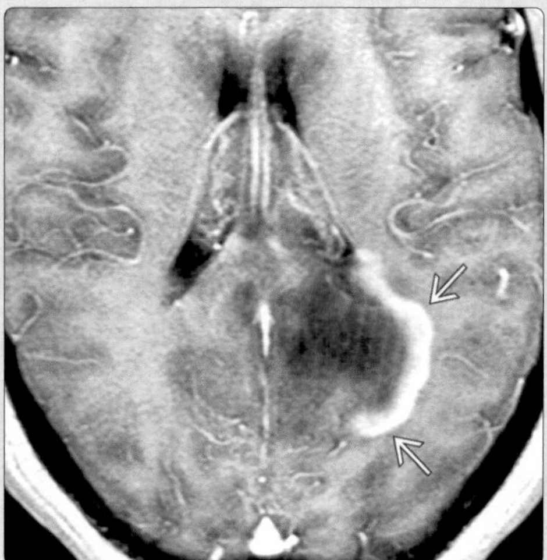

Hypercellularity, Demyelinating Disease

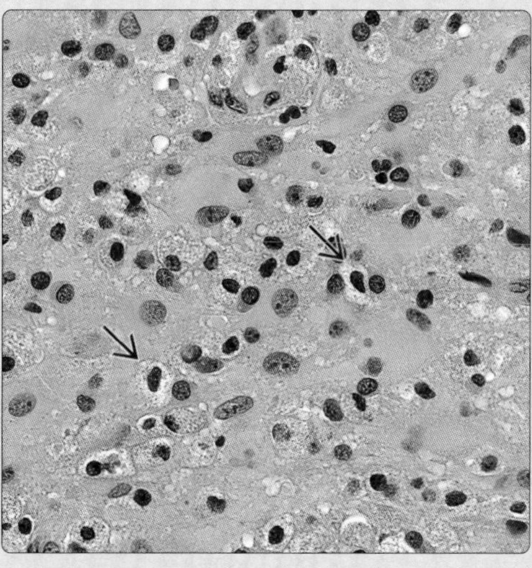

(Left) *The enhancing rim of demyelinating plaques ➔ is typically "open" rather than closed and complete as seen in abscesses and malignant gliomas. This is sometimes referred to as the open ring sign. (Courtesy M. Mirfakhree, MD.)* **(Right)** *A high index of suspicion helps identify foamy macrophages ⇨ in a lesion that otherwise closely resembles an infiltrating glioma.*

Smear, Demyelinating Lesion Macrophages

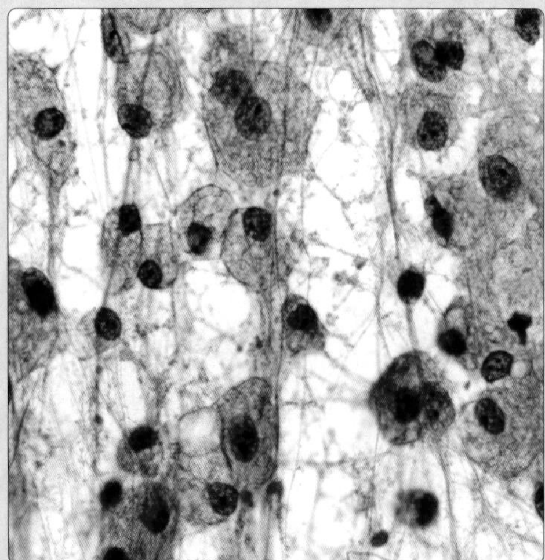

MS With Brain Atrophy at Autopsy

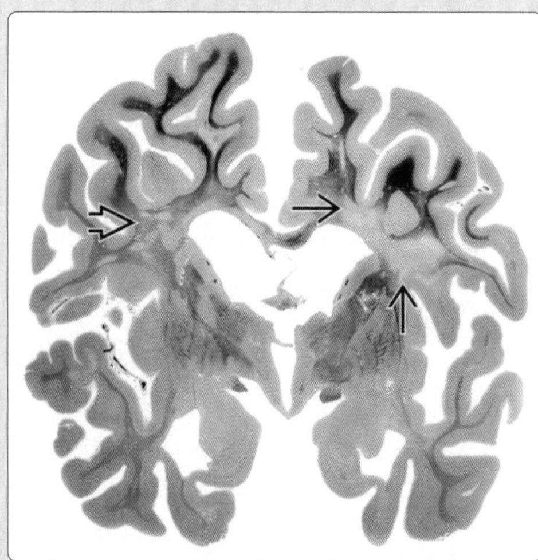

(Left) *Identification of numerous foamy macrophages on smear preparation at the time of intraoperative consultation should prompt 1st consideration of acute demyelinative lesion or infarct, not tumor.* **(Right)** *Biopsies represent early phases of MS, unlike autopsies. Whole mount autopsy brain section from an MS patient demonstrates multifocal loss of "robin's egg blue" myelin in periventricular sites ⇨ and as ovoid plaques in deeper white matter ⇨. There is severe brain atrophy in the late stages of the disease, as seen here.*

TERMINOLOGY

Abbreviations

- Multiple sclerosis (MS)

Definitions

- Large, usually solitary, lesion > 2 cm in size or lesion with significant mass effect, edema, or ring enhancement
  - May be mistaken on neuroimaging studies for tumor or abscess
- Most patients with acute demyelinating disease prompting biopsy eventually develop relapsing-remitting MS (Pittock et al)
  - Clinical course of MS in most patients with tumefactive-like lesions similar to that of "ordinary" MS patients, i.e., not more severe or monophasic

CLINICAL ISSUES

Epidemiology

- Age
  - Median age at onset: 30-40 years
- Sex
  - Slightly more common in females

Presentation

- Patients polysymptomatic
  - Motor, cognitive, sensory symptoms
- Symptom onset-biopsy interval usually about 2 months
  - Clinical expressions prompting biopsy initial neurological events in majority of cases
- Prior history of relapsing remitting MS (in some cases)
- History of progressive disease (rare)

Treatment

- Surgical approaches
  - Stereotactic biopsy (most cases)
  - Open biopsy
    - Aggressive resection potentially associated with new or increased neurological deficit
- Adjuvant therapy
  - Plasma exchange (PLEX)
    - Ring-enhancing lesions &/or mass effect associated with beneficial response to PLEX

Prognosis

- Good, but variable
- Does not portend aggressive subsequent downhill clinical course
- Median time to 2nd attack of demyelination ~ 5 years
- Large lesions (> 5 cm) associated with slightly more clinical dysfunction

IMAGING

MR Findings

- Large, confluent lesion(s), often periventricular or subcortical
- Contrast enhancement
  - Common in acute phase
  - "Open ring" or horseshoe-shaped configuration highly suggestive
  - Inconsistent with pathological diagnosis of grade II infiltrating gliomas
- Perilesional edema
  - Variable, but may be prominent with larger lesions
- Multiple lesions on prebiopsy scan in ~ 70%
- Rare variant, Balo sclerosis, shows concentric globe appearance with alternating bands of myelin loss and preservation

MACROSCOPIC

General Features

- Acute plaques with somewhat ill-defined margins, tan-yellow, granular
- Chronic inactive plaques usually have sharply defined margins, gray, glistening, depressed
- Often periventricular, gray-white junction, or deep white matter
  - Perivenular orientation at angles of lateral ventricles, with extension along veins: "Dawson fingers"
- Balo sclerosis not easily detected on gross tissue examination
  - Diagnosis requires correlation with MR imaging

MICROSCOPIC

Histologic Features

- Borders
  - Usually discrete in chronic inactive plaques
  - Somewhat more irregular, but still microscopically well defined, in acute/active plaques
- Perivenular orientation
  - More obvious in autopsy specimens
- Macrophages
  - Principal component
  - Frequent perivascular concentration
  - Contents
    - Foamy to granular
    - Luxol fast blue (LFB) (+), acute
    - Periodic acid-Schiff (+), subacute to chronic
- Reactive astrocytes
  - Evenly dispersed
  - Long tapering cytoplasmic processes
  - Large nuclei, prominent nucleoli, and vesicular nuclei when highly reactive
  - Multinucleate (Creutzfeldt cell)
    - Common but not specific
- Loss of myelin
  - LFB/H&E, LFB/PAS
- Axonal loss
  - Axonal swellings in acute examples
  - Proportionally less than that of myelin
- Perivascular inflammation
  - Variable, not always present
  - T cells predominate
- Little if any cavitation
- Mitoses
  - Granular
    - Exploding pattern of chromosomes in cells with copious cytoplasm
    - Presumed precursor of Creutzfeldt cell

- Conventional
  - Occasional

ANCILLARY TESTS

Cytology

- Macrophages
  - Sharp cell borders
  - Foamy or granular cytoplasm
  - Cytologically bland
- Reactive astrocytes
  - Conventional, can simulate astrocytoma
  - Multinucleated (Creutzfeldt cell)
- Granular mitoses

Histochemistry

- Modified Bielschowsky, Bodian stains
  - Reactivity: Axons
  - Staining Pattern: Preservation relative to myelin loss

Immunohistochemistry

- GFAP
  - Reactive astrocytes strongly (+)
- Macrophage markers
  - HAM56
    - Specific macrophage marker
    - Qualitatively and quantitatively less staining than with CD68
  - CD68
    - Lysosomal, rather than specific macrophage, marker
    - All phagocytes (+)
- Axonal markers
  - Neurofilament protein, especially phosphorylated, e.g., SMI-31
    - Axons generally preserved
    - Some reduction and fragmentation but less than in infarcts
- Antibodies directed against myelin basic protein (MBP), proteolipid protein (PLP)
- Aquaporin-4 IHC recently recognized as method to identify acute demyelinative lesions related to neuromyelitis optica (NMO)/NMO spectrum disorder
  - Should be followed up with subsequent AQP4-IgG testing to confirm NMO/NMO spectrum disorder

DIFFERENTIAL DIAGNOSIS

Astrocytoma, Oligodendroglioma

- Few if any macrophages
- Cytoplasm of neoplastic oligodendrocytes artifactually clear, not foamy or granular
- Little if any perivascular inflammation, except for gemistocytic astrocytomas
- IDH-1 and Olig2(+), almost all cases

Glioblastoma

- More variable nuclear size, shape, and hyperchromatism
- Often more variable cell distribution, greater cellularity
- Pseudopalisading necrosis
- Microvascular proliferation
- Macrophages and microglia, but not in large numbers or sheets
- EGFR, EGFRVIII(+), in some cases
- IDH-1(+), in secondary glioblastoma (GBM), small subset of all GBMs

Lymphocytic Vasculitis

- Transmural, not perivascular, lymphocytes
- Vessel wall distortion, destruction
- Associated infarction in some cases
- Angiographic features of vasculitis in some cases

Infarct

- Loss of axons and myelin in near equal proportions
- Cavitation in subacute and chronic phases
- Lesions in vessel distribution
- Little if any perivascular chronic inflammation

Acute Disseminated Encephalomyelitis

- Perivenous, rather than confluent, demyelination
- Microglial activation and aggregation without cortical demyelination
- Depressed level of consciousness, headache, meningismus, cerebrospinal fluid pleocytosis, or multifocal enhancing magnetic resonance imaging abnormalities more common

Steroid-Treated Central Nervous System Lymphoma

- Sheets of macrophages, reactive astrocytes, variable numbers of nonneoplastic lymphocytes
  - Residual lymphocytes often nonneoplastic CD3(+) T cells
  - Greater disruption of background neuropil, "empty bed"
- Apoptosis, acutely prominent post steroids

Neuromyelitis Optica/Neuromyelitis Spectrum Disorder

- Can present as acute demyelinative lesion
- May have eosinophils in biopsy (rare in MS)
- AQP4 immunoreactivity lost
- AQP4-IgG serum test (+), unlike multiple sclerosis
- Myelin vacuolation, vascular hyalinization, macrophages containing GFAP(+) debris may be present

Balo Sclerosis

- Considered rare variant of MS, not fully separate disorder
- May present acutely, prompting biopsy
- Diagnosis requires correlation with MR imaging of "concentric globe" appearance
- Requires histochemistry for LFB/PAS or IHC for MBP, PLP to detect concentric myelin loss and preservation

DIAGNOSTIC CHECKLIST

Pathologic Interpretation Pearls

- May closely resemble astrocytoma or oligodendroglioma in H&E sections due to hypercellularity
- Recognition of macrophages on touch and smear preparations during intraoperative consultation aids in diagnosis
- Absence of inflammation does not negate diagnosis
- Periventricular, perivenular location typical

SELECTED REFERENCES

1. Lucchinetti CF et al: The pathology of an autoimmune astrocytopathy: lessons learned from neuromyelitis optica. Brain Pathol. 24(1):83-97, 2014

Plaque Components

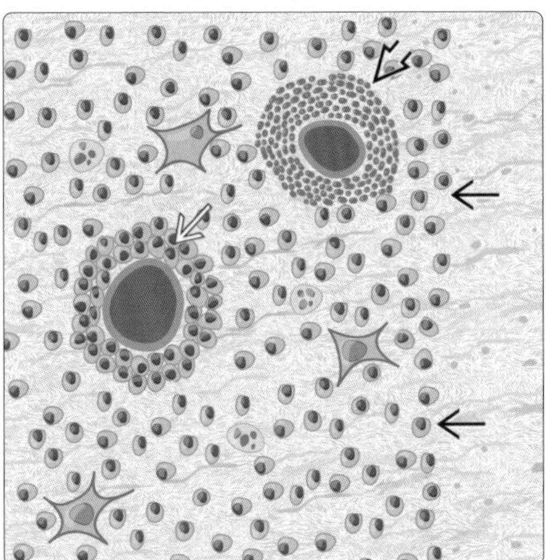

Sharp Demarcation, Demyelinative Plaque

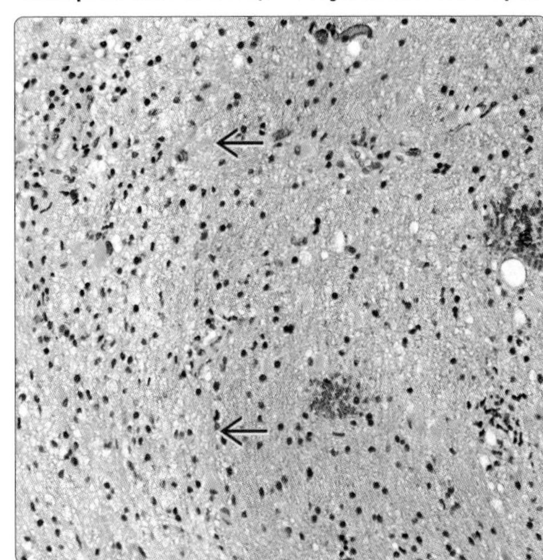

(Left) *In H&E sections, demyelinating plaques typically have (1) sharp borders ➡, (2) macrophages, both interstitial & perivascular ➡, & (3) perivascular chronic inflammation ➡. Scattered large stellate reactive astrocytes complete the picture.* **(Right)** *Even a subtle sharp border ➡ between the pale lesion on the left and the darker normal white matter on the right is highly suspicious for demyelinating disease. This interface is easy to overlook, however. Note the lesion's glioma-like hypercellularity.*

Sharp Interface, Plaque

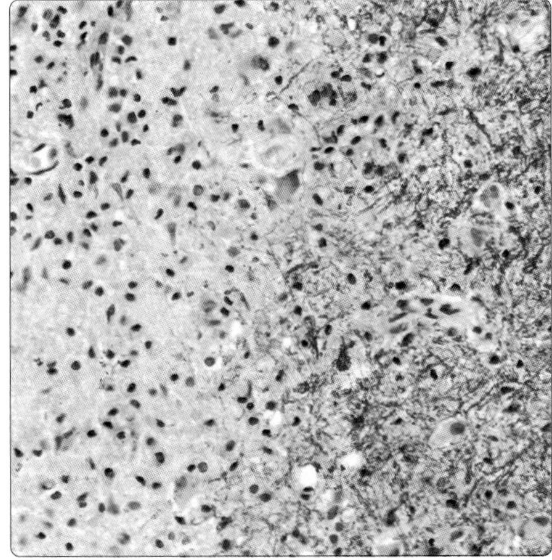

Myelin Basic Protein, Edge of Plaque

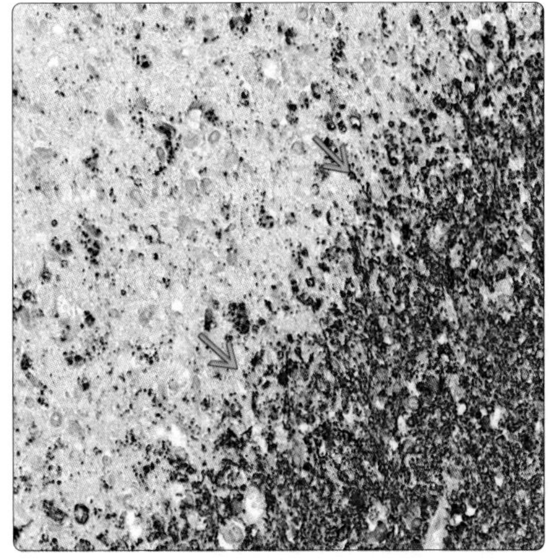

(Left) *H&E/Luxol fast blue stain emphasizes sharp interface between lesion and normal parenchyma, typical of most demyelinating plaques, unless they possess significant remyelination.* **(Right)** *Immunostains for myelin basic protein can be used to highlight the sharp border ➡ between areas of myelin loss and preservation. Staining for axons, either histo- or immunohistochemically, could then be employed to confirm the suspected relative preservation of axons.*

Macrophages, Edge of Chronic Active Plaque

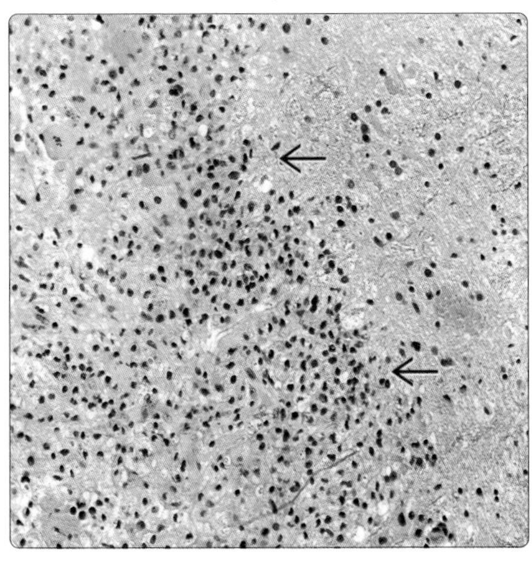

Macrophages, Chronic Active Plaque Edge

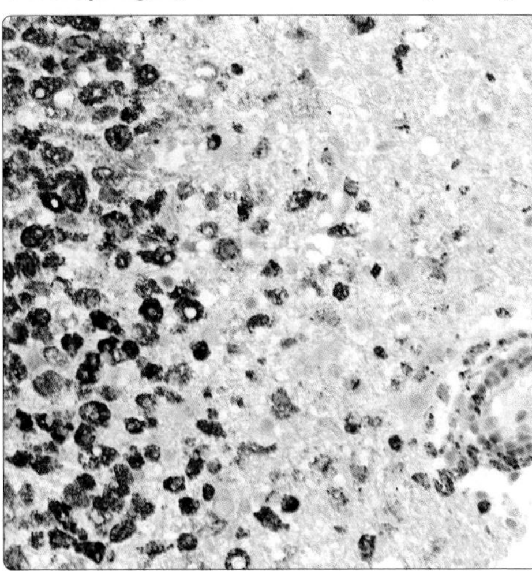

(Left) *Macrophages crowding along the edge of plaque ➡ emphasize the lesion's typically sharp border and are seen in chronic active (smoldering) lesions.* **(Right)** *CD68(+) macrophages stop abruptly at the margin of a demyelinated plaque. Staining of relatively preserved axons would establish the presence of demyelination.*

(Left) *Immunostaining for neurofilament protein shows axons ⇒ are relatively preserved in this lesion that was almost devoid of myelin. Macrophages sit in the background.* **(Right)** *Axonal preservation is often not complete, as evidenced by fragmentation and swelling in some cases.*

Axonal Preservation

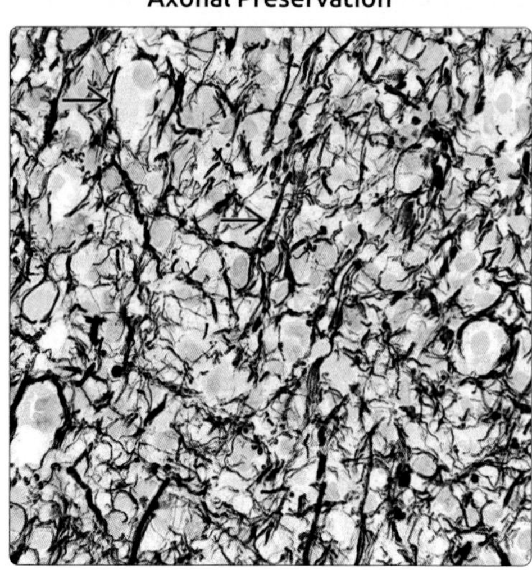

Axonal Preservation Incomplete

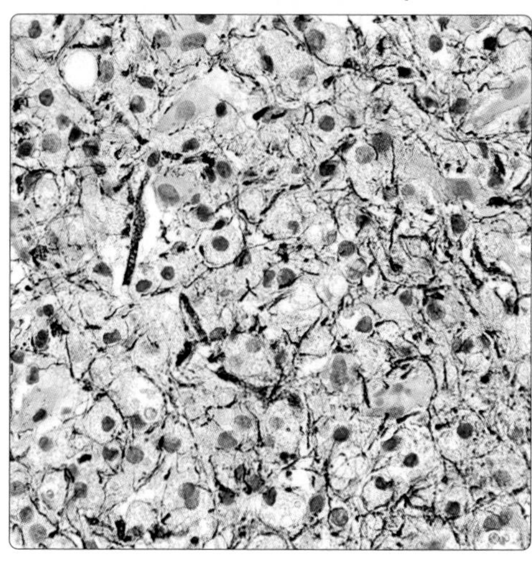

(Left) *Some biopsies of tumefactive demyelination have profuse perivascular lymphocytic cuffing that raises concern for vasculitis or even CNS lymphoma. Note the absence of vessel wall destruction ⇒ and small lymphocytes devoid of cytological atypia.* **(Right)** *While not specific, perivascular lymphocytes should suggest the possibility of demyelinating disease, even without obvious macrophages, as in this case. Note the eosinophils ⇒; these can suggest neuromyelitis optica (NMO).*

Perivascular Lymphocytic Cuffing

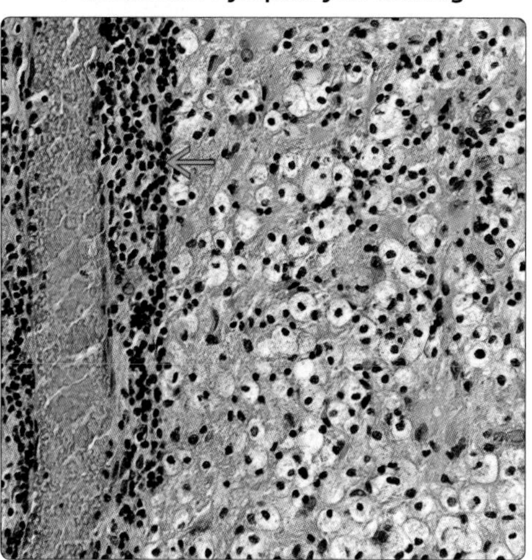

Rare Eosinophils: Rule Out Neuromyelitis Optica

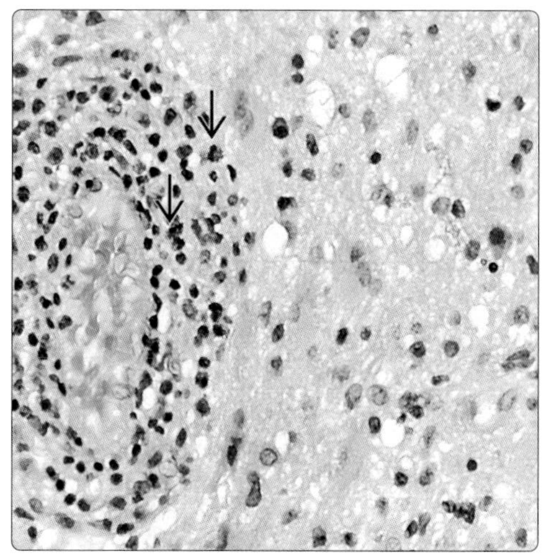

(Left) *The presence of macrophages may not come to mind, especially if clinical concerns are focused on the possibility of a glioma. Gemistocytes are evenly distributed, however, as is expected of a reactive, nonneoplastic process.* **(Right)** *Active demyelinating plaques may be mistaken for an infiltrating glioma, whether astrocytic, oligodendroglial, or mixed. When a single macrophage ⇒ is recognized, others rapidly become apparent.*

Gemistocytic Astrocytes, Demyelinative Plaque

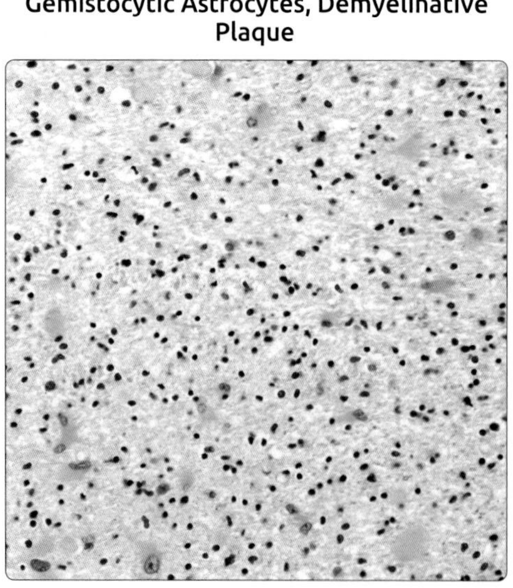

Hypercellular Plaque, Active

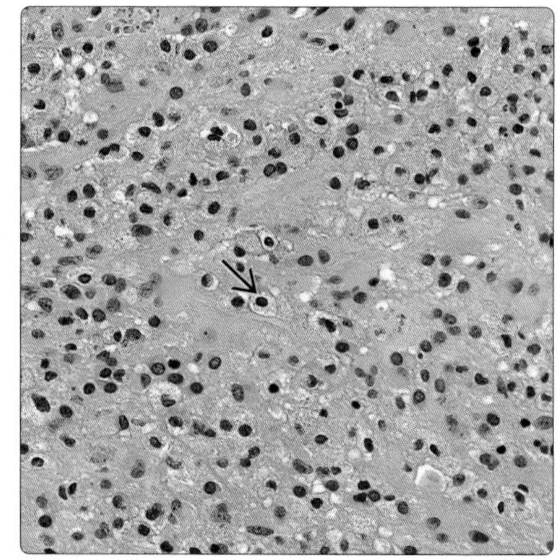

Nuclear Hyperchromatism, Astrocytes in Plaque

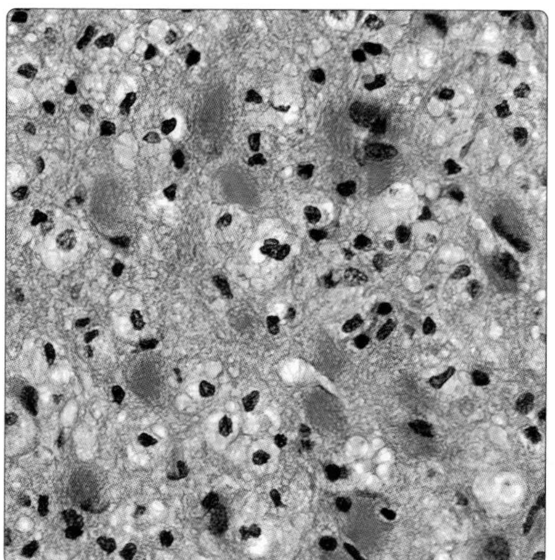

Macrophages Obscured by H&E Pallor

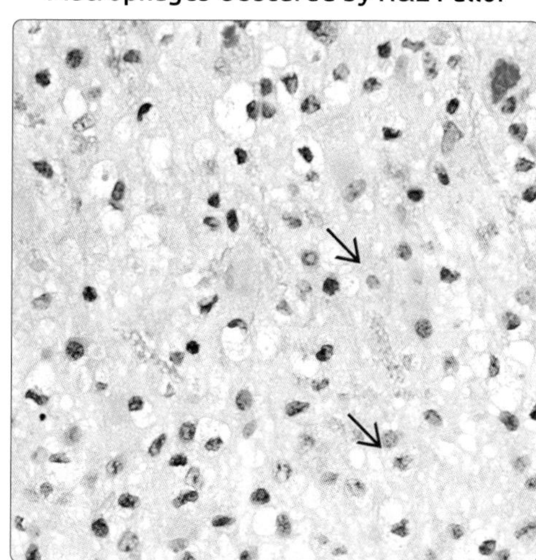

(Left) *A degree of nuclear hyperchromatism and pleomorphism, not uncommon in demyelinating disease, should not in itself be interpreted as evidence of neoplasia.* **(Right)** *Macrophages ⇒ can be overlooked easily in pale-stained sections. Other features of demyelination, such as a sharp border, may be present.*

Macrophages Simulating Oligodendrocytes

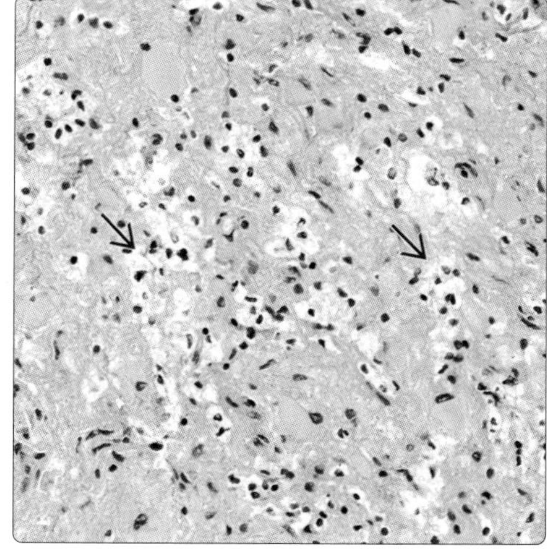

Macrophages Obscured, Core of Plaque

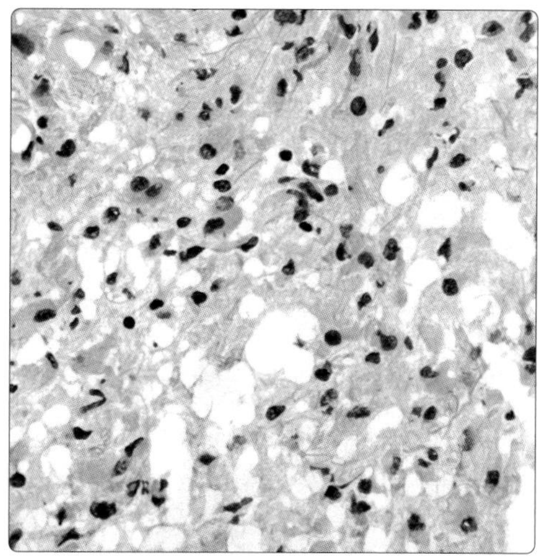

(Left) *Macrophages (here the clear cells ⇒) can be overlooked or interpreted as oligodendrocytes, leading to a misdiagnosis of glioma.* **(Right)** *The core of demyelinating disease plaques may have a nonspecific appearance in which macrophages are difficult to recognize, even if suspected. Positive staining with macrophage markers such as HAM56 or CD68, will resolve the issue.*

Granular Mitoses

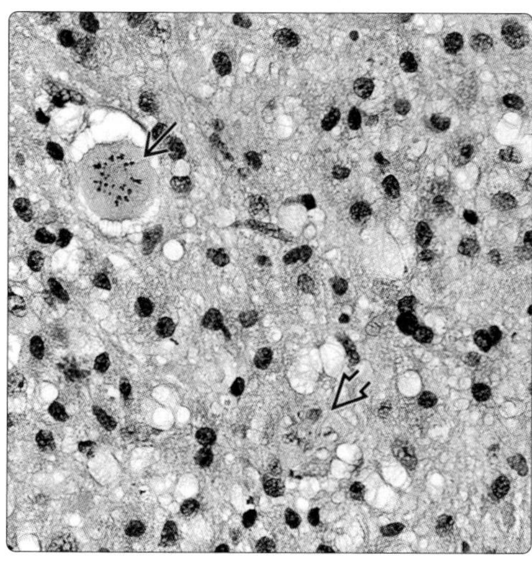

Frozen Section Obscuring Diagnosis

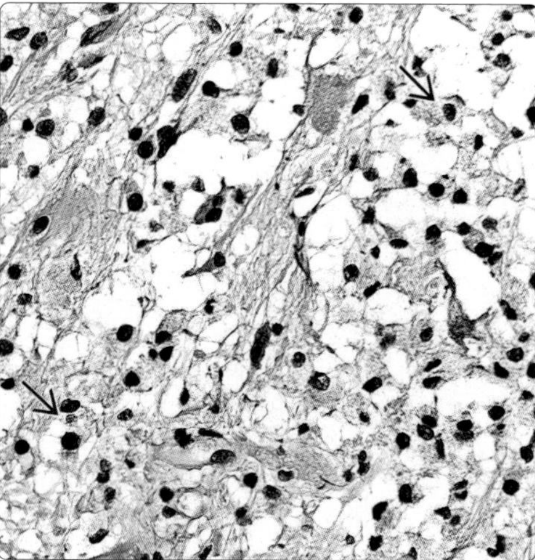

(Left) *In the context of a macrophage infiltrate, a reactive astrocyte with an exploding "granular mitosis" ⇒ and its sequel, a multinucleated Creutzfeldt cell ⇒, should generate strong suspicions of demyelinating disease.* **(Right)** *Since macrophages ⇒ may be difficult to recognize in frozen sections, use of concomitant smear preparations at the time of intraoperative frozen section is recommended.*

Perivascular Macrophages

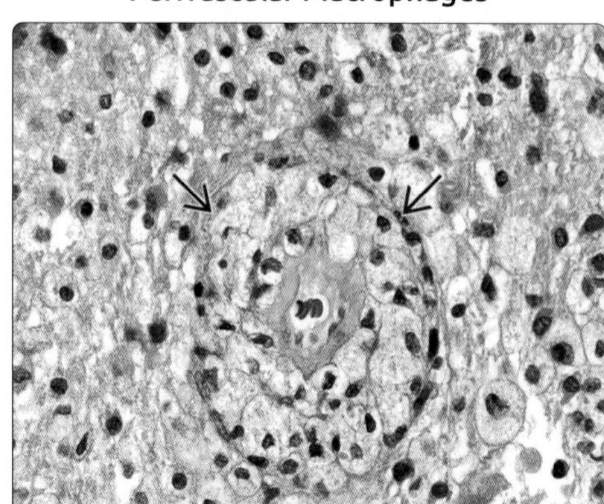

Macrophage Clusters

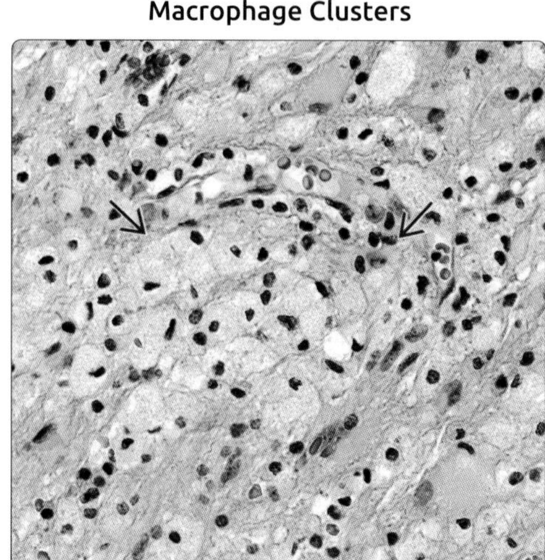

(Left) *A perivascular cuff of macrophages → is highly suspicious for demyelinating disease or infarct. Intraparenchymal phagocytes are present here as well.* **(Right)** *As tumefactive demyelination lesions evolve, macrophages → with their burden of phagocytized myelin debris migrate to vessels and may form clusters.*

Reactive Stellate Astrocytes

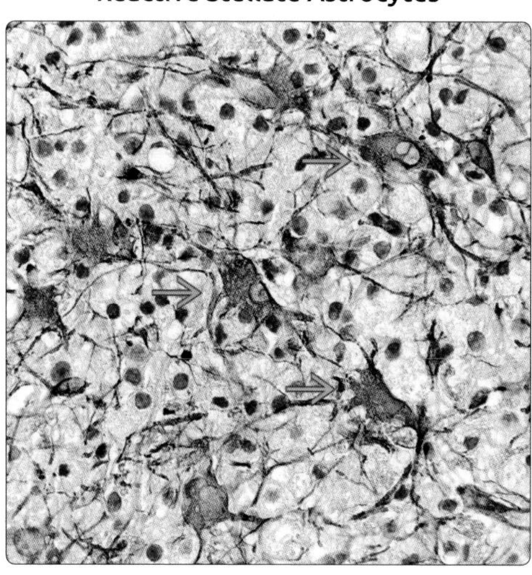

Smear, Macrophages

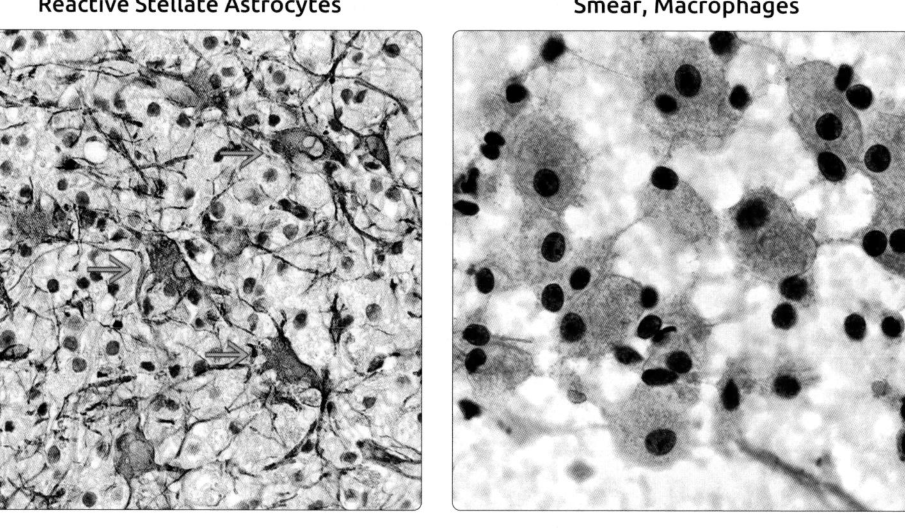

(Left) *Reactive astrocytes → with long thin tapering processes are highlighted by immunostaining for GFAP. Unlike tumoral astrocytes, these reactive forms are evenly spaced and often show features that match their neighboring astrocytes, including stellate cytoplasm. Macrophages fill the interstices.* **(Right)** *Macrophages in a rapidly fixed smear are easy to identify and distinguish from tumor cells. Characteristic features are roundness, sharp cell borders, bland nuclei, and variably granular or foamy contents.*

Smear, Granular Mitosis

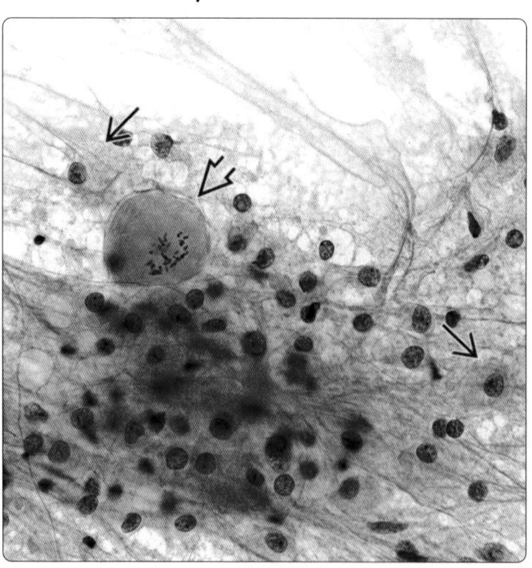

Smear, Large Reactive Astrocytes

(Left) *While not specific, granular mitoses → in astrocytes are particularly common in demyelinating disease, as seen here in a smear preparation. Such dispersed chromosomes condense to form the multinucleated Creutzfeldt cell. Macrophages → are more readily identified when spread apart.* **(Right)** *Exaggerated hypercellularity created by heaped up tissue fragments, when combined with large astrocytes →, may misrepresent demyelinating disease as glioma on a smear preparation.*

Smear, Vacuolated Macrophages

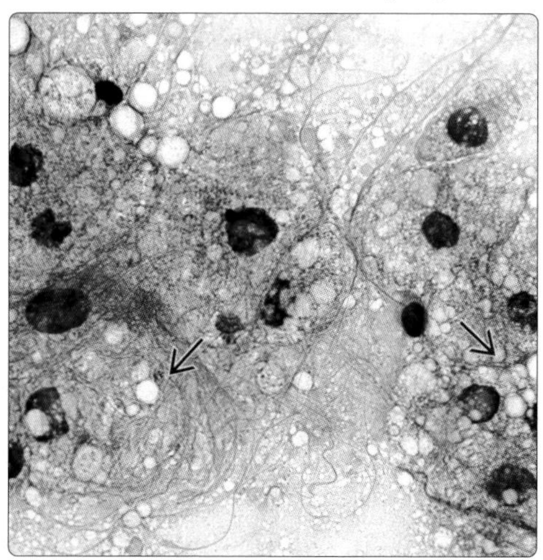

Smear, Dried, Suboptimal

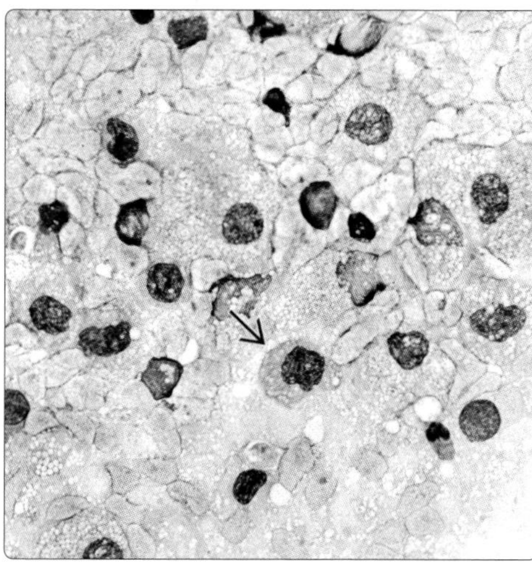

(Left) *Macrophages can be recognized in smear preparations in part by their vacuolation ➡. Large numbers of these cells are also common in evolving infarcts.* **(Right)** *Misinterpretation as a neoplasm is possible when drying in smears robs macrophages of their distinctive cytological features. The cells' typically sharp borders ➡ are retained here focally, however.*

Chronic Inactive Plaque, Persistent Scant Perivascular Inflammation

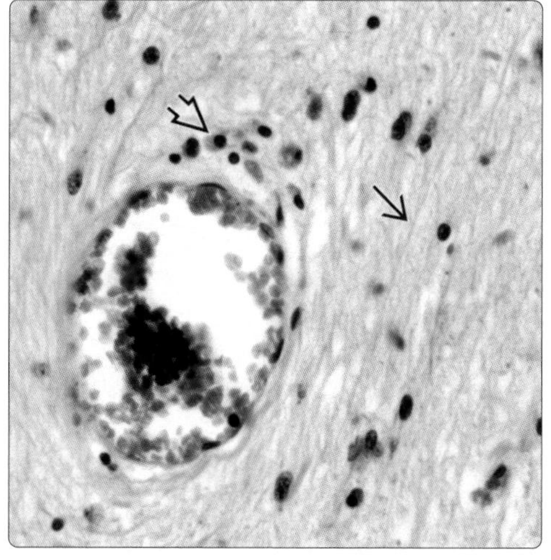

Multiple Sclerosis, Chronic Inactive, Preserved Axons

(Left) *A few perivascular lymphocytes and plasma cells ➡ linger around small blood vessels in chronic inactive plaques. Axons ➡ are preserved relative to myelin that, in this case, was totally lost.* **(Right)** *Although demyelinated axons are usually discernible in H&E sections, specific axonal stains, such as Bodian ➡ or immunohistochemistry for neurofilament protein, are required for diagnostic certainty.*

Plaque Edge, Myelin Sheaths

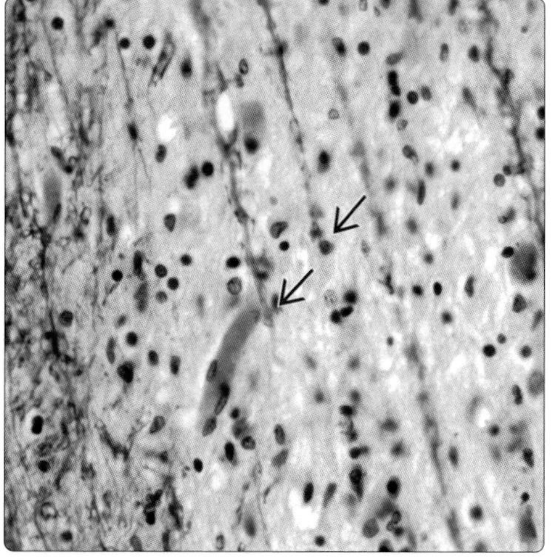

Multiple Sclerosis, Gray-White Junction Plaques

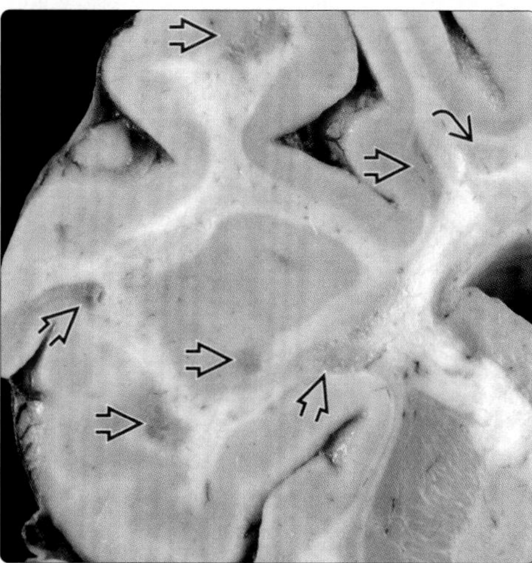

(Left) *As is characteristic, myelin sheaths may end abruptly ➡ near the edge of a plaque.* **(Right)** *Patients with tumefactive demyelination may later be diagnosed with MS or may have known MS at the time of biopsy. Gross brain from an MS patient shows a periventricular, gray-white junction ➡ and white matter plaques ➡.*

KEY FACTS

TERMINOLOGY

- Cerebritis: Ill-defined area of inflammation without capsule
- Brain abscess: Later stage of localized purulent infection with fibrous capsule

IMAGING

- Enhancing rim, often uniform but may be thinner on medial, deeper aspect
- Hypointense (dark) rim corresponding to fibrous tissue in capsule on T2WI MR
- Bright (restricted diffusion)

MICROSCOPIC

- Capsule is granulation tissue
- Fibroblasts, sometimes with mitoses, form granulation tissue, may suggest neoplasm
- Organisms found within necrotic areas, not capsule or surrounding gliotic brain
  - May be difficult to find

ANCILLARY TESTS

- Culture often necessary to document organism(s)
- Pyrosequencing new technique for subtyping organisms, including *Nocardia* species
- Uncommon *Nocardia* species increasingly identified as causes of brain abscess with newer techniques
- Culture negative in rare instances but diagnosis possible with molecular techniques

DIAGNOSTIC CHECKLIST

- Retarded capsule formation on deep aspect may enable formation of "daughter abscess"

Thin Rim Enhancement

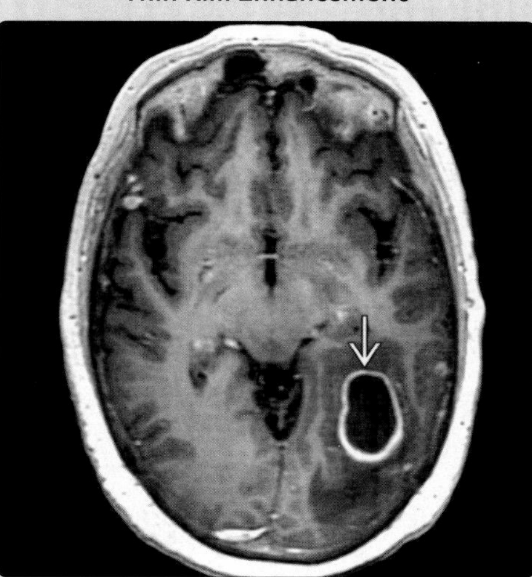

Dark Collagen-Rich Capsule on T2

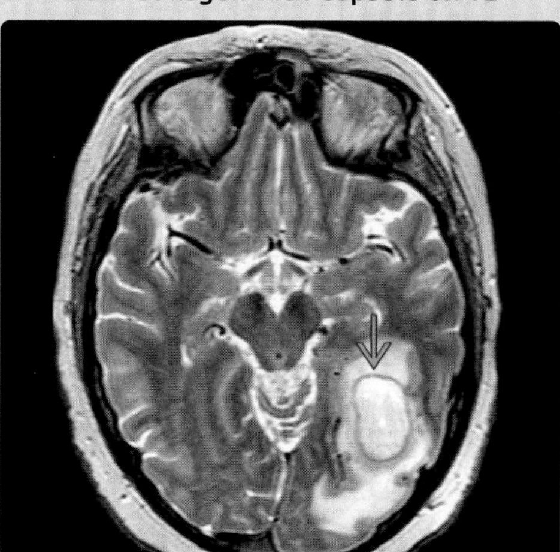

(Left) *The developed abscess has a complete rim of enhancing tissue ➡ surrounding a nonenhancing core. The rim lacks the irregular, shaggy profile of high-grade tumors such as glioblastoma.* **(Right)** *On T2WI MR, mature abscesses have hypointense, dark, collagen-rich capsules ⇨ that surround a hyperintense (white) core of purulent material. The bright signal of edema surrounds the lesion.*

Hyperemic Rim

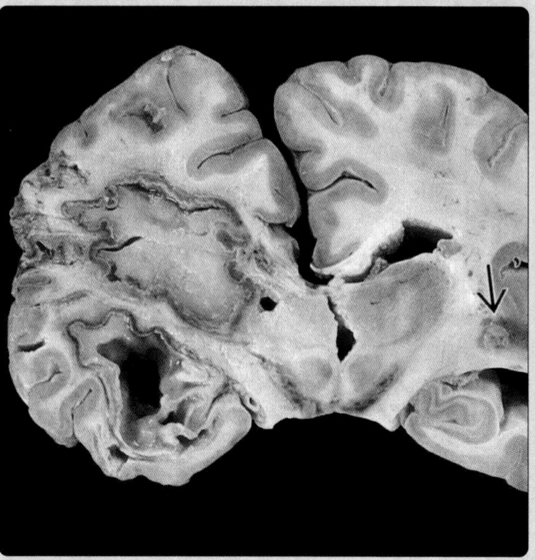

Gram-Positive Cocci

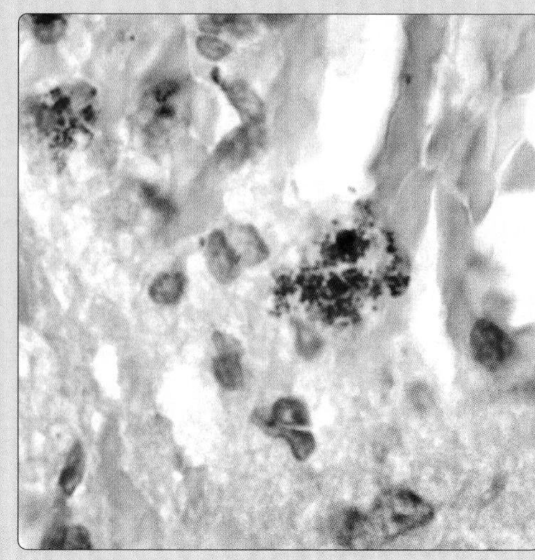

(Left) *Brain abscesses usually manifest hyperemic, reddish-colored, thin rims with centers containing yellow to white necrotic debris. Although, this may be less apparent in smaller examples ⇨.* **(Right)** *Brain abscesses are usually caused by bacteria, especially in immunocompetent hosts. Numerous gram-positive cocci are shown here.*

TERMINOLOGY

Definitions

- Focal pyogenic infection with (abscess) or without (cerebritis) well-formed surrounding fibrous capsule

ETIOLOGY/PATHOGENESIS

Infectious Agents

- Hematogenous dissemination of bacteria, usually from pulmonary source
- Direct extension from sinusitis, otitis, mastoiditis, recent dental work

CLINICAL ISSUES

Epidemiology

- Incidence
  - 1/100,000 in developed countries
  - *Nocardia* brain abscess relatively rare
    - More common in immunocompromised patients

Presentation

- Headache/vomiting
- Focal neurological deficits
- Confusion/disorientation
- Fever, some cases

Treatment

- Surgical drainage and culture
- Antibiotic choice dependent on organism(s)

Prognosis

- Mortality: < 10%
  - Considerably higher with *Nocardia* abscesses if not promptly diagnosed and treated (> 30%)

IMAGING

MR Findings

- T1WI with contrast
  - Enhancing rim, often uniform but may be thinner on deeper aspect
  - Unlike irregular, shaggy profile of high-grade gliomas
  - Dark, nonenhancing core
- T2WI: Hypointense (dark) rim corresponding to fibrous tissue in capsule
- Perilesional edema, usually pronounced, and mass effect
- Diffusion-weighted imaging
  - Bright (restricted diffusion)
  - Dark on ADC map

MACROSCOPIC

General Features

- Liquified, greenish, purulent center
- Capsule
  - Hyperemic
  - Firm and gray when mature
  - Thinner on deep aspect near ventricle
- Cerebritis hyperemic, more poorly defined than abscess

MICROSCOPIC

Histologic Features

- Central necrosis
- Central neutrophils and neutrophilic debris
- Fibrous capsule formed by reticulin fibers and collagen
- Source of collagen is fibroblasts in leptomeninges and blood vessels
- Thickness of capsule often greatest near leptomeninges or cortex
- Mitoses and high Ki-67 index in evolving capsule
- Lymphoplasmacytic infiltrate
- Macrophages, may be prominent
- Organisms
  - Within necrotic areas, not capsule or surrounding gliotic brain
  - Bacteria usually not visible on H&E except filamentous bacteria or clusters of gram-positive cocci
  - Identification of most bacteria requires Gram stain, sometimes still difficult to find
  - Filamentous bacteria also seen with Fite and Grocott methenamine silver stains
- Edema and gliosis in surrounding brain

Cytologic Features

- Inflammatory cells
- Plump fibroblasts, sometimes with mitoses, from granulation tissue; may suggest neoplasm

DIFFERENTIAL DIAGNOSIS

Necrotic Primary Brain Tumor

- Highly necrotic glioblastoma
  - Neoplastic cells
    - Presence may be difficult to identify histologically
    - IDH-1(+) in secondary glioblastoma
  - No collagenous capsule
- Highly necrotic glioblastoma with mesenchymal differentiation ("gliosarcoma")
  - GFAP(+) tumor
  - More atypia, more mitoses in mesenchymal tissue than in abscess capsule

Metastatic Tumor

- Tumor cells
- Little acute inflammation

DIAGNOSTIC CHECKLIST

Clinically Relevant Pathologic Features

- Retarded capsule formation on deep aspect

Pathologic Interpretation Pearls

- Highly necrotic glioblastomas with acute necrosis may mimic cerebritis, especially on frozen sections

SELECTED REFERENCES

1. Bonfield CM et al: Pediatric intracranial abscesses. J Infect. 71 Suppl 1:S42-6, 2015
2. Moazzam AA et al: Intracranial bacterial infections of oral origin. J Clin Neurosci. 22(5):800-6, 2015
3. Lin YJ et al: Nocardial brain abscess. J Clin Neurosci. 17(2):250-3, 2010

(Left) *Cerebritis is focal but note the well-delimited purulent inflammation with surrounding hyperemia.* **(Right)** *The central region in cerebritis contains purulent, necrotic material with considerable nuclear debris and intact neutrophils.*

Early Stage of Abscess Formation

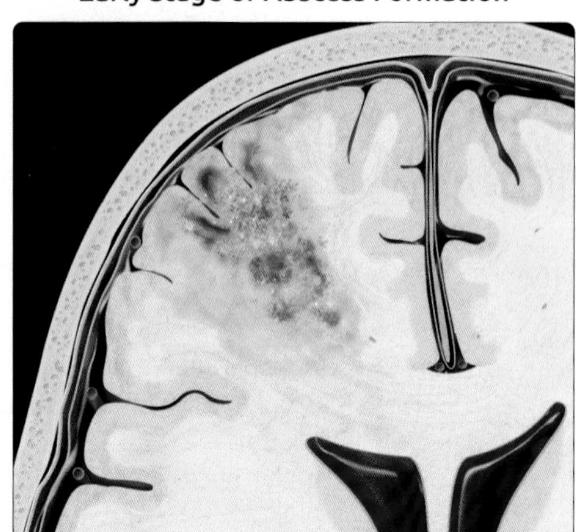

Cerebritis

(Left) *Abscesses are dangerous expansile lesions, as in this example in the basal ganglia that compresses the lateral ventricle. The capsule is thinner on its deep aspect near the ventricle →.* **(Right)** *Early abscess capsule has a hyperemic rim due to congested proliferating capillaries.*

Thin Capsule Wall, Deeper Aspect

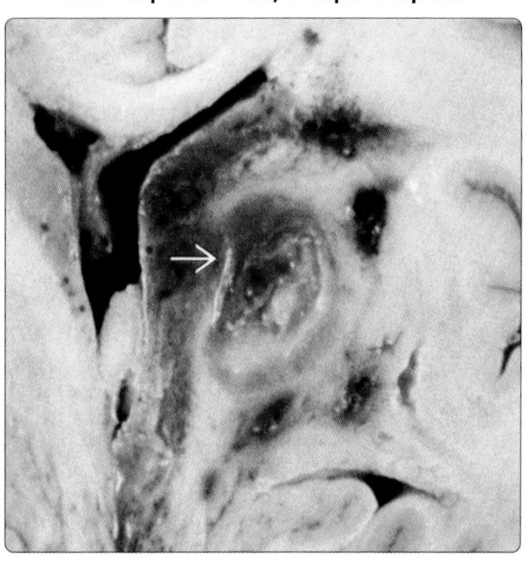

Hyperemic Rim

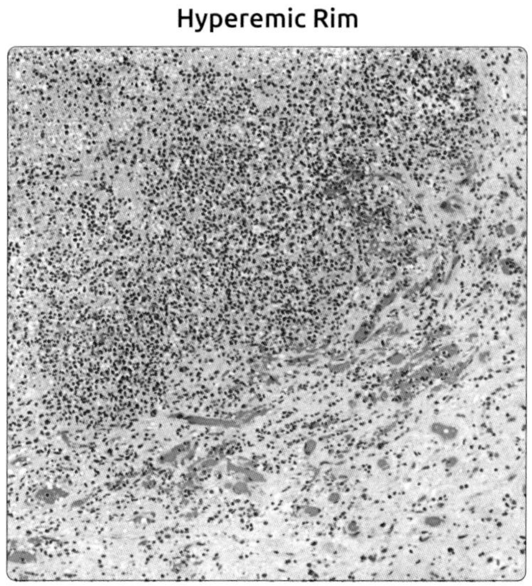

(Left) *Proliferating fibroblasts → during early stages of abscess encapsulation are admixed with neutrophils as is typical of granulation tissue.* **(Right)** *Well-formed abscess has increased mass effect, here with expansion of the frontal lobe, gyral expansion, and sulcal narrowing. Confluent necrosis is encircled by a well-defined hyperemic capsule.*

Proliferating Fibroblasts

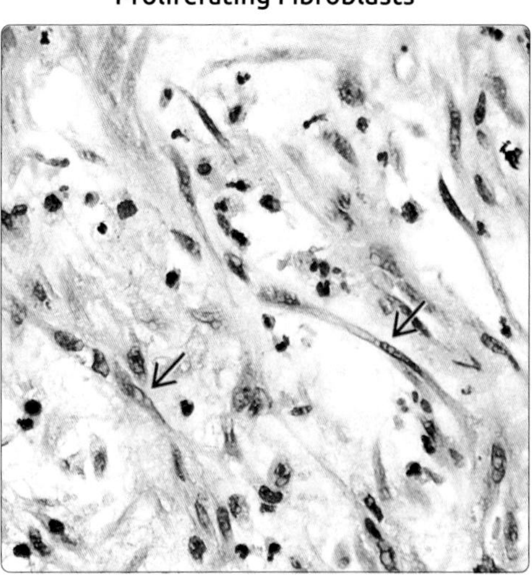

Well-Formed Abscess

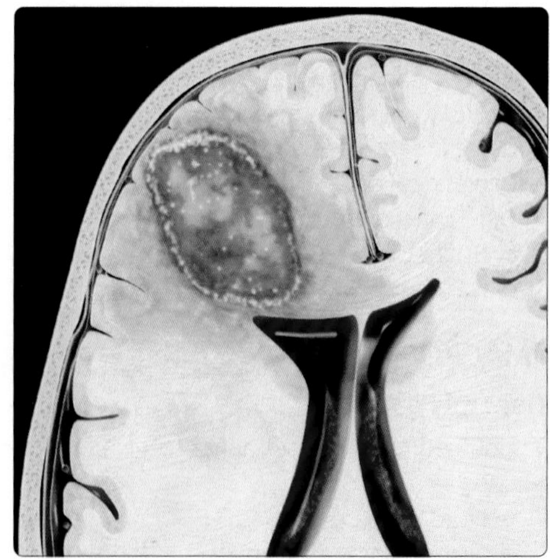

Herniation Due to Brain Abscesses

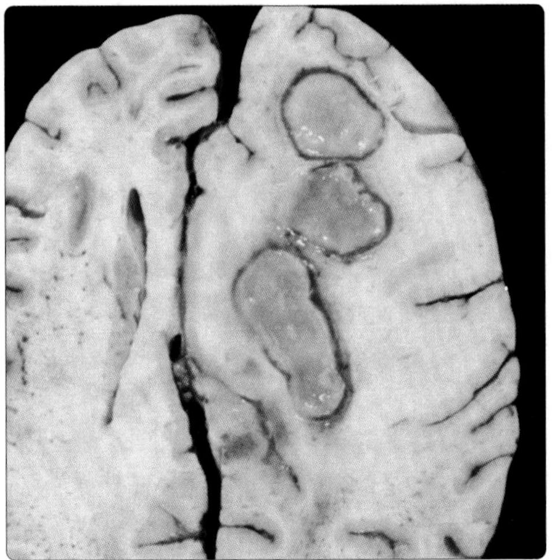

Capsule Wall With Proliferated Small Vessels

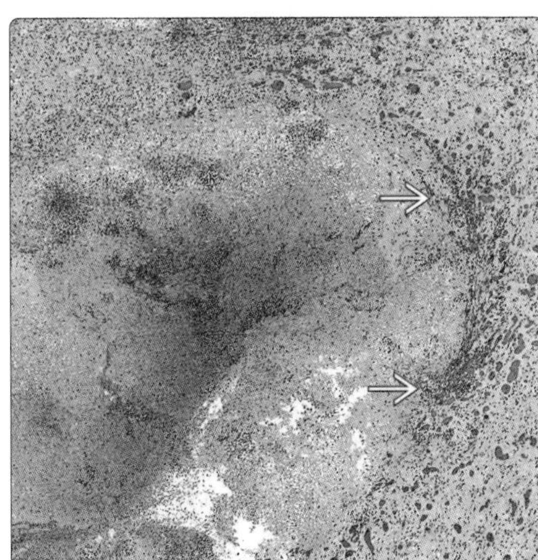

(Left) *Axial brain specimen from a patient with longstanding bronchiectasis has 3 contiguous abscesses with hyperemic rims. The ultimately lethal combined mass effect is evidenced by the pronounced right-to-left shift.* **(Right)** *The capsular hyperemia of an abscess seen macroscopically corresponds to a fairly discrete, narrow rim of granulation tissue within the evolving capsule. Note the numerous small congested vessels ➡.*

Capsule Wall, Reticulin

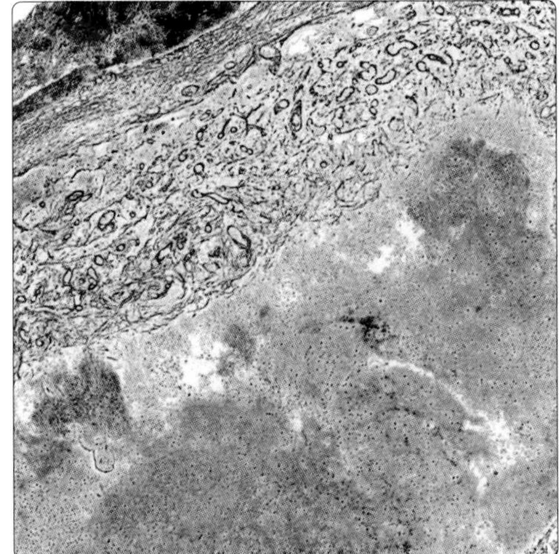

Capsule Wall, Reticulin

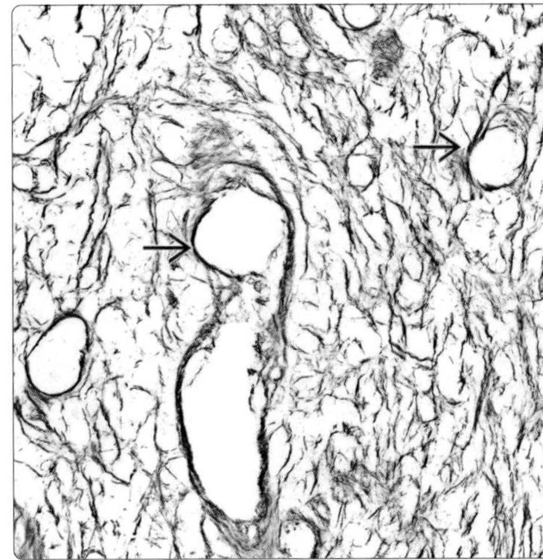

(Left) *Reticulin fibers generated by perivascular fibroblasts ultimately coalesce to form the dense fibrotic capsule characteristic of the mature abscess.* **(Right)** *Derived from perithelial fibroblasts, reticulin fibers abound in the developing abscess capsule. Vessel profiles are easily discerned ➡.*

Capsule Wall, Trichrome

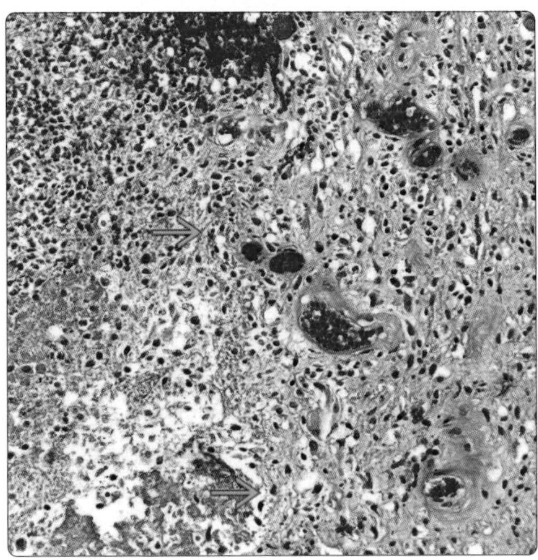

Mitotic Activity, Inflammation

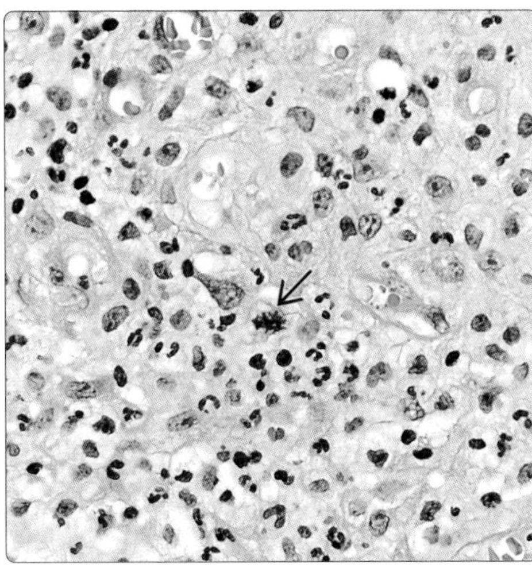

(Left) *The capsule contains collagen fibers that coalesce to form a dense wall. Note the interface ➡ between pus at the left and the hyperemic, collagen-rich (blue-stained) capsule at the right.* **(Right)** *Parts of the abscess capsule during early stages of formation have neutrophils as well as chronic inflammatory cells. Mitotic figures may be present ➡.*

(Left) *Granulation tissue at the edge of an abscess during early stages of capsule formation contains a variety of cell types, including plump fibroblasts with basophilic cytoplasm. Note the dense pink background in the capsule corresponding to newly formed collagen.* **(Right)** *The abscess capsule later often contains hyalinized small vessels, plasma cells, and lymphocytes.*

Early Capsule Wall, Granulation Tissue

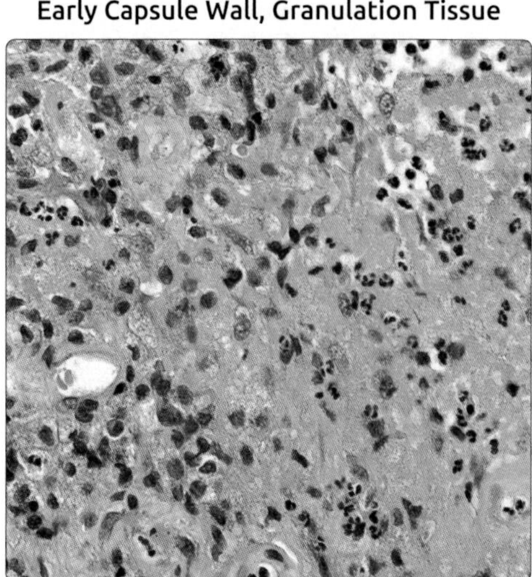

Well-Formed Capsule Wall

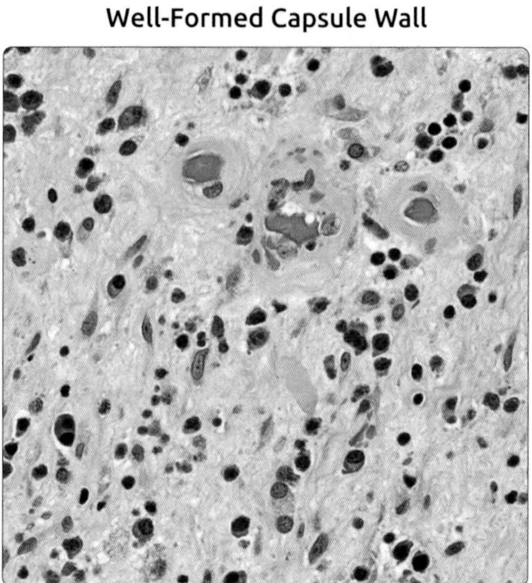

(Left) *Macrophage-rich tissue adjacent to the abscess capsule may be misinterpreted as a neoplasm.* **(Right)** *Bacteria can seldom be identified in abscesses by hematoxylin and eosin staining alone unless they are large and filamentous. Actinomyces, seen here, often forms dense clusters of fuzzy-appearing bacteria.*

Numerous Nearby Macrophages

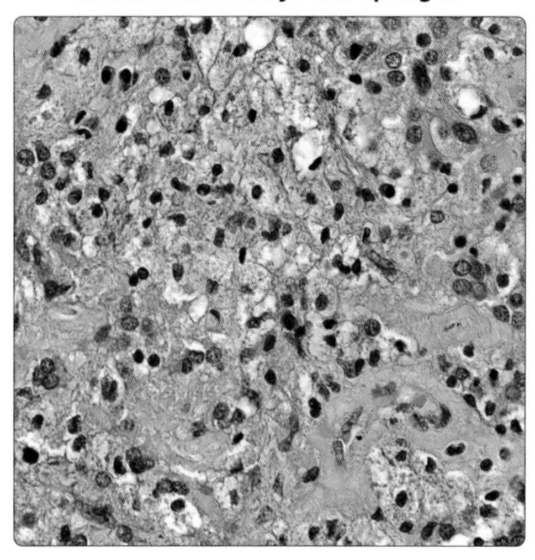

Actinomyces

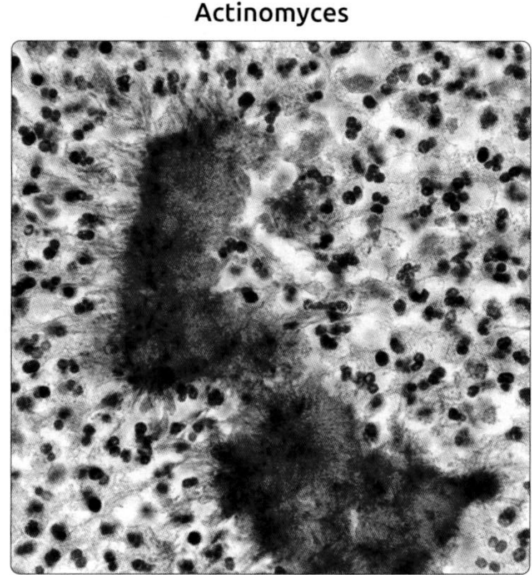

(Left) *Gram-positive cocci in an abscess can be best identified with special bacterial stains, such as the Gram method.* **(Right)** *This abscess in a patient with lung disease has mixed flora, including both gram-positive cocci (dark blue) ⇒ and larger gram-negative bacilli (red) ⇒.*

Gram-Positive Cocci

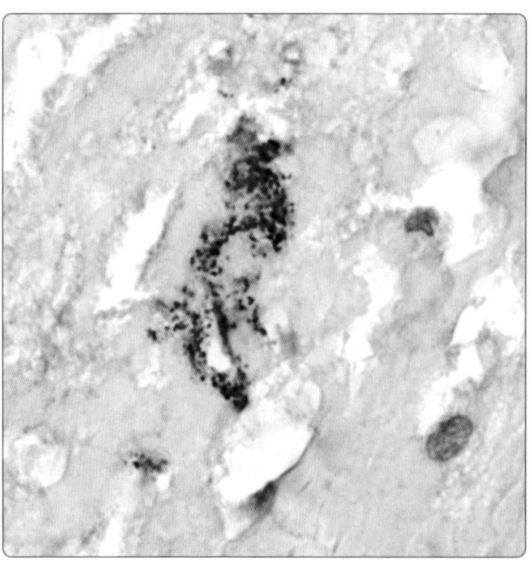

Mixed Flora

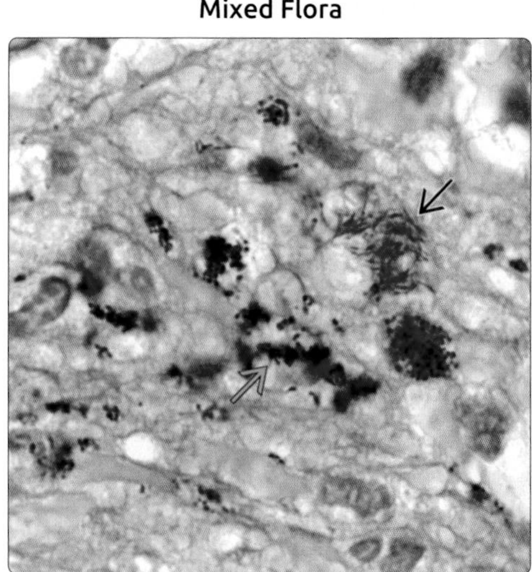

Listeria

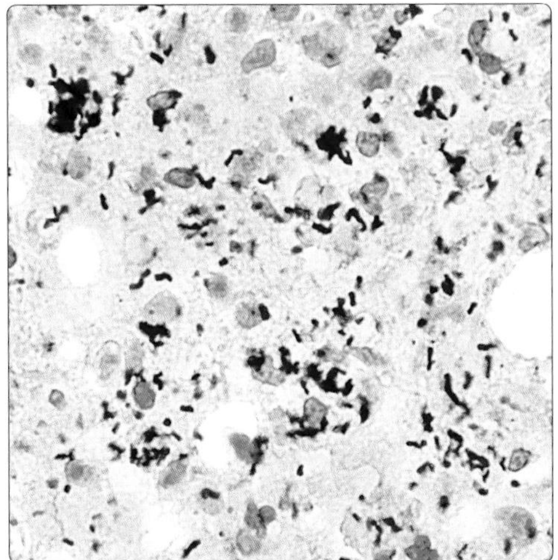

***Listeria*, Culture Plate**

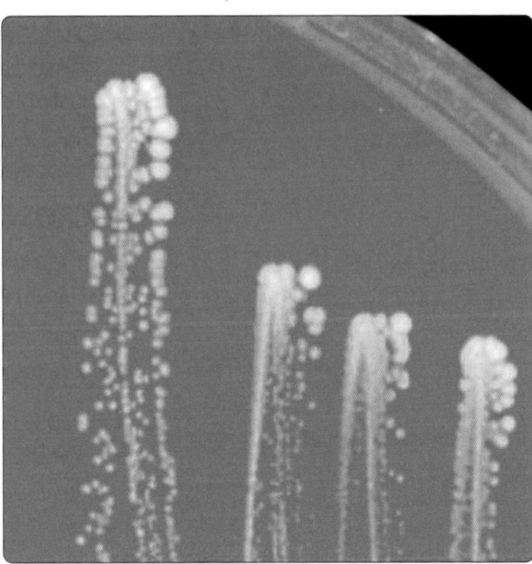

(Left) *Listeria appears as small plump rods that can be difficult to identify in histological sections of an abscess, although the gram-positive organisms are obvious here.* **(Right)** *This culture plate containing Listeria monocytogenes represents positive confirmation of Listeria as the cause of a brainstem abscess in a young child. Although Gram stain of the tissue must be performed, culture is ultimately necessary to confirm specific bacterial type. (Courtesy Dr. P. Boyer.)*

***Listeria*, Agar Tube**

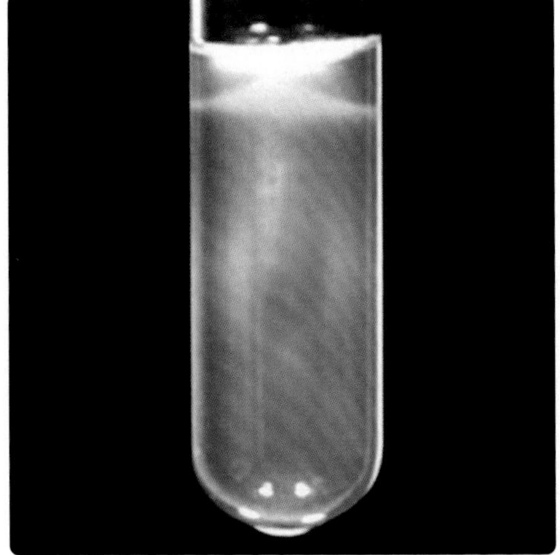

***Nocardia*, Gram Stain**

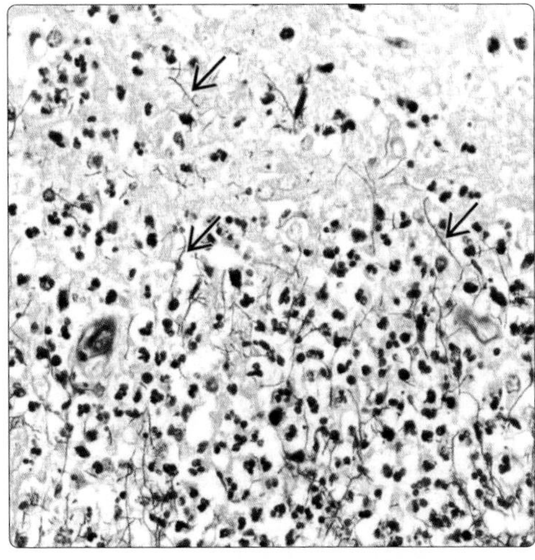

(Left) *Listeria, shown here as an umbrella-shaped growth in a stab agar tube, was successfully cultured from a brainstem abscess in a child. (Courtesy Dr. P. Boyer.)* **(Right)** *Nocardia species are nearly impossible to identify within a brain abscess by H&E staining and can even be overlooked in a Gram stain. Note the delicate gram-positive filamentous organisms ⇒.*

***Nocardia*, Fite Stain**

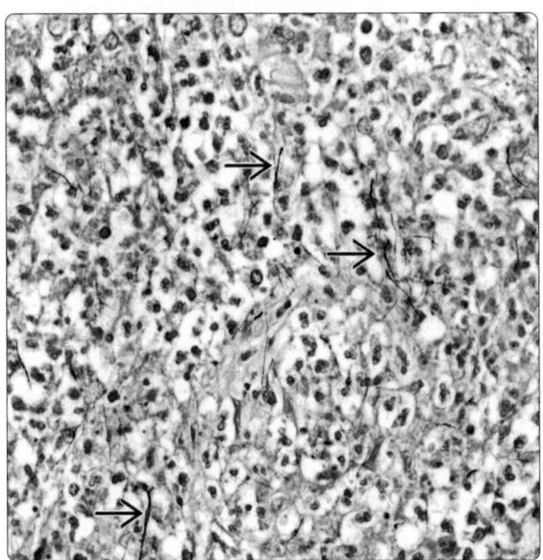

***Nocardia*, Grocott Methenamine Silver**

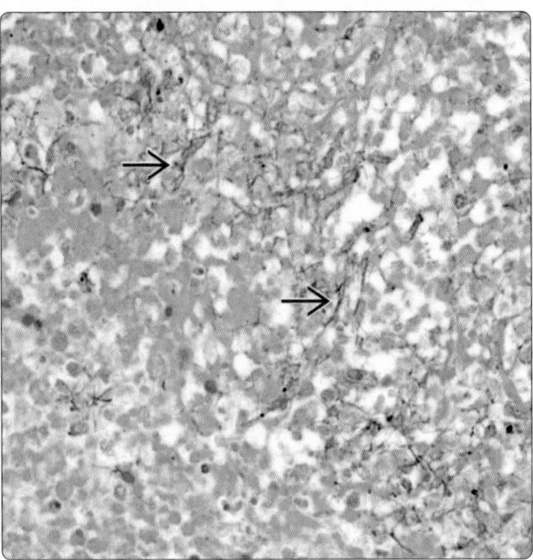

(Left) *Nocardia are partially acid fast on Fite staining. These delicate, fuschia-colored, single, filamentous bacteria ⇒ may be overlooked in the debris in the center of an abscess. A beaded profile will be apparent at high magnification (oil immersion).* **(Right)** *Nocardia can be identified with fungal stains such as Grocott methenamine silver (GMS), as shown here in the inflammatory exudate of an abscess. These delicate filamentous bacteria ⇒ are far thinner than fungi.*

Whipple Disease

KEY FACTS

TERMINOLOGY

- Chronic, multisystemic disorder characterized by migratory polyarthralgias, chronic diarrhea, fever
  - 5% of patients present with CNS symptoms
  - More patients develop symptoms later
- CNS presenting site in 5% of cases

ETIOLOGY/PATHOGENESIS

- Bacterial infection by *Tropheryma whipplei*
- Inert material surrounding bacteria within macrophages is PAS(+) 110-kDa glycoprotein-containing sialic acid
  - Glycosylation likely impairs host antibody-mediated immune recognition
- No ↑ in patients with AIDS, renal transplant recipients, and other major immunodeficiency states

CLINICAL ISSUES

- Cognitive changes, supranuclear palsy, altered consciousness, psychiatric features, hypothalamic dysfunction
- Predilection for periaqueductal gray matter, hypothalamus, hippocampus, cerebral cortex

MICROSCOPIC

- Inflammatory foci containing macrophages with sickle-shaped cytoplasmic PAS(+) material
- Organism-filled macrophages have grayish cytoplasm

ANCILLARY TESTS

- Biopsy may be from non-CNS sites, especially small bowel
- PCR higher sensitivity and specificity than light microscopy

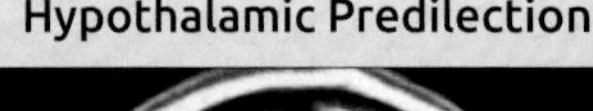

Hypothalamic Predilection

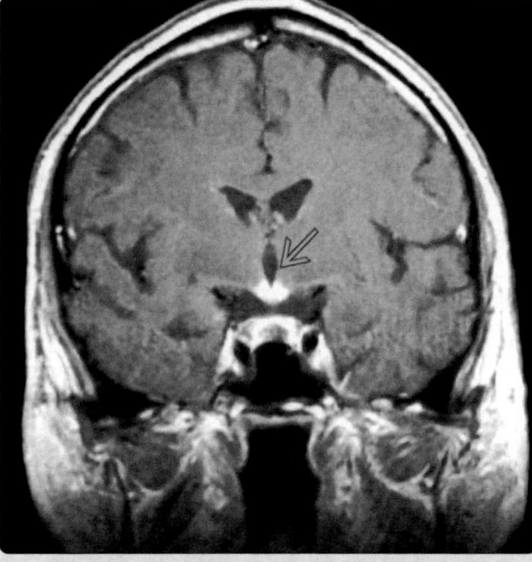

Hypothalamic, Mesial Temporal Lobe Disease

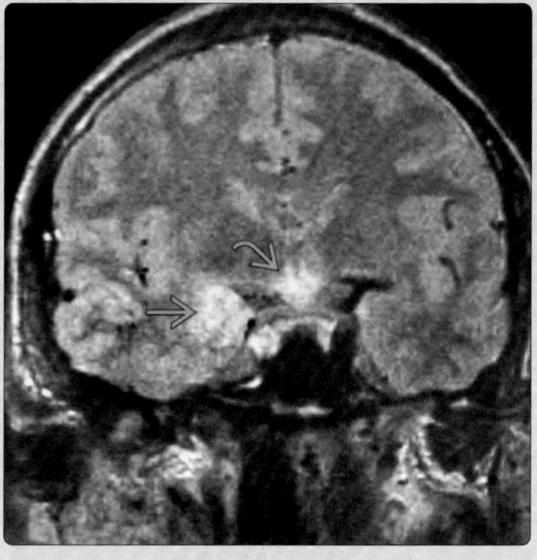

(Left) *Contrast-enhanced T1-weighted MR shows typical hypothalamic enhancement ➡ in a patient with CNS Whipple disease.* **(Right)** *Coronal FLAIR MR at level of optic chiasm demonstrates hyperintense signal within the hypothalamus ➡ and mesial right temporal lobe ➡. There is no significant mass effect. but expansion of right amygdala is apparent.*

Macrophages Stuffed With Bacilli

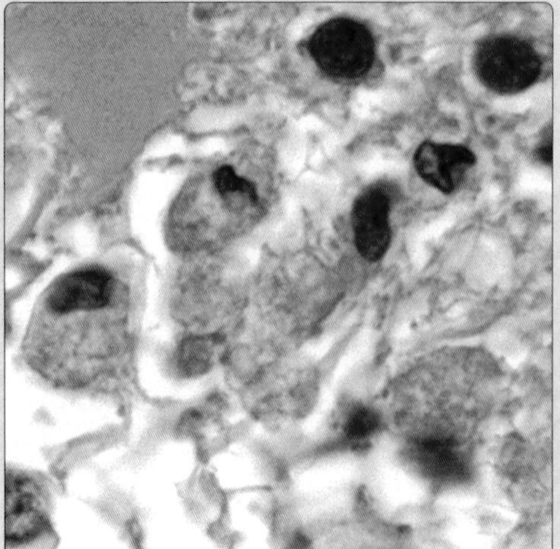

PAS-Positive Bacilli

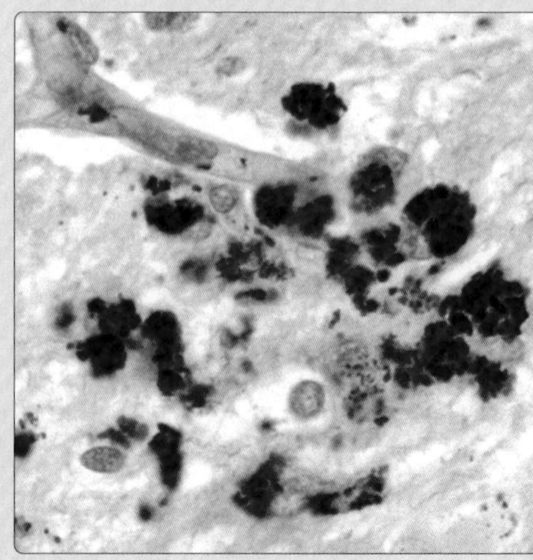

(Left) *Macrophages stuffed with large numbers of bacilli can display a blue-gray tincture on H&E.* **(Right)** *Clumped intracytoplasmic bacilli are intensely positive for PAS. Individual organisms are difficult to resolve within the clumps.*

TERMINOLOGY

Definitions

- Chronic, multisystemic disorder characterized by migratory polyarthralgias, chronic diarrhea, fever; 5% of patients present with CNS symptoms; more patients develop symptoms later

ETIOLOGY/PATHOGENESIS

Environmental Exposure

- Bacterial DNA of *Tropheryma whipplei* found in individuals without symptoms
- Bacterial DNA detected in sewage water, normal stool

Infectious Agents

- Bacterial infection by *T. whipplei*

CLINICAL ISSUES

Epidemiology

- Incidence
  - Uncommon disease, especially isolated CNS Whipple type
  - Patients coming to CNS biopsy often with limited systemic symptoms &/or negative biopsies from more accessible sites (small bowel or lymph node)
  - No increase in patients with AIDS, renal transplant recipients, and other major immunodeficiency states
- Age
  - Mean: 50 years
- Sex
  - Strong male predominance

Site

- Periaqueductal gray matter, hypothalamus, hippocampus, cerebral cortex, basal ganglia, cerebellum

Presentation

- Cognitive change, supranuclear palsy, altered consciousness, hypothalamic dysfunction, cranial nerve palsies
- Non-CNS symptoms: Weight loss, diarrhea, arthralgia/arthritis, adenopathy absent in some CNS cases

Treatment

- Drugs
  - Antibiotics, usually ceftriaxone
  - 40% CNS Whipple patients unresponsive to trimethoprim-sulfamethoxazole
  - Reduced penetration of drugs into CNS may be responsible for relapses

Prognosis

- Fatal if untreated
- Clinical course can be fulminant
- Outcome for CNS form can be adverse even with therapy

IMAGING

MR Findings

- Varied neuroimaging features; common sites of involvement hypothalamus, midbrain, mesial temporal lobes although some have normal MR
- Atrophy of brain; mass lesions seen in some patients, often with minimal enhancement

MACROSCOPIC

General Features

- Atrophy
- Small scattered chalky nodules

MICROSCOPIC

Histologic Features

- Small loose aggregates of histiocytes, lymphocytes, plasma cells
- Grayish-tinged macrophage cytoplasm on H&E
- Macrophages with PAS(+), GMS(+)
- Surrounding astrocytosis
- CNS histologic involvement frequent even in patients without neurological symptoms
- Little, if any, granulomatous inflammation

ANCILLARY TESTS

Cytology

- CSF histiocytes with PAS(+) granular or sickle-shaped cytoplasmic particles

Immunohistochemistry

- Antibodies to *T. whipplei* (+)

PCR

- High sensitivity and specificity
- Can be performed on small bowel, lymph node, or CNS biopsies, and CSF
- 70-80% patients have (+) CSF PCR

DIFFERENTIAL DIAGNOSIS

Mycobacterial Infections

- Acid-fast organisms
- Caseating necrosis

Histoplasmosis

- Intracytoplasmic organisms are round to oval

DIAGNOSTIC CHECKLIST

Clinically Relevant Pathologic Features

- Diagnosis established by tissue biopsy or PCR
- Biopsy sites: Small intestine, lymph nodes, CNS

Pathologic Interpretation Pearls

- Grayish-tinged macrophages with PAS(+) contents
- Large numbers of intracytoplasmic organisms obscure bacterial shape

SELECTED REFERENCES

1. Balasa M et al: Clinical and neuropathological variability in clinically isolated central nervous system Whipple's disease. Brain Pathol. 24(3):230-8, 2014
2. Compain C et al: Central nervous system involvement in Whipple disease: clinical study of 18 patients and long-term follow-up. Medicine (Baltimore). 92(6):324-30, 2013
3. Mohamed W et al: Isolated intracranial Whipple's disease–report of a rare case and review of the literature. J Neurol Sci. 308(1-2):1-8, 2011

(Left) *Stereotypical features of CNS Whipple disease include loose aggregates of histiocytes, lymphocytes, and plasma cells, all with surrounding reactive astrocytosis ➡. When only focal, organism-filled macrophages may be inconspicuous.* **(Right)** *Features of CNS Whipple disease include multifocal small aggregates of histiocytes, lymphocytes, and plasma cells. Compact granulomas, as in sarcoidosis, are generally not present.*

Loose Aggregates of Histiocytes

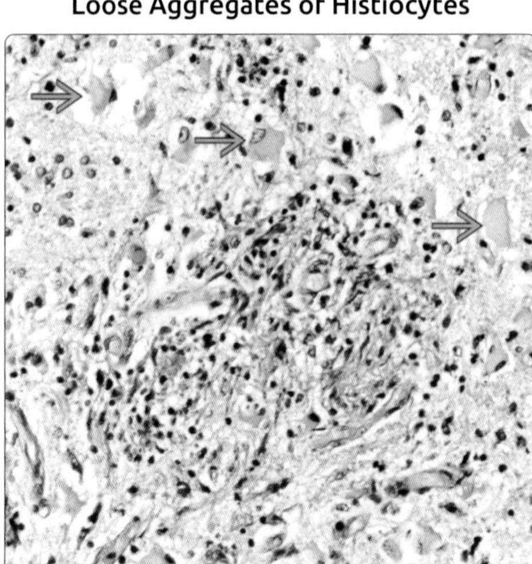

Absence of Compact Granulomas

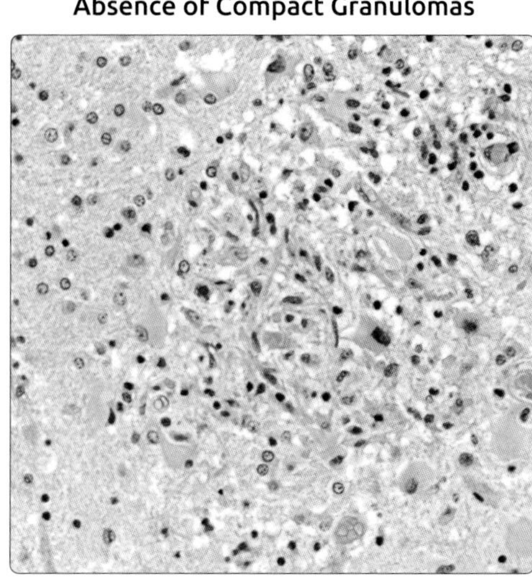

(Left) *Large, clustered, perivascular macrophages are eye catching because of their blue-gray tint ➡.* **(Right)** *Loose aggregates of macrophages with paler gray contents ➡ are classic features. Biopsies of CNS Whipple disease are uncommon since the diagnosis is usually made from jejunal biopsies or PCR of CSF.*

Macrophages With Blue-Gray Contents

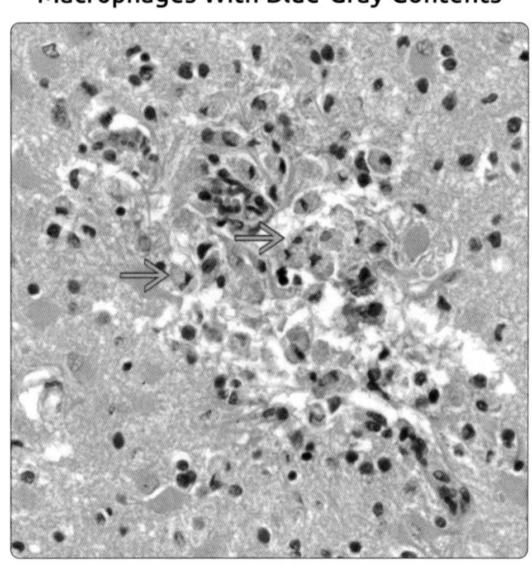

More Subtle Numbers of Intracellular Bacilli

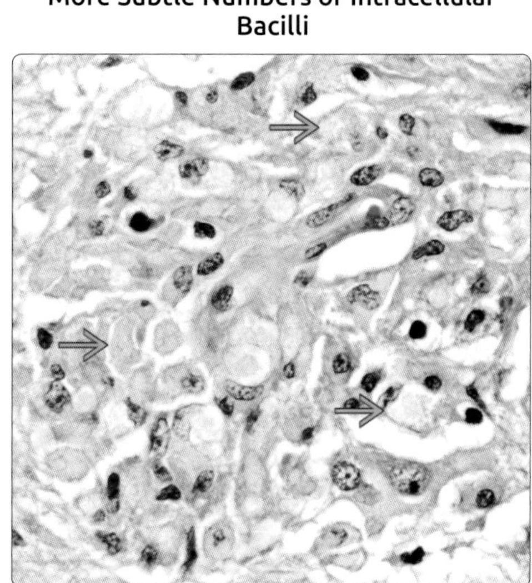

(Left) *Inflammation in CNS Whipple disease consists of microglia ➡, lymphocytes, plasma cells, and histiocytes. The latter may be obvious when filled with bacteria, but inconspicuous when not.* **(Right)** *Lymphoplasmacytic infiltrates may be quite scant, and only a few organism-containing macrophages ➡ may be present.*

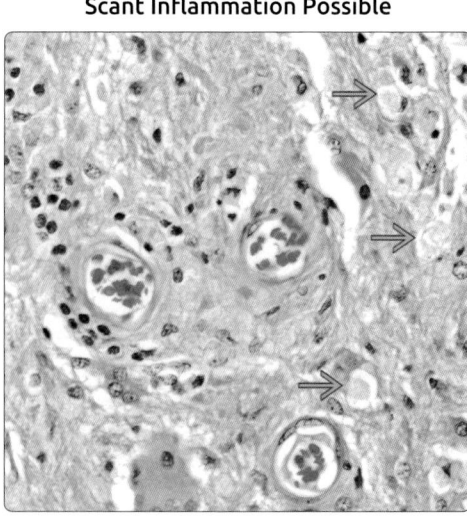

Scattered Microglia

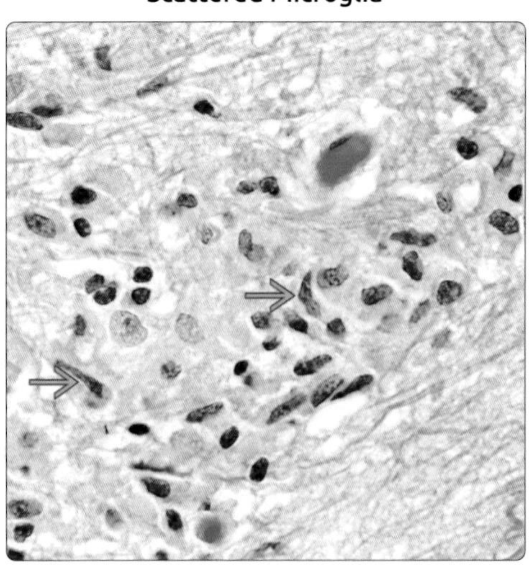

Scant Inflammation Possible

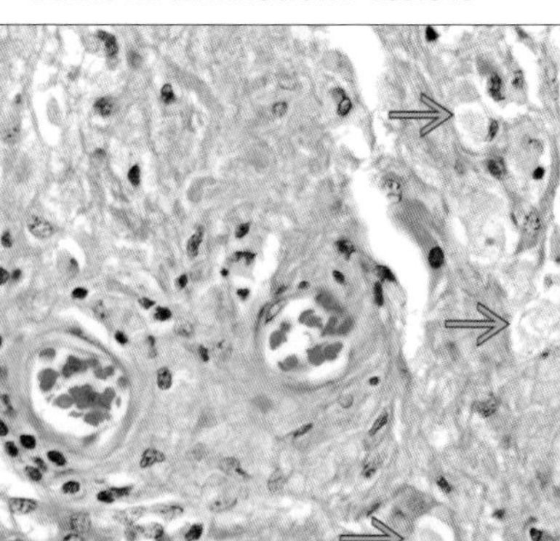

Copious Bacteria in Macrophages

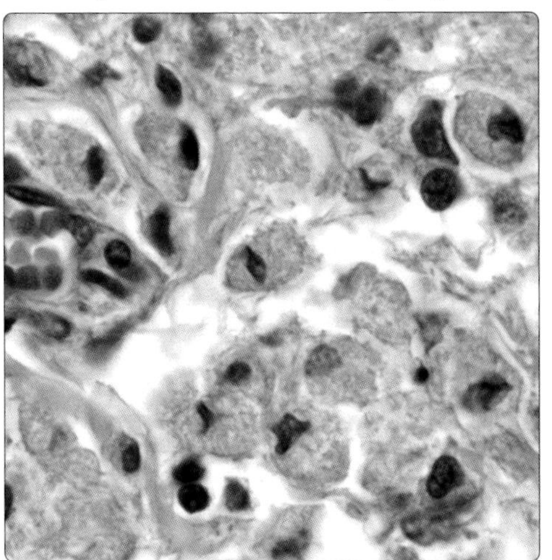

PAS-Positive Bacteria in Macrophages

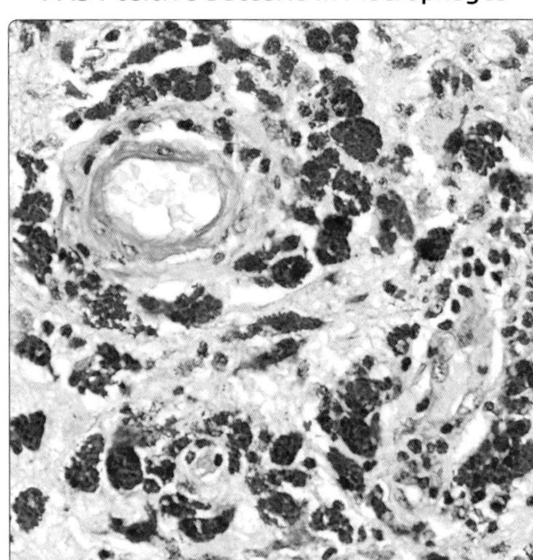

(Left) *A grayish tinge is helpful when suspecting that the cytoplasms of macrophages are filled with organisms rather than generic phagocytized debris. Organisms are so numerous that they cannot be individually resolved. This should not be mistaken for an artifact or a storage disorder.* **(Right)** *PAS-diastase is the best histochemical stain for disclosing bacteria that fill the cytoplasm of histiocytes. These positive conglomerates are likened to sickle shapes. Individual bacteria are usually impossible to resolve.*

Individual Bacteria

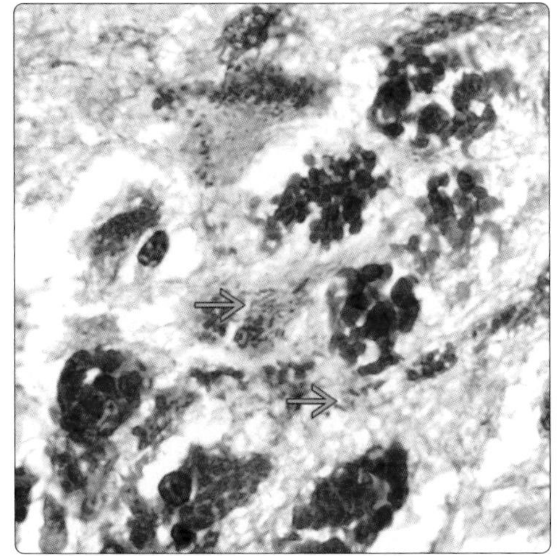

Bacteria, GMS

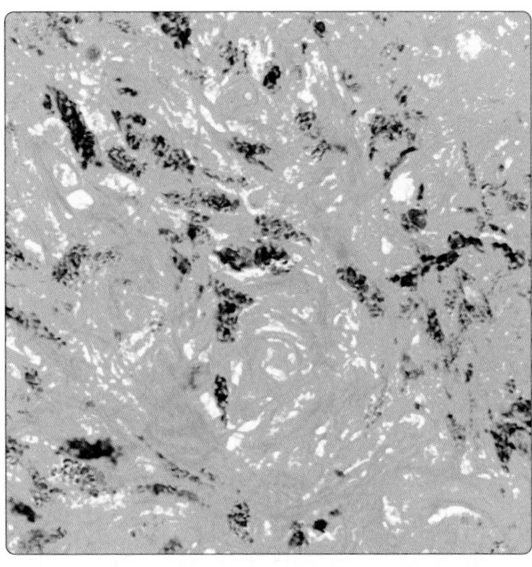

(Left) *High-power view of a PAS-stained section of CNS Whipple disease shows the intensely fuschia-colored cytoplasmic clumps of bacteria. These dense, sickle-shaped inclusions obscure detail, and only in areas of lesser density are individual bacteria resolved ➡.* **(Right)** *Bacteria of Whipple disease are positive on GMS stains. Because of the GMS(+), they somewhat simulate fungi, but lack yeast or hyphal shapes. They are also too small to represent a yeast, even histoplasma.*

Immunostaining for Bacteria

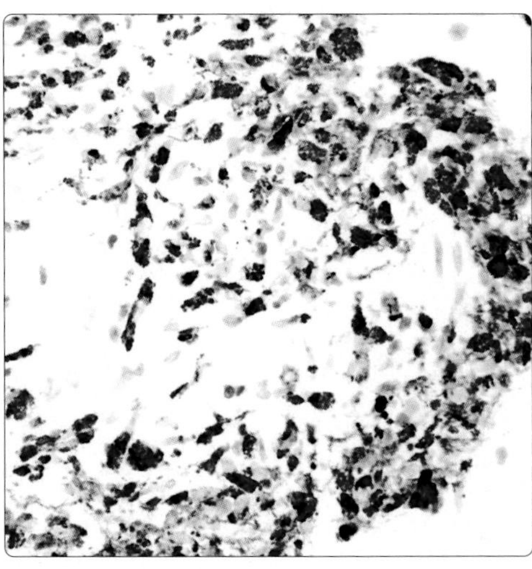

Immunostaining

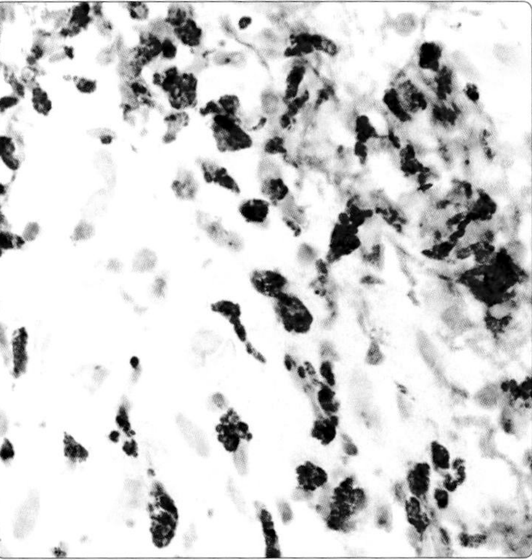

(Left) *Immunostaining for the bacteria Tropheryma whipplei is a definitive diagnostic test.* **(Right)** *Immunostaining for the bacteria in CNS Whipple disease identifies the pathogenetic agent.*

Tuberculosis

KEY FACTS

TERMINOLOGY

- Diffuse meningeal (meningitis) or localized (tuberculoma) infection by mycobacteria, usually *Mycobacterium tuberculosis*
- Localized, largely histiocytic lesion with infection by *Mycobacterium avium-intracellulare* in immunocompromised patient, mycobacterial spindle cell pseudotumor
- Skeletal tuberculosis (TB)
  - Spinal form: Tuberculous spondylitis/Pott disease

CLINICAL ISSUES

- TB meningitis more common, but tuberculomas most likely to be biopsied
- Several forms of disease may coexist, especially meningitis and tuberculomas

MICROSCOPIC

- Tuberculomas
  - Caseous central necrosis and surrounding histiocytes, multinucleated cells, chronic inflammation
- Rare pseudotumors composed of epithelioid histiocytes containing overwhelming numbers of *Mycobacterium avium-intracellulare* seen in immunocompromised patients
- Skeletal forms associated with bony destruction

DIAGNOSTIC CHECKLIST

- Diligent search often required to find organisms, most always confined to necrotic areas
  - Tissue PCR testing may be necessary
  - Granulomas without acid-fast bacilli are suggestive of disease in correct clinical setting &/or patients with indications of TB infection by systemic testing
    - Positive TB skin test, etc.
- Mycobacterial pseudotumor response more histiocytic than granulomatous

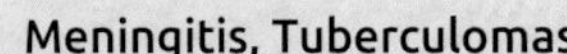

Meningitis, Tuberculomas | **Necrotizing Granulomatous Inflammation**

(Left) *Coronal T1 contrast-enhanced MR shows basilar tuberculous meningitis around middle cerebral artery → and enhancing tuberculomas →. Note subtle low signal in left basal ganglia secondary to arteritis with ischemia.* **(Right)** *Necrotizing granulomatous inflammation, usually with giant cells, is the histological hallmark of tuberculosis caused by infection with M. tuberculosis.*

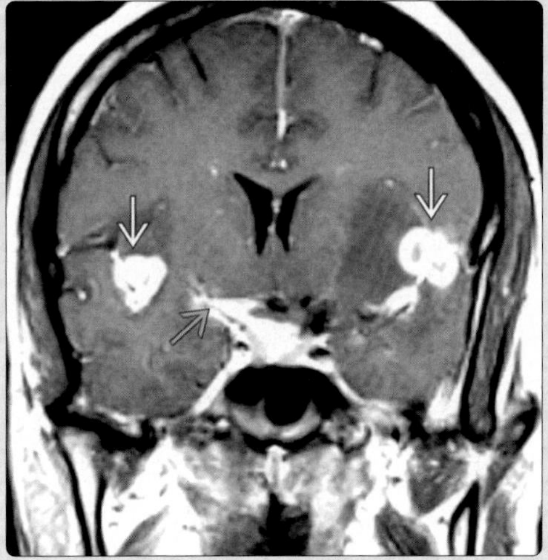

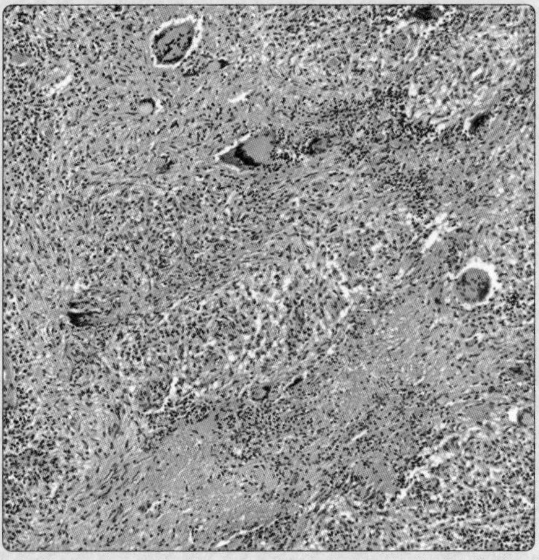

Tuberculoma, Cerebellum | **Skeletal TB, Spinal Cord Compression**

(Left) *Discrete tuberculoma in the cerebellum → shows a central dense eosinophilic area of caseating necrosis →.* **(Right)** *Tuberculosis of the spine, caused by M. tuberculosis, can distort the spinal cord →. This example occurred in a young HIV(+) woman who had been living in a refugee camp in Zambia for the last 18 years; she presented with a history of at least 1 year of bilateral lower extremity weakness.*

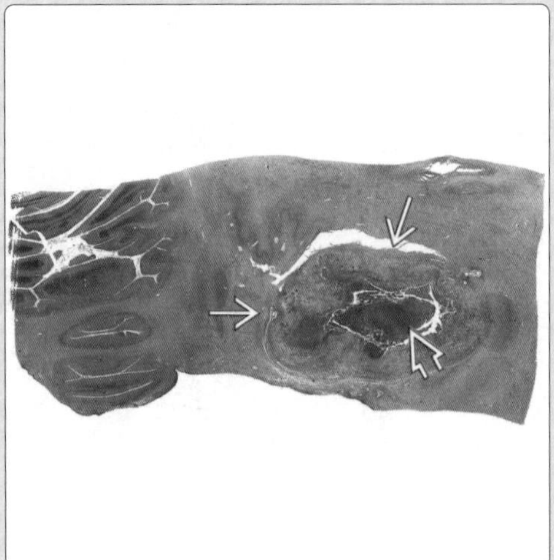

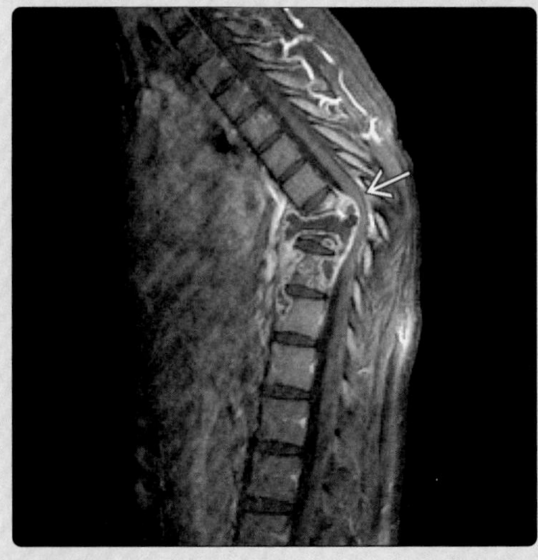

TERMINOLOGY

Abbreviations

- Tuberculosis (TB)

Definitions

- Diffuse meningeal (meningitis) or localized (tuberculoma) infection by mycobacteria
  - Usually *Mycobacterium tuberculosis*
- Localized, largely histiocytic lesion with infection by *Mycobacterium avium-intracellulare* in immunocompromised patient, mycobacterial spindle cell pseudotumor
- Skeletal/spinal tuberculosis

ETIOLOGY/PATHOGENESIS

Environmental Exposure

- Endemic in many developing countries
- Most cases secondary to hematogenous spread, usually from lung
- Reemergence in developed countries due to increased incidence in HIV(+) patients
- Occasionally seen in patients on immunosuppressive medications
- Emergence of drug-resistant strains

CLINICAL ISSUES

Epidemiology

- Incidence
  - CNS 10-15% of all TB infections
  - Tuberculomas 10-30% of brain masses in endemic countries (e.g., India, Pakistan)
  - Miliary form 1% of all TB
    - Widespread hematogenous dissemination of organisms
    - CNS involvement in approximately 1/5 of miliary TB cases, usually meningitis
  - Unusual manifestations of CNS involvement and types of tuberculous organisms can occur in patients with acquired immunodeficiency syndrome
  - Disadvantaged groups or those with limited access to medical care may be at higher risk for morbidity and mortality

Presentation

- Most common overall CNS manifestation is meningitis, not tuberculoma
- Children most likely to present with meningitis
- Less common nervous system manifestations
  - Tuberculous abscess, rare
  - Spinal intramedullary
  - Tuberculomas in cavernous sinus mimicking meningioma
- Skeletal tuberculosis
  - Spine involved in up to 50% of skeletal TB cases
    - May present in advanced stages due to indolent nature of infection
    - Often low index of suspicion for skeletal involvement in TB in non-TB endemic areas
  - Pott disease of spine associated with potential paraplegia from cord compression
- Several forms of disease may coexist, especially meningitis and tuberculomas
- Meningioma-like mycobacterial spindle cell pseudotumor in immunocompromised

Treatment

- First-line 4-drug regimen
  - Isoniazid
  - Rifampin
  - Pyrazinamide
  - Ethambutol
- Dexamethasone for some meningitis patients or those with papilledema, myelitis
- Surgical intervention for spinal TB, with debridement, decompression of spinal cord, spinal stabilization

Prognosis

- Variable depending on promptness of treatment
- Most improve with therapy
- Concomitant HIV infection reduces survival rate in TB meningitis

IMAGING

MR Findings

- Basilar meningitis
- Tuberculomas caseating or noncaseating show variable signal intensities
- Majority (2/3) in cerebral hemispheres, especially frontoparietal and basal ganglia
- Dural-based, meningioma-like mass with mycobacterial spindle cell pseudotumor
- Skeletal disease can be present, with up to 50% of those cases having spine involvement (tuberculous spondylitis, Pott disease)
  - Spinal deformity
  - May be associated with spinal cord edema on MR &/or paravertebral and epidural abscesses

CT Findings

- Solid or ring enhancing on contrast-enhanced scans

MACROSCOPIC

General Features

- Tuberculomas up to 6 cm in size
  - Majority < 2.5 cm
- Necrotic center

MICROSCOPIC

Histologic Features

- Central caseation necrosis
- Surrounding epithelioid histiocytes, lymphocytes, plasma cells, and multinucleated giant cells
- Multinucleated giant cells, generally Langhans type
- Plasma cells may be large and binucleate due to chronic stimulation
- Acid-fast bacilli may be difficult to demonstrate
- Mycobacterial spindle cell pseudotumor
  - Sheets of histiocytes rather than granulomas
  - Little necrosis
  - Innumerable intracellular organisms

- *M. avium-intracellulare*
- Bony destruction in cases of skeletal infection

ANCILLARY TESTS

Cytology

- Multinucleated cells
- Epithelioid cells

PCR

- Tissue PCR testing for organisms may be necessary, especially in granulomas

DIFFERENTIAL DIAGNOSIS

Neurosarcoid

- No large, geographic areas of necrosis, but possible within individual granulomas
- Granulomas in varying stages of fibrosis
- No organisms

Bacterial Brain Abscess

- Except for nocardia, brain abscesses not surrounded by histiocytes
- Liquefactive necrosis with neutrophils and neutrophilic debris
- Bacteria, by culture or Gram stain

Fungal Granulomatous Infection

- Share multinucleated giant cells with tuberculosis
- Share central necrosis within granuloma(s), as can be seen in tuberculosis
- Requires identification of specific causative fungus responsible for the granulomatous infection on histochemical stains
  - Supplemented by culture results, identification by polymerase chain reaction (PCR) testing
  - Histoplasmosis (*Histoplasma capsulatum*)
    - Small yeast forms on Grocott methenamine silver (GMS) or Periodic acid-Schiff (PAS) stains
    - Appear much smaller on H&E than on GMS or PAS stains
    - Even in endemic areas not a frequent cause of CNS granulomas
      - More likely to affect lung and dissemination usually confined to spleen and liver
  - Blastomycosis (*Blastomyces dermatitidis*)
    - Larger yeast forms with broad-based bud
    - Multiple nuclei seen on hematoxylin and eosin in well-fixed tissues
    - Even in endemic areas, not a frequent cause of CNS granulomas
      - More likely to affect lung
  - Coccidioidomycosis (*Coccidioides immitis*)
    - Large sporangia containing sporangiospores (endospores); spherule used for intermediate forms between released endospores and sporangium
    - Spherules may lie within multinucleated giant cells
    - May affect CNS even in immunocompetent patients

DIAGNOSTIC CHECKLIST

Clinically Relevant Pathologic Features

- Organisms may be scarce

Pathologic Interpretation Pearls

- Diligent search often required to find organisms
- Organisms almost always confined to necrotic areas
- Mycobacterial spindle cell pseudotumor response more histiocytic than granulomatous

SELECTED REFERENCES

1. Barr LK et al: Intraventricular granulomatous mass associated with Mycobacterium haemophilum: A rare central nervous system manifestation in a patient with human immunodeficiency virus infection. J Clin Neurosci. 22(6):1057-60, 2015
2. Francisco NM et al: TNF-dependent regulation and activation of innate immune cells are essential for host protection against cerebral tuberculosis. J Neuroinflammation. 12:125, 2015
3. Gao Z et al: A population-based study of tuberculosis case fatality in Canada: do Aboriginal peoples fare less well? Int J Tuberc Lung Dis. 19(7):772-9, 2015
4. Jiang T et al: Outcomes and treatment of lumbosacral spinal tuberculosis: a retrospective study of 53 patients. PLoS One. 10(6):e0130185, 2015
5. Kilborn T et al: Pediatric and adult spinal tuberculosis: imaging and pathophysiology. Neuroimaging Clin N Am. 25(2):209-31, 2015
6. Maitra A et al: Tackling tuberculosis: insights from an international TB Summit in London. Virulence. 1-12, 2015
7. Spanos JP et al: Microglia are crucial regulators of neuro-immunity during central nervous system tuberculosis. Front Cell Neurosci. 9:182, 2015
8. Tanaka T et al: Central nervous system manifestations of tuberculosis-associated immune reconstitution inflammatory syndrome during adalimumab therapy: a case report and review of the literature. Intern Med. 54(7):847-51, 2015
9. Garg RK et al: Neurological complications of miliary tuberculosis. Clin Neurol Neurosurg. 112(3):188-92, 2010
10. Jansen M et al: The role of biopsy in the diagnosis of infections of the central nervous system. Ir Med J. 103(1):6-8, 2010
11. Lu M: Imaging diagnosis of spinal intramedullary tuberculoma: case reports and literature review. J Spinal Cord Med. 33(2):159-62, 2010
12. Tinsa F et al: Central system nervous tuberculosis in infants. J Child Neurol. 25(1):102-6, 2010
13. Ramdurg SR et al: Spinal intramedullary tuberculosis: a series of 15 cases. Clin Neurol Neurosurg. 111(2):115-8, 2009
14. Morrison A et al: Mycobacterial spindle cell pseudotumor of the brain: a case report and review of the literature. Am J Surg Pathol. 23(10):1294-9, 1999

Basilar Meningitis, Infarcts

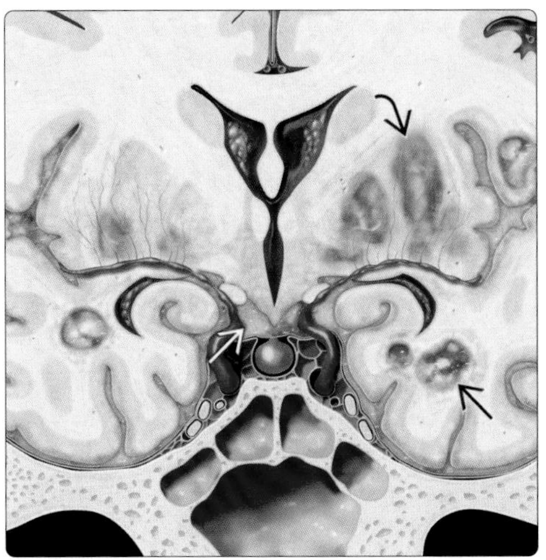

Caseous Necrosis

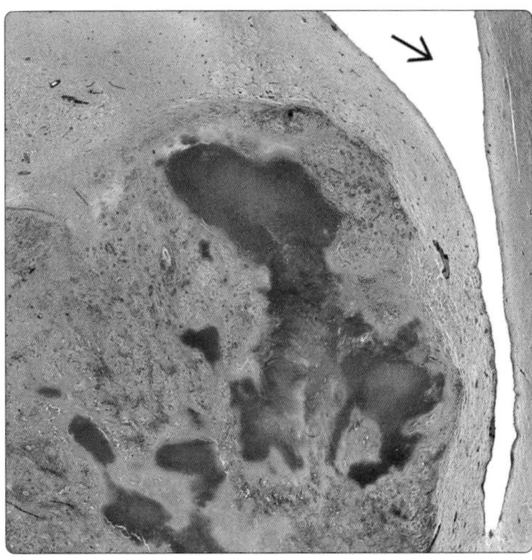

(Left) *Basilar TB meningitis ➡ and tuberculomas ➡ often coexist in infections with M. tuberculosis. Note the affected middle cerebral artery and the resultant basal ganglia infarcts ➡.* **(Right)** *This tuberculoma of the hypothalamus caused by M. tuberculosis infection has central caseous necrosis with distinctive serpiginous borders and, in some cases, a blue hue due to karyorrhectic debris. This lesion causes severe edema and tissue bulges into the 3rd ventricle ➡.*

Rim of Multinucleated Giant Cells

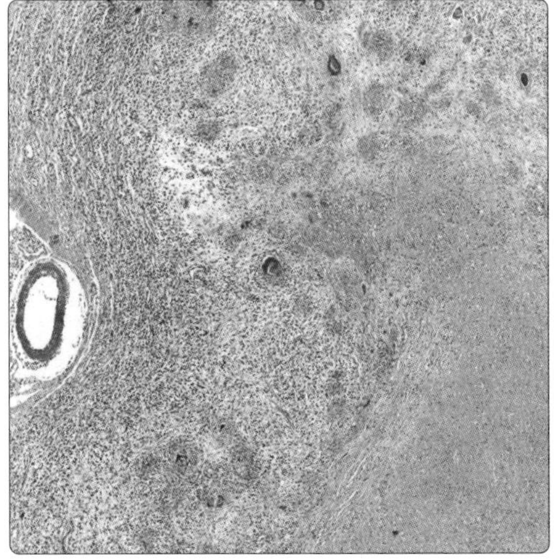

Small Tuberculous Granuloma

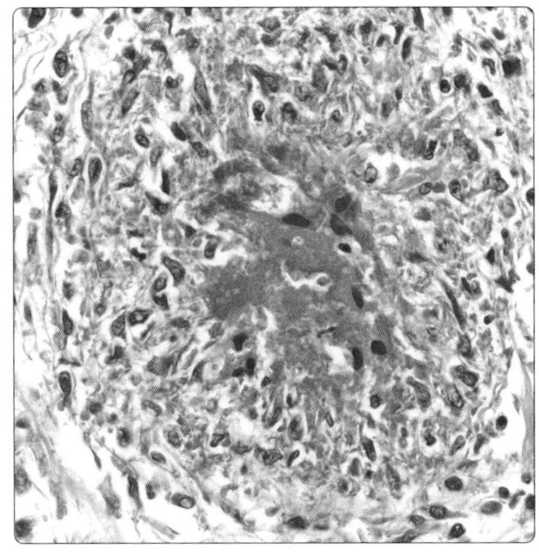

(Left) *Lesions such as this, with chronic inflammation and extensive central caseation necrosis, are highly suspect for tuberculosis caused by M. tuberculosis and very unlikely to be sarcoidosis. Note the numerous multinucleated giant cells.* **(Right)** *Caseation necrosis is seen here as densely eosinophilic necrotic debris within a small tuberculous granuloma caused by M. tuberculosis. Intragranuloma necrosis also can occur in sarcoidosis but is usually less extensive than in TB.*

Langhans Giant Cell

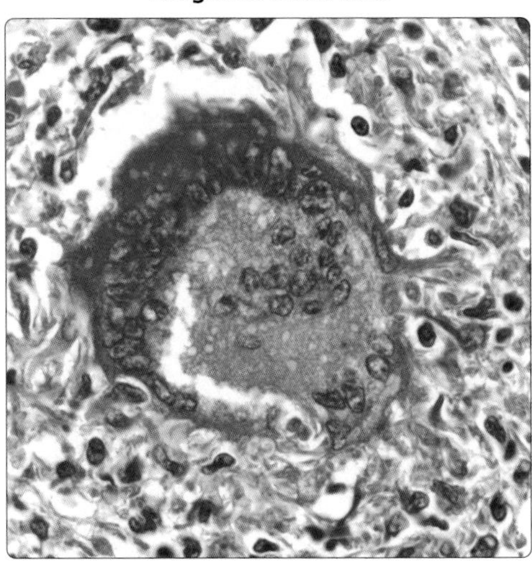

Fibrous Capsule

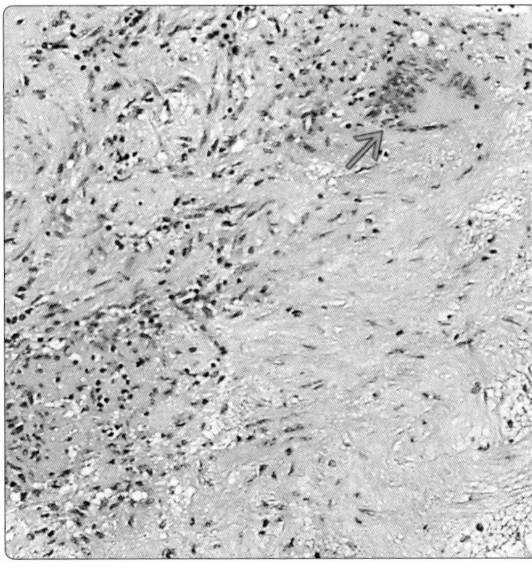

(Left) *Nuclei in tuberculosis caused by M. tuberculosis are often concentrated at the periphery in giant cells of the so-called Langhans type.* **(Right)** *The edge of a developed tuberculoma is a fibrous capsule containing multinucleated giant cells ➡ and a chronic inflammatory cell infiltrate.*

Nonnecrotic Granuloma

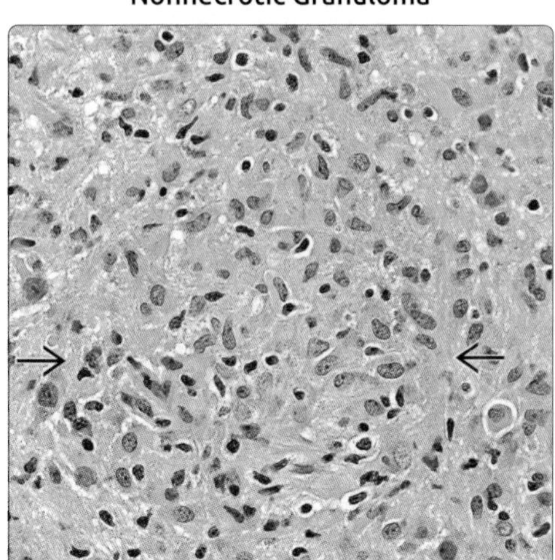

Plasma Cells

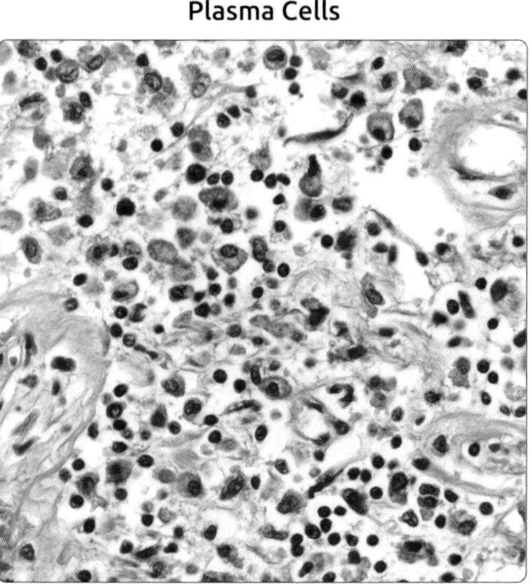

(Left) *Granulomas in tuberculosis in infections caused by M. tuberculosis may be subtle and nonnecrotic* →. *Distinguishing these cases from those of sarcoidosis is impossible without culture or PCR evidence of tuberculous infection.* **(Right)** *Plasma cells are admixed with lymphocytes at the edge of a tuberculoma, but eosinophils are generally inconspicuous, unlike parasitic infections, in which they may be numerous.*

Binucleate Plasma Cells

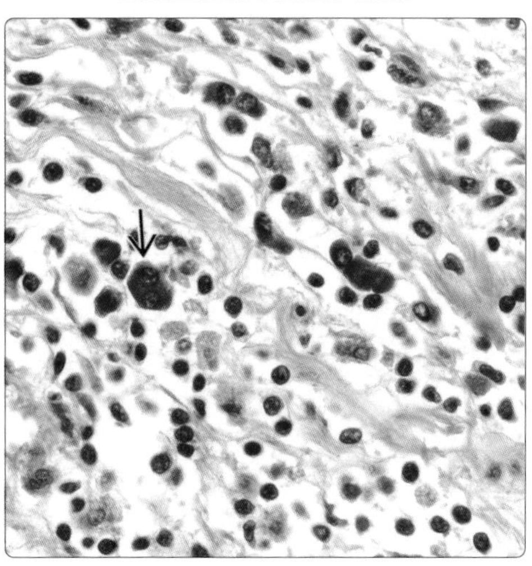

Rim Enhancement

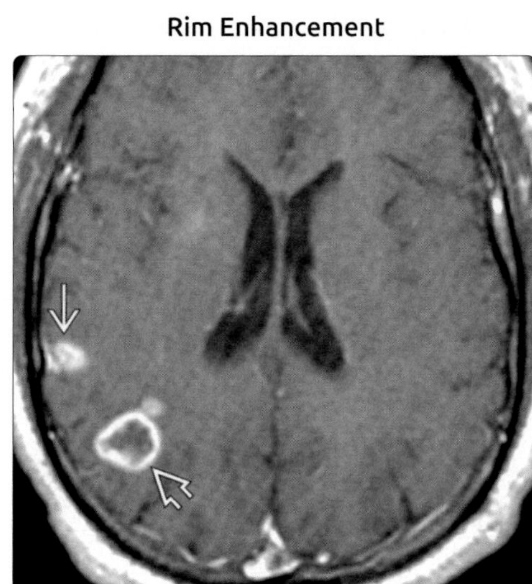

(Left) *Plasma cells within the capsule of a tuberculoma caused by M. tuberculosis can have features of activation, i.e., large, even binucleate nuclei* → *and darkly basophilic cytoplasm.* **(Right)** *Axial T1 C+ MR shows homogeneous, nodular enhancement typical of noncaseating tuberculoma* → *and rim enhancement with central necrosis in a caseating counterpart* →, *due to M. tuberculosis infection.*

Rare Acid-Fast Bacillus

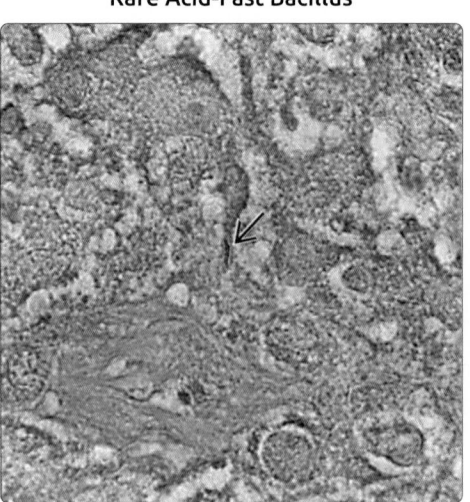

Numerous Acid-Fast Bacilli

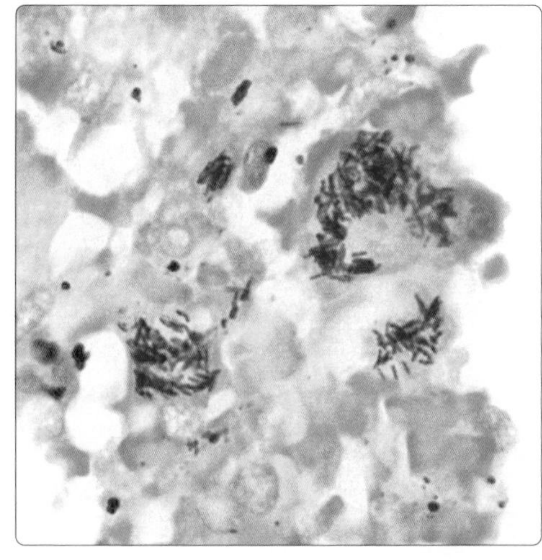

(Left) *Acid-fast organisms of M. tuberculosis can be difficult, if not impossible, to locate in CNS tuberculosis, especially in tuberculomas where the infection is well contained. The single organism in this microscopic field* → *could be easily overlooked.* **(Right)** *Numerous acid-fast bacilli are the exception, not the rule, in most cases of infection with M. tuberculosis unless the host is experiencing an overwhelming infection due to poor host defense.*

Pott Disease

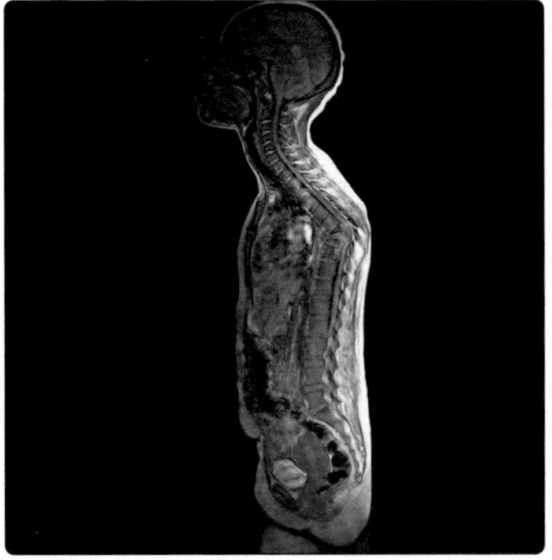

Thoracic TB

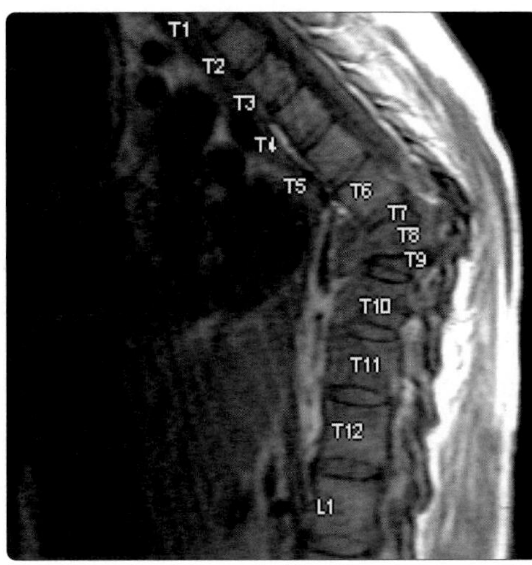

(Left) *Pott disease is a form of tuberculous infection caused by M. tuberculosis that involves the spine, causing collapse of vertebral bodies and deformity known as gibbus. A high index of suspicion is necessary for TB diagnosis, especially in nonendemic areas of the world.* **(Right)** *This example of tuberculosis of the spine caused by M. tuberculosis resulted in severe damage to thoracic vertebrae T7, T8, and T9. Spine is involved in a high percentage of skeletal TB cases.*

Multinucleated Giant Gell

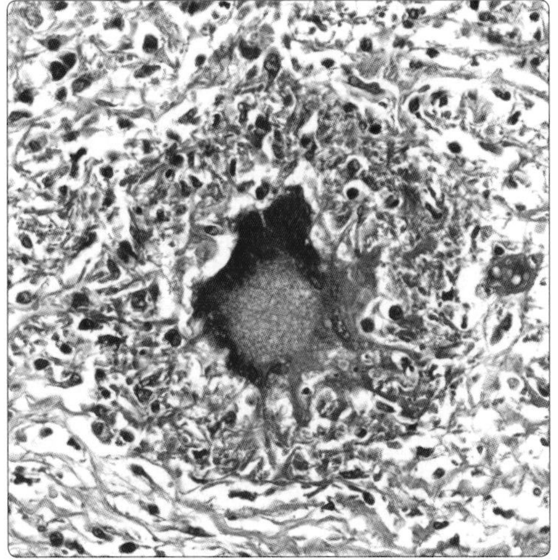

Mycobacterial Pseudotumor

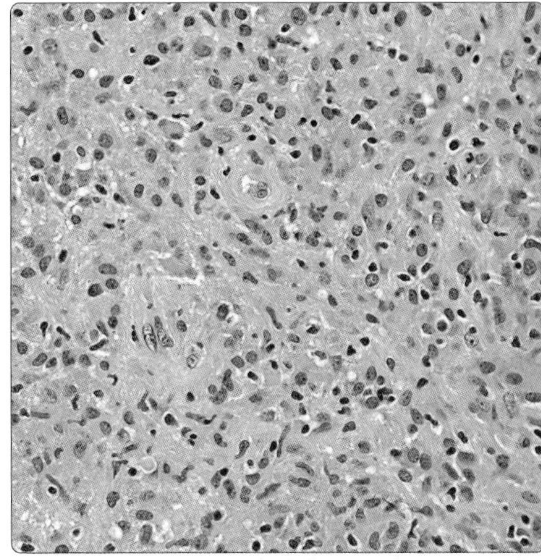

(Left) *Langhans-type multinucleated giant cells can be seen in tuberculous granulomas caused by M. tuberculosis, including those infections in skeletal sites.* **(Right)** *Occasionally, Mycobacterium other than M. tuberculosis are the cause of a CNS lesion. This pseudotumor in the CNS was composed of sheets of epithelioid histiocytes and contained innumerable Mycobacterium avium-intracellulare.*

Epithelioid Histiocytes

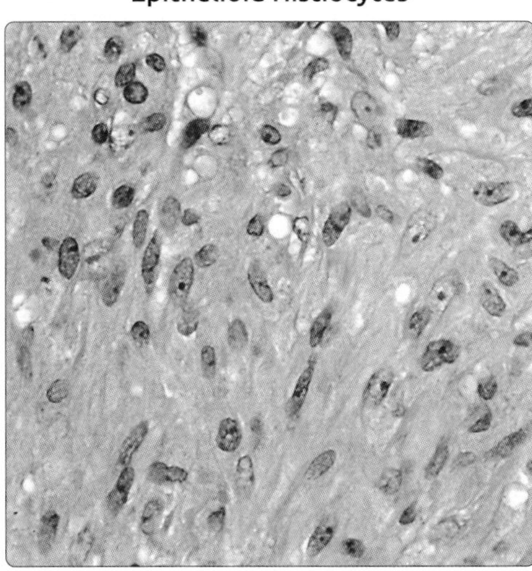

M. avium-intracellulare

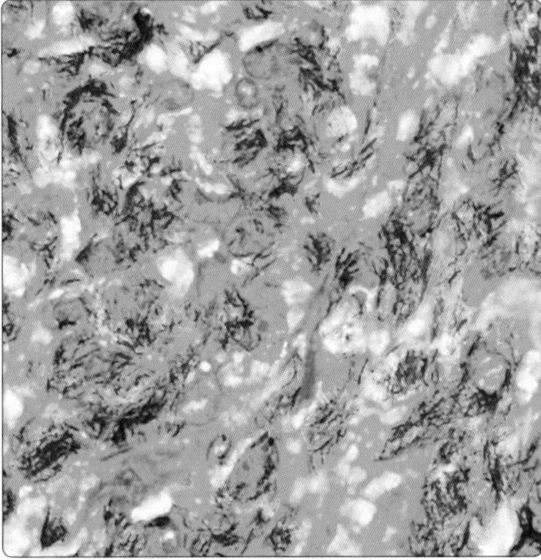

(Left) *This type of infectious pseudotumor in the CNS is composed of sheets of epithelioid histiocytes with distinct nucleoli, open nuclear chromatin, and abundant eosinophilic cytoplasm. These histiocytes often contain innumerable Mycobacterium avium-intracellulare.* **(Right)** *Acid-fast bacilli in large numbers fill histiocytes in this CNS mycobacterial spindle cell pseudotumor in a patient with AIDS. The organisms in this variant of tuberculosis are M. avium-intracellulare, not M. tuberculosis.*

Herpes Simplex Encephalitis

KEY FACTS

ETIOLOGY/PATHOGENESIS

- Herpes simplex virus (HSV) encephalitis is a hemorrhagic, necrotizing central nervous system infection by HSV
- Most common cause of sporadic fatal encephalitis
- Most patients immunocompetent

CLINICAL ISSUES

- Most cases show fever, focal neurological deficits, significant alteration in level of consciousness, psychiatric symptoms, cognitive defects

IMAGING

- MR is more sensitive than CT, shows hyperintense medial temporal, inferior frontal lobe involvement
- Limbic system involved including cingulate gyri, insular cortex, with basal ganglia sparing
- Bilateral involvement usual but may be asymmetric

MICROSCOPIC

- Hemorrhagic, necrotizing encephalitis
- Neutrophilic, lymphocytic, microglial influx with tissue destruction
- Viral inclusions, with Cowdry A owl's eye herpetic inclusion classic
- Later stages of disease may show mostly macrophages, rare viral inclusions
- End stages of disease show rarefaction, cavitation of tissue
- Pseudoischemic form seen in overwhelming infections in immunocompromised individuals

ANCILLARY TESTS

- CSF PCR diagnostic gold standard for diagnosis
  - Test may be negative early in course of HSV; repeat testing should be considered if HSV suspected
- Use of CNS biopsy has been largely obviated by CSF PCR testing

TOP DIFFERENTIAL DIAGNOSES

- Other types of viral encephalitis

Asymmetric Involvement

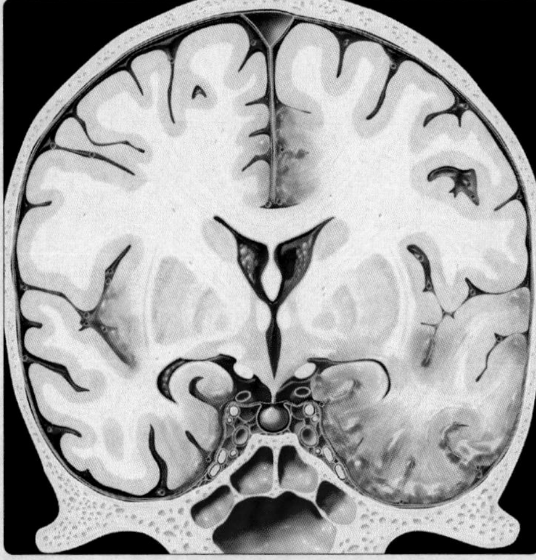

Owl's Eye Herpetic Inclusions

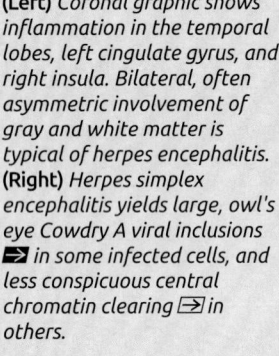

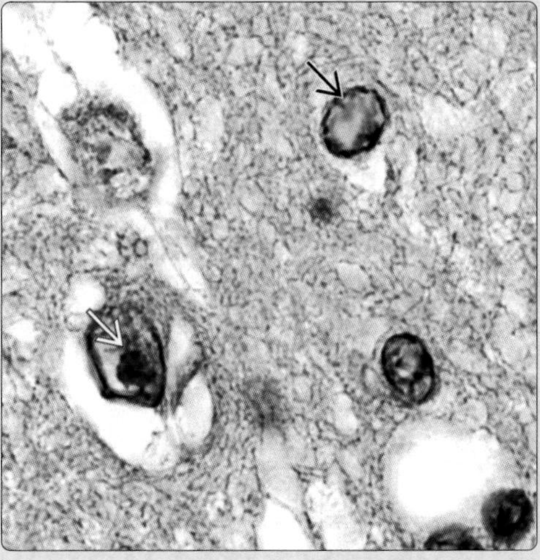

(Left) *Coronal graphic shows inflammation in the temporal lobes, left cingulate gyrus, and right insula. Bilateral, often asymmetric involvement of gray and white matter is typical of herpes encephalitis.* **(Right)** *Herpes simplex encephalitis yields large, owl's eye Cowdry A viral inclusions* ➡ *in some infected cells, and less conspicuous central chromatin clearing* ⇨ *in others.*

Herpes Simplex Virus Immunostaining

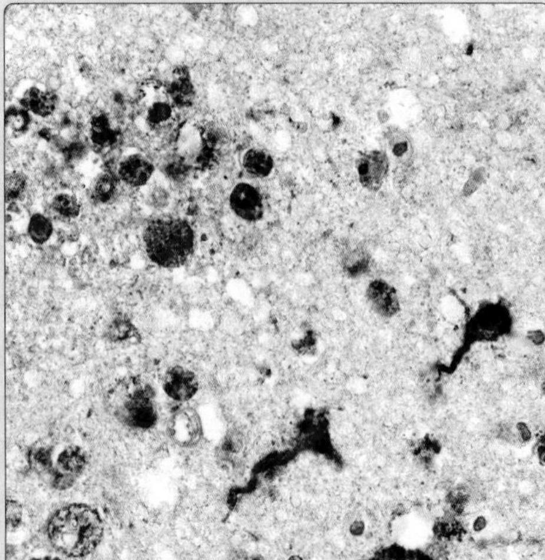

Inclusion Immunoreactive by HSV IHC

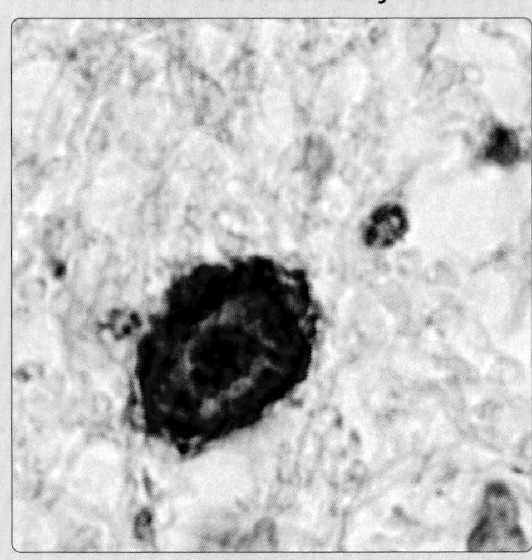

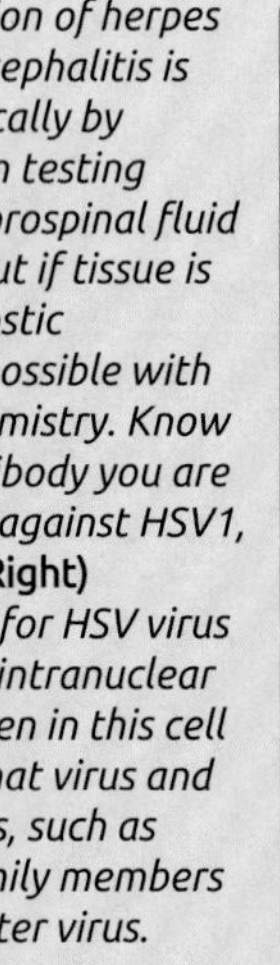

(Left) *Confirmation of herpes simplex virus encephalitis is often made clinically by polymerase chain testing (PCR) from cerebrospinal fluid (CSF) samples, but if tissue is obtained, diagnostic confirmation is possible with immunohistochemistry. Know whether the antibody you are using is directed against HSV1, HSV2, or both.* **(Right)** *Immunostaining for HSV virus verifies that the intranuclear viral inclusion seen in this cell is produced by that virus and not another virus, such as other herpes family members like varicella zoster virus.*

Herpes Simplex Encephalitis

TERMINOLOGY

Abbreviations

- Herpes simplex virus (HSV) encephalitis

Definitions

- Hemorrhagic, necrotizing central nervous system infection by herpes simplex virus

ETIOLOGY/PATHOGENESIS

Infectious Agents

- Herpes simplex virus type 1 (HSV1): Most common cause of HSV
- Disease typically caused by reactivation of virus in immunocompetent patients
- HSV relatively uncommon in HIV(+) population

CLINICAL ISSUES

Epidemiology

- Incidence
  - HSV most frequent cause of sporadic viral encephalitis
  - No seasonal predilection; no animal or insect vector
  - Patients usually not immunocompromised, although more severe forms of HSV occur in severely immunocompromised patients, including those with HIV(+)

Site

- HSV shows predilection for frontal, temporal lobes, limbic system including cingulate gyri and insular cortex
- Disease usually bilateral but may be asymmetric
  - Asymmetrical or atypical locations more likely to prompt biopsy
- Brainstem predominance uncommon

Presentation

- HSV encephalitis
  - Encephalopathy or focal neurological symptoms, plus fever
  - Encephalitis shows more significant alterations in level of consciousness, more psychiatric symptoms and cognitive defects than viral meningitis
  - Usually caused by HSV1
  - Atypical presentations in immunocompromised patients: Fewer focal neurological deficits, diffuse nonnecrotizing encephalitis involving hemispheres and brainstem
- Brainstem infection
  - Neuroophthalmologic findings in most patients
  - Cranial nerve deficits in majority
  - Fever in majority
  - Quadriplegia unusual
  - Usually caused by HSV1 but much less frequent than frontal/temporal lobe type
- Herpes simplex meningitis (formerly recurrent Mollaret meningitis)
  - Infection due to HSV2
  - Usually in adults
  - Aseptic meningitis occurs in ~ 1/3 of females with primary HSV2 genital infection
- Fetal intrauterine or perinatal infection
  - HSV2 genital herpetic infection transmitted during vaginal birth
    - Risk to fetus reduced with cesarean section
  - Rare, but devastating
  - May be disseminated systemic infection or encephalitis only
  - Risk only 1% if mother is HSV2 seropositive but without genital infection

Treatment

- Drugs
  - Acyclovir
    - Should be started immediately if HSV suspected

Prognosis

- HSV devastating disorder
  - 1/2 of patients either die or left with major neurological deficits
- HSV aseptic meningitis mild, self-limited
  - Minority of patients require hospitalization

IMAGING

MR Findings

- Best imaging tool; usually positive 24-48 hours earlier than CT
- Hyperintense medial temporal, inferior frontal cortex involvement
- Involvement of other limbic areas such as cingulate gyrus, insular region highly suggestive of diagnosis
- Involvement of contralateral temporal lobe highly suggestive of diagnosis
- Disease may be asymmetrical
- Basal ganglia sparing is typical
- Subacute blood products may be seen in later stages of infection
- Neonatal encephalitis may be focal or multifocal, involving any lobe(s)

CT Findings

- CT often normal early in disease course

MACROSCOPIC

General Features

- Temporal lobe necrosis, hemorrhage
- Temporal lobe rarefaction, cavitation in advanced cases

MICROSCOPIC

Histologic Features

- HSV: Hemorrhagic, necrotizing parenchymal infection
- Neutrophilic and lymphocytic meningeal infiltrates, may be intense
  - Perivascular lymphocytes, some highly activated
  - Diffuse permeation of necrotic parenchyma by neutrophils
- Parenchymal necrosis
  - Immunocompromised patients: Widespread "red-dead" neurons with scant/absent inflammation simulate infarction (pseudoischemic form)
- Profuse microglial influx in response to tissue damage
  - Neuronophagia

- Neuronal apoptosis results from direct viral injury, not dependent on inflammatory T-cell responses
- Inflammation and tissue destruction predominantly cortical but may extend into subgyral white matter
- Viral inclusions in neurons, astrocytes, oligodendrocytes
- Viral inclusions confined to acute and subacute phases
    - Remote stages of disease with loss of viral inclusions
- Subset of larger cells show Cowdry A, owl's eye herpetic inclusions without cell enlargement (i.e., without cytomegaly as in cytomegalovirus infections)
- Infected oligodendrocytes show violaceous viral inclusions with beading of nuclear membrane and virus filling nucleus without discrete inclusions
- Cavitation in late stages of disease, with variably persistent lymphocytic inflammation

ANCILLARY TESTS

Cytology

- Viral inclusions yield nuclear enlargement and eosinophilic owl's eye Cowdry A herpetic inclusions

Immunohistochemistry

- Usually positive for HSV1
    - Significantly larger numbers of cells immunopositive than those with viral inclusions
    - Most immunoreactivity in inclusions and nucleus, but some in cytoplasm as cell lysis begins
- Many commercial antibodies are directed against HSV1 or HSV2, not both; recognize this when ordering immunostain

PCR

- Diagnostic gold standard is cerebrospinal fluid (CSF) HSV PCR
- In CSF: 96-98% sensitive
- In cases with negative results but high clinical suspicion, should be repeated in CSF after 3-7 days, since testing may be negative in 1st days of illness
- In 1 large study, 7.6% of 1,224 CSF specimens were positive for HSV DNA
    - CSF HSV DNA positive patients had meningitis (52%), encephalitis (26%), neonatal infection (17%), or nonclassifiable disease (5%)
    - 17% of HSV patients had mild or atypical disease characterized by absence of focal findings and slow progression in absence of antiviral therapy

Serologic Testing

- HSV serology may help define whether HSV is primary or reactivated infection, although clinical features, therapy, and prognosis are similar

DIFFERENTIAL DIAGNOSIS

Paraneoplastic Limbic Encephalitis

- Usually neuronal antibodies in serum and CSF
- More protracted clinical course than HSV, less fever
- Usually seen with carcinoma of lung in adult patients

Other Viral Encephalitides

- Usually lack frontal/temporal, limbic distribution
- Negative for CSF HSV PCR
- Negative for positive immunohistochemical reaction for antibodies against HSV1/2

Acute Infarction

- Lacks intense leptomeningeal, perivascular inflammation
- CSF PCR (HSV)(-)
- IHC against HSV1/2(-)
- Vascular distribution of involvement (i.e., in territory of middle, posterior cerebral artery or branches)
- Unassociated with fever or flu-like illness

DIAGNOSTIC CHECKLIST

Pathologic Interpretation Pearls

- Especially in immunocompromised patients, HSV can present with pseudoischemic appearance due to widespread "red-dead" neurons
    - Inflammation in such cases can be limited

SELECTED REFERENCES

1. Ericsdotter AC et al: Reactivation of herpes simplex type 1 in pneumococcal meningitis. J Clin Virol. 66:100-2, 2015
2. Hebant B et al: Absence of Pleocytosis in Cerebrospinal Fluid does not Exclude Herpes Simplex Virus Encephalitis in Elderly Adults. J Am Geriatr Soc. 63(6):1278-9, 2015
3. Lo Presti A et al: Herpes simplex reactivation or postinfectious inflammatory response after epilepsy surgery: Case report and review of the literature. Surg Neurol Int. 6:47, 2015
4. Pfender N et al: Reactivation of herpesvirus under fingolimod: A case of severe herpes simplex encephalitis. Neurology. 84(23):2377-8, 2015
5. Christman MP et al: Recurrence of herpes simplex encephalitis associated with temozolomide chemoradiation for malignant glioma: a case report and review of the literature. Oxf Med Case Reports. 2014(1):1-4, 2014
6. George BP et al: Encephalitis hospitalization rates and inpatient mortality in the United States, 2000-2010. PLoS One. 9(9):e104169, 2014
7. Sermer DJ et al: Herpes simplex encephalitis as a complication of whole-brain radiotherapy: a case report and review of the literature. Case Rep Oncol. 7(3):774-9, 2014
8. Tan IL et al: Atypical manifestations and poor outcome of herpes simplex encephalitis in the immunocompromised. Neurology. 79(21):2125-32, 2012
9. Fernandes AF et al: Extra-temporal involvement in herpes simplex encephalitis. J Clin Neurosci. 17(9):1221-3, 2010
10. Livorsi D et al: Brainstem encephalitis: an unusual presentation of herpes simplex virus infection. J Neurol. 257(9):1432-7, 2010
11. Bale JF Jr: Fetal infections and brain development. Clin Perinatol. 36(3):639-53, 2009
12. Big C et al: Viral infections of the central nervous system: a case-based review. Clin Med Res. 7(4):142-6, 2009
13. Baringer JR: Herpes simplex infections of the nervous system. Neurol Clin. 26(3):657-74, viii, 2008
14. Berger JR et al: Neurological complications of herpes simplex virus type 2 infection. Arch Neurol. 65(5):596-600, 2008
15. Elbers JM et al: A 12-year prospective study of childhood herpes simplex encephalitis: is there a broader spectrum of disease? Pediatrics. 119(2):e399-407, 2007
16. Naito K et al: Herpes simplex virus type-1 meningoencephalitis showing disseminated cortical lesions. Intern Med. 46(11):761-3, 2007
17. Tyler KL: Herpes simplex virus infections of the central nervous system: encephalitis and meningitis, including Mollaret's. Herpes. 11 Suppl 2:57A-64A, 2004
18. DeBiasi RL et al: Central nervous system apoptosis in human herpes simplex virus and cytomegalovirus encephalitis. J Infect Dis. 186(11):1547-57, 2002
19. DeBiasi RL et al: Use of PCR for the diagnosis of herpesvirus infections of the central nervous system. J Clin Virol. 25 Suppl 1:S5-11, 2002
20. Erdem G et al: Intracranial hemorrhage in herpes simplex encephalitis: an unusual presentation. Pediatr Neurol. 27(3):221-3, 2002
21. Kleinschmidt-DeMasters BK et al: Polymerase chain reaction as a diagnostic adjunct in herpesvirus infections of the nervous system. Brain Pathol. 11(4):452-64, 2001

Basal Ganglia Sparing

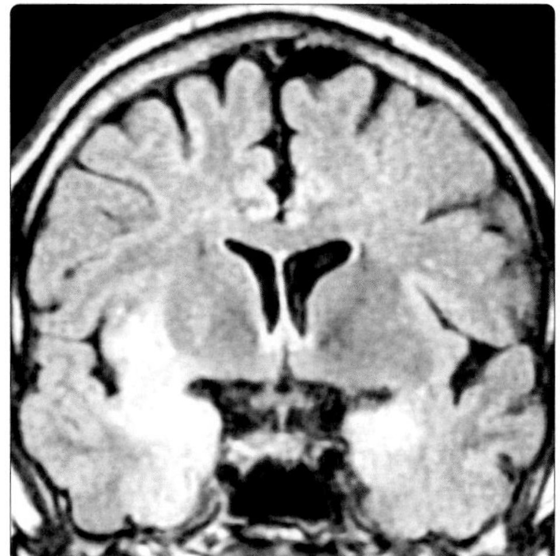

Asymmetric Enhancement

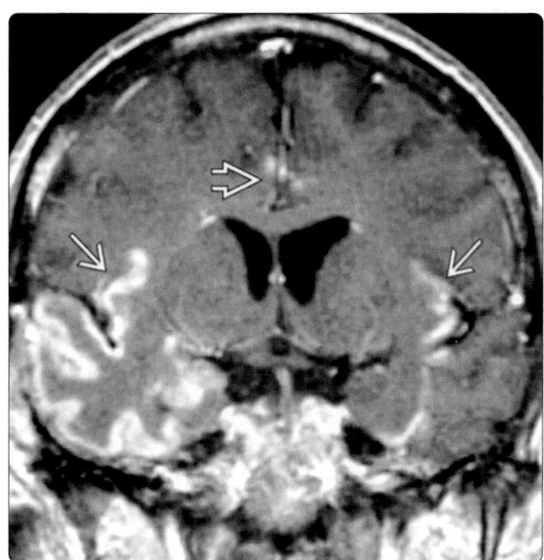

(Left) *Coronal FLAIR MR shows classic bilateral, asymmetric involvement of the medial temporal lobes and right insula in this 46-year-old woman with herpes encephalitis. Basal ganglia sparing is typical.* **(Right)** *Coronal T1 C+ MR shows striking bilateral but asymmetric enhancement in the temporal lobe and insular cortex ➡. Subtle lesions in the cingulate gyri ➡ are classic for HSV.*

Intense Microgliosis

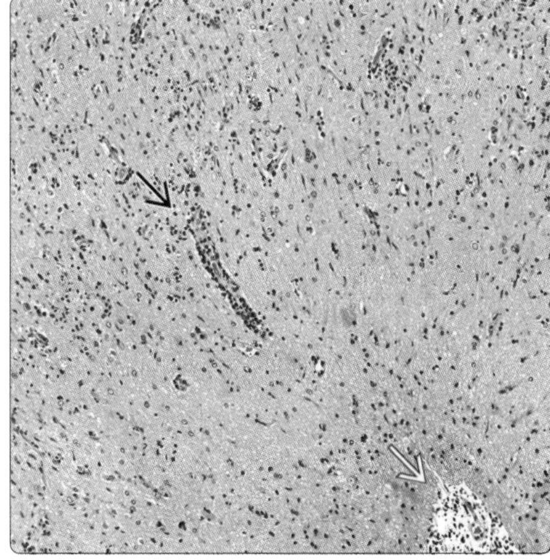

Microglial Cluster

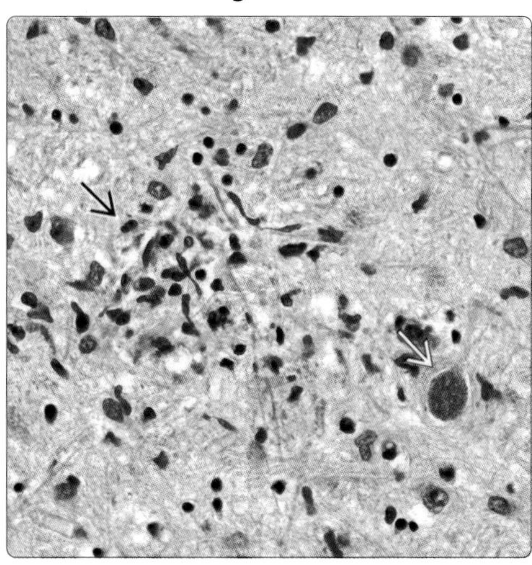

(Left) *Early phases of infection can produce intense microgliosis and perivascular lymphocytic infiltrates ➡. The pial surface in the section of the temporal lobe is at bottom right ➡.* **(Right)** *HSV infection occasionally involves the brainstem, as in this section of the pontine tegmentum. Note the microglial cluster ➡ typical of most viral encephalitides. A large intact neuron is present ➡.*

Necrotizing, Hemorrhagic Encephalitis

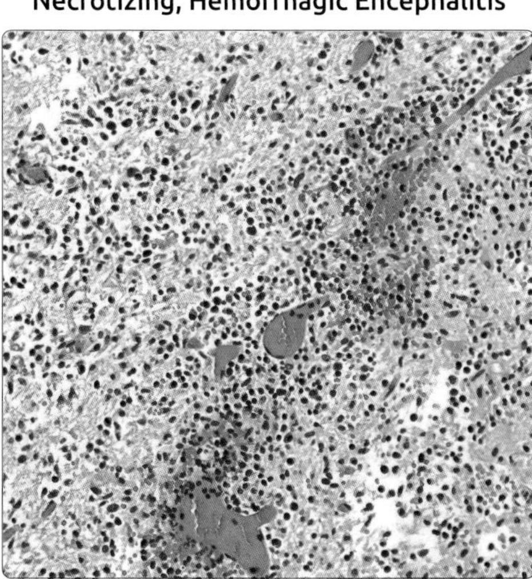

Neutrophilic Response in Viral Infection

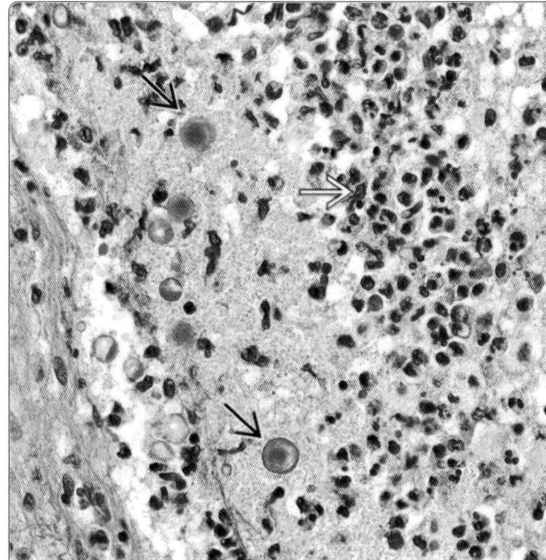

(Left) *HSV is a necrotizing, hemorrhagic parenchymal infection, potentially with severe tissue destruction.* **(Right)** *HSV may elicit an intense neutrophilic infiltrate ➡, not to be confused with a pyogenic response to a bacterium. Subpial corpora amylacea ➡ caught up in the process should not be mistaken for infectious organisms such as the Coccidioides species.*

(Left) *Vascular necrosis is common in HSV with extensive neutrophilic infiltrates* ➡*. This is not a primary vasculitis since the necrotic vessel lies within a zone of parenchymal necrosis* ⇨*.* **(Right)** *In overwhelming HSV infections, especially those in immunocompromised patients, pauciinflammatory necrosis of parenchyma is accompanied by "red-dead" neurons* ⇨ *simulating those of an infarct. This is the so-called pseudoischemic form of infection.*

Vascular Necrosis

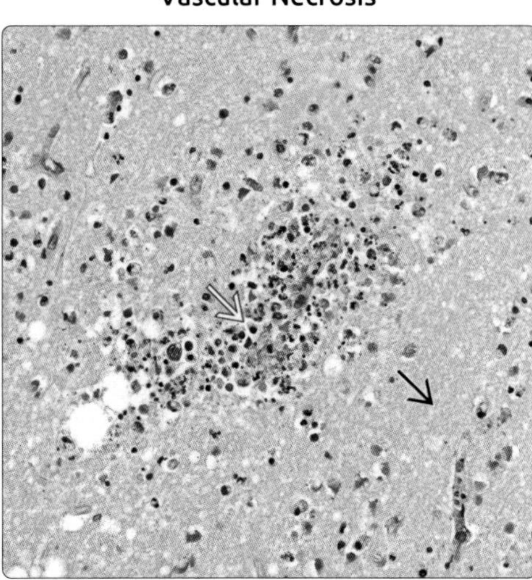

Simulating Infarct, Immunocompromised Hosts

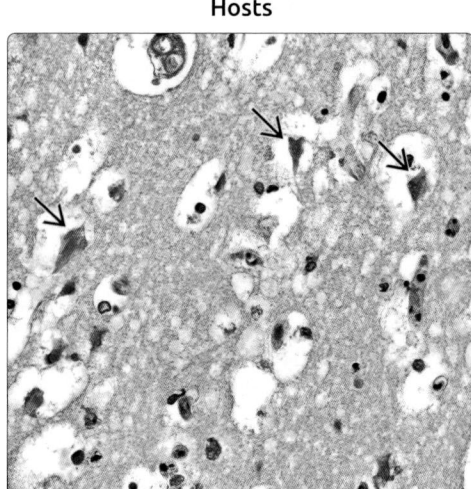

(Left) *HSV produces intense inflammation that can be sufficiently profuse to prompt consideration of vasculitis, or even lymphoma.* **(Right)** *Highly reactive immunoblasts* ⇨ *and plasmacytoid lymphocytes* ➡ *in HSV may create confusion with lymphoma.*

Striking Perivascular Inflammation

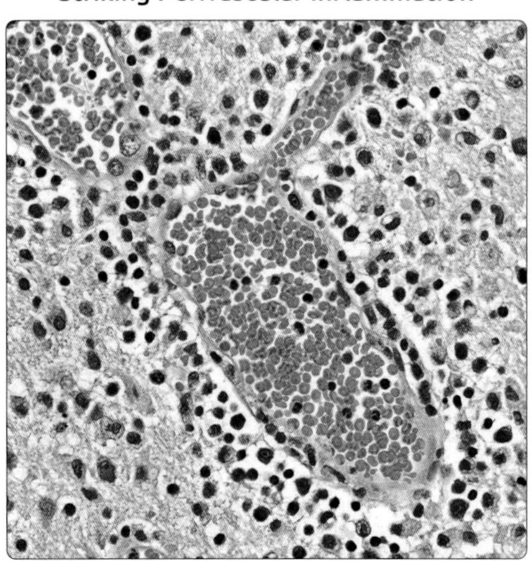

Immunoblasts Simulating Lymphoma

(Left) *In HSV, cells that are identified in later stages of infection just prior to cell lysis can have fragmented host nuclear chromatin and viral particles that fill the nucleus, yielding a violaceous, less discrete, non-Cowdry A inclusion* ⇨*.* **(Right)** *In HSV, peripheralization and beading of host cell nuclear chromatin* ⇨ *are present in some infected cells, while others have discrete Cowdry A inclusions* ➡*.*

Infected Cell, Later Stages of Infection

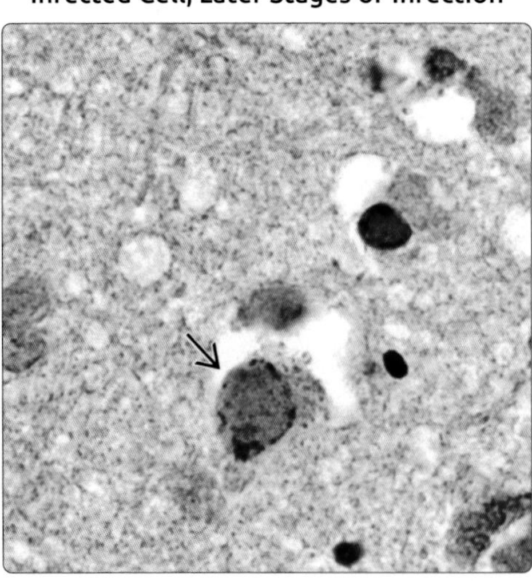

Viral Inclusions

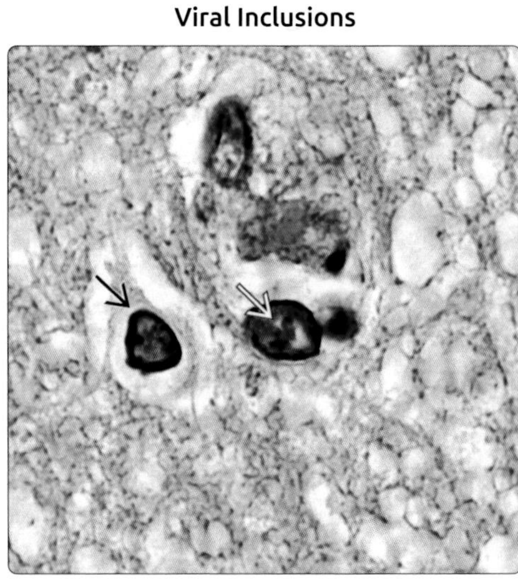

Cowdry A Inclusions, Immunohistochemistry

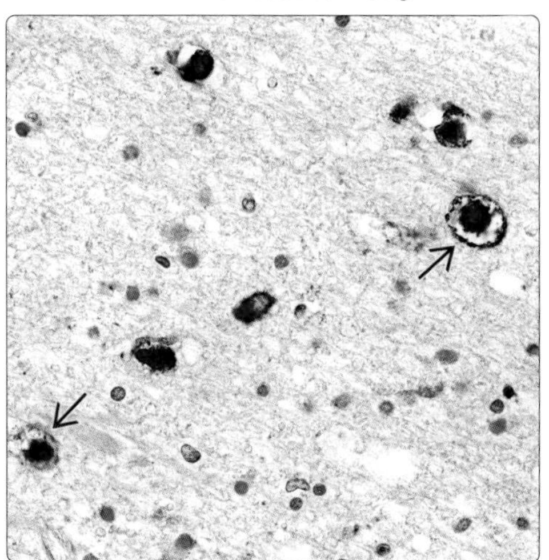

Cytoplasmic Immunostaining

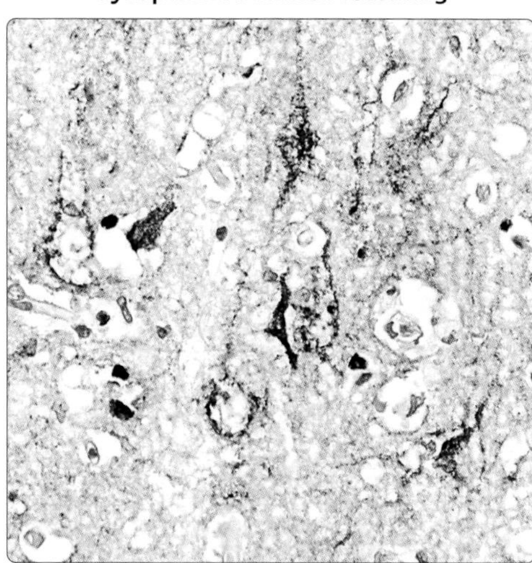

(Left) *Multiple cells, 2 with Cowdry A inclusions* ⇒, *are immunopositive for HSV.* **(Right)** *In overwhelming HSV infections seen in immunocompromised patients, the so-called pseudoischemic form of disease, "red-dead" neurons may be filled with HSV1/2 IHC(+) particles, both intranuclear and intracytoplasmic, just antecedent to cell lysis.*

CD68(+) Microglial Activation

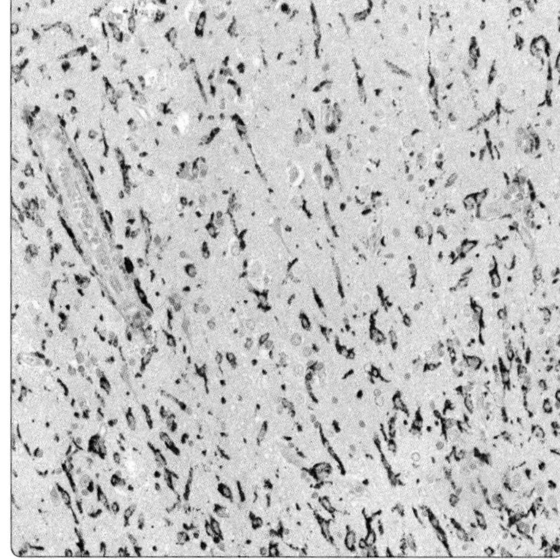

CD68(+) Macrophages

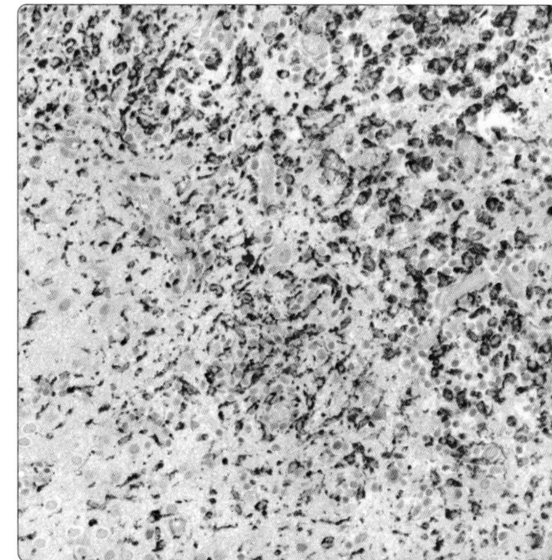

(Left) *Activated, and hence CD68 immunoreactive, microglia are prominent during early stages of HSV.* **(Right)** *CD68(+) macrophages are active in areas of tissue necrosis in HSV.*

Remote Herpes Simplex Virus Encephalitis

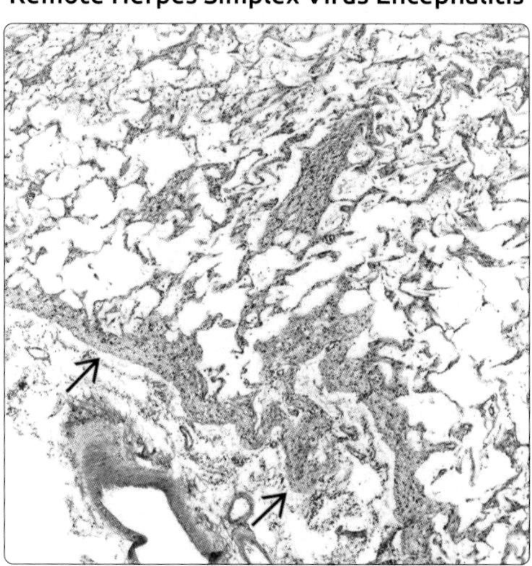

Tissue Rarefaction

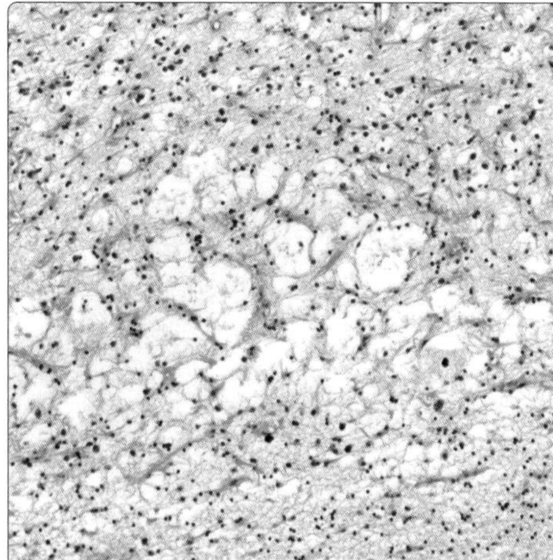

(Left) *Extensive temporal lobe tissue cavitation characterizes the late-stage disease of HSV encephalitis, in which only leptomeningeal vessels and a thin layer of most superficial cerebral cortex beneath the pial surface* ⇒ *remain.* **(Right)** *Nonspecific loose, spongy tissue remains in the chronic state of HSV.*

Progressive Multifocal Leukoencephalopathy

KEY FACTS

TERMINOLOGY

- CNS demyelinating disorder caused by lytic viral infection of oligodendrocytes by John Cunningham (JC) polyomavirus

ETIOLOGY/PATHOGENESIS

- Due to reactivation of latent infection by JC neurotropic virus, usually in immunocompromised host

CLINICAL ISSUES

- Sensory deficits, hemianopsia, cognitive dysfunction, aphasia, gait disturbance
- Seizures less common

IMAGING

- Multifocal white matter lesions predominantly in subcortical cerebral white matter, cerebellar peduncles
- Gray matter lesions in basal ganglia, thalamus

MACROSCOPIC

- Small ovoid, yellow-tan lesions maximal near cortical gray-white matter junction
- Later lesions coalescent, large, depressed

MICROSCOPIC

- Demyelination, oligodendrocyte loss, nuclear oligodendrocyte inclusions
- Virally infected cells often Ki-67(+), p53(+)
- Cytologically bizarre enlarged astrocytes in context of high Ki-67 and p53 staining indices can suggest high-grade glioma

ANCILLARY TESTS

- Detection of JC virus DNA in cerebrospinal fluid establishes diagnosis

(Left) *As illustrated in a noncontrast T1WI image ➔, the white matter-based lesions of progressive multifocal leukoencephalopathy (PML) exert little mass effect.* **(Right)** *Axial FLAIR MR in a patient with PML shows right subcortical hyperintensity sparing adjacent gray matter (GM) ➔ without mass effect and a 2nd small lesion ➔.*

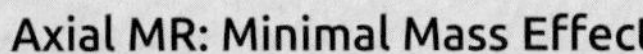

Axial MR: Minimal Mass Effect

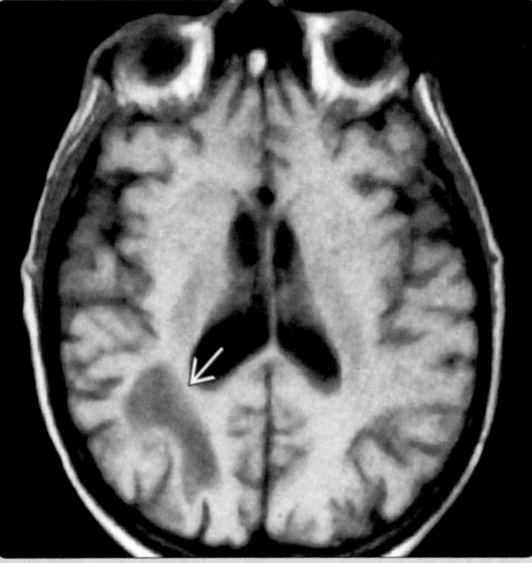

Axial MR: Multiple Lesions

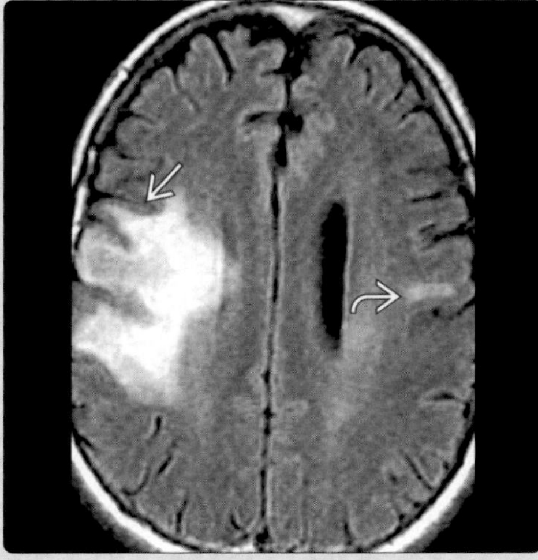

(Left) *Homogenized nuclei of oligodendrocytes are a classic expression of viral infections, such as PML.* **(Right)** *When more dense and hyperchromatic rather than washed-out, infected nuclei may suggest a neoplasm or a glioma, rather than an infectious process.*

Oligodendroglial Viral Inclusions

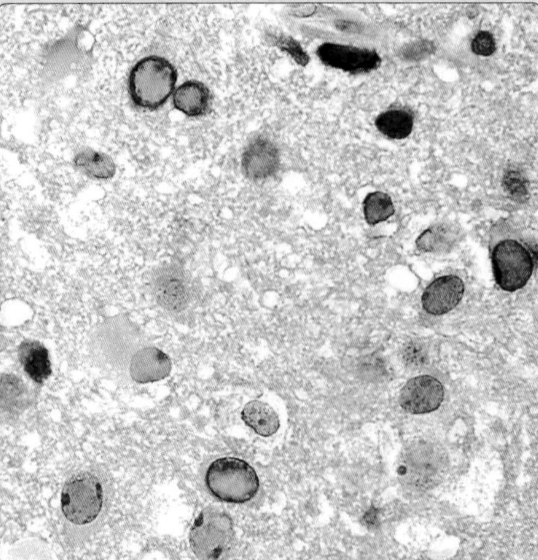

Progressive Multifocal Leukoencephalopathy Simulating Glioma

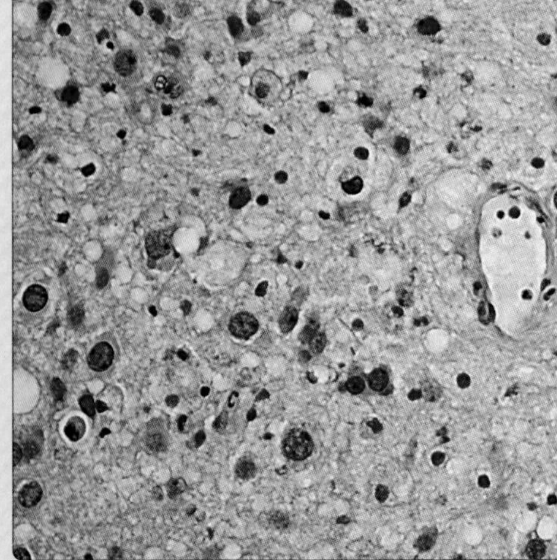

TERMINOLOGY

Abbreviations

- Progressive multifocal leukoencephalopathy (PML)

Definitions

- Opportunistic viral infection of oligodendrocytes by John Cunningham (JC) polyomavirus, resulting in central nervous system demyelination

ETIOLOGY/PATHOGENESIS

Environmental Exposure

- Archetype virus
  - Circulates widely in environment
    - Found in sewage
  - May transform to neurotropic virus via deletion or duplication gene event(s)
- Asymptomatic primary viral infection in childhood
- After initial viral infection, virus thought to be latent in kidneys, bone marrow, lymphoid tissue

Infectious Agents

- Disease caused by reactivation of latent virus, usually in immunocompromised host
- Virus named JC after 1971 isolation of virus from autopsied brain of patient John Cunningham

Impaired Immune Status

- Progressive multifocal leukoencephalopathy most frequently identified in patients with AIDS
  - Estimated to be present in ~ 80% of cases in AIDS patients
- Also occurs in patients on immunosuppressive medications
  - Natalizumab (α4β1 and α4β7 integrin inhibitor)
    - Progressive multifocal leukoencephalopathy can occur with monotherapy
    - Risk of progressive multifocal leukoencephalopathy increases with duration of exposure to natalizumab over first 3 years of treatment
  - Rituximab, usually in combination with other medications
- Collagen vascular diseases
  - Rare in systemic lupus erythematosus, autoimmune vasculitis
  - Very rare in rheumatoid arthritis, multiple sclerosis (without natalizumab), Sjögren disease, solid organ transplantation
- Cancer
  - Originally recognized in patients with hematological malignancies

Immunocompetent Patient

- Rare in this context

CLINICAL ISSUES

Presentation

- Changes in cognition, personality
- Motor deficits, aphasia, gait difficulties, homonymous hemianopsia
- Seizures in small percentage of patients

Treatment

- Plasma exchange or immunoabsorption to hasten clearance of natalizumab (otherwise natalizumab remains active for several months)
  - **I**mmune **r**econstitution **i**nflammatory **s**yndrome (IRIS) may develop days to weeks after plasma exchange, may be severe

Prognosis

- AIDS patients
  - Progressive multifocal leukoencephalopathy fatal prior to advent of AIDS drugs
    - Highly active antiretroviral therapy (HAART)
  - Substantial incidence of stability or improvement after HAART therapy
  - AIDS patients with IRIS (after AIDS drugs) may survive decade(s) without progressive multifocal leukoencephalopathy recurrence
- Majority of patients with progressive multifocal leukoencephalopathy from natalizumab survive
  - Need drug withdrawal and plasma exchange therapy
  - Survivors potentially left with residual defects dependent on lesion location

IMAGING

General Features

- Multiple lesions common
- Subcortical hemispheric white matter or cerebellar peduncle involvement frequent
- Multifocal white matter lesions predominantly in subcortical cerebral white matter, cerebellar peduncles
- Gray matter lesions seen in basal ganglia, thalamus
- Distributions of lesions do not correspond to vascular territories

MR Findings

- Hyperintensities on T2-weighted and FLAIR images
- Hypointensities on T1-weighted images
- Classic lesions devoid of edema, mass effect, contrast enhancement
- Contrast enhancement, edema, mass effect with immune reconstitution syndrome

MACROSCOPIC

Early Stage

- Small, ovoid, yellow-tan demyelinating lesion maximal at cortical gray-white matter junction

Intermediate Stage

- Small lesions coalesce, occupy large volumes of white matter
- Demyelination, preferentially in frontal and parietooccipital regions
- Lesions sometimes in cerebellum, brainstem

Late Stage

- Large depressed lesions in white matter
- Seldom fully cavitated as infarcts

MICROSCOPIC

Histologic Features

- Demyelination
  - Ranges from myelin pallor to severe loss
  - Variably visible on H&E, histochemical stains (e.g., Luxol fast blue), immunohistochemical preparations (e.g., antimyelin basic protein)
  - Associated with loss of oligodendrocytes
- Axonal injury
  - Axonal swellings in severe, early examples
  - Axonal loss (Bielschowsky stain, antineurofilament immunohistochemistry) less than myelin loss
  - No cavitation as in infarct
- Macrophages
  - In areas with marked myelin loss
  - Dispersed throughout areas of active myelin breakdown, perivascular in later stages
  - May be subtle background feature
- Viral inclusions
  - Large, round, infected oligodendrocytes with violaceous nuclear inclusions
    - Viral inclusion fills nucleus
    - Some oligodendrocytes manifest cleared nucleoplasm centrally, marginated chromatin, nuclear enlargement
    - No cytoplasmic inclusions
  - Inclusion-bearing cells maximal at periphery of demyelinating lesions, fewer centrally
  - Inclusions may be lacking in burnt-out cases, or posttreatment with IRIS
  - Virally infected cells often Ki-67(+), p53(+)
- Some large oligodendrocytes with hyperchromatic nuclei with little homogenization
- Lymphocytic inflammation
  - Limited in patients with severe immunocompromise
  - Severe inflammation with few viral inclusions in patients with IRIS
- Neuronal infection (rare)
  - Cerebellar granular neurons
  - Cerebral neurons
    - Fulminant JC virus encephalopathy

ANCILLARY TESTS

Cytology

- Purple ground-glass intranuclear inclusions, oligodendrocytes
- Some large oligodendrocytes with hyperchromatic nuclei with little homogenization
- Large, bizarre nuclei of astrocytes
- Macrophages
- Creutzfeldt cells
  - Multinucleated reactive astrocytes

Immunohistochemistry

- Infected oligodendrocytes, but less so atypical astrocytes, positive for JC or SV40 virus
- Virally infected cells with high Ki-67(+) and p53(+) index

In Situ Hybridization

- Viral inclusions, and to lesser extent atypical astrocytes, positive for JC virus probes

PCR

- Detection of JC virus DNA in cerebrospinal fluid establishes diagnosis

DIFFERENTIAL DIAGNOSIS

Multiple Sclerosis

- No viral inclusions
- Immunohistochemistry and in situ hybridization negative for JC virus
- Burnt-out cases of progressive multifocal leukoencephalopathy may be difficult to distinguish from multiple sclerosis
  - Multiple sclerosis not preferentially seen in immunocompromised patients
- Multiple sclerosis more likely to affect certain anatomical sites
  - Spinal cord
  - Optic nerve
  - Periventricular regions
  - Gray matter, with lesions at gray-white junction (leukocortical) and within gray matter as perivenular or subpial bands of demyelination
    - Immunostaining for myelin basic protein, proteolipid protein necessary to identify most intracortical demyelinative lesions
  - Perivenular and subpial plaques characteristic in most anatomical sites

Infarct

- No viral inclusions
- Ischemic, "red-dead" neurons in acute phase
- Loss of both axons and myelin
- Cavitation in chronic phase
- More cortical based

High-Grade Glioma

- No viral inclusions
- Extensive myelin destruction with macrophage influx rare in untreated tumor
- Cytologically bizarre cells more numerous and associated with other cytologically atypical glial cells

Post-Natalizumab Immune Reconstitution Inflammatory Syndrome

- Occurs in patient receiving natalizumab who develops progressive multifocal leukoencephalopathy, then receives plasma exchange or other therapy to clear the drug
- Occasionally reported in patients after natalizumab discontinued
- IRIS develops, with clearing of virus but can leave large destructive areas of tissue damage
- Large areas of demyelination may be devoid of residual viral inclusions
- Residual viral inclusions often difficult to identify
  - Utilize immunohistochemistry for John Cunningham virus or SV40 virus

Other Virally Mediated Demyelinating Disorders

- Varicella-zoster virus (VZV) encephalitis
  - Viral inclusions in multiple cell types
  - Immunopositive for VZV
  - Immunonegative for SV40, JC virus
  - Usually smaller, less coalescent areas of demyelination
- Human immunodeficiency virus related demyelination

DIAGNOSTIC CHECKLIST

Clinically Relevant Pathologic Features

- Deep white or gray matter location of lesions may lead to negative cerebrospinal fluid JC virus on PCR testing in some patients
- Progressive multifocal leukoencephalopathy has been associated with therapy using several different specific monoclonal antibodies, including
  - Natalizumab
  - Efalizumab
  - Rituximab
- Progressive multifocal leukoencephalopathy due to disturbances of adaptive immunity affecting
  - B cells
  - Antibodies
  - CD4(+) &/or CD8(+) T cells
- No specific therapy for progressive multifocal leukoencephalopathy
- Treatment consists of attempts to reconstitute immune function
  - Progressive multifocal leukoencephalopathy-IRIS may result after drug withdrawal
  - Extensive CD8(+) T cell infiltrates, numerous macrophages within, few or no virally infected cells seen in IRIS lesions

Pathologic Interpretation Pearls

- High Ki-67 and p53 indices, cytologically bizarre astrocytes simulate high-grade astrocytoma

SELECTED REFERENCES

1. Al-Tawfiq JA et al: Progressive multifocal leukoencephalopathy (PML) in a patient with lymphoma treated with rituximab: A case report and literature review. J Infect Public Health. 8(5):493-7, 2015
2. Jelcic I et al: Immunology of progressive multifocal leukoencephalopathy. J Neurovirol. ePub, 2015
3. Vermeer NS et al: Drug-induced progressive multifocal leukoencephalopathy: Lessons learned from contrasting natalizumab and rituximab. Clin Pharmacol Ther. ePub, 2015
4. Fine AJ et al: Progressive multifocal leukoencephalopathy after natalizumab discontinuation. Ann Neurol. 75(1):108-15, 2014
5. Killestein J et al: PML-IRIS during Fingolimod Diagnosed after Natalizumab Discontinuation. Case Rep Neurol Med. 2014:307872, 2014
6. Wüthrich C et al: Natalizumab-associated progressive multifocal leukoencephalopathy in a patient with multiple sclerosis: a postmortem study. J Neuropathol Exp Neurol. 72(11):1043-51, 2013
7. Kleinschmidt-DeMasters BK et al: Update on PML and PML-IRIS occurring in multiple sclerosis patients treated with natalizumab. J Neuropathol Exp Neurol. 71(7):604-17, 2012
8. Metz I et al: Pathology of immune reconstitution inflammatory syndrome in multiple sclerosis with natalizumab-associated progressive multifocal leukoencephalopathy. Acta Neuropathol. 123(2):235-45, 2012
9. Amend KL et al: Incidence of progressive multifocal leukoencephalopathy in patients without HIV. Neurology. 75(15):1326-32, 2010
10. Clifford DB et al: Natalizumab-associated progressive multifocal leukoencephalopathy in patients with multiple sclerosis: lessons from 28 cases. Lancet Neurol. 9(4):438-46, 2010
11. Di Lernia V: Progressive multifocal leukoencephalopathy and antipsoriatic drugs: assessing the risk of immunosuppressive treatments. Int J Dermatol. 49(6):631-5, 2010
12. Lima MA et al: Clinical outcome of long-term survivors of progressive multifocal leukoencephalopathy. J Neurol Neurosurg Psychiatry. 81(11):1288-91, 2010
13. Lysandropoulos AP et al: Demyelination as a complication of new immunomodulatory treatments. Curr Opin Neurol. 23(3):226-33, 2010
14. Paues J et al: Fatal progressive multifocal leukoencephalopathy in a patient with non-Hodgkin lymphoma treated with rituximab. J Clin Virol. 48(4):291-293, 2010
15. Shishido-Hara Y: Progressive multifocal leukoencephalopathy and promyelocytic leukemia nuclear bodies: a review of clinical, neuropathological, and virological aspects of JC virus-induced demyelinating disease. Acta Neuropathol. 120(3):403-17, 2010
16. Sidhu N et al: Unmasking of PML by HAART: unusual clinical features and the role of IRIS. J Neuroimmunol. 219(1-2):100-4, 2010
17. Tan CS et al: JC virus latency in the brain and extraneural organs of patients with and without progressive multifocal leukoencephalopathy. J Virol. 84(18):9200-9, 2010
18. Tan CS et al: Progressive multifocal leukoencephalopathy and other disorders caused by JC virus: clinical features and pathogenesis. Lancet Neurol. 9(4):425-37, 2010
19. Vaklavas C et al: Progressive multifocal leukoencephalopathy in a patient without apparent immunosuppression. Virol J. 7:256, 2010
20. Carson KR et al: Monoclonal antibody-associated progressive multifocal leucoencephalopathy in patients treated with rituximab, natalizumab, and efalizumab: a Review from the Research on Adverse Drug Events and Reports (RADAR) Project. Lancet Oncol. 10(8):816-24, 2009
21. Oberdorfer P et al: Progressive Multifocal Leukoencephalopathy in HIV-Infected Children: A Case Report and Literature Review. Int J Pediatr. 2009:348507, 2009
22. Calabrese LH et al: Progressive multifocal leucoencephalopathy in the rheumatic diseases: assessing the risks of biological immunosuppressive therapies. Ann Rheum Dis. 67 Suppl 3:iii64-5, 2008
23. Kleinschmidt-DeMasters BK et al: Progressive multifocal leukoencephalopathy complicating treatment with natalizumab and interferon beta-1a for multiple sclerosis. N Engl J Med. 353(4):369-74, 2005

(Left) *Early lesions are ovoid, yellow-tan demyelinated foci along the cortical gray-white junction ➡. There is no cavitation.* **(Right)** *Older, grayish lesions of PML are coalescent and depressed ➡.*

Early Lesions

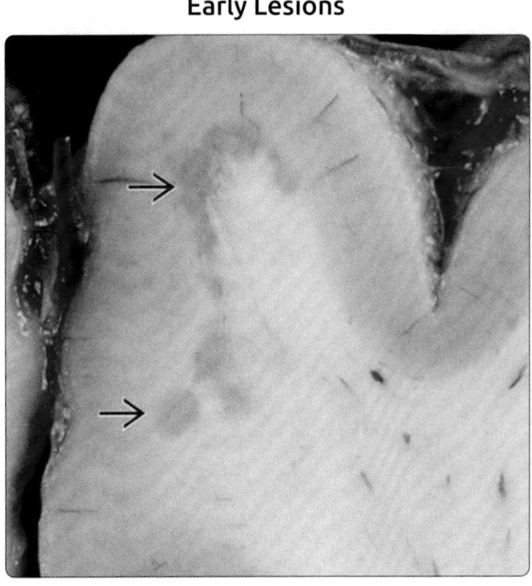

Older Lesions

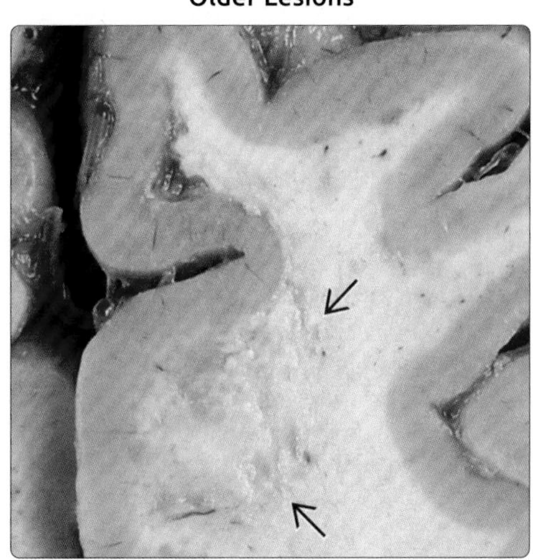

(Left) *Small lesions may be subtle, pale-staining foci in H&E stained sections, with darkly stained nuclei of infected oligodendroglia ➡ serving as clues to the nature of the disease.* **(Right)** *Individual foci ➡ are best identified at low magnification in sections stained for myelin (here, Luxol fast blue).*

Subtle Early Lesions

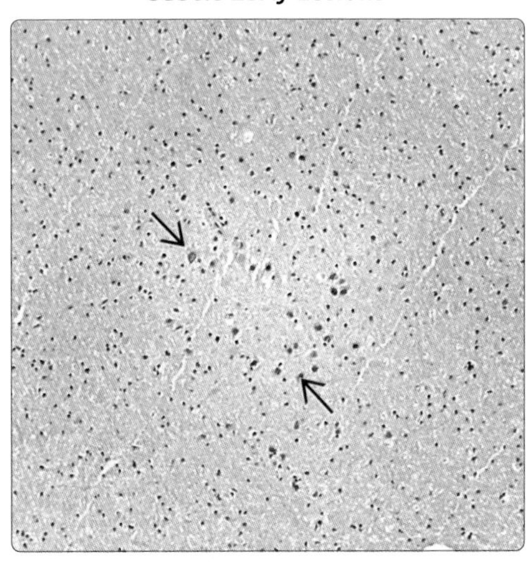

Individual Small Ovoid Lesions

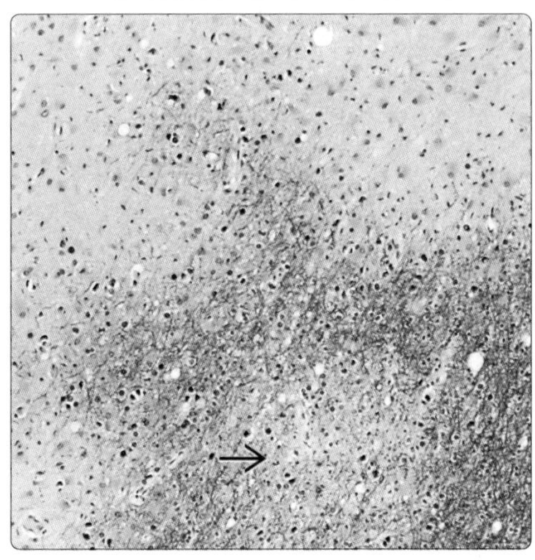

(Left) *Dark, infected oligodendrocytes ➡ that have not yet lysed remain at the edge of demyelinated foci.* **(Right)** *Inclusion-bearing, enlarged nuclei in virally infected oligodendrocytes ➡ typically sit at the periphery of demyelinated foci. Note the peripheral displacement of native nuclear chromatin ➡ and admixed macrophages.*

Inclusions at Lesion Edge

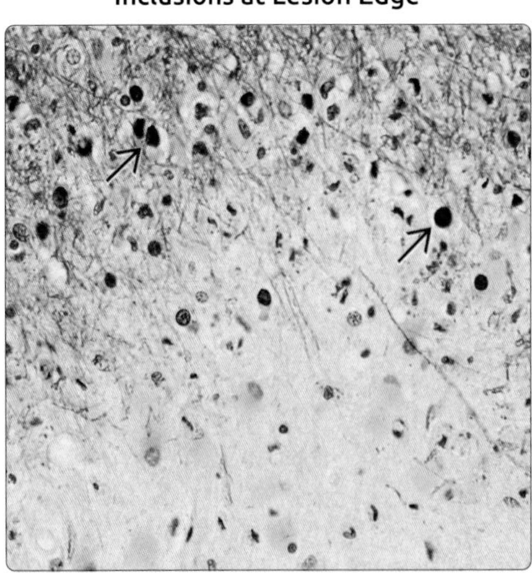

Displaced Nuclear Chromatin

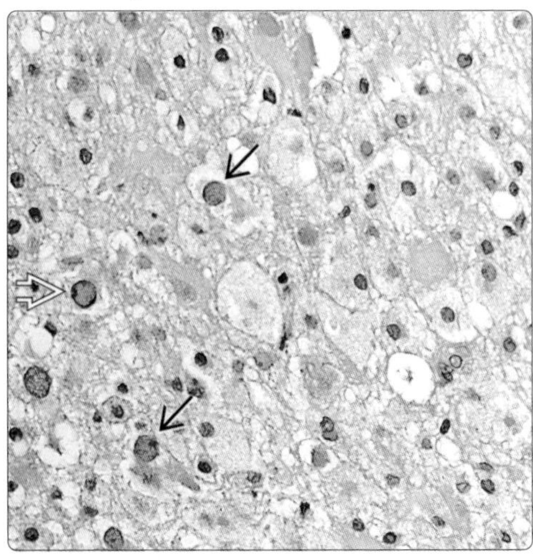

Viral Inclusion

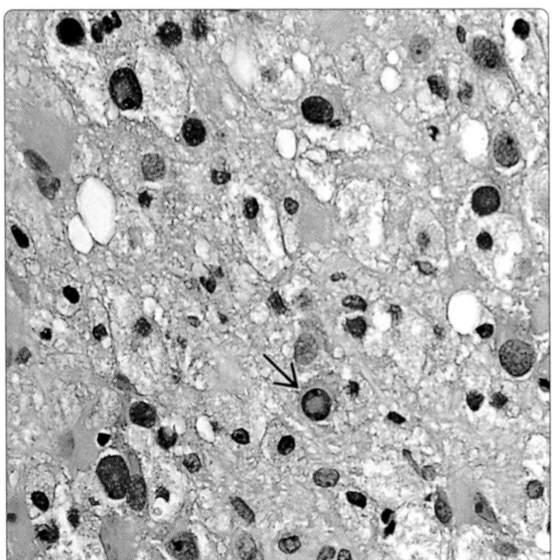

Pleomorphic Astrocytes

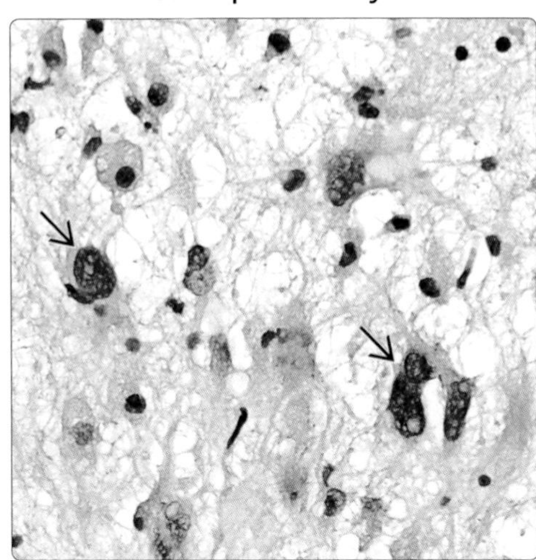

(Left) *Macrophages and a hyperchromatic, inclusion-bearing cell* ➡ *are clues that this is PML, not astrocytoma.* **(Right)** *Nuclear pleomorphism and atypia of astrocytes* ➡ *can be misinterpreted as evidence of a high-grade glioma in PML lesions.*

Viral Inclusions Mixed With Macrophages

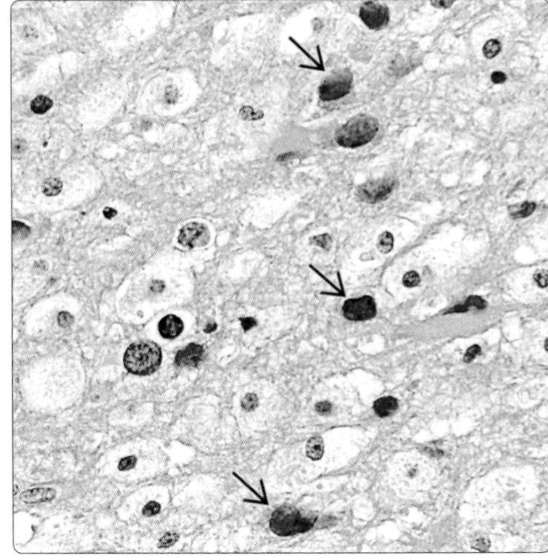

Inconspicuous Macrophages

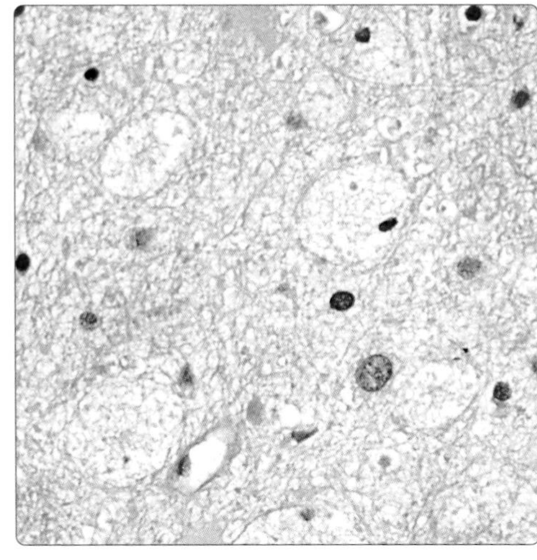

(Left) *The histological diagnosis is easier when macrophages are admixed with cells with viral inclusions* ➡*.* **(Right)** *Macrophages often blend into the background with seemingly little tendency to migrate to vessels and leave a cavity. This subtle population of scavenger cells is more typical of PML than back-to-back arrangement of foamy cells, which is more characteristic of a demyelinating disease, such as multiple sclerosis.*

Numerous Macrophages

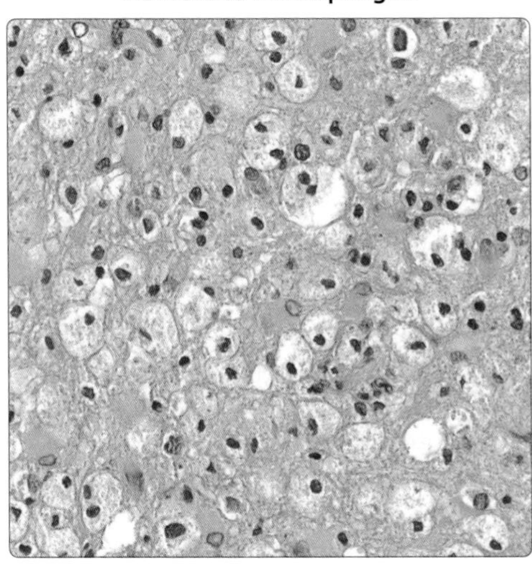

Central Area of Lesion

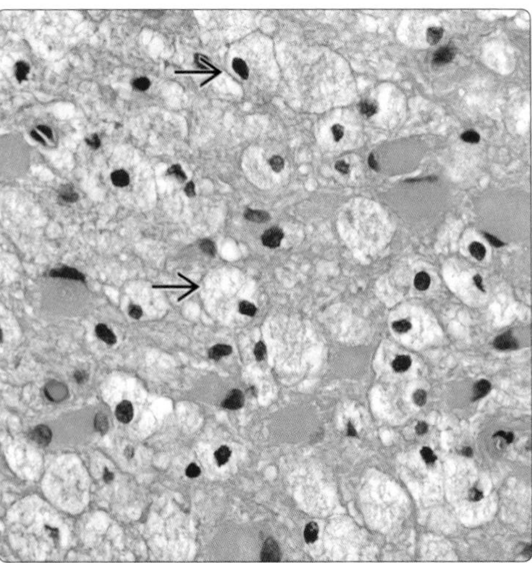

(Left) *Macrophages in PML sometimes collect in dense aggregates similar to those in other demyelinating diseases, such as multiple sclerosis.* **(Right)** *The central area of a PML lesion is often devoid of inclusions. As oligodendrocyte nuclei are lysed by the virus of PML, inclusion-bearing cells are lost centrally in the lesion, macrophage influx increases* ➡ *and reactive astrocytosis becomes brisk. Viral inclusion-bearing cells should be sought at the lesion periphery.*

(Left) *As macrophages clear out the myelin debris, they aggregate around perivascular spaces* ➔. *Perivascular macrophages are seen in several types of demyelinating disorders and are not specific for PML.* **(Right)** *At highest power, the myelin debris within macrophages often displays a linear appearance. Note the admixed reactive astrocytes* ➔ *in the lesion.*

Perivascular Macrophages

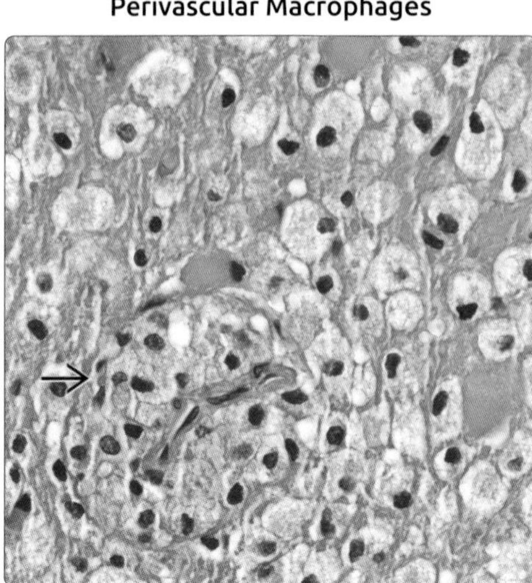

Macrophage Debris

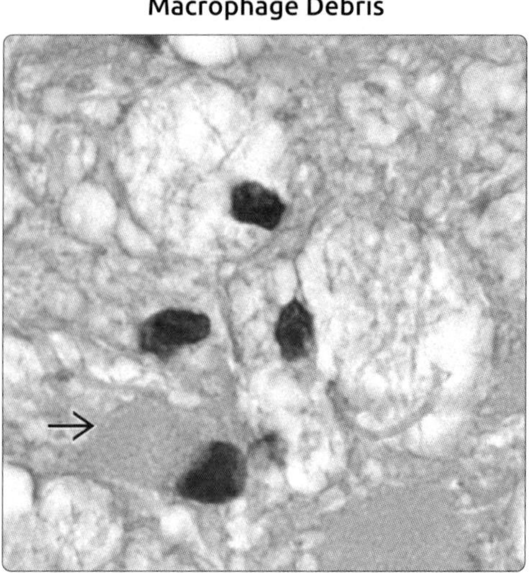

(Left) *LFB/PAS staining can be utilized to identify the age of myelin debris. Acutely digested myelin is LFB(+), whereas subacute myelin breakdown products are PAS(+), as seen here in intraparenchymal and perivascular macrophages.* **(Right)** *Antineurofilament protein immunostaining identifies preserved axons in demyelinated foci. Note the intercalated macrophages.*

Subacute Myelin Debris

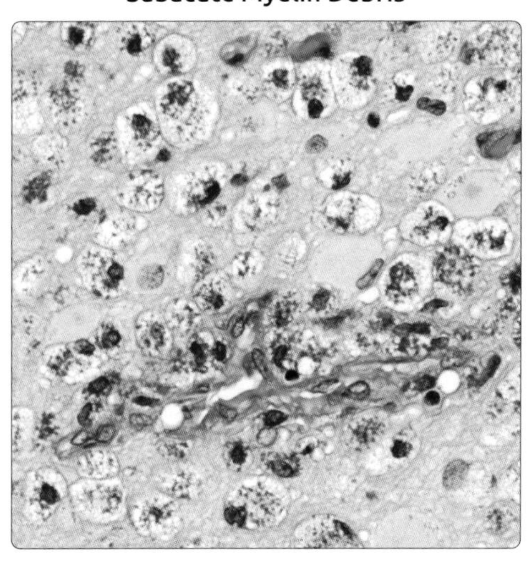

Axonal Preservation

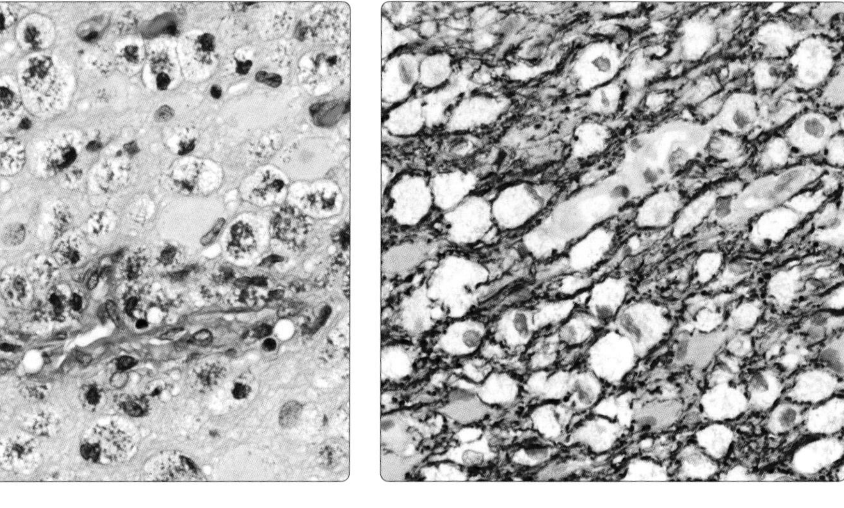

(Left) *Occasional cases of PML elicit significant host lymphoplasmacytic inflammation, although this is more commonly seen after treatment in the immune reconstitution inflammatory syndrome (IRIS). In such situations, any viral inclusions that are still present may be very rare and easily overlooked.* **(Right)** *Inflammatory PML can contain large numbers of plasma cells* ➔. *This should not be misinterpreted as a plasma cell disorder or other type of infectious process.*

Occasional Lymphoplasmacytic Inflammation

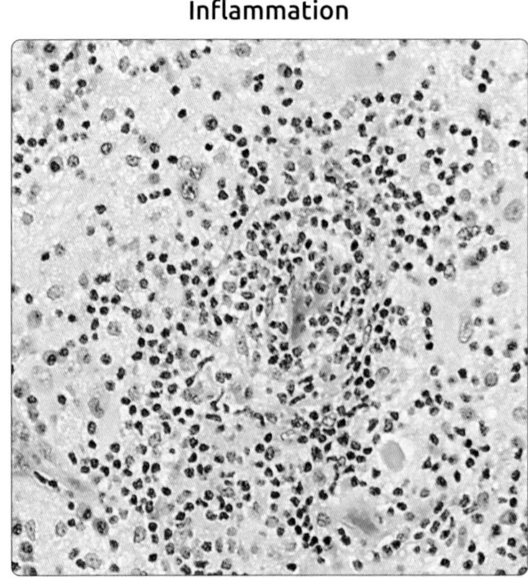

Plasma Cells

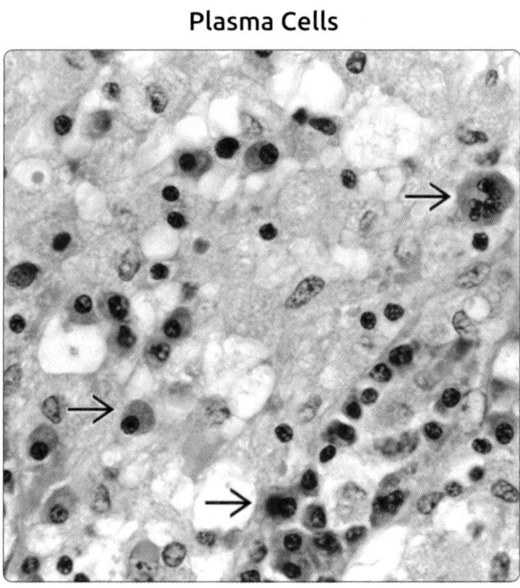

Immunostaining for Virus

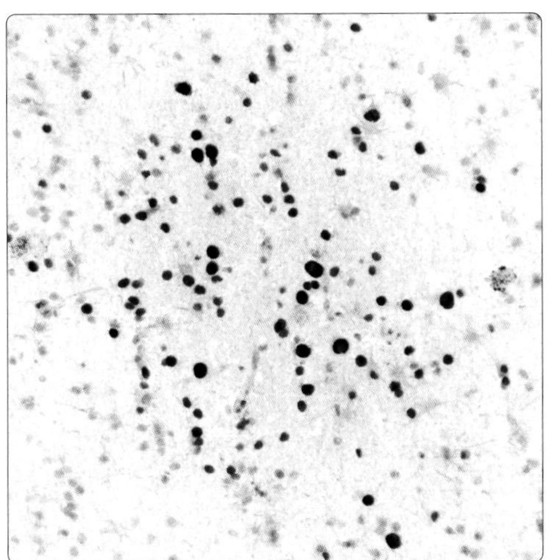

Ki-67 Mimicking Tumor

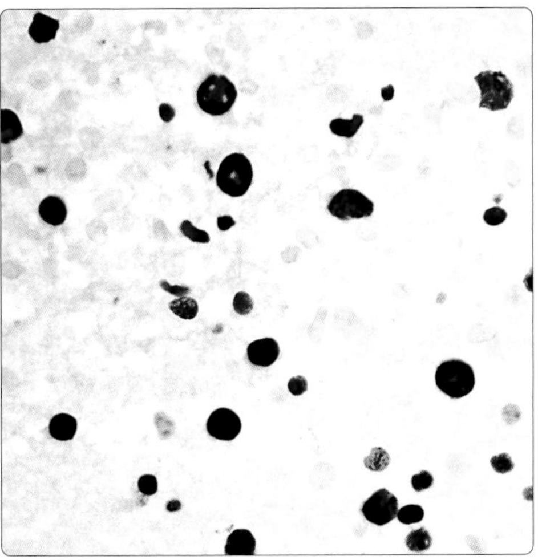

(Left) *Immunostaining for SV40 allows identification of infected oligodendrocytes, as seen in this small early lesion.* **(Right)** *The high Ki-67 rate of infected cells may raise concern about a high-grade infiltrating glioma. The same cells are also immunoreactive for p53.*

p53 Mimicking Tumor

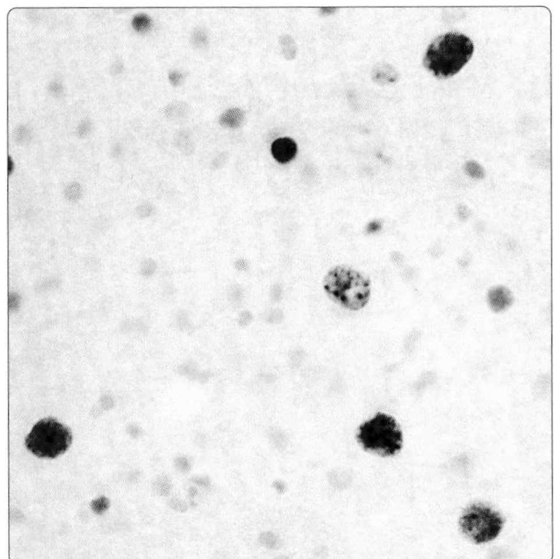

Smear, Inclusions, Multinucleated Astrocyte

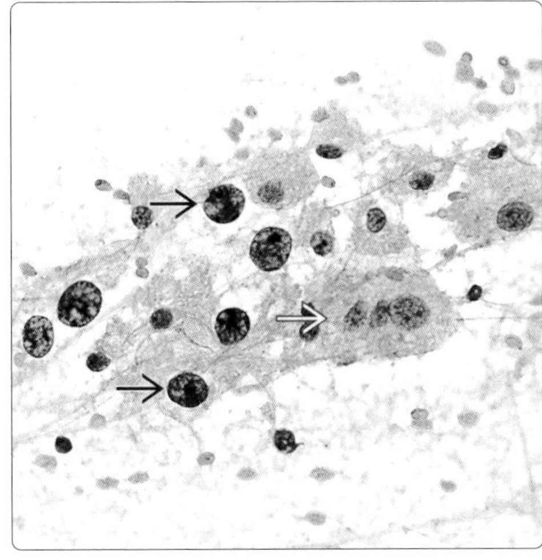

(Left) *Virally infected cells in PML demyelinating lesions bind p53 and demonstrate nuclear immunoreactivity; this can cause the pathologist to mistake a PML lesion for a p53(+) glioma.* **(Right)** *Intraoperative smear preparation captures enlarged oligodendrocytic nuclei with characteristic viral inclusions, although the latter may not have the diffuse nuclear homogenization classic for PML ⇒. A multinucleated reactive astrocyte (Creutzfeldt cell), common in macrophage-rich demyelinating lesions, is also present ➡.*

Smear, Pleomorphic Astrocytes

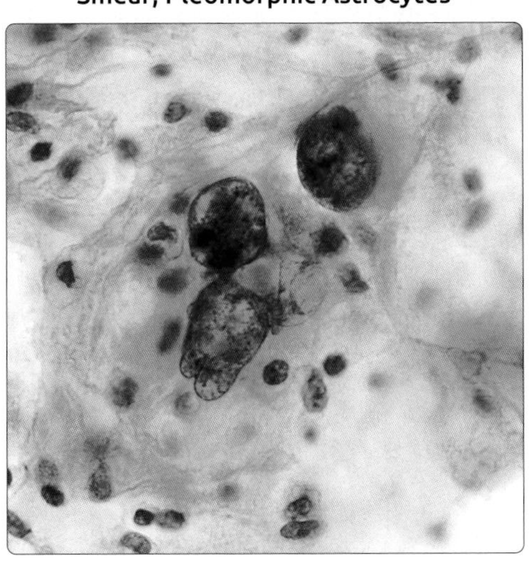

Advanced Cavitated Lesions

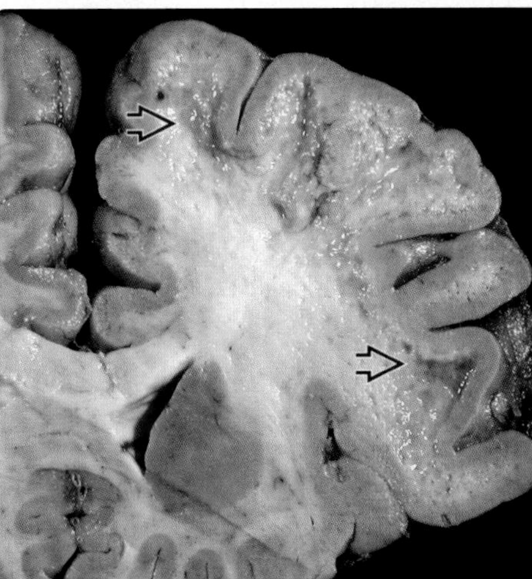

(Left) *Malignant glioma-like pleomorphic astrocytes in a smear preparation misrepresent the lesion as high-grade astrocytoma.* **(Right)** *In advanced stages of PML, large areas of cerebral white matter can be occupied by depressed, cavitated areas ⇒. Note the granular appearance of the damaged tissue.*

HIV Encephalitis

KEY FACTS

TERMINOLOGY

- Infection of CNS by HIV virus, with microglial, macrophage, or astrocytic reaction and presence of HIV virus proven by immunohistochemistry or in situ hybridization

CLINICAL ISSUES

- Impaired concentration, memory loss, confusion
- Apathy, agitation, hallucinations, withdrawal, dementia [still present in highly active retroviral therapy (HAART) era], psychosis
- Prognosis dependent on stage of disease treated with HAART

IMAGING

- FLAIR: Bilateral and symmetric periventricular white matter hyperintensities

MACROSCOPIC

- Atrophy, ventricular enlargement in later stages
- Diffuse fusiform intracranial aneurysms, especially in pediatric HIV(+) patients
  - Infarctions, hemorrhages

MICROSCOPIC

- Microglial activation with clusters; monocytes
- Multinucleated giant cells, often perivascular, may be scanty
- Myelin pallor and vacuolization, astrocytosis
- Basal ganglia calcification, especially in pediatric HIV encephalitis (HIVE)
- Cerebral aneurysms

ANCILLARY TESTS

- Risk of HIV dementia correlates with cerebrospinal fluid viral loads
- Nadir CD4 cell count below 50/mL has greatest risk of neurocognitive impairment

Advanced HIV White Matter Damage

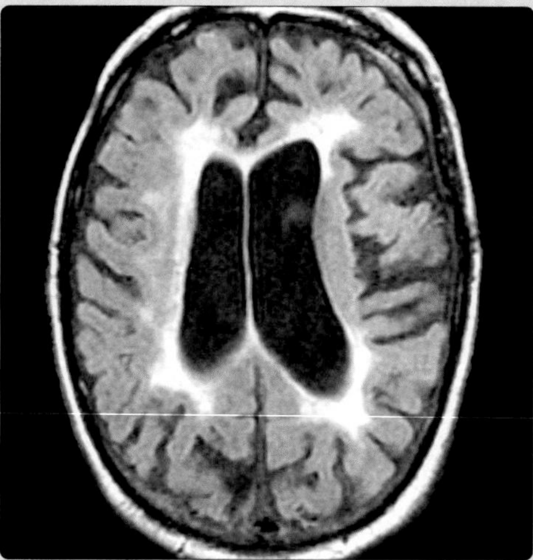

Minimal Abnormalities at Autopsy

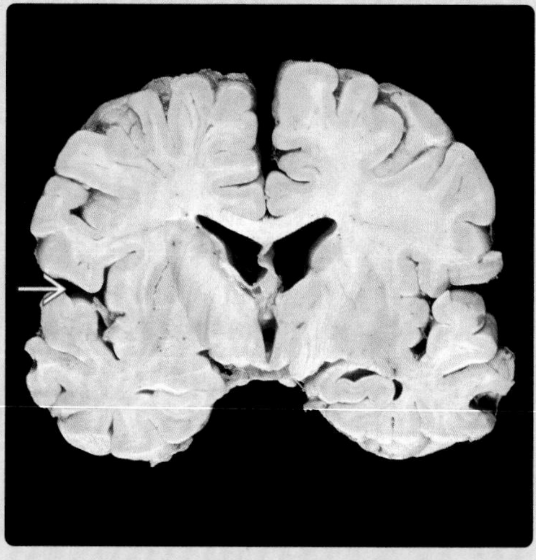

(Left) *Cortical atrophy, bilateral and symmetric periventricular white matter hyperintensities, and ventriculomegaly characterize advanced HIV encephalitis (HIVE), as shown in this axial FLAIR MR.* **(Right)** *Many patients succumbing to advanced stages of an HIV infection without CNS opportunistic infections have minimal abnormalities at the time of gross autopsy examination, except for atrophy; note the widening of the insula* ➡.

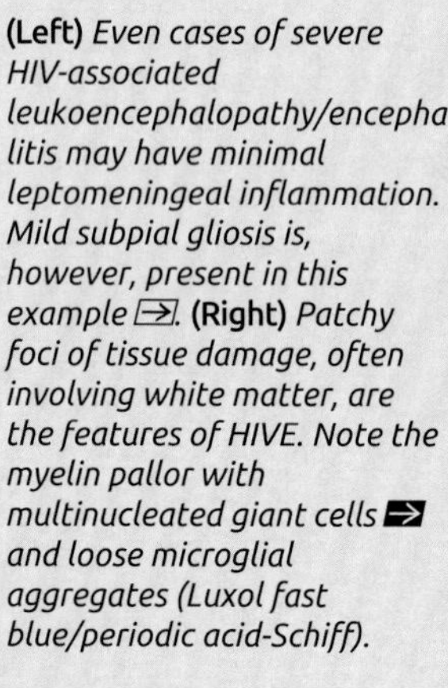

(Left) *Even cases of severe HIV-associated leukoencephalopathy/encephalitis may have minimal leptomeningeal inflammation. Mild subpial gliosis is, however, present in this example* →. **(Right)** *Patchy foci of tissue damage, often involving white matter, are the features of HIVE. Note the myelin pallor with multinucleated giant cells* ➡ *and loose microglial aggregates (Luxol fast blue/periodic acid-Schiff).*

Minimal Leptomeningeal Inflammation

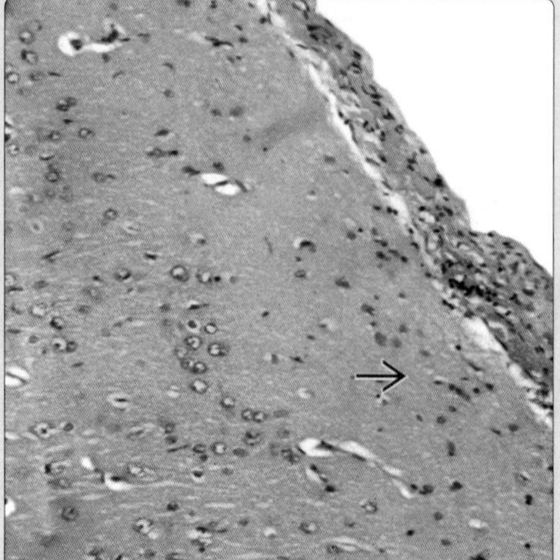

Patchy Foci of Tissue Damage

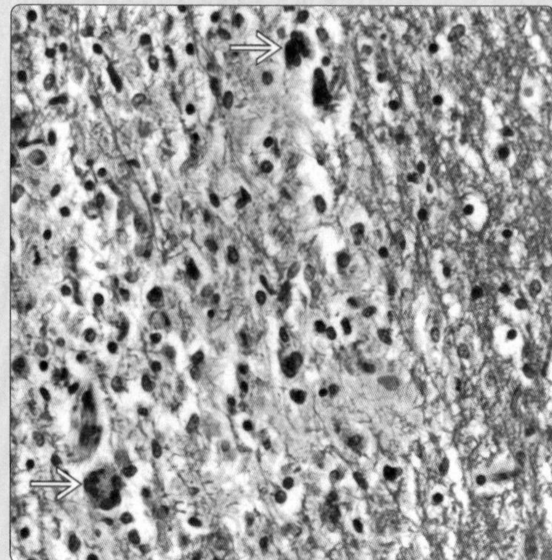

TERMINOLOGY

Abbreviations

- HIV encephalitis (HIVE)

Synonyms

- HIV-associated neurocognitive disorder
- Acquired immunodeficiency syndrome dementia complex

Definitions

- HIVE: Multiple disseminated foci composed of microglia, macrophages, and multinucleated giant cells
  - If multinucleated giant cells cannot be found, must show HIV antigen or nucleic acid by immunohistochemistry (IHC) or in situ hybridization
- HIV leukoencephalopathy (HIVL): Diffuse white matter damage seen in HIV(+) patients thought to be separate process from HIVE and due to secondary damage of white matter as result of infected macrophages and giant cells
  - Diffuse pallor of white matter, centrum semiovale
  - Spares subcortical U-fibers, corpus callosum, internal capsule
- HIVE and HIVL often occur in same brain (i.e., combination of multiple disseminated foci of damage in gray and white matter and diffuse white matter pallor)

ETIOLOGY/PATHOGENESIS

Infectious Agents

- T cells are major site of viral infection
- HIV type 1 (HIV-1) enters brain early in course of infection, presumably via infected microglia, macrophages
- HIV-1 persists in brain perivascular macrophages, microglia
- Does not seem to directly infect neurons
  - Possible neuronal death from inflammatory chemokines
  - Possible neuronal death due to neurotoxic viral proteins, including viral transactivator
  - May be alterations in brain protein turnover in proteasome system
- Antiviral approaches may not be effective in fully suppressing viral replication in CNS

CLINICAL ISSUES

Presentation

- Neurocognitive impairment
  - Asymptomatic early stage
  - Mild-intermediate stage
  - HIV-associated dementia
- Highly active retroviral therapy (HAART) introduced in 1990s
  - Prevents or delays progression to full HIV-associated dementia
  - Dementia, especially mild-moderate degree, still prevalent
  - HIV dementia becoming most common neurologic complication of HIV infection in countries that use HAART
  - Opportunistic infections most common, CNS infections in areas without HAART
- Early stages
  - Impaired concentration, memory loss, confusion
  - Apathy, agitation, hallucinations, withdrawal
- Late stages
  - Dementia, psychosis

Treatment

- Asymptomatic patients: HAART suppresses HIV-1 in cerebrospinal fluid (CSF), reduces incidence of symptomatic dementia
- Patients with dementia: HAART prevents neurological progression, leads to variable recovery

Prognosis

- Dependent on stage of disease treated with HAART

IMAGING

MR Findings

- Cortical atrophy variable
- FLAIR: HIVL shows bilateral and symmetric periventricular white matter hyperintensities

CT Findings

- Cortical atrophy (variable)
- Nonenhancing diffuse hypodensity in deep, periventricular white matter
- Ventricular enlargement (variable)
- Bilateral, symmetrical calcifications in basal ganglia, especially in children

MACROSCOPIC

General Features

- Early stages
  - Normal-appearing brain
- Advanced stages
  - Atrophy
  - Bilateral ventricular enlargement (hydrocephalus ex vacuo)

MICROSCOPIC

Histologic Features

- HIVE characterized by disseminated foci of white or gray matter damage, often coalescent
  - Small aggregates of inflammatory cells: Histiocytes, multinucleated giant cells, microglia, few lymphocytes
- Multinucleated giant cells
  - Often perivascular
  - Represent fused monocytes
  - Immunoreactive for HIV proteins, including gp120, p24
  - Immunoreactive for cytokines, including IL-1β, IL-1, caspase-1
- Activated microglia
- Microglial clusters
  - Degree of microglial activation similar in pre- and post-HAART era
  - Suggestion of more basal ganglia involvement in pre-HAART era
  - More hippocampal involvement in post-HAART era
- Monocytes, macrophages
  - CD163 normally expressed by blood-derived monocytes or macrophages but not resident microglia in CNS
  - CD163(+) cells increased in HIVE

- Immunoreactive for HIV proteins, including gp120, p24
- No tight epithelioid granulomas (as are present in sarcoidosis or fungal infections)
- Reactive gemistocytic astrocytosis
  - Immunoreactive for inducible nitric oxide synthase
- Lymphocytes
  - Meningeal
  - Predominantly T cells, often CD8(+) cytotoxic cells
- Patchy myelin pallor, vacuolization
- No viral inclusions
- Neuronal loss
  - Frontal cortex, substantia nigra, cerebellum, putamen
- Decreased synaptic and dendritic density
- Endothelial hypertrophy
- Basal ganglia calcifications, most common in children
- HIVL characterized by ill-defined, diffuse myelin pallor best appreciated on larger sections of tissue
  - Most prominent in centrum semiovale, poorly demarcated edges of myelin loss

ANCILLARY TESTS

Cerebrospinal Fluid Viral Load

- Risk of HIV dementia correlates with CSF viral loads

CD4 Count

- Nadir CD4 cell count below 50/mL has greatest risk of neurocognitive impairment

DIFFERENTIAL DIAGNOSIS

Progressive Multifocal Leukoencephalopathy

- Discrete ovoid areas of myelin loss, many macrophages
- Viral intranuclear inclusions
- Immunohistochemistry for John Cunningham virus (+)

Varicella-Zoster Virus Encephalomyelitis

- May affect white matter with mixed ischemic-demyelinative lesions
- Viral intranuclear inclusions
- IHC(+) for varicella-zoster virus (VZV) antigen
- May have associated hemorrhage
- Not confined to HIV(+) patients

DIAGNOSTIC CHECKLIST

Pathologic Interpretation Pearls

- Gross brain usually normal in early stages
- Even large areas of demyelination often difficult to identify macroscopically
- Perivascular multinucleated cells may be scanty

SELECTED REFERENCES

1. Gelman BB: Neuropathology of HAND with suppressive antiretroviral therapy: encephalitis and neurodegeneration reconsidered. Curr HIV/AIDS Rep. 12(2):272-9, 2015
2. Tauber SC et al: HIV encephalopathy: glial activation and hippocampal neuronal apoptosis, but limited neural repair. HIV Med. ePub, 2015
3. George BP et al: Encephalitis hospitalization rates and inpatient mortality in the United States, 2000-2010. PLoS One. 9(9):e104169, 2014
4. Hellmuth J et al: Interactions between ageing and NeuroAIDS. Curr Opin HIV AIDS. 9(6):527-32, 2014
5. Nightingale S et al: Controversies in HIV-associated neurocognitive disorders. Lancet Neurol. 13(11):1139-51, 2014
6. De Broucker T et al: Acute varicella zoster encephalitis without evidence of primary vasculopathy in a case-series of 20 patients. Clin Microbiol Infect. 18(8):808-19, 2012
7. Nath A et al: Eradication of HIV from the brain: reasons for pause. AIDS. 25(5):577-80, 2011
8. Goldstein DA et al: HIV-associated intracranial aneurysmal vasculopathy in adults. J Rheumatol. 37(2):226-33, 2010
9. Gras G et al: Molecular mechanisms of neuroinvasion by monocytes-macrophages in HIV-1 infection. Retrovirology. 7:30, 2010
10. Johnson T et al: Neurological complications of immune reconstitution in HIV-infected populations. Ann N Y Acad Sci. 1184:106-20, 2010
11. King JE et al: Mechanisms of HIV-tat-induced phosphorylation of N-methyl-D-aspartate receptor subunit 2A in human primary neurons: implications for neuroAIDS pathogenesis. Am J Pathol. 176(6):2819-30, 2010
12. Nguyen TP et al: Persistent hijacking of brain proteasomes in HIV-associated dementia. Am J Pathol. 176(2):893-902, 2010
13. Sanada M et al: Multiple cerebral aneurysms caused by HIV-associated vasculopathy. Intern Med. 49(18):2029-30, 2010
14. Xing HQ et al: In vivo expression of proinflammatory cytokines in HIV encephalitis: an analysis of 11 autopsy cases. Neuropathology. 29(4):433-42, 2009
15. Yadav A et al: CNS inflammation and macrophage/microglial biology associated with HIV-1 infection. J Neuroimmune Pharmacol. 4(4):430-47, 2009
16. Fischer-Smith T et al: Monocyte/macrophage trafficking in acquired immunodeficiency syndrome encephalitis: lessons from human and nonhuman primate studies. J Neurovirol. 14(4):318-26, 2008
17. Modi G et al: Human immunodeficiency virus associated intracranial aneurysms: report of three adult patients with an overview of the literature. J Neurol Neurosurg Psychiatry. 79(1):44-6, 2008
18. Price RW et al: Antiretroviral therapy and central nervous system HIV type 1 infection. J Infect Dis. 197 Suppl 3:S294-306, 2008
19. Smith AB et al: From the archives of the AFIP: central nervous system infections associated with human immunodeficiency virus infection: radiologic-pathologic correlation. Radiographics. 28(7):2033-58, 2008
20. Hamilton DK et al: Subarachnoid hemorrhage and diffuse vasculopathy in an adult infected with HIV. Case report. J Neurosurg. 106(3):478-80, 2007
21. Tipping B et al: Stroke caused by human immunodeficiency virus-associated intracranial large-vessel aneurysmal vasculopathy. Arch Neurol. 63(11):1640-2, 2006
22. Zhao ML et al: Expression of inducible nitric oxide synthase, interleukin-1 and caspase-1 in HIV-1 encephalitis. J Neuroimmunol. 115(1-2):182-91, 2001
23. Budka H et al: HIV-induced central nervous system pathology. In Atlas of Neuropathology of HIV Infection. F. Gray, ed. Oxford: Oxford Science Publications.1-46, 1993
24. Budka H: Cerebral pathology in AIDS: a new nomenclature and pathogenetic concepts. Curr Opin Neurol Neurosurg. 5(6):917-23, 1992
25. Budka H et al: HIV-associated disease of the nervous system: review of nomenclature and proposal for neuropathology-based terminology. Brain Pathol. 1(3):143-52, 1991
26. Budka H: Neuropathology of human immunodeficiency virus infection. Brain Pathol. 1(3):163-75, 1991
27. Petito CK et al: Neuropathology of acquired immunodeficiency syndrome (AIDS): an autopsy review. J Neuropathol Exp Neurol. 45(6):635-46, 1986

Perivascular Multinucleated Cells

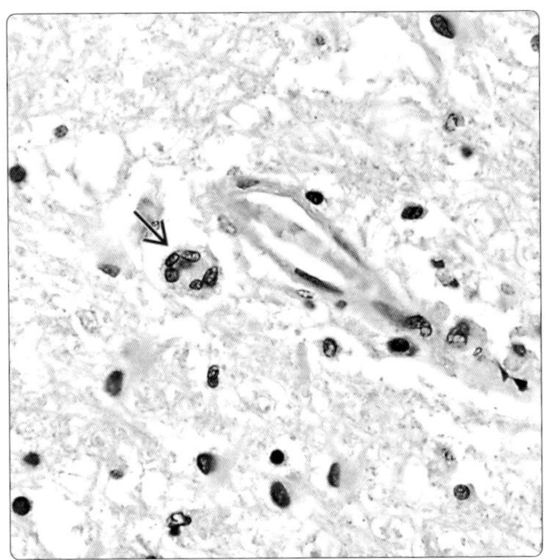

Fused Monocytes

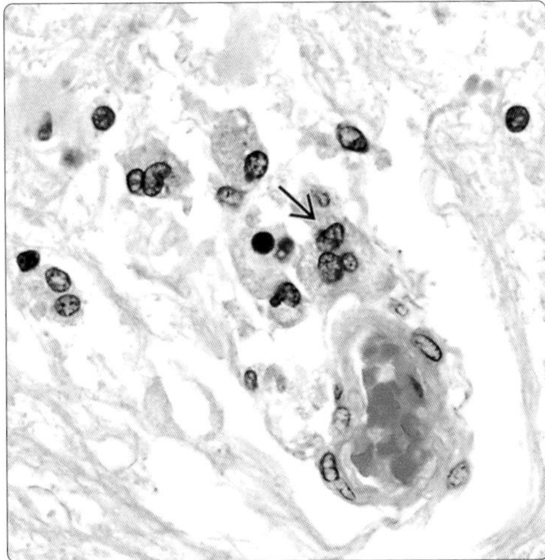

(Left) *Perivascular multinucleated cells ⮕ and reactive astrocytosis are typical of HIVE. Note the sharp outline and abundant cytoplasm of the multinucleated cell.* **(Right)** *Multinucleated giant cells ⮕ in HIVE are fused monocytes. The loose aggregates of these cells should be contrasted with tight aggregates of epithelioid histiocytes in granulomas of sarcoidosis and some mycoses. Note the absence of a significant chronic inflammatory cell infiltrate.*

gp120 Immunohistochemistry for Envelope Protein

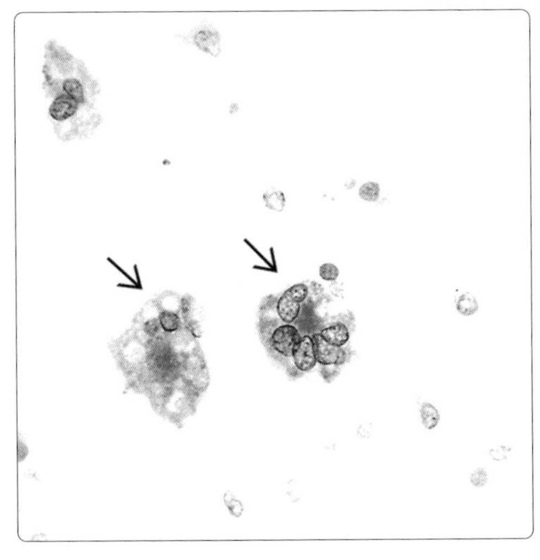

Basal Ganglia Calcifications

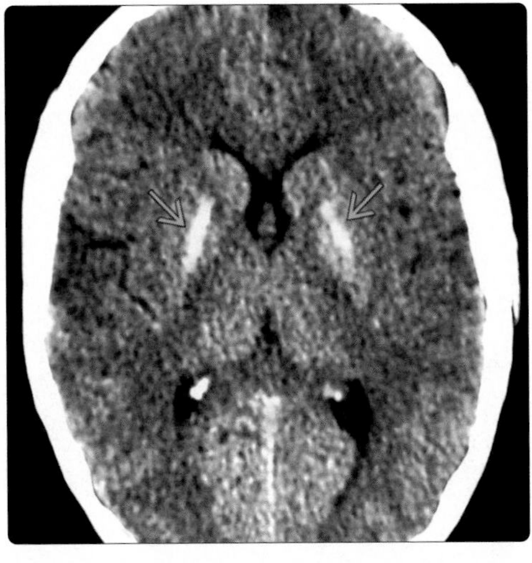

(Left) *Multinucleated giant cells in HIVE contain viral antigens and are immunoreactive for envelope protein gp120 ⮕. Immunostaining can also be performed for gp4. (Courtesy C. Pardo, MD.)* **(Right)** *Bilateral and symmetrical calcifications in the basal ganglia, especially the globus pallidus, are present in some cases of HIVE ⮕, as shown in this nonenhanced CT scan. Calcifications may also be present in the hippocampus and centrum semiovale.*

Basal Ganglia Calcifications

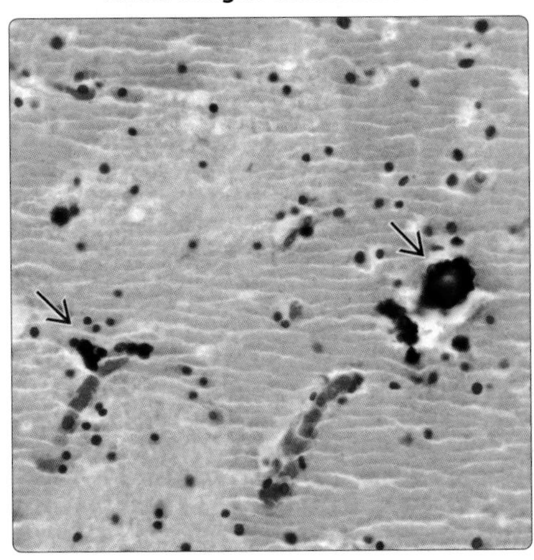

HIV-Associated Aneurysm Formation

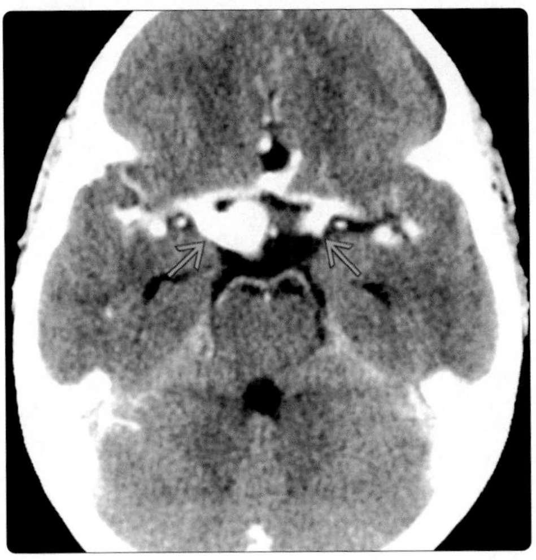

(Left) *Especially in children with HIVE, small basophilic calcifications ⮕ are often present in the basal ganglia.* **(Right)** *Diffuse aneurysmal formation, in the form of dilated arteries ⮕, is more common in pediatric than adult HIV(+) patients, as shown in this axial contrast-enhanced CT.*

KEY FACTS

TERMINOLOGY

- CNS viral infections
  - Environmental contact
    - Arboviruses, enteroviruses
  - Reactivation in immunocompromised host
    - Varicella-zoster virus, cytomegalovirus
  - Smoldering viral infection with inability of host to completely clear virus
    - Subacute sclerosing panencephalitis (SSPE)

ETIOLOGY/PATHOGENESIS

- Enteroviruses, arboviruses common causes of sporadic CNS meningitis, encephalitis
- Herpes family viruses often seen in immunocompromised host, e.g., AIDS

MACROSCOPIC

- Early stages of meningitis, encephalitis yield normal or near-normal gross brain appearance
- May have only edema, hyperemia

MICROSCOPIC

- Signature feature of meningitis
  - Leptomeningeal lymphocytes, often sparse
- Signature feature of encephalitis
  - Perivascular lymphocytes, parenchymal gliosis, microglial clusters, often sparse
- Most sporadically occurring viral infections lack viral inclusions
  - Diagnosis made by serological testing or IHC
- Viral inclusions usually seen with herpesvirus family, measles virus
  - Also seen in rare adenovirus infections

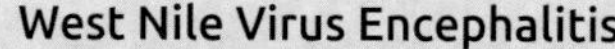

West Nile Virus Encephalitis

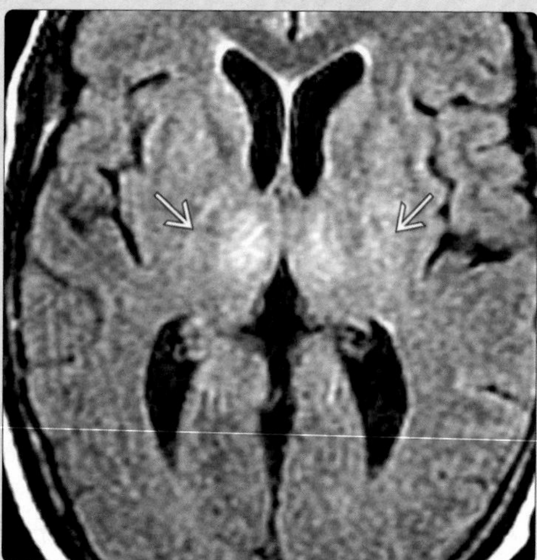

Intense T-Cell Meningeal Infiltrates

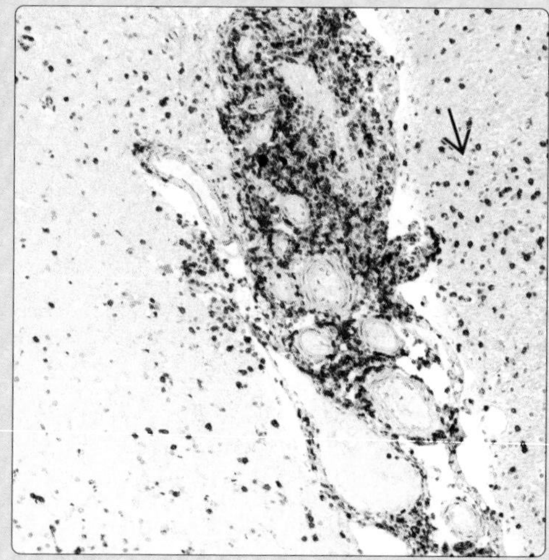

(Left) *Axial FLAIR MR in a patient with West Nile viral encephalitis shows bilateral, symmetric, high signal foci in the thalami, basal ganglia, and right internal capsules ➡.* **(Right)** *The hallmark of viral meningoencephalitis, at least in immunocompetent patients, is perivascular and leptomeningeal lymphocytic inflammation, often with some individual T cells permeating the parenchyma ➡. It is often not this intense, however.*

CD68(+) Microglial in West Nile Virus Myelitis

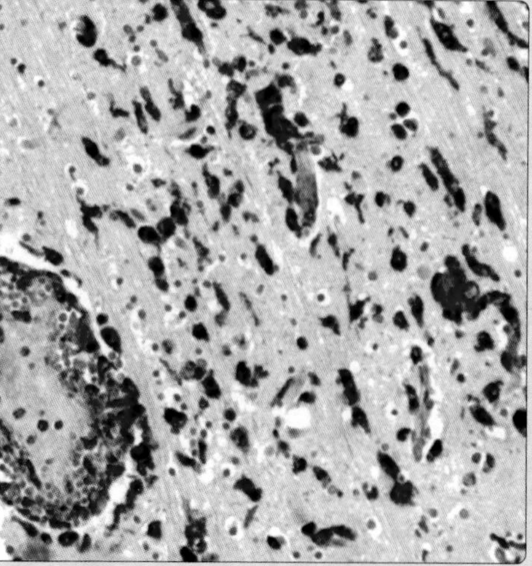

Varicella-Zoster Virus Ependymal Inclusions

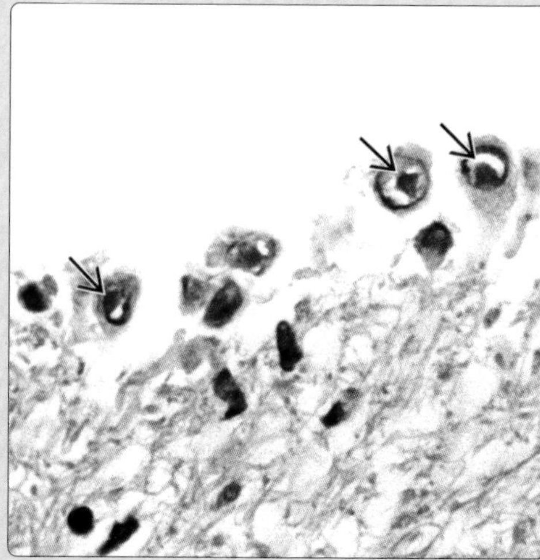

(Left) *As highlighted by immunohistochemistry for CD68, an influx of microglia is a common feature of CNS viral infections of all types; West Nile myelitis is seen here.* **(Right)** *Occasionally varicella-zoster virus (VZV) encephalitis can manifest extensive ependymal cell infection, with resultant ventriculitis. Such cases usually occur in immunocompromised patients. In this case, note Cowdry A inclusions ➡ but absence of cellular enlargement (cytomegaly), as would be expected in cytomegalovirus (CMV) infection.*

TERMINOLOGY

Definitions

- CNS viral infection, either meningitis (leptomeningeal inflammation), encephalitis (parenchymal inflammation), or both (meningoencephalitis)

ETIOLOGY/PATHOGENESIS

Infectious Agents

- Arbovirus (arthropod-borne vectors) infections
  - Transmitted by mosquito bite
    - Examples: West Nile virus (WNV) meningitis/encephalitis, eastern equine encephalitis (EEE), St. Louis encephalitis (SLE), Western equine encephalitis (WEE), California (La Crosse) encephalitis
    - Exception: Tick bite for Colorado tick fever and Powassan fever
    - Small mammal and bird reservoirs
  - In North America, fewer than 10 arboviruses that cause significant neurological disease
  - Strong seasonal predilection for summer/early fall
  - Strong geographic predilection/environmental exposure
    - SLE: Entire USA
    - WEE: Western 2/3 of USA
    - EEE: Atlantic and Gulf Coasts
    - California: Eastern and Upper Midwest/Central USA
  - Asymptomatic infections associated with seroconversion outnumber cases of neuroinvasive disease by 100–1,000:1
  - Common cause of sporadic viral encephalitis
    - Most arboviral neuroinvasive infections cause encephalitis rather than meningitis
    - West Nile virus (WNV) meningitis also common
  - Hosts usually immunocompetent
    - Disease more devastating in immunocompromised hosts (AIDS, transplant recipients, elderly, debilitated)
- Enterovirus
  - 75-80% of all viral meningitis caused by enteroviruses
    - Examples: Echoviruses, coxsackieviruses A and B, polioviruses, enteroviruses 70 and 71
  - Person-to-person transmission
    - Fecal/oral route usual
    - Respiratory less common
  - Strong human contact/environmental exposure
  - Seasonal predilection for summer/early fall
- Herpes family infections
  - Reactivation in immunocompromised hosts, usually AIDS
  - Cytomegalovirus (CMV): Subacute encephalitis, ventriculitis, retinitis
  - Varicella-zoster virus (VZV): Meningoencephalitis, vasculopathy, demyelination, myelitis
  - Epstein-Barr virus (EBV): Meningoencephalitis
  - No seasonal predilection
- Subacute sclerosing panencephalitis (SSPE)
  - Rare, chronic neurodegenerative encephalitis due to measles virus
  - Patients usually had early primary measles infection at < 2 years of age
    - Virus incompletely cleared
    - Smoldering infection results
    - SSPE manifests 6-8 years later

CLINICAL ISSUES

Presentation

- Meningitis
  - Fever, headache, altered mental status in immunocompetent patients
    - Potential for systemic symptoms depending on virus
    - Malaise, myalgia, anorexia, nausea, vomiting, abdominal pain, diarrhea
  - Febrile response less likely in immunocompromised patients
- Encephalitis
  - Immunocompetent patients have many of same symptoms as patients with meningitis
  - Also focal neurological signs/symptoms, seizures
- Acute flaccid paralysis
  - Most frequent with WNV infections
  - Less frequent with several other arboviruses (Dengue, St. Louis encephalitis, Powassan, Eastern equine encephalitis)

Treatment

- Usually supportive care only
  - No antiviral drugs are approved for treatment of arbovirus infection

Prognosis

- Variable, but most meningitis and encephalitis cases not fatal
- Poor prognosis of some encephalitis cases in immunocompromised patients
  - WNVE poor outcome in transplant recipients, AIDS patients, elderly
  - Herpes family virus infections: Poor prognosis in AIDS and other immunocompromised patients
- SSPE: Relentless progression
  - 95% die within 5 years

IMAGING

General Features

- West Nile neurological disease (WNVE)
  - Patients may have normal neuroimaging studies
    - Frequency of acute MR abnormalities < 50%
    - Yield increased if FLAIR and diffusion-weighted imaging used in addition to standard MR work-up, T2-weighted sequences
  - T2-weighted images: Foci of increased signal intensity in basal ganglia, thalamus, cerebellum, brainstem
  - Frequency of abnormalities higher in later stage disease (2-4 weeks post onset)
- Other types of encephalitis
  - Imaging often nonspecific
  - Abnormal T2 hyperintensities in gray &/or white matter, basal ganglia
  - Abnormal periventricular signal in ventriculitis
- SSPE
  - T2-weighted scans may be normal early; develop mild asymmetric leukoencephalopathy
  - Abnormal T2-weighted signal in cortex, basal ganglia

MACROSCOPIC

General Features

- Early stages: Most cases of meningitis and encephalitis exhibit near-normal gross appearance
  - Congestion/hyperemia; absence of meningeal purulent exudate
  - Edema, possible focal petechiae
- Late stages: Foci of gray matter softening in some cases
- CMV ventriculitis can have periventricular necrosis
  - Dystrophic mineralization in late stages
- VZVE can have white matter lesions
- SSPE late stages: Cerebral atrophy, white matter discoloration

MICROSCOPIC

Histologic Features

- Meningitis
  - Involvement of leptomeninges/subarachnoid and perivascular spaces by lymphocytes
  - Lymphocytes may be sparse, ill distributed
  - Some fulminant cases have meningeal neutrophils
  - Unlike encephalitis, no parenchymal gliosis, microgliosis, microglial clusters, neuronophagia
- Encephalitis
  - Involvement of brain by parenchymal gliosis, perivascular lymphocytes, microgliosis, microglial clusters, variable neuronal loss, and neuronophagia
  - May be focal and in select anatomical regions, depending on virus
    - Involvement of spinal cord (myelitis)
- Meningoencephalitis (encephalitis + meningitis)
- Meningomyeloencephalitis (encephalitis + meningitis + spinal cord involvement)
- Arbovirus
  - Perivascular lymphocytic cuffing
    - Mainly CD4(+) and CD8(+) T cells with occasional B cells
  - Mononuclear and polymorphonuclear cells
  - Microglial clusters, neuronophagia of infected cells
  - Heavy concentration of lesions in brain stem of fatal cases
  - Involvement of spinal anterior horns (myelitis) especially characteristic of WNVE
    - Also thalamic, hippocampal involvement in WNVE
  - No viral inclusions
    - Diagnosis by clinical or serological findings for viral antigens
    - Immunohistochemistry variably available
- CMV
  - In immunosuppression, AIDS, or as congenital infection
  - Distribution
    - Retinitis
    - Ventriculitis (may be hemorrhagic, necrotizing)
    - Encephalitis (hemorrhagic/necrotizing foci or multifocal microglial nodules)
    - Myelitis
  - Cowdry A viral inclusions: Large, discrete, intranuclear
    - Less distinct cytoplasmic inclusions
    - Cytoplasmic replication yields viral accumulation, cytomegaly
  - Immunohistochemistry for viral antigens widely available
  - Congenital infection, if severe, often leads to hearing loss, microcephaly, abnormalities in gyral migration (especially polymicrogyria)
- VZVE
  - Causes chickenpox (varicella), usually in childhood and with few, if any, neurologic sequelae
    - Virus latent in neurons of cranial and spinal ganglia
    - Reactivation produces shingles (zoster) in elderly, immunocompromised individuals
    - Postherpetic neuralgia after resolution of zoster in many elderly patients
    - Uncommon spread of virus to large cerebral arteries causing spectrum of damage, ranging from vasculopathy to vasculitis, with resultant stroke
    - Potential for deeper tissue penetration of virus in immunocompromised individuals, especially in malignancy and AIDS
  - Virus in neurons, oligodendrocytes, meningeal cells, ependymal cells, or blood vessel wall in immunocompromised patients
    - Detection often requires combination of morphologic, immunohistochemical, in situ hybridization, PCR
    - Deep penetration can cause meningoencephalitis, myelitis, small-vessel vasculopathy, ventriculitis
    - White matter lesions ovoid, usually smaller, less coalescent than progressive multifocal leukoencephalopathy (PML)
  - Cowdry A viral inclusions
    - No cytoplasmic inclusions, no cytomegaly
    - Immunohistochemistry for viral antigens variably available
- SSPE
  - Scattered perivascular and leptomeningeal lymphocytes; microglial clusters
  - Disease may affect mainly gray or white matter
  - Glassy intranuclear viral inclusions without distinct owl's eye Cowdry A appearance

ANCILLARY TESTS

Serologic Testing

- Rapid serum or cerebrospinal fluid IgM antibody capture ELISA assays available for diagnosis of acute infection for all North American arboviruses

PCR

- Cerebrospinal fluid (CSF) PCR for herpesvirus CNS infections
- Sensitivity of CSF PCR for diagnosis of arboviral infections significantly below that reported for both enteroviruses and herpesviruses for which this is method of choice
- Quantitative CSF PCR can be useful in distinguishing CNS EBV-mediated lymphoma from other EBV-related disorders
  - Primary CNS EBV-mediated lymphoma: High EBV load, low leukocyte counts
  - EBV-mediated encephalitis: High EBV load, high leukocyte counts

- Patients with postinfectious EBV complications: Low EBV load, high leukocyte counts

CSF Profile

- Serologically confirmed WNV meningitis and WNVE produce similar degrees of CSF pleocytosis, frequently associated with substantial CSF neutrophils
- All viral meningitis, encephalitis in immunocompetent patients characterized by CSF mononuclear cells, elevated protein, and usually normal glucose
  - Contrasts with CSF profile of bacterial and fungal infections (low glucose, greater protein elevation, often culture positive)

DIFFERENTIAL DIAGNOSIS

Rasmussen Encephalitis

- Immunocompetent children usually affected
- Clinical course longer than viral encephalitis
- Unrelated to direct viral infection
  - Serology, CSF PCR, immunohistochemistry negative for viral infection
- Lymphocytic infiltrates, microglial clusters, neuronophagia, but no viral inclusions

Paraneoplastic Encephalitis

- Adults with occult carcinoma usually affected
- Clinical course more protracted than viral encephalitis
- Unrelated to direct viral infection
  - Serology, CSF PCR, immunohistochemistry negative for viral infection
- Lymphocytic infiltrates, microglial clusters, neuronophagia, but no viral inclusions

DIAGNOSTIC CHECKLIST

Pathologic Interpretation Pearls

- Viral encephalitides, especially arboviral infections, have overlapping, nonspecific histological features
  - Arbovirus infections: No viral inclusions; viral antibodies for IHC not widely available
  - Diagnosis of almost all arbovirus infections based on serum &/or CSF serology
    - Acute infections: 50% of patients have virus-specific IgM antibodies by IgM capture ELISA at time of hospitalization; > 90% have antibody after 1 week of symptoms
    - Check laboratory results for premortem serological testing
    - Save blood sample(s) for postmortem serological testing in suspected CNS viral infection
    - Culture of virus from blood/CSF difficult, not routinely performed
- Little inflammation in viral infections in immunocompromised patients
- Viral infections in immunocompromised patients often feature viral inclusions
  - Inclusions may be few in late-stage disease
- Results of tissue-based PCR examination for herpesviruses must be interpreted cautiously, since this sensitive technique may detect portions of viral genomic material in absence of active viral infection

SELECTED REFERENCES

1. Danthanarayana N et al: Acute meningoencephalitis associated with echovirus 9 infection in Sri Lanka, 2009. J Med Virol. ePub, 2015
2. Johnson MG et al: Seasonality and survival associated with three outbreak seasons of West Nile virus disease in Oklahoma-2003, 2007, and 2012. J Med Virol. ePub, 2015
3. Pan M et al: Human infection with a novel highly pathogenic avian influenza A (H5N6) virus: Virological and clinical findings. J Infect. ePub, 2015
4. Solbrig MV et al: Current neurological observations and complications of dengue virus infection. Curr Neurol Neurosci Rep. 15(6):29, 2015
5. Suwantarat N et al: Risks to healthcare workers with emerging diseases: lessons from MERS-CoV, Ebola, SARS, and avian flu. Curr Opin Infect Dis. 28(4):349-61, 2015
6. Vora SB et al: Cytomegalovirus in immunocompromised children. Curr Opin Infect Dis. 28(4):323-9, 2015
7. Halloran ME et al: Emerging, evolving, and established infectious diseases and interventions. Science. 345(6202):1292-4, 2014
8. Salazar R et al: Varicella zoster virus ischemic optic neuropathy and subclinical temporal artery involvement. Arch Neurol. 68(4):517-20, 2011
9. Gutierrez J et al: Subacute sclerosing panencephalitis: an update. Dev Med Child Neurol. 52(10):901-7, 2010
10. Levi ME et al: Impact of rituximab-associated B-cell defects on West Nile virus meningoencephalitis in solid organ transplant recipients. Clin Transplant. 24(2):223-8, 2010
11. Sabella C: Measles: not just a childhood rash. Cleve Clin J Med. 77(3):207-13, 2010
12. Vincentelli C et al: 35-year-old HIV-positive woman with Basal forebrain mass. Brain Pathol. 20(1):265-8, 2010
13. Blakely PK et al: Disrupted glutamate transporter expression in the spinal cord with acute flaccid paralysis caused by West Nile virus infection. J Neuropathol Exp Neurol. 68(10):1061-72, 2009
14. Cheeran MC et al: Neuropathogenesis of congenital cytomegalovirus infection: disease mechanisms and prospects for intervention. Clin Microbiol Rev. 22(1):99-126, Table of Contents, 2009
15. Huppatz C et al: Encephalitis in Australia, 1979-2006: trends and aetiologies. Commun Dis Intell. 33(2):192-7, 2009
16. Souraud JB et al: Adult fulminant subacute sclerosing panencephalitis: pathological and molecular studies--a case report. Clin Neuropathol. 28(3):213-8, 2009
17. Tyler KL: Emerging viral infections of the central nervous system: part 1. Arch Neurol. 66(8):939-48, 2009
18. Tyler KL: Neurological infections: advances in therapy, outcome, and prediction. Lancet Neurol. 8(1):19-21, 2009
19. Davis LE et al: North American encephalitic arboviruses. Neurol Clin. 26(3):727-57, ix, 2008
20. Rafailidis PI et al: Severe cytomegalovirus infection in apparently immunocompetent patients: a systematic review. Virol J. 5:47, 2008
21. Davis LE et al: West Nile virus neuroinvasive disease. Ann Neurol. 60(3):286-300, 2006
22. Tyler KL et al: CSF findings in 250 patients with serologically confirmed West Nile virus meningitis and encephalitis. Neurology. 66(3):361-5, 2006
23. Kleinschmidt-DeMasters BK et al: Naturally acquired West Nile virus encephalomyelitis in transplant recipients: clinical, laboratory, diagnostic, and neuropathological features. Arch Neurol. 61(8):1210-20, 2004
24. Barkovich AJ et al: Fetal brain infections. Childs Nerv Syst. 19(7-8):501-7, 2003
25. DeBiasi RL et al: Central nervous system apoptosis in human herpes simplex virus and cytomegalovirus encephalitis. J Infect Dis. 186(11):1547-57, 2002
26. DeBiasi RL et al: Use of PCR for the diagnosis of herpesvirus infections of the central nervous system. J Clin Virol. 25 Suppl 1:S5-11, 2002
27. Weinberg A et al: Quantitative CSF PCR in Epstein-Barr virus infections of the central nervous system. Ann Neurol. 52(5):543-8, 2002
28. Kleinschmidt-DeMasters BK et al: Polymerase chain reaction as a diagnostic adjunct in herpesvirus infections of the nervous system. Brain Pathol. 11(4):452-64, 2001
29. Kleinschmidt-DeMasters BK et al: Varicella-Zoster virus infections of the nervous system: clinical and pathologic correlates. Arch Pathol Lab Med. 125(6):770-80, 2001
30. Gilden DH et al: Neurologic complications of the reactivation of varicella-zoster virus. N Engl J Med. 342(9):635-45, 2000
31. Anders KH et al: Adenovirus encephalitis and widespread ependymitis in a child with AIDS. Pediatr Neurosurg. 16(6):316-20, 1990

(Left) *Viral encephalitis usually features perivascular lymphocytic cuffing ⇨, as well as a microglial influx ⇨. Either or both may be patchy in gray matter. No tight microglial clusters are present here.* **(Right)** *The hallmark of viral encephalomyelitis is perivascular lymphocytic cuffing, mainly by CD3(+) T cells, as seen here in the anterior spinal horn of a patient infected with West Nile virus.*

Perivascular Lymphocytic Cuffing, Microglial Influx

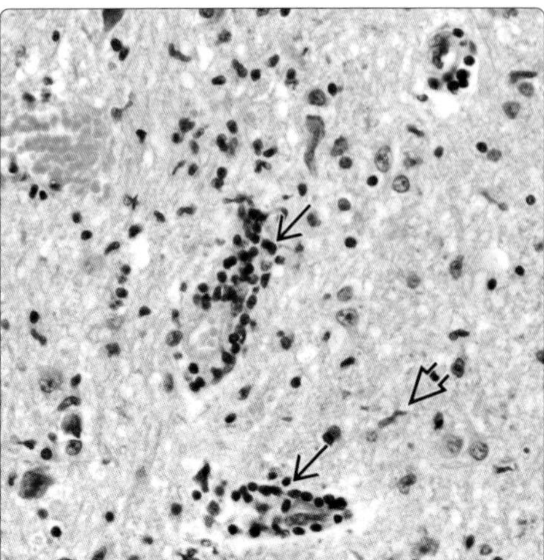

Perivascular Lymphocytic Cuffing

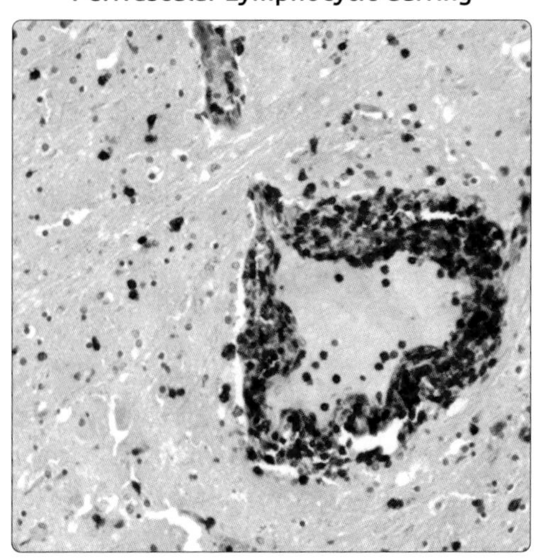

(Left) *Viral meningoencephalitis typically has moderate numbers of leptomeningeal lymphocytes ⇨ and parenchymal gliosis, as seen here. Microglial clusters were present in other sections. As is often the case, the presumptive diagnosis was never confirmed by identification of an organism.* **(Right)** *This example of viral meningitis exhibited only scant meningeal lymphocytic infiltrates ⇨.*

Leptomeningeal Lymphocytes, Meningoencephalitis

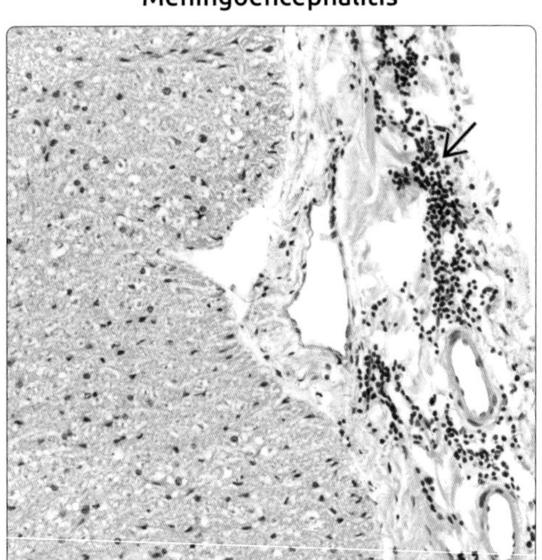

Scant Meningeal Inflammation Possible

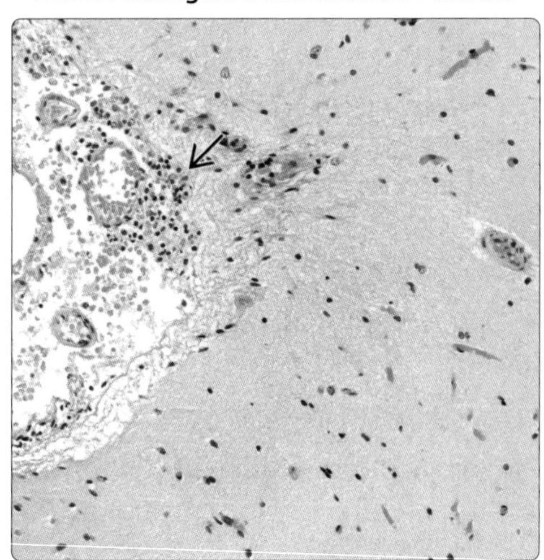

(Left) *In the face of only patchy perivascular lymphocytic infiltrates, the diagnosis of Eastern equine encephalitis would be impossible without corroborating clinical history &/or other CNS findings.* **(Right)** *Immunostaining for the arbovirus of Eastern equine encephalitis permitted a specific diagnosis in this example of viral encephalitis. (Courtesy S. Zaki, MD.)*

Eastern Equine Encephalitis

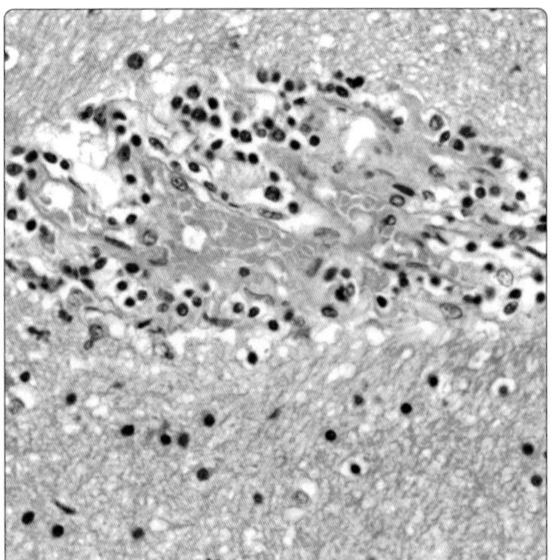

Eastern Equine Encephalitis, IHC

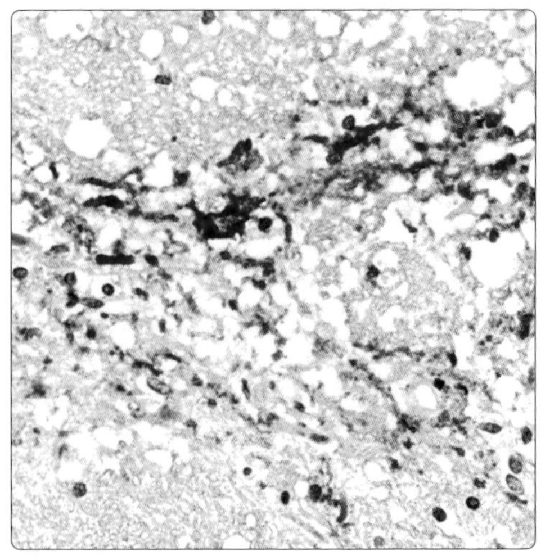

Trigeminal Neuralgia, Varicella-Zoster Virus

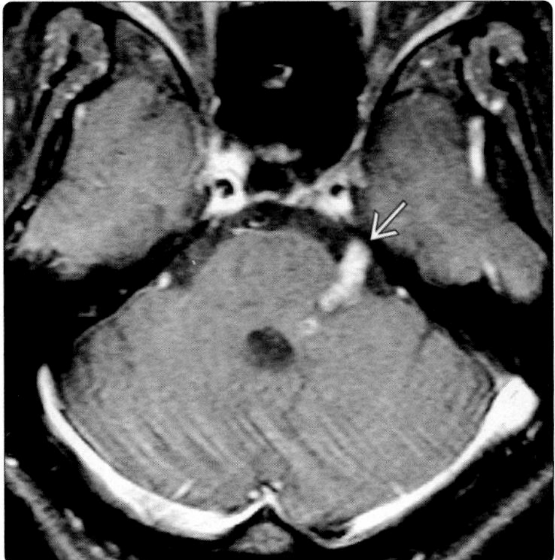

Trigeminal Neuralgia, Cranial Zoster

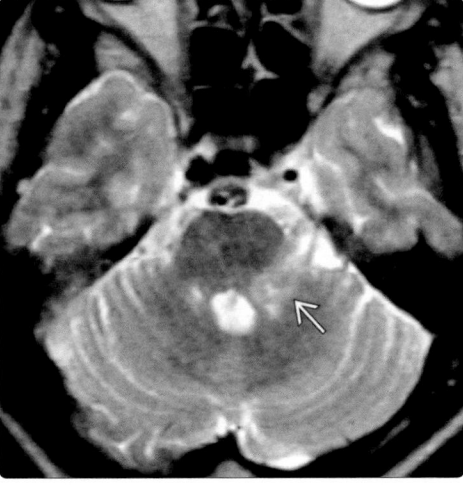

(Left) *Axial T1WI C+ MR scan shows enhancement of the CN5 root entry zone ➡ and brachium pontis in a patient with trigeminal neuralgia due to VZV infection. The most common form of cranial zoster involves the ophthalmic branch (V1). This usually develops in immunocompetent patients.* **(Right)** *Axial T2WI MR in a patient with numbness of the tongue and trigeminal neuralgia from cranial zoster (caused by reactivation of varicella-zoster virus) shows abnormal hyperintensity in a brachium pontis ➡ in the region of the CN5 entry zone.*

Varicella-Zoster Virus Spinal Cord Damage

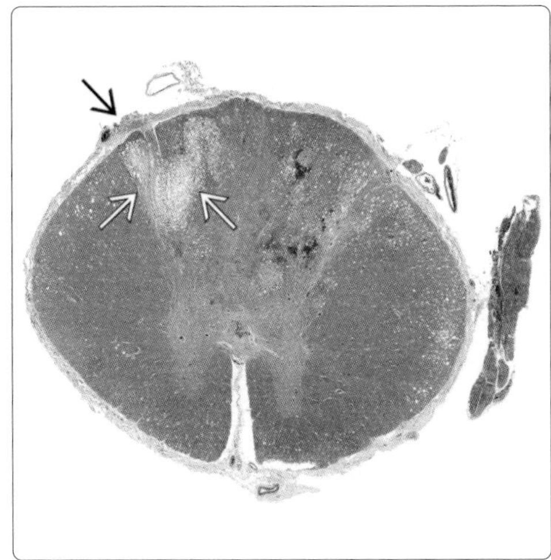

Varicella-Zoster Virus Necrotizing Vasculitis

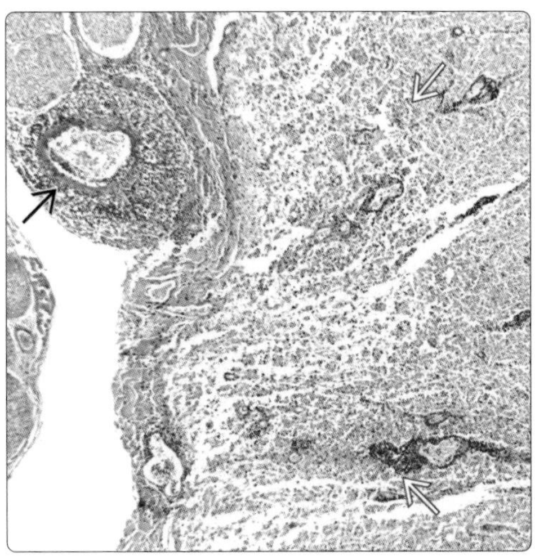

(Left) *Varicella-zoster virus encephalitis (VZVE) can cause arteritis in leptomeningeal vessels, near the spinal dorsal root entry zone ⇨, as is seen in this case where it is associated with an underlying wedge-shaped hemorrhagic infarct ➡.* **(Right)** *VZVE can be associated with necrotizing vasculitis ⇨, usually in the leptomeninges near CN5 or, as in this case, the dorsal horn of the spinal cord. There is underlying hemorrhagic necrosis ➡.*

Fibrinoid Vascular Necrosis, Varicella-Zoster Virus

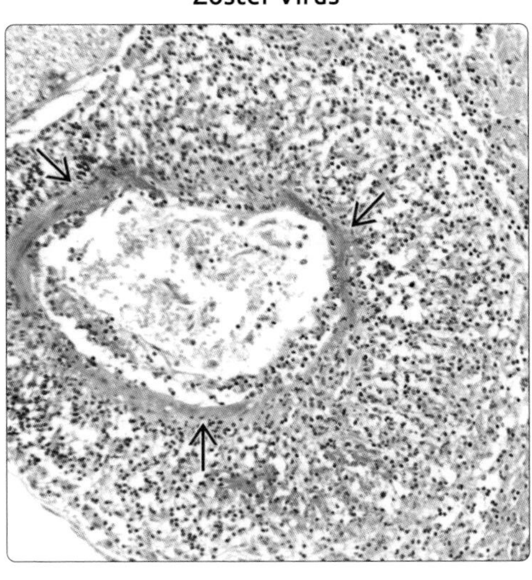

Varicella-Zoster Virus, Granulomatous Arteritis

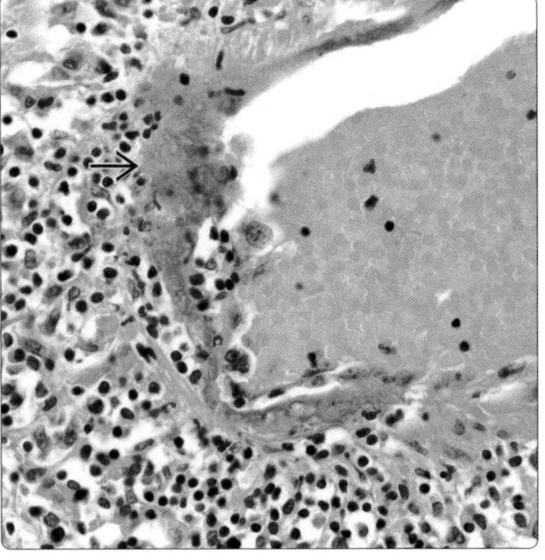

(Left) *As seen here, VZVE can cause necrotizing arteritis of leptomeningeal vessels, with fibrinoid vascular necrosis ⇨ and intense inflammation. Large vessel involvement is often associated with a wedge-shaped zone of hemorrhagic necrosis.* **(Right)** *Varicella-Zoster virus can cause a spectrum of vascular damage, including granulomatous arteritis and inflammation without fibrinoid necrosis. Severe vasculitis with fibrinoid necrosis ⇨ and mononuclear inflammation was the result in this case.*

(Left) *Severely immunocompromised patients, such as those with AIDS, may have VZV intraparenchymal small vessel vasculitis indicating deep tissue penetration of the organism.* **(Right)** *VZV spreading into CNS parenchyma may result in small vessel vasculitis and resultant ovoid mixed ischemic-demyelinative lesions concentrated at the gray-white junction →. These discrete foci are usually less coalescent than those in progressive multifocal leukoencephalopathy.*

Varicella-Zoster Virus, Immunocompromised Patient

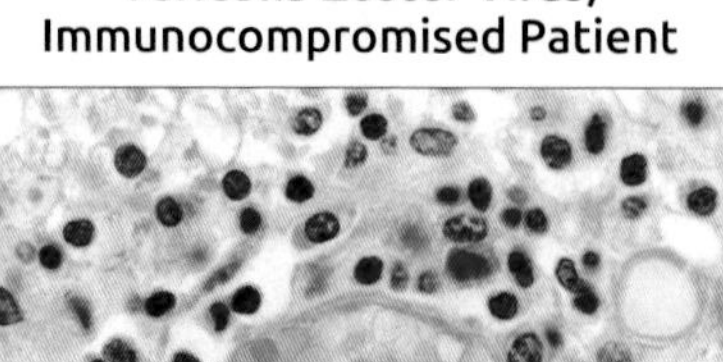

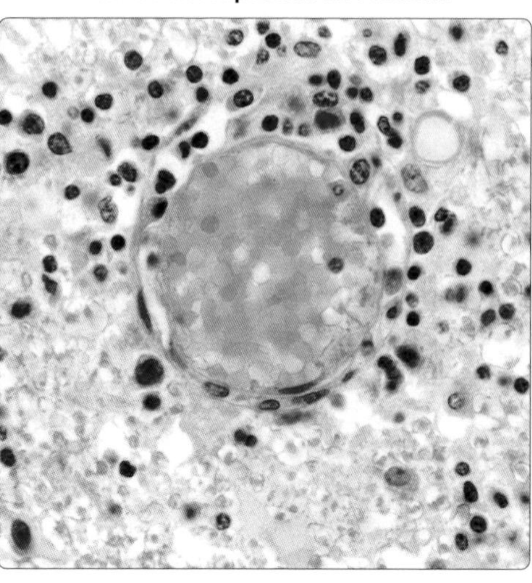

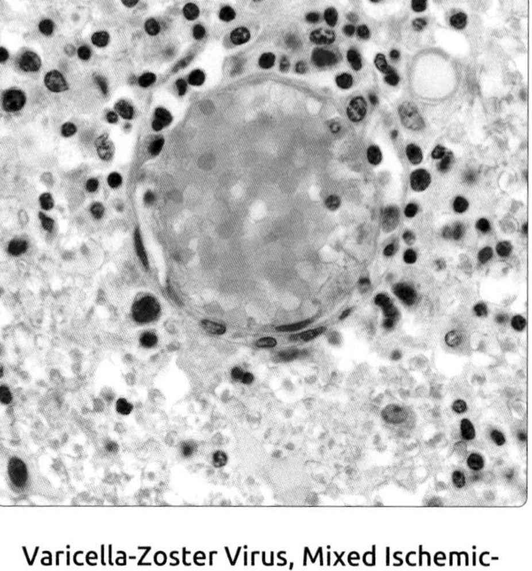

Varicella-Zoster Virus, Mixed Ischemic-Demyelinative Lesions

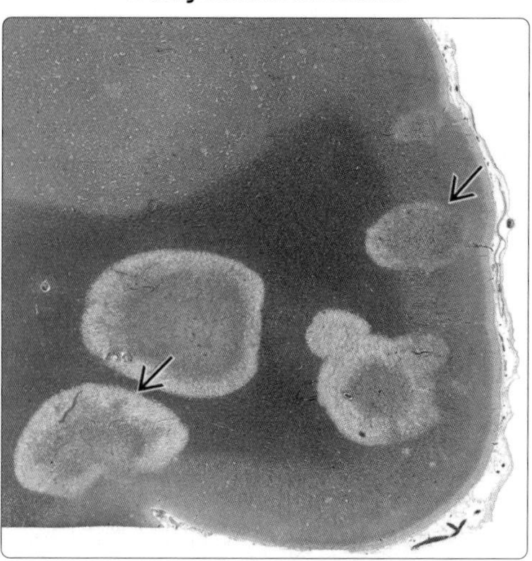

(Left) *VZVE in AIDS can spread into small parenchymal vessels and glia, causing ovoid lesions. Note the central area of infarction → and a peripheral rim of demyelination ➡ that is seen here.* **(Right)** *VZVE in AIDS patients includes significant infection in glial cells, both astrocytes and oligodendrocytes. The latter results in myelin loss, vacuolization, and intranuclear inclusions →.*

Varicella-Zoster Virus, Mixed Ischemic-Demyelinative Lesions

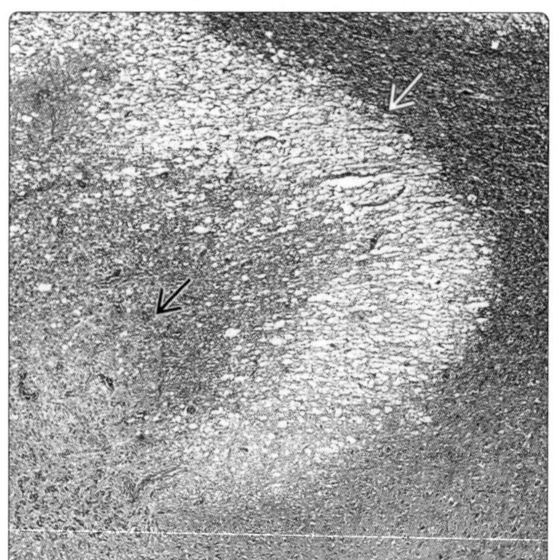

Varicella-Zoster Virus, Viral Inclusions

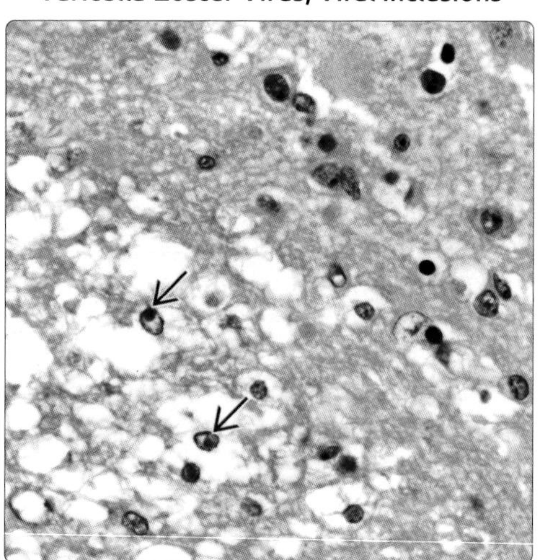

(Left) *Axial T1WI C+ MR scan of CMV encephalitis in an immunocompromised adult shows ependymal ➡ and periventricular ➡ enhancement. While CMV encephalitis often produces hemorrhagic, necrotic lesions, it can also cause a more subtle micronodular encephalitis.* **(Right)** *Note the scant inflammatory cells →, loss of ependymal cells ⇨, and cytomegalic glia ➡ in the CMV ventriculitis seen here in an AIDS patient. Intranuclear inclusions are difficult to identify at low magnification.*

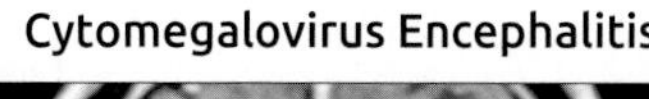

Cytomegalovirus Encephalitis

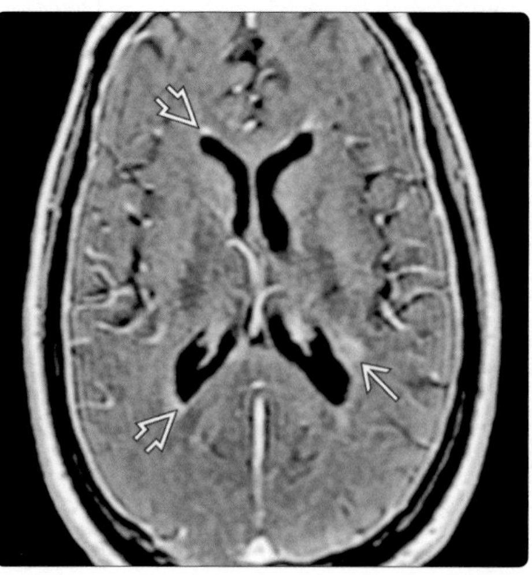

Cytomegalovirus Ventriculitis, AIDS Patient

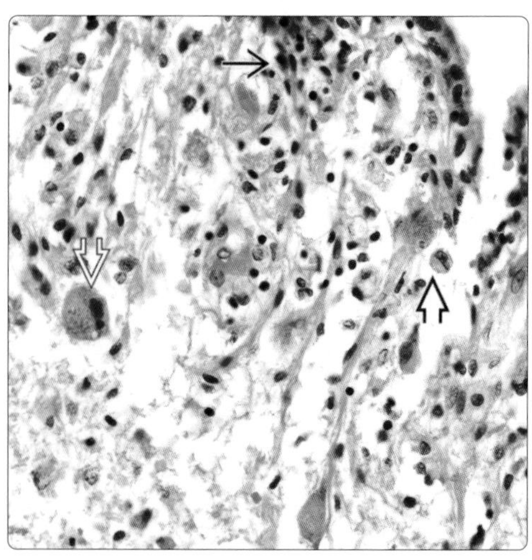

Cytomegalovirus, Periventricular Predilection

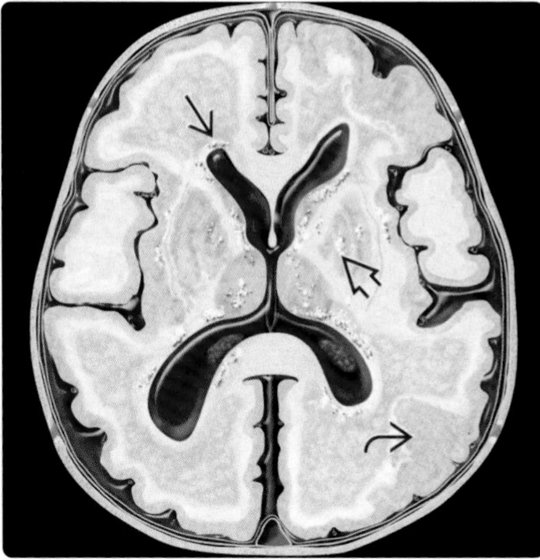

Cytomegaly

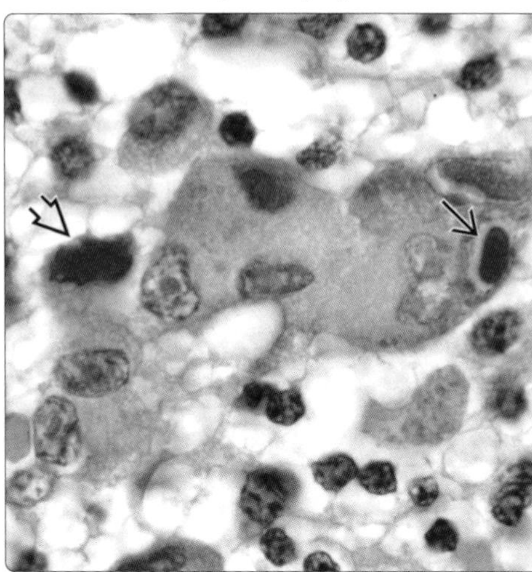

(Left) *Axial graphic of congenital CMV shows periventricular ⇒ and basal ganglia ⇒ calcification. Hydrocephalus ex vacuo is due to white matter loss. Note the cortical malformation ⇒. The brain malformation in congenital CMV infection is usually micropolygyria.* **(Right)** *Cytomegaly and Cowdry A owl's eye intranuclear inclusions ⇒ are easily seen at high power and are typical of CMV infection. Inclusions are less discrete when virions fill the entire nucleus ⇒.*

Cytomegalovirus, Endothelial Cells

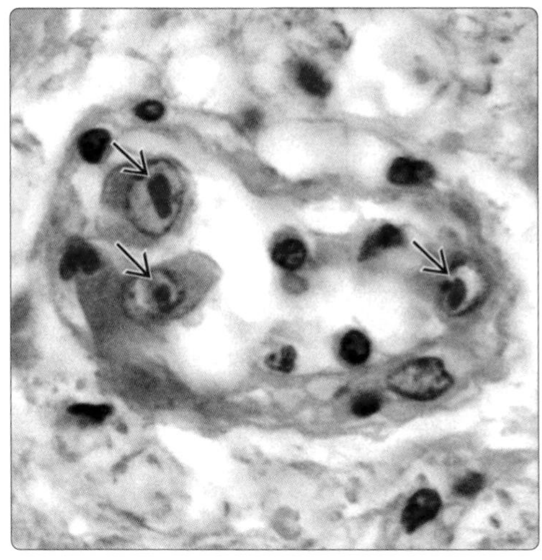

Congenital Cytomegalovirus Infection

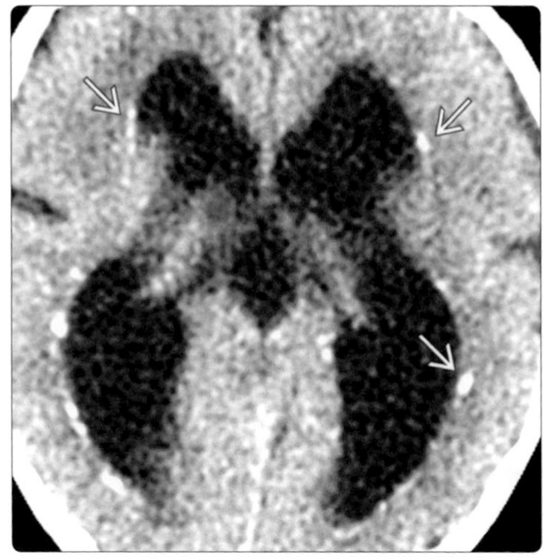

(Left) *In an AIDS patient with CMV myelitis, endothelial cells have classic Cowdry A nuclear inclusions ⇒. Note the classic clearing and peripheral margination of chromatin from the host endothelial cell.* **(Right)** *Coronal nonenhanced CT of congenital CMV shows scattered periventricular calcifications ➡. Ventriculomegaly reflects loss of periventricular white matter.*

Congenital Cytomegalovirus Infection

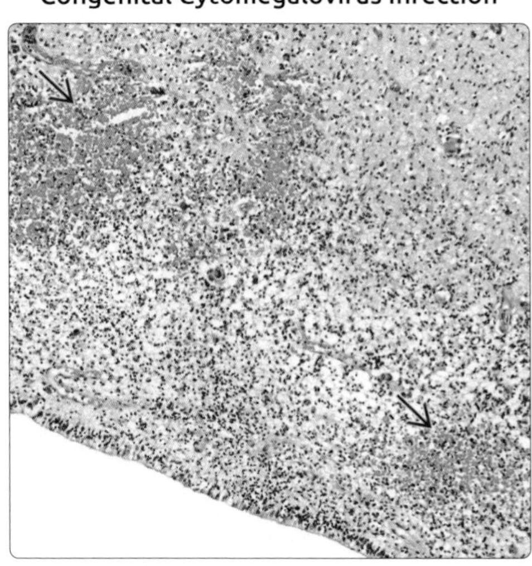

CMV, Immunohistochemistry

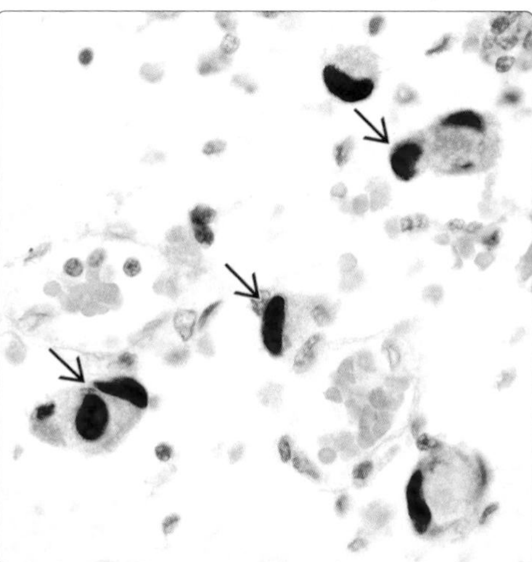

(Left) *Severe congenital CMV infection occurs when the virus is transmitted early in gestation. Note the hemorrhagic necrosis ⇒ that is seen here.* **(Right)** *In this case, CMV encephalitis is suggested by large cells with Cowdry A nuclear inclusions. A specific tissue diagnosis requires immunohistochemistry ⇒.*

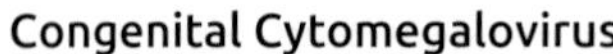

(Left) *Congenital CMV infection causes severe ventriculitis and periventriculitis with late-stage dystrophic periventricular mineralization ➜. Note the adjacent choroid plexus ➜ in this case.* **(Right)** *Congenital CMV infection shows a predilection for periventricular areas and disrupts the germinal matrix with resultant micropolygyria. Note the undulating, 4-layer cortex ➜; note also the narrow 4th layer separated by the zone of pallor ➜.*

Congenital Cytomegalovirus

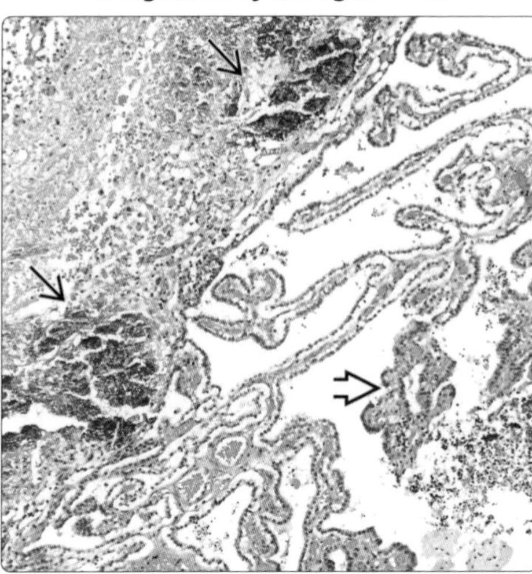

Congenital Cytomegalovirus

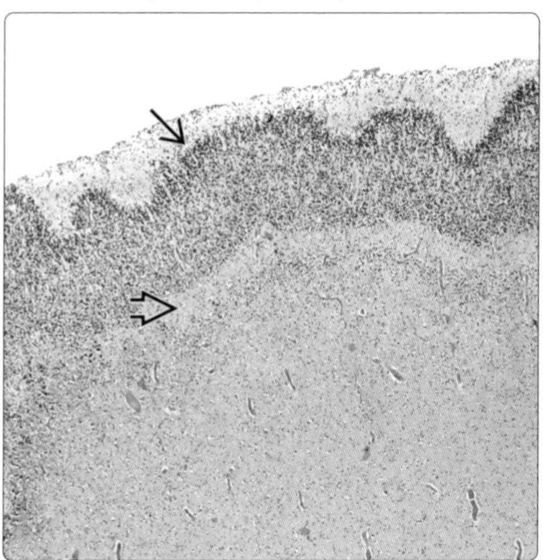

(Left) *As with other forms of viral encephalomyelitis, microglial clusters may be the principal finding in EBV encephalomyelitis in AIDS. While it is a herpes family virus, EBV does not produce intranuclear inclusions in either glia or neurons. Identification requires immunohistochemistry or in situ hybridization on tissue sections, or PCR of cerebrospinal fluid.* **(Right)** *This is an example of EBV CNS infection in an AIDS patient. Microglial clusters are highlighted by immunostaining for CD68.*

Epstein-Barr Virus Encephalomyelitis, AIDS

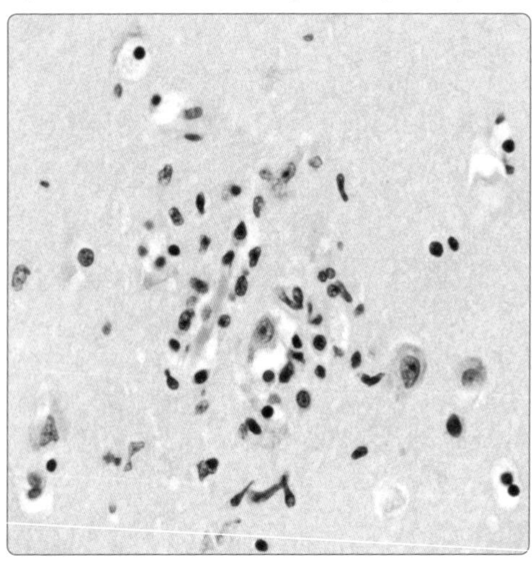

Epstein-Barr Virus Encephalomyelitis, AIDS

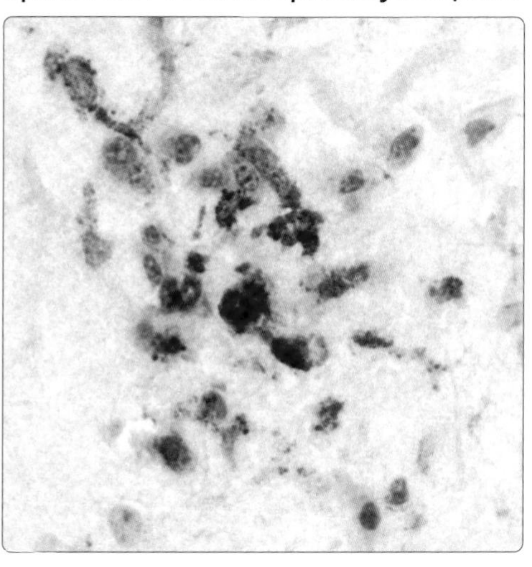

(Left) *An axial T2WI MR scan in subacute sclerosing panencephalitis (SSPE) shows subcortical white matter hyperintensities ➜ with ill-defined margins. SSPE usually follows a latent period of months to years after an initial infection with measles at age 2 years or less. A smoldering viral encephalitis ensues since patients are unable to clear the virus.* **(Right)** *Axial T2WI MR scan shows extensive SSPE with confluent areas of abnormal hyperintensity ➜ in white matter and ventriculomegaly.*

Subacute Sclerosing Panencephalitis

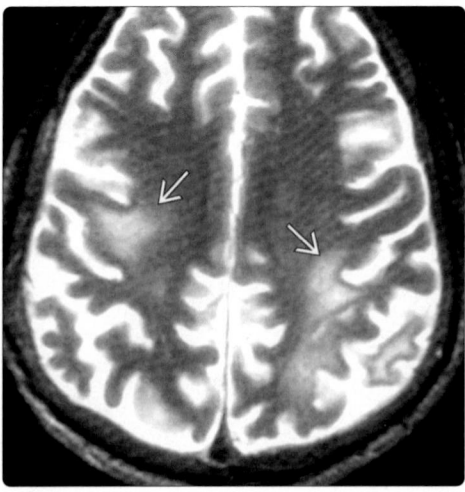

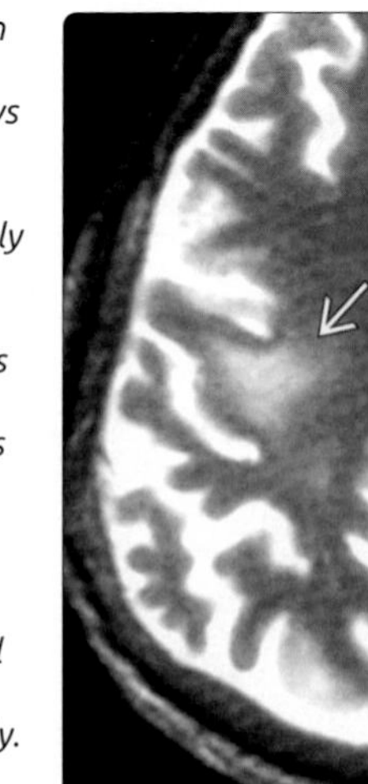

Subacute Sclerosis Panencephalitis

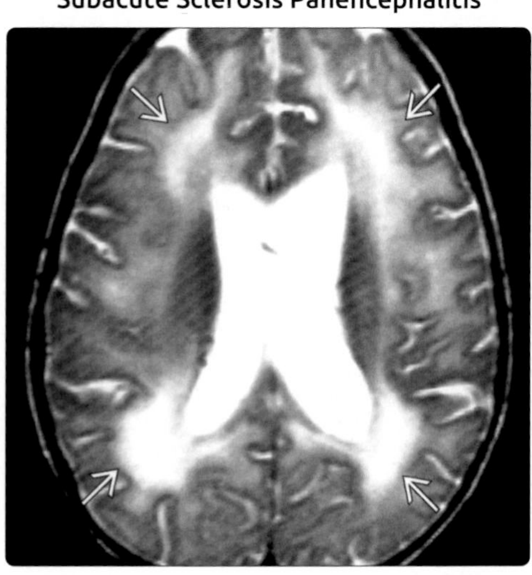

Subacute Sclerosing Panencephalitis, Microgliosis

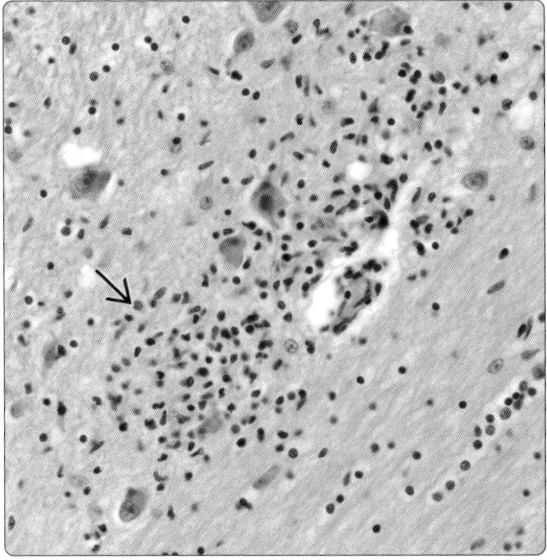

Subacute Sclerosing Panencephalitis, Perivascular Lymphocytic Cuffing

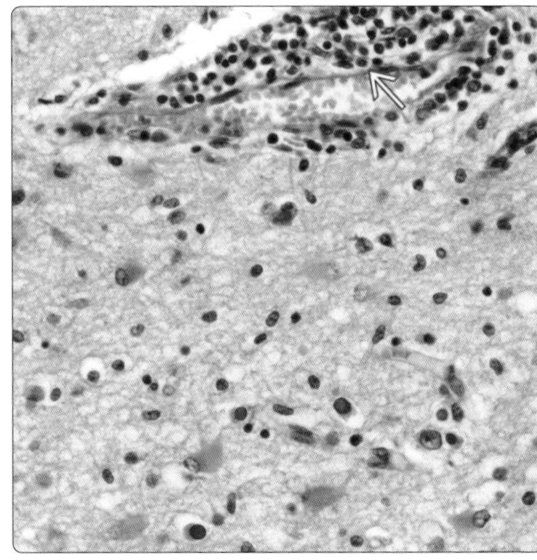

(Left) *SSPE is a slowly progressive encephalitis with parenchymal gliosis, neuronal loss, microglial infiltrates ⇨, neuronophagia, and tight microglial clusters.* **(Right)** *SSPE also has nonspecific features of viral encephalitis, including perivascular lymphocytic cuffing ➡ and intense gliosis.*

Subacute Sclerosing Panencephalitis, Viral Inclusions

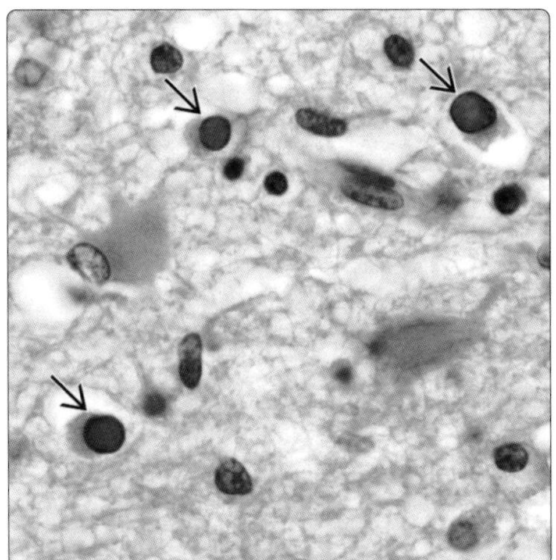

Subacute Sclerosing Panencephalitis, White Matter Damage

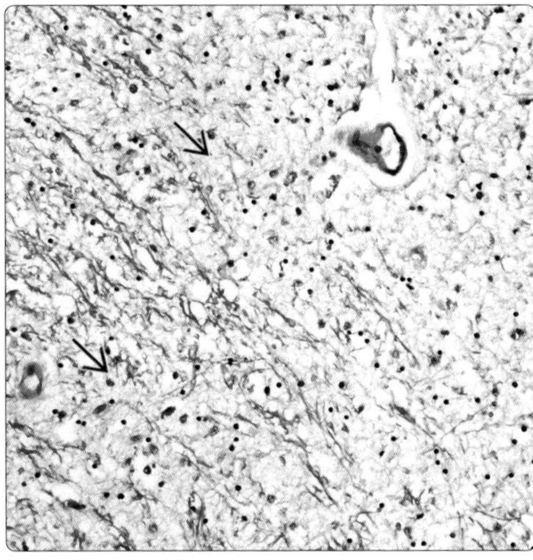

(Left) *Glassy nuclear viral inclusions ⇨ are typical of SSPE, and discrete Cowdry A inclusions are rare. SSPE predominantly affecting gray matter was historically termed "Dawson" subacute inclusion body encephalitis.* **(Right)** *SSPE predominantly affecting white matter was referred to as "van Bogaert" subacute inclusion body encephalitis. Note the patchy myelin loss ⇨ seen here.*

Subacute Sclerosing Panencephalitis, Diffuse Atrophy

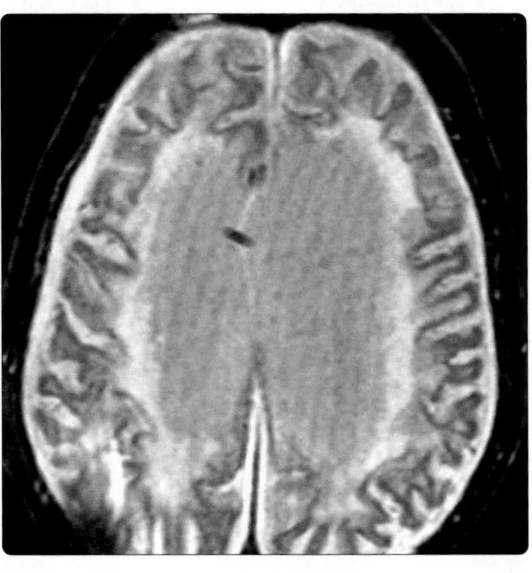

Subacute Sclerosing Panencephalitis Neurofibrillary Tangles

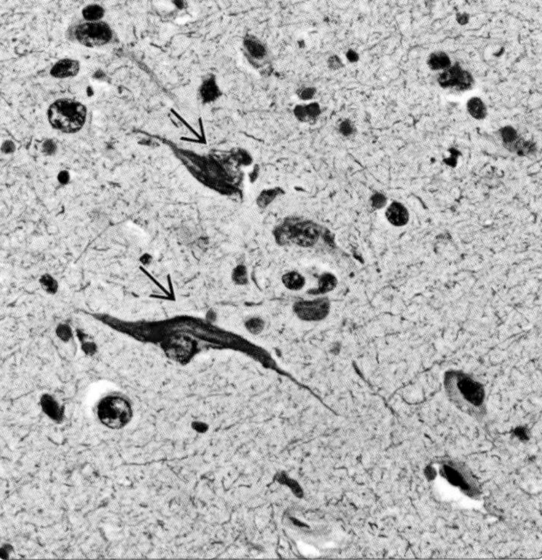

(Left) *SSPE typically appears in childhood and early adolescence, being rare in adults. Progressive diffuse atrophy, as in this case, is a late finding. Almost no white matter remains in severe cases.* **(Right)** *Large neurons in late-stage SSPE may have neurofibrillary tangles ⇨, as seen here after staining with the Bodian method.*

Fungal Infections

KEY FACTS

TERMINOLOGY

- Central nervous system (CNS) infection by pathogenic or opportunistic fungi

CLINICAL ISSUES

- Common: Basal meningitis, hydrocephalus, space-occupying lesions (cerebral abscesses and granulomas), and stroke
  - Basal meningitis
  - Hydrocephalus
  - Space-occupying lesions (abscesses, granulomas)
  - Stroke
- Less common
  - Orbito-rhino-cerebral syndromes
  - Spinal infection

MICROSCOPIC

- Yeasts: *Blastomyces, Histoplasma, Cryptococcus*
- Yeast and pseudohyphae: *Candida*
- Hyphae: *Aspergillus, Zygomycetes*
- Sporangium and endospores: *Coccidioides*
- Yeasts not vasoinvasive
  - Usually do not cause infarctions, hemorrhages
- Hyphae and pseudohyphae vasoinvasive
  - May cause infarctions, hemorrhages
- Focal confined infections [granuloma(s)] if host relatively immunocompetent
- Meningitis more common if host immunocompromised

DIAGNOSTIC CHECKLIST

- Do not mistake normal corpora amylacea for fungal forms
  - Corpora amylacea also PAS(+)
  - Corporal amylacea also (GMS)(+)
  - Corpora amylacea usually not within macrophages
  - Corpora amylacea often congregate in subpial, perivascular locations
- Necrotic fungi within tissue do not show as pristine morphological features as they do in culture

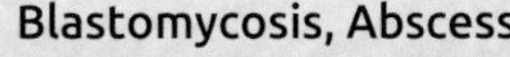

Blastomycosis, Abscess

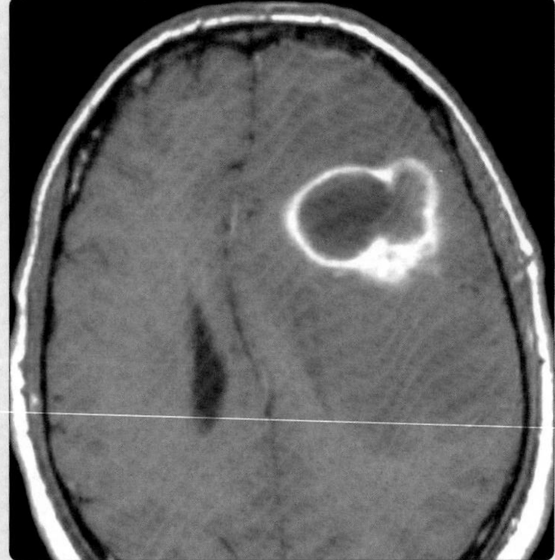

***Blastomyces* Species, Double Contour Wall**

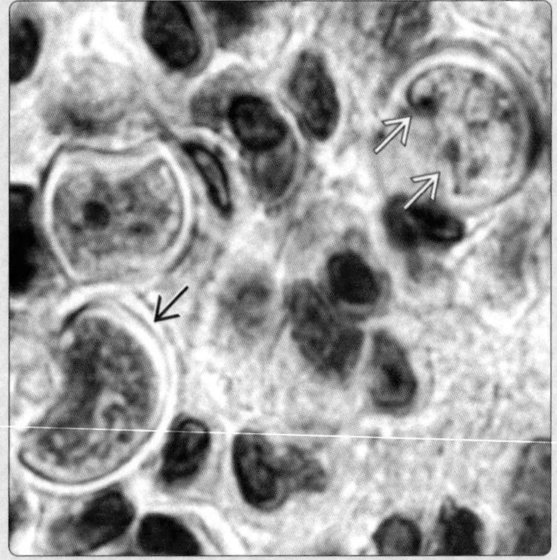

(Left) *Intracerebral blastomycosis abscesses are expansile, edema eliciting, and ring enhancing, as shown in this axial T1 C+ MR.* **(Right)** *Blastomyces species have thick, "double contour" walls ⇨ and multiple nuclei ➡. Note the flattened profiles that may represent recent sites of broad-based budding.*

***Blastomyces* Species, GMS**

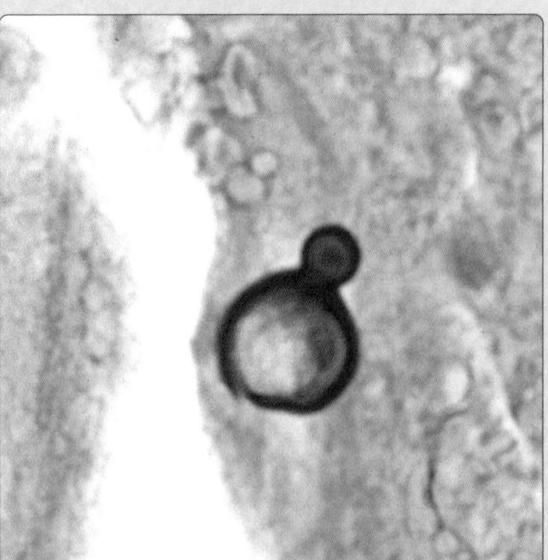

***Histoplasma* Meningitis, AIDS**

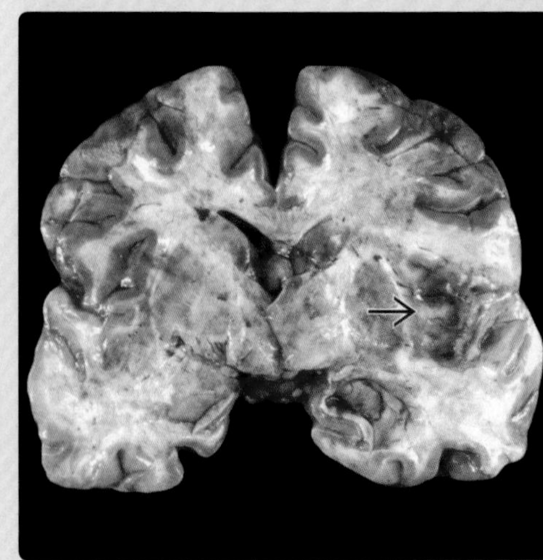

(Left) *Methenamine silver stain illustrates the relatively broad-based budding typical of Blastomyces species.* **(Right)** *Coronal brain section from a woman with AIDS and to Histoplasma meningitis shows areas of infarction ⇨ and widespread hyperemia and swelling. Disseminated disease can occur in immunocompromised hosts.*

TERMINOLOGY

Synonyms

- Blastomycosis: Gilchrist disease, Chicago disease
- Coccidioidomycosis: Valley fever
- Cryptococcosis: Torulosis

Definitions

- Central nervous system (CNS) infection by opportunistic or pathogenic fungi

ETIOLOGY/PATHOGENESIS

Environmental Exposure

- Most fungi acquired through inhalation
  - Most present in soil
    - Exception is *Candida* species, which is normal constituent of human gut flora
    - Several related to bird feces (e.g., *Cryptococcus, Histoplasma*)
  - Most ubiquitous in environment, worldwide occurrence
    - Exception: Coccidioidomycosis occurs in areas with low rainfall and high summer temperatures
    - Coccidioidomycosis endemic in southern California, Arizona, New Mexico, southwestern Texas, Mexico, Central and parts of South America
    - Exception: Histoplasmosis and blastomycosis occur in watershed areas with moist soil
    - Histoplasmosis: Ohio and Mississippi River valleys
    - Blastomycosis: Regions that border Great Lakes and St. Lawrence River, Ohio and Mississippi River valleys
- Many CNS infections preceded by pulmonary infection
  - Pulmonary infection may be dominant type of infection (e.g., blastomycosis, histoplasmosis)
  - Pulmonary infection may be clinically overlooked or absent at time of CNS disease (e.g., cryptococcosis)
- Fungi reach CNS via hematogenous route, usually from lung
- Pathogenic infections: Organism has capability of producing disease in any individual following exposure to sufficient numbers of fungi
  - Blastomycosis, histoplasmosis usually pathogenic and infection usually confined to lung
  - Focal granulomatous disease in immunocompetent hosts
  - Disseminated disease including CNS involvement occurs in immunocompromised hosts (e.g., AIDS)
- Opportunistic infections: Organism causes disease in patients with lowered resistance
  - Candidiasis, *Zygomycetes*, cryptococcal infections usually opportunistic
  - Coccidioidomycosis, aspergillosis in both immunocompetent and immunocompromised hosts
- Risk factors that lower host resistance
  - Neutropenia
  - Steroids
  - Impaired cell-mediated immunity
  - Impaired integument (e.g., *Candida* species)
  - Diabetic ketoacidosis (e.g., *Zygomycetes* species)

Infectious Agents

- *Blastomyces dermatitidis*
- *Histoplasma capsulatum*
- *Coccidioides immitis*
- *Aspergillus fumigatus*
- *Cryptococcus neoformans*
- *Zygomycetes* species *(Rhizopus, Mucor, Absidia)*
- *Candida albicans*
- Numerous very rare fungi, e.g., pigmented fungi
- Rare dematiaceous fungi are emerging agents for cerebral mycosis
  - *Cladophialophora (Cladosporium) bantiana, Fonsecaea monophora* examples

CLINICAL ISSUES

Presentation

- CNS mycoses present as focal parenchymal or diffuse meningeal disease
  - Focal infections: Discrete granulomas
    - Seizures, focal neurological deficits, variable fever
  - Diffuse infections: Meningitis
    - Headache, meningeal irritation signs, mental status changes
    - Hydrocephalus
- Fungi variably vasoinvasive; may cause stroke
  - Yeasts not vasoinvasive, e.g., *Histoplasma, Blastomyces, Cryptococcus*
  - Hyphal and pseudohyphal fungi vasoinvasive, e.g., *Candida, Aspergillus, Zygomycetes*, occasionally *Coccidioides*

Treatment

- Drugs
  - Amphotericin B
  - Voriconazole, fluconazole, itraconazole

Prognosis

- Dependent on prompt diagnosis and treatment, degree of underlying immunosuppression
- Outcome poor in many patients, even with treatment

MACROSCOPIC

General Features

- Basilar meningitis, focal granulomatous parenchymal lesion, hemorrhagic infarction(s), hemorrhage: Depending on type of fungus, degree of host immunocompetency

MICROSCOPIC

Histologic Features

- *Blastomyces dermatitidis*
  - Uncommon CNS infection, even in endemic areas
    - Usually pathogenic infection
    - Most infections pulmonary, not CNS
    - Rare CNS examples, usually localized granuloma
    - In recent study, CNS blastomycosis manifested as epidural abscess (1 of 22), meningitis (7 of 22), intracranial mass lesions (10 of 22), concomitant intracranial mass lesions and meningitis (4 of 22)
  - Yeast, 8-15 μm, with broad-based bud
    - Multiple nuclei seen in well-fixed tissues
    - Mucicarmine (-) or shows thin outline, contrasting with thick (+) capsule in *Cryptococcus*

  - Fontana-Masson (-)
  - Positive with GMS, PAS
- *Histoplasma capsulatum*
  - Uncommon CNS infection in endemic areas
  - Most infections in reticuloendothelial system
    - Infection usually confined to lung, yields small discrete localized granulomas
    - Dissemination usually limited to spleen and liver
    - Dissemination in immunocompromised hosts, e.g., AIDS patients; may produce CNS disease
    - CNS disease manifests as meningitis, sometimes with secondary CNS infarction due to vasculitis in leptomeninges
  - Localizing granulomas in immunocompetent patients
  - Disseminated disease in AIDS patients
  - Yeast (difficult to identify in H&E sections)
  - 2-4 μm, intracellular within macrophages
  - Not encapsulated
  - Appear much smaller on H&E than on PAS or GMS
    - Fixation causes retraction of protoplasm from rigid cell wall, leaving clear space
    - Retraction artifact can produce "pseudocapsule"
    - Uninucleate, contrasting with multinucleate *Blastomyces dermatitidis*
- *Coccidioides immitis*
  - Usually occurs as meningitis in both immunocompetent and AIDS patients
    - Subacute, granulomatous meningitis
    - Often basilar meningitis
  - Brain abscesses less common
  - Disseminated disease in minority of immunocompetent patients, but predilection for CNS
  - Systemic organ involvement possible in addition to CNS: Skin, bones, joints
  - Histiocytes, multinucleated giant cells
  - Caseous material more common in lung than CNS lesions
  - 30-60 μm sporangia contain 1-5 μm sporangiospores (endospores)
    - Term "spherule" used for intermediate forms between released endospores and sporangium
    - Intact sporangia elicit granulomatous reaction
    - Spherules may lie within multinucleated giant cells
  - Hyphal forms exceedingly rare in CNS (arthrospores)
- *Aspergillus fumigatus*
  - Uncommon infection in healthy individuals
    - In farmers exposed to silage
    - In some relatively healthy patients with only risk factor such as steroid use for asthma
    - Orbito-rhinal infections
  - In immunocompromised patients, most commonly in debilitated patients
    - Steroids, neutropenia principal risk factors
    - Impaired integument
    - Chronic pulmonary disease, hematological malignancies, bone marrow transplantation recipients, burn victims
    - Uncommon in AIDS patients
    - *A. fumigatus* uncommon in patients with solid systemic organ neoplasms
    - Other species: *Aspergillus flavus, Aspergillus niger*
    - *Aspergillus terreus* may be more common pathogen in metastatic, primary brain tumor patients with lymphopenia
  - Dichotomous, branching hyphae
  - Acute angle branching
  - Hyphae permeate vessel wall
  - Septate hyphae radiate from center of thrombosed vessel
  - Hyphae positive with PAS, GMS
  - Hyphae may be bulbous, distorted in tissue sections
  - Neutrophilic reaction in acute infections, uncommon in immunocompetent host
  - Granulomatous to absent reaction in immunocompromised host
  - Thrombosis leads to hemorrhagic infarction, overt hemorrhage
  - Cannot distinguish *Aspergillus* species on tissue features; culture required
- *Cryptococcus neoformans*
  - Usually opportunistic infection
  - Most common fungal CNS infection in AIDS patients
  - Primary infection thought to be pulmonary but rarely clinically recognized
  - Widely disseminated disease may affect multiple organs, CNS most severely
  - Meningitis, often with minimal host inflammatory response
  - Occasional focal granulomatous response
  - Yeast, 4-7 μm
  - Mucinous capsule, mucicarmine stain (+) (carminophilic); Alcian blue (+)
  - Capsule 3-5 μm thick
  - Yeast in old fibrotic, caseous lesions have diminished carminophilia
  - Yeast PAS(+), GMS(+)
- *Zygomycetes* species *(Rhizopus, Mucor, Absidia)*
  - Usually opportunistic infection
  - Diabetic ketoacidosis
  - Patients with malignancy
  - Broad hyphae
    - 10-15 μm diameter
    - Branching irregular compared to *Aspergillus* species
    - Only rare septations; folds may mimic septations
    - Vasoinvasive, leads to infarction
    - Classic is vasoinvasion large vessels at base of brain, with rhino-cerebral disease
  - Most infections due to *Rhizopus* species, but cannot distinguish types in tissue sections; culture required
  - Often minimal inflammatory host response
  - Sometimes seen better on H&E than PAS, GMS
- *Candida* species
  - Opportunistic infection
  - Patients often with prolonged antibiotic therapy, abdominal operations, catheters, etc.
  - CNS involvement usually late in disseminated disease
  - Higher incidence of CNS fungal infection by *Candida* species at autopsy
  - Yeast (+) pseudohyphae ("noodles and eggs")
    - 3-4 μm
    - Vasoinvasive: Hemorrhagic infarctions

- Usually minimal inflammatory host response
- Dematiaceous fungi
  - Brown by H&E

Cytologic Features

- Cryptococci may abound in cerebrospinal fluid (CSF) but is easy to overlook if not specifically sought
- Some cases with fungal meningitis, ventriculitis may have histiocytes, lymphocytes, multinucleated giant cells in CSF

ANCILLARY TESTS

Cultures

- Necessary to document species, sometimes type of fungal infection

DIFFERENTIAL DIAGNOSIS

Histoplasma From *Toxoplasma*

- *Toxoplasma* smaller, not in macrophages
- *Toxoplasma* negative for PAS, GMS fungal stains
- Immunohistochemistry for *Toxoplasma*(+)

Histoplasma From *Pneumocystis carinii*

- *Pneumocystis* (+) on GMS, but *P. carinii* infection does not affect CNS

Cryptococcus From *Blastomyces*

- *Blastomyces* slightly carminophilic, but contains multiple nuclei
- *Cryptococcus* thicker carminophilic, Alcian blue (+), capsule
- *Cryptococcus* Fontana-Masson (+), *Blastomyces* Fontana-Masson (-)

Histoplasma From *Cryptococcus*

- *Histoplasma*, smaller; pseudocapsule due to retraction artifact, not true capsule
- *Histoplasma* usually nearly invisible on H&E, *Cryptococcus* is gray-blue in H&E sections, more visible due to thick capsule
- *Histoplasma* mucicarmine (-)

DIAGNOSTIC CHECKLIST

Clinically Relevant Pathologic Features

- Hyphal forms often vasoinvasive, with risk for infarction

Pathologic Interpretation Pearls

- *Histoplasma* smaller on H&E than on PAS, GMS fungal stains due to fixation-induced retraction of protoplasm from rigid wall
  - *Histoplasma* nearly invisible on H&E
- *Cryptococcus* species Fontana-Masson (+) and stronger mucicarmine (+); *Blastomyces* species Fontana-Masson (-)
- Rare true septations in hyphae do not exclude diagnosis of *Rhizopus* species; exclude folds in broad hyphae

SELECTED REFERENCES

1. Garcia RR et al: Fusarium brain abscess: case report and literature review. Mycoses. 58(1):22-6, 2015
2. Gonzalez-Duarte A et al: Cryptococcal meningitis in HIV-negative patients with systemic connective tissue diseases. Neurol Res. 37(4):283-7, 2015
3. Henao-Martínez AF et al: Cryptococcosis in solid organ transplant recipients. Curr Opin Infect Dis. 28(4):300-7, 2015
4. Naik V et al: Intracranial Fungal Granulomas: A Single Institutional Clinicopathologic Study of 66 Patients and Review of the Literature. World Neurosurg. 83(6):1166-1172, 2015
5. Hocevar SN et al: Microsporidiosis acquired through solid organ transplantation: a public health investigation. Ann Intern Med. 160(4):213-20, 2014
6. Murthy JM et al: Fungal infections of the central nervous system. Handb Clin Neurol. 121:1383-401, 2014
7. Bariola JR et al: Blastomycosis of the central nervous system: a multicenter review of diagnosis and treatment in the modern era. Clin Infect Dis. 50(6):797-804, 2010
8. Glick JA et al: Candida meningitis post Gliadel wafer placement successfully treated with intrathecal and intravenous amphotericin B. Ann Pharmacother. 44(1):215-8, 2010
9. Joshi NS et al: Epidemiology of cryptococcal infection in hospitalized children. Pediatr Infect Dis J. 29(12):e91-5, 2010
10. Mathisen G et al: Coccidioidal meningitis: clinical presentation and management in the fluconazole era. Medicine (Baltimore). 89(5):251-84, 2010
11. Mazumder SA et al: Cryptococcal meningitis after neurosurgery. Am J Med Sci. 339(6):582-3, 2010
12. Pruitt AA: Central nervous system infections in cancer patients. Semin Neurol. 30(3):296-310, 2010
13. Raman Sharma R: Fungal infections of the nervous system: current perspective and controversies in management. Int J Surg. 8(8):591-601, 2010
14. Raparia K et al: Cerebral mycosis: 7-year retrospective series in a tertiary center. Neuropathology. 30(3):218-23, 2010
15. Saccente M et al: Clinical and laboratory update on blastomycosis. Clin Microbiol Rev. 23(2):367-81, 2010
16. Tai YF et al: Central nervous system histoplasmosis in an immunocompetent patient. J Neurol. 257(11):1931-3, 2010
17. Zhu LP et al: Cryptococcal meningitis in non-HIV-infected patients in a Chinese tertiary care hospital, 1997-2007. Med Mycol. 48(4):570-9, 2010
18. Drake KW et al: Coccidioidal meningitis and brain abscesses: analysis of 71 cases at a referral center. Neurology. 73(21):1780-6, 2009
19. Kleinschmidt-Demasters BK: Disseminated Fusarium infection with brain abscesses in a lung transplant recipient. Clin Neuropathol. 28(6):417-21, 2009
20. Damek DM et al: Aspergillus terreus brain abscess mimicking tumor progression in a patient with treated glioblastoma multiforme. Clin Neuropathol. 27(6):400-7, 2008
21. Saccente M: Central nervous system histoplasmosis. Curr Treat Options Neurol. 10(3):161-7, 2008
22. Dotis J et al: Central nervous system aspergillosis in children: a systematic review of reported cases. Int J Infect Dis. 11(5):381-93, 2007
23. Crum-Cianflone NF et al: Unusual presentations of coccidioidomycosis: a case series and review of the literature. Medicine (Baltimore). 85(5):263-77, 2006
24. Schestatsky P et al: Isolated central nervous system histoplasmosis in immunocompetent hosts: a series of 11 cases. Scand J Infect Dis. 38(1):43-8, 2006
25. Davis LE et al: Central Nervous System Coccidioides immitis Infections. Curr Treat Options Neurol. 7(2):157-165, 2005
26. Pagano L et al: Fungal CNS infections in patients with hematologic malignancy. Expert Rev Anti Infect Ther. 3(5):775-85, 2005
27. Wheat LJ et al: Diagnosis and management of central nervous system histoplasmosis. Clin Infect Dis. 40(6):844-52, 2005
28. Kleinschmidt-DeMasters BK: Central nervous system aspergillosis: a 20-year retrospective series. Hum Pathol. 33(1):116-24, 2002
29. Friedman JA et al: Meningoencephalitis due to Blastomyces dermatitidis: case report and literature review. Mayo Clin Proc. 75(4):403-8, 2000
30. Kleinschmidt-DeMasters BK et al: Coccidioidomycosis meningitis with massive dural and cerebral venous thrombosis and tissue arthroconidia. Arch Pathol Lab Med. 124(2):310-4, 2000

(Left) *Blastomyces often elicit a granulomatous response with multinucleated giant cells. The yeast-form organism* → *is often easily identified.* **(Right)** *Blastomyces dermatitidis usually elicits a brisk inflammatory reaction. Note the thick walls* → *of these large yeast-form organisms. Although not illustrated here, the inflammatory reaction may be granulomatous.*

***Blastomyces*, Granulomatous Response**

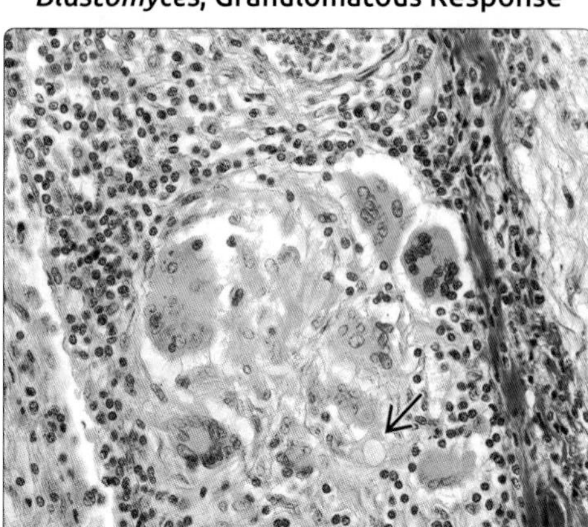

***Blastomyces*, Organisms**

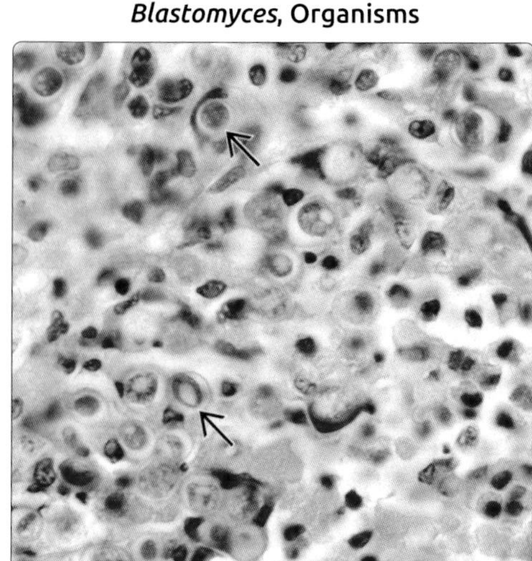

(Left) *Blastomyces are large, round, generally uniformly sized cocci that are here engulfed by multinucleated giant cells.* **(Right)** *Methenamine silver stain illustrates the relatively broad-based budding typical of the Blastomyces species.*

***Blastomyces*, GMS, Engulfed by Giant Cells**

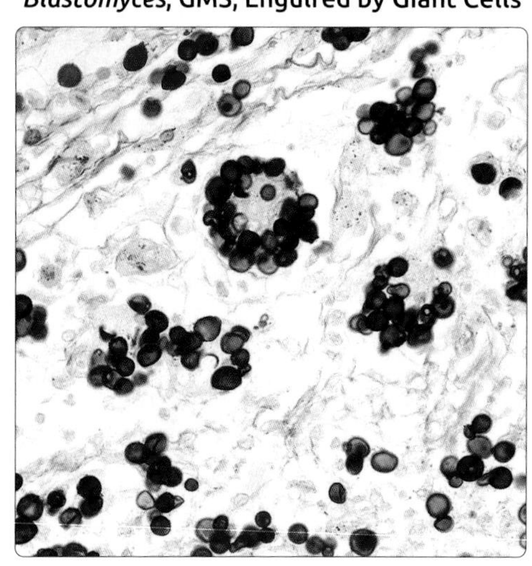

***Blastomyces*, Broad-Based Budding**

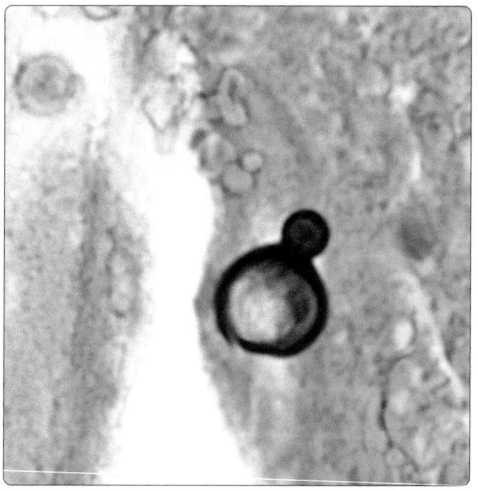

(Left) *Bilateral multifocal airspace opacities* → *due to inhalational histoplasmosis appeared in a patient who felled a tree populated by many birds. Histoplasmosis may be clinically silent, or restricted to pulmonary disease, in immunocompetent hosts.* **(Right)** *Histoplasma meningitis can be associated with secondary vasculitis with intimal proliferation* →*. As with leptomeningeal tuberculosis, cerebral infarctions can result from this infectious vasculitis.*

Histoplasmosis

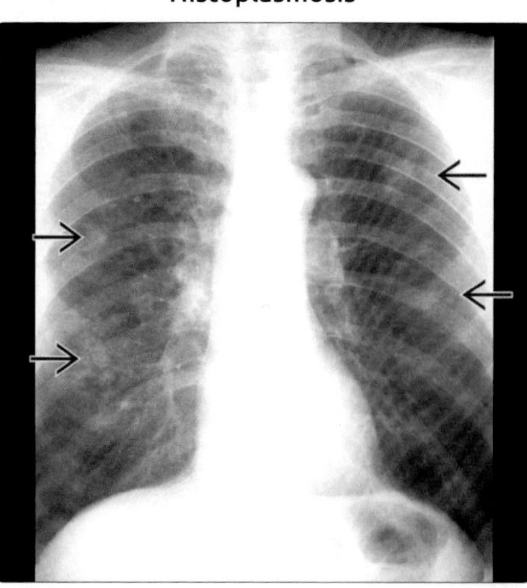

***Histoplasma* Meningitis, Secondary Vasculitis**

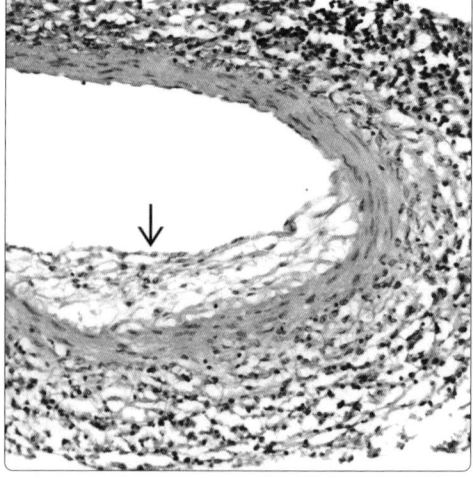

Histoplasma, Yeasts

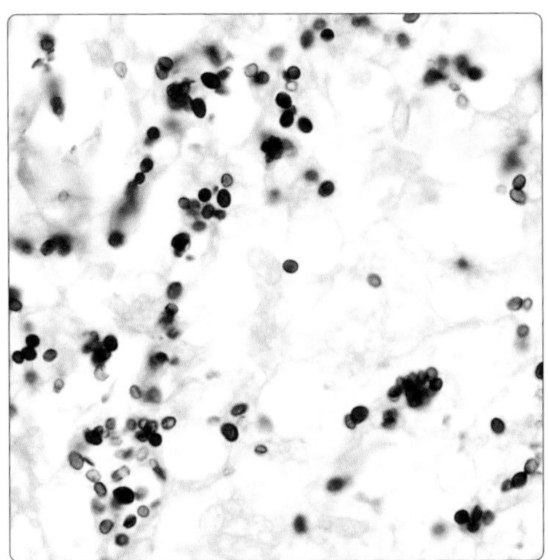

Histoplasma, Narrow-Neck Budding

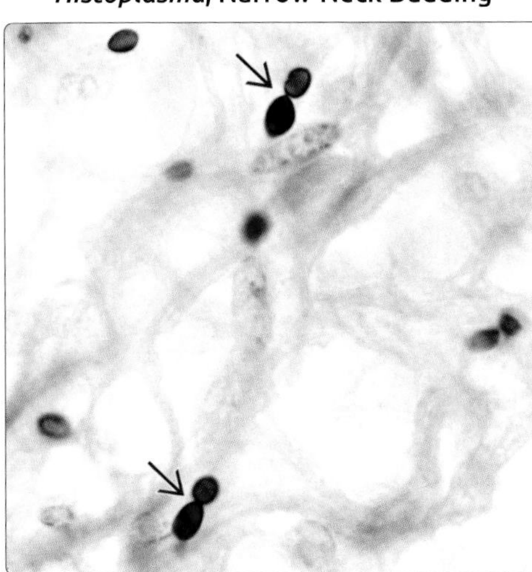

(Left) *Large numbers of Histoplasma capsulatum can be found in fungal meningitis in patients with severe immunosuppression, such as AIDS. The yeasts are often extracellular, i.e., not within macrophages.* **(Right)** *Narrow-neck budding ➡ is classic for Histoplasma capsulatum, an organism that, in spite of its name, is not truly encapsulated. Fungal stains, such as methenamine silver, are generally required for identification, as this small yeast is difficult to detect in H&E sections.*

Coccidioidomycosis

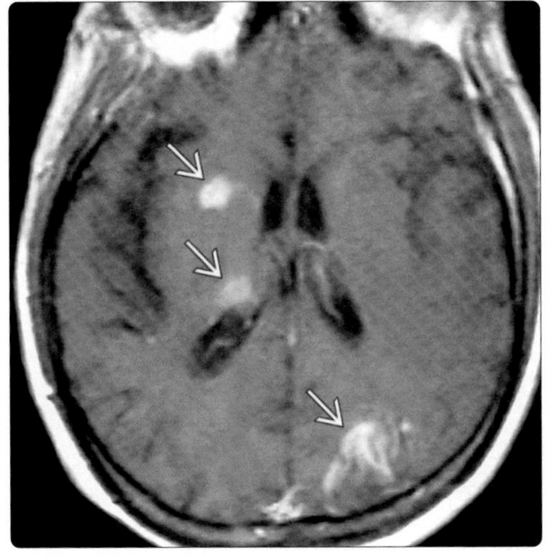

Endospores

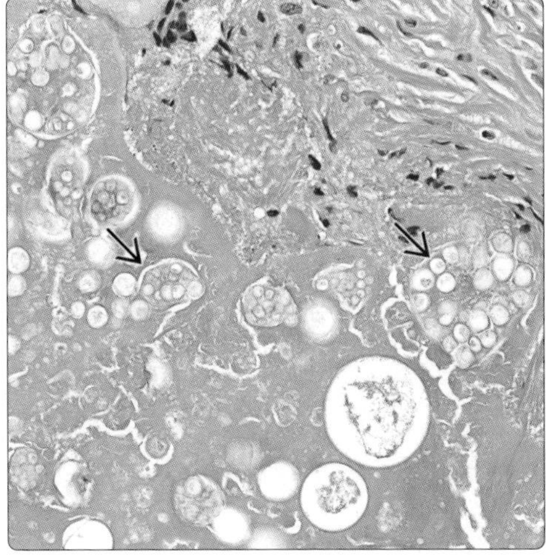

(Left) *As active areas of acute and chronic inflammation, lesions of coccidioidomycosis ➡ are understandably contrast enhancing. Axial T1 C+ MR shows involvement of the right basal ganglia, right thalamus, and left occipital lobe.* **(Right)** *Degenerating sporangia containing endospores (sporangiospores) ➡ are easily seen in the center of this granuloma produced by the Coccidioides species.*

Coccidioides immitis

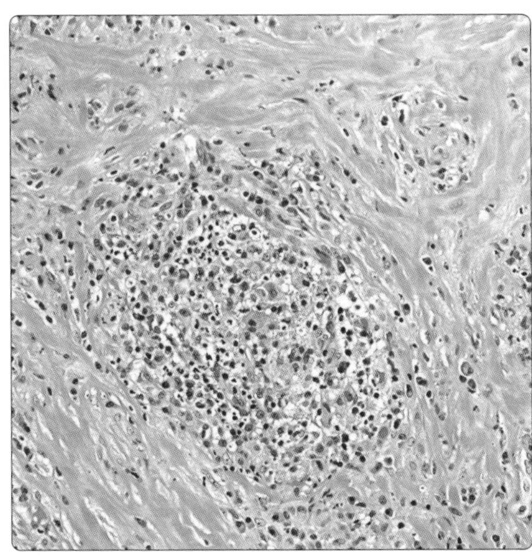

Coccidioides immitis, Focal Necrosis

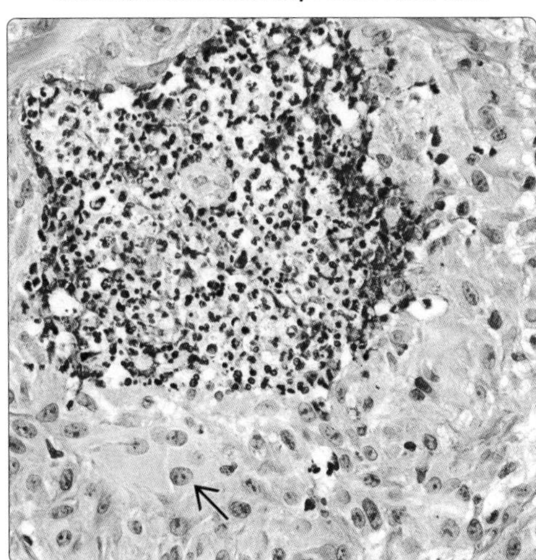

(Left) *Coccidioides immitis may produce small tight granulomas in tissue sections.* **(Right)** *Identification of foci of necrosis within granulomas filled with epithelioid histiocytes ➡ should prompt thorough search for infectious organisms, including fungi. This example was produced by Coccidioides immitis, although the spherules are not visible here.*

(Left) *A fractured sporangiospore wall* ⇨ *of Coccidioides immitis retracts from its former contents of sporangiospores. Released intermediate forms are sometimes referred to as spherules* ⇨. **(Right)** *Most fungi can also be seen on periodic acid-Schiff staining. Note the fracturing of the sporangium wall* ⇨ *with release of endospores* ➡ *of Coccidioides immitis. Endospores should not be mistaken for large yeast forms, such as Blastomyces species.*

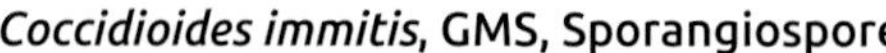

***Coccidioides immitis*, GMS, Sporangiospore**

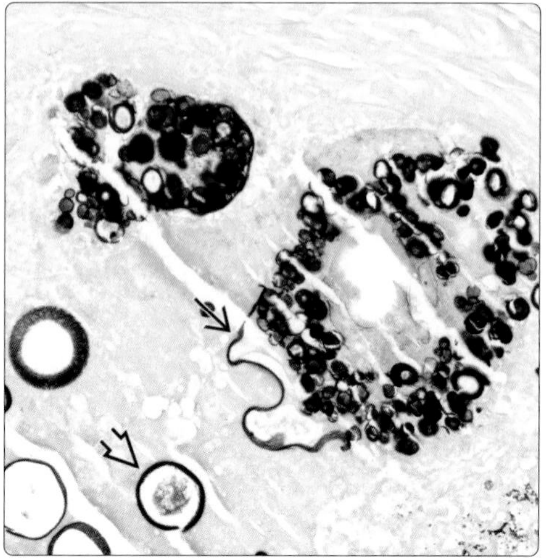

***Coccidioides immitis*, PAS**

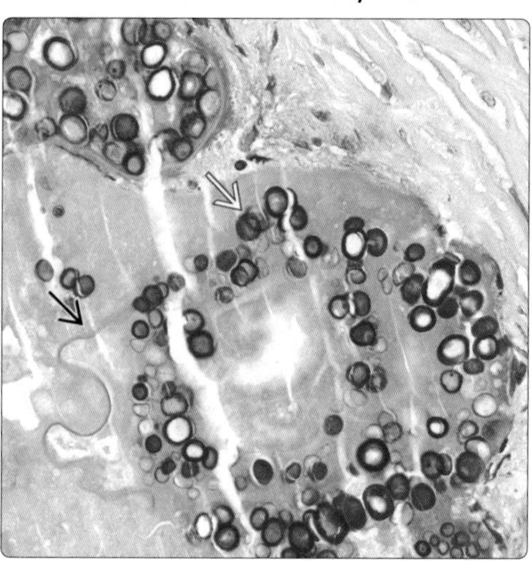

(Left) *The angioinvasive potential of the Aspergillus species is apparent here, as dense colonies* ⇨ *penetrate these leptomeningeal vessels.* **(Right)** *Methenamine silver stains best demonstrate angioinvasive Aspergillus hyphae* ⇨. *Yeast-form organisms typically are not vasoinvasive.*

***Aspergillus* Species, Angioinvasion**

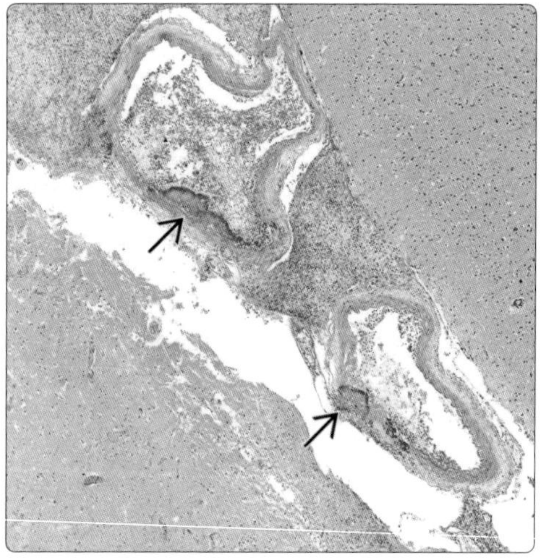

***Aspergillus* Species, GMS, Angioinvasion**

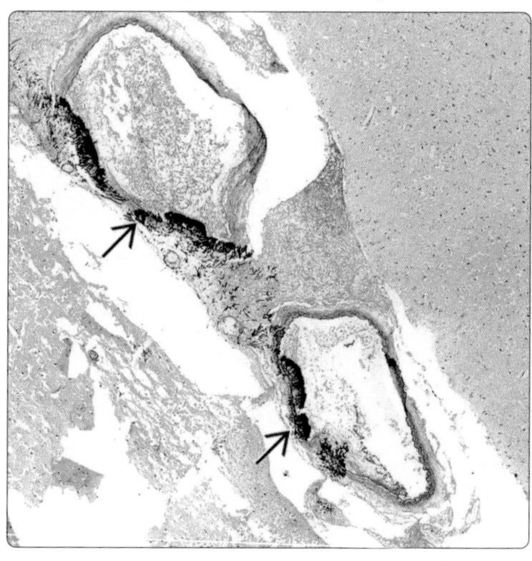

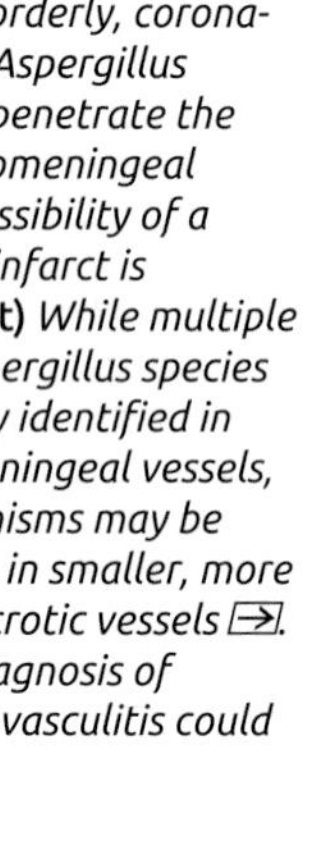

(Left) *Dense, orderly, corona-like arrays of Aspergillus species fungi penetrate the wall of a leptomeningeal vessel. The possibility of a parenchymal infarct is obvious.* **(Right)** *While multiple hyphae of Aspergillus species may be readily identified in large leptomeningeal vessels, isolated organisms may be inconspicuous in smaller, more peripheral necrotic vessels* ⇨. *A mistaken diagnosis of noninfectious vasculitis could be made.*

***Aspergillus* Species, Corona-Like Array**

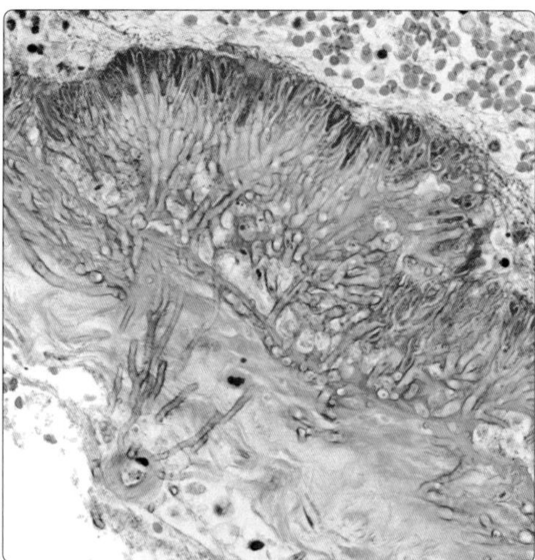

***Aspergillus* Species Infection Mimicking Noninfectious Vasculitis**

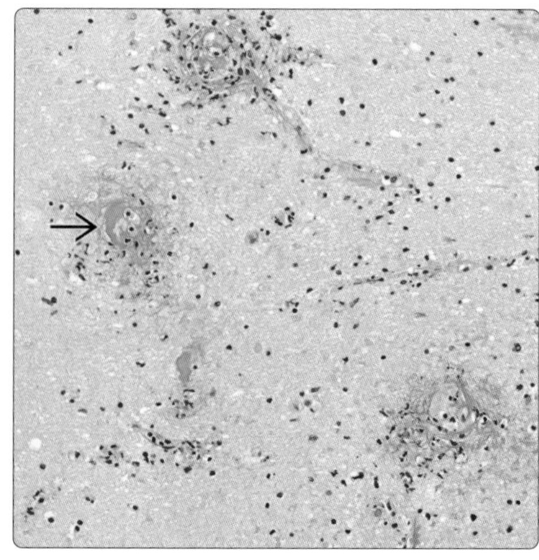

Aspergillus Species, GMS

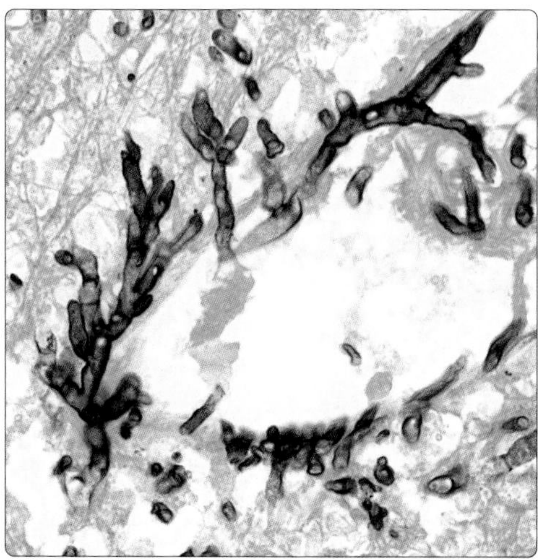

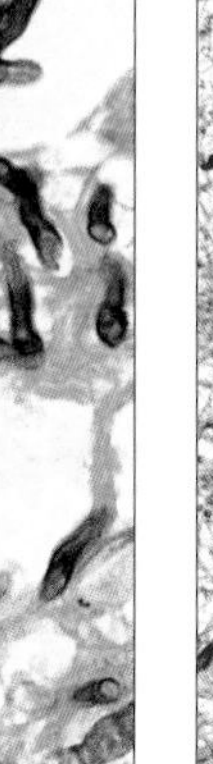

Splendore-Hoeppli Phenomenon

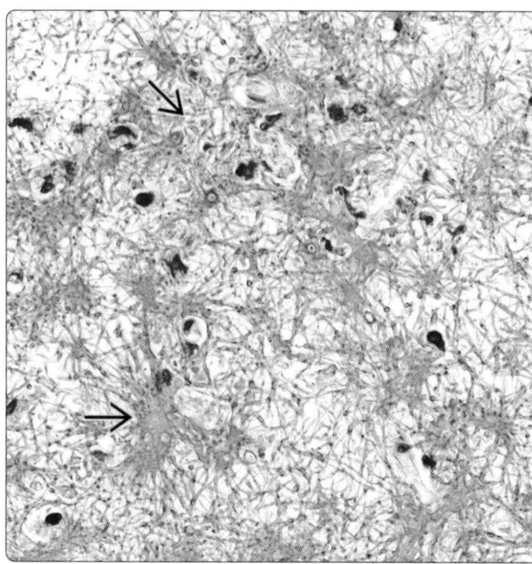

(Left) *Aspergillus species has dichotomous, septate hyphae that branch at regular intervals.* **(Right)** *Splendore-Hoeppli phenomenon consists of amorphous, eosinophilic material around pathogenic organisms ⊡ as the result of a local antigen-antibody reaction. It occurs in both fungal and parasitic infections, but is present here with Aspergillus. Often it is dense globular material, but here it is a radiating, starburst, astrocyte-like pattern of filament-like protein strands.*

Cerebrospinal Fluid Multinucleated Giant Cell

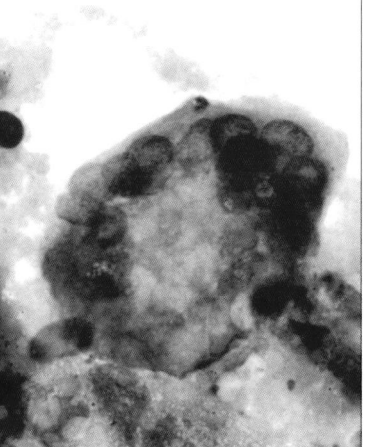

Fungal Organisms, Cerebrospinal Fluid From Ventriculoperitoneal Shunt

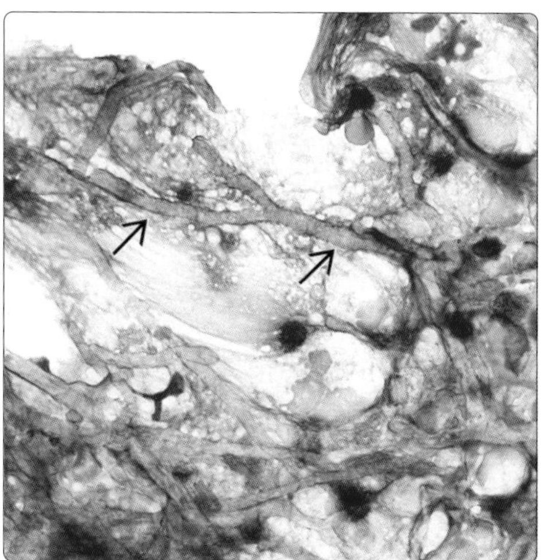

(Left) *Fungi themselves are rarely seen in cerebrospinal fluid, although inflammatory cells, such as the multinucleated giant cells here, are occasionally encountered.* **(Right)** *CSF cytology found this branching, septated fungus ⊡ that cerebrospinal fluid (CSF) culture identified as Scedosporium species. The debilitated patient had multiple shunt revisions for hydrocephalus. This fluid came from a shunt.*

Fusarium

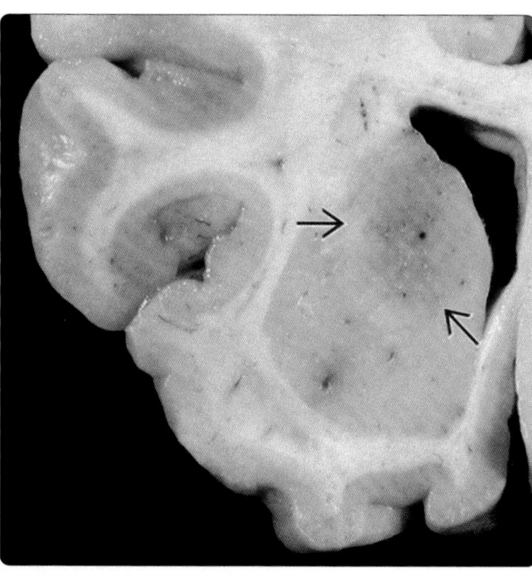

Fusarium, GMS

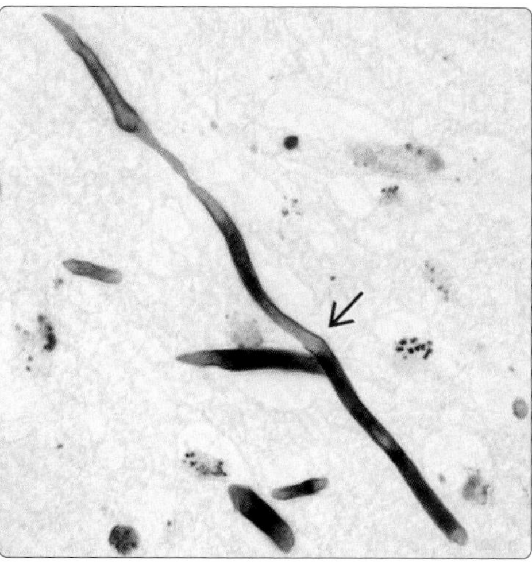

(Left) *An ill-defined focus of greenish discoloration in the caudate nucleus ⊡ is present in a coronal section from a lung transplant recipient who succumbed to disseminated Fusarium species mycosis.* **(Right)** *Identification of a fungus often requires culture. This GMS-stained tissue shows the Fusarium species with long tapering hyphae and focal branching ⊡, albeit with less regularity than Aspergillus species.*

Candida Species

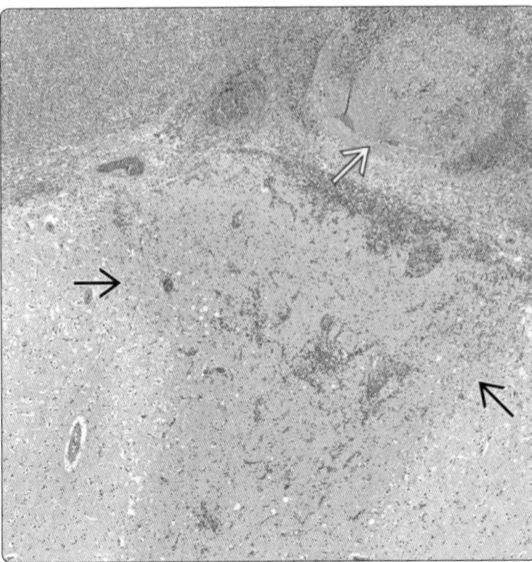

Candida Species, GMS

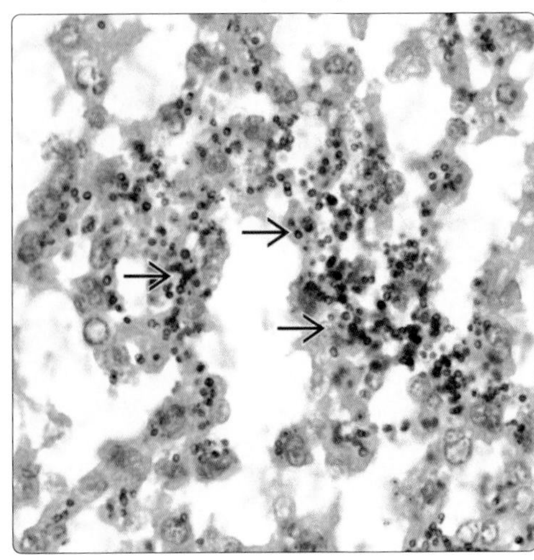

(Left) *Several types of vasoinvasive hyphal and pseudohyphal fungi can produce infarction. This example, with Candida species, is due to the large thrombosed leptomeningeal vessel* ➡ *above the acute, wedge-shaped area of necrosis* ➡*. Note the typical exuberant acute inflammatory response to Candida.* **(Right)** *Myriad small GMS(+) yeast forms of Candida species* ➡ *populate a cerebral infarct due to embolism from an infected rheumatic mitral valve.*

Mucor Species

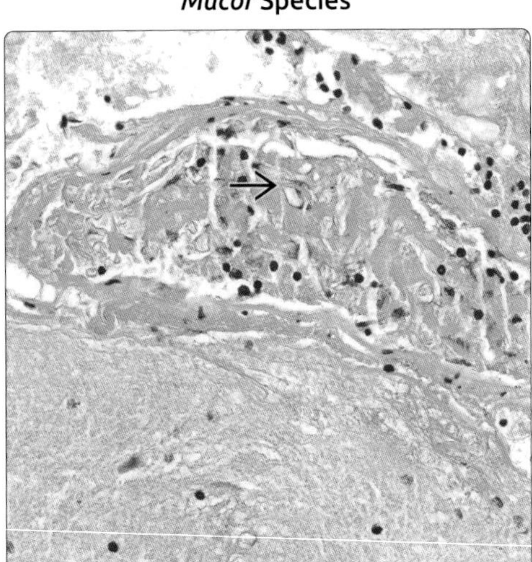

Mucor Species, PAS

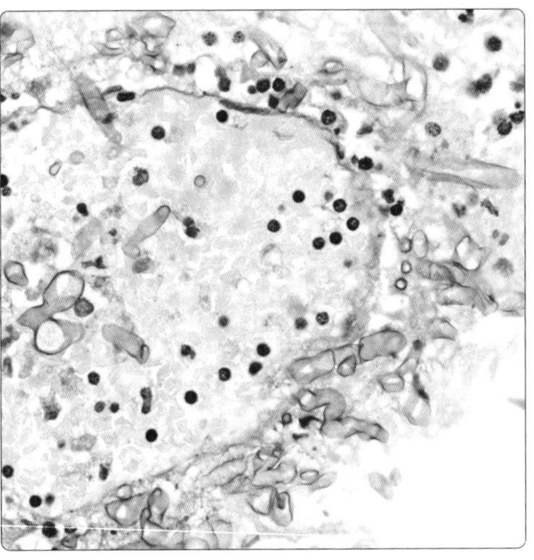

(Left) *An elderly man requiring intensive treatment for small cell lymphoma developed a large, acute infarct due to occlusion of the M1 branch of the left-middle cerebral artery. Brain biopsy revealed thrombosed blood vessels packed with ill-defined hyphae consistent with Mucor* ➡*. CSF showed 1068 WBCs with mostly neutrophils; Gram stain and cultures were negative.* **(Right)** *PAS staining highlights broad angioinvasive hyphae consistent with the Mucor species. Note the paucity of septations.*

Mucor Species, GMS

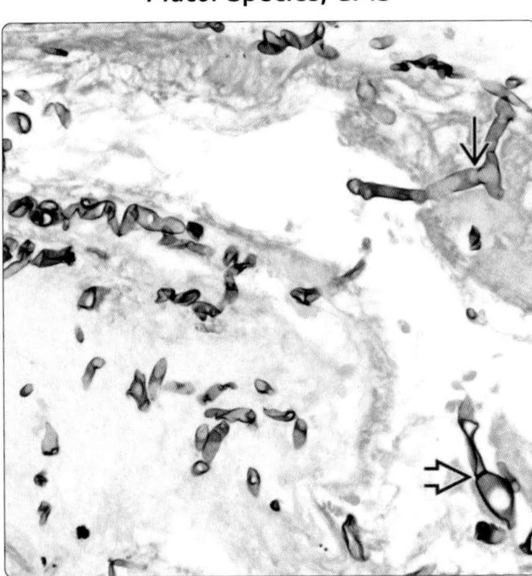

Pigmented Fungi

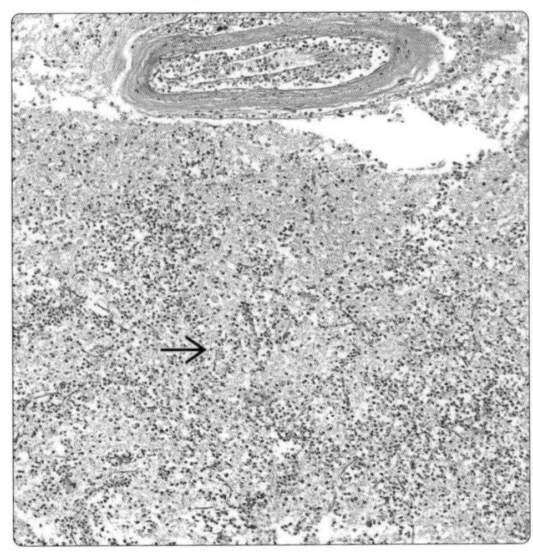

(Left) *GMS staining may recognize Mucor species in tissue sections. Broad hyphae, with a paucity of regular branching, are atypical of Aspergillus species. Very rare, probable septa* ➡ *do not exclude the diagnosis; more often there is only folding* ➡*, not true septation.* **(Right)** *Pigmented fungi are increasingly encountered as a cause of fungal cerebritis. This example, caused by Cladophialophora bantiana, has individual fungi* ➡ *in the inflamed parenchyma.*

Pigmented Fungi

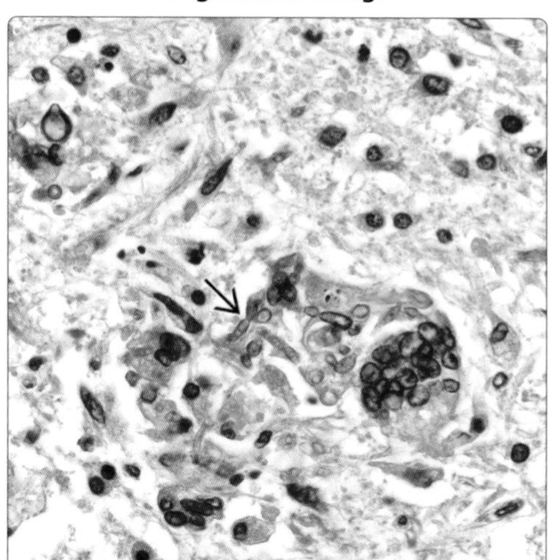

Cladophialophora* (*Cladosporium*) *bantiana

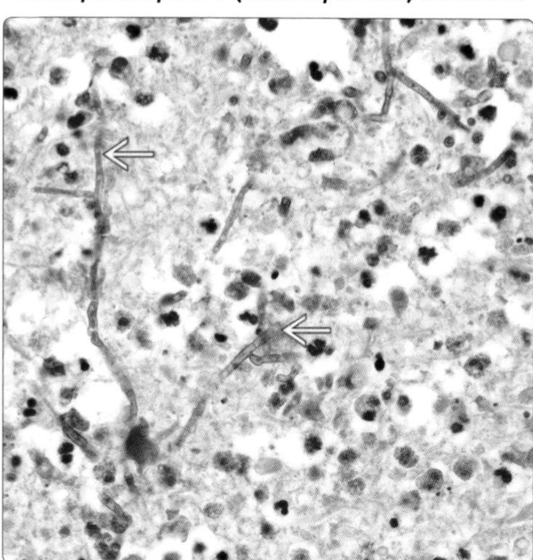

(Left) *Their pigment makes brown fungi ⇨, such as Cladophialophora bantiana, easily identifiable in H&E sections. Note the multinucleated giant cells.* **(Right)** *Hyphal forms of brown fungi ➡, in this case Cladophialophora (Cladosporium) bantiana, are the occasional causes of fungal cerebritis. Dematiaceous fungal cerebritis may arise in both immunosuppressed and immunocompetent patients.*

Cryptococcosis

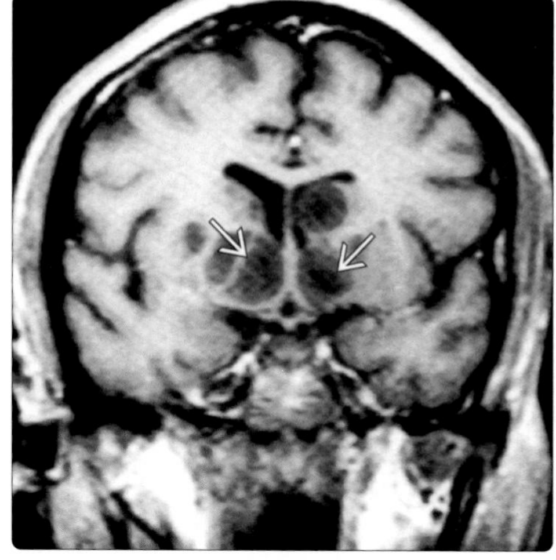

Cryptococcosis, Pseudocysts

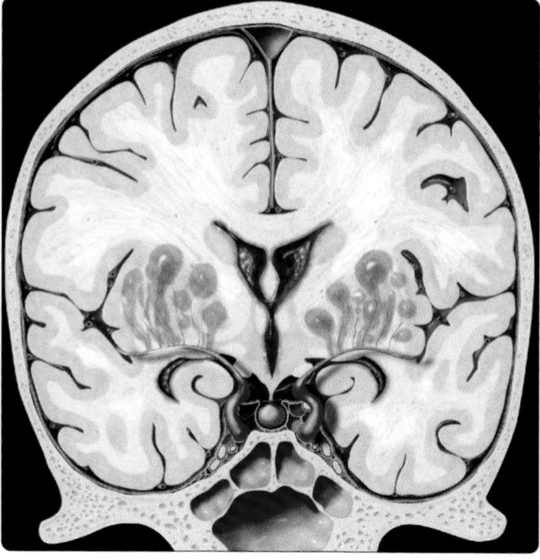

(Left) *Bilateral nonenhancing, hypointense gelatinous pseudocysts within perivascular spaces of the basal ganglia ➡ are typical of CNS cryptococcosis.* **(Right)** *Involvement of basilar perivascular spaces produces gelatinous pseudocysts in leptomeningeal cryptococcosis.*

Cryptococcosis

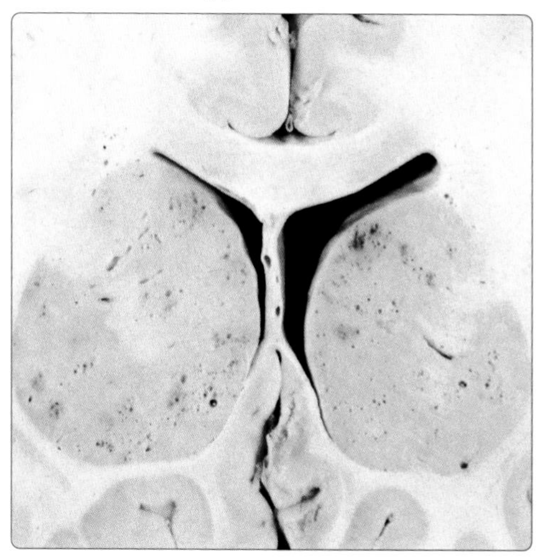

Cryptococcosis

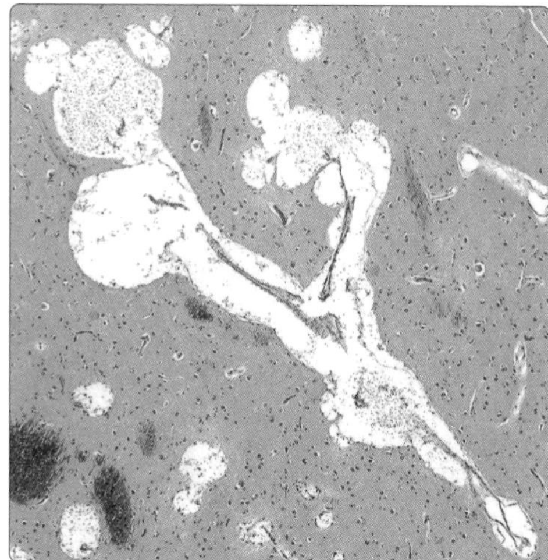

(Left) *Enlarged perivascular spaces filled with cryptococci give a pathognomonic spongy appearance to the corpus striatum.* **(Right)** *Vessels, largely in longitudinal section, sit in spaces filled with cryptococci.*

(Left) *Small, centrally placed vessels* → *are surrounded by myriad minute, pale cryptococci* ⇨. *The absence of inflammatory response in this patient with AIDS is obvious even at low magnification.* **(Right)** *Gelatinous pseudocysts due to Cryptococcus, as seen on neuroimaging or gross examination, are perivascular spaces filled with encapsulated, mucicarmine (+) yeasts. Note the small blood vessel* → *and absence of inflammatory response in this section of basal ganglia.*

Cryptococcosis, Absent Inflammatory Response

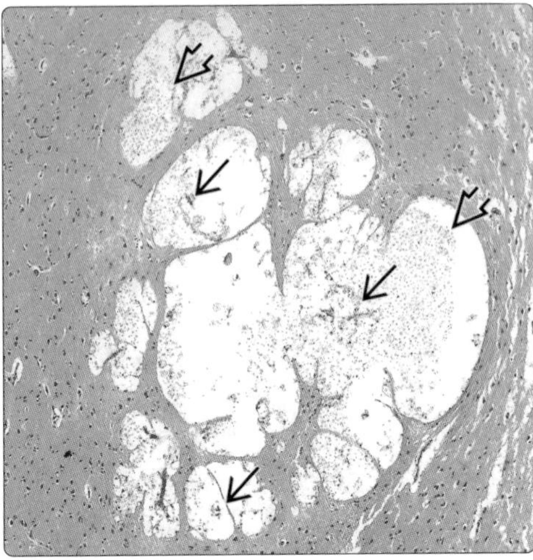

Cryptococcosis, Mucicarmine

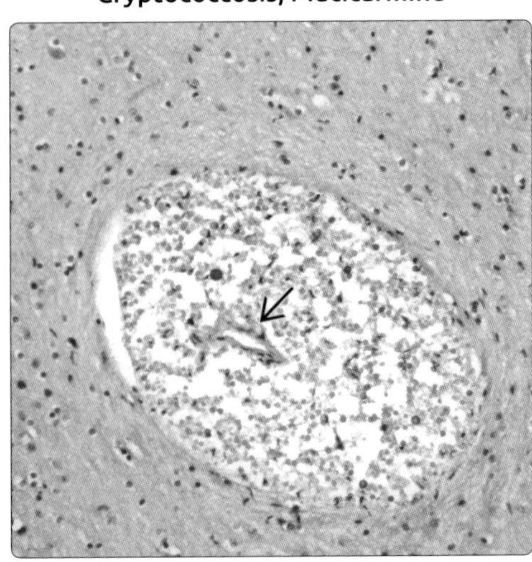

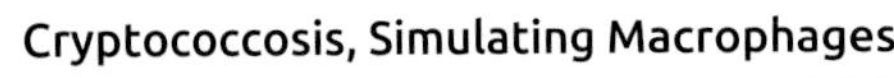

(Left) *Perivascular spaces in the basal ganglia are filled with pale organisms* → *that sometimes resemble macrophage at low magnification. Cryptococcus is the most common fungal CNS infection in AIDS patients.* **(Right)** *Alcian blue staining highlights the myriad of cryptococcal yeasts in this immunocompromised patient.*

Cryptococcosis, Simulating Macrophages

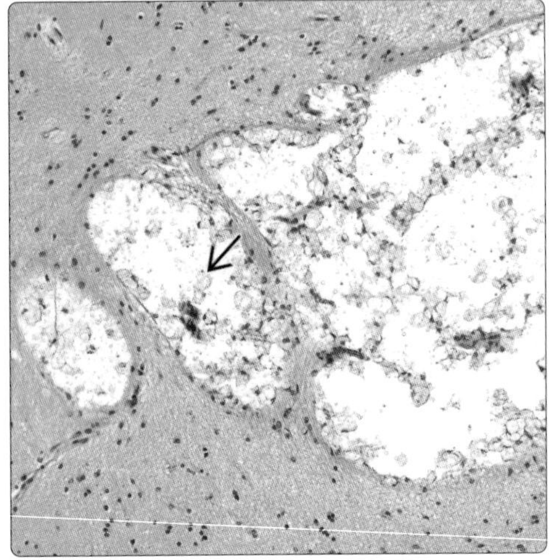

Cryptococcosis, Alcian Blue

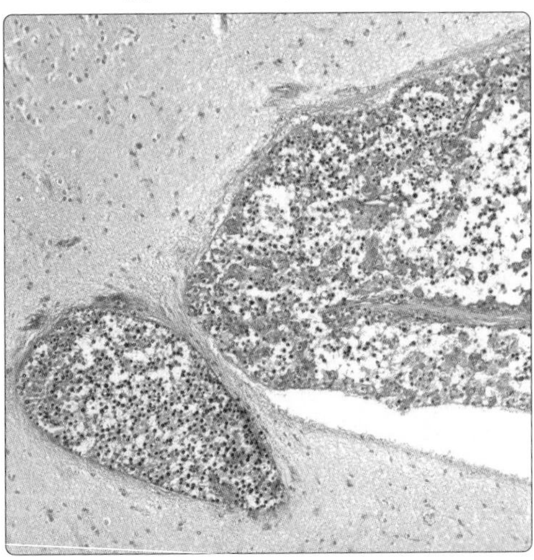

(Left) *Easy to overlook, cryptococcal leptomeningitis, as here in an AIDS patient, is often little more than a gelatinous thickening. Cryptococcus immitis is the only truly encapsulated common human pathogenic yeast.* **(Right)** *A subtle leptomeningeal opacification* → *is the macroscopic appearance of Cryptococcal leptomeningitis. A mucoid quality is present when organisms abound.*

Cryptococcosis, Meningitis

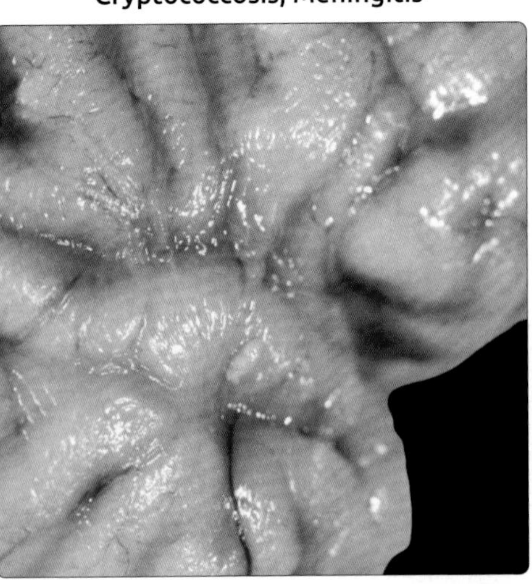

Cryptococcosis, Basilar Meningitis

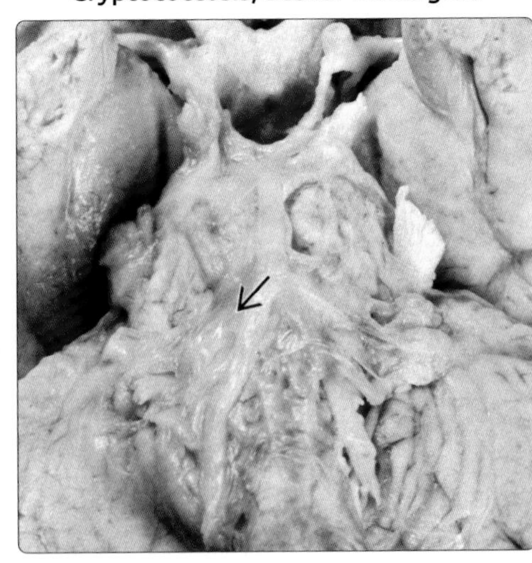

Cryptococcosis, Leptomeninges

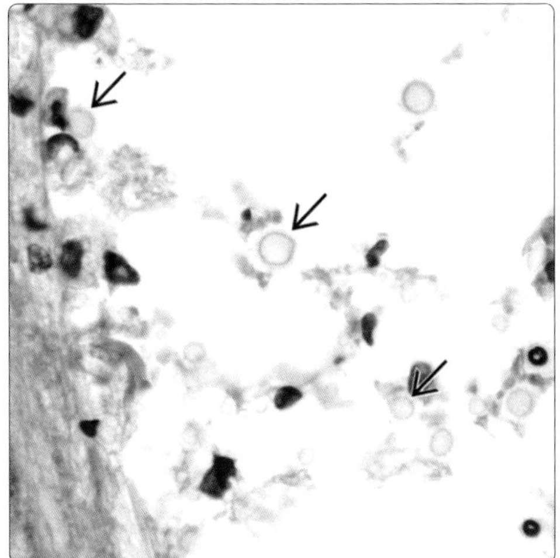

Cryptococcosis, Alcian Blue

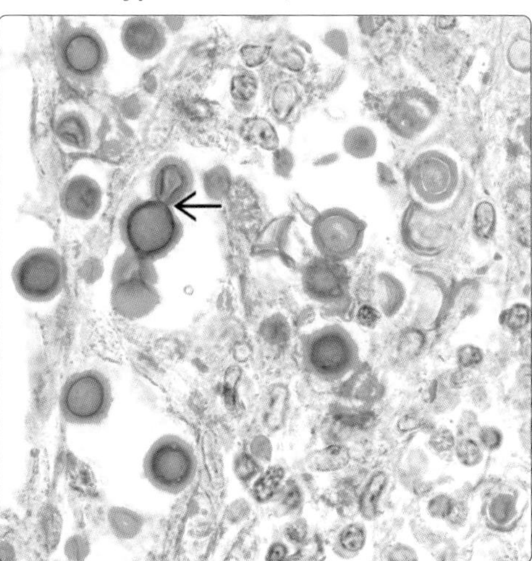

(Left) *Typically inconspicuous in H&E sections ➙, pale-staining cryptococci usually elicit little inflammation due to the immunocompromised status of the host.* **(Right)** *The cell wall and some of the capsule stain vividly with Alcian blue. Note the narrow-neck budding ➙, typical of Cryptococcus.*

Cryptococcosis, Multinucleated Giant Cell

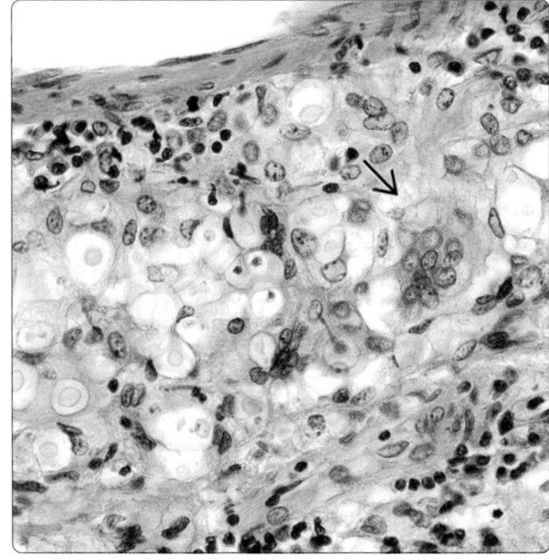

Cryptococcosis, Organisms in Giant Cells

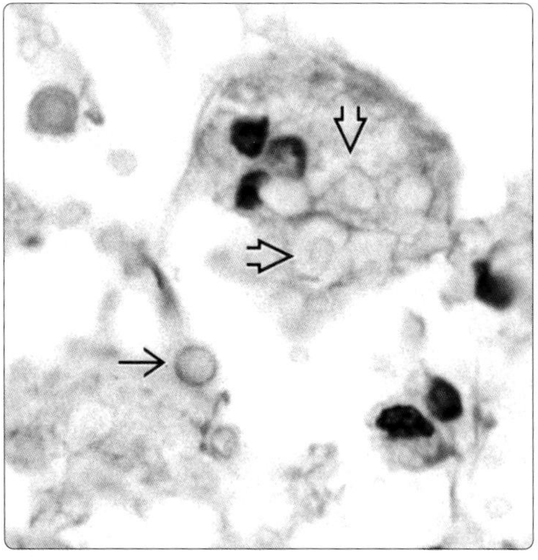

(Left) *The pale gray, encapsulated organisms typically elicit little inflammatory response. An engulfing multinucleated giant cell ➙ is present in this case, however.* **(Right)** *Cryptococcus species, usually found extracellularly ➙ in the subarachnoid or perivascular spaces, are gray-blue in H&E sections. Some organisms are ingested by macrophages ⇨.*

Cryptococcosis, Cerebrospinal Fluid, PAP Stain

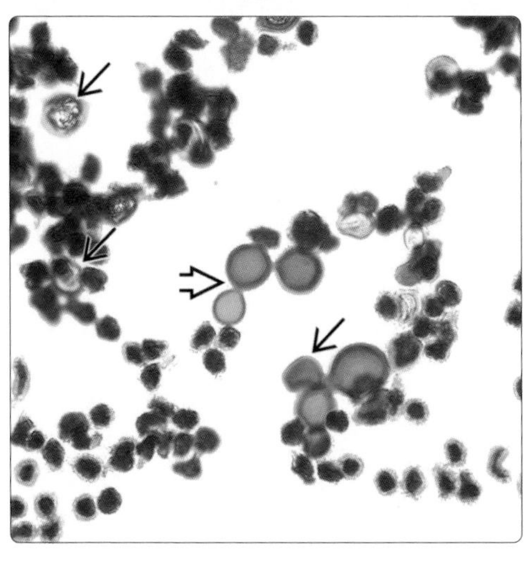

Cryptococcosis, Cerebrospinal Fluid, India Ink

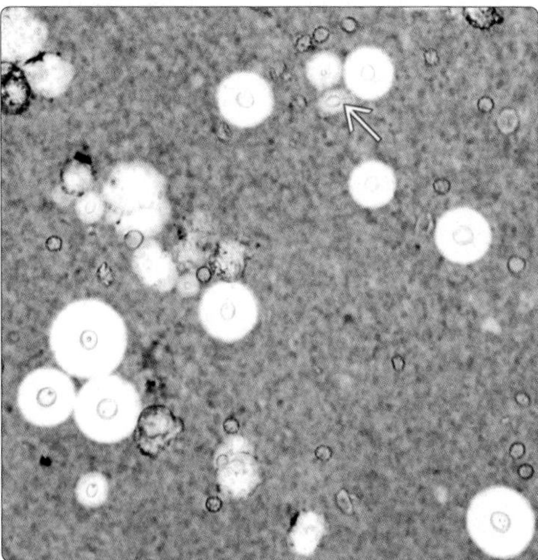

(Left) *Cryptococci assume varying appearances in Papanicolaou-stained samples of CSF ➙. Some organisms are solid and blue, others ring-shaped with more obvious cell walls. They can be easy to overlook, especially when there is little inflammatory response to suggest the possibility of infectious disease. Budding occurs with a narrow neck ⇨.* **(Right)** *The full extent of a Cryptococcus' capsule is best seen in an India ink preparation. A small budding organism is present ➙.*

Toxoplasmosis

KEY FACTS

TERMINOLOGY

- CNS infection caused by intracellular protozoal parasite, *Toxoplasma gondii*
- Symptomatic infection usually in immunocompromised patient
- Congenital toxoplasmosis: Wide spectrum of lesions from extensive necrotizing lesions to intraparenchymal calcifications

CLINICAL ISSUES

- Most frequent mass lesion in AIDS patients prior to advent of highly effective antiretroviral therapy (HAART)
- Diminished frequency with advent of HAART

IMAGING

- Ring-enhancing lesions, often multiple, often in basal ganglia
- Acute lesions with surrounding edema and mass effect

MACROSCOPIC

- Acute necrotizing, organizing, chronic abscesses
- Different stages of disease may coexist in same patient

MICROSCOPIC

- Necrotizing lesions of varying sizes (dirty necrosis)
- Fibrinoid vascular necrosis
- Limited or absent lymphocytic inflammation
- Ventriculitis (uncommon)
- Diffuse encephalitic form (uncommon)
- Classic lesion: Coagulation necrosis of vessels and parenchyma with little, if any, inflammation
- Recognition of organisms is important
    - Tachyzoites, most suggestive of active infection
    - Tissue cysts containing bradyzoites, mostly along periphery of necrotizing abscesses

ANCILLARY TESTS

- Immunohistochemistry for organisms valuable in diagnosis

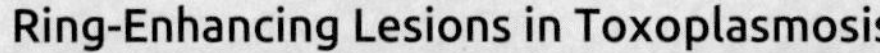

Ring-Enhancing Lesions in Toxoplasmosis

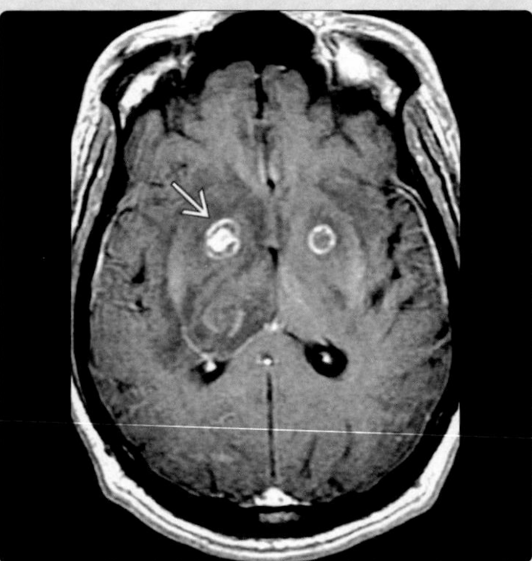

Toxoplasma Abscess, Significant Edema

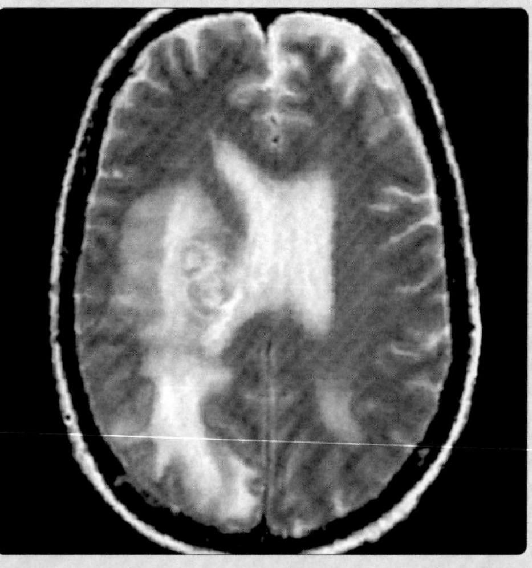

(Left) *The typically ring-enhancing lesions are often positioned in gray matter, such as cerebral cortex or basal ganglia ➡. Bilateral lesions in the latter site are especially characteristic.* **(Right)** *Axial T2WI MR shows lesions with hypointense rim and surrounding vasogenic edema, consistent with toxoplasmosis abscess.*

Encysted Organisms of Toxoplasmosis

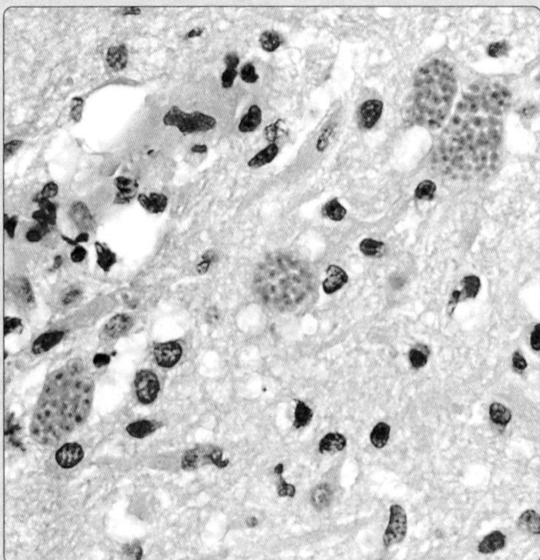

Toxoplasma, Free Tachyzoites, Immunohistochemistry

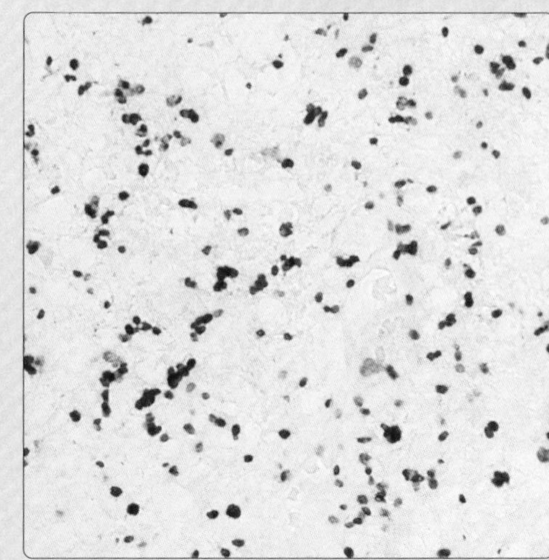

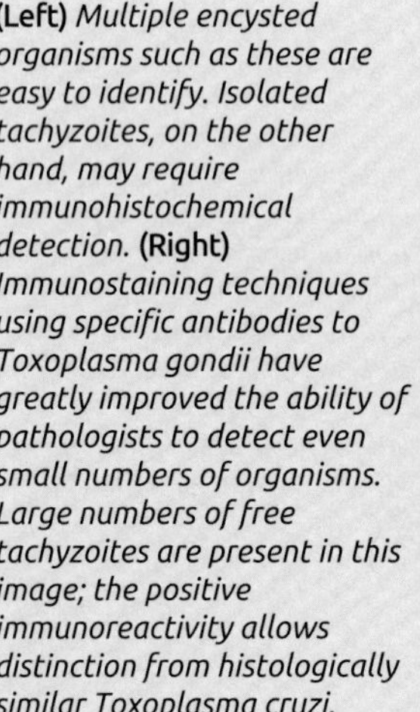

(Left) *Multiple encysted organisms such as these are easy to identify. Isolated tachyzoites, on the other hand, may require immunohistochemical detection.* **(Right)** *Immunostaining techniques using specific antibodies to Toxoplasma gondii have greatly improved the ability of pathologists to detect even small numbers of organisms. Large numbers of free tachyzoites are present in this image; the positive immunoreactivity allows distinction from histologically similar Toxoplasma cruzi.*

TERMINOLOGY

Definitions

- Central nervous system infection by *Toxoplasma gondii*, almost always in immunocompromised patients

ETIOLOGY/PATHOGENESIS

Environmental Exposure

- Humans infected by ingestion of oocysts or tissue cysts (bradyzoites)
  - Consumption of cysts in undercooked meat, particularly pork and lamb, is major risk factor
  - Ingestion of oocysts in contaminated soil and water; oocytes shed in cat feces
- Only definitive host is cat; cat only source of infectious oocysts
  - Life cycle of parasite: Sexual phase occurs in cat; oocysts secreted in cat feces survive 1 or more years
  - After oocyst ingestion by human or animal, sporozoites released in intestine enter circulatory system and spread hematogenously
  - Once sporozoite gains access to cell, transforms into tachyzoites
  - Tachyzoites form tissue cysts containing bradyzoites

Infectious Agents

- *T. gondii* is intracellular protozoal parasite
- Found in almost all geographical areas; cysts can be identified in most warm-blooded animals

CLINICAL ISSUES

Presentation

- Neurologic disease
  - Focal lesions in immunocompromised patients; prior to antiretroviral therapy, most common focal cerebral lesion in AIDS patients
    - ~ 1/2 of *Toxoplasma*-seropositive patients
    - Marked decrease incidence after highly active antiretroviral therapy (HAART)
    - Focal neurological deficits (e.g., seizures, hemiparesis)
    - Fever
  - Diffuse encephalitic form
    - Mental status changes, rapid global neurological deterioration
    - Nonlocalizing symptoms
  - Mild to subclinical meningoencephalitis in immunocompetent patient
    - Disease usually resolves spontaneously without clinical sequelae
    - Symptomatic disease: Infectious mononucleosis-type illness with adenopathy &/or fever with maculopapular rash
    - Identifiable structural CNS lesions uncommon; presents as mild meningoencephalitis
  - Ventriculitis
    - Symptoms referable to hydrocephalus
- Congenital toxoplasmosis
  - Frequently with ocular involvement
  - Acquired in utero, damage to fetus maximal in midterm infections, minimal effects in late gestation
  - Microcephaly in severe cases
- Chorioretinitis
- Immune reconstitution syndrome (IRIS) may develop after HAART therapy

Treatment

- Drugs
  - Pyrimethamine plus sulfadiazine (P+S)
  - Trimethoprim-sulfamethoxazole in resource-poor settings where P+S not available

Prognosis

- Prior to introduction of HAART, median survival > 1 year
  - With reinstitution of HAART therapy, may see IRIS in infected patients
- Infections with *Toxoplasma* not currently preventable by immunization
- Postnatal therapy of infected neonates substantially improves outcome

IMAGING

MR Findings

- Smooth rim enhancement
- Central targetoid, low-density area corresponding to necrosis
- Perilesional edema
- Often multifocal
- Bilateral lesions in basal ganglia especially characteristic

CT Findings

- Ring-enhancing hypodense lesions in basal ganglia or cortical gray matter
- CT often underrepresents number of lesions found pathologically

MACROSCOPIC

General Features

- Multifocal abscesses with appearance dependent on stage
  - Usually involve cerebral hemisphere, especially basal ganglia
  - Most prominent near cortical gray-white junction
  - Also in cerebellum
  - Brainstem and spinal cord involvement infrequent and usually in association with heavy disease burden in cerebral hemispheres
- Necrotizing abscesses, poorly circumscribed, softened necrotic tissue, petechiae, surrounding edema
- Organizing abscesses better demarcated, central yellow necrosis, hyperemic border, peripheral yellow capsule
- Chronic abscesses well demarcated, central yellow necrosis, minimal edema
- Ventriculitis with necrotic yellow exudate, periventricular petechiae

MICROSCOPIC

Histologic Features

- Multifocal discrete necrotizing lesions
  - 3 morphological stages (different stages and sizes of lesions can coexist in same patient)

- Necrotizing: Coagulative necrosis, *Toxoplasma* cysts, and numerous free tachyzoites, usually minimal host inflammatory response, small arteries with fibrinoid necrosis, endothelial damage, thrombosis
- Organizing: Central eosinophilic, acellular, coagulative necrosis, periphery with histiocytes containing lipid and hemosiderin, variable inflammation, astrocytosis, microglial proliferation
- Chronic: More demarcated capsule, often hemosiderin and intense reactive gliosis at periphery; organisms may not be found, especially after treatment (burnt out cases)

- Ventriculitis
  - Periventricular necrosis, petechial hemorrhages or hemosiderin, usually minimal patient inflammatory response, numerous *Toxoplasma* free tachyzoites
- Diffuse encephalitic form
  - Multifocal cysts and free tachyzoites
  - Diffuse cortical microglial nodules
  - No necrosis
- Chorioretinitis
  - Retinal necrosis, histiocytes, organisms

ANCILLARY TESTS

Immunohistochemistry

- Monoclonal antibodies specific for organism
- Immunohistochemistry for organism diagnostic and especially highlights free tachyzoites
  - Organisms may be difficult or impossible to identify post treatment with antibiotics

Serologic Testing

- *Toxoplasma* serum antibodies

DIFFERENTIAL DIAGNOSIS

Dystrophic Microcalcifications/Mineralizations

- Basophilic structures lack substructure of *Toxoplasma* cysts
- *Toxoplasma* immunohistochemistry (-)

Trypanosoma cruzi

- Cysts identical to those of toxoplasmosis
- *Toxoplasma* immunohistochemistry (-)

Histoplasma capsulatum

- Small yeasts similar in size to *Toxoplasma* free tachyzoites but lack elongate shape
- Organisms intracellular (histiocytes)
- Positive for fungal histochemical stains (Grocott methenamine silver, periodic acid-Schiff)
- Negative for *Toxoplasma* immunohistochemistry

Other TORCH Infections

- TORCH: Toxoplasmosis, other (syphilis, varicella-zoster, parvovirus B19), rubella, cytomegalovirus (CMV), and herpes
- Viral inclusions in congenital CMV
- Congenital toxoplasmosis may cause extensive brain destruction, calcification, few residual organisms
- Examine eye for organisms

Necrotizing Vasculitis

- Fibrinoid necrosis of blood vessels
- Perivascular inflammation
- No organisms or focal abscesses

Radiation Necrosis

- History of irradiation
- White matter localization
- Telangiectatic vessels
- No organisms

DIAGNOSTIC CHECKLIST

Pathologic Interpretation Pearls

- Organisms most frequent at periphery of necrotic areas and near blood vessels
- Necrotizing vasculitis may be most eye-catching feature
- Fulminant cases contain more tachyzoites than cysts
- Few if any organisms post treatment

SELECTED REFERENCES

1. Campos FA et al: Incidence of congenital toxoplasmosis among infants born to HIV-coinfected mothers: case series and literature review. Braz J Infect Dis. 18(6):609-17, 2014
2. Caniglia EC et al: Antiretroviral penetration into the CNS and incidence of AIDS-defining neurologic conditions. Neurology. 83(2):134-41, 2014
3. Galván-Ramírez Mde L et al: The role of hormones on Toxoplasma gondii infection: a systematic review. Front Microbiol. 5:503, 2014
4. Elmore SA et al: Toxoplasma gondii: epidemiology, feline clinical aspects, and prevention. Trends Parasitol. 26(4):190-6, 2010
5. Martin-Blondel G et al: Toxoplasmic encephalitis IRIS in HIV-infected patients: a case series and review of the literature. J Neurol Neurosurg Psychiatry. Epub ahead of print, 2010
6. Talabani H et al: Factors of occurrence of ocular toxoplasmosis. A review. Parasite. 17(3):177-82, 2010
7. Abedalthagafi M et al: Asymptomatic diffuse "encephalitic" cerebral toxoplasmosis in a patient with chronic lymphocytic leukemia: case report and review of the literature. Int J Clin Exp Pathol. 3(1):106-9, 2009
8. Kur J et al: Current status of toxoplasmosis vaccine development. Expert Rev Vaccines. 8(6):791-808, 2009
9. Nissapatorn V: Toxoplasmosis in HIV/AIDS: a living legacy. Southeast Asian J Trop Med Public Health. 40(6):1158-78, 2009
10. Weiss LM et al: Toxoplasmosis: A history of clinical observations. Int J Parasitol. 39(8):895-901, 2009
11. Dedicoat M et al: Management of toxoplasmic encephalitis in HIV-infected adults (with an emphasis on resource-poor settings). Cochrane Database Syst Rev. 3:CD005420, 2006
12. Mueller-Mang C et al: Imaging characteristics of toxoplasmosis encephalitis after bone marrow transplantation: report of two cases and review of the literature. Neuroradiology. 48(2):84-9, 2006
13. Gray F et al: The changing pattern of HIV neuropathology in the HAART era. J Neuropathol Exp Neurol. 62(5):429-40, 2003
14. Mele A et al: Toxoplasmosis in bone marrow transplantation: a report of two cases and systematic review of the literature. Bone Marrow Transplant. 29(8):691-8, 2002
15. Scaravelli F et al: Opportunistic infection. In Gray: Atlas of the Neuropathology of HIV Infection. Oxford, UK: Oxford University Press. 103-117, 1993
16. Navia BA et al: Cerebral toxoplasmosis complicating the acquired immune deficiency syndrome: clinical and neuropathological findings in 27 patients. Ann Neurol. 19(3):224-38, 1986
17. Petito CK et al: Neuropathology of acquired immunodeficiency syndrome (AIDS): an autopsy review. J Neuropathol Exp Neurol. 45(6):635-46, 1986

Deep Basal Ganglia Predilection

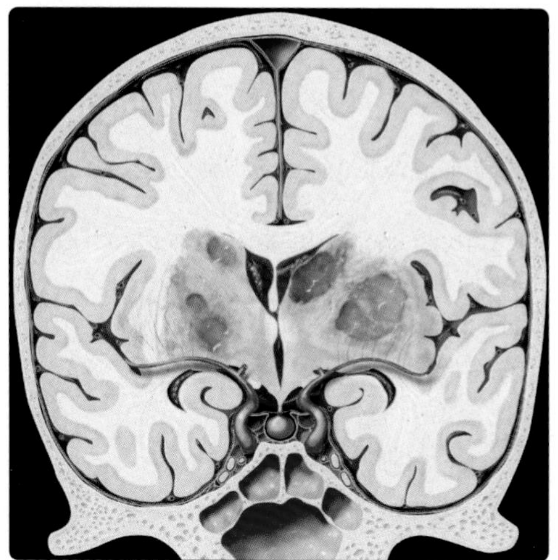

Toxoplasmosis, Highly Necrotic

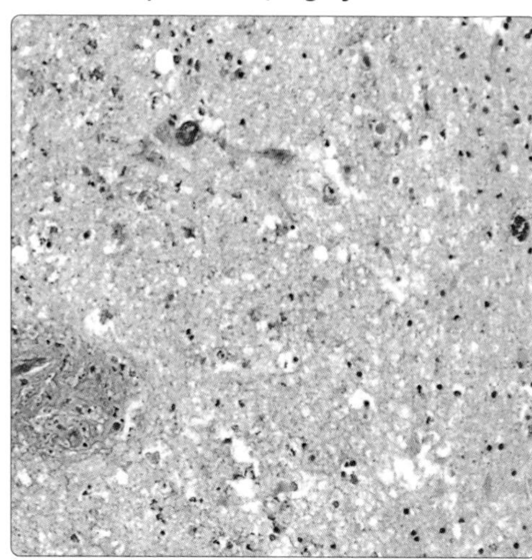

(Left) *Toxoplasma necrotizing foci are most commonly identified in deep basal ganglia.* **(Right)** *Toxoplasma necrotizing lesions in severely immunocompromised patients, such as those with AIDS, are largely necrotic, with little or no inflammatory response.*

Fibrinoid Vascular Necrosis

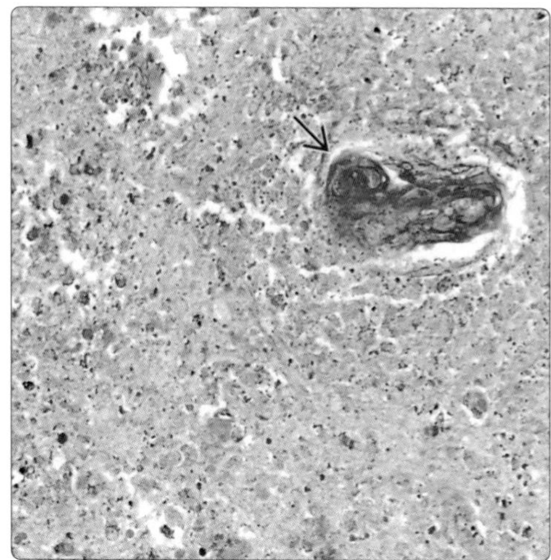

Free Tachyzoites

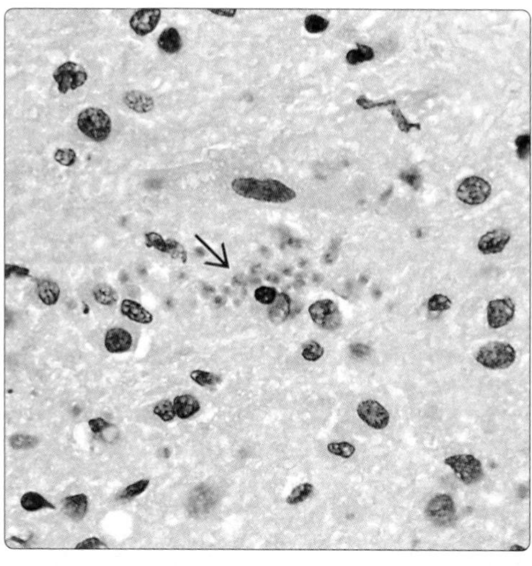

(Left) *Fibrinoid vascular necrosis is a cardinal feature of toxoplasmosis necrotizing foci ⇒. Vasculitic inflammation may be present if the patient is able to mount an inflammatory response.* **(Right)** *Lesions of toxoplasmosis usually contain larger numbers of small, basophilic, free tachyzoites ⇒ than encysted forms. Note the substructure to the tachyzoites that allows distinction from microcalcifications.*

Encysted Forms

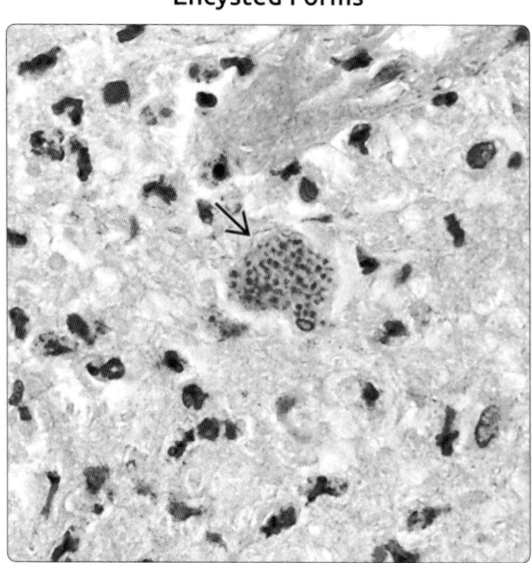

Toxoplasma gondii, IHC

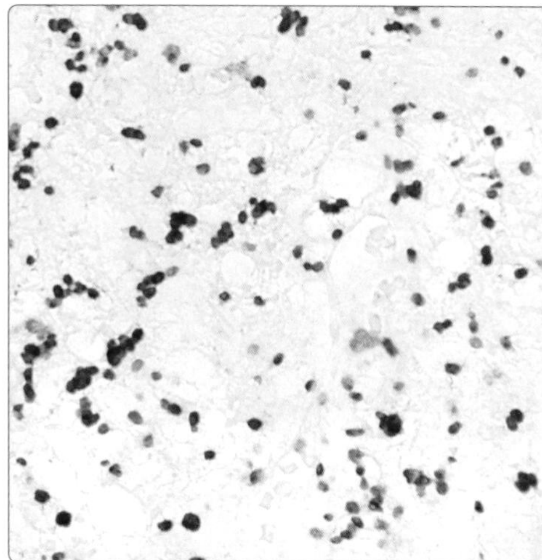

(Left) *There are fewer encysted forms ⇒ than free tachyzoites in severely immunocompromised individuals.* **(Right)** *Antibodies to Toxoplasma gondii have greatly improved the ability of pathologists to detect even small numbers of organisms. Large numbers of free tachyzoites are present in this image. Their immunoreactivity allows distinction from histologically similar Trypanosoma cruzi.*

Amebiasis

KEY FACTS

TERMINOLOGY

- Primary amebic meningoencephalitis (PAM)
  - Caused by infection with *Naegleria fowleri*
- Granulomatous amebic encephalitis (GAE)
  - Caused by *Acanthamoeba* species
  - Name GAE may be misnomer for some acute *Balamuthia* infections without granulomas

ETIOLOGY/PATHOGENESIS

- PAM in immunocompetent children and young adults swimming in fresh water or inadequately chlorinated pools
- PAM maximal in hot summer months
- *Acanthamoeba* seen in immunosuppressed or debilitated hosts
- *Acanthamoeba* and *Balamuthia* infections: No seasonal predilection
- *Balamuthia* infections in persons with soil exposure

MICROSCOPIC

- Necrotizing, hemorrhagic, neutrophilic fibropurulent meningoencephalitis in PAM
  - Numerous trophozoites, no cysts of *Naegleria fowleri*
  - Severe angiitis
- Granulomatous infection with *Acanthamoeba* species
  - Trophozoites and cysts
- Range of acute, chronic, and granulomatous inflammatory response in *Balamuthia mandrillaris* CNS infection

TOP DIFFERENTIAL DIAGNOSES

- Cerebral infarct
- Demyelinating disease
- Neurotuberculosis
- Primary angiitis of central nervous system

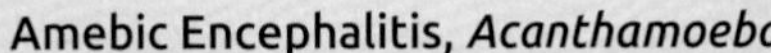

Amebic Encephalitis, *Acanthamoeba*

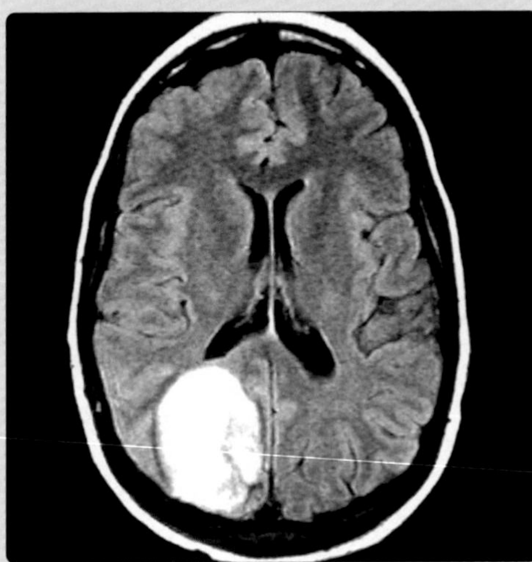

Acanthamoeba

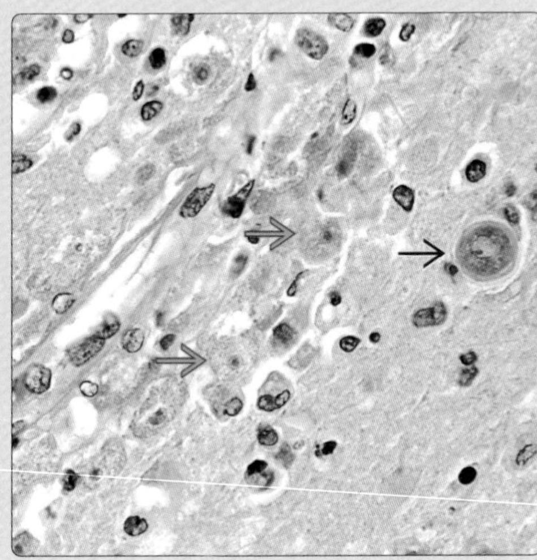

(Left) *Axial FLAIR MR in a patient with cardiac transplantation and granulomatous amebic encephalitis (Acanthamoeba species) shows an hyperintense lesion of the right occipital lobe. (Courtesy A. Yachnis, MD.)* **(Right)** *Amebic encephalitis caused by Acanthamoeba has both encysted organisms ➔ and trophozoites ⇨. The latter closely resemble macrophages.*

Balamuthia mandrillaris

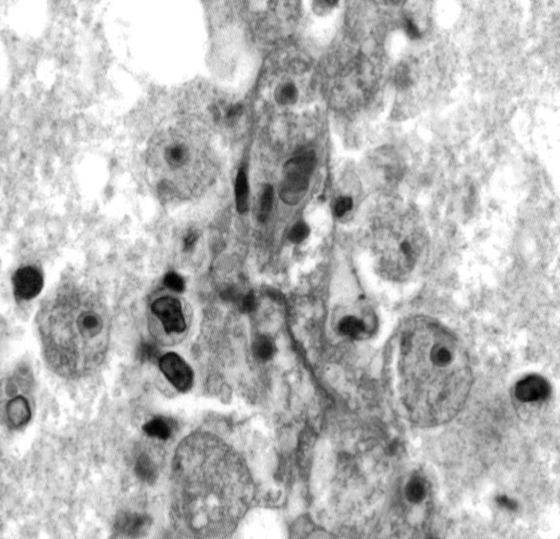

Naegleria fowleri

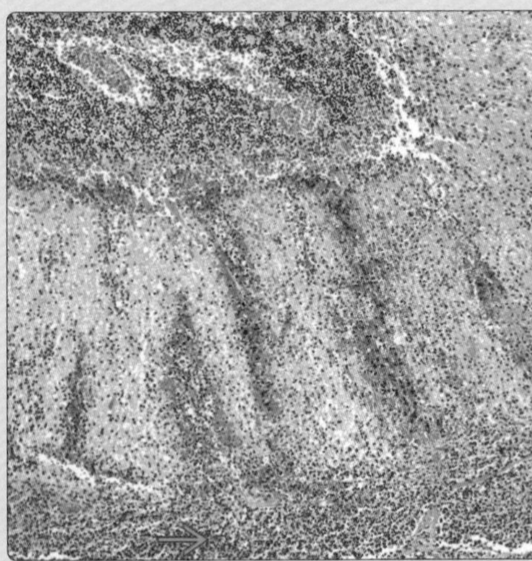

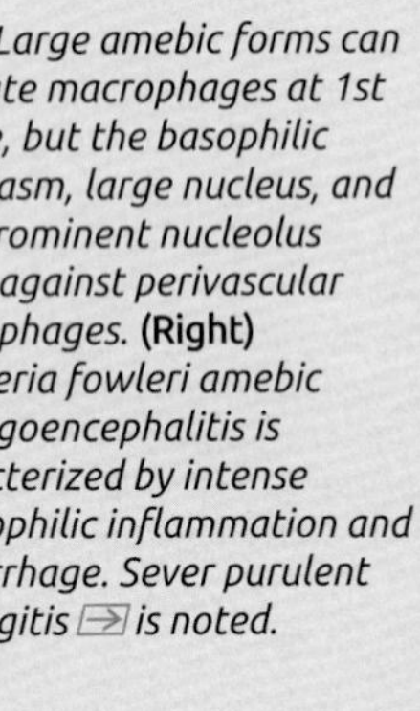

(Left) *Large amebic forms can simulate macrophages at 1st glance, but the basophilic cytoplasm, large nucleus, and very prominent nucleolus argue against perivascular macrophages.* **(Right)** *Naegleria fowleri amebic meningoencephalitis is characterized by intense neutrophilic inflammation and hemorrhage. Sever purulent meningitis ➔ is noted.*

TERMINOLOGY

Synonyms

- Granulomatous amebic encephalitis (GAE) due to opportunistic infection by *Acanthamoeba* species or *Balamuthia mandrillaris*
- Primary amebic meningoencephalitis (PAM) due to infection by *Naegleria fowleri*

Definitions

- Brain infection due to various ameba species

ETIOLOGY/PATHOGENESIS

Environmental Exposure

- Exist as free-living organisms
- Ubiquitous
- Occur worldwide
- *Acanthamoeba* species in soil, fresh and brackish water, heating and air conditioning units, hot tubs, hydrotherapy pools, dialysis machines, dental irrigation units, dust, contact lens gear
- *Balamuthia mandrillaris* in soil
- *Naegleria fowleri* in soil and fresh water; can tolerate temperatures up to 45° C and proliferate during warmer months
- *Entamoeba histolytica* cysts in fecally contaminated food or water
- Up to 10% of world population infected with *Entamoeba histolytica* but CNS disease rare

Naegleria fowleri

- Only species of *Naegleria* to cause primary amebic encephalitis
- Acute, fulminant, necrotizing, hemorrhagic meningoencephalitis
- Healthy children and young adults swimming in warm fresh water
- In hot summer months
- Enters through olfactory epithelium

Acanthamoeba Species

- > 6 species cause disease
- Chronic disease with usual insidious course
- Immunocompromised hosts
  - HIV/AIDS, organ transplantation
- Debilitated hosts
  - Chronically ill, diabetic, rarely immunocompetent
- No seasonal predilection
- *Acanthamoeba* CNS infections in South American patients may follow skin lesions; often no antecedent skin lesion in North American patients

Balamuthia mandrillaris

- Only *Balamuthia* species to cause granulomatous amebic encephalitis
- Variable clinical course from acute to subacute/chronic over 2 weeks to 2 years
- Healthy children and immunocompromised patients
- Common risk may be exposure to soil
  - Gardening, playing with dirt, inhalation of cysts in soil
  - May enter through break in skin or possibly olfactory epithelium
- May be increased risk for infection in Hispanic persons
  - Often those employed in agrarian jobs with soil exposure
- No seasonal predilection

Brain Abscess Due to *Entamoeba histolytica*

- Rare in Western countries
- Patients in endemic areas usually have intestinal infection, 90% asymptomatic
  - Dysentery, watery, sometimes bloody stool, and abdominal pain in symptomatic patients
  - CNS disease rare even in endemic areas
  - Hepatic abscess most common extraintestinal manifestation
- May be single brain abscess

CLINICAL ISSUES

Site

- Brain parenchyma
- Meninges

Presentation

- Meningitic symptoms for *Naegleria fowleri* primary amebic meningoencephalitis
  - Headache, neck stiffness, lethargy, altered mental status, nausea, emesis, fever
  - Onset usually 5-7 days after exposure to water (swimming, diving, immersing head)
  - Death soon after clinical onset
- Meningitic ± focal symptoms for granulomatous encephalitis with *Balamuthia mandrillaris* and *Acanthamoeba* species
  - Altered mental status, stiff neck, low-grade fever, cerebellar ataxia, seizures, hemiparesis, facial palsy with numbness
  - Clinical history: Weeks to months in infection with *Acanthamoeba* species
  - Range of presentation, including fulminant, in infection with *Balamuthia mandrillaris*
- Brain abscess due to *Entamoeba histolytica*
  - Headache, altered mental status, meningitis in ~ 1/2
  - Cranial nerve palsies
  - Once CNS disease develops, duration of 10-15 days to death if untreated

Treatment

- Rare GAE patients successfully treated with combination pentamidine, sulfadiazine, flucytosine, and fluconazole or itraconazole
- 1 child with PAM successfully treated with amphotericin B, miconazole, rifampin
- Good response to metronidazole for *Entamoeba histolytica* brain abscess ± surgical resection

Prognosis

- PAM caused by *Naegleria fowleri* almost always fatal
- GAE usually fatal
- Brain abscess due to *Entamoeba histolytica* responds to drug plus surgical excision

IMAGING

MR Findings

- Meningeal enhancement
  - Basilar in location especially with primary amebic meningoencephalitis
- Multiple ring-enhancing lesions

MACROSCOPIC

General Features

- Hemorrhagic meningeal necrosis and fibrinopurulent exudate in PAM
  - Maximal in orbitofrontal, temporal lobes, hypothalamus, brain stem, upper cord
- Olfactory bulbs hemorrhagic and necrotic in PAM
- Multifocal hemorrhagic, necrotic abscesses in GAE
- Severe cerebral edema

MICROSCOPIC

Histologic Features

- PAM caused by *Naegleria fowleri*
  - Necrotizing, hemorrhagic meningitis
  - Neutrophilic exudate
  - Necrotizing angiitis and perivascular hemorrhage
  - Numerous trophozoites around vessels and in tissue
  - No cysts due to fulminancy of process
- GAE caused by *Acanthamoeba* species
  - Predominantly granulomatous inflammation
  - Multinucleated giant cells
  - Trophozoites
  - Cysts seen in some cases; positive cyst wall with Grocott methenamine silver
  - PAS stain
  - Meningitis, frequent
- GAE caused by *Balamuthia mandrillaris*
  - Wide spectrum of histological features, possibly related to host immune status
  - Some cases with granulomatous inflammation
  - Others only mixed acute and chronic inflammation without granulomas
  - Acute neutrophilic inflammation in fulminant cases
  - Trophozoites
  - Cysts more often in granulomatous cases; usually not in acute cases
  - Meningitis, often
- Brain abscess due to *Entamoeba histolytica*
  - Trophozoites best seen at edge of abscess
  - Trophozoites slightly better seen with PAS

Cytologic Features

- Trophozoites frequently found in CSF in PAM with *Naegleria fowleri*
- Trophozoites almost never found in CSF in GAE
- Trophozoites of *Entamoeba histolytica* may be seen on direct smear of fluid from brain abscess

DIFFERENTIAL DIAGNOSIS

Cerebral Infarct

- Macrophages
- Ischemic ("red-dead") neurons
- Generally preserved vessels
- Little inflammation

Demyelinating Disease

- Largely white matter
- Demyelinating
  - Loss of myelin (myelin stain, such as H&E/Luxol fast blue)
  - Macrophages
  - Preserved axons
  - No acute inflammation
  - No granulomas
- Minimal (if any) meningitis

Neurotuberculosis

- No trophozoites and amebic cysts
- Usually more granulomatous, with caseating necrosis
- Acid-fast organisms by stains, culture, or PCR
- Usually not associated with neutrophilic angiitis or significant hemorrhage

Primary Angiitis of Central Nervous System

- Vasculitis involves larger caliber blood vessels
- No organisms
- More ischemic, less necrotizing and hemorrhagic

DIAGNOSTIC CHECKLIST

Pathologic Interpretation Pearls

- Macrophages similar to ameba but
  - No nucleoli
  - CD68(+) and HAM56(+)
- Ameba best identified using specific immunostaining at reference laboratories
- PCR methods available for identifying ameba in paraffin sections at reference laboratories
- *Balamuthia mandrillaris* infections may be more necrotizing and hemorrhagic than granulomatous

SELECTED REFERENCES

1. Satlin MJ et al: Fulminant and fatal encephalitis caused by Acanthamoeba in a kidney transplant recipient: case report and literature review. Transpl Infect Dis. 15(6):619-26, 2013
2. Bravo FG et al: Balamuthia mandrillaris amoebic encephalitis: an emerging parasitic infection. Curr Infect Dis Rep. 14(4):391-6, 2012
3. Yoder JS et al: The epidemiology of primary amoebic meningoencephalitis in the USA, 1962-2008. Epidemiol Infect. 138(7):968-75, 2010
4. Schuster FL et al: Under the radar: balamuthia amebic encephalitis. Clin Infect Dis. 48(7):879-87, 2009
5. Fung KT et al: Cure of Acanthamoeba cerebral abscess in a liver transplant patient. Liver Transpl. 14(3):308-12, 2008
6. Yagi S et al: Demonstration of Balamuthia and Acanthamoeba mitochondrial DNA in sectioned archival brain and other tissues by the polymerase chain reaction. Parasitol Res. 102(2):211-7, 2008
7. Guarner J et al: Histopathologic spectrum and immunohistochemical diagnosis of amebic meningoencephalitis. Mod Pathol. 20(12):1230-7, 2007
8. Perez MT et al: Fatal amebic encephalitis caused by Balamuthia mandrillaris in an immunocompetent host: a clinicopathological review of pathogenic free-living amebae in human hosts. Ann Diagn Pathol. 11(6):440-7, 2007
9. Salles JM et al: Invasive amebiasis: an update on diagnosis and management. Expert Rev Anti Infect Ther. 5(5):893-901, 2007

Amebic Meningoencephalitis, *Balamuthia mandrillaris*

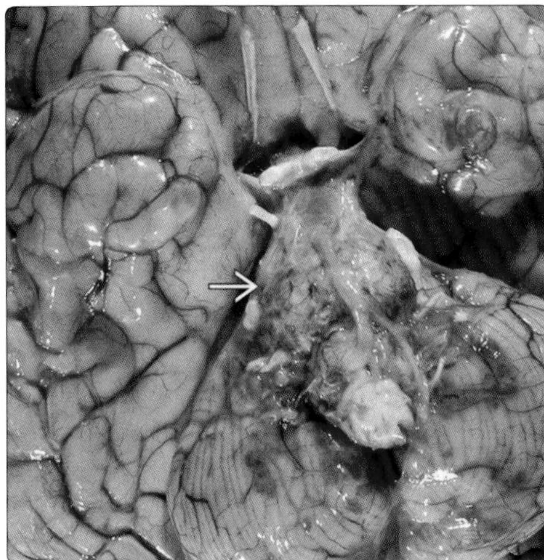

Amebic Meningoencephalitis, *Balamuthia mandrillaris*

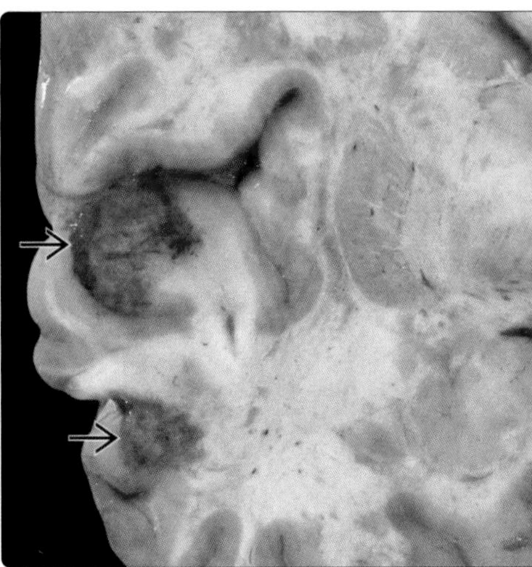

(Left) *Amebic meningoencephalitis caused by Balamuthia mandrillaris has hemorrhagic exudates surrounding the brainstem and cerebellum ➡.* **(Right)** *Parenchymal foci of amebic infection are hemorrhagic and necrotic ➡, as are these in the temporal lobe of a child who succumbed to the disease caused by Balamuthia mandrillaris.*

Amebic Meningoencephalitis, *Balamuthia mandrillaris*

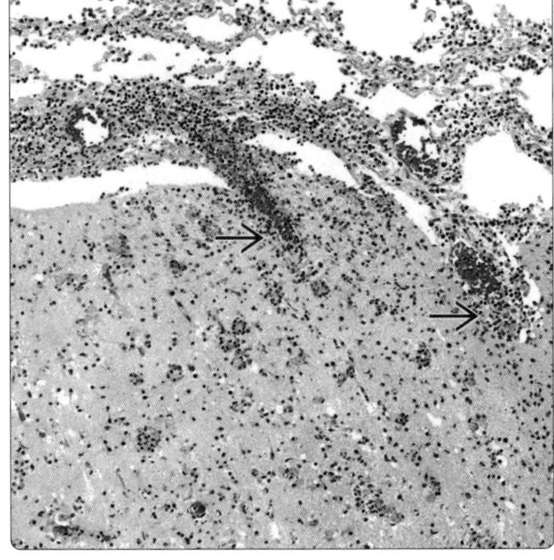

***Balamuthia mandrillaris*, Trophozoites**

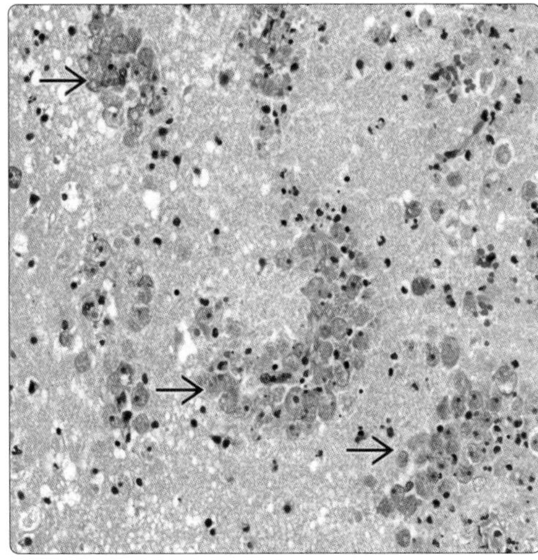

(Left) *Inflammatory cells extend along Virchow-Robin spaces ➡ in this intense amebic meningoencephalitis due to Balamuthia mandrillaris.* **(Right)** *Balamuthia mandrillaris in fulminant cases with large numbers of ameba can overwhelm host response and be minimally inflammatory in some areas. Although perivascular trophozoites ➡ can easily be mistaken for macrophages, the cytoplasm is considerably more amphophilic than that of a phagocyte.*

Trophozoite Simulating Macrophage

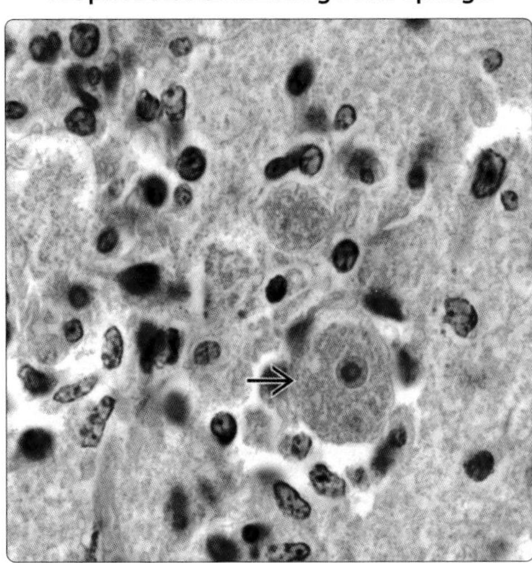

Prominent Nucleolus Unlike Macrophage

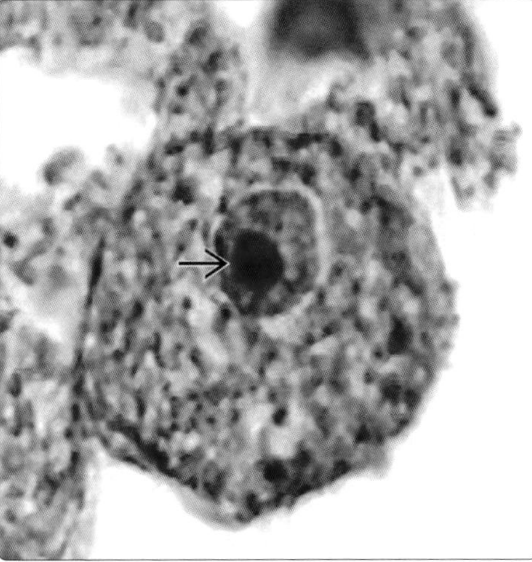

(Left) *In contrast to macrophages, amebic trophozoites ➡, here of Balamuthia mandrillaris, have lower nuclear:cytoplasmic ratios, smaller and rounder nuclei, and more prominent nucleoli.* **(Right)** *As is characteristic, a trophozoite of Balamuthia mandrillaris has granular cytoplasm and an especially prominent nucleolus ➡, the latter helping to distinguish the organism from a macrophage.*

(Left) *Necrotizing angiitis ➡, a characteristic of fulminant amebic meningoencephalitis, may distract the eye from the pathogenic agents ➡.* **(Right)** *Acute angiitis in amebic meningoencephalitis involves a full range of vessels, including small parenchymal vessels, as illustrated here.*

Necrotizing Angiitis

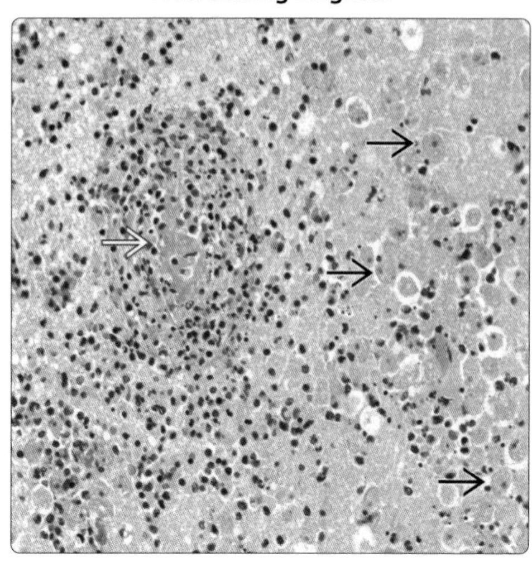

Necrotizing Angiitis

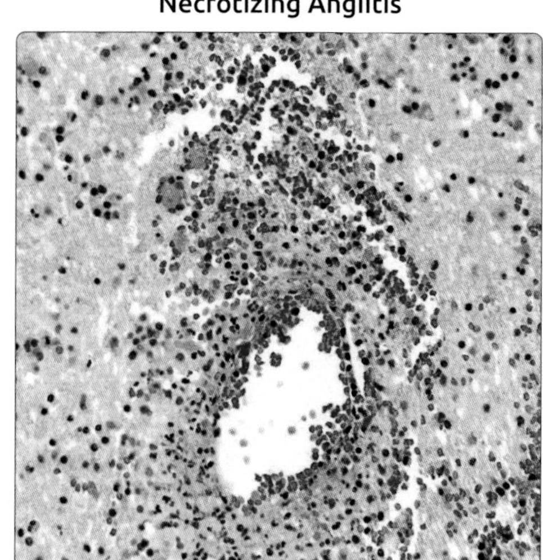

(Left) *Vessels often bear the brunt of the inflammatory response in amebic meningoencephalitis. Similar angiitis occurs with toxoplasmosis encephalitis. No amebae are present in this field.* **(Right)** *Reactive gliosis is intense in overt inflammatory lesions, such as amebic meningoencephalitis, as seen on this GFAP immunostain. Balamuthia mandrillaris was the cause. Note the perivascular inflammation ➡.*

Vascular Inflammation

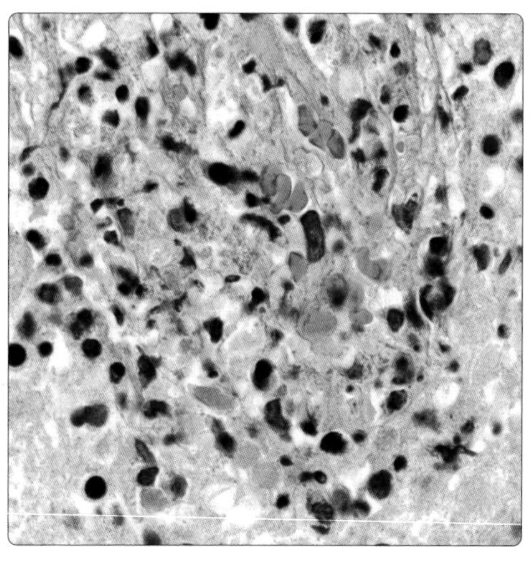

Reactive Gliosis

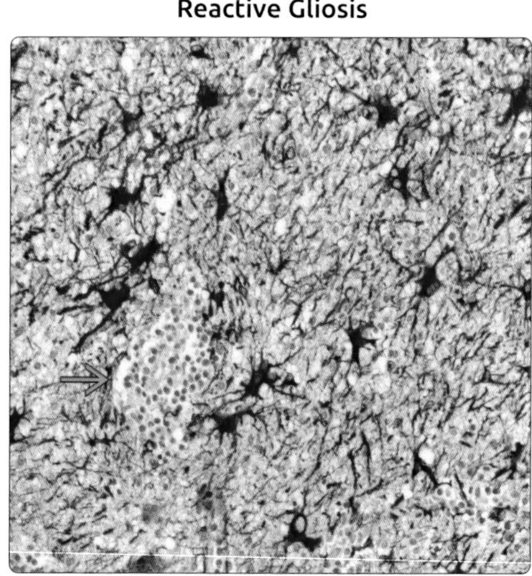

(Left) *Chronic and granulomatous inflammation is characteristic of granulomatous amebic encephalitis due to the Acanthamoeba species. Some cases of Balamuthia mandrillaris meningoencephalitis can also elicit a mixed acute and chronic inflammatory infiltrate.* **(Right)** *Perivascular and scattered parenchymal inflammatory cells in amebic meningoencephalitis ➡ are best identified by CD45 immunostain.*

Intense Inflammation

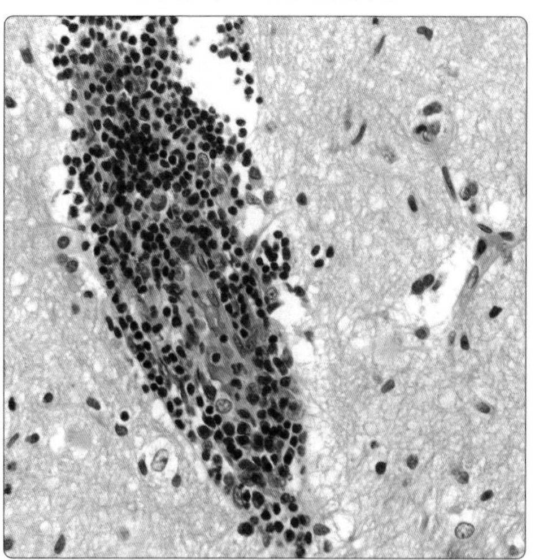

Intense Perivascular Inflammation

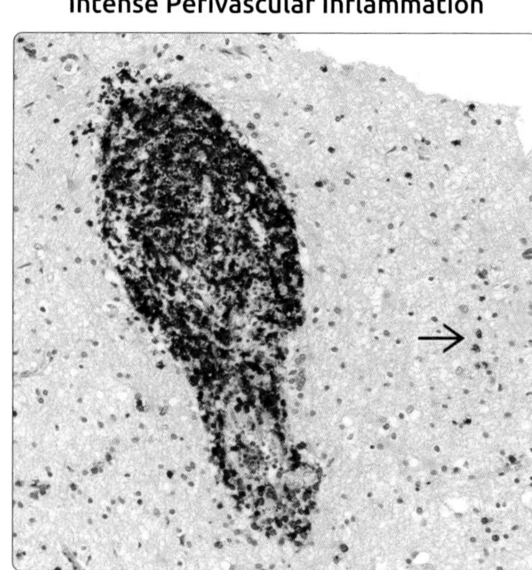

Granulomatous Inflammation

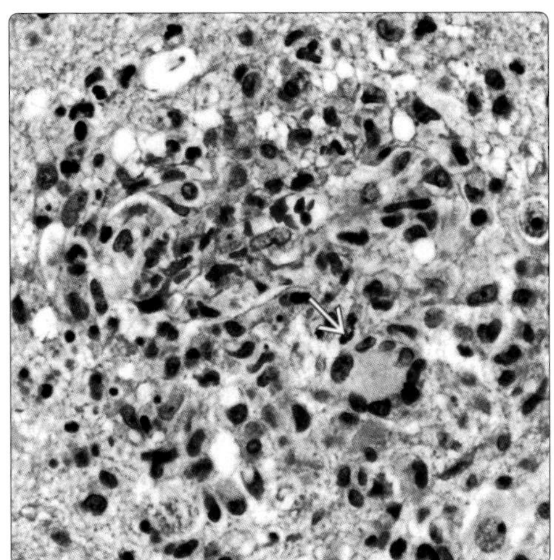

***Acanthamoeba*, Encysted Form**

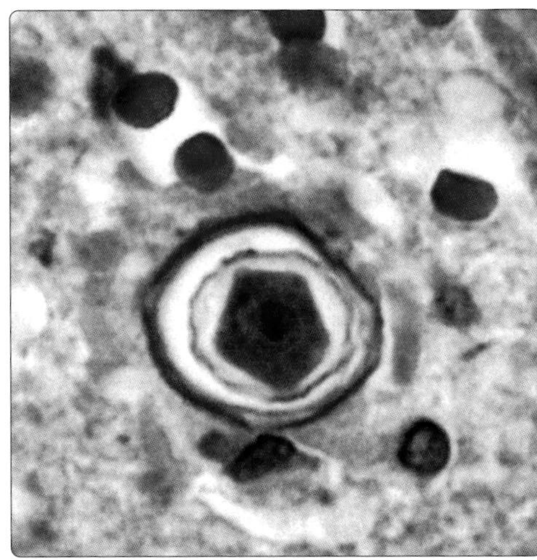

(Left) *Encephalitis caused by Acanthamoeba species may be granulomatous, with multinucleated giant cells ➡. (Courtesy A. Yachnis, MD.)* **(Right)** *Shrinkage artifact produces the artifactual pentagonal shape in an encysted Acanthamoeba. (Courtesy A. Yachnis, MD.)*

Cyst Wall, Grocott Methenamine Silver

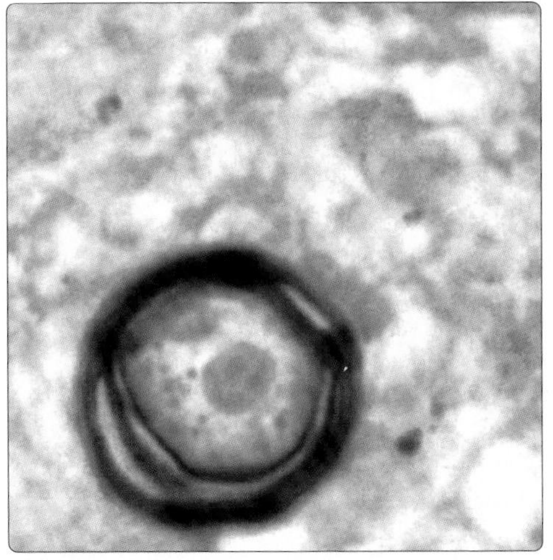

***Naegleria fowleri*, Meningoencephalitis**

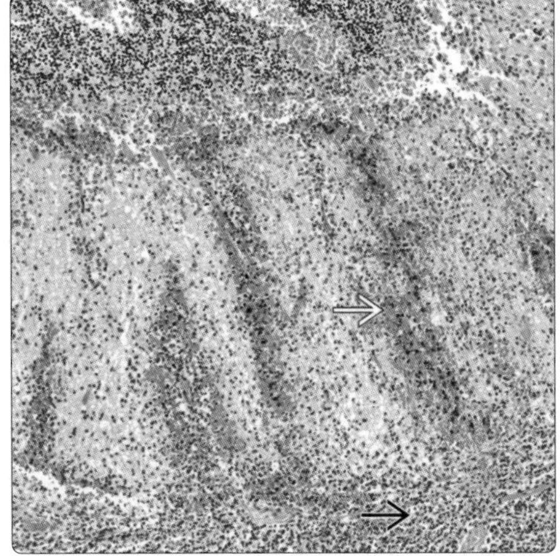

(Left) *GMS stain highlights the cyst walls of the Acanthamoeba species. Cysts are often found in chronic GAE due to Acanthamoeba, occasionally in chronic examples due to Balamuthia mandrillaris, and almost never in fulminant primary amebic meningoencephalitis due to Naegleria fowleri. (Courtesy A. Yachnis, MD.)* **(Right)** *Meningoencephalitis due to Naegleria fowleri typically has intense neutrophilic inflammation ➡ and hemorrhage ➡.*

***Naegleria fowleri*, Trophozoites**

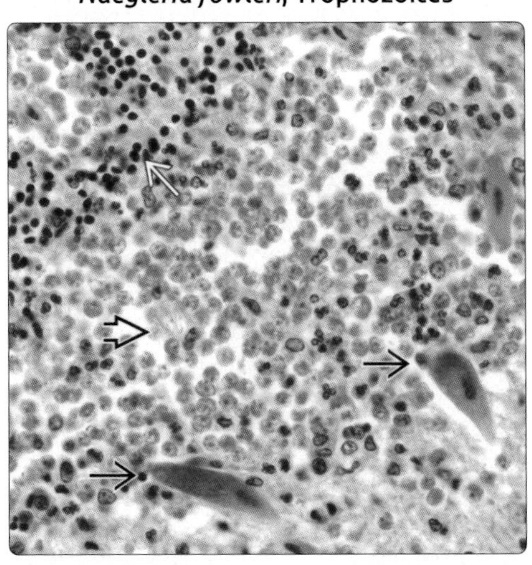

***Naegleria fowleri*, Nonencysted Forms**

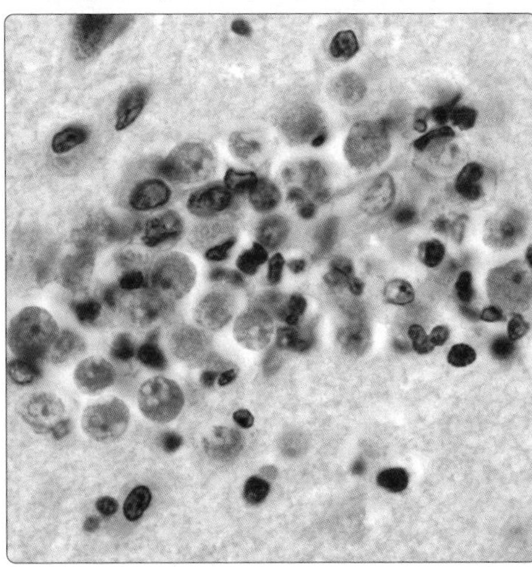

(Left) *A homogeneous layer of trophozoites ➡ displaces Purkinje cells ➡ from the edge of the cerebellar granule cell layer ➡. Note the absence of host inflammatory response in this case of amebic meningoencephalitis due to Naegleria fowleri.* **(Right)** *Naegleria fowleri are similar cytologically to other ameba, but are smaller and almost never encysted. Immunohistochemistry is necessary for specific identification.*

Cysticercosis

KEY FACTS

ETIOLOGY/PATHOGENESIS

- Neurocysticercosis (NCC) is brain infection by larval form of *Taenia solium*

CLINICAL ISSUES

- Major cause of seizures in developing world
- Treatment with antihelminthic drugs
- Surgical resection may be necessary for intraventricular cysts
- Ventriculoperitoneal shunting for hydrocephalus

MACROSCOPIC

- Cysts in subarachnoid space, ventricles, brain/spinal cord parenchyma
- Viable cysts round, discrete, filled with translucent fluid; may see single scolex
- Degenerating cysts have opaque fluid
- Later stages of degenerating cysts devoid of identifiable larvae, surrounded by fibrous capsule, chronic inflammation including eosinophils

MICROSCOPIC

- 3-layered cyst wall may be only portion of larva available for histological review; scolex may not be seen
- Cyst wall unlike any human tissue; no resemblance to neuroepithelial cysts
- Single scolex, 4 large suckers
- Rostellum with double row of large and small acid-fast hooklets
- Racemose cysts lack scolex; cyst wall more folded
- Long-dead organism with fibrosis sometimes difficult to distinguish from nonspecific scar or sclerotic vascular malformation

(Left) *Intracerebral cysticercosis is usually in the form of small, circular, enhancing foci near the gray-white junction ➡ or in other gray matter structures, such as basal ganglia.* **(Right)** *CT shows widespread calcifications throughout the brain due to remote neurocysticercosis (NCC). Ventricular cysts can lead to ependymal scarring and gliosis with obstruction to cerebrospinal fluid (CSF). flow and hydrocephalus.*

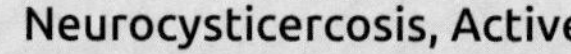

Neurocysticercosis, Active

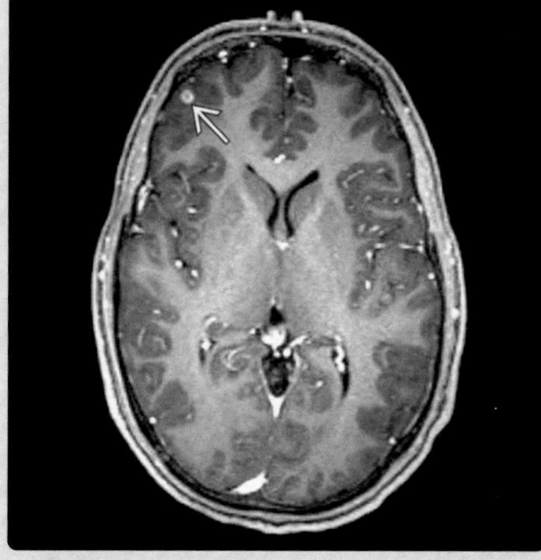

Neurocysticercosis, Remote, Widespread Calcifications

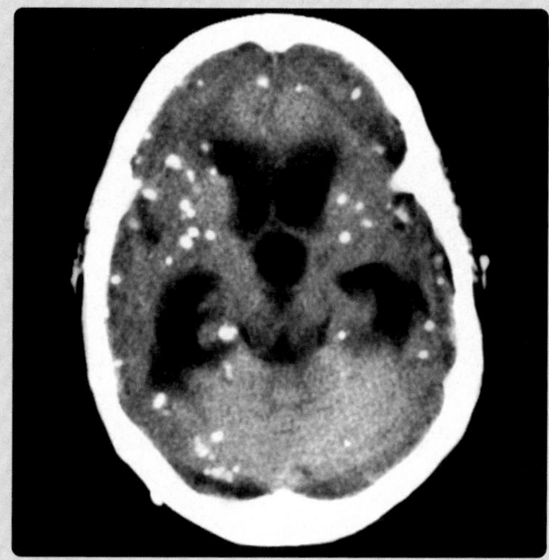

(Left) *A large, clear, translucent colloidal cyst seen in the lateral ventricle at autopsy shows the tiny, single, discrete scolex diagnostic for neurocysticercosis ➡. (Courtesy R. Breeze, MD.)* **(Right)** *Resected lesion from a seizure patient shows translucent cyst with a characteristic, single, invaginated pearly white scolex, diagnostic of neurocysticercosis ➡. (Courtesy B. Cremin, MD.)*

Neurocysticercosis, Intraventricular Cyst

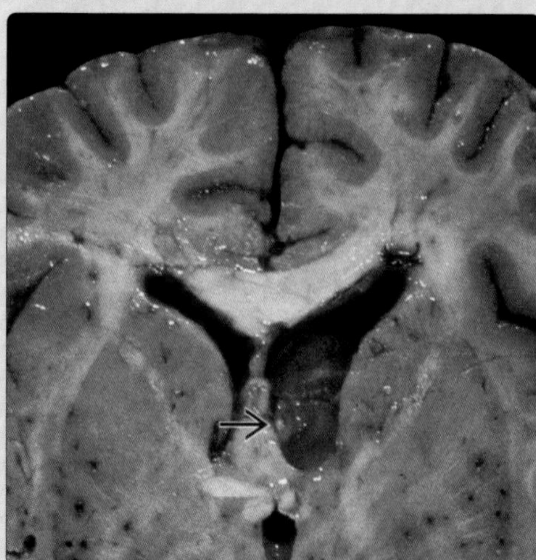

Neurocysticercosis, Scolex

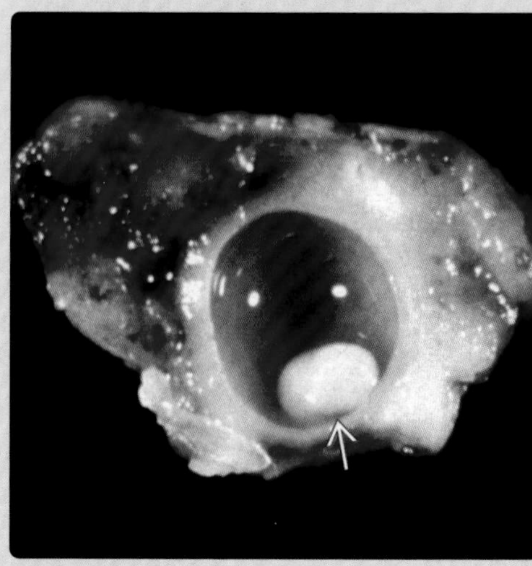

TERMINOLOGY

Synonyms

- Neurocysticercosis (NCC)

Definitions

- CNS infection by larval stage of pork tapeworm *Taenia solium*
- Cysticercus: Larva that migrates to tissues, especially skeletal muscle, brain, eye
- Scolex: Head-like part of tapeworm, bearing hooks and suckers
  - In adult tapeworm, serves as attachment site to host intestine
  - In larval form, invaginated into 1 end of cyst (bladder)

ETIOLOGY/PATHOGENESIS

Environmental Exposure

- Due to ingestion of embryonated eggs &/or gravid proglottids of *T. solium*
  - Adult intestinal tapeworm sheds gravid proglottids/eggs in feces
  - Eggs inadvertently ingested by 2nd (or same) person hatch into oncospheres, cross intestinal wall, enter bloodstream, reach tissues, and develop into larvae
    - CNS symptoms from inflammatory response to dead larvae or blockage of ventricular system by larval cyst(s)
  - Ingested eggs acquired from several sources
    - Contaminated water or food
    - Symptom-free tapeworm carrier in household (most common source)
    - Food handlers harboring adult tapeworm in intestine, with improper handwashing after toilet
    - Autoinfection (larva and adult tapeworm in same person) (minority of NCC)
- Ingestion of undercooked pork with cysticerci (larvae) causes intestinal tapeworm (taeniasis) not NCC

CLINICAL ISSUES

Epidemiology

- Incidence
  - Most common CNS parasitic infection worldwide, responsible for almost 1/2 of seizures in developing world
- Age
  - Older children, adults

Site

- Brain/cord parenchyma, especially cerebral hemispheres at junction of gray and white matter and basal ganglia, ventricles, subarachnoid space
- Often coexistent muscle disease; can have ocular disease

Presentation

- Seizures (~ 3/4 of patients), focal neurological signs, intracranial hypertension (especially racemose form), encephalitis in some young children

Treatment

- Surgical approaches
  - Resection or endoscopic aspiration: Intraventricular cysts
  - Ventriculoperitoneal shunt: Hydrocephalus
  - Surgical excision: Ocular, spinal cysts
- Drugs
  - Praziquantel, albendazole
  - Antiparasitic drugs contraindicated in encephalitis, arachnoiditis, angiitis: Steroids only

Prognosis

- Drugs destroy 60-85% viable intracranial cysticerci

MACROSCOPIC

General Features

- Cysts
  - Intraparenchymal, usually < 20 mm
    - Vesicular wall and pearly white 2-3 mm scolex
    - Maximal in cerebral cortex, basal ganglia due to high vascular supply
  - Cortical sulci
  - Subarachnoid cysts in basal cisterns, can be > 50 mm
    - Racemose cysts are large, translucent, grape-like, or soap bubble-like
    - Usually no scolex identifiable
- Viable cysts translucent; discrete 2-3 mm scolex in vesicular phase
- Involuting/degenerating cysts with opaque vesicular fluid, irregular edges of cyst (colloidal phase)
- Remote stage of degenerating cysts small calcified nodule(s) (calcified stage)
- All stages not coexistent in same individual

MICROSCOPIC

Histologic Features

- Vesicular cyst wall with 3 distinct layers: Outer cuticular, middle cellular with pseudoepithelial appearance, small dark uniform nuclei; inner fibrillary or reticular
- Viable larva: Scolex with rostellum, hooklets, suckers
- Later stage of degeneration: Absence of larva, fibrotic capsular wall similar to any type of abscess, variable numbers of lymphocytes, plasma cells, eosinophils
- Dystrophic calcified nodule(s) with remote infection

DIFFERENTIAL DIAGNOSIS

Coenurosis (*Taenia multiceps*)

- Larger cysts, numerous scolices (not just 1)

Chronic Vascular Malformation

- May be difficult to distinguish; no organism parts

DIAGNOSTIC CHECKLIST

Clinically Relevant Pathologic Features

- Common cortical involvement expressed as seizures

Pathologic Interpretation Pearls

- 3-layered larval cyst wall unlike any human tissue; unlike developmental/neurenteric cyst wall

SELECTED REFERENCES

1. Del Brutto OH: Neurocysticercosis. Semin Neurol. 25(3):243-51, 2005

(Left) *Coronal graphic shows subarachnoid and ventricular cysts of NCC. Note the small scolices within some of the cysts.* **(Right)** *Sagittal STIR MR shows multiple hyperintense cysts in the quadrigeminal cistern and basal subarachnoid spaces related to racemose NCC. Note the typical lack of a scolex. (Courtesy E. Bravo, MD.)*

Neurocysticercosis, Cysts

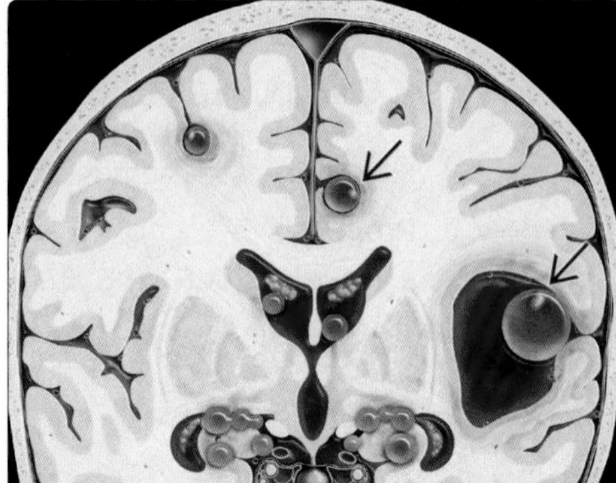

Racemose Cysts

(Left) *In its racemose form, NCC consists of meningeal or intraventricular clear cysts without scolices. Involvement of basal cisterns is commonly associated with hydrocephalus. (Courtesy R. Hewlett, PhD.)* **(Right)** *The head, neck, and body of the larva are condensed in a discrete nodule that is invaginated within the cyst.*

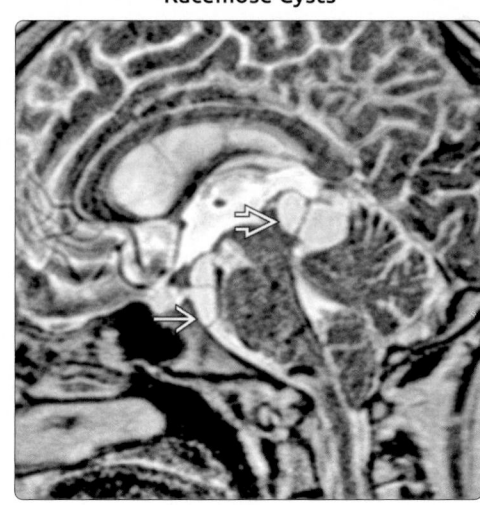

Racemose Cysts

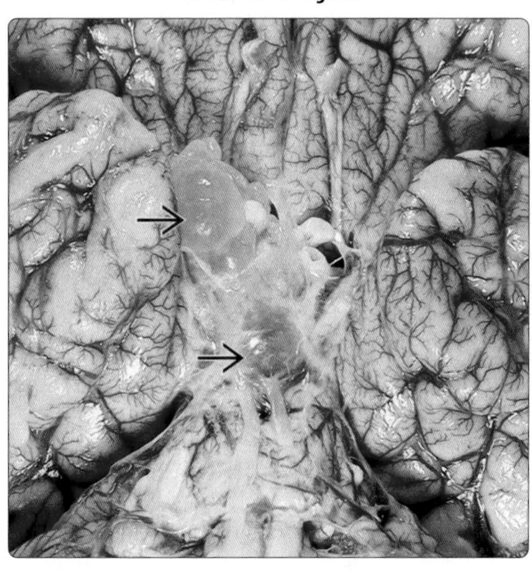

Cyst With Discrete Nodule

(Left) *Intraventricular and subarachnoid cysts are seen in this coronal autopsy brain section from a patient with NCC. Close inspection is necessary to discern whether the cysts are in brain parenchyma or if they are actually within the subarachnoid space with the adjacent gyri "sealed" around them. (Courtesy R. Breeze, MD.)* **(Right)** *The intact organism of NCC has a thin-walled cyst and focal white nodule representing the scolex, neck, and remaining body, all invaginated within the cyst or bladder.*

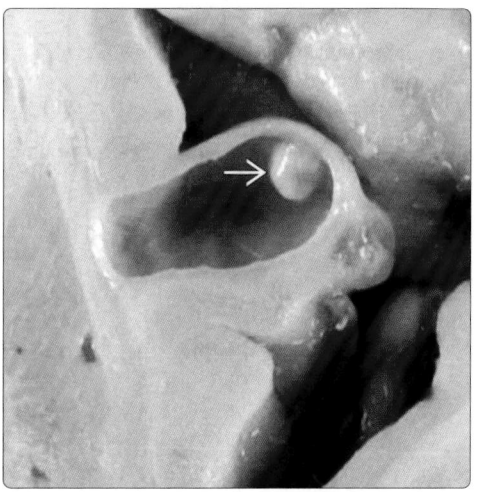

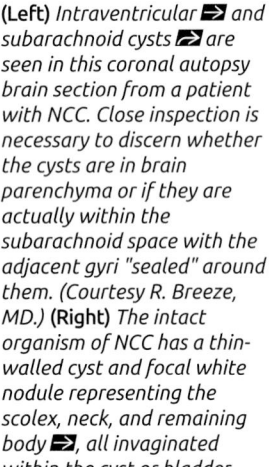

Intraventricular, Subarachnoid Cysts

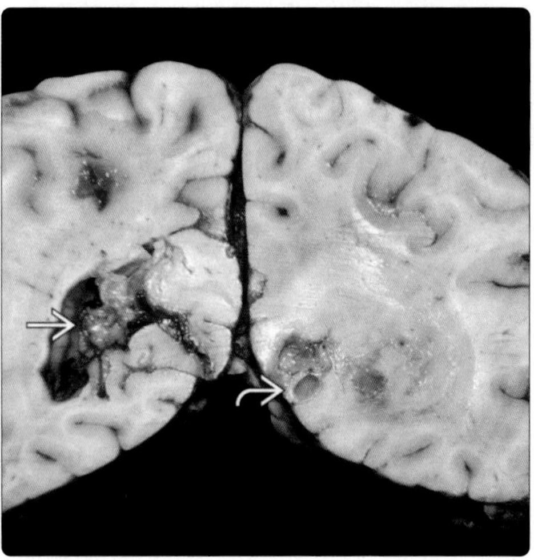

Focal Nodule Representing Scolex, Neck, Remaining Body

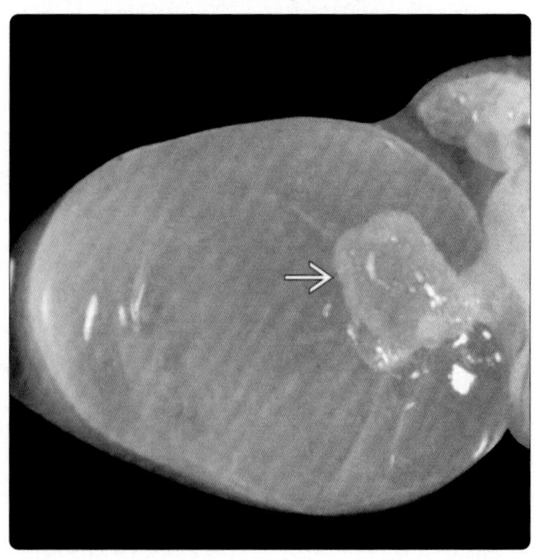

Neurocysticercosis, Larva

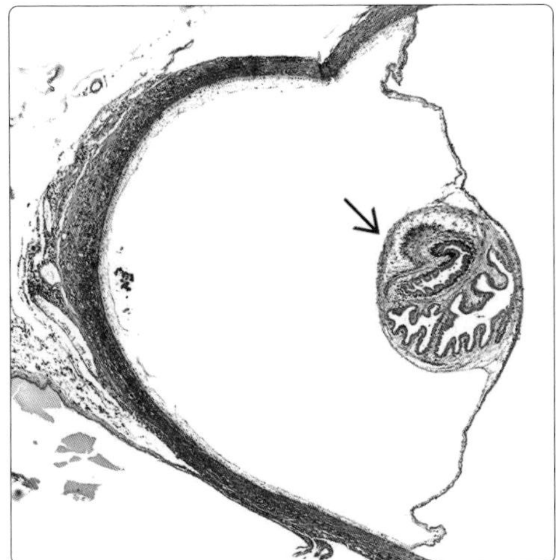

Scolex, Spiral Canal

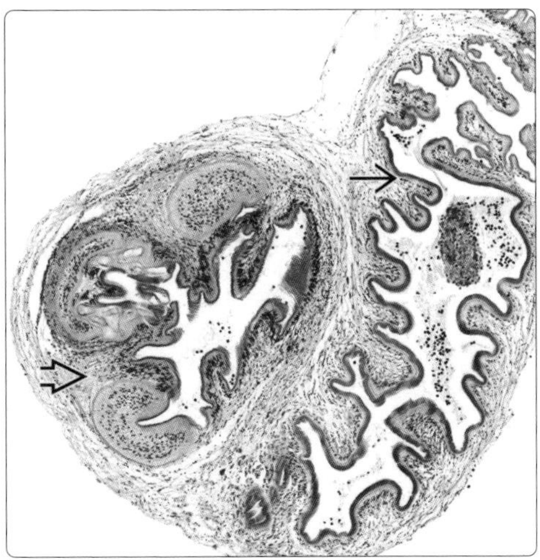

(Left) *The larva ⇒, including the serrated spiral canal, lies within the thin-walled cyst, also known as the bladder. In its functional state within the intestine, the head and body evaginate so that the former can attach to the gut wall.* **(Right)** *Fortuitous sections from a cysticercus (larval form of Taenia solium) capture both the spiral canal ⇒ and scolex ⇨. The latter is basically the head of the larva and morphologically similar to the head of the adult tapeworm.*

Hooklets

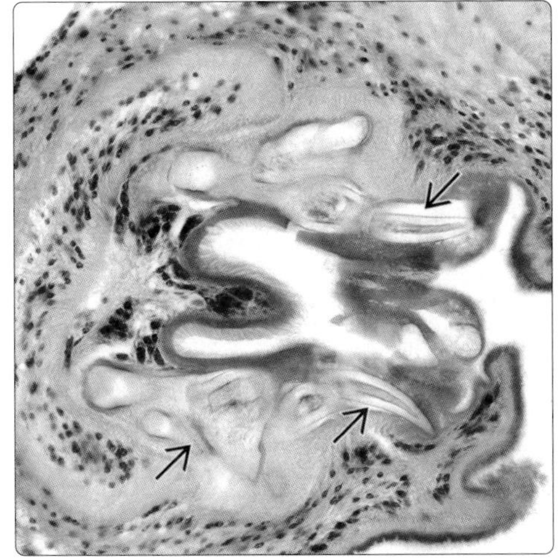

Hooklets, Acid Fast

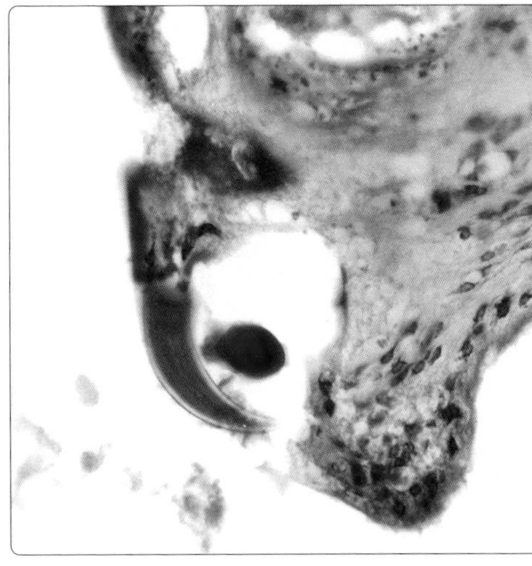

(Left) *Multiple hooklets ⇒, in a double row, are apparent in favorable sections of the scolex in NCC.* **(Right)** *Hooklets are acid fast, as illustrated here, one in longitudinal and another in the cross section in this case of NCC.*

Sucker

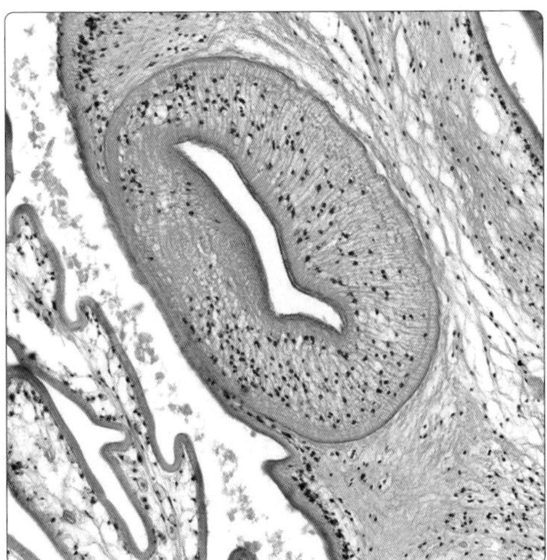

Cyst Wall

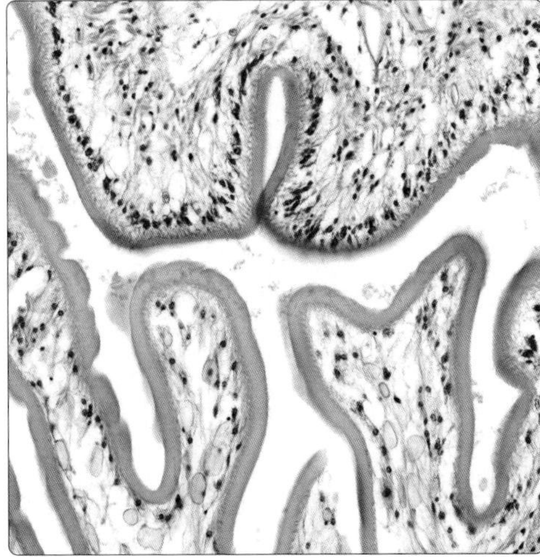

(Left) *Suckers are muscular structures used to attach the organism to the intestinal wall in NCC.* **(Right)** *The cyst wall in NCC varies in the extent to which layers remain. It is distinctive in any case and dissimilar to any normal human tissue.*

(Left) *Well-preserved microtriches (microvilli) → on the tegument of the cysticercus cysts look like little hairs.* **(Right)** *Calcified bodies are common in NCC. Note also the tubular, hyphae-like excretory canaliculi →; these should not be mistaken for fungi.*

Microtriches

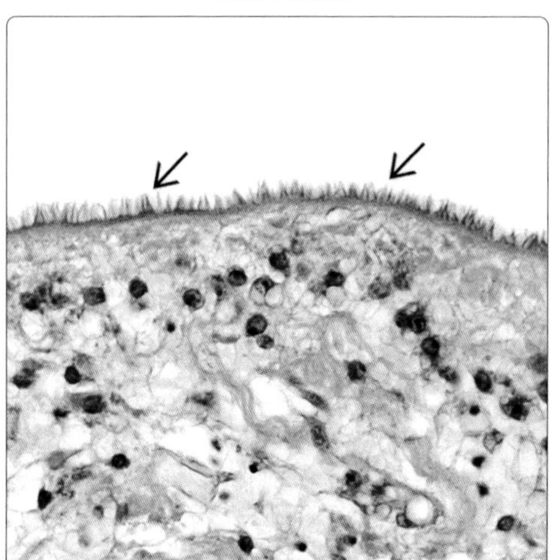

Excretory Canaliculi

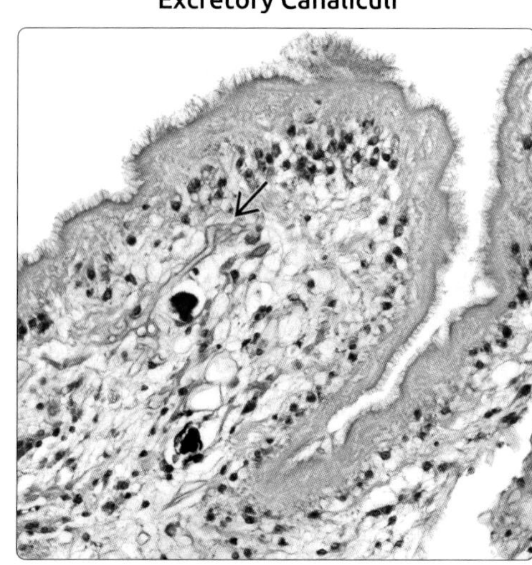

(Left) *The outer portion of the cyst ⇨, tegument, contains microtriches lined with a glycocalyx. The cyst wall itself shows 3 layers: Outer eosinophilic cuticular layer beneath which are bundles of muscle fibers ➡, cellular layer containing uniform small dark nuclei →, and inner reticular layer containing loosely arranged fibrils ➡.* **(Right)** *Microtriches (microvilli) ➡ on the surface of the cyst wall appear as little hairs. Note also the excretory canaliculi in the reticular layer →.*

Cyst Wall, 3 Layers

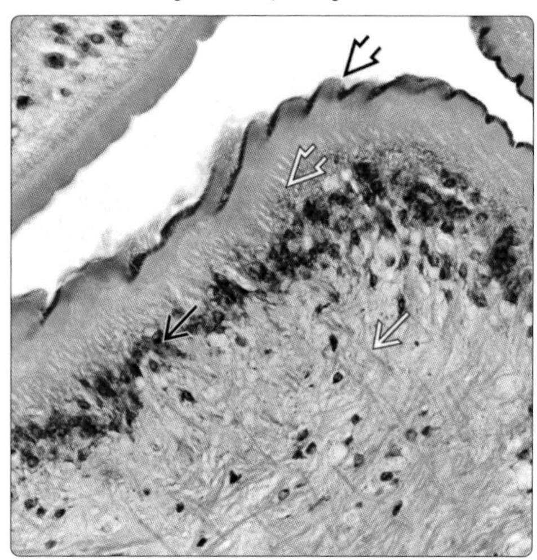

Surface of Cyst Wall

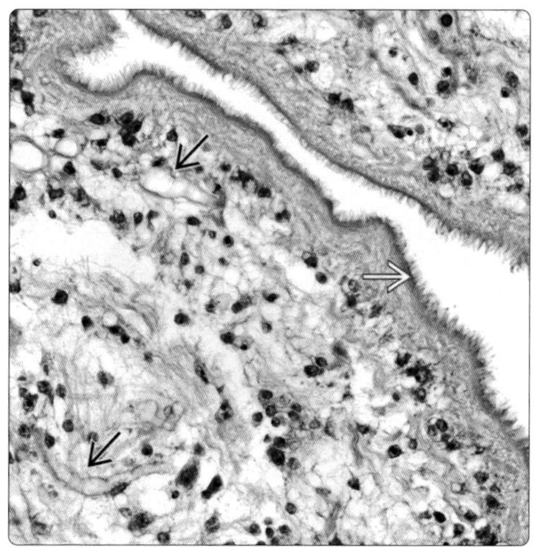

(Left) *Excretory canaliculi → in the reticular layer of cysticercosis resemble fungi, especially Rhizopus species.* **(Right)** *Racemose cysts (Latin racemus meaning a bunch of grapes) are larger than the cysticercus cysts and, unlike the latter, do not contain scolices. The cyst wall of a racemose cyst, illustrated here, is more folded and convoluted with knobby surface protrusions →.*

Excretory Canaliculi Simulating Fungi

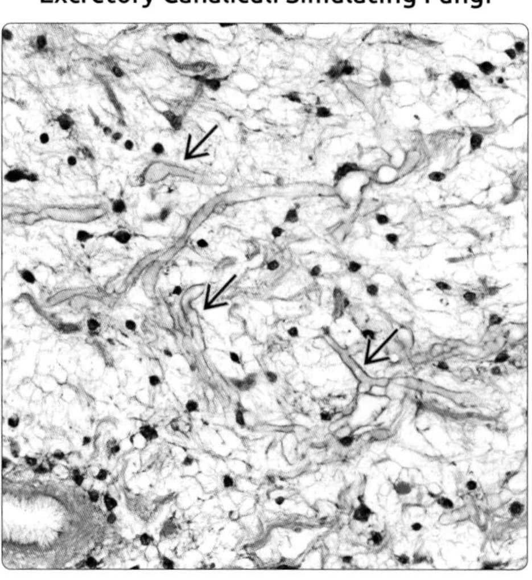

Racemose Cyst Wall

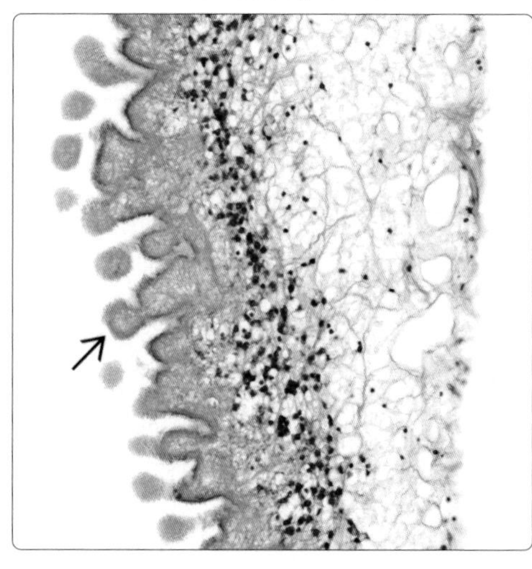

Inner Reticular Layer, Cyst Wall

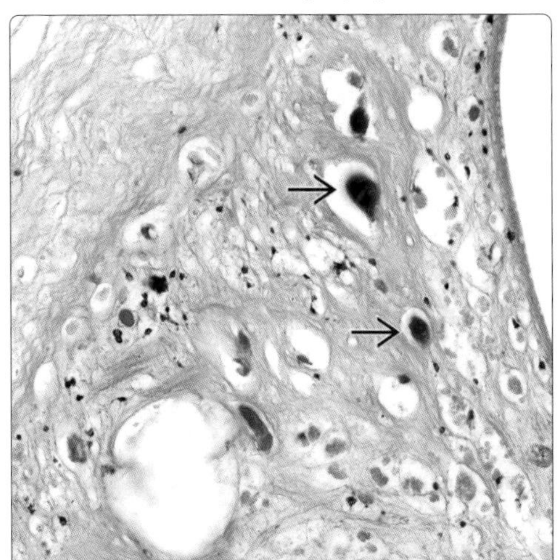

"Mummified," Dead Larvae in Later Stages

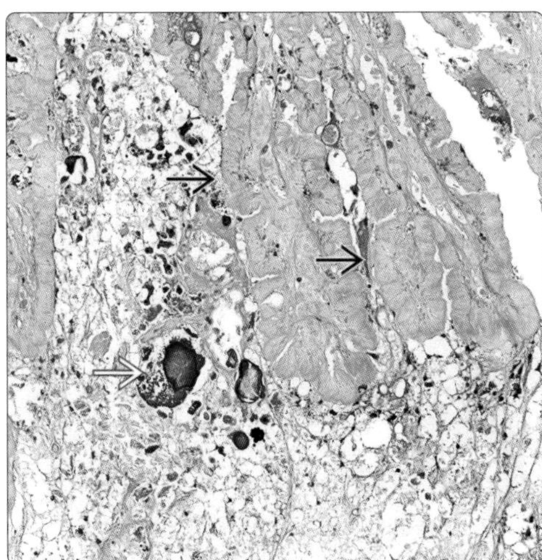

(Left) *The inner reticular layer of the cyst wall in NCC contains several small oval-to-round calcified corpuscles ➔.* **(Right)** *Only the outline of the dead larva is discernible ➔ in later stages of NCC. Dystrophic calcifications are common ➔.*

Fibrotic Nodule, Late Stage Neurocysticercosis

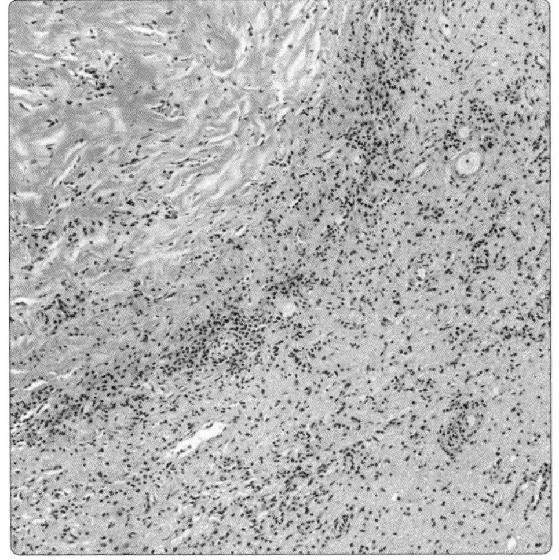

Intense Reaction After Larval Death

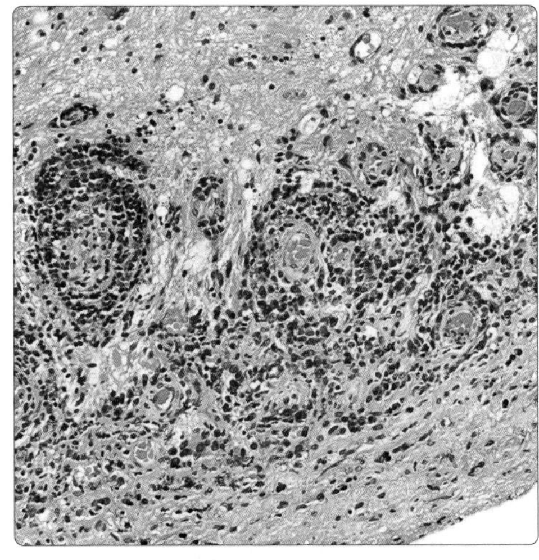

(Left) *A fibrotic nodule, often with dystrophic calcification, forms in the site of the degenerating intraparenchymal cysticercus. Histological findings are not specific for NCC at this stage. Seroconversion (for IgG antibody) between acute and convalescent sera is strong evidence of recent infection.* **(Right)** *After larval demise, an intense inflammatory host response is elicited, as seen in this wall that surrounded a dead organism in NCC.*

Plasma Cells

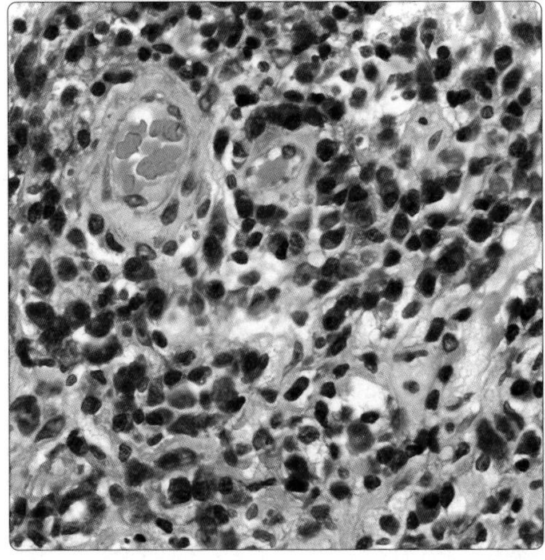

Eosinophils

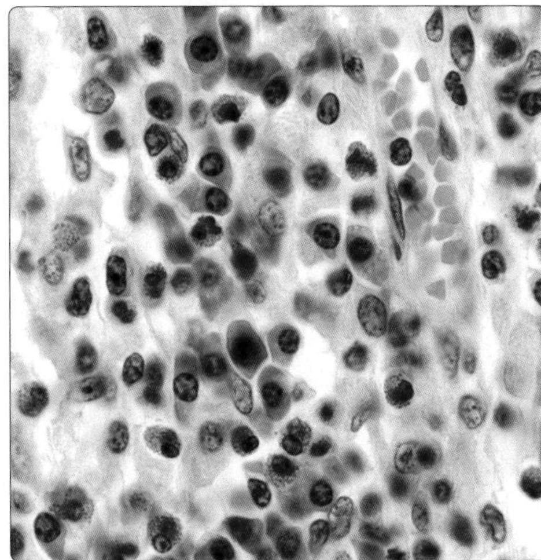

(Left) *The degenerating organism may elicit a dense inflammatory response in which plasma cells may predominate. This should not be mistaken for a plasma cell dyscrasia.* **(Right)** *Eosinophils, as well as plasma cells, may participate in the inflammatory response to dead larvae in NCC.*

Miscellaneous Parasitic Infections

KEY FACTS

ETIOLOGY/PATHOGENESIS

- Cerebral malaria acquired by mosquito bite
- Schistosomiasis acquired by exposure to snail-infested waters
- Paragonimiasis acquired by ingestion of
  - Raw, undercooked, marinated crabs or crayfish in endemic areas

MACROSCOPIC

- Brain with cerebral malaria shows variable edema, congestion, petechial hemorrhages
- Schistosomiasis and paragonimiasis
  - Usually chronic diseases with granulomas surrounding eggs

MICROSCOPIC

- Cerebral malaria with sequestration of erythrocytes in numerous blood vessels
  - Usually little or no inflammation except Dürck granuloma
  - Erythrocytes devoid of hemoglobin
    - Digested hemoglobin leaves dark brown hemozoin (malarial pigment) in RBCs
  - Petechial ring or punctate hemorrhages
- Schistosomiasis, paragonimiasis
  - Granulomatous reaction to eggs
    - Often with surrounding eosinophils
  - Lesions in early stages of chronic infection filled with eggs in varying states of degeneration
  - Later stages fibrotic and calcified

TOP DIFFERENTIAL DIAGNOSES

- For malaria: Other conditions with white matter petechiae
  - Fat embolism, carbon monoxide poisoning, acute hemorrhagic leukoencephalitis
  - No parasites or malarial pigment

Malaria / **Schistosomiasis**

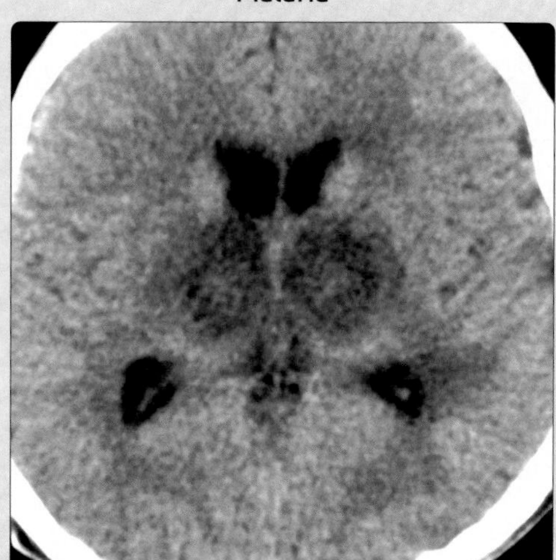

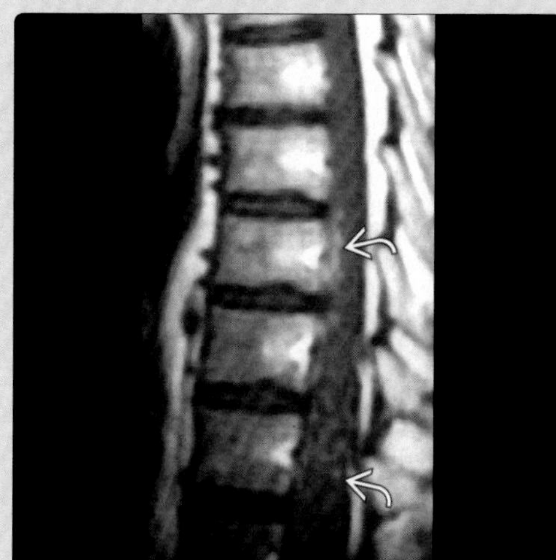

(Left) *Axial NECT shows symmetric, bilateral thalamic hypodensity in a young patient with malaria and severely altered consciousness. (Courtesy R. Ramakantan, MD.)* **(Right)** *Sagittal T1WI C+ MR shows enhancement of distal thoracic cord ➔ due to schistosomiasis. Cerebrospinal fluid (CSF) examination shows inflammatory pattern with increased protein and mononuclear cells in 90% of cases ± IgG against schistosomal antigens. (Courtesy R. Mendonca, MD.)*

Paragonimiasis, Eggs / ***Echinococcus* (Hydatid Disease)**

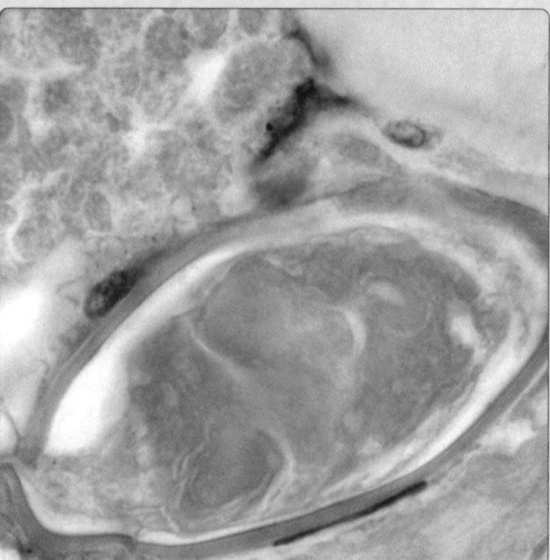

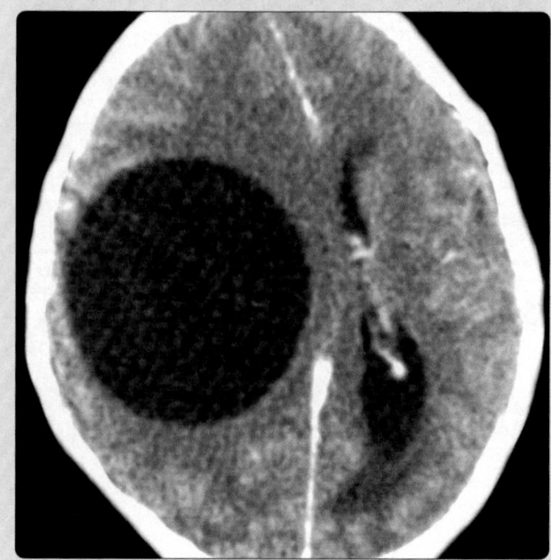

(Left) *Paragonimiasis eggs in tissue are large and display a highly refractile, thick wall.* **(Right)** *Axial CECT of a patient from Turkey shows a unilocular cyst with no surrounding edema or enhancement, typical of Echinococcus (hydatid disease). Note the significant mass effect.*

TERMINOLOGY

Synonyms

- Schistosomiasis (bilharziasis), Katayama fever (acute schistosomiasis)

Definitions

- Nervous system infection by pathogenic parasites, usually acquired by immunocompetent host living or traveling in endemic regions

ETIOLOGY/PATHOGENESIS

Infectious Agents

- Cerebral malaria
  - *Plasmodium falciparum* most virulent species, causes cerebral malaria
  - Susceptible hosts: Children, nonimmune travelers, pregnant women
  - Malaria transmitted from person to person by bite of female anopheline mosquitoes
  - Parasitizes erythrocytes at any stage, multiple parasites per RBC
- Schistosomiasis
  - Trematode infection
  - Humans acquire infection through contact with water-harboring infected snails
    - Snails release fork-tailed motile larvae (cercariae)
    - Cercariae penetrate human skin (may cause itching and cutaneous irritation)
    - Once cercariae penetrate epidermis of skin, tail drops off; parasite is then schistosomulum
    - Schistosomula migrate through tissues, penetrate blood vessels, mature into male and female forms in hepatic portal venules
    - Adult worms migrate to small venules of intestine and rectum (*Schistosoma mansoni*, *Schistosoma japonicum*), and urinary bladder (*Schistosoma hematobium*)
    - Mature worms release eggs
    - Eggs either penetrate bladder (*S. hematobium*) or intestine (*S. mansoni*, *S. japonicum*), shed in urine or feces
    - Eggs enter water, develop into miracidia in water, return to snail, cycle complete
    - Eggs that do not successfully penetrate bladder or intestine remain in walls of these organs &/or are carried to ectopic sites
    - Eggs hematogenously borne to brain or spinal cord causing neuroschistosomiasis
  - *Schistosoma hematobium* endemic in Africa, especially upper basin Nile River
  - *Schistosoma mansoni* endemic in Africa, especially lake plateau region in midcontinent
    - Most widely distributed schistosome; also found in South America, Caribbean islands
  - *Schistosoma japonicum* endemic in China, especially Yangtze River valley
  - *Schistosoma mekongi* endemic in Far East
- Paragonimiasis
  - Trematode infection
  - Multiplies and develops in snail, parasites invade crustaceans, humans infected by eating undercooked crustaceans
  - *Paragonimus westermani*: Southeast Asia, Central and South America
  - CNS paragonimiasis is primarily pediatric disease, especially adolescent males

CLINICAL ISSUES

Presentation

- Cerebral malaria diffuse, rapid, but potentially reversible encephalopathy
  - Seizures, confusion, stupor, coma
  - Occasional cerebellar syndrome
  - Progression to coma and death may occur within 1-2 days after symptom onset
- Neuroschistosomiasis
  - Acute or chronic disease
    - Acute disease: Katayama fever 4-8 weeks after infection
    - Katayama fever: Fever, arthralgias, urticaria, abdominal pain, vomiting, diarrhea
    - Chronic disease: Result of granulomatous reaction to eggs in cerebrum or spinal cord
    - May see peripheral eosinophilia, cerebrospinal fluid (CSF) pleocytosis with acute disease
  - Cerebral disease: Seizures, ± visual, sensory, motor deficits
  - Spinal cord disease: Acute transverse myelitis, subacute myeloradiculopathy (*S. mansoni*)
  - Systemic symptoms: Urinary (*S. hematobium*), intestinal (*S. mansoni, S. japonicum*) often absent in chronic neuroschistosomiasis
  - Chronic disease: 75% of patients lack eggs in rectal biopsy, stool, urine
- Paragonimiasis
  - Acute disease with meningitis, headache, vomiting seen in only small subset of people
  - Chronic cerebral disease: Seizures, visual changes
    - CSF can be normal; eggs in CSF very rare
  - Chronic spinal cord involvement uncommon, usually extradural space of lower thoracic region
  - Pulmonary infection often precedes CNS infection by several months
    - History of rust-colored sputum, chest pain suggestive of diagnosis
    - Sputum, gastric aspirate, stool may contain eggs

Treatment

- Cerebral malaria
  - Antimalarial drugs, supportive care
- Neuroschistosomiasis
  - Schistosomicidal drugs, steroids in acute cases
  - Decompression laminectomy for spinal disease refractory to medical management
- CNS paragonimiasis
  - Antihelminthic drugs, supportive care
  - Surgical treatment for spinal disease refractory to medical management

Prognosis

- Cerebral malaria
  - Mortality, especially pediatric disease, cited as 10-50% in treated patients
  - Neurological deficits in up to 10% of recovered patients
- Schistosomiasis
  - Cerebral disease: Variable, may be relatively asymptomatic and discovered only postmortem
  - Severe spinal cord disease may result in permanent deficits
- CNS paragonimiasis
  - Usually favorable response to antihelminthic drugs

IMAGING

MR Findings

- Cerebral malaria
  - Punctate and ring hemorrhages
  - Minimal edema early in course
  - Hypointensities in severe cases
- Schistosomiasis
  - Hyperintense cerebral masses
  - Spinal cord enhancement
- Paragonimiasis: Hemorrhages, granuloma simulating neoplasm, late calcification

MACROSCOPIC

General Features

- Cerebral malaria causes congestion and variable cerebral edema
  - Numerous white matter petechiae seen in patients who survived for several days in medical care
- Schistosomiasis
  - Focal meningeal and parenchymal firm masses
  - Old lesions may be calcified
- Paragonimiasis
  - Focal meningeal and parenchymal firm masses
  - Old lesions may be calcified

MICROSCOPIC

Histologic Features

- Cerebral malaria
  - Blood vessels occluded by parasitized RBCs ("sequestration") in active/acute cases
    - Parasites remain intravascular
    - Cerebral malaria not inflammatory, i.e., not encephalitis
    - Usually little or no lymphocytic meningeal or perivascular inflammation
    - Sequestered RBCs may be absent in patients who die after prolonged illness or after treatment
    - Parasites ingest and catabolize host hemoglobin as nutrition and release breakdown product of small dark brown refractile pigment granules (hemozoin or malarial pigment)
  - Hemorrhages, either punctate or ring
    - Ring hemorrhages relatively specific, with early stage showing small central blood vessel with parasitized RBCs, surrounding pallor of brain parenchyma, then outer ring of uninfected RBCs
    - Next stage of ring hemorrhage is central necrosed blood vessel, surrounded by inner ring of uninfected RBCs and outer ring of parasitized RBCs, free pigment, host monocytes
    - Dürck granuloma still later stage of ring hemorrhage, with surrounding host microglial and astroglial response
    - Axonal injury associated with hemorrhages by β-amyloid precursor protein (immunohistochemistry)
  - Neuronal ischemic damage rare and related to cardiorespiratory arrest
    - Brain intact surrounding small vessels filled by parasitized RBCs
  - Tissue damage thought to be due to release of cytokines, tumor necrosis factor-α, nitric oxide
- Schistosomiasis
  - Eggs elicit granulomatous inflammatory reaction, with edema, mass effect
  - *S. japonicum* frequently involves brain, meninges
  - *S. mansoni* and *S. hematobium* more frequently involve spinal cord than brain
  - Schistosome eggs only slightly birefringent
  - Degenerating eggs in tissue may crenate and distort, making species classification difficult
  - *S. japonicum* egg: No spine
  - *S. hematobium* egg: Terminal spine
  - *S. mansoni* egg: Lateral spine
  - Eosinophils in surrounding tissue
  - Eggs eventually encased in fibrous tissue; may calcify in late stages
- Paragonimiasis
  - Eggs elicit granulomatous inflammatory reaction, causing mass effect, edema
  - Lesions usually in brain
  - Egg features
    - Brilliantly birefringent compared to those of schistosomes
    - Lack spine, larger than schistosome eggs
    - Thick walled, yellow-brown, have flattened operculum at 1 end

DIFFERENTIAL DIAGNOSIS

For Malaria: Other Conditions With White Matter Petechiae

- Fat embolism, carbon monoxide poisoning, acute hemorrhagic leukoencephalitis
- No parasites or malarial pigment

Schistosomiasis, Paragonimiasis

- Distinguished by geography, epidemiology, egg size, birefringence, absence/presence/location of spine, especially in stool, urine, sputum specimens

SELECTED REFERENCES

1. Christensen SS et al: Cerebral malaria as a risk factor for the development of epilepsy and other long-term neurological conditions: a meta-analysis. Trans R Soc Trop Med Hyg. 109(4):233-8, 2015
2. Seydel KB et al: Brain swelling and death in children with cerebral malaria. N Engl J Med. 372(12):1126-37, 2015
3. Jauréguiberry S et al: Acute schistosomiasis, a diagnostic and therapeutic challenge. Clin Microbiol Infect. 16(3):225-31, 2010

Cerebral Malaria, Absence of Inflammation

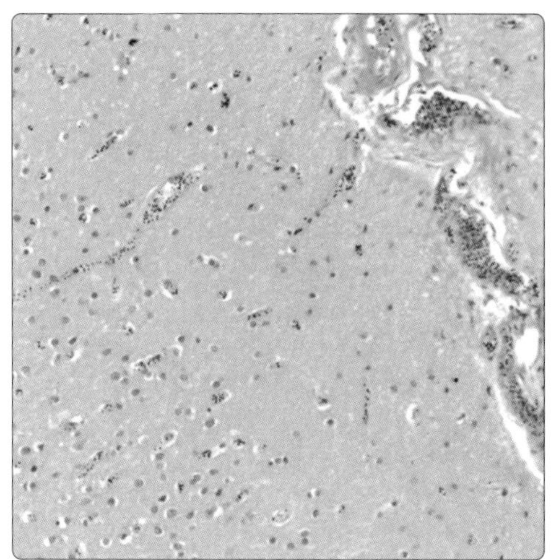

Hemozoin (Malarial) Pigment

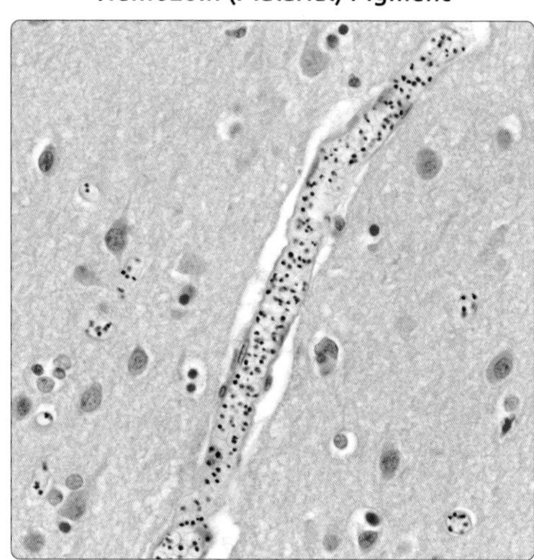

(Left) *As an intravascular rather than inflammatory process, there are no leukocytes from which to infer an infectious nature. Parasites infect red blood cells that preferentially localize in deep vascular beds, such as those in the brain, in a process known as sequestration.* **(Right)** *In cerebral malaria, parasites convert metabolized hemoglobin to hemozoin (malarial pigment).*

Neurons Appear Normal

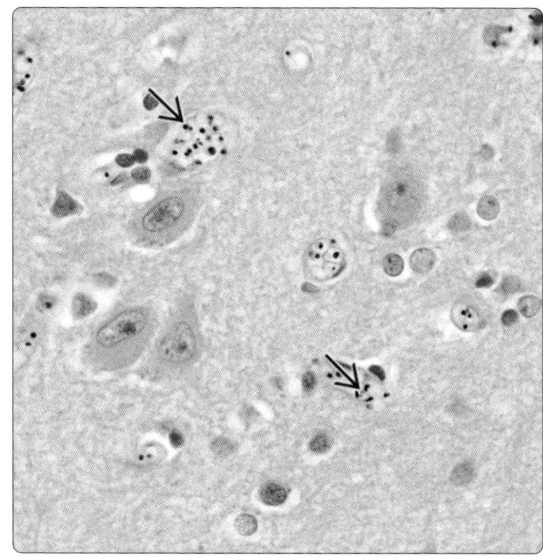

Black Malarial Pigment

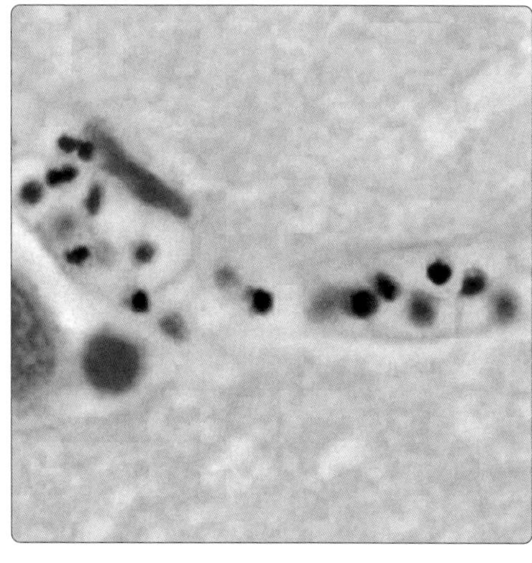

(Left) *In cerebral malaria, cortical neurons may be devoid of anoxic change or any other evidence of injury by light microscopy. Note the malarial pigment* ⇒. **(Right)** *Sequestered RBCs infected with Plasmodium falciparum are depleted of hemoglobin in RBCs. Note the diagnostic black malarial pigment (hemozoin bodies).*

Schistosomiasis

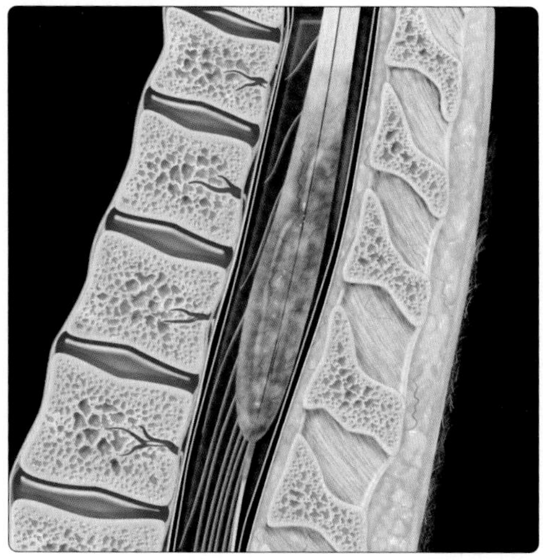

Schistosomal Myelitis

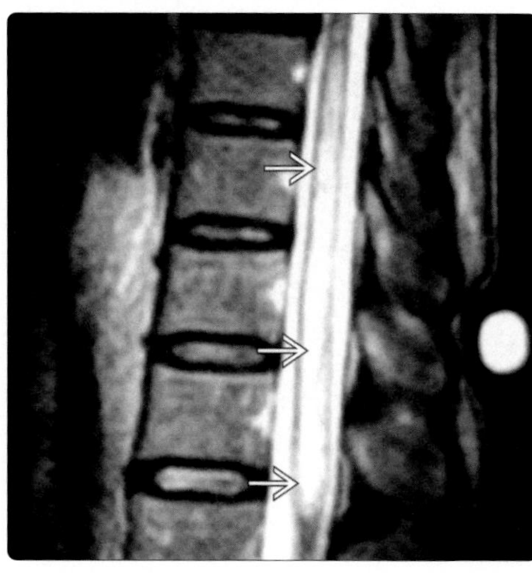

(Left) *Granulomatous inflammatory response to schistosomiasis can produce an expansile pseudotumor, as here in the conus medullaris.* **(Right)** *Sagittal STIR MR depicts diffuse hyperintensity in an enlarged distal cord and conus* ➡. *Schistosomal myelitis occurs early after infection and is more likely to be symptomatic than its intracranial counterpart. (Courtesy A. El-Razek, MD.)*

(Left) *Cerebral schistosomiasis appears as multiple discrete leptomeningeal and superficial parenchymal granulomas surrounded by an intense inflammatory response.* **(Right)** *Schistosome eggs elicit a granulomatous response.*

Cerebral Schistosomiasis

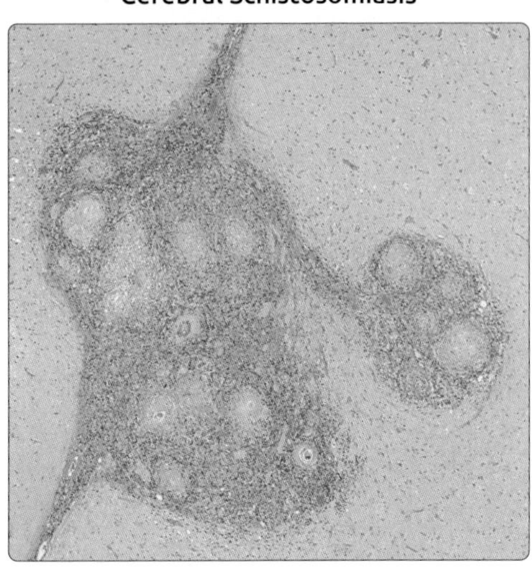

Cerebral Schistosomiasis

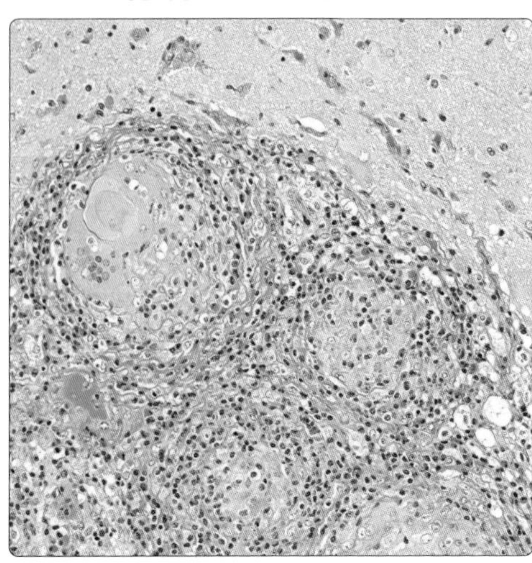

(Left) *Eggs of Schistosoma mansoni have a characteristic lateral spine ⮕, but the latter may not be as evident in degenerating eggs within tissue. Note the encompassing serrated zone of eosinophilic material: Splendore-Hoeppli phenomenon.* **(Right)** *A multinucleated giant cell engulfs a schistosome egg whose small nuclei are still visible.*

Splendore-Hoeppli Phenomenon

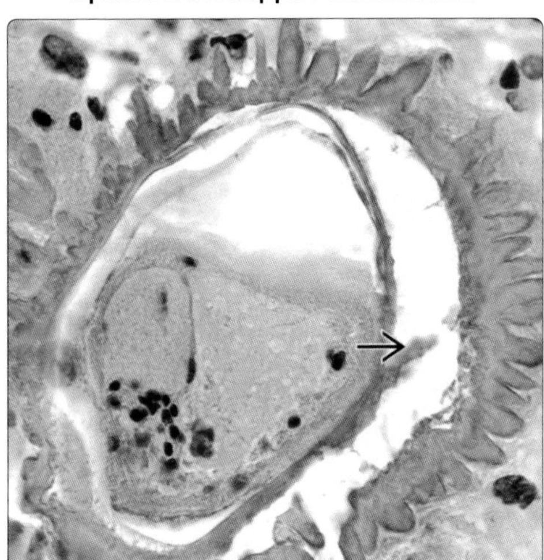

Schistosomiasis, Egg

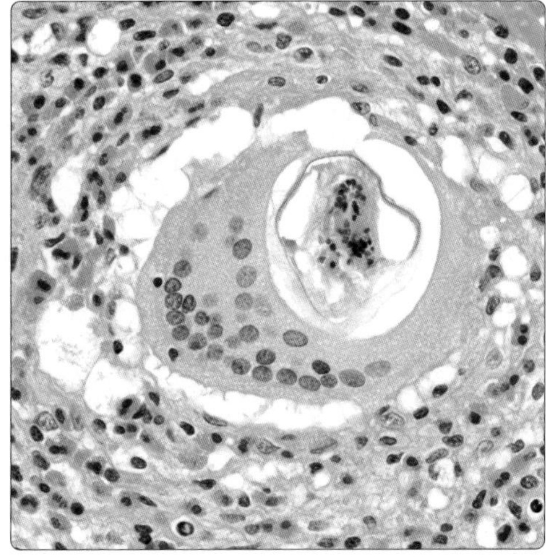

(Left) *An engulfed schistosome egg remains only as a fragmented cell wall ⮕. Note the surrounding eosinophilic reaction.* **(Right)** *Schistosome eggs in an advanced state of degeneration are crenated and distorted, although multiple small nuclei persist in some ⮕.*

Schistosomiasis, Fragmented Egg Wall

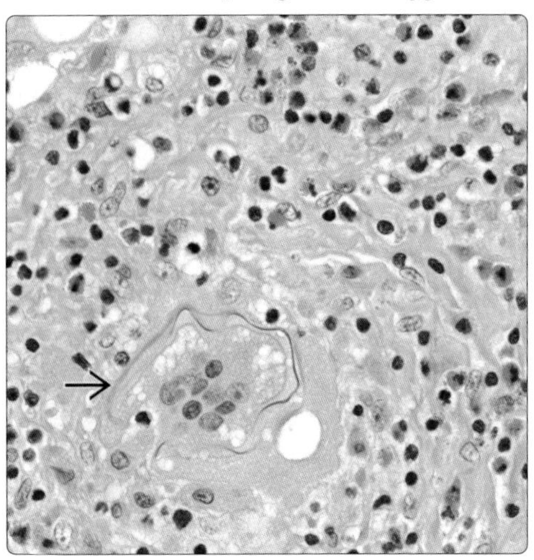

Schistosomiasis, Advanced Stage of Egg Degeneration

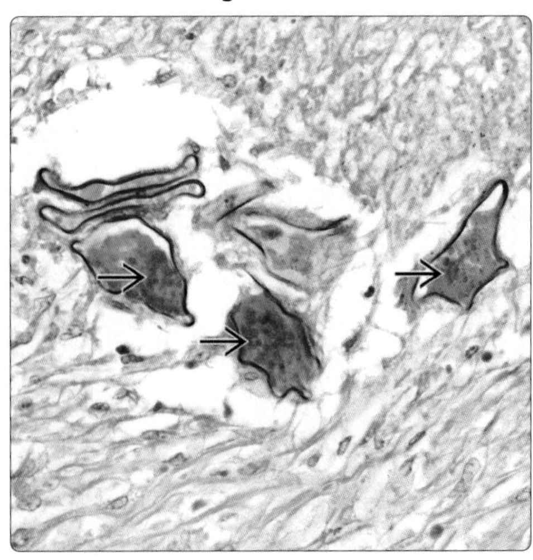

Paragonimiasis

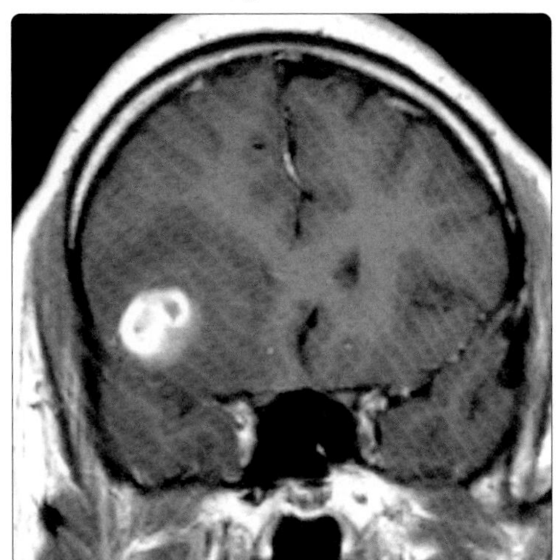

Paragonimiasis

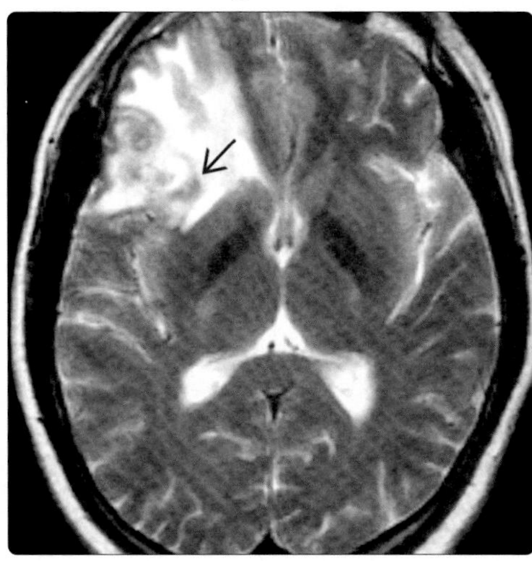

(Left) *As seen in a contrast-enhanced MR, a ring-enhancing lesion of paragonimiasis with marked surrounding edema closely resembles a high-grade glioma. Calcification and contraction will appear in the chronic state.* **(Right)** *Axial T2WI MR shows a heterogeneous lesion in the right frontal lobe with mass effect and surrounding edema in this patient from East Asia. Note the dark sector of fibrous tissue* ⇨ *that often accompanies chronic inflammation of any etiology.*

Paragonimiasis, Granuloma

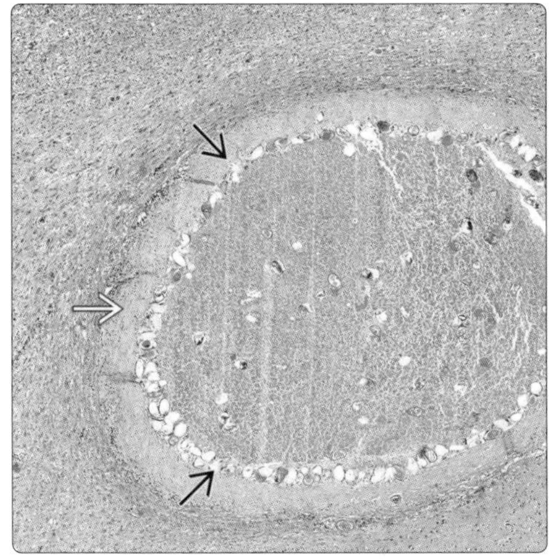

Paragonimiasis, Eggs

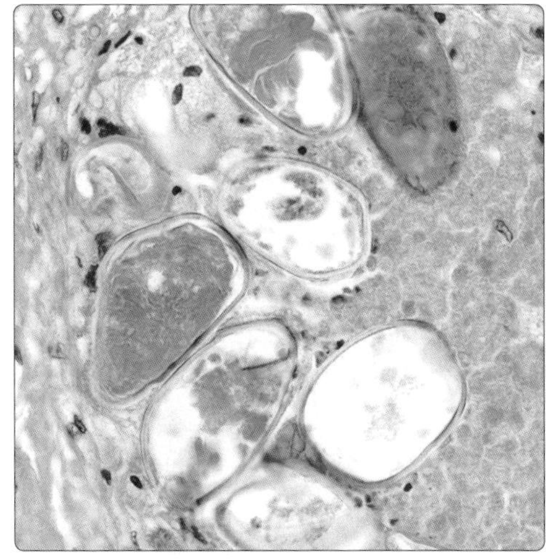

(Left) *A CNS paragonimiasis granuloma is a reaction to eggs that marginate along the thick fibrotic wall* ➡ *and appear as clear oval spaces* ⇨*.* **(Right)** *Thick-walled, yellow-brown Paragonimus eggs at the edge of a fibrotic granuloma are shown. The degenerating eggs retain varying amounts of internal material.*

Paragonimiasis, Giant Cell

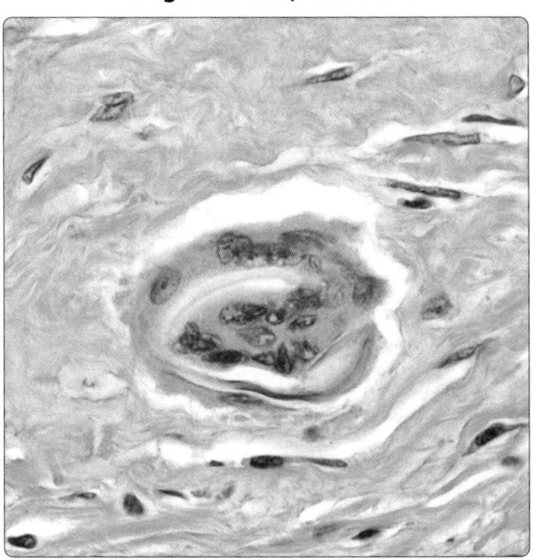

Paragonimiasis, Hemosiderin, Gliosis

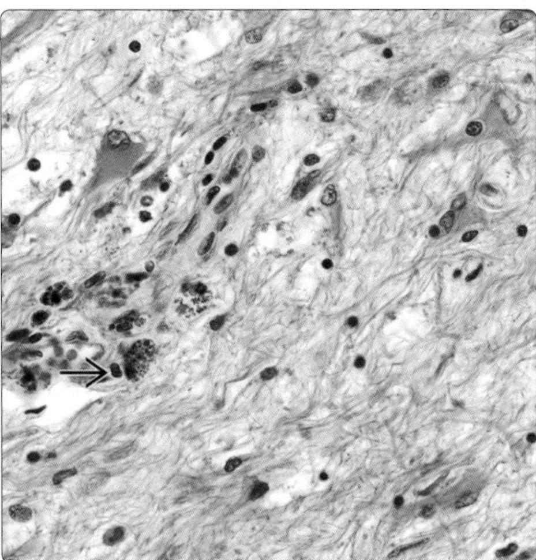

(Left) *A multinucleated giant cell engulfs a brown egg remnant of Paragonimus species, likely westermani.* **(Right)** *Intense gliosis and sometimes hemosiderin pigment* ⇨ *may surround granulomas of CNS paragonimiasis.*

Sarcoidosis

KEY FACTS

TERMINOLOGY

- Neurosarcoidosis
  - CNS or PNS involvement by inflammatory disorder of unknown cause, characterized by compact, small, noncaseating granulomas and no identifiable organism(s)

ETIOLOGY/PATHOGENESIS

- Unknown
- Disease more common in African Americans than Caucasian Americans

CLINICAL ISSUES

- Protean clinical features
  - Disease may be asymptomatic, indolent
- Usual presentation is cranial nerve palsy, optic neuritis, acute or chronic aseptic meningitis, mass lesion(s) with focal neurological deficits, seizures

IMAGING

- Dural, leptomeningeal, parenchymal lesions of brain, cranial nerves, spinal cord
  - Basal cisterns, optic chiasm, hypothalamus especially affected
- Solitary or multifocal CNS masses with enhancement
  - Hypothalamus > brainstem > cerebral hemisphere > cerebellar hemisphere
- May be associated with abnormal chest x-ray

MICROSCOPIC

- Discrete, noncaseating, nonnecrotic granulomas
- Nodular aggregates of epithelioid histiocytes, with variable numbers of multinucleated giant cells
- Surrounding nonneoplastic lymphocytes and plasma cells

Neurosarcoidosis: Ventricular Involvement

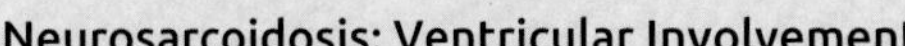

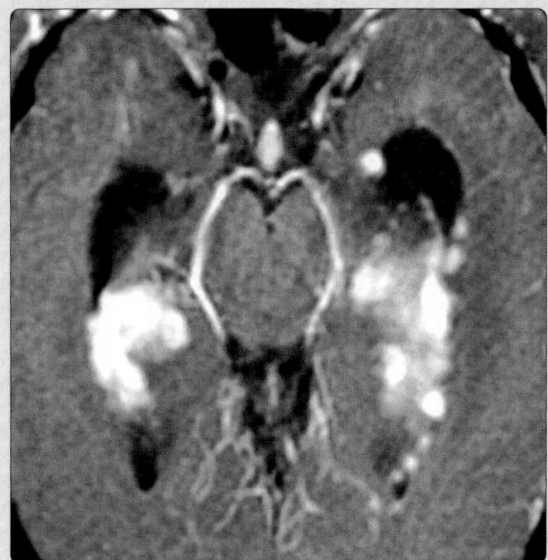

Hypothalamus: Infundibulum Often Involved

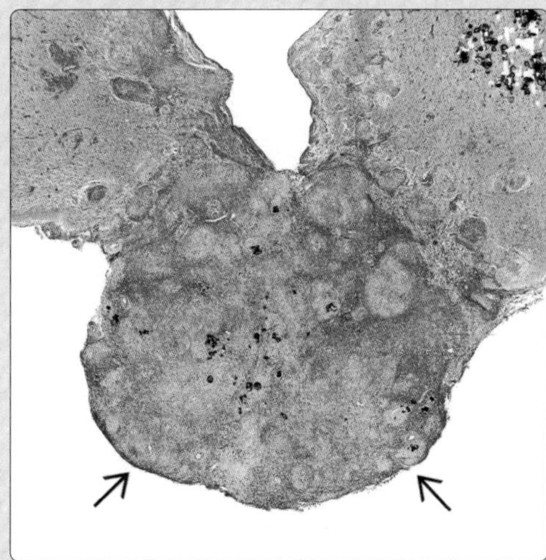

(Left) *Axial T1 C+ fat saturation shows multiple enhancing neurosarcoid lesions involving the choroid plexus, ependymal surfaces, and infundibulum. Hydrocephalus is also noted.* **(Right)** *The hypothalamus is a favored site for sarcoidosis, as in this lesion seen post mortem that expands the 3rd ventricular floor and proximal infundibulum ⇨.*

Leptomeningeal Lymphocytes: Inconspicuous Small Granulomas

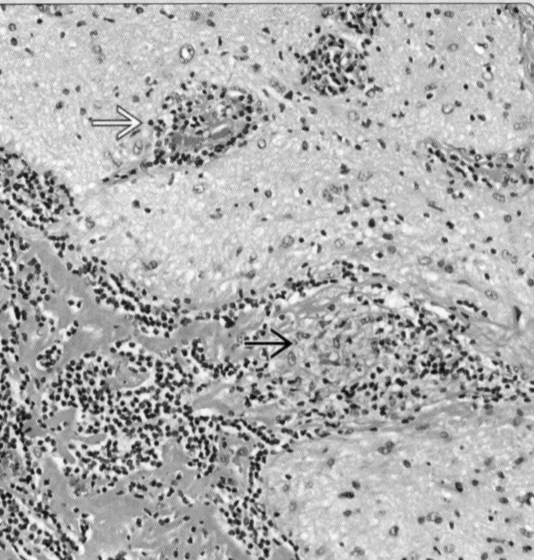

Piloid Gliosis Near Sarcoid Granulomas

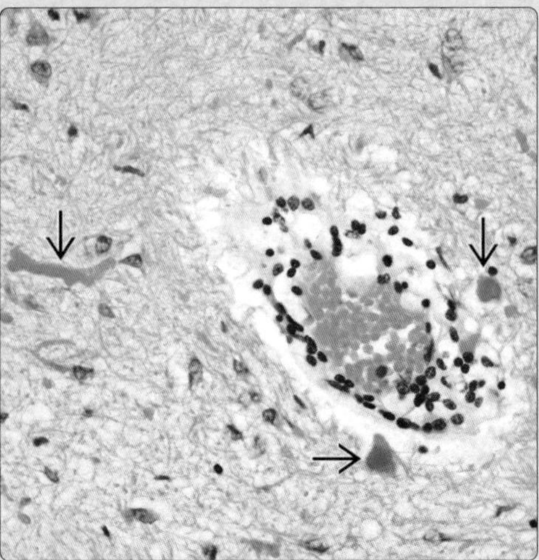

(Left) *Granulomas may be quite small ⇨, irregularly distributed, and inconspicuous. Note the extension of the meningeal lymphocytic inflammation along the Virchow-Robin spaces ➡. Unlike viral infections, intraparenchymal microglial clusters are not seen in neurosarcoidosis.* **(Right)** *Scant perivascular lymphocytic inflammation is not a specific finding, and, when associated with numerous Rosenthal fibers ⇨, the piloid gliosis of neurosarcoidosis closely simulates pilocytic astrocytoma.*

TERMINOLOGY

Synonyms

- Neurosarcoidosis

Definitions

- Multisystem inflammatory disorder of uncertain etiology characterized by discrete, typically noncaseating granulomas
- Diagnosis of exclusion; stains and cultures negative
- Neurosarcoidosis: Part of systemic disease or, rarely, confined to CNS
  - ~ 25% of patients with systemic disease have CNS involvement, although often subclinical
  - 5-15% have clinical neurosarcoidosis

ETIOLOGY/PATHOGENESIS

Environmental Exposure

- Unknown
  - Thought to result from exposure of genetically susceptible hosts to unknown environmental factors
    - Infectious and noninfectious triggers postulated to account for occasional clustering of cases

CLINICAL ISSUES

Epidemiology

- Incidence
  - 1-50 cases per 100,000 individuals, varying among ethnic and racial groups
    - Most common among African Americans, Northern Europeans
  - Occurs worldwide; up to 90% of patients have lung involvement
- Age
  - Typically affects adults

Site

- Dural mass(es), simulating meningioma
- Brain
  - Parenchyma, leptomeninges
  - Hypothalamus favored
  - Optic nerve
- Spinal cord: Parenchyma, leptomeninges

Presentation

- Cranial nerve palsy, especially facial
- Optic neuritis with subacute loss of central vision, retrobulbar pain, and papilledema
- Aseptic meningitis, acute or chronic
  - Fever, headache, neck rigidity, sterile cerebrospinal fluid (CSF)
- Mass lesions: Small or large, single or multiple
  - Seizures with meningeal or cortical brain parenchymal lesions
  - Endocrine dysfunction with hypothalamic/pituitary region lesions
- Myelopathy with weakness &/or sensory abnormalities
- Myopathy
  - Myalgia, weakness proximal > distal
  - Symptomatic muscle involvement uncommon
- Peripheral nerve involvement
  - Chronic sensory motor neuropathy and mononeuropathy multiplex most common presentations
  - Some patients have painful neuropathy or chronic inflammatory demyelinating polyneuropathy
- Disease often indolent or even asymptomatic

Treatment

- Drugs
  - Long-term treatment: Prednisone &/or other immunomodulators (azathioprine, methotrexate, or mycophenolate mofetil)
    - Steroids initial drug of choice
  - Rituximab

Prognosis

- Steroids suppress inflammation, but symptoms recur in subset of patients treated at lower doses
- Steroid-related side effects significant
- Other drugs have 60-80% response rates

IMAGING

MR Findings

- Enhancing multifocal, dural-based lesions
- Basal cisterns often involved
- Lesions common in choroid plexus, ependymal regions, hypothalamus/infundibulum
- Orbit often involved
- Presentation as isolated CNS mass without systemic findings rare

MACROSCOPIC

Gross Findings Protean

- Dural thickening
- Leptomeningeal thickening, especially basilar
- Hypothalamic/pituitary region mass(es)
- Single or multifocal, large or small, discrete firm granulomas

MICROSCOPIC

Histologic Features

- Widespread anatomic distribution
- Dural, meningeal, brain, and spinal cord parenchymal lesions are small, discrete, usually nonnecrotizing granulomas
- Granulomas show central aggregates of epithelioid histiocytes, variable numbers of multinucleated giant cells
  - Epithelioid histiocytes have abundant eosinophilic cytoplasm, vesicular nuclei
  - Multinucleated giant cells represent fusion of macrophages, are CD68(+)
  - Giant cells may or may not have Langhans giant cell morphology
    - Langhans cells, after German pathologist Theodor Langhans; not to be confused with Langerhans cell, after German physician Paul Langerhans
    - Langhans cells with multiple peripheral nuclei
- Granulomas often associated with vessels
- Asteroid or Schaumann bodies only occasionally present

- Neither necessary nor specific for diagnosis
- Asteroid body: Stellate-like inclusion often within vacuole in giant cell
- Schaumann body: Calcified, proteinaceous inclusion
- Epithelioid granulomas surrounding nonneoplastic lymphocytes and plasma cells
  - Fibroblasts at periphery laying down collagen; fibrosis becoming progressively more prominent
  - Longstanding cases often with dense perivascular, meningeal fibrosis
- Necrosis, focal, in some cases
  - Usually within individual granulomas
  - Not geographic areas encompassing tissue parenchyma and vasculature as in tuberculosis
- Microglial clusters, in CNS parenchyma, absent
- No fungal or mycobacterial organisms by H&E, histochemical or immunohistochemical stains, culture
- Peripheral nerve, muscle may be involved by small granulomas
  - Noncaseating granulomas variably present in nerve, both nerve and muscle, or muscle alone
  - Loss of myelin in nerve and fibrosis in advanced sarcoid neuropathy

ANCILLARY TESTS

Immunohistochemistry

- No specific immunohistochemical stain
- Brain biopsy is safe, effective diagnostic technique

Cerebrospinal Fluid Abnormalities Usually Nonspecific

- Mild pleocytosis, high protein, sometimes slightly low glucose
- 1/3 of patients with neurosarcoidosis have normal CSF findings
- CSF findings overlap with patients with other diseases, including multiple sclerosis, systemic lupus erythematosus
- Angiotensin-converting enzyme in CSF high in > 1/2 of patients with neurosarcoidosis
  - Elevated levels not specific to neurosarcoidosis

Cytology

- Cytologically bland histiocytes, lymphocytes, plasma cells

DIFFERENTIAL DIAGNOSIS

Fungal or Tuberculous Meningitis

- Identification of causative organisms by special histochemical, immunohistochemical stains

Primary Angiitis of Central Nervous System

- Immunopositive for varicella-zoster virus, in some cases
- Absence of brain parenchymal granulomas or systemic organ involvement
- Distinction difficult in some cases

Amyloid Angiopathy With Granulomatous Response

- Congo red (+) and immunostains for amyloid (+) in vessels

Pilocytic Astrocytoma

- Especially in cases of hypothalamic involvement with piloid gliosis
- Absence of granulomas
- Loose, spongy microcystic tissue (in most cases)

Hypophysitis

- Lymphoplasmacytic inflammation centered on, and destructive of, adenohypophysis (in most cases)
- Frequent relationship to pregnancy
- Systemic sarcoidosis or CNS granulomas elsewhere must be excluded in cases of granulomatous hypophysitis

Rheumatoid Arthritis

- Positive serology

Wegener Granulomatosis

- Usually fewer discrete granulomas, more vasocentric chronic inflammation; fragmented vessels in center of necrosis
- Usually restricted to dura

DIAGNOSTIC CHECKLIST

Pathologic Interpretation Pearls

- Piloid tissue with Rosenthal fibers in gliosis surrounding longstanding neurosarcoid granulomas not to be mistaken for pilocytic astrocytoma
- Most patients with neurosarcoidosis do not require CNS biopsy; those that do have little or no systemic disease; diagnosis may be unsuspected clinically
- Don't mistake fibrosis in peripheral nerve in late stages of sarcoidosis for amyloidosis
- Small foci of necrosis in granulomas should encourage search for organisms, but necrosis does not preclude diagnosis of sarcoidosis

SELECTED REFERENCES

1. Berrios I et al: A case of neurosarcoidosis secondary to treatment of etanercept and review of the literature. BMJ Case Rep. 2015:bcr2014208188, 2015
2. Agnihotri SP et al: Neurosarcoidosis. Semin Neurol. 34(4):386-94, 2014
3. Bomprezzi R et al: A case of neurosarcoidosis successfully treated with rituximab. Neurology. 75(6):568-70, 2010
4. Das DK et al: Sarcoidosis diagnosed on transbronchial fine needle aspiration smears: a case report with new information on asteroid bodies. Acta Cytol. 54(2):225-8, 2010
5. Kimball MM et al: Neurosarcoidosis presenting as an isolated intrasellar mass: case report and review of the literature. Clin Neuropathol. 29(3):156-62, 2010
6. Lee CH et al: Hydrocephalus as a presenting manifestation of neurosarcoidosis : easy to misdiagnose as tuberculosis. J Korean Neurosurg Soc. 48(1):79-81, 2010
7. Scott TF et al: Neurosarcoidosis mimicry of multiple sclerosis: clinical, laboratory, and imaging characteristics. Neurologist. 16(6):386-9, 2010
8. Stern BJ et al: Neurologic presentations of sarcoidosis. Neurol Clin. 28(1):185-98, 2010
9. Vargas DL et al: Neurosarcoidosis: diagnosis and management. Semin Respir Crit Care Med. 31(4):419-27, 2010
10. Wong SH et al: Brain biopsy in the management of neurology patients. Eur Neurol. 64(1):42-5, 2010
11. Pawate S et al: Presentations and outcomes of neurosarcoidosis: a study of 54 cases. QJM. 102(7):449-60, 2009
12. Vital A et al: Sarcoid neuropathy: clinico-pathological study of 4 new cases and review of the literature. Clin Neuropathol. 27(2):96-105, 2008
13. Nemoto I et al: Tumour-like muscular sarcoidosis. Clin Exp Dermatol. 32(3):298-300, 2007
14. Burns TM et al: The natural history and long-term outcome of 57 limb sarcoidosis neuropathy cases. J Neurol Sci. 244(1-2):77-87, 2006
15. Hoitsma E et al: Neurosarcoidosis: a clinical dilemma. Lancet Neurol. 3(7):397-407, 2004
16. Zisman DA et al: Sarcoidosis involving the musculoskeletal system. Semin Respir Crit Care Med. 23(6):555-70, 2002

Neurosarcoidosis Simulating Meningiomas

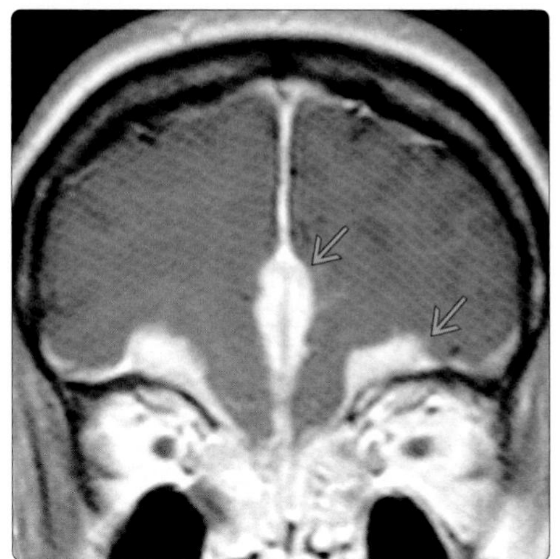

Dural Thickening

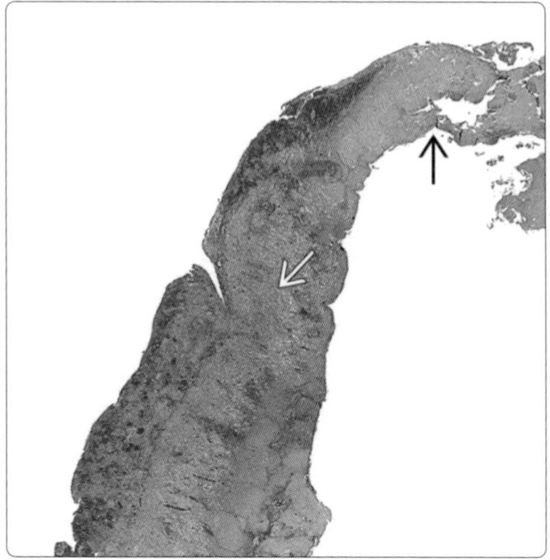

(Left) *Intracranial sarcoidosis often appears as dural-based masses ⇨ that can simulate meningiomas.* **(Right)** *Even at low magnification, the lesion has the look of a diffuse inflammatory lesion, rather than a discrete neoplastic lesion. Sarcoidosis ➡ has here thickened the normal dura ⇨ 3x.*

Predilection for Optic Nerve

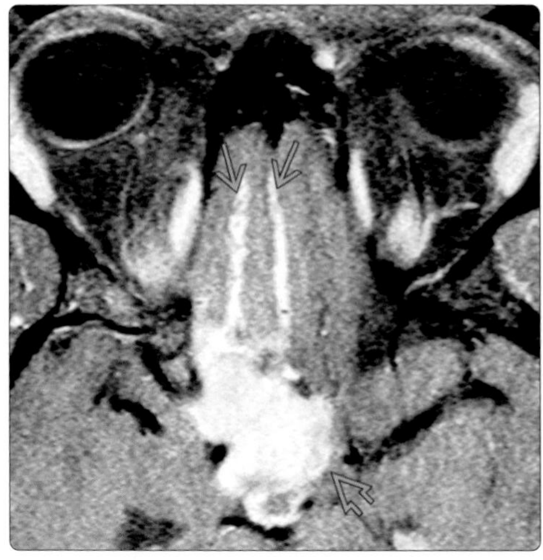

Optic Nerve: Extension Along Fibrovascular Septa

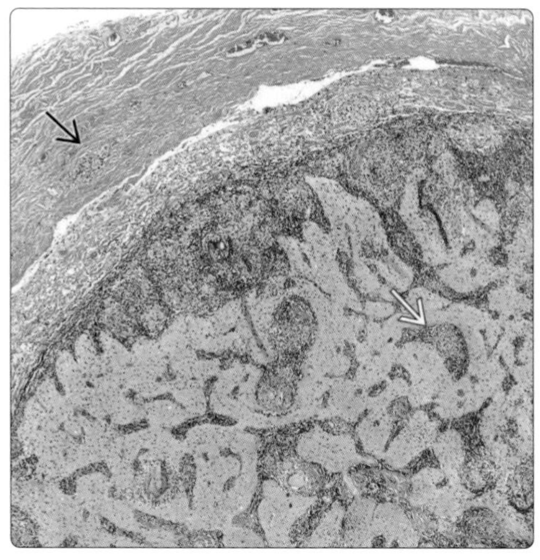

(Left) *Neurosarcoidosis has a predilection to involve the optic nerve. Axial T1 C+ and fat saturation show a thick, enhancing process that envelops the optic chiasm ⇨ and extends along the rectus gyri ⇨.* **(Right)** *Sarcoid infiltrates and granulomas of the optic nerve extend along the fibrovascular septa ➡. A small granuloma is present in the dura ⇨.*

Leptomeningeal Predilection

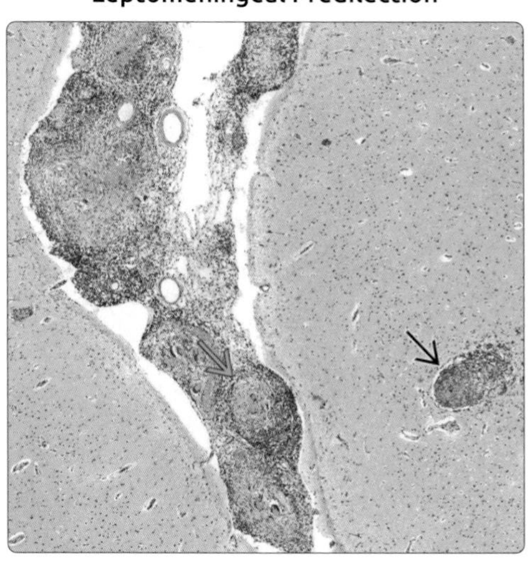

Small Granulomas

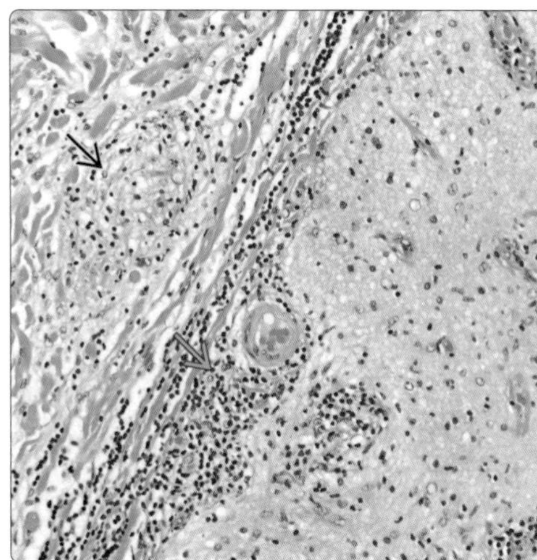

(Left) *Neurosarcoidosis favors the leptomeninges, here with granulomatous inflammation ⇨ extending into Virchow-Robin spaces ⇨.* **(Right)** *Neurosarcoidosis can have small leptomeningeal granulomas ⇨ associated with leptomeningeal and intraparenchymal perivascular lymphocytic infiltrates ⇨.*

(Left) *A small, ovoid granuloma ⇒ is nestled in a sulcus in association with a scant meningeal lymphocytic infiltrate.* **(Right)** *Granulomas in neurosarcoidosis are often related to blood vessels ⇒, potentially raising considerations of infectious granulomatous vasculitis, such as that of varicella-zoster virus or primary angiitis of the nervous system of the granulomatous type. The latter would not show the discrete granulomas elsewhere in brain or spinal cord parenchyma expected in neurosarcoidosis.*

Inconspicuous Small Granuloma

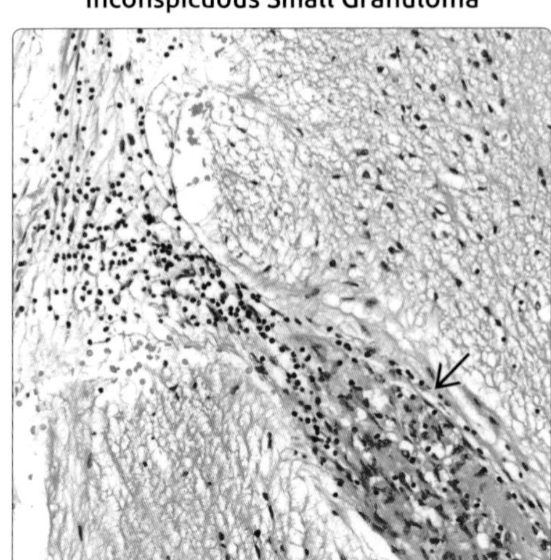

Granulomas Often Around Vessels

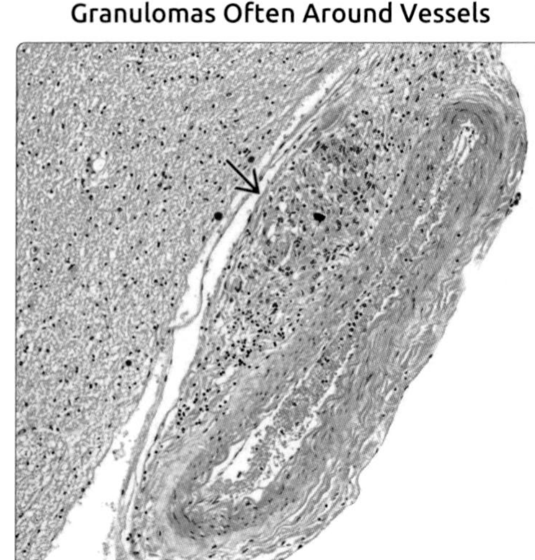

(Left) *Sarcoidosis is characterized by compact, noncaseating epithelioid granulomas.* **(Right)** *This small, discrete, well-demarcated granuloma in the brain parenchyma is composed of epithelioid histiocytes centrally ⇒ and multinucleated giant cells peripherally ⇒. The surrounding brain is gliotic.*

Compact: Noncaseating Granulomas

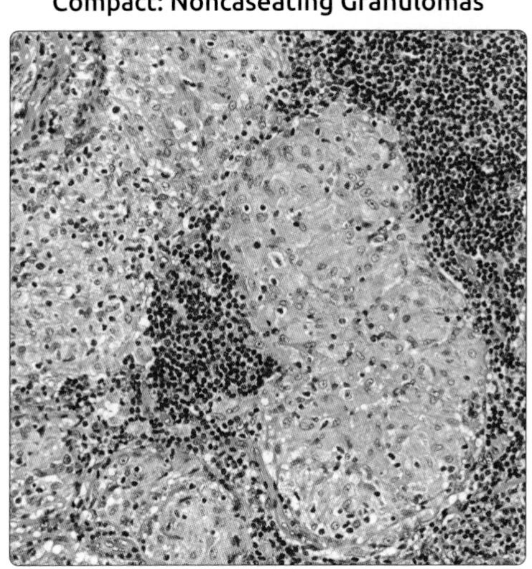

Occasional Multinucleated Giant Cells

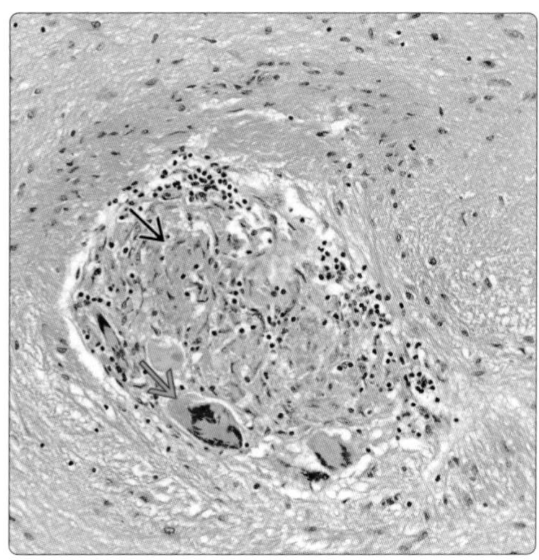

(Left) *The typical epithelioid granuloma of sarcoidosis is discrete and nonnecrotizing.* **(Right)** *Some multinucleated giant cells in sarcoidosis contain vacuoles ⇒ that should not be mistaken for Coccidioides species or other fungi, such as Blastomyces. Stellate asteroid bodies sometimes fill these spaces.*

Epithelioid Granuloma

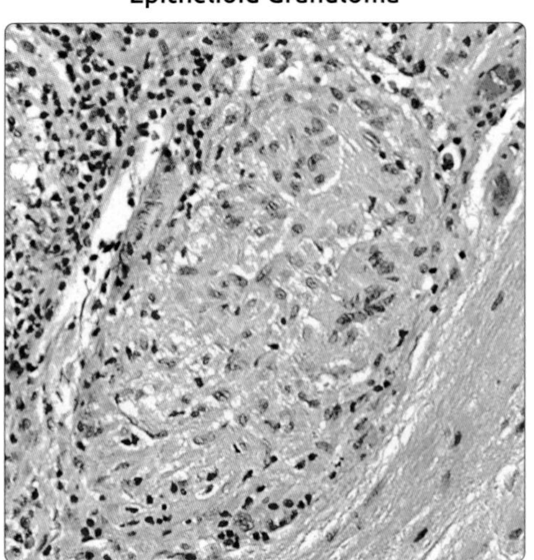

Vacuoles in Giant Cells Simulating Fungi

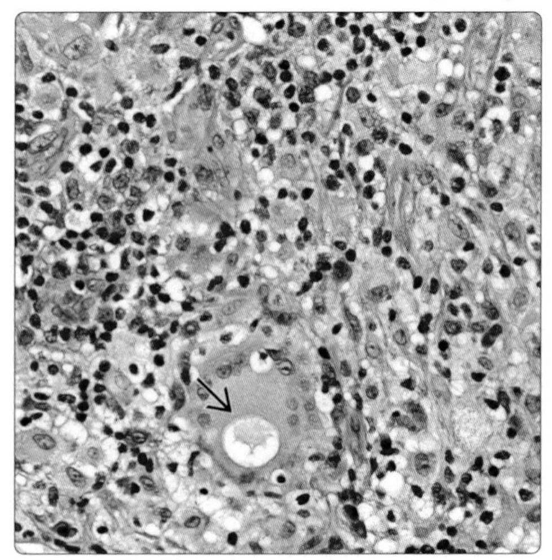

Langhans Giant Cell

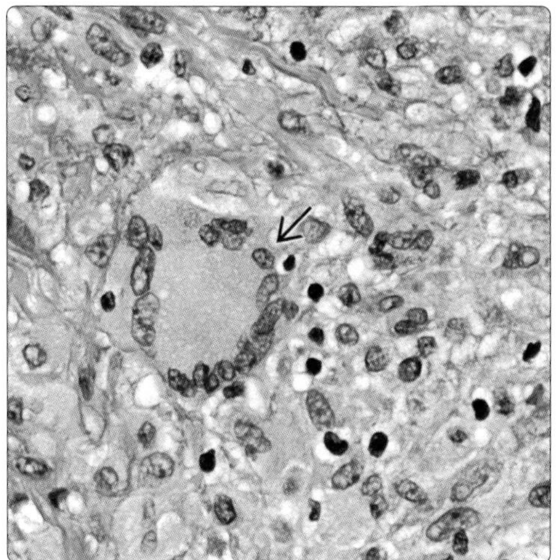

CD68: Giant Cell

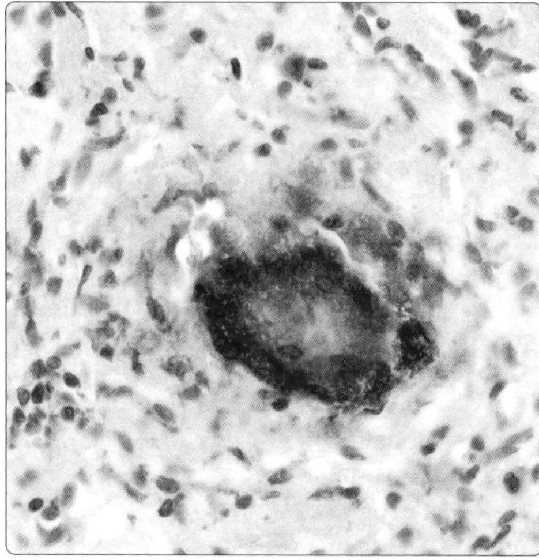

(Left) *Langhans giant cell ⇒ is the best-known type of multinucleated giant cell in sarcoidosis. This cell is not specific for sarcoidosis, however, and can be found in almost any type of granulomatous disease.* **(Right)** *As fused histiocytes, multinucleated giant cells in sarcoid granulomas maintain the expected immunoreactivity for CD68.*

Schaumann Body

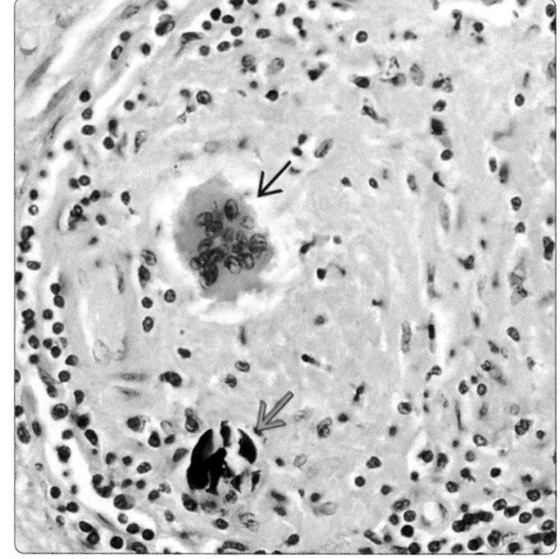

Small Foci of Necrosis

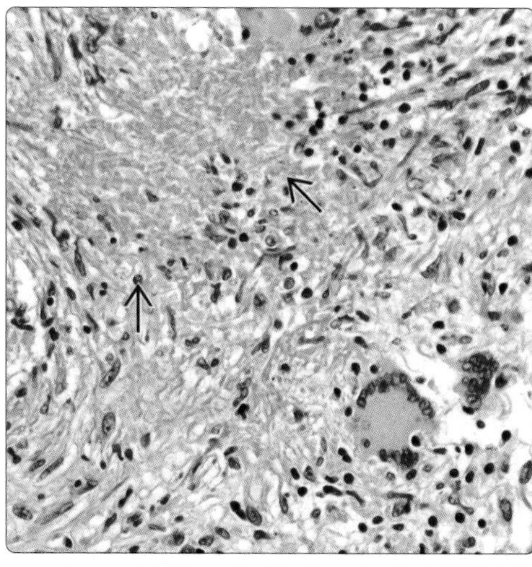

(Left) *The typically discrete granulomas of sarcoidosis are often gradually replaced by fibrous tissue. A giant cell ⇒ and a Schaumann body ⇒ persist in this case.* **(Right)** *Small areas of necrosis ⇒ do not preclude a diagnosis of sarcoidosis, but large caseating zones would make the same diagnosis much less tenable.*

Peripheral Nerve Involvement

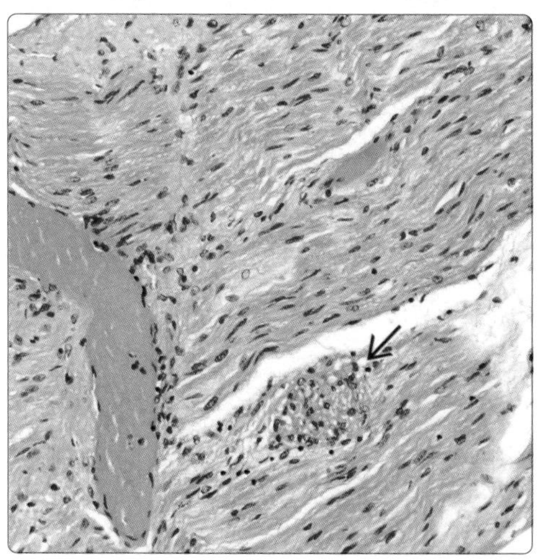

Peripheral Nerve Fibrosis

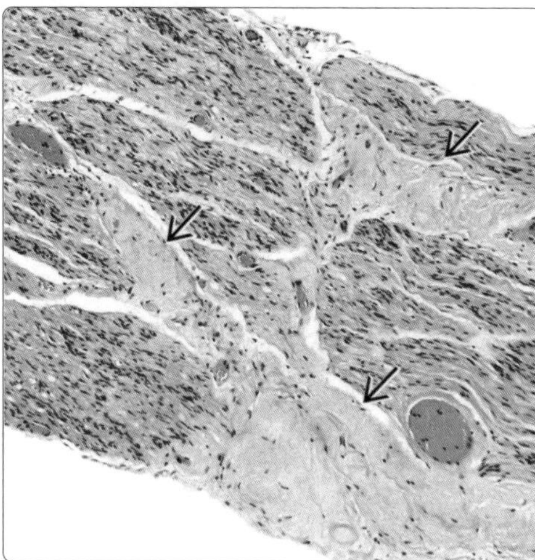

(Left) *Peripheral nerves may be biopsied in the diagnosis of neurosarcoidosis. Small isolated granulomas may be inconspicuous ⇒.* **(Right)** *Peripheral nerves in longstanding cases of sarcoidosis unresponsive to medications may develop significant damage, including fibrosis ⇒. These deposits should not be mistaken for amyloidosis in the nerve.*

Rasmussen Encephalitis

KEY FACTS

TERMINOLOGY

- Rare, unilateral, inflammatory disorder usually of childhood with intractable focal epilepsy and neurological deficits

ETIOLOGY/PATHOGENESIS

- Viral etiology never proven
- Probable immune etiology: Humoral, cell mediated, or both

CLINICAL ISSUES

- Seizures: Epilepsia partialis continua characteristic, but not always seen
- Hemiparesis, hemianopia, cognitive deficits

IMAGING

- Unilateral T2/FLAIR signal changes and hemiatrophy with epicenter in frontotemporal and insular, periinsular regions
- Signal abnormalities progressively spread toward occipital lobe
- Atrophy of ipsilateral caudate head

MICROSCOPIC

- Patchy microglial clusters earliest microscopic feature
- Progressive perivascular T-lymphocytic infiltrates, neuronal loss, astrocytosis, cavitation
- No viral inclusions
- Gyral segments with rarefaction, chronic cases

ANCILLARY TESTS

- No single diagnostic laboratory test

DIAGNOSTIC CHECKLIST

- Do not mistake microglial cells in encephalitis for gliomatosis cerebri
- Do not mistake gliomatosis cerebri for autoimmune or viral encephalitis

(Left) *Axial FLAIR MR shows increased T2 signal ➔ in the cortex and subcortical white matter in a stage 1 Rasmussen encephalitis (RE). Unilateral cerebral involvement is typical of RE.* **(Right)** *Axial T1WI MR shows the focal atrophy involving the left frontal and temporal lobes of the ipsilateral ventricle. This represents a later stage of RE.*

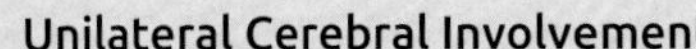

Unilateral Cerebral Involvement

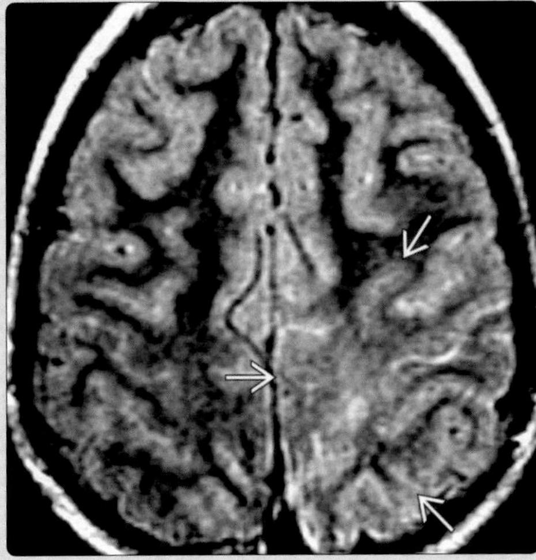

Late-Stage Atrophy

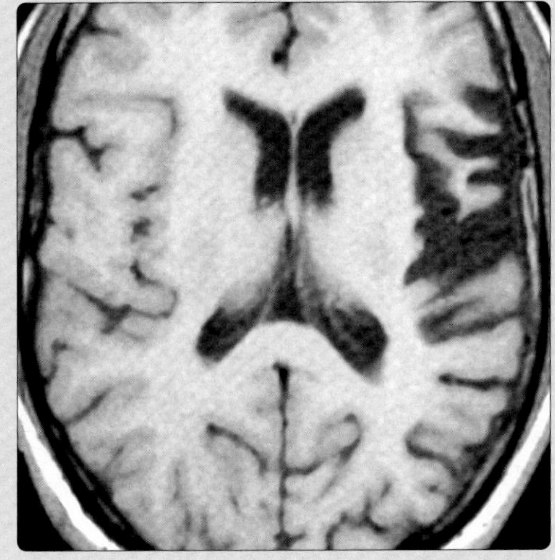

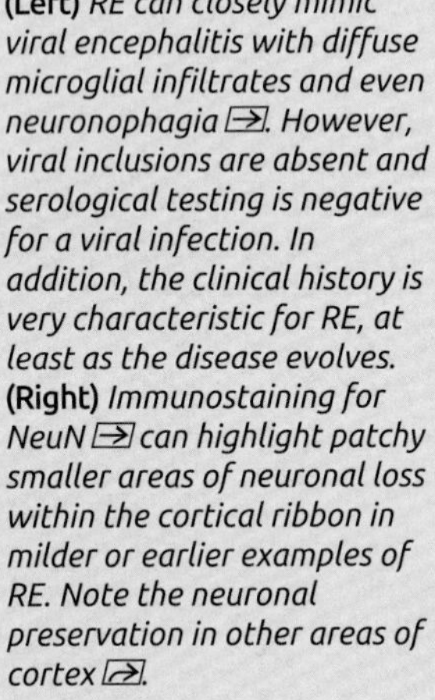

(Left) *RE can closely mimic viral encephalitis with diffuse microglial infiltrates and even neuronophagia ➔. However, viral inclusions are absent and serological testing is negative for a viral infection. In addition, the clinical history is very characteristic for RE, at least as the disease evolves.* **(Right)** *Immunostaining for NeuN ➔ can highlight patchy smaller areas of neuronal loss within the cortical ribbon in milder or earlier examples of RE. Note the neuronal preservation in other areas of cortex ➔.*

Neuronophagia

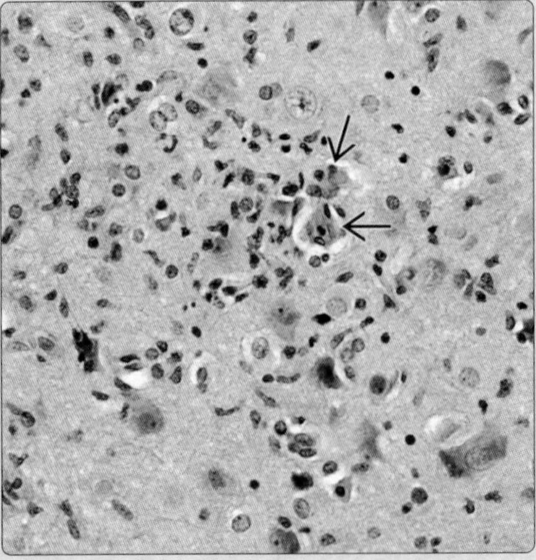

NeuN Showing Patchy Neuronal Loss

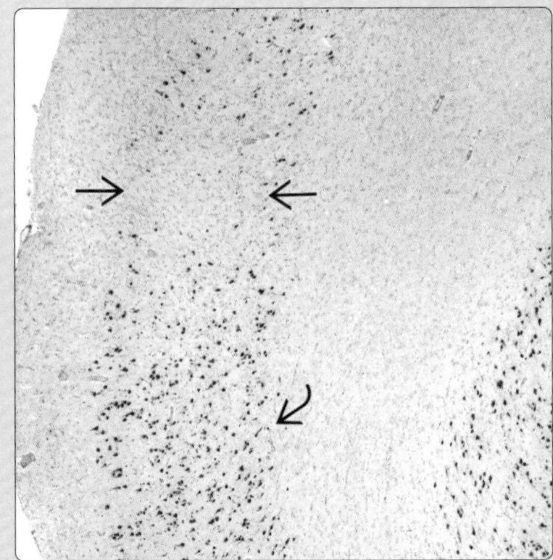

TERMINOLOGY

Abbreviations

- Rasmussen encephalitis (RE)

Definitions

- Rare, chronic, progressive, inflammatory, unilateral, epileptic brain disorder of uncertain etiology

ETIOLOGY/PATHOGENESIS

Infectious Agents

- No proven infectious etiology
  - Numerous studies inconclusive for viral etiology
    - Including polymerase chain reaction (PCR) studies
- By definition, serological cerebrospinal fluid (CSF) studies negative for neurotropic viruses such as herpes simplex 1 and 2, cytomegalovirus, and EBV
- Most similar to Russian spring-summer meningoencephalitis
  - Flavivirus infection confined to Siberia, transmitted by tick bites
  - RE diagnosis would be excluded by (+) antibody reaction against virus &/or brain biopsy showing viral inclusion bodies
  - No evidence RE caused by flavivirus infection

Sporadic

- No strong genetic component

Immune Pathogenesis

- Humoral autoimmunity linked to anti-GluR3 autoantibodies (Ab)
  - Anti-GluR3 Ab not present in all patients
    - Also found in other epilepsy types in comparable percent of patients
  - Antigen GluR3 is N-methyl-D-aspartate glutamate receptor
  - Testing done on both serum and cerebrospinal fluid
  - Subset of patients show autoantibodies to Munc18-1
    - 20% of patients
    - This subset shows B cells and plasma cells in resection material
- T cell-mediated cytotoxicity
  - Local immune response includes restricted T-cell populations
  - Granzyme B-mediated cytotoxic T-lymphocyte reaction targeting neurons and astrocytes, inducing apoptosis
- Focal seizures postulated to disrupt blood brain barrier (BBB)
  - Allow humoral compounds to reach neurons and cause damage
  - Vicious circle set up, with more damage leading to more focal seizures and focal BBB disruption
  - BBB disruption explains spread of neuronal damage from epicenter in frontotemporal/insular regions

CLINICAL ISSUES

Site

- Unilateral, cerebral hemisphere
- Frontotemporal and periinsular regions usually involved
  - Damage to unilateral cerebral hemisphere spreads from frontotemporal to occipital regions over time
  - Spread pattern correlates with march of the epileptic focus across the hemisphere
- Fewer patients present with occipital or parietal lobe involvement

Presentation

- Intractable focal epilepsy and slowly progressive unilateral neurological deficits
  - Hemiparesis, hemianopia, cognitive deterioration
  - Aphasia if dominant hemisphere is affected
- Childhood onset typical
  - Median age: 6 years
  - Normal development before onset of seizures
  - Adolescent and adult cases
    - More protracted, milder clinical course than in childhood onset cases
    - Fewer residual functional deficits; more frequent occipital lobe onset
    - Identical clinical, pathological features to childhood onset cases
- Epilepsy polymorphic in given patient, frequently occurs as epilepsia partialis continua, medically intractable
  - Simple partial motor seizures involving 1 side of body most common
    - Followed by secondarily generalized tonic-clonic seizures, complex partial seizures, postural seizures, and somatosensory seizures
  - Epilepsia partialis continua (EPC) seen in 56-91% of RE patients at some time during disease course
    - EPC not influenced by anticonvulsive drugs; no tendency to spread or stop after short time compared to other focal motor seizures
- Uveitis in subset of patients
  - Ipsilateral to involved cerebral hemisphere
  - May occur at any time during course of disease
- Clinical disorder occurs in 3 stages
  - Stage 1: Nonspecific prodromal stage
    - Relatively low seizure frequency, rarely mild hemiparesis
    - Median duration: 7 months (range: 0 months-8 years)
  - Stage 2: Acute stage
    - May be initial stage in up to 1/3 patients
    - Frequent seizures, often EPC
    - Neurological deterioration
    - Median duration 8 months (range: 4-8 months)
  - Stage 3: Residual stage
    - Many seizures but less frequent than in acute stage
    - Neurological deficits permanent and stable
    - Not all patients hemiplegic
    - Hemiparesis most useful marker of disease since most consistently identified deficit

Laboratory Tests

- No single diagnostic test
- Presence or absence of GluR3 autoantibodies should not be used to select or exclude treatment options
- In 1/2 of patients, CSF cell counts and protein levels in normal range
- Oligoclonal bands may be present in CSF

Treatment

- Surgical approaches
  - Surgery only cure for disease progression
  - Focal resections not effective
  - Full anatomic hemispherectomies used in past had higher morbidity, mortality
  - Current procedures involve functional hemispherectomy, hemidecortication, hemispherotomy
  - Timing of surgery controversial
    - Some advocate early in disease course
  - Timing of surgery dependent on dominance of hemisphere involved, weighing of surgery-related neurological deficits vs. seizure reduction
- Adjuvant therapy
  - Corticosteroids
    - Boluses for status epilepticus
  - Intravenous immunoglobulin (IVIG)
  - Plasmapheresis
  - Protein A IgG immunoadsorption
  - Tacrolimus
- Drugs
  - Antiepileptic drugs at all stages

Prognosis

- Immunotherapy used for patients with neurological deterioration
  - Immunomodulatory treatments slow but do not halt disease progression
    - Also do not change eventual outcome
- Surgical excision halts disease

IMAGING

MR Findings

- Serial MRs show progression of disease
- Most patients have unilateral enlargement of ventricular and subarachnoid CSF compartments by 4 months into disease
- Atrophy most accentuated in insular and periinsular regions
- Increased cortical &/or subcortical T2/FLAIR signal
- Atrophy of ipsilateral head of caudate nucleus in majority
- Spread of signal changes and atrophy within affected hemisphere over time
- Additional PET, SPECT, and magnetic resonance spectroscopy can confirm unihemispheric nature in early cases

MACROSCOPIC

General Features

- Cavitation and cortical destruction seen in late stages

MICROSCOPIC

Histologic Features

- Dependent on disease duration
- Earliest stages
  - Numerous microglial clusters ± neuronophagia, perivascular lymphocytes, or astrocytosis
- Early-intermediate stage
  - Microglial clusters, cuffs of perivascular lymphocytes
- Later intermediate stage
  - Neuronal loss, gliosis, abundant perivascular lymphocytes, fewer microglial clusters
- Late stage
  - No or few microglial clusters, mild perivascular inflammation, variable and sometimes segmental neuronal loss, gliosis, and rarefaction
- Dual pathology in minority of cases
  - Dual pathology usually nonballoon cell type focal cortical dysplasia, i.e., not focal cortisol dysplasia (FCD) type IIb
- No viral inclusions
  - IHC(-) for infectious agent

Cytologic Features

- Neurons show dysmorphism (i.e., cortical dysplasia) only in cases with dual pathology

ANCILLARY TESTS

Immunohistochemistry

- Lymphocytes predominantly CD3(+) T cells, mostly CD8(+) T suppressor cells
- CD68(+), Iba1(+), or HLA-DR(+) microglia predominate
  - Numerous parenchymal macrophages nearly exclude diagnosis
  - HLA-DR IHC may highlight more microglial cells than CD68
  - Iba1(+) microglial cells more numerous than in cortical dysplasia
- Newly described, uncommon subset of RE typified by CD20(+) B cells, CD138(+) plasma cells

DIFFERENTIAL DIAGNOSIS

Diagnosis Rests on Clinical, Electrophysiological, and Morphological Studies

- For most chronic patients with symptoms > 1 year duration
  - Few differential diagnoses exist
- In early cases, consensus criteria established to make diagnosis
  - Either all 3 of the following must be present
    - Focal seizures (± epilepsia partialis continua and unilateral cortical deficits)
    - Unihemispheric EEG slowing
    - Unihemispheric focal cortical atrophy and either gray or white matter T2/FLAIR hyperintense signal or hyperintense signal or atrophy of ipsilateral caudate head
  - Or, 2 of the following 3 must be present
    - Epilepsia partialis continua or progressive unilateral cortical deficits
    - Progressive unihemispheric focal cortical atrophy by MR
    - T cell-dominated encephalitis with activated microglial cells (typically, but not necessarily forming microglial nodules) and astrocytosis

Chronic Viral Encephalitides

- Virus identified by serology, viral inclusions, or IHC evidence of productive viral infection

Paraneoplastic Encephalitis

- Systemic tumor identified

- Most paraneoplastic encephalitis in children is due to opsoclonus-myoclonus in patients with neuroblastoma, not limbic encephalitis that would be confused with RE
- Positive paraneoplastic antibody panel (e.g., anti-Hu)
- Usually occurs in adults with lung cancer
    - Adults uncommonly develop RE

Gliomatosis Cerebri

- Cytologically atypical, infiltrating neoplastic cells
- Neoplastic astrocytes often in background of CD68(+) activated microglia, but neoplastic glial cells are CD68 immunonegative

DIAGNOSTIC CHECKLIST

Clinically Relevant Pathologic Features

- Not all RE cases require brain biopsy for diagnosis
- Brain biopsy can give false, nonspecific results in burnt-out cases
- Small (e.g., stereotactic) biopsies may not be diagnostic
    - Sampling error likely due to close juxtaposition of normal and abnormal tissues
- Open biopsy recommended, to include meninges, gray and white matter
- Biopsies should be taken from noneloquent areas with increased T2/FLAIR signal on MR
    - Can use PET or SPECT to determine favorable biopsy site if MR does not show clear lesions

Pathologic Interpretation Pearls

- Exclusionary histological features
    - Numerous parenchymal macrophages, granulomas
    - Numerous CD20(+) B cells
        - Exception: Cases with anti-Munc18-1
    - Prominent CD138(+) plasma cells
        - Exception: Cases with anti-Munc18-1
    - Viral inclusion bodies
    - IHC(+) for any virus
        - i.e., evidence of productive lytic viral infection
    - Tissue-based PCR may be positive for low copy level of virus but does not prove viral etiology
- Autoantibodies against Munc18-1 in 20% of patients with biopsy-proven RE
    - Subset with striking perivascular accentuated infiltration of B lymphocytes and plasma cells
- CD8(+) suppressor T cells predominate in all types of encephalitis, including paraneoplastic and RE
    - Subtyping of T cells is not specifically diagnostic for any type of encephalitis
- Do not mistake elongated individual tumor glial cells in gliomatosis cerebri for encephalitis
    - Gliomatosis cerebri should not have neuronophagia or tight microglial clusters
    - Neoplastic gliomatosis cerebri tumor cells often in background of CD68(+) activated microglia, but neoplastic glial cells are CD68 immunonegative
- Do not mistake elongated microglial cells or lymphocytes for gliomatosis cerebri tumor cells
    - Distinguish by CD68/CD3/CD45 immunohistochemistry

SELECTED REFERENCES

1. Casciato S et al: Epilepsy surgery in adult-onset Rasmussen's encephalitis: case series and review of the literature. Neurosurg Rev. 38(3):463-71, 2015
2. Owens GC et al: Evidence for the involvement of gamma delta T cells in the immune response in Rasmussen encephalitis. J Neuroinflammation. 12(1):134, 2015
3. Liu J et al: Evidence for mTOR pathway activation in a spectrum of epilepsy-associated pathologies. Acta Neuropathol Commun. 2:71, 2014
4. Varadkar S et al: Rasmussen's encephalitis: clinical features, pathobiology, and treatment advances. Lancet Neurol. 13(2):195-205, 2014
5. Irislimane M et al: Serial MR Imaging of adult-onset Rasmussen's encephalitis. Can J Neurol Sci. 38(1):141-2, 2011
6. Kashihara K et al: Twenty-one-year course of adult-onset Rasmussen's encephalitis and bilateral uveitis: case report. J Neurol Sci. 294(1-2):127-30, 2010
7. Muto A et al: Nationwide survey (incidence, clinical course, prognosis) of Rasmussen's encephalitis. Brain Dev. 32(6):445-53, 2010
8. Takei H et al: Dual pathology in Rasmussen's encephalitis: a study of seven cases and review of the literature. Neuropathology. 30(4):381-91, 2010
9. Schwab N et al: CD8+ T-cell clones dominate brain infiltrates in Rasmussen encephalitis and persist in the periphery. Brain. 132(Pt 5):1236-46, 2009
10. Wirenfeldt M et al: Increased activation of Iba1+ microglia in pediatric epilepsy patients with Rasmussen's encephalitis compared with cortical dysplasia and tuberous sclerosis complex. Neurobiol Dis. 34(3):432-40, 2009
11. Alvarez-Barón E et al: Autoantibodies to Munc18, cerebral plasma cells and B-lymphocytes in Rasmussen encephalitis. Epilepsy Res. 80(1):93-7, 2008
12. Gambardella A et al: Limited chronic focal encephalitis: another variant of Rasmussen syndrome? Neurology. 70(5):374-7, 2008
13. Basheer SN et al: Hemispheric surgery in children with refractory epilepsy: seizure outcome, complications, and adaptive function. Epilepsia. 48(1):133-40, 2007
14. Bauer J et al: Astrocytes are a specific immunological target in Rasmussen's encephalitis. Ann Neurol. 62(1):67-80, 2007
15. Bien CG et al: Slowly progressive hemiparesis in childhood as a consequence of Rasmussen encephalitis without or with delayed-onset seizures. Eur J Neurol. 14(4):387-90, 2007
16. Buenz EJ et al: Mechanisms of action of IVIG in adult onset Rasmussen's encephalitis. Can J Neurol Sci. 34(1):108-9, 2007
17. Villani F et al: Adult-onset Rasmussen's encephalitis: anatomical-electrographic-clinical features of 7 Italian cases. Epilepsia. 47 Suppl 5:41-6, 2006
18. Bien CG et al: Pathogenesis, diagnosis and treatment of Rasmussen encephalitis: a European consensus statement. Brain. 128(Pt 3):454-71, 2005
19. Bien CG et al: T-cells in human encephalitis. Neuromolecular Med. 7(3):243-53, 2005
20. Freeman JM: Rasmussen's syndrome: progressive autoimmune multi-focal encephalopathy. Pediatr Neurol. 32(5):295-9, 2005
21. Larionov S et al: MRI brain volumetry in Rasmussen encephalitis: the fate of affected and "unaffected" hemispheres. Neurology. 64(5):885-7, 2005
22. Bien CG et al: The natural history of Rasmussen's encephalitis. Brain. 125(Pt 8):1751-9, 2002
23. Mantegazza R et al: Antibodies against GluR3 peptides are not specific for Rasmussen's encephalitis but are also present in epilepsy patients with severe, early onset disease and intractable seizures. J Neuroimmunol. 131(1-2):179-85, 2002
24. Farrell MA et al: Chronic encephalitis associated with epilepsy: immunohistochemical and ultrastructural studies. Acta Neuropathol. 89(4):313-21, 1995
25. Vinters HV et al: Herpesviruses in chronic encephalitis associated with intractable childhood epilepsy. Hum Pathol. 24(8):871-9, 1993

(Left) *Early stages of RE are characterized by modest perivascular nonneoplastic lymphocytic cuffing* ⇨ *and microglial clusters* ➡. *These changes are indistinguishable from those of viral encephalitis, except for the absence of viral inclusion bodies.* **(Right)** *Microglial influx in RE takes the form of both microglial clusters (a.k.a. microglial stars)* ⇨ *and more subtle diffuse microglial influx by individual cells* ➡.

Early Stage DIsease Mimicking Viral Encephalitis

Microglial Clusters

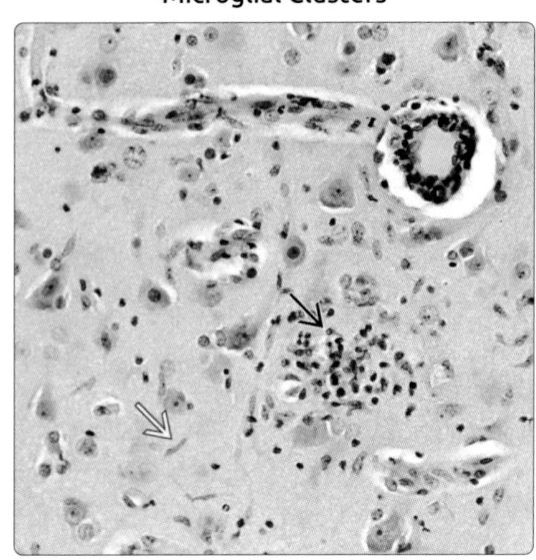

(Left) *Microglial cells* ⇨ *may be involved with neuronophagia in RE.* **(Right)** *Immunohistochemistry for CD68 highlights microglial cells that diffusely infiltrate the parenchyma* ➡. *Note the negative immunostaining for the small T lymphocytes* ⇨.

Neuronophagia

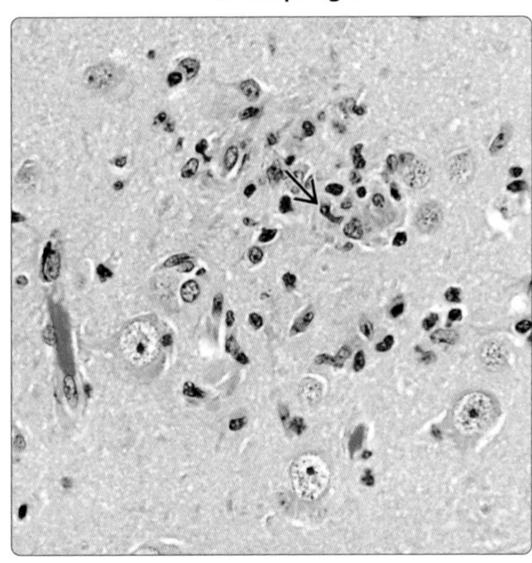

CD68 Highlights Diffuse Microgliosis

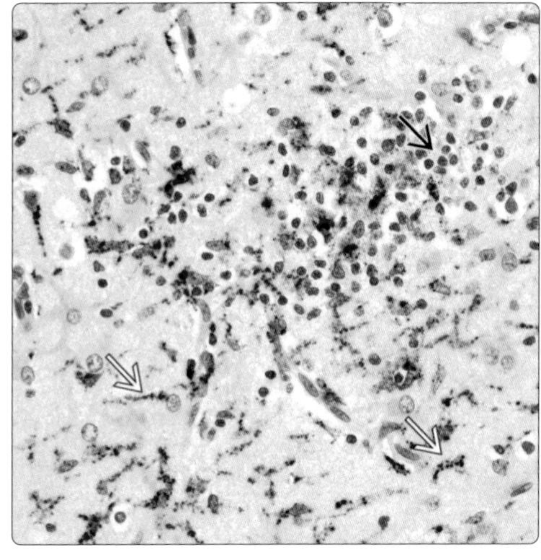

(Left) *T lymphocytes* ⇨ *are admixed with microglia* ➡, *supporting the hypothesis that a cytotoxic T-lymphocyte reaction targets neurons and astrocytes, inducing apoptosis.* **(Right)** *Immunohistochemistry for CD3 verifies that T lymphocytes in RE are present in the parenchyma, not just perivascular regions.*

T Lymphocytes

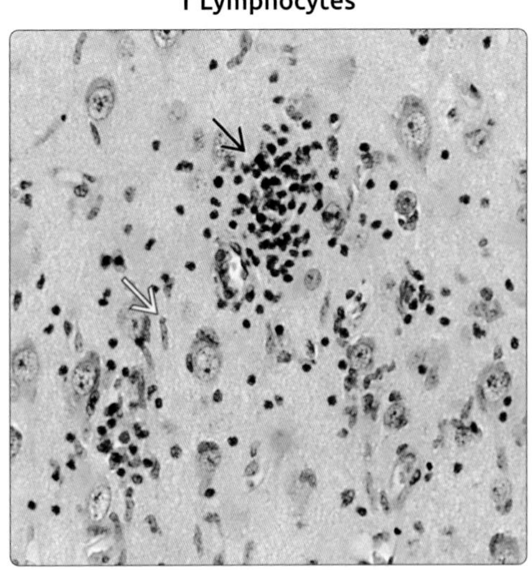

T Cells in Parenchyma

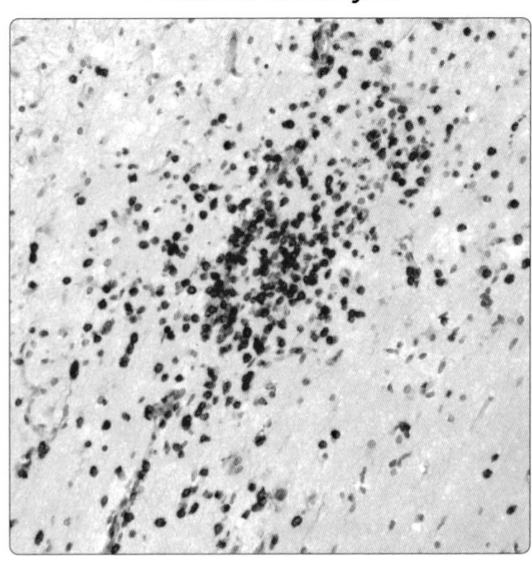

Elongate Microglia Simulating Gliomatosis Cerebri

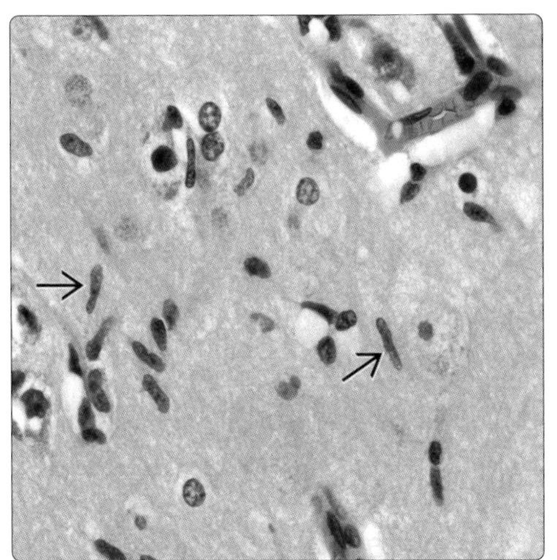

Diffuse Microglial Infiltrates

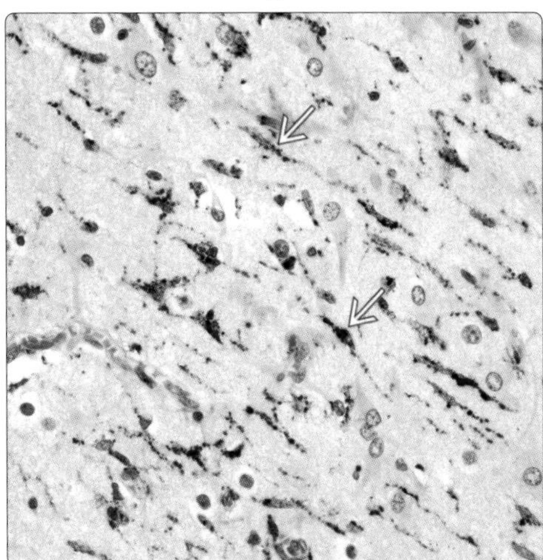

(Left) *Elongated microglial cells ⇒ should not be mistaken for infiltrating tumor astrocytes as in gliomatosis cerebri. Note the relatively uniform shape of the microglia as well as absence of hyperchromasia.* **(Right)** *CD68 IHC proves that the elongated cells individually permeating parenchyma are microglia ⇒ and not neoplastic astrocytes. Note, however, that gliomatosis cerebri can be accompanied by CD68(+) microgliosis as tumor infiltrates the brain. However, the tumor cells themselves are not CD68(+).*

Reactive Astrocytosis

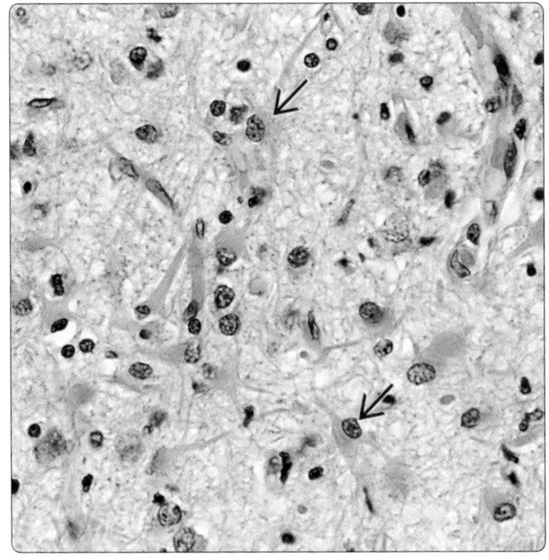

GFAP, Intense Gliosis

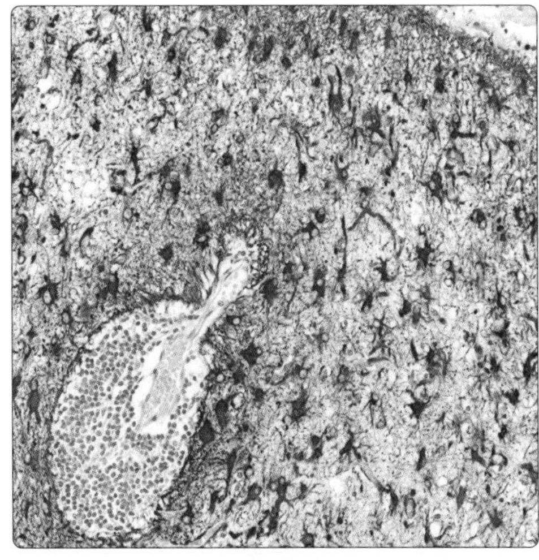

(Left) *Intense reactive astrocytosis with eosinophilic cytoplasm and stellate tapering processes ⇒ can be present in later stages of the disease when there is more pronounced neuronal loss.* **(Right)** *GFAP IHC underscores intense reactive astrocytosis in later stages of RE. Note the uniform distribution of the reactive astrocytes and long tapering processes. These features are typical of reactive, not neoplastic, astrocytic conditions. Note the intense perivascular lymphocytic cuffing.*

Rarefaction, Partial Cavitation

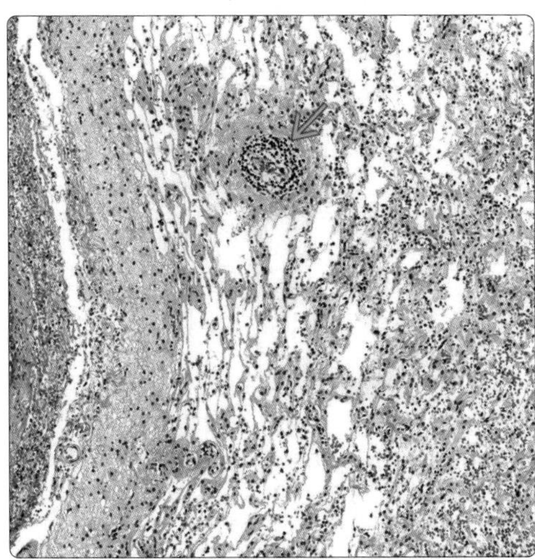

Severe Cortical Damage

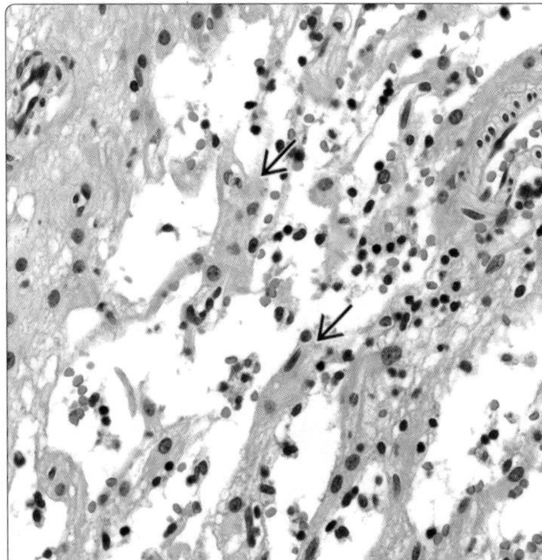

(Left) *Late stages of RE can have patchy, severe loss of neurons and parenchyma. Leptomeninges are at the left. Unlike an infarction, this tissue damage does not correspond to vascular territories of supply. Also note the perivascular lymphocytic cuffing ⇒, a relatively uncommon feature in remote infarctions.* **(Right)** *Severe cortical damage, with only strands of densely gliotic tissue ⇒ may remain in chronic lesions.*

KEY FACTS

TERMINOLOGY

- Rare neurological disorders developing in cancer patients, not attributable to CNS or PNS metastases

ETIOLOGY/PATHOGENESIS

- Autoimmune disorders
- Targets are onconeuronal antigens, proteins shared by tumor cells and nervous system

CLINICAL ISSUES

- Paraneoplastic disorders often precede detection of underlying cancer

IMAGING

- Limbic encephalitis: Abnormal hyperintensity in medial temporal lobes on T1-weighted scan
- Paraneoplastic cerebellar degeneration: MR often normal

MACROSCOPIC

- Normal to focal atrophy of limbic system, cerebellar cortex

MICROSCOPIC

- Lymphocytic, microglial infiltrates
- No viral inclusions, negative testing for infectious agents

ANCILLARY TESTS

- Must perform testing for onconeuronal antibodies in serum/cerebrospinal fluid

TOP DIFFERENTIAL DIAGNOSES

- Viral encephalitis
  - Negative for onconeural antibodies, usually shorter clinical duration
- Rasmussen encephalitis
  - Negative for onconeural antibodies; unilateral disease centered in fronto-temporal, insular regions; usually in children

Paraneoplastic Limbic Encephalitis

Cerebellar Paraneoplastic Encephalitis

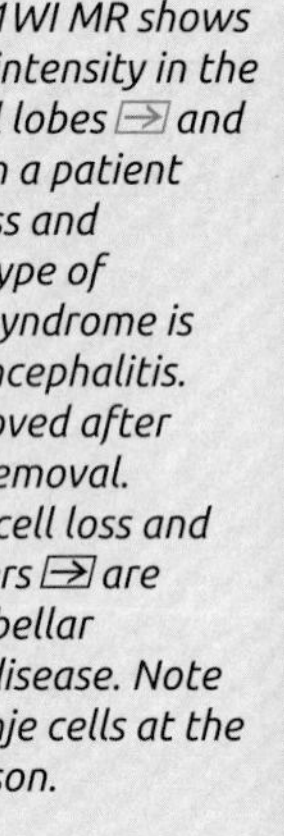

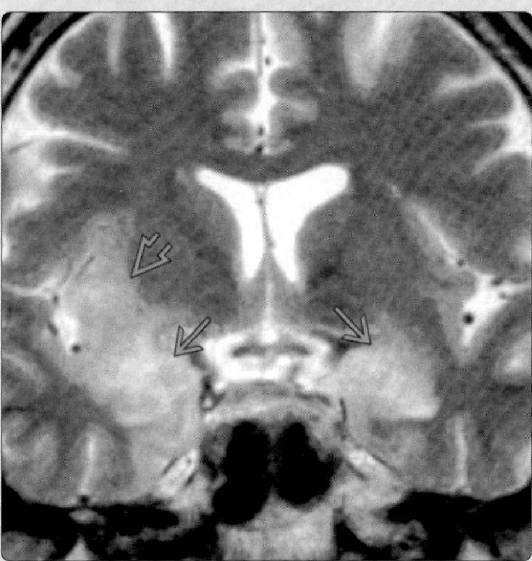

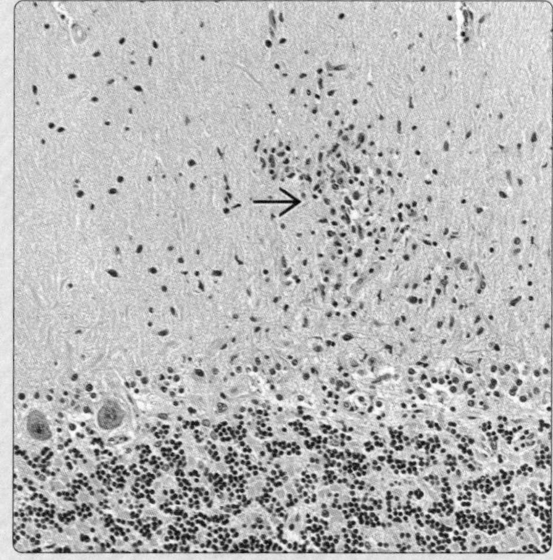

(Left) *Coronal T1WI MR shows abnormal hyperintensity in the medial temporal lobes → and right insula → in a patient with memory loss and dementia. This type of paraneoplastic syndrome is termed limbic encephalitis. Symptoms improved after primary tumor removal.* **(Right)** *Purkinje cell loss and microglial clusters → are common in cerebellar paraneoplastic disease. Note the intact Purkinje cells at the left for comparison.*

Microglial Clusters Characteristic but Not Specific

CD68 Highlights Microglial Influx

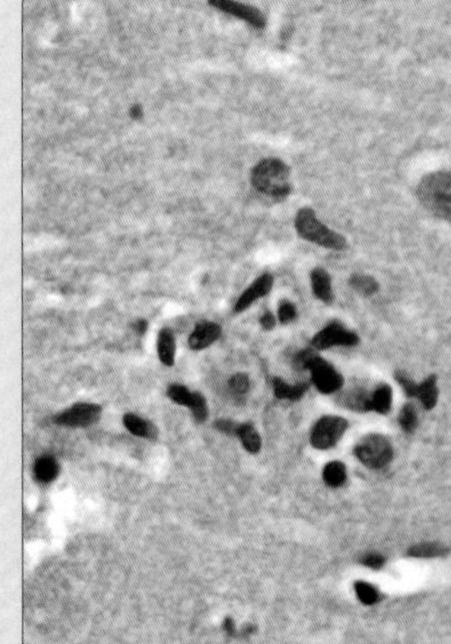

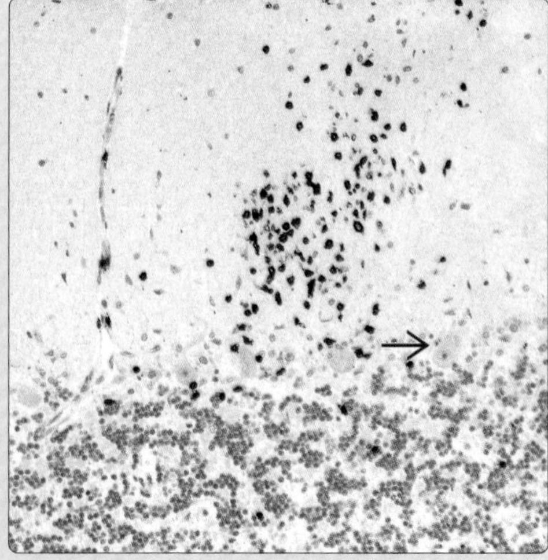

(Left) *Microglial clusters are characteristic in most types of paraneoplastic encephalomyelitis. However, they are not specific for paraneoplastic encephalitis and can also be found in viral encephalitis and Rasmussen encephalitis, the 2 chief disorders in the differential diagnosis.* **(Right)** *Immunostaining for CD68, or other microglial/macrophage markers, highlights the infiltrates. Purkinje cells → are preserved in this area of involved cerebellum.*

TERMINOLOGY

Definitions

- Neurological signs and symptoms associated with malignancy, which are not explained by direct tumor invasion, metastasis, or previous therapy

ETIOLOGY/PATHOGENESIS

Autoimmune

- Response to neural antigens ectopically expressed by tumor; immune attack directed at own CNS or PNS
- Contributions of cell-mediated vs. humoral-mediated nervous system damage differ among syndromes

CLINICAL ISSUES

Presentation

- Adult cases usually associated with small cell lung cancer, Hodgkin lymphoma, gynecological tumors (adenocarcinoma of breast, ovary), testicular cancer, or thymoma
  - Many CNS paraneoplastic syndromes T-cell mediated
  - Subacute sensory neuronopathy: Pain, sensory loss, and ataxia
  - Cerebellar degeneration: Subacute ataxia
  - Lambert–Eaton syndrome: Fatigable weakness, dysautonomia
  - Encephalomyelitis: Subacute confusion, brainstem signs, myelitis
  - Limbic encephalitis: Short-term memory loss, hallucination, psychiatric features
- Childhood opsoclonus-myoclonus associated with neuroblastoma
  - Mediated by receptor/ion channel autoantibodies
  - Opsoclonus-myoclonus ataxia: Eye-movement disorders, myoclonic jerks, and limb or gait ataxia
- Rare overall: Seen in < 0.01% of all cancer patients
  - Higher incidence in patients with thymoma, small cell lung cancer
- Paraneoplastic disorders often appear well in advance of cancer detection
  - Clinical diagnoses difficult, need high index of suspicion
  - Not all paraneoplastic disorders with positive onconeuronal antibodies in serum or cerebrospinal fluid (CSF)

Treatment

- Identify, eliminate underlying malignancy
- Immunomodulatory treatment when underlying tumor not identified
- Plasmapheresis, intravenous immunoglobulins may be effective in patients with receptor/ion channel autoantibodies

Prognosis

- Variable

IMAGING

MR Findings

- Limbic encephalitis: Abnormal hyperintensity in medial temporal lobes on T1-weighted scan
- Limbic encephalitis: Subtle patchy enhancement of medial temporal lobes, usually unilateral

MICROSCOPIC

Histologic Features

- Limbic encephalitis, cerebellar degeneration
  - Inflammatory infiltrates, perivascular CD4(+) T cells, B cells
  - Parenchymal CD8(+) T cells, microglia
  - Variable neuronal loss

ANCILLARY TESTS

Serum, CSF Onconeuronal Antibodies

- Immunoprecipitation assays most sensitive
- Paraneoplastic neurological syndromes present in 82% of cancer patients seropositive by immunoprecipitation
- Classic onconeuronal antibodies: Anti-Hu, Yo, Ma2, CRMP-5, amphiphysin, Ri
- Antibodies directed against cell-surface antigens: Anti-N-methyl D-aspartate, anti-voltage-gated potassium channel, anti-acetylcholine receptor

DIFFERENTIAL DIAGNOSIS

Viral Encephalitis

- Usually shorter clinical duration
- Symptoms of infection (e.g., meningitis, fever)
- Positive serological testing for virus &/or positive immunohistochemistry, culture in tissue
- Onconeuronal antibodies negative

Rasmussen Encephalitis

- Unilateral inflammatory disorder, classically in children
- Disease centered in fronto-temporal, insular regions
- Progressive seizures, neurological deficits, unilateral brain atrophy
- Onconeuronal antibodies negative

DIAGNOSTIC CHECKLIST

Clinically Relevant Pathologic Features

- Limbic encephalitis resembles direct viral infection of temporal lobes
- Need to put histological features together with clinical information and negative testing for infectious agents

Pathologic Interpretation Pearls

- Negative testing for onconeuronal antibodies does not rule out paraneoplastic syndrome

SELECTED REFERENCES

1. Ariño H et al: Paraneoplastic neurological syndromes and glutamic acid decarboxylase antibodies. JAMA Neurol. ePub, 2015
2. Berger B et al: "Non-classical" paraneoplastic neurological syndromes associated with well-characterized antineuronal antibodies as compared to "classical" syndromes - More frequent than expected. J Neurol Sci. 352(1-2):58-61, 2015
3. Storstein A et al: Onconeural antibodies: improved detection and clinical correlations. J Neuroimmunol. 232(1-2):166-70, 2011
4. Blaes F et al: Paraneoplastic neurological disorders. Expert Rev Neurother. 10(10):1559-68, 2010
5. Gozzard P et al: Which antibody and which cancer in which paraneoplastic syndromes? Pract Neurol. 10(5):260-70, 2010

Textiloma (Muslinoma, Gauzoma, Gossypiboma)

KEY FACTS

TERMINOLOGY

- Textiloma
  - Used for all resorbable and nonresorbable materials
- Gossypiboma
  - Used only for reaction to retained cotton

ETIOLOGY/PATHOGENESIS

- Localized tissue reaction surrounding retained surgical hemostatic material

MICROSCOPIC

- Foreign body giant cells
- Lymphoplasmacytic infiltrates
- Eosinophilic response to some materials, especially Avitene
- Histology of inert material varies depending on type
- Some retained hemostatic materials polarize; others do not
- Cotton
  - Linear fibers, extracellular or engulfed by giant cells
  - Polarizable
- Surgicel
  - Oxidized, knitted, polymer gauze
  - Macroscopically, piece of white mesh
  - Empty ghost fibers when degenerated
  - Nonpolarizable
- Gelfoam
  - Whipped foam
  - Basophilic spicules in smears and sections
  - Nonpolarizable

TOP DIFFERENTIAL DIAGNOSES

- Recurrent tumor
- Abscess
- Radiation necrosis

DIAGNOSTIC CHECKLIST

- Use polarized light to help identify cotton fibers

Textiloma Mimicking Recurrent Tumor

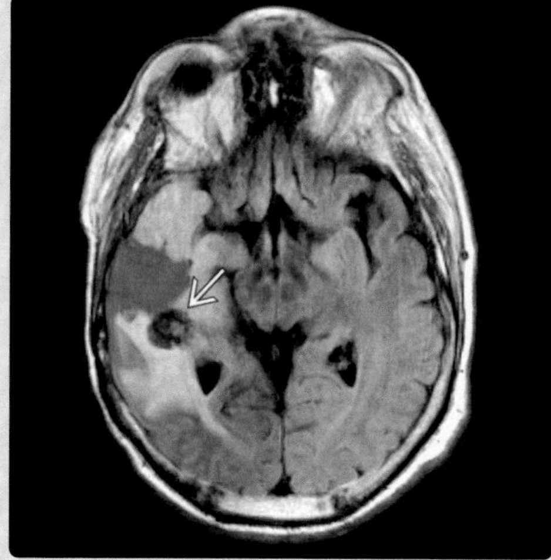

Cotton Ball Textiloma, Enhancement

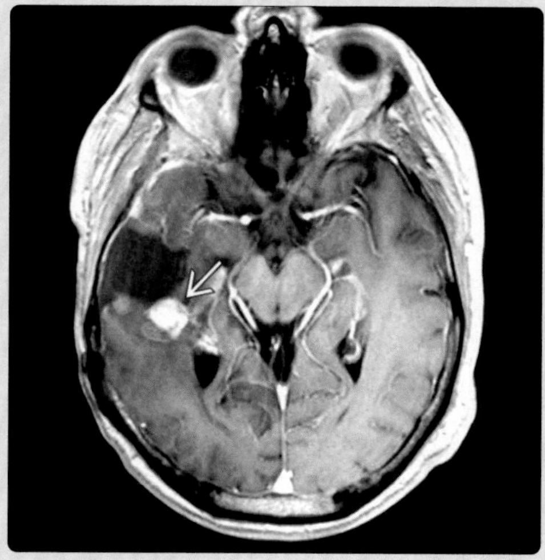

(Left) *A retained cotton ball textiloma ➔ can be misinterpreted as a residual or recurrent tumor, although the darkness of the lesion in a FLAIR would be unusual for a glioma.* **(Right)** *As textilomas, cotton balls may be enhancing ➔, but some are dark in postcontrast T1W images.*

Surgicel Granuloma

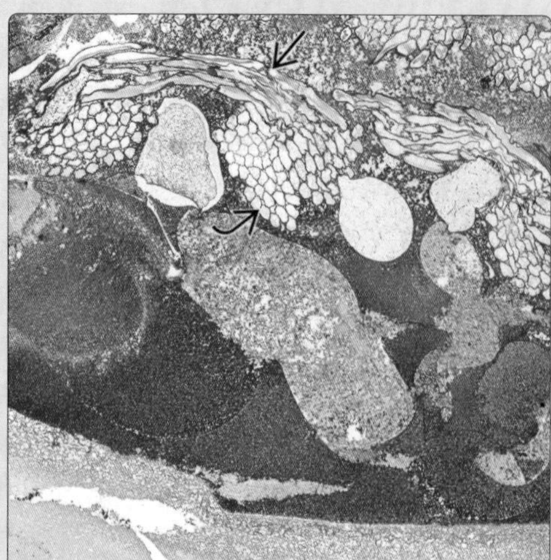

Avitene Granuloma, Eosinophils

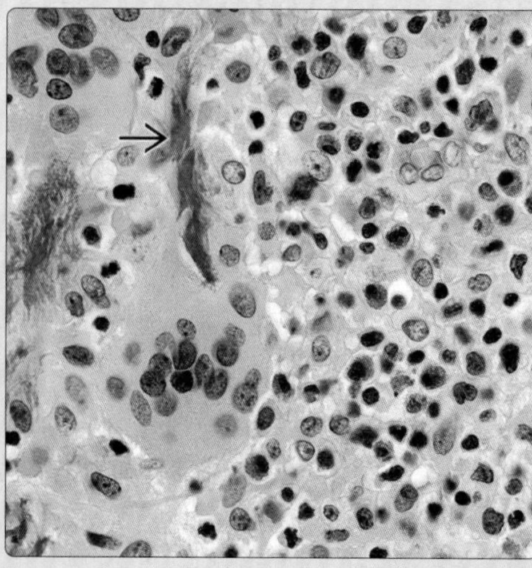

(Left) *Large amounts of Surgicel hemostatic material, seen in longitudinal ➔ and cross section ➔, fill the central cavity of this textiloma.* **(Right)** *Retained Avitene hemostatic material can elicit not only giant cell response, with engulfment of the foreign body material ➔, but prominent influx of eosinophils.*

TERMINOLOGY

Synonyms

- Gossypiboma, muslinoma, gauzoma

Definitions

- Retained, inflamed, foreign surgical material, used for hemostasis, resulting in symptomatic mass lesion
- Gossypiboma from Latin: *Gossypium* (genus of cotton plants), reaction to cotton fibers
- Pure use of terms gossypiboma, muslinoma, and gauzoma should refer to retained nonresorbable cotton materials
- Textiloma more broadly encompasses response to any surgical material, including resorbable materials

ETIOLOGY/PATHOGENESIS

Environmental Exposure

- CNS examples develop 1-7 months or longer after initial surgical resection; usually found on postoperative follow-up MR scans
- Nonresorbable hemostatic aids: Cotton, rayon (cottonoids and kites)
- Resorbable hemostatic aids: Gelfoam and Surgicel (both oxidized cellulose), Oxycel, Avitene (microfibrillar collagen), rayon

CLINICAL ISSUES

Epidemiology

- Incidence
  - Likely underestimated
  - Examples reported in 2004 review
    - 45 intracranial
    - 24 intra- or paraspinal
    - 24/24 intra- or paraspinal due to cotton from nonresorbable cotton swabs

Site

- Previous surgical resection bed

Presentation

- Symptoms similar to original tumor
- Asymptomatic neuroradiological finding

Treatment

- Surgical approaches
  - Resection

Prognosis

- Same as original neoplasm or condition for which hemostatic material employed
- No adverse effects after removal

IMAGING

MR Findings

- Cavity surrounded by ring enhancement
- Center of cotton ball sometimes dark in T2W/FLAIR images
- Center variably enhancing, some nonenhancing due to compact retained foreign material

MACROSCOPIC

General Features

- Surgically excised specimen may show central inert material

MICROSCOPIC

Histologic Features

- Foreign body giant cells and histiocytes, especially with cotton
- Chronic lymphoplasmacytic inflammation
- Intense gliosis &/or surrounding tumor
- Cotton fibers
  - Unstained with hematoxylin and eosin
  - Hollow
  - Bright with polarized light
- Surgicel
  - Solid fibers
  - No birefringence
- Oxycel
  - Hollow twisted tubules
  - No birefringence
- Gelfoam
  - Gelatin sponge
  - Branching spicule-like shapes
  - No birefringence
- Avitene
  - Microfibrillary collagen
  - Frayed strands of fibers
  - Birefringent

Cytologic Features

- Foreign body giant cells
- Macrophages
- Inert fiber material
  - Cotton: Hollow, intensely birefringent
- Lymphocytes, plasma cells; brisk eosinophil reaction with Avitene

DIFFERENTIAL DIAGNOSIS

Recurrent Tumor

- Neoplastic cells identified
- No retained foreign hemostatic material

Abscess

- No retained foreign hemostatic material
- Usually acute and chronic inflammation
- Infectious organism by culture or microscopy

Radiation Necrosis

- Amorphous necrosis with minimal inflammatory response
- Calcifications
- Vessels with fibrinoid vascular necrosis and hyalinization
- No retained foreign material

SELECTED REFERENCES

1. Ribalta T et al: Textiloma (gossypiboma) mimicking recurrent intracranial tumor. Arch Pathol Lab Med. 128(7):749-58, 2004

(Left) *Cotton fibers (here in a smear preparation from a textiloma) polarize intensely, whereas resorbable materials, such as Surgicel and Gelfoam, do not.* **(Right)** *The granulomatous, foreign body response to cotton fibers in a textiloma is well illustrated in a smear preparation, wherein a multinucleated cell responds to a cotton fiber →.*

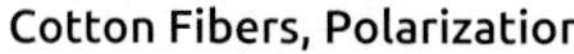

Cotton Fibers, Polarization

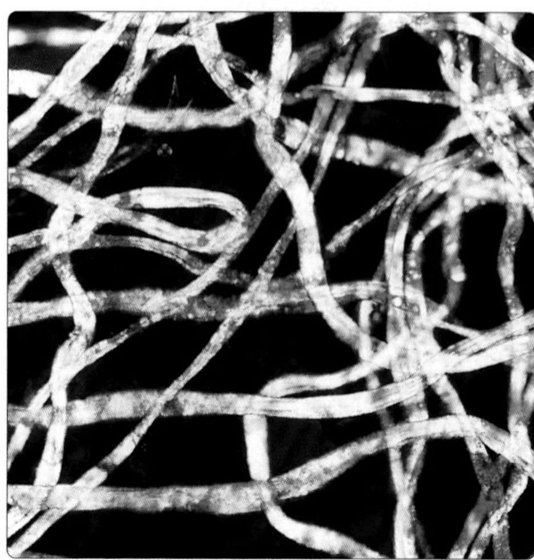

Smear, Multinucleated Giant Cells

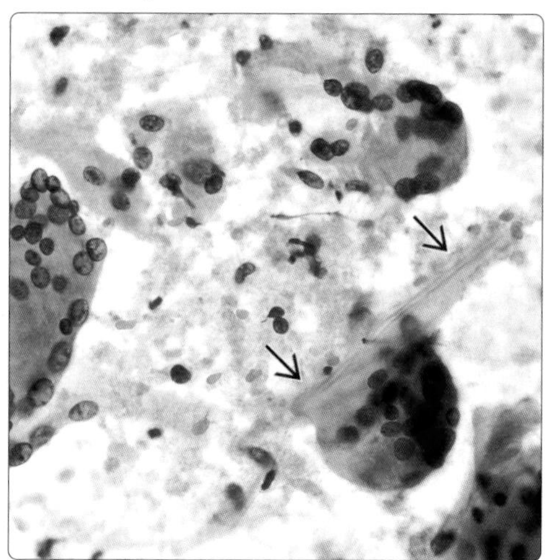

(Left) *A foreign body multinucleated giant cell engulfs gray cotton fibers. Combined, the cotton and inflammatory response form the mass of the textiloma.* **(Right)** *Cotton fibers may be overlooked in the absence of an inflammatory response in a gossypiboma. The hollow, gray fibers → are unstained in H&E sections.*

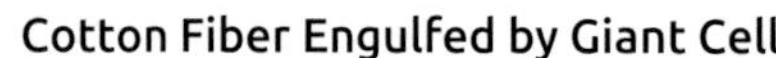

Cotton Fiber Engulfed by Giant Cell

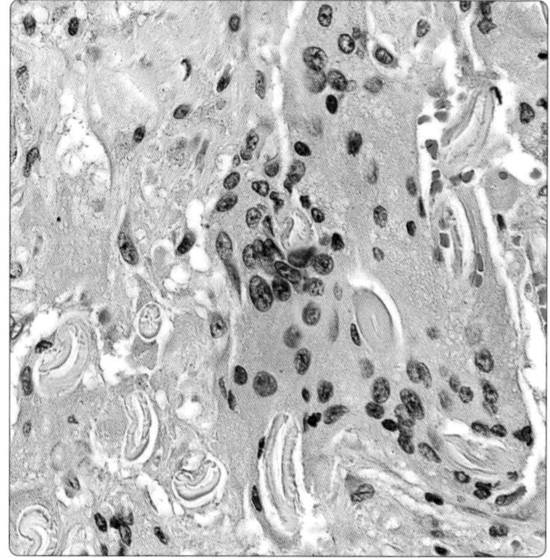

Cotton Fibers Mimicking Artifact

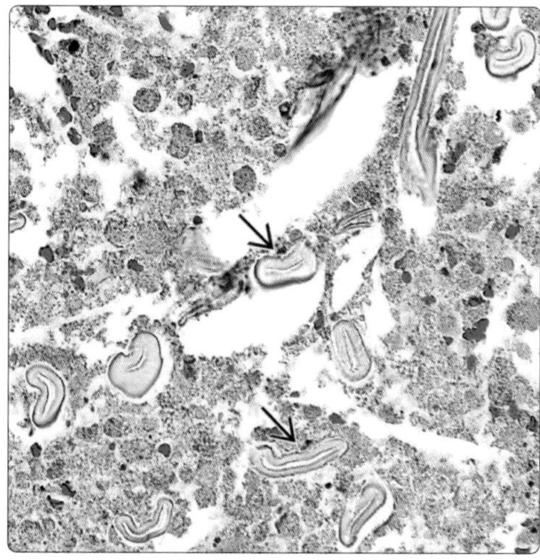

(Left) *Foreign body multinucleated giant cells in this gossypiboma contain opaque, nonstained, short cotton fibers →.* **(Right)** *Cotton fibers polarize after tissue processing in histological section as they do in smear preparations. The number of fibers in sections of a textiloma is often much greater than one might suspect. This can be seen by comparing polarized and nonpolarized images of the same section.*

Gray Cotton Fibers Engulfed by Giant Cells

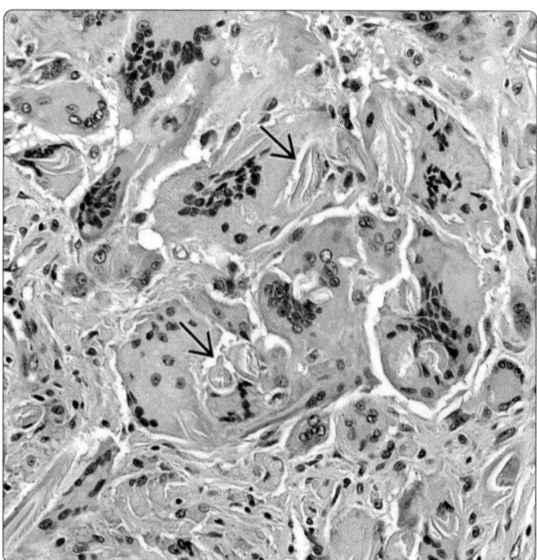

Cotton Fibers, Polarization

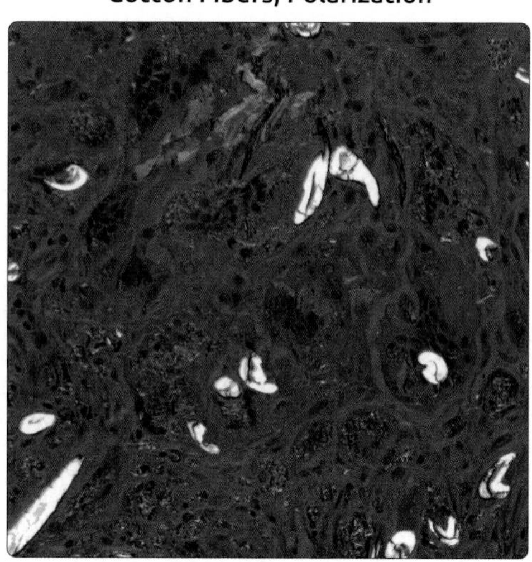

Gelfoam, Surgicel

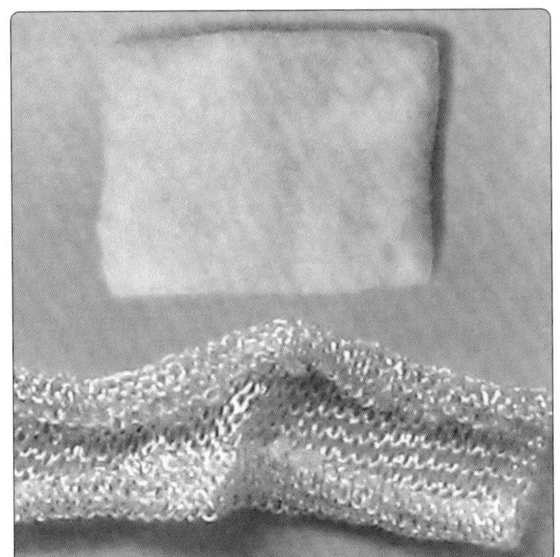

Gelfoam, Low-Power Magnification

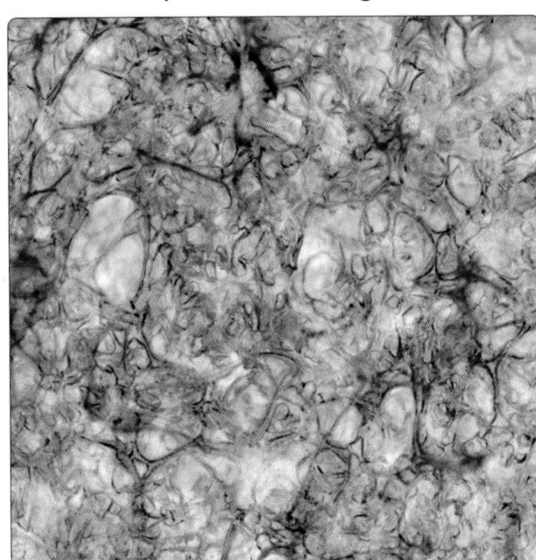

(Left) *The square, tan, sponge-like quality of Gelfoam (top) is to be compared to the silvery, woven, fabric-like meshwork of Surgicel (bottom). Both are resorbable materials sometimes responsible for textilomas.* **(Right)** *Microscopically on low-power magnification, amorphous Gelfoam has a spicule-like appearance quite different from than that of Surgicel, although both are oxidized cellulose.*

Gelfoam, in Tissue

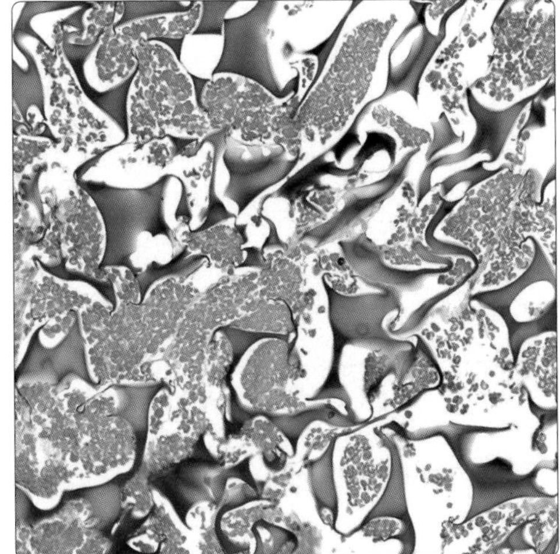

Gelfoam Spicules, in Tissue

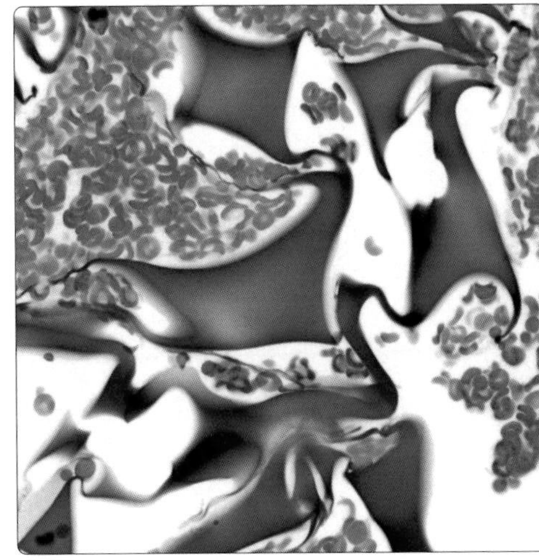

(Left) *Gelfoam is readily recognized in tissue sections by its distinctive purple, spicule-like, jigsaw shapes. Hemostatic agents are often interspersed with blood, reminding the pathologist of their use. Gelfoam is more common as an incidental finding than as the cause of a textiloma.* **(Right)** *Amorphous Gelfoam spicules, as seen here at high power, may be innocent incidental findings in patients reoperated for reasons other than a textiloma.*

Surgicel, Low-Power Magnification

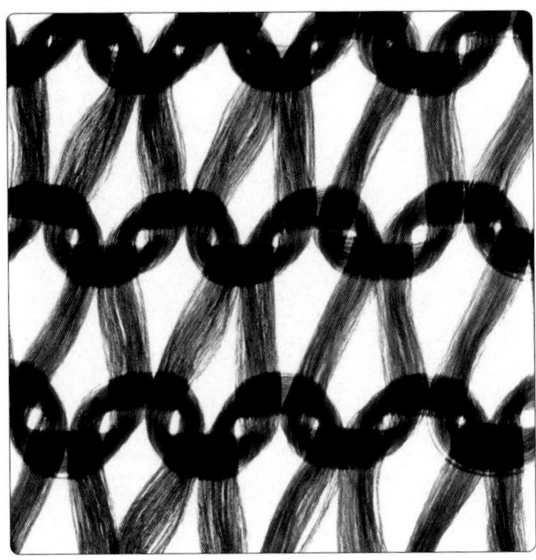

Surgicel, High-Power Magnification

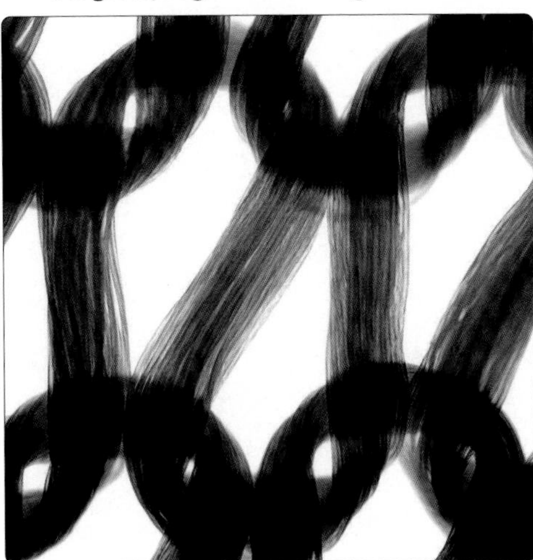

(Left) *Under low-power magnification, Surgicel is a beautifully uniform knitted meshwork.* **(Right)** *High magnification of Surgicel resolves the finely fibrillar makeup of this inert hemostatic material.*

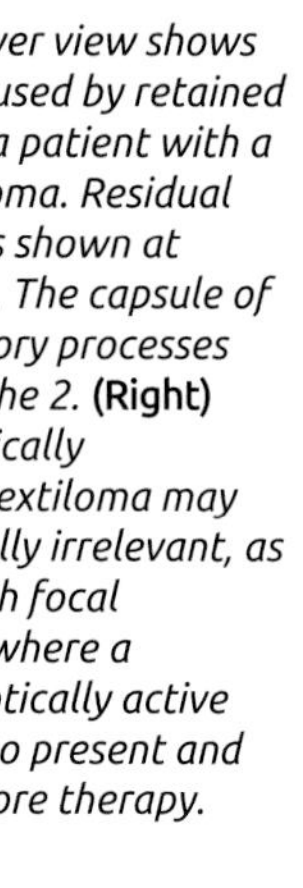

(Left) *Low-power view shows a textiloma caused by retained Surgicel* ⇒ *in a patient with a high-grade glioma. Residual glioblastoma is shown at lower right* ➡. *The capsule of the inflammatory processes* ➡ *separates the 2.* **(Right)** *While histologically interesting, a textiloma may be prognostically irrelevant, as in this case with focal glioblastoma, where a recurrent, mitotically active* ⇒ *tumor is also present and may require more therapy.*

Surgicel Granuloma, in Tissue

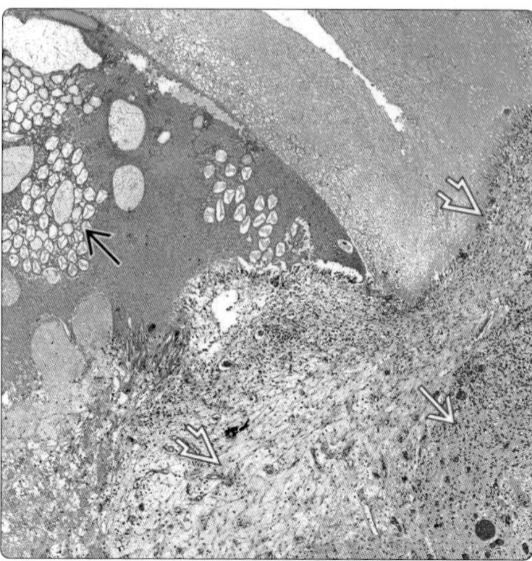

Residual Nearby Glioblastoma

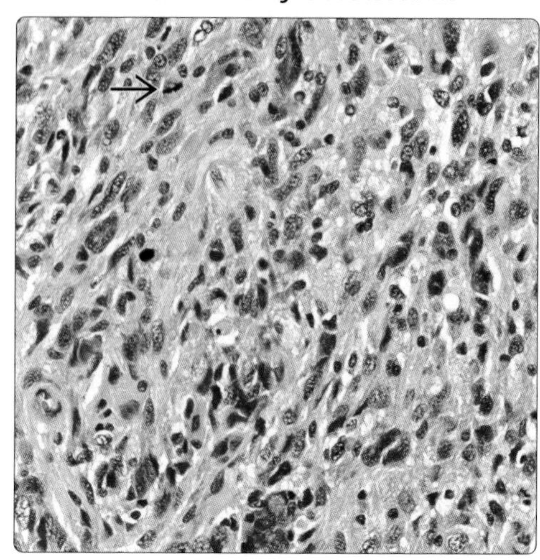

(Left) *Surgicel is composed of solid fibers and, in this area, unassociated with adjacent inflammatory cells. Well-preserved, nondegenerated Surgicel is seen here in cross* ⇒ *and longitudinal sections.* **(Right)** *Degenerating Surgicel fibers are hollow tubules, although the overall fiber-like arrangement is retained. Note the fibrinous protein threads/strands in the upper left.*

Surgicel, in Tissue

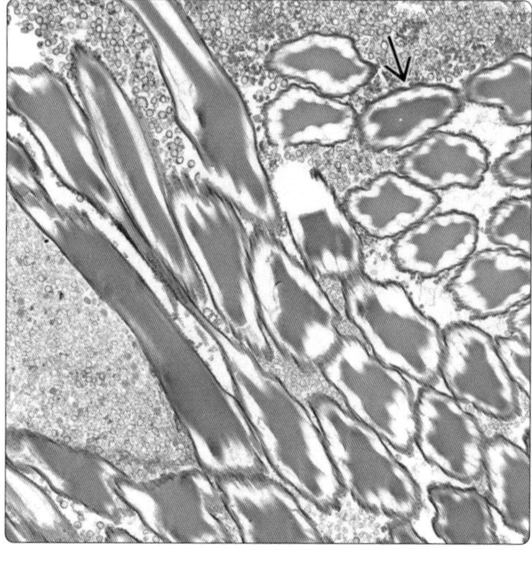

Surgicel Hollow Tubes in Tissue

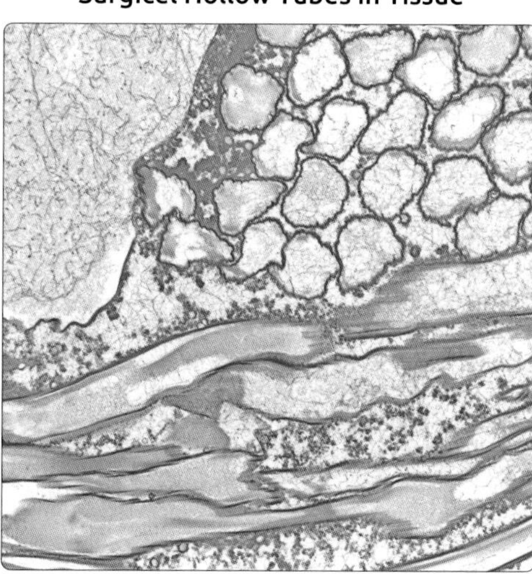

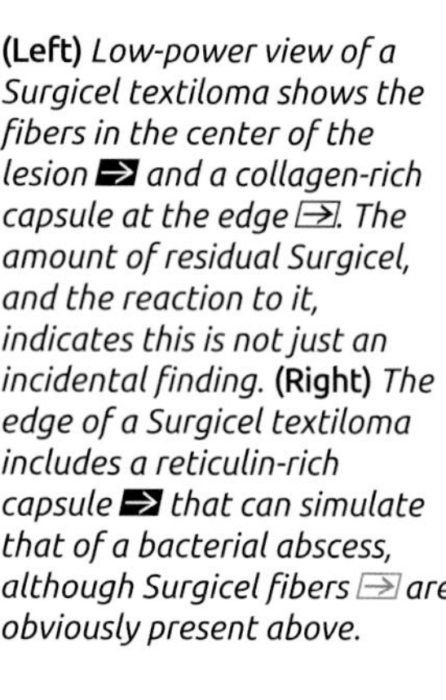

(Left) *Low-power view of a Surgicel textiloma shows the fibers in the center of the lesion* ➡ *and a collagen-rich capsule at the edge* ⇒. *The amount of residual Surgicel, and the reaction to it, indicates this is not just an incidental finding.* **(Right)** *The edge of a Surgicel textiloma includes a reticulin-rich capsule* ➡ *that can simulate that of a bacterial abscess, although Surgicel fibers* ⇒ *are obviously present above.*

Surgicel Textiloma, Abundant Residual Material

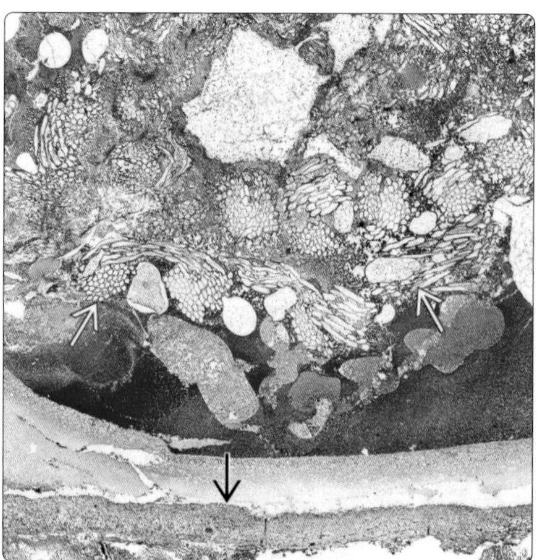

Reticulin-Rich Capsule

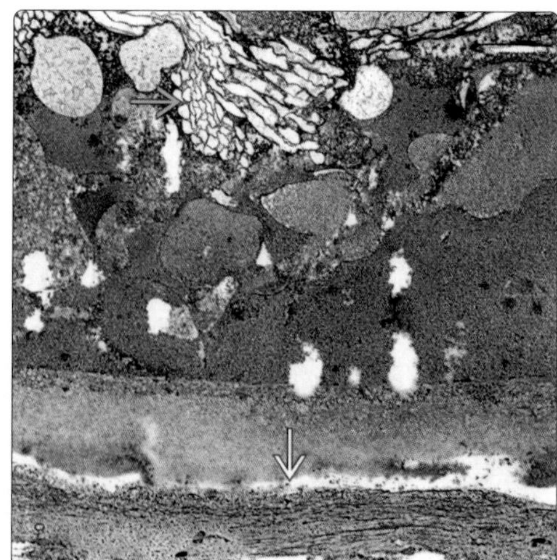

Peripheral Chronic Inflammation

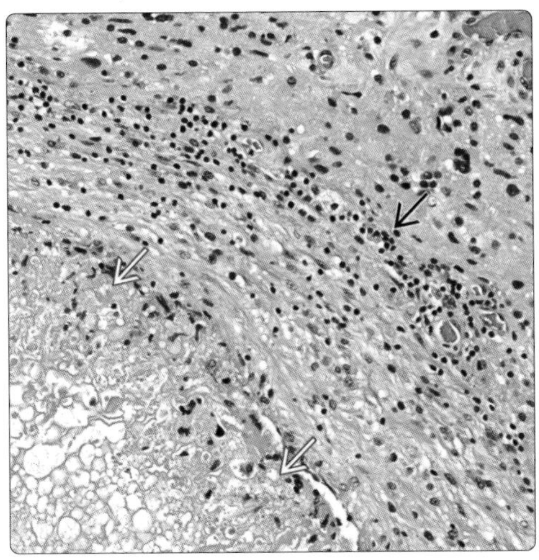

Simulating Granulomatous Infection

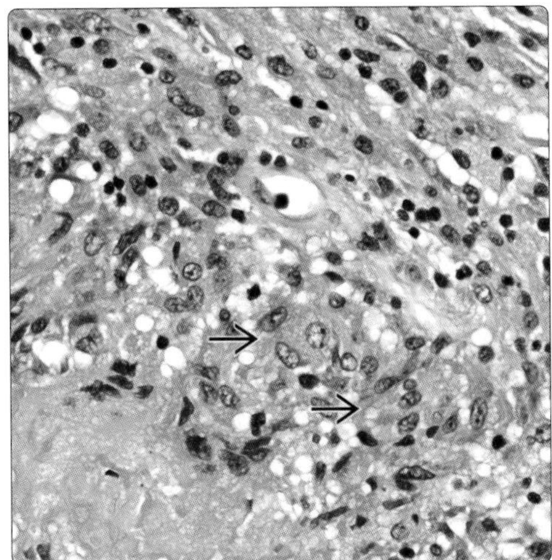

(Left) *The edge of a Surgicel textiloma has central amorphous debris ➔, a peripheral palisade of histiocytic nuclei, a fibrous capsule, and surrounding chronic inflammation ➔.* **(Right)** *This Surgicel textiloma contains epithelioid histiocytes ➔ that could suggest an infectious granulomatous process. Identification of residual Surgicel in central parts of the lesion is necessary for correct diagnosis. Surgicel is less likely to recruit eosinophils than other hemostatic materials, such as Avitene.*

Multinucleated Giant Cell

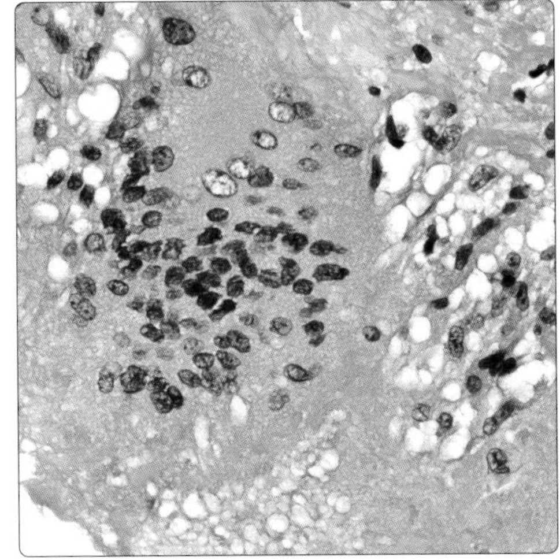

Avitene Granuloma

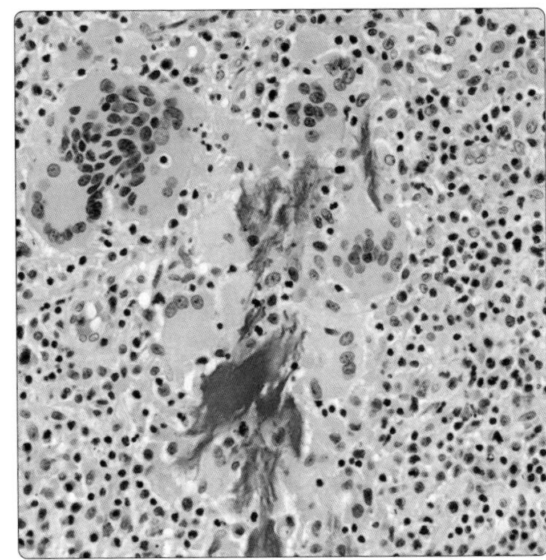

(Left) *Multinucleated giant cells may be part of the granulomatous response to Surgicel in a textiloma.* **(Right)** *The amorphous residual Avitene hemostatic material is surrounded, and sequestered, by multinucleated giant cells. Note the nearby eosinophils in the mixed inflammatory cell response.*

Comparison With Radiation Necrosis

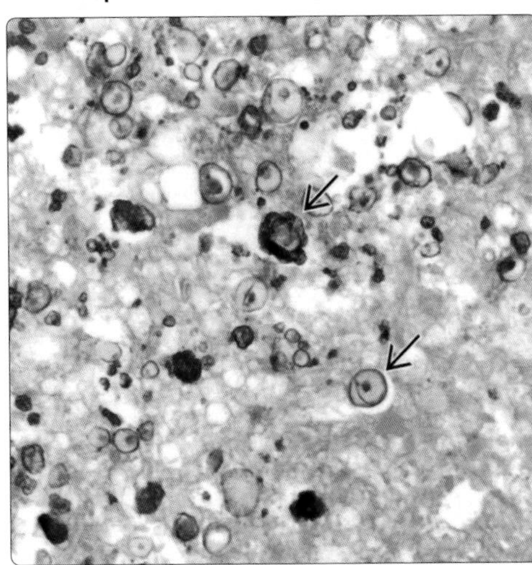

Comparison With Radiation Fibrinoid Necrosis

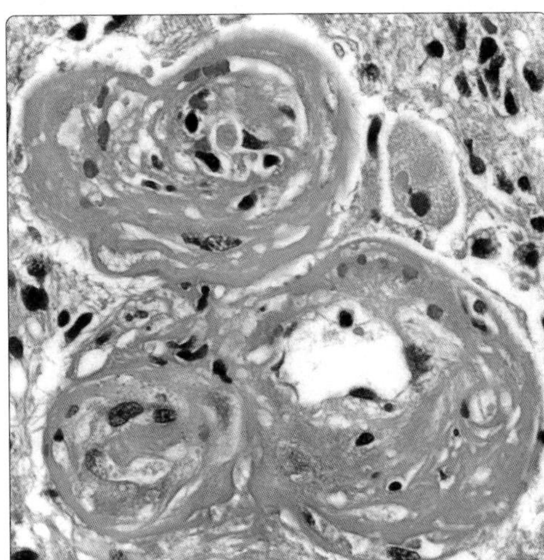

(Left) *Textilomas may simulate radiation necrosis by neuroimaging studies. Unlike textilomas, however, radiation necrosis often contains dystrophically calcified necrotic axons ➔, as shown here for comparison.* **(Right)** *Unlike textilomas, radiation injury often produces vascular fibrinoid necrosis, as shown here for comparison.*

Inflammatory Pseudotumors

KEY FACTS

ETIOLOGY/PATHOGENESIS

- Many patients with inflammatory pseudotumors (IPTs) have other concomitant systemic inflammatory diseases
- Some suggest that subacute systemic inflammatory state can predispose to locally exuberant inflammatory mass
- IgG4-associated IPTs have been reported in numerous sites

IMAGING

- Predilection for basal meninges
- Diffusely enhancing mass with focal area of meningeal thickening
- Occasionally displays peritumoral edema on T2-weighted or FLAIR images

MICROSCOPIC

- Prominent inflammatory infiltrate composed of lymphocytes and plasma cells
- Less prominent histiocytic, neutrophilic, and eosinophilic infiltrates, and Russell bodies
- Sclerotic, collagenous stroma

TOP DIFFERENTIAL DIAGNOSES

- Inflammatory myofibroblastic tumor
  - Perform ALK IHC, consider testing for clonal rearrangement of ALK receptor tyrosine kinase gene on Chr 2p23
- Meningioma, lymphoplasmacytic-rich type
  - Search for meningioma component by light microscopy, IHC
    - May be difficult to differentiate inflammatory pseudotumor from this type of meningioma
- Lymphoma
  - Should have cytological atypia, clonal tumor cell population
- Plasmacytomas
  - Should have cytological atypia, light chain restriction

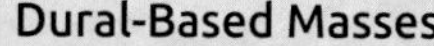

Dural-Based Masses

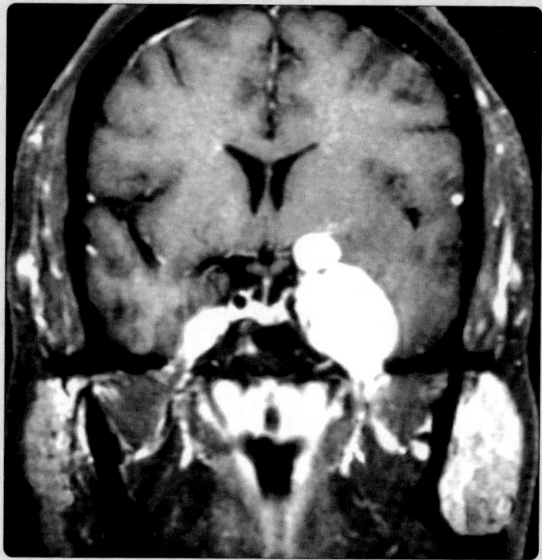

Prominent Histiocytes, Plasma Cells

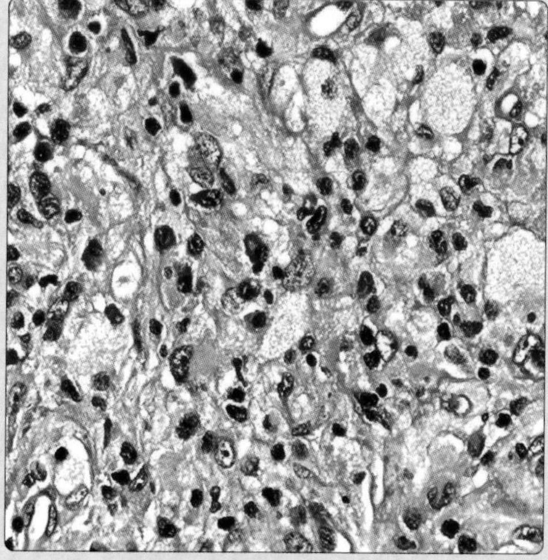

(Left) *Inflammatory pseudotumors (IPTs) are contrast-enhancing, typically dural-based masses with a predilection for the base of the brain.* **(Right)** *Prominent foamy histiocytes are seen in this inflammatory pseudotumor, along with a mixed lymphocytic and plasmacytic cell inflammatory infiltrate.*

Collagenous Stroma, Hyalinized Vessels

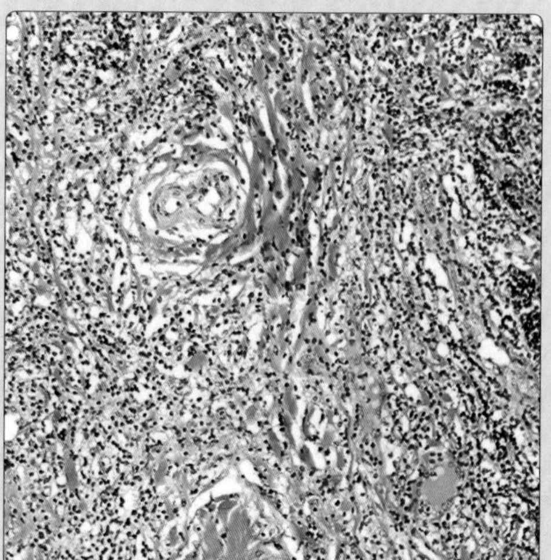

CD45, Mixed Infiltrates

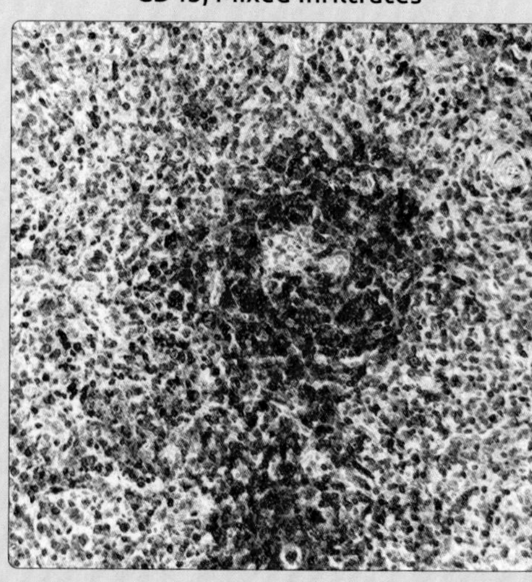

(Left) *IPTs demonstrate a mixed inflammatory infiltrate against a collagenous stroma and occasionally hyalinized vessels.* **(Right)** *Immunohistochemical studies of IPTs demonstrate the nature of the mixed infiltrate with most cells staining for CD45. Almost all are mature T cells.*

TERMINOLOGY

Abbreviations

- Inflammatory pseudotumor (IPT)

Synonyms

- Plasma cell granuloma

Definitions

- Not a specific diagnostic entity, includes diverse lesions
- Pseudoneoplasm composed of mixed, nongranulomatous inflammatory reaction
- Often contains fibrosis and granulation tissue
- True neoplasms, such as inflammatory myofibroblastic tumor, sometimes included in this category

ETIOLOGY/PATHOGENESIS

Infectious Agents

- EBV infection, in some cases
- Some suggest infectious etiology

Inflammatory Etiology

- Some patients with concomitant systemic inflammatory diseases
- Subacute systemic inflammatory states may predispose to locally exuberant inflammatory mass
- IgG4-associated IPTs occur in numerous sites

CLINICAL ISSUES

Presentation

- Fever, weight loss, and pain are frequent complaints
- Site determines symptoms and presentation
- Rarely asymptomatic

Treatment

- Surgical excision
- Rituximab, in some cases

IMAGING

MR Findings

- Iso- or hypointense mass on either T1W or T2W images
- Diffusely enhancing mass with focal meningeal thickening
- Occasionally perilesional edema on T2W or FLAIR images
- Predilection for basal meninges

CT Findings

- Enhancing, often dural-based mass

MICROSCOPIC

Histologic Features

- Prominent inflammatory infiltrate composed of lymphocytes and plasma cells
- Less prominent histiocytic, neutrophilic, and eosinophilic infiltrates and Russell bodies
- Variable number of spindle cells
- Sclerotic, collagenous stroma
- Rarely focally myxoid background
- No atypical lymphocytes
- No granulomas
- Focal vasculitis, some necrotizing in some cases
- IgG4-related lesions (hyper IgG4 disease)
    - Varying degrees of fibrosis and intense lymphoplasmacytic infiltrates
    - Scattered neutrophils, eosinophilic aggregates
    - Significant increase in IgG4(+) plasma cells
    - Majority of lymphocytes CD8(+) and CD4(+)
    - Small vessel vasculitis and obliterative arteritis, some cases

DIFFERENTIAL DIAGNOSIS

Inflammatory Myofibroblastic Tumor

- Neoplastic proliferation of fibroblasts or so-called myofibroblasts
- Clonal rearrangement of ALK receptor tyrosine kinase gene on Chr 2p23
- More closely related to inflammatory fibrosarcoma
- Spindle cells ALK(+)
- Nodular fasciitis-type is most commonly confused with IPT

Meningioma, Lymphoplasmacyte-Rich Subtype

- Occasional whorls and psammomatous calcifications
- Spindle cells often meningothelial
    - EMA(+) and PR(+)
- Distinction from meningeal hyperplasia in IPT difficult
    - Meningeal component small in IPT

Malignant Lymphoma

- Perivascular arrangement of malignant cells
- Numerous mitoses
- Atypical lymphocytes(+), CD20(+), CD79-a(+)
- Typically intraaxial
- Clonal tumor cell population

Plasmacytoma

- Light chain restriction
- Atypical plasma cells
- Limited number of inflammatory infiltrates
- Atypical/neoplastic cells CD138(+)

SELECTED REFERENCES

1. Schneider C et al: Primary intracranial plasma cell granuloma responsive to rituximab. Neurology. 83(12):1119-20, 2014
2. Nishino T et al: IgG4-related inflammatory pseudotumors mimicking multiple meningiomas. Jpn J Radiol. 31(6):405-7, 2013
3. Gandhi RH et al: Intraventricular inflammatory pseudotumor: report of two cases and review of the literature. Neuropathology. 31(4):446-54, 2011
4. Szabo B et al: Idiopathic orbital inflammatory pseudotumor: case report and review of the literature. Rom J Morphol Embryol. 52(3):927-30, 2011
5. Mauermann ML et al: Inflammatory pseudotumor of nerve: clinicopathological characteristics and a potential therapy. J Peripher Nerv Syst. 15(3):216-26, 2010
6. Gonzalez-Duarte A et al: Inflammatory pseudotumor associated with HIV, JCV, and immune reconstitution syndrome. Neurology. 72(3):289-90, 2009
7. Yamamoto H et al: Inflammatory myofibroblastic tumor versus IgG4-related sclerosing disease and inflammatory pseudotumor: a comparative clinicopathologic study. Am J Surg Pathol. 33(9):1330-40, 2009
8. Swain RS et al: Inflammatory myofibroblastic tumor of the central nervous system and its relationship to inflammatory pseudotumor. Hum Pathol. 39(3):410-9, 2008
9. Lee JH et al: Concomitant inflammatory pseudotumor of the temporal bone and lung: a case report. Ear Nose Throat J. 86(10):614-6, 2007
10. Wong S et al: Hypophysitis presented as inflammatory pseudotumor in immunoglobulin G4-related systemic disease. Hum Pathol. 38(11):1720-3, 2007

Lymphocytic Hypophysitis

KEY FACTS

TERMINOLOGY
- Rare, autoimmune, usually lymphocytic inflammatory disorder of pituitary gland leading to variable destruction, mass effect, and hormone deficiency
- Humoral autoimmunity also involved

ETIOLOGY/PATHOGENESIS
- May be associated with pregnancy, pre- or postpartum
- Increasingly recognized in males and nonpregnant females
- Drug-related with cytotoxic T-lymphocyte antigen 4 (CTLA4): Ipilimumab

CLINICAL ISSUES
- Headache, hormonal deficits, visual deficits
- Treatment: Steroids and hormone supplementation as needed

IMAGING
- Symmetrically enlarged, contrast-enhancing anterior pituitary gland
- May show signal abnormality in anterior lobe or, less often, in posterior lobe, infundibulum, or all 3

MICROSCOPIC
- T-cell lymphocytes in primary lymphocytic hypophysitis
- Histiocytes and multinucleated giant cells in granulomatous hypophysitis variant
- No organisms on special stain
- Xanthogranulomatous reaction/hypophysitis different entity than lymphocytic hypophysitis (LYH)

ANCILLARY TESTS
- Antipituitary antibodies often not positive or specific for lymphocytic hypophysitis; diagnosis rests on clinical suspicion &/or biopsy

TOP DIFFERENTIAL DIAGNOSES
- Germinoma
- Langerhans cell histiocytosis
- Sarcoidosis

Thickened Pituitary Stalk

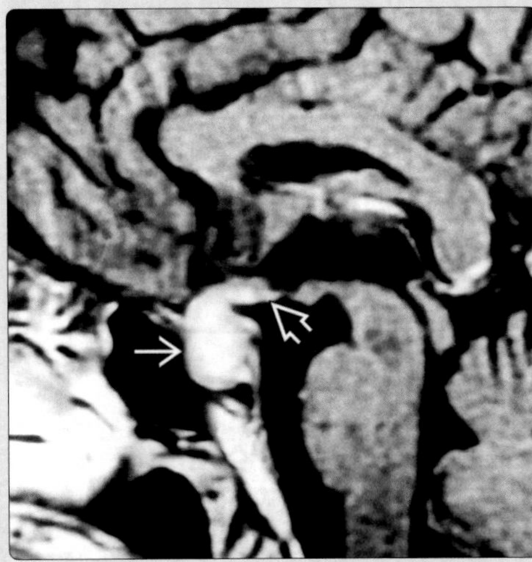

Involvement of Infundibulum and Anterior Lobe

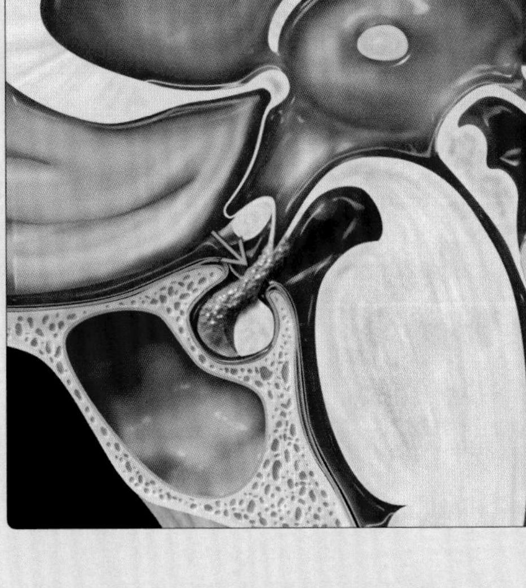

(Left) *Sagittal T1 C+ MR shows enlarged pituitary gland ➡ with thickened stalk ➡ extending upward to the median eminence of the hypothalamus.* **(Right)** *Sagittal graphic shows lymphocytic hypophysitis (LYH). Note the thickened infundibulum as well as infiltration into the anterior lobe of the pituitary gland ➡.*

Lymphoplasmacytic Infiltrates

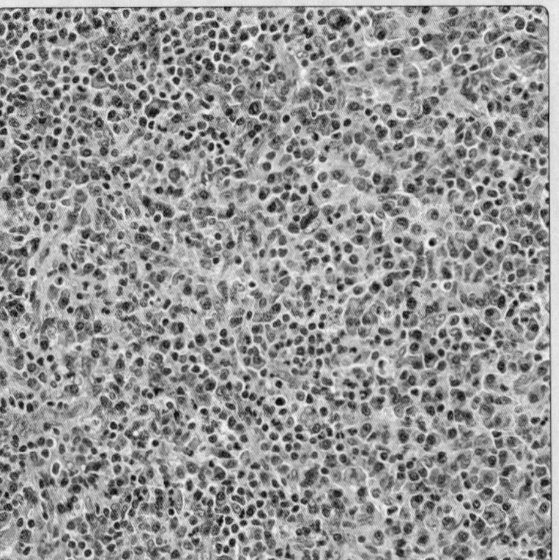

T Lymphocytes

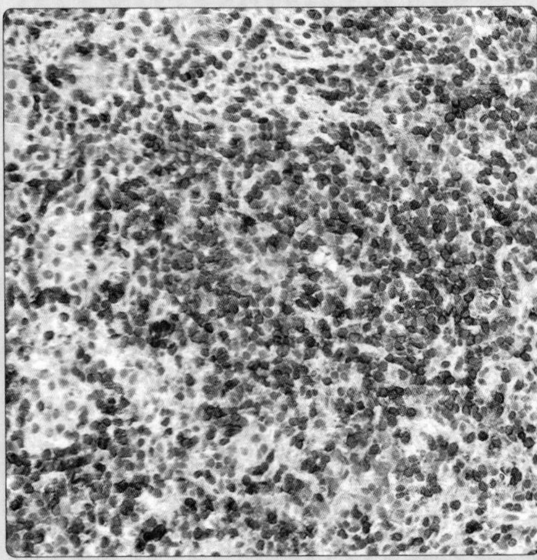

(Left) *Lymphoplasmacytic infiltrates in lymphocytic adenohypophysitis may obscure the underlying anterior lobe architecture.* **(Right)** *CD3(+) T cells in adenohypophysitis characterize primary LYH, an autoimmune disease.*

TERMINOLOGY

Abbreviations

- Lymphocytic hypophysitis (LYH)
  - Lymphocytic adenohypophysitis (LAH)
  - Lymphocytic infundibuloneurohypophysitis (LINH)

Definitions

- Rare, humoral, and lymphocytic inflammatory autoimmune disorder of pituitary gland leading to variable parenchymal destruction, hormonal deficits, and occasionally mild mass effects

ETIOLOGY/PATHOGENESIS

Lymphocytic Adenohypophysitis of Autoimmune or Presumed Autoimmune Origin

- Associated with pregnancy, pre- or postpartum in some cases
  - Gland may become more accessible to immune system during pregnancy due to changes in blood flow
  - Reestablishment of immune competence in late pregnancy/postpartum period
  - Antipituitary antibodies target α-enolase and coreact with both pituitary gland and placenta
- Associated with systemic autoimmune disorders
  - ~ 1/4 of patients with LAH have coexistent systemic inflammatory/autoimmune disease
  - Most common association is thyroiditis; thyroid peroxidase antibodies may be positive (e.g., Hashimoto disease)
  - Also described in polymyositis, type 1 diabetes, psoriasis

Nonlymphocytic Adenohypophysitis

- Granulomatous
  - Less frequent than primary lymphocytic hypophysitis
  - Possibly autoimmune
  - More equitably affects men and women
- Plasmacytic
  - IgG4-rich lymphocytic infiltrate
  - Associated with autoimmune disease, especially pancreatitis

CLINICAL ISSUES

Epidemiology

- Incidence
  - Rare
- Sex
  - LAH mainly affects females
    - 30-60% of female patients present in association with pregnancy
    - Usually occurs in last month of pregnancy or first 2 months postpartum
    - No adverse effect on fetus

Presentation

- Hypopituitarism
  - May be partial or total
  - Adrenocorticotrophic hormone (ACTH) deficits often earliest
  - Hormone deficits may be selective, e.g., ACTH, PRL
- Mass lesion simulating pituitary adenoma
  - Headache
  - Visual deficits
- Hyperprolactinemia due to stalk compression or release of hormone from tissue destruction
  - 1/3 of patients
- LINH (extensive disease variant) may be associated with diabetes insipidus
- Presumptive clinical diagnosis based on onset of hypopituitarism in late gestation or early postpartum period, hypopituitarism disproportionate to size of pituitary mass, and relatively rapid onset hypopituitarism

Treatment

- Replacement of deficient pituitary hormones
- Biopsy only
  - Surgical excision of too much pituitary tissue to be avoided except for patients with visual deterioration requiring decompression
- Steroids most effective in lymphocytic hypophysitis
  - Decreases pituitary size
  - Less effective in granulomatous hypophysitis
- Conservative management during pregnancy
- Rare examples treated by radiosurgery
- Drug-related hypophysitis [cytotoxic T-lymphocyte antigen 4 (CTLA4): Ipilimumab] usually requires steroid therapy only

Prognosis

- Excellent
- Pregnancy can occur after primary LAH, either spontaneously or with induction of ovulation
- No increased risk for developing LAH in subsequent pregnancies
- Subset of patients develop multiple endocrinopathies

IMAGING

MR Findings

- Contrast enhancement
- Enhancing dural tail (in some cases)
- Late stage, empty sella (in some cases)
- Pituitary enlargement with diffuse midline thickening of pituitary stalk
- Loss of neurohypophyseal bright spot

MACROSCOPIC

General Features

- Early phase nonspecific; chronic phase pale and firm

MICROSCOPIC

Histologic Features

- LAH
  - Inflammation predominantly or exclusively of anterior gland
  - Mainly T lymphocytes; B lymphocytes uncommon
  - Equal ratio of CD4(+) helper to CD8(+) suppressor T cells
  - High numbers of activated CD8(+) T cells especially seen in LYH presenting during pregnancy
  - T-cell lymphocytes characterization as helper vs. regulatory may differentiate subsets of LYH

- Varying anterior lobe destruction and fibrosis
- Reactive lymphoid follicles in some cases
- LINH
  - LAH does not usually involve neurohypophysis, but LINH involves both neuro- and adenohypophysis
- Granulomatous hypophysitis
  - Multinucleated giant cells, histiocytes
  - Variable numbers of plasma cells, lymphocytes
  - No necrosis
  - Infectious organisms lacking

ANCILLARY TESTS

Serologic Testing

- Antipituitary or hormone-specific antibodies in some
- Cerebrospinal fluid (CSF): Lymphoplasmacytic pleocytosis in some

Cytology

- Lymphocytes not atypical

DIFFERENTIAL DIAGNOSIS

Germinoma

- Large, PAS(+), CD117(+), and OCT4(+) tumor cells (may be sparse)
- Noncaseating granulomas (occasional)

Langerhans Cell Histiocytosis

- Langerhans cells, S100 protein (+), CD1a(+), langerin (+)
- Eosinophils

Pituitary Adenoma

- Monomorphic endocrine-appearing cells
- Usually no lymphocytic infiltrates
- Immunoexpression of ≥ 1 pituitary hormones, not all hormone types as in normal anterior lobe
- Disruption of normal acinar pattern (reticulin staining)
- Synaptophysin (+) (all pituitary adenomas positive, but normal anterior lobe cells also positive; inflammatory cells negative)

Pituitary Apoplexy

- Small, dark, anterior pituitary cells due to crush artifact, acute necrosis with karyolysis
- Crushed anterior pituitary cells immunoreactive for cytokeratin (CAM5.2), synaptophysin, negative for CD3

Lymphoma

- Cytologic atypia
- Immunohistochemistry, usually CD20(+)

Inflammatory Response to Ruptured Adamantinomatous Craniopharyngioma or Rathke Cleft Cyst

- Xanthogranulomatous reaction (xanthogranulomatous, xanthomatous hypophysitis)
  - Cholesterol clefts with foreign body reaction
  - Lipid-rich foamy histiocytes
  - Smaller numbers of lymphocytes, plasma cells, occasionally eosinophils
  - Wet keratin (when associated with craniopharyngioma)
  - Hemosiderin
  - Fibrosis
  - Epithelium (may be absent or focal feature)

Bacterial Infections

- Pyogenic: Organisms by stain &/or culture
- Mycobacterial: Organisms by stain &/or culture

Sarcoidosis

- Overlaps with granulomatous hypophysitis
- Centered on neurohypophysis/stalk
- More discrete, often hyalinizing, noncaseating granulomas

DIAGNOSTIC CHECKLIST

Clinically Relevant Pathologic Features

- Hypophysitis may not be suspected clinically; diagnosis may be made by pathologist
  - Intraoperative diagnosis of hypophysitis critical to avoid excessive resection of presumed adenoma or craniopharyngioma

Pathologic Interpretation Pearls

- Crushed anterior pituitary cells can simulate lymphocytes or small cell carcinoma
- Prolactinoma treated with dopamine agonist may show severe cytoplasmic reduction in adenoma cells, resemble lymphocytes

SELECTED REFERENCES

1. Faje A: Immunotherapy and hypophysitis: clinical presentation, treatment, and biologic insights. Pituitary. ePub, 2015
2. Hunn BH et al: Idiopathic granulomatous hypophysitis: a systematic review of 82 cases in the literature. Pituitary. 17(4):357-65, 2014
3. Imber BS et al: Hypophysitis: a single-center case series. Pituitary. ePub, 2014
4. Kleinschmidt-DeMasters BK et al: Update on hypophysitis and TTF-1 expressing sellar region masses. Brain Pathol. 23(5):495-514, 2013
5. Karaca Z et al: Pregnancy and pituitary disorders. Eur J Endocrinol. 162(3):453-75, 2010
6. Rumana M et al: Lymphocytic hypophysitis with normal pituitary function mimicking a pituitary adenoma: a case report and review of literature. Clin Neuropathol. 29(1):26-31, 2010
7. Carpinteri R et al: Pituitary tumours: inflammatory and granulomatous expansive lesions of the pituitary. Best Pract Res Clin Endocrinol Metab. 23(5):639-50, 2009
8. Gonzalez-Cuyar LF et al: Sudden unexpected death in lymphocytic hypophysitis. Am J Forensic Med Pathol. 30(1):61-3, 2009
9. Janeczko C et al: Hypophysitis secondary to ruptured Rathke's cyst mimicking neurosarcoidosis. J Clin Neurosci. 16(4):599-600, 2009
10. Karaca Z et al: Empty sella may be the final outcome in lymphocytic hypophysitis. Endocr Res. 34(1-2):10-7, 2009
11. Abe T: Lymphocytic infundibulo-neurohypophysitis and infundibulo-panhypophysitis regarded as lymphocytic hypophysitis variant. Brain Tumor Pathol. 25(2):59-66, 2008
12. Gellner V et al: Lymphocytic hypophysitis in the pediatric population. Childs Nerv Syst. 24(7):785-92, 2008
13. Murakami M et al: Granulomatous hypophysistis associated with rathke's cleft cyst: a case report. Minim Invasive Neurosurg. 51(3):169-72, 2008
14. Molitch ME et al: Lymphocytic hypophysitis. Horm Res. 68 Suppl 5:145-50, 2007
15. Gutenberg A et al: Primary hypophysitis: clinical-pathological correlations. Eur J Endocrinol. 155(1):101-7, 2006
16. Rivera JA: Lymphocytic hypophysitis: disease spectrum and approach to diagnosis and therapy. Pituitary. 9(1):35-45, 2006
17. Caturegli P et al: Autoimmune hypophysitis. Endocr Rev. 26(5):599-614, 2005
18. Gutenberg A et al: Immunopathology of primary hypophysitis: implications for pathogenesis. Am J Surg Pathol. 29(3):329-38, 2005
19. Leung GK et al: Primary hypophysitis: a single-center experience in 16 cases. J Neurosurg. 101(2):262-71, 2004

Recognizable Acinar Pattern, Normal Cell Types

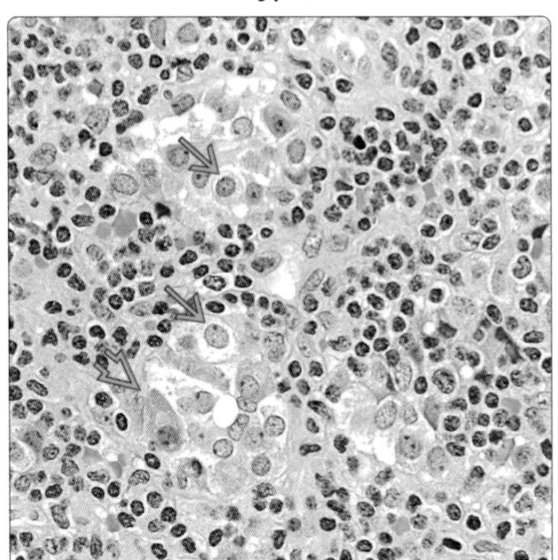

Reticulin Stain Reveals Preserved Acini

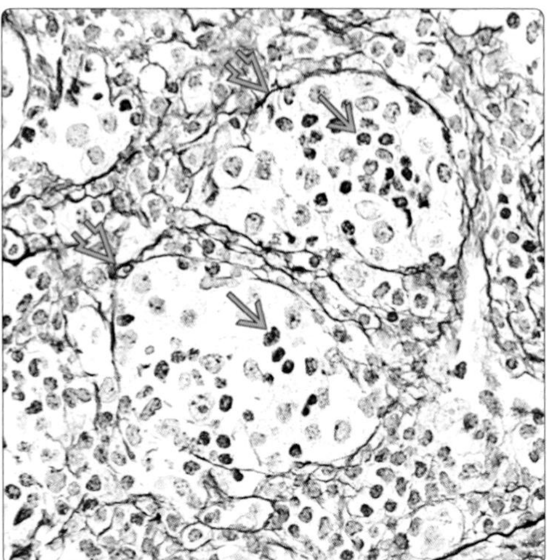

(Left) *In lymphocytic adenohypophysitis (LAH), the anterior pituitary maintains its normal, nested acinar pattern with the expected admixture of acidophils ⇒, basophils, and chromophobes →. As is typical, intraacinar lymphocytes appear to attack acinar cells.* **(Right)** *Reticulin staining helps identify acini ⇒. The acinar pattern would be lost in a pituitary adenoma. Intraacinar lymphocytes are present →.*

Anterior Pituitary Cells Difficult to Find

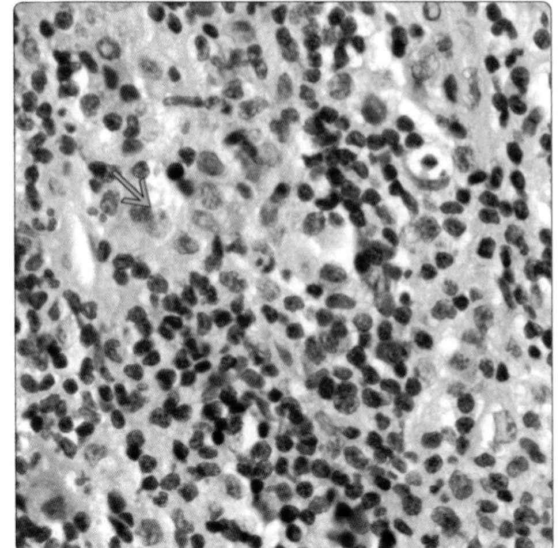

Completely Obscured Architecture

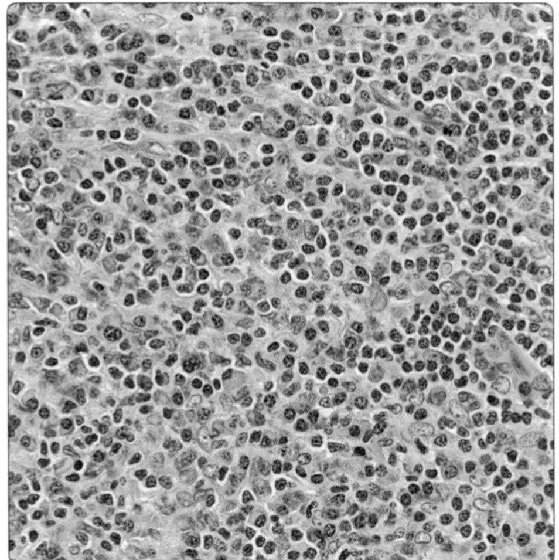

(Left) *Pale-staining adenohypophyseal cells → may be difficult to distinguish from histiocytes by H&E staining.* **(Right)** *LAH is typified by numerous, infiltrating, cytologically benign lymphocytes and plasma cells overrunning the gland. Few, if any, adenohypophysial cells may be seen in maximally affected areas.*

Predominantly T Cells

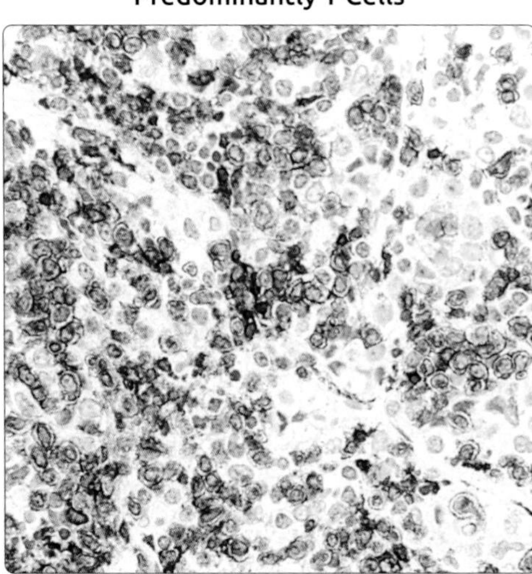

Focal Plasma Cells

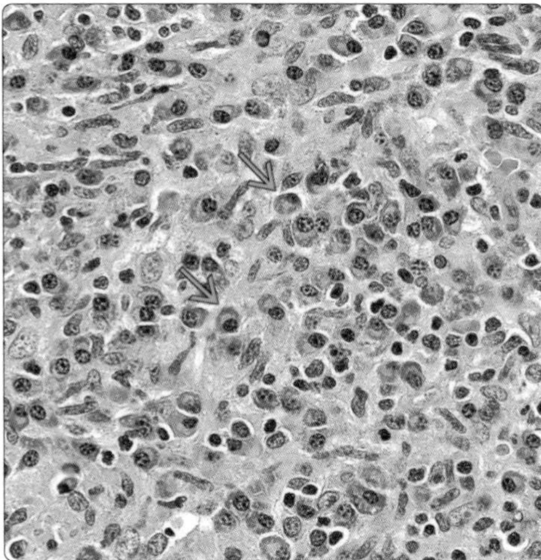

(Left) *Small CD3 immunoreactive T lymphocytes predominate in an adenohypophyseal infiltrate in which CD20(+) B cells are uncommon.* **(Right)** *While the lesion is predominantly lymphocytic, plasma cells → may be focally prominent.*

KEY FACTS

TERMINOLOGY

- Rosai-Dorfman disease (RDD): Sinus histiocytosis with massive lymphadenopathy
- May be only in CNS at presentation

ETIOLOGY/PATHOGENESIS

- No known etiology; no infectious cause known

CLINICAL ISSUES

- Benign condition
- Usually curable by surgery alone

IMAGING

- Most CNS cases dural-based mass(es)
- Often involves both sides of dura
- Mimics meningioma(s)

MACROSCOPIC

- Dural mass
- Mimics meningioma

MICROSCOPIC

- Fibrosis: May obscure histiocytes
- Histiocytic infiltrates
- Emperipolesis, but absence does not exclude diagnosis of RDD
- No tight granulomas
- Eosinophils inconspicuous
- RDD histiocytes with round nuclei, no longitudinal nuclear grooves
- RDD histiocytes S100(+), CD1a(-)

ANCILLARY TESTS

- Unlike many cases of Erdheim-Chester disease and Langerhans cell histiocytosis, RDD usually negative for BRAF VE1 (paralleling absence of *BRAF V600E* mutation)

(Left) *Coronal T1-weighted contrast-enhanced MR shows multiple, homogeneously enhancing, dural-based masses in a patient with known sinus histiocytosis with massive lymphadenopathy [Rosai-Dorfman disease (RDD)].* **(Right)** *CNS RDD usually presents as 1 or more meningioma-like dural masses. The dura ⇒ is easily identified at the edge of the lesion but relatively obscured where it courses through the middle of this mass.*

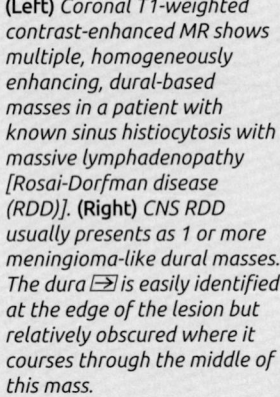

Rosai-Dorfman Disease Simulating Meningiomas

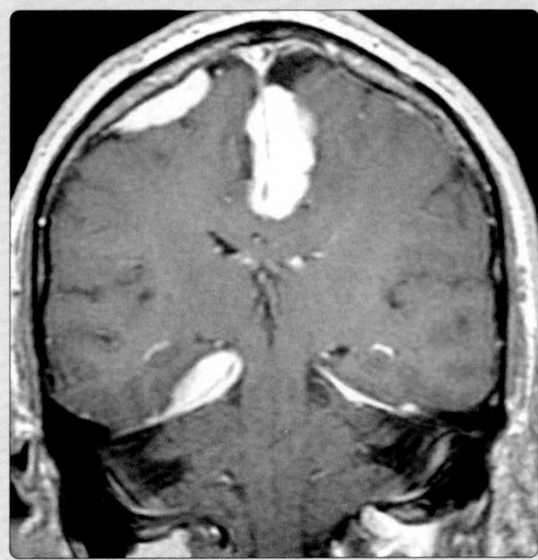

Dural Mass

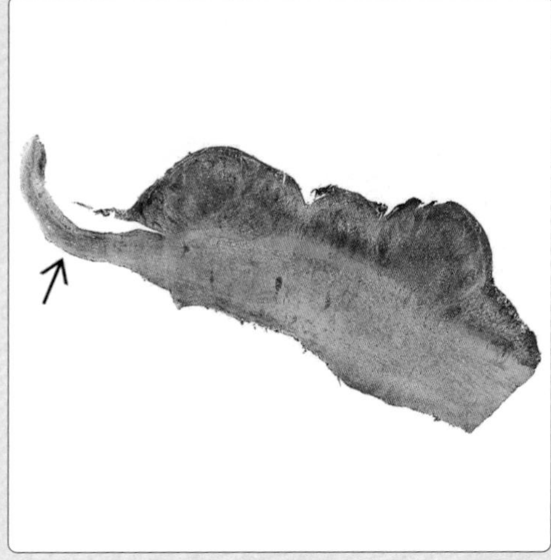

(Left) *Laid out in a smear preparation are large histiocytes containing viable lymphocytes ⇒ engulfed in the phenomenon known as emperipolesis.* **(Right)** *RDD may contain large foamy histiocytes admixed with variable numbers of lymphocytes and plasma cells. Unlike Langerhans cell histiocytosis, the histiocytes lack grooved nuclei, and eosinophils are usually absent.*

Engulfed Lymphocytes

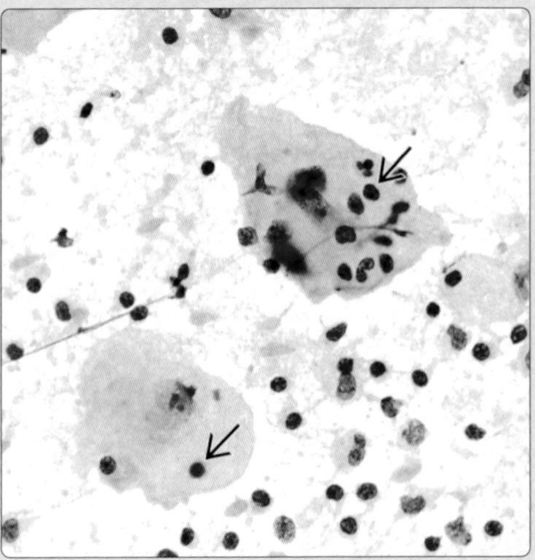

Large Histiocytes

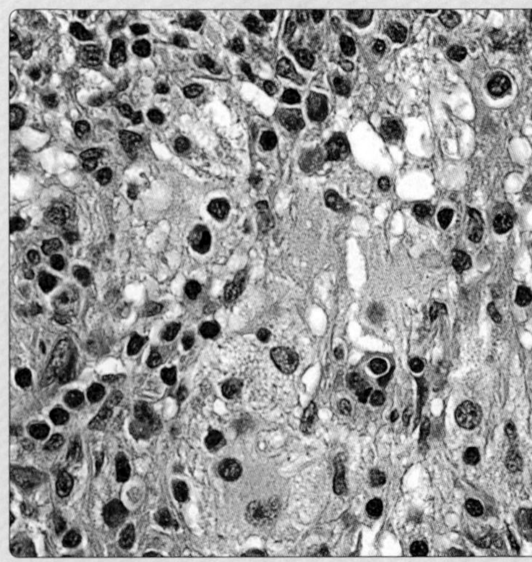

TERMINOLOGY

Abbreviations

- Rosai-Dorfman disease (RDD)

Synonyms

- Sinus histiocytosis with massive lymphadenopathy

Definitions

- Benign lymphoproliferative disorder with massive cervical lymphadenopathy, fever, polyclonal hypergammaglobulinemia; may appear only in CNS at presentation

ETIOLOGY/PATHOGENESIS

Environmental Exposure

- No known etiology
- No infectious cause known

CLINICAL ISSUES

Site

- Dura, usually skull base
- Orbits
- May involve both sides of dura

Presentation

- CNS cases: Weakness, headache, visual loss; fever often absent

Treatment

- Surgical excision of dural mass(es)
- Rare cases respond to steroids

Prognosis

- Good
- Benign condition, curable by surgery

IMAGING

MR Findings

- Dural-based mass(es)
- Mimics meningioma

MACROSCOPIC

General Features

- Thickened dura
- Mimics meningioma or other inflammatory dural process
- May involve both sides of dura (i.e., transdural)

MICROSCOPIC

Histologic Features

- Thickened fibrotic dura: Fibrosis may obscure histiocytes
- Diffuse lymphoplasmacytic infiltrates
- Histiocytes of both usual and RDD type
- Lymphophagocytosis without cell destruction (emperipolesis), but not all cases
- Stains for organisms negative
- No tight granulomas
- No caseating necrosis
- RDD histiocytes sometimes multinucleated
- RDD histiocytes S100(+), CD1a(-)

Cytologic Features

- RDD histiocytes
  - Sometimes multinucleated
  - Larger, more hyperchromatic nuclei than usual histiocytes
  - Abundant pale pink cytoplasm
  - Emperipolesis
- Lymphocytes, plasma cells

ANCILLARY TESTS

Immunohistochemistry

- RDD histiocytes S100(+), CD1a(-)
- Unlike many cases of Erdheim-Chester disease and Langerhans cell histiocytosis (LCH), RDD usually negative for BRAF VE1 (paralleling absence of *BRAF V600E* mutation)

DIFFERENTIAL DIAGNOSIS

Lymphoplasmacyte-Rich Meningioma

- Meningioma in background of intense inflammation
- Epithelial membrane antigen (+)

Langerhans Cell Histiocytosis

- LCH histiocytes with longitudinally grooved reniform nuclei
- No emperipolesis
- LCH histiocytes CD1a(+), S100(+), langerin (+)
- Often BRAF VE1(+)
- Eosinophils prominent

Wegener Granulomatosis

- Granulomatous inflammation
- Histiocytes S100(-)
- Necrotizing vascular damage
- Fragments of vascular elastica lamina

Neurosarcoidosis

- Tight, well-formed granulomas, usually nonnecrotizing
- Asteroid bodies
- Histiocytes S100(-)

Plasma Cell Granuloma

- No RDD histiocytes
- Histiocytes C68(+), S100(-)

DIAGNOSTIC CHECKLIST

Pathologic Interpretation Pearls

- 30% of CNS RDD devoid of emperipolesis
- Lymphocytes and plasma cells may overshadow RDD histiocytes
- Fibrosis may obscure RDD histiocytes
- Detection of RDD histiocytes aided by immunohistochemistry for S100

SELECTED REFERENCES

1. Bubolz AM et al: Potential clinical implications of BRAF mutations in histiocytic proliferations. Oncotarget. 5(12):4060-70, 2014
2. Haroche J et al: High prevalence of BRAF V600E mutations in Erdheim-Chester disease but not in other non-Langerhans cell histiocytoses. Blood. 120(13):2700-3, 2012

Nodular Transdural Mass

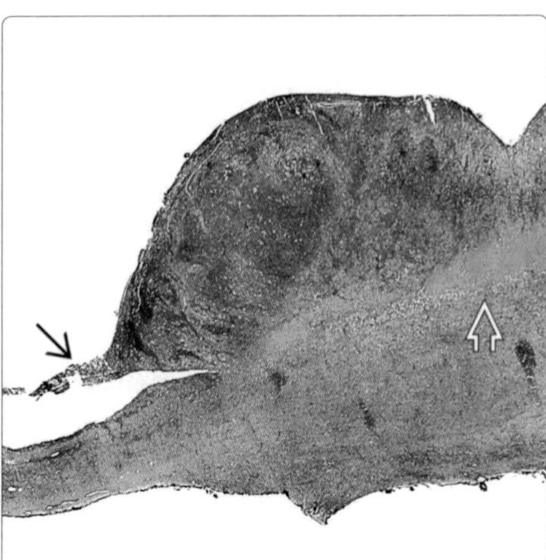

Subdural Rosai-Dorfman Disease

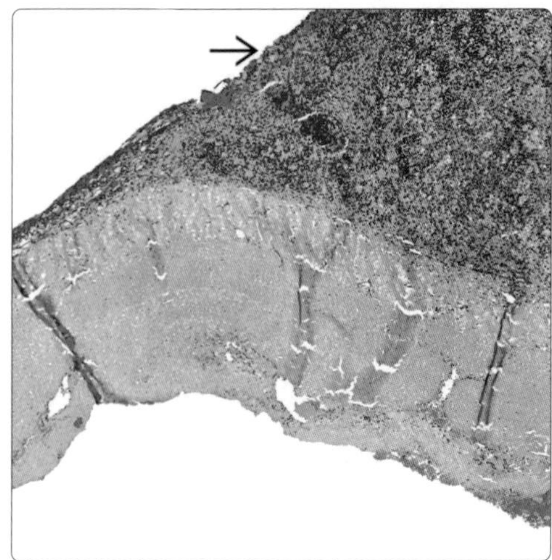

(Left) *CNS RDD usually presents as 1 or more meningioma-like dural masses. The dura ➡ runs through the middle of this mass that is thus both subdural and epidural. Note the small dural tail ➡, a feature similar to that in meningioma.* **(Right)** *It is easy to see how RDD can resemble meningioma, both radiologically and macroscopically. This example affects only the subdural ➡ compartment.*

Rosai-Dorfman Disease With Nonspecific Lymphoplasmacytic Infiltrates

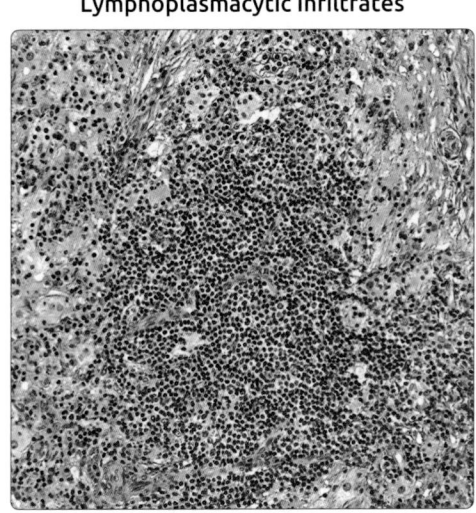

Hyalinized Connective Tissue

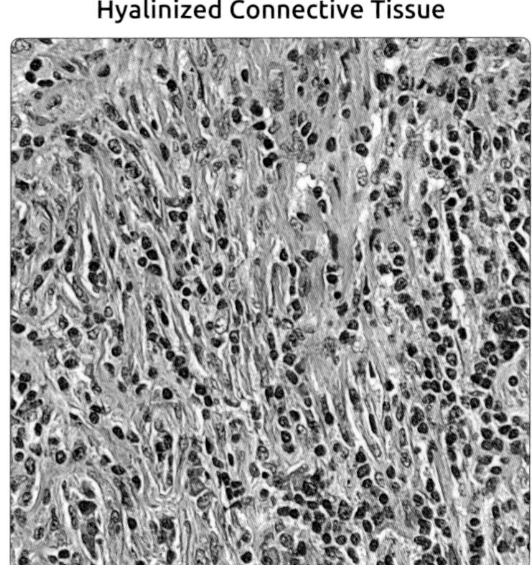

(Left) *RDD may be largely a nonspecific lymphoplasmacytic infiltrate. Composed largely of small cytologically normal lymphocytes, it is not malignant lymphoma, e.g., marginal zone type that occurs on the dura.* **(Right)** *Hyalinized connective tissue from the dura can dominate the lesion or areas thereof.*

Large Pale Histiocytes

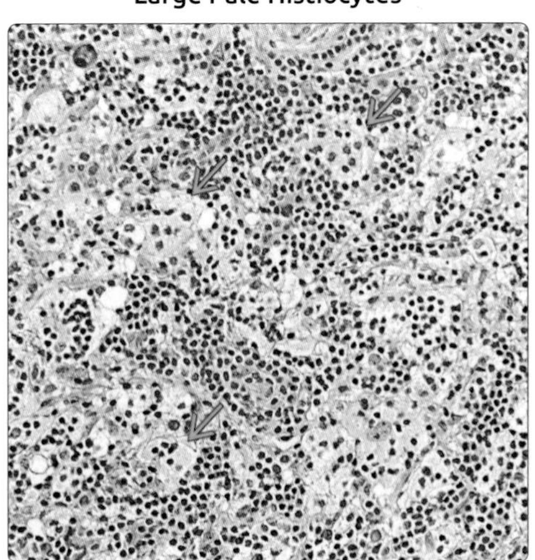

Histiocytes With Frothy Cytoplasm

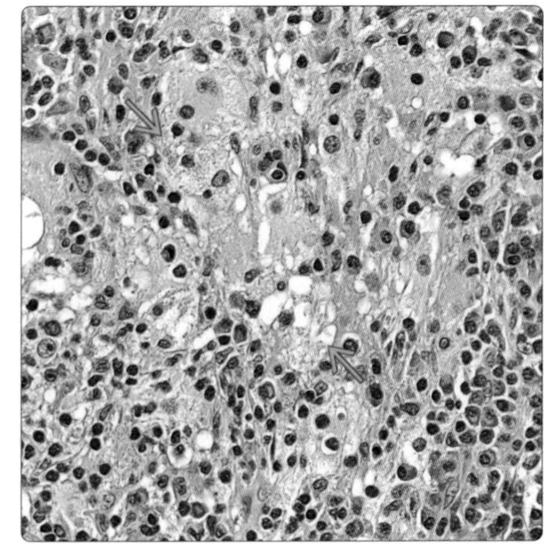

(Left) *RDD has lymphocytes, plasma cells, and groups of large pale histiocytes ➡. Unlike Langerhans cell histiocytosis, eosinophils are inconspicuous.* **(Right)** *Rosai-Dorfman histiocytes, with frothy cytoplasm, often occur in small groups and clusters ➡.*

Emperipolesis

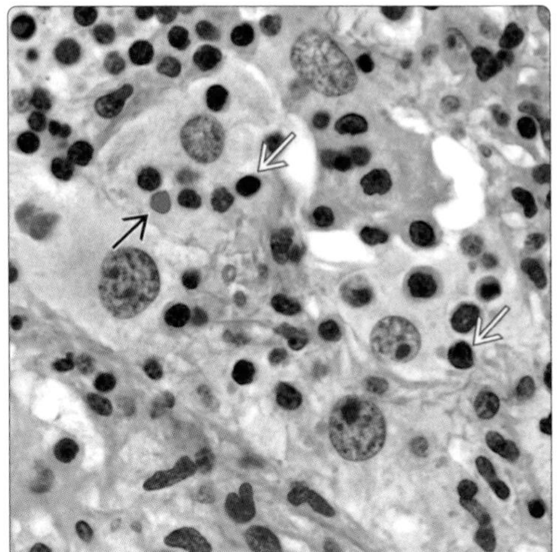

Plasma Cells

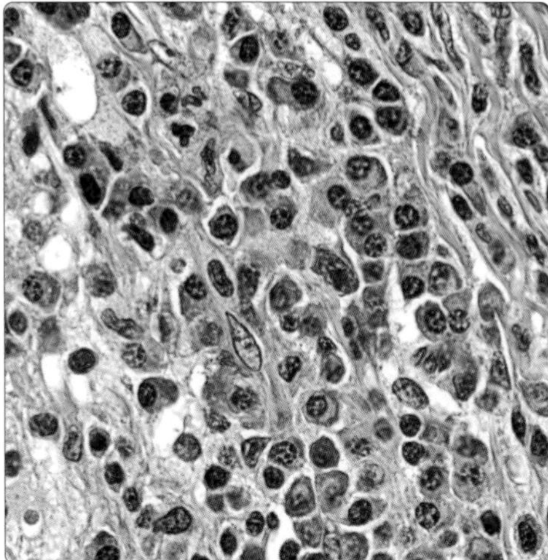

(Left) *RDD histiocytes engulf lymphocytes ➡, plasma cells, and rarely even erythrocytes ⇨. This is known as emperipolesis. Note the round, nongrooved nuclei with prominent nucleoli. (Courtesy A. Yachnis, MD.)* **(Right)** *In the absence of RDD histiocytes, focal sheets of plasma cells put plasma cell granuloma high on the differential diagnosis list for a dural-based, meningioma-like mass.*

S100 Immunoreactive Histiocytes

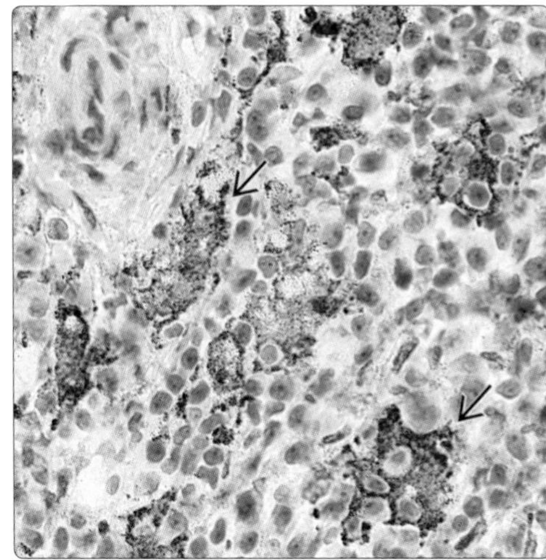

S100 Outlining Engulfed Lymphocytes

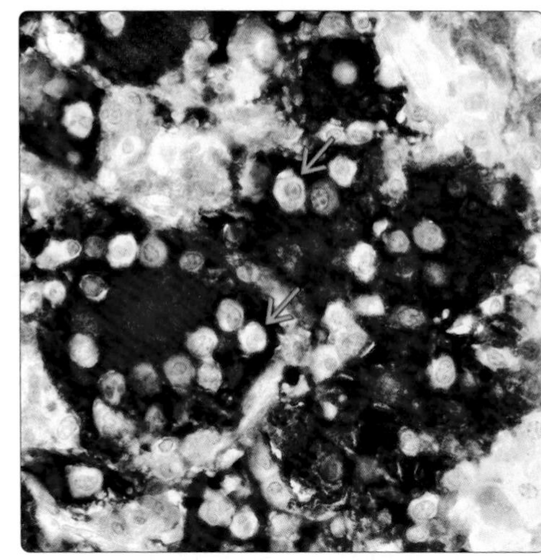

(Left) *Histiocytes of RDD are immunoreactive for S100 protein ⇨, whereas conventional histiocytes are not.* **(Right)** *Engulfed lymphocytes stand in relief against the S100(+) cytoplasm of RDD histiocytes ⇨. (Courtesy A. Yachnis, MD.)*

CD68 Immunoreactive Histiocytes

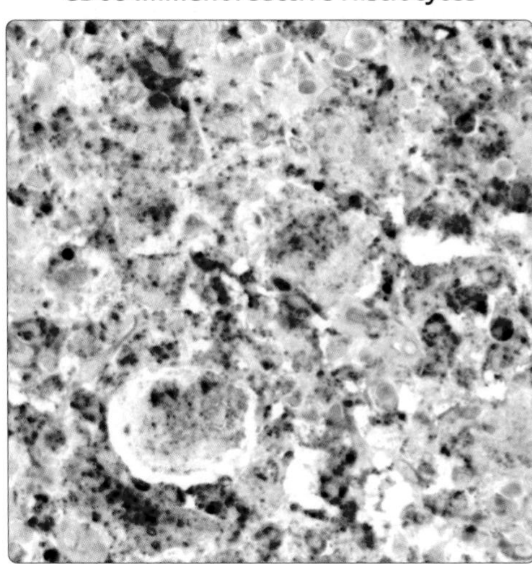

Negative CD1a

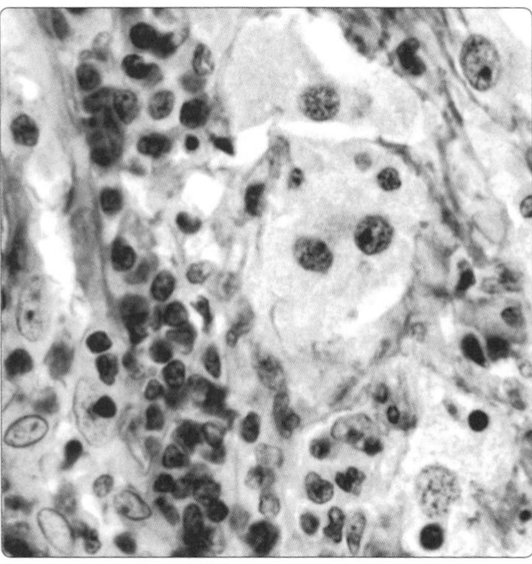

(Left) *RDD of the central nervous system contains conventional CD68(+) histiocytes. (Courtesy A. Yachnis, MD.)* **(Right)** *As illustrated in a negative immunostain for CD1a, nuclei of RDD histiocytes have round profiles, not the kidney bean-shaped, grooved contours typical of Langerhans cells. The latter also would be positive for CD1a.*

KEY FACTS

TERMINOLOGY

- Perivascular proliferation of spindled cells and small blood vessels in meninges and superficial cortex, ± associated overlying calcification or meningioma

ETIOLOGY/PATHOGENESIS

- Both sporadic and meningioma-associated cases
- Some cases associated with neurofibromatosis type 2 (NF2); may be multifocal in this setting

CLINICAL ISSUES

- Refractory seizures &/or headache in sporadic type

IMAGING

- Thickened cortex; overlying calcified sulcal mass, some cases
- Dark, sinuous, "gyriform" signal of affected cortex in T2WI

MACROSCOPIC

- Plaque-like or nodular mass ± sulcal calcific mass

MICROSCOPIC

- Leptomeningeal and intracortical perivascular cells, variably meningothelial, fibroblastic, with transitions
  - More fibroblastic and less meningothelial-appearing in deeper cortical layers
- Islands of entrapped cortex contain large ganglion cells
  - Neurofibrillary tangles in occasional trapped ganglion cells

TOP DIFFERENTIAL DIAGNOSES

- Brain-invasive meningioma (WHO grade II)
  - More pushing invasion of parenchyma, rather than extensive perivascular spread as in meningioangiomatosis

(Left) *Axial T2WI MR demonstrates the collagen-rich dark cortex ➡ and bright signal of underlying white matter typical of meningioangiomatosis (MA).* **(Right)** *The interface ➡ between the cortical-based MA (below the arrows) and the subjacent white matter ➡ is remarkably discrete.*

Collagen-Rich Dark Cortex

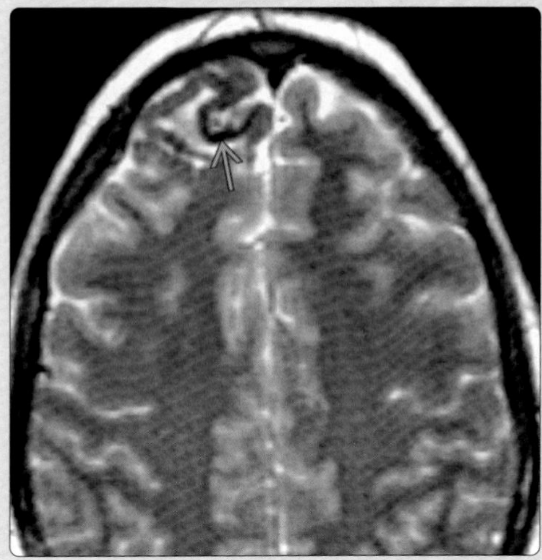

Cortical-Based Meningioangiomatosis

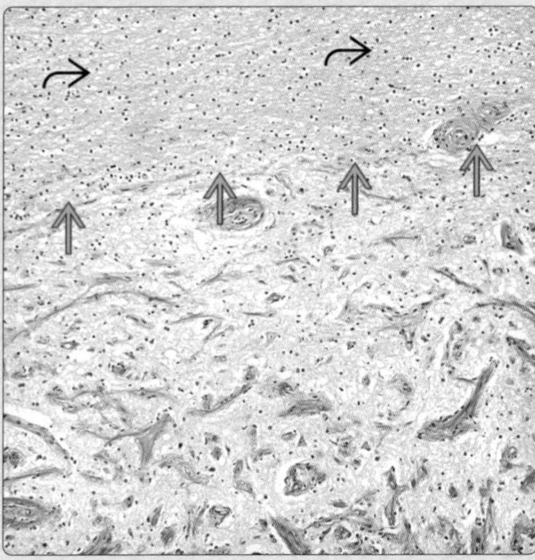

(Left) *Perivascular cells, cytologically intermediate between meningothelial cells and fibroblasts, ensheathe intracortical vessels. A purple psammoma body supports a meningothelial origin of the lesion.* **(Right)** *Light microscopy shows ➡ mildly dysmorphic neurons within the intervening neuropil.*

Spindle Cells Ensheathing Intracortical Vessels

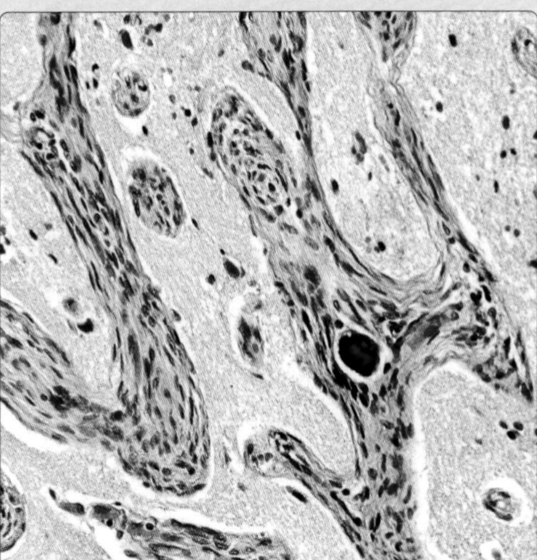

Interspersed, Minimally Dysmorphic Neurons

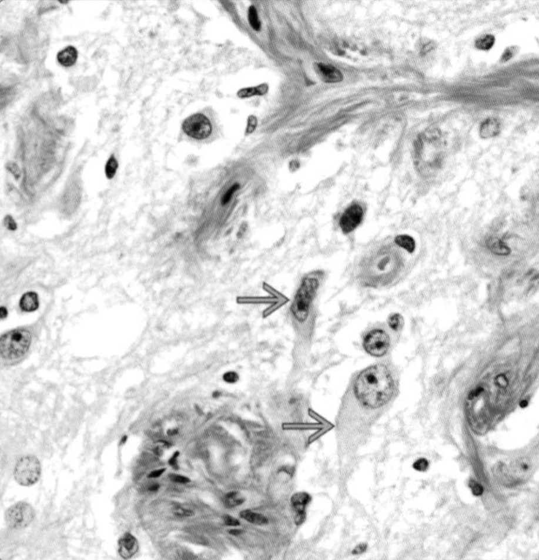

TERMINOLOGY

Definitions

- Proliferation of small blood vessels and accompanying spindled cells involving meninges and superficial cortex, ± associated overlying calcific mass or meningioma

CLINICAL ISSUES

Epidemiology

- Incidence
  - Rare
  - Sporadic or neurofibromatosis type 2 (NF2) associated
    - Ratio 4:1
  - Associated with overlying meningioma in minority of cases
- Age
  - Children and young adults

Site

- Cerebral cortex and leptomeninges
- Usually frontal &/or temporal
- Solitary in sporadic cases
- Multiple in NF2

Presentation

- Sporadic: Refractory seizures &/or headache
- NF2 associated: Often asymptomatic, incidental finding

Treatment

- Antiepileptic drugs
- Resection

Prognosis

- Variable effect upon seizures

IMAGING

General Features

- Best diagnostic clue
  - Thickened leptomeninges, overlying calcified mass in sulcus
- Location
  - Cerebral cortex (frontal and temporal)
  - Rarely in
    - 3rd ventricle
    - Thalami
    - Brainstem
    - Cerebellum
- Size
  - Generally small (1-3 cm)

MR Findings

- Dark, sinuous, "gyriform" signal in affected cortex on T2WI
- Surrounding bright signal of edema on T2WI
- Variable contrast enhancement
- Occasionally cystic due to subcortical malacia

CT Findings

- Solitary or multifocal process with hypo- or isodensity round lesion(s)
- Gyriform intracortical calcification(s)

MACROSCOPIC

General Features

- Plaque-like or nodular, firm intracortical
  - Sporadic: Solitary lesion
  - NF2 associated: Usually multifocal
- Intracortical with focal leptomeningeal thickening
- Adherent calcific mass (calcifying pseudoneoplasm of the neuraxis) in overlying sulcus, uncommon
- Sometimes "cystic" due to subcortical malacia

MICROSCOPIC

Histologic Features

- General features
  - Leptomeningeal and intracortical perivascular cells, variably meningothelial and fibroblastic, with transitions
    - Pronounced in superficial cortex, less prominent in deeper levels
    - More fibroblastic and less meningothelial in deeper cortical layers
  - Islands of cortex, with large ganglion cells, isolated by thickened vessels
    - Neurofibrillary change (tangles) in trapped ganglion cells
    - May be associated with focal cortical dysplasia
  - Gliosis
  - Psammoma bodies (occasional)
  - No perivascular chronic inflammation
  - No hemosiderin
- Associated lesions
  - Meningioma
    - Broad attachment to cortical surface
    - Grade I or II
    - Filling of perivascular spaces with meningothelial cells, often with transition to more fibroblastic cells in mid- and deep-level cortex; such perivascular extension not to be equated with cortical invasion
  - Calcifying pseudoneoplasm of neuraxis, both ± NF2
    - Hypocellular fibrillar mass with peripheral "ropey" cords
    - Amorphous to finely fibrillar core
    - Chondroid matrix
    - Variable superficial rind of spindle to epithelioid cells (cortical layer)

ANCILLARY TESTS

In Situ Hybridization

- Loss of *NF2* gene in meningioangiomatosis (MA) associated with meningioma but not lost in sporadic MA
  - 1 smaller study: Loss of *NF2* locus (22q12) in both meningioma and underlying meningioangiomatosis
  - Loss of heterozygosity (LOH) on either chromosome 22q12 or 9p21 in sporadic MA

Immunohistochemistry

- EMA
  - Overlying meningioma (+)
  - Intracortical perivascular and leptomeningeal, meningothelial cells (+); usually (-) in fibroblast-like cells
- Ki-67

- Intracortical component, ± associated meningioma: < 1%
  - Higher in associated meningioma

Electron Microscopy

- Interdigitating processes joined by desmosomes, consistent with a meningothelial lesion
- Paired helical filaments (neurofibrillary tangles) in occasional trapped neurons

Genetic Testing

- Sporadic lesions lack mutations in *NF2* gene

DIFFERENTIAL DIAGNOSIS

Conventional Meningioma With Cortical Invasion

- Usually older patients
- No (or minor) superficial involvement of cortex
  - More pushing invasion of parenchyma than extensive perivascular spread
  - Invading component more obviously meningothelial
- Ki-67 labeling of invasive component same as rest of tumor

Vascular Malformation

- Telangiectasis
  - Small, thin-walled vessels
  - Normal intervening parenchyma
  - No perivascular meningothelial proliferation
  - No psammoma bodies
- Cavernous angioma
  - Hyalinized, nondescript vessels
    - Often occluded
  - No perivascular meningothelial proliferation
  - No psammoma bodies
  - Perilesional hemosiderin
- Arteriovenous malformation
  - Large caliber vessels including arteries, veins, and transitional forms
  - Not restricted to cortex

Ganglion Cell Tumor

- Discrete, nonplaque-like lesion
- Cytologically abnormal, often binucleate ganglion cells
- Less perivascular thickening
- No perivascular meningothelial proliferation
- Calcospherites but not laminated psammoma bodies
- Glial element; often resembles pilocytic astrocytoma
- Eosinophilic granular bodies
- Perivascular lymphocytes common

DIAGNOSTIC CHECKLIST

Clinically Relevant Pathologic Features

- Cortical involvement with resultant seizures
- May be associated with focal cortical dysplasia

Pathologic Interpretation Pearls

- Grossly: Plaque-like or nodular
- Microscopically: Proliferation of small blood vessels ensheathed by meningothelial and fibroblast-like cells
- May resemble vascular malformation
- Do not interpret perivascular spread in meningioma-associated type as evidence of grade II meningioma

SELECTED REFERENCES

1. Bulut E et al: Meningioangiomatosis of the cerebellum: radiopathologic characteristics of a case. Acta Neurochir (Wien). 157(8):1371-2, 2015
2. Grabowski MM et al: Focal cortical dysplasia in meningioangiomatosis. Clin Neuropathol. 34(2):76-82, 2015
3. Li P et al: Multicystic meningioangiomatosis. BMC Neurol. 14:32, 2014
4. Chen YY et al: Sporadic meningioangiomatosis-associated atypical meningioma mimicking parenchymal invasion of brain: a case report and review of the literature. Diagn Pathol. 5:39, 2010
5. Fedi M et al: Cystic meningioangiomatosis in neurofibromatosis type 2: an MRI-pathological study. Br J Radiol. 82(979):e129-32, 2009
6. Kim NR et al: Allelic loss on chromosomes 1p32, 9p21, 13q14, 16q22, 17p, and 22q12 in meningiomas associated with meningioangiomatosis and pure meningioangiomatosis. J Neurooncol. 94(3):425-30, 2009
7. Kim SH et al: A case of infantile meningioangiomatosis with a separate cyst. J Korean Neurosurg Soc. 46(3):252-6, 2009
8. Saad A et al: Meningioangiomatosis associated with meningioma: a case report. Acta Cytol. 53(1):93-7, 2009
9. Kobayashi H et al: Cystic meningioangiomatosis. Pediatr Neurosurg. 42(5):320-4, 2006
10. Jallo GI et al: Meningioangiomatosis without neurofibromatosis: a clinical analysis. J Neurosurg. 103(4 Suppl):319-24, 2005
11. Perry A et al: Insights into meningioangiomatosis with and without meningioma: a clinicopathologic and genetic series of 24 cases with review of the literature. Brain Pathol. 15(1):55-65, 2005
12. Sinkre P et al: Deletion of the NF2 region in both meningioma and juxtaposed meningioangiomatosis: case report supporting a neoplastic relationship. Pediatr Dev Pathol. 4(6):568-72, 2001
13. Izycka-Swieszewska E et al: Meningioangiomatosis with a predominant fibrocalcifying component. Neuropathology. 20(1):44-8, 2000
14. Jallo GI et al: Meningioangiomatosis. Pediatr Neurosurg. 32(4):220-1, 2000
15. Giangaspero F et al: Meningioma with meningioangiomatosis: a condition mimicking invasive meningiomas in children and young adults: report of two cases and review of the literature. Am J Surg Pathol. 23(8):872-5, 1999
16. Wiebe S et al: Meningioangiomatosis. A comprehensive analysis of clinical and laboratory features. Brain. 122 (Pt 4):709-26, 1999
17. Mokhtari K et al: Atypical neuronal inclusion bodies in meningioangiomatosis. Acta Neuropathol. 96(1):91-6, 1998
18. Stemmer-Rachamimov AO et al: Meningioangiomatosis is associated with neurofibromatosis 2 but not with somatic alterations of the NF2 gene. J Neuropathol Exp Neurol. 56(5):485-9, 1997
19. Prayson RA: Meningioangiomatosis. A clinicopathologic study including MIB1 immunoreactivity. Arch Pathol Lab Med. 119(11):1061-4, 1995
20. Goates JJ et al: Meningioangiomatosis: an immunocytochemical study. Acta Neuropathol. 82(6):527-32, 1991
21. Liu SS et al: Meningioangiomatosis: a case report. Surg Neurol. 31(5):376-80, 1989
22. Sakaki S et al: Meningioangiomatosis not associated with von Recklinghausen's disease. Neurosurgery. 20(5):797-801, 1987
23. Halper J et al: Meningio-angiomatosis: a report of six cases with special reference to the occurrence of neurofibrillary tangles. J Neuropathol Exp Neurol. 45(4):426-46, 1986

Simulating Vascular Malformation

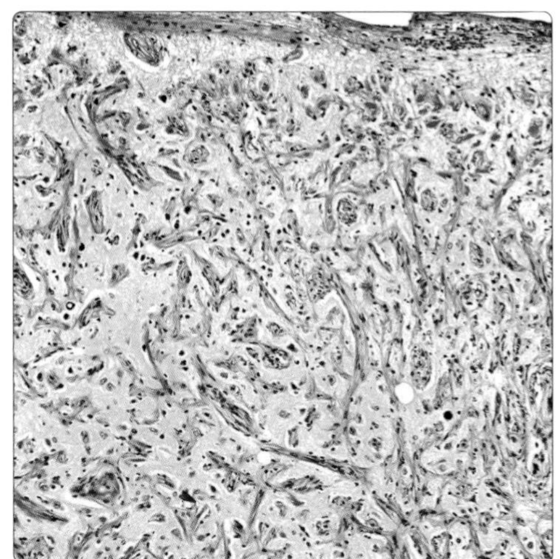

Psammoma Bodies

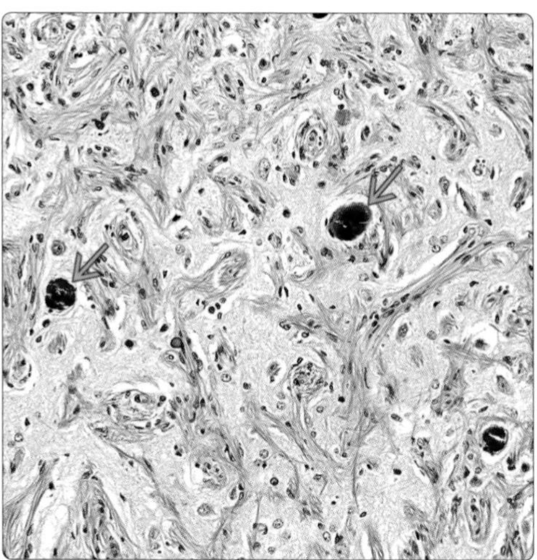

(Left) *With its numerous thickened intracortical blood vessels, MA can resemble a vascular malformation. Vessels are, however, too thick to be those of telangiectasis, yet too thin, small, and numerous to be cavernous angioma.* **(Right)** *Almost all vessels, large and small, show nonspecific thickening. Psammoma bodies ➙, however, suggest the presence of a meningothelial element. Fibroblastic features are also present and areas with transitional features can also be present.*

Thickening of Vessels

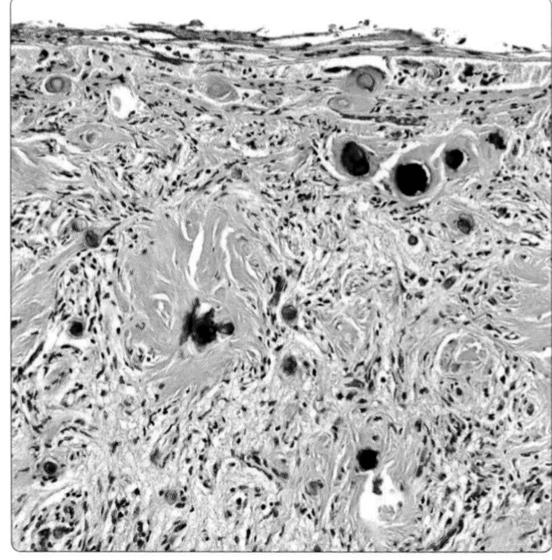

Psammoma Bodies Suggest Meningothelial Origin

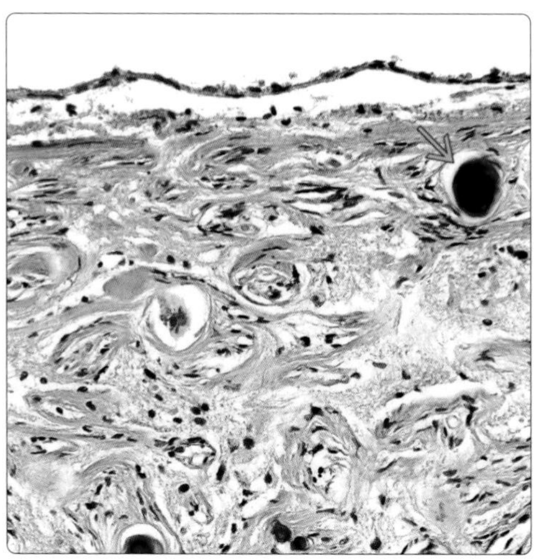

(Left) *Vessels in MA are thickened and associated with psammoma bodies. Intervening cortex may be intact but may be hypercellular and disorganized enough to suggest a glioma.* **(Right)** *Usually, there is little evidence other than the presence of psammoma bodies ➙ to suggest that the lesion is meningothelial in nature. Most of the areas appear fibroblastic.*

Simulating Brain-Invasive Meningioma

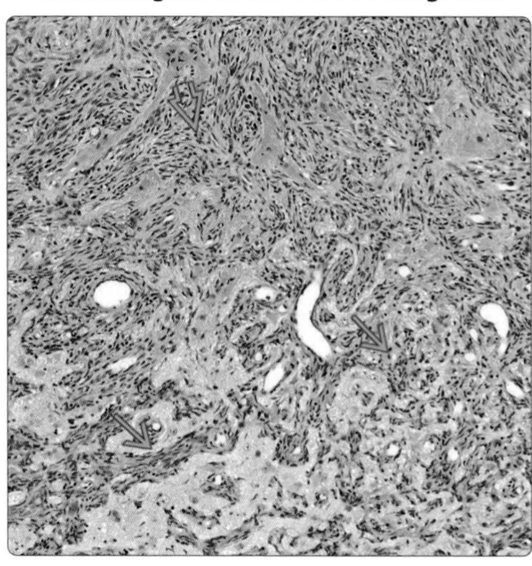

Surrounding Intracortical Small Vessels

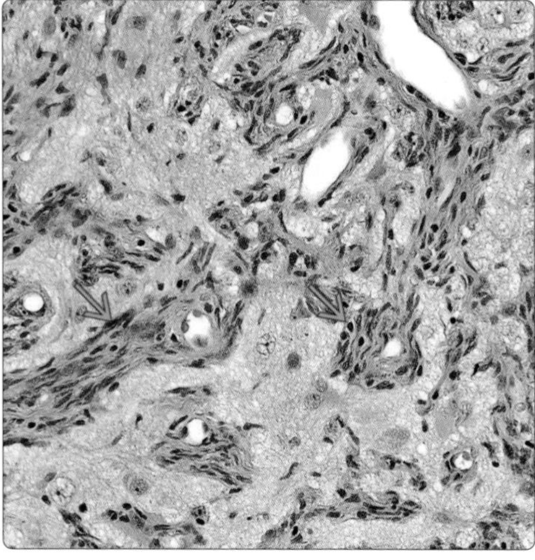

(Left) *A meningioma ➙ spreads around intracortical vessels ➙ in 1 form of MA. Unlike a conventional invasive meningioma, there is extensive involvement of multiple small vessels, some deep within the cortex.* **(Right)** *Short spindle cells with features suggesting a meningothelial origin, yet at the same time somewhat fibroblastic, surround the intracortical vessels ➙ in this case of MA associated with an overlying meningioma. This dual meningothelial-fibroblastic morphology is characteristic.*

Vasocentricity Obscured

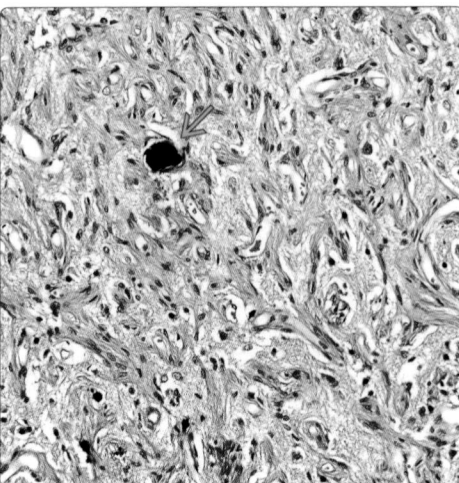

Meningothelial Cells

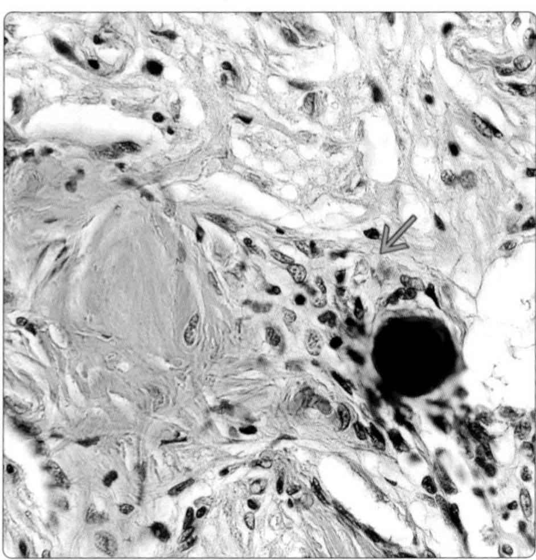

(Left) *Extensive involvement of small vessels results in a high degree of cellularity, partially obscuring the lesion's signature vasocentricity. Psammoma bodies are a common feature →.* **(Right)** *A nest of meningothelial cells → and a psammoma body are clear expressions of meningothelial differentiation. Often, however, especially in deeper cortical layers, the lesion is phenotypically fibroblastic with little to suggest meningothelium.*

Whorl-Like Arrangement

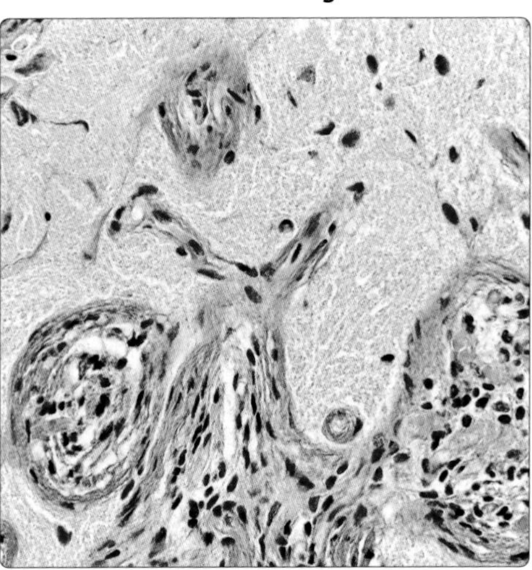

Minimal Adjacent Gliosis

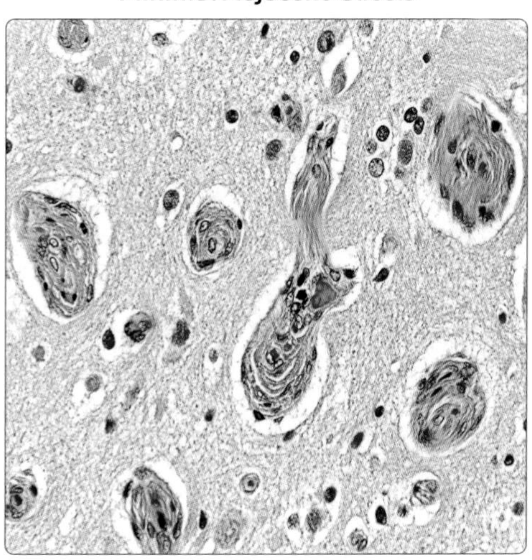

(Left) *While nonspecific, the whorl-like arrangement of perivascular cells is highly suspicious for MA.* **(Right)** *Vascular thickening in MA may appear nonspecific. There is little gliosis in such mildly affected areas.*

Whorl-Like Pattern in Fibroblastic-Appearing Areas

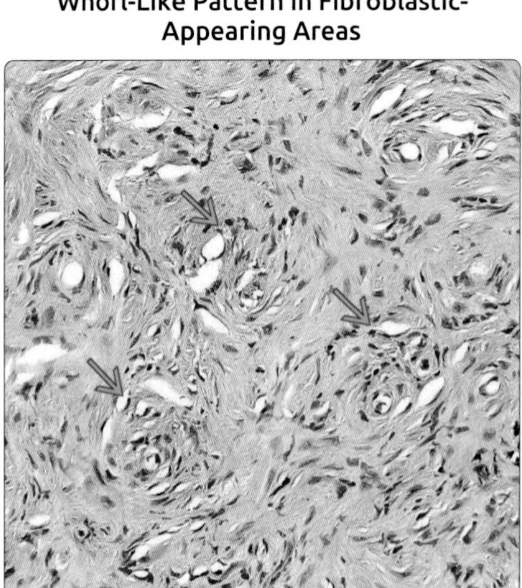

Simulating Infiltrating Glioma

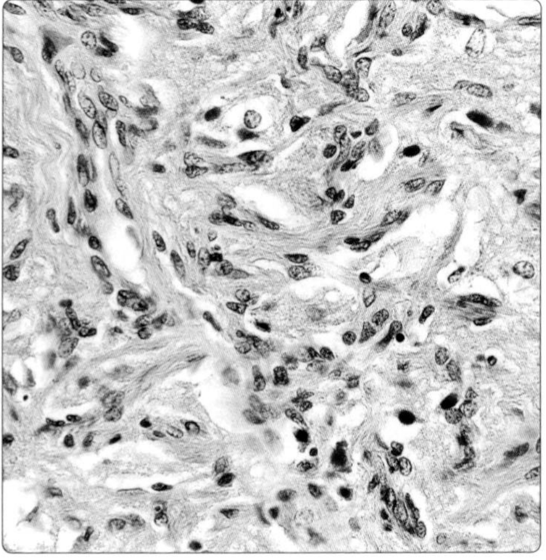

(Left) *Small vessels surrounded by cells, sometimes more fibroblastic than meningothelial in appearance, create a whorl-like pattern →.* **(Right)** *Taken out of context at high magnification, more cellular areas of MA may resemble infiltrating glioma.*

Hybrid Fibroblast-Meningothelial Features

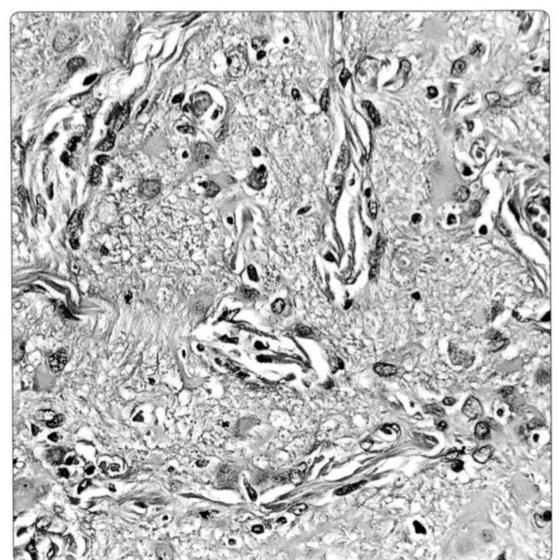

Scant Perivascular Cells

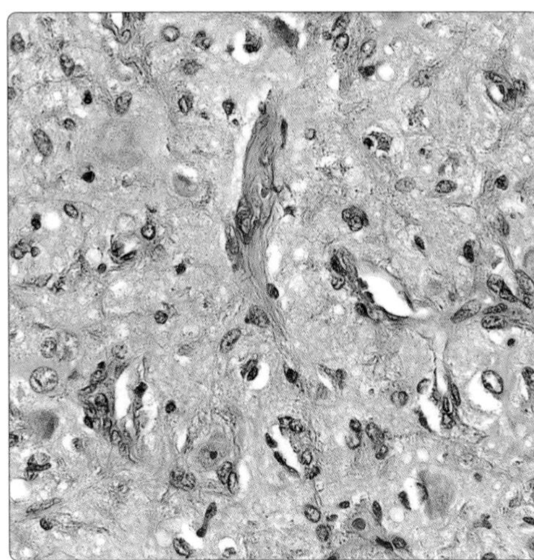

(Left) *Cells with hybrid fibroblast-meningothelial cell qualities surround the vessels in MA.* **(Right)** *There may be few seemingly nonspecific perivascular cells in deeper cortical levels of MA.*

Entrapped Neurons

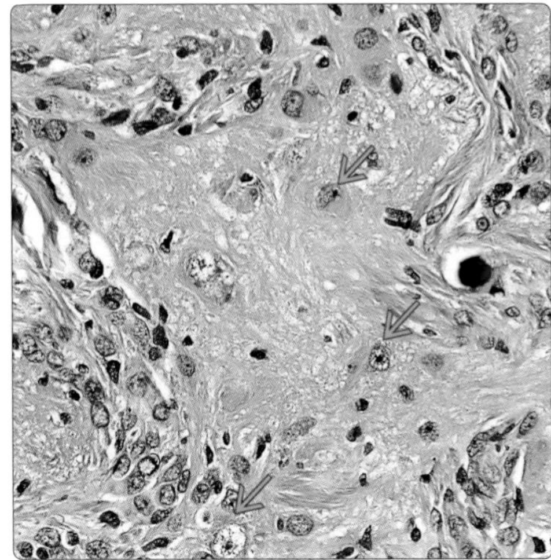

Neurofibrillary Tangle Formation

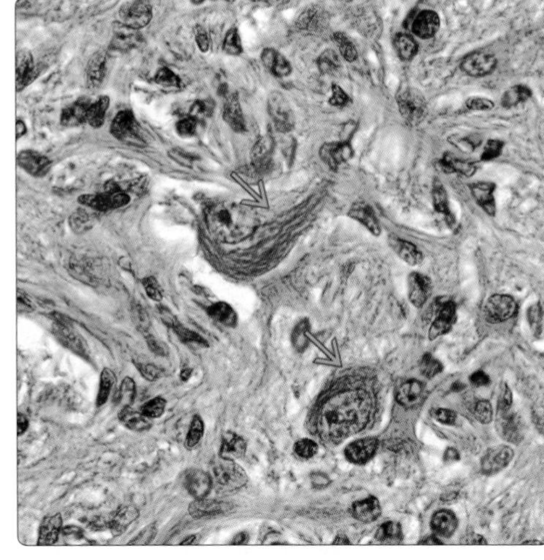

(Left) *Plump perivascular cells and a psammoma body are clues to the nature of the lesion. Neurons ➙ trapped in the cortical MA may be difficult to recognize.* **(Right)** *Trapped ganglion cells in MA are prone to neurofibrillary tangle formation ➙. Positive immunohistochemistry for TAU would be confirmatory.*

TAU, Neurofibrillary Tangles

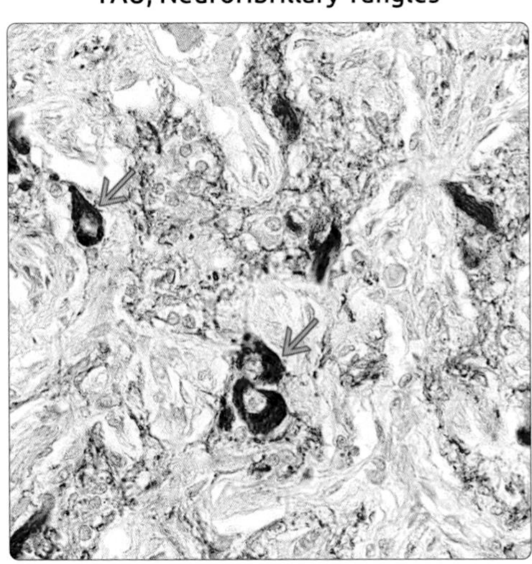

EMA(+) in Meningothelial Areas

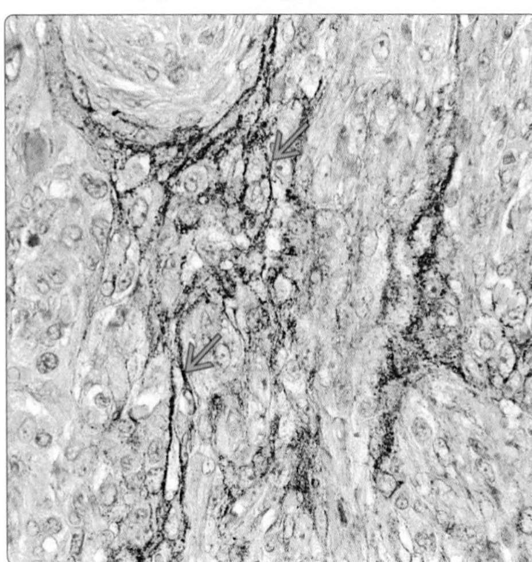

(Left) *Neurofibrillary tangles ➙ in MA are immunoreactive for TAU protein.* **(Right)** *Meningothelial areas, or associated meningiomas, are often immunoreactive for epithelial membrane antigen ➙. Fibroblastic areas are typically not.*

KEY FACTS

ETIOLOGY/PATHOGENESIS

- Cerebrospinal fluid (CSF) leak

CLINICAL ISSUES

- Often assumed preoperatively to be metastatic tumor or inflammation/infection
- Often history of surgery, CSF drainage (shunting or lumbar tap)
- Occasionally spontaneous

IMAGING

- Diffuse dural, nonleptomeningeal, enhancement

MICROSCOPIC

- Narrow band of capillaries on inner aspect of dura, often inconspicuous at low (and even high) magnification
- Sometimes micronodules of hyperplastic meningothelial cells

TOP DIFFERENTIAL DIAGNOSES

- Subdural hematoma
- Dural metastatic tumor
- Dural inflammatory disorder
- Normal dura
  - No proliferating vessels
  - No hyperplastic meningothelial cells
- Meningioma
  - Mass, not isolated micronodules of meningothelial cells among few delicate vessels

DIAGNOSTIC CHECKLIST

- More obvious radiologically than histologically
- Radiologically impressive but functionally harmless

(Left) *New vessels on the inner aspect of the dura create the impressive diffuse meningeal enhancement that is dural ⇨, not leptomeningeal.* **(Right)** *Multiple small, thin-walled vessels ➡ are the basis of the radiological finding in the meningeal response to intracranial hypotension.*

Diffuse Dural Enhancement

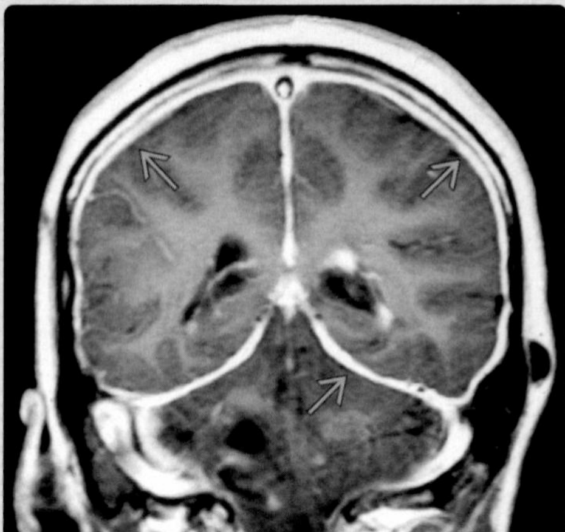

Multiple Thin-Walled Vessels

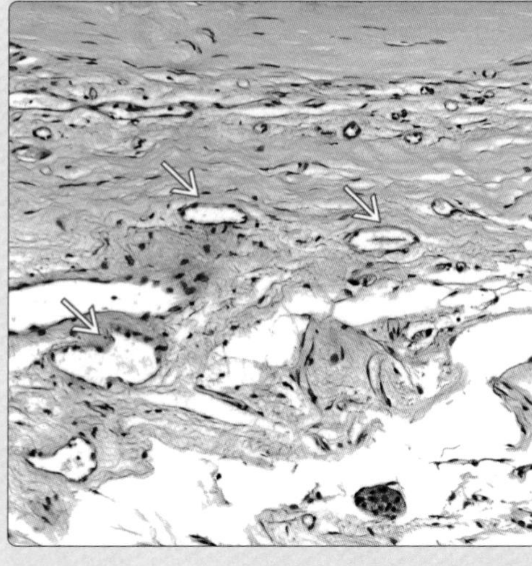

(Left) *Micronodules of meningothelial cells* ⇨ *are present among delicate vessels.* **(Right)** *While prominent in some cases, nodules of hyperplastic meningothelial cells* ⇨ *do not attain meningioma proportions.*

Nodules of Meningothelial Cells

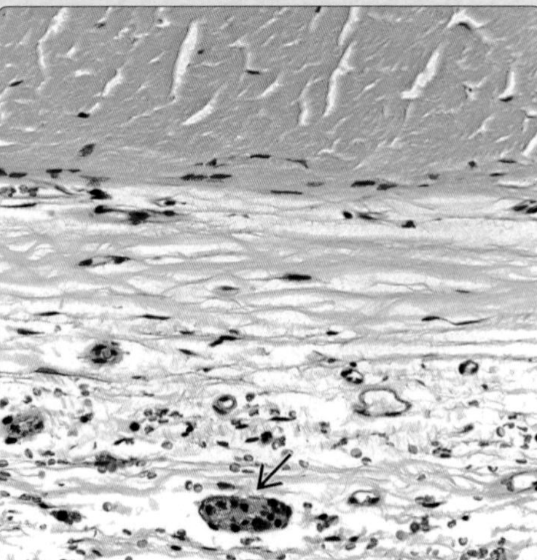

Prominent Hyperplastic Meningothelial Cells

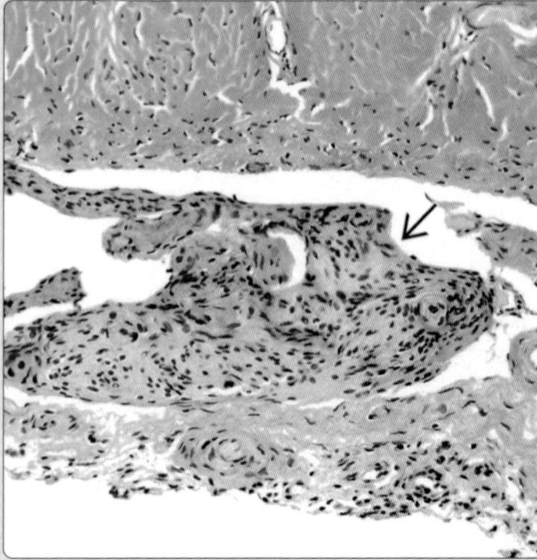

ETIOLOGY/PATHOGENESIS

Intracranial Hypotension

- Postsurgical, post-cerebrospinal fluid (CSF) drainage (shunt, spinal tap)
  - Adults and children
- Post traumatic
  - Adults and children
- Spontaneous
  - Adults

CLINICAL ISSUES

Presentation

- Headache, especially orthostatic
- Dizziness, especially orthostatic
- Neck stiffness

IMAGING

MR Findings

- Diffuse dural enhancement, usually just intracranial
- Downward displacement of brain, some cases

MACROSCOPIC

General Features

- Minimal, if any, visible dural thickening

MICROSCOPIC

Histologic Features

- Thin, sometimes very thin, band of capillaries on inner aspect of dura
- Clusters of trapped, sometimes hyperplastic, meningothelial cells

DIFFERENTIAL DIAGNOSIS

Normal Dura

- No proliferating vessels
- No hyperplastic meningothelial cells

Dural Metastatic Tumor

- May be clinical diagnosis
- Anaplastic tumor
- Usually lepto- rather than pachymeningeal when diffuse ("meningeal carcinomatosis")

Dural Inflammatory Disease

- Sometimes clinical diagnosis
- When dural, usually focal "lumpy/bumpy" rather than diffuse and thin
- Most diffuse meningeal inflammatory diseases leptomeningeal rather than dural
- Specific lesions
  - Rosai-Dorfman
    - 1 or more dural-based masses
    - Both sides of dura simultaneously
    - Dense lymphoplasmacytic infiltrate
    - Large, S100 protein-immunoreactive histiocytes engaged in emperipolesis
  - Sarcoid
    - Dural or leptomeningeal
    - Bulky
    - Granulomatous inflammation
    - Lymphocytic infiltrate
  - Infection
    - Cellular, acute, chronic, or granulomatous
    - Organisms

Vascular Malformation

- Mass, not layer of delicate vessels
- Larger vessels
- Hyalinization
- Hemosiderin

Meningioma

- Mass, not isolated micronodules of meningothelial cells among few delicate vessels

Subdural Hematoma

- More localized
- Mass of blood
- Organization in subacute phase
- Somewhat similar in chronic stage, but with
  - Membranes, inner and outer
  - Hemosiderin staining

DIAGNOSTIC CHECKLIST

Clinically Relevant Pathologic Features

- Radiologically impressive but functionally harmless
- Index of intracranial hypotension
  - Usually post surgery, shunt, or spinal tap
  - Occasionally spontaneous

Pathologic Interpretation Pearls

- More obvious radiologically than histologically
- Changes inconspicuous at low magnification
- Dural, not leptomeningeal, process
  - New vessels on inner aspect of dura create impressive diffuse meningeal enhancement that is dural, not leptomeningeal

SELECTED REFERENCES

1. Mokri B: Spontaneous CSF leaks: low CSF volume syndromes. Neurol Clin. 32(2):397-422, 2014
2. Mea E et al: Clinical features and outcomes in spontaneous intracranial hypotension: a survey of 90 consecutive patients. Neurol Sci. 30 Suppl 1:S11-3, 2009
3. Su CS et al: Clinical features, neuroimaging and treatment of spontaneous intracranial hypotension and magnetic resonance imaging evidence of blind epidural blood patch. Eur Neurol. 61(5):301-7, 2009
4. Couch JR: Spontaneous intracranial hypotension: the syndrome and its complications. Curr Treat Options Neurol. 10(1):3-11, 2008
5. Fuh JL et al: The timing of MRI determines the presence or absence of diffuse pachymeningeal enhancement in patients with spontaneous intracranial hypotension. Cephalalgia. 28(4):318-22, 2008
6. Smirniotopoulos JG et al: Patterns of contrast enhancement in the brain and meninges. Radiographics. 27(2):525-51, 2007
7. Hochman MS et al: Intracranial hypotension. Neurology. 47(2):612-3, 1996
8. Mokri B et al: Meningeal biopsy in intracranial hypotension: meningeal enhancement on MRI. Neurology. 45(10):1801-7, 1995
9. Good DC et al: Pathologic changes associated with intracranial hypotension and meningeal enhancement on MRI. Neurology. 43(12):2698-700, 1993
10. Hochman MS et al: Spontaneous intracranial hypotension with pachymeningeal enhancement on MRI. Neurology. 42(8):1628-30, 1992

KEY FACTS

TERMINOLOGY

- Defined region of parenchymal necrosis following irradiation
  - Complication
- Postirradiation interval of usually 1-2 yr
- Radiation necrosis must be distinguished from histologically similar tissue in and around bed of previously irradiated tumor, usually high-grade glioma
- Overlap between desired therapeutic necrosis (treatment effect) and mass-like necrosis requiring debulking (complication)

CLINICAL ISSUES

- Prognosis good, but lesion may continue to evolve

IMAGING

- Thin, generally uniform, enhancing rim following contours of cortical ribbon
- Mass effect

MACROSCOPIC

- Granular, coagulative necrosis, principally of white matter and deep cortical laminae
- Expansile in acute phase
- Contractile in chronic phase
- Calcifications in chronic phase

TOP DIFFERENTIAL DIAGNOSES

- Toxoplasmosis
- Infarct
- Vasculitis

DIAGNOSTIC CHECKLIST

- Eventually self-limiting but may continue to evolve
- Significant mass effect may require surgical decompression

(Left) *Delayed radionecrosis in its early phase is expansile and enhancing, as in this example that appeared 19 months after irradiation of a skull base chondrosarcoma.* **(Right)** *An almost 50% increase in size in the hemisphere on the right attests to the potential expansile quality of delayed radionecrosis in its early, and in this case lethal, phase. Note the near-total loss of robin's egg blue myelin in the white matter of the affected right cerebral hemisphere.*

Delayed Radionecrosis, Early Phase, Expansile

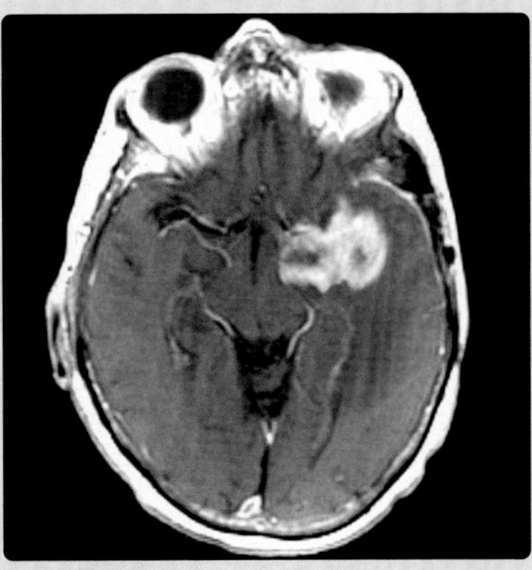

Delayed Radionecrosis, Early Phase, White Matter Predilection

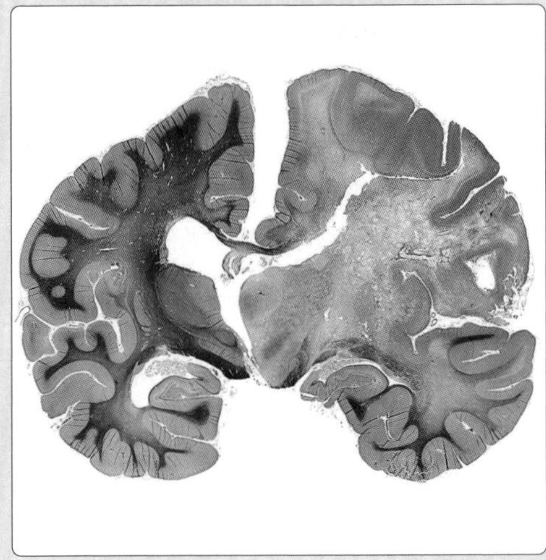

(Left) *An amorphous eosinophilic coagulum with a paucity of inflammatory or macrophage influx is the classic feature of radiation necrosis.* **(Right)** *Delayed radionecrosis in late phases often contains dystrophic calcifications in areas of remote necrosis, as well as thickened hyalinized blood vessels, the end stage of fibrinoid vascular necrosis.*

Paucity of Macrophages

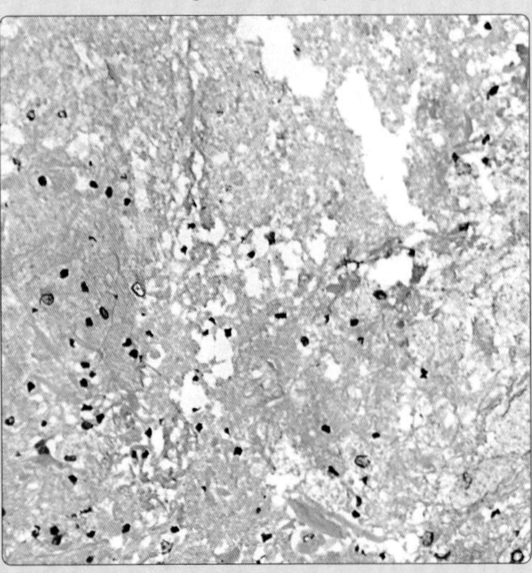

Dystrophic Mineralization

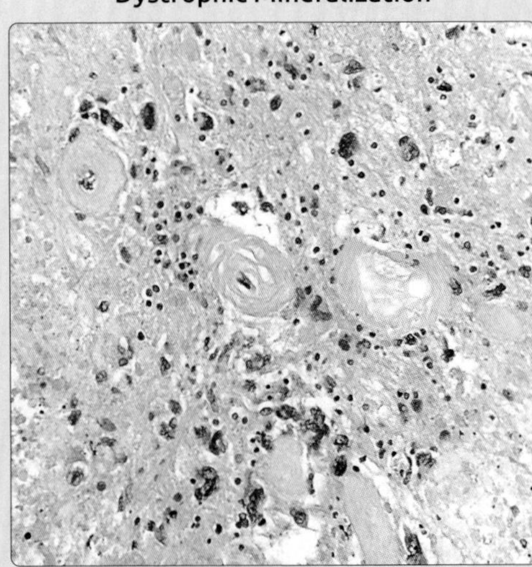

TERMINOLOGY

Synonyms

- Delayed or late delayed radionecrosis
- Radiation myelopathy or myelitis (spinal cord)
- Pseudoprogression
  - Occurs in irradiated neoplasm that develops clinical and neuroimaging features simulating apparent recurrence of tumor
    - Histologic features in pseudoprogression are those of tissue necrosis alone due to therapy **or** varying combinations of therapy-induced necrosis + tumor
      - Necrosis + active viable tumor (active tumor: Highly cellular and similar to pretreatment)
      - Necrosis + quiescent tumor (quiescent tumor: Paucicellular, mildly pleomorphic, amitotic)
      - Mixture of active and quiescent tumor

Definitions

- Defined region of parenchymal necrosis following irradiation of extracranial or pituitary neoplasm
  - Radiation necrosis is more easily distinguishable from necrosis in original tumor than in situation of radiation therapy given to glioma
  - Postirradiation interval usually 2 yr or more; occasionally decade or more
- Expansile mass of necrosis following irradiation of intracranial lesions
  - High-grade neoplasm, e.g., glioblastoma
    - Tumor progression post therapy vs. pseudoprogression is important clinical problem
    - Posttreatment interval usually < 6 months
    - Radiation-induced demise of tumor is desirable but overlap between desired therapeutic necrosis (treatment effect) and mass-like necrosis of surrounding brain that requires debulking
    - Pathogenetic synergy between radiation and chemotherapy to create radiation necrosis
  - Low-grade neoplasm
    - Development of radiation necrosis is complication, not intrinsic behavior of most low-grade neoplasms
  - Vascular malformation
    - Development of radiation necrosis is complication, not intrinsic behavior of any vascular malformation

ETIOLOGY/PATHOGENESIS

Environmental Exposure

- Iatrogenic cause: Occurs after physician delivery of therapeutic irradiation to tumor or other lesion
  - Brain, usually occurs when > 50 Gy delivered
  - Spinal cord, usually occurs when > 45 Gy delivered
  - Radiation necrosis occurs within portals/field that therapeutic radiation is given
  - May occur after external beam irradiation or stereotactic radiation
  - Enhanced by radiosensitizers
- Chemotherapy, often synergistic with radiation in cases of pseudoprogression

CLINICAL ISSUES

Site

- Brain
- Spinal cord

Presentation

- Mass effect
- Focal symptoms dependent on site
- Seizures

Treatment

- Surgical: Decompression
- Medical
  - Bevacizumab (Avastin): Common treatment
  - Steroids: Common treatment to reduce mass effect
  - Hyperbaric oxygen
  - Vitamin E
  - Pentoxifylline

Prognosis

- Good, but lesion may continue expanding; some cases fatal
- Dependent on nature of irradiated intraparenchymal lesion in cases of pseudoprogression

IMAGING

MR Findings

- Expansile in early stages
- White matter predominantly affected
- Thin, generally uniform, enhancing rim that may follow contours of cortical ribbon
- Perilesional edema

MACROSCOPIC

General Features

- Acute phase
  - Expansile, erythematous
- Necrosis
  - Principally of white matter and deep cortex
    - Granular
    - Yellow-tan with petechiae
    - Coagulative necrosis
- Chronic lesions
  - Contractile
  - Cystic
  - Calcified

MICROSCOPIC

Histologic Features

- Necrosis
  - Principally affects white matter and deep cortex
  - Mosaic pattern with coalescing foci of necrosis
  - Coagulative
    - Vessels and parenchyma involved
    - Some surviving cells occur in midst of necrosis or fibrinous exudate, partial necrosis
    - Few macrophages, except at periphery
    - Amorphous, sometimes calcified coagulum in chronic cases

- Intraparenchymal fibrinous exudate
- Inflammation of chronic type, typically mild
- Vascular changes
  - Fibrinoid necrosis
  - Hyalinization
  - Sclerosis
  - Vascular thrombosis
  - Telangiectasis
  - Microvascular proliferation, loose glomeruloid type
- Chronic lesion
  - Contracting, cystic change, calcifications
  - Radiation atypia of astrocytes, usually mild
- Pseudoprogression
  - Necrosis only or
  - Necrosis plus tumor
    - Active tumor: Highly cellular and similar to pretreatment
    - Quiescent tumor: Paucicellular, mildly pleomorphic, amitotic
    - Mixture of active and quiescent tumor

DIFFERENTIAL DIAGNOSIS

Toxoplasmosis

- Confluent rather than mosaic-like necrosis
  - Overall similar appearance, but dirty blue
- Perivascular inflammation
- Organisms, most numerous near necrosis-viable tissue interface
- Immunocompromised host

Infarct

- Prominent cortical involvement
- Macrophage-rich rather than coagulative necrosis
- Vessels preserved and hyperplastic
- Calcifications rare

Vasculitis

- Less parenchymal necrosis
- Many macrophages in infarcted area
- Not largely restricted to white matter
- Vascular inflammation
  - Neutrophil predominant (necrotizing)
  - Lymphocytic
  - Granulomatous

DIAGNOSTIC CHECKLIST

Clinically Relevant Pathologic Features

- Eventually self-limiting but may continue to evolve
- Fibrinoid vascular necrosis is key feature
  - Severe damage to vessels makes it nearly impossible for circulating monocytes/macrophages to gain access to necrotic areas or to clean up debris
- Later stage vessels may manifest severe vascular hyalinization, including medium- and small-size vessels
  - Occasional vessel wall nuclei show cytological nuclear atypia
- Cavernous malformation-like vascular changes occur in some cases
  - Radiation-induced cavernous malformation is poor mimic of sporadic cavernous malformations
    - More fibrinoid necrosis in radiation-induced examples than sporadic ones
    - Younger patients and those who received larger dose of radiation are at increased risk of radiation-induced cavernous malformations

SELECTED REFERENCES

1. Cutsforth-Gregory JK et al: Characterization of radiation-induced cavernous malformations and comparison with a nonradiation cavernous malformation cohort. J Neurosurg. 122(5):1214-22, 2015
2. McDonald MW et al: Dose-volume relationships associated with temporal lobe radiation necrosis after skull base proton beam therapy. Int J Radiat Oncol Biol Phys. 91(2):261-7, 2015
3. Miyatake S et al: Pathophysiology, diagnosis, and treatment of radiation necrosis in the brain. Neurol Med Chir (Tokyo). 55(1):50-9, 2015
4. Sneed PK et al: Adverse radiation effect after stereotactic radiosurgery for brain metastases: incidence, time course, and risk factors. J Neurosurg. 1-14, 2015
5. Di Giannatale A et al: Natural history of cavernous malformations in children with brain tumors treated with radiotherapy and chemotherapy. J Neurooncol. 117(2):311-20, 2014
6. Foster KA et al: Bevacizumab for symptomatic radiation-induced tumor enlargement in pediatric low grade gliomas. Pediatr Blood Cancer. ePub, 2014
7. Gujral DM et al: Clinical features of radiation-induced carotid atherosclerosis. Clin Oncol (R Coll Radiol). 26(2):94-102, 2014
8. Boothe D et al: Bevacizumab as a treatment for radiation necrosis of brain metastases post stereotactic radiosurgery. Neuro Oncol. 15(9):1257-63, 2013
9. Wang Y et al: Reversal of cerebral radiation necrosis with bevacizumab treatment in 17 Chinese patients. Eur J Med Res. 17:25, 2012
10. Vinchon M et al: Radiation-induced tumors in children irradiated for brain tumor: a longitudinal study. Childs Nerv Syst. 27(3):445-53, 2011
11. Liu Y et al: Cerebral cavernoma: an emerging long-term consequence of external beam radiation in childhood. Clin Endocrinol (Oxf). 73(5):555-60, 2010
12. Keezer MR et al: Radiation-induced cavernous hemangiomas: case report and literature review. Can J Neurol Sci. 36(3):303-10, 2009
13. Brandsma D et al: Clinical features, mechanisms, and management of pseudoprogression in malignant gliomas. Lancet Oncol. 9(5):453-61, 2008
14. Yoshii Y: Pathological review of late cerebral radionecrosis. Brain Tumor Pathol. 25(2):51-8, 2008
15. Chen HI et al: Recurrent late cerebral necrosis with aggressive characteristics after radiosurgical treatment of an arteriovenous malformation. Case report. J Neurosurg. 105(3):455-60, 2006
16. Perry A et al: Cancer therapy-associated CNS neuropathology: an update and review of the literature. Acta Neuropathol. 111(3):197-212, 2006
17. Ruben JD et al: Cerebral radiation necrosis: incidence, outcomes, and risk factors with emphasis on radiation parameters and chemotherapy. Int J Radiat Oncol Biol Phys. 65(2):499-508, 2006
18. Forsyth PA et al: Radiation necrosis or glioma recurrence: is computer-assisted stereotactic biopsy useful? J Neurosurg. 82(3):436-44, 1995

Delayed Radionecrosis, Early Phase, Mosaic-Like Appearance

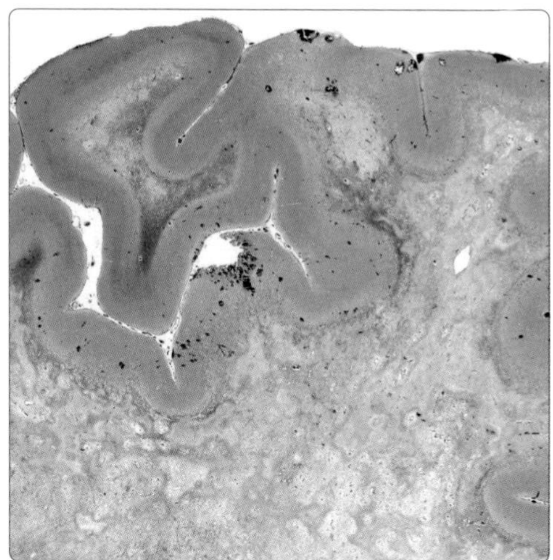

Delayed Radionecrosis, Later Phase, Coagulum

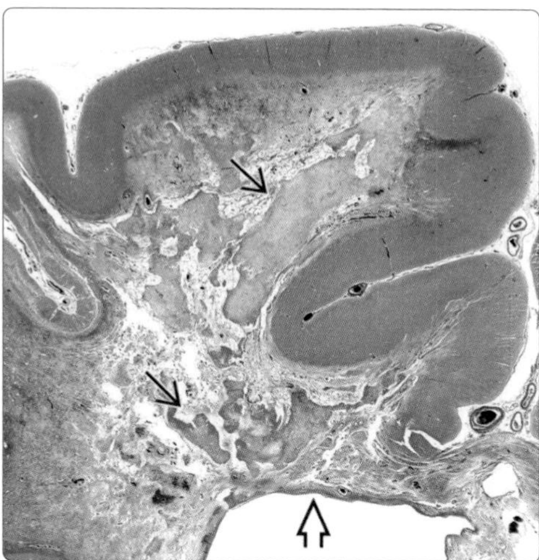

(Left) *In its early, expansile phase, delayed radionecrosis is a confluent area of necrosis that is largely confined to white matter. The lesion's location relative to white and gray matter and its characteristic mosaic-like appearance are best seen at low magnification.* **(Right)** *Rarefaction and islands of coagulum mark the chronic lesion ➙. Note the cortical sparing. The chronic lesion's destructive nature is apparent in the compensatory dilatation (hydrocephalus ex vacuo) of the adjacent frontal horn ➙.*

Coalescent Amorphous Necrosis

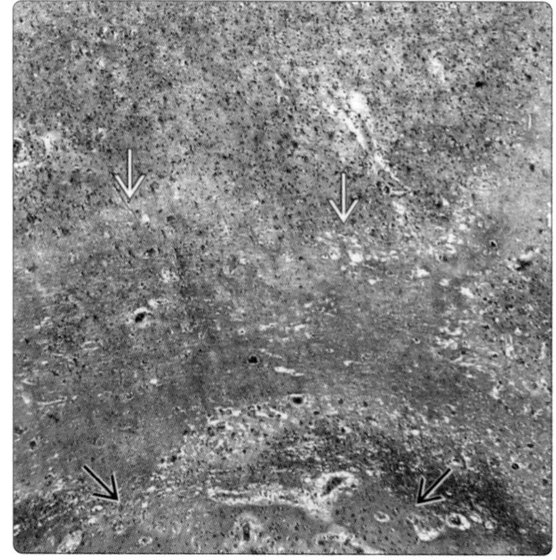

Patchy Individual Foci of Necrosis

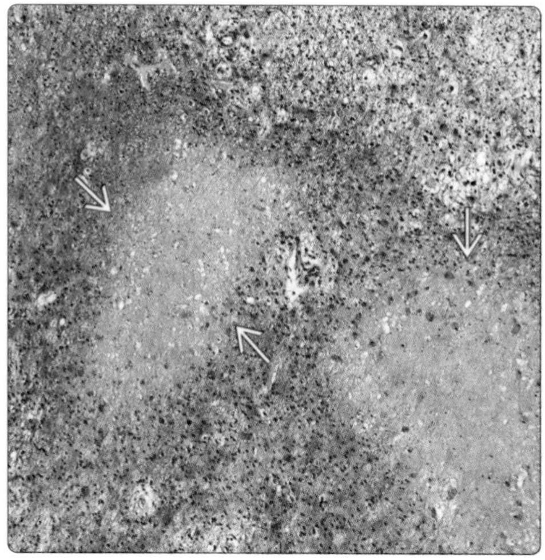

(Left) *Presumed to be ischemic in origin, radiation necrosis begins as individual foci of amorphous coagulation necrosis ➙. Cortex, or at least its upper laminae, is spared ➙.* **(Right)** *Freestanding discrete foci of necrosis mark less-involved regions ➙. With confluence and coalescence, large macroscopically evident lesions are produced. As is typical of radiation necrosis, macrophages are sparse.*

Discrete Borders

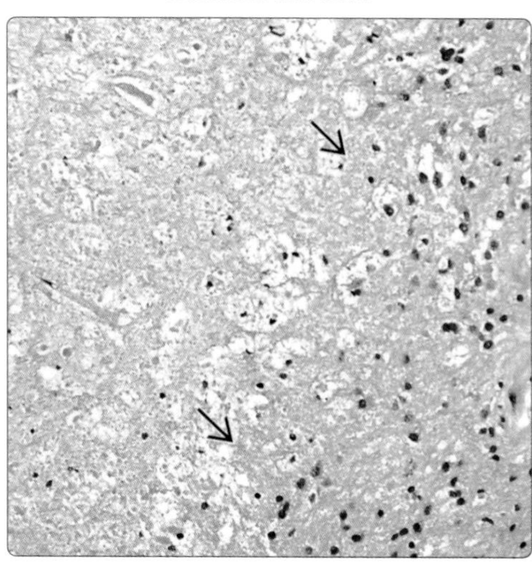

Foci With Subtotal Cell Loss

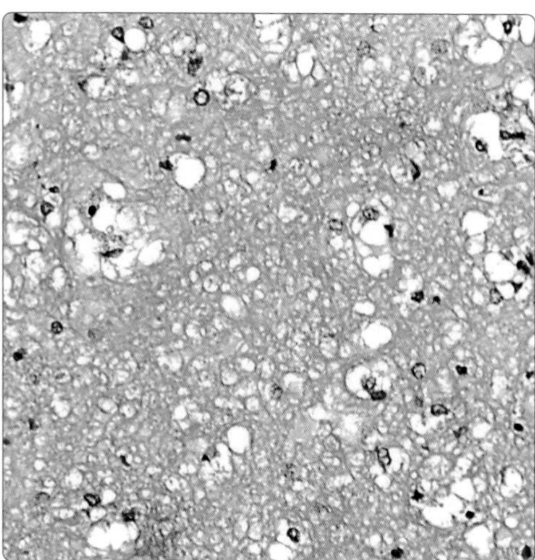

(Left) *Necrotic foci often have discrete borders ➙. Only a few macrophages survive in the midst of necrotic tissue. In contrast to radionecrosis, necrosis in infarcts and demyelinating disease is macrophage rich and generally spares vessels.* **(Right)** *In this area, some cells survived radiation injury, but others did not. Such partially depopulated parenchyma is common in delayed radionecrosis. Discrete foci of total coagulative necrosis are usually present as well.*

(Left) *Radiation necrosis can be total, including parenchyma and vasculature, leaving eosinophilic zones devoid of intact nuclei.* **(Right)** *Coagulative necrosis with few macrophages is typical of radiation necrosis, as in this example of radiation myelopathy or myelitis. Note the swollen axons in the spinal cord* →.

Total Cell Loss

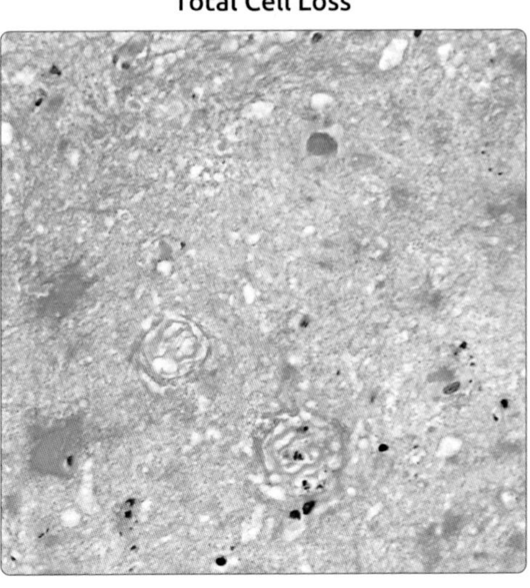

Radiation Myelopathy

(Left) *It can be difficult to determine whether viable perivascular tissue is gliosis or persistent glioma. This is gliosis; there was no history of glioma. Tissue with the changes of radionecrosis in and around previously irradiated tumors is responsible for the phenomenon of pseudoprogression.* **(Right)** *This tissue is nonspecific yet highly suggestive of radionecrosis, with an amorphous, almost fibrinous background, loss of some but not all cells, and a thickened vessel* →.

Radiation-Induced Gliosis-Simulating Glioma

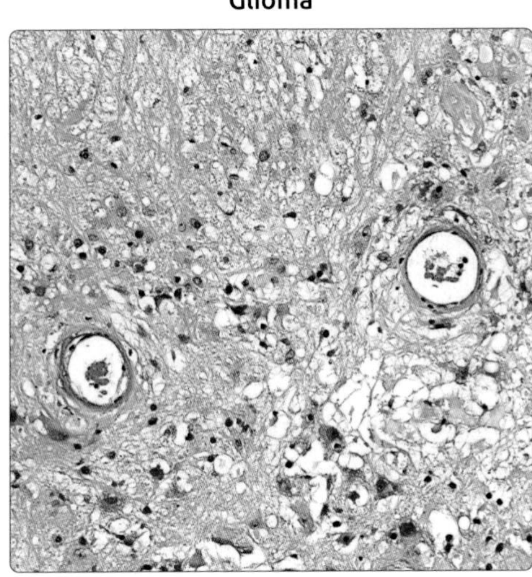

Thickened Vessels

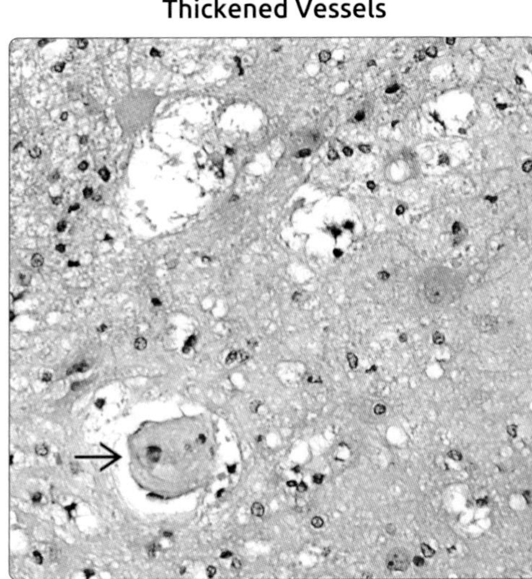

(Left) *Macrophages are often conspicuously absent in areas of total necrosis. Note the necrotic vessel* → *typical of delayed radionecrosis. Similar complete tissue necrosis, although usually with some associated inflammation, can be seen in toxoplasmosis.* **(Right)** *Areas of necrosis are often sharply defined from surrounding brain* →. *This form of necrosis attracts few macrophages, unlike an infarct.*

Necrotic Vessel

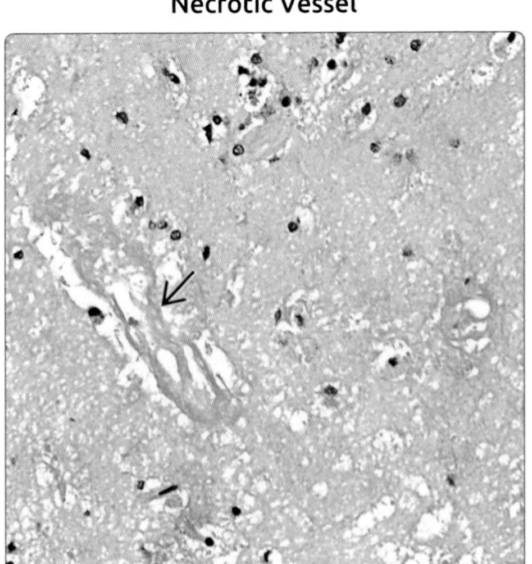

Sharp Demarcation

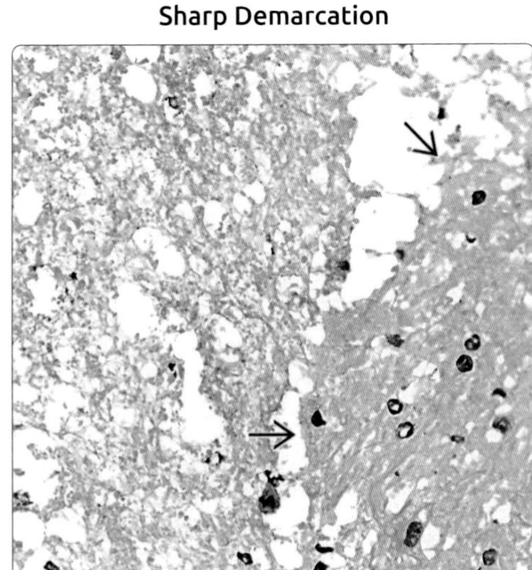

Fibrinous Exudate From Necrotic Vessels

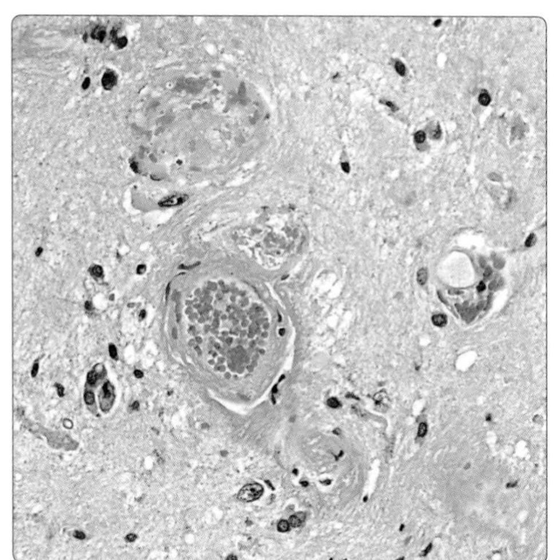

Fibrinoid Vascular Necrosis

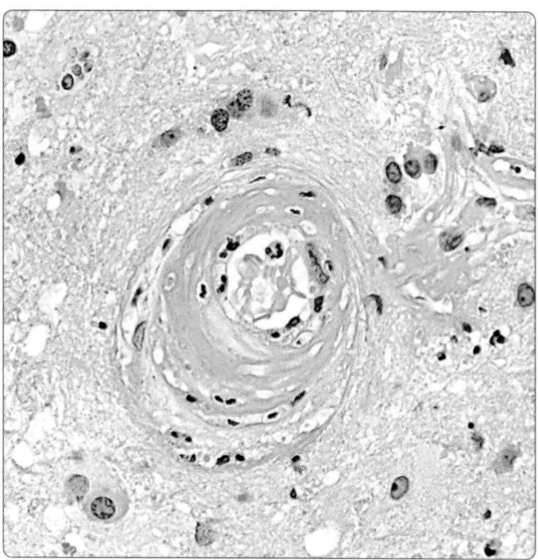

(Left) *Fibrin exudes into brain parenchyma from necrotic vessels. While not specific, this change is highly suspicious for delayed radiation injury.* **(Right)** *Vessels with fibrinoid necrosis may be present in perinecrotic tissue. A necrotizing, nonirradiation-associated vasculitis is another diagnostic possibility. Most necrotizing vasculitis from nonirradiation causes, however, is associated with neutrophilic inflammatory reaction.*

Radiation-Induced Vascular Damage

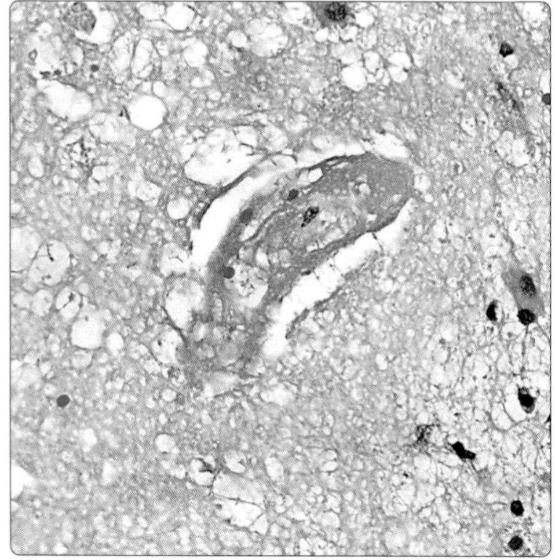

Telangiectasia, Late-Phase Delayed Radionecrosis

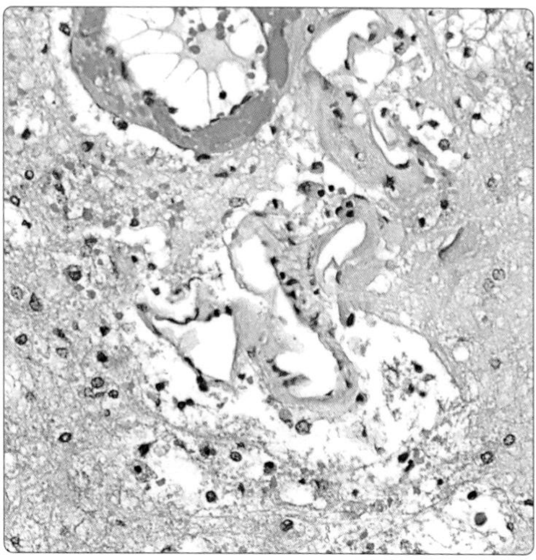

(Left) *Vessels often participate in radiation necrosis; in infarcts, vessels are often spared. Infarcts are rich in macrophages, whereas radiation necrosis is not.* **(Right)** *Vessel duplication and telangiectases are common variants of vasculopathy in late delayed radiation necrosis.*

Pseudoprogression

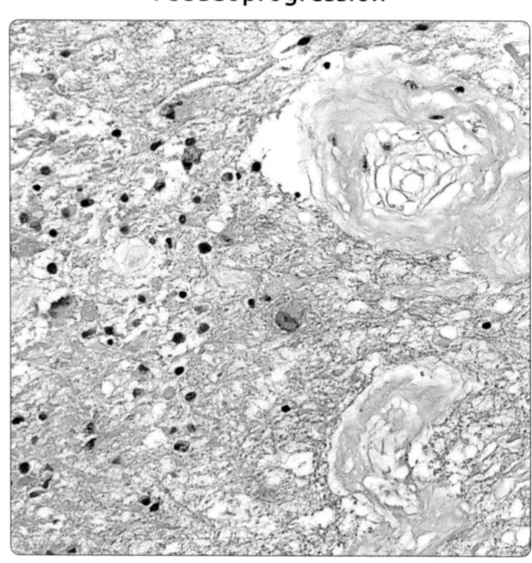

Glomeruloid Vascular Proliferation Simulating High-Grade Glioma

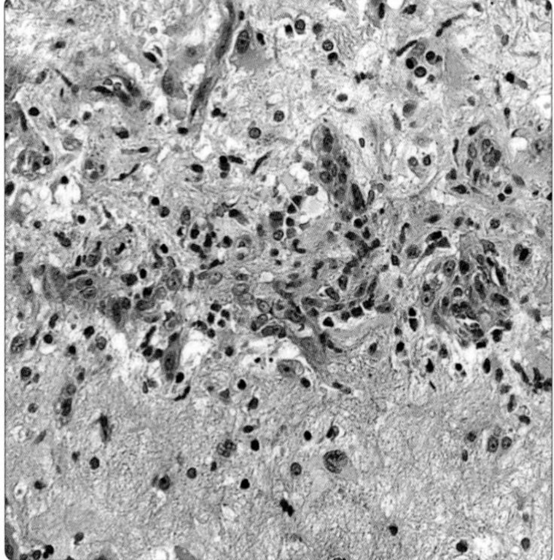

(Left) *In the context of a treated neoplasm, symptomatic &/or radiologically apparent radionecrosis is known as pseudoprogression. There is nothing in this treated lesion to suggest recurrent glioblastoma. In other cases of pseudoprogression, proliferating active glioma and radionecrosis coexist, in varying proportions.* **(Right)** *Glomeruloid vascular proliferation can, particularly in a case of pseudoprogression such as this, misrepresent the lesion as active high-grade glioma.*

(Left) *Densely calcified tissue may persist for the duration, unlike necrosis in other forms of injury such as infarcts, wherein necrotic debris is engulfed by macrophages and transported to vessels. Encephalomalacia is what remains in chronic infarcts, not the dense coagulum with superimposed dystrophic mineralization, as seen here.* **(Right)** *Well-circumscribed, brightly eosinophilic areas of coagulation necrosis mark the chronic lesion* ➙*. This is from the cerebellum; note the small dark blue nuclei of the granule cell neurons.*

Densely Calcified Tissue, Late Phases, Delayed Radionecrosis

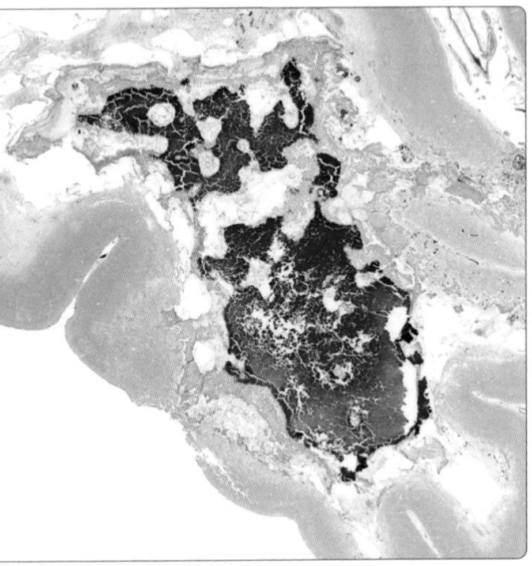

Eosinophilic Coagulum

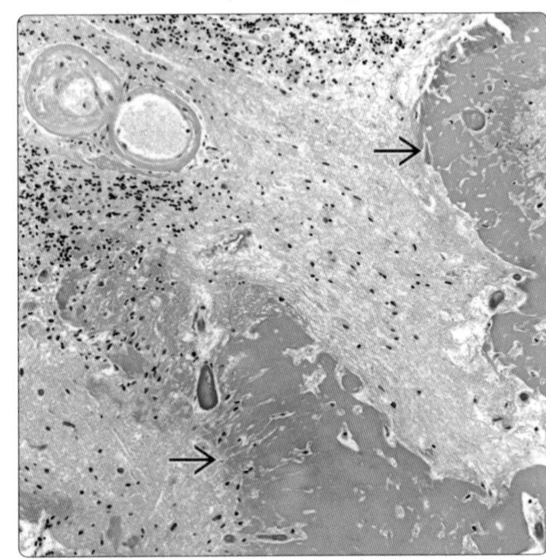

(Left) *Unresorbed, brightly eosinophilic areas of necrosis with a fibrinous quality* ➙ *may survive for years. Note the dilated vessels.* **(Right)** *Previously irradiated high-grade gliomas, such as this glioblastoma, may have only scattered pleomorphic cells* ➙ *in a somewhat fibrinous background. If neoplastic, they are inactive, not evidence of tumor regrowth.*

Unresorbed Fibrinous Exudate

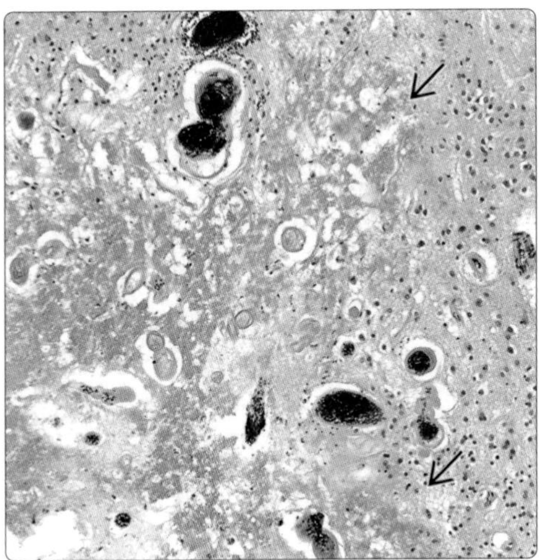

Residual Pleomorphic Cells

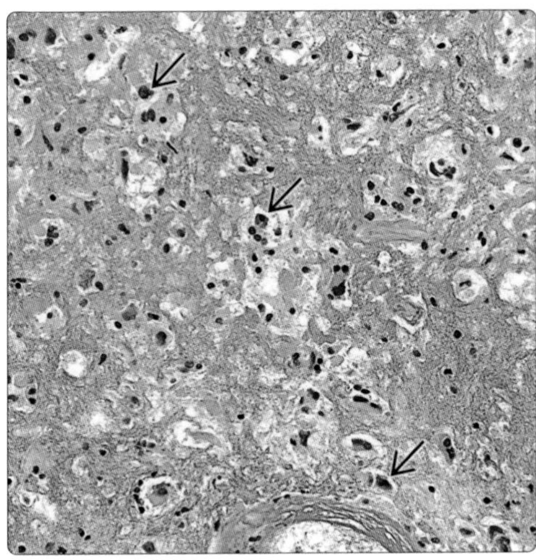

(Left) *An irradiated astrocytoma has a sharply defined area of necrosis, typical of radiation effect. While potentially so large and edema producing as to require debulking, the presence of such foci is not necessarily a complication. Note the absence of surrounding pseudopalisading tumor cells, in contrast to tumor-induced necrosis.* **(Right)** *It can be difficult to determine whether irradiated tissue contains tumor or just gliosis. The suspect cells* ➙ *in this case closely resemble those of the original astrocytoma.*

Absence of Pseudopalisading

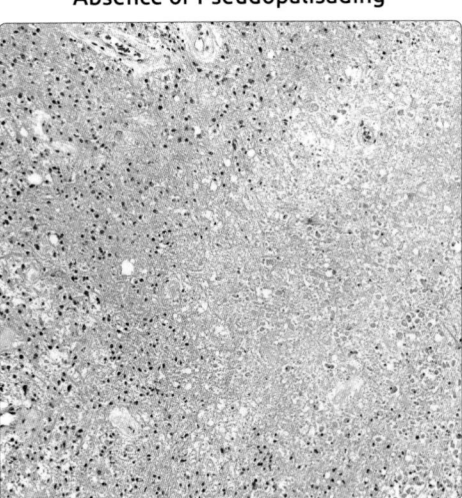

Tumor or Reactive Glia

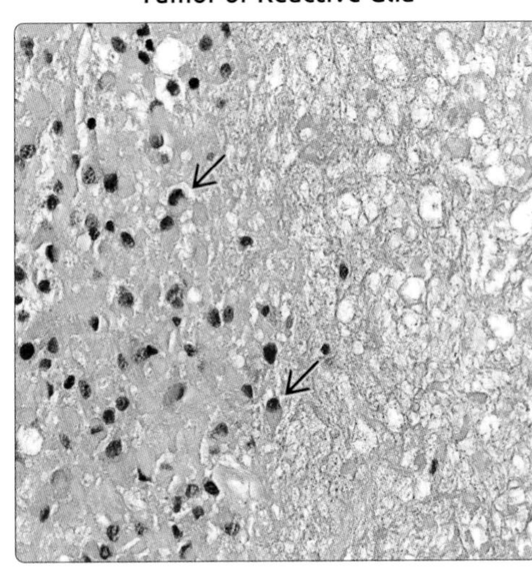

Radiation-Induced Cavernoma-Like Lesion

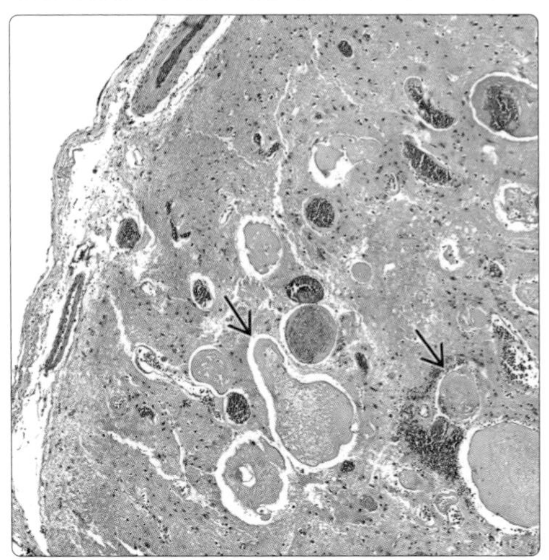

Radiation-Induced Cavernoma-Like Lesion

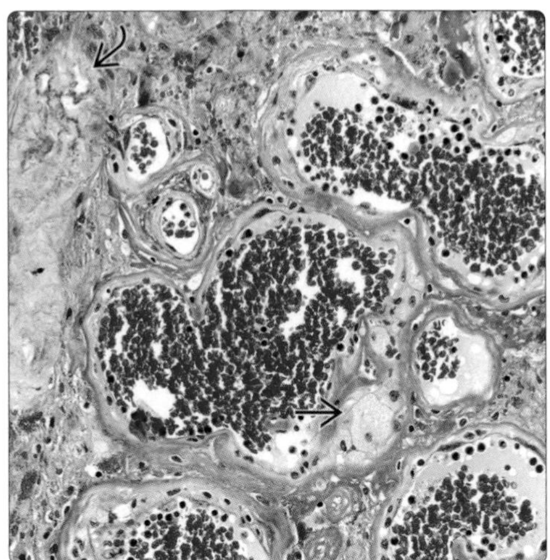

(Left) *Radiation can have, as a late effect, such severe vascular damage that cavernous malformation-like lesions develop in brain, although they are poor mimics of spontaneous cavernomas. Note that many of the vessels have lumina obliterated by remote fibrinoid vascular necrosis* →. **(Right)** *Radiation-induced cavernomas (cavernous malformation) are poor mimics of their sporadic counterparts. Note the macrophages trapped within the wall of these hyalinized vessels* →*, some of which are devoid of lumina* ↗.

Small-Vessel Hyalinization

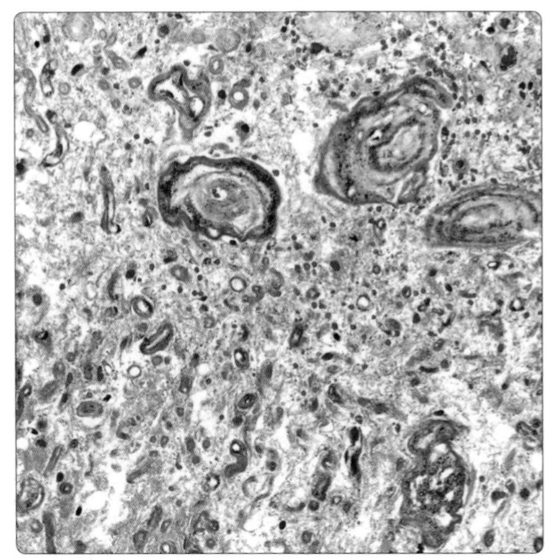

Radiation-Induced Atherosclerosis

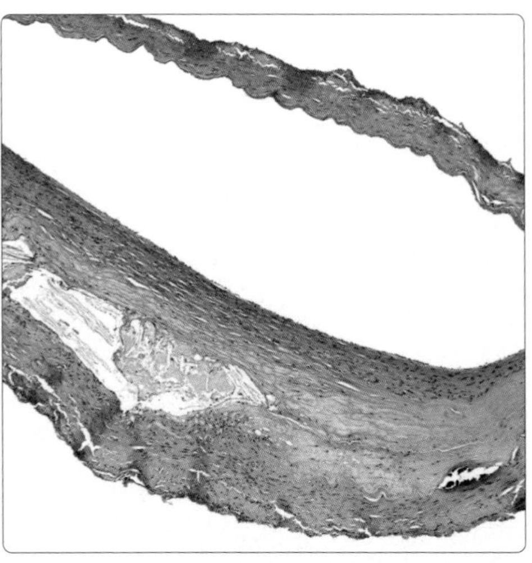

(Left) *Vessels of nearly all sizes can suffer hyalinization or damage as a late effect of radiation therapy; note the very small and medium-sized vessels with hyalinization in this trichrome-stained example.* **(Right)** *Radiation therapy can affect large vessels of the brain, including those from the circle of Willis, as in this example seen at autopsy. There are no distinctive histological features of radiation-induced vs. spontaneous atherosclerosis.*

Original Glioblastoma Prior to Radiation

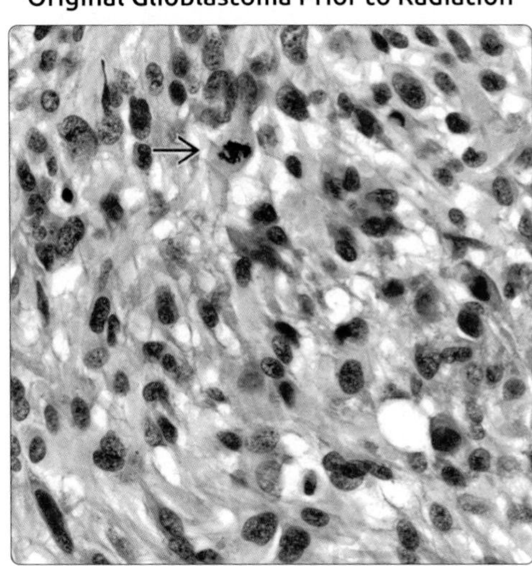

Glioblastoma, Postradiation Cytological Atypia

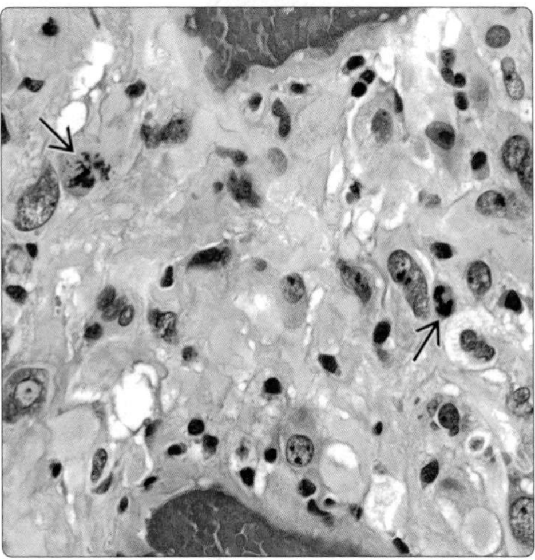

(Left) *This tumor prior to radiation therapy showed cytological atypia and numerous mitotic figures* →. **(Right)** *The glioblastoma seen in the previous image was rebiopsied 3 months later after recent completion of therapy. Note that, while a few mitotic figures persist* →*, there now is severe nuclear pleomorphism. The latter develops due to paralyzation of the mitotic apparatus, resulting in increased ploidy.*

Calcifying Pseudoneoplasm of the Neuraxis

KEY FACTS

TERMINOLOGY

- Discrete, chondrocalcific, sometimes ossified, mass with variable surface layer of epithelioid, presumably meningothelial, cells

CLINICAL ISSUES

- Leptomeningeal location
- Cured by resection

IMAGING

- Dark, often black, on T2W MR imaging

MACROSCOPIC

- Discrete, hard
- Most extraaxial
- Ostensibly intraparenchymal if intrasulcal

MICROSCOPIC

- Hypocellular fibrillar mass with peripheral "ropey" cords
- Amorphous to finely fibrillar core
- Chondroid matrix
- Variable superficial rind of spindle to epithelioid cells

ANCILLARY TESTS

- Surface cells variably EMA(+)

TOP DIFFERENTIAL DIAGNOSES

- Osteosarcoma
- Chondrosarcoma
- Tumoral calcinosis
- Meningioma with extensive calcifications

DIAGNOSTIC CHECKLIST

- Distinctive, "seen one, you've seen them all" appearance
- Spinal extradural examples probably different entity, e.g., tumoral calcinosis
- Considered nonneoplastic
- Discreteness aids in surgical excision, which is usually curative

Calcifying Pseudoneoplasm, Edema

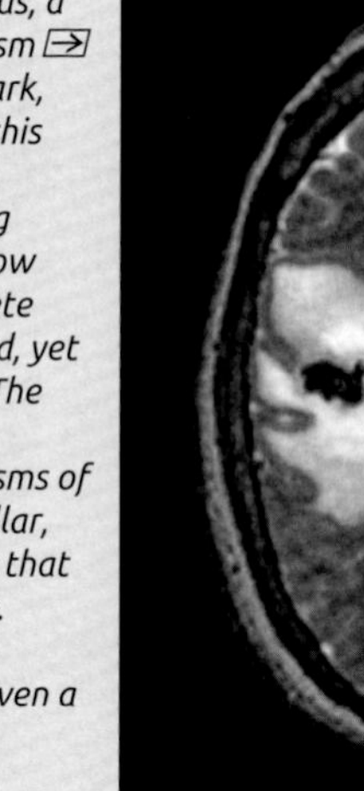

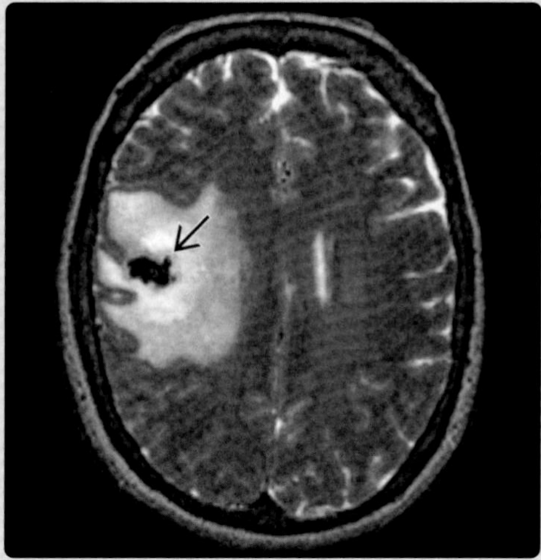

Classic Fibrillar Center, Calcifying Pseudoneoplasm

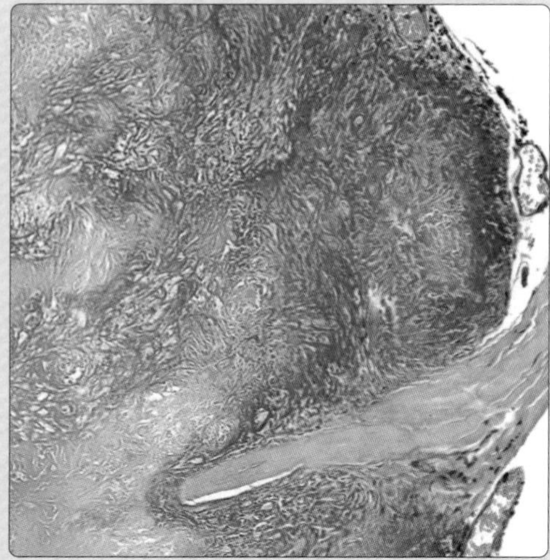

(Left) *Deep within a sulcus, a calcifying pseudoneoplasm → generates its typically dark, usually black profile on this T2WI MR. There is considerable surrounding edema.* **(Right)** *Even at low magnification, the discrete mass has an unstructured, yet distinctive, appearance. The central areas of classic calcifying pseudoneoplasms of the neuraxis have a fibrillar, haphazard linear quality that is seen in no other entity. When this obvious, chondrosarcoma is not even a consideration.*

Sharply Demarcated, Prominent Cortical Cells at Edge

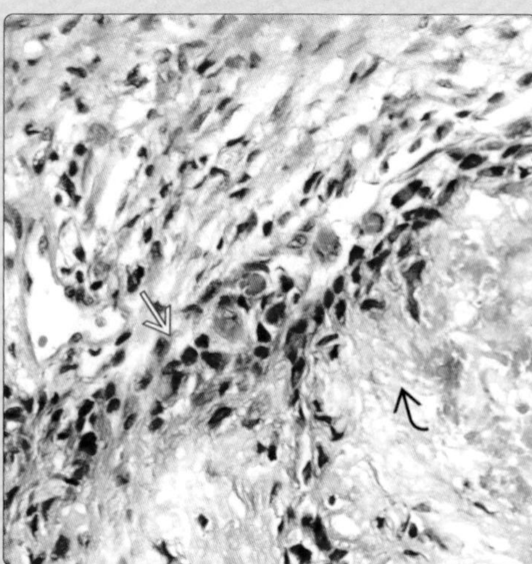

Inconspicuous Cortical Cells

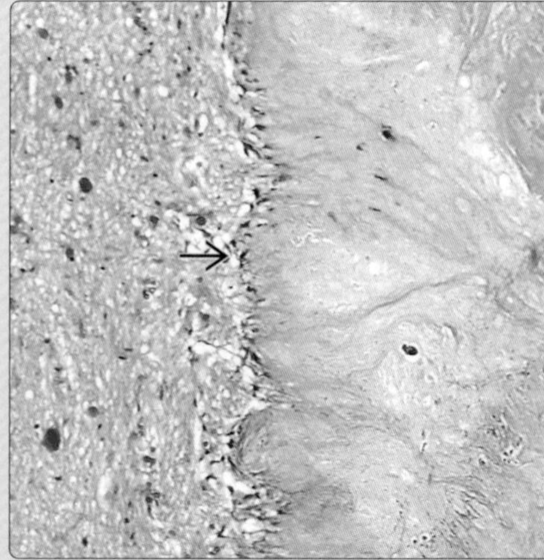

(Left) *Calcifying pseudoneoplasm of the neuraxis is sharply demarcated, with a variably prominent coating of cells at the edge called cortical cells →. They are prominent in this area. Note the characteristic finely fibrillar core →.* **(Right)** *The lesion can somewhat resemble fibrocartilage. Cortical cells are inconspicuous along the brain-lesion interface in this case →. True single cell invasion is not a feature of this well-circumscribed lesion. Note the finely fibrillar core in this image.*

TERMINOLOGY

Synonyms

- Calcifying pseudotumor
- "Crudoma"

Definitions

- Discrete, chondrocalcific, sometimes ossified, mass with variable surface layer of epithelioid, presumably meningothelial, cells

ETIOLOGY/PATHOGENESIS

Sporadic

- Overwhelming majority; etiology unknown

In Neurofibromatosis 2

- Small percentage of all cases
- Incidence of calcifying pseudoneoplasm in this syndrome unknown

CLINICAL ISSUES

Epidemiology

- Age
    - Adults

Site

- Meninges
    - Supratentorial
        - Dura, especially falx
        - Leptomeninges; some ostensibly intraparenchymal, but actually intrasulcal
    - Intraspinal
- Spine
    - Often differs histologically from lesion described here (more granulomatous)
    - May be different entity, e.g., tumoral calcinosis

Presentation

- Site dependent
    - Seizures, intracranial
    - Cranial nerve signs and symptoms, intracranial
    - Back pain, intraspinal
- With meningioangiomatosis in neurofibromatosis 2, rare
- May be incidental microscopic finding associated with other processes, e.g., ependymoma, dysembryoplastic neuroepithelial tumor

Treatment

- Surgical approaches
    - Resection

Prognosis

- Excellent
- Cured by resection

IMAGING

MR Findings

- Discrete
- Variable enhancement
    - Usually peripheral
- Dark, often black, on T2WI MR
- Accompanying large cyst, some cases
- Little mass effect
- Perilesional edema
    - Variable
    - May be extensive

MACROSCOPIC

General Features

- Discrete, hard
- White
- Granular, gritty

MICROSCOPIC

Histologic Features

- Well circumscribed
- Hypocellular fibrillar mass with peripheral "ropey" cords
- Amorphous to finely fibrillar core
- Chondroid matrix
- Variable superficial rind of spindle to epithelioid cells (cortical layer)
- Mature bone (some cases)
- Mature adipose tissue (some cases)
- Spherical calcifications (some cases)

ANCILLARY TESTS

Immunohistochemistry

- Surface cells variably EMA(+)

DIFFERENTIAL DIAGNOSIS

Osteosarcoma

- High cellularity, anaplasia, mitoses
- Osteoid
- No radiating peripheral structures

Chondrosarcoma

- Hyaline cartilage
- Mitoses, high-grade examples
- No radiating peripheral structures

Meningioma

- Mass of meningothelial cells, hyalinized vessels
- No fibrillar/chondroid matrix
- No radiating peripheral structures

Tumoral Calcinosis

- Extradural, spine
- Histiocytic and granulomatous response
- No cortical cells
- No radiating peripheral structures

SELECTED REFERENCES

1. Stienen MN et al: Calcifying pseudoneoplasms of the neuraxis (CAPNON): clinical features and therapeutic options. Acta Neurochir (Wien). 155(1):9-17, 2013
2. Aiken AH et al: Calcifying pseudoneoplasms of the neuraxis: CT, MR imaging, and histologic features. AJNR Am J Neuroradiol. 30(6):1256-60, 2009

(Left) *The rind of plump cortical cells ⇒ is not always as obvious as it is in this case. While nonspecific, the finely fibrillar core is characteristic.* **(Right)** *Calcifying pseudoneoplasm of the neuraxis is sharply demarcated, with a variably prominent coating of cells at the edge called cortical cells ⇒. They are prominent in this area. Note the characteristic fibrillar core ⇒.*

Obvious Cortical Cells

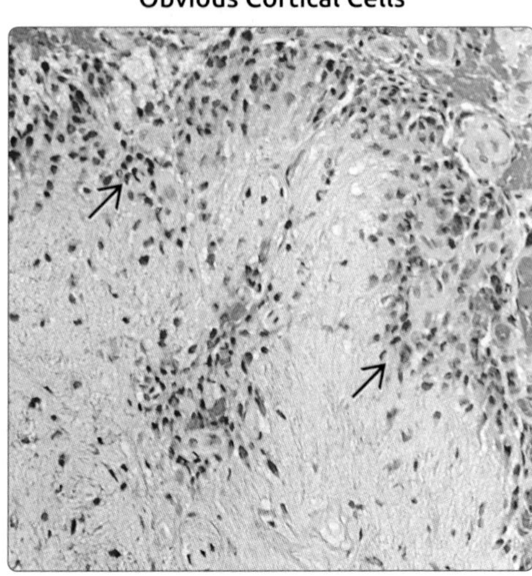

Sharp Demarcation

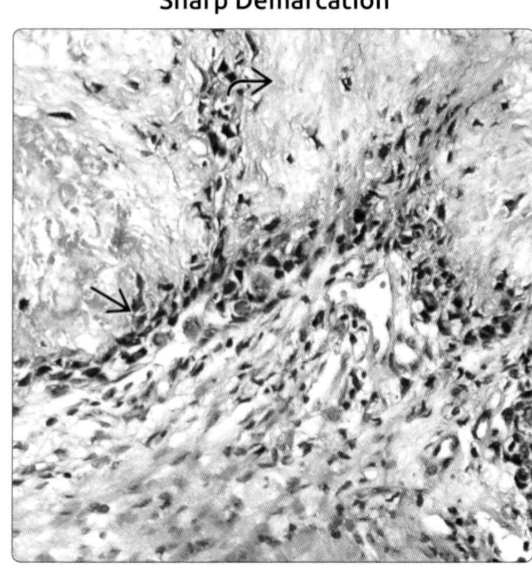

(Left) *An interrupted cortical layer ⇒ overlies a basophilic core in a classic calcifying pseudoneoplasm. Overall, it is a largely unstructured, but also rather distinctive, entity.* **(Right)** *The linear quality of the fibrillar core and the paucity of nuclei is characteristic of calcifying pseudotumor (CAPNON).*

Cortical Layer Overlying Basophilic Core

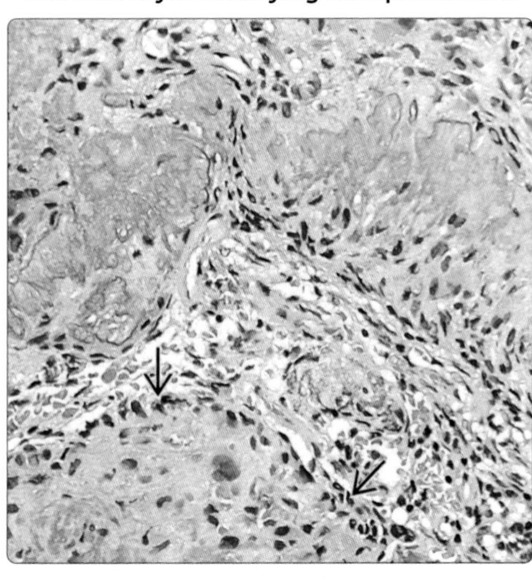

Fibrillar Core

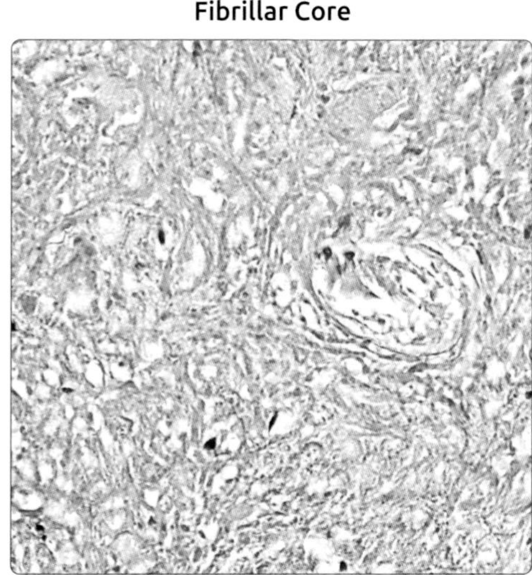

(Left) *The core of this example is lumpy and congealed, rather than finely fibrillar. The superficial cells ⇒ are not continuous enough to be considered a layer in this case.* **(Right)** *Lumpy eosinophilic cords ⇒ radiating to the surface are distinctive and characteristic features of calcifying pseudoneoplasm. Individually, they bear a resemblance to Rosenthal fibers.*

Less Finely Fibrillar Core

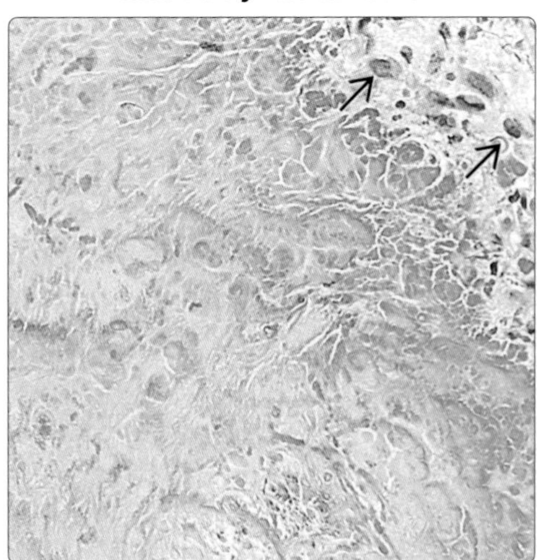

Lumpy Eosinophilic Cords

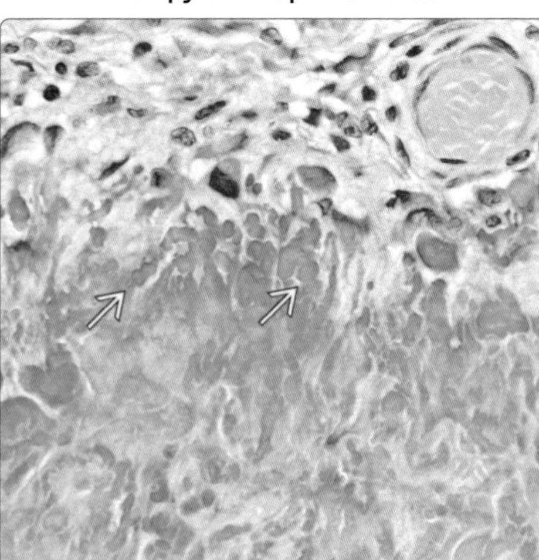

Vaguely Chondroid Areas

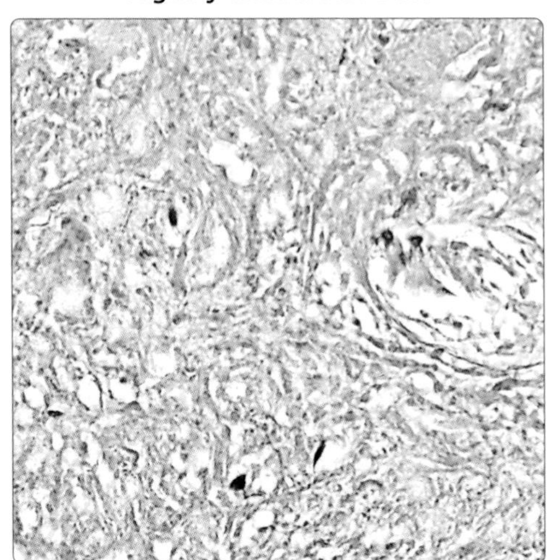

Calcified Spherules

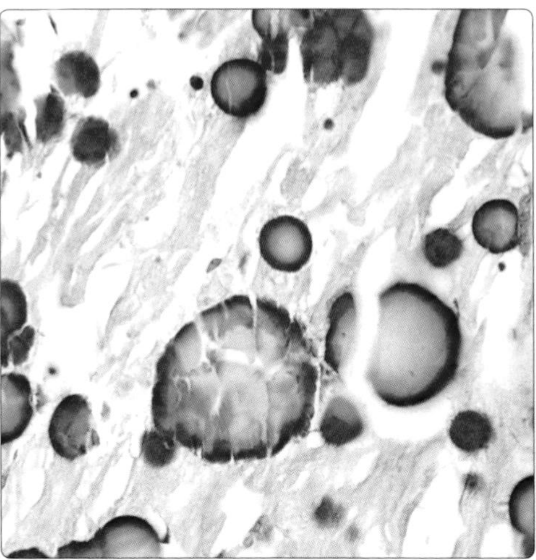

(Left) *Unstructured, amorphous, vaguely chondroid areas, such as this, are in themselves, only "consistent with" calcifying pseudoneoplasm. Chondrosarcoma and chondroma would be considerations, although the tissue is fibrillar in this image, not hyaline.* **(Right)** *Suspended calcified spherules enliven some examples. The structures somewhat resemble psammoma bodies but lack the latter's laminated architecture and origin within a whorl.*

Occasional Lamellar Bone

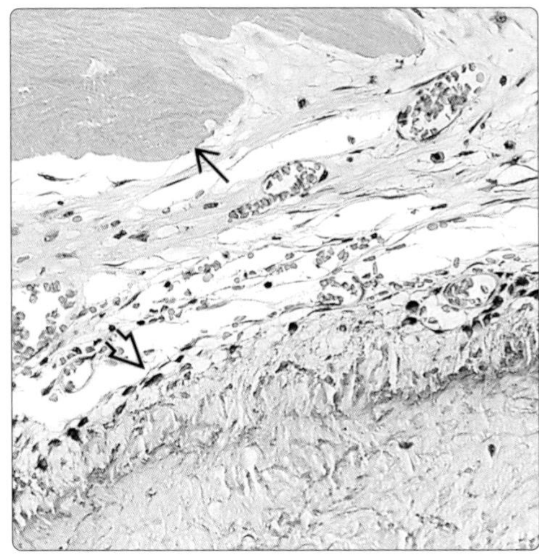

Coexistent Adipose Tissue

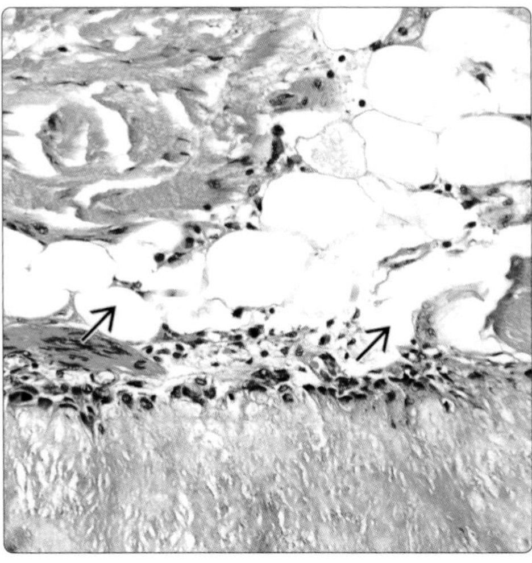

(Left) *Lamellar bone ➙ is occasionally present in this longstanding, slowly growing lesion. Note the interrupted layer of cortical cells ➙.* **(Right)** *Calcifying pseudoneoplasms may be associated with mature adipose tissue ➙. The finely fibrillar amorphous tissue at the bottom is typical of this uncommon, generally leptomeningeal lesion.*

EMA(+) Cortical Cells, Prominent

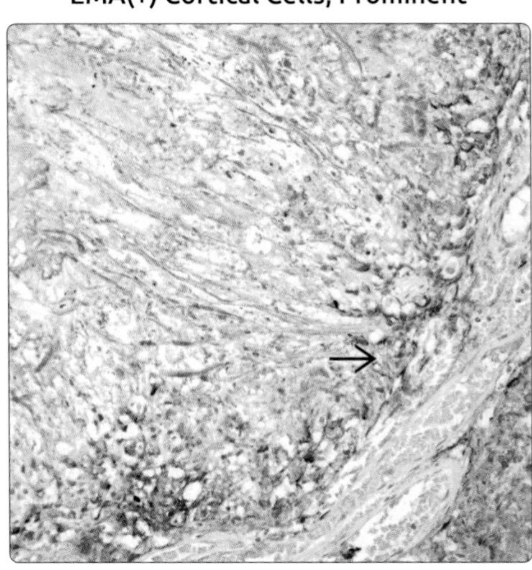

EMA(+) Suggests Meningothelial Origin

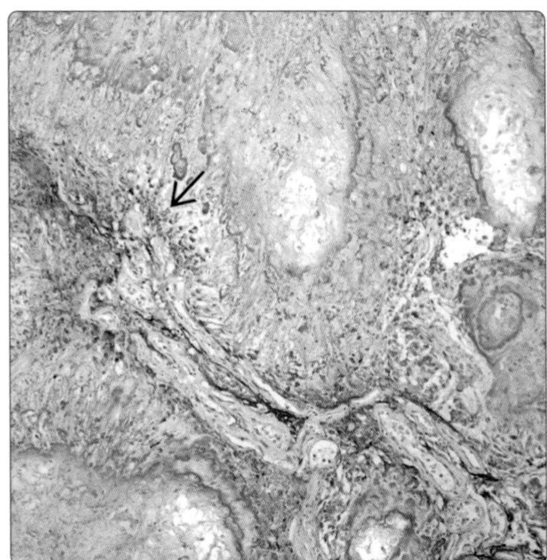

(Left) *Lobules in CAPNON are defined by their EMA(+) cortical cells ➙. While prominent in this case, such immunoreactive cells are sometimes sparse.* **(Right)** *Fine surface staining of cells within the superficial layer with EMA ➙ is consistent with a meningothelial origin. The extent and intensity for EMA varies from case to case.*

PART II
SECTION 3
Vascular Diseases

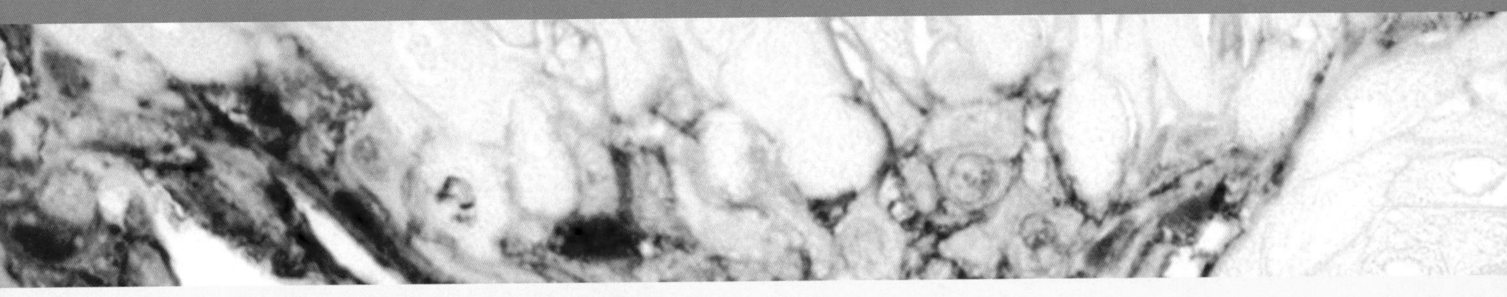

Vascular Malformations and Neoplasms

Vascular Lesions

Vasculitis and Vasculopathy

Telangiectasis

KEY FACTS

ETIOLOGY/PATHOGENESIS

- Sporadic, common
- No known etiology
- No known genetic association
- Only very rarely seen in association with hereditary hemorrhagic telangiectasia syndrome
- Hereditary hemorrhagic telangiectasia syndrome more likely to be associated with brain arteriovenous malformations or pulmonary arteriovenous malformations

CLINICAL ISSUES

- Asymptomatic, incidental
- Almost never requires biopsy

MACROSCOPIC

- Small, subtle hyperemic, discrete lesion(s)
- Most common in basis pontis
- Usually solitary but may be multiple
- Usually < 1 cm in diameter
- No mass effect
- No surrounding hemosiderin staining
- No associated hemorrhage
- Occasional small venous component, and then overlap with venous angioma

MICROSCOPIC

- Thin-walled, closely clustered, dilated capillaries
- No thrombosis, hyalinization, or calcification
- Intervening brain parenchyma histologically normal

DIAGNOSTIC CHECKLIST

- Incidental finding, unassociated with acute, subacute, or chronic blood products

(Left) *Axial T2* GRE MR shows mildly decreased signal intensity ➔. As is typical, this telangiectasis has no mass effect. The lesion is almost always an incidental finding.* **(Right)** *A blush of enhancement ➔ is usually the solitary radiological finding. As here, most telangiectases occur in the pons.*

Axial MR: Pontine Location

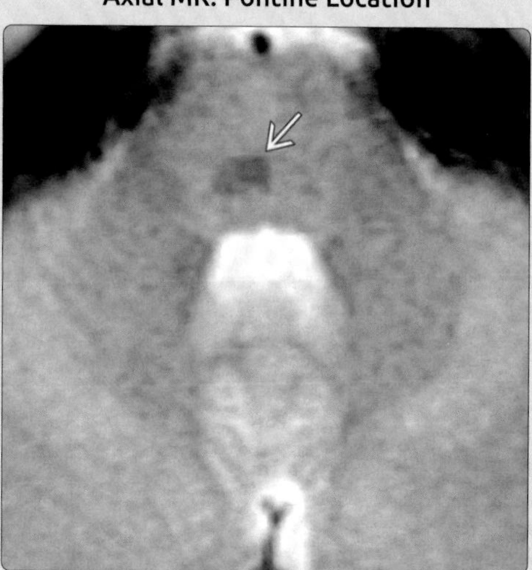

Axial MR: Blush of Enhancement

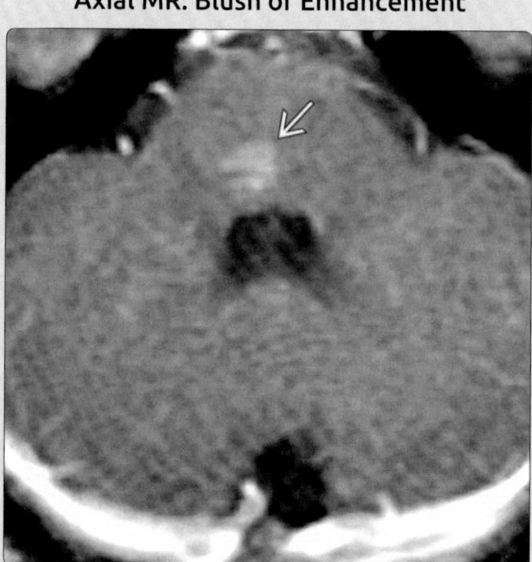

(Left) *Telangiectasias within the cortex can mimic a metastatic tumor grossly. Compare the vascular malformation to the normal cortex with normal vascular density ➔.* **(Right)** *Telangiectasias are neither prone to bleeding or thrombosis; the parenchyma surrounding these dilated capillaries is normal.*

Cortical Telangiectasia

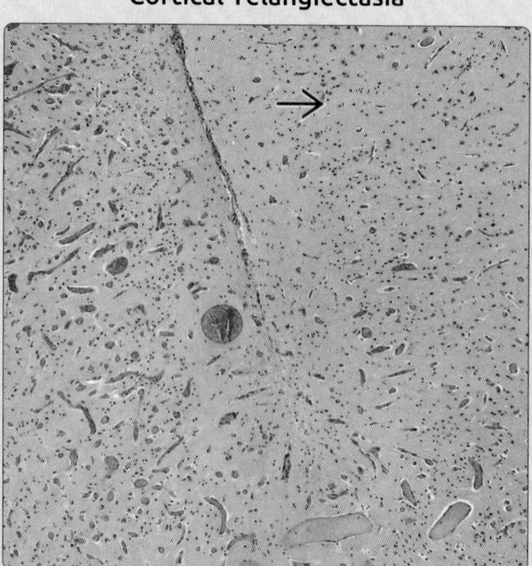

Surrounding Normal Parenchyma

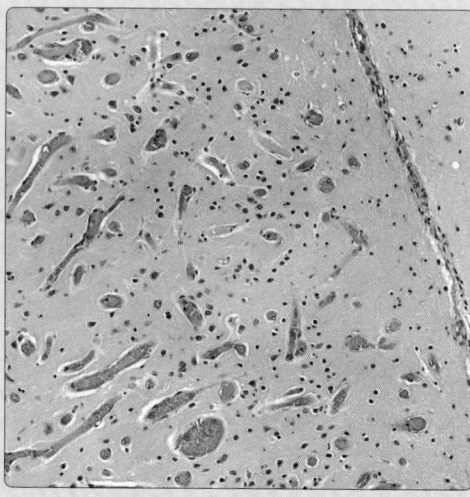

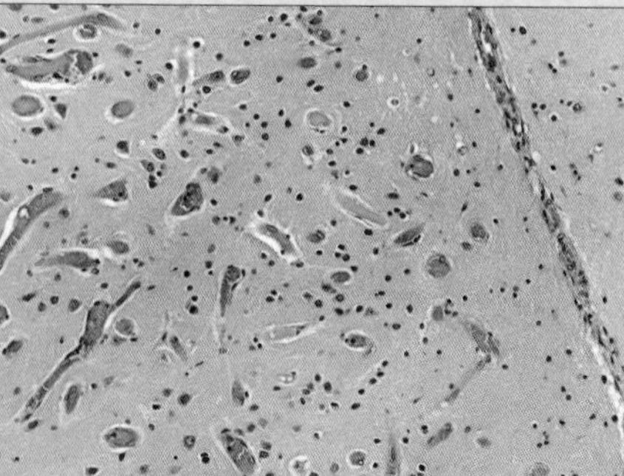

TERMINOLOGY

Synonyms

- Capillary telangiectasia, brain capillary telangiectasia (BCT)

Definitions

- Vascular malformation with clusters of thin-walled, mildly dilated capillaries and normal intervening brain parenchyma

ETIOLOGY/PATHOGENESIS

Developmental Anomaly

- Sporadic vascular anomaly
- May be multiple
- No genetic association for vast majority
- Rare in hereditary hemorrhagic telangiectasia (HHT, Rendu-Osler-Weber syndrome)
  - Hereditary hemorrhagic telangiectasia syndrome more likely to be associated with brain arteriovenous malformations or pulmonary arteriovenous malformations

CLINICAL ISSUES

Epidemiology

- Incidence
  - Common incidental finding, neuroimaging or autopsy
  - Constitutes 15-20% of all vascular malformations

Site

- Pons, usually basis pontis
- Spinal cord
- Subcortical cerebral white matter
- Medulla
- Midbrain

Presentation

- Asymptomatic, incidental
- Very rarely bleeds or becomes symptomatic

Treatment

- None required

Prognosis

- Excellent; little or no chance for spontaneous hemorrhage
- No role for embolization

IMAGING

MR Findings

- Minimal/subtle hypointense T2WI bright lesion
- Faint blush of homogeneous enhancement (some cases)
- T1W images without contrast usually normal
- No mass effect
- Normal angiogram

MACROSCOPIC

General Features

- Usually small (2 mm to < 1 cm) hyperemic area
- Ill-defined borders
- No surrounding acute hemorrhage
- No hemosiderin staining

MICROSCOPIC

Histologic Features

- Thin-walled, closely clustered, mildly dilated capillaries with small amount of normal intervening brain parenchyma
- Vessel walls devoid of calcification or hyalinization
- No thrombosis
- No hemosiderin

DIFFERENTIAL DIAGNOSIS

Small, Hyperemic Metastasis

- Neoplastic cells

Focal Petechial Hemorrhage

- Absence of increased numbers of capillaries, presence of red blood cells in parenchyma

Cavernous Malformation

- Larger, more closely juxtaposed vascular caverns with hyalinized walls
- Hemosiderin staining and gliosis
- Thrombosis, recent and remote
- 80% supratentorial, although occasionally present in pons

Venous Angioma (Developmental Venous Anomaly)

- Venous angioma more likely to be located at angle of ventricle near frontal horn or adjacent to 4th ventricle
- Dilated veins more widely dispersed within brain parenchyma
- Fewer vessels per unit area
- Caput medusa imaging profile

DIAGNOSTIC CHECKLIST

Clinically Relevant Pathologic Features

- Incidental finding, unassociated with acute, subacute, or chronic blood products

Pathologic Interpretation Pearls

- Thin-walled capillaries with small amount of intervening brain parenchyma but no surrounding hemosiderin staining
- Almost never requires biopsy

SELECTED REFERENCES

1. Alvarez H et al: Genetic markers and their influence on cerebrovascular malformations. Neuroimaging Clin N Am. 25(1):69-82, 2015
2. Beukers RJ et al: Pontine capillary telangiectasia as visualized on MR imaging causing a clinical picture resembling basilar-type migraine: a case report. J Neurol. 256(10):1775-7, 2009
3. Abla A et al: Developmental venous anomaly, cavernous malformation, and capillary telangiectasia: spectrum of a single disease. Acta Neurochir (Wien). 150(5):487-9; discussion 489, 2008
4. Morinaka S et al: Abrupt onset of sensorineural hearing loss and tinnitus in a patient with capillary telangiectasia of the pons. Ann Otol Rhinol Laryngol. 111(9):855-9, 2002
5. Castillo M et al: MR imaging and histologic features of capillary telangiectasia of the basal ganglia. AJNR Am J Neuroradiol. 22(8):1553-5, 2001
6. Clatterbuck RE et al: The juxtaposition of a capillary telangiectasia, cavernous malformation, and developmental venous anomaly in the brainstem of a single patient: case report. Neurosurgery. 49(5):1246-50, 2001
7. Scaglione C et al: Symptomatic unruptured capillary telangiectasia of the brain stem: report of three cases and review of the literature. J Neurol Neurosurg Psychiatry. 71(3):390-3, 2001
8. McCormick WF et al: Vascular malformations ("angiomas") of the brain, with special reference to those occurring in the posterior fossa. J Neurosurg. 28(3):241-51, 1968

(Left) *Telangiectases are most common in the pons, specifically the base →. There is no mass effect, hemorrhage, or surrounding hemosiderin staining in these lesions that are most always asymptomatic incidental findings, whether radiological or pathological (post mortem).* **(Right)** *Pontine telangiectasia is often an incidental finding at autopsy; the blush of discoloration can be misinterpreted as a pontine hemorrhage or as a vascular metastasis. (Courtesy AFIP.)*

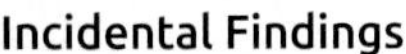

Incidental Findings

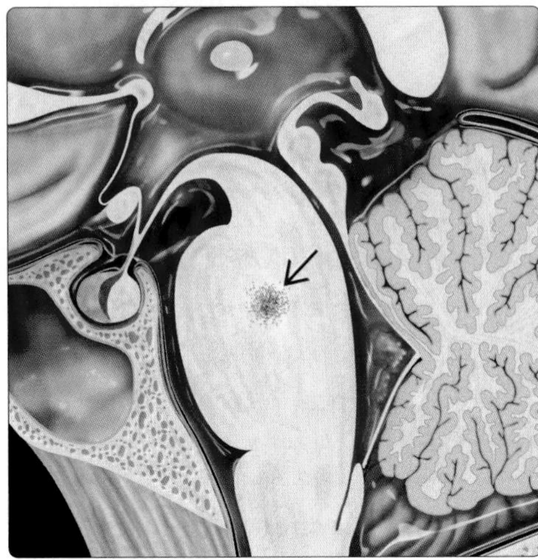

Tissue Discoloration

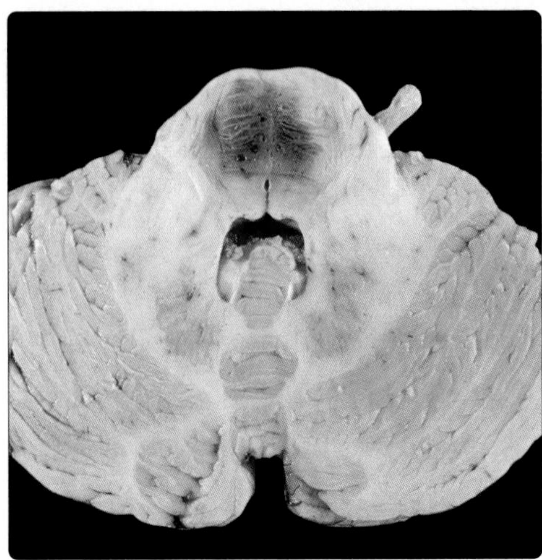

(Left) *The capillary aggregates in a telangiectasis are often more apparent at low magnification.* **(Right)** *Capillary telangiectases are nothing more than scattered, thin-walled, generally uniform, delicate vessels. Normal brain parenchyma is interspersed with the telangiectasis.*

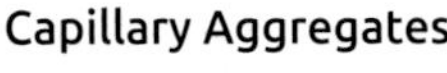

Capillary Aggregates

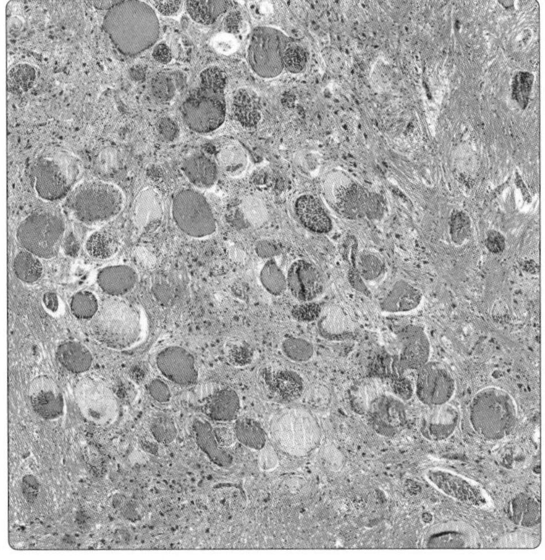

Uniform Delicate Vessels

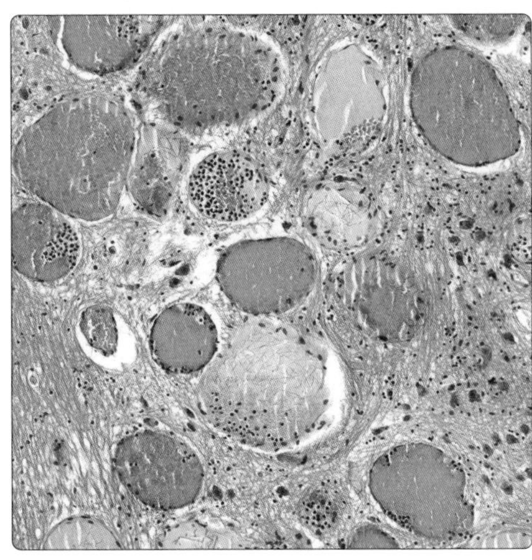

(Left) *Intravascular protein threads or strands can be misconstrued as fungal hyphae, although the latter are more uniform. Grocott methenamine silver staining will be negative as well. Such conglomerates often marginate in small and medium-caliber vessels, including those of a telangiectasis.* **(Right)** *Neutrophils may congregate harmlessly in the small caliber vessels of a telangiectasis.*

Protein Threads

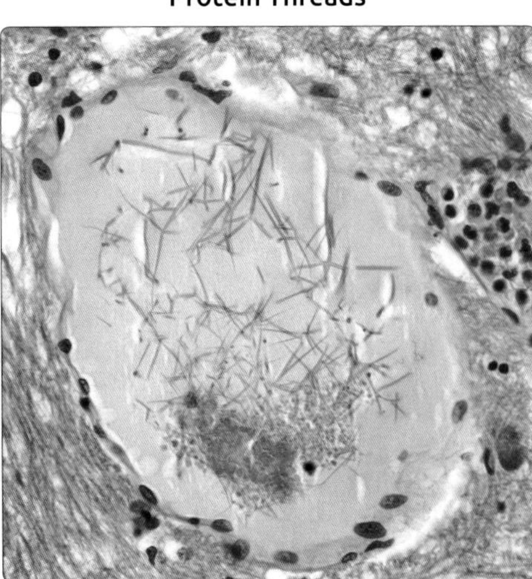

Neutrophil Margination

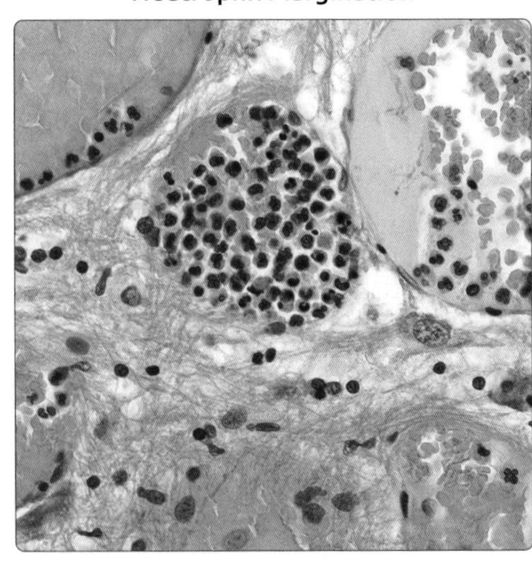

Venous Angioma

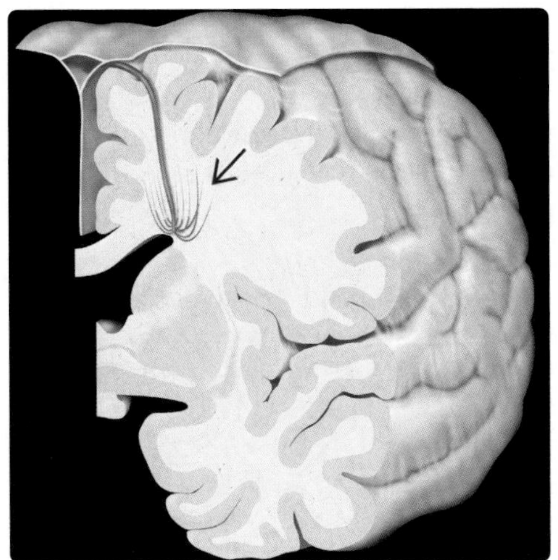

Medusa-Head Architecture

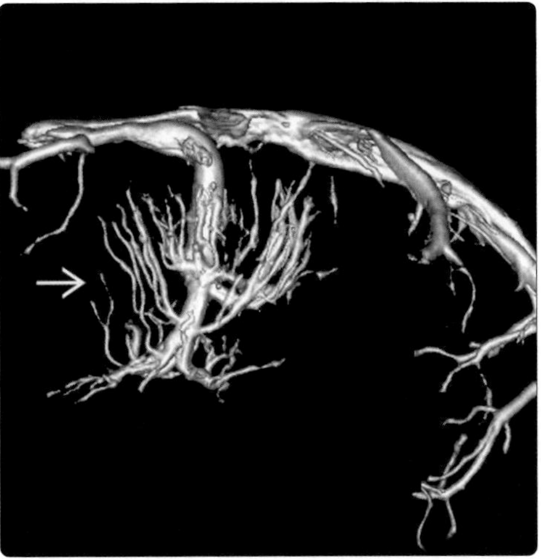

(Left) *Coronal oblique graphic of a developmental venous anomaly (venous angioma) shows a tuft-like Medusa head group of mature, dilated veins ➡ draining into a single major venous trunk. The lesion is depicted in its most common location, near the lateral aspect of the lateral ventricle.* **(Right)** *Developmental venous angioma can be reconstructed in a 3D fashion (3D DSA angio) to show the exquisite Medusa head-like ➡ architecture. (Courtesy P. Lasjaunias, MD.)*

Incidental Venous Angioma

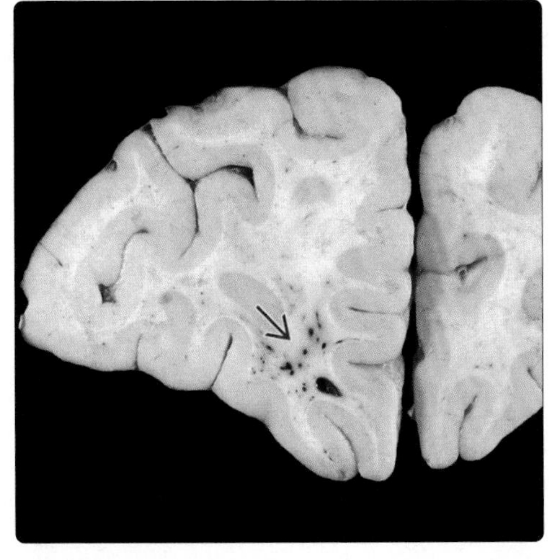

More Compact

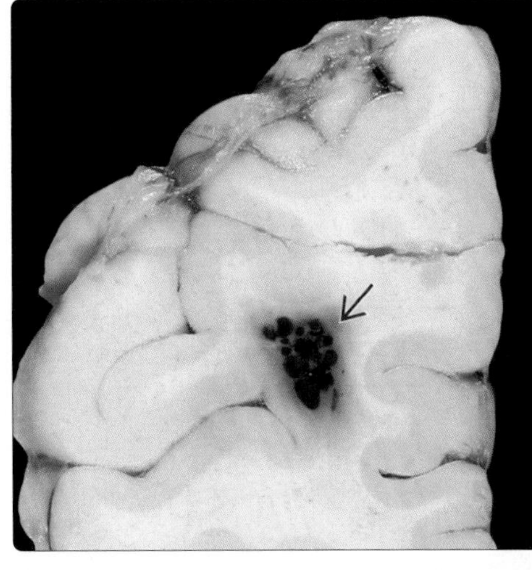

(Left) *This venous angioma is an incidental finding; it is composed of a loose aggregate of slightly dilated veins of varying calibers ➡ and located near the cortical gray-white junction.* **(Right)** *Occasional lesions ➡ are more compact than the usual venous angioma, but composed of normal veins, not the hyalinized vessels of a cavernoma. As with the classic dispersed venous angiomas, these difficult-to-classify lesions are unassociated with hemosiderin deposition.*

Veins Patent

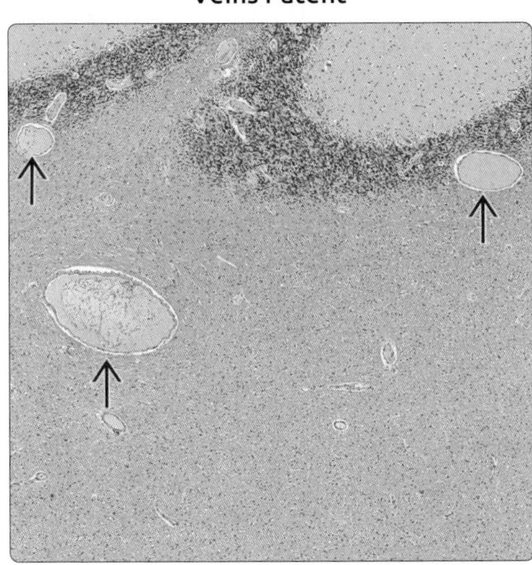

Simulating Intravascular Fungi

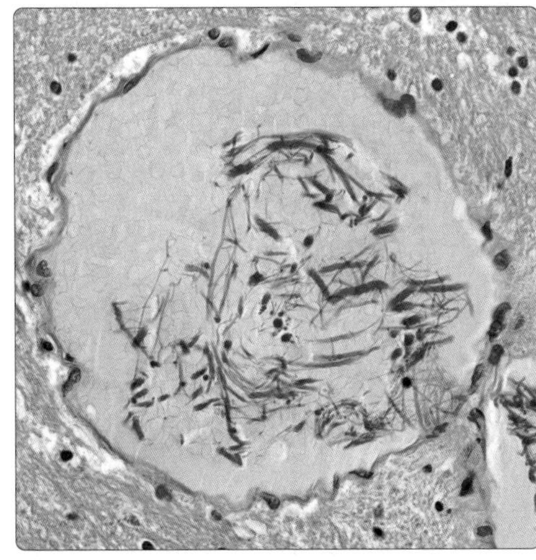

(Left) *Venous angiomas are composed of dilated, patent delicate veins ➡ separated by expanses of normal intervening brain parenchyma. Note the absence of blood products or rarefaction of the interspersed white matter.* **(Right)** *Other than dilatation, component veins of a venous angioma are unremarkable. They may contain protein strands (protein threads) that should not be mistaken for fungi. Protein threads lack the homogeneity of size and shape expected of infectious organisms.*

Cavernous Angioma

KEY FACTS

TERMINOLOGY

- Mulberry-like aggregate of hyalinized vascular caverns

ETIOLOGY/PATHOGENESIS

- Developmental anomaly
  - Multiple lesions should prompt consideration of familial form or history of cranial radiation therapy
- Environmental exposure
  - Radiation-induced cavernous malformations arise years after receipt of radiation, often in childhood

CLINICAL ISSUES

- Most common mutation in persons of Hispanic American ethnicity is CCM1 (*KRIT1*)

MACROSCOPIC

- Tight mulberry-like aggregate of hyalinized blood vessels
- Peripheral hemosiderin staining
- Discrete

MICROSCOPIC

- Usually have repeated subclinical bleeding episodes leading to varying ages of blood products
- Often calcified
- Intense gliosis and surrounding hypercellularity
- Ferrugination of surrounding parenchyma

DIAGNOSTIC CHECKLIST

- Discrete nature allows for surgical cure
- Compact, hyalinized vessels without features of arteries or veins
- Hemosiderin stained and gliotic surrounding parenchyma

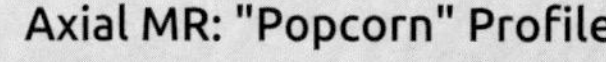

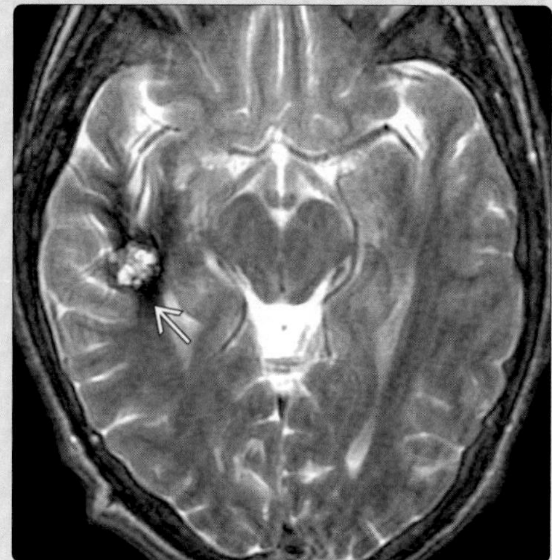

Familial Cavernous Angioma Syndrome

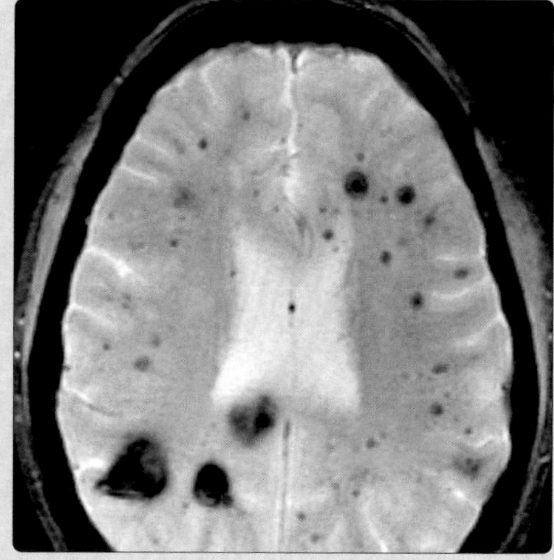

(Left) *Cavernomas have multinodular "popcorn" profiles and surrounding rims of dark signal due to hemosiderin ➔ in T2W and FLAIR images.* **(Right)** *Axial T2* GRE MR in a patient with familial syndrome of multiple cavernomas shows innumerable foci of "blooming" signal loss caused by ferromagnetic blood products.*

Closely Juxtaposed Hyalinized Channels

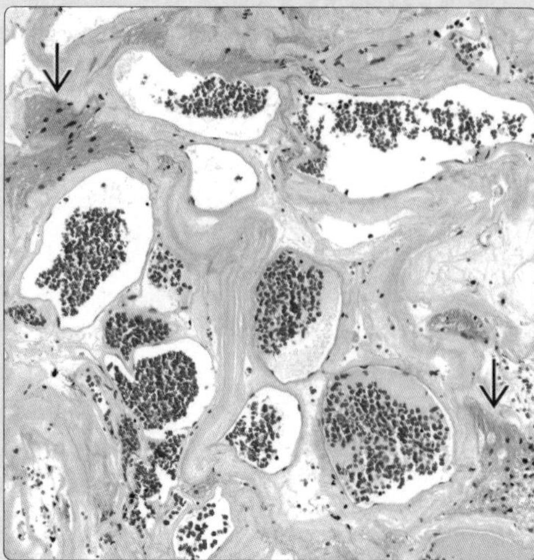

Surrounding Hemosiderin

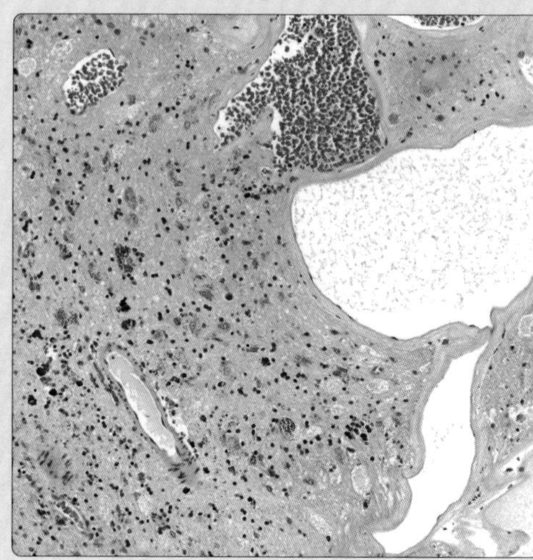

(Left) *Cavernous angiomas (synonymous with cavernoma) are composed of closely juxtaposed, hyalinized vascular channels. There is no arterial component. Only a small amount of interspersed brain tissue is present ⇨.* **(Right)** *Cavernous malformations are low-flow vascular malformations that often leak blood repetitively. They are usually surrounded by hemosiderin pigment.*

TERMINOLOGY

Synonyms

- Cavernous malformation, cerebral cavernous malformation (CCM), cavernoma

Definitions

- Vascular disorder of brain characterized by abnormal vascular spaces lined by single layer of endothelium without intervening neural parenchyma or identifiable mature vessel wall elements (Gunel definition)

ETIOLOGY/PATHOGENESIS

Developmental Anomaly

- Congenital vascular malformation with low pressure
- Isolated lesion in sporadic form of disease
- Multiple lesions in familial form
- New lesions develop over time at rate of 0.4 lesions per patient per year in familial form
- Etiology in familial forms consistent with "2-hit hypothesis," with germline mutation in 1 gene and somatic mutation in 2nd gene within vascular endothelial cells
- Adjacent venous angioma in some cases

Environmental Exposure

- Radiation-induced examples
  - Form years or decades after irradiation
  - More common in patients irradiated during childhood
  - May be multiple

CLINICAL ISSUES

Epidemiology

- Incidence
  - Incidence of 0.00056% in adults (age > 16 years) in Scottish Intracranial Vascular Malformation Study
  - Autosomal dominant inheritance in familial form
  - 3 genes identified to date: CCM1 (*KRIT1*), CCM2 (malcavernin, *C7orf22*), CCM3 (programmed cell death 10, *PDCD10*)
  - Penetrance in patients with CCM1 estimated at 60-88%, in CCM2 100%, in CCM3 63%
  - Increasing cumulative incidence in long-term survivors of medulloblastoma at 3, 5, and 10 years after radiation, but most do not require intervention
- Ethnicity
  - CCM1 mutation seen in virtually all persons of Hispanic American heritage with cavernomas
  - CCM1 mutation in Spanish American kindreds known to be due to founder mutation in common ancestor

Site

- Throughout CNS, including spinal cord

Presentation

- Seizures: Usual presentation
- Recurrent headache
- Focal motor/sensory deficits
- Lesions symptomatic in 60% with familial form

Treatment

- Resection for diagnosis, hemorrhage, enlargement, or seizures

Prognosis

- Excellent following resection
- Incidence of symptomatic hemorrhage: 1.1% per year

IMAGING

MR Findings

- Popcorn ball appearance of mixed hyper- and hypointense blood-containing channels in T1WI
- "Blooming" artifact due to iron (hemosiderin) in T2W gradient-echo images
- Little blood flow

MACROSCOPIC

General Features

- Most (80%) supratentorial
- Mulberry-like cluster of tightly compacted dilated vessels
- Heterogeneous discoloration due to admixed acute and subacute blood products, hemosiderin, gliosis, myelin breakdown in surrounding brain

MICROSCOPIC

Histologic Features

- Closely juxtaposed, dilated vascular channels, little or no intervening brain parenchyma
- Variable vascular hyalinization and absence of muscularis or well-developed venous or arterial features
- "Knots" of hyalinization representing remote thrombosis, as well as ongoing thrombosis
- Calcification
- Peripheral hemosiderin, gliosis, and rarely Gamna-Gandy bodies
- Iron-induced axonal spheroids in surrounding parenchyma
- Endothelial cells attenuated but cytologically normal despite possible somatic mutation

DIFFERENTIAL DIAGNOSIS

Arteriovenous Malformation

- Large, wedge-shaped when occurring in cerebral cortex with broad base on leptomeningeal surface
- True veins and smaller numbers of arteries with latter identifiable by elastic stains
- Vessels usually lack thrombosis unless embolized

Capillary Telangiectasia

- Capillary-sized blood vessels devoid of thrombosis or surrounding hemosiderin or acute/subacute blood products
- Small amount of normal intervening brain parenchyma
- Most located in basis pontis
- Almost never seen as surgical specimen

SELECTED REFERENCES

1. Gault J et al: Cerebral cavernous malformations: somatic mutations in vascular endothelial cells. Neurosurgery. 65(1):138-44; discussion 144-5, 2009

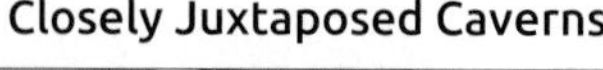

Closely Juxtaposed Caverns

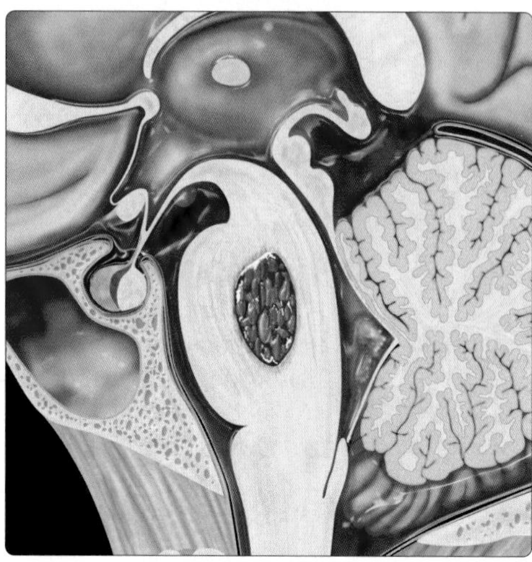

Discrete Red Masses

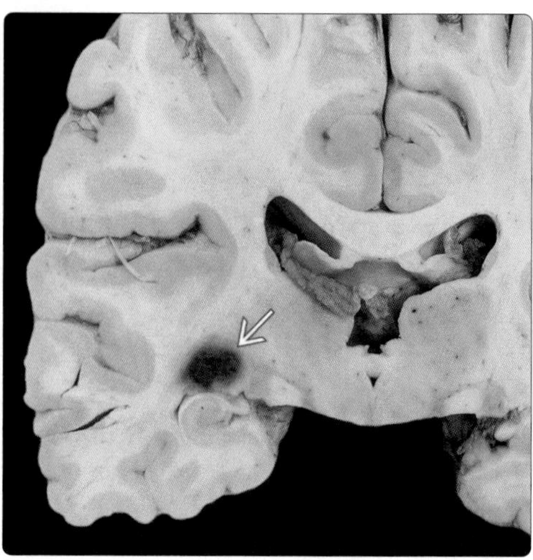

(Left) *Cavernomas, here in the pons, are composed of multiple closely juxtaposed caverns that contain blood products in varying stages of degradation. The thin brown rim is hemosiderin-stained parenchyma.* **(Right)** *Cavernomas are discrete, red masses* ➡ *that, on distant view, can be mistaken for small hematomas. The packed vascular channels that compose cavernous malformations may not be discernible without close inspection.*

Bleeding in Critical Location

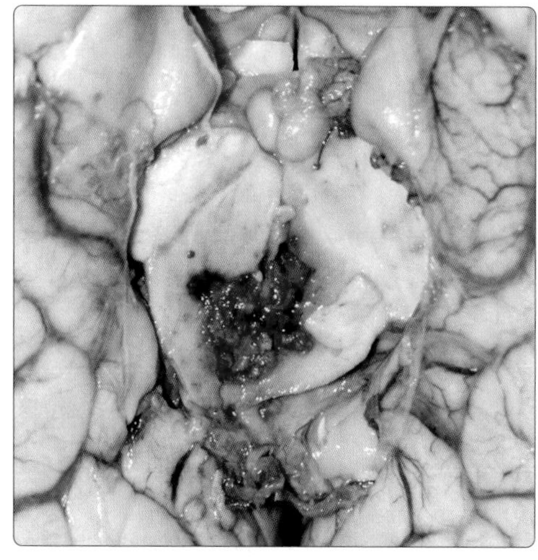

Multiple Cavernomas

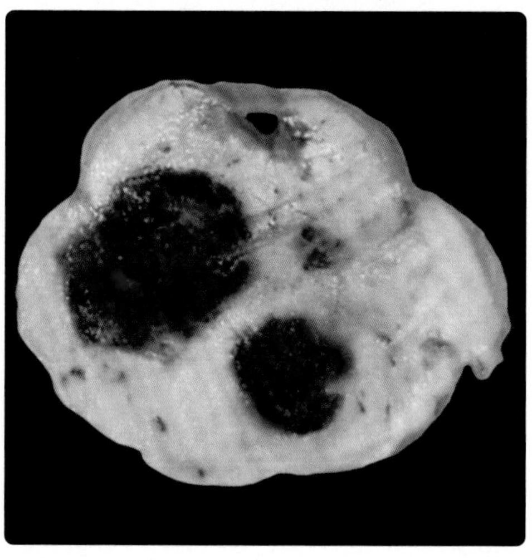

(Left) *Although most patients with cavernous malformations do not succumb to lesional hemorrhage, bleeding in critical locations, such as the brainstem, may prove fatal.* **(Right)** *Multiple pontine cavernous angiomas can occur in the disease's familial form. Surgical resection is possible for more favorably placed lesions given cavernomas' usually discrete nature.*

Juxtaposed Vascular Channels

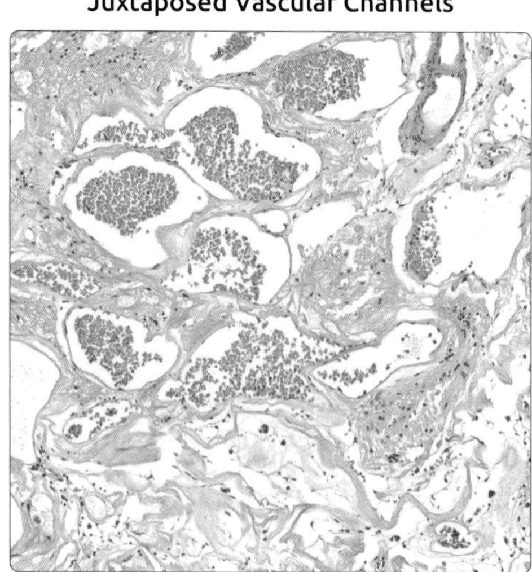

Surrounding Gliosis

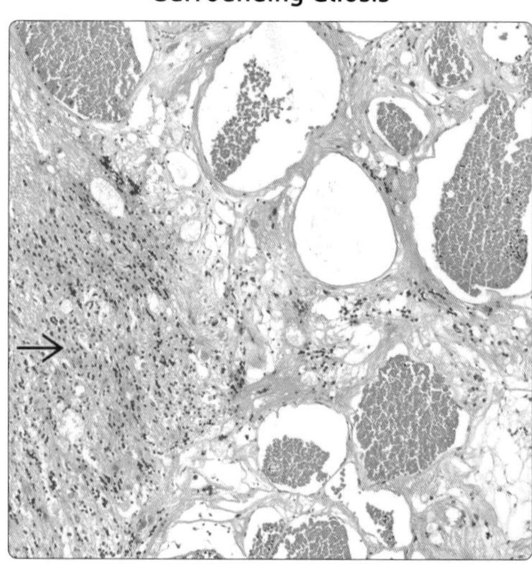

(Left) *The typical cavernoma has tightly juxtaposed abnormal vascular channels that are hyalinized and never include arteries or usually even recognizable veins.* **(Right)** *Cavernous malformations can be surrounded by intense gliosis that often leads to considerable hypercellularity* →*. This reactive gliosis should not be mistaken for a glioma, especially oligodendroglioma.*

Remote Thromboses

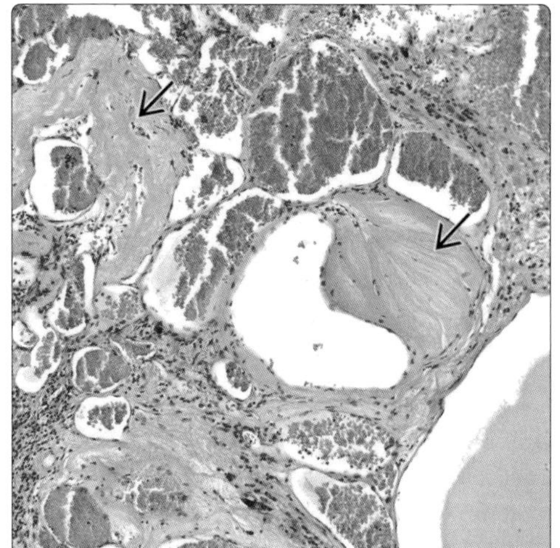

Calcified

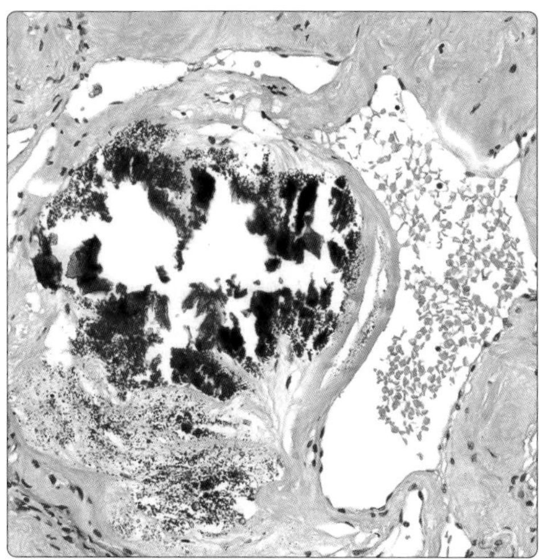

(Left) *As the result of remote thrombosis, cavernous malformations usually contain hyalinized "knots" in vessel walls* ⇒*. As is typical, although not always the case, there is only a scant amount of intervening parenchyma. Cavernomas undergo constant vascular remodeling.* **(Right)** *Remote thrombi (hyalinized knots) in cavernomas may be dystrophically calcified. Tiny dot-like calcifications should not be misinterpreted as toxoplasma.*

Encrusted Small Vessels

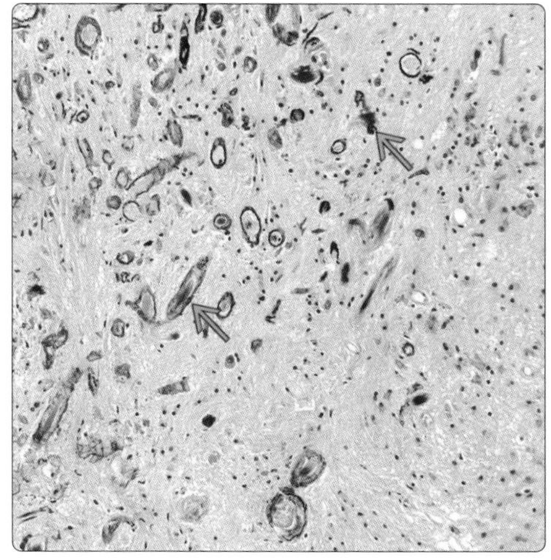

Disrupted Cell Processes

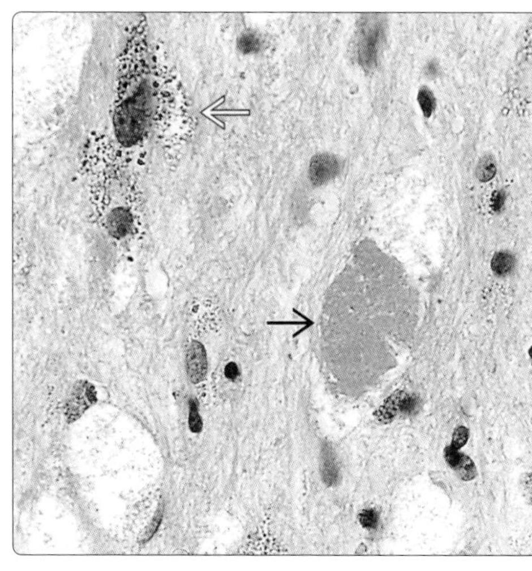

(Left) *With repetitive bleeding, perilesional small-caliber vessels around cavernomas may become encrusted with calcium salts* ⇒*.* **(Right)** *Gliotic parenchyma around a cavernous angioma may contain eosinophilic, spheroidal, disrupted cell processes* ⇒*, not to be mistaken for eosinophilic granular bodies. Note the astrocyte with hemosiderin deposition* ➡*.*

Hemosiderin

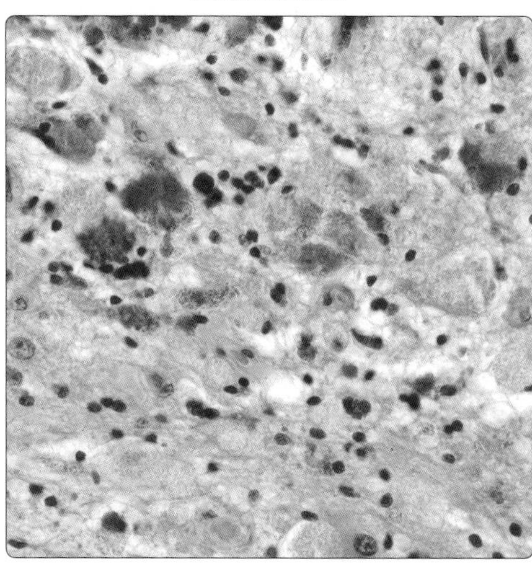

Gamna-Gandy Bodies

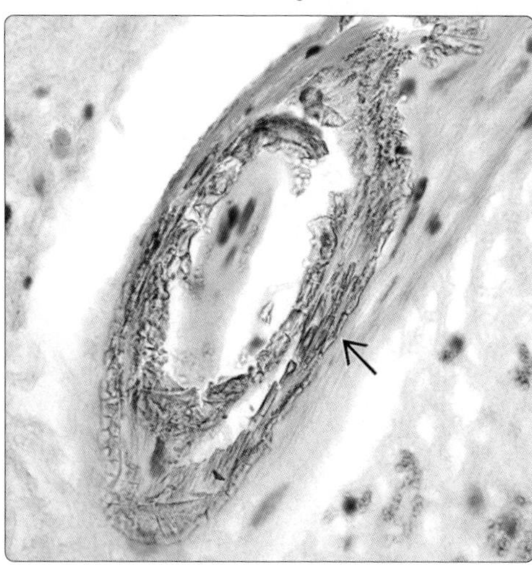

(Left) *Hemosiderin-stained gliotic tissue is usually at the perimeter of cavernous malformations due to the repeated subclinical episodes of bleeding.* **(Right)** *Due to repeated episodes of bleeding, Gamna-Gandy bodies may form in the parenchymal vessels adjacent to a cavernoma. These bamboo-like, yellow-brown, refractile deposits* ⇒*, originally described in spleen, are mineral-encrusted collagenous and elastic fibers. They should not to be misconstrued as hyphae.*

Arteriovenous Malformation

KEY FACTS

ETIOLOGY/PATHOGENESIS

- Most sporadic

CLINICAL ISSUES

- Usually present with brain hemorrhage in patients ages 20-40 years

IMAGING

- Flow voids (high-flow) on T1WI and, especially, T2WI
- Enlarged arterial feeders, nidus of tight-packed vessels, dilated draining veins, shunting (angiography)

MACROSCOPIC

- Superficial AVMs: Wedge-shaped aggregates of closely juxtaposed, abnormal, dilated veins; fewer arteries
- Most supratentorial

MICROSCOPIC

- Combination of arteries and veins by light microscopy and special stains
- Arteries with duplicated elastic lamina
- Dilated, hyalinized, calcified, and occasional thrombosed vessels
- Usually many more veins than arteries

ANCILLARY TESTS

- Trichrome stain shows hyalinization of veins, loss of muscularis
- Elastic stain highlights arterial component
    - Usually fewer arteries than veins in AVMs
- Elastic stain may also show duplicated elastic lamina in arteries

DIAGNOSTIC CHECKLIST

- Do not confuse artifactually compacted normal leptomeningeal vessels with AVM
- Clinically, radiologically, and pathologically distinct from cavernous angioma

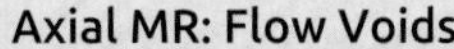

Axial MR: Flow Voids

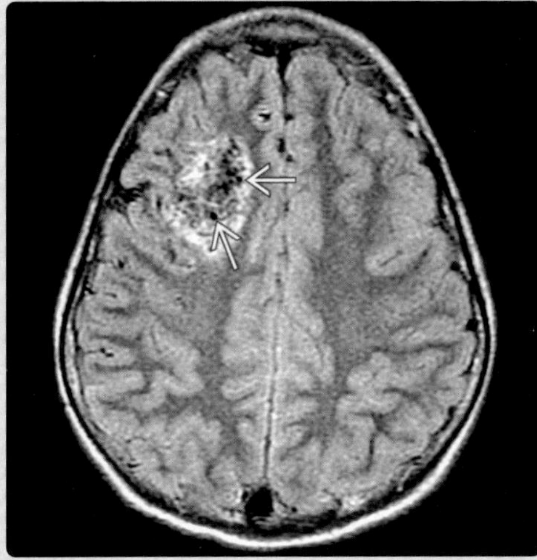

Axial MR: Large Draining Veins

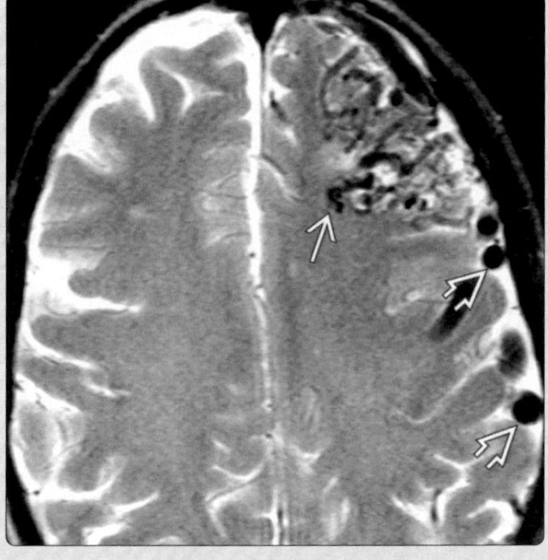

(Left) *Axial FLAIR MR shows a large, nonhemorrhagic right frontal AVM with flow voids ➡ and gliosis (bright signal) in surrounding brain tissue. This patient presented with seizures.* **(Right)** *Axial T2WI MR shows a large conglomeration of flow voids in the left frontal lobe, characteristic of a high-flow AVM nidus ➡. Note the large leptomeningeal draining veins ➡.*

Wedge Shape

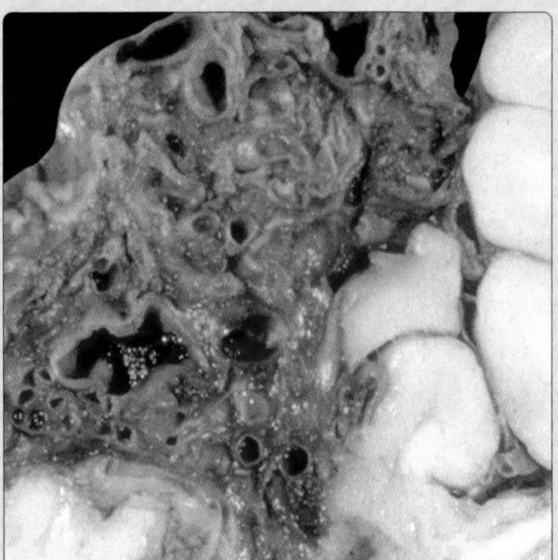

Dystrophic Calcification

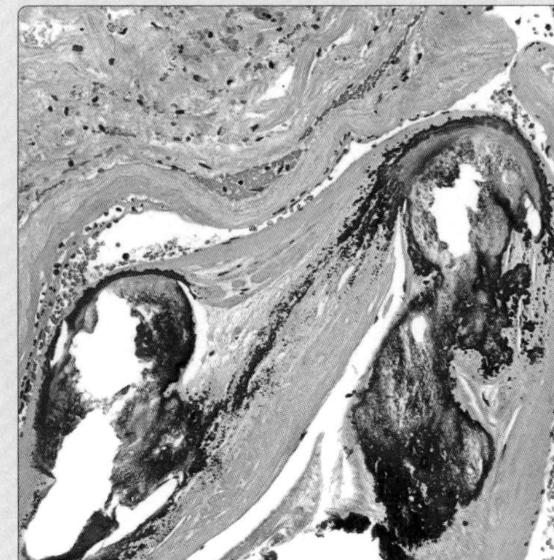

(Left) *Close-up view of arteriovenous malformation at autopsy illustrates classic wedge shape, with the AVM extending to the leptomeningeal surface. Note the numerous dilated veins. (Courtesy P. Boyer, MD, PhD.)* **(Right)** *Dystrophic calcification of the vessel walls, usually in the hyalinized veins, is often present in longstanding AVMs.*

TERMINOLOGY

Abbreviations

- Arteriovenous malformation (AVM)

Synonyms

- Brain arteriovenous malformation (BAVM)

Definitions

- Vascular malformation with arteries shunting directly into tangle of veins, without intervening capillary bed
- Focal abnormal conglomerations of dilated arteries and veins within brain parenchyma
  - Lack of intervening capillary bed results in abnormal arteriovenous shunting
  - Relatively well-circumscribed center of lesion known as nidus

ETIOLOGY/PATHOGENESIS

Developmental Anomaly

- Congenital origin is traditional view, but development of acquired AVMs has also been infrequently reported
  - Children documented with previously normal neuroimaging later found by neuroimaging to have AVM
- Possible increased susceptibility and risk for rupture linked to various genetic factors
- Small percentage associated with hereditary hemorrhagic telangiectasia syndrome (Rendu-Osler-Weber)
  - HHT is systemic disorder characterized by mucocutaneous telangiectasias, epistaxis, and AVMs
  - Caused by mutations in transforming growth factor-beta signaling genes (*ENG, ALK1, SMAD4*)
  - Patients often have multiple brain AVMs, which is highly predictive of diagnosis of HHT
  - Recent study suggests risk of AVM rupture same in HHT pts (< 2.5% per year) as that for sporadic brain AVM cohorts (2.3% per year)

CLINICAL ISSUES

Epidemiology

- Incidence
  - < 1% of population (0.1-0.2%)
  - 1-4% of brain masses
  - Majority sporadic
  - Hemorrhage of AVM accounts for 1-2% of all strokes
    - Majority of intracerebral bleeds in pediatric population caused by ruptured AVM
  - Patients may have coassociated saccular aneurysm of feeding vessels
    - Aneurysms may be multiple
- Age
  - Peak clinical presentation: 20-40 years old
  - Vein of Galen arteriovenous malformation (aneurysm) most frequent type of AVM found in infants and neonates
    - Presents with high-output cardiac failure due to shunting or hydrocephalus
    - Can be life-threatening if not diagnosed and treated early
    - Most diagnosed in 1st year of life
  - Stroke rare in pediatric patients, and AVMs less common than in adults, but most intracerebral bleeds in childhood due to ruptured AVM
  - Mean age of AVM presentation in children is 11 years
- Sex
  - No strong gender predilection

Site

- Intracranial
- Intraspinal
- Extradural shunting nidus in some cases

Presentation

- Cerebral hemorrhage
  - Once AVM has presented with bleed, much higher incidence of bleeding recurrence
  - Risk for hemorrhage in pediatric AVMs associated with nidus size, periventricular nidus location, deep venous drainage, associated aneurysm
- Seizures
- Mass effect/headache
- Ischemic tissue damage due to steal of blood flow and hypoperfusion of adjacent brain

Treatment

- Embolization
- Resection
- Radiosurgery

Prognosis

- Risk of hemorrhage
  - 2-4% per year
- Hemorrhage associated with
  - 5-10% chance of death
  - 30-50% chance of permanent neurological deficits

IMAGING

General Features

- Can be obscured by hematoma

Radiographic Findings

- Enlarged arterial feeders, nidus of tight packed vessels, dilated draining veins, shunting (angiography)

MR Findings

- Highly vascular
- Larger, less compact than cavernoma
- Flow voids (high-flow) on T1WI and, especially, T2WI
- Hemorrhage (some cases)

MACROSCOPIC

General Features

- Superficial AVMs often wedge-shaped with broad base near surface
- Focal aggregate of tangled blood vessels of varying caliber and thickness
- Deep AVMs drain into deep venous system
- May see intravascular embolization material or coils
- Often not hemosiderin stained
- Larger, more intermingled with brain than cavernoma

MICROSCOPIC

Histologic Features

- Multiple abnormal vessels
- Veins more numerous and larger than arteries
- Veins hyalinized, calcified, occasionally thrombosed
- Duplication of arterial internal elastic lamina
- Gliotic brain in and around lesion due to ischemic "steal"
- Generally little parenchymal hemosiderin
- Occasional examples present de novo with large obliterating hemorrhage
  - Search surgically resected brain clot diligently for entrapped abnormal vessels
- Eosinophilic, neutrophilic, mononuclear, and multinucleated giant cell reaction in some embolized AVMs
  - Embolization material may be amorphous gray-blue color or jet-black

DIFFERENTIAL DIAGNOSIS

Normal, Artifactually Compacted Vessels

- Confined to leptomeninges
- Vessels individually normal
- Calcification absent in vessel walls
- Vessels even with arteriosclerosis usually not as severely hyalinized as in AVM

Cavernous Angioma

- Well-circumscribed compact mass
- Abnormal vessels, no normal arteries or veins
  - Hyalinized
  - Usually more closely packed than in AVM
- Almost always with surrounding hemosiderin

Aneurysm

- Dilatation of single vessel, usually arteries on Circle of Willis
- No venous component

DIAGNOSTIC CHECKLIST

Clinically Relevant Pathologic Features

- Thin-walled vessels with high flow prone to rupture
- Intervening parenchyma and varying caliber of vessels, plus arteries and veins, rules out cavernous malformation

Pathologic Interpretation Pearls

- Clinically, radiologically, and pathologically distinct from cavernous angioma
- Check surgically resected brain clots for entrapped abnormal vessels to rule out ruptured AVM
- Recognize intraluminal embolization material
  - Jet-black onyx
  - May occasionally see inflammation in tissue from previously embolized AVMs
- Arteries are less frequent than veins in arteriovenous malformations
  - Veins hyalinized, calcified, occasionally thrombosed
- Either unruptured or embolized AVMs may be surrounded by tissue rarefaction, gliosis

SELECTED REFERENCES

1. De Beritto T et al: Vein of Galen Arteriovenous Malformation in a Neonate. Pediatr Ann. 44(10):e243-6, 2015
2. Ding D et al: Cortical plasticity in patients with cerebral arteriovenous malformations. J Clin Neurosci. ePub, 2015
3. Kim H et al: Hemorrhage rates from brain arteriovenous malformation in patients with hereditary hemorrhagic telangiectasia. Stroke. 46(5):1362-4, 2015
4. Ma L et al: Periventricular Location as a Risk Factor for Hemorrhage and Severe Clinical Presentation in Pediatric Patients with Untreated Brain Arteriovenous Malformations. AJNR Am J Neuroradiol. 36(8):1550-7, 2015
5. Nakamura M et al: De Novo AVM Growth Secondary to Implantation of Genetically Modified Allogeneic Mesenchymal Stem Cells in the Brain. Neurosurgery. ePub, 2015
6. Nicolato A et al: Leksell Gamma Knife for pediatric and adolescent cerebral arteriovenous malformations: results of 100 cases followed up for at least 36 months. J Neurosurg Pediatr. 1-12, 2015
7. Park JC et al: Growing Organized Hematomas Following Gamma Knife Radiosurgery for Cerebral Arteriovenous Malformation : Five Cases of Surgical Excision. J Korean Neurosurg Soc. 58(1):83-8, 2015
8. Reinard KA et al: Surgical Management of Giant Intracranial Arteriovenous Malformations: A Single Center Experience over 32 years. World Neurosurg. ePub, 2015
9. Stein KP et al: Associated aneurysms in supratentorial arteriovenous malformations: impact of aneurysm size on haemorrhage. Cerebrovasc Dis. 39(2):122-9, 2015
10. von der Brelie C et al: Seizure Outcomes in Patients With Surgically Treated Cerebral Arteriovenous Malformations. Neurosurgery. ePub, 2015
11. Yan J et al: Outcome and complications of endovascular embolization for vein of Galen malformations: a systematic review and meta-analysis. J Neurosurg. 123(4):872-90, 2015
12. Yeo JJ et al: Pediatric de novo cerebral AVM: report of two cases and review of literature. Childs Nerv Syst. 31(4):609-14, 2015
13. Kim H et al: Untreated brain arteriovenous malformation: patient-level meta-analysis of hemorrhage predictors. Neurology. 83(7):590-7, 2014
14. Lummus S et al: Histopathologic features of intracranial vascular involvement in fibromuscular dysplasia, ehlers-danlos type IV, and neurofibromatosis I. J Neuropathol Exp Neurol. 73(10):916-32, 2014
15. Morales-Valero SF et al: Are parenchymal AVMs congenital lesions? Neurosurg Focus. 37(3):E2, 2014
16. Murphy PA et al: Constitutively active Notch4 receptor elicits brain arteriovenous malformations through enlargement of capillary-like vessels. Proc Natl Acad Sci U S A. 111(50):18007-12, 2014
17. Toulgoat F et al: Vascular malformations of the brain. Handb Clin Neurol. 112:1043-51, 2013
18. Kim H et al: Brain arteriovenous malformation biology relevant to hemorrhage and implication for therapeutic development. Stroke. 40(3 Suppl):S95-7, 2009
19. Kim H et al: Common variants in interleukin-1-Beta gene are associated with intracranial hemorrhage and susceptibility to brain arteriovenous malformation. Cerebrovasc Dis. 27(2):176-82, 2009
20. Leblanc GG et al: Biology of vascular malformations of the brain. Stroke. 40(12):e694-702, 2009
21. Kim H et al: Genetic considerations relevant to intracranial hemorrhage and brain arteriovenous malformations. Acta Neurochir Suppl. 105:199-206, 2008
22. Achrol AS et al: Association of tumor necrosis factor-alpha-238G>A and apolipoprotein E2 polymorphisms with intracranial hemorrhage after brain arteriovenous malformation treatment. Neurosurgery. 61(4):731-9; discussion 740, 2007
23. Friedlander RM: Clinical practice. Arteriovenous malformations of the brain. N Engl J Med. 356(26):2704-12, 2007
24. Chen Y et al: Interleukin-6 involvement in brain arteriovenous malformations. Ann Neurol. 59(1):72-80, 2006
25. Folz BJ et al: Manifestations of hereditary hemorrhagic telangiectasia in children and adolescents. Eur Arch Otorhinolaryngol. 263(1):53-61, 2006
26. Katzman GL et al: Incidental findings on brain magnetic resonance imaging from 1000 asymptomatic volunteers. JAMA. 282(1):36-9, 1999
27. Yamamoto M et al: Gamma knife radiosurgery for cerebral arteriovenous malformations: an autopsy report focusing on irradiation-induced changes observed in nidus-unrelated arteries. Surg Neurol. 44(5):421-7, 1995
28. Elisevich K et al: Neuropathology of intracranial arteriovenous malformations following conventional radiation therapy. Stereotact Funct Neurosurg. 63(1-4):250-4, 1994

AVM, Associated Saccular Aneurysm

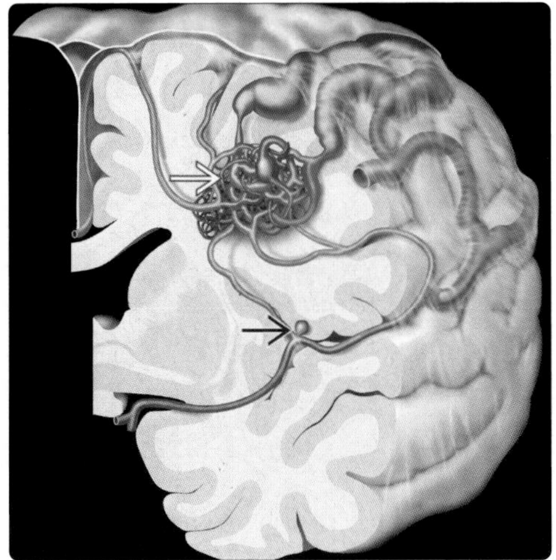

Surface of AVM

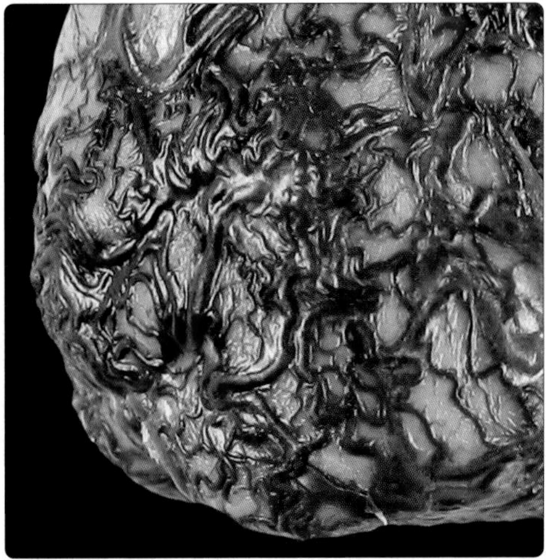

(Left) *The core of the AVM is a compact tangle of abnormal arteries and veins ➡. This intraparenchymal nidus has both enlarged feeding arteries and dilated draining veins that extend to the pial surface. Small saccular aneurysms ➡ are present in some cases.* **(Right)** *Superficial AVMs are tangled masses of jumbled, large-caliber leptomeningeal vessels. The shunting portion of the lesion (i.e., nidus) may be intraparenchymal.*

Large, Dilated, Thin-Walled Veins

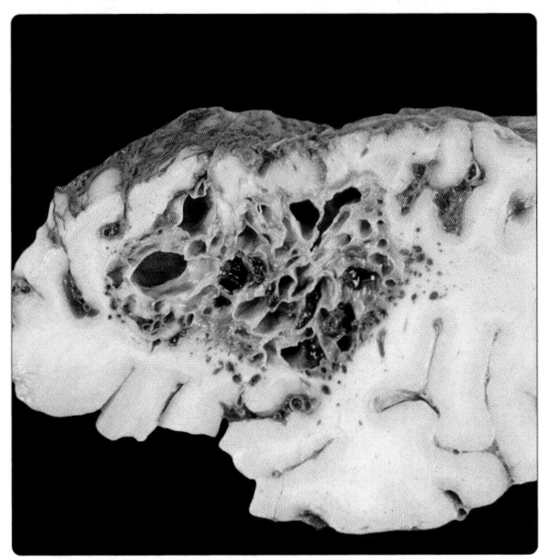

Unruptured AVM, Large-Caliber Veins

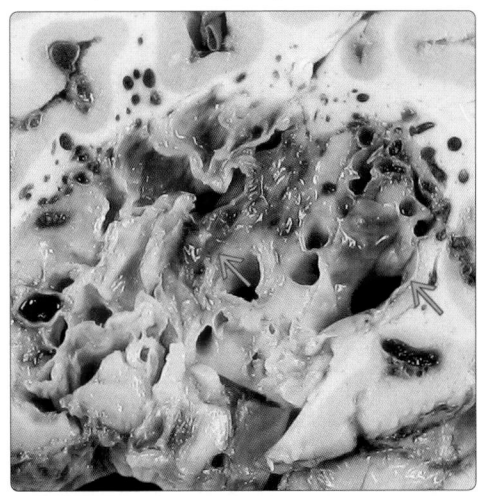

(Left) *AVMs are localized masses of patent vessels of varying size.* **(Right)** *An unruptured AVM has the translucent vessel walls of the larger caliber veins ➡. Note the varying amounts of interspersed brain parenchyma between the vessels that are part of the lesion. Unlike the situation with cavernous angiomas, brain parenchyma around AVMs is generally not hemosiderin stained.*

Large-Caliber Vessels, Mostly Veins

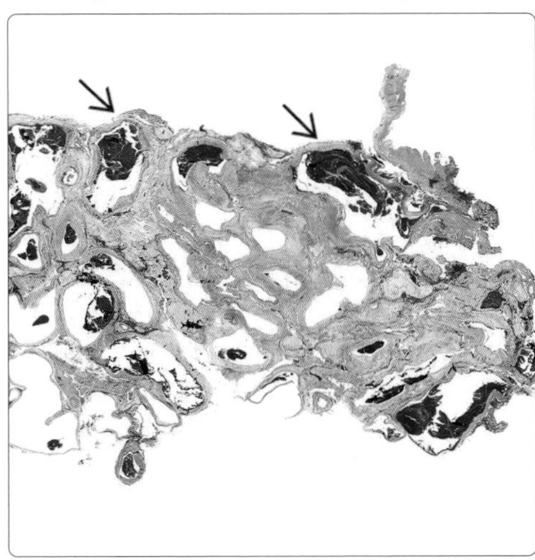

Patent, Abnormal Large-Caliber Vessels

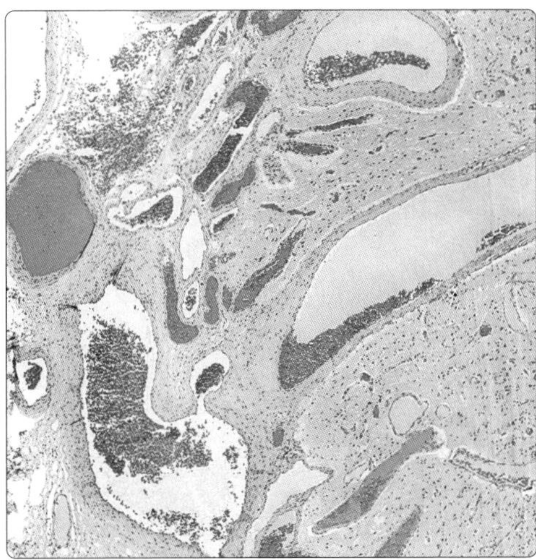

(Left) *Trichrome stain of a whole mount section of AVM emphasizes the variably sized, patent blood vessels, some of which are leptomeningeal ➡.* **(Right)** *This surgically excised AVM has the typical malformed, jumbled vessels, both veins and arteries, separated by variable amounts of intervening parenchyma. Unlike those of the cavernoma, vessels are typically patent in the absence of embolization.*

(Left) *Trichrome stain of an AVM emphasizes the venous nature of most large vessels. Unlike the cavernoma, there is little, if any, intraparenchymal hemosiderin but intervening parenchyma is present. Patency of vessels is another distinguishing feature since cavernomas often contain thromboses.* **(Right)** *Elastic fibers of the internal elastic lamina* → *are often duplicated and disrupted in AVMs.*

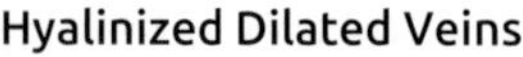

Hyalinized Dilated Veins

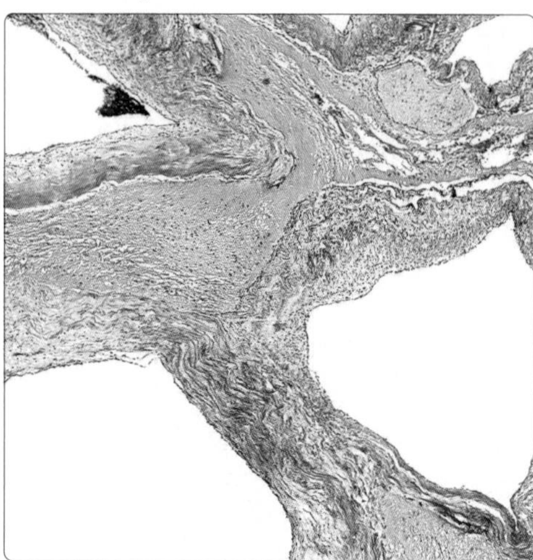

Duplicated Elastic Lamina

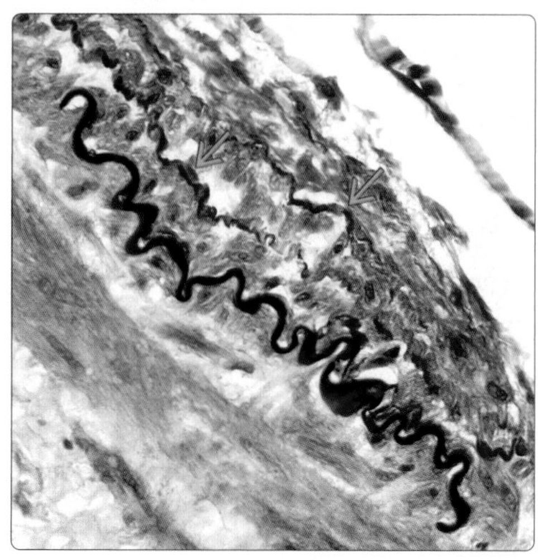

(Left) *This patient received 3 preoperative embolizations with n-BCA (N-butyl cyanoacrylate) "glue" to aid in resection. As is typical, not all vessels of this AVM were filled.* **(Right)** *Blue embolic material, polyvinyl alcohol, fills the vessels in an AVM and elicits a foreign body giant cell response.*

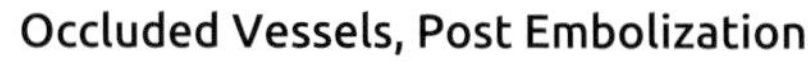

Occluded Vessels, Post Embolization

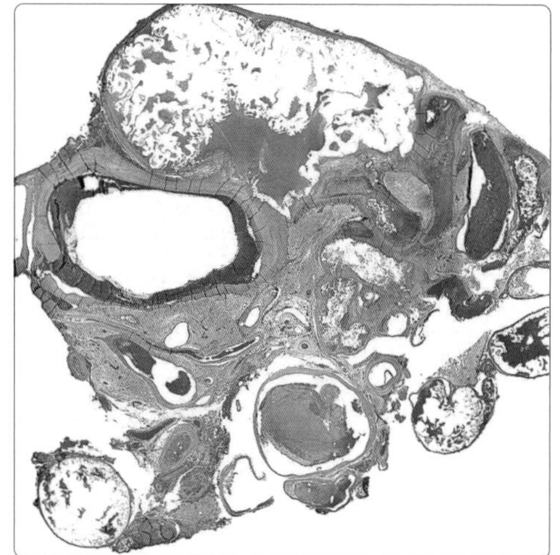

Foreign Body Giant Cells, Post Embolization

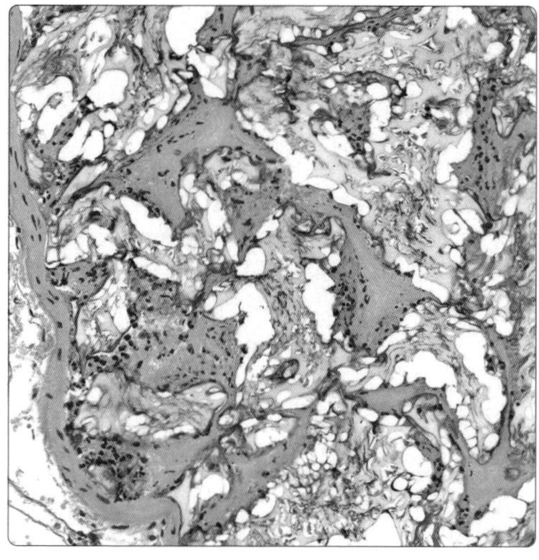

(Left) *Embolization with onyx [tantalum powder as a radiopaque marker + ethylene-vinyl alcohol copolymer dissolved in dimethyl-sulfoxide (DMSO)] fills some, but not all, vessels of this AVM with granular jet-black material* →*. Embolization is due to diffusion of the DMSO out of solution and copolymerization.* **(Right)** *Embolization of an AVM, especially when repeated, can elicit a histiocytic* → *and eosinophilic response to the foreign material.*

Post Onyx Embolization

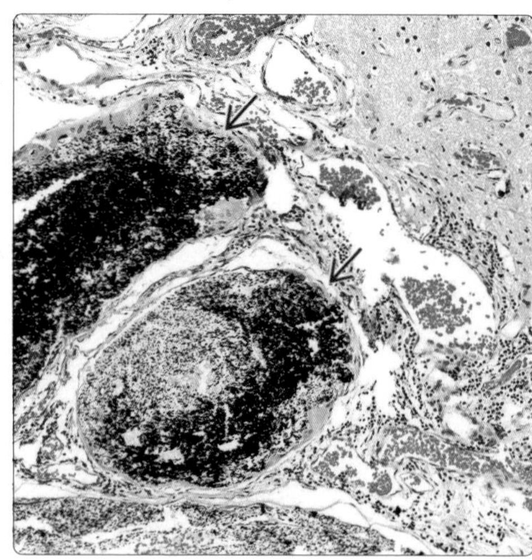

Eosinophilic Response, Post Embolization

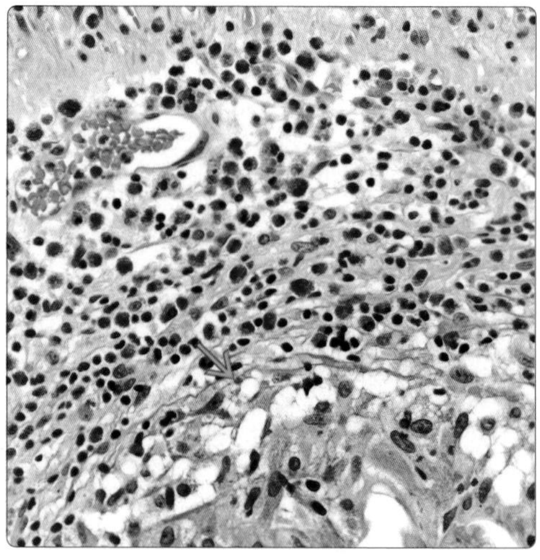

AVM Obscured by Acute Hemorrhage

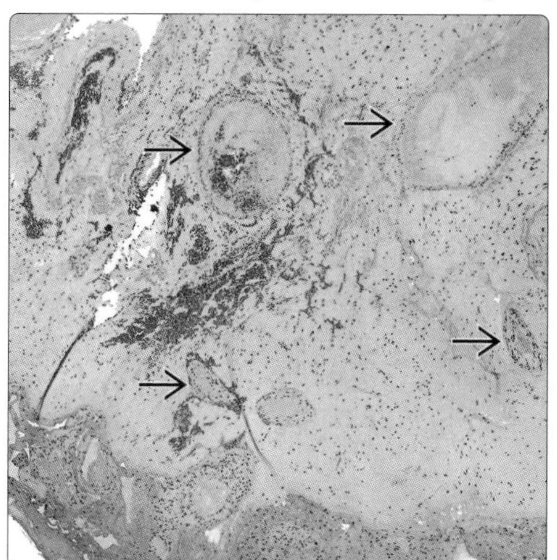

Brain Clot, Hemostatic Material

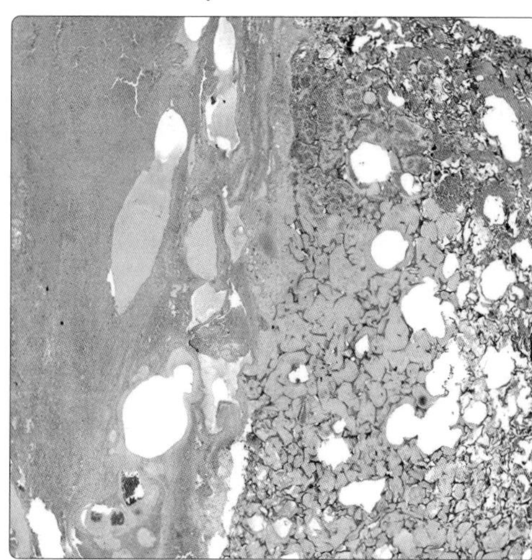

(Left) *This man presented with an acute brain hemorrhage; careful inspection showed that a ruptured AVM (not previously known to exist until the bleed) was the culprit. Note the large-caliber vessels in parenchyma* ➙*.* **(Right)** *This brain clot with inert hemostatic material at right contained one tissue fragment that proved to be an underlying AVM as the cause of the bleed. Note that the AVM is not present in this image.*

Axial CT: Sturge-Weber Syndrome

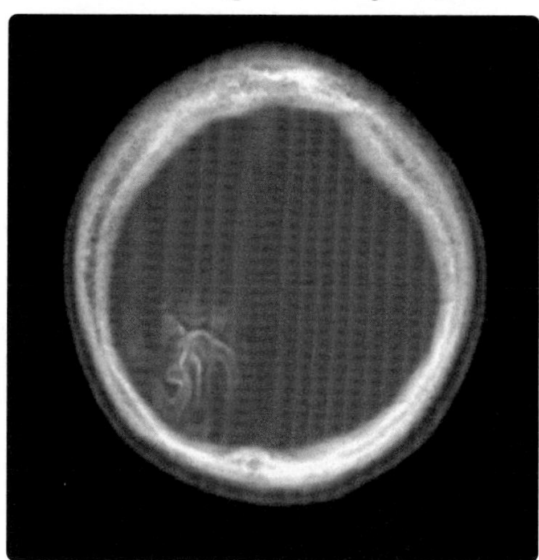

Sturge-Weber Syndrome

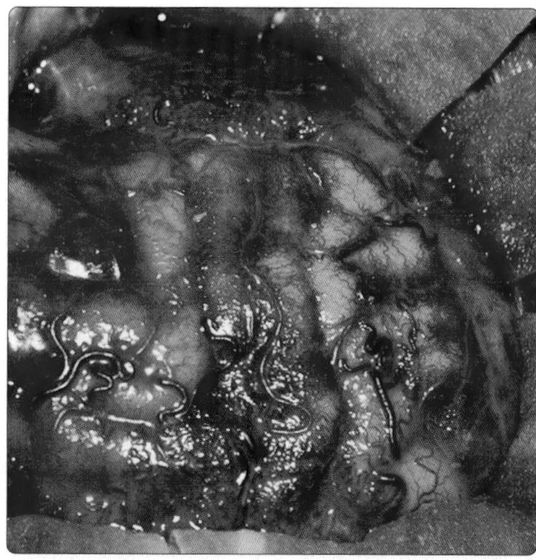

(Left) *The vascular malformation in Sturge-Weber is not a true AVM; no arterial component is present in the angiomatosis. Instead, there are numerous, thin-walled, back-to-back, ectatic vessels within leptomeninges. Underlying cortex shows extensive dystrophic calcification; the latter is highlighted here on CT.* **(Right)** *The angiomatosis of Sturge-Weber disease can be appreciated intraoperatively, or on a gross specimen, as a feltwork of densely tangled, matted, small-caliber vessels covering the surface of brain.*

Angiogram: Vein of Galen Aneurysm

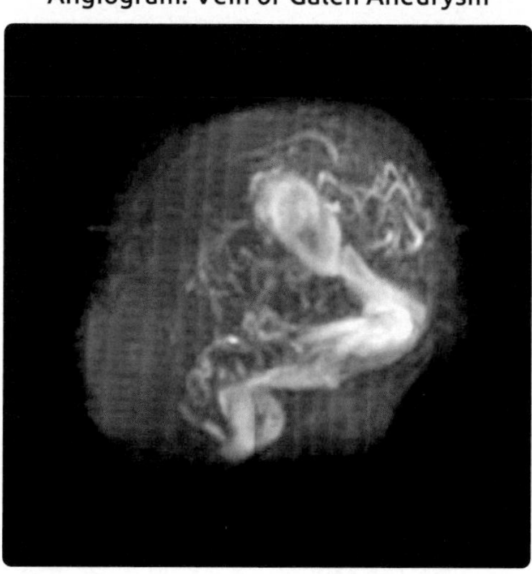

Vein of Galen

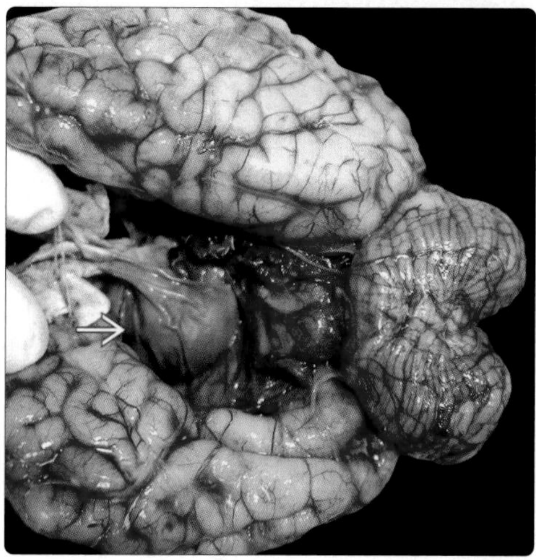

(Left) *Vein of Galen aneurysm is a special type of congenital AVM encountered in newborns with cardiomegaly and congestive heart failure. The rapid shunting of blood from the feeding arteries leads to massive dilatation of the large draining vein of Galen, part of the deep draining venous system, as seen in this angiogram.* **(Right)** *Although unusual, this infant succumbed to his vein of Galen aneurysm, a special type of congenital AVM. Note the cerebral edema and the large bulbous draining vein* ➙*.*

Capillary Hemangioma

KEY FACTS

TERMINOLOGY

- Abbreviations
  - Lobular hemangioma (LH)
- Definition
  - Benign vascular tumor formed of multiple capillary-sized vessels with large feeding vessel

CLINICAL ISSUES

- Site
  - Intraspinal in most cases
    - Nerve root (common)
  - Intracranial (uncommon)

IMAGING

- MR
  - Discrete
  - Contrast enhancing, homogeneous

MICROSCOPIC

- Histologic features
  - Lobular
  - Multiple small capillaries with draining vessel
    - Flat or plump but not notably atypical endothelial cells
    - Scattered mitoses

TOP DIFFERENTIAL DIAGNOSES

- Cavernous angioma
- Hemangioblastoma
- Solitary fibrous tumor/hemangiopericytoma
- Papillary endothelial hyperplasia of Masson

DIAGNOSTIC CHECKLIST

- Do not interpret mitoses and brisk Ki-67 index as evidence of malignancy

(Left) *In its common intradural extramedullary location, the discrete, lobular red lesion is often attached to a nerve root* ➡. **(Right)** *Capillary hemangiomas are masses of closely apposed capillaries that feed into larger draining veins* ➡*.*

Attached to Nerve Root

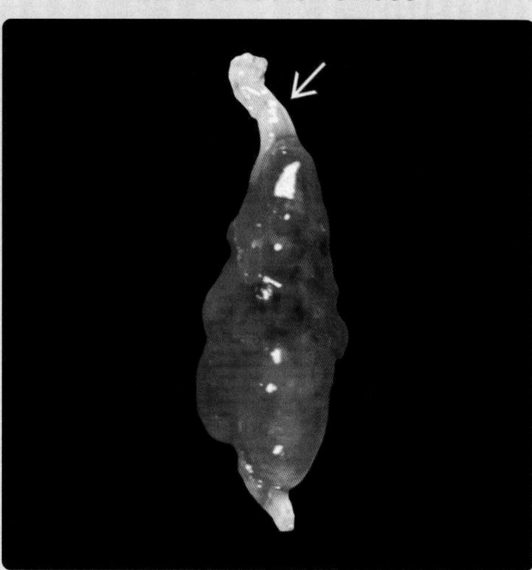

Masses of Capillaries

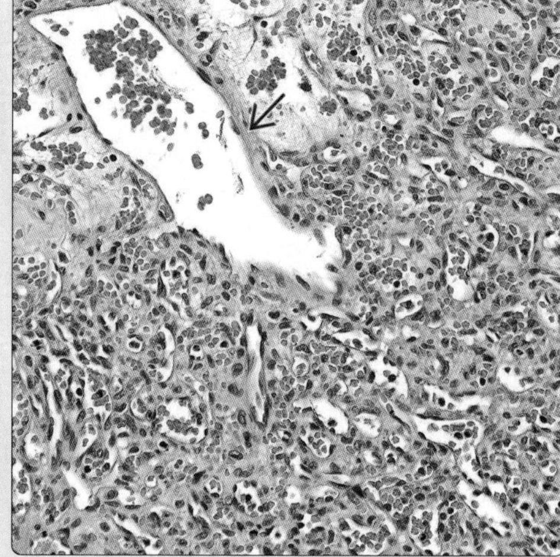

(Left) *The large number of component capillaries is sometimes less apparent in compact areas.* **(Right)** *Component vascular cells are diffusely immunoreactive for vascular markers, such as CD34. Note the characteristic large draining vessel* ➡*.*

Compact Areas

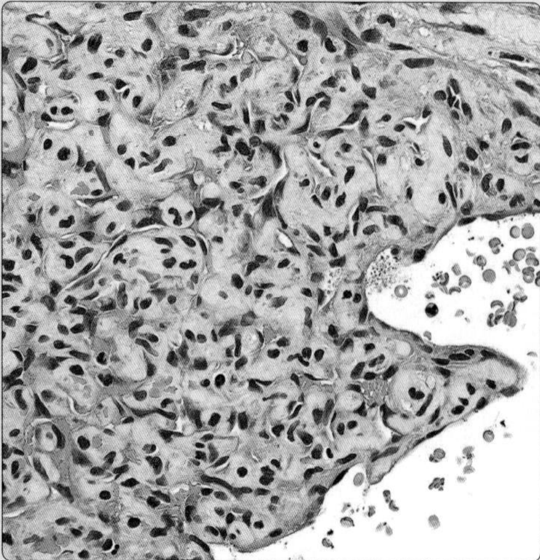

Large Draining Veins

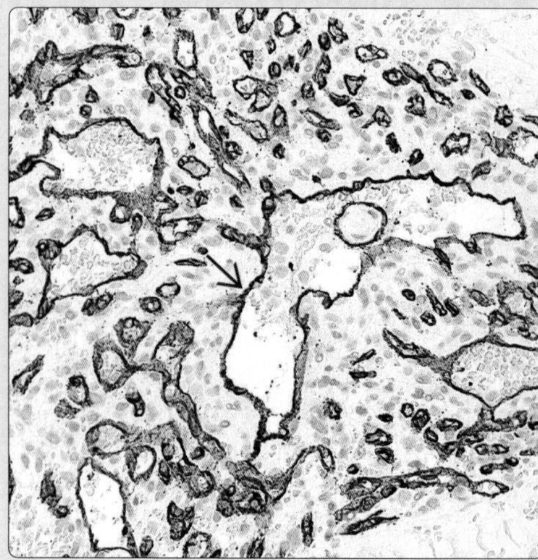

TERMINOLOGY

Synonyms

- Lobular hemangioma (LH)

Definitions

- Benign vascular tumor formed of multiple capillary-sized vessels with large feeding vessel

CLINICAL ISSUES

Site

- Intraspinal in most cases
  - Nerve root (common)
  - Spinal cord
    - Periphery, pial surface
    - Intramedullary (rare)
- Intracranial (rare)

Presentation

- Intraspinal
  - Progressive sensorimotor deficits, pain, no spontaneous hemorrhage
- Intracranial
  - Mass effects, seizures

Treatment

- Surgical approaches
  - Complete resection curative

Prognosis

- Excellent
  - Recurrence possible after subtotal resection

IMAGING

MR Findings

- Spinal lesions usually intradural extramedullary
- Discrete
- Contrast enhancing, homogeneous
- No evidence of acute or remote hemorrhage

Angiography

- Discrete, highly vascular

MACROSCOPIC

General Features

- Well circumscribed, globular
- Red or purple

MICROSCOPIC

Histologic Features

- Well circumscribed by delicate pseudocapsule
- Lobular masses of capillary-sized vessels
- Small muscularized feeding arteries
- Large, thin-walled draining vessels
- Multiple small capillaries
  - Flat or plump but not notably atypical endothelial cells
  - Scattered mitoses
- Highly cellular, compact areas, focal
- Fibroepithelial papillae; focal in some cases
- Loose intralobular stroma
  - Occasional mitoses

ANCILLARY TESTS

Histochemistry

- Reticulin
  - Reactivity: Positive
  - Staining Pattern: Pericapillary

Immunohistochemistry

- CD31(+), CD34(+), and FVIIIRAg(+) endothelial cells
- Smooth muscle in supplying arterioles smooth muscle actin (+)
- Ki-67, brisk rate

DIFFERENTIAL DIAGNOSIS

Cavernous Angioma

- Component vessels
  - Larger, hyalinized
  - Thrombosed, chronically
- Evidence of prior hemorrhage
  - Hemosiderin
  - Positive iron stain
- Calcification
- Gliosis

Hemangioblastoma

- Interstitial, extravascular cells
  - Vacuolated (lipidized)
  - Inhibin-α (+)

Solitary Fibrous Tumor/Hemangiopericytoma

- Alobular
- Highly cellular, nonlobular
- Slit-like ("stag horn") vessels
- Parenchymal, not just vascular, cells CD34(+)
- Extravascular tumor cells

Papillary Endothelial Hyperplasia of Masson

- Relation to large vessel
- Associated thrombus
- More papillary

DIAGNOSTIC CHECKLIST

Pathologic Interpretation Pearls

- Do not interpret mitoses and brisk Ki-67 index as evidence of malignancy

SELECTED REFERENCES

1. Mirza B et al: Strawberries on the brain–intracranial capillary hemangioma: two case reports and systematic literature review in children and adults. World Neurosurg. 80(6):900.e13-21, 2013
2. Morace R et al: Intracranial capillary hemangioma: a description of four cases. World Neurosurg. 78(1-2):191.E15-21, 2012
3. Chung SK et al: Capillary hemangioma of the thoracic spinal cord. J Korean Neurosurg Soc. 48(3):272-5, 2010
4. Abe M et al: Capillary hemangioma of the central nervous system: a comparative study with lobular capillary hemangioma of the skin. Acta Neuropathol. 109(2):151-8, 2005
5. Kelleher T et al: Intramedullary capillary haemangioma. Br J Neurosurg. 19(4):345-8, 2005
6. Abe M et al: Capillary hemangioma of the central nervous system. J Neurosurg. 101(1):73-81, 2004

Subdural Hematoma

KEY FACTS

TERMINOLOGY

- Subdural hematoma (SDH)
  - Acute (aSDH), subacute (sSDH), chronic (cSDH)

ETIOLOGY/PATHOGENESIS

- Tearing of bridging veins traversing subdural space
- Capillaries in granulation tissue can rebleed with little or no additional trauma

CLINICAL ISSUES

- aSDH: 6 hours-3 days old
- sSDH: ± 3 days-3 weeks old
- sSDH: ± > 3 weeks old

IMAGING

- Crescentic extraaxial collections by CT
- Varying signal characteristics depending on age of blood
- Dural neoplasms can mimic SDH

MACROSCOPIC

- Acute clot in aSDH
- Neomembranes in chronic subdurals

MICROSCOPIC

- Granulation tissue can appear highly vascular and reactive
- Eosinophils, basophils, or extramedullary hematopoiesis in granulation tissue
- Rare primary brain tumors, brain cysts associated with subdural hematomas

DIAGNOSTIC CHECKLIST

- Examine hematoma carefully for occult tumor cells in cancer patients
- Plump mitotically active fibroblasts can suggest neoplasm

Axial CT: Chronic Subdural

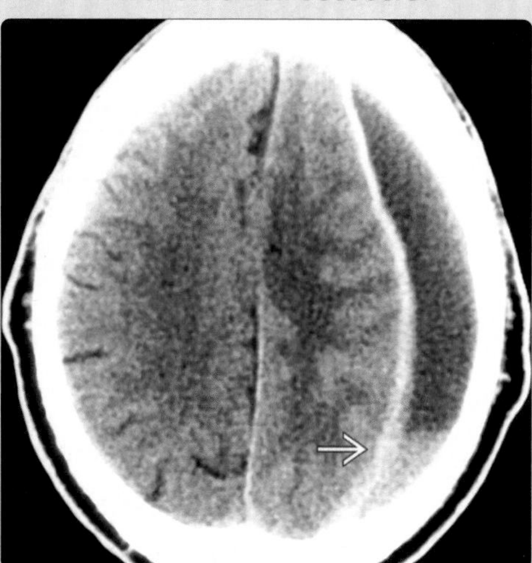

Chronic Subdural

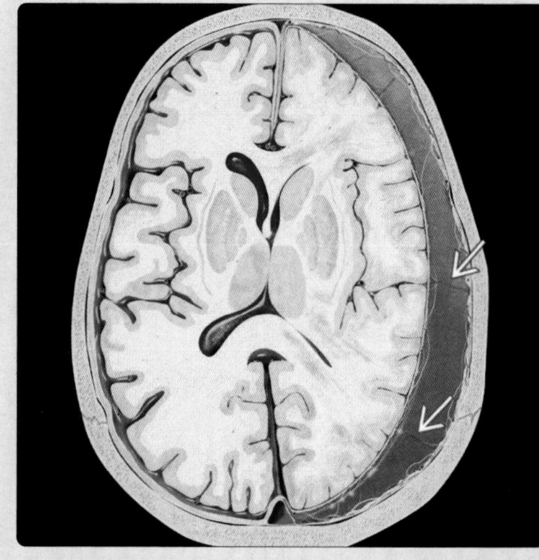

(Left) *Axial NECT shows hemispheric chronic subdural hematoma, largely cerebrospinal fluid (CSF) density, with interval rebleed ➔ producing a separated appearance or hematocrit level.* **(Right)** *Chronic subdural hematomas form internal membranes (tan septations) and show intact bridging veins that traverse the blood-filled subdural space ➔.*

Acute Subdural

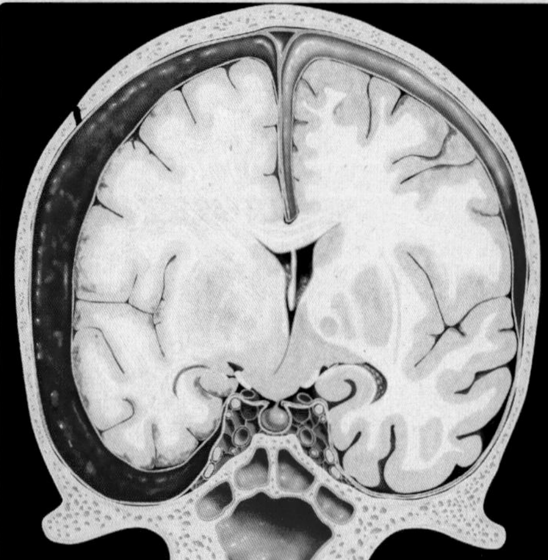

Post Biopsy Small Acute Subdural

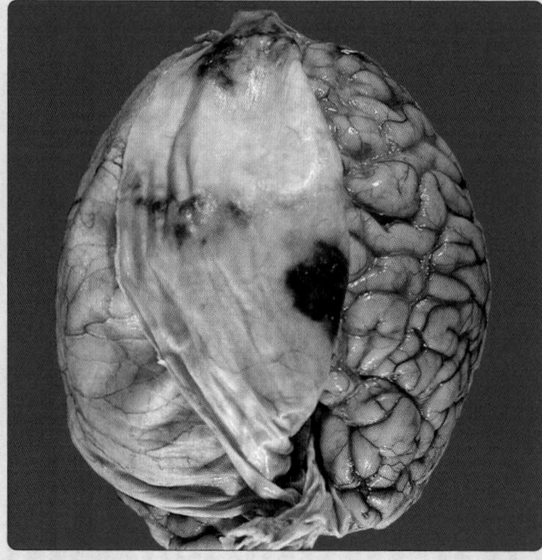

(Left) *This acute subdural hematoma is occurring in a patient with a subacute bleed in the opposite subdural compartment.* **(Right)** *Small acute subdural hematomas occurring after a surgical procedure, such as the premortem brain biopsy in this patient, are to be expected. The small volume is unassociated with clinical sequelae.*

TERMINOLOGY

Abbreviations

- Subdural hematoma (SDH)
  - Acute (aSDH), subacute (sSDH), chronic (cSDH)

Synonyms

- Subdural bleed

Definitions

- Collection of acute, subacute, or chronic blood and blood products in subdural space

ETIOLOGY/PATHOGENESIS

Environmental Exposure

- Acute head trauma
  - SDH in young children raises suspicion of nonaccidental trauma

Cancer Patients

- Dural metastases may coexist with SDH
  - Prostate, breast carcinomas, hematological malignancies
- Coagulopathies in cancer patients due to thrombocytopenia more common cause of SDH than dural metastases
  - Thrombocytopenia from bone marrow infiltration by tumor or chemotherapy

Patients With Brain Atrophy

- Stretching of bridging cortical veins as they cross subdural space to enter dural venous sinuses
- Bleeding into subdural space without associated trauma

Coagulopathy

- Often associated with hemorrhages elsewhere in CNS or systemic organs

CLINICAL ISSUES

Presentation

- Chronic subdural
  - Elderly patients ± known neurodegenerative disorder
  - Nonlocalizing symptoms
- Acute subdural
  - Acute posttrauma hemorrhage with mass effect
  - Requires surgical drainage

Treatment

- Surgical approaches
  - Drainage in acute/large examples
  - Observation only in many chronic subdurals
  - Excision of chronic neomembranes in some cases to prevent leakage and rebleeding from delicate vessels in granulation tissue

Prognosis

- Chronic
  - Recurrence possible
- Acute
  - Variable, depending on hematoma size and comorbidities; may be lethal

IMAGING

CT Findings

- Crescentic extraaxial collection over convexity
- Hyperdense crescent in aSDH
- Iso- to hypointense signal in crescent in sSDH
- Multiseptated collection with enhancing surrounding membranes in cSDH
- Other traumatic brain lesions in most patients with aSDH

MACROSCOPIC

General Features

- Acute clot in aSDH
- Neomembranes stripped in sSDH or cSDH (some cases)

MICROSCOPIC

Histologic Features

- Organizing hematoma in subacute phase
- Granulation tissue
  - Usually isolated, long, slender myofibroblasts
  - Sometimes masses of shorter, cytologically atypical, mitotically active cells with high Ki-67 index
  - Many macrophages
  - Ki-67 high during active organization of clot
- Extramedullary hematopoiesis
  - Erythroblastic cells positive for CD43, glycophorin A, erythropoietin A
  - Very high Ki-67 index
- Eosinophils, sometimes abundant and with Charcot-Leyden crystals
- Blood clot only with acute hematoma
- Potential for occult tumor cells in cancer patients
- Purulent exudate when superinfected

Cytologic Features

- Granulation tissue fibroblasts with plump nuclei, prominent nucleoli, basophilic cytoplasm
- Mitoses

DIAGNOSTIC CHECKLIST

Clinically Relevant Pathologic Features

- Delicate capillaries in granulation tissue can rebleed with little or no additional trauma

Pathologic Interpretation Pearls

- Plump, mitotically active fibroblasts can suggest neoplasm
- Extramedullary hematopoiesis can simulate small cell carcinoma or hematopoietic neoplasm
- Examine hematoma for occult tumor cells in cancer patients

SELECTED REFERENCES

1. Grisold W et al: Stroke and cancer: a review. Acta Neurol Scand. 119(1):1-16, 2009
2. Matschke J et al: Nonaccidental head injury is the most common cause of subdural bleeding in infants
3. Kuhn E et al: Extramedullary erythropoiesis in chronic subdural hematoma simulating metastatic small round cell tumor. Int J Surg Pathol. 15(3):288-91, 2007

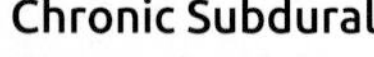

(Left) *Chronic subdural hematomas can be focal or extensive. Rebleeding in this large example was derived from delicate vessels in granulation tissue of the neomembrane. Little or no trauma may be needed to precipitate this event.* **(Right)** *Patients with cSDH may show severe distortion of the brain, but may present with surprisingly few neurological deficits.*

Chronic Subdural

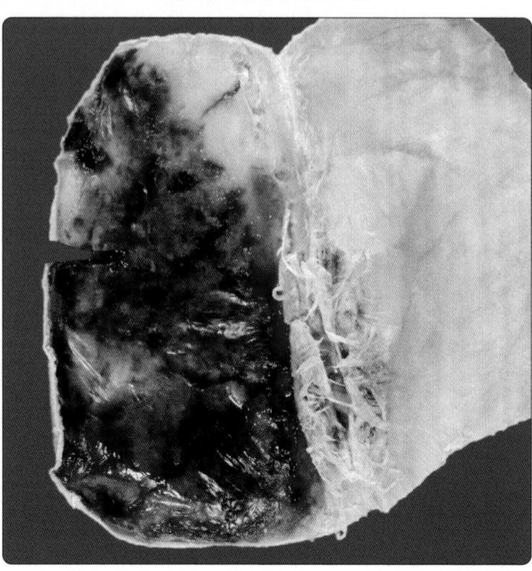

Severe Distortion From Chronic Subdural

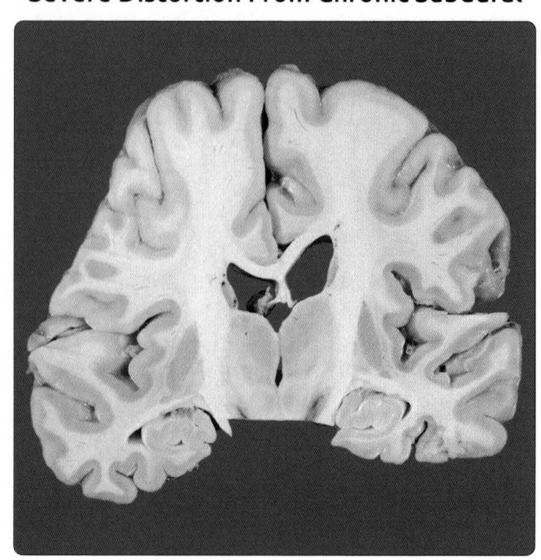

(Left) *The hypocellular inner membrane, nearest the brain, from a cSDH is composed of fibroblasts, but no proliferative capillaries.* **(Right)** *Organization of the clot from the outer membrane of a SDH involves granulation tissue composed of proliferative capillaries and reactive fibroblasts. The highly cellular combination is potentially misinterpreted as a neoplasm.*

Hypocellular Neomembrane

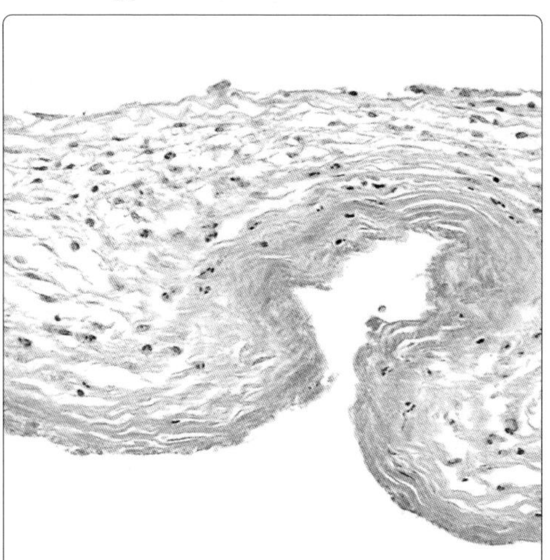

Organizing Subdural

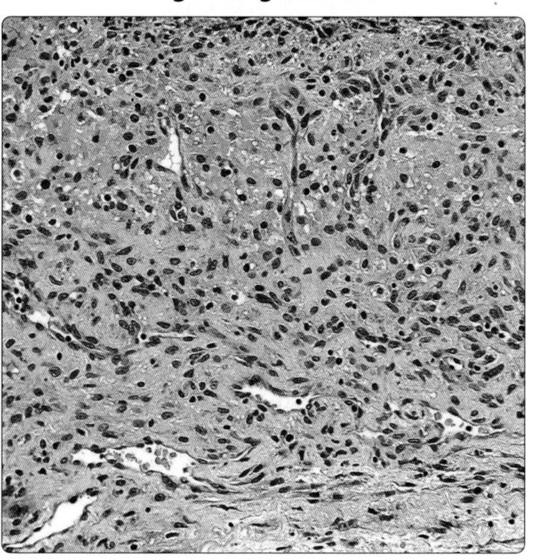

(Left) *A subdural hematoma in the subacute phase contains mitotically active cells ➡ and hemosiderin.* **(Right)** *The inner surface of the neomembrane of a SDH contains reactive cells with vesicular nuclei, prominent nucleoli, and basophilic cytoplasm, all features of metabolically active cells. Their cytological features can resemble those of a neoplasm.*

Mitosis in Organizing Subdural

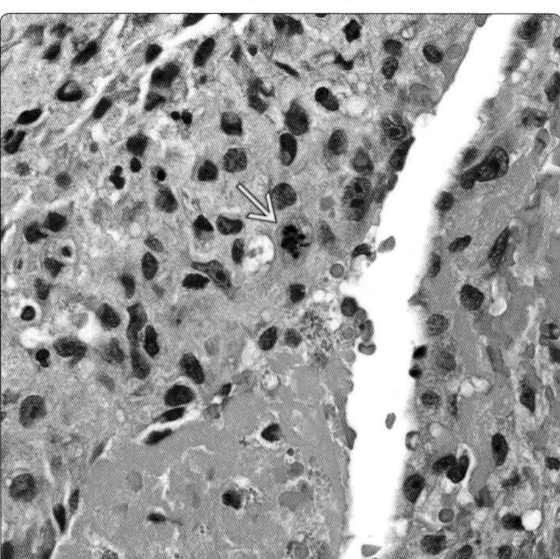

Simulating Neoplasm

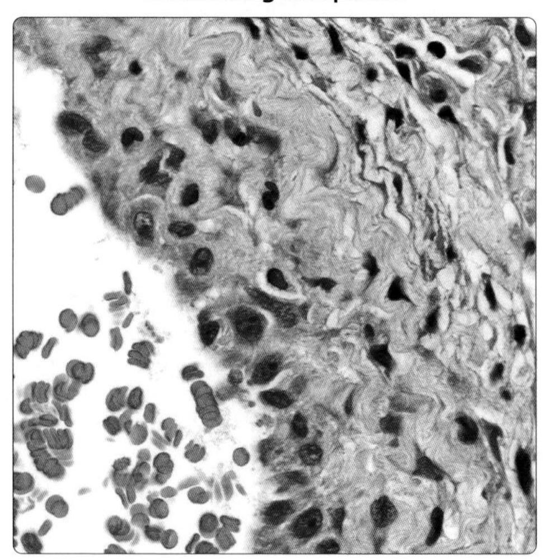

Ki-67 in Granulation Tissue

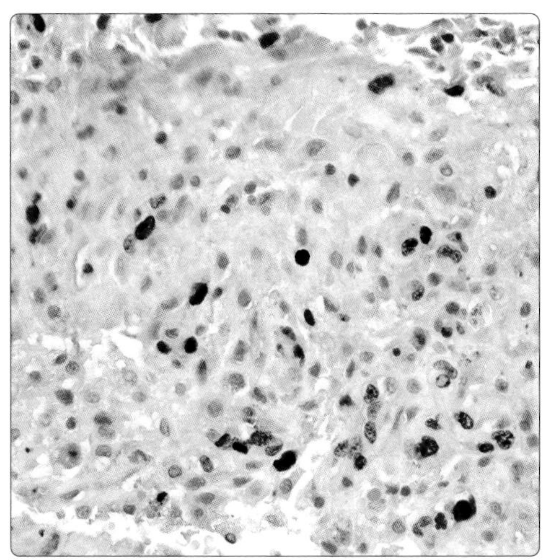

Macrophages in Granulation Tissue

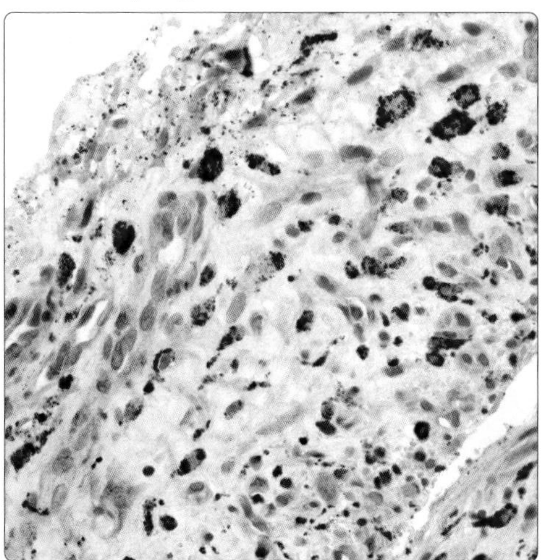

(Left) *The Ki-67 rate is high in granulation tissue, such as that in SDH neomembranes.* **(Right)** *A CD68 immunostain for macrophages illustrates the number of the latter cells in a subacute hematoma.*

Progressive Fibrosis of Neomembrane

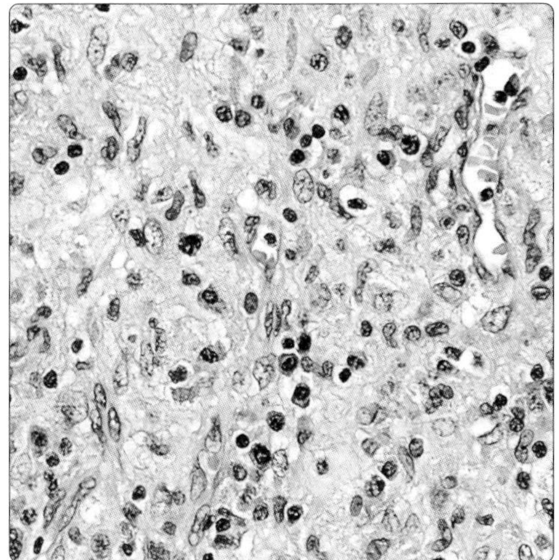

Extramedullary Hematopoiesis

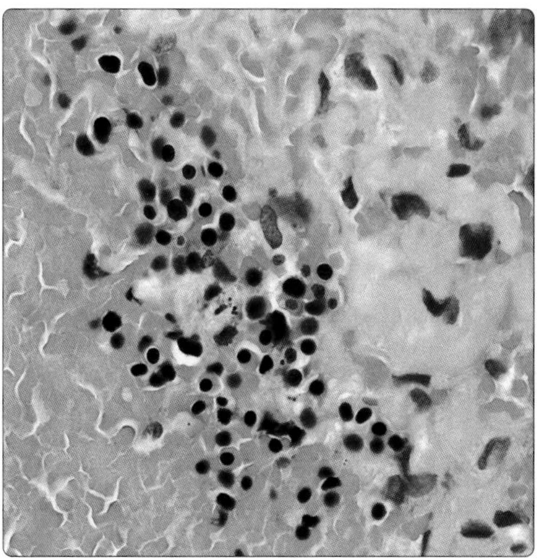

(Left) *As the degenerating blood is organized in a SDH, neomembranes become more fibroblastic and acquire scattered lymphocytes and plasma cells. This inflammatory component is not an index of bacterial superinfection.* **(Right)** *Extramedullary hematopoiesis can be irregularly scattered throughout the granulation tissue in a neomembrane of an SDH. The eosinophilic cytoplasm of the immature erythrocytes helps in their distinction from lymphocytes.*

Eosinophils

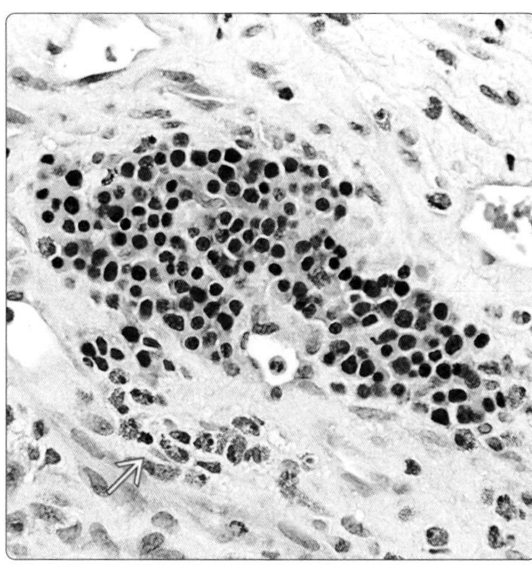

Charcot-Leyden Crystals

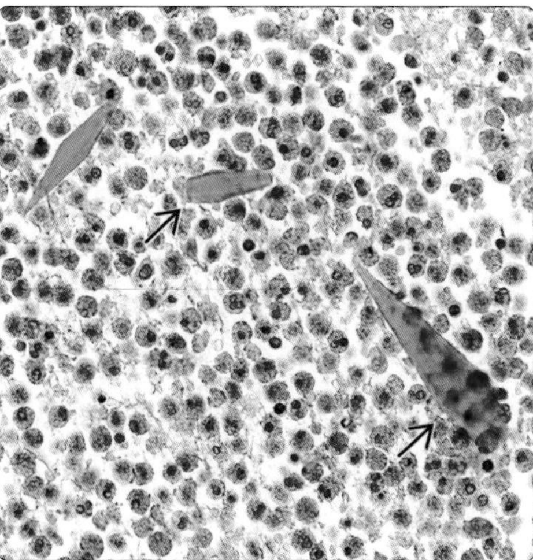

(Left) *One of the most striking features of chronic and subacute subdural hematomas is the presence of eosinophils* ➔ *and foci of extramedullary hematopoiesis. The latter should not be mistaken for small cell carcinoma or hematopoietic malignancy.* **(Right)** *Eosinophil-rich subdural membranes in SDHs can develop refractile, needle-like, Charcot-Leyden crystals* ➔ *composed of lysolecithin acylhydrolase synthesized by eosinophils.*

(Left) *Axial graphic shows a subacute subdural hematoma with traversing bridging veins* ➡*. The inset focuses on developing membranes* ⇨ *that encase the hematoma.* (Right) *A subacute subdural hematoma is often hemosiderin stained at its periphery. This small discrete example was incident to a recent neurosurgical biopsy.*

Subacute Subdural

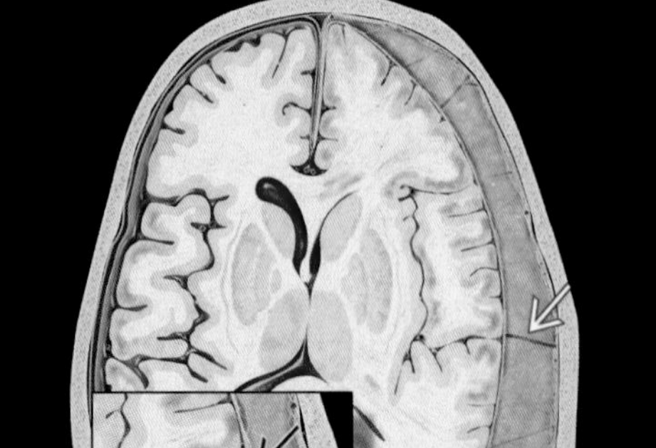

Subacute Subdural

(Left) *A resolving, subacute subdural hematoma neomembrane has a layer of clot and a layer of proliferative granulation tissue.* (Right) *Proliferating capillaries in a resolving subacute subdural hematoma have the large, plump nuclei typical of reactive endothelial cells.*

Subacute Subdural

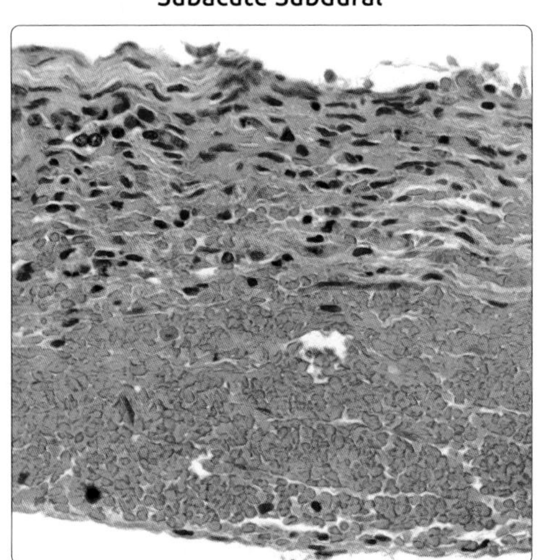

Subacute Subdural

(Left) *Resolving, subacute subdural hematomas contain brown hemosiderin pigment* ➡ *and delicate congested capillaries.* (Right) *Hemosiderin is abundant in resolving subdural hematomas, as is best identified with an iron stain, such as Perls.*

Hemosiderin

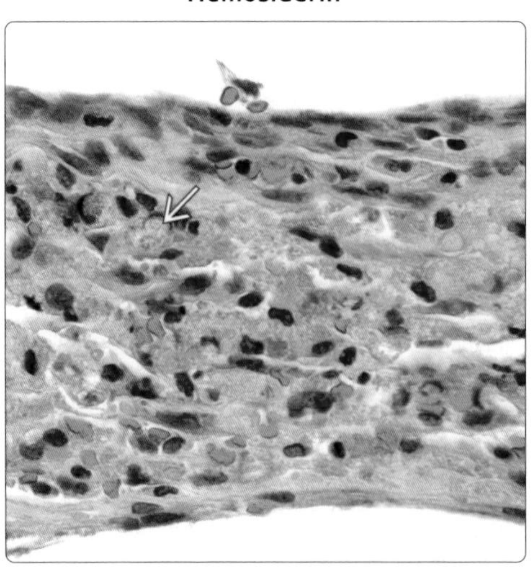

Perls Iron

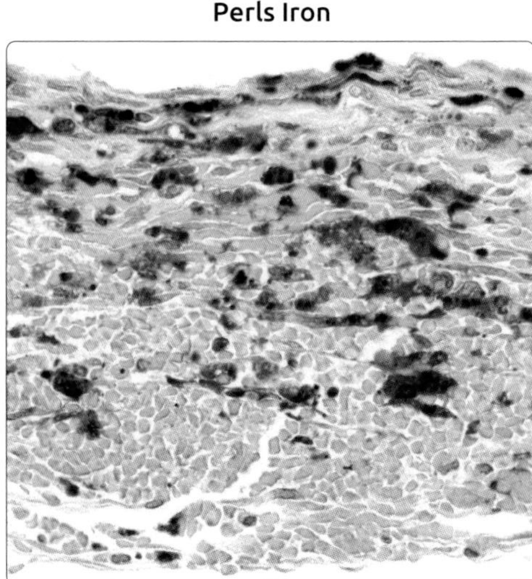

Acute Subdural

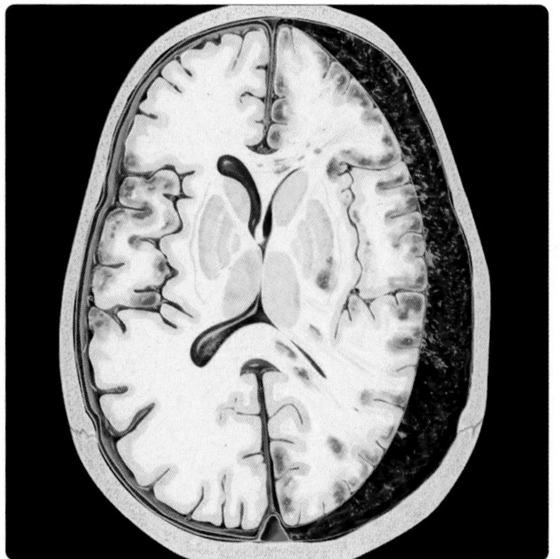

Acute Subdural

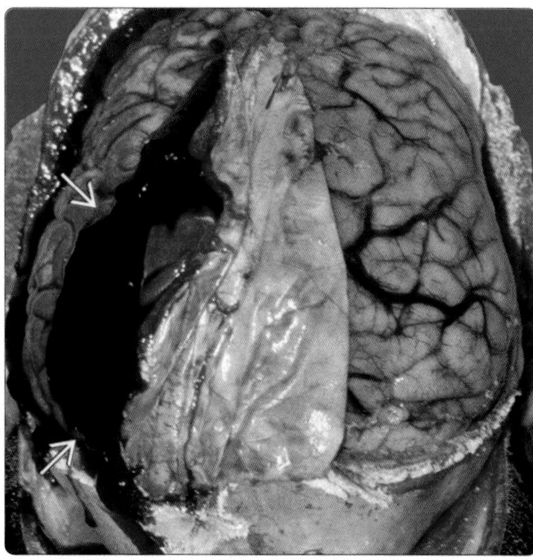

(Left) *Multiple proximate and remote contusions are often associated with traumatic aSDH.* **(Right)** *Falling from a ladder, this child sustained an acute left-sided SDH ➡. Note the severe cerebral edema with sulcal obliteration and gyral flattening. Unlike subarachnoid blood, subdural clot can be freely wiped away from the underlying brain.*

Early Organization

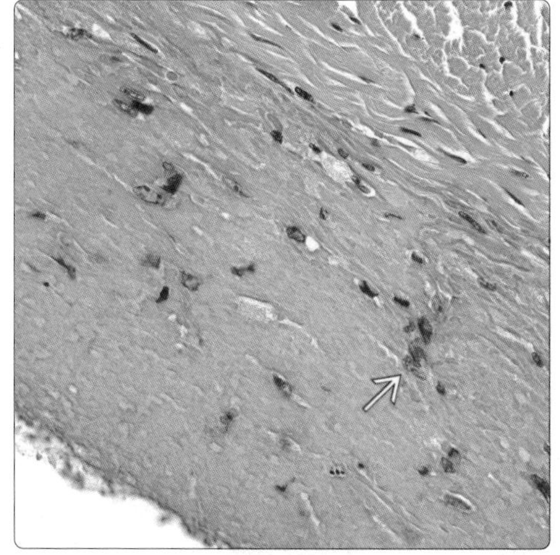

Dural Metastasis

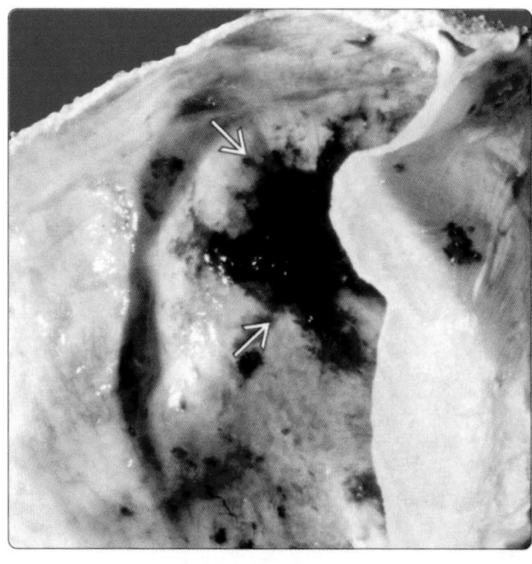

(Left) *This acute to early subacute subdural hematoma shows early organization, with influx of capillaries ➡.* **(Right)** *Most SDHs seen in patients with cancer result from secondary coagulopathies and thrombocytopenia, but are occasionally due to metastatic subdural tumor itself. This patient, with stomach cancer, had a fall-induced SDH ➡ with focal metastatic tumor.*

Dural Metastasis With Subdural

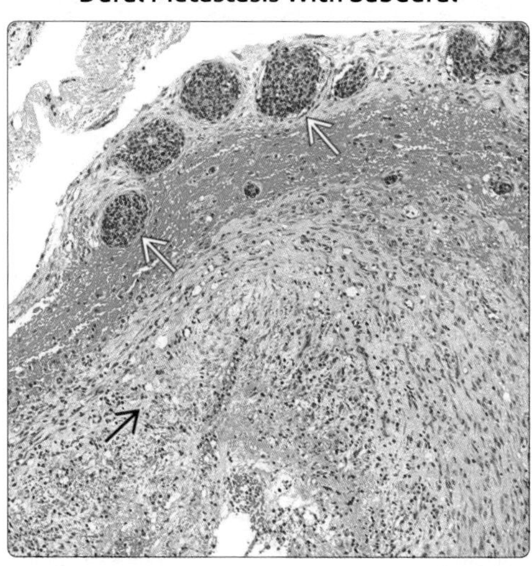

Clusters of Metastatic Tumor

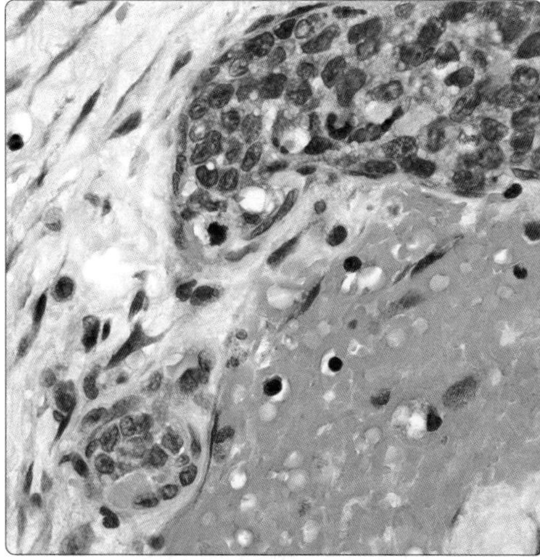

(Left) *SDHs from patients with cancer should be studied for metastatic dural tumor. A posttraumatic neomembrane in a patient with stomach cancer has nests of metastatic tumor ➡ as well as granulation tissue of the neomembrane ➡.* **(Right)** *A neomembrane in a cSDH from a patient with stomach cancer has nests of mitotically active metastatic cells. If necessary, immunostains can help exclude the possibility that these are only of exuberant capillaries.*

Infarct

KEY FACTS

ETIOLOGY/PATHOGENESIS

- Uncommon as surgical specimen
  - Unusual features
    - Young age, absence of sudden onset of symptoms, atypical vascular distribution
  - When acute, can simulate tumor, especially in posterior fossa
  - More frequent hematologic causes than in older patients

IMAGING

- Diffusion-weighted imaging
  - Hyperacute, within 6 hours
  - Hyperintense (bright) in contrast to dark signal with most malignant gliomas and metastases

MACROSCOPIC

- No definite gross changes until 6-8 hours
- Cracking of gray from white matter due to advanced tissue necrosis, 3-4 days

MICROSCOPIC

- Acute (12-24 hours)
  - "Red-dead," acutely ischemic neurons
- Subacute
  - Progressive influx of microglia and macrophages
- Chronic (weeks to months)
  - Progressive removal of necrotic debris by macrophages, cavitation

DIAGNOSTIC CHECKLIST

- Contracted "red-dead" neurons may be inconspicuous
- Hypertrophic and hyperplastic vascular cells often clue to nature of lesion but also can simulate vascular changes in malignant glioma

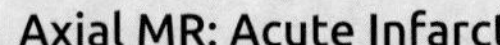

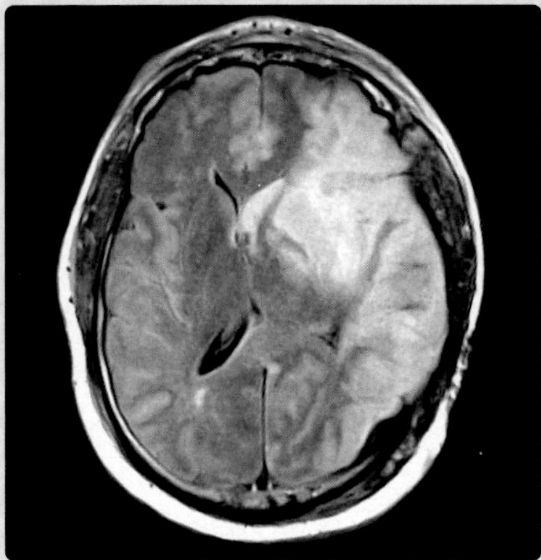

Acute and Chronic Infarcts

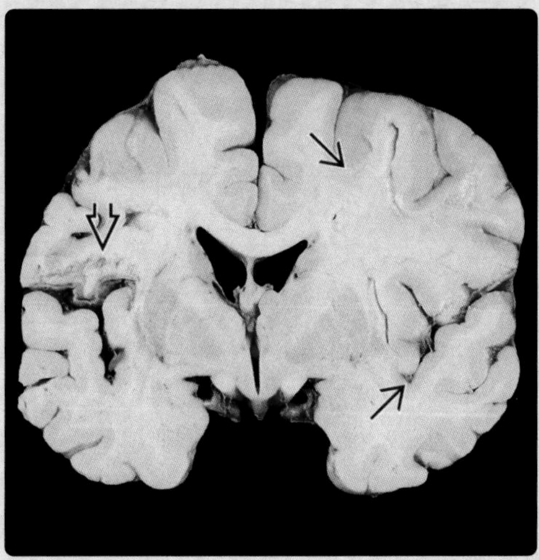

(Left) *Increased signal in this FLAIR represents a massive, expansile acute infarct in the distribution of the left middle cerebral artery.* **(Right)** *An acute middle cerebral artery infarct is a glistening lesion → with, in this case, enough mass effect to compress the adjacent ventricle. There is also a contralateral contracted old infarct ⇨.*

Prominent Endothelial Cells

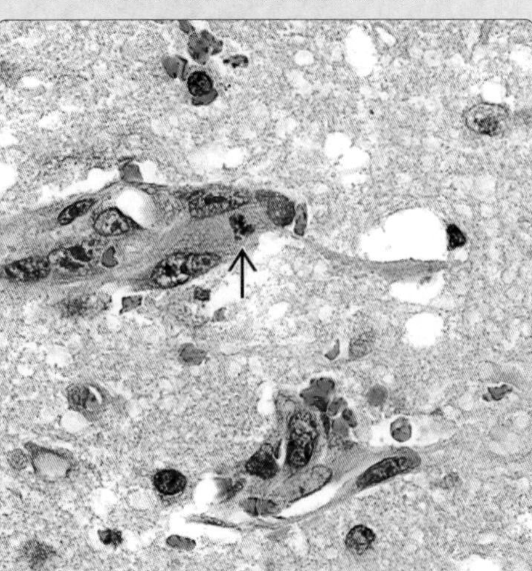

Remote Hemosiderin-Stained Infarct

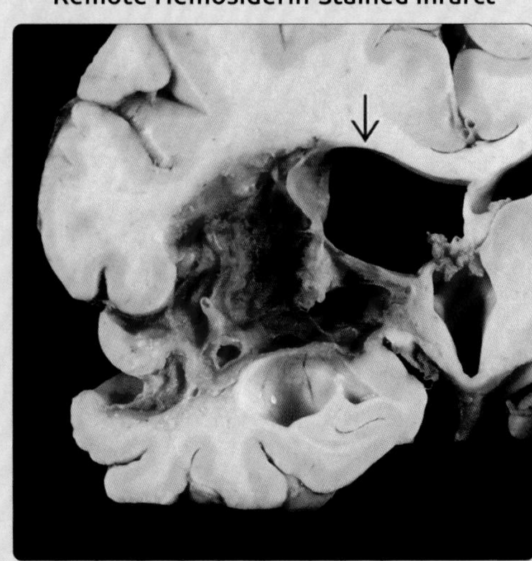

(Left) *The diagnosis of infarct is usually made at autopsy, but in the uncommon scenario when an infarct comes to surgical biopsy, the prominent endothelial cells in reactive blood vessels in late acute/early subacute tissue necrosis can simulate tumor vessels. Note the mitosis →.* **(Right)** *This remote, cavitated, hemosiderin-stained infarct is associated with secondary hydrocephalus ex vacuo →.*

TERMINOLOGY

Synonyms

- Cerebrovascular accident (CVA)

Definitions

- Loss of blood supply, and hence oxygen and nutrients, to a given area of brain due to blood vessel occlusion, resulting in tissue necrosis

ETIOLOGY/PATHOGENESIS

Nonmodifiable Risk Factors

- Increasing age, male > female
- Race (lower risk for white North Americans/Europeans), family history

Treatable Risk Factors

- Hypertension (most important risk)
- Lipid disorders (high total cholesterol, low-density lipoprotein [LDL])
- Smoking, diabetes mellitus, obesity (relatively small risk after correction of other problems)
- Alcoholism (low intake decreases risk, high intake increases risk)
- Stimulant use/abuse

Common Proximate Causes

- Atherosclerosis with thrombosis
- Embolic occlusion
  - Source of embolism often heart or atherosclerotic carotid arteries
  - Cardiac disease: Atrial fibrillation, valvular defects, patent foramen ovale, atrial septal defect
- Hypoperfusion (profound systemic hypotension, shock)
  - May combine with regional atherosclerosis to produce lesion in single vessel distribution

Uncommon Proximate Causes

- Fibromuscular dysplasia
  - Women in 30s and 40s; associated with arterial dissection, aneurysms
- Moyamoya disease
  - Focal occlusion of middle cerebral artery, nonatherosclerotic, usually in children or women in 30s and 40s
- Spontaneous arterial dissection (traumatic or nontraumatic)
- Hematological disorders (more associated with venous infarction than arterial)
  - Protein C, protein S, factor V, Leiden, prothrombin gene, antithrombin (formerly antithrombin III) gene
  - Sickle cell anemia, coagulopathies associated with malignancies
  - Oral contraceptives
  - Postpartum (usually venous infarction, day 3-5)
  - Antiphospholipid syndrome
- Migraine (vasospasm, increased platelet aggregation)
- Vasospasm after subarachnoid hemorrhage

Rare Causes

- Intravascular lymphoma
- Angioimmunoproliferative lesion (lymphomatoid granulomatosis)
- Emboli from atrial myxoma
- Primary CNS angiitis
- Radiation vasculopathy

Infectious Causes

- Septic emboli, infected cardiac valve
- Vasoinvasive fungi, *Aspergillus, Rhizopus* (mucormycosis)
- Meningovascular syphilis (usually smaller vessel infarcts)

Infarct as Surgical Specimen

- Uncommon
- Unusual features: Young patient age, absence of sudden onset of symptoms, atypical vascular distribution
- When acute, can simulate tumor, especially in posterior fossa
- More frequent hematologic causes than in older patients
- Exclude primary CNS angiitis
- Subacute superficial infarct in epilepsy patients after grid placement

CLINICAL ISSUES

Epidemiology

- Incidence
  - Rare between ages 45-55 years; more common in elderly
  - ~ 800,000 cases per year in USA
  - Major cause of adult disability in USA
  - 3rd leading cause of mortality
  - Increasing incidence in developing world

Presentation

- Sudden onset of neurological deficit
  - Large vessel infarct in middle cerebral artery may cause hemiparesis, hemisensory loss, homonymous hemianopsia contralateral to vessel occlusion
  - Small vessel infarct (e.g., lacunar infarction) yields more isolated motor or sensory deficit

Treatment

- 1st few hours: Recombinant tissue plasminogen activator (TPA)
- Risk reduction: Aspirin, antiplatelet drugs, anticoagulants
- Endarterectomy for high-grade (70-90%) carotid stenosis

Prognosis

- Tissue damage irreversible
- Outcome/residual neurological deficits dependent on size and location of lesion

IMAGING

MR Findings

- Diffusion-weighted imaging
  - Hyperacute, within 6 hours
  - Hyperintense (bright) with diffusion weighted imaging, in contrast to dark signal with most malignant gliomas and metastases
- Mild to moderate FLAIR hyperintensity, especially gray matter, acute
- Wedge shape in cortical infarcts, after 1-2 days
- Enhancement, cortical gyriform, develops within 1 week, persists as long as infarction undergoing resolution
- Cystic, chronic state

CT Findings

- Unremarkable in 1st few hours after stroke unless hemorrhagic
- Hypodense beginning at 24 hours

MACROSCOPIC

General Features

- Acute
  - 1st feature: Blurring of gray-white matter junction, congested vessels, tissue softening, 1-2 days
  - Cracking of gray from white matter due to advanced tissue necrosis, 3-4 days
  - Progressive softening and cavitation during subacute resolving stage
  - Bland ischemic infarct: Little or no blood or blood pigments
  - Hemorrhagic, often embolic or venous: Blood or blood pigments, especially in gray matter
  - No definite gross changes until 6-8 hours
- Remote
  - Cavity with variable degree of collapse
  - In territory of supply of occluded vessel

MICROSCOPIC

Histologic Features

- Acute, 8-12 hours
  - Neurons histologically normal
- Acute, 12-24 hours
  - "Red-dead," acutely ischemic neurons
    - Shrunken, sometimes extremely so
    - Hypereosinophilic cytoplasm
    - Karyolysis
  - Background vacuolization of neuropil
  - Occluded vessel, some cases
- Subacute
  - Progressive influx of microglia and macrophages
  - Vessels usually spared
    - Unlike diffuse coagulation necrosis in malignant glioma
  - Hypertrophy and hyperplasia of capillary vascular cells
    - Scattered mitoses
  - Plump reactive astrocytes at perimeter
- Chronic: Weeks to months, progressive removal of necrotic debris by macrophages, cavitation, strands of residual glial tissue, and traversing blood vessels

ANCILLARY TESTS

Cytology

- Macrophages
- Ischemic, "red-dead" neurons
- Abnormal capillaries

DIFFERENTIAL DIAGNOSIS

Malignant Glioma

- Neoplastic cells
  - Very focal, some in extensively necrotic glioblastomas
  - Deeper sections and immunohistochemistry may be necessary for detection
- Overt vascular proliferation, glomeruloid and true endothelial

Demyelinating Disease

- Restricted largely to white matter
- Often at angles of lateral ventricles
- Preserved axons (demyelination)
- No ischemic "red-dead" neurons
- Better preservation of axons

Herpes Simplex Encephalitis

- Inferofrontal-temporal, often bilateral
- Intranuclear inclusions
- Immunohistochemistry for HSV(+)

DIAGNOSTIC CHECKLIST

Pathologic Interpretation Pearls

- Contracted "red-dead" neurons may be inconspicuous
- Hypertrophic and hyperplastic vascular cells often a clue to nature of lesion but can also simulate vascular changes in malignant glioma

SELECTED REFERENCES

1. Decker D et al: Vascular and ischemic disorders. In Perry et al: Practical Neuropathology. Philadelphia: Churchill Livingston. 527-50, 2010
2. Murakami M et al: Cerebellar infarction caused by primary central nervous system angiitis of childhood: case report. J Stroke Cerebrovasc Dis. 19(1):77-80, 2010
3. Edlow JA et al: Diagnosis and initial management of cerebellar infarction. Lancet Neurol. 7(10):951-64, 2008
4. Schmidt JM et al: Frequency and clinical impact of asymptomatic cerebral infarction due to vasospasm after subarachnoid hemorrhage. J Neurosurg. 109(6):1052-9, 2008
5. Salih IS et al: Lacunar stroke attributable to radiation-induced intracranial arteriopathy. Eur J Neurol. 14(8):937-9, 2007
6. Caplan LR: Cerebellar infarcts: key features. Rev Neurol Dis. 2(2):51-60, 2005
7. Raco A et al: Management of acute cerebellar infarction: one institution's experience. Neurosurgery. 53(5):1061-5; discussion 1065-6, 2003
8. Chuaqui R et al: Histologic assessment of the age of recent brain infarcts in man. J Neuropathol Exp Neurol. 52(5):481-9, 1993

Acute Infarct, Ventricular Compression

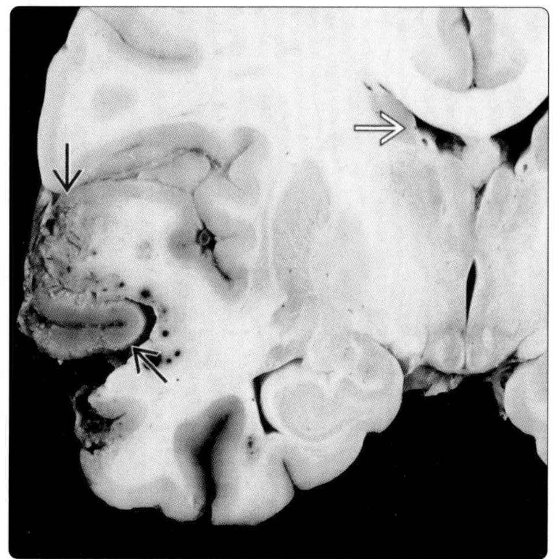

Cerebellar Acute Infarct

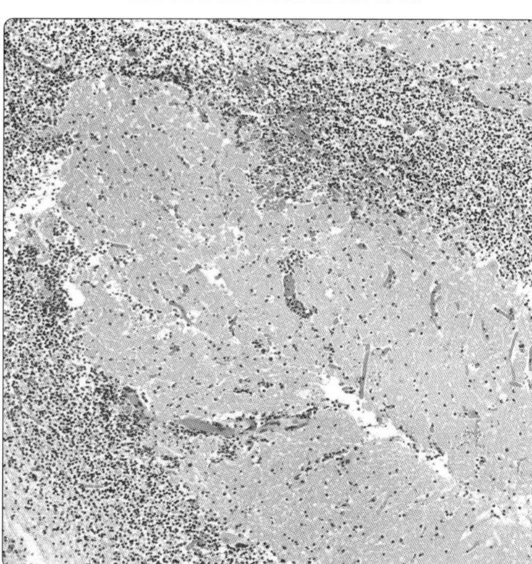

(Left) *An acute infarct, of the type that may come to biopsy, is a soft, swollen, variably hemorrhagic mass ⇨ that can compress an adjacent ventricle ➡. **(Right)** This cerebellar acute infarction was surgically removed because of concern about a neoplasm. Vessels are congested, the tissue is somewhat fragmented, and there are ischemic, "red-dead" Purkinje cells (seen with difficulty at this low magnification).*

Pale Acute infarct

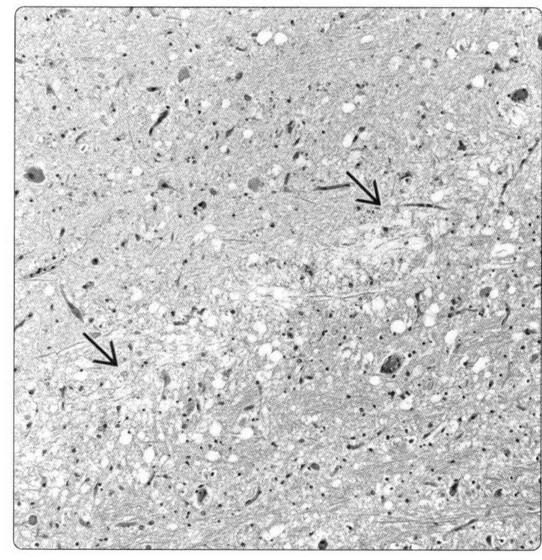

"Red-Dead" Neuron

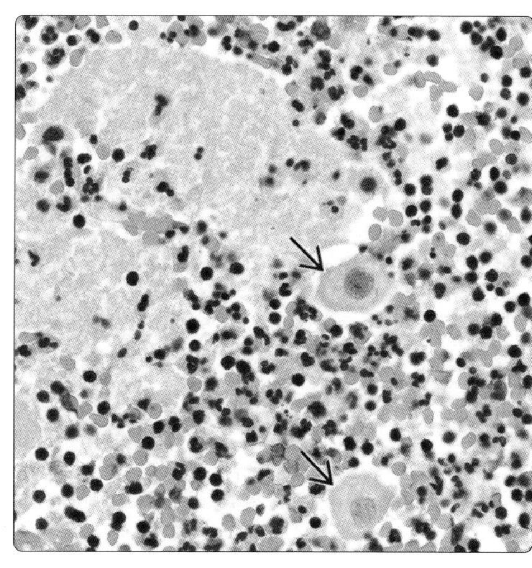

(Left) *Acute infarcts are pale and often vacuolized, especially at the perimeter near the junction with intact brain ⇨. **(Right)** In this acute cerebellar infarct excised as a surgical specimen, early karyolysis in the Purkinje cells ⇨ is a principal finding indicative of ischemia. Neutrophils are also part of the early response.*

"Red-Dead" Neuron

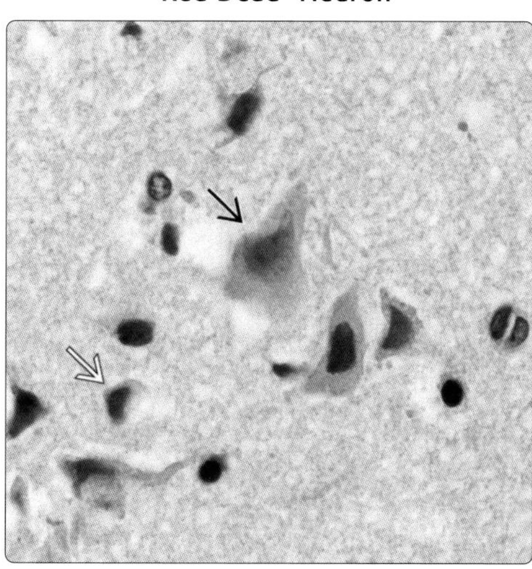

Neuronophagia

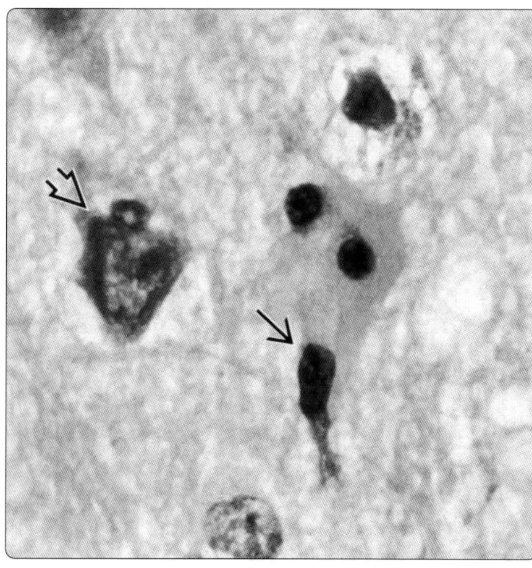

(Left) *Irreversible acute anoxic injury causes "red-dead" neurons with karyolytic nuclei, refractile eosinophilic cytoplasm, and concave borders ⇨. Smaller "red-dead" neurons ➡ sometimes are so small that they are difficult to recognize as neurons. **(Right)** If the infarction is several days old, resting tissue phagocytes (i.e., microglial cells) and blood-borne monocytes begin to phagocytose dead neurons ⇨. Note the nearby viable neuron ⇨ for comparison.*

(Left) *Small groups of neutrophils ⇨ are common in infarcts of several days duration. Note the red necrotic neurons with karyolytic nuclei.* **(Right)** *As a result of reperfused necrotic vessels, acute infarcts due to emboli or secondary to herniation often contain petechiae.*

Neutrophils

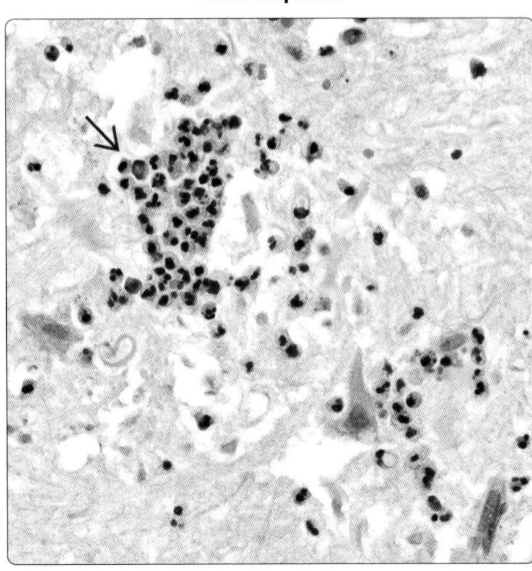

Petechiae

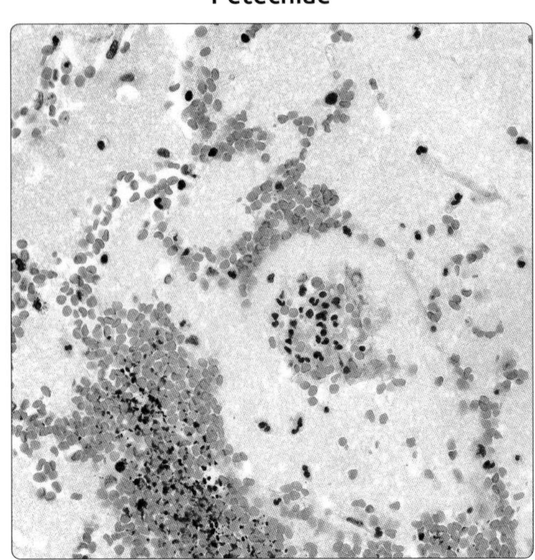

(Left) *Vascular cells in the early infarct are hypertrophic and sometimes in mitotic division ⇨. A "red-dead" neuron ⇨ helps in the diagnosis.* **(Right)** *Macrophages are the principal product of smearing in the subacute phase of an infarct. An ischemic "red-dead" neuron ⇨ helps distinguish this lesion from demyelinating disease.*

Prominent Reactive Vessels

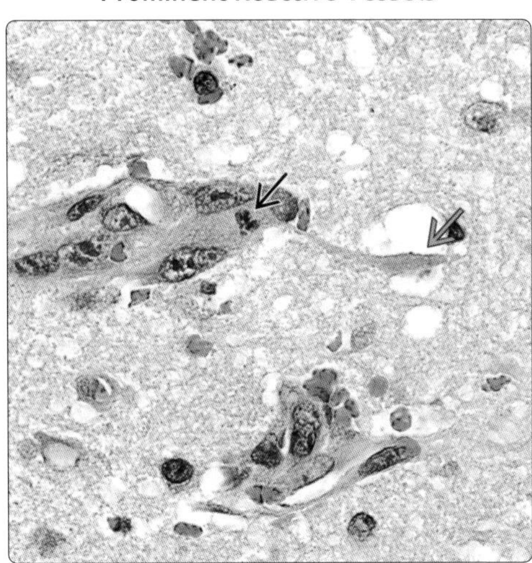

Macrophages

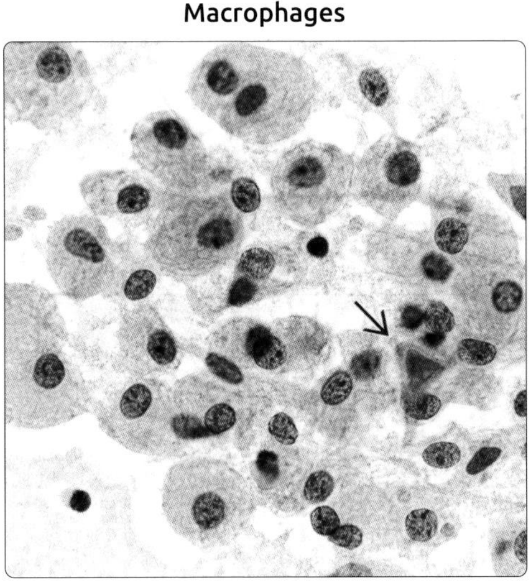

(Left) *Axial NECT obtained 48 hours after presentation demonstrates the classic appearance of a late acute/early subacute cerebral infarct. Note the wedge-shaped, low-density area involving both the gray and white matter in the left main cerebral artery (MCA) distribution ⇨.* **(Right)** *Axial NECT obtained 1 week after ictus demonstrates gyriform areas of slightly increased attenuation ➡ in keeping with hemorrhagic transformation. This typically occurs between 48 and 72 hours after onset.*

Axial CT: Late Acute Infarct

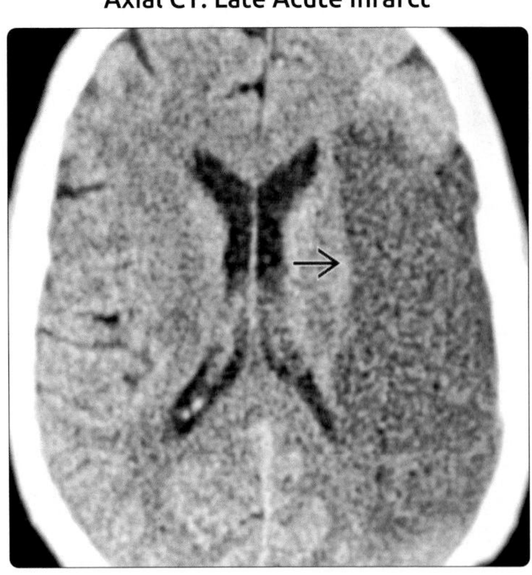

Axial CT: 1-Week Infarct

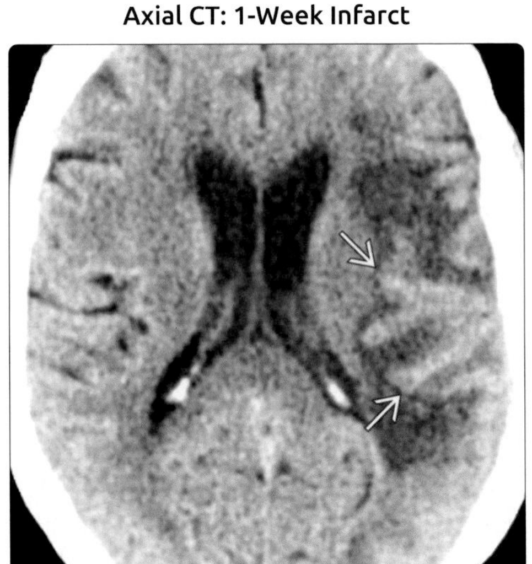

1-Week Infarct

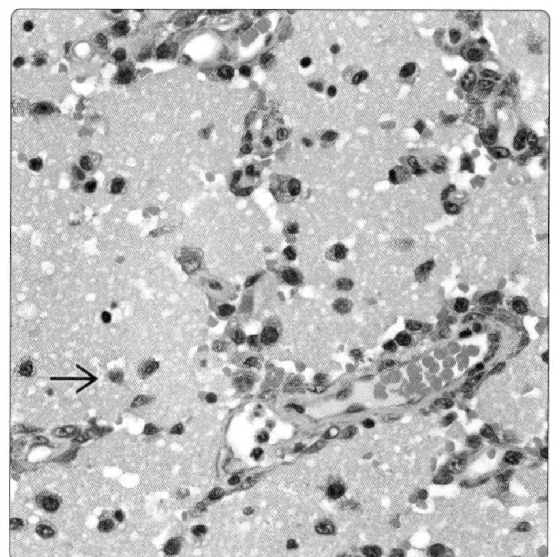

Early Macrophage Influx

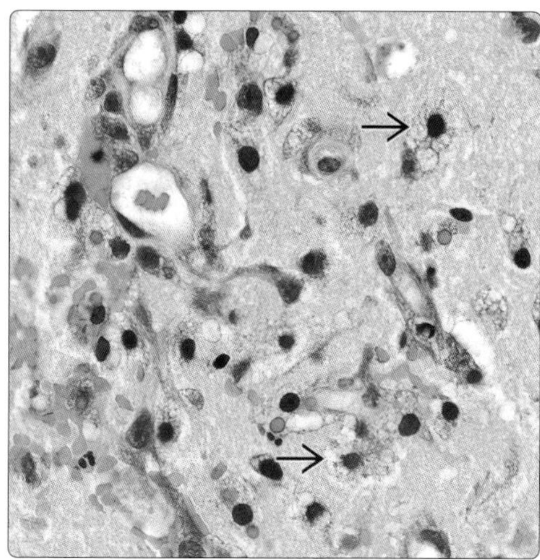

(Left) *During the 1st week after tissue infarction, neurons are progressively removed and "red-dead" neurons become barely discernible ➙. The basophilia of the proliferative vasculature reflects the high metabolic rate of these cells, but can be worrisome to the surgical pathologist.* **(Right)** *Proliferating capillaries facilitate the entry of blood monocytes, which become phagocytic macrophages with bubbly cytoplasm and small dark nuclei ➙.*

Prominent Macrophage Influx

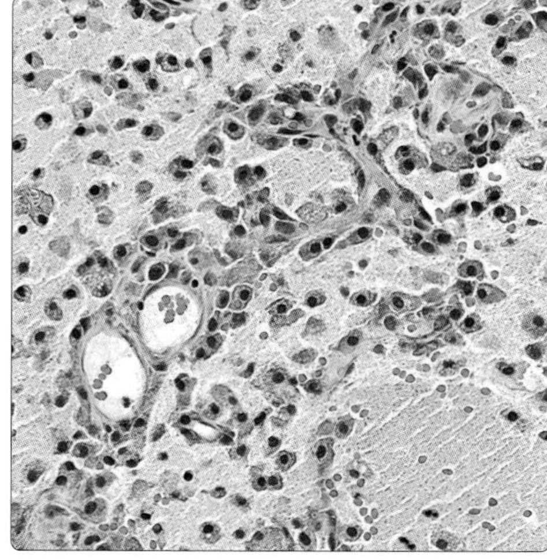

Plump Endothelial Cells

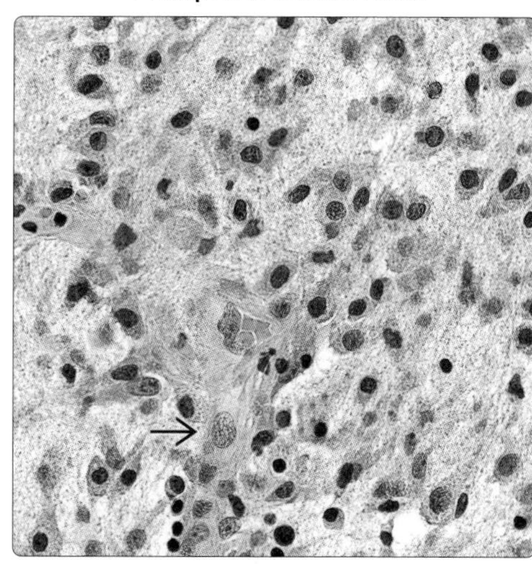

(Left) *By the end of the 1st week, the macrophage influx is well underway as these cells move beyond the immediate perivascular areas toward the center of the necrotic zone. The phagocytes persist for as long as necrotic debris remains, usually months in the case of a large lesion.* **(Right)** *When macrophages are abundant in an infarct, they may give the impression of a glioma due to the hypercellularity. This is especially true when they occur along with plump endothelial cells ➙.*

Early Cavitation

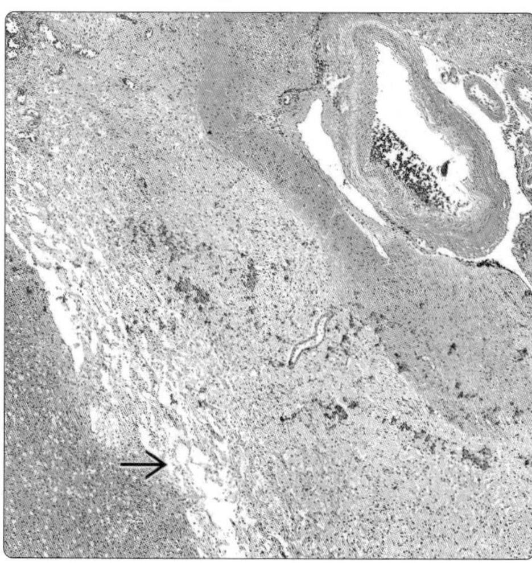

Progressive Cavitation

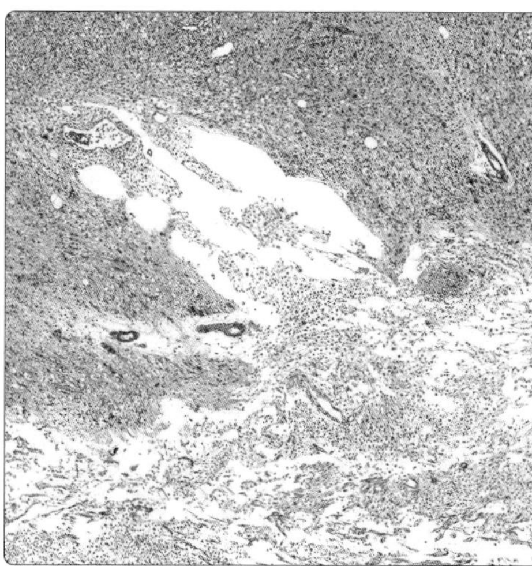

(Left) *Progressive removal of necrotic debris over weeks to months leads to early cavitation ➙.* **(Right)** *Progressive cavitation of an infarct appears over weeks to months.*

(Left) *Macrophages in a subacute or chronic evolving infarct are interspersed with strands of glial tissue and delicate blood vessels.* **(Right)** *The central area of a remote, years-old infarction contains little other than glial strands and delicate surviving vessels.*

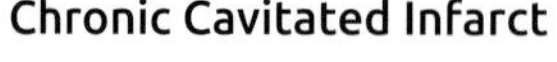

Chronic Cavitated Infarct

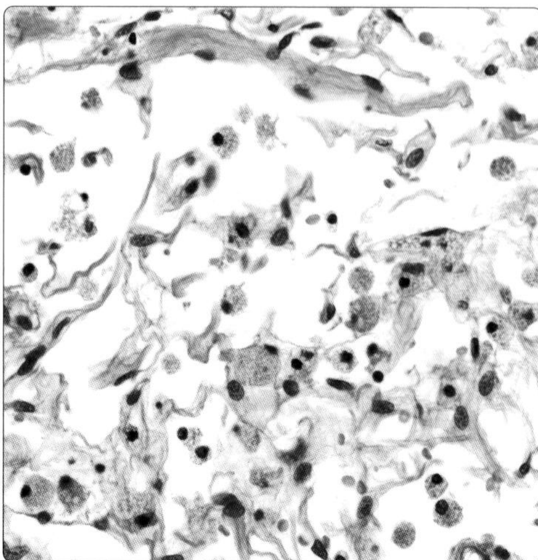

Chronic Cavitated Infarct

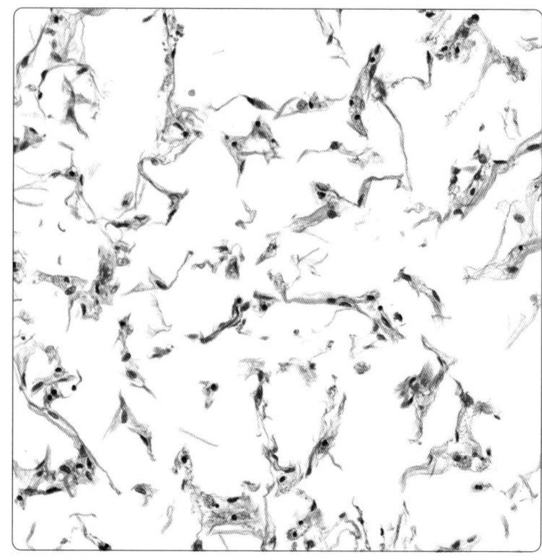

(Left) *A remote, cavitated infarction in the territory of the MCA exhibits the typical irregular, "ratty" edge of an old infarct and a very large cavitated hole.* **(Right)** *A 10-year-old boy had left-sided weakness from a right middle cerebral artery infarct discovered in infancy. The remote infarct was resected for seizure control. Note the nodular gliotic walls of the cystic cavity. Highly gliotic remote infarcts can simulate tumor.*

Chronic Infarct

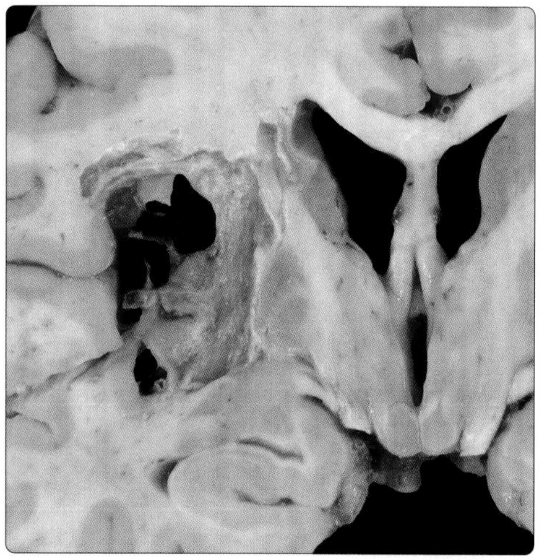

Gliotic Infarct Mimicking Tumor

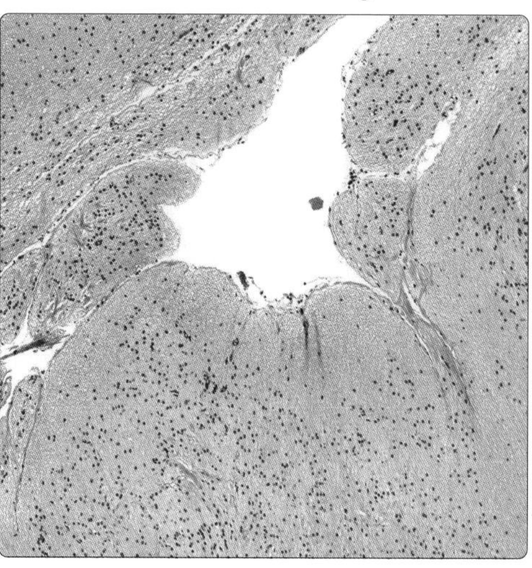

(Left) *Axial T1WI C+ MR shows a 19-year-old woman admitted to the hospital with pyelonephritis. History of headache prompted MR imaging, which revealed this right-sided, nonenhancing cystic lesion. Concern for a cystic tumor led to resection of this remote stroke, likely intrauterine or perinatal.* **(Right)** *Unlike demyelinating disease, axons are severely depleted and fragmented in infarcts, as illustrated here on immunostaining for neurofilament protein.*

Remote Cystic Infarct Simulating Tumor

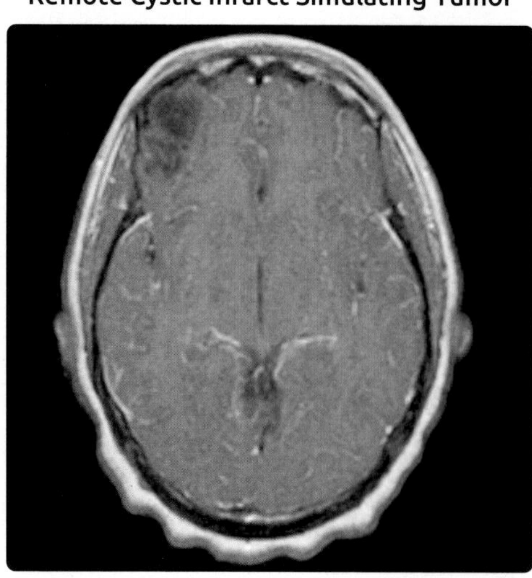

Severe Axonal Damage

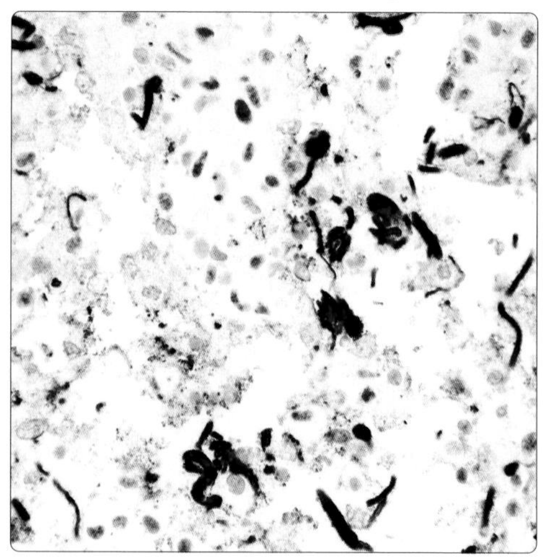

Lacunar Infarct

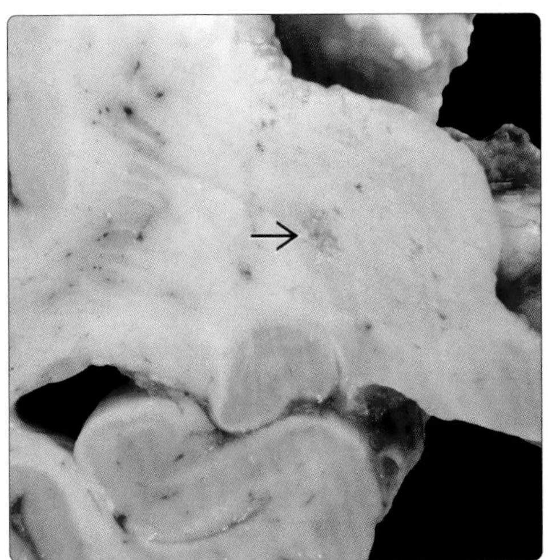

Posterior Inferior Cerebellar Artery Territory

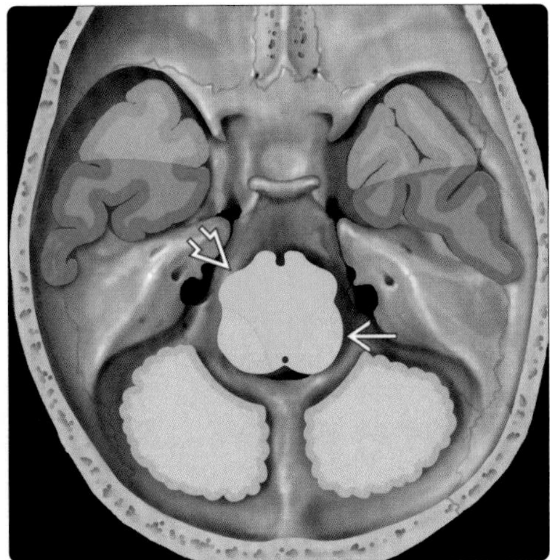

(Left) *Small infarctions 1 cm or less in size are often related to chronic hypertension and arteriolosclerosis and are often found in thalamus ➙, basal ganglia, deep white matter of the cerebral hemispheres, and basis pontis.* **(Right)** *Axial graphic shows the primary posterior inferior cerebellar artery (PICA) territory of the lateral medulla ➙ and inferior cerebellum in tan. Penetrating arteries from the vertebral and anterior spinal arteries supply the remainder of the medulla ➙.*

Axial MR: PICA Infarct

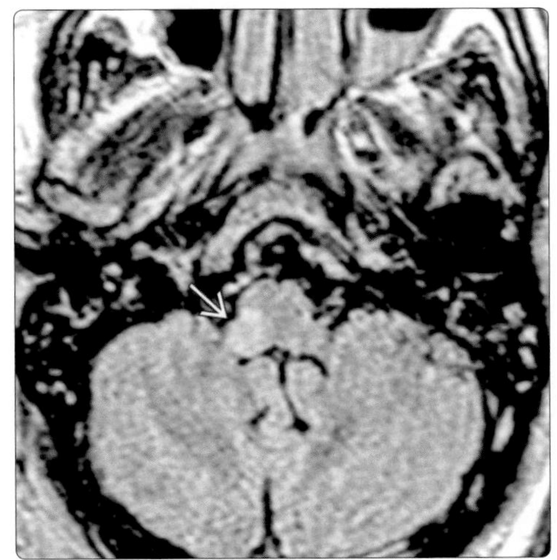

Lateral Medullary Infarct

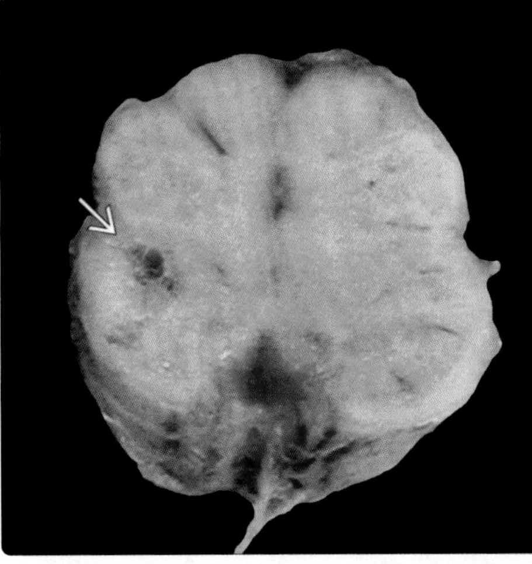

(Left) *Axial FLAIR MR shows hyperintensity in the lateral medulla ➙ related to a PICA infarct in this patient with Wallenberg syndrome, with the clinical triad of Horner syndrome, ataxia, and contralateral hemisensory findings. Lateral medullary infarcts are typically related to vertebral artery disease, including dissection.* **(Right)** *Gross specimen from an 83-year-old man with an infarct in the lateral medulla ➙ is shown. Symptoms included unilateral decreased sensation and movement.*

Axial MR: Amphetamine Abuse

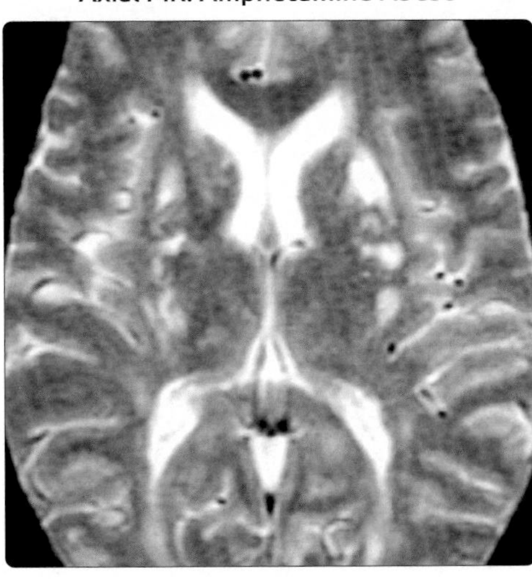

Superficial Tissue Necrosis, Post-Seizure Monitoring

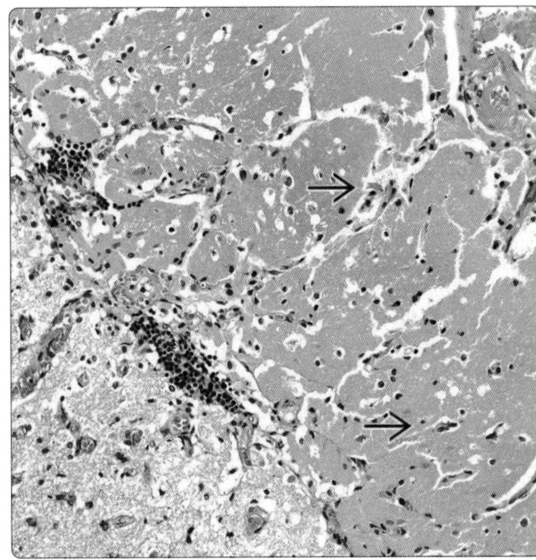

(Left) *Axial T2WI MR shows multiple areas of increased signal intensity in basal ganglia consistent with infarcts caused by amphetamine use.* **(Right)** *Strip-like areas of tissue necrosis are found in superficial cortex directly underlying the site of grid placement in patients who undergo monitoring prior to seizure resection surgery. The eosinophilic necrotic tissue shows capillary proliferation ➙, but the tissue damage lacks the wedge shape seen in typical infarcts.*

KEY FACTS

CLINICAL ISSUES

- Difficult clinical diagnosis
  - Usual presentation
    - Stroke, headache, encephalopathy
- Recent clinical contribution is recognition of reversible cerebral vasoconstriction syndromes (RCVS) that mimic primary angiitis of central nervous system (PACNS), but lack vessel wall inflammation

MICROSCOPIC

- Multinucleated giant cells, lymphocytic, monocytic inflammation in granulomatous angiitis of nervous system (GANS)
- Vessel wall necrosis lacking in granulomatous, lymphocytic types of PACNS
  - Present in necrotizing form of PACNS
- Intimal proliferation, luminal occlusion in healing phases

ANCILLARY TESTS

- Exclude infectious causes by culture/serology
  - Infections producing vasculitis
    - Varicella-zoster virus
    - HIV
    - Syphilis
    - Lyme disease
    - Rickettsial disease
    - Fungal infections
    - Bacterial infections
- Need to exclude systemic causes of vasculitis with CNS involvement
  - Systemic lupus erythematosus, scleroderma, rheumatoid arthritis, Sjögren
  - Rule out antiphospholipid syndrome, cryoglobulinemia, polyarteritis nodosa ± hepatitis infection
- Exclude A-β-related angiitis by special stains for amyloid

(Left) *Lateral digital subtraction angiography internal carotid injection shows multiple alternating arterial stenoses → with focal fusiform dilatations ⇨ typical for primary angiitis of the central nervous system (PACNS).* **(Right)** *Epithelioid histocytes, multinucleated giant cells →, and lymphocytes overrun and narrow vessels in PACNS. Granulomatous PACNS should be distinguished from neurosarcoidosis, if possible.*

Arterial Stenoses, Dilatations

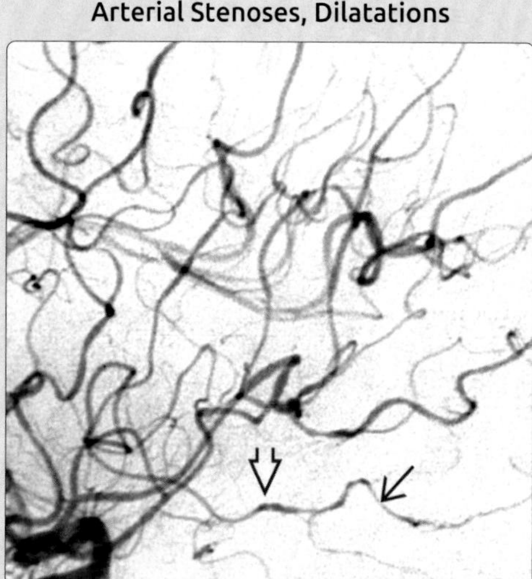

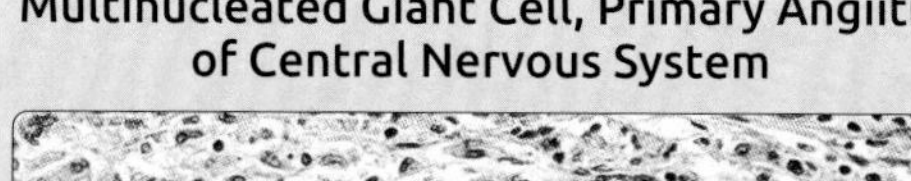

Multinucleated Giant Cell, Primary Angiitis of Central Nervous System

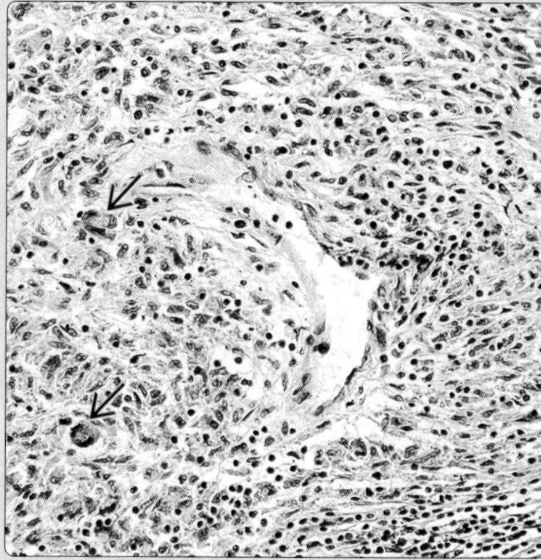

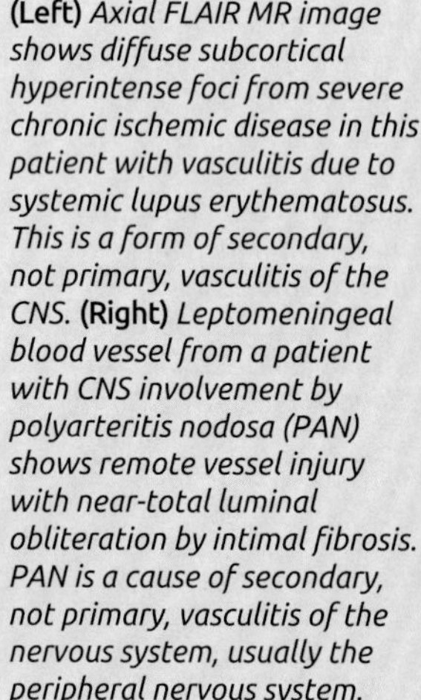

(Left) *Axial FLAIR MR image shows diffuse subcortical hyperintense foci from severe chronic ischemic disease in this patient with vasculitis due to systemic lupus erythematosus. This is a form of secondary, not primary, vasculitis of the CNS.* **(Right)** *Leptomeningeal blood vessel from a patient with CNS involvement by polyarteritis nodosa (PAN) shows remote vessel injury with near-total luminal obliteration by intimal fibrosis. PAN is a cause of secondary, not primary, vasculitis of the nervous system, usually the peripheral nervous system.*

Axial MR: Secondary Vasculitis

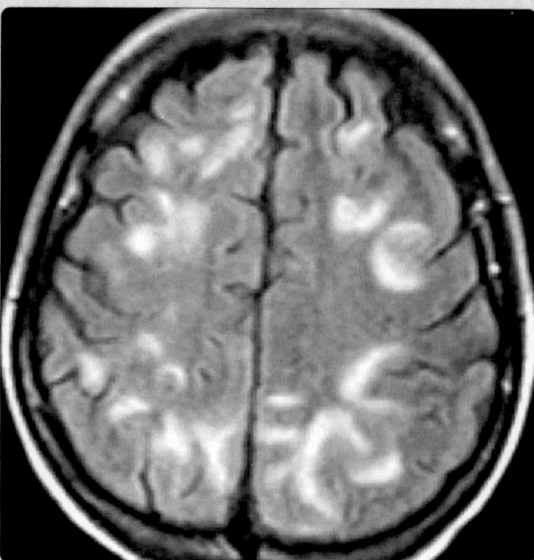

Polyarteritis Nodosa

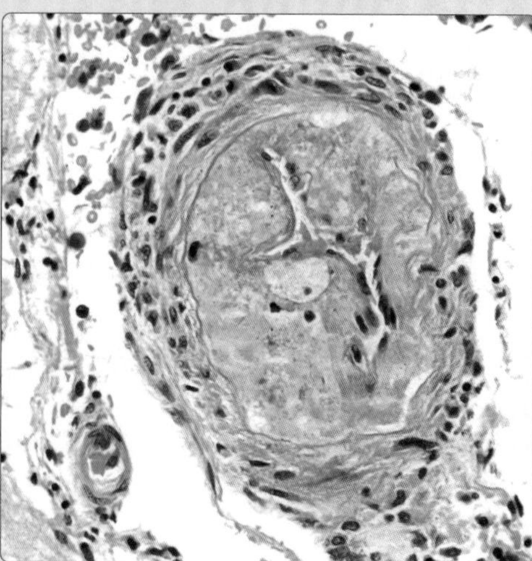

TERMINOLOGY

Abbreviations

- Primary angiitis of the central nervous system (PACNS)

Synonyms

- Isolated angiitis of CNS
- Primary CNS vasculitis

Definitions

- Vasculitis restricted to vasculature of brain and spinal cord, without evidence of systemic vasculitis
- Newly acquired neurological deficit with angiographic **or** histological evidence of CNS vasculitis, after excluding another systemic condition that could explain findings

ETIOLOGY/PATHOGENESIS

Infectious Agents

- Varicella-zoster virus (VZV)
  - Difficult to differentiate from noninfectious PACNS without immunohistochemistry, in situ hybridization, PCR testing

Etiology Unknown

- Probably heterogeneous disorder
- Childhood and adult forms may differ
- Subset of PACNS is granulomatous angiitis of nervous system (GANS) angiopathy
  - GANS in older adults often associated with amyloid angiopathy

CLINICAL ISSUES

Epidemiology

- Incidence
  - Rare
- Age
  - Adults, 4th and 5th decades
  - Pediatric cases increasingly recognized
- Sex
  - Slight male predominance in adults

Presentation

- Fluctuating or stepwise progressive course
- Symptoms often develop over weeks
- Headache, encephalopathy
- Stroke
  - Focal symptoms in < 20% of patients at onset
- Seizures, myelopathy
- Diagnosis of exclusion
  - Many patients have other diseases
  - Diagnosis to be established histologically if angiography (-)
- Uncommon subset with rapid clinical course
  - Bilateral, large infarctions

Treatment

- Drugs
  - Prednisone
  - Cyclophosphamide, other immunosuppressive medications

Prognosis

- Variable, but relapses, mortality possible
- Survival in majority, in recent years

IMAGING

General Features

- Vascular irregularities, stenoses, occlusions in pattern atypical for atherosclerosis
- Conventional angiography gold standard
  - Digital subtraction angiography (DSA) when clinical suspicion is high, regardless of MR findings

MR Findings

- Multifocal deep gray and subcortical hypointensities on T1WI
  - Most patients with some MR abnormality, but usually nonspecific
- Patchy enhancement, in some cases
- MR angiography changes with large vessel involvement

MACROSCOPIC

General Features

- May be minimal
- Multifocal strokes with large vessel involvement

MICROSCOPIC

Histologic Features

- Granulomatous
  - Arteries and veins
  - Mononuclear inflammatory infiltrates
    - Histiocytes, lymphocytes, plasma cells
  - Multinucleated giant cells
  - Intimal proliferation
  - Luminal narrowing and occlusion
- Acute necrotizing
  - Least frequent subtype of PACNS
  - Fibrinoid vascular necrosis in acute phases
  - With intracranial hemorrhage, in some cases
  - Morbidity and mortality not necessarily higher than in other forms of PACNS
  - Need to exclude polyarteritis nodosa with systemic involvement
- Lymphocytic
  - Difficult, practical, and conceptual distinction from chronic inflammation, in some cases
  - 2nd most common form in adults
  - PACNS almost exclusively lymphocytic in children
  - Definition of PACNS
    - Fibrinoid vascular necrosis not present in this form of PACNS
    - Criteria suggest need for minimum of 2 layers of lymphocytes within or around vessel walls
    - Need for structural alterations of vessel walls, such as prominent endothelial cells
    - Criteria does not require fibrinoid vascular necrosis in all forms of PACNS
    - Alternate diagnoses, such as viral encephalitis, should be excluded before diagnosis of PACNS rendered

- Not all PACNS cases are granulomatous (giant cell) (GANS) vasculitis
- Lymphocytic, necrotizing forms of vasculitis exist
- Fibrocellular intimal proliferation may be seen in healed vasculitis, in absence of inflammatory cell infiltrates
- Steroid therapy modifies number, types of inflammatory cells in biopsy/at autopsy

ANCILLARY TESTS

Serologic Testing

- Rule out infection by varicella-zoster virus, *Borrelia burgdorferi* (Lyme disease), neurosyphilis, HIV, rickettsial, or fungal infection
- Markers of systemic vasculitides to be negative
  - Hepatitis B, C
  - ANCA, MPO
  - Cryoglobulins
  - Rheumatoid factor, SS-A, SS-B, Sm, SCL-70, anticardiolipin IgG, IgM, or IgG antiphospholipid antibodies
  - Positive ANA permitted, but not other features of systemic autoimmune disease
- Serum findings usually normal

Cerebrospinal Fluid

- Modest, nonspecific elevations in protein &/or white blood cell count

DIFFERENTIAL DIAGNOSIS

Granulomatous Arteritis Caused by Varicella-Zoster Virus

- Antecedent zoster rash, positive serology for VZV, in some cases
- IHC, in situ hybridization, or PCR evidence of virus in vessels

Neurosarcoidosis

- Granulomas
  - Often in systemic organs as well
  - Not as angiocentric, throughout parenchyma, more dispersed
  - Discrete, well formed, often fibrotic
- But distinction between angiocentric sarcoidosis and GANS not always possible

Granulomatous Arteritis Associated With Amyloid Angiopathy (A-β-Related Angiitis)

- Amyloid by IHC, Congo red staining

Arteritis Associated With HIV

- Diffuse fusiform intracranial aneurysms of large vessels in HIV(+) children
  - Rare examples in HIV(+) adults
- Arteritis in HIV(+) persons may be multifactorial
  - Often associated with infection or lymphoproliferative disorder

Septic Vasculitis

- Usually known embolic source, e.g., cardiac valve, lung
- Cultures or stains (+)

Systemic Vasculitides

- Systemic involvement
- Serological testing positive for collagen vascular disorder in CNS secondarily affected by systemic lupus erythematosus, scleroderma, rheumatoid arthritis, Sjögren syndrome, Behçet disease

Drug-Related Central Nervous System Vasculitis

- Cocaine use associated with ischemic and hemorrhagic stroke
- Cocaine causes vasoconstriction, not vasculitis
- Cause of vasculitis often multifactorial
- Seek clinical history, systemic organ/skin involvement, or serum testing evidence of drug abuse

Reversible Cerebral Vasoconstrictive Syndromes (Clinical Differential)

- Abnormal angiography but no vasculitis
- More likely in young females (middle-aged male predominance with PACNS)
- Often acute onset of severe headache
  - Adult PACNS usually chronic progressive headaches
- Normal cerebrospinal fluid
  - Adult PACNS has moderate CSF leukocytosis, elevated protein

Angioimmunoproliferative Lesion (Lymphomatoid Granulomatosis)

- Angiocentric, angiodestructive pleomorphic lymphocytic disorder
- Additional involvement of lung, other systemic sites, but occasionally restricted to CNS
- Cases with lung and systemic involvement often mediated by Epstein-Barr virus (EBV)
  - Positive in situ hybridization for EBV-encoded small RNAs (EBER ISH)
- Isolated CNS examples often EBV(-)
- Immunoglobulin *IGH* gene rearrangement studies sometimes positive
- Vasocentric, pleomorphic population of mononuclear cells, histiocytes
  - Not granulomatous inflammation with tight granulomas
- Cytologically atypical B-cell lymphocytes in variable numbers
  - Classified into 3 subtypes based on numbers of neoplastic B-cell lymphocytes
- Vessel wall necrosis

Primary Central Nervous System Lymphoma

- Cytologically atypical lymphocytes, usually B cells
- High Ki-67 rate
- Usually EBV mediated in setting of immunocompromise: EBER ISH(+)
- Clonality usually established by gene rearrangement studies
- Tumor cells, but not inflammatory cells, often lysed by preoperative steroids

DIAGNOSTIC CHECKLIST

Clinically Relevant Pathologic Features

- Yield greater for targeted lesional biopsies versus biopsies from nonlesional sites, as determined by neuroimaging

Pathologic Interpretation Pearls

- Brain and meningeal biopsy gold standard
  - Specimen sampling should obtain all 3 superficial layers of brain tissue: Leptomeninges, gray matter/cortex, subcortical white matter
  - Dura seldom involved
- Biopsy results may be influenced by prolonged time to biopsy, prior steroid treatment, sampling issues
- Distribution of changes focal or segmental; thus, 25-50% of biopsies nondiagnostic
  - Nondiagnostic biopsies more often from nonlesional sites
- Steroid treatment can severely alter features of angioimmunoproliferative lesion, primary CNS lymphoma
  - Ascertain history of preoperative steroids
  - Residual vasocentric nonneoplastic lymphocytes and histiocytes, but few if any neoplastic cells
- Exclude systemic polyarteritis nodosa in necrotizing CNS vasculitis
- Nearly 1/2 of all granulomatous examples of PACNS associated with β-amyloid in some studies
- Lymphocytic PACNS with transmural inflammation, vessel wall injury to be distinguished from chronic perivascular inflammation
  - May be difficult
- Perivascular inflammation, nonspecific gliosis, and infarction(s) insufficient alone for definitive histological diagnosis of vasculitis

SELECTED REFERENCES

1. Rodriguez-Pla A et al: Primary angiitis of the central nervous system in adults and children. Rheum Dis Clin North Am. 41(1):47-62, viii, 2015
2. de Boysson H et al: Primary angiitis of the central nervous system: description of the first fifty-two adults enrolled in the French cohort of patients with primary vasculitis of the central nervous system. Arthritis Rheumatol. 66(5):1315-26, 2014
3. Nouh A et al: Amyloid-Beta related angiitis of the central nervous system: case report and topic review. Front Neurol. 5:13, 2014
4. Suri V et al: Primary angiitis of the central nervous system: a study of histopathological patterns and review of the literature. Folia Neuropathol. 52(2):187-96, 2014
5. Salvarani C et al: Rapidly progressive primary central nervous system vasculitis. Rheumatology (Oxford). 50(2):349-58, 2011
6. Berlit P: Diagnosis and treatment of cerebral vasculitis. Ther Adv Neurol Disord. 3(1):29-42, 2010
7. Cellucci T et al: Central nervous system vasculitis in children. Curr Opin Rheumatol. 22(5):590-7, 2010
8. Elbers J et al: Brain biopsy in children with primary small-vessel central nervous system vasculitis. Ann Neurol. 68(5):602-10, 2010
9. Goldstein DA et al: HIV-associated intracranial aneurysmal vasculopathy in adults. J Rheumatol. 37(2):226-33, 2010
10. Gupta T et al: Isolated central nervous system involvement by lymphomatoid granulomatosis in an adolescent: a case report and review of literature. Pediatr Hematol Oncol. 27(2):150-9, 2010
11. Hajj-Ali RA: Primary angiitis of the central nervous system: differential diagnosis and treatment. Best Pract Res Clin Rheumatol. 24(3):413-26, 2010
12. Hunder GG et al: Primary central nervous system vasculitis: Is it a single disease? Ann Neurol. 68(5):573-4, 2010
13. Hutchinson C et al: Treatment of small vessel primary CNS vasculitis in children: an open-label cohort study. Lancet Neurol. 9(11):1078-84, 2010
14. Birnbaum J et al: Primary angiitis of the central nervous system. Arch Neurol. 66(6):704-9, 2009
15. Lucantoni C et al: Primary cerebral lymphomatoid granulomatosis: report of four cases and literature review. J Neurooncol. 94(2):235-42, 2009
16. Melica G et al: Primary vasculitis of the central nervous system in patients infected with HIV-1 in the HAART era. J Med Virol. 81(4):578-81, 2009
17. Miller DV et al: Biopsy findings in primary angiitis of the central nervous system. Am J Surg Pathol. 33(1):35-43, 2009
18. Elbers J et al: Central nervous system vasculitis in children. Curr Opin Rheumatol. 20(1):47-54, 2008
19. Guillevin L: Vasculitides in the context of HIV infection. AIDS. 22 Suppl 3:S27-33, 2008
20. Ishiura H et al: Lymphomatoid granulomatosis involving central nervous system successfully treated with rituximab alone. Arch Neurol. 65(5):662-5, 2008
21. Nishihara H et al: Immunohistochemical and gene rearrangement studies of central nervous system lymphomatoid granulomatosis. Neuropathology. 27(5):413-8, 2007
22. Kossorotoff M et al: Cerebral vasculopathy with aneurysm formation in HIV-infected young adults. Neurology. 66(7):1121-2, 2006
23. Scolding NJ et al: Abeta-related angiitis: primary angiitis of the central nervous system associated with cerebral amyloid angiopathy. Brain. 128(Pt 3):500-15, 2005
24. Alrawi A et al: Brain biopsy in primary angiitis of the central nervous system. Neurology. 53(4):858-60, 1999
25. Calabrese LH et al: Primary angiitis of the central nervous system: diagnostic criteria and clinical approach. Cleve Clin J Med. 59(3):293-306, 1992
26. Lie JT: Primary (granulomatous) angiitis of the central nervous system: a clinicopathologic analysis of 15 new cases and a review of the literature. Hum Pathol. 23(2):164-71, 1992
27. Calabrese LH et al: Primary angiitis of the central nervous system. Report of 8 new cases, review of the literature, and proposal for diagnostic criteria. Medicine (Baltimore). 67(1):20-39, 1988

(Left) *Coronal graphic illustrates alternating segmental areas of narrowing and dilation, as well as infarction* ➙*, within underlying brain in PACNS.* **(Right)** *Granulomatous angiitis, the most frequent form of PACNS, has inflammatory infiltrates composed of epithelioid cells, lymphocytes, plasma cells, and variable numbers of multinucleated giant cells. The lumen may be narrowed* ➙*.*

Primary Angiitis of Central Nervous System

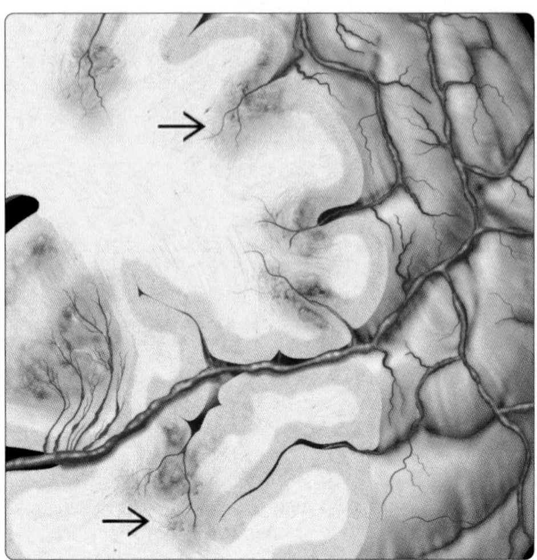

Granulomatous Primary Angiitis of Central Nervous System

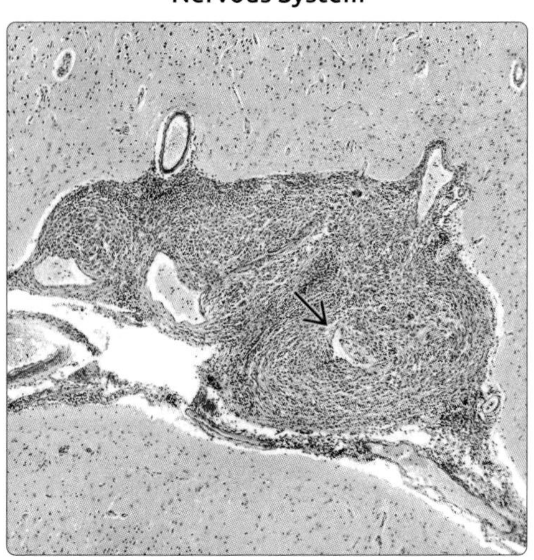

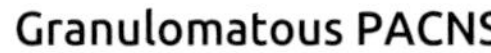

(Left) *Granulomatous angiitis of the central nervous system (GANS) of leptomeningeal vessels in later stages manifests intimal injury with fibroblastic intimal proliferation causing severe stenosis* ➙*.* **(Right)** *Small parenchymal granulomas may occur in GANS, but the vessel may not be evident in the plane of section. Cases of GANS must be distinguished not only from neurosarcoidosis (NS) but also from cerebral amyloid angiopathy with granulomatous inflammation (A-β-related angiitis).*

Granulomatous PACNS

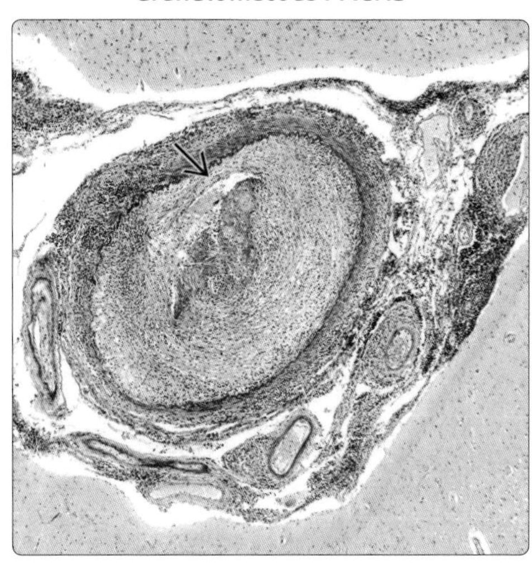

Overlap With Neurosarcoidosis

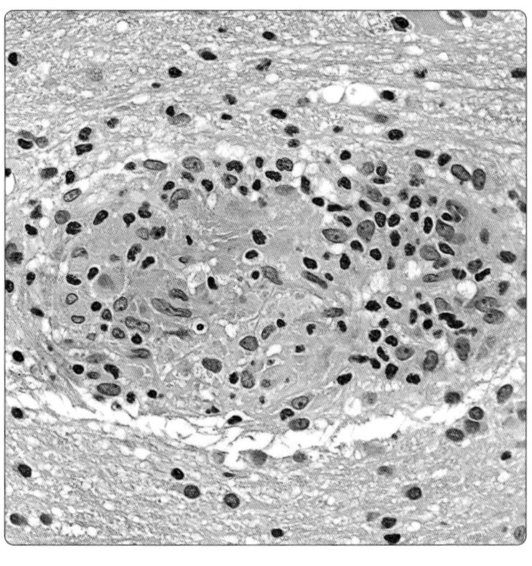

(Left) *NS should be a strong consideration in cases of GANS, such as this with relatively discrete, tight granulomas. NS usually has more parenchymal CNS involvement and more well-formed granulomas than PACNS. The distinction may be impossible in some cases especially in small specimens.* **(Right)** *Granulomatous inflammation in the GANS variant of PACNS contains predominantly mononuclear epithelioid histiocytes. Multinucleated giant cells may be rare to absent.*

Overlap With Neurosarcoidosis

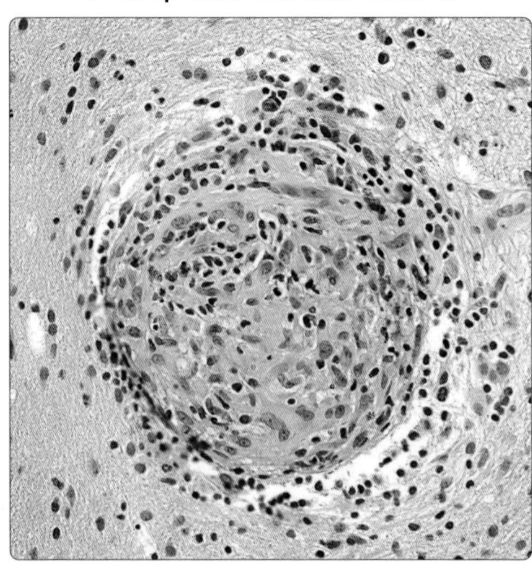

Mononuclear Histiocytes

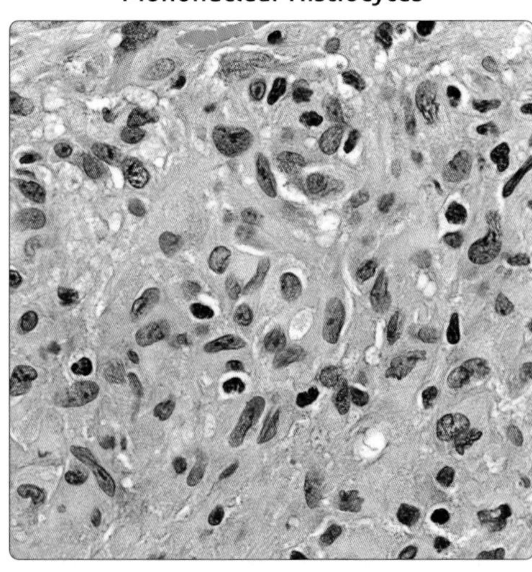

Amyloid Angiopathy as Cause of GANS

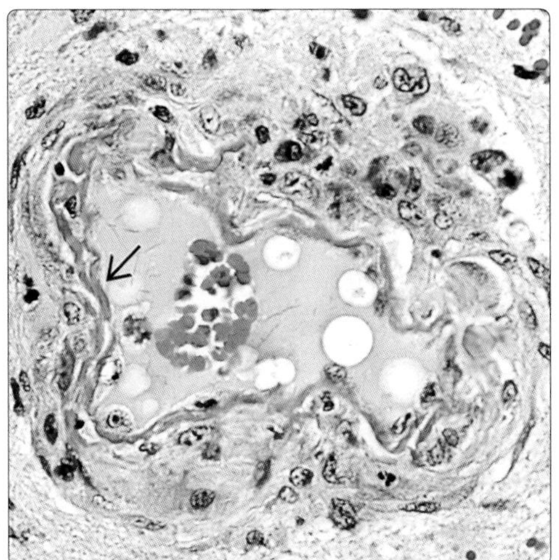

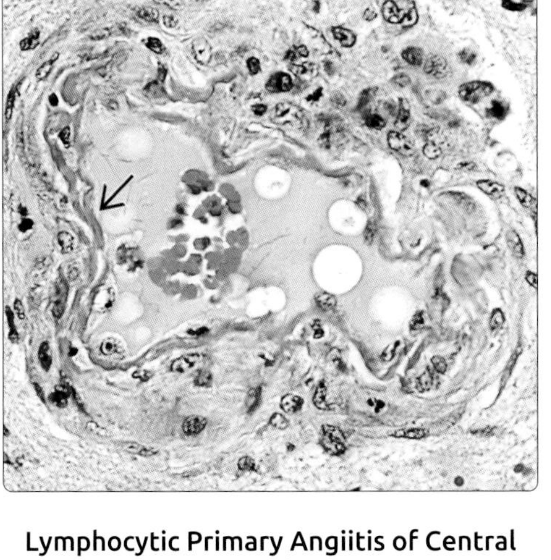

Lymphocytic Primary Angiitis of Central Nervous System

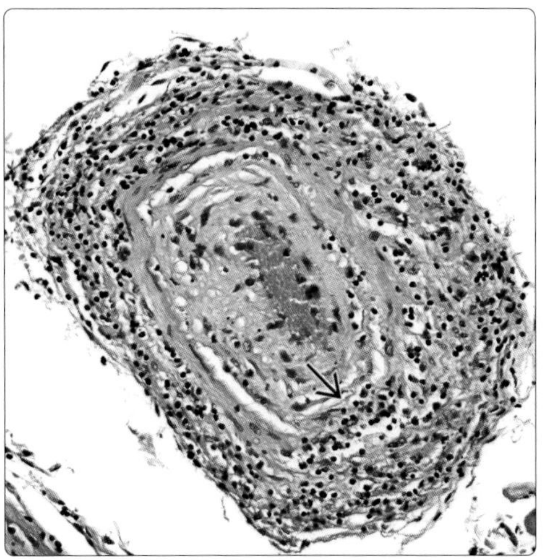

(Left) *A common form of GANS is amyloid angiopathy with a granulomatous response. Hypereosinophilic amyloid* ⇒ *may be associated with granulomatous inflammation in a subset of patients.* **(Right)** *Low-power image from the autopsy of a patient with multifocal T2W and FLAIR hyperintensities shows intimal proliferation and medial wall injury, as well as medial* ⇒ *and adventitial inflammatory changes that are sufficient for the diagnosis of lymphocytic CNS vasculitis.*

Lymphocytic Primary Angiitis of Central Nervous System

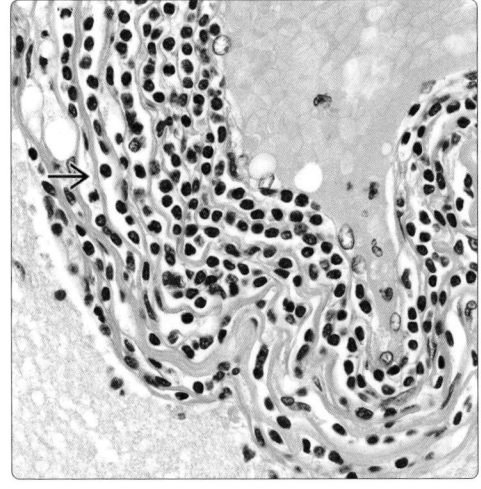

Axial MR: Cocaine Abuse

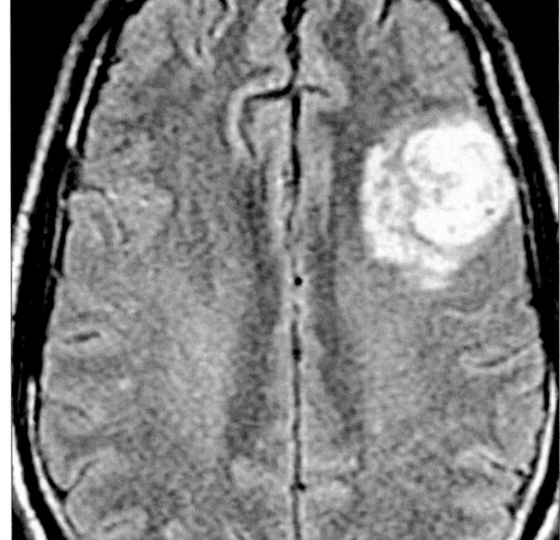

(Left) *Lymphocytic vasculitis shows transmural inflammation by cytologically normal lymphocytes. Fibrinoid vascular necrosis is absent in the lymphocytic form of PACNS. Eccentric proliferation of reticulin fibers indicates vessel wall distortion and damage* ⇒. **(Right)** *Vascular complications of cocaine abuse include infarcts, apparent in this axial FLAIR MR as a hyperintense, rounded frontal lobe lesion in a 22 year old.*

Axial MR: Amphetamine Abuse

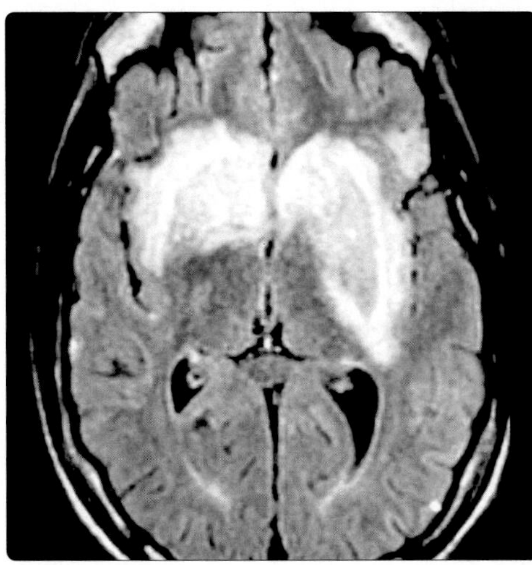

Post Steroid Treatment

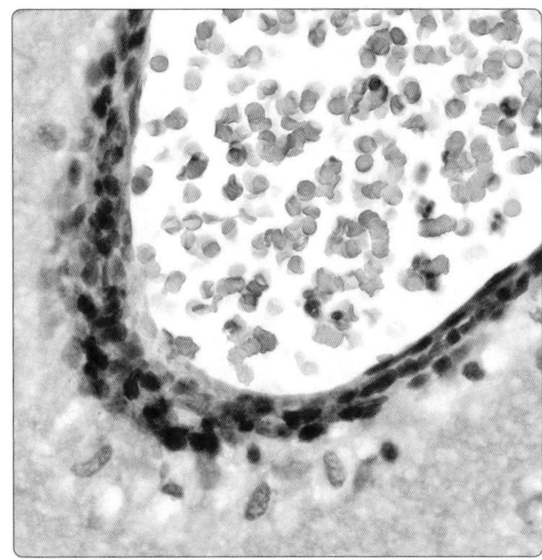

(Left) *Axial FLAIR MR in a patient with a history of amphetamine abuse shows bilateral basal ganglia edema related to vasculitis. A corresponding angiogram showed the typical beaded appearance of vasculitis.* **(Right)** *This 18-year-old woman had steroid-responsive CNS symptoms for 9 months; her biopsy showed moderate numbers of lymphocytes and subacute and remote infarcts. Preoperative steroids may have modified number, or type, of inflammatory cells.*

(Left) *Biopsy tissue from an 18-year-old woman with fluctuating neurological symptoms responsive to steroids shows scant transmural nonneoplastic lymphocytes. The steroids may have modified the number or type of inflammatory cells.* **(Right)** *This 18-year-old, HIV(-) woman with recurrent CNS symptoms was biopsied for suspected vasculitis; her biopsy shows a partially cavitated ➡ infarct with macrophages and surrounding gliosis ➡.*

Post Steroid Treatment

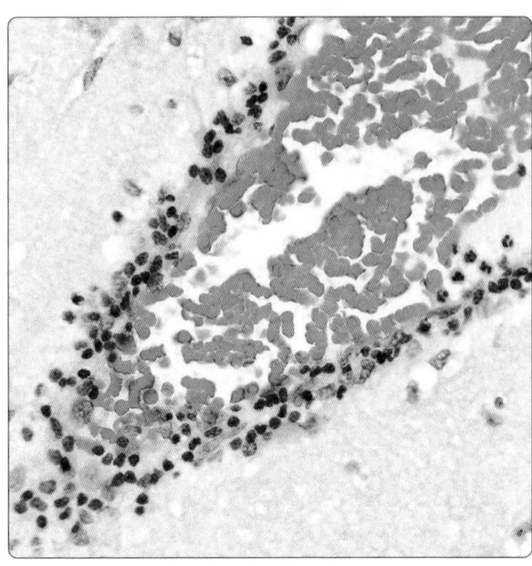

Infarct

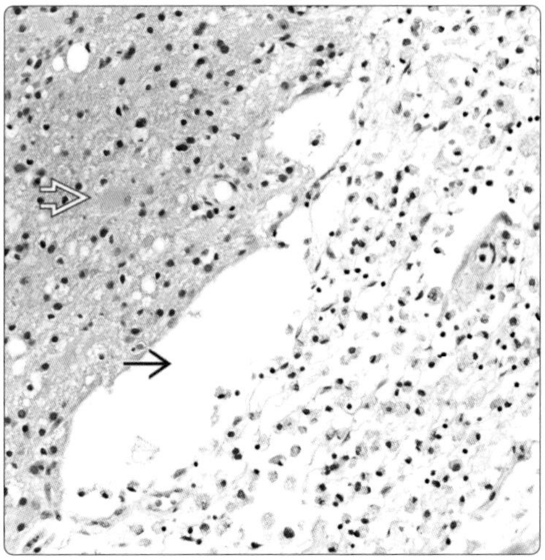

(Left) *This necrotizing vasculitis occurred in a middle-aged male without systemic vasculitis at autopsy. Note the small vessel fibrinoid vascular necrosis ➡ and obliteration of architectural features. Extensive work-up for infection was negative, including IHC for herpes simplex and EBV and PCR testing for varicella-zoster virus.* **(Right)** *Leptomeningeal CNS blood vessels in a patient with known systemic PAN show recent and remote ➡ vasculitis.*

Necrotizing Primary Angiitis of Central Nervous System

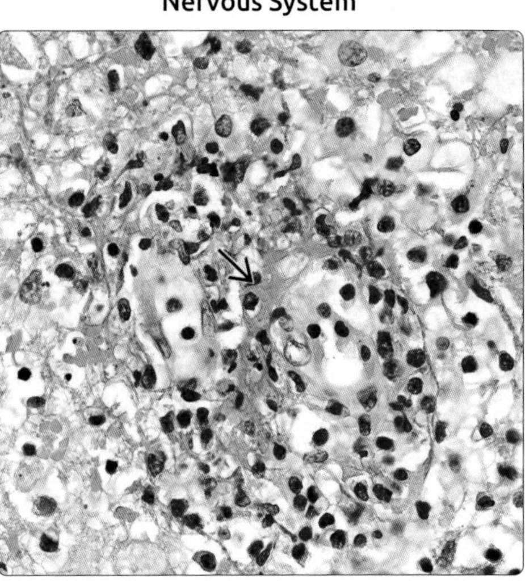

Secondary Angiitis, Polyarteritis Nodosa

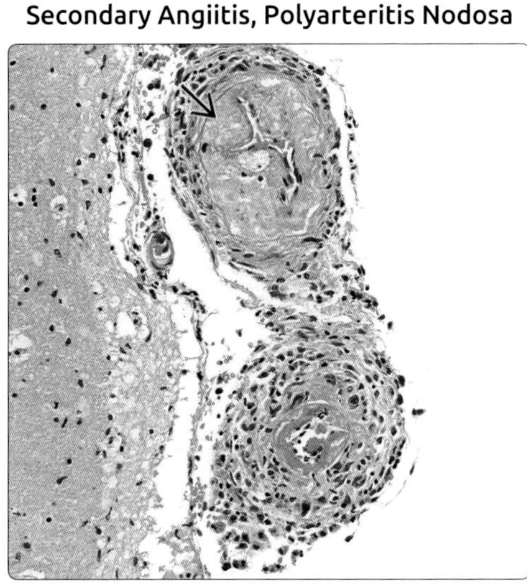

(Left) *CNS vessels can be involved in patients with PAN and show features similar to PAN elsewhere in the body, including fibrinoid vascular necrosis ➡. The peripheral nervous system is more frequently involved in PAN than the central.* **(Right)** *Fibrinoid necrosis ➡ with smudgy, amorphous fibrinous material and obliteration of vascular architecture is typical of PAN. CNS involvement is uncommon.*

Fibrinoid Necrosis, Polyarteritis Nodosa

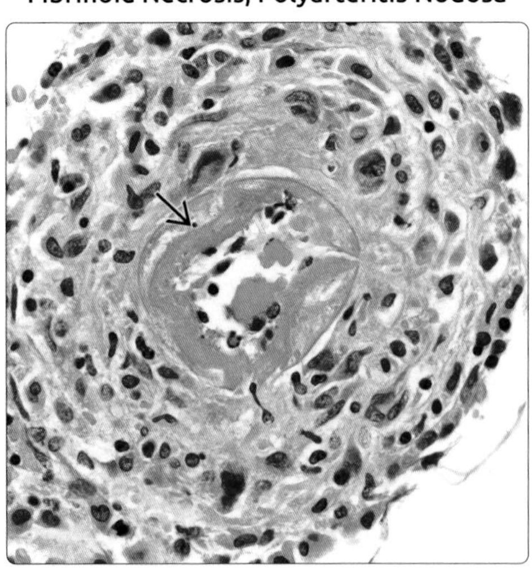

Uncommon Central Nervous System Involvement, Polyarteritis Nodosa

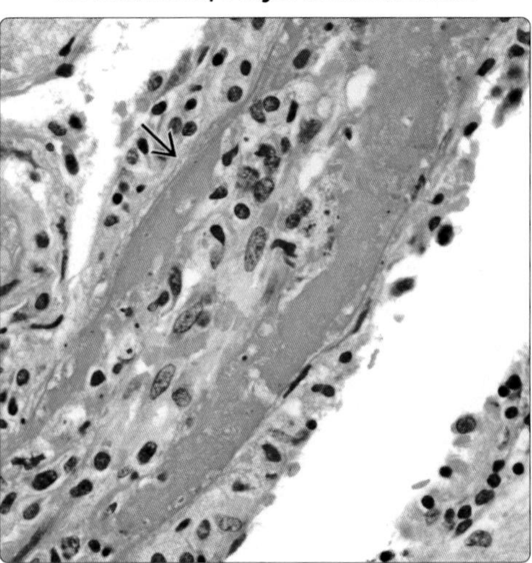

Secondary Vasculitis, SLE

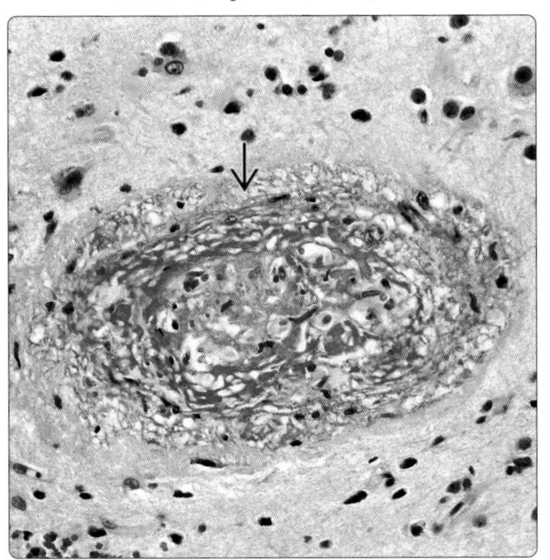

Primary CNS Lymphoma

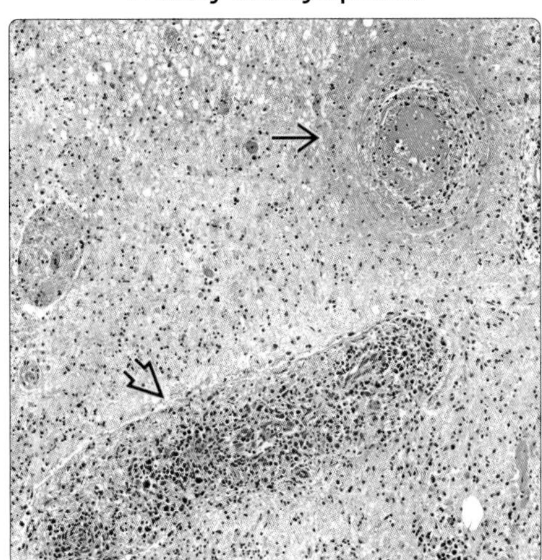

(Left) *Intracranial complications of systemic lupus erythematosus are more often related to treatment effects, but intracranial vessels may show damage due to SLE; necrotizing angiitis ➡, however, is rare.* **(Right)** *This example of primary CNS B-cell lymphoma (PCNSL) occurred in a renal transplant recipient. Note CNS vessels with necrosis ➡ and inflammatory infiltrates ➡. Such necrotic changes are not expected in the more common, sporadic form of PCNSL.*

Primary B-Cell Lymphoma

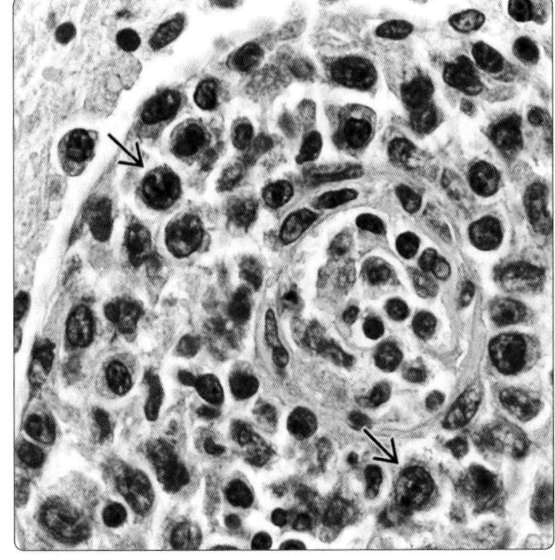

CD20

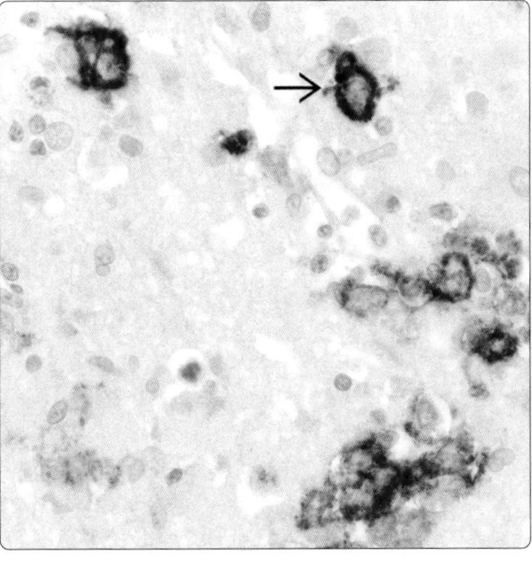

(Left) *Angiocentric/angiodestructive primary CNS B-cell lymphomas can resemble angiitis, but not when cytologically atypical cells ➡ are as obvious as they are here. This example occurred in a renal transplant recipient on immunosuppressive therapy.* **(Right)** *Immunohistochemistry for B-cell marker CD20 helps identify tumor cells ➡ in primary CNS lymphoma, even when present in small numbers.*

EBER

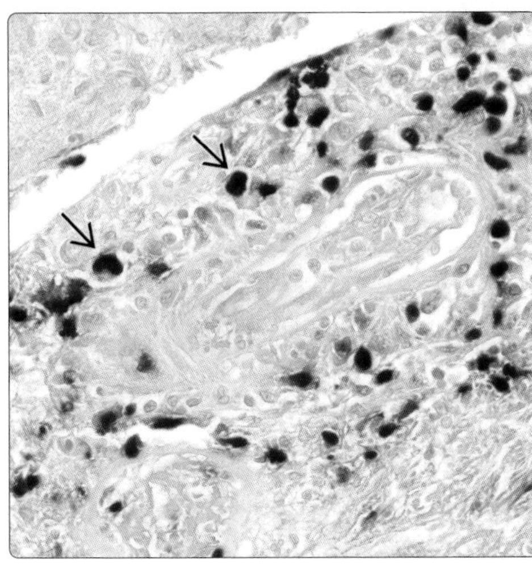

HIV Vasculitis/Vasculopathy

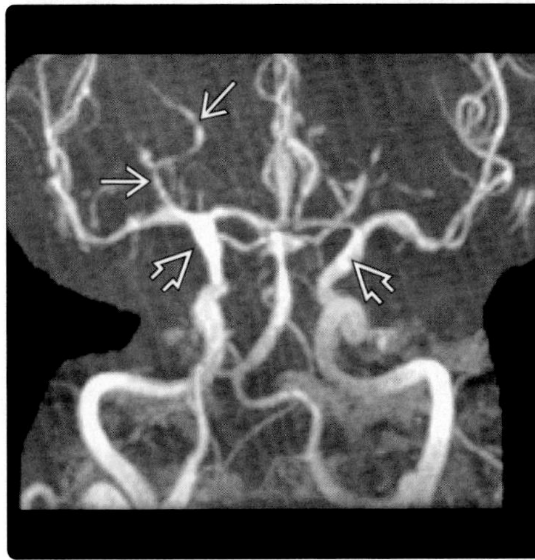

(Left) *Primary CNS lymphomas that arise in the context of immunosuppression are almost uniformly EBV-driven, as evidenced by strong signal for EBV small RNA (EBER) by in situ hybridization ➡.* **(Right)** *MR angiography shows multifocal areas of alternating vessel constriction ➡ and dilatation ➡ in this HIV(+) patient with severe vasculitis/vasculopathy.*

Amyloid (Congophilic) Angiopathy

KEY FACTS

TERMINOLOGY

- Synonyms
  - Cerebral amyloid angiopathy (CAA)
  - Congophilic angiopathy
- Amyloid isolated to CNS

CLINICAL ISSUES

- Lobar and microhemorrhages, small infarctions, differing ages and sizes

MICROSCOPIC

- Amyloid deposition earliest/maximal in leptomeningeal and superficial cortical blood vessels
- Medium to small arteries, arterioles preferentially affected

TOP DIFFERENTIAL DIAGNOSES

- Vessels with electrocautery artifact can appear smudgy, eosinophilic, and congophilic
  - Electrocauterized vessels do not polarize on Congo red stain
- Cerebral amyloid angiopathy (CAA) often incidental finding in patients without cerebral hemorrhage(s)
- Rule out other causes of hemorrhage
  - Coagulopathy
  - Thrombocytopenia
  - Neoplasm

DIAGNOSTIC CHECKLIST

- Use Congo red or immunohistochemistry to rule out presence of amyloid in all cases of clot evacuation in elderly persons if fragments of cortex &/or leptomeninges are present
- Assess surgical specimen for presence of neuritic plaques and tangles by modified Bielschowsky silver stain or TAU immunohistochemistry

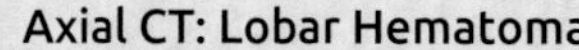

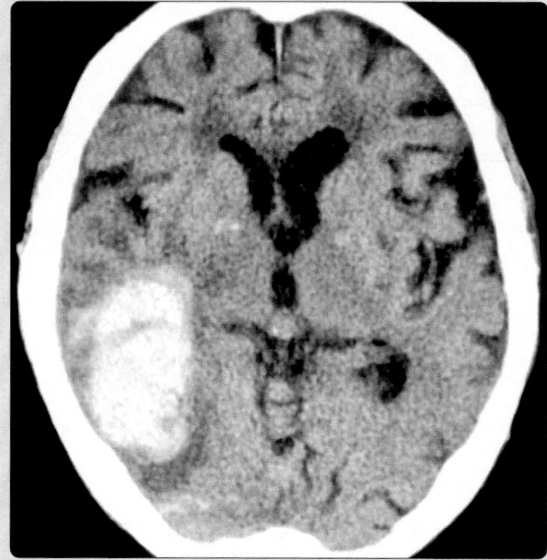

Multifocal Hematomas

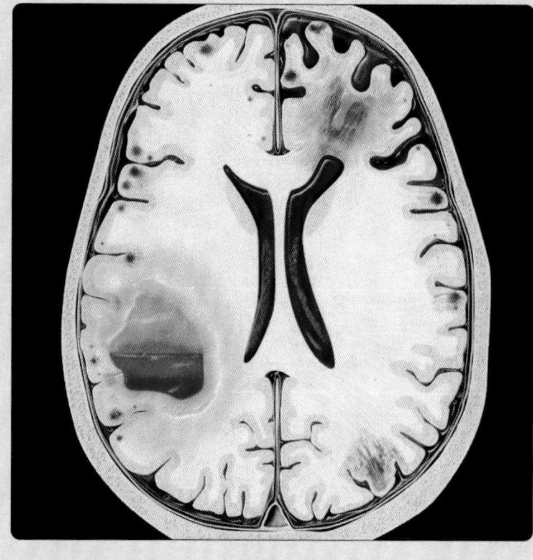

(Left) *Axial nonenhanced CT shows an acute lobar hematoma in this normotensive patient with known "congophilic angiopathy." The cortical atrophy and ventricular dilatation are consistent with the patient's advanced age.* **(Right)** *Axial graphic depicts cerebral amyloid angiopathy (CAA), with multifocal large lobar and microhemorrhages of differing ages. Bleeds tend to be more superficially located than chronic hypertensive bleeds.*

Severe Cerebral Amyloid Angiopathy

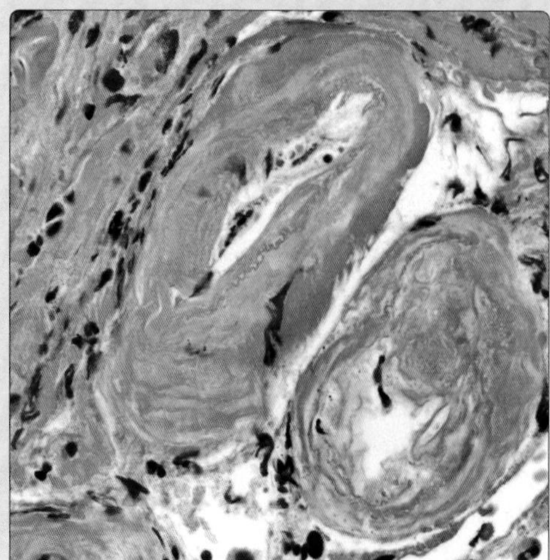

Aβ-Related Angiitis

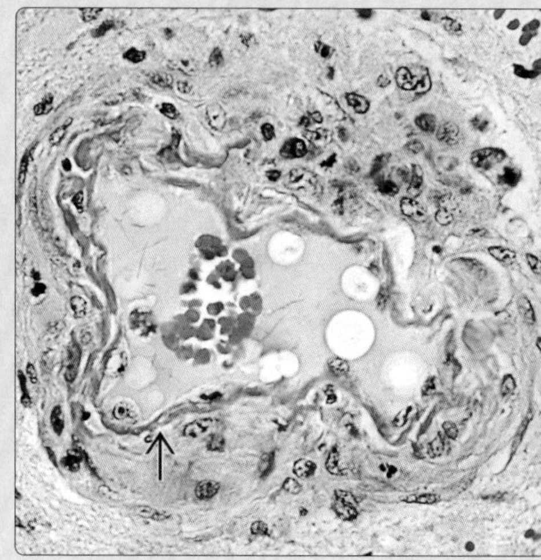

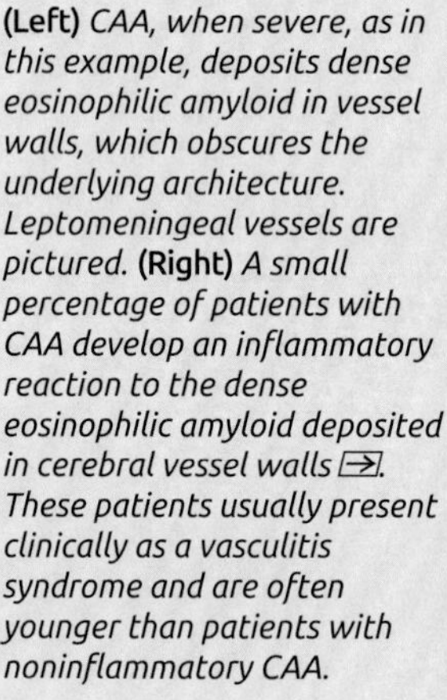

(Left) *CAA, when severe, as in this example, deposits dense eosinophilic amyloid in vessel walls, which obscures the underlying architecture. Leptomeningeal vessels are pictured.* **(Right)** *A small percentage of patients with CAA develop an inflammatory reaction to the dense eosinophilic amyloid deposited in cerebral vessel walls →. These patients usually present clinically as a vasculitis syndrome and are often younger than patients with noninflammatory CAA.*

TERMINOLOGY

Synonyms

- Cerebral amyloid angiopathy (CAA)
- Congophilic angiopathy

Definitions

- Amyloid deposition in wall of leptomeningeal and cortical vessels, preferentially medium to small arteries and arterioles, without associated amyloid deposition in blood vessels of systemic organs

ETIOLOGY/PATHOGENESIS

Sporadic Cerebral Amyloid Angiopathy

- Precursor protein
  - Amyloid precursor protein (APP)
    - Protein is amyloid beta peptide (Aβ)
- Amyloid also present in cores of neuritic plaques in Alzheimer disease (AD)
- Most common form cerebral amyloid

Cerebral Amyloid Angiopathy in Down Syndrome

- Precursor protein
  - APP

Hereditary Forms

- Hereditary cerebral hemorrhage with amyloid (HCHWA)
  - Dutch, Italian, Flemish/British, Icelandic types
    - Only Dutch type has Aβ deposition

CLINICAL ISSUES

Epidemiology

- Incidence
  - CAA lobar hemorrhages
    - 5-20% of all nontraumatic cerebral hemorrhages in elderly patients
  - Apolipoprotein epsilon 4 (APOE4) genotype influences risk of CAA-related hemorrhage
  - Most patients with Alzheimer disease have some degree of CAA
- Age
  - Sporadic CAA
    - Usually patients > 55 years old
  - CAA in Down syndrome
    - May be seen by 40-50 years of age
  - Hereditary forms
    - Onset usually between 45-50 years of age
  - Hereditary Icelandic form related to cystatin C
    - Onset between 20-30 years of age
- Ethnicity
  - Hereditary forms
    - Small numbers of families affected within ethnic group bearing disorder name

Site

- Supratentorial, all lobes
- Subarachnoid bleeds
- Superficial cortical bleeds
  - Bleeds spare deep gray matter (basal ganglia, thalamus), rarely involve cerebellum

Presentation

- Recurrent lobar hemorrhages
- Focal neurological deficits

Treatment

- No specific treatment
  - Treat chronic hypertension
- Intracranial surgical procedures carry risk of rebleeding

Prognosis

- Guarded, due to risk for repeated hemorrhage

IMAGING

MR Findings

- Recurrent large lobar and microhemorrhages of varying ages
- Small infarction(s)
- Ischemic white matter damage

MACROSCOPIC

General Features

- Surgical specimen
  - Acute clot with small fragments of admixed brain parenchyma
- Autopsy
  - Major lobar hemorrhages in frontal or frontoparietal areas
  - Cortical petechial hemorrhages
  - Small infarcts
  - White matter ischemic lesions

MICROSCOPIC

Histologic Features

- Smudgy, eosinophilic thickening of leptomeningeal and cortical vessels
  - Full circumferential or segmental vascular amyloid deposition
  - Severe examples have
    - Vessel splitting ("lumen within lumen")
    - Thrombosis
    - Aneurysmal change
  - Lobar hemorrhage correlates with severity of CAA
  - Mild CAA focally distributed, most often seen as incidental finding
- On Congo red, CAA vessels congophilic with birefringence after polarization
- Sporadic, Down-, and AD-associated CAA
  - Aβ(+) by immunohistochemistry
- Variable amounts parenchymal amyloid, neuritic plaques, neurofibrillary tangles, dystrophic neurites
- CAA with granulomatous inflammation/Aβ-angiitis (uncommon)
  - Multinucleated giant cells with intracytoplasmic Aβ(+) amyloid
  - Epithelioid histiocytes, lymphocytes
  - Perivascular to transmural inflammation
  - Fibrinoid vascular necrosis in some cases

DIFFERENTIAL DIAGNOSIS

Hemorrhages Due to Other Causes

- Neoplasm (primary or metastatic)
  - No amyloid, unless incidental finding
- Chronic hypertension
  - Bleeds usually involve basal ganglia, thalamus, basis pontis, cerebellar white matter
  - Arteriolosclerosis
- Coagulopathy related
  - Often associated with systemic organ hemorrhages

Primary Central Nervous System Angiitis

- No amyloid

DIAGNOSTIC CHECKLIST

Clinically Relevant Pathologic Features

- Recurrent lobar hemorrhages

Pathologic Interpretation Pearls

- CAA maximal in cortical and leptomeningeal vessels; rare in white matter vessels

SELECTED REFERENCES

1. Esiri M et al: Cerebral amyloid angiopathy, subcortical white matter disease and dementia: literature review and study in OPTIMA. Brain Pathol. 25(1):51-62, 2015
2. Thal DR et al: Capillary cerebral amyloid angiopathy identifies a distinct APOE epsilon4-associated subtype of sporadic Alzheimer's disease. Acta Neuropathol. 120(2):169-83, 2010
3. Keage HA et al: Population studies of sporadic cerebral amyloid angiopathy and dementia: a systematic review. BMC Neurol. 9:3, 2009
4. Revesz T et al: Genetics and molecular pathogenesis of sporadic and hereditary cerebral amyloid angiopathies. Acta Neuropathol. 118(1):115-30, 2009
5. Pezzini A et al: Cerebral amyloid angiopathy-related hemorrhages. Neurol Sci. 29 Suppl 2:S260-3, 2008
6. Scolding NJ et al: Abeta-related angiitis: primary angiitis of the central nervous system associated with cerebral amyloid angiopathy. Brain. 128(Pt 3):500-15, 2005
7. O'Donnell HC et al: Apolipoprotein E genotype and the risk of recurrent lobar intracerebral hemorrhage. N Engl J Med. 342(4):240-5, 2000
8. Vonsattel JP et al: Cerebral amyloid angiopathy without and with cerebral hemorrhages: a comparative histological study. Ann Neurol. 30(5):637-49, 1991

Incidental Cerebral Amyloid Angiopathy

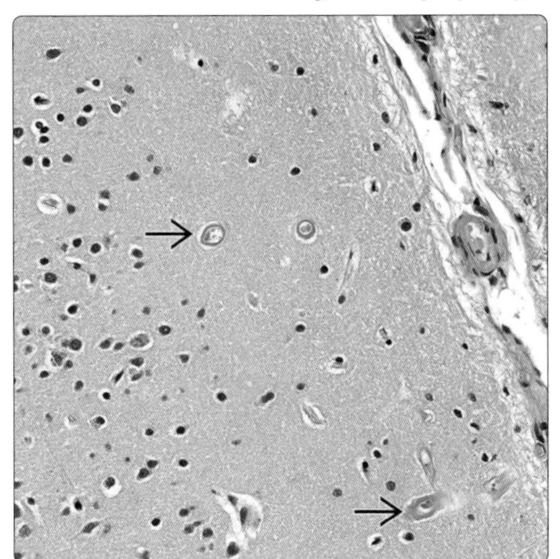

Severe Cerebral Amyloid Angiopathy

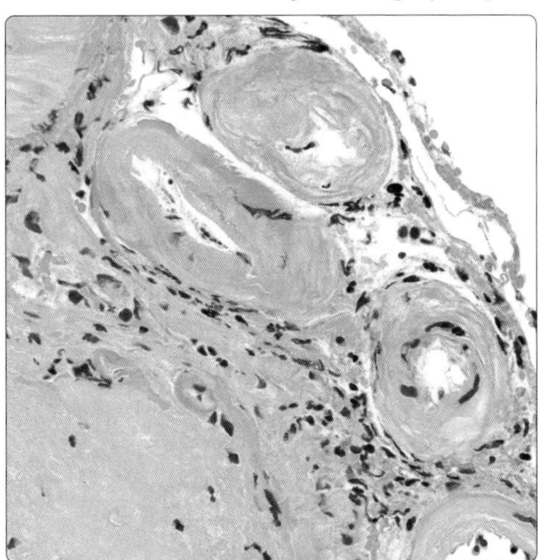

(Left) *Incidental CAA is common and demonstrates mildly thickened, pipe-like leptomeningeal and small superficial cortical vessels* ➙. *Amyloid is usually more prominent in cases with hemorrhage.* **(Right)** *Surgical specimens from patients with intracerebral hemorrhage due to CAA usually contain severely thickened vessels with a smudgy eosinophilic appearance. Severe cases can manifest vessel splitting, fibrinoid necrosis, or thrombosis.*

Smudgy Thickened Vessel Wall

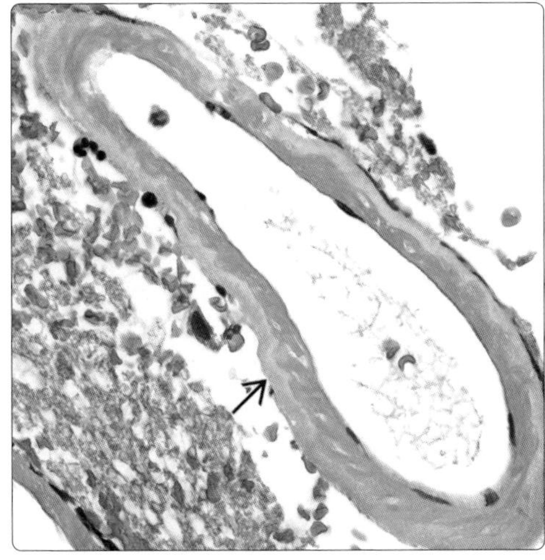

Small Intraparenchymal Vessel

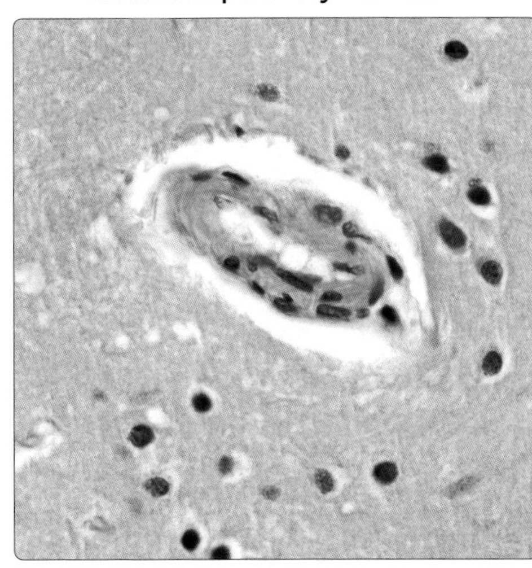

(Left) *Surgically drained clots from older persons should be carefully searched for cortical brain tissue fragments that might contain thickened blood vessels. Note the smudgy eosinophilic wall* ➙ *in this case of CAA. Amyloid is circumferential in this example.* **(Right)** *Small intraparenchymal cortical vessels may be only minimally thickened in CAA. The full extent of amyloid deposition is best appreciated histochemically or immunohistochemically.*

β-A4-Amyloid

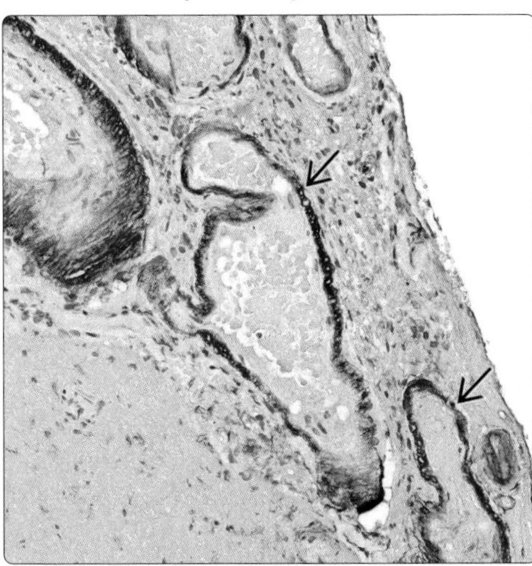

β-A4-Amyloid

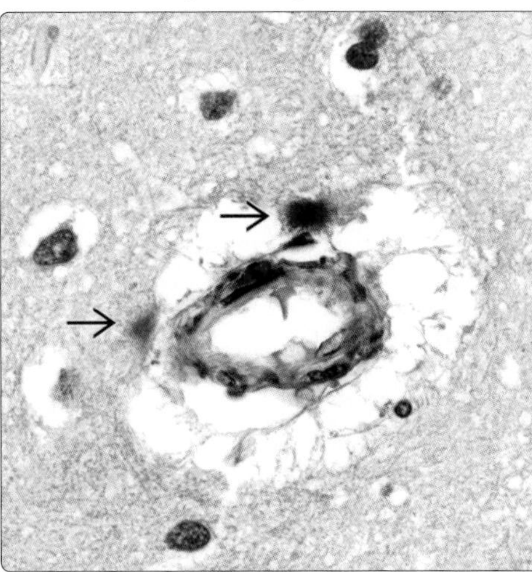

(Left) *CAA is best appreciated with immunohistochemistry for β-A4-amyloid* ➙. *Amyloid deposition is circumferential here, but may be segmental in less severe examples.* **(Right)** *A small superficial parenchymal vessel with segmental amyloid deposition on immunostaining for β-A4-amyloid is illustrated. Note the nearby perivascular deposits of the same amyloid* ➙.

Neuritic Plaque With Amyloid Core

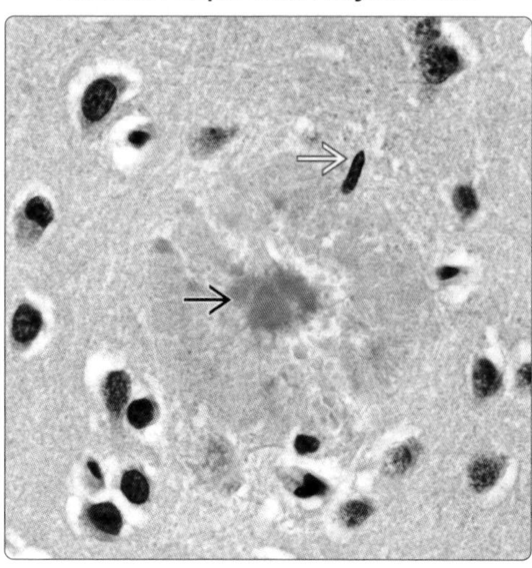

β-A4-Amyloid in Neuritic Plaque

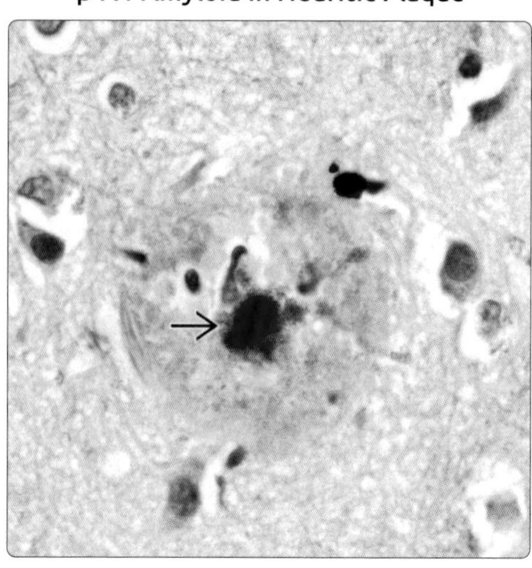

(Left) *Patients with CAA often have neuritic plaques, neurofibrillary tangles, and dystrophic neurites sufficient for diagnosis of Alzheimer disease. Note the prominent amyloid core in this neuritic plaque* ⇨*. Amyloid, in this case, can be easily seen on H&E, as can an adjacent microglial cell* ➡ *that is part of the plaque.* **(Right)** *Immunohistochemistry for β-A4-amyloid highlights the amyloid-rich core* ⇨ *in neuritic plaques. Alzheimer disease is found in some patients with CAA.*

Aβ-Related Angiitis

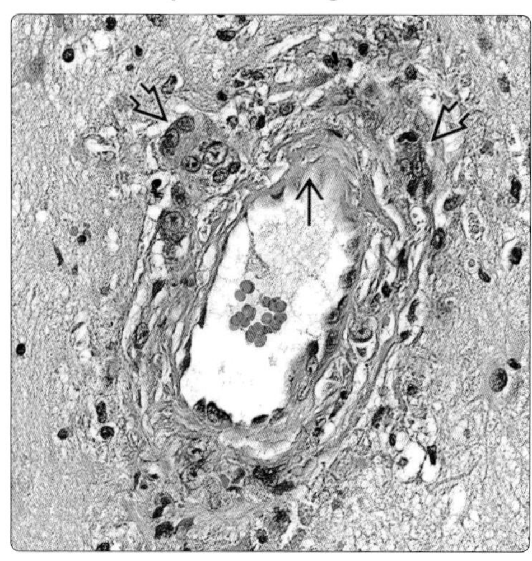

Multinucleated Giant Cell

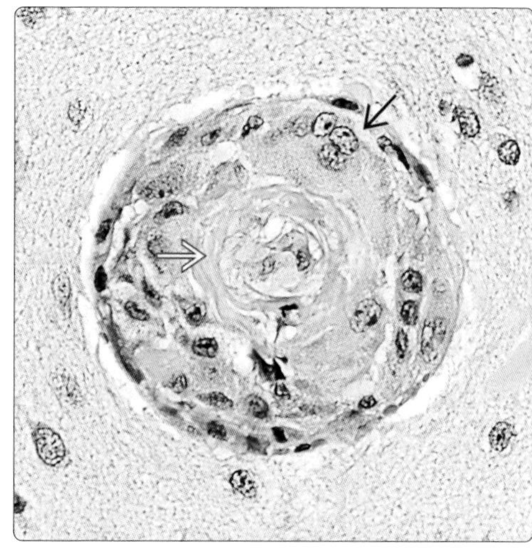

(Left) *In CAA associated with granulomatous inflammation, affected vessels* ⇨ *attract multinucleated giant cells* ⇨ *and epithelioid histiocytes. Aβ-related angiitis patients tend to be younger than those with sporadic noninflammatory CAA.* **(Right)** *A smudged, amyloid-containing vessel* ➡ *has attracted epithelioid cells and at least 1 multinucleated giant cell* ⇨*. Aβ-related angiitis is clinically more similar to primary CNS angiitis than to noninflammatory CAA.*

Congo Red, Aβ-Related Angiitis

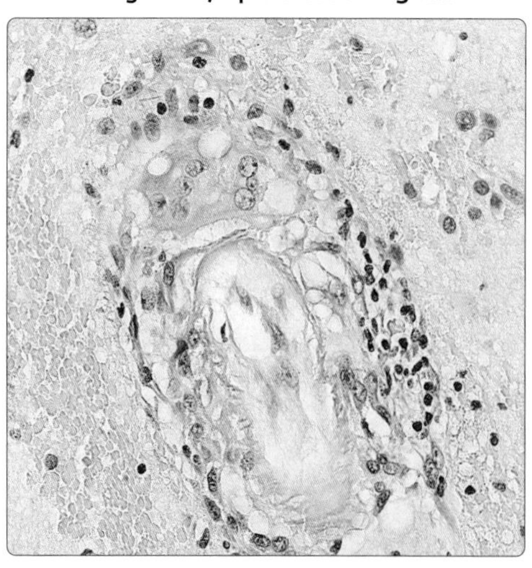

Polarization, Aβ-Related Angiitis

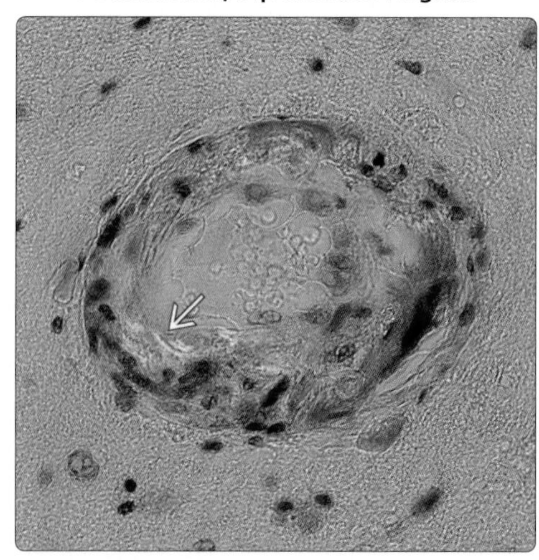

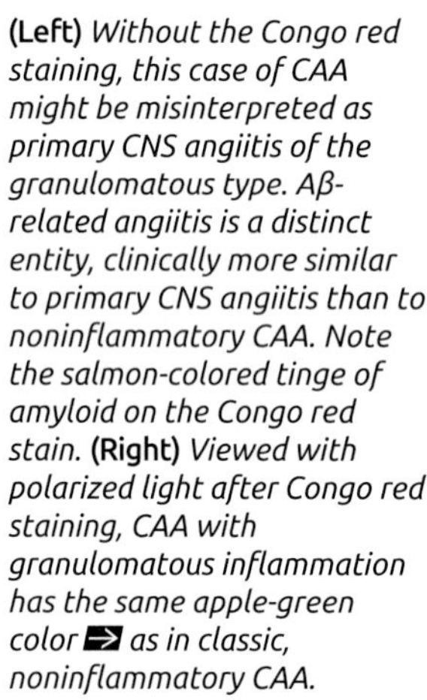

(Left) *Without the Congo red staining, this case of CAA might be misinterpreted as primary CNS angiitis of the granulomatous type. Aβ-related angiitis is a distinct entity, clinically more similar to primary CNS angiitis than to noninflammatory CAA. Note the salmon-colored tinge of amyloid on the Congo red stain.* **(Right)** *Viewed with polarized light after Congo red staining, CAA with granulomatous inflammation has the same apple-green color* ➡ *as in classic, noninflammatory CAA.*

Acute Bleed

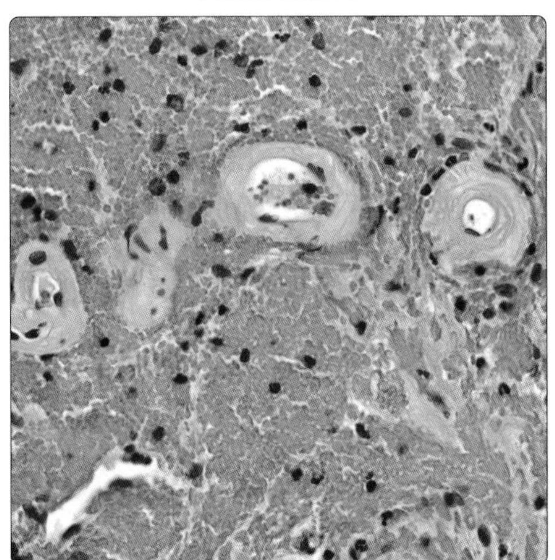

Simulating Electrocautery Artifact in Surgical Specimen

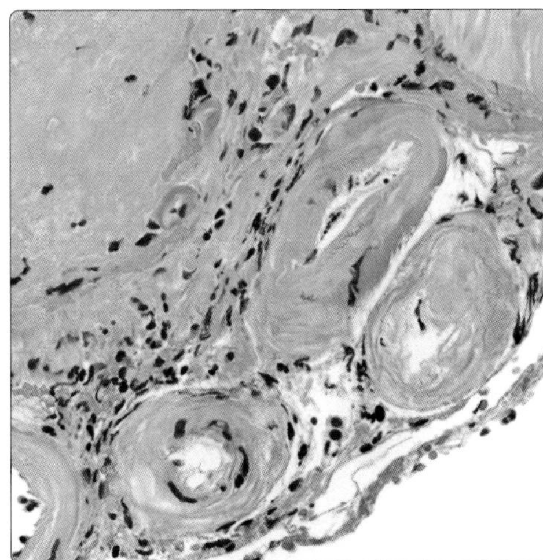

(Left) *Any acute cerebral bleed, especially in an older person, should be examined carefully for entrapped blood vessels with CAA.* **(Right)** *To the unwary, cerebral vessels with dense eosinophilic smudgy material that obscures vessel wall details can be mistaken for electrocautery artifact from the surgical instruments.*

Congophilia

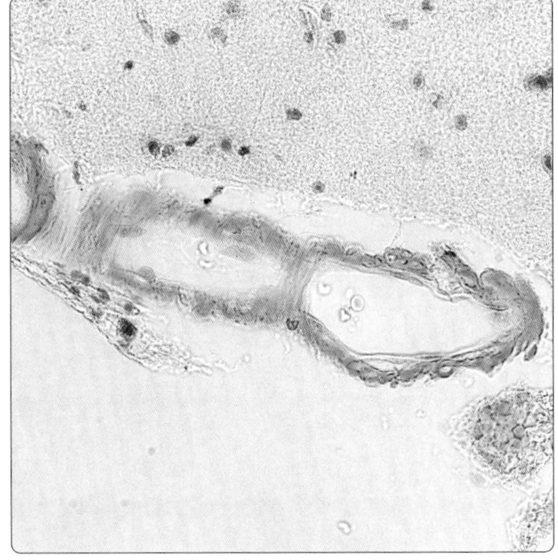

Congo Red

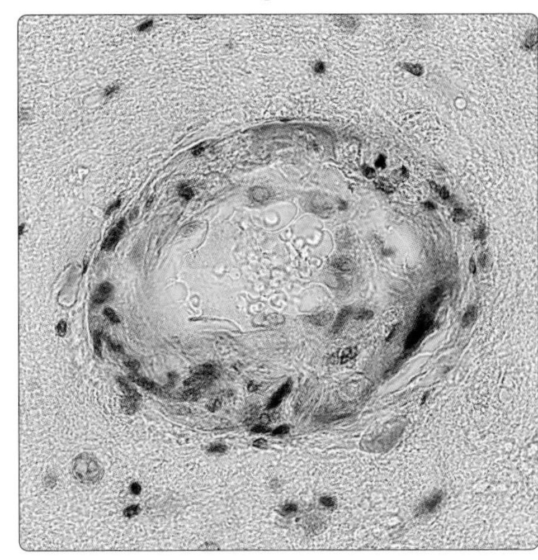

(Left) *CAA stained with Congo red is characterized by blood vessels with orangish colored congophilia. Particularly affected are medium and small-sized arteries and arterioles in leptomeninges (illustrated here) and cortex. The white matter is not affected.* **(Right)** *Before performing polarization for suspected CAA, make certain that the Congo red histochemical stain demonstrates congophilia. Collagen also polarizes, albeit with a less apple-green tint.*

Circumferential Amyloid

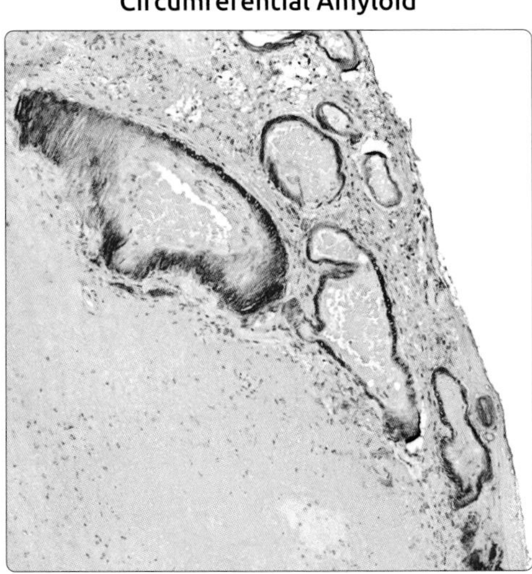

Segmental Amyloid

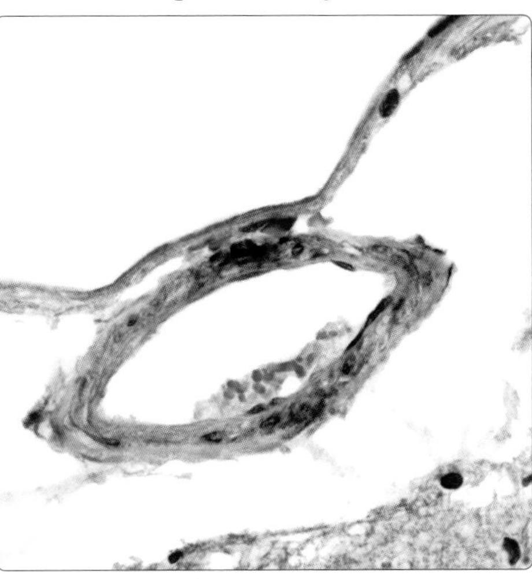

(Left) *Leptomeningeal vessels are immunoreactive for beta amyloid, which can occur in either a focal segmental or circumferential pattern. The latter is seen here.* **(Right)** *Immunostaining for β-A4-amyloid best allows one to appreciate the focal, segmental amyloid deposition that can occur in CAA.*

PART II
SECTION 4
Cortical Dysplasia

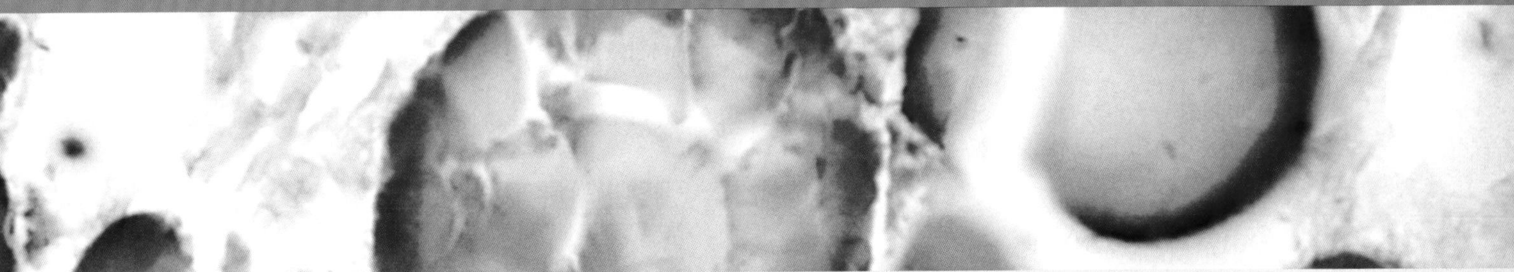

Cortical Dysplasia

KEY FACTS

TERMINOLOGY

- Localized area of cortical maldevelopment with varying degrees of dyslamination, immature or giant neurons, dysmorphic neurons, balloon cells

CLASSIFICATION

- Interobserver concordance for International League Against Epilepsy (ILAE), Palmini classification systems best for focal cortical dysplasia (FCD) type IIb
- Classification systems may not fully encompass all types of cortical dysplasia

ETIOLOGY/PATHOGENESIS

- Developmental migrational defect
- Type III associated with early acquired lesion: Hippocampal sclerosis, low-grade neoplasm, vascular malformation, ischemic/traumatic/encephalitic brain injury

CLINICAL ISSUES

- Surgical resection principal treatment for drug-resistant FCD
- 60% seizure free at 1 year postoperatively

ANCILLARY TESTS

- Histochemistry, immunohistochemistry to identify neuronal pattern, individual neuronal distribution and cytology; gliosis; myelin loss

TOP DIFFERENTIAL DIAGNOSES

- Ganglioglioma
  - Neoplasm with mass effect
  - Significant glial population
  - May have calcifications, microcysts, eosinophilic granular bodies, Rosenthal fibers, complex vasculature
  - Not confined to cortex

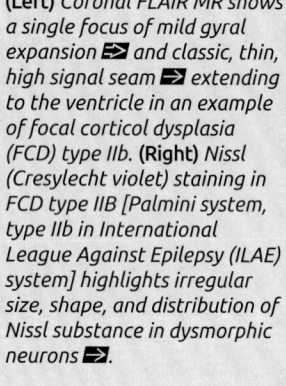

(Left) *Coronal FLAIR MR shows a single focus of mild gyral expansion ➡ and classic, thin, high signal seam ➡ extending to the ventricle in an example of focal corticol dysplasia (FCD) type IIb.* **(Right)** *Nissl (Cresylecht violet) staining in FCD type IIB [Palmini system, type IIb in International League Against Epilepsy (ILAE) system] highlights irregular size, shape, and distribution of Nissl substance in dysmorphic neurons ➡.*

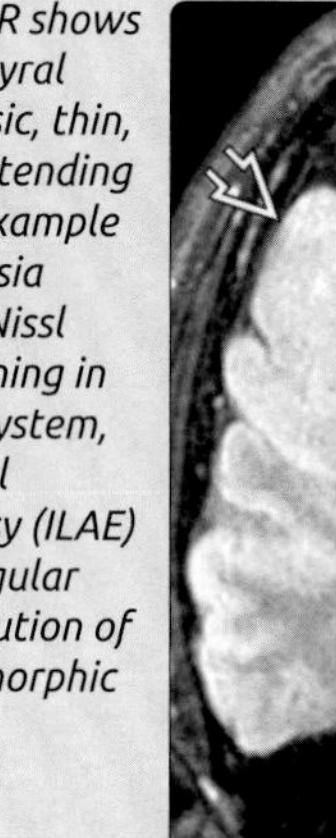

Coronal MR: Focal Corticol Dysplasia Type IIb

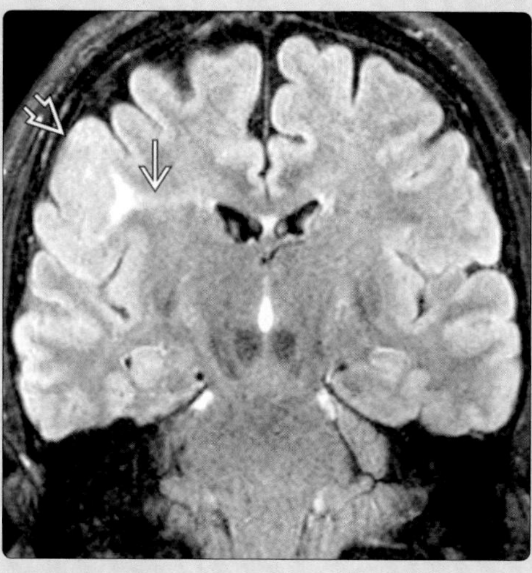

Focal Corticol Dysplasia Type IIb

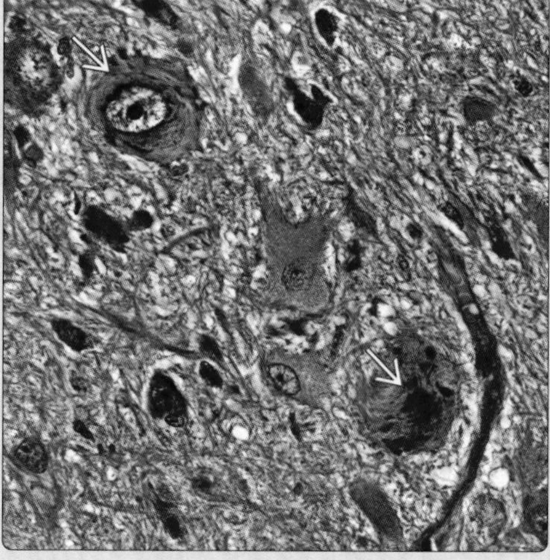

(Left) *Balloon cells are pathognomonic of focal cortical dysplasia, type IIb and are usually maximal near the cortical gray-white matter junction. The pale eosinophilic cytoplasm with rounded cytoplasmic borders are typical of balloon cells. These cells can be easily overlooked or mistaken for macrophages.* **(Right)** *Abnormal clusters of neurons, either purely in vertical columns (uncommon), tangentially (more common), or both (more common), can best be appreciated on NeuN immunohistochemistry.*

Balloon Cells, Focal Corticol Dysplasia Type IIb

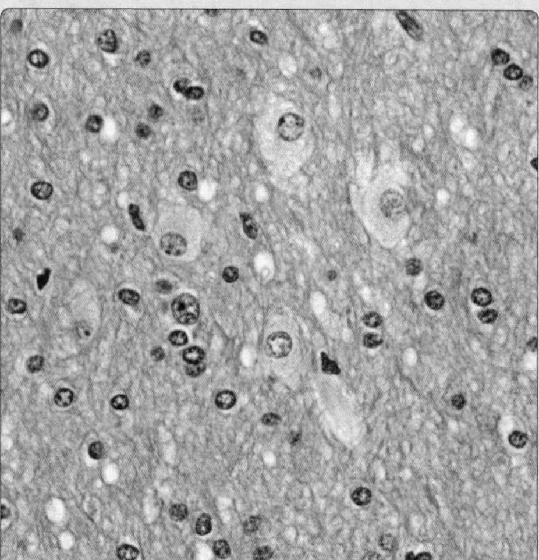

Cortical Dyslamination

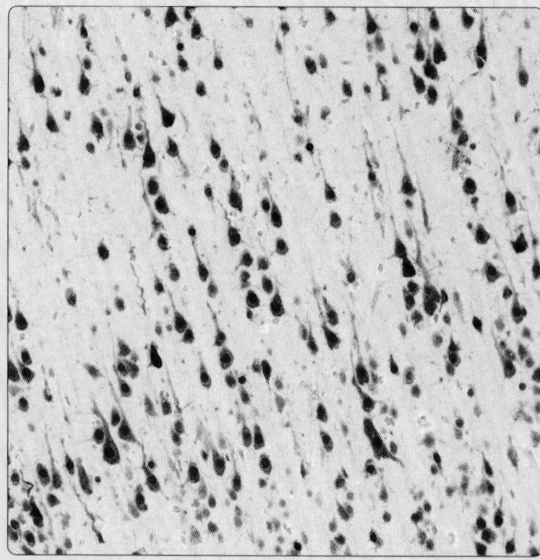

TERMINOLOGY

Synonyms

- Focal cortical dysplasia (FCD)

Definitions

- Developmental abnormality of neuronal migration that is strictly, or mostly, intracortical

ETIOLOGY/PATHOGENESIS

Developmental Anomaly

- Neuronal migrational abnormality; etiology unknown

CLINICAL ISSUES

Presentation

- FCD type I in young children with severe epilepsy and psychomotor retardation
- FCD type II (a.k.a. Taylor-type FCD) most frequent

Treatment

- Surgical approaches
  - Surgical excision of epileptogenic focus (foci)
  - Temporal lobectomy for temporal lobe lesions

Prognosis

- 60% seizure free at 1 year postoperatively
- Children and adults equally likely to benefit from surgery
- Complete resection, temporal lobe location favorable prognostic indicators of seizure-free outcome

IMAGING

MR Findings

- FCD type I: Often multilobar
  - Nonenhancing
- FCD type II: Most frequent in extratemporal locations, especially frontal lobe
  - Hyperintense juxtacortical T2 signal
  - Transmantle sign with abnormal signal in subgyral white matter tapering from depth of gyrus toward ventricle
  - FLAIR more sensitive than T2

MICROSCOPIC

Histologic Features

- International League Against Epilepsy (ILAE) classification
  - FCD type I: Abnormal neuronal layering of neocortex, affecting single or multiple lobes
    - Aberrant radial lamination (type Ia) (microcolumns of > 8 neurons aligned vertically)
    - Aberrant tangential lamination (type Ib); often missing distinctive layers 2 or 4
    - Aberrant radial and tangential lamination (type Ic)
  - FCD type II: Cortical dyslamination with dysmorphic neurons
    - Type IIa: Without balloon cells
    - Type IIb: With balloon cells (boundary of gray with white matter always blurred)
  - FCD types I, II not associated with any other structural brain lesion (isolated FCD)
  - FCD type III: In combination with structural lesion
    - Histopathological features very similar to those observed in type I
    - FCD type IIa or IIb in combination with structural lesion = "dual pathology"
    - FCD type IIIa: In combination with hippocampal sclerosis
    - FCD type IIIb: In combination with epilepsy-associated tumors
    - FCD type IIIc: Adjacent to vascular malformations
    - FCD type IIId: In association with other epileptogenic lesions obtained in early life (e.g., traumatic injury, ischemic injury, encephalitis)
- Older Palmini system similar, except
  - FCD type IA in Palmini not subdivided into tangential and radial lamination subtypes
  - FCD type IIB in Palmini specifies presence of abnormal lamination, plus giant or immature neurons
  - FCD type III, in combination with structural lesion, not recognized

ANCILLARY TESTS

Histochemistry

- Nissl for neurons, Luxol fast blue for myelin
  - Nissl
    - Dyslamination, dysmorphic neurons, neuronal loss, or individual ectopic neurons
  - Luxol fast blue
    - Myelin pallor in subgyral white matter, especially with type IIb

Immunohistochemistry

- NeuN: Dyslamination, dysmorphic neurons; neuronal loss or individual ectopic neurons
- Gliosis GFAP(+)
- Dysmorphic neurons cytoplasm neurofilament protein (+)

DIFFERENTIAL DIAGNOSIS

Ganglioglioma

- Neoplasm with mass effect
- Not confined to cortex
- More cellular neuronal and glial populations
- Calcifications, microcysts, perivascular nonneoplastic lymphocytes (in some cases)

Infiltrating Intracortical Glioma

- More cellular, mitoses (in some cases)
- Increased glial cell population, nuclear atypia
- Variably (+) for Ki-67, nuclear p53, cytoplasmic IDH-1

SELECTED REFERENCES

1. Blümcke I et al: Neuropathological work-up of focal cortical dysplasias using the new ILAE consensus classification system - practical guideline article invited by the Euro-CNS Research Committee. Clin Neuropathol. 30(4):164-77, 2011
2. Blümcke I et al: The clinicopathologic spectrum of focal cortical dysplasias: a consensus classification proposed by an ad hoc Task Force of the ILAE Diagnostic Methods Commission. Epilepsia. 52(1):158-74, 2011
3. Chamberlain WA et al: Interobserver and intraobserver reproducibility in focal cortical dysplasia (malformations of cortical development). Epilepsia. 50(12):2593-8, 2009
4. Palmini A et al: Terminology and classification of the cortical dysplasias. Neurology. 62(6 Suppl 3):S2-8, 2004

(Left) *Heterotopic neurons within the molecular layer ⇨ can be seen in isolation in mild malformations of cortical development (mMCD) or in combination with cortical dyslamination in several types of FCD. A densely fibrillar layer, known as Chaslin subpial gliosis, underlies the pial surface ➡. This latter, nonspecific finding is often seen in patients with longstanding seizures.* **(Right)** *NeuN highlights large numbers of heterotopic neurons in the molecular layer ⇨.*

Heterotopic Neuron, Molecular Layer

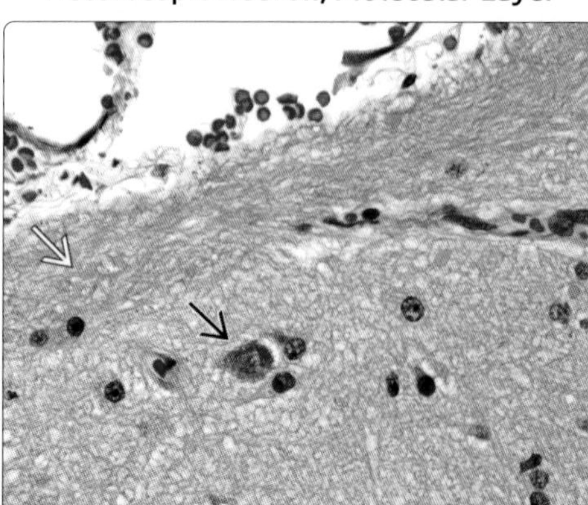

Heterotopic Neurons, NeuN Stain

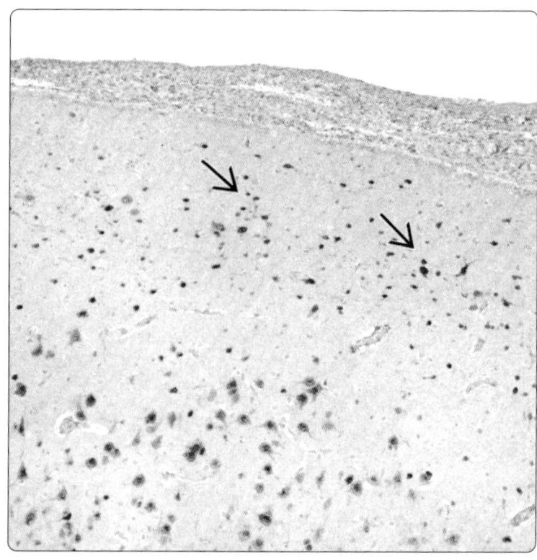

(Left) *Heterotopic single neurons in white matter ➡, also a normal finding, tend to be more frequent in epilepsy specimens and represent a form of mMCD.* **(Right)** *FCD type I in both epilepsy classification systems manifests cortical dyslamination without neuronal dysmorphism. If there is abnormal radial cortical lamination with microcolumns of 8 or more small-diameter neurons crowded together ➡, this is FCD type IA (Palmini system, type Ia in ILAE).*

Heterotopic Neuron, White Matter

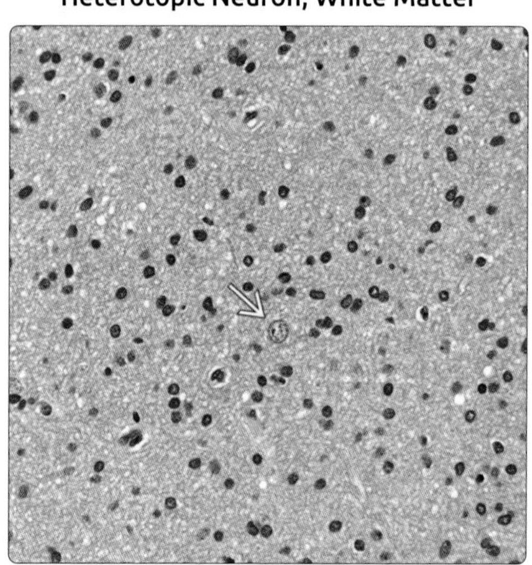

Dyslamination

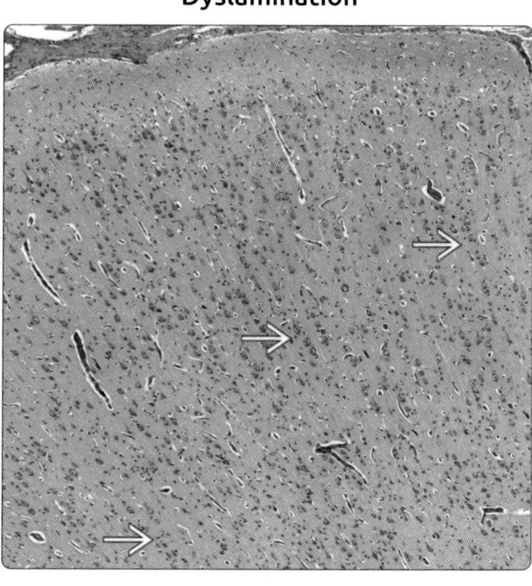

(Left) *In FCD type Ia (ILAE system), microcolumns of 8 or more neurons ⇨ should be identified on 4-micron thick paraffin sections with NeuN immunohistochemistry in a region perpendicular to the pial surface. These columns of 8 or more small neurons are felt to recapitulate embryonic cells migrating along radial glia.* **(Right)** *FCD type Ib (ILAE system) shows tangential cortical disorganization ➡ with irregularly clustered clumps of neurons within roughly the same horizontal layer.*

Dyslamination, NeuN Stain

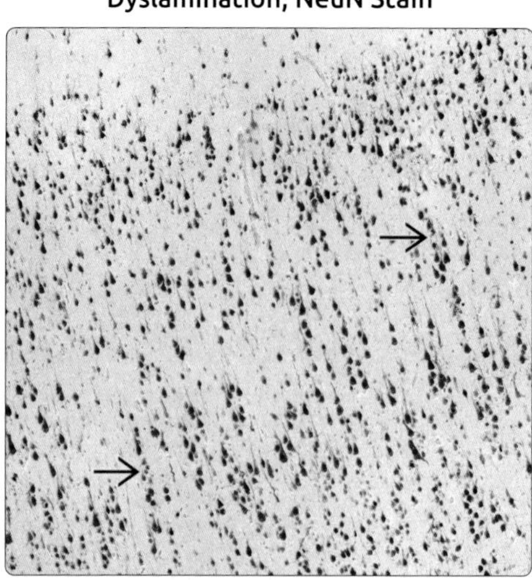

Dyslamination

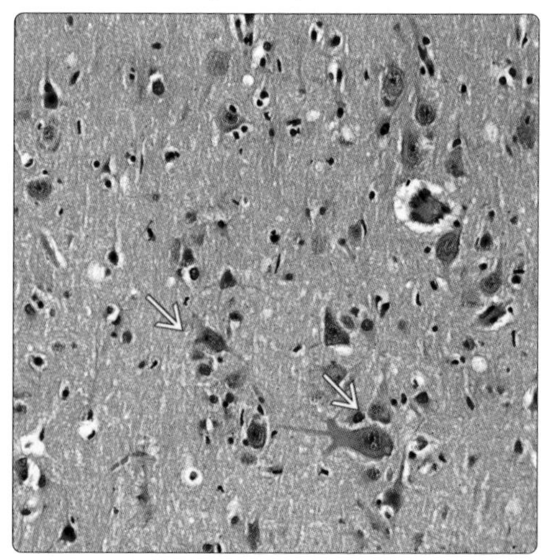

Immature Neurons

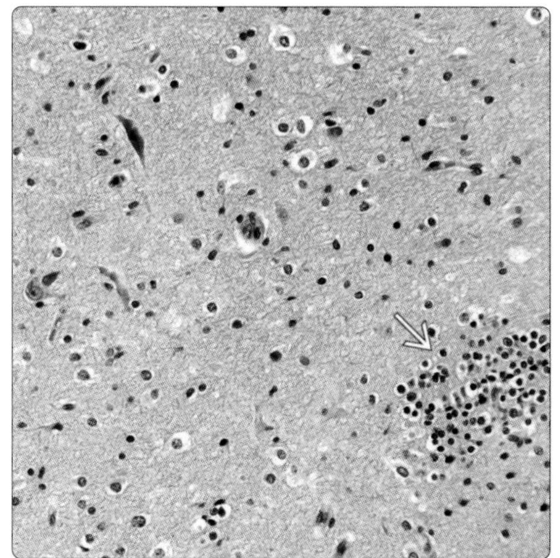

Immature Neurons Simulating Lymphocytes

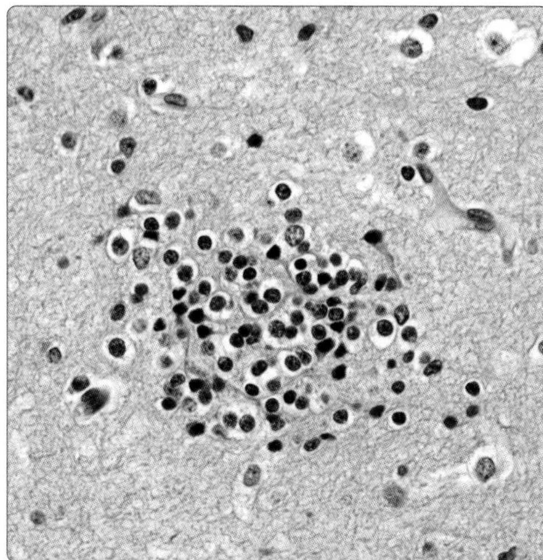

(Left) *Clusters of immature neurons ➡ (sometimes called microdysgenesis or glioneuronal hamartias) are found in FCD type IB in the Palmini system and can be present in FCD type Ia, Ib, or Ic of the ILAE system. These can simulate lymphocytes.* **(Right)** *Immature neurons can resemble oligodendrocytes or lymphocytes. These are often negative for neuronal or glial lineage IHC markers, but cells manifest antiapoptotic marker Bcl-2, suggesting they are immature cells that have failed to regress.*

Giant Neurons, Monotonous Population

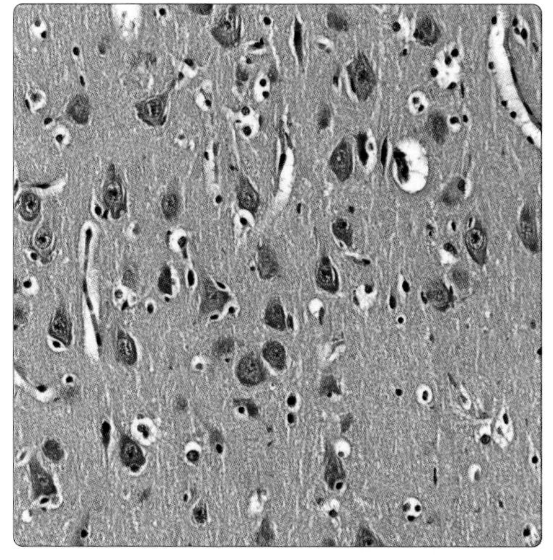

Dyslamination, NeuN Stain

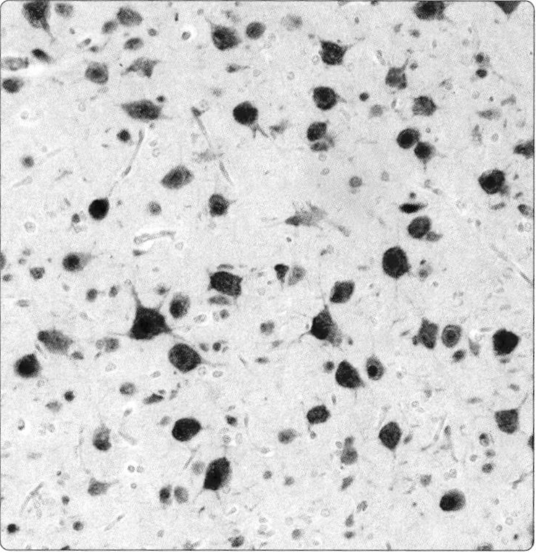

(Left) *Giant (hypertrophic pyramidal) neurons outside of cortical layer 5 are a signature feature of FCD type IB (Palmini) and can be found in any of the 3 types of FCD type I (types Ia, Ib, Ic) in the ILAE system. These cells are not dysmorphic, by definition, in FCD type I. Note how all the cells share the same size.* **(Right)** *NeuN highlights the cortical dyslamination that is present in FCD type IIB (Palmini system).*

Large But Not Dysmorphic Neurons

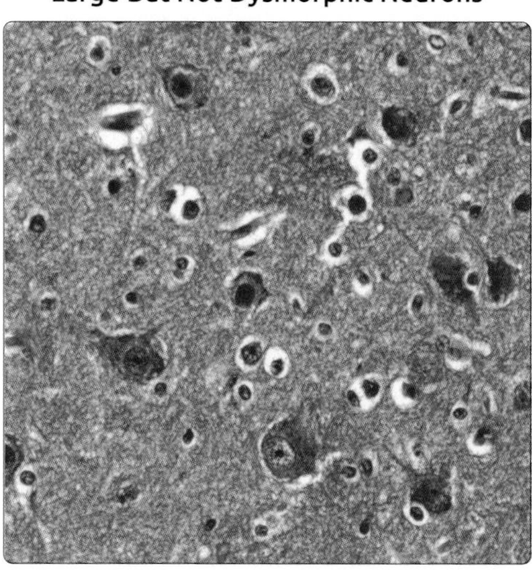

Cortical Neurons Without Increased Neurofilament Immunostaining

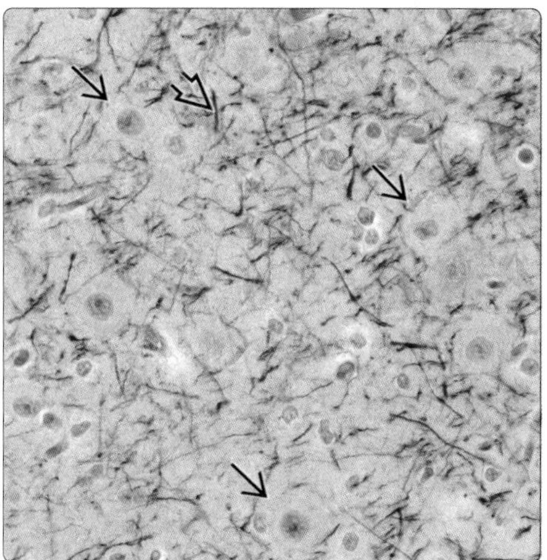

(Left) *Nissl (Cresylecht violet) section in FCD type IB (Palmini) verifies that the giant neurons seen outside of layer 5 have normal distribution of Nissl substance and are not dystrophic.* **(Right)** *Antineurofilament protein immunohistochemistry highlights the numerous normal, linear, intracortical axonal processes ⇨ in FCD type IIB (Palmini), but does not show abnormal increased neurofilament distribution within the cytoplasm of the nondysmorphic neurons →.*

(Left) *Coronal T2WI MR of FCD type IIb shows a juxtacortical high signal ➡ with a thin "seam" of high signal ➡ tracking along the expected course of the radial glial fibers to the subependymal margin. This imaging feature is now realized to be pathognomonic for FCD type IIb.* **(Right)** *Pallor near the cortical gray-white matter junction ➡ is typically seen in FCD type IIB (Palmini system). This results in blurring of the gray-white junction on T1-weighted images and increased white matter signal on T2 and FLAIR images.*

Coronal MR: Focal Cortical Dysplasia Type IIb

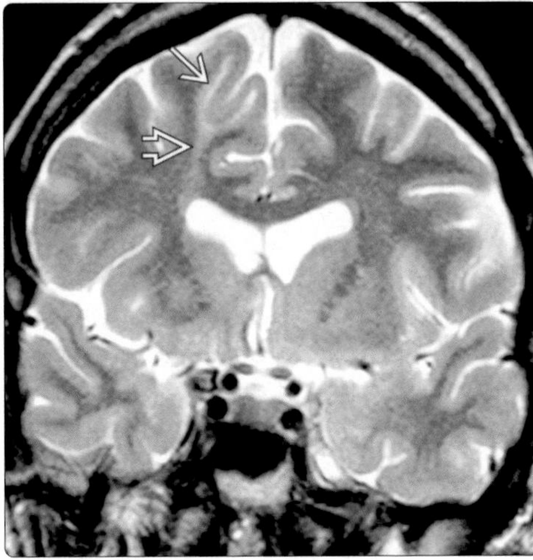

Pallor at Cortical Gray-White Junction, Focal Cortical Dysplasia Type IIb

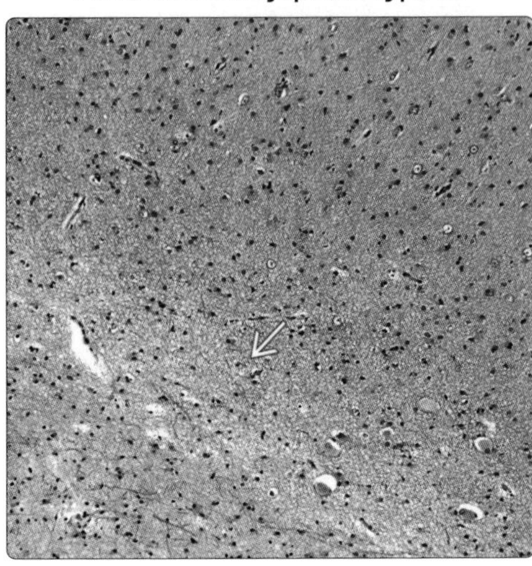

(Left) *NeuN immunostaining illustrates that severe dyslamination occurs in FCD type IIb, with dysmorphic neurons ➡ usually randomly scattered throughout the cortex.* **(Right)** *FCD types IIA and IIB in Palmini system (types IIa, IIb in ILAE) show dysmorphic neurons in the cortex with irregular shapes, sizes, and distribution of Nissl substance ➡.*

Cortical Dysplasia, NeuN Stain

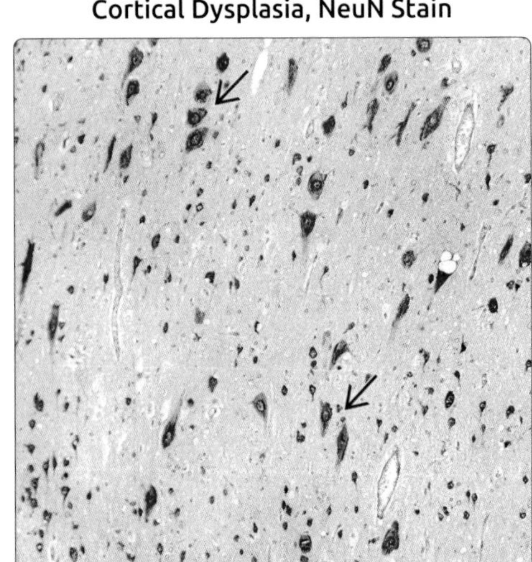

Cortical Dysplasia, H&E

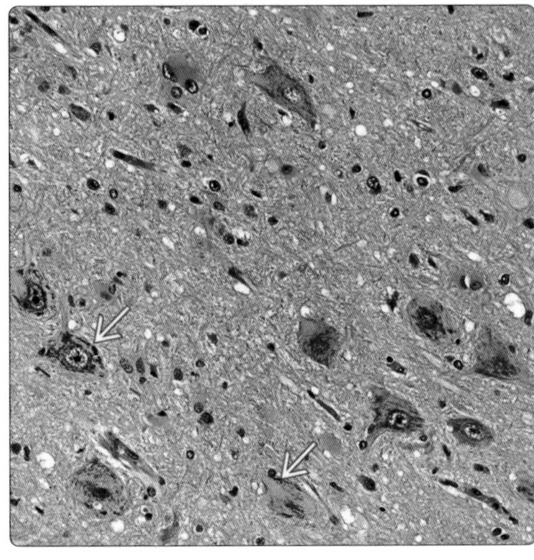

(Left) *A Nissl (Cresylecht violet) stained section in FCD type II highlights cortical dyslamination and abnormal distribution of Nissl substance in the dysmorphic neurons ➡.* **(Right)** *NeuN immunostaining highlights abnormal distribution of Nissl substance ➡ in dysmorphic neurons in FCD type II.*

Cortical Dysplasia, Cresyl Fast Violet Stain

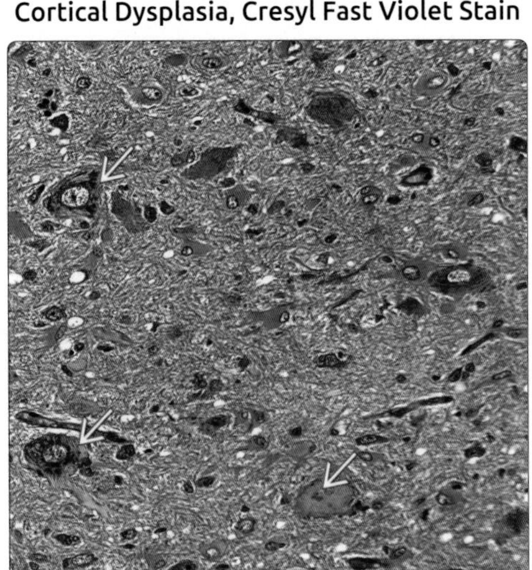

Cortical Dysplasia, NeuN Stain

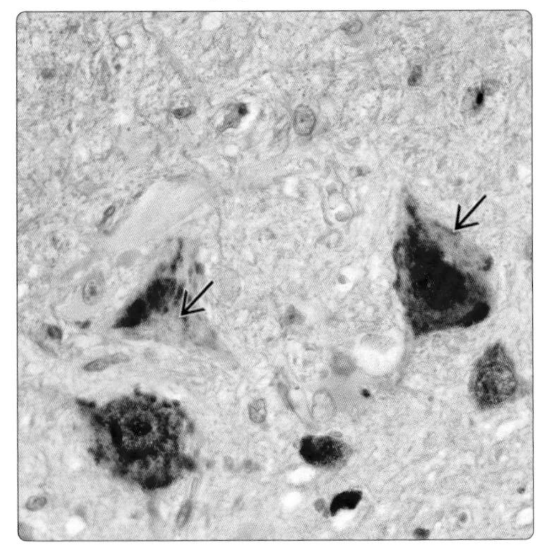

Cortical Dysplasia, NFP Stain

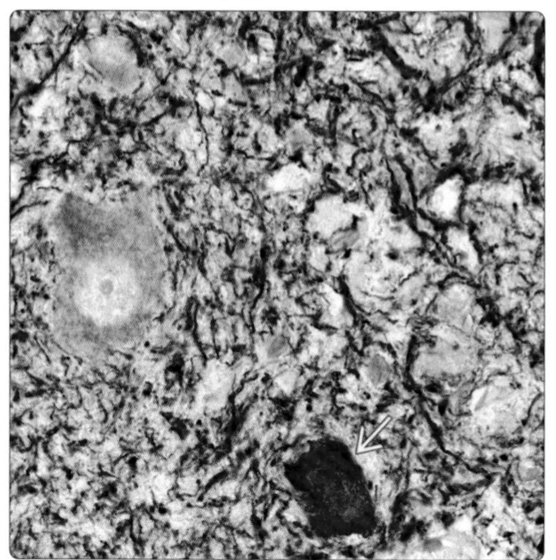

Cortical Dysplasia, GFAP Stain

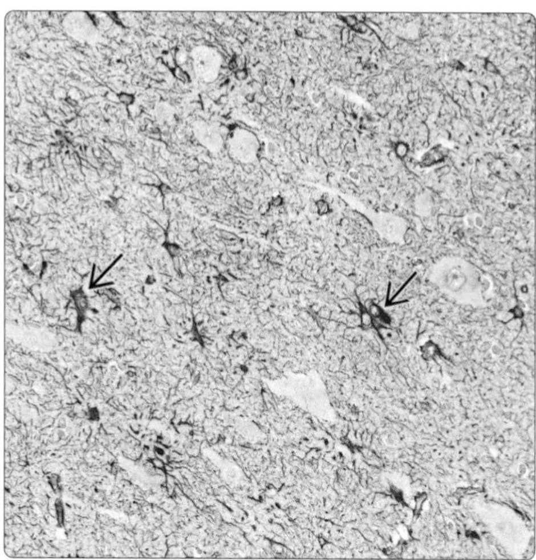

(Left) *Antineurofilament immunohistochemistry highlights the abnormal distribution of neurofilaments* ➡ *in dysmorphic neurons in FCD type II.* **(Right)** *Reactive astrocytes* ➡ *are often identified on GFAP immunostaining within the dysplastic cortex of FCD type II.*

Cortical Dysplasia, H&E

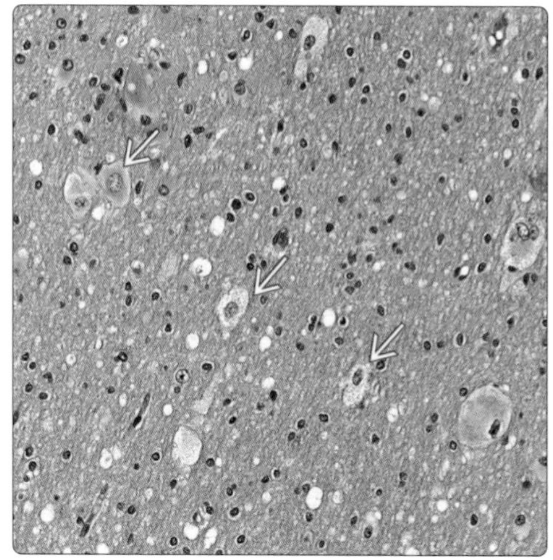

Cortical Dysplasia, H&E

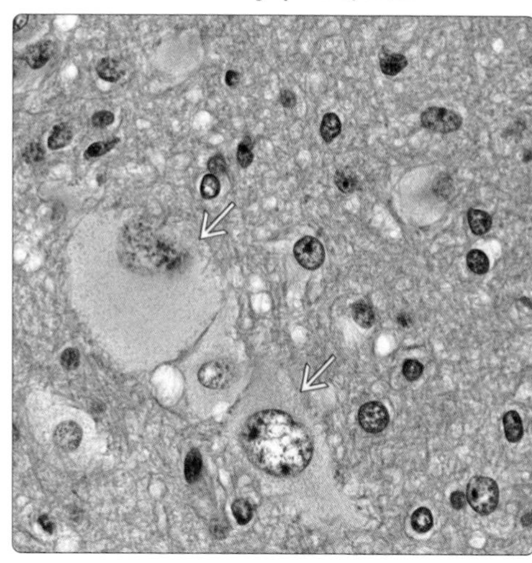

(Left) *Balloon cells with glassy eosinophilic cytoplasm* ➡ *are scattered irregularly throughout the white matter in FCD type IIB (Palmini system, type IIb in ILAE system).* **(Right)** *Balloon cells* ➡ *are often found near the cortical gray-white matter junction in FCD type IIB (Palmini system, type IIb in ILAE). They often lack immunoreactivity for specific glial or neuronal immunomarkers, but may show immunostaining for more immature cell markers such as vimentin, CD34, or nestin.*

Cortical Dysplasia, GFAP Stain

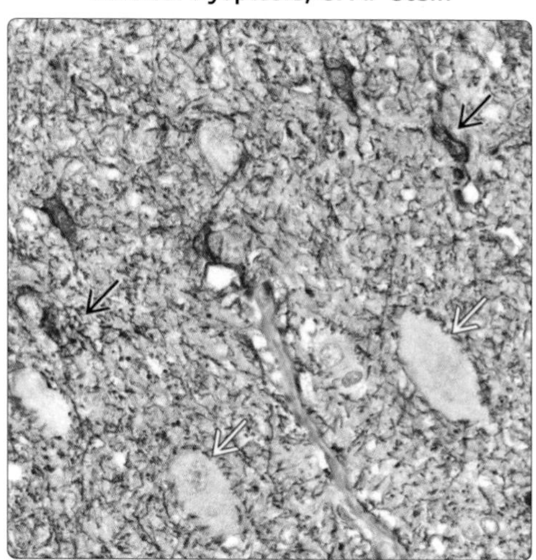

NFP Stain

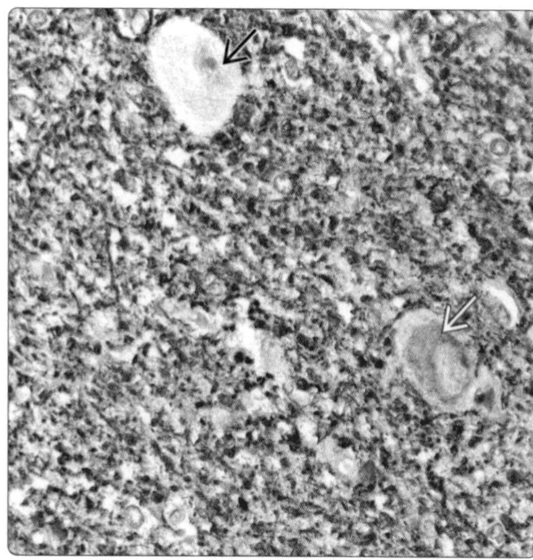

(Left) *Balloon cells* ➡ *are usually not immunoreactive for GFAP. Interspersed reactive astrocytes are positive* ➡. **(Right)** *Antineurofilament immunostains usually do not highlight the cytoplasm in balloon cells* ➡*, but occasional ones will be mildly positive* ➡. *Balloon cells are more often immunoreactive for more immature cell markers, such as vimentin, CD34, or nestin.*

INDEX

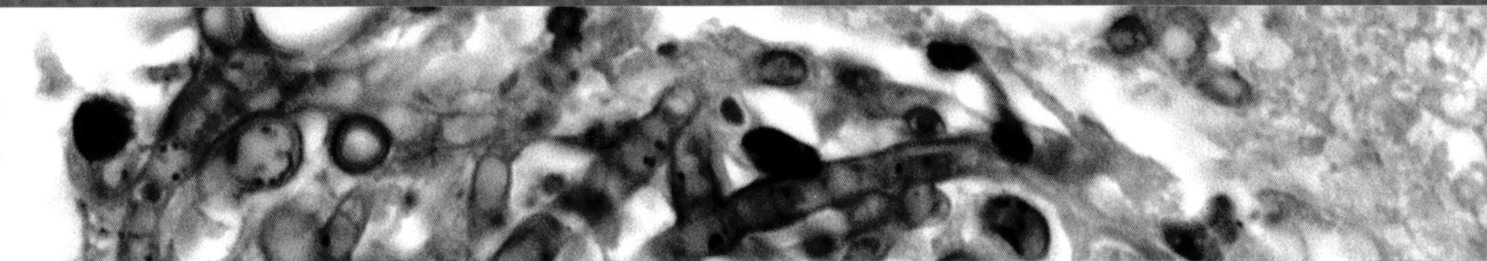

A

INDEX

INDEX

B

INDEX

C

INDEX

INDEX

INDEX

INDEX

D

E

INDEX

F

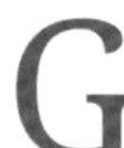

INDEX

H

INDEX

I

INDEX

J

K

L

INDEX

M

INDEX

INDEX

INDEX

N

INDEX

O

P

R

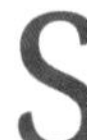

T

U

V

W

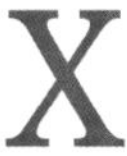

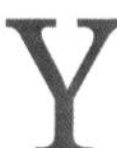

Z

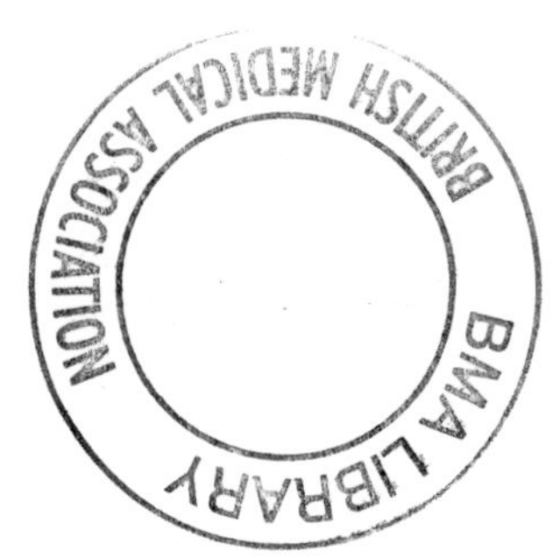